PROCEDURES

Fundamentals of Contemporary Nursing Practice

Fundamentals of Contemporary Nursing Practice

Carol A. Lindeman, PhD, RN, FAAN
Dean and Professor Emeritus
School of Nursing
Oregon Health Sciences University

Marylou McAthie, EdD, RN
Professor Emeritus
Department of Nursing
Sonoma State University

W.B. SAUNDERS COMPANY
A Division of Harcourt Brace & Company
Philadelphia London Toronto Montreal Sydney Tokyo

W.B. SAUNDERS COMPANY
A Division of Harcourt Brace & Company

The Curtis Center
Independence Square West
Philadelphia, Pennsylvania 19106

Library of Congress Cataloging-in-Publication Data

Lindeman, Carol Ann.
Fundamentals of contemporary nursing practice / Carol A. Lindeman, Marylou McAthie.—1st ed.

p. cm.

ISBN 0-7216-3527-X

1. Nursing—Practice. I. McAthie, Marylou. II. Title.
[DNLM: 1. Nursing. 2. Nursing Care. WY 16L743f 1999]

RT86.7.L56 1999 610.73—dc21

DNLM/DLC 98-36263

FUNDAMENTALS OF CONTEMPORARY NURSING PRACTICE ISBN 0-7216-3527-X

Printed in the United States of America.

Last digit is the print number: 9 8 7 6 5 4 3 2 1

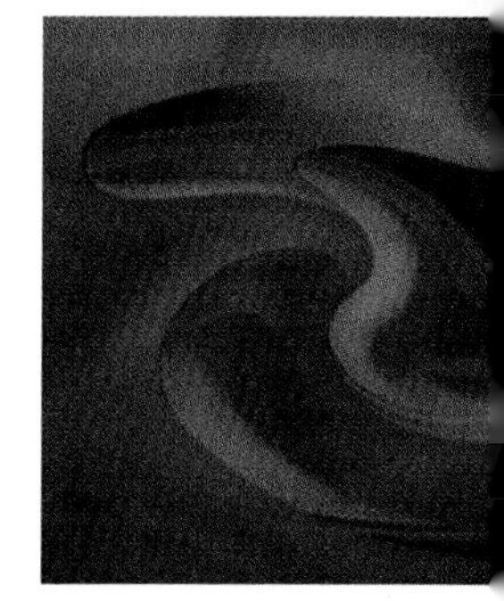

Contributors

Irene B. Alyn, PhD, RN

Professor and Chair, Department of Nursing
Cedarville College
Cedarville, Ohio
28 Skin Integrity

Dr. Alyn is Professor and Chair, Department of Nursing at Cedarville College where she also teaches Introduction to Nursing, Nutrition and Pharmacology. Her current research interests include outcome assessment and innovative teaching methods.

"Maintaining skin integrity in patients is a key independent responsibility for nursing students and registered nurses. Nurses have conducted research in maintenance of skin integrity and clearly have opportunities to continue to advance this key responsibility of professional nursing."

Lori J. Andreas, MSN, RN, CNS, AOCN

Clinical Manager, Adult Oncology, Inpatient and
Outpatient Bone Marrow Transplant
Clinical Nurse Specialist Comfort Care Team
Oregon Health Sciences University
Portland, Oregon
35 Care of the Dying

Lori Andreas has been the Clinical Manager of the Adult Oncology and Inpatient and Outpatient Adult Bone Marrow Transplant Program at Oregon Health Sciences University in Portland, Oregon for the last 5 years. She has also owned a temporary staffing agency as well as Adult Foster Homes. She also is the Clinical Nurse Specialist with the Comfort Care Team at OHSU.

"I encourage student nurses and new Registered Nurses to reach for the stars! Nursing has so much to offer. Find your strengths and develop them!"

Laura J. Armstrong, EdD, RN, MPH

Chief, Community Health Nursing Division
Hawaii State Department of Health
Honolulu, Hawaii
6 Determinants of Health and Illness

Charold Baer, PhD, RN, FCCM, CCRN

Professor, Acute Care & Director of the ACNP Program
School of Nursing
Oregon Health Sciences University;
Faculty Clinician in Nephrology and Critical Care
Oregon Health Sciences University Hospital
Portland, Oregon
Appendix

Pauline Beecroft, PhD, RN, FAAN

Nurse Researcher
Editor, *Clinical Nurse Specialist: The Journal for Advanced Nursing Practice*
Childrens Hospital, Los Angeles, California
16 Pharmacology and Medication Administration: Administering Medication by Intramuscular Injection

Pauline C. Beecroft's interest in intramuscular (IM) injections was sparked when a clinical nurse specialist presented an article on the complications of injecting children's thighs. As chairperson of the hospital Procedure Committee she could not change practice based on a single article. After a significant review of the literature she found more questions than answers about IM injections. In this chapter she shares over ten years of work in this area.

Judith A. Berg, PhD, RN, WHNP

Assistant Professor
University of Arizona College of Nursing, Tucson, Arizona
Women's Health Nurse Practitioner
Planned Parenthood of Southern Arizona, Tucson, Arizona
33 Sexual Health Protection and Health Promotion

Judith A. Berg is an Assistant Professor at the University of Arizona College of Nursing, teaching graduate students in nurse practitioner options. She has provided primary care services to women as a Women's Health Nurse Practitioner for more than 25 years. Her research focus is symptom management strategies for mid-life women negotiating the perimenopausal transition.

"Students are encouraged to consider sexual health assessment within the broader context of male and female health assessment and to include sexual health promotion strategies whenever health education is provided to clients."

Beth P. Black, MSN, RN

Research Assistant Professor
University of North Carolina at Chapel Hill,
Chapel Hill, North Carolina
35 *Care of the Dying*

Ms. Black is currently the director of the Maternal Symptom Management (MSM) Grant at the University of North Carolina at Chapel Hill. This research project is testing the efficacy of an in-home nursing intervention aimed at reducing symptom distress and increasing early recognition of infection in HIV-positive African American mothers of young children.

Ms. Black has clinical experience both in home health and in hospice nursing, providing in-home care for the dying and their families.

"To new nursing students: My hope for each of you is that you find in this marvelous profession of nursing the deep joy that I have found in following your heart to exquisite places of human need, courage and strength. Hang on for a real-life adventure!"

Sandra Blake-Von Behren, MS, RN

Infection Control Epidemiologist
Loyola University Medical Center
Maywood, Illinois
17 *Sterile Technique and Infection Control*

Sandra Blake-Von Behren is the Infection Control Epidemiologist at Loyola University Medical Center in Maywood, Illinois, with 23 years of active experience in infection control practice. Her areas of special interest and responsibility include the development and implementation of processes for the collection and analysis of data on the incidence of nosocomial infection; the use of process control charts to report infection control findings; and the review and evaluation of newly published research on infection control so that health care policies and procedures can be consistent with current findings.

"As you begin your nursing career, I urge you to remember that apathy cannot exist in nursing practice. In today's health care environment, nurses are continually challenged to do more with less—a situation that can lead to stress, exhaustion, and burn out. Face this time as a challenge by developing new and more efficient ways to perform responsibilities; however, also allow time to take care of yourself to assure that you are a rested and healthy provider of care."

Fay Bower, DNSc, RN, FAAN

Nurse Consultant
Bower Consulting
Clayton, California
21 *Respiration*

Fay Bower's last position was as President of Clarkson College in Omaha, NE. Its programs include nursing (baccalaureate and master's), radiology, occupational therapy, physical therapy, medical imaging, health service management, and business for health providers. Thus, she considers herself an expert about what health care providers need as a theoretical base for practice. She also taught research and advanced nursing practice to master's students and occasionally professionalism to the undergraduate students. She has also authored books about fundamentals and consulted with nursing programs about how to develop curricula for nursing skills courses. Her own research has focused on outcome assessment.

"This text presents a new way to learn fundamental skills for the practice of nursing because it provides the student with the most current research about each skill. The nurse of today cannot afford to be without the material presented in this text for it provides the nurse with current, safe, and well tested approaches to nursing care."

Julia Brown, PhD, RN, MA

Professor Emeritus
Oregon Health Sciences University School of Nursing
Portland, Oregon
36 *Health Promotion and Self-Care*

Rosemary Campos, PhD, RN

Adjunct Faculty, Holy Name College
Oakland, California:
Assistant Research Psychologist
Institute of Human Development
University of California, Berkeley, California;
Hospice Nurse, Kaiser Permanente
Walnut Creek, California
32 *Touch*

Rosemary Campos is a hospice nurse with Kaiser Permanente of Northern California, as well as Assistant Research Psychologist at the University of California, Berkeley. Her research centers on comfort interventions for infant pain. That research led to an enduring interest in the application of touch in clinical nursing.

Carolyn E. Carlson, PhD, RN, MA

Professor, Department of Nursing
Cedarville College
Cedarville, Ohio
28 *Skin Integrity*

Dr. Carlson is a Professor of Nursing at Cedarville College, Cedarville, OH, where she teaches Nursing Research as well as Clinical Nursing to BSN students. Recently, she was a member of the AHCRP panel that developed the guidelines for prevention and for treatment of pressure ulcers. She continues her research interests initiated at the Rehabilitation Institute of Chicago where she was the Associate Director of Research and Evaluation.

Anita Catlin, DNSc, RN, FNP
Professor of Nursing
Napa Valley College
Napa, California
26 *Personal Hygiene*

Dr. Catlin holds a certificate degree in ethics consultation. She writes for *Pediatric Nursing* and serves on the editorial board of *Image*. Her recent research is on physician decision making and ethical issues in maternal-child health.

"Set your goals and know you can meet them. Find nurses who inspire you and stay in contact. Let them guide you in career growth. Think, contemplate, study, and never give up your ideals about how to provide good nursing care."

Katherine Crabtree, DNSc, RN
Associate Professor of Nursing
Department of Primary Health Care Nursing
Oregon Health Sciences University School of Nursing
Portland, Oregon
Adult Nurse Practitioner
Pacific University
College Health Service
Forest Grove, Oregon
36 *Health Promotion and Self Care*

Katherine Crabtree coordinates the Adult Nurse Practitioner pathway in the master's program at OHSU.

Marilee I. Donovan, PhD, RN
Adjunct Faculty
Oregon Health Sciences University School of Nursing;
Project Director/Clinical Nurse Specialist
Regional Pain Management Program
Kaiser Permanente Northwest
Portland, Oregon
27 *Pain and Comfort*

Since 1994, Marilee Donovan, PhD, RN, has been the Director of the Multidisciplinary Chronic Pain Management Program for Kaiser Permanente Northwest Region where she is responsible for improving the management of chronic pain for the HMO's 500,000 members. This is the culmination of 25 years of teaching, writing, and research devoted to improving pain management for those with cancer, acute pain, and/or chronic pain. Her research on factors related to poor pain management is ongoing.

"Pain is the second most common reason for visits to healthcare settings. Recent scientific findings suggest that poorly controlled acute pain is a root cause of the development of chronic pain syndromes. Nurses with their broad knowledge of pathophysiology, psychosocial modifiers, and cultural variability are uniquely prepared to improve the identification and control of pain in a variety of settings and to minimize the creation of disabling chronic pain."

Loretta Filitske, BSN, RN, CRNP
Pittsburgh, Pennsylvania
24 *Urinary Elimination*

Nancy Fugate Woods, PhD, RN, FAAN
Professor and Dean, School of Nursing
University of Washington
Seattle, Washington
33 *Sexual Health Protection and Health Promotion*

Nancy Fugate Woods is a widely respected authority and nursing scholar in the field of women's health. Author of numerous books and research articles, she has focused her research attention on perimenstrual syndromes and other women's health issues. Among her many honors are citations from the American Nursing Foundation, the Institute of Medicine, and the American Psychological Association. She is currently dean of and professor at the School of Nursing, University of Washington, Seattle.

Pamela Hellings, PhD, RN, CPNP
Associate Professor and Chair, Department of Primary Care
Oregon Health Sciences University
Portland, Oregon
15 *Patient Assessment*

Pam Hellings is an Associate Professor at the Oregon Health Sciences University where she serves as Chair, Department of Primary Care and Director, Breastfeeding Service. She has been an educator in nurse practitioner programs for over 25 years. Her current practice and research activities involve studying and working with complex breastfeeding problems and the knowledge and attitudes of nurse practitioners and nurse midwives about breastfeeding.

"There is no more critical aspect of working with patients than complete and accurate assessment. Understanding this process will serve you well throughout your professional life."

Marguerite Jackson, PhD, RN, FAAN, CIC
Administrative Director, Nursing Research and Education & Epidemiology Unit
University of California San Diego Medical Center
and
Associate Clinical Professor of Family & Preventive Medicine
UCSD School of Medicine
San Diego, California
18 *Personal Safety in Nursing Practice*

Rosemarie B. King, PhD, RN
Research Assistant Professor, Northwestern University School of Medicine
Adjunct Assistant Professor, University of Illinois at Chicago, College of Nursing
Senior Research Associate, Rehabilitation Institute of Chicago
Chicago, Illinois
28 Skin Integrity

Dr. King's current position is Research Assistant Professor, Northwestern University School of Medicine, Department of Physical Medicine and Rehabilitation. She also holds a Senior Research Associate position at the Rehabilitation Institute of Chicago. Dr. King has been the recipient of federal, foundation, and professional organization funding for studies related to physical disability. Recently, she was a co-principal investigator for a descriptive study funded by NINR on prevention of pressure ulcers in spinal cord injury (SCI). Currently, she is principal investigator for an intervention study on prevention of pressure ulcers in SCI that is funded by the CDC. Additional current research projects include an intervention study of caregivers, and a longitudinal descriptive study of stroke survivors and their caregivers.

Sheila Kodadek, PhD, RN
Professor
Oregon Health Sciences University School of Nursing
Portland, Oregon
6 Determinants of Health and Illness

Diane Krasner, PhD, RN, CETN, CWS
Wound Care Consultant;
Adjunct Associate Professor
School of Nursing
Johns Hopkins University
Baltimore, Maryland
23 Intestinal Elimination; 24 Urinary Elimination

Diane Krasner is an ET nurse with extensive experience in wound, skin, and incontinence care. She lectures and publishes extensively and serves on numerous editorial and corporate advisory boards. Dr. Krasner's research interests include wound-related pain, the assessment of wound healing, wound care trends and practice, and Heideggerian Hermeneutic phenomenology.

*"The more you are prepared,
The more you can anticipate,
The more you can use your common sense,
The better you will be at meeting patient and family needs, resulting in positive outcomes."
"Chance favors the prepared mind."—Louis Pasteur*

Ellen Kreighbaum, PhD
Professor & Department Head, Department of Health and Human Development
Montana State University
Bozeman, Montana
20 Biomechanics and Mobility

Dr. Ellen Kreighbaum has taught and researched kinesiology and biomechanics topics for over 25 years. She is internationally known for her successful textbook, *Biomechanics,* a qualitative approach for studying human movement, which is in its fourth edition. She is also co-editor and author of *Sports and Fitness Equipment Design.* Dr. Kreighbaum has served as president of the International Society for Biomechanics in Sports and continues to serve on its board of directors. Her research interests are in lower extremity alignments during weight bearing and the biomechanics of mobility in the older adult. Dr. Kreighbaum currently serves as department head of Health and Human Development at Montana State University.

Kathryn A. Lee, PhD, RN, FAAN
Professor, Department of Family Health Care Nursing
University of California
San Francisco, California
25 Rest and Sleep

Kathryn A. Lee joined the faculty in the Department of Family Health Care Nursing at the University of California, San Francisco in 1988, and she is currently Professor and the James and Marjorie Livingston Chair in Nursing. For the past 10 years her program of research has focused on women's health with an emphasis on sleep patterns, circadian rhythms, and fatigue. Studies have included childbearing women, women with HIV/AIDS, and midlife women. She is very active in the Symptom Management Nursing Faculty Group at UCSF School of Nursing and the Sleep Research Society.

Anita Lohman, PhD, MA, BBA
Private practice psychotherapy
Clinical Psychologist
Portland, Oregon
19 Health of the Nursing Student

Christine Lush, MN, RN
Learning and Development Consultant
Kaiser Permanente of Northern California
Oakland, California
14 Documentation

"This is an exciting time to be a part of the health care industry. As a clinical nurse educator and consultant, I consistently find a need for references that address issues encountered today and in the new millenium. This text gives learners access to the insights of a diverse group of experts who share their knowledge and experiences. Nurses must continue to work collaboratively so that we can be assured of exemplary practice and achievements."

Mary Lush, PhD, RN

Senior Consultant, Division of Nursing Services
Kaiser Permanente Medical Care Plan
Oakland, California
14 Documentation

Dr. Lush has presented nationally and internationally on the use of data collected during the course of patient care to evaluate the processes and outcomes of that care. Her publications have focused on the requirements for outcome infrastructures sensitive to the independent practice of the nurse. Dr. Lush also directs the development of human response concepts for inclusion in an evolving convergent health care terminology planned for continuum of care clinical information systems.

"An outcomes infrastructure based on data collected during care provides the foundation for the multidisciplinary team to evaluate the processes and outcomes of patient care. Nurses in all settings of care are encouraged to look on documentation as the vehicle through which the impact of their independent practice on health outcomes can be quantified."

Margaret A. Martin, MSN, RN, CETN

Manager, Clinical Programming
Genesis ElderCare
Kennett Square, Pennsylvania
23 Intestinal Elimination

Margaret Martin has 28 years of Clinical Nursing experience in a variety of specialties and in all sites of care (acute, home, and long-term). She worked for ten years as an Enterostomal Therapy Nurse providing care to persons with ostomies, wounds, and incontinence. In her current position as a Clinical Nurse Specialist in Gerontology, she designs, develops, and implements Clinical Nursing Care Programs for ElderCare, a large long-term care corporation.

Margaret S. Miles, PhD, RN, FAAN

Professor
School of Nursing, University of North Carolina at Chapel Hill
Chapel Hill, North Carolina
34 Grief; 35 Care of the Dying

Margaret Shandor Miles is presently a Professor of Nursing at the University of North Carolina at Chapel Hill. She also is conducting research examining the process of parenting a critically ill infant, parenting a prematurely born child, and an intervention study helping African American mothers with HIV cope with and manage their illness. She has written and lectured extensively about grief and death. This chapter is an adaptation of a lecture she has given undergraduate students at two different universities over the past 20 years because of her commitment to helping student nurses become comfortable with care of the dying.

"Caring for dying patients and grieving families, whether they are young or old, is both challenging and rewarding. It is challenging because we are forced to confront our own feelings and fears about death at a time when we are called upon to help highly distressed patients and their families. It is rewarding because if we learn to help patients and their families through this important life transition, we will have helped them grow and mature as individuals and as a family. In addition, we will have learned valuable lessons ourselves as professionals and as individuals. Nurses have an important, a critical role in helping with the process of dying and with helping families with their grief after death."

Christine A. Nelson, MS, RN

Research Associate
School of Nursing
Center for Ethics in Health Care
Oregon Health Sciences University
Portland, Oregon
29 Social Support

Christine Nelson, MS, RN, is a Research Associate in the Oregon Health Sciences University (OHSU) School of Nursing and the OHSU Center for Ethics in Health Care. In her 15 years as a nurse researcher she has served as a Research Assistant, Research Associate, or Project Director on seven NIH-funded research teams at OHSU and at the University of California, San Francisco. She currently serves as a Research Associate with the Program of Research on Ethics and End-of-Life Care at OHSU. As part of this research team, she has served on four different research projects relating to end-of-life care. She is the Project Director on a National Institute of Nursing Research funded grant to explore the impact of family decision making when life-sustaining treatments are withdrawn from decisionally incapacitated family members.

Hob Osterlund, MS, RN, CHTP

Clinical Coordinator, Pain Management Services
The Queen's Medical Center, Honolulu, Hawaii
32 Touch

Ms. Hob Osterlund is the Clinical Coordinator for Pain Management Services at The Queen's Medical Center in Honolulu, Hawaii, where she has integrated Healing Touch as a significant part of the pain management options. As the first hospital in the country to fully integrate an energy modality into acute care, Queen's has offered thousands of HT treatments and supports research in this work. Ms. Osterlund is co-investigator for research on Healing Touch and post-op mastectomy pain and is principal investigator for Healing Touch and acute back injuries in Queen's Medical Center employees. Ms. Osterlund is also well-known for her work in humor and health care, and is the creator of acclaimed comedy character *Ivy Push, RN.*

"Nursing calls for the most steadfast of individuals. I encourage you to have the courage to find the peaceful zone that integrates caring wholeheartedly and staying fully detached from the pain of other's lives. Bless you on your journey."

Margaret A. Ovitt, MS, RN, MLA

President
Western Illinois Land Design, Inc.
Macomb, Illinois
30 Environment and Health

Margaret Ovitt went on from her nursing career to obtain a graduate degree in landscape architecture, with the intention of "building a garden in the intensive care unit." Her masters thesis study with intensive care nurses contributed to the knowledge base on the stress-reducing properties of nature.

"When I was in nursing, I became very interested in the relationship between the environment and health. I observed that the natural environment could be restorative and healing, and that having some sort of access to nature was important to patients, staff, and visitors. In my chapter, I attempted to introduce nursing students to the far-reaching effects of the physical environment, and that it indeed matters how we shape and treat our environment. Including nature in the high-tech hospital environment is becoming more important as the research demonstrates. Of course, I hasten to add that the research is supporting what Florence Nightingale observed in the nineteenth century: the patient needs fresh air, a view, a quiet environment, and the sight of flowers to promote healing."

Mariann Piano, PhD, RN

Associate Professor, Medical Surgical Nursing
Coordinator, Acute Care Nurse Practitioner Graduate Program
University of Illinois School of Nursing
Chicago, Illinois
16 Pharmacology and Medication Administration

Dr. Mariann Piano is an Associate Professor at the University of Illinois at Chicago. Dr. Piano is involved in many aspects of the graduate acute care nurse practitioner option and some of her responsibilities include the coordination and teaching of advanced physiology and health care management of acutely ill patients. Dr. Piano's research and scholarly writing has focused in the area of alcoholic heart muscle disease, heart failure, and cardiovascular physiology and nursing.

"It is critical that nurses understand the fundamentals of pharmacology, such as the mechanism of drug action. This is because nurses are responsible for the administration of the pharmacologic agent as well as monitoring the patient's response to therapy."

Lisa Pompeii, MS, RN, COHN-S

Research Associate
University of North Carolina at Chapel Hill
Chapel Hill, North Carolina
18 Personal Safety in Nursing Practice

Sarah E. Porter, PhD, RN, MPH

Associate Professor of Mental Health Nursing
Associate Dean of Student and International Affairs
School of Nursing
Oregon Health Sciences University
Portland, Oregon
19 Health of the Nursing Student

Sarah Porter is the Associate Dean for Student and International Affairs for the Oregon Health Sciences University School of Nursing. She creates or supports policies, procedures, and processes for students that promote the development of their leadership, assertiveness, self-advocacy, and professional growth. She finds working with a widely diverse group of students enriching and exciting. Her research with ethnic-minority nursing students provides the nursing community with a framework for understanding the unique stressors and identifying useful coping strategies for all students who are under-represented.

"As nursing students you have much more power and control to influence positive changes in your life than you may realize. Seek out your nursing school faculty to assist you in gaining skills in negotiation and conflict resolution. More than anything else, take care of yourself. In the long run, it will be your health and vitality that will enable you to provide a caring and healing environment for your clients."

Bonnie Rogers, DrPh, RN, COHN-S, FAAN

Associate Professor of Nursing and Public Health
Director, Occupational Health Nursing
School of Public Health
University of North Carolina at Chapel Hill;
President, American Association of Occupational Health Nursing;
Chapel Hill, North Carolina
18 Personal Safety in Nursing Practice

In addition to her academic responsibilities, Bonnie Rogers is currently president of the American Association of Occupational Health Nurses. Her research interests are mainly focused on hazards to health care workers and ethical issues in occupational health.

"For all of us, it is vitally important to concern ourselves with the health and safety of our own work. Our lives will be enriched through our own personal caring for our patients, colleagues, work environment, and ourselves. Understanding workplace health will enhance the well being of those you serve and your own."

Thérése Rymer, RN, CFNP, COHN-S

Director, Clinical Services
University of California San Diego Center for Occupational and Environmental Medicine
University of California San Diego Medical Center
San Diego, California
18 Personal Safety in Nursing Practice

Dorie Schwertz, PhD, RN

Associate Professor, Medical-Surgical Nursing and Pharmacology
University of Illinois at Chicago
Chicago, Illinois
Chair, Illinois Council of Nurse Researchers
Co-Chair, Physiologic Research Subsection
Midwest Nursing Research Society
Sigma Theta Tau
16 *Pharmacology and Medication Administration*

Dorie W. Schwertz is an Associate Professor in Medical Surgical Nursing at the University of Illinois at Chicago. She holds an adjunct appointment in the Department of Pharmacology. She is a current member of the National Institutes of Health, Nursing Research Study Section and present Chair of the Illinois Council of Nurse Researchers. Dr. Schwertz conducts research in two focus areas. One is investigation of ischemia-induced changes in cell signaling and the role of these changes in myocardial cell injury. The other is examination of sex differences in myocardial function and response to drugs.

"The holistic base of the nursing profession includes physiologic, cellular, and molecular aspects of your patients. In learning pharmacology it is nearly impossible to memorize the actions of all drugs. Moreover, the specific drugs that are available for therapeutic intervention will change over the course of a nurse's career. For these reasons, I recommend that you learn the basic principles of pharmacology (pharmacokinetics and pharmacodynamics) because these principles can be applied to aid in the understanding of any new drug that the nurse encounters."

Diana L. Taylor, PhD, RN, FAAN, NP

Associate Professor
School of Nursing;
Co-Director, Center for Collaborative Innovation in Primary Care
University of California, San Francisco
San Francisco, California
33 *Sexual Health Protection and Health Promotion*

Diana Taylor, nurse practitioner, educator and researcher, is an Associate Professor in the University of California, San Francisco Department of Family Health Care Nursing and formerly the Director of the Women's Primary Care Program, the first women's health training program in California. Most recently, she was appointed Co-director of the Center for Collaborative Innovations in Primary Care to advance interdisciplinary practice, teaching, and research at UCSF. She has focused much of her clinical and research work on the understanding of the biopsychosocial and lifespan factors that affect the health and illness of women within the context of cyclic changes across the menstrual cycle. She is the co-author of the book *Menstruation, Health & Illness.* Her current research projects focus on testing alternative and complementary therapies for women's health conditions, developing women's health promotion programs, and studying symptom management for complex women's health conditions.

"We hope that this chapter will challenge you to think about men's and women's health beyond the usual reproductive or genitourinary disease perspectives. Sexual health promotion, as a combined system of health and illness care practices, integrates gender, culture, family, and community. Nursing practice includes the skill, knowledge, and responsibility to apply the biopsychosocial, multicultural, lifespan, activist, and gender-centric frameworks to health protection and promotion for men and women."

Virginia P. Tilden, DNSc, RN, FAAN

Youmans Spaulding Professor & Associate Dean for Research, School of Nursing
Associate Director, OHSU Center for Ethics in Health Care
Director, Program of Research on Ethics and End of Life Care
Oregon Health Sciences University, School of Nursing
Adjunct Faculty, School of Medicine
Portland, Oregon
29 *Social Support*

Virginia P. Tilden, DNSc, RN, FAAN is a Youmans Spaulding Professor and Associate Dean for Research, School of Nursing; and an Associate Director for the Center for Ethics in Health Care at Oregon Health Sciences University. Her research focus is on reducing the suffering of patients and their families near the time of death and the design of improvements in end-of-life care in order to meet unmet comfort-care needs of families and dying patients.

May Timmons, EdD, RN

Associate Professor & Director of the Graduate Nursing Program
Clarkson College
Omaha, Nebraska
21 *Respiration*

Mae E. Timmons is currently an Associate Professor and Director of the Graduate Nursing Program at Clarkson College in Omaha, Nebraska. Dr. Timmons has taught undergraduate students in Adult Health Theory and clinical as well as Theory and Laboratory courses related to Professional Nursing Skills. In addition to her administrative responsibilities, Dr. Timmons currently teaches Nursing Research to the undergraduate students, serves as a thesis chairperson to graduate students, and coordinates the Graduate Thesis Development course. Dr. Timmons has conducted clinical as well as educational research with her life-long mentor, Dr. Fay L. Bower.

"I'd like to emphasize the importance of reading and critiquing current nursing research to guide clinical practice. Without nursing research we would still be treating pressure ulcers with a sugar mixture and directly exposing the affected area to a heat lamp."

Margaret Topf, PhD, RN
Associate Professor
School of Nursing, University of Colorado Health Sciences Center
Denver, Colorado
30 Environment and Health

Margaret Topf, PhD, RN, is an Associate Professor at the University of Colorado Health Sciences Center School of Nursing. Her PhD is in Social-Environmental Psychology. Her research focuses on environmental hazards and health. Her current interest is in noise pollution, coping, and health in patients and nurses occupying hospital critical care units.

"With the increased national interest in the physical environment and health it is clear that the future will call for nurses to engage in environmental activism. As part of interdisciplinary teams nurses will plan and implement interventions to reduce environmental hazards and enhance restorative/aesthetic surroundings for patients and community members in the hospital, the home, schools, and the workplace as well as other settings."

Sandra J. Weiss, PhD, RN, DNSc, FAAN
Professor, Department of Community Health Systems
School of Nursing, University of California at San Francisco
San Francisco, California
32 Touch

Dr. Weiss is a Professor in the Department of Community Health Systems at UCSF School of Nursing. Her background in the fields of biological psychology and child/family nursing lays the foundation for her clinical and theoretical expertise regarding touch. Dr. Weiss' program of research related to touch spans 25 years. Over that time, her NIH-funded studies have examined the effects of touch on the neurobehavioral development and health status of high-risk infants, the relationship between parental touch and body image in children, and the psychophysiological impact of touch used in clinical care of cardiovascular patients.

"To the students: Your understanding of the role of touch in health and health care, and the skill and sensitivity with which you use touch in your nursing practice will be critical determinants of whether you provide 'good nursing care'!"

Joan Stehle Werner, DNS, RN
Professor, Department of Adult Health Nursing
School of Nursing
University of Wisconsin-Eau Claire
Eau Claire, Wisconsin
31 Stress and Anxiety

Dr. Joan Stehle Werner has taught at the School of Nursing, University of Wisconsin-Eau Claire (UWEC) for the past 17 years. She currently holds the position of Professor, Department of Adult Health Nursing. She has also served as Research Facilitator at UWEC. Dr. Werner's research and scholarly writing has focused in the areas of occupational stress, patient/client stress and coping, long-term care stress and quality of care, and, educationally, critical thinking and synthesis.

Dr. Werner advocates the weaving of research into every nursing endeavor. She would like students of nursing to be ever mindful of the words of Virginia Henderson (1987): "When nurses' sensitivity to human needs (their intuition) is joined with the ability to find and use expert opinion, with the ability to find reported research and apply it to their practice, and when they themselves use the scientific method of investigation, there is no limit to the influence they might have on health care worldwide."

PROCEDURES

Paula Riemar Milner, MS, RN, CS
Medical-Surgical Clinical Educator
Scottsdale Healthcare Osborn
Scottsdale, Arizona

Mary Ann Wells, BSN, RN, MSEd
Educator
Scottsdale Healthcare
Scottsdale, Arizona

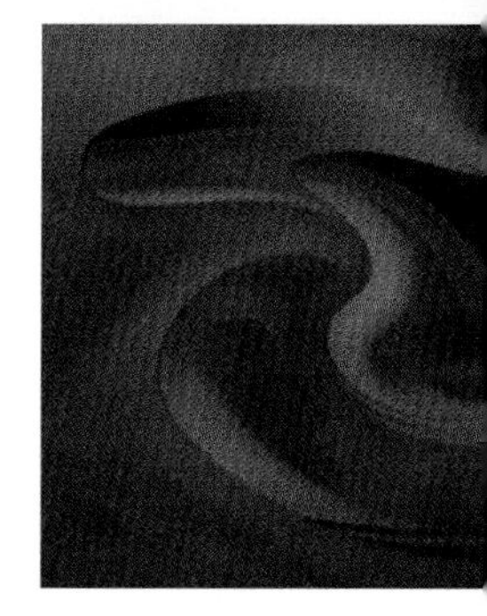

Reviewers

Connie S. Austin, MSN, RN, MAEd
Associate Professor
Azusa Pacific University
Azusa, California

Janice M. Beitz, PhD, RN, CS, CNOR, CWOCN
Graduate Program Director
School of Nursing
LaSalle University
Philadelphia, Pennsylvania

Margaret W. Bellak, MN, RN
Indiana University of Pennsylvania
Indiana, Pennsylvania

Elisa A. Bianchi-Smak, MS, RN, CS, NP-C
Raritan Bay Medical Center
Perth Amboy, New Jersey

Elizabeth Muncey Blunt, MSN, CEN
Allegheny University of the Health Sciences
Philadelphia, Pennsylvania

Sharon E. Bolin, MS, RN, EdD
Executive Director, Doctors on Call for Service
Saint Simons Island, Georgia

Dianne Booth-McCormack, MSN, RN, PHN
Golden West College
Huntington Beach, California

Barbara Brillhart, PhD, RN, CRRN, FNP-C
College of Nursing
Arizona State University
Tempe, Arizona

Bonita F. Broyles, BSN, RN, MA, EdD
Piedmont Community College
Roxboro, North Carolina

Mary M. Callahan, EdD, RN
Long Beach City College
Long Beach, California

V. Christine Champagne, MSN(R), RN, CS, ANP
Midwest Chest Consultants
St. Charles, Missouri

Marianne Chiafery, MS, RN, PNP, CCRN
Strong Memorial Hospital
University of Rochester
Rochester, New York

Susan H. Davis, EdD, RN
Bellarmine College
Louisville, Kentucky

Patricia Ann Durham-Taylor, PhD, RN
Truckee Meadows Community College;
St. Mary's Hospital
Reno, Nevada

Chris Eaton, MS, RN, MA, CETN
Hartnell College
Salinas, California

Margaret Hanna Ederer, MSN, RN, CEAP
SSM Behavioral Medicine
St. Louis, Missouri

Mildred DuBois Fennal, PhD, RN, CCRN
South Carolina State University
Orangeburg, South Carolina

Peggy Hawkins-McWilliams, MN
Assistant Professor of Nursing
School of Nursing
University of Mississippi
Jackson, Mississippi

Amy Zlomek Hedden, MS, RN, CNS, NP
California State University Bakersfield;
Bakersfield Family Medical Center
Bakersfield, California

Dickie L. Hale Gerig, MS, RN, CPR-ARC
Grayson County College
Denison, Texas

Joyce M. Johnson, MN, RN, FNP
South Carolina State University
Columbia, South Carolina

Susan S. Johnson, MSN, RN
Guilford Technical Community College
Jamestown, North Carolina

Kathleen A. Kick, MS
Purdue University Calumet
Calumet, Illinois

Judith Ann Kilpatrick, MSN
School of Nursing
Widener University
Chester, Pennsylvania

Eloise R. Lee, MSN, RN, EdD
Cedar Crest College
Allentown, Pennsylvania

Margo Payne Leithead, MSN, RN
School of Nursing
Pennsylvania State University/Geisinger Health System
Danville, Pennsylvania

Laurie Jean Maidl, BSN, RN, CETN
Mayo Clinic
Rochester, Minnesota

Susan E. Majerus, MSN, FNP
Mayo Clinic
Rochester, Minnesota

Ann H. Martinick, MSN, RN, CNS
Mercy Hospital School of Nursing
Pittsburgh, Pennsylvania

Jeanne M. McHale, MSN, RN
Beth Israel Deaconess Medical Center
Boston, Massachusetts

Patricia L. Newland, MS, RN
Broome Community College
Binghamton, New York

Patricia Ann O'Leary, DSN, RN
School of Nursing
Middle Tennessee State University
Murfreesboro, Tennessee

Netha O'Meara, MSN, RN
Wharton County Junior College
Wharton, Texas

Barbara L. Ogden, MSN, RN, CCRN
Gainesville VA Medical Center
Gainesville, Florida

Susan L. Olson, BSN, RN, CNN
Shady Grove Adventist Hospital
Rockville, Maryland

Gloria R. Perry, PhD, RN
Professor Emeritus
Southern Illinois University at Edwardsville
Edwardsville, Illinois

Linda P. Picklesimer, MSN, RN
Greenville Technical College
Greenville, South Carolina

Karen A. Piotrowski, MSN
D'youville College
Buffalo, New York

Priscilla W. Ramsey, PhD, RN, CS
East Tennessee State University
Johnson City, Tennessee

Roger L. Ready, BSN, RN
Mayo Medical Center
Rochester, Minnesota

Barbara Ridley, MS, RN, CRRN
Alta Bates Medical Center
Berkeley, California

Christine M. Rosner, PhD, RN
Division of Nursing
Holy Family College
Philadelphia, Pennsylvania

Mary E. Sampel, MSN, RN
Saint Louis University
St. Louis, Missouri

Susan M. Schlesselman, MSN, RN, OCN
Augusta State University
Augusta, Georgia

Barbara J. Schroeder, MS, RN
Mayo Clinic
Rochester, Minnesota

Marsha Johnson Schulte, MSN, RN, CS
Adult Nurse Practitioner
St. Charles Clinic
St. Peters, Missouri

Lisa K. Anderson-Shaw, MSN, RN, MA
College of Nursing
University of Illinois at Chicago
University of Illinois Medical Center
Chicago, Illinois

Sharon P. Shipton, PhD, RN, AS
Associate Professor
Youngstown State University
Youngstown, Ohio

Thomas J. Smith, PhD, APN-G
Nicholls State University
Thibodaux, Louisiana

Zelda Suzan, MA, RN
Phillips Beth Israel School of Nursing
New York, New York

Charleen Tachibana, MN, RN
Virginia Mason Medical Center
Seattle, Washington

Sharon C. Wahl, MS, RN, EdD
School of Nursing
San Jose State University
San Jose, California

Kathleen H. Werle, MSN, RN
Victor Valley College
Victorville, California

Denise D. Wilson, PhD, RN, CS, FNP
Associate Professor
Mennonite College of Nursing;
Clinical Practice, Medical Hills Internists
Bloomington, Illinois

Ann Windsor, DNS, RN
University of Wisconsin-Madison
Madison, Wisconsin

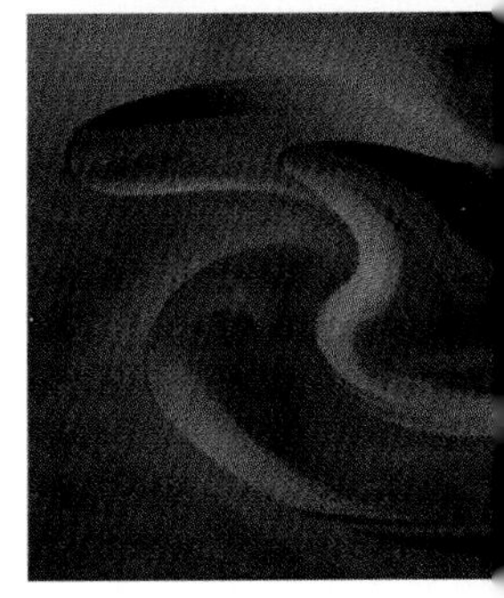

Preface

TO THE STUDENT

With this textbook you will be taking the first and perhaps the most important steps toward joining the nursing profession. You may be coming to the profession through the example or influence of a mentor or family member; you may be coming from another profession, or from a lifetime spent raising a family; or nursing may in fact be the very first career choice you've made. Your impression of health care and nursing may have been formed by personal experiences or by books, movies, and television. Whatever your personal situation, this preface explains that the profession you are entering is quite changed from the one that welcomed the nurses now practicing. If you don't already have some impression of how health care and nursing were until just a few years ago, you might do well to skip to the part of this preface headed "Organization and Content" and then come back to the first part after getting introduced to the health care system as part of your course.

TO THE INSTRUCTOR

This preface sets forth the values and beliefs that underlie this textbook. We do this so that you, the instructor, can determine whether this is the right text for you and your students. We believe that profound changes have taken place in health care and in nursing, which have not by any means run their course. We believe these changes must affect—in equally profound ways—how we educate future generations of nurses. We hope that you find that this preface and this textbook accurately reflect the current trends in health care and nursing and that you find using this textbook with your students an exciting new means of addressing the challenges that these trends pose for us all.

Fundamentals of Contemporary Nursing Practice is intended for use at the beginning of the nursing curriculum for registered nurses. Its inception and development stem from a distinct set of values and beliefs about professional nursing practice and education. Those values and beliefs are described in this Preface under the heading "Contemporary Nursing Practice and Education." The content of the book and the rationale for its organization are presented under the heading "Organization and Content." Other features of the textbook are discussed under the headings "Text Features" and "Teaching and Learning Package."

CONTEMPORARY NURSING PRACTICE AND EDUCATION

Health Care

The United States health care system is undergoing a paradigm shift, or a fundamental and radical change in the assumptions and principles by which it operates. No one single factor or event triggered the shift; instead, it can be attributed to the interaction of scientific, technological, sociological, and economic developments. Of all these developments, it is the economic forces that seem currently to be producing the most dramatic system-wide changes. Steven Schroeder, president of The Robert Wood Johnson Foundation, offers this analysis (1997, p. 3):

> . . . the United States has opted for the market, not government, as a way to address escalating medical costs. Indeed, the story of medical care for the past two years could be labeled the triumph of the market. Enrollment in managed care plans is surging; for-profit hospitals and health plans are expanding at a much greater rate than their not-for-profit competitors; and federal, state, and local politicians of both parties promote managed care as the best way to control Medicare and Medicaid costs. *The market has emerged as our de facto national health policy* (emphasis added).

The Pew Health Professions Commission (1995, p. v) describes the changes as follows:

> American health care is experiencing fundamental change. What was recently conceived as a set of policy changes for reform is now being lent the form and weight of institutional reality by the enormous power of the trillion dollar health care market. In five brief years the organizational, financial, and legal frameworks of much of the U.S. health care industry have been transformed to emerging systems of integrated care that combine primary, specialty, and hospital services. These systems attempt to manage the care delivered to enrolled populations in such a manner as to achieve some combination of cost reduction, enhanced patient and consumer satisfaction, and improvement of health care outcomes.

The Pew Commission believes that all contemporary health care providers must have these competencies (pp. xii–xvi):

- Care for the community's health
- Expand access to effective care
- Provide clinically competent care
- Emphasize primary care
- Participate in coordinated care
- Ensure cost-effective and appropriate care
- Practice prevention
- Involve patients and families in the decision-making process
- Promote healthy lifestyles
- Assess and use technology appropriately
- Improve the health care system
- Manage information
- Understand the role of the physical environment
- Provide counseling on ethical issues
- Accommodate expanded accountability
- Participate in a racially and culturally diverse society
- Continue to learn

Competencies required in this new world of health care include but are not limited to:

- Relationship skills
- Critical thinking
- Cultural competence
- Consumer empowerment
- Assessment of individuals, families, and communities
- Care management (right care, right time, right setting, and right cost)
- Primary care
- Communication/negotiation
- Community/population prevention skills
- Intervention skills
- Development and use of databases
- Epidemiological methodology
- Use of information systems
- Use of technology as extension of self
- Evaluation of technology
- Assessment of cost-effectiveness of care
- Identification and measurement of appropriate outcomes of care

It is this dynamic new world of health care that we, the authors, had in mind in creating this textbook.

Nursing Practice

Nurses everywhere are having to deal with a health care system characterized by complexity, conflict, and above all change. Just as health care is undergoing a radical change, so is nursing practice. The emerging changes in nursing practice can be portrayed as follows:

FROM	TO
Nursing imperative (do *everything* possible for *everyone*)	Cost-effective imperative
Needs drive	Resource drive
Discipline-specific	Interdisciplinary
Explicit roles/job descriptions	Blurred roles/team expectations
Provider judgment	Practice guidelines and provider judgment
Reductionist view (problems and diagnoses)	Holistic view (person as an entity and as part of a family and community
Linear problem-solving	Critical thinking
Episodic care	Care over a continuum
Moderate technology	High technology and de-skilling
Paradigm (textbook) cases	Population-based/individualized care
Process	Outcomes
Doing my job the way I was taught	Caring, daring, sharing

The opportunities in this new world of health care for the profession of nursing are truly exciting. Realization of those opportunities does require nurses to give up the old and accept the challenge of the new. As stated by one set of nurse leaders (Vicenzi et al, 1997, p. 31) "You have a newly positive, proactive attitude about your professional future. At the same time [you continue to advocate for patients and nursing's role in the new health care system], you're promoting a new, invigorated image of nurses as pioneers who are interdependent with the other major players in the system—not isolated defenders of the status quo. Instead of being pulled reluctantly into the future, you're riding the tide of change."

Nursing Research

Since the 1960s, the discipline of nursing has accepted the importance of developing a scientific base for practice. Today we can be proud of the quality and quantity of research produced by members of the discipline. We can also be proud of the integration of science from other disciplines into the knowledge base for nursing practice.

In a market-driven health care system, care based on research and evidence is critical. As patients (or "consumers") are forced to take more control over their own health care, they will demand that what health care professionals do for them is effective. They will want to know that, as much as possible, research supports the connection between a particular intervention and a particular outcome. Therefore, a new health care system requires an even greater alignment among theory, research, and practice. All nurses—from the beginning of their education and throughout their career—will be expected to know how to use research findings in practice, whether from the natural sciences or the humanistic sciences.

Research is a process driven by inquiry. The practice of nursing must inform that inquiry at the same time practice is informed by existing research. The problems studied, the methods used, and the perspectives taken will vary from inquiry to inquiry, but the interplay between practice and research must remain at the core. As the discipline of nursing is still maturing, all nurses should, in the ideal, approach their practice with this same spirit of inquiry. The strong presentation of research from nursing and other disciplines throughout this text is meant in part to foster that spirit among beginning students.

Nursing Education

Nursing educators are experiencing the stress of change in almost every aspect of the faculty role. Faculty are being asked to make major curriculum changes to reflect changes in the health care system. They are being asked to use the community rather than the hospital as the primary clinical teaching setting. They are asked to address the needs of students who are more heterogeneous in terms of age, culture, life experiences, and values than the students of the past. They are asked to do more with less.

Most germane to this textbook is the shift from the focus on teaching to a focus on learning—and a shift from process to outcomes. The focus on teaching gave the teacher control of the classroom and the educational inputs. The teacher, as "the sage on the stage," controlled the reading list, guest lecturers, content, and learner objectives. The teacher expected all students to progress through the faculty-determined sequence of learning experiences. Roles of teacher and student were clearly differentiated, and both teacher and student understood who had more power than the other.

In this current era, the focus of the public is on learning and outcomes. The public wants to know what an educational program will cost, and what it will enable a student to do upon its completion. This shift to learning and outcomes has occurred at the same time science has produced new insights about learning and technology and has given both teacher and student new tools. In this era, the teacher is expected to be a "guide on the side"

- assisting students to benefit from the rich array of inputs available through the Internet and other technologies;
- allowing students to progress through different learning paths;
- empowering learners to be active in the design of the course/curriculum;
- facilitating creating knowledge between the learner and the known;
- allowing roles to be flexible;
- treating the classroom as a community; and
- creating a learning community where people learn together beyond the classroom

Along with the fundamental changes in health care, nursing practice, and nursing research, these major changes in nursing education also fed the impetus to create this textbook.

ORGANIZATION AND CONTENT

In one sense a fundamentals textbook is the most important nursing textbook a student will use. From this first resource the beginning student develops an understanding of the nature of nursing practice. The fundamentals textbook establishes the base for the more specialized knowledge and competencies developed later in the curriculum and for the student's future practice as a registered nurse. The textbook must reflect contemporary nursing practice and developments in the profession. It must present the complexity of nursing practice but in a manner appropriate to the novice. In addition to presenting the appropriate content, it must develop an understanding about the relationship between knowing, thinking, and doing. It must prepare the student to be a dynamic and flexible practitioner who will work in a constantly changing system.

Influence of Virginia Henderson

The organization and context of this book reflect Virginia Henderson's beliefs about nursing practice. Henderson believed that thinking and doing should be one (Chinn, 1996). She talked about nursing practice as a continuous, unbroken spectrum of thought and action involving patterned thought, i.e., the ability to connect detail and generality into a meaningful whole (Evans, 1980). Henderson rejected the notion that nursing is a set of prescribed skills and behaviors; she believed, rather, that nursing is a complex practice (Bishop and Scudder, 1996). She also believed that the meaning of nursing should come from the study of nursing practice.

Henderson was one of the first to challenge the adequacy of the nursing process for nursing practice. She stated (1982, p. 109)

> while the nursing process recognizes the purpose of the problem-solving aspects of the nurses' work, a habit of inquiry and the use of investigative techniques in developing the scientific basis for nursing, it ignores the subjective or intuitive aspect of nursing and the role of the experience, logic and expert opinion as bases for practice. In stressing a dominant and independent function for the nurse, it fails to stress the value of collaboration of health professionals and particularly the importance of developing the self-reliance of clients.

Henderson's connection of thinking with doing is comparable to the current view of the nurse as a "knowledge worker." Knowledge workers are individuals valued in the workplace because of the knowledge they bring, as opposed to the tasks they are capable of performing. Their knowledge is their capital asset. Henderson's view of nursing also has similarities to Schon's (1983) view of the reflective practitioner. The reflective practitioner is more than a conduit for the transmission of scientific knowledge. The reflective practitioner uses multiple sources of information including that embedded within the practice situation itself. The reflective practitioner learns by reflecting on practice, entering each encounter with a spirit of inquiry, and remaining intellectually alive during the encounter.

These beliefs of Virginia Henderson led us, the authors, to require practice-oriented objectives throughout the text, to include information about other health care providers, to emphasize clinical decision making that includes but is not limited to the cognitive skills involved in the nursing process, to recognize the various sources of knowledge used in practice, and to highlight the research base for practice.

Henderson's definition of nursing and conception of basic nursing practice were used to organize the clinical content of this text. Henderson (1969, p. 4) stated that the unique function of the nurse is "to assist the individual, sick or well, in the performance of those activities contributing to health or its recovery (or to a peaceful death) that he would perform unaided if he had the necessary strength, will, or knowledge. And to do this in such a way as to help him gain independence as rapidly as possible." Included in the components of basic nursing are (Henderson, 1969, p. 12–13): nutrition, respiration, elimination, mobility, sleep and rest, vital signs, personal hygiene, emotionally and physically safe environments, communication, spirituality, social well-being, and education and information. The chapters in Unit III were designed to encompass this view of basic nursing care.

Wolf et al (1994) identified four critical changes occurring in nursing practice:

- Practice must evolve from a needs-driven model of care to one that is sensitive to limited resources.
- There is a direct correlation between critical thinking and quality, not between manpower and quality.
- Standardization and routines for patient care will be replaced by individualization and creativity.
- Accountability, responsibility, and authority for clinical decision making will evolve from the manager to the practitioner, in partnership with the patient.

The authors believe these changes describe what is happening in nursing practice. Therefore, in this text, these themes are emphasized:

- Clinical decision making
- Research base for practice
- Future trends
- Individual differences
- Technology as a complement to practice
- Financial and ethical considerations
- The nurse as a knowledge worker
- Promoting self-care, health promotion, and the interdependence of the patient, family, community, and nurse
- Education and relationship-centered care as powerful nursing interventions

Organization

The textbook consists of 36 chapters organized into four units: *The Context for Nursing Practice, The Process of Nursing Practice, Special Considerations Basic to Nursing Practice,* and *The Content of Basic Nursing Care.*

Nursing practice does not occur in a vacuum. It is influenced by contextual factors such as the technology explosion, changing demographics, and changing policies regarding the financing and delivery of health care. The chapters in the first unit provide the student with facts and concepts related to the current context for nursing practice as well as historical and futuristic perspectives. To highlight the dynamic nature of these topics, each chapter contains a discussion of a "Current Controversy." The chapters in the first unit cover the nature of nursing practice, the nature of nursing knowledge, the health care system, health care finance, technology and nursing practice, determinants of health and illness, leadership and management, legal aspects, and ethics.

Some reviewers believed that beginning students did not need information on health care finance. The authors chose to include that chapter, believing that everyone in health care—including students—needs to understand basic issues regarding the financing of health care. The minute a nurse sets foot on a clinical unit today, issues of cost, resources (including time), and reimbursement arise to influence the kind of care to be provided. The beginning student cannot be ignorant of this aspect of the context of nursing practice.

The authors also believed that contemporary nursing practice requires an understanding of epidemiological principles and data. This content is included in the discussion of the determinants of health and illness.

Although both the context and content (specific nursing actions) for nursing practice will change over time, there are core elements of practice that will remain. Five core elements were identified that apply to nursing regardless of where it is practiced, and these are discussed in Unit II. These elements of practice are also ones mentioned frequently by patients and families when they discuss quality: the helping relationship, caring, clinical decision making, patient and family education, and documentation.

Health care providers work in settings where there is a high risk for stress and injury. Likewise, patients are cared for in environments that hold some risk for them. A knowledge of infection control, personal safety, and biomechanics and mobility is important to reducing these risks. The chapters in Unit III address these and other universal considerations basic to nursing care, such as assessment, the health of the nurse, and pharmacology and medication administration.

While some reviewers of the chapter on "Health of the Nursing Student" wondered about including negative data about nurses and their health behaviors, we believed that it is important to alert beginning students to health risks and assist them in developing healthy life styles. Health promotion is important for everyone—including nurses themselves.

To facilitate student learning and to ensure that the intent of the textbook was fulfilled, contributors for the final unit were asked to follow a standard outline:

A *Case Study* describes a typical patient situation, highlighting the area of nursing practice covered in the chapter. The case study will help the student visualize the specific area of practice as well as set the stage for the section on clinical decision-making.

A *Scope of Practice* overview discusses the importance of this area of nursing practice. *Objectives* state the nursing practice outcomes expected after the student has mastered the chapter contents.

The *Knowledge Base* section summarizes relevant basic science information and highlights the research and theory base for practice. Classic research and current studies relevant to practice are included.

Factors Affecting Clinical Decisions include information on factors that influence this specific aspect of practice such as age, gender, values, and culture. Also addressed are influence of setting, and ethical and financial considerations. Understanding these factors will help the student individualize care.

Future Developments identify changes anticipated in the future that will affect nursing practice. Some areas considered are the impact of managed care, health care reform, technology, and changing demographics.

Nursing Care Actions are divided into two sections. The first, *Principles and Practices,* covers specific nursing principles and practices, showing students the "whats" and "hows." Information on assessment and interventions is included. *Procedures* are presented in the second section.

The clinical content covered in the final unit are respiration, nutrition and fluids, intestinal elimination, urinary elimination, rest and sleep, personal hygiene, comfort, skin integrity, social support, environment and health, stress and anxiety, touch, sexual health protection and promotion, grief, care of the dying, and health promotion and self-care.

TEXT FEATURES

The text includes various features that enhance and expand on the narrative. By highlighting important concepts and issues, these features help the student learn and quickly reference key information.

As discussed earlier, a ***Case Study*** at the beginning of each "clinical" chapter (Chapters 15–36) presents a detailed, realistic clinical scenario pertinent to the chapter's content. This case presentation gives the student an immediate, "real world" context for the material covered in the chapter. It also serves as "touchstone" throughout the chapter, as it is periodically revisited to help remind the student how such factors as financial considerations, cultural/ethnic/socioeconomic differences, ethical principles, spiritual/religious beliefs, and care setting (hospital, home, or other facility) affect clinical decision making and nursing care.

The ***Clinical Decision Making*** feature is also included in each clinical chapter, and builds on the case presentation and its subsequent revisitations throughout the chapter text, providing a specific illustration of how the nurse applies critical thinking skills to arrive at sound nursing practice decisions.

Patient Education boxes also appear throughout the clinical chapters. These focus on instructions that nurses provide to patients and their families to help them learn sound health promotion and disease prevention practices, or to cope with life changes caused by illness.

Research Highlights boxes, included in nearly every chapter, provide synopses of recent nursing research articles and other scientific articles applicable to nursing. Each box provides a summary of the article and a discussion of possible implications for nursing practice. This feature helps the student identify the strengths and weaknesses of the research and see how research can help guide nursing practice. This feature complements the thorough grounding of each and every chapter on the large body of nursing and health science research, and thus supports the text's theme of research and science as the foundation for sound nursing practice.

Current Controversy boxes highlight "in the news" issues associated with nursing care, the health care system, and other health-related topics. A typical feature presents an excerpt from a newspaper or magazine article exploring a controversial topic—for example, HMO gag rules or health care rationing. Besides providing students with insight into how various factors both inside and outside of the health care system affect nursing and health care, this feature also raises ethical and other questions that further encourage the student to think critically about important issues of the day.

Finally, ***Nursing Procedures*** are found in most of the clinical chapters. These step-by-step presentations, complete with rationales for each nursing action, are liberally illustrated with photographs and line drawings. Also included as part of the standard format of each procedure are objectives and expected outcomes, pertinent terminology, critical elements and risk factors to consider, instructions for preparation of equipment and the patient, guidelines for evaluation and documentation, and patient teaching concerns. The selection of procedures for this textbook was based on a survey of nurse educators and education directors in health care facilities. A review of other texts led to the identification of 216 skills that could be included in the text. Respondents were asked to rank each skill in terms of frequency of occurrence, importance in care, and level of nurse assigned to implement the skill. Those skills rated by the majority as above average in frequency and importance and associated with the beginning student are included in this text. The authors recognize that many of the procedures included in this text are now done under the supervision of the registered nurse rather than by the registered nurse. Supervision requires the nurse to know how the procedure should be performed. Therefore, whether the nurse does the procedure or supervises another doing it, the same knowledge base is required.

TEACHING AND LEARNING PACKAGE

A complete and innovative teaching and learning package is available to those who use this text.

- The *Instructor's Resource Manual* consists of a printed manual and a CD-ROM. The printed manual contains selected reprints of important articles that will provide the instructor with a practical, in-depth introduction to the perspective from which this textbook was written. For each chapter the printed manual also contains learning objectives, teaching strategies, "writing to learn" assignments, case studies, and references for instructor enrichment. The CD-ROM will contain the entire text of the printed manual, plus presentation visuals for classroom use.
- The *Study Guide,* available for purchase by students, contains not only traditional activities for knowledge review and knowledge synthesis but also more open-ended activities that encourage *reflective learning* on the student's part. These encourage students to assess their own learning on a regular basis (Bartels, 1998). The *Study Guide* also includes a CD-ROM containing NCLEX-style chapter review questions and interactive tutorials on four key areas in nursing fundamentals: fluids and electrolytes, medication administration, basic IV therapy, wound care and dressing changes, and nutrition and tube feeding.
- A *Test Bank* is available to adopters of the text, and contains over 700 questions in NCLEX format. The Test Bank is also available on the ExaMaster 99 software program for test generation and classroom management.

ACKNOWLEDGMENTS

First and foremost we must thank the contributors who wrote the chapters and parts of chapters in this book. Distinguished nurse educators and clinicians from many different parts of the country gave generously of their time, expertise, and scholarship to help fulfill the vision of a book that would help set nursing practice on a new foundation of research-based, scientific, and humanistic principles.

We also thank the reviewers and consultants who provided us with invaluable advice on how to improve the content and make it more applicable to beginning nursing students.

The authors wish to acknowledge Thomas Eoyang of W.B. Saunders Company who had the initial inspiration and motivation to produce a research-based fundamentals textbook. His belief that beginning nursing students needed to be exposed to the most current knowledge and research was critical to the development of this book. We thank Thomas and all of his staff who contributed to producing this textbook.

We also thank our family and friends who listened to our complaints and supported us along the way.

REFERENCES

Bartels, J.E. (1998). Developing reflective learners—student self-assessment as learning. *Journal of Professional Nursing, 14*(3), 135.

Bishop, A.H., Scudder, J.R. (1996). "And Gina Sews": A tribute to Virginia Henderson, 1989–1996. *Advances in Nursing Science, 19*(1), 1–2.

Chinn, P.L. (1996). From the Editor. *Advances in Nursing Science, 19*(1), viii.

Evans, D.L. (1980). Everynurse as a researcher: An argumentative critique of principles and practice of nursing. *Nursing Forum, 19*(4), 335–349.

Henderson, V. (1969). Basic Principles of Nursing Care. Geneva, Switzerland: International Council of Nurses.

Henderson, V. (1982). The nursing process—is the title right? *Journal of Advanced Nursing, 7*, 103–109.

Pew Health Commission (1995). Critical Challenges: Revitalizing the health professions for the twenty-first century. San Francisco: UCSF Center for the Health Professions.

Schroeder, S.A. (1997). The Triumph of the Market. The Robert Wood Johnson Foundation Annual Report 1996. Princeton, NJ: The Robert Wood Johnson Foundation.

Schon, D.A. (1983). The Reflective Practitioner. New York: Basic Books.

Vicenzi, A.E., White, K.R., Begun, J.W. (1997). Chaos in nursing: Make it work for you. *American Journal of Nursing, 97*(10), 26–32.

Wolf, G.A., Boland, S., Aukerman, M. (1994). A transformation model for the practice of nursing. *Journal of Nursing Administration, 24*(4), 51–57.

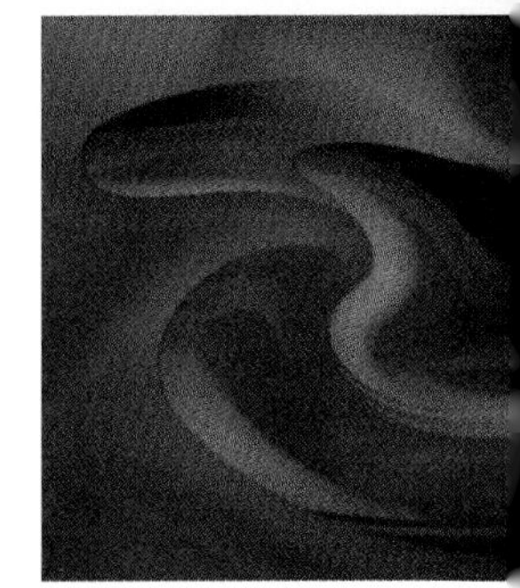

About the Authors

Carol Ann Lindeman, PhD, RN, FAAN

During her career, Dr. Carol A. Lindeman has served as President of Sigma Theta Tau and the National League for Nursing, as a board member of the American Nurses Association and the Association of Colleges of Nursing, as Chair of the Western Institute of Nursing, and as an officer of various state nursing associations. Various institutions and boards of higher education across the United States and Canada have benefited from her expertise as a consultant and program reviewer. She was appointed by the Secretary of the United States Department of Health and Human Services to serve on the Advisory Council for Nursing Education, becoming the first member of the Council to co-chair the Council.

Dr. Lindeman has been cited for her vision for nursing education and her contributions to nursing research by more than a dozen educational institutions and by both the National League for Nursing and the American Nurses Association. Her contributions to the community have been recognized by the League of Women Voters and the Institute for Managerial and Professional Women.

Among Dr. Lindeman's many awards and honors, her citation from the University of Minnesota as one "who is committed to increasing the scientific base of nursing practice and improving the health of the public" typifies the qualities that underlie the vision of this textbook. Dr. Lindeman began her nursing education at Deaconess Hospital in Milwaukee, Wisconsin. She obtained her baccalaureate and master's degrees at the University of Minnesota and her PhD at the University of Wisconsin, Madison.

Dr. Lindeman worked as a staff nurse, private duty nurse, and head nurse before beginning her career in nursing education. She served on the faculty at the University of Wisconsin, Eau Claire and as Dean and Professor at the School of Nursing, Oregon Health Sciences University, Portland. She worked as a nurse researcher at a community hospital in Wisconsin and directed the Regional Program for Nursing Research Development at Western Institute for Higher Education.

Marylou McAthie, EdD, RN

Administrator, consultant, teacher: Dr. Marylou McAthie has filled these roles during her years in nursing. Dr. McAthie began her nursing career as a head nurse and a supervisor in nursing service. She then became a nurse educator, first at Presbyterian–St. Luke's Hospital in Chicago and then at California State University in Sacramento. She then managed the nursing service and other related departments at San Joaquin Medical Services in Stockton, California, where she forged a close working relationship with medical and public health services that broadened her vision regarding coordinated community nursing services.

Dr. McAthie next joined the Division of Nursing of the Health Resources Administration, United States Public Health Service (USPHS), as a nursing consultant in San Francisco. She served as a consultant to nursing services and nursing educational institutions in the western United States and the American Pacific basin including American Samoa, Guam, and the American Trust Territory, and later to the emerging nations of the Republic of Palau, Federated States of Micronesia, and Republic of the Marshall Islands. She initiated many new programs in these regions, including the American Pacific Nursing Leadership Council.

Dr. McAthie then returned to teaching, joining the faculty of the Department of Nursing at Sonoma State University, Rohnert Park, California. As Professor of Nursing, she began a graduate program in nursing administration and taught at both the undergraduate and graduate levels.

Among Dr. McAthie's many honors are the USPHS regional award for excellent performance; the USPHS Special Recognition Award for significant contributions to improving the quality of nursing personnel and services in the United States Pacific Insular areas; the Jo Eleanor Elliot Award for outstanding leadership to the Western Council of Higher Education, Western Institute for Nursing; and the California Nurses Association Lulu Hassenplug Award for an outstanding contribution by a registered nurse to nursing education in the state of California. She is certified as an Ambassador of the Government of Guam Legislature and has received a Special Recognition Award for outstanding service to the government of Guam. She also has received special merit awards from the American Pacific Nurses Leadership Council.

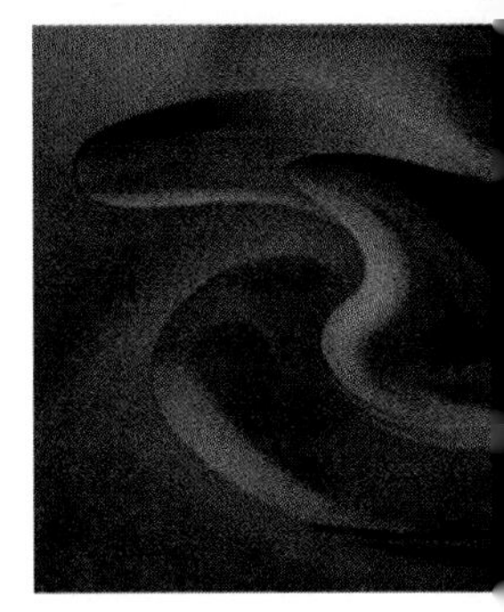

Contents

NOTICE

UNIT I

The Context for Nursing Practice

We have entered a new era of civilization—one in which change is the defining feature. Everywhere one turns there is a sense of conflict between what was, what is, and what is evolving. The view of the world as predictable and controllable has been replaced by the view as constantly changing, unpredictable, complex, and turbulent. In today's world there is an acknowledgment of the interaction between the context of our lives and the actions we take. Nursing practice does not occur in a vacuum. It is shaped through interactions with the context of today's health care system, which in turn is influenced by change drivers such as the information explosion, technology explosion, and changing demographics. Contemporary nursing practice requires that the nurse understand the context in which that practice occurs. Each of the nine chapters in this Unit addresses one critical aspect of the context for nursing practice. The student is provided with facts and concepts relevant to the current context as well as a historical or futuristic perspective.

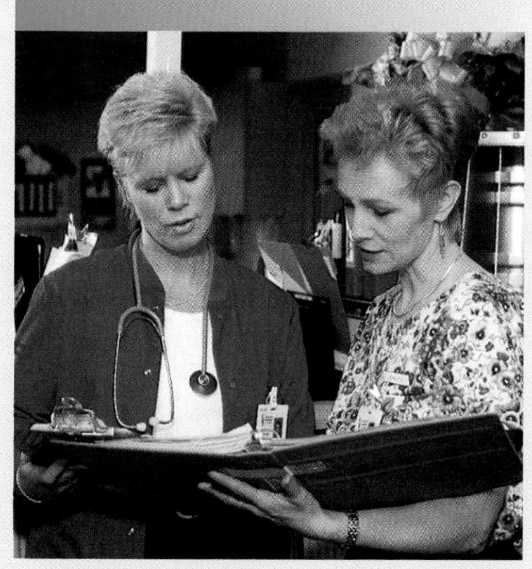

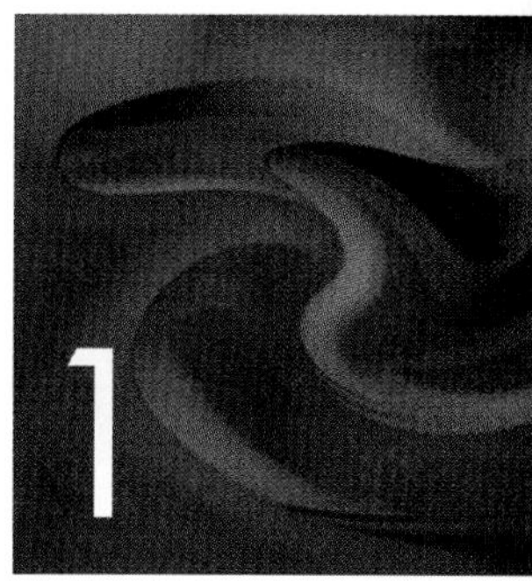

1

The Nature of Contemporary Nursing Practice

Marylou McAthie

Individuals choose to follow a specific career path for many different reasons. In general, those deciding to enter the nursing profession have in common the desire and commitment to care for and contribute to the well-being of another. Caring for and contributing to the well-being of others are key components in contemporary nursing. What, then, is *nursing* and what are the elements that make up nursing?

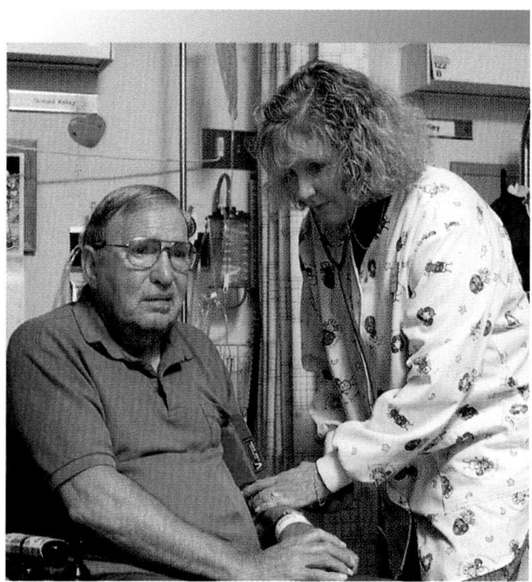

OBJECTIVES

After studying this chapter, the student will have:

- **explored the historical roots of nursing**
- **reviewed the definitions of nursing**
- **discussed society's impact on nursing**
- **explored the unique role and functions of the nurse**
- **defined the art and science of nursing**
- **described the settings in which nursing is practiced**
- **examined nursing as a profession**
- **reviewed standards of nursing practice**

THE EVOLUTION OF NURSING

To understand nursing as it is practiced today, one must consider nursing's historical roots. Over the years, the issues surrounding nursing have included:

- the evolution of different definitions of nursing
- the changing role and nature of nursing practice
- the levels of educational preparation of nurses
- the development of the nursing profession

According to Dock and Stewart (1938, p. 3):

> No occupation can be intelligently followed or understood unless it is, at least to some extent, illuminated by the light of history interpreted from the human standpoint. The origin of our various activities, the spirit animating the founders of a profession, and the long struggle toward an ideal as revealed by a search in the past—these vivify and ennoble the most prosaic labors, clarify their relation to all else that humanity is doing, and give to workers an unfailing inspiration in the consciousness of being one part of a great whole.

They further wrote (1938, p. 4):

> We must know how our work of nursing arose; what lines it has followed and under what direction it has developed best. Possessing this knowledge, each one may help it guide and influence its future in harmony with its historical mission.

Early Developments

Little is written about nursing in early historical accounts because the care of the sick was considered an ordinary event–it seems that it was not important enough to record. In all ages, nursing has been influenced by religious beliefs and practices. Even the oldest of religions were concerned with sickness and health. Some religions fostered cruelty and intolerance, others tenderness, hospitality, charity, and compassion. The latter groups fostered the care of the sick. For many centuries nursing was regarded as a calling and could be practiced only by those who removed themselves from worldly activities. To care for the sick required sacrifice and was a penitence endured only by those who had renounced materialism. To become a nurse required a pious devotion, or being remorseful or repentant, and atoning for a sin (Dock and Stewart, 1938).

PREHISTORIC EVENTS

In prehistoric ages, nursing and medicine seem to have been one and the same. Women gathered and dispensed herbs, roots, and leaves to those who were ailing. As time progressed, activities were divided into the medicine-giver and the caregiver. A woman, a nurturer, tended to fulfill the caregiver role. The men tended to become the medicine-givers. The male became the physician who was called in emergencies, prescribed treatments, and conducted ceremonies of magic or religion to banish evil spirits. The physician assumed a monopoly on theoretical and scientific knowledge and authority and relegated practical handwork to the caregiver assistants (Dock and Stewart, 1938).

Religion and medicine were united very early, with medicine men, and later physicians, becoming priests. Many persons believed that sickness was a punishment for committing a sin. This concept led to many strange methods of treating diseases, with such procedures as pommeling, beating, and starving being used to drive out evil spirits.

EARLY CHRISTIAN PERIOD

After the advent of the Christian church, nursing continued to be practiced and to advance through establishment of religious orders of sisterhoods and deaconesses. Philanthropy was considered a religious exercise, as was nursing. Nursing brotherhoods also thrived. Christian hospitals were established, as were hospitals in Arabian countries.

Medical science continued to expand during the early Christian period (to the end of the fifth century); however, during the Middle Ages the Church's attitude changed and metaphysics gradually transformed medicine into mysticism. Monasteries controlled medical practice and limited research and progress because there was widespread opposition to dissection of the human body. Clerical powers were opposed to the performing of surgery. The fortunes of nursing waxed and waned with those of medicine.

REFORMATION PERIOD

During the Reformation in the sixteenth century, monasteries were suppressed, church hospitals fell into disrepair, and the quality of nursing care given to patients declined. Governmental agencies such as cities assumed the responsibility of providing care. Nursing care fell into the hands of the unskilled servant class, whose work was inadequate at best. The political conditions of the period induced a general apathy and indifference to suffering. The hospitals erected by the cities were cheerless and dreary places, airless and unsanitary. The subjection of women was almost absolute during the seventeenth and eighteenth century (Dock and Stewart, 1938). Protestantism was narrowly intolerant toward women; witch-baiting and burning were prevalent. The withholding of education was deliberate and intentional. Avenues of self-support for women were closed, preventing them from making an organized revolt.

Monasteries for the sick in England and throughout Europe were closed. Hospital nursing was at its lowest ebb. Nurses were illiterate, harsh, venal, and overworked. Their time was divided between housework, laundry, scrubbing floors, and a semblance of nursing at its roughest (Dock and Stewart, 1938).

The dark period in nursing and patient care descended in the late 1600s and continued until changes were gradually initiated in the 1800s. This period lasted for over 300 years. It was during this time that Charles Dickens wrote about the character "Sairey Gamp," a secular nurse who was illiterate, heavy-handed, overworked, and frequently intoxicated. Gradually, religious orders such as the Daughters of Charity,

Protestant Deaconesses, and physicians in many European countries realized the need for skilled hospital personnel (Dock and Stewart, 1938).

REVIVAL OF NURSING

By the start of the nineteenth century, the changes in societal attitudes toward patient care started to improve. Several prominent women in England wrote of the degraded position of women and the need for human rights to be impartially applied to women. Others such as Elizabeth Fry, a member of the Society of Friends, became associated with the revival of nursing and the improvement of conditions in prisons (Jamieson and Sewall, 1944).

By the mid 1800s, several organizations had initiated programs to train nurses. An example was Pastor Theodor and Friederike Fliedner, who started a hospital and training program for nurses in Kaiserwerth, Germany. The Fliedner organization became a model for other deaconess facilities. The training program for the deaconesses consisted of rotations through a variety of different services, including the apothecary's room, office of the chapel, kitchen, laundry, sewing room, writing room, garden, communicable disease unit, and convalescent unit (Jamieson and Sewall, 1944). Students arose at 5 o'clock in the morning and worked and studied until 9 at night. Once a week they were expected to work for 24 straight hours. Uniforms, aprons, and a white hood-like cap with ruffles around the face and a bow under the chin were worn. The program served as a model for other institutions involved in training nurses.

Changes were gradually being initiated in English hospitals as a result of the interest of Elizabeth Fry and like-minded individuals. The pace of change was very slow and the quality of patient care remained poor. A series of sisterhoods under the English church was begun. The sisterhoods maintained control of the nursing activities; however, the new orders were not adequate to fill the needs of the public, in either numbers or training (Jamieson and Sewall, 1944). Nursing preparation was still lacking and the situation in majority of the hospitals remained unchanged.

THE NIGHTINGALE INFLUENCE

Florence Nightingale (Fig. 1–1), a member of English society, developed an interest in social reform and in improving nursing care. She determined to learn the methods being used to prepare nurses at Kaiserwerth. Her interest in social work and reform led her to become involved in meeting people with similar concerns. Her desire to become a nurse was realized when she obtained her family's consent to "train" with Fliedner's program. Miss Nightingale completed a course of study at Kaiserwerth. She also traveled to other countries and visited hospitals to observe the methods being used to improve patient care. She used her knowledge to improve nursing in England.

As a result of Nightingale's efforts, schools of nursing were established in England. One of the revolutionary features of

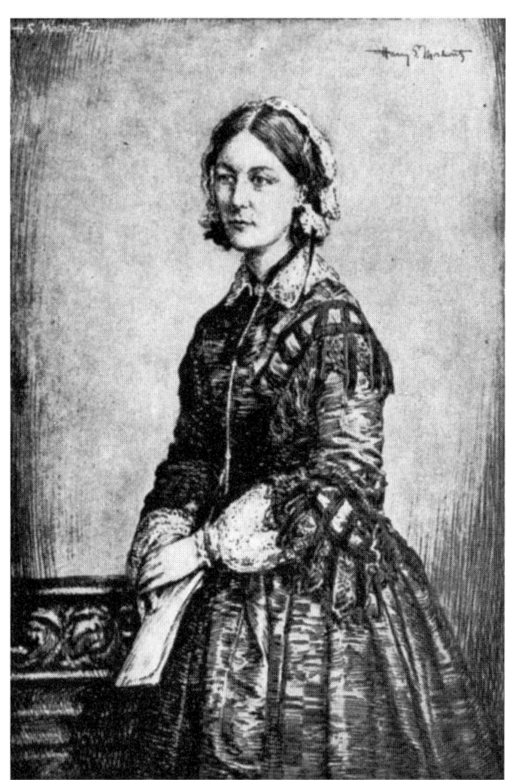

Figure 1-1. Florence Nighingale. (From Jamieson, E.M., Sewall, M.F., Suhrie, E.B. [1966]. *Trends in Nursing History.* Philadelphia: W.B. Saunders.)

the Nightingale plan for nursing was a positive mandate that the control of nursing rest with a trained, competent nurse and not be supervised by hospital non-nurse managers or physicians. English schools expanded and the supply of nurses increased. The concepts included in the Nightingale schools served as the basis for the development of schools of nursing in the United States. Miss Nightingale has become known as the primary founder of modern-day nursing.

NURSING IN THE UNITED STATES

The development of nursing in the United States began in the mid 1800s and, as stated above, was strongly influenced by the programs established in England by Florence Nightingale. During the century, both religious and secular hospitals of various sizes greatly increased in numbers in the United States. Epidemics of yellow fever, cholera, and other contagious diseases were rampant.

Medical science progressed to the extent of the recognition that:

- diseases were spread by germs
- inoculation for smallpox was a reality
- scurvy was preventable by eating citrus fruits
- quinine was effective in controlling malaria

Knowledge of anatomy and physiology had increased, and instruments such as the stethoscope, mercury thermometer, microscope, and x-rays were being used. Physicians were being directed to diagnose symptoms and observe disease patterns. It was determined that some illnesses were better treated and the spread of diseases was reduced when patients were separated from the general public. Surgery also was expanded as a result of the application of sterile techniques.

The changes in technology created a need for hospital staff to be adequately prepared. Training programs were established in some hospitals, both large and small. There were no existing standards to follow; almost all of the programs were of poor quality, with few educational classes offered. The training provided was the on-the-job apprentice type. In the late 1850s, Elizabeth Blackwell, the first American woman to become a physician, was instrumental in starting a rudimentary program to train nurses at the New York Infirmary, a hospital totally staffed by women. Her work inspired the development of comparable efforts in other cities such as Philadelphia and Boston.

Blackwell was a personal friend of Florence Nightingale and knew of Nightingale's success in starting nursing programs in England. Through Blackwell's efforts, Nightingale's work in nursing became known in the United States. An attempt was made to start a school of nursing at the New England Hospital for Women and Children in Boston in the early 1860s. The effort at first failed but became more successful when the Kaiserwerth methods of training were introduced. Linda Richards (Fig. 1–2) was the first nurse to graduate from the program in 1873. She has become known as the "first trained nurse in America."

Elizabeth Blackwell was also involved in organizing efforts to train nurses for duty in the battlefields during the Civil War. Also tied to the training of nurses during the war was Dorothea Dix, a woman who was already well known for her work in assisting in establishing asylums for the humane care of the insane. The lack of properly trained nurses caused many unnecessary deaths of soldiers.

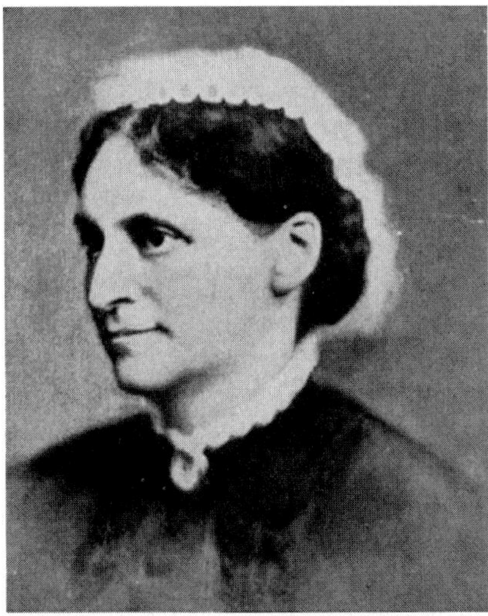

Figure 1–2. Linda Richards. (From Jamieson, E.M., Sewall, M.F., Suhrie, E.B. [1966]. *Trends in Nursing History.* Philadelphia: W.B. Saunders.)

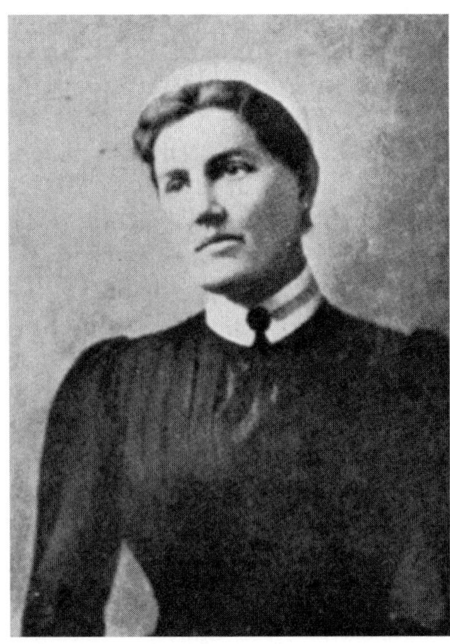

Figure 1–3. Isabel Hampton Robb. (From Jamieson, E.M., Sewall, M.F., Suhrie, E.B. [1966]. *Trends in Nursing History.* Philadelphia: W.B. Saunders.)

After the war there was a growing recognition that nurses needed to be better trained. The president of the American Medical Association, Dr. S. D. Gross, in 1868, stated:

> It seems to me to be just as necessary to have well-trained, instructed nurses, as to have intelligent and skillful physicians. I have long been of the opinion that there ought to be in all the principal towns and cities of the Union, institutions for the education of persons whose duty it is to take care of the sick (quoted in Bullough and Bullough, 1969, p. 128).

As a result of the speech, a committee was formed in 1869 that recommended the establishment of district schools. Publications such as women's magazines started to agitate for reform in attitudes toward nursing. Efforts to change the image of the nurse were intensified. By 1873, three schools of nursing were opened: The first was at Bellevue Hospital in New York, the second and third at Connecticut Training School in New Haven and at the Boston Training School at Massachusetts General Hospital (Bullough and Bullough, 1969).

The Bellevue School was the first to adopt the Nightingale system, and through its program prepared many of the future leaders in American nursing. One of these was Isabel Hampton Robb (Fig. 1–3), who organized schools in Illinois and at Johns Hopkins Hospital. She wrote the first book recognized as a standard for other nursing texts. Another graduate was Lavinia Dock, who held administrative positions in several hospitals and schools. She wrote the first text in *Materia Medica* (pharmacology) and with Adelaide Nutting the first text on the history of nursing (Jamieson and Sewall, 1944).

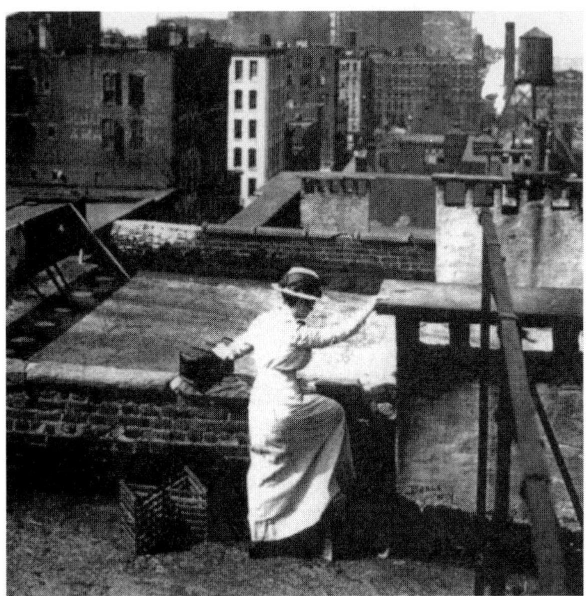

Figure 1–4. A visiting nurse in the tenements of New York City, about 1910. (Courtesy of the Visiting Nurse Association of America.)

Hospitals and nursing training schools were proliferating throughout the United States. Student nurses were being used to staff hospitals and private duty nurses were being used in homes, particularly among the rich. The poor had little care available at home. Lillian Wald and Mary Brewster moved into this void by starting the Henry Street Settlement in the slums of New York City in 1893. All of the problems of the people living within the tenements became nursing problems. Nurses visiting the people in their homes recognized social causes of illness underlying the physical and bacterial causes (Fig. 1–4). Public health issues were identified, and visiting nursing was established as an important part of health care (Jamieson and Sewall, 1944).

The increasing number of schools led to many problems; there were no standards for courses of study or for the legal distinction between trained nurses and those with little or no training. Nursing leaders realized that efforts would have to be made to develop and implement some type of controls. Nursing organizations began to emerge.

EMERGENCE OF ORGANIZED NURSING

The issues of how nurses should be educationally prepared and the need to set standards for schools were discussed by Isabel Hampton Robb in an address to The International Congress of Charities, Correction, and Philanthropy in Chicago in 1893. She stated that "the teaching methods of no two schools were alike" and that "each school was a law unto itself." Further, the term trained nurse "may mean anything, everything, or next to nothing." She later stated that "the criticisms of us as a profession are constant, severe and searching" (Roberts, 1954, pp. 22, 49).

The meeting had been mutually planned by Robb and Mrs. Bedford Fenwick from England and marked the beginning of nursing organizations in America. Mrs. Fenwick was also instrumental in starting organized nursing in England. The seeds for starting international organizations were sewn. The Congress was a milestone in American nursing history. As a result of the meeting, the American Society of Superintendents of Training Schools for Nurses in Canada and the United States was formed in 1894. The name was changed in 1912 to the National League for Nursing Education. The International Council of Nurses (ICN) was established in 1899.

In 1896, the Society of Superintendents brought together alumnae from various schools and initiated the Nurses' Associated Alumnae of the United States and Canada, an organization for professional nurses. The name was change to the American Nurses' Association (ANA) in 1911.

The American Red Cross (ARC) was established in 1881. A national committee on Red Cross nursing services, headed by Jane Delano, was appointed in 1909. In cooperation with the American Nurses' Association, a system was established for nurses to enroll in the ARC. Membership in the ARC nursing service required professional preparation beyond the minimum of many state nursing licensure requirements.

Box 1–1 lists important events in nursing from 1900 to the present day.

NURSING DEFINED

The definition of nursing has changed over the years and reflects society's changing perceptions of the nurse. The meaning of the word *nurse* varies depending upon the source but the definitions are usually found in dictionaries, in legislative statutes, or professional nursing publications.

DICTIONARY DEFINITIONS

Dictionaries describe the word *nurse* in many different ways. Early definitions (before the 1950s) gave various usages of the term. Examples are:

- one who cares for or suckles a child
- one who looks after and fosters
- worker or social insect that cares for its young
- an assistant to the physician and surgeon

Only the last statement relates to the practice of nursing and is restricted in that it identifies the relationship of the nurse to the physician. It does not describe the nursing role.

Recent dictionaries have modified the definition to reflect the same generalized descriptions but have expanded the description to declare that the nurse is "a person formally educated and trained in the care of the sick or infirm, especially a registered nurse" (*Webster's Collegiate Dictionary,* 1995, p. 799). The definition suggests that the nurse carries out *inde-*

BOX 1-1
SIGNIFICANT EVENTS IN NURSING IN THE TWENTIETH CENTURY

1900	American Journal of Nursing, a publication owned and operated by the American Nurses' Association (ANA) was founded.
1901	U.S. Army Nurse Corps started.
1903	First state nursing legislative act in the U.S. was passed in North Carolina, followed by New York and Virginia.
1907	Courses for graduate nurses were initiated at Teacher's College, Columbia University, New York City.
1908	National Association of Colored Graduate Nurses was started.
1908	Navy Nurse Corps began.
1909	University of Minnesota established the first university school of nursing. Students were awarded a diploma, not a degree.
1910	Flexner report recommending changes in medical education published.
1912	The National Organization for Public Health Nursing was formed by visiting nurses and public health nurses. The first president was Lillian Wald.
1917	United States declared war against Germany and its allies. American nurses were sent overseas to Europe to care for the wounded. A shortage of trained nurses existed in the U.S.
1918	United States Army School of Nursing with Annie Goodrich as Dean opened. World War I ended in November 1918.
1919–1923	The Committee for the Study of Nursing Education, funded by the Rockefeller Foundation, conducted a study of nursing and nursing education. The study, conducted by Josephine Goldmark, reported on the preparation of nurses and problems confronting hospitals with schools of nursing. Financial support for university-based nursing educational programs was recommended.
1923–1934	Series of reports and studies conducted to establish standards and criteria for nursing education and nursing services.
1925	Frontier Nursing Service started in mountains of Kentucky by Mary Breckinridge.
1929–1935	A major economic depression in the U.S. created massive unemployment of nurses. Hospitals were underutilized, and public clinics and facilities were overutilized. The National Recovery Act in 1933 provided funds for employing public health nurses. The Social Security Act of 1935 also expanded nursing services.
1937	Curriculum Guide for Schools of Nursing published by the National League for Nursing Education.
1941–1945	United States enters World War II. The National Nursing Council for War Service was formed. The U.S. Cadet Nurse Corps was initiated by the U.S. Public Health Service to provide nurses for the war effort. Nurses served in every service and in all war theaters.

continued on next page

pendent functions—examples include the supervision of a patient including the whole management of care, requiring the application of the principles of biologic, physical, and social sciences—or the performing of nursing procedures and techniques. The definition also implies that the nurse is *solely responsible* for the independent functions because the definition does not specify that the nurse is under the control of the physician. However, there are nursing activities, for example, prescribing medications, that are *dependent* upon the orders of a physician.

The independent and dependent nursing functions serve as legal basis for nursing practice. The law and regulations of state and territorial governments of the United States determine which activities are considered to be medical practice and which are nursing practice.

LEGAL DEFINITIONS

In the United States, nursing functions are defined by the laws and regulations of each of the states and territories. Legal restrictions on nursing and medical practice are also prevalent in many countries in the world.

The development of nursing as a profession in the United States began in the mid 1800s and was influenced by Florence Nightingale's work in England. Nightingale recognized that caring for the sick was complex and required caregivers who had adequate educational preparation. As previously discussed, Nightingale founded schools of nursing in England. Hospitals in the United States followed her lead and developed nurse training schools. There was uncontrolled growth of hospitals and nursing schools over the ensuing years. Many of the nursing programs were of questionable quality. For example, in 1896, 220 schools were known to exist, and by 1898, there were over 500 (Goodnow, 1937). Hospitals realized that students were a source of inexpensive labor. Lack of supervision of students in the schools resulted in ill-prepared nurses. Entrance requirements for applicants to the schools were minimal and all types of students were accepted. Working on the patient wards had priority over classroom lectures. Students were often too tired to comprehend what was being taught. There was little assurance provided to the public who hired the graduates that safe nursing care was being practiced (Bullough and Bullough, 1969). In addition to the hospital schools of nursing, there were also short-term private and correspondence schools

BOX 1-1 (cont'd)
SIGNIFICANT EVENTS IN NURSING IN THE TWENTIETH CENTURY

continued from previous page

1946	Hospital Survey and Construction (Hill-Burton Act) passed in the U.S. Congress. Hospital construction flourished. A shortage of nurses continued and became more severe.
1948	Publication of Brown report on nursing education recommending that nursing education programs be based in universities not hospitals.
1950	Korean War started. Mobile army surgical hospital (MASH) units were placed as close to the front lines as possible. Nurses were an integral part of the hospital staff.
1951	Concept of 2-year nursing programs based in community colleges proposed by Mildred Montag. First eight programs founded between 1952 and 1956.
1952	National League for Nursing Education, Association of Collegiate Schools of Nursing, and National Organization of Public Health Nursing merged to become the National League for Nursing.
1953	National Student Nurses' Association founded.
1956	Federal funding for nursing research began.
1963	Surgeon General's Report, Toward Quality in Nursing, recommended recruitment of nurses and increased focus on advanced educational preparation for nurses. Federal funding for nursing increased.
1965	ANA issued its first Position Paper on Education for Nursing stating that minimal educational entry for the profession nurse should be at the baccalaureate level, and for the technical nurse at the associate degree level.
1967	Role of the nurse practitioner emerges in experimental programs started in Kansas and Colorado.
1970s	Series of studies and reports on nursing conducted and completed.
1970–1980s	Shortage of nurses continues.
1973	American Academy of Nursing started by ANA.
1978	National Council of State Boards of Nursing established.
1980	ANA publishes Nursing: A Social Policy Statement.
1985	ANA House of Delegates votes to support use of title of "registered nurse" for baccalaureate degree–prepared nurses and "associate nurse" for associate degree–prepared nurses.
1986	National Center for Nursing Research established at the National Institutes of Health in Bethesda, Maryland.
1990s	National health care legislation fails to pass in the U.S. Congress. Major shifts occur in health care agencies with the emergence of health maintenance organizations. Role of nurses in constant flux with "re-engineering" changing nursing practice.

preparing nurses. A nursing diploma could be procured from a correspondence school for $13.00!

By the early 1900s, nursing leaders were actively seeking to control nursing education and practice. It was believed that the public needed to be protected from nurses who were not adequately prepared. Legislation to control medical practice had already been in existence in several states. In 1901, at the first meeting of the International Council of Nurses, a resolution was passed stating that it was the duty of the nursing profession of every country to work for suitable legislation to regulate the education of nurses and protect the public interest by securing state examinations, public registration, and a system to enforce the legislation by establishing penalties for breaking the law.

American nursing leaders worked diligently to comply with the Council's resolution. Legislation to regulate the practice of nurses was first passed in 1903 after much discussion as to who should be eligible for licensure. Some leaders thought that all persons calling themselves nurses should be included. Some thought that only persons who had graduated from certain types of schools should qualify. Other disagreements involved the membership of the boards that were to control nursing legislation. Another area of discussion was the decision as to what the title of the nurse was to be. Because of the difficulties in reaching agreement within the various factions, it took years before all of the states and territories adopted nursing laws.

The laws in each of the states include regulations and define the functions of the nurse. The laws, entitled Nurse Practice Acts, determine the scope of practice of the nurse in the state or territory and vary from state to state and territory to territory. The scope of practice specifies the parameters and functions that the qualified nurse can legally perform within the individual state. Nursing practice acts and the scope of nursing practice will be further discussed in Chapter 8.

NURSING DEFINED BY NURSES AND THE NURSING PROFESSION

It is important that a professional group adopt a definition to identify the group's sphere of practice. The definition gives guidance to identify the goals and focus the activities of the group. The definition also serves to give direction to the educational preparation of the members of the profession.

Early definitions of nursing put forth by the profession were general in nature and could be applied to any other health professional group. The statements reflected the legal rather than the practice aspects of nursing. For example, the ANA in 1937 stated that nursing was

> A blend of intellectual attainment, attitudes, and mental skills based upon the principles of scientific medicine acquired by means of prescribed course in a school of nursing affiliated with a hospital, recognized by the state and practiced in conjunction with curative and preventive medicine by an individual licensed to do so by the state.

The ANA changed the statement several times and in 1980 stated that "nursing is the diagnosis and treatment of human responses to actual or potential health problems" (American Nurses' Association, 1980). This definition has been criticized for its inattention to health and health promotion activities, which are considered an integral part of nursing care. The definition has not been accepted by many in the profession (Orlando, 1987; Schlotfeldt, 1987). The ANA revised the Social Policy Statement in 1995. The statement recognizes the changes that have occurred in nursing since 1980 by stating that since 1980, nursing philosophy and practice have been influenced by a greater elaboration of the science of caring and its integration with the traditional knowledge base for diagnosis and treatment of human responses to health and illness. As such, definitions of nursing more frequently acknowledge four essential features of contemporary nursing practice:

- attention to the full range of human experiences and responses to health and illness without restriction to a problem-focused orientation
- integration of objective data with knowledge gained from an understanding of the patient or group's subjective experience
- application of scientific knowledge to the processes of diagnosis and treatment
- provision of a caring relationship that facilitates health and healing

Florence Nightingale, considered the founder of modern-day nursing, was one of the first to define the nursing role. She proposed that a nurse is to "have charge of the personal health of somebody . . . What nursing has to do is to put the patient in the best condition for nature to act upon him" (Nightingale, 1860). She also focused on nursing care for patients being given by nurses who had received training rather than by unprepared individuals; on nurses doing nursing care and menial jobs being assigned to others; and on nurses being formally educated in high-quality nursing schools.

A widely accepted definition of nursing, and one that will be used in this text, was proposed originally in 1955 by Virginia Henderson (Box 1–2):

> The unique function of the nurse is to assist the individual, sick or well, in the performance of those activities contributing to health or its recovery (or to a peaceful death) that he would perform unaided if he has the necessary strength, will or knowledge. And to do this in such a way as to help him gain independence as rapidly as possible (Henderson, 1969, p. 4).

Henderson also commented, "This aspect of her work, this part of her function, she initiates and controls; of this she is master" (Henderson, 1969, p. 4). The definition has been adopted in the United States and throughout the world as the clearest statement describing the role of the nurse. Although formulated in 1955, the implementation of the concept in practice has gradually evolved and been further amplified by Henderson and others. The statement implies that nurses initiate, control, and become responsible and accountable for their own actions. In addition, the nurse helps the patient carry out the therapeutic plan of the physician. The relationship with the patient is interactive. The nurse assists the patient in becoming whole, complete, and independent and "gets inside the skin" of the patient to determine what the patient wants and also what is needed to maintain life and regain health. The essence of nursing lies in its personal, individualized, and humane character. The nurse is a member of a team and helps other members plan and conduct a total program for the improvement of the health of the patient, recovery from illness, or support in death. All members of the team should consider the patient as the central figure and realize that they are primarily all assisting him or her. Nursing is an intimate, demanding, but rewarding service to those in need (Henderson, 1969).

Henderson and Nightingale shared a common belief that an integral part of nursing is assisting patients to become agents for their own health care management. They both emphasize the environment as an important aspect in nursing care, and the importance of nursing being both an art and a science.

The definition of nursing continues to emerge. The perceptions and expectations of society are changing, and therefore the roles and functions of nurses will continually be altered to reflect these shifts.

Nursing and Social Expectations

According to Henderson (1980), nursing can be discussed as an element in the work of all societies. The essence of nursing can be understood only in relation to the society in which it exists. Societies range in any age from primitive to civilized. Nursing differs from one group to another, from one country to another, and from one era to another. Nursing is an important part of society. Social conditions affect nursing and have varied over the years. Some examples of specific changes that have affected nurses include the following:

- The educational status of the population, particularly women, has improved over the past several decades.
- The social status of women in western societies has been altered by greater equality being attained in male-female relationships.

BOX 1-2
NURSING LEADER VIRGINIA HENDERSON
1898–1996

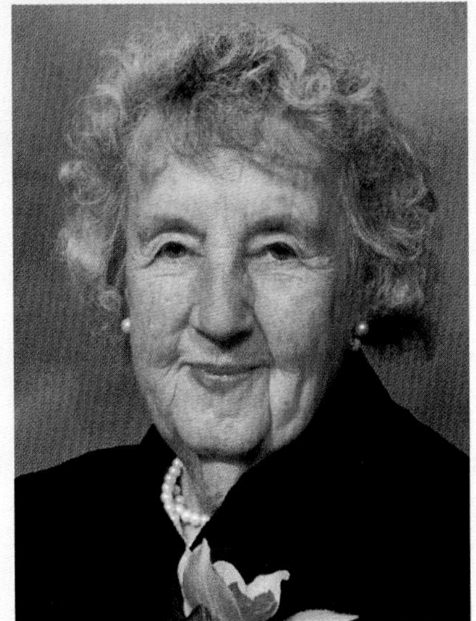
Virginia Henderson. (Courtesy of Sigma Theta Tau.)

Virginia Henderson was one of the most renowned and respected nurses in American nursing. She was known for her many contributions, specifically for providing a definition of nursing and for her authorship of nursing textbooks. Her work is known worldwide. She wrote, with Bertha Harmer, five revisions of the text *The Principles and Practice of Nursing* and a sixth revision with Gladys Nite. She has also authored *Nursing Research, A Survey and Assessment* with Leo Simmons and *the Nature of Nursing,* which has been translated into Japanese and Hebrew. Her nursing texts have been translated into 25 languages. She helped nursing become a respected independent profession. She is known as the mother of modern nursing.

Miss Henderson was born in Kansas City, Missouri, and was named for her mother's home state. She was educated in a boys' school run by her grandfather. She entered the Army School of Nursing at Walter Reed Hospital in Washington. She has been impressed with the work of Florence Nightingale, but she entered nursing at a time in which nurses were still considered to be handmaidens of the physician. In the 1920s she became a public health nurse. She became an educator and a nurse researcher at Teacher's College, Columbia University, in the 1930s and 1940s and then at Yale University, New Haven, Connecticut. She started writing nursing texts in 1939. Nineteen years were spent in gathering, classifying, and cross-referencing the material included in the nursing research survey.

Miss Henderson received nine honorary degrees. She has received the Mary Adelaide Nutting Award from the National League for Nursing; honorary Fellowship in the American Academy of Nursing; honorary membership in the Association of Integrated and Degree Courses in Nursing, London; honorary Fellowship in the Royal College in England; and the Sigma Theta Tau International's Mary Tolle Wright Founders Award.

A prolific writer, Miss Henderson contributed many, many articles for nursing journals and other publications. A great deal of her efforts were directed to the issue of providing a definition of nursing. She also, in her clear, fearless fashion, spoke out on issues relating to nursing. She was an avid believer in tax-supported health care for American people.

- The increasing numbers of women in medicine and men in nursing have changed stereotypical ideas regarding roles.
- The numbers and types of health care workers have increased remarkably over the years since World War II, resulting in an expanded number and types of activities assumed by nurses.
- Technological advances, rising health care costs, and increased consumer sophistication have raised societal expectations regarding the role of the nurse and the quality of nursing care to be received.
- Shifts in disease patterns, lifestyle changes, and increased numbers of elderly individuals have altered the sites and settings where health care is provided.

According to Henderson, the nature of nursing and role of the nurse depend on the value attached to health by the public and to the prevalent ideas about therapeutic practices—the state of the science and its art (Henderson, 1980). One method that can be used to determine societies' perceptions of nurses is to review current magazines and newspapers for the type of articles published. For example, increased attention is being paid in the media to nurse practitioners and nurse-midwives involved in providing primary care nursing. In general, the public today expects that the nurse will be well educated, intellectually capable, highly skilled, and have exceptional personal qualities exhibited in the way in which they care for others.

Nursing Roles and Functions

The ministering of nursing care requires that the nurse be involved in many different roles and perform a variety of functions. For example, at any one time the nurse may be attempting to ease a patient's pain, comfort members of the patient's family, and perform a nursing procedure. The roles and functions of the decision maker, comforter, and skilled caregiver are intertwined.

From its earliest beginnings, nursing has been about caring for others and was founded on a desire to provide care for those in need. The lifestyle of the nurse and activities performed by nurses today little resemble "duties" assigned to nurses 100 or even 50 years ago. The contemporary job description of a registered nurse comprises:

- planning the nursing care of a group of patients either alone as the primary caregiver or in a team relationship with assistive nursing personnel

- participating in giving care
- documenting care
- evaluating the care given

The other elements included in the nurse's daily activities are conferring with the physician in planning and providing for the patient. Physicians write specific medical orders for each patient. The nurse incorporates the orders into a nursing care plan that also includes nursing orders. The nurse coordinates all aspects of the care with other health care professionals working in a team relationship. The nurse may serve as a case manager, assuming the responsibility of bringing all aspects of information about the patient into a comprehensible format that is used by all members of the health care team.

The nurse interacts with family members providing support and assistance. Teaching the family how to assume responsibility for caring for the patient at home or in other settings is also an important function of the nurse. Family members should receive detailed information about all aspects (especially any clinical procedures) of the care to be given by them.

The work of the professional nurse today is focused on the assessment of health care needs, making decisions based on the clinical information attained during the assessment process, and implementing and evaluating a therapeutic plan of care that has been formulated for the individual patient.

Functions and roles of nurse are affected by various disparate elements:

- Technological advances. The increasing developments in medical technology have caused drastic changes in methods used in surgical operations, emergency care, obstetrics, etc. Nursing care practices have also changed to incorporate the new technology; for example, the increasing use of monitoring machines and computers in clinical and in home settings (Fig. 1–5). New nursing skills must constantly be learned.
- Changes in licensing regulatory acts. Many states are reviewing state nursing licensure laws to determine whether nurse practitioners can be allowed to prescribe medications and whether advanced practice nursing should require advanced licensure. Changes in state nursing laws affect how nursing is allowed to function in the work setting.
- Increasing advanced educational opportunities. Increasing demands for skilled nurses has led to the development of various types of educational programs including categories of clinical nurse specialists, adult nurse practitioners, family nurse practitioners, and many others.
- Increasing availability of a variety of different types of health care workers. Redesigning of the work in the health care setting appears to be causing a reduction of the functions assigned to nurses and increasing the use of unlicensed assistive personnel. The role of the nurse is changing to become more managing and less active caregiving.

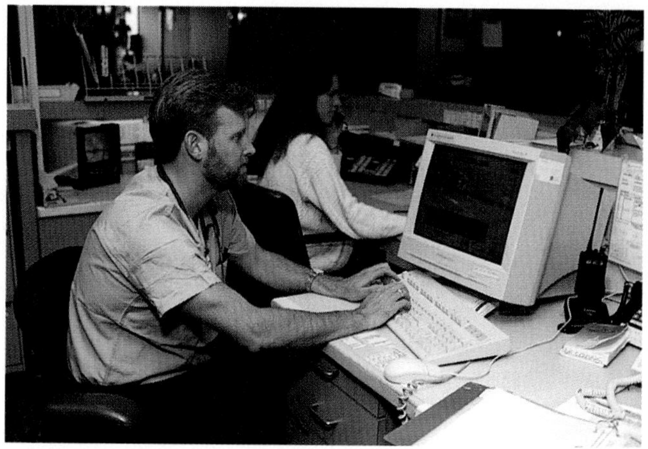

Figure 1–5. A modern-day professional nurse documenting patient care at a computer terminal.

A philosophical and conceptual framework for the role and functions of nurses has been constructed by Virginia Henderson. These are the basic assumptions that guide the administering of nursing care. According to Henderson (1969), nursing has its roots in the fundamental needs of all people, whether sick or well. Humans need food, protection from the environment (shelter, clothing), love and approval, feeling of being useful, and the opportunity to participate in meaningful and significant human relationships. In addition, each person needs recognition of his or her own personal being and consideration as to his or her own ethnic, cultural, and religious practices. Each individual has the right to expect a style of living, a set of values, and ethical principles that are unique and will be accepted by those administering nursing care.

Patients receiving nursing care have the right to participate in the decisions being made about their care. The nurse may need to intervene in some situations. However, changes in the way care is given may have to be made to allow the patient freedom to make his or her own decisions. Only in situations where the patient may be in danger or unable to communicate his or her desires would a nurse decide for rather than with the patient.

Nursing has its own unique functions, separate and distinct from other health professional groups including physicians. Nursing practice is divided into those functions that are conducted in the *direct* presence of the patient and those that are considered *indirect* and performed for but away from the immediate presence of the patient. The basic components present in all situations and settings in which direct nursing care is given including helping the patient:

- with respiration
- with eating and drinking
- with elimination

- maintain desirable posture in walking, sitting, lying, and moving from one position to another
- rest and sleep
- select clothing, dress, and undress
- maintain body temperature within normal range
- keep the body clean and well groomed and protect the integument
- avoid dangers in the environment and protecting others from any potential danger from the patient, such as infection or violence
- communicate with others—to express needs and feelings
- practice his or her religion or conform to his or her concept of right or wrong
- with work, or productive occupation
- with recreational activities
- learn

In addition to these unique functions, nurses assume responsibility for assisting the patient in carrying out the physicians' plan of care.

Certain functions are crucial in the administration of indirect nursing care and are an integral part of contemporary nursing practice:

- Coordination. Nurses are part of the health care team and serve to coordinate the patient care activities of all team members. Nurses have the responsibility for the total care of the patient.
- Advocacy. The nurse is the advocate for patients, especially when patients are unable to speak for themselves.
- Management. Nurses assume responsibility for providing for the therapeutic and personal needs of the patient by arranging for adequate resources such as equipment and supplies. Nurses assure that patients receive effective, high-quality care from all members of the nursing team.
- Communication. Nurses document and communicate all pertinent information about the patient to appropriate sources. Confidential information about the patient is always protected. Nurses provide information to the family and significant others to ensure that the patient will be knowledgeable about care to be continued in the absence of nursing and medical staff.

Nurses as individuals assume many different roles. There are those that have to do with their own personal lives in which they may be sisters or brothers, daughters or sons, spouses, parents, or primary economic providers, to name but a few. The nurse brings his or her personal self into each situation where nursing care is being given.

The roles assumed by nurses while giving nursing care take many different forms. For example, in one instance the nurse may be serving as a caregiver involved in the most highly technical procedure such as the insertion of an intravenous catheter (tube) into the vein of a critically injured patient. In another situation, the nurse may be a teacher imparting information to a patient soon to be discharged from an acute care hospital setting to home with no one to assist in giving injections for the patient's diabetes. Under other circumstances, the nurse could be discussing with a physician a plan of care for a patient who is to be cared for at home where medical equipment needs to be procured for the use of the patient at home (Fig. 1–6). It is the self, the being, or behavior of the nurse that will make a difference in how successful and how artfully the role is played. Henderson (1964) stated that the relationship between the patient and the nurse is of such sensitivity that the nurse is

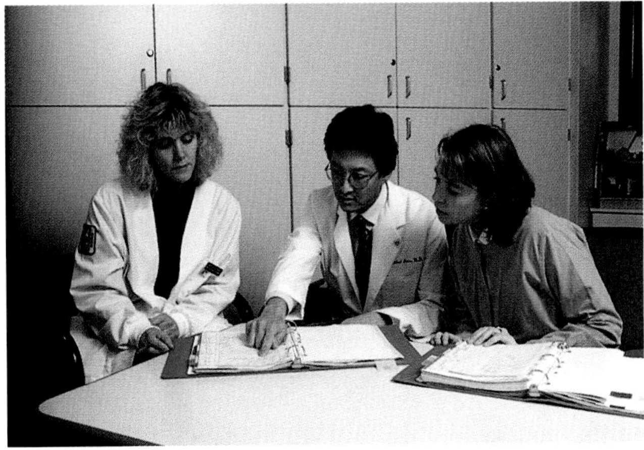

Figure 1–6. A nurse collaborating with other members of the interdisciplinary health care team, discussing a patient's case.

- temporarily the consciousness of the unconscious
- the love of life for the suicidal
- the leg of the amputee
- the eyes of the newly blind
- a means of locomotion for the infant
- knowledge and confidant for the young mother
- the "mouthpiece" for those too weak or withdrawn to speak.

It is the application of both the art and the science of nursing that determines the quality of the nursing care that is given.

THE ART AND SCIENCE OF NURSING

Dock and Stewart, as early as 1938, cited three elements that need to be present in any person giving nursing care:

- a humanitarian instinct
- expertness gained through education
- knowledge based upon science

The statement can be paraphrased and amplified to reflect nursing practice today. Nursing is the blending of:

- the humaneness of the caregiver
- the expert application of technical skills attained through education and practice
- the utilization of a knowledge base to make sound clinical decisions

Knowledge is acquired through both formal education and practice. The knowledge base includes knowledge gained from the sciences and knowledge gained through other avenues such as intuition and tradition. The application of the art and the science of nursing ideally occurs simultaneously in nursing practice.

The Art of Nursing

Art is defined as skilled performance acquired by experience, study, or observation. It is also described as a systematic application of knowledge or skill used to attain a desired result. The art of nursing is the skill with which nursing activities are practiced (Jennings, 1986). The art of nursing incorporates the dimensions of:

- intuition, the power to attain direct knowledge without rational thought or inference or quick and ready insight
- expression, making known one's feelings by facial expressions, body movements, or vocal intonation
- humaneness, the demonstration of consideration, kindness, and sympathy toward others
- subjectivity, impressions arising from conditions within the brain or sense organs and not directly caused from external stimuli
- holism, the organic and functional relation between the parts and the whole. In nature, the whole is greater than the sum of the individual parts.

The primary instrument in the art of nursing is the nurse.

Nurses interact with patients when the patient may be most vulnerable. The nurse assists the patient in facing life-threatening situations and plays a vital role in sustaining life and assisting in recovery. The self of the nurse is presented as a concerned, caring, compassionate, competent person. Expressions of the values nurses hold are embedded in gestures, what is said, and in the "tender touch," which is the ability to convey caring and concern through human contact with the patient.

Nursing practice includes many techniques, procedures, and skills that require dexterity and deftness in execution. Mastery of the skills, procedures, and techniques can become artistic in nature when performed with precision, with confidence, and with concentration by the nurse. Nurses who are very skilled in administering nursing care will convey self-confidence, which assists the patient in developing a sense of trust and confidence in the nurse.

The art of nursing is highly personal because each nurse is different and each interaction with the patient is different. It is also imprecise and nonscientific. The art of nursing is bound only by the limits of the nurse's conscience and professional ethics (Peplau, 1988). The art of nursing cannot be separated from the science of nursing.

Dock and Stewart (1938) state that to be a nurse requires the person to have a spirit that prompts a feeling of caring for those that are suffering or helpless, but in addition a certain degree of skill and expertness must also be attained. Without this, love or care would not suffice to nurture health or overcome disease. Even among primitive people we find great manual dexterity in the carrying out of many nursing and medical procedures. Although all arts require certain inborn qualities (which sometimes amount to genius), they do not reach perfection without careful training and experience.

Dock further states that nursing arts, as with medical arts, are based on science, or knowledge of true facts and principles.

The words of Effie Taylor (1934), a leader in nursing, summarizes the art of nursing: The real depth of nursing can only be made known through ideals, love, sympathy, knowledge, and culture, expressed through artistic practice.

The Science of Nursing

Synonyms for the word *science* are knowledge, information, lore, and wisdom. Science has several definitions. For example, it is stated to be:

- a branch of knowledge of study dealing with a body of facts
- systematic knowledge of the physical or material world gained through observation and experimentation
- any of the branches of natural or physical science
- knowledge, as of facts or principles, gained by systematic study

The scientific method is described as the principles and procedures for the systematic pursuit of knowledge. It involves specific steps:

- Recognize and define a problem.
- Gather relevant data.
- Formulate a hypothesis.
- Test the hypothesis.
- Gather and analyze the data (*Webster's College Dictionary,* 1996, p. 1201).

The scientific method is also referred to as the *research process.*

Scientific or research methods are used by all sciences to build and add to their knowledge base. For example, in the field of medicine, studies are conducted to learn more about diseases such as cancer, diabetes, and cardiac problems. In nursing, studies are being conducted in pain management, sleeplessness, and care of low–birth weight babies. The conducting of research studies serves as the basis for knowledge development in all scientific fields. Advances resulting from medical science and space research have provided major technological breakthroughs in developing new techniques and equipment for the care of patients.

Nursing research provides the basis for developing new theories, new clinical practice techniques, and new methods for teaching in the academic world. Many other areas are also being explored as nursing strives to develop its own knowledge base. The conducting of nursing research studies is an essential component of nursing practice to assure the future of nursing. Research is to be incorporated in the practice of all nurses.

Sciences are divided into many categories. Among them are the natural sciences, biologic sciences, physical sciences, and psychological and social sciences. In addition, the knowledge base used in many specific disciplines (fields of study) such as medicine and nursing is based on scientifically developed principles.

The knowledge base of the nurse is grounded in the information learned from nursing as a discipline and from other sciences and disciplines, for example, the biologic and physical sciences (i.e., anatomy and physiology, chemistry, physics), psychological and social sciences (i.e., psychology, sociology), and medical sciences.

The discipline of nursing involves the discovery, creation, structuring, testing, and refining of knowledge needed to practice nursing (Boykin and Schoenhofer, 1993). Nursing uses the information generated in other fields but also develops its own science. Its knowledge is based in the scientific process and the life experiences found in the nursing practice situation. To explain in another way, it is the amalgamation of knowledge from other fields, the use of scientific inquiry, and the use of experiences from the daily practice of nursing that provides the content for nursing practice. The aim of nursing science is to build an ever-increasing body of knowledge that moves nurses into increasingly sound nursing practices.

The practice of nursing unites and weds the science of nursing with the art of nursing. Nursing knowledge is based on scientific inquiry but also incorporates the everyday life experiences, traditions, intuition, and lore present in nursing practice situations. The skillful practitioner uses a blend of scientific inquiry, knowledge of the patient situation, and technical skills to care for patients.

The development of nursing as a science is advancing slowly. Many of the practices, nursing skills, routines, and techniques used in clinical settings today are based on trial and error methods. For example, many of the rituals such as each patient requiring a daily bed bath are based upon traditions and not the individual requirements of the patients. Research studies have demonstrated that certain patients such as the elderly with dry skin should not be bathed daily but instead have treatment for the skin dryness. Nursing practices need to be systematically studied to determine if better ways to give care to patients can be devised. There will be further discussion of the nursing science and nursing research in subsequent chapters.

Decision Making in Contemporary Nursing Practice

The blending of the art and science of nursing provides for a different approach in the way in which the knowledge base is operationalized in planning for and giving patient care. If one were to use only the scientific inquiry method, a step-by-step linear thought process would be used to make decisions about patient care. If one uses a different thought process based on a combination of information gained from academic knowledge; clinical experiences; intuition; problem solving; creativity; and collection, analysis, and synthesis of data; then a less linear decision-making process results. In current nursing practice, the decisions made by nurses in planning for and implementing patient care are based on the latter model. Contemporary nursing practice requires that making nursing decisions and nursing judgments be an interactive process wherein all components of the thought process are integrated into a conceptual whole that allows the nurse to formulate the best solution to a problem. The nurse needs to see knowledge as dynamic and possess the intellectual and psychomotor skills that facilitate its application in rapidly changing practice settings.

The scientific knowledge base of nursing and clinical decision-making models for nursing practice will be further explored in subsequent chapters in the text. The knowledge base of nursing is general in nature and is used by nurses in many different settings. Clinical decision making is a component in every nursing interaction. Further discussion of nursing decision making is found in Chapter 12, Clinical Decision Making.

Settings for Nursing Practice

The settings in which nursing is practiced are unlimited. The movement for reform of the health care industry has and will create new opportunities for nurses to practice in even a greater variety of different arenas.

The primary practice site for nursing professionals for the last 50 years has been at the patient's bedside in the acute care hospital. Patients within hospitals are sicker than in the past and require more complex care. The functions of nurses within hospitals and community health services have expanded, with many different roles being assumed. For example, the nurse who is assigned as an information specialist designing nursing computer programs; the case manager; the infection control program nurse; the inservice educator; the nurse recruiter; the critical care nurse; the research nurse; and nurse specialists in cancer, pain control, cardiac care, etc. In addition, nurses function in the emergency department, operating room, obstetrics, pediatrics, and clinics. Nurses with graduate educational preparation practice as clinical specialists and nurse practitioners and are used in gerontology, critical care, midwifery, burn units, and women's health, to name but a few.

Although the hospital continues to be the largest employer of nursing services, many other different settings are being used. Hospital patients are being discharged earlier in their illness and therefore are more acutely ill. This change has resulted in more patients being sent to long-term care facilities. Home care programs have also increased. Many patients are discharged requiring extensive highly technological nursing care, which may be provided either in the nursing home or at home. Nurses providing care to these patients must be highly skilled in assessing the patients' condition and in providing hands-on care.

The development of outpatient services independent from hospitals has created other sites where nursing services are utilized. Many different procedures including invasive surgery are done and the patient discharged home. These sites include surgical centers, maternity centers, and mental health centers. Nurses employed in these settings usually have advanced nursing practice skills. One of the functions of the nurse is to teach the patient and family members the specific nursing care procedures to be completed after discharge.

Nursing services have been used in tax-supported public health agencies for many years. The nursing role has changed significantly over the years and will continue to as health care changes. Public health nursing is universal, supported by the World Health Organization, federal governments, and state and local governments.

Nursing is practiced in settings such as schools, industries, privately owned clinics, and physician's offices. There are many nurse entrepreneurs who have an individual practice and clients, or own their own business.

The development of health maintenance organizations has had a profound effect on the role and functions of nurses in many hospital settings. Increasingly, nurses in hospitals are faced with changes in their daily activities. For example, increasing the numbers of unlicensed assistive personnel has placed the nurse in the role of overseeing health care workers who have had limited training. The nursing staff have more administrative functions and less opportunity to interact directly with the patient.

It is significant that the opportunities for nurses to expand practice to other settings are without limits. New avenues for nursing practice are occurring with increasing frequency. Recent examples are the use of nurses as expert witnesses in lawsuits and in assisting insurance companies to make decisions regarding the appropriateness of payments for medical care already administered to enrollees or to be administered. The discussion regarding settings where nursing is practiced will be pursued in Chapter 3, The Health Care System.

THE NURSING PROFESSION

Nursing As a Profession

There are many different ways in which professions have been defined. Huber (1996) indicates a "profession is composed of a system of roles that are socially defined. Changes in society influence professions." Professions are an important element of and are granted autonomy and prestige by social institutions. Concomitant with societies bestowing of prestige and autonomy is the necessity for the profession to uphold the public trust by competently carrying out duties and responsibilities.

There are economic and psychological reasons for wanting an occupational group to be recognized as a profession. Individuals in professional groups usually are given greater prestige and earn higher incomes. Persons associated with professions also seem to have higher self-actualization and greater self-identity.

The advent of the information age and the increasing number of institutions providing human services as their product have spawned many new groups of occupations and professions and have changed the way in which "professions" are described. There is confusion as to what a "profession" really is, and there are many different approaches in trying to define "professional."

A **profession** is defined as "a vocation requiring extensive education in science or the liberal arts and often specialized training, any vocation or business, or the body of persons engaged in an occupation." A **professional** is described as "following an occupation as a means of livelihood; pertaining to a profession; engaged in one of the learned professions, as law or medicine; following as a business something usually regarded as a pastime, as a professional golfer; or something done by a professional expert." **Professionalism** is "professional character, spirit, or methods; or the standing, practice, or methods of a professional as distinguished from those of an amateur" (*Webster's College Dictionary,* 1996, p. 1077).

Professionalism as defined by Huber (1996) is also a dynamic process whereby a group moves from being a nonprofessional occupation to professional status.

The question as to whether nursing is a profession continues to be asked. Nursing is considered by some to be an occupation and by others to be a profession. It is essential that nurses consider that nursing is a profession and that they perform in a professional and ethical manner.

INDIVIDUAL COMMITMENT OF A PROFESSIONAL

As stated in the beginning of this chapter, nursing is about the desire and commitment to care for others. In the early days of nursing, it was felt that nursing was a "calling." Those who became nurses were expected to spend most of their waking hours in nurturing and providing care to others. The nurses of today are expected to have a personal dedication to their patients and to their profession but not at the expense of their own well-being. It is assumed that the nurse has not only desirable personal attributes but is also technically competent and knowledgeable. The nurse has a responsibility to self, patients, and the profession to

- preserve and enhance the image of the profession. The conduct of the professional is observed by both peers and the public as reflecting the presence or absence of personal standards of behavior. The behavior of one member of a profession will reflect on all members of that group. Above all, the nurse must maintain high ethical standards.
- respect the interests of the public. All individuals who require the services of health professionals have the

right to expect that the nurse will be competent and caring in clinical nursing practice.
- maintain competency by continued learning. Professionals recognize that technology is advancing at a very rapid rate, requiring the practitioner to maintain competency by constantly learning and applying new methods of treatment.
- continue to be of service to the public and the profession. Maintaining a high professional standard of competency and conduct and contributing to the welfare of the community and the profession should serve as the altruistic aim of all nurses (adapted from Moore, 1970).

Nurses individually and collectively are an integral part of the health care system. Nurses personally have a great impact on the organization of nursing functions in their own sphere of influence. Participating in organizational activities in the work setting is important to ensure that nurses as a group are represented in the decision making of the institution. Playing an active role ensures that both patients' and nurses' interests will be served.

DEVELOPMENT OF THE PROFESSION THROUGH ORGANIZATIONS

The importance of each nurse's participation cannot be overstated. However, the concerted effort of individual nurses banding together to accomplish a common goal can and did have great influence and impact on the development of the nursing profession. Early nursing leaders recognized the need to organize nursing to enable nurses to speak with one voice and further the aims of nursing. It was to this end that nursing leaders decided that one solution to nursing's problems was the development of an organization that would represent the total nursing group.

As previously discussed, nursing organizations were started in the United States in 1893 when one of nursing's early leaders, Isabel Hampton Robb, was appointed chairman of a committee to arrange a congress of nurses at the Chicago World's Fair. Mrs. Robb decried the poor nursing education and lack of standards in nursing programs in the United States. A major theme of the Congress was the need for nurses to organize and to improve nursing education in schools of nursing. Shortly after the Congress ended, the American Society of Superintendents of Training Schools for Nursing was initiated. Linda Richards, the first trained nurse in America, was elected president. The name of the organization was later changed to the National League of Nursing Education (which later, in combination with other nursing organizations, became the National League for Nursing).

By 1895, Isabel Hampton Robb and other nurses who had attended the 1893 Congress recognized the need for a separate and different kind of organization dedicated to furthering the profession for the nurse and nursing. Particular focus was placed on influencing public opinion. In 1896, delegates from nursing school alumnae associations met and formed the Nurses' Associated Alumnae of the United States and Canada. In 1911 the name was changed to the American Nurses' Association. Isabel Hampton Robb was elected as the first president. A major problem identified in the early meetings was the need for nursing licensure so that standards for nursing education programs could be developed and the interests of the public protected. Another major issue was a need to develop a method for communicating within nursing. This was accomplished by establishing a nursing publication. The *American Journal of Nursing* was published in 1900 and licensure established a few years later.

The concerns of the pioneers in nursing were also directed not only to developing but to maintaining quality in schools of nursing and in nursing practice. The efforts of the early leaders were accomplished through the activities of the organizations. Such issues as registered nurse licensure, economic welfare of nurses, the status of nurses in the military services, development of funding sources to support the research efforts of nurses, establishing accreditation programs for maintaining standards for schools of nursing, and credentialing for advanced nursing practitioners are but a few of the accomplishments of nursing organizations such as the American Nurses' Association and the National League for Nursing.

Many other nursing associations have been formed over the years. Examples include the National Student Nurses' Association, founded in 1953; the National Black Nurses Association, formed in 1971; and the National Hispanic Nurses Association, founded in 1974. Organizations exist at local, state, national, and international levels. Many organizations are dedicated to specific types of clinical nursing services such as pediatric nursing, obstetrics and gynecological nursing, operating room nursing, and others.

The International Council of Nurses formed in 1899 has had a major impact on the development of nursing worldwide. It serves to improve the standards of nursing and status of nursing in nations through out the world. It is the major international organization to promote the nursing profession and aid and assist nursing and nurses' causes through the world. It speaks for all nurses. Another international organization is Sigma Theta Tau, a nursing honor society started in 1922 at the University of Indiana. It is an association that promotes nursing research and leadership.

As previously stated, developing and maintaining quality in education and in practice were among the purposes of the organizations. Over the years efforts have been directed to improving the care of patients by maintaining high standards of nursing practice and enhancing the role of the professional nurse to function in the highly technical health care system.

Standards of Clinical Nursing Practice

The concern for maintaining high-quality patient care has existed since Florence Nightingale initiated efforts to improve care for British soldiers during the Crimean War. She was

BOX 1-3
AMERICAN NURSES' ASSOCIATION STANDARDS OF CARE

ASSESSMENT

The nurse collects health care data.

DIAGNOSIS

The nurse analyzes the assessment data in determining diagnoses.

OUTCOME IDENTIFICATION

The nurse identifies expected outcomes individualized to the patient.

PLANNING

The nurse develops a plan of care that prescribes interventions as identified in the plan of care.

EVALUATION

The nurse evaluates the client's progress toward attainment of outcomes.

American Nurses' Association [1991]. *Standards of Clinical Nursing Practice*. Kansas City: American Nurses' Association.

BOX 1-4
AMERICAN NURSES' ASSOCIATION STANDARDS OF PROFESSIONAL PRACTICE

QUALITY OF CARE

The nurse systematically evaluates the quality and effectiveness of nursing practice.

PERFORMANCE APPRAISAL

The nurse evaluates his or her nursing practice in relation to professional practice standards and relevant statutes and regulations.

EDUCATION

The nurse acquires and maintains current knowledge in nursing practice.

COLLEGIALITY

The nurse contributes to the professional development of peers, colleagues, and others.

ETHICS

The nurse's decisions and actions on behalf of clients are determined in an ethical manner.

COLLABORATION

The nurse collaborates with the client, significant others, and health care providers in providing client care.

RESEARCH

The nurse uses research findings in practice.

RESOURCE USE

The nurse considers factors related to safety, effectiveness, and cost in planning and delivering client care.

American Nurses' Association [1991]. *Standards of Clinical Nursing Practice*. Kansas City: American Nurses' Association.

among the first to gather data and develop standards for reducing noise and improving cleanliness, housing, and food.

The first step in improving the quality of patient care is to establish standards by which to evaluate. This is known as standard setting. Standards are defined as authoritative statements that describe a common level of care or performance by which the quality of practice can be determined or measured. Standards help define professional practice (Huber, 1996). Standards are set by professional groups and by agencies outside of the professions. The latter groups include the federal government through Medicare or Medicaid regulations, state licensing boards, and private accreditation groups such as the JCAHO.

One of the major professional nursing organizations concerned with the development and maintaining of standards of nursing care is the ANA. The ANA Congress for Nursing Practice stated in 1973 that "a profession that does not maintain confidence of the public will soon cease to be a social force." A profession must provide for the safety of the public. This goal is accomplished by controlling practice. The nursing profession provides control by establishing standards. The ANA, in 1991, revised and published the *Standards of Clinical Nursing Practice*. The standards serve as the basis of practice for all nurses. The nurse's performance and decision making will be compared against the standards to ensure that safe nursing care has been provided. The standards are divided into two sections: standards of care (Box 1–3) and standards of professional performance (Box 1–4).

The standards are applicable in all situations where nursing care is being administrated. Adherence to the standards is of utmost importance to the individual nurse because nurses are held accountable for ensuring that competent nursing care is being provided. The use of the standards has a great impact on judging the nurse's performance. Legal implications of using the standards are discussed in Chapter 8.

The National League for Nursing (NLN) assumes the responsibility for determining and accrediting schools of nursing in the United States. It is an organization dedicated to improving the quality of nursing education and therefore the quality of nursing practice. The accreditation process is voluntary. Faculty members in schools of nursing decide whether their school will participate. Accreditation of the program ensures that high-quality education is being provided. The NLN also serves individual members through a variety of special interest councils.

In 1996, the membership of the American Association of Colleges of Nursing (AACN) supported the development of the Commission on Collegiate Nursing Education (CCNE). The CCNE is an autonomous accrediting agency contributing to the improvement of the public's health by ensuring the quality and integrity of baccalaureate and graduate education programs. Baccalaureate and graduate programs may elect both NLN and AACN accreditation or select one or the other.

CURRENT CONTROVERSY

DEFINING OUR FUTURE, DIVIDING OUR RESOURCES

By Virginia Trotter Betts, JD, MSN, RN
President, American Nurses' Association

Some among us would like to make the consideration of—and even the discussion of—certain topics politically incorrect within the American Nurses' Association (ANA). Career security, restructuring, managed care, work-force redesign, collective bargaining, workplace advocacy, collaboration and enhanced membership options are among a variety of topics that appear so emotionally laden that ANA leaders are pressured not to discuss them openly.

I, on the other hand, believe that many of these concepts are so critical in today's nursing and association climates that they require open dialogue and debate. Clear thinking and decisions about much of nursing's environment must be made by nurses' analysis of their relative merits in order to act together to achieve or oppose them with the ANA. An essential purpose of the ANA is to forecast trends in nursing and health care that impact nurses and nursing associations and then to ensure both remain relevant, valued, and valuable over time.

By ANA's current analysis, the work life of the nurse will likely change as dramatically as the health delivery marketplace. Among our predictions are increased acuity in hospitals and long-term care facilities; less hospital care and more community care; more care delivered in organized systems that manage quality and cost across multiple sites; an increased focus on primary health care and prevention; and an increased need for health services with a constricted resource base.

Nursing has a historic focus on patients, their families, and communities during times of both health and illness. Nurses have always met patient needs through continuity of care and a continuum of services. Thus, we are ideally equipped to address these projected delivery changes. However, positioning all of us there is time-, energy-, and resource-intensive even when we're very focused. When our emotions prevent dialogue, analysis and good planning we do our members a disservice and our resources are expended without positive results on members' behalf.

The stark realities of the health marketplace of the moment cause us all pain. However, if we entrench ourselves in the past; if we insist that the core of nursing care is illness services in hospitals; and if we demand that the American Nurses' Association and state nursing associations invest all their resources in fighting for jobs most familiar to nursing, I fear we will lose the momentum to step through the narrowing window of opportunity for nursing to be an essential player in the rapidly altering delivery system.

Nurses are health professionals fundamentally connected by our philosophical beliefs about health and the value of the quality of human life and by our commitment to care and to service the public. As members of state nursing associations and the American Nurses' Association, let us define our professional future by spending our resources of effort, dues and deliberation to effectively confront the current and future realities of health care and to ensure that nurses are valued, valuable, and essential providers in all practice settings.

Betts, Virginia Trotter (1995). President's Perspective: Defining our Future, Dividing our Resources. *The American Nurse,* October 16.

The art and science of nursing incorporates both the knowledge base and a mastery of skills performed by a caring, competent person. Nursing is practiced in an ever-increasing array of settings, from hospitals to homes, to schools, to clinics, and other more esoteric sites.

The nurse of today will need to participate in professional activities in his or her own work setting and in professional organizations dedicated to improving the quality of care provided to patients. These latter activities are particularly important in this era in which the numbers of professional registered nurses caring for patients in institutions are being reduced. The expert nurse will use accepted standards of practice to guide his or her daily nursing care activities. Today's nurse will combine scientific knowledge and a mastery of nursing skills to provide the highest quality of nursing care.

CHAPTER HIGHLIGHTS

- Knowledge of the history of nursing promotes an understanding and appreciation of the development of the profession.
- Nursing is defined by legislation, the general public, and by the profession. A definition of nursing by Virginia Henderson has gained worldwide acceptance.
- The essence of nursing is understood only in relation to the society in which it exists.
- Nurses participate in many different roles and have many different functions. Nurses perform both independent and dependent functions and provide direct and indirect patient care.
- Nursing is both an art and a science.
- The practice of nursing is conducted in many varied settings.
- The nursing professional blends intellect, creativity, and caring, and participates in activities that foster the profession.
- The profession of nursing promulgates adherence to standards of quality nursing care.

REFERENCES

American Nurses' Association (1937). Professional nursing defined. *American Journal of Nursing*, 37(5), May, 518.

American Nurses' Association (1980). *Nursing, A Social Policy Statement*. Kansas City: American Nurses' Association.

American Nurses' Association (1991). *Standards of Clinical Nursing Practice*. Kansas City: American Nurses' Association.

American Nurses' Association (1995). *Nursing, A Social Policy Statement*. Washington, D.C.: American Nurses' Association.

Boykin, A., Schoenhofer, S. (1993). *Nursing, A Model for Transforming Practice*. New York: National League for Nursing.

Bullough, V.L., Bullough, B. (1969). *The Emergence of Modern Nursing*. London: Macmillan, pp. 128–130.

Dock, L., Stewart, I.M. (1938). *A Short History of Nursing*. New York: G.P. Putnam.

Goodnow, M. (1937). *Outlines of Nursing History* (5th ed.). Philadelphia: W.B. Saunders, p. 197.

Harmer, B., Henderson, V. (1955). *Textbook of the Principles and Practices of Nursing*. New York: Macmillan.

Henderson, V. (1964). The nature of nursing. *American Journal of Nursing, 6* (8), 61–68.

Henderson, V. (1969). *Basic Principles of Nursing Care*. Switzerland: Basel; published for the International Council of Nurses.

Henderson, V. (1978). The concept of nursing. *Journal of Advanced Nursing, 3*, 121–122.

Henderson, V. (1980). Nursing—Yesterday and tomorrow. *Nursing Times*, May 22, 905–906.

Huber, D. (1996). *Leadership and Nursing Care Management*. Philadelphia: W.B. Saunders, p. 29.

Jamieson, E., Sewall, M. (1944). *Trends in Nursing History* (2nd ed.). Philadelphia: W.B. Saunders, pp. 351–355, 430–434, 438–439.

Jennings, P.M. (1986). Nursing science: More promise than threat. *Journal of Advanced Nursing, 11*, 105.

Moore, W.E. (1970). *The Professions: Roles and Rules*. New York: Russell Sage Foundation, pp. 240–242.

Nightingale, F. (1860). *Notes on Nursing: What It Is and What It Is Not*. Reproduction of First American Edition. New York: Appleton.

Orlando, I. (1987). Nursing in the 21st century: Alternate paths. *Journal of Advanced Nursing, 12*, 405–412.

Peplau, H. (1988). The art and science of nursing: Similarities, differences, and relations. *Nursing Science Quarterly*, 1, Winter, pp. 8–15.

Roberts, M. (1954). *American Nursing: History and Interpretation*. New York: Macmillan, pp. 22, 49.

Schlotfeldt, R.M. (1987). Defining nursing: A historic controversy. *Nursing Research, 36* (1), 64–67.

Webster's College Dictionary (1996). New York: Random House.

Webster's Collegiate Dictionary (1995). Springfield, MA: Merriam Co.

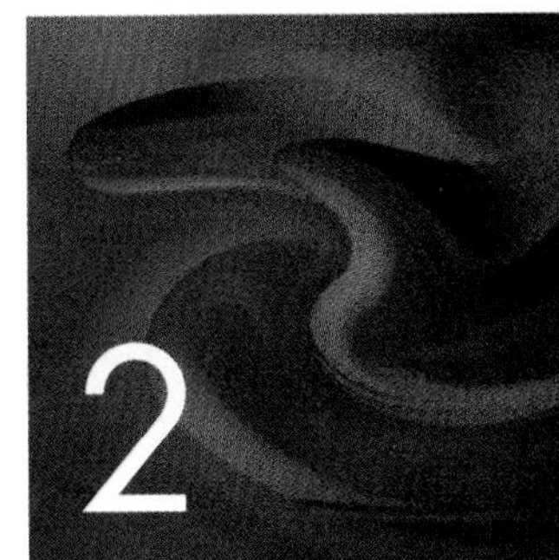

The Nature of Nursing Knowledge

Carol Lindeman

Imagine that you are assigned to take care of a newly admitted patient who is experiencing severe back pain. The physician has ordered an array of diagnostic tests to determine the cause of the pain and eventual treatment. The physician has also ordered medication for pain. How do you know what care the patient needs from you? What knowledge do you use to guide your practice?

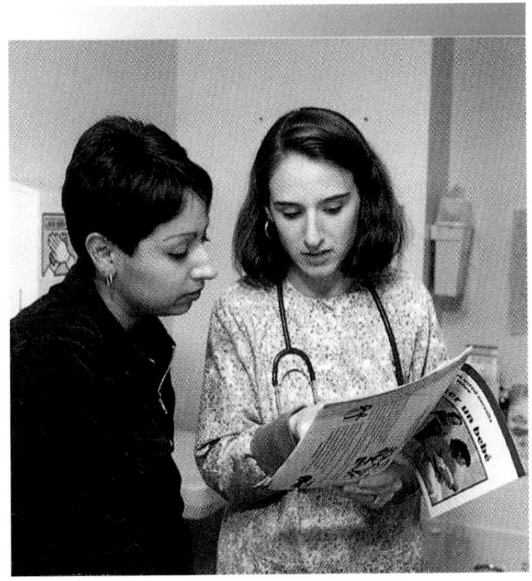

Chapter 1 described the nature of nursing practice. This chapter describes the sources of knowledge required for that practice. As the practice of nursing becomes more complex, so does the knowledge base required for that practice. Furthermore, as the practice of nursing becomes less dependent on physicians' orders and more dependent on professional judgment, the knowledge base of the nurse becomes more important in determining the outcomes of care.

OBJECTIVES

After studying this chapter, students will be able to:

- **reflect on the sources of knowledge used in every-day clinical activities**
- **evaluate their own use of all possible sources of knowledge**
- **develop a personal position on the relationship between knowing and doing within the practice of nursing**

NURSES AS KNOWLEDGE WORKERS

Drucker (1994), a futurist and management guru, describes the dramatic changes taking place in our society. He points out that the very nature of work and the workforce are changing quantitatively and qualitatively from what they were in the first part of this century and also from what has existed at any other time in history. He describes the growth of the knowledge worker in a knowledge society—a society where knowledge is the important capital. He distinguishes knowledge from information by stating that information becomes knowledge only when *applied* in action. He concludes, "In the knowledge society *knowledges* are tools, and as such are dependent for their importance and position on the tasks to be performed."

Naisbitt (1982) describes the information society that we live in as a society where economic value is associated with the acquisition and use of knowledge. For the nurse, as for other professionals, the creation, processing, distribution, and use of information is the job. Naisbitt also describes the plight of the overwhelmed knowledge worker with statistics about the rapid growth of information. For example, he mentions that 6000 to 7000 scientific articles are written each day and that knowledge doubles every 5.5 years.

In the language of Drucker's knowledge society and Naisbitt's information society, the nurse is a knowledge worker. This does not mean that the nurse will not be involved in implementing procedures and working with technology. Rather it means that it is the knowledge nurses have that makes it possible for them to use techniques and technology to the benefit of the patient. Just as a neurosurgeon is a knowledge worker even though it is the psychomotor skills that are visible, so the nurse is a knowledge worker.

At first, the image of the nurse as a knowledge worker may seem in conflict with the public's image of the nurse. The public tends to define nursing by what they see the nurse **do.** The nurse gives a pain medication when needed. The nurse carries out the physician's orders. The nurse does this, the nurse does that. You yourself may actually have chosen to enter nursing because of what you saw nurses **doing.** What is not evident in that portrayal of nursing is the knowledge and thought that surrounds every action. There is nothing in nursing practice that can be done safely without knowledge and thought. High-quality nursing care requires the nurse to consciously use knowledge while implementing and evaluating each and every nursing action.

Consider the nurse about to administer a pain medication. That nurse must have knowledge about the medication, the

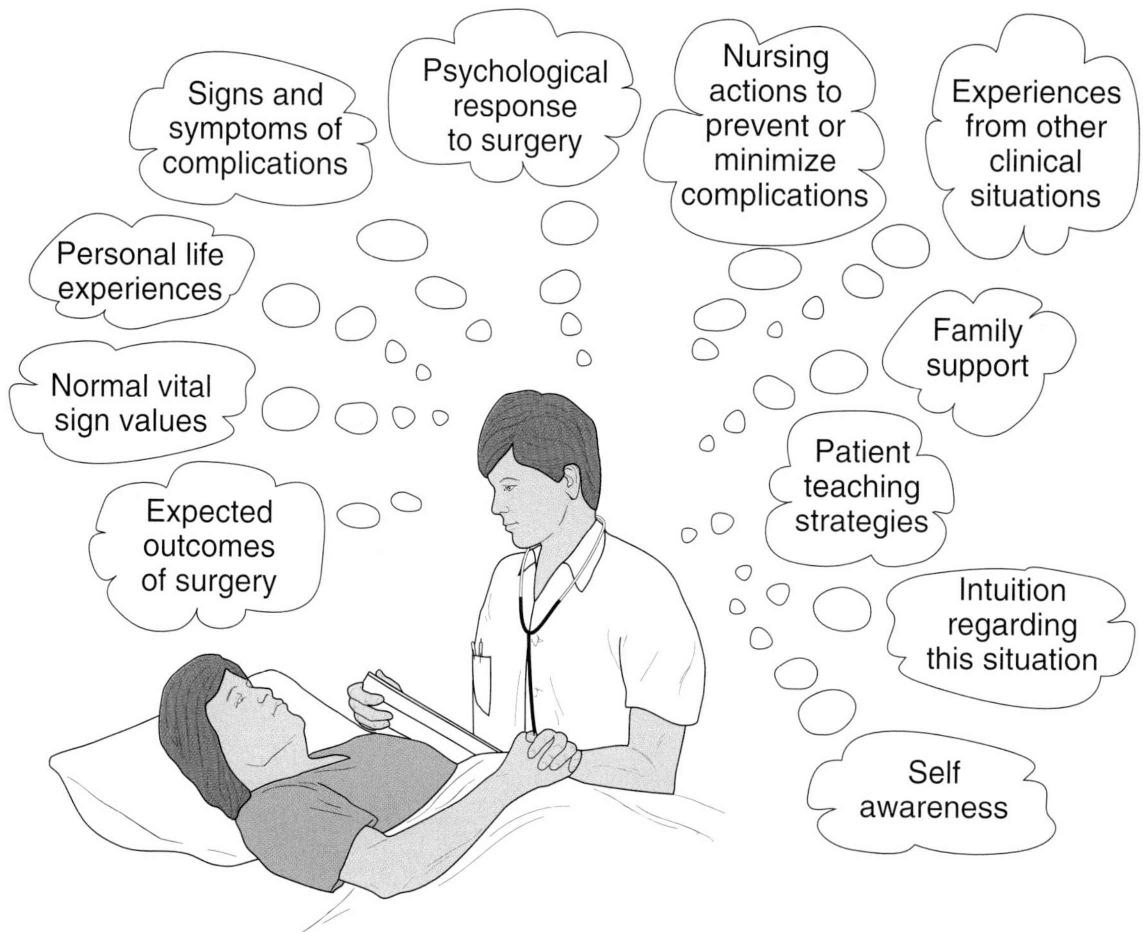

Figure 2-1. Nursing knowledge is multifaceted.

person receiving the medication, the technology used to administer the medication, interpersonal techniques, evaluation procedures, how to use that knowledge to obtain the best results for the individual in pain, and how to share the knowledge of that situation.

Consider the nurse caring for the patient who has just been wheeled out of the operating room. The nurse must know anatomy and physiology; signs and symptoms associated with normal respiration and circulation; actions that can be implemented to enhance respiration and circulation; measurement and interpretation of vital signs (e.g., temperature, pulse, respiration, and blood pressure); reassurance techniques; and signs and symptoms associated with successful surgery (Fig. 2–1). Again, the nurse must not only know the textbook information but also be able to apply that knowledge to the particular individual being cared for.

Many other illustrations could be given that would emphasize the breadth and depth of knowledge that is needed by today's nurse. With every illustration one could raise the question "In that situation would you want to be cared for by a nurse who did not have knowledge or who did not know how to use that knowledge? Would you want to be cared for by a nurse who was intellectually dead?" No one wants to be cared for by an intellectually dead nurse. The importance of knowledge and the ability to use knowledge to benefit patients is obvious.

THE RELATIONSHIP BETWEEN KNOWING AND DOING

Earlier in the twentieth century, nurses were trained through the use of an apprenticeship model. A student learned by imitating the practice of a registered nurse. Although students attended some classes, their content dealt with personal care procedures and implementing medical orders. In the apprenticeship model of nursing practice, knowing and doing are one and the same, because what one learns is exactly what one does. This model is shown in Figure 2–2.

In the second half of the twentieth century, nursing viewed itself as an applied science. Nursing practice was therefore the application of science in practice. Nursing research and theory, the building blocks of science, determined nursing practice. Within the framework of nursing as an applied science was a set of basic beliefs about research. Research was to be free of bias, time and context free, and done to discover the laws of nature or cause and effect. With this view of research it seemed logical to assume that if nursing practice was based on research, it would be care of the highest quality. In this model of nursing practice, knowing and doing are isolated processes conducted with the assumption that research and theory will determine practice. This model is shown in Figure 2–3.

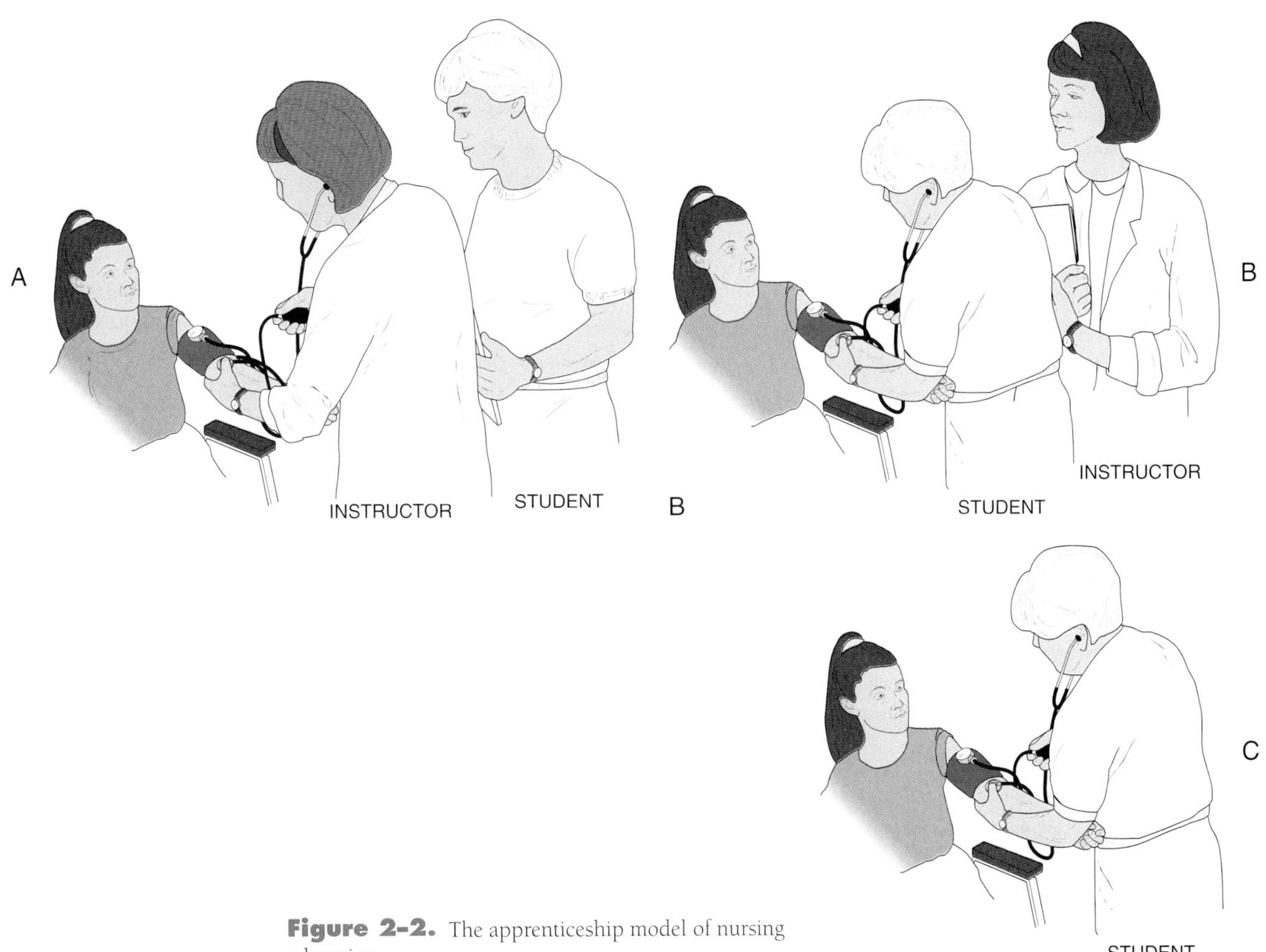

Figure 2–2. The apprenticeship model of nursing education.

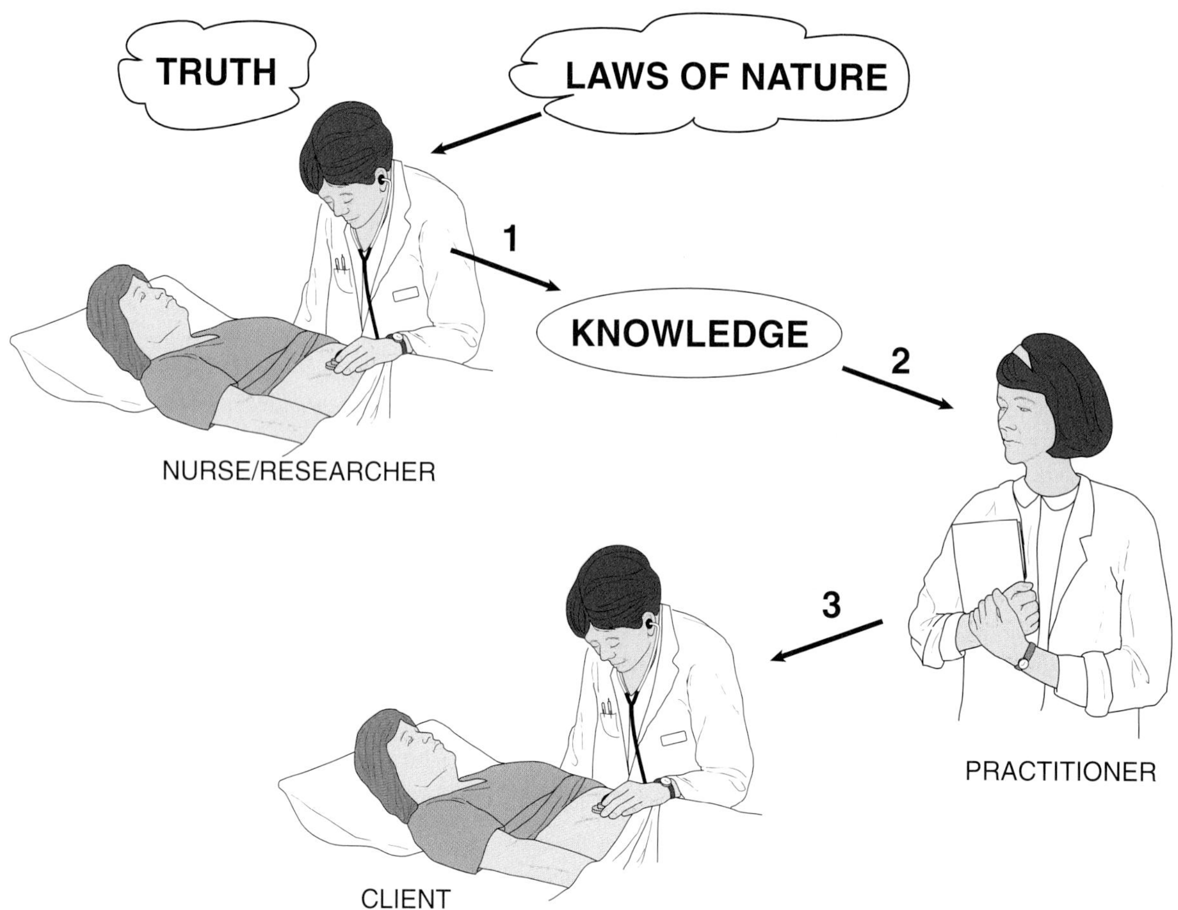

Figure 2–3. The applied science model of nursing practice. 1 = Research process; 2 = educational process; 3 = care process.

The process for linking knowing and doing in the applied science model of nursing practice is called the *nursing process*. The nursing process is a problem-solving process similar to the research process. The nursing process will be described more fully in Chapter 12.

In the 1980s many disciplines including nursing began looking toward new models of practice. The applied science view was too restrictive for a rapidly changing, diverse world. It did not work as well in human sciences as it did in the natural sciences. Professionals found themselves in situations of uncertainty, uniqueness, and value conflict in which research was only marginally helpful. The "Reflective Practitioner" model described by Schon (1987) and the "Expert Practitioner" model described by Benner (1984) are two of the new models of practice.

Schon (1987) describes the relationship between knowledge and practice as follows:

- Inherent in the practice of highly competent professionals is a core of artistry.
- Artistry is an exercise of intelligence, a kind of knowing, although different in crucial respects from the applied science model of knowing and doing.
- In the terrain of professional practice, applied science and research-based technique occupy a critically important though limited territory, bounded on several sides by artistry. An art of *problem framing*, an art of *implementation*, and an art of *improvisation* are all necessary to mediate the use in practice of applied science and technique.

Benner (1984) distinguishes theoretical knowledge—"knowing that"—from practical knowledge—"knowing how." Clinical "knowing how" develops through experience. An example of clinical knowing is the nurse who can use past experiences with patients to recognize subtle physiologic changes in a patient being cared for now and intervene to prevent a serious problem.

In the models that are emerging, knowledge is viewed as relative to the specific situation. Instead of laws of nature that remain forever true, there is an assumption of continuous change and complex interactions. In these emerging models of nursing practice, knowing and doing are interactive processes with the assumption that knowledge comes from many sources, not just research and theory. Research does not dictate practice—instead it offers choices and guides that can be used by both the nurse and the patient. This model of practice is diagramed in Figure 2–4. Clinical decision making is the process used to link knowing and doing. Clinical decision making is fully explained in Chapter 12.

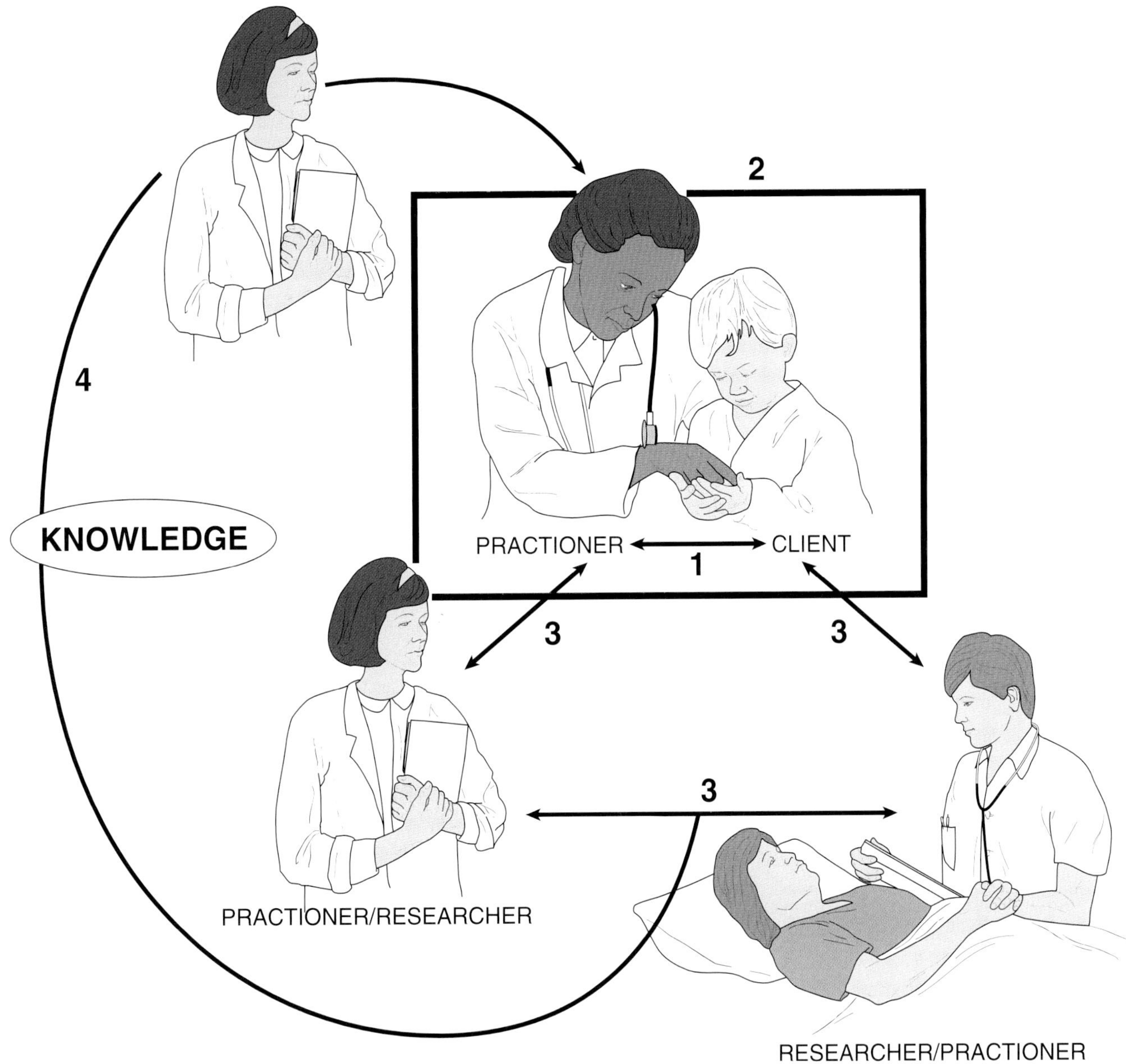

Figure 2-4. The reflective practitioner model of nursing practice. 1 = Interactive care process for helping people help themselves. 2 = Context surrounding practitioner and client. 3 = Reasearch process and integration of multiple sources of knowledge. 4 = Educational process of both practitioner and client.

It is important to remember that no matter what model of nursing practice is in place today, tomorrow another will evolve. That is the nature of human society. Research and theory will always be an important base for practice. The challenge is how that knowledge is used.

SOURCES OF NURSING KNOWLEDGE

Nurses use knowledge from the basic sciences such as anatomy and physiology, the human sciences such as sociology and psychology, as well as nursing science and theory. The history of nursing, including the rituals and routines of nursing practice, is a part of a nurse's knowledge base. Practice itself is a source of knowledge. Knowledge regarding technology and ethics is a growing component of nursing knowledge.

Nursing Science

Nursing science refers to the body of knowledge generated through the application of the research process to events of concern to the discipline of nursing. Because the science that nurses use includes a broad range of facts, concepts, and theories, many research approaches can produce knowledge for nursing practice. The positivist and naturalist are the most common frameworks for inquiry in nursing. A third framework, complexity, is growing in popularity (Maliski and Holditch-Davis, 1995).

The positivist view of science assumes that the role of research is to uncover the laws of nature. It includes the assumption of truth, which is a single, knowable objective reality; the ability to generalize from sample to population; and cause and effect.

The naturalist viewpoint assumes the existence of multiple realities that are subjective and humanly constructed; assumes that all knowledge is time and context bound; and assumes that it is difficult to distinguish cause and effect.

The complexity framework seeks to understand patterns of phenomena within their context. It emphasizes irregular patterns, variability, interactions within systems, and nonlinear change. It assumes an external reality but also assumes that this reality changes continuously. Cause and effect are not important.

It is important to know the researcher's framework when reading and evaluating a research report. The criteria to determine the scientific merit or credibility of the research vary from framework to framework. For example, in the positivist framework it is important to conduct the research with unbiased, objective methods. With a naturalist framework, this is not a criterion. Studies must be conducted and evaluated by criteria appropriate to the framework used.

The information that follows about the research process reflects the positivist framework, as this remains the most frequently used framework in nursing research.

THE RESEARCH PROCESS

The research process can be thought of as a series of steps beginning with a statement of the problem and ending with conclusions and recommendations (Table 2–1). This step-by-step approach to research has value, because it makes an abstract concept (e.g., the research process) a set of observable behaviors that can be learned. The steps in the research process include steps related to the scientific component of the investigation, i.e., the "what" and "why." Other steps in the process relate to the structure and rigor of the investigation, i.e., the "how." The way in which these steps are implemented affects the ultimate credibility of the research.

Formulating the Research Question. As mentioned, the research process begins with a statement of the problem that will be addressed by the research. This is the most important step in the process. It sets the stage for every other step. Developing a statement of the problem is an individual, creative, intellectual adventure. It involves many hours of intensive thought and literature review. It reflects current knowledge as well as the insights and intuition of the individual researcher. This statement should link the proposed research to nursing practice.

The process of developing a statement of the problem concludes with specific research questions or hypotheses. A research question should meet the following three criteria:

1. **The question can be answered by collecting observable evidence or data.** The question "What are the effects of preoperative teaching of deep breathing and coughing techniques on postoperative ability to do deep breathing and coughing?" can be answered by observable data. The question "Should nurses do preoperative teaching?" does not lend itself to being answered through observable data. "Should" questions usually involve value judgments and opinion and therefore are not good research questions.
2. **The question contains reference to two or more variables (a characteristic, property, or behavior that varies under varying circumstances).** The question "What is the effect of preoperative teaching?" has only one variable—preoperative teaching. To create a researchable question, the investigator would have to identify the variable(s) affected by preoperative teaching such as postoperative complications or length of hospital stay.

TABLE 2–1 The Whys and Hows of the Research Process

Research Process	Scientific Steps	Technical Steps
Formulate the problem	Formulate the problem	
Review the literature	Review the literature	
Formulate the framework of theory	Formulate the framework of theory	
Formulate hypotheses	Formulate hypotheses	
Define the variables	Define the variables	
Determine how variables will be quantified		Define how variables will be quantified
Determine the research design		Determine the research design
Delineate the target population		Delineate the target population
Select and develop a method for collecting data		Select and develop a method for collecting data
Formulate a method of analyzing the data		Formulate a method of analyzing the data
Determine how results will be interpreted (generalized)	Determine how results will be interpreted (generalized)	
Determine a method of communicating results		Determine a method of communicating results

3. **The question follows from what is already known or offers sound argument for an alternate approach.** If no one had collected data on the effects of teaching patients deep breathing and coughing techniques as a means of decreasing respiratory and circulatory complications following surgery, an investigator would have to conduct an exploratory study to first determine if such a relationship existed. It would be premature to design an experimental study testing the effects of teaching. The importance of building on what is known cannot be overemphasized.

Defining Key Terms. Next the investigator needs to develop definitions of all major terms and variables. These definitions are called operational definitions, literally meaning the specific way the terms are defined or operationalized for the particular study. Using dictionary definitions or general statements is not adequate. The definition must make the variable observable and measurable.

Selecting Methods. The investigator has now completed the steps of the research process that relate to the "what" and "why" and is ready to move to those steps that relate to the "how" of the research process. Although each step in the "how" must be thought out independently, the decisions must be compatible across all steps. For example, the investigator cannot decide to use a hospital setting if data are to be collected on healthy subjects. The steps in this part of the process include:

- specifying the data needed to answer the question(s)
- selecting the research design—e.g., experimental or nonexperimental, control group or not, random assignment or not
- determining how the treatment or intervention will be implemented if the study is experimental (who, how, when)
- selecting setting, subjects, and sample
- planning data analysis

Each of these steps involves judgment and in-depth knowledge of the research process.

Interpreting Data. Once the data are collected and statistically summarized and analyzed, the investigator begins the process of interpreting the data. Interpretation requires the investigator to consider the data from the current study in relationship to the literature and the insight and experiences that led to the development of the study (Fig. 2–5). This is a very intensive, thoughtful process. Unfortunately, many investigators treat this step lightly and rely on the statistical analysis for interpretation. This step ends with the statement of conclusions and recommendations.

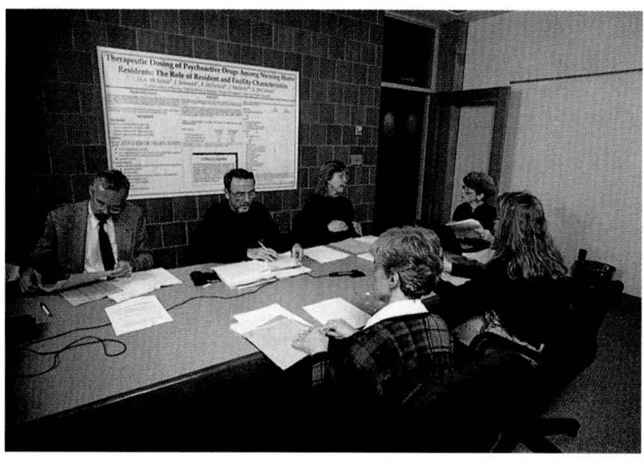

Figure 2–5. A group of nurse researchers interpreting study results.

ETHICAL ISSUES

The design and conduct of research requires consideration of three basic ethical principles:

- **Respect for persons.** Individuals are to be treated as autonomous agents, and people with diminished autonomy are entitled to protection. This principle is implemented in the research process through informed consent. Informed consent necessitates that information be presented in such a manner that the individual comprehends his or her role in the research and that participation is voluntary and can be withdrawn at any time.
- **Beneficence.** This principle is frequently described as (1) do no harm, and (2) maximize possible benefits and minimize possible harms. This principle is enacted in the research process when the investigator determines the "risk-benefit ratio." The risk-benefit ratio is not a number but answers to the following questions:
  What are the risks to the subjects?
  What are the benefits to society?
  What is the social significance of the research?
  Do the benefits outweigh the risks?
- **Justice.** This principle is a question of who should receive the benefits of research and who should bear the burden of research. In the research process, this principle is implemented in the selection of subjects and in the selection of the research question. In recent years, concern regarding the lack of research on women's health has been expressed. Concern has also been expressed that poor people or minority populations may serve as research subjects more often than do others.

It is a privilege to be allowed to conduct research with human subjects. The investigator must design the best possible study and implement it in a scientifically meritorious and ethically sound manner. Furthermore, as part of that privilege the investigator must share the completed research with those who can benefit from the knowledge. Presentations and publications from the research are not options but requirements. These and other ethical issues are discussed in Chapter 9.

RESEARCH AS INQUIRY

The research process is first and foremost an act of inquiry. The most important instrument in that process is the mind of the investigator. At each step the investigator must analyze the logic and arguments for and against the proposed approach. Sources of error must be eliminated or accounted for in the analysis of the data. The investigator must display the raw data and the processes by which they were compressed and rearranged to make the conclusions credible. Although some investigations will follow well-established formal procedures, some investigations need to be free-ranging and speculative in their initial stages.

An example of nursing practice research follows. This example demonstrates the research process as well as its link to nursing practice.

EXAMPLE OF THE RESEARCH PROCESS

This research was conducted by Lindeman (Lindeman and Van Aernam, 1971) and has been used over the years as a good example of the research process applied to nursing practice. The study was conducted at Luther Hospital in Eau Claire, Wisconsin.

Formulating the Research Question. As early as the 1940s, nurses were encouraged to initiate selected activities **pre**operatively as a means of enhancing **post**operative recovery. Through the years thoughtful nurses have attempted to do this, referring to those activities as preoperative preparation or preoperative teaching. Usually this preoperative preparation was based on the trial-and-error practice of the individual nurse or on intuition. Data to document the benefit of these activities were not collected. Therefore, despite decades of doing preoperative preparation, nurses still did not know the effectiveness of this nursing practice. They did not know the best way to do it. The knowledge base supporting that nursing practice was an inadequate guide to safe, effective care.

Therefore the surgical nurses in one community hospital decided to conduct a series of studies to improve postoperative recovery through preoperative teaching. The first study was designed to answer the question, "Does the structured preoperative teaching of deep breathing, coughing, and bed exercises influence postoperative recovery?"

The nursing staff formulated the following principles to make their beliefs about patient teaching explicit:

- Patient teaching is an important aspect of nursing practice.
- Patients are reasonable, rational human beings capable of learning in the preoperative period.
- Patients should be **active** participants in their care and recovery to the point they choose and are able.
- Patients have the right to obtain the information and guidance **they** believe is necessary.
- Effective educational methods and technology should be used in patient education.
- Educational programs for patients should be well organized to promote and support learning.

As the staff members applied these principles to the teaching of deep breathing, coughing, and bed exercises, they decided to consider these exercises "skills" and to use guidelines that emphasized learning to *do*. This meant that the educational program had to be based on an analysis of the exercises from the standpoint of the learner, had to begin with a demonstration of the exercises, had to guide the initial practice verbally and physically, had to provide for practice, had to provide the learner knowledge about his or her performance, and had to aid the learner to evaluate his or her own performance.

Because the preoperative teaching program was basically teaching the skills of effective breathing and coughing, it was decided to collect data regarding ventilatory function (i.e., vital capacity and forced expiratory flow rate). Data on length of hospital stay were also to be collected as another indicator of postoperative recovery.

The following hypotheses were stated:

- Structured preoperative teaching will significantly increase the adult surgical patient's ability to cough and deep breathe as measured by vital capacity, maximum expiratory flow rate, and forced expiratory volume.
- Structured preoperative teaching will significantly reduce average length of hospital stay for the adult surgical patient.

Defining Key Terms. For the purpose of this study, the following definitions were agreed to (only selected ones are provided as examples):

- Length of hospital stay is the number of days the patient is hospitalized. Day of admission is counted as a day; day of discharge is not counted.
- Deep breathing is used interchangeably with diaphragmatic breathing and refers to the flattening of the dome of the diaphragm during inspiration with a resulting enlargement of the upper abdomen as the air rushes in. The abdominal muscles and diaphragm are consciously contracted during expiration.

Selecting the Method. The design that was selected is labeled "static group pretest/posttest." Static group means that all qualified subjects during a specified period will receive the same research treatment. Pretest/posttest refers to the collection of data both before and after the implementation of the research treatment. For this particular study, all adult surgical patients admitted during a specified period received the typical preoperative preparation, labeled "unstructured preoperative teaching," for the research study. Data were collected on each patient before the teaching and then again in the postoperative period. When data collection was completed, hospital personnel were instructed in structured preoperative teaching. Structured preoperative teaching was then formally introduced into routine nursing practice. Data were again collected preoperatively and postoperatively. The structured teaching was done by the same nurses who had done the unstructured teaching months earlier. Data were collected by staff of the Respiratory Therapy Department.

Interpreting Data. The difference between preoperative and postoperative scores on all tests of ventilatory function was calculated and a statistical test of significance applied to the mean difference scores, comparing the unstructured teaching group with the structured teaching group. On all measures of ventilatory function and length of hospital stay, the patients receiving structured preoperative teaching did significantly better. The statistical data, coupled with the clinical observations of the nursing staff, led to two conclusions: (1) The ability of patients to deep breathe and cough postoperatively was significantly improved by structured preoperative teaching. (2) The mean length of hospital stay was significantly reduced by structured preoperative teaching. The nursing staff recommended that structured preoperative teaching of deep breathing, coughing, and bed exercises become an accepted part of nursing practice. And so it did, to the benefit of all surgical patients.

The study just described was conducted in the 1960s and is considered a classic study. Today the nursing research literature contains thousands of studies producing knowledge for nursing practice. Throughout this text, nursing research is presented as part of the knowledge base needed for contemporary nursing practice.

NURSING RESEARCH JOURNALS

Although many nursing journals carry research articles, the journals devoted solely to research include *Nursing Research, Advances in Nursing Science, Research in Nursing and Health, Scholarly Inquiry for Nursing Practice,* and *The Western Journal of Nursing Research.*

The *Annual Review of Nursing Research,* started in 1983, is an excellent summary of research in given practice areas. It is also an excellent critique of research.

RESEARCH UTILIZATION

The nursing literature contains thousands of research studies. Yet nursing practice frequently lags behind nursing research. As the information society unfolds and 6000 to 7000 scientific articles are produced daily and knowledge doubles every 5 to 6 years, practice may lag even further behind research. The issue of how research is used is therefore an important topic. Merely publishing research reports or presenting findings at conferences is no guarantee that research will be used in practice.

Research Utilization Models. In the 1970s, out of concern for the growing gap between research and practice, the federal government funded two major nursing research utilization projects. The goals for these two projects were to increase the use of research in practice, and to test a particular model of research utilization. The first of these projects was housed at the Western Council on Higher Education for Nursing (WCHEN). Nurses from any setting in the 13 Western states could request to be involved. Those nurses selected as participants attended a workshop on research utilization, received consultation on their specific plan, and had the opportunity to share their success with others.

In that project, the individual nurse was seen as the key to research utilization. The method that was used to promote utilization was a modified problem-solving process. Participants were asked to link research findings to problems they encountered in practice. The nurse identified a problem in the real world clinical setting and then searched for research that might offer a solution. Once promising research was found, the nurse designed an explicit plan for changing practice.

This problem-solving approach was an effective means of increasing the use of research in practice. Its success was linked to the significance of the initial problem/need; the adequacy of the plan; and the interest and motivation of the individual clinician.

The second research utilization project was housed at the Michigan Nurses Association. It focused on the system rather than on the individual clinician. In this model the clinical agency created a committee or committees to systematically identify patient care problems and identify, assess, and select relevant research-based knowledge. The research-based knowledge was translated into a practice protocol/innovation. The innovation was implemented and tested before being adapted. This model is referred to as the CURN (Conduct and Utilization of Research in Nursing) model and is still used today.

A recent research utilization model introduced in nursing is the Stetler (1994) model. This model is based on four assumptions:

- The formal organization may or may not be involved in an individual's utilization of research.
- Research usually provides us with probabilistic information, not absolutes.
- Experiential and theoretical information are more likely to be combined with research information than they are to be ignored.
- Lack of knowledge regarding research utilization can inhibit appropriate, effective use of research.

The Stetler model is a prescriptive, individual-oriented approach designed to increase the role of critical thinking in practice.

Another recent model for nursing research utilization is the Iowa Model of Research in Practice. It uses the concept of "triggers" as the basis for change. A trigger could come from problems in practice or it could come from new knowledge. This model uses a process of planned change.

White et al (1995) have compared the CURN, Stetler, and Iowa models. The critical characteristics of the three models are shown in Table 2–2.

Research Utilization Example. McCollam (1995) described the use of the CURN model in a project to reduce

TABLE 2-2 Characteristics of Three Research Utilization Models

	CURN Project	Stetler Model	Iowa Model
Origin	Inductively developed to bridge gap between research and practice	Inductively developed to bridge gap between research and practice	Inductively developed outgrowth of the Quality Assurance Model Using Research
Goal	Change practice	Facilitate application of research findings	Change practice
Stimulus	Problem focused	Problem focused	Knowledge or problem focused
Perspective	Organizationally focused	Individually focused	Organizationally focused
Assumptions	1. Organization must be committed to the process 2. Visible, potent, and enduring mechanisms must be in place, i.e., standing committees, policies and procedures, and so forth 3. Substantive resources including personnel, equipment, time, and funds must be provided 4. Planned change is essential 5. Two or more studies are required to support practice change	1. Formal organization may or may not be involved 2. Research usually provides probabilistic information, not absolutes 3. Experiential and theoretical information are more likely to be combined with research information 4. Lack of knowledge regarding utilization can inhibit appropriate, effective use 5. User of model must have sound research knowledge of the research process, research utilization process, and substantive area under review	1. Research can be applied to practice 2. A link between academia and practice potentiates success of use of this model 3. Creating an environment where inquiry and critical thinking are valued enhances the effectiveness of this model 4. Expectations of involvement in research activities must be communicated in job descriptions, clinical ladders, and merit programs
Process	1. Systematic identification of patient care problems 2. Identification and assessment of research base 3. Transformation of the knowledge into a solution or clinical protocol 4. Clinical trial and evaluation 5. Decision 6. Develop means to extend or diffuse the new practice 7. Develop mechanisms to maintain the innovation over time	1. Preparation 2. Validation 3. Comparative evaluation 4. Decision making 5. Translation/application 6. Evaluation	1. Identification of problem or knowledge-focused triggers 2. Assemble relevant research literature 3. Critique 4. Determine sufficiency of research base 5. If insufficient, conduct research, consult with experts, and determine scientific principles 6. If sufficient, identify outcomes, design intervention(s), conduct pilot and evaluation, and modify as needed 7. Decision making 8. Change practice 9. Monitor outcomes
Evaluation	1. Determination as to whether predicted result was obtained	1. Informal self-monitor of individual patient responses 2. Ongoing assessment at the individual level 3. Formal monitoring of effectiveness of innovation	1. Impact on patient and family 2. Impact on staff 3. Fiscal implications

CURN = Conduct and Utilization of Research in Nursing.
From White, J.M., Leske, J.S., Pearcy, J.M. (1995). Models and processes of research utilization. In M. Titler and C. Goode (eds.): The Nursing Clinics of North America: Research Utilization. Philadelphia, W.B. Saunders, pp. 409–420.

patient falls. The nursing staff at the Portland Veterans Affairs Medical Center were concerned about the high incidence of patient falls. They believed that improved identification of fall-prone patients was one way to decrease falls. Using the CURN criteria they searched for a falls identification assessment tool. The one that met the criteria was the Morse Fall Scale (MFS). The Research in Practice Committee at the Hospital decided to pilot test the MFS. The pilot study was designed to answer three questions: (1) Does the MFS accurately identify patients at risk for falling? (2) Can the MFS be used reliably by nursing staff? (3) Is the MFS practical to use routinely in the clinical setting?

The MFS was used over a 3-month period on a Cardiology–General Medicine Unit. The MFS successfully identified 22 out of 23 fallers. Nurses were able, once trained in the use of the scale, to use it reliably. The MFS was considered easy to use by the majority of the nursing staff and took 1 minute or less to score. Ironically, the use of the Scale did not decrease the number of falls but did decrease the number of severe falls. The author concludes, "The MFS is a research-based practice innovation designed to identify patients at risk for falling. With careful selection of falls cut-off scores, it offers an effective method for identifying most patients at risk for falling. It is important to remember that a falls assessment instrument needs to be accompanied by a strong falls prevention program."

To date there is no evidence to suggest that one research utilization model is significantly better than any other model. The important point is that research exists to be used. Nursing research can only improve patient care if it is used in practice.

Barriers to Research Utilization. There are barriers to research utilization. Funk et al (1995) summarize data from 924 nurses holding clinical positions regarding barriers. They report the following as major barriers:

- Lack of awareness of the research
- Being isolated from knowledgeable colleagues
- Insufficient authority to change patient care procedures
- Insufficient time on the job to implement new ideas
- Research has not been replicated
- Uncertainty about the believability of the results
- Statistical analyses are not understandable
- The relevant literature is not compiled in one place

They conclude, "Nurses see substantial barriers to the use of research findings in practice. Limitations in the setting, the nurse's research values and skills, how the research is communicated, and the quality of the research itself can all interfere with our ability to inform practice through our research."

Additional Ideas for Research Utilization. In addition to formal models of research utilization, research utilization occurs any time research-based knowledge is consciously used in practice. Reading about a particular study might stimulate thinking about another area of practice, it might help develop insight into a complex clinical issue. A particular study may lead you to try an innovation in the clinical setting to see if it works for you—or with a particular clinical population. Reading about the research may help you understand the nature of current practice. There are many ways to use research—all should be encouraged.

Tanner et al (1989) offer guidelines for evaluation of research for use in practice. Their guidelines are linked with the potential uses of the research. Their guidelines for evaluating the clinical relevance of research are shown in Box 2–1. This set of guidelines is very appropriate for the novice learning to use research in practice.

Certainly in the clinical setting research can help improve practice. Contemporary nursing practice requires the nurse to compare current practice with the research literature and implement change as warranted. Reading research reports will also aid clinical judgment. For example, the research report may contain information about cues associated with clinical conditions or information about risk factors. Research reports are filled with the rich thoughts of the investigator as well as the testing of patient care interventions. Reading the research literature will lead you to valid and reliable data gathering

BOX 2-1
EVALUATION FOR CLINICAL RELEVANCE

TYPE OF STUDY:

1. Is the purpose of the study primarily (a) to describe a phenomenon of concern to nursing or (b) to test the effects of one or more independent variables, such as a nursing intervention?
2. Is the kind of data collected primarily quantitative or qualitative?

POTENTIAL USE IN PRACTICE THROUGH DIRECT APPLICATION:

1. What was the clinical problem that was studied? Does this study have the potential to help solve a problem which you currently face in your practice?
2. Does the study have the potential to help you with any of the following types of decisions?
   Deciding on appropriate observations to make in order to infer both patient problems and strengths.
   Identifying the extent to which patients may be at risk for certain problems or complications.
   Deciding on the intervention most likely to produce desired outcomes and/or reduce the probability of complications.
3. Is a theory or proposition which might serve to guide practice generated, developed, or tested by the study? What kinds of clinical nursing decisions might be guided by this theory?
4. How did the investigator measure the dependent variables or outcomes? Do you see the potential for using any of these measures in your practice?

OTHER USES FOR RESEARCH: ENLIGHTENMENT

Please describe any other aspect of the research report which you particularly appreciate or find enlightening. What applications of the research do you see that the investigator did not see? What are applications other than the categories described above?

PAUSE FOR REFLECTION:

If the answer to any of the above questions is positive, then the study deserves further consideration. It has potential for use in practice. If you answered no to *all* of the questions, then the study is probably not relevant to your practice and there is no need to evaluate it further (unless you are reviewing the study for other reasons).

From Tanner, C.A., Imle, M., Stewart, B. (1989). Guidelines for evaluation of research for use in practice. In C.A. Tanner and C.A. Lindeman (eds.): Using Nursing Research. New York: National League of Nursing, pp. 35–60.

CURRENT CONTROVERSY
IS THEORY IMPORTANT TO NURSING PRACTICE?

Myra Levine was a nurse theorist, a pioneer in the nursing theory movement, and professor emerita at the University of Illinois College of Nursing. She saw theory as the intellectual life of nursing and as an essential part of nursing knowledge. Levine was critical of those who minimize the importance of theory for guiding practice. She was also critical of those who believe one theory can be used to guide all of nursing practice. Both points are controversial. She had this to say in "The Rhetoric of Nursing Theory", *Image*, Spring 1995, pp. 11–14:

- In the 1970s and 1980s nursing theory was seen as critical to the development of the discipline of nursing. Yet in the 1990s many nursing faculty question its relevance in the nursing curriculum.
- Many nurses are in practice today who were educated by countless instructors to believe that there is a chasm between theory and practice. The curriculum listed the two aspects of a clinical course separately. Two separate grades which often conflicted with each other reinforced the distance between book learning and hands-on practice.
- Exploring a variety of nursing theories ought to provide nurses with new insights into patient care, opening nursing options otherwise hidden, and stimulating innovative interventions. But it is imperative that there be a variety—for there is no global theory of nursing that fits every situation.

devices such as questionnaires that could be helpful in practice. Keeping up with research is also a way to continue one's own professional growth. Expert clinicians never lose the sense of inquiry.

CLINICAL PRACTICE GUIDELINES

In 1989 the federal government created the Agency for Health Care Policy and Research (AHCPR) to enhance the quality, appropriateness, and effectiveness of health care services and access to those services. AHCPR carries out its mission in a variety of ways, one of which is the development and dissemination of clinical practice guidelines. These guidelines are developed in formats suitable for providers, consumers, educators, and scientists.

Guidelines are systematically developed statements to assist provider and consumer decisions about appropriate health care for specific clinical conditions. They are developed by an independent, multidisciplinary panel of clinicians and other experts. The panel uses scientific methodology and expert clinical judgment to develop statements on assessment and management of a particular clinical condition. The guidelines reflect the current state of knowledge on effective and appropriate care. Guidelines undergo peer review and field testing before release. AHCPR also encourages and funds studies to implement and evaluate guidelines.

Guidelines for specific conditions and treatments include:

- Acute low back problems
- Acute pain
- Benign prostatic hyperplasia
- Cataracts in adults
- Sickle cell disease
- Depression
- Early HIV infection
- Heart failure
- Management of cancer pain
- Otitis media
- Pressure ulcers in adults
- Quality determinants of mammography
- Treatment of pressure ulcers
- Urinary incontinence

Guidelines are available for the clinician and the patient. To obtain copies, write to AHCPR, Publications Clearinghouse, Box 8547, Silver Spring, MD 20907.

Reimbursement for health care funded by the federal government may be linked to the use of Clinical Practice Guidelines. Therefore these guidelines cannot be ignored. Clinicians must be aware of them and incorporate them into practice as appropriate. Relevant guidelines are incorporated in this text; for example in the skin and elimination chapters. An example of the use of the pain guidelines in practice is provided by Bach (1995).

NURSING THEORY

The word *theory* has multiple meanings and connotations. In science, theory refers to the carefully formulated analysis of a set of facts or concepts in their relation to one another. Many college students studying introductory psychology become familiar with Maslow's Hierarchy of Needs theory or Skinner's theory linking rewards and behavior. Both of these theories fit the definition of theory just given. Theory is constructed as a guide for action. Theory and practice, like knowing and doing, are intertwined.

The knowledge base for nursing practice includes theory developed by nurses for nursing as well as theory borrowed from other disciplines.

Linking nursing theory to nursing practice is a relatively underdeveloped aspect of nursing knowledge. This is due in part to the abstract nature of some early nursing theories. Clinicians did not see the relevance of the concepts in those theories to the in-practice reality. Furthermore nurses thought they had to pick one theory over another and became lost trying to find the "right" theory. For a period of time it seemed that nursing theory was useful for curriculum development but not for nursing practice. Today undergraduate nursing students study nursing and other relevant theory and are guided in its use in practice. It is obvious that humans use theory in their day-to-day activities. We may use a theory from psychology to explain a friend's behavior. We may use an economic theory to pass judgment on an act taken regarding the raising or lowering of taxes. We may create a theory of our own to explain or predict some upcoming event such as the outcome of an athletic event. Just as the use of theory and creation of theory are important in our everyday life, they are essential in nursing practice.

Today's nurse must be able to analyze a clinical situation in terms of known theory and, if that is inadequate, create and test new theory. Although some theory is developed using very abstract concepts, theory also exists at less abstract levels. It is at the less abstract level that the clinical nurse may make great contributions to theory.

Theory Development. In general, theory is developed through either inductive or deductive processes. In reality, theory is developed using both processes but in a variety of different sequences. Inductive approaches to theory development begin without known constructs. One uses observation of normally occurring events as the raw material from which constructs are identified and labeled. For example, a nurse might observe that when parents are allowed to care for their hospitalized child, both child and parent are less anxious. The nurse might use those observations to formulate a theory regarding positive outcomes of parent empowerment.

Deductive approaches to theory development begin with constructs assumed to be significant and then testing those assumptions. For example, a nurse is trying to facilitate a teenager in changing her lifestyle because she is diagnosed as diabetic. She is uncertain what educational approach might be best. She decides to view the situation through Skinner's theory of stimulus and reward and use behavioral conditioning to achieve the desired outcomes. In doing so she begins with the constructs and labels created by Skinner but modifies them in terms of the complex lifestyle changes required in this type of patient education situation.

Observation, labeling, isolating features, comparing and contrasting, defining, and analysis of ideas at both the conceptual and empirical realms are all part of theory development.

Examples of Nursing Theory. Nursing theories can be contrasted around four topics: the nature of nursing; the individual recipient of care; society and environment; and health (Fawcett, 1984). In nursing theories, the nature of nursing is usually represented as an interpersonal, helping, or caring process. Thereafter theorists emphasize different constructs. Most nursing theories treat the recipient of care from a holistic perspective. Society and environment are treated differently in different theories. As our understanding of the role of environment on health deepens, this will undoubtedly receive more attention in nursing theory. Nursing theories agree that health is the focus of nursing. However, the way in which health is conceptualized differs among theories.

This text reflects Henderson's conceptions of nursing. However it is important to hold a pluralistic approach to nursing theory. All contribute to the understanding of nursing practice. Two major nursing theories are described briefly to provide a sense of this aspect of nursing knowledge.

Since the late 1950s Dorothea Orem has been perfecting the "self-care deficit theory of nursing." The focus is self-care, defined as those activities that people perform to maintain life, health, and well-being. Self-care requirements include such activities as maintaining sufficient intake of air, water, and food; getting adequate rest and sleep; and the prevention of hazards. When individuals cannot maintain continuous self-care or independent care due to health or health-related factors, they experience self-care deficits. Nursing practice includes identifying self-care requirements and designing and implementing actions to meet those requirements. Society and environment are not major factors in the theory.

Part of the popularity of this theory is attributable to the current popularity of self-care. Having experienced the consequences of the "eat, drink, be merry, and hope your doctor can cure you" era, Americans are now very conscious of what they eat and drink and of their need for physical exercise. The theory is also popular because Orem continues to perfect its major constructs to ensure its relevance to contemporary nursing practice. Of concern to some is its failure to clearly define crucial terms such as self-care agency.

Another well-known theory is the Roy Adaptation Theory. In developing this nursing theory, Roy drew heavily on nonnursing experts in the field of adaptation. The concept of person as a biopsychosocial being in constant interaction with a changing environment is critical. Another crucial conception is that health and illness are different points on a single continuum. This view of health and illness as a single continuum differs from those who see health as more than the absence of illness. According to Roy, nursing is needed when external or internal factors make the individual unable to adapt or cope.

The popularity of this theory has been negatively affected by the lack of clarity of key terms such as *cognator* and *regulator coping mechanisms*. Nonetheless, nurses are finding it useful in practice situations.

Nursing theories are a component of nursing knowledge. Their use in practice would be greatly enhanced if the crucial concepts were labeled or defined in terms common to the practice of nursing.

PRACTICE AS A SOURCE OF KNOWLEDGE

In recent years, the nursing profession has pursued the view that the practice situation is in itself a source of knowledge (Fig. 2–6). For example, Benner's (1984) contrast of the novice and expert clinician highlighted practice as a critical source of knowledge. For the expert clinician, practice is

CURRENT CONTROVERSY
IS INTUITION AN IMPORTANT NURSING PRACTICE TOOL?

In recent years nursing leaders have emphasized the scientific base for nursing practice. Yet expert nursing clinicians have credited their intuition for lifesaving nursing actions. Is intuition important for nursing practice? Can it be taught and learned?

Carolyn Kresse Murry is a rehabilitation nurse who graduated from nursing school in the early 1980s. She shared her insight into the importance of intuition in an article titled "Go Back . . . Something's Wrong" published in the July 1994 issue of the *American Journal of Nursing*. Here are some of her statements:

- I learned that good nursing requires an astute awareness of the things that aren't always visible, audible, or palpable.
- Intuition is the ability to perceive or know things without conscious reasoning, as if by instinct. What nurse hasn't followed the hunch that—despite a patient's normal blood pressure, strong pulse, even respirations, good color, and alert level of consciousness—something isn't quite right? That extra trip to the bedside to appease the nagging feeling may find a nasogastric tube that had been fine 20 minutes ago now draining bright red blood.
- [Intuition] needs to be openly acknowledged and discussed.
- We need to support our colleagues' intuitive urges.
- We need to recognize, nurture, and encourage our own powers of intuition by heeding the voice inside that says "Go back . . . something's wrong."

much more than repetitive doing or perfecting performance through experience. The expert nurses in Benner's study created new knowledge from their patient encounters. They used that knowledge as they cared for others.

How can practice be a source of knowledge? There are many ways of knowing, and therefore there are many sources of knowledge. Intuition is one type of knowing associated with practice. Expert clinicians will describe a feeling they experienced—a feeling that something was about to happen to a patient and they needed to take certain actions. This feeling is thought of as intuition based on previous experiences. An example of expert clinician intuition follows.

A small group of nurses working in a long-term care facility were troubled that the medical staff were no longer trying to rehabilitate a group of residents. The physicians had concluded that no further recovery was possible and the residents should just be left as they were. The nurses had a feeling that some recovery was still possible. Because of their feeling and their courage, they asked and were allowed to create a nurse-managed unit. On this unit the nursing staff had the authority to manage the total care for this group of residents. The nurses decided to emphasize independence and socialization in their care routines. Instead of leaving residents in bed for meals, they had them get out of bed and eat in a common dining room. A number of the residents had been tube fed for years—some for as long as 12 to 14 years. The nurses felt that these residents could learn to swallow once again and that they did not have to be tube fed. Resident by resident they began removing the nasogastic tube and teaching the residents to swallow and chew. Not once did they make an error in judgment. All residents who had the tube removed were able to learn to eat either by themselves or with minor assistance. Imagine the courage it required of that nursing staff to undertake such an intervention! But these nurses trusted their intuition—intuition that came from practice.

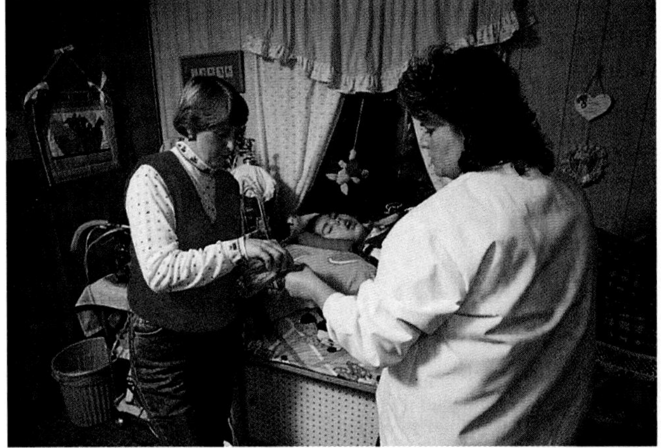

Figure 2-6. The expert nurse creates new knowledge from each patient encounter, then uses that knowledge in caring for other patients.

The practice situation is a source of knowledge for another reason. Most of the knowledge produced through research is based on aggregate data or group averages. Research usually requires a reductionist approach, that is, the isolation of the factor thought to be most important for study. It minimizes the importance of individual differences. Nursing practice, on the other hand, is a holistic approach that attends to individual differences. Therefore the research knowledge that the nurse brings to the situation must be augmented by the knowledge the nurse learns while in the situation. Isn't scientific knowledge a better base for practice than knowledge created in the practice situation?

Expert nurses are the first to point out that it is not an "either-or" in terms of a knowledge base. Nursing practice is complex and requires many ways of knowing—many sources of knowledge. To create knowledge in practice in isolation of existing knowledge is inadequate. To assume that scientific knowledge is adequate and ignore the knowledge in the practice situation is equally inadequate. Knowledge, irrespective of how it was created, has value if it serves as a guide to effective action in the day-to-day reality. Contemporary nursing practice requires the use of all sources of knowledge in the moment-to-moment reality of a patient care situation.

THE SCHOLARLY CLINICIAN

This chapter began with a description of the nurse as a knowledge worker—a person who is required to consciously use knowledge while providing nursing care. Nursing practice requires constant interaction between the processes of knowing and processes of doing. The nurse who practices this way is called a scholarly clinician.

The current world of nursing practice involves caring for individuals, families, and communities where the health care problems are complex. There are few if any "standard" patients. The nurse deals with uncertainty, uniqueness, instability, and value conflicts. Violence, substance abuse, stress, poverty, and aging are examples of the complex social and health care issues that confront nurses today. Before the nurse can engage in any problem-solving activities, the patient and the nurse must agree on the naming and framing of the problem. The patient may state that she has an ear infection. The nurse may believe the woman has been physically abused. Unless both agree to the problem (naming and framing of it), any prescribed treatment may be ineffective. In this context nursing practice becomes a very special art form in which the nurse is an active participant in the development and application of knowledge. In the process of providing care, the nurse must conceptualize and reconceptualize the patient's circumstances in light of available knowledge. As necessary, the nurse will have to create and test new theory. In this way the nurse is a researcher and theoretician while being the clinician.

This view of the nurse is not new. It was advocated by such nurse leaders as Florence Nightingale and Virginia Henderson. However it is a view that has been lost for the last two decades. During those decades nursing practice was seen as instrumental problem solving made rigorous by the application of scientific theory and technique. Researchers would generate the knowledge; practitioners would use the knowledge; patients would get well. The goal of nursing science was to develop standardized solutions to standardized problems that could be implemented through standardized nursing interventions. That goal may have been reasonable in the 1950s and 1960s when it seemed that health problems had a specific cause and cure. It is not a goal that matches today's reality.

The nurse of today needs to know the research and theory base for practice. That nurse also needs to create knowledge in the situation to enable effective use of existing research and theory and to guide nursing actions where the research and theory base are inadequate. The nurse of today is a knowledge worker. The expert nurse of today is a scholarly clinician.

CHAPTER HIGHLIGHTS

- Contemporary nursing practice is a complex process based on continuous interactions between knowing and doing.
- Research from nursing and other disciplines is an important source of nursing knowledge.
- Utilization of research in practice occurs in many different ways: for example, it could occur through the use of a research-based protocol or a guide to nursing actions.
- Clinical practice guidelines are another important source of nursing knowledge.
- Practice itself is a source of knowledge associated with the evolution of the nurse from novice to expert.
- In recent years, intuition has been accepted as a source of nursing knowledge.
- The nurse must be intellectually alive and a lifelong learner.

REFERENCES

Bach, D.M. (1995). Implementation of the agency for health care policy and research postoperative pain management guidelines. In M. Titler and C. Goode (eds.): *The Nursing Clinics of North America: Research Utilization.* Philadelphia: W.B. Saunders, pp. 515–528.

Benner, P. (1984). *From Novice to Expert.* Menlo Park, CA: Addison-Wesley.

Drucker, P. (1994). The age of social transformation. *The Atlantic Monthly, 11,* 54–78.

Fawcett, J. (1984). *Analysis and Evaluation of Conceptual Models of Nursing.* Philadelphia: F.A. Davis.

Funk, S.G., Tornquist, E.M., Champagne, M.T. (1995). Barriers and facilitators of research utilization: An integrative review. In M. Titler and C. Goode (eds.): *The Nursing Clinics of North America: Research Utilization.* Philadelphia: W.B. Saunders, pp. 395–408.

Lindeman, C.A. (1984). *Issues in Professional Nursing Practice. 3. The Relationship of Research and Theory to Practice.* (A monograph) American Nurses' Association, Washington, D.C.

Lindeman, C.A., Van Aernam, B. (1971). Nursing interventions with the pre-surgical patient—the effects of structured and unstructured preoperative teaching. *Nursing Research, 20,* 319–332.

Maliski, S.L., Holditch-Davis, D. (1995). Linking biology and biography: Complex nonlinear dynamical systems as a framework for nursing inquiry. *Complexity and Chaos in Nursing, 2*(1), 25–35.

McCollam, M.E. (1995). Evaluation and implementation of a research-based falls assessment innovation. In M. Titler and C. Goode (eds.): *The Nursing Clinics of North America: Research Utilization.* Philadelphia: W.B. Saunders, pp. 507–514.

Meleis, A.I. (1985). *Theoretical Nursing*. Philadelphia: J.B. Lippincott.

Naisbitt, J. (1982). *Megatrends.* Ten New Directions Transforming Our Lives New York: Warner Books, Inc.

Schon, D.A. (1987). *Educating the Reflective Practitioner.* San Francisco: Jossey-Bass.

Stetler, C. (1994). Refinement of the Stetler/Marram model for application of research findings to practice. *Nursing Outlook 42,* 15–25.

Tanner, C.A., Imle, M., Stewart, B. (1989). Guidelines for evaluation of research for use in practice. In C.A. Tanner and C.A. Lindeman (eds.): Using Nursing Research. New York: National League for Nursing, pp. 35–60.

Urinary Incontinence Guideline Panel: *Urinary Incontinence in Adults: Clinical Practice Guidelines.* AHCPR Pub. No. 92-0038. Rockville, MD: Agency for Health Care Policy and Research, Public Health Service, U.S. Department of Health and Human Services, March 1992.

White, J.M., Leske, J.S., Pearcy, J.M. (1995). Models and processes of research utilization. In M. Titler and C. Goode (eds.): *The Nursing Clinics of North America: Research Utilization.* Philadelphia: W.B. Saunders, pp. 409–420.

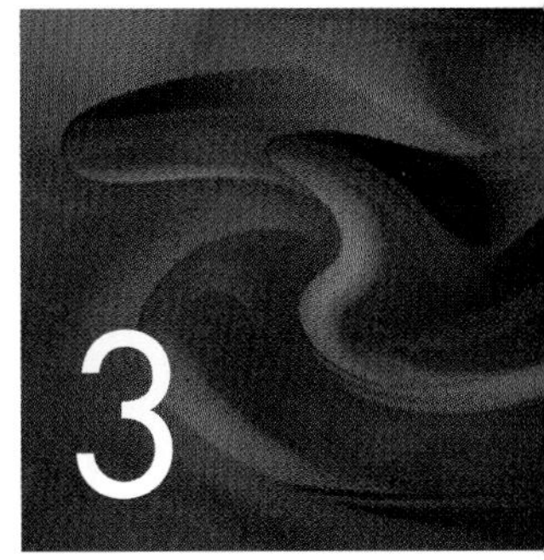

The Health Care System 3

Carol Lindeman

What picture comes to mind when you hear the phrase "health care system?" If you are like the majority of Americans, you may picture a doctor's office or a community hospital—distinct settings where many receive health care. That picture is a fairly accurate portrayal of the U.S. health care system. It consists of a variety of settings that can be pieced together to provide the services required. It also consists of a range of health care providers that form a team to deliver services in a cost-effective manner.

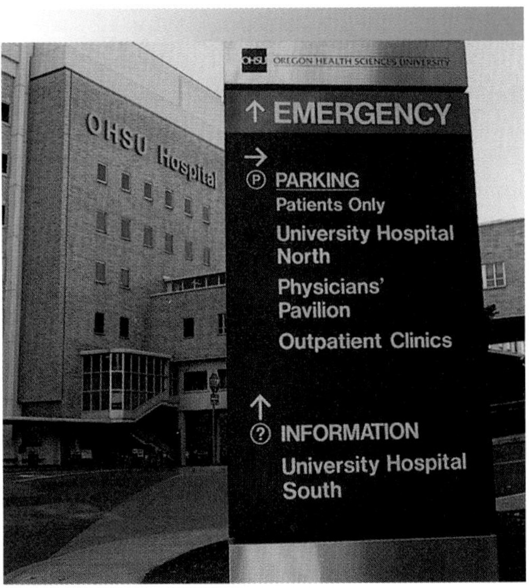

According to a 1994 national opinion survey sponsored by the W. K. Kellogg Foundation, over two thirds of U.S. citizens do not think the health care system meets the needs of most Americans! They also believe that the future system should make greater use of family doctors, nurses, and other basic health care providers rather than medical specialists.

Our health care system is undergoing dramatic change. Mergers of hospitals and other health care settings are common. Public hospitals including academic health centers are being purchased by hospital systems in the for-profit sector. More and more care is being delivered in the home and in ambulatory settings.

Contemporary nursing practice requires that the nurse know which setting is most cost-effective in caring for a particular patient at various points in time. For example, when should a patient leave the hospital after a heart attack? If a patient needs a blood transfusion, should it be done in the person's home, in the hospital, or in an ambulatory care setting?

OBJECTIVES

After studying this chapter, students will be able to:

- **understand the role of the major settings and providers in the health care system**
- **participate in discussions regarding the settings for caring for their patients**

OVERVIEW OF THE U.S. HEALTH CARE SYSTEM

Although both the professional and lay literature include references to the U.S. health care system, no such single entity exists. In reality, there are different systems for different populations, e.g., the military, veterans, Native Americans, the insured, the uninsured, and the poor. Individuals with or without coordination from a health care provider must put together sets of services and settings to meet their unique requirements. Depending on the services required, this can be extremely difficult for the average person.

The System for Insured Persons

The individual with good health care insurance or personal wealth obtains *primary health care* from a private health care provider (physician, nurse practitioner, or physician assistant) in that provider's office. Primary health care includes health education, nutrition counseling, maternal and child health services, immunizations, treatment of common diseases and injuries, provision of essential drugs, and routine health screening. Should the individual require more intensive or extensive services such as surgery, or monitoring and treatment for acute coronary disease, the individual would be admitted to a community hospital. If more specialized, unique services are required, the individual would be admitted as a private patient to a university-based teaching hospital. Such individuals may be discharged to their home with or without home care services or discharged to a nursing home and then to their home. Thereafter, care would be available through the provider in his or her office.

The System for Uninsured Persons

Individuals who are uninsured or underinsured (that is, their health insurance may not cover the particular service or may cover it at a level that a provider will not accept) use county health clinics for primary care or wait until a serious problem develops and then use the hospital emergency room. If more intensive or extensive services are required, the individual is admitted to a county hospital or a teaching hospital subsidized to provide care to those who cannot pay. Access to other services is limited.

The System for Veterans

The United States maintains a system for providing health care to veterans. Although the system consists primarily of acute care hospitals, new services are being developed to correspond to the changing health care needs of the aging veteran population. Physicians working in this system are employees with an annual salary; they are not part of the fee-for-service approach to medical care. Some of the hospitals in this system are considered "Deans' Hospitals," a designation that means a close affiliation with a medical school. Some of these hospitals are also forming partnerships with a nursing school and/or dental school. The assumption (proven true over the years) is that these affiliations with academic institutions lead to higher quality of care for the veteran.

The System for Active Military Personnel

Military personnel receive all of their health care through yet another system, which some consider as the only real *system* of care in the United States. A full array of services is available to the military personnel and their families by contacting the appropriate person at their base. The system emphasizes health promotion and disease prevention. Services such as routine physicals and immunizations are mandatory.

Public Health Services

Local, state, and federal taxes are also used to support a system of public health services. In general, public health services are what we do collectively to assure the conditions in which people can be healthy. Control of epidemic diseases, safe food and water, proper sanitation, and maternal and child health services are typical public health concerns. Immediate crises such as the AIDS epidemic, deaths from measles, and toxins in the environment are also issues of public health. Each day people living in this country benefit from public health services. Yet in recent years, services have deteriorated due to confusion over the mission of public health, government's role in fulfilling the mission, and the responsibilities unique to each level of government. The Institute of Medicine's report *The Future of Public Health* (1988) considers the deterioration in services so severe that one chapter is titled "The Disarray of Public Health: A Threat to the Health of the Public."

The Health Care System As an Industry

In its totality, health care constitutes big business and has many characteristics of an industry. In 1987, 8.5 million persons were employed in the health services industry, or about 7 percent of the total U.S. employment. Between 1990 and 1996 the number of civilians employed in health service sites increased by 19 percent to 11.2 million persons compared with a 7-percent increase in total civilian employment (Public Health Service Centers for Disease Control and Prevention and National Center for Health Statistics, 1997). In 1996, national health care expenditures totaled $1.035 trillion, an average of over $2.84 billion per day and an average of $3,633 per person per year (Levit et al, 1998). Stated another way, in 1996, the United States spent 13.6 percent of its gross domestic product on health (Levit et al, 1998).

HEALTH CARE SETTINGS

In this section, five health care settings are described: acute care hospital, nursing home/long-term care facility, home health/community care, ambulatory care, and the nursing center. The focus is on these settings because for each one, nurses are crucial to the services provided.

Acute Care Hospital

Today the hospital is the scientific, technological, and educational hub of the medical care system (Fig. 3–1). Acute care hospitals account for the largest single expenditure of health care dollars. But hospitals were not always as they are today. The first hospitals in the United States were established primarily as almshouses for the poor over 200 years ago. The care of the sick in these settings was incidental to that primary purpose. Early hospitals were described as follows (Raffel, 1980, pp. 202–203):

> Up to this century, hospitals were not objects of public esteem. They were founded as shelters for the aged and infirm, orphans, vagrants, and the maimed; as part of the charitable program of religious and welfare organizations; as protection for the inhabitants of a community from communicable diseases and from the dangerously insane; and as emergency quarters to accommodate wounded and sick soldiers, sailors, and marines during wartime. . . . The earliest American hospitals were crowded and unsanitary; medical care was meager and largely ineffective. Their poor reputation deterred people from entering them voluntarily. The hazards to health were usually greater in the hospital than in the home. Admission to these institutions was frequently regarded as a disgrace.

During the latter half of the nineteenth century many developments were made in the biological sciences that physicians found useful in diagnosis and treatment. The development of anesthesia by individuals such as Long, Wells, and Montor, of antisepsis by Holmes and Semmelweiss, and of bacteriology by Pasteur are examples of these scientific advances. These developments, along with those of thousands of other scientists, laid the groundwork for today's modern hospital. It is important to note that the term hospital now refers to an institution that has as its *primary* function the care of the sick and infirm.

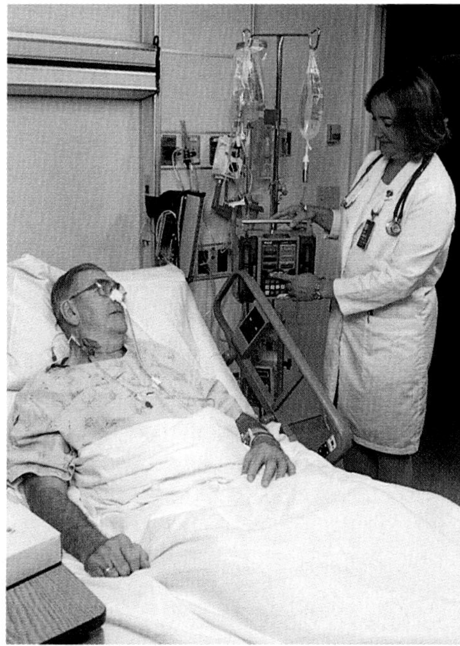

Figure 3–1. A nurse caring for a patient in an acute care hospital.

Today's hospitals are diverse, including very small and very large facilities; teaching and nonteaching hospitals; nonprofit and for-profit hospitals; church owned, community owned, federally owned, and state owned; and general as well as specialty hospitals. In this era of rapid change in health care financing and delivery, the hospital is also changing dramatically. Many are downsizing, i.e., reducing the number of beds in operation. Some are closing. Some are eliminating services such as pediatrics or maternity. In 1990 health care professionals viewed the hospital as the hub of the health care system. By 1995 health care administrators viewed the hospital negatively as an expensive "cost center"—a setting where patients were to be placed as the last resort. The role of the hospital in a re-formed health care system is yet to be determined.

Hospital Nursing Workforce. According to findings from the March 1996 National Sample Survey of Registered Nurses, conducted by the Division of Nursing, Bureau of Health Professions, Health Resources and Services Administration, approximately 60 percent of the employed registered nurses in the United States work in hospitals (Fig. 3–2). This percentage has been steadily declining over recent years and likely will continue to do so, given the trend toward hospital downsizing. In the near future it is likely that only 33 to 40 percent of registered nurses will be working in the acute hospital setting. This is a national average—the percentages differ in different regions of the country. For example, an environmental scan of nursing supply and demand in the Minneapolis–St. Paul, Minnesota, area (Metropolitan Healthcare Council, 1995) showed that only 47 percent of registered nurses were now employed in acute hospital settings.

Nursing Home/Long-Term Care Facility

Just as the hospital is the primary setting for acute care, the nursing home is considered the primary setting for long-term care (Fig. 3–3). Like hospitals, nursing homes also originated in the county poorhouses of the 1700s and 1800s. Local governments established these institutions to care for the poor, the homeless, invalids, mentally ill, mentally retarded, and other incurables or undesirables. In some states, these poorhouses were located on sites that enabled the inhabitants to work to help pay for their care. In Wisconsin, for example, the poorhouses were connected to a county-owned farm and the residents worked on the farm. Local governments funded these facilities at the base minimum.

Nursing homes were created under sponsorships other than state or local governments. Church groups and fraternal groups developed homes for their elderly members. In the 1930s, for-profit nursing homes were created with the

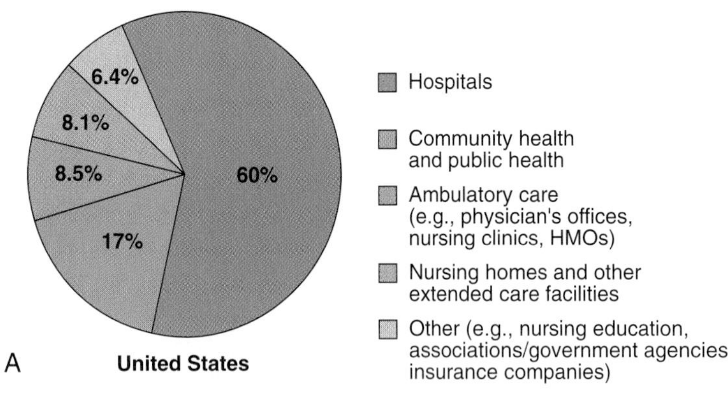

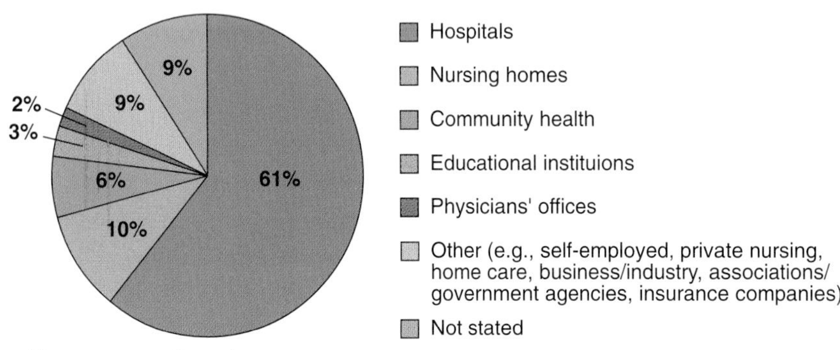

Figure 3-2. *A* and *B*, Registered nurse employment in various health care settings, the United States and Canada. (Data from Health Resources and Services Administration, Bureau of Health Professions, Division of Nursing [1996]. National Sample Survey of Registered Nurses, March 1996. Rockville, MD, and Statistics Canada [1995]. Registered Nurses Management Data. Ottawa.)

thought that residents could use welfare payments available to them through the Social Security Act of 1935 to pay for care.

Although nursing homes have improved since their inception in the 1700s, the same problems plague them today. Funding of nursing homes is still at bare minimum levels resulting in inadequate staffing levels, low salaries, and crowded conditions. Although they are the object of review by regulatory bodies, care and conditions cannot improve without improved financing.

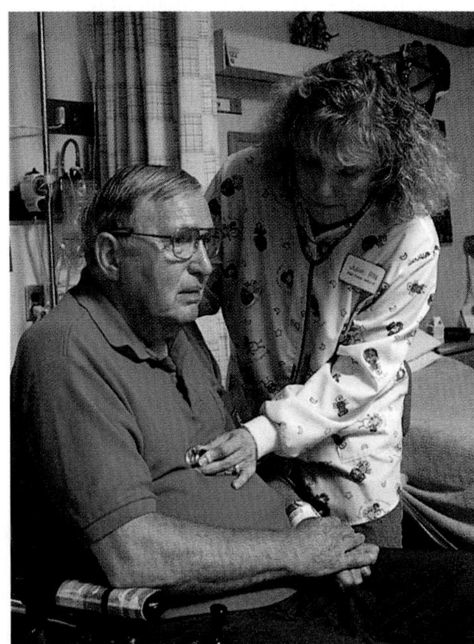

Figure 3-3. A nurse caring for a patient in a nursing home.

The current demand for nursing home beds exceeds the supply and it is anticipated that the need will become more critical. The population is aging, more people are living longer with chronic diseases as a result of advanced technology, and family units are smaller and more mobile, making it difficult to care for the elderly at home. Also, patients are discharged from the hospital at earlier points in their recovery.

Today nursing homes are still our almshouses caring for the poor, the chronically ill, the mentally ill, the retarded, and the elderly. They are also settings used to provide care to patients discharged from the hospital but not quite ready for discharge home. The introduction of the Medicare Prospective Payment System has increased this role of the nursing home and underscored the need for a continuous system of health care. Health professionals and the lay public frequently hold negative views of the nursing home and fail to realize two principles: the important contributions to health care these settings make and the need to ensure funding levels commensurate with the services provided.

In addition to nursing homes, other long-term care facilities include chronic disease hospitals, rehabilitation hospitals, psychiatric hospitals, and institutions for the mentally retarded.

In contrast to data describing growth and utilization of the short-stay hospital, the number of nursing homes and beds increased during the 1980s to 15,385 homes with 1.6 million beds in 1988. This trend is projected to continue. Also in contrast to data describing ownership of short-stay hospitals, for-profit nursing homes dominate, accounting for 74 percent of the nursing homes operating.

Nursing Home Nursing Workforce. Nursing homes employ an average of 0.88 workers per bed, with church-related homes having the highest ratio of employees to beds, and for-profit homes the lowest ratio. Major differences between the two are in the number of direct care personnel, including registered nurses. According to the Division of Nursing's 1996 National Sample Survey, an estimated 8.1 percent of the registered nurse workforce is employed in nursing homes (see Fig. 3–2).

Home Health/Community Care

Home health care is another rapidly growing component of the health care system (Fig. 3–4). The home has the longest history as a setting for providing health care. In the early 1900s most people were born at home, died at home, and in between were treated for maladies at home. As hospitals became safer settings and as medical technology expanded, it became more efficient and effective to provide illness care in the hospital instead of the home. In recent years, particularly since the federal government introduced a fixed fee payment schedule for hospital care (Medicare Prospective Payment System) and the development of health care technology with instruments that can be transported and used in the home, the home is again becoming a major setting in the health care system.

Today home health care agencies operate with various organizational ties; they may be an independent agency, hospital operated, or part of a health department. They may offer very specialized services or a range of services. Most offer nursing services, other professional services such as physical therapy, and nonprofessional services such as homemaker services. Some agencies combine services of volunteers, such as people delivering meals, with services of a paid staff. The funding for home health care is under serious review, with agencies claiming that the current reimbursement system is focused on acute or short-term problems whereas most patients have chronic

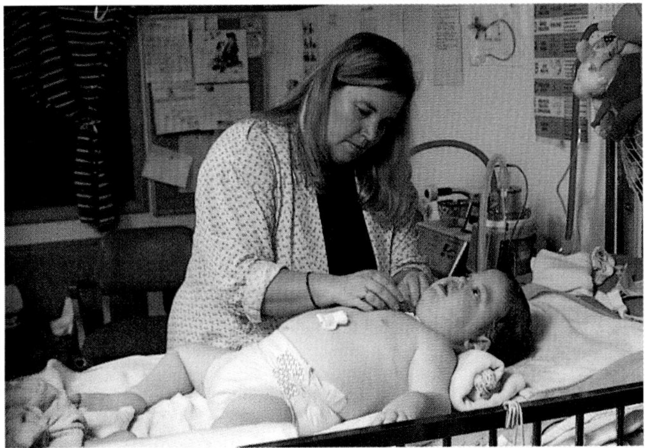

Figure 3–4. The home care setting may include high-tech patient care equipment.

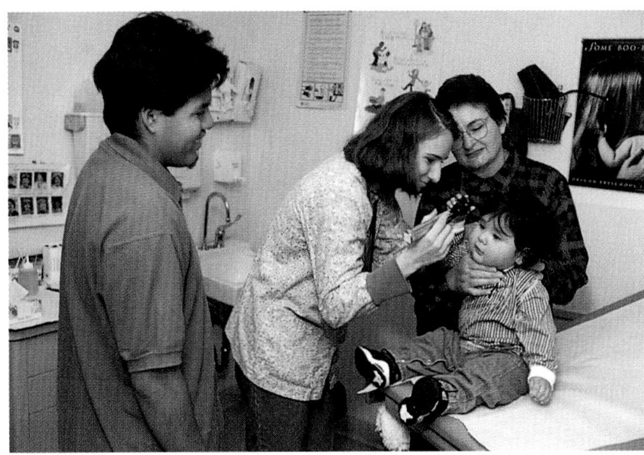

Figure 3–5. An increasing number of nurses are employed in ambulatory care settings.

or long-term needs. To the extent that reimbursement policies and the health care needs of the clientele are mismatched, the home health care component of our health care delivery system will not fulfill its potential.

Community-based nursing services such as those of public health and school nurses are important supplements to home health care. Some public health nurses provide direct patient care whereas others engage in health promotion and disease prevention activities. School nursing also varies, with some nurses providing direct care to children in the classroom whereas others perform routine assessments such as vision screening and health protection activities such as immunizations. Although these are very significant areas of nursing practice, they did not show significant growth during the 1990s.

Home Health/Community Care Nursing Workforce. In 1989, there were 8,105 home health agencies operating nationwide. This was 53 percent more than the number operating in 1986. Almost three fourths of the agencies are relatively small businesses with revenues of less than $1 million. It is difficult to obtain accurate measures of the size and composition of the workforce for these agencies. The workforce includes a high percentage of part-time employees, and the composition changes daily depending on service demands.

The 1996 National Sample Survey estimates that some 17 percent of employed registered nurses are working in non–hospital-based home health agencies, such as visiting nursing services; hospital-based home care agencies; and other community health settings. This setting experienced the largest growth in registered nurse employment since the last survey in 1992.

Ambulatory Care

Ambulatory care includes services provided in a physician's office, hospital outpatient clinic, free-standing clinics, ambulatory surgical centers, and health maintenance organizations (Fig. 3–5). There is considerable growth in size and services available in this component of the system. These changes are related to the high costs of hospital care and advancing technology. Providers are being pushed to use the hospital only when absolutely necessary. Surgical procedures that once required hospital stays of over a week, such as cataract surgery, are now performed in ambulatory care settings.

Ambulatory Care Nursing Workforce. The number of nurses employed in these settings continues to increase. According to the 1996 Sample Survey, approximately 8.5 percent of employed registered nurses work in ambulatory care settings (see Fig. 3–2).

Nursing Centers

Nursing centers are a unique component of the U.S. health care system. The major services provided in nursing centers include case finding and outreach, comprehensive assessment, care coordination, primary health care services, maintenance/surveillance, and health promotion and disease prevention (Fig. 3–6). The key elements of a nursing center are (Aydelotte et al, 1989):

- The client has direct access to nursing services.
- Nurses diagnose and treat and promote health and optimal functioning.
- Services are client-centered.
- Services should be reimbursed.
- Accountability and responsibility for client care remains with the nurse.
- Overall accountability for the center remains with the nurse executive.

The National League for Nursing (NLN) Council for Nursing Centers (1993) defines a nursing center as:

> An organization managed individually or as a group practice which offers clients the opportunity to contract directly with professional nurses for health care services rendered in community settings. A range of services are provided. Nursing centers are managed by nurses and staffed by advanced practice nurses, such as clinical specialists and nurse practitioners who function and/or are certified as defined by the State Nurse Practice Act where those nurses are licensed to practice.

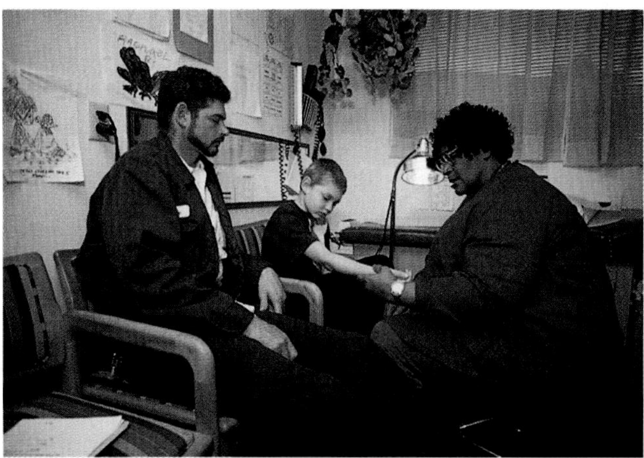

Figure 3–6. A nurse interacting with a patient in a nursing center.

Nursing centers can trace their origin to the Henry Street Settlement founded by Lillian Wald in 1893. Today's nursing center is also an outgrowth of the nurse practitioner role established in 1965. In the 1970s some university schools of nursing created nursing centers to provide settings for faculty practice and research, community service, and student learning experiences. In the 1980s there was a growth of many types of nursing centers—academic based, hospital based, and free-standing.

The NLN (1993) estimates that there are 250 nursing centers in the United States. About 56 percent of the centers are affiliated with a school of nursing, hospital, or other health care agency. The other 44 percent are free-standing. Staffing at the centers varies from a staff of one nurse to a staff of 115 nurses. The majority of the centers have five or fewer staff members. Budgets range from $1500 per year to $40,000,000. The median budget is $222,500. The centers tend to care for the most needy people including vulnerable populations such as the elderly, children, the homeless, and people with AIDS.

THE ROLE OF THE FEDERAL GOVERNMENT

The health care system receives support and consultation from agencies supported through the federal government. One such agency, the Food and Drug Administration (FDA) is described in Chapter 5. Another important agency is the Centers for Disease Control (CDC). The CDC was created to protect the health of the public. Today it has six bureaus: the Center for Preventive Services, the Center for Environmental Health, the National Institute for Occupational Health, the Center for Health Promotion and Education, the Center for Professional Development and Training, and the Center for Disease Investigation and Diagnosis.

It is impossible to describe the role of the federal government with any certainty because it changes depending on the philosophy of Congress and the White House. Programs currently funded through the federal government such as childhood immunizations, family planning, migrant health centers, and venereal disease control may or may not remain federally funded programs.

HEALTH CARE PROVIDERS

There are six major groups of health care providers that make the system work: allied health, dentistry, public health, pharmacy, medicine, and nursing.

Allied Health

Blayney and Fitz (1990) report between one and four million allied health professionals in practice. The reason the figure is

CURRENT CONTROVERSY

MOST HEALTH INSURANCE DOES NOT COVER SO-CALLED ALTERNATIVE THERAPIES SUCH AS HERBAL REMEDIES, MASSAGE, MEDITATION, AND ACUPUNCTURE. AS OF JANUARY 1, 1996, THE STATE OF WASHINGTON MANDATES THAT THEY MUST. IS THIS A GOOD MOVE IN TERMS OF THE HEALTH OF THE PUBLIC?

From the **New York Times,** *in the* **San Francisco Chronicle,** *Wednesday, January 3, 1996*

SEATTLE TO HAVE NATION'S FIRST TAX-SUPPORTED NATURAL HEALTH CLINIC

Most of the time, the people who write the laws for the most populous county in the Pacific Northwest talk about tax increments and zoning variances. But for a few days during the past year, the King County Council has been rhapsodizing about garlic pills and the healing power of the ginkgo tree extract.

In voting to establish the nation's first government-subsidized natural medicine clinic, the Republican-dominated council sounded like a therapy group discussing wonder cures.

One member said he owed his good health to a dietary supplement of enzymes and vitamins. Another said acupuncture cured her migraine headaches. A third member said she used botanical fluid to help her relax.

The council, which governs the greater Seattle area, has voted unanimously to establish the naturopathic health clinic, in which diet, exercise, vitamins and treatments such as acupuncture take precedence over drugs and the tools of traditional medicine.

The council hopes to use state or federal money for a two-year pilot project beginning some time this year.

Natural medicine, long considered to be on the fringe of health care, is reaching the mainstream, and to no greater extent than in Washington state. The new clinic will put the alternative treatments, which have been the province of better-educated and more affluent Americans, within reach of the poor.

And as of Monday, Washington state began requiring health insurance to cover treatments such as acupuncture, massage therapy and other forms of licensed health care.

No other state has gone as far in requiring coverage for such a broad variety of alternative medicine, said state Insurance Commissioner Deborah Senn. Senn, a Democrat, said she used acupuncture along with traditional medicine.

Natural medicine, despite strong opposition from many experts who view it as quackery, is quickly taking root, supporters say.

"This clinic we're trying to set up here will be the Starbucks of the health care world," Merilly Manthey said, drawing an analogy between the first coffee bar set up in Seattle by Starbucks Co. and the fledgling King County clinic.

Still, establishing the nation's first taxpayer-subsidized natural health clinic has not been easy. Although the County Council has voted twice in the last year to go ahead with the clinic, officials have yet to figure out whether state, federal or county money will be used to pay for the estimated $1 million to $2 million annual operating costs.

The clinic has taken on symbolic importance beyond its size, which is to consist of several naturopaths working with medical doctors.

Supporters say institutions that have the most to lose by the growth of natural medicine—pharmaceutical companies and the medical establishment—are fighting to keep alternative health care at the fringe of the market.

"You can blame the trillion-dollar medical-industrial complex for the delay," said Joseph E. Pizzorno, president of Bastyr University. The school will help run the clinic. "Fundamentally, if you can teach people how to take care of themselves, they don't need doctors, and that's seen as a threat by many people."

Naturopaths emphasize diet and exercise for preventive care, and recommend vitamins, herbal remedies, massage, meditation, and acupuncture for other problems.

Some medical doctors say that many claims of natural medicine are overblown, unproven or even outright fraud and that it is a mistake for governments to subsidize it in any form.

so vague is the difficulty in defining this group of professionals. The definition offered by the Committee on Allied Health Education and Accreditation defines allied health practitioners as:

> a large cluster of health care–related professions and personnel whose functions include assisting, facilitating, or complementing the work of physicians and other specialists in the health care system, and who choose to be identified as allied health personnel.

The allied health professions have evolved and expanded with the development of new technologies in health care. Examples of the occupations that fall into this category are:

- emergency medical technician
- medical illustrator
- medical technologist
- occupational therapist
- respiratory therapist
- physician assistant

Many allied health professions are technology driven (e.g., magnetic resonance imagers, who use specialized technology for visualizing parts of the body) and therefore have very limited scopes of practice. There is the possibility that new technology will reduce the need for these workers (the deskilling described in Chapter 5). They are likely to be replaced with an allied health worker who is multicompetent or with another type of generalist, e.g., a registered nurse (Paavola et al, 1993).

Dentistry and Dental Hygiene

Dental care focuses on oral health and oral function. This care is provided through general dentists, dental specialists, and dental hygienists. Although it is more and more difficult to separate oral health from the rest of the individual's health state (for example, if you have dental problems and cannot chew food, your overall nutrition is affected), this group of providers remains separate from the main health care system. The care that they provide is usually not covered by the individual's health insurance plan. Instead, the care is paid by a dental insurance plan or by the individual's personal money.

Dental care has changed significantly in the last quarter of this century. Initially, dental care focused on the treatment of dental caries and its effects with tooth restoration or prosthetic devices. Today the focus is on preventive aspects of oral health care. The public is interested in prevention of dental disease, good occlusion, pain-free joint and jaw function, good lip function for speech, and skeletal harmony in their faces for a normal appearance (White and Formicola, 1990).

In the future, dentists may become part of large health care systems linking clinical records about oral health to the records about physical and mental health. They would also be part of the health care team providing holistic care. Another challenge facing the field of dentistry is the growing elderly population with chronic illnesses who now expect to maintain good oral health. Dentists must understand more about the overall health status of an individual in order to provide safe, effective dental care.

Also in the future, the role of the dental hygienist is likely to expand as early preventive oral health services are emphasized by insurers. Dental hygienists have demonstrated their effectiveness in this arena with children in schools and with the elderly in nursing homes.

Public Health

The focus of public health professionals is the promotion of health and prevention of disease in communities. This is accomplished by a multidisciplinary approach to research, teaching, and public service. At a program level, public health is equated with the investigation and treatment of venereal diseases; with the investigation and treatment of epidemics such as food poisoning; with major environmental issues such as hazardous waste, the greenhouse effect, radon, pollution of air and water; and health and safety in the work place. Public health professionals have contributed to the health of the world by uncovering environmental and personal risk factors, in formulating national and local public health policies, and in establishing and evaluating prevention programs (Ibrahim and Osborn, 1990).

Like allied health, public health is diffuse and poorly defined. Core elements of the discipline include epidemiology, biostatistics, and management and organizational policies of health care. Beyond those areas, public health professionals have varied backgrounds and interests.

The future programs developed by public health professionals need to reflect the changes in the demographics of the population, the changes in the conditions affecting the public, and the changes in the health care system. The AIDS epidemic has underscored the need for a strong contemporary public health system. The respective roles of the federal, state, and local governments and the private sector in creating this strong contemporary public health system will be the subject of future debate.

Pharmacists

As with all other health care professionals, the role of the pharmacist is changing. Until recently, the major focus of the pharmacist was dispensing prescription and nonprescription drugs. This included assuring adequate drug supplies, filling prescriptions correctly, detecting overdoses, recognizing forged prescriptions, and maintaining accurate records. While fulfilling those responsibilities, the pharmacist retained a passive attitude toward the drug therapy ordered by the physician. The new role that has emerged requires the pharmacist to assume a major responsibility for drug therapy (Cole and Goyan, 1990).

The increase in the number of drugs available as well as in the number of drugs taken by a given individual are factors associated with this new role. In addition, the scientific base for pharmacology is growing dramatically (see Chapter 16). As pharmacists move into the realm of clinical pharmacy (drug therapy), their dispensing role will undoubtedly be done by technicians or through automation. This latter change will require changes in state regulatory law. It is also likely that these changes will reduce the number of pharmacists required by the health care system.

The relationship between medicine and pharmacy and nursing and pharmacy is affected by the new role for pharmacists. Neither medicine nor nursing is willing to relinquish its role in drug therapy. Yet both disciplines understand the specialized knowledge the pharmacist brings. The process of clarifying these new roles and relationships is taking place through discussions at professional meetings and published papers.

Medicine

The role of the physician is the diagnosis and treatment of disease. The ability to do this has been greatly improved with advances in biomedical science and technology (Whitcomb and Tosteson, 1990). Although the role of the physician is not likely to change as a result of the changes in the health care system, **how** that role is **implemented** is changing.

Because many of these changes are described in the next chapter, only a brief example is included here. In some capitated managed care systems (a system in which the physician is paid a flat monthly fee to provide care to those enrolled in the plan), the physician must receive approval from the insurance company before a patient can be referred to a specialist. A case manager (frequently a nurse) charged with resource management makes the decision about the referral. The physician can always challenge the decision but cannot overturn it. Likewise, these same systems develop guidelines regarding drugs that can be prescribed and a physician is not free to order something not on the list. These are significant changes in how physicians have practiced medicine.

Perhaps the greatest current controversy regarding the discipline of medicine and its future is whether too many physicians, and also the wrong types, are being trained. This issue is clearly portrayed by Richard Lamm (1994) (see the Current Controversy Box).

Nursing

Nurses are significant members of the health care team. The Division of Nursing (a federal agency located within the Department of Health and Human Services) provides national leadership to ensure an adequate nursing workforce. To assist in accomplishing that mission, the Division collects data through sample surveys of the registered nurses in this country. The last such survey was conducted in 1996. The results can be summarized as follows:

- An estimated 2,239,816 individuals had current licenses to practice as registered nurses (RNs) and were living in the 50 states and the District of Columbia. This is a 35 percent increase since 1980.
- Eighty-three percent of these individuals were employed in nursing.
- Four and three-tenths percent of the working registered nurses were men. The number of male RNs is growing at a faster rate than the total number of RNs.
- About 9 percent of the total RN population is from racial/ethnic minority backgrounds. This percentage has not increased in recent years.
- The average age of RNs has increased from 40.3 in 1980 to 43.1 in 1992. Even with the growth in the total number of RNs, the number under 30 has declined from 418,000 in 1980 to about 246,000 in 1992.
- The average age at graduation from a basic nursing program is 29.8 years. Fifteen years ago the average age at graduation was 22.7 years.
- About 72 percent of all registered nurses are married; 16.5 percent are widowed, divorced, or separated; and 11 percent were never married.
- Some 21 percent of the total RN workforce has completed additional academic preparation since graduation from their basic program.
- In 1992, 34 percent had the diploma as the highest educational level, 28 percent the associate degree, 30 percent the baccalaureate degree, and 8 percent the master's or doctoral degree. The percentage of those with diploma preparation continues to decline as the percentages of those with other degrees all continue to increase.

New Nursing Roles. As with the other health professions, the nature of nursing is not likely to change, but the roles or jobs that nurses fill will. One role that is increasing in importance as the health care system moves into managed care is the role of *case manager.* It should be noted that many but not all case managers are nurses.

Case Manager. The basic concept of case management is the timely coordination of high-quality services to meet an individual's specific health care needs in a cost-effective manner (Smith et al, 1995). The definition of case management approved by the Case Management Society of America is a collaborative process which assesses, plans, implements, coordinates, monitors, and evaluates options and services to meet an individual's health needs through communication and available resources to promote quality cost-effective outcomes.

Settings for case management services include:

- acute-care hospitals
- corporations
- public insurance programs, such as Medicare
- private insurance (i.e., casualty, auto, accident and health)
- managed care organizations
- independent case management companies
- government-sponsored programs, such as those in maternal–child health
- provider agencies and facilities (e.g., home health and mental health)

Case managers are powerful people within the health care system. They have the authority to allocate or deny resources for care. They have the responsibility to use health care dollars effectively. Over the years, case managers have demonstrated their value to patients and insurers. The demand for well-prepared case managers is increasing because they have proven their worth and because the system needs to control costs.

In the near future, case managers are likely to be used as gatekeepers to the system as well. One scenario has the case manager assigned to an aggregate of people (enrolled in the same managed care plan) with the same chronic illness such as diabetes. The case manager will hold meetings with that group of people, facilitating their social support of each other and the exchange of information about **living** with a chronic illness. By implementing these sessions that emphasize health promotion and the prevention of complications, costly visits to the physician or hospital should be avoided. If the case manager determined that a member of the group needed **medical** care, the person would be referred to the physician.

Telephone Triage Nurse. Another new role is the telephone triage nurse. This new role was described in a recent

CURRENT CONTROVERSY

IS AMERICA TRAINING THE WRONG NUMBERS AND TYPES OF HEALTH PROFESSIONALS? RICHARD LAMM, AN EXPERT ON HEALTH POLICY AND THE FORMER GOVERNOR OF COLORADO, THINKS SO

By Richard Lamm in the **Healthcare Forum Journal,** *Sept./Oct. 1994*

AMERICA IS TRAINING THE WRONG NUMBERS AND THE WRONG TYPES OF HEALTH PROFESSIONALS

American taxpayers pay for most medical school education and virtually all graduate medical education. But we have not been training the right numbers, nor the right types, nor the right mix of those professionals. I chair the Pew Health Professions Commission and the closer we look at this issue the larger it becomes.

We are using taxpayer dollars to prepare a generation of young professionals for careers that will not fit the market. We have produced too many doctors and not enough nurse practitioners or physician assistants. We have trained too many specialists and not enough primary health providers. Dr. John E. Wennberg warns, "if the hiring practices of prepaid HMOs had been enforced throughout the United States in 1988, more than half of all specialists would now be unemployed."

This is both a private and public tragedy. It means that some of the medical students today are going to have a hard time professionally. And if present trends continue, the 25 billion public dollars we devote to support health professions education each year will continue to give us many professionals we simply do not need.

Given the complexity of medical student career decisions, it is not reasonable to hold medical schools exclusively accountable for the career choices of their graduates. Yet, medical schools must take responsibility for influences within their own sphere: inappropriate and outdated institutional missions, admissions and recruitment policies, and curriculum and faculty role models.

Given the repeated calls for an increase of primary-care physicians along with warnings of an oversupply of many medical subspecialties, it is scandalous for medical schools and residency programs to continue to promote fields that may become obsolete, or for which there is little or no public need.

Much of what we do in healthcare serves the interests of a profession or an institution, rather than the broader interests of the public. Medical schools almost inevitably perpetuate the unbalanced makeup of their faculty. What if your local fire department produced three arson specialists for every firefighter? What if your local police department produced three forgery experts for every cop on the beat? What if United Airlines produced three pilots for every ground mechanic?

We will not have comprehensive healthcare reform without workforce reform. All systems are ultimately anchored in the skills and competence of the people who run them.

Medical schools and academic health centers cannot continue to be all things to all people: instead they must focus their training programs more effectively on the needs of the communities in which they reside—rather than on the financial health or technological interests of a teaching faculty, or on their research interests. Such a shift in focus would require making the following changes:

1. Create health teams that include a more general mix of allied health professionals.
2. Reduce the size of the physician entering class, probably by 25 percent.
3. Produce a 50–50 physician workforce balance between generalists and specialists, in the shortest time possible.
4. Change the service orientation of the teaching hospital to reflect the primary-care needs of most people.
5. Balance biomedical research with broader preventive, behavioral, and health services research.
6. Double the number of physician assistants and nurse practitioners, and start to train technicians to perform many functions now performed by specialists.

article in the *New York Times* (Gilbert, 1995). Health maintenance organizations and other managed care insurers have given patients access to toll-free telephone lines staffed by registered nurses, most operating 24 hours a day and 7 days a week. The goal is to reduce unnecessary doctor visits by having the nurses determine whether the caller needs medical help or can get by with self-care. Nurses do not make diagnoses but rather assess how serious the situation is. They ask detailed questions and also give detailed information. Data collected to date indicate that this saves from $46 to $184 a member per year and that the callers are very happy with the system.

RESEARCH REGARDING THE HEALTH CARE SYSTEM

Research regarding the delivery of health care is increasing in importance as the public demands to know more about the efficacy and outcomes of care. Although some view this field of research as relatively new, the literature leads to the conclusion that health care providers have always struggled over issues of quality. For example, Florence Nightingale used a set of outcome standards to assess care provided during the Crimean War. She compared mortality rates for hospitalized British soldiers with those of civilians. The point was made forcefully that soldiers were the victims of atrocious care. Her report resulted in improved environmental and health conditions for the armed forces—and obtained strong support for nurses as important health care providers.

Quality Assurance Framework

In the 1960s, Donabedian (1969) proposed a framework for evaluating quality of care within a health care agency or delivery system. That framework continues to be used by quality assurance committees and by health service researchers. The framework consists of three categories of factors that could be used to evaluate care: structure, process, and outcomes. **Structure** refers to characteristics of a health care agency such as experience and qualifications of staff, staff-patient ratios, hours of nursing care, conditions of the physical plant, and the adequacy of equipment. **Process** refers to the interactions between the provider(s) and the patient such as the specific services offered, the criteria used to select services, and the length of treatment. **Outcome** refers to the effect of care upon the patient such as morbidity rates, birth weights of infants, knowledge about disease, health status, and health-related behaviors (smoking, substance abuse).

Nurse researchers studying structure in relation to quality have focused on variables such as cost, ownership of institution, resources, amount of nursing care available, type of nursing personnel, clinical competency, roles of personnel, and organizational variables. In the 1960s and early 1980s, nurse researchers attempted to develop tools to measure quality in practice/process. Although several tools were developed, each has serious problems for use in the real world. Nursing research focusing on outcome measures is increasing. The research on preoperative teaching presented in Chapter 2 is an example of outcome research.

Example of a Quality Assurance Program

Many health care agencies have quality assurance committees that use process criteria for measuring quality. Few agencies have programs that include criteria on structure, process, and outcomes. The Coordinated Home Care Program (CHCP) introduced in Alberta in 1978 is one such agency (Sorgen, 1986). Services provided by the CHCP include nursing care, physiotherapy, occupational therapy, respiratory therapy, speech therapy, homemaker/home helper, handyman services, meals-on-wheels, wheels-to-wheels, transportation, friendly visiting, heavy housework services, and volunteers.

The CHCP formed a Home Care Standards Committee to develop the quality assurance program. The committee first developed explicit standards related to the organization and delivery of home care services (structure standards). These included standards regarding staff development, staffing ratios, performance appraisals, records, equipment and supplies. General case coordination process standards were developed and incorporated into an audit tool for use in assessing the process of care as described in the problem-oriented record.

The Committee then began the most difficult task of creating outcome measures. After several years of research they developed a set of valid, reliable, and sensitive outcomes measures. The measures were pain management, symptom control, physiological health status, activities of daily living, activities of household management, application of knowledge, satisfaction with services, and family strain.

This comprehensive approach to assuring quality enables the agency to see the relationship between changes in structure and process on outcomes. It also provides patient, provider, and funder with the most important data—the outcomes of care.

Example of Quality Assurance Nursing Research

The example of health care research selected for inclusion in the chapter concerns the delivery of nursing services. The researchers compare two approaches for delivering nursing care: primary nursing and team nursing. This topic was selected because it represents the single most frequently studied topic by nurse researchers focusing on the delivery system. A conservative estimate of the studies in this area is well over 250; there were 150 reports in the 1970s alone. Also, this research was selected because it illustrates the evaluation of the effects of structure/process on outcomes. This is the type of research emphasized in the current health care system.

Gardner (1989) reported a five-year study conducted at Rochester (New York) General Hospital comparing the effects of primary versus team nursing. The investigator believed that deficiencies in previous research and major changes in the health care system supported the importance of a systematic evaluation of primary nursing. The research was designed to compare the two systems in terms of (1) quality of patient care, (2) effect on nursing staff, and (3) costs.

Definition of Primary Nursing. The three major characteristics that the nursing staff designed their primary nursing delivery system around were 24-hour responsibility, individualized care, and direct communication. Primary nursing was defined as one nurse who is responsible for the patient within 24 hours of admission until discharge from the unit. This nurse has a 24-hour responsibility for the overall assessment, planning, and evaluation of the nursing care rendered to the patient.

In addition, whenever the nurse is working, he or she is either giving direct patient care or is responsible for the nursing care given for that shift. The primary nurse coordinates nursing communications regarding nursing care to their patients, their patients' families, other nurses, and other health care professionals.

Another major activity of the primary nurse is to promote an effective and therapeutic nurse-patient relationship. This relationship facilitates the nurse to individualize the patient's care, and to ensure that the patient's needs are addressed.

Primary nurses assign themselves to patients. It is expected that each primary nurse will have an average of four primary patients. Specific primary nursing responsibilities include:

- Introduces self to primary patients and provides patient with explanation form; explains role and what the primary nurse-patient relationship means.
- Provides direct or indirect nursing care to primary patients each day on duty.
- Establishes a healthy, trusting relationship with patient/family in which all feel free to communicate with one another.
- Acts as a patient advocate by investigating and gaining insight into problems/complaints and attempting to work them out with the patient; evaluates progress and interacts with other health care givers on the patient's behalf.
- Reviews the nursing diagnosis and care plan if these have already been started. Adds to the care plan if necessary; co-initials any updates.
- Establishes nursing diagnosis and goals of the new nursing diagnoses when necessary and updates and writes new goals and orders when necessary.
- Is the patient's nursing care planner and has final say on what is written on the care plan. Other staff members are encouraged to add to the patient's care plan, but the primary nurse can change what is written if appropriate.
- Evaluates plan of care for primary patients with other members or staff via patient care conferences and/or discharge patient conferences.
- Begins discharge planning on admission and communicates this via the care plan.
- Informs primary patients of the goals whenever possible. Some goals need patient cooperation if they are to be met.
- Communicates patient's needs to other health care givers verbally and in writing via the care plan. Other nurses are expected to follow the primary nurse's plan of care.
- Assures when leaving the unit that another nurse is informed of critical patient issues.

It is expected that each primary nurse's responsibility is to maintain a minimum number of primary patients. When going on vacation, it is the primary nurse's responsibility to arrange coverage for continuity of care for his or her primary patients. When the primary nurse is not working, another registered nurse, called the "RN associate nurse," is assigned to the patient. This person is responsible for communicating pertinent information to the primary nurse. All licensed practical nurses and nursing assistants work under the registered nurse's direction if the primary nurse is not present.

On a shift-by-shift basis, nursing staff members are responsible for completing their daily assignments. Except for nights, the nursing staff is expected to provide most of the patient care. Nursing assistants are available to help under the registered nurse's supervision.

Only registered nurses who have successfully worked more than 6 months on the unit are eligible to be primary nurses. A specific primary nurse orientation is planned. Nurses who work fewer than 20 hours per week are not eligible to be primary nurses.

There is no "charge nurse" on the primary nursing unit. Instead, a registered nurse is designated as "shift coordinator." This person provides overall direction regarding staffing issues on a shift-by-shift basis and ensures that all patients who are eligible have a primary nurse. In addition to these responsibilities, the shift coordinator provides direct care to patients. The nurse manager designates the shift coordinator. Each unit has an assignment board. This board has the patient's room number, patient's name, primary nurse's name, and physician's name. This board is placed in a central visible place on the unit.

It is expected that all members of the unit nursing staff be available to assist the primary nurse in planning and evaluating the patient's care. With the above description, the staff believes that primary nurses should have sufficient authority and autonomy to practice primary nursing.

Definition of Team Nursing. There are approximately 12 patients per team. Each day and evening shift has a charge nurse, team leaders (3), and team members: registered nurse (RN), licensed practical nurse (LPN), nursing assistant (NA), and one nurse assigned to medication administration. Each skill level of staff has designated specific responsibilities.

Assignments are made at the team level by the charge nurse. Each team decides on a shift-by-shift basis how it is going to work together. Approximately midway through the shift, each team has a multidisciplinary (RNs, LPNs, and NAs) conference. The purposes of these conferences are to assess patients' needs, plan care, and make alternate patient assignments. Members of the team are expected to discuss their working relationships at these meetings.

Each registered nurse is to give evidence of successful orientation to team leadership before she or he can assume these responsibilities. These responsibilities include:

- coordinating the patient care on the team
- routinely checking on all patients on the team
- providing direct care to patients
- monitoring clinical data and any appropriate interventions for all patients on the team
- leading team conferences and working with the charge nurse
- serving as a resource person to the team
- giving a report to the next shift

The charge nurse on the unit verifies all orders, assigns staff to the teams, coordinates all emergencies, coordinates staffing within the shift, assures that all unit base documentation is completed for that shift, works with the team leaders, and coordinates routine communication for the shift to the other departments and professionals.

BOX 3–1
QUALITY OF PATIENT CARE SCALES

The Quality of Patient Care Scales (Qualpacs) is a 68-item rating scale that measures quality of nursing care through direct observation and chart review. The 68 items fall into six subscales:

- psychosocial individual
- psychosocial group (not used in this study)
- physical
- general
- communication
- professional implications.

The nurse observer rates the care given a specific patient by each member of the nursing staff who interacts with the patient over a 2-hour period. Each of the 68 items is rated on a 5-point scale from best to poor.

It is expected that all members of the unit nursing staff will work cooperatively together as a team in providing nursing care.

Measurement of the Outcomes of Care. Instruments used to measure quality of care were the Quality of Patient Care Scales (Box 3–1), Nursing Support Scale (Box 3–2), and Hospital Stress Rating Scale (Box 3–3). The impact on nursing personnel was measured with the Nursing Stress Scale. Cost data were obtained from the budget and census reports. Demographic characteristics of the staff were also included in the analysis.

Data collection was conducted over a 4-year period. Nursing personnel self-selected to work on either a primary or team unit. Patients were randomly assigned. Four units were initially included in the study; a fifth unit was added midway through the study.

Data Analysis and Conclusions. Analysis of data from the Quality Patient Care Scale showed statistically significant higher scores for patients receiving primary nursing care. Initially all scores improved but then team nursing scores remained stable and primary nursing continued to improve.

The primary nurses reported the primary nursing intervention system as more challenging and professionally rewarding than the team approach. They also felt the opportunities to increase their nursing competencies were more available as primary nurses. The retention of all nursing staff on the primary units was higher than the team units at the end of one, two and three years by 23%, 31%, and 18%, respectively. Unexpectedly, the cost to the hospital for nursing care was lower for the primary units than for the team units. The lower cost per patient per day for nursing services in the primary units cumulatively resulted in a cost-saving of $279,709 over 36 months. The cost savings realized were attributed to at least three factors: fewer nurse administrators on primary units, higher patient-staff ratios and less use of agency nurses (Gardner, 1989).

Recommendations. As a result of this study, the investigator recommended that primary nursing be utilized to delivery high-quality care, promote professional-based nursing practice, and retain registered nurses.

BOX 3–2
NURSING SUPPORT SCALE

The **perception** of nurse support is a measure of quality of care. Nurses can function competently on behalf of patients and yet not generate a sense of support. Two intrinsic elements in primary nursing, continuity of care and an emphasis on the nurse-patient relationship, were combined to generate the hypothesis that patients in primary care units would perceive greater support than patients in team units. The Nursing Support Scale was used to test this hypothesis.

Here is an illustration of the items on the Scale.

PATIENT NUMBER
CODE _____

Nursing Support Scale
By K. Gardner and E. Wheeler

Nurses vary on how often they are able to do these nursing activities.

Please indicate *how often* you have received the following nursing activities. Opposite the nurse activity, please write the number that corresponds to *how often* you have received each nursing activity during this hospitalization.

HOW OFTEN

SCALE: 1—Never
2—Rarely
3—Somewhat Infrequently
4—Neither Frequently or Infrequently
5—Frequently
6—Very Frequently
7—Always

	How Often	For Office Use Only
1. Gave advice to me.	_____	18
2. Was friendly to me.	_____	19
3. Included my family to participate in my plan of care.	_____	20
4. Spent time with my family.	_____	21
5. Helped me to solve problems.	_____	22
6. Helped me to establish realistic goals.	_____	23
7. Explained procedures and medications.	_____	24
8. Helped to reduce my anxiety.	_____	25
9. Responded positively to my attempts at being friendly.	_____	26

Published as part of the Gardner (1989) study.

BOX 3-3
HOSPITAL STRESS RATING SCALE

The Hospital Stress Rating Scale is a 49-item tool based on stressful hospital events identified by patients, lay people, physicians, and nurses. The 49 items fall into nine subscales:

- unfamiliarity of surroundings
- loss of independence
- separation from spouse
- financial problems
- isolation from other people
- lack of information
- threat of severe illness
- separation from family
- problems with medications

CHALLENGES TO THE CURRENT U.S. HEALTH CARE SYSTEM

The current literature is filled with articles critical of health care in the United States. Data show that we spend more for health care than other industrialized nations but health status indicators are poorer (Lamm 1994; National League for Nursing, 1992). The percentage of the population without health insurance continues to grow; in 1995, 15.4 percent were without coverage (PHS, 1997). In addition, health care is perceived by consumers as fragmented, depersonalized, confusing, and poorly coordinated (Ginsburg and Prout, 1990). Consumers do not know what services to expect, from whom, and where. To the consumer, the health care industry seems to exist to benefit the provider of services rather than the consumer and the community (Yankelovich and Immerwahr, 1991).

The American public have read or heard statistics such as the following (Chambliss and Reier, 1990):

- About 35 percent of all surgical deaths and 50 percent of postoperative complications, such as infections, are probably preventable.
- As many as one fourth of all patients who die in hospitals may have been misdiagnosed by physicians.
- Up to 35 percent of all hospital admissions are not needed.
- Some 15 percent to 30 percent of diagnostic tests do not help or are not even looked at.
- Forty-four percent of bypass surgeries are unwarranted or questionable.
- One fourth of hospital days, one fourth of procedures, and two fifths of medications could be done without.

Health Care Reform Initiatives

Health professionals must play a central role in reforming and redesigning the health care system. Berwick (1994) from the Institute for Healthcare Improvement identifies social needs in four basic categories as the motivation for health care reform: (1) to improve the health status of populations and the clinical outcomes of care; (2) to improve the experience of care for patients, families, and communities; (3) to reduce the total economic burden of care and illness; and (4) to improve social justice and equity in the health status of Americans.

Berwick has identified 11 plausible goals based on health services research:

1. Reduce inappropriate surgery, hospital admissions, and diagnostic tests.
2. Reduce key underlying root causes of illness (smoking, handgun violence, and so on).
3. Reduce cesarean section rates.
4. Reduce the use of unwanted medical procedures at the end of life.
5. Simplify pharmaceutical use, especially for antibiotic use and for the elderly.
6. Increase active patient participation in therapeutic decision making.
7. Decrease waiting time in health settings.
8. Reduce inventory levels in health care agencies.
9. Record only useful information only once.
10. Consolidate and reduce the total supply of high-technology medical and surgical care.
11. Reduce the racial gap in infant mortality and low birth weight.

Berwick believes that these reforms are totally possible if clinicians across disciplines join together with a commitment to making reform occur (Boxes 3–4 and 3–5).

The National Commission on Nursing Implementation Project (1988 p. 1) states that in addition to providing excellent care for acute episodes of disease, the reformed health care system must:

- enable individuals to better understand and assume more control over their own health and well-being—and, in the process, conserve finite health care resources
- ensure, in a cost-containment environment, that all citizens have access to basic health care
- promote the use of more cost-effective health care alternatives of equal quality
- provide suitable and cost-effective care for a rapidly growing elderly population and citizenry with significant health problems related to chronic illness
- guide consumers through an increasingly complex health care maze, coordinating the services they may receive from a variety of caregivers who practice in different types of sites

Health Care Innovations

In addition to changes that will occur because of health care reform initiatives, the system will change because of innovations. For example, the Institute for Alternative Futures

BOX 3-4

DURING NURSES' WEEK IN 1991, MAJOR NURSING ORGANIZATIONS UNVEILED NURSING'S AGENDA FOR HEALTH CARE REFORM

THE FRAMEWORK FOR CHANGE

Nurses strongly believe that the health care system must be restructured, reoriented, and decentralized in order to guarantee access to services, contain costs, and ensure quality care. Our plan—the product of consensus building within organized nursing—is designed to achieve this goal. It provides central control in the form of federal minimum standards for essential services and federally defined eligibility requirements. At the same time, it makes allowances for decentralized decision making which will permit local areas to develop specific programs and arrangements best suited to consumer needs.

Nursing's plan is built around several basic premises, including the following:

- All citizens and residents of the United States must have equitable access to essential health care services (a core of care).
- Primary health care services must play a very basic and prominent role in service delivery.
- Consumers must be the central focus of the health care system. Assessment of health care needs must be the determining factor in the ultimate structuring and delivery of programs and services.
- Consumers must be guaranteed direct access to a full range of qualified health care providers who offer their services in a variety of delivery arrangements at sites which are accessible, convenient, and familiar to the consumer.
- Consumers must assume more responsibility for their own care and become better informed about the range of providers and the potential options for services. Working in partnership with providers, consumers must actively participate in choices that best meet their needs.
- Health care services must be restructured to create a better balance between the prevailing orientation toward illness and cure and a new commitment to wellness and care.
- The health care system must assure that appropriate, effective care is delivered through the efficient use of resources.
- A standardized package of essential health care services must be provided and financed through an integration of public and private plans and sources.
- Mechanisms must be implemented to protect against catastrophic costs and impoverishment.

The cornerstone of nursing's plan for reform is the delivery of primary health care services to households and individuals in convenient, familiar places. If health is to be a true national priority, it is logical to provide services in the places where people work and live. Maximizing the use of these sites can help eliminate the fragmentation and lack of coordination which have come to characterize the existing health care system. It can also promote a more "consumer friendly" system where services such as health education, screening, immunizations, well-child care, and prenatal care would be readily accessible.

At the same time, consumers must be the focus of the health care system. Individuals must be given incentives to assume more responsibility for their health. They must develop both the motivation and capability to be more prudent buyers of health services. Promotion of healthy lifestyles and better informed consumer decisions can contribute to effective and economical health care delivery.

Finally, in implementing reforms, attention must be directed to the unique needs of special population groups whose health care needs have been neglected. These individuals include children, pregnant women, and vulnerable groups such as the poor, minorities, AIDS victims, and those who have difficulty securing insurance because of preexisting conditions. Lack of preventive and primary care for this sector has cost the nation enormously—both in terms of lives lost or impaired and dollars spent to treat problems that could have been avoided or treated less expensively through appropriate intervention.

Access to care alone may not be sufficient to resolve the problems of these vulnerable groups. For those individuals whose health has been seriously compromised, a "catch up" program characterized by enriched services is justified. Coverage of pregnant women and children is critical. This first step represents a cost effective investment in the future health and prosperity of the nation.

It is this set of values that distinguishes nursing's plan from other proposals and offers a realistic approach to health care reform.

Nursing's Agenda for Health Care Reform (1991) Publication No. 41-2505 American Nurses Publishing Kansas City, MO 64108.

(1995) has identified the following trends shaping health care and innovation:

- Systems approaches to disease management—The shift is from a focus on the components of therapy, e.g., a specific drug, to a focus on the therapeutic or disease management system as a whole.
- Accountability supported by (clinical) outcomes.
- Cost-effectiveness.
- Reinvention of drug and device regulation—Drug and device regulation are likely to face further pressure for change, as well as an environment in which their public policy goals can be better achieved.
- Changing biomedical research platform—The platform for biomedical research will change and research without clearly anticipatable outcomes will receive less funding.

BOX 3-5

IN 1993 THE NATIONAL LEAGUE FOR NURSING RELEASED ITS VISION FOR NURSING EDUCATION. THE ASSUMPTION BEHIND THE VISION WAS THAT IF HEALTH CARE WAS TO CHANGE SO WOULD NURSING EDUCATION.

A VISION FOR NURSING EDUCATION

Executive Summary

Nursing's vision for a health care system that ensures access, quality, and cost containment through a new approach to the delivery of care is within reach. The nursing education system required by that new approach must move quickly to provide adequate numbers of appropriately prepared nurses.

Successful implementation of nursing's approach to health care delivery requires:

1. Significant increases in the numbers of advanced nurse practitioners prepared to provide primary health care to communities and primary care services in group and interdisciplinary practices.
2. A shift in emphasis for all nursing education programs to ensure that all nurses—whatever their basic and graduate education and wherever they choose to practice—are prepared to function in a community-based, community-focused health care system.
3. An increase in the numbers of community nursing centers and their increased utilization as model clinical sites for nursing students.
4. An increase in the number of nursing faculty prepared to teach for a community-based, community-focused health care system.
5. A shift in emphasis for nursing research and an increase in the numbers of studies concerned with health promotion and disease prevention at the aggregate and community levels.
6. Targeted national initiatives to recruit and retain nurse providers, faculty, administrators and researchers from diverse racial, cultural, and ethnic backgrounds.

A Vision for Nursing Education, National League for Nursing, 61 Broadway, NY, NY 10006.

- Information technology advances—The information revolution for health—centered on the development of sophisticated expert systems, extensive and accessible knowledge databases, and personal body function profiles—will allow greater productivity due to dramatic changes in the nature of medical records, health care delivery, medical education, and medical research.
- Biochemically unique medical care—Genetic and biomedical research will lead health care providers to focus on the biochemically unique nature of each of us, and to develop protocols that can deal with uniqueness. This creation of subgroups in the population will dramatically change health care delivery and drug regulation.
- The "predict, prevent, and manage paradigm"—Health care is moving from treating symptoms to anticipating changes in health status, preventing morbidity that can be avoided, and optimally managing the morbidity that does occur.
- Changing industry roles—Pharmaceutical companies will function as health companies rather than mere drug companies.
- Community focus for health—Health care providers will increasingly share the responsibility for the health outcomes of the communities they serve, independent of the individuals they treat.
- Alternative therapies—Interest among consumers and a growing number of health care providers in alternative and complementary approaches to health care holds the potential for generating new knowledge and therapies from homeopathic, acupuncture, nutritional, behavioral, and spiritual approaches.

The Institute for Alternative Futures sees these as the trends. They are quick to point out that identifying trends is only a beginning point. What is required is the **vision** that deals with the preferred future one wants to create.

THE BOTTOM LINE FOR THOSE ENTERING NURSING

Whatever the health care system is today is not what it will be tomorrow. Change of the magnitude predicted for the health care system is difficult for those in the profession of nursing and for those entering the profession. For both groups it is essential to be clear on the core values that the health care system should demonstrate. How important is universal access? How important is personal choice of provider? Should the community have a greater voice in health care resource allocations? Should the health care system be a for-profit business? These are the type of value-oriented questions you will deal with while you are a student and throughout your nursing career. Individually and collectively nurses must be part of the solution—not a part of the problem.

CHAPTER HIGHLIGHTS

- Although more care is being delivered in the home and community settings, the hospital continues to be the primary setting for delivering care.
- New roles for nurses are evolving in all health care settings. These new roles are usually in addition to the roles nurses have traditionally held.
- Futurists predict major changes in health care delivery and the roles and relationships of health care providers.

REFERENCES

A Vision for Nursing Education (1993). Available from the National League for Nursing, 61 Broadway, NY, NY 10006.

Aydelotte, M.K., Gregory, M.S. (1989). Nursing practice: Innovative models. In *Nursing Centers: Meeting the Demand for Quality Health Care.* New York: National League for Nursing Press, pp 1–20.

Berwick, D.M. (1994). Eleven worthy aims for clinical leadership of health system reform. *Journal of the American Medical Association, 272,* 797–802.

Blayney, K.D., Fitz, P.A. (1990). The allied health professions: A critical resource in the future of health care. In E.H. O'Neil (ed.): *Perspectives on the Health Professions.* Durham, NC: Pew Health Professions Programs, pp. 5–22.

Chambliss, L., Reier, S. (1990). How doctors have ruined health care. *Financial World,* January 9, 46–52.

Cole, J.R., Goyan, J.E. (1990). The profession of pharmacy. In E.H. O'Neil (ed.): *Perspectives on the Health Professions.* Durham, NC: Pew Health Professions Program, pp. 71–88.

Donabedian, A. (1969). Part II—Some issues in evaluating the quality of nursing care. *American Journal of Public Health, 59,* 1833–1836.

Gardner, K.G. (1989). The effects of primary versus team nursing on quality of patient care and impact on nursing staff and costs. *Pew Charitable Trusts Reference Number: 860506HE.* Published by The Rochester General Hospital, Rochester, NY.

Gilbert, S. (1995). In the 90s, house calls are to nurses, by phone. *The New York Times,* November 8.

Ginsburg, J.A., Prout, D.M. (1990). Access to health care. *Annals of Internal Medicine, 112*(9), 641–644.

Health Resources and Services Administration (1990). *Health Resources and Services Administration: Seventh Report to the President and Congress on the Status of the Health Personnel in the United States.* (HRS-P-OD-90-1). Washington, DC: U.S. Government Printing Office.

Ibrahim, M.A., Osborn, J.E. (1990). Future of the public health profession. In E.H. O'Neil (ed.): *Perspectives on the Health Professions.* Durham, NC: Pew Health Professions Programs, pp. 35–44.

Institute for Alternative Futures (1995). IAF scenarios for health care innovation in 2010. 100 North Pitt Street, Suite 235, Alexandria, VA 22314.

Lamm, R.D. (1994). Healthcare heresies. *Healthcare Forum Journal,* September/October, 45–61.

Levit, K.R., Lazenby, H.C., Braden, B.R., et al. (1998). National health expenditures, 1996. *Health Care Financing Review, 19,* 161–200.

Metropolitan Healthcare Council (1995). *Human Resource Planning. Environmental Scan: Nursing Supply and Demand.* St. Paul, MN.

Moses, E.B. (1992). *The Registered Nurse Population.* (ISBN 0-16-042616-2). Washington, D.C.: U.S. Government Printing Office.

National Commission on Nursing Implementation Project (1988). *The Nation's Nurses: A Credible Profession Doing An Incredible Job.* Milwaukee, WI.

National League for Nursing. (1992). Comparison of national health care systems. *Nursing & Health Care, 13,* 202–203.

Nursing's agenda for health care reform. (1991). Pub. No. 41–2505. American Nurses Publishing, Kansas City, MO.

Nursing centers (1993). *Prism The NLN Research and Policy Quarterly, 1,*(1), 1,3.

Paavola, F.G., Brand, M.K., Schwab, P.M., Clark, N.L. (1993). Developments in the national workforce policy: Challenges for allied health education. *Journal of Allied Health,* Summer, 229–237.

Public Health Service (PHS) Centers for Disease Control and Prevention and National Center for Health Statistics (1997). *Health, United States, 1996–97.* Washington DC: U.S. Government Printing Office.

Raffel, M. (1980). *The U.S. Health System: Origins and Functions.* New York: John Wiley and Sons, Inc.

Smith, D.S., Boling, J., Ferretti, C.K., et al. (1995). Standards of practice for case management. *The Journal of Care Management, 1,* 7–16.

Sorgen, L.M. (1986). The development of a home care quality assurance program in Alberta. *Home Health Care Services Quarterly, 70,* 13–28.

What the public values in its health care system. (1994). W.K. Kellogg Foundation, One Michigan Ave., Battle Creek, MI 49017.

Whitcomb, M.E., Tosteson, D.C. (1990). Medical education in the context of the changing American health care system. In E.H. O'Neil (ed.): *Perspectives on the Health Professions.* Durham, NC: Pew Health Professions Programs, pp. 45–54.

White, R.P., Formicola, A.J. (1990). Dentistry and the health care system issues and challenges. In E.H. O'Neil (ed.): *Perspectives on the Health Professions.* Durham, NC: Pew Health Professions Programs, pp. 23–34.

Williams, S., Torrens, P. (eds.) (1988). *Introduction to Health Services.* New York: John Wiley and Sons, Inc.

Yankelovich, D., Immerwahr, J. (1991). A perception gap. *Health Management Quarterly, XIII,* Third Quarter, 11–14.

4 Health Care Financing

Carol Lindeman

OBJECTIVES

After studying this chapter, students will be able to:

- **identify nursing care in keeping with the philosophy of a patient's health insurance plan**
- **consider cost and effectiveness when implementing the independent functions of nursing**
- **maintain job satisfaction in a cost-sensitive environment**
- **actively participate in discussions regarding health care financing policies**

In 1993 the United States public learned about Angela and Amy Lakeberg—the twins who came into the world joined at the heart. For one twin to live, the other would have to die on the operating room table. The quality and length of life for the remaining twin was uncertain. Their story is illustrative of the complex issues surrounding the financing of health care in this country.

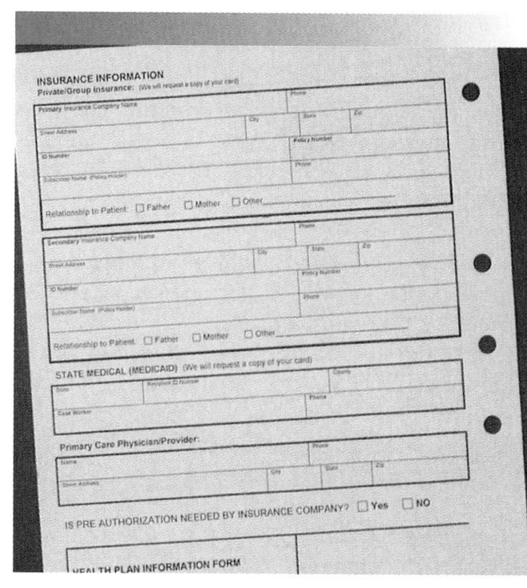

According to syndicated columnist Ellen Goodman (1994), Reitha and Kenneth Lakeberg, the parents, were told that Reitha was carrying conjoined twins and an abortion was offered. The parents chose not to have the abortion, and the twins were born at Loyola University Hospital in Chicago. The doctors there decided not to operate because the odds were that the remaining twin would not survive for very long.

The Lakebergs found another hospital and a team of doctors that would perform the surgery. Amy died and Angela lived. Angela lived in an intensive care unit fed through tubes and attached to a respirator for 10 months. Then Angela died.

By the time of Angela's death, the medical care costs were more than $1.3 million dollars. Three states, two hospitals, and one Medicaid program were arguing over who should pay for what and who should be reimbursed for what. The only item that was clear was that one way or another, the U.S. public would pay.

At the same time the public would pay the costs for giving Angela 10 months of life with marginal quality, 37 million Americans were denied the benefits of health insurance and primary health care such as immunizations, health screening, tests to detect cancer, and care for minor illnesses.

The issues surrounding health care financing are complex. Americans have seen a rapid growth of public responsibility for personal health care spending For example, the federal government's share of the nation's health care bill rose from 28.1 percent in 1990 to 31.7 percent in 1993 (Levit et al, 1994). Also, from 1990 to 1993, federal and state Medicaid funding in creased at a

16 percent average annual rate, a rate almost twice the increase in overall spending (Levit et al, 1994). During this same period the number of uninsured continued to rise; the uninsured nonelderly population grew from 16.6 percent in 1991 to 17.4 percent in 1992, indicating an increase in the lack of affordable private health insurance (Levit et al, 1994). In comparison to the United States, other industrialized countries have healthier citizens and lower costs (Lamm, 1994). Few Americans are satisfied with the current system, yet there is little agreement on how the system should change (Yankelovich and Immerwahr, 1991).

Contemporary nursing practice requires all nurses to understand the complex issues of health care financing and the impact on health care delivery. The need to contain increases in health care costs to match those of inflation has resulted in an era of intense cost consciousness. Nurses in every clinical setting are expected to participate in identifying and implementing cost-containment measures. Nurses are being told to avoid waste, delegate nonnursing tasks, identify less expensive nursing interventions (without cutting quality), increase efficiency, teach self-care early, and to do nothing that is not absolutely necessary and directly related to improved outcomes of care. In many settings nurses are asked to monitor the progress or care and the use of resources through the use of **critical pathways** (see Chapter 11 for a discussion of critical pathways). If too many resources are being used or a patient is not progressing as projected, the nurse is expected to intervene. The goal is cost-effective care, not just quality care. Cost consciousness based on an understanding of health care financing is a mandatory aspect of contemporary nursing practice.

HOW MUCH MONEY IS SPENT ON HEALTH CARE?

In 1996, the U.S. spent $1.035 trillion on health care, up 4.4 percent from 1995 (Levit et al, 1998). This increase stands in sharp contrast to the double-digit growth rate experienced in the 1980s. Managed care health insurance policies offering lower premiums through tighter controls on costs and utilization are credited with producing this dramatic turn-around in expenditures. Figure 4–1 shows how national health expenditures grew as a percentage of the gross domestic product for the years 1960 through 1996.

We spend significantly more money on health care than any other country in the world. For example, the U.S. spends 40 percent more per capita than Canada; 91 percent more than Norway; 127 percent more than Japan; and 158 percent more than Denmark (Brown, 1992). These differences tended to increase as other countries held growth in health care expenditures in check while ours increased faster than inflation (Schieber et al, 1992). Today the U.S. still spends more money on health care than other countries, but the rate of growth is being contained.

WHAT IS THE MONEY SPENT ON?

National health expenditures fall into two broad categories: health services and supplies (those services and products that are **currently** consumed) and research and construction. In 1996, $1,003.6 trillion was spent on health services and supplies while $31.5 billion was spent on research and construction (Levit et al, 1998). Health services and supplies can be

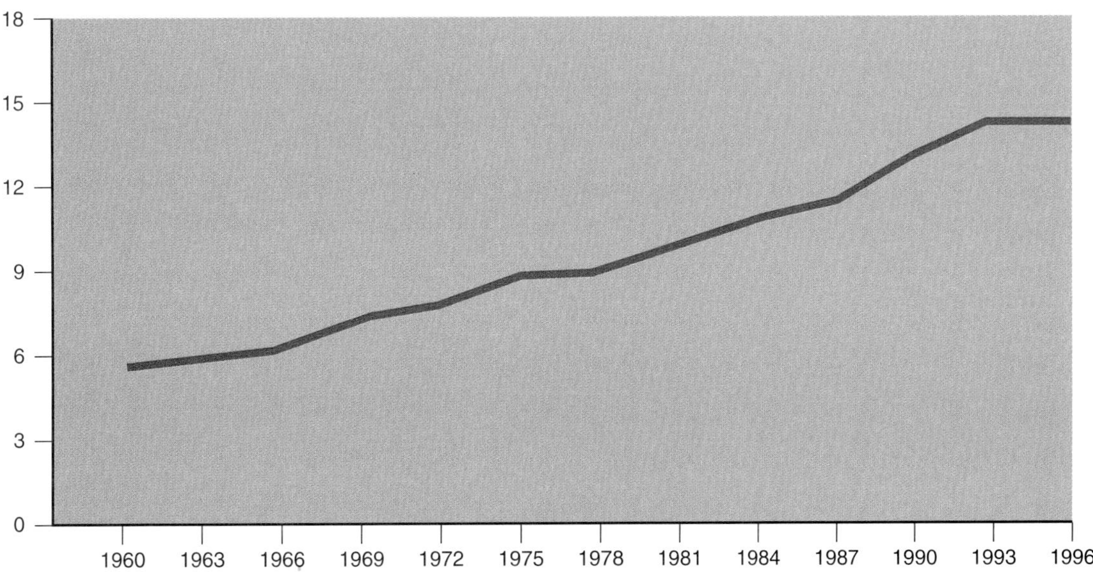

Figure 4–1. National health care expenditures as a percentage of gross national product, 1960–1993.

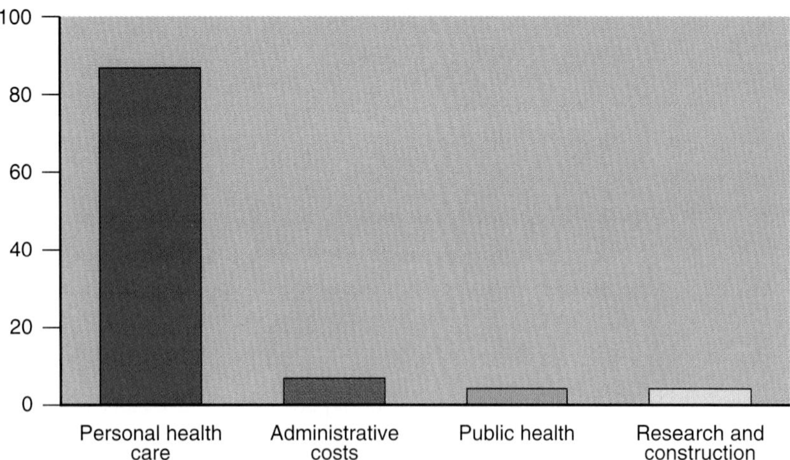

Figure 4–2. How the health care dollar is spent.

further broken down into those dollars spent on personal health care, administration of public programs, and government public health activities.

In 1993, 88 cents of every health care dollar went for personal health care, 6 cents went for administrative costs of public and private insurance, 3 cents went for government public health activities, and 3 cents went for research and construction (Fig. 4–2). When viewed this way, the use of the health care dollar has been fairly constant over the last 50 years (Levit et al, 1991; Levit et al, 1994). It is of interest that in 1996 there were significant differences in program administration and net cost of insurance between fee-for-service capitated payment arrangements. Under fee-for-service, 1.9 percent of expenditures fell in that category in contrast to 9.1 percent for capitated arrangements (Levit et al, 1998).

However, the use of the health care dollar within the category of personal health care has changed. Table 4–1 shows the use of personal health care funds for three time periods (Bovbjerg et al, 1993). Clearly shown is the significant use of personal health care funds for hospital care and physician care.

From 1990 to 1993, growth slowed in every health care category except dental services. Concern over the spread of AIDS increased purchases of supplies leading to increased charges for services (Levit et al, 1994). In 1996, the only area *not* experiencing decelerated growth was nondurable medical products, e.g. over-the-counter medicines, medical sundries, and prescription drugs (Levit et al, 1998). The slowed growth in hospital expenditures and physician services is attributed to pressure from insurance companies, managed care, and changes in the Medicare payment system.

TABLE 4–1 U.S. Total Health Care Spending Uses of Funds for 1940, 1960, 1990

	1940		1960		1990		
	Amount	*Share*	*Amount*	*Share*	*Amount*	*Share*	**Change**
Uses of Funds for Health Care	4.0	100%	27.2	100%	666.1	100%	
Health Services and Supplies	3.9	97%	25.5	94%	643.3	97%	-0-
Personal Health Care	3.5	89%	23.9	88%	585.3	88%	−1%
Hospital Care	1.0	25%	9.3	34%	256.0	38%	+13%
Physician Services	1.0	24%	5.3	19%	125.7	19%	−5%
Dental Services	0.4	11%	2.0	7%	34.0	5%	−6%
Other Professional Services	0.2	4%	0.6	2%	31.6	5%	+1%
Home Health Care		0%	0.0	0%	6.9	1%	+1%
Drugs and Other Medical Non-Durables	0.6	16%	4.2	15%	54.6	8%	−8%
Vision Products and Medical Durables	0.2	5%	0.8	3%	12.1	2%	−3%
Nursing Home Care	0.0	1%	1.0	4%	53.1	8%	+7%
Other Personal Health Care	0.1	3%	0.7	3%	11.3	2%	−1%
Administrative Costs of Public and Private Insurance	0.2	4%	1.2	4%	38.7	6%	+2%
Government Public Health Activities	0.2	4%	0.4	1%	19.3	3%	−1%
Research and Construction	0.1	3%	1.7	6%	22.8	3%	-0-
Research	0.0	0%	0.7	3%	12.4	2%	+2%
Construction	0.1	3%	1.0	4%	10.4	2%	−1%

WHERE DOES THE MONEY COME FROM?

In 1990, 23 percent of personal health care costs were paid directly by the individual (Bovbjerg et al, 1993). Costs paid this way are called *out-of-pocket payments*. The remaining 77 percent of costs were paid by third-party payers, i.e., neither the party receiving the care nor the party giving the care. **Private** third-party payers such as Blue Cross paid 36 percent of health care costs. Federal, state, and local **governments** paid the remaining 41 percent of the costs. The governments' payments were associated primarily with the Medicare program for persons 65 and older and the Medicaid program for persons with incomes below the poverty level and the disabled.

This distribution of responsibility for financing health care represents a dramatic change from the beginning of the century when people paid for almost all of their health care costs themselves. It was not until the 1930s that health insurance even seemed a viable idea. Even then health insurance seemed of limited value because the costs of health care were rather small in comparison with income. Figure 4–3 illustrates the changes in the financing of personal health care costs.

The trend toward more government responsibility for financing health care continues. In 1996 personal health care costs were financed as follows:

- The amount spent by governments increased to 47 percent of all expenditures.
- Private funding (i.e., private health insurance and philanthropy) remained at approximately 36 percent.
- Out-of-pocket purchases decreased to 17 percent (Levit et al, 1998).

HISTORICAL PERSPECTIVE

It is easy to forget that only 100 years ago health care providers were doctors and nurses in private practice with a bag of herbs and tonics caring for middle-class Americans in their homes. Hospitals were charity wards where people with no one to care for them went to die. As a result of research and establishing professional standards and licensure requirements, a famed Harvard professor commented that by 1912, ". . . for the first time in human history, a random patient with a random disease consulting a doctor chosen at random stands a better than 50/50 chance of benefiting from the encounter" (Bovbjerg et al, 1993).

Developments in health insurance are reflective of advances in medical science. Initially workers were provided a **sickness** insurance, which was really a form of **income protection.** The main purpose of the insurance was to make up for lost pay; it was not designed to pay the costs of medical care. In its simplest form it consisted of collecting small monthly contributions from members of a work group in return for the

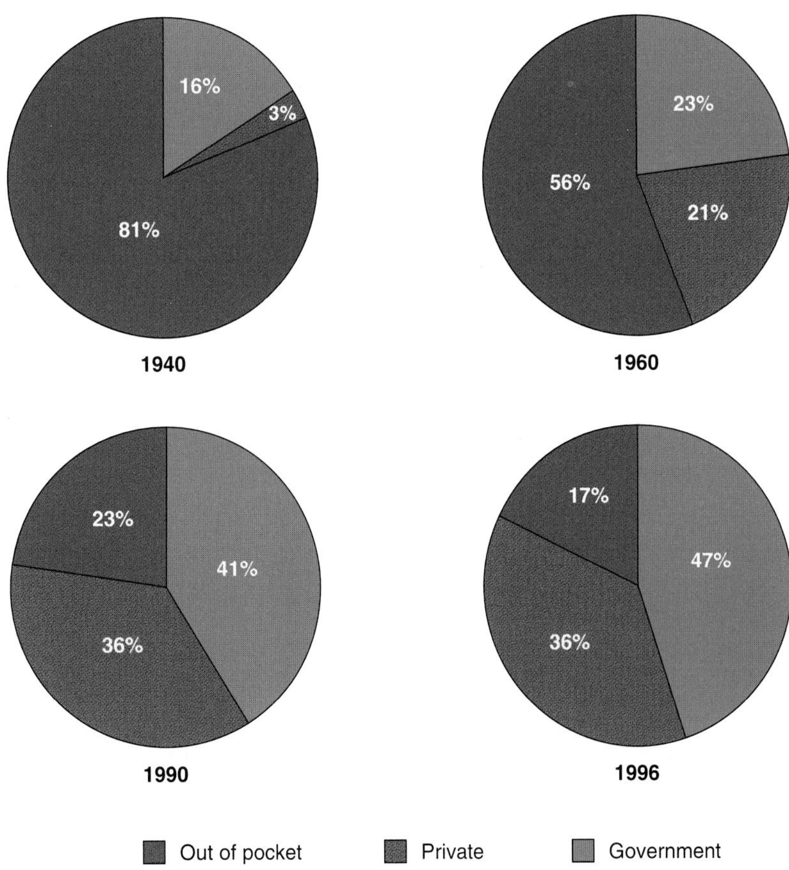

Figure 4–3. Changes in the financing of personal health care costs.

promise to pay a cash benefit if an accident or death occurred. It was a protection against the loss of income associated with the unpredictable need for health care.

Private Sector Health Insurance

Health insurance as we know it today appeared in the late 1920s. Elk City, Oklahoma, created the first prepaid, community-based health insurance plan in 1929. This plan and others like it (1) accepted preset premiums, (2) had their own salaried physicians, and (3) owned their own hospitals. At the same time in Dallas, a group of school teachers contracted with Baylor University Hospital to provide room, board, and a set of health services for a set monthly fee. Hospitals liked this arrangement as it bolstered their occupancy rates in the aftermath of the country's Great Depression.

In the 1930s this hospital-based health insurance plan grew in popularity. Hospitals banded together and developed plans under the title Blue Cross. In a parallel move, physicians banded together and created Blue Shield plans. Both the Blue Cross and Blue Shield plans (Blues) had strong ties to the hospital and medical societies. The plans established by the Blues were the dominant pattern for health insurance for most of the twentieth century.

These health insurance plans offered:

- Free choice of provider, meaning persons could choose almost any provider they wanted.
- Few if any out-of-pocket costs at the time service was provided. Providers received retrospective fee-for-service payment.
- All services the provider determined as medically necessary.
- Fees to the provider that the providers determined as reasonable.
- Costs and eligibility determined by the insurance company.

The insurance company became known as the "third party" because it was neither the provider nor the patient. Because these plans were seen as having a social good over and above ordinary insurance plans, they were often given tax benefits and subject to different regulatory rules. Initially these plans worked well because few people were covered, medical costs were low, and medical technology was in its infancy.

In the 1940s and 1950s private health insurance grew rapidly. This growth was an outcome of the improving economy, advances in medical science, and the ability of the unions to negotiate benefits for organized workers.

Medicare and Medicaid

In the 1960s the government expanded its role in subsidizing health care by creating medical entitlement programs for the poor, frail, and elderly. In 1965 Congress amended the Social Security Act, adding the programs of Medicare and Medicaid. Medicare is a health insurance program for citizens age 65 and older irrespective of income, health, or wealth. It consists of two parts: Part A and Part B. Part A provides benefits for hospital care, skilled nursing home care, and home health care. Part B provides Supplementary Medical Insurance for items such as physician fees and outpatient and emergency department services. Medicare was created with two parts as a cost-saving measure for both the insured and the government. Individuals could purchase what they needed and/or could afford. In 1972, Medicare provisions were modified to make the program available to selected disabled persons under the age of 65. The Medicaid program is a federal-state financed program to pay for the health services for those defined as categorically financially and medically needy. The federal government determines the definition of financially and medically needy. If you fit into that category, you have all the benefits of the program.

Prospective Payment System

In the 1970s and 1980s costs for health care continued to rise faster than the rate of inflation. This meant that governments at the state and federal levels were using more and more of their resources to pay for health care. In addition, the rising costs of care resulted in decreased coverage for those insured through the Medicaid program in terms of numbers covered and in terms of services provided. The economic downturn in the late 1980s added to the problem as people lost their jobs and therefore their health insurance.

In 1983 the United States Congress enacted amendments to the Social Security program in an attempt to limit the rate of increase in health care expenditures. One aspect of these amendments mandated a prospective payment system (PPS) for Medicare reimbursement to hospitals. Medical diagnoses and/or treatment procedures were grouped in terms of the "ordinary" expenses associated with treatment. Those with similar expenditures were put into the same category. The categories are called diagnosis-related groups (DRG). Under the PPS approach a hospital would receive a flat fee for providing care to a patient on Medicare irrespective of the actual amount spent. Unlike the previous retrospective, cost-reimbursement financing in which there were few incentives for cost saving, this approach provided an incentive *if* the hospital spent less than the government paid for a given DRG. This financing of hospital care for patients on Medicare continues, but its impact on costs has not been as dramatic as hoped.

The Uninsured

The system for financing health care in the United States does not assure universal access or coverage for all Americans. The number of Americans without health insurance is significant. During the 1980s, the number of uninsured grew from 12.5 to 15 percent of the population. In 1991, a total of 36.9 million people were uninsured (Center for Health Economics Research, 1993). In 1992, 17.4 percent of the population or 46.6 million people were uninsured (Levit et al, 1994). In

1995 (perhaps associated with an improved U.S. economy) the percentage decreased to 15.4 (PHS, 1997).

Who are the uninsured? Many of them are employed or the dependents of employees. However, health care insurance is not a fringe benefit offered by their employers. Some of them are self-employed. They are poor—too poor to pay for their care out-of-pocket. The uninsured are disproportionately African American and Hispanic:

- One out of every three Hispanics is uninsured.
- One out of every four African Americans is uninsured.
- One out of every eight whites is uninsured (Center for Health Economics Research, 1993).

The uninsured are also disproportionately young; people aged **18 to 24** account for almost **half** of the uninsured (Center for Health Economics Research, 1993).

Traditionally, the uninsured received charity care. However, the increased financial strain on health care agencies has resulted in limits placed on the amount of charity care available. The uninsured tend to use hospital emergency departments for care and they tend to delay care until an illness is severe. Both of these practices actually increase the cost of health care to society.

Issues

In the 60 years from 1930 to 1990 this country saw rapid expansion of health insurance, moving from a period when health insurance was held by a few to where it was the expectation of the majority. Associated with this expansion was

- the increased percentage of the gross national product used for health care
- the shift from health care payment as a personal responsibility to health care payment as a public responsibility
- significant growth in the role of the federal and state governments as payers
- significant increases in the number of uninsured

COMPARISONS WITH OTHER COUNTRIES

National Health Insurance

With the exception of the United States and South Africa, all industrialized nations have a form of national health insurance that provides coverage to most or all citizens. Health insurance as a feature of industrialized societies began in 1883 in Germany. Chancellor Bismarck implemented a system of insurance for working men. The plan provided sickness insurance and funeral benefits. Employees paid two thirds of the costs and the employer one third. The major result of the plan was an obvious improvement of the health of the workers. The success of the plan in improving the health of the workforce and therefore its productivity was so clear that within a few decades 10 other European countries had adopted some form of compulsory health insurance.

Today the health care systems of Canada and major European countries have some similarities and some differences. For example, both Canada and Germany have achieved universal access, very high health status outcomes from care, high-volume care, and partially effective cost controls. The Canadian system is a single-payer system financed through federal and provincial general revenues. Germany has a multiple-payer system and relies on social health insurance linked to employment supplemented by public general revenue funds. In both systems, global budgets for health care are prospectively determined. In both systems, providers (essentially physicians) are private, independent contractors with the relevant health ministry acting as third-party payer—the sole purchaser and reimburser of health services (Koch, 1993).

The national health service model, in which the government owns the facilities and employs providers (doctors) directly, is growing in popularity in Europe. The United Kingdom, Denmark, Spain, Italy, Greece, and Portugal have national health service systems (Koch, 1993).

National health care systems vary in the amount of money spent on administration. Countries with single-payer systems spend less money on administrative costs than countries with multiple payers. For example, administrative costs in Canada are about 4 percent. In the United States, administrative costs are about 20 percent (Shindul-Rothschild and Gordon, 1994). Shindul-Rothschild and Gordon (1994) point out an interesting relationship between level of administrative costs and level of money spent on nursing. Countries with low administrative costs spend more on nursing. Norway, New Zealand, Ireland, Australia, and Canada spend the most on nursing. When comparing total expenditures on nursing in 17 industrialized countries, the United States ranks second to the bottom. Only Turkey spends less on nursing than the United States.

METHODS/PHILOSOPHIES FOR PAYMENT FOR HEALTH CARE SERVICES

At the present time there are two primary methods for paying for health care services: fee-for-service (FFS) and managed care. The FFS method dominated for most of the latter half of the twentieth century. However, since the early 1990s, managed care plans have been rapidly penetrating the market. In 1994, cities such as San Francisco, Los Angeles, Miami, Boston, and Minneapolis were considered high managed care cities. Atlanta, Dallas, Houston, Indianapolis, and Pittsburgh were low managed care cities (Hall, 1996).

The FFS method is frequently equated with free choice, i.e., individual enrollees may **choose** their provider and ask for the services **they** desire. The ability of the person to change providers at will is seen as an advantage in that it gives the individual economic clout over the provider. Providers like FFS because they are reimbursed according to the outputs of services. The more they do, the more they are paid.

Prior to the advent of health insurance most physicians and hospitals had a sliding FFS scale for payments. They charged the rich more than they charged the poor. The costs of caring for the poor were shifted to the rich. Today payments are more regulated and there is likely to be one schedule used for all payers—rich or poor, out-of-pocket, or third party. Payments in the FFS method may be based on a "relative value scale" (RVS), a "usual, customary, and reasonable" (UCR) fee, or a preset fixed amount (contract). The RVS is a point system in which each service/procedure is rated according to its technical difficulty and time cost. Each point is worth a set number of dollars. In the UCR, the fee must be usual for that practice, customary in that community, and reasonable in terms of the range of fees in that community. In the fixed fee approach, a preset amount is determined for a service and that is what the provider is paid. Variations of these three payment mechanisms are used to control costs and protect the insurers from unlimited liability. As a further cost-control mechanism, the people insured are asked to pay for part of the costs of the services. These payments are called *copayments* and are intended to reduce consumer misuse of the system.

Managed care (Box 4–1) is a generic term used to describe a health care plan that uses a prepayment, capitated approach for a defined, enrolled population. The concepts incorporated into managed care are an integrated delivery system (the hospital, ambulatory care setting, and provider's office are all part of the same system), providing incentives and reducing barriers to contain costs, an administrative structure that manages the enrolled population's use of services, and reduced paperwork for the enrolled person.

The person enrolled in a managed care plan must use the providers and facilities that are part of that plan. In most managed care plans the person is assigned or chooses a primary care provider (PCP). The PCP is the gatekeeper to the services of the plan. For example, access to a specialist is controlled by the PCP. Managed care plans have minimal copayment requirements.

Think back to the opening paragraphs about Angela and Amy. Their parents were undoubtedly in a fee-for-service plan. When the first hospital refused to do the surgery, they went to another hospital and found another team of surgeons. There

BOX 4–1
MANAGED CARE TERMINOLOGY

Capitation—A method of payment for health services in which an individual or institutional provider is paid a fixed (usually monthly) amount for each person served without regard to the actual number or nature of services provided to each person. (Generally characteristic of HMOs.)

Closed Panel—A health care plan in which the beneficiaries are allowed to obtain services only from those providers specifically approved by the health care plan.

Fee-For-Service—A method of charging whereby a physician bills for each encounter or service rendered.

Gatekeeper System—A plan where the enrollee selects a primary care physician (case manager) from among the physician pool at the time of enrollment. The enrollee must then seek primary care services and authorization for referrals to specialists from that selected physician.

Global Budgeting—Generally refers to a state or national cap on total health care expenditures. It is designed to force providers, patients, and payers to cut costs and make hard choices. Some Democrats are proposing global budgeting through a national commission which would recommend a budget to Congress, covering public and private health care spending and capital outlays.

Group Model HMO—The HMO contracts with a group practice to provide physician services. The HMO generally pays the group a negotiated per capita rate and the physicians are paid by the group practice on a salary plus incentive basis.

Health Maintenance Organization (HMO)—An organized system for providing health care in a geographic area. The entity provides or otherwise assures the delivery of an agreed upon set of basic and supplemental health maintenance and treatment services to a voluntarily enrolled group. The HMO is reimbursed for those services through a per enrollee capitated fee.

Indemnity Insurance—Traditional health insurance coverage offered by insurance companies, wherein the patient or the provider is directly reimbursed after the medical encounter occurs.

Independent Practice Association (IPA)—An association of physicians in both solo and group practices. The IPA is reimbursed by a managed care plan at a negotiated per capita rate, on a flat retainer rate, or on a negotiated discounted fee-for-service basis. Frequently, the IPA puts the physicians "at risk" by withholding a portion of their fees as an incentive to contain costs. If utilization targets are met, the IPA then releases the impounded funds. Unlike the group model HMO, IPA physicians provide services in their own offices.

Integrated Network—A consolidated group of providers (hospitals, physicians, etc.) focusing on continuous and coordinated organization, delivery, and management of care. Also referred to as a "seamless" organization.

Managed Care—AMA defines this as systems or techniques generally used by third-party payers or their agents to affect access to and control payment for health care services. Most managed care plans include one or more of the following:

- financial incentives or disincentives related to the use of specific providers, services, or service sites;

continued on next page

were no restrictions on where they could go and what they could ask for. The costs were paid by the public even though the public had no input. Had Angela and Amy been in a managed care plan, their parents would have been limited to the set of providers and facilities of that plan. If denied services, they would have had access only by paying for the care themselves.

Essentially in an FFS plan, providers earn more if they do more, and because of the way fees are set, they earn more if they do more procedures. Initially there was little worry about the incentives in this system because of public trust in physicians. In recent years the public has seen the misuse of these incentives in the form of unnecessary surgical procedures and diagnostic tests.

In a managed care system the incentives are designed to decrease use of services. The managed care plan makes more money if less of the capitated fee is used for services. Initially the public supported this approach, thinking it would lead to greater emphasis on health promotion and disease prevention. Physicians would be paid to keep people healthy rather than to care for them when they were sick. In recent years the public has questioned the wisdom of giving the control over access to services to those that will make more money if fewer services are used. Access can be curtailed through waiting time for an appointment (one may have to wait several weeks to see a PCP), number of visits to a specialist (one might be restricted to just one visit with a dietitian), tighter guidelines for high-cost procedures (one might not be allowed to have cataract surgery because of one's age), and reducing the length of time for an office visit (one's PCP may have to see a new patient every 8 minutes).

The research to date shows that costs are lower and quality higher under managed care plans (Hall, 1996). For example, in Oakland, California, a city with high managed care penetration, hospital costs are 46.3 percent below the national average. In Houston, Texas, a city with low managed care penetration, hospital costs are 32.8 percent above national averages. On average, cities with high managed care penetration had hospital costs 11.2 percent below the U.S. benchmark. After adjusting for severity of cases, high managed care penetration areas had mortality rates 5.25 percent better than the national average.

Despite the positive research evaluations of managed care costs and outcomes, neither the public nor physicians are pleased with some aspects of that method of paying for health services.

BOX 4-1 (cont'd)
MANAGED CARE TERMINOLOGY

continued from previous page

- prior, concurrent, and retrospective review of the medical necessity and appropriateness of services and/or sites of services;
- contracts with selected health care professionals or providers;
- controlled access to and coordination of services by a case manager; and
- payer efforts to identify treatment alternatives and modify benefit restrictions for high-cost patient care.

Managed Care Organization (MCO)—An organization which engages in managed care activities.

Managed Competition—A regulated free market approach to controlling health care costs. Current national plan calls for individuals to buy health insurance as part of large groups, organized by sponsors. A state or county could be a sponsor. At least one of the sponsor's plans would offer free, basic coverage. Generally, managed competition plans are funded by a payroll tax on employers or employees. Insurers would get a fixed fee for each enrollee.

Network Model HMO—An HMO contracts with one or more independent multi-specialty group practices and/or individual physicians to provide care in return for a monthly capitated fee. Income is distributed to physicians according to a prearranged agreement.

Physician Care Organization (PCO)—A capitated contractual arrangement whereby a physician agrees to provide medical services to Medicaid recipients through a medical assistance program.

Primary Care Physician (PCP)—The physician responsible for providing care and for authorizing and channeling care to specialists and other providers in a gatekeeper system. Also referred to as a "gatekeeper" or "case manager."

Preferred Provider Organization (PPO)—An entity representing a group of physicians and/or hospitals that contracts with employers, insurance carriers, or third party administrators to provide comprehensive medical services on a fee-for-service basis to subscribers. The PPO contracts with physicians and hospitals to provide services at an established fee, generally at a discount from their usual charges.

Staff Model HMO—An HMO which employs physicians who are compensated on a salary basis.

Utilization Review (UR)—An evaluation of the medical necessity, appropriateness, and efficiency of medical services, procedures, and facilities. In a hospital this includes concurrent and retrospective review of the appropriateness of admissions, services ordered and provided, length of stay, and discharge practices. Often required by HMOs in conjunction with quality assurance (QA) programs intended to assure the quality of care in a defined medical setting.

Data from the Oregon Medical Association.

CURRENT CONTROVERSY

WHAT ARE THE EFFECTS OF CHANGE TO A CAPITATED SYSTEM ON THE QUALITY OF HEALTH CARE?

By Michael Quint, in the **New York Times,** *Dec. 12, 1995*

CLIENT SUES AETNA HEALTH PLANS, CALLING FLAT-FEE SYSTEM ILLEGAL

A customer of Aetna health plans of New York filed a lawsuit in a Federal court yesterday to stop the health plan from adopting new arrangements to pay some doctors a flat fee for each patient rather than a fee based on the services they provide.

The complaint by Maria Maltz, who has two children with a chronic intestinal disease, said that the widely used flat fees violated a Federal law that covers group-health insurers. Mrs. Maltz, who lives in North Bellmore, L.I., contended that her children were being harmed because the flat-fee arrangement, known as a capitation agreement, was forcing her doctor to leave the Aetna plan, and would effectively limit the amount of medical care that the children received.

Whitney Seymour, Jr., a partner at Brown & Seymour, the New York law firm representing Mrs. Maltz, said the complaint marked the first attempt to block capitation arrangements on the ground that they violate the Employee Retirement Income Security Act of 1974. ERISA covers all group health-insurance contracts—where employers buy health coverage from companies such as Aetna Health Plans, based in San Bruno, Calif. ERISA requires that the insurers act "solely in the interest of the participants and beneficiaries."

The flat-fee arrangements, Mr. Seymour said, "are in the interest of the insurer, not the participants and beneficiaries."

Mrs. Maltz said that her pediatrician for the last 16 years, Dr. Marvin L. Sussman, told her of the impending change in Aetna's fees and said that as a result, he would drop out of the Aetna plan.

Before she learned of the impending change at Aetna, Mrs. Maltz said in an interview yesterday, she was very satisfied with the Aetna group insurance plan.

"It was much cheaper for us," she said, noting that the plan required her to pay only $15 per doctor visit, with the rest of the bill paid by Aetna. But after her doctor explained the change in the way he would be paid, she said, "I became concerned that we would not get the quality care we need."

Aetna officials said the New York health plan has been converting many doctor contracts from fee-for-service arrangements to flat-fee arrangements. The flat fees "are perfectly legal" said Walter L. Cherniak, a spokesman for Aetna Health Plans. Among the thousands of doctors already paid flat fees there was "no evidence of any adverse effect on the quality of care patients receive," he said.

Dr. Sussman said in an interview that Aetna's proposed fee of $5 to $6 per patient per month "is not enough to pay my overhead, never mind make a living." Like many other doctors, he also objected to the plan because "it rewards doctors for not seeing patients, for not making tests and for not making referrals."

CURRENT CONTROVERSY

WHAT ARE THE EFFECTS OF HMO "GAG RULES" ON COMMUNICATION WITH PATIENTS?

By Robert Pear, in the **New York Times,** *Dec. 21, 1995*

DOCTORS SAY HMOs LIMIT WHAT THEY CAN TELL PATIENTS

Washington, Dec. 20—Doctors across the country say that health maintenance organizations routinely limit their ability to talk freely with patients about treatment options and HMO payment policies, including financial bonuses for doctors who save money by withholding care.

In interviews over the last three weeks, many doctors said such restrictions interfered with their ethical and legal duty to provide patients with information about the benefits, risks and costs of various treatments.

Ill feeling over the restrictions is growing as more and more Americans join HMOs and employers encourage their use to control costs. Typically, HMOs offer a wide range of services in return for a fixed monthly premium. They recommend a select list of doctors and hospitals, and patients must pay more if they go outside that network.

HMOs may limit access to certain tests and treatments and require doctors to obtain permission from the HMO to offer them. Doctors may receive bonuses or other financial rewards from the HMO if they control costs and help restrain the use of health care.

But patients are often unaware of these financial arrangements because many contracts between doctors and HMOs prohibit the doctors from disclosing them. Increasingly, doctors are objecting to these confidentiality clauses, which they call "gag clauses," and they say that patients are entitled to such information.

For their part, HMOs say that some of the restrictions are intended to protect trade secrets and proprietary information. Susan M. Pisano, a spokeswoman for the Group Health Association of America, which represents managed care companies, said another purpose was to "discourage doctors from disparaging HMOs and encourage them to discuss their concerns about payment and treatment policies with doctors and physical managers in the health plan, rather than with patients."

CURRENT CONTROVERSY

SHOULD A STATE'S ELECTORATE BE ABLE TO PREVENT CAPITATION AND DICTATE WHICH CATEGORIES OF HEALTH CARE PROVIDERS MUST BE COVERED BY HEALTH PLANS?

By Patrick O'Neill, in the **Oregonian,** *Nov. 27, 1995*

VOTERS GET Rx FOR HEALTH CARE

Oregon voters could shake the foundation of the state's health care system in November 1996 if two proposed measures make it onto the ballot.

Two initiative petitions—one planned and the other now circulating—could force massive changes in the way much of the health care is delivered to more than 1.2 million members of health maintenance organizations in Oregon.

The initiatives address how doctors are paid and how patients choose a health care provider. They come at a time when HMOs rapidly are gaining ground throughout the United States. Oregon, with 40 percent of the population covered by HMOs, is the nation's leader.

Petitioners say their objectives are to promote high-quality health care and to give patients a choice of providers.

But officials of managed-care organizations say the initiatives are motivated by the economic self-interest of some physicians and alternative care providers. Moreover, they say, the initiatives would wreck Oregon's successful attempts to hold down health care costs. They say the measures would restrict, not enhance, consumer choice.

At issue are two cost-cutting strategies heavily used in health maintenance organizations. HMOs strive for savings:

- By giving physicians a financial incentive to keep the cost of medical treatment down. The details of the incentives vary widely from plan to plan. But generally, the less it costs to keep patients well, the more money the physicians can earn.

THE OREGON EXPERIMENT

Discussions regarding the financing of health care usually focus on the national level and the U.S. Congress. Although states do not contribute as much as the federal government to the financing of health care, it is possible that effective solutions to the crisis in health care financing will evolve at the state level. The Oregon Health Plan is presented as one illustration of a state initiative to control health care expenditures while providing universal access.

The Oregon Health Plan was created because of the failure of Medicaid. The Oregon State legislature was faced with escalating health care costs, a weakening economic base, and no health care policy to guide its decisions. In 1987 the legislature was faced with $48 million in immediate social program needs but had only $21 million to allocate. As it deliberated the issues, it decided to discontinue state Medicaid funding for most organ transplants and instead to fund more prenatal care. It was argued that putting the money into organ transplants would help 30 people, putting the money into prenatal care would help 3000 people. Although this decision was known, it did not receive much publicity until a young boy with leukemia was denied Medicaid funds for a bone marrow transplant. He died while private funds were being raised.

The case prompted a request for the legislature to release money to fund transplants for eight people in immediate need. The request was denied—not because the legislature was opposed to transplants but because the issue was framed in a new way. The legislature had to consider its decisions in light of limited resources and social good versus individual good. Should a few Oregonians have access to all health care services while an increasing number had access to no services? It was easy to list the benefits of providing services. But now the legislature had to identify the consequences of *not* providing services as well. They realized that they were accountable for what they did as well as for what they did not do.

The legislature was supported in its efforts to develop an explicit policy on funding of health care through the work of a citizen-based organization called Oregon Health Decisions (OHD). During the mid 1980s, the OHD implemented a systematic approach to obtain grass roots community input into policy decisions about health care. The approach called for (1) identifying and training community volunteers who would organize and lead meetings in their areas, (2) conducting small group meetings, (3) holding town hall meetings, (4) analyzing the identified problems/issues, (5) formulating resolutions, (6) leading a citizens' health care forum, (7) releasing a final report, and (8) initiating activities to implement the resolutions.

Over 30 community volunteers held 300 small group meetings and 17 town hall meetings. Some 5000 Oregonians gave input. The following are the five areas of general agreement:

- The autonomy and dignity of sick and dying patients need better protection.
- Much greater emphasis should be placed on disease prevention and health promotion.
- Everyone should have access to an adequate level of health care.
- Health care costs must be brought under control.
- Rationing and allocation decisions must be made openly and fairly.

These values became the core of the Oregon Plan.

For most Oregonians, the Oregon Plan is a way to provide access to health care. In addition to providing universal access, the plan defines a basic benefit package, addresses the reality of financial limits, makes affordable coverage available, includes cost-containment provisions, and provides for broad-based consensus on health policy.

The goal of the Oregon Plan is to keep all Oregonians healthy. Key principles underlying the plan are:

- Health can be maintained only if investments in a number of related areas are kept balanced.
- There must be clear accountability for allocating public funds and for the consequences of those decisions.
- All Oregonians must have access to a basic level of health care.
- There must be an explicit process to determine what constitutes a basic level of care.
- Society has the responsibility to provide the resources to finance a basic level of care for those who cannot afford to pay.
- The criteria used to determine the basic package of health care must be publicly debated, reflect social values, and consider the common good of society.

An analysis of the uninsured showed that they fell into three categories: those unemployed but still not poor enough to qualify for Medicaid, those employed by businesses that did not provide health insurance as a benefit, and those denied insurance because they were considered at high risk. Three bills were passed by the legislature to extend coverage to each of these groups. The legislation expanding Medicaid has received the most national attention. It makes Medicaid benefits available to everyone at or below the federal poverty level. The benefits are specified in a basic benefit package. The benefit package is the result of a ranking of health care services from most to least important to the population and funding decisions by the legislature. Although more people have access, the services to which they have access are limited.

The most difficult and controversial aspect of this legislation is the requirement that health care services be prioritized in terms of medical effectiveness and social values. The Commission appointed to this task finally published a list of 709 diagnosis/treatment services grouped into 17 categories. The categories are prioritized. For example, category 1 is labeled "acute fatal" and defined as treatment that prevents death and allows full recovery. It includes such services as appendectomy for appendicitis; nonsurgical treatment for whooping cough; and repair of deep, open wound of the neck. Category 2 is maternity care, including most disorders of the newborn. These two categories of services plus the following six categories are considered essential care: preventive care for children, chronic fatal, reproductive services, comfort care, preventive dental care, and proven effective preventive care for adults. In the seventeenth category, labeled "fatal or nonfatal," treatment produces minimal or no improvement in the quality of life. Aggressive treatment for people at the end stage of their disease falls into this category.

The Oregon Plan was implemented in February of 1994. It is administered somewhat like a managed care system. Some time must elapse before an evaluation can determine the full success of the plan. However, enrollment in the plan has exceeded expectations and access to health care has increased. Although the Oregon Plan has been modified since its inception, its core values remain.

POLICY ISSUES

Policy issues have been alluded to throughout this chapter. Although formal debate on health care ended with the 103rd Congress, the issues continue. Should all citizens have equal access to basic/essential health services? If so, what are those services? Who should pay for basic health services? Who should bear the financial risk for health services? Should health care rationing be with the first dollar (as many states do with Medicaid and eligibility criteria) or last dollar (the Oregon experiment)? What is the balance between cost and quality and who should set those standards?

All citizens need to be involved in debating these issues. However, health care professionals must be willing and able to provide information and leadership to resolve them.

IMPACT ON NURSING PRACTICE

Changes in the method and philosophy of payment for health care have transformed health care. Today the system is a **medical** care system. Tomorrow it will be a **health** care system. Today almost two thirds of nurses work in hospitals. Tomorrow, two thirds will work in outpatient, community, and home settings. Today the system focuses on what is best for the individual. Tomorrow the system will care for individuals from a population focus. Today most care is illness care. Tomorrow most care will be directed at wellness and quality of life.

The practice of nursing is affected by every one of these changes. For example, under a FFS/cost reimbursement philosophy, a "needs" approach to nursing assessment worked well. The nurse assessed the patient to determine all possible illness problems. Following that, the nurse developed and implemented a nursing plan of care to meet those needs. In doing so the nurse focused on the individual with the intent of doing everything known to assist the individual become well. After discharge, the clinical agency billed the insurance company for all the care provided.

Under a managed care philosophy, the nurse weighs the cost-effectiveness of every action. The nurse is aware that resources are limited and that priorities based on outcomes of care must be set. The nurse will still do an assessment, but then, rather than attending to **all** needs, the nurse will limit care to those actions that influence specific health outcomes. The plan of care will be interdisciplinary and will also emphasize self-care and prevention. The nurse will spend relatively more time teaching the individual and family and less time providing direct care. The relationship between a patient and nurse does not end at "discharge" because the individual is a part of that managed care plan. The nurse thinks longitudinally rather than in terms of an acute episode.

In today's health care environment nurses are expected to:

- limit the expenditure of resources while providing effective care
- understand the pressures clinical agencies are experiencing as they adjust to changing financial incentives
- advocate for the patient in terms of outcomes of care, and
- broker resources for cost effective care

CHAPTER HIGHLIGHTS

- Health care expenditures represent 13.6 percent of the country's gross domestic product.
- The federal government is the major health care payer.
- The United States has repeatedly rejected national health insurance plans that provide care to all citizens.
- Capitated approaches to funding health care costs are advocated as a means of reducing health care expenditures while retaining quality.
- Contemporary nursing practice requires the nurse to consider cost and outcomes of nursing interventions.

REFERENCES

Bauman, H. (1992). Verging on national health insurance since 1910. In R.P. Huefner and M.P. Battin (eds.): *Changing to National Health Care: Vol. 4. Ethics in a Changing World.* Salt Lake City: University of Utah Press, pp. 29–49.

Bovbjerg, R.R., Griffin, C.C., Carroll, C.E. (1993). *The Journal of Law, Medicine and Ethics,* Summer, 141–160.

Brown, E.R. (1992). Problems of insurance coverage and health care costs in the United States. In Pan American Health Organization (eds.): *International Health: A North-South Debate.* Washington, D.C.: Pan American Health Organization, pp. 87–101.

Center for Health Economics Research (1993). *Access to Health Care Key Indicators for Policy.* Princeton, NJ: The Robert Wood Johnson Foundation.

Fein, R.F. (1992). Health care reform: Is it time for our medicine? *Modern Maturity, 35* (4), 22–35.

Goodman, E. (1994). An easy choice was made hard. *Boston Globe,* June 19, p. B3.

Hall, C.T. (1996). Area hospitals low in cost. *San Francisco Chronicle,* February 1, B 1, 2.

Koch, A.L. (1993). Financing health services. In S.R. Williams and P.R. Torrens (eds.): *Introduction to Health Services,* 4th ed. Albany, NY: Delmar, pp. 299–331.

Lamm, R.D. (1994). Healthcare heresies. *Healthcare Forum Journal,* September/October, 45, 46, 59–61.

Levit, K.R., Lazenby, H.C., Cowan, C.A., Letsch, S.W. (1991). National health expenditures, 1990. *Health Care Financing Review, 13* (1), 29–54.

Levit, K.R., Sensenig, A.L., Cowan, C.A., et al. (1994). National health expenditures, 1993. *Health Care Financing Review, 16* (1), 247–294.

Levit, K.R., Lazenby, H.C., Braden, B.R. (1998). National health expenditures, 1996. *Health Care Financing Review, 19* (1), 161–200.

McCabe, M.S. (1993). The ethical context of health care reform. *Oncology Nursing Forum, 20* (10) (Supplement), 35–43.

Public Health Service (PHS) Centers for Disease Control and Prevention and National Center for Health Statistics (1997). *Health, United States, 1996–97.* Washington, D.C.: U.S. Government Printing Office.

Question on health care costs . . . [editorial] (1993). *The Washington Post,* December 28.

Reinhardt, U.W. (1991). Rationing the health-care surplus: An American tragedy. In P.R. Lee and C.L. Estes (eds.). *The Nation's Health,* 3rd ed. Boston: Jones and Bartlett, pp. 104–111.

Schieber, G.J., Poullier, J., Greenwald, L.M. (1992). U.S. health expenditure performance: An international comparison. *Health Care Financing Review, 13,* 1–88.

Shindul-Rothschild, J., Gordon, S. (1994). Single-payor versus managed competition: Implications for nurses. *Journal of Nursing Education, 33* (5), 198–207.

Sonnefeld, S.T., Waldo, D.R., Lemieux, J.A., McKusick, D.R. (1991). Projections of national health expenditures through the year 2000. *Health Care Financing Review, 13* (1), 1–15.

Starr, P. (1982). Transformation in defeat: The changing objectives of national health insurance, 1915–1980. *American Journal of Public Health, 72* (1), 7–17.

Terris, M. (1992). The health situation in the Americas. In Pan American Health Organization (eds.): *International Health: A North-South Debate.* Washington, D.C.: Pan American Health Organization, pp. 71–85.

Weissenstein, E. (1992). U.S. health spending soars 11%. *Modern Healthcare,* January 6, p. 3.

Yankelovich, D., Immerwahr, J. (1991). A perception gap. *HMO, Third Quarter,* 11–14.

5 Technology and Nursing Practice

Carol Lindeman

OBJECTIVES

After studying this chapter, students will be able to:

- **discuss the major effects of technology on health care delivery and nursing practice**
- **understand what they and their patients must do to use technology safely and effectively**
- **identify ethical issues imbedded in the use of specific technologies**
- **obtain information about new technology**

Picture this scenario of a "paperless" hospital. A nurse enters a patient's room carrying something that looks like a remote control for a television set. The nurse moves toward the patient and points the device first at the bar code on her staff badge and then at the bar code on the patient's wristband. She then punches into the device's keypad the patient's temperature, pulse, respiration, blood pressure, and fluid balance as shown on the monitoring equipment. Prior to giving the patient his medication, she scans the bar-coded labels affixed to the medication container. The device is connected with a central database that is programmed to verify medication orders as well as check for contraindications and drug interactions. A green light appears so the nurse gives the patient the medication. If an error had been detected, a red light would have appeared. All data from the interaction are entered simultaneously in the patient's financial record, chart, and the quality assurance review committee records.

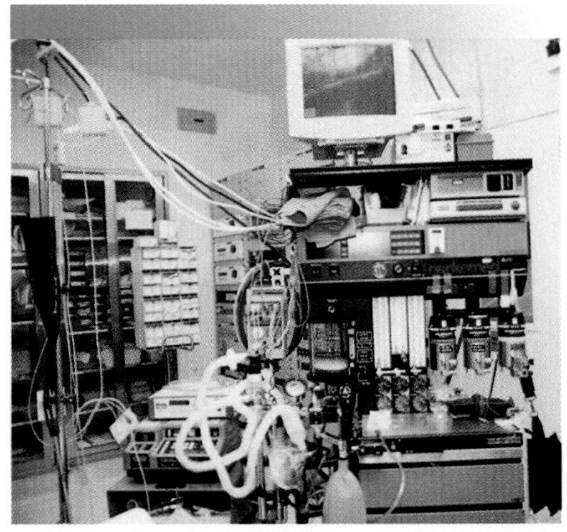

Although devices such as the one described are still in the developmental stage, the paperless hospital will be a reality in the near future (Coile, 1990). Some benefits from this type of automation are speed, accuracy, improved records, rapid access to relevant patient data, and elimination of redundant entry. Under the current nonautomated system nurses spend as much as 50 percent of their time charting and completing forms for reimbursement. With automation as described here, nurses will have more time for direct care.

Some dramatic effects of technology on nursing practice were highlighted in a presentation at the 1995 National Student Nurses Association Annual Convention. Dr. Margaret McClure (McClure, 1995), one of the United States' foremost nursing administrators, offered these observations about tomorrow's workplace:

- Technology will continue to enable the migration from inpatient to outpatient care. Increasingly, treatment will occur in Day Surgery and short procedure units.

- Robots like HANK will be available to assist nurses and patients. HANK is a trade name for a camera-equipped computer/robot that has been developed for patients who need minor home care. HANK can remind its owner to take a medication and at the same time deliver through an opened drawer the correct dose. HANK can also monitor items like a pacemaker and wound healing. The data HANK collects are sent to a central station where a nurse receives, interprets, and acts on the data. The nurse does not have to travel to the home to obtain information.
- User-friendly computers will be available at the point of care and provide data from across settings. Technological advances will enable health care generalists such as nurses to do the work currently done by specialized workers. For example, technicians working in hospital departments such as the laboratory or x-ray will no longer be necessary.

Even the Walt Disney organization is involved in exploring the use of technology and health care delivery. A Walt Disney planned community called Celebration Health is scheduled to open in the near future. Within that community the latest technology will be used to provide access to health care for the residents. Every home is wired with a fiberoptics network allowing residents to have access to health care information, participate in self-help groups, and communicate with health care providers. In the clinic setting, providers will carry hand-held computers that allow them to update medical records immediately and send prescriptions immediately to the pharmacy (Nelson, 1997).

The growth of technology in health care is phenomenal. It is affecting every setting in which care is delivered as well as every aspect of care per se. This growth is a reflection of the amount of money invested in research and technology development and the value placed on health care.

Is this growth of technology good? What are the implications for nursing practice? Does it detract from or enhance nursing care?

DEFINITION OF HEALTH CARE TECHNOLOGY

Technology is a broad concept referring to *the systematic application of scientific or other organized knowledge to practical tasks.* Technology is culturally, morally, and politically neutral. It provides tools independent of the organizations and humans that may eventually use those tools. In reality, technology does not exist in a vacuum. The phrase *technology-practice* is used when referring to the application of technology. Specifically, technology-practice is defined as "the application of scientific and other knowledge to practical tasks by ordered systems that involve people and organizations, living things and machines" (Pacey, 1984).

Health care technology encompasses everything from bandages to open heart surgery, from cough syrup to complex pharmaceuticals, from the furniture in a patient's room to the design of emergency vehicles, and from the equipment used to record nurses' notes to that used in discharge teaching. The breadth of technology used in health care today is reflected in the multiple classification systems used. For example, a technology can be classified by its state of development: innovation, clinical trial, and the like. A technology could also be classified in terms of its health care objective: diagnostic (x-ray), illness management (blood glucose monitor), or prevention (immunization). The Food and Drug Administration (FDA) simply distinguishes between drugs and medical devices because that is how the laws were written.

As with technology in general, health care technology is considered neutral. Issues arise with health care technology-practice. For example, the needle and syringe is an important part of health care delivery. Many lifesaving medications are delivered with this technology. Yet, a needle and syringe can be used by a drug abuser with the exact opposite outcome. The next sections of this chapter focus on technology development and assessment. Implications for nursing practice are then discussed, followed by a section on ethical issues.

HEALTH CARE TECHNOLOGY DEVELOPMENT

Where do new technologies originate? How do they become part of practice? The process of creating a new technology and the process of adaptation take many different forms. The process reflects the uniqueness of the innovator, device, and institution. It is also much less rigorous than most people realize. The profession of nursing determined the lack of rigor surrounding medical technologies was a serious problem in this country. *Nursing's Agenda for Health Care Reform* (1991) proposed that providers would be reimbursed only for those medical technologies in which there was objective evidence supporting efficacy.

McKinlay (1981), based on his review of several different innovations, identified seven stages in the career of a medical innovation:

- The Stage of the "Promising Report." Ideas for new health care technology come from a variety of sources. Drug companies spend millions of dollars annually on the development of new pharmaceutical products. Equipment companies have research development centers that focus on improving existing products and creating new ones. Health care practitioners generate ideas from their own practices. Occasionally patients will develop better approaches for their own care. Researchers at academic health centers are major contributors to new health care technology.

Usually the person who conceives of a new technology develops, tests, and reports on its success. That individual may contract with others and may also seek funding for the work involved. This stage in the process typically ends with a presentation that can be labeled the "Promising Report." That label was used by McKinlay to suggest that testing to date is probably minimal, ranging from anecdotal data and case studies to uncontrolled pilot studies. The label also implies that the enthusiasm about the new technology by its creator is evident throughout the report.

- The Stage of Professional and Organizational Adoption. Following the presentation or publication of a promising report, there is adoption in practice by some members of the discipline or by some institutions. Adoption may be the result of peer pressure, the opportunity to deliver improved care, wanting to be seen as up-to-date, or financial benefit. The latter seems a more important motivator for institutions than for individual practitioners.
- The Stage of Public Acceptance and Endorsement by Insurance Companies. As the number of practitioners and institutions adopting the innovation grow, there is pressure to have the innovation recognized by the public and by insurers or other official endorsement agencies. This is particularly important for innovations reimbursed through insurance plans. McKinlay found that pressure to endorse an innovation occurred even though the innovation has had minimal formal evaluation. The claims of people rather than sound scientific data are the basis for acceptance at this stage.
- The Stage of "Standard Procedure" and Observational Reports. Once recognized by the public and insurers, the innovation becomes standard procedure by practitioners and institutions. Faculty teach the innovation to students as the standard procedure. The innovation (which is no longer an innovation) is seen as the most appropriate way of proceeding with a particular problem or issue. Jacox (1990) reports that 80 to 90 percent of all medical procedures are estimated to be inadequately assessed.
- The Stage of the Randomized Controlled or Clinical Trial (RCT). Although one might think rigorous testing of an innovation would occur before public acceptance, that is not true for most health care technology. The randomized clinical trial remains the most powerful method of determining the efficacy of a new technology. (In a random clinical trial, subjects who consent to participate and who meet explicit criteria are randomly assigned to receive either the new treatment or some type of placebo. Neither the provider nor the patient [research subject] know whether or not the patient is receiving the innovation. This research method eliminates factors that could otherwise influence the results of the study.) Yet health care researchers concerned about the legal and ethical issues surrounding randomization are reluctant to use the methodology. Furthermore, although the RCT is a powerful research design for dealing with innovations that can reduce the human being to a cause-and-effect situation (e.g., Does this drug reduce pain?), it is less powerful when testing an innovation that involves complex human responses (e.g., a treatment program to stop drug abuse).

  The RCT is also very expensive, as it requires a large number of subjects. The end result is the dissemination of health care technologies that are inadequately assessed.
- The Stage of Professional Denunciation. Following the stage of additional testing that may include an RCT comes the stage of skepticism and denunciation. The advocates for a particular innovation criticize the research, usually through letters to the editor of the journal that published the research. During this stage professional journals are used by both the advocates and the skeptics to make their points.
- The Stage of Erosion and Discreditation. This stage usually occurs about a decade after the "Promising Report." It occurs only when a replacement procedure becomes available—through the presentation of a new "Promising Report."

The concerns regarding the **lack** of objective, accurate assessment of new technology are shared by many. For example, Abele (1991), in an editorial directed at cardiologists, stated, "The issue of credible presentations on new technology is an embarrassment at many medical meetings and courses. Some of the poor science and self-serving exaggerations would not pass high school standards."

McKinlay would correct this situation with the following requirements for services paid for by government or insurance companies:

- Determine in some objective manner the nature and magnitude of human needs in our society.
- Evaluate objectively all services before they are introduced.
- Begin a systematic evaluation of all existing technologies.
- Implement incentives that encourage the use of only those services proven effective.

Needless to say, there is not universal support for these recommendations nor agreement on how to finance the research and evaluation.

HEALTH CARE TECHNOLOGY ASSESSMENT

Think back to some of the old western movies you have seen on television. Remember the medicine man who would ride into town with his wagon? He would sell his homemade remedies and then quickly leave town before people demanded their money back! We laugh when we see it on television. It was not a laughing matter in the early 1900s. In fact, the federal government created the first food and drug regulatory agency because of unsafe, falsely advertised products of the home remedy type being offered to the public.

The Role of the Food and Drug Administration

Federal regulation of food, drugs, and medical devices is authorized by the Food, Drug and Cosmetic Act passed in 1906. That act authorized the creation of the Food and Drug Administration (FDA) with the responsibility to regulate the marketing of drugs and foods for safety. The Act was amended in 1938, requiring more rigorous testing of drugs for safety. In 1962, the Act was further amended to require that the efficacy as well as safety of drugs be established prior to marketing. In 1976, the Act was amended to also regulate the marketing of medical devices for safety and efficacy.

The FDA remains the major agency for medical technology assessment. It requires that firms manufacturing drugs and medical devices demonstrate the efficacy and safety of a product. It does this by developing product standards, regulating testing, developing and/or approving clinical protocols, evaluating technical and clinical evidence, and carefully regulating product labeling. It is important to note that the FDA evaluates products *in terms of the claims on their labels and not in comparison with other products.*

The Role of Federally and Privately Funded Research

Throughout this century, the U.S. Congress has created other agencies to promote the public's best interest in health care. For example, the National Institutes of Health (NIH) sponsors clinical trials and conducts consensus conferences on practice issues. The National Institute for Nursing Research is an Institute within NIH that nurse researchers look to for funding for clinical trials and technology assessment.

An example of nursing technology assessment is the research reported by Goode et al (1991). The researchers surveyed hospitals to determine the procedure used to maintain patency, decrease phlebitis, and increase duration of peripheral heparin locks. A heparin lock is a special vein needle and rubber diaphragm used to administer selected medications intermittently. They found that different hospitals used different solutions (heparin or saline) as well as different concentrations of saline. They also found 17 studies in the research literature that were conducted and reported in a manner that allowed combining findings across studies. By analyzing data across studies, a more powerful analysis is possible. The following conclusions were reached:

- Saline is as effective as heparin in maintaining patency, preventing phlebitis, and increasing duration of the lock.
- Using saline to flush the lock promotes overall quality of care.
- Using saline could result in yearly savings of \$109,100,000 to \$218,200,000.

There are an increasing number of nursing research studies evaluating nursing technologies. These reports are published in research journals as well as clinical journals.

The Role of the Office of Technology Assessment

Until September 1995, the Office of Technology Assessment (OTA) served as a research and advisory body for Congress. That Office defined health care technology as the drugs, devices, and procedures used in the delivery of health care *and the organizational or administrative systems that support its use.* It was closed as part of the restructuring of the federal government. An example of that Office's contribution to technology assessment is the monograph *Nurse Practitioners, Physician Assistants, and Certified Nurse-Midwives: A Policy Analysis* (1986). That monograph is an analysis of research comparing the effectiveness of these three groups of providers with the effectiveness of physicians. It is this analysis that led to the conclusion that nurse practitioners could do 80 percent of what a generalist physician does as well or better than generalist physicians. Since that policy analysis, the federal government has been quite positive about funding nurse practitioner and nurse midwifery programs.

The Office of Health Technology Assessment

The Office of Health Technology Assessment within the Agency for Health Care Policy and Research (AHCPR) publishes brief evaluations of health technologies. The evaluation of a particular ventilator illustrates the use of unsafe treatment as well as the role of AHCPR in technology assessment. The following evaluation was published in the Agency's digest "Research Activities" (1994).

Intermittent positive pressure breathing (IPPB) ventilators, which are pressure-cycled respirators, were developed during World War II to help high-altitude pilots breathe in unpressured cabins. Soon IPPB attained widespread use in medical settings to treat patients with chronic obstructive pulmonary disease and other respiratory conditions. IPPB became one of the most common procedures performed in respiratory therapy departments before its efficacy was called into question in the early 1980s. (IPPB refers both to the ventilator and to treatment using this device.) Today, consensus in the medical literature is that IPPB is both ineffective for most indications and potentially dangerous. It is expensive as well, not only because of its direct costs but also because of the complications it can cause. However, findings from a recent study by AHCPR's Center for General Health Services Intramural Research, Division of Provider Studies, indicate that, although IPPB use declined considerably in the past decade, it has not ceased, and rates of use and decline have varied among hospital types. Further, while fewer hospital inpatients receive IPPB, the distribution across diagnoses of patients on whom it is used have remained virtually constant.

For emphasis:

- An innovation developed for use in an airplane cockpit was used to treat patients with lung problems without sufficient research to support that use.
- The use of that treatment continued for over 20 years before the necessary research base was available for full assessment of the treatment.
- The research showed that the treatment is ineffective and unsafe.
- The treatment is still being used.
- People with diagnoses that were treated with IPPB in the early 1960s when the treatment was thought to be safe and effective are still likely to be treated with IPPB even though it is now known to be unsafe and ineffective.

The Role of the Private Sector

There are other governmental agencies that could be listed and new ones that will be created. The public sector, e.g., the American Medical Association and the American Hospital Association, has also created agencies that focus on premarket approval of new medical technologies. The American Medical Association sponsors the Diagnostic and Therapeutic Technology Assessment program designed to educate its members about the appropriate use of technologies. The American Hospital Association has a Hospital Technology Series that educates hospital administrators about hospital devices and technology. The task of protecting the public from unsafe and/or ineffective drugs and medical devices is a large one given our high-technology, interventionist health care system.

A Case Study of a Health Technology Innovation

Societal Need. Nurses and other health care workers are very concerned about an occupational risk called *needle stick.* Needle stick refers to an accidental stick by a contaminated needle (a needle that has been used). The incidence of needle-stick injuries is from 7.5 to 16 per 100 employees and from 4.27 to 12.4 per 100 registered nurses (deCarteret, 1987). This may be an underestimation because up to two thirds may not be reported (Armstrong, 1991). Another estimate of the incidence of needle-stick injuries in raw numbers is 600,000 to one million annually (Constans, 1991). An exposé on the needle-stick epidemic cites one million needle sticks each year, with one health care worker each week on average becoming infected with the HIV virus (Holding and Carlsen, 1998). The reporters claim that technology exists to greatly reduce these statistics.

Armstrong (1991) synthesized several research studies to present a full picture of the costs of needle-stick injuries. One study hospital had 340 reported needle sticks and an estimated 680 unreported sticks. The full cost for the treatment of those injured was estimated at $246,823 without considering the treatment costs of hepatitis or other diseases transmitted by the needle, the cost of litigation, or the costs of psychological counseling for those injured. Armstrong believes affordable, safer technology should be available to health care workers.

The Innovation. The Biojector 2000 Needle-free Injection Management System is one such technology. The Biojector is a pressure-powered device that rapidly administers vaccines, local anesthetics, antibiotics, and other common medications **without** a needle. The Biojector allows health care professionals to inject medications through the skin, both intramuscularly and subcutaneously, without a needle. The Biojector 2000 system consists of two components: a hand-held, reusable jet-injector; and a sterile, single-use disposable syringe. The injector is powered by a CO_2 cartridge that provides the energy source for the injector. The system is capable of delivering variable dose needle-free injections up to 1 ml.

This needle-free system is not so much new technology as improved technology. Jet injection equipment had been used for mass immunizations in the past. These earlier systems were cumbersome, painful, and impractical. They could give only a fixed dosage of one type of medication and they also risked cross contamination across patients. The key was to develop a lightweight, portable, and sterile needleless system.

The product that was developed, the Biojector 2000 system, contains the jet-injector on one end and a sterile plastic container (the syringe) of medication on the other (Fig. 5–1). With the pull of an activator on the jet-injector, enough CO_2 pressure is released to push the plunger on the syringe and thereby force a stream of medication out of a minuscule hole in the syringe and through the patient's skin in less than one half of a second. By the time the patient hears the whooshing sound of the CO_2, the medication is in the tissue.

Clearly technology such as the Biojector is of benefit to health care providers and patients. The manufacturer, Bioject Inc., claims it eliminates the risk of cross contamination compared with traditional needle injection systems because there are no contaminated needles. They also list the following characteristics of the Biojector: a faster and easier delivery;

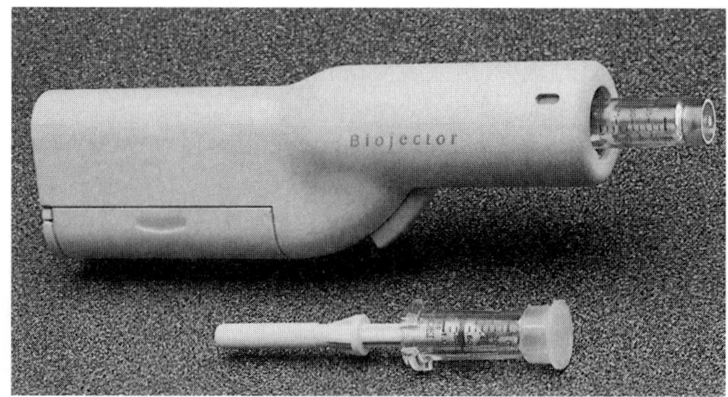

Figure 5–1. The Biojector 2000 needle-free injection system. (Courtesy of Bioject Inc., Portland, OR.)

proven depth of penetration; a unique, portable design; easy to learn to use; safer, cost-effective disposal (the needle-free syringe can be disposed of in regular medical waste versus a sharps container for needles); and daily maintenance not required.

FDA Approval. Before a product can be marketed it must be cleared or approved by the FDA. This process assures that products are safe and effective and that the manufacturing practices offer quality assurance of their products.

The Biojector system is currently classified by the FDA as class II, i.e., devices that do not pose an unreasonable risk of illness or injury. As a class II technology it is subject to a premarket notification process called 510(k) in order to distribute and sell the product in the United States. Under this process Bioject Inc. submitted to the FDA performance data, product labeling, and information which demonstrated that the product for which the premarket clearance is requested is substantially equivalent to a legally marketed product. This notification process can be very lengthy. The most recent 510(k) submission for the Biojector took 2 years for review and clearance. With clearance by the FDA the Biojector is considered safe for clinical use.

For each new or significantly modified existing product, Bioject must submit additional 510(k) premarket notifications. Products that do not qualify for the 510(k) notification process, e.g., class III technologies, which present a high potential risk of illness or injury, require a premarket approval (PMA). The PMA application is much more complex, requires extensive performance testing, and may have a much longer approval timeframe!

Bioject's manufacturing facilities are routinely subject to inspection by the FDA. The company is required to keep specific records and maintain procedures relating to various operations and processes related to the manufacture of the Biojector. FDA inspections of the facility, which are unannounced, include review of such records and procedures for accuracy and completeness. This compliance surveillance by the FDA is another means of assuring that companies not only design safe and effective products but also manufacture quality products over time for the consumer.

Reports from Users. The Biojector system has been used in many different settings, with different age groups and with different medications. The anecdotal and research reports are positive. For example, an emergency room nurse reported an experience with a combative patient in which a contaminated needle and syringe went flying across the room and almost hit his arm. The hospital decided to evaluate the use of the Biojector system. After a 2-week trial, the hospital purchased the system for its emergency department and since then has made it available elsewhere in the hospital.

Reports from Researchers. Greenberg and colleagues reported their research using the Biojector at the 1994 annual meeting of the American Society of Anesthesiologists. The researchers hypothesized that midazolam administered using the Biojector needle-free injection system would effectively and rapidly sedate children before general anesthetic. Achieving this outcome has been a problem using traditional routes for delivering the medication. The data collected from 40 children under 9 months of age supported the hypothesis.

Baer and her colleagues (1996) conducted a study of the effectiveness of a jet injection system in administering morphine and heparin to healthy adults. She designed the study to build on the existing unpublished research regarding the efficacy of the Biojector system. The research question was whether or not the Biojector system delivered the drug in a clinically useful way. She used a research design in which each subject received injections in both the needle and needleless routes. The data collected supported the conclusion that the Biojector provided equivalent plasma drug concentrations to a conventional needle and syringe when administering intramuscular morphine and low-dose subcutaneous heparin.

Training. Bioject offers several types of training programs for those using the system. The company has created various publications, brochures, and video training materials that are available to the users of its products. The company also provides onsite inservice education on the Biojector. Training is provided for each customer who purchases the Biojector system. In addition, Bioject offers a certification program for injection administration via jet injection. This is available to all customers and includes an examination and certificate of completion. Customers also receive telephone support through Bioject Customer Service.

Summary. This case study demonstrates a current innovation that responds to a true health care need. Needle-stick injuries are a serious health problem. Disposing of contaminated waste materials is a major health problem. Dealing with fears of needle sticks particularly in young children has concerned nurses for years and is the subject of numerous nursing research studies.

The published and unpublished research supports the effectiveness of this innovation. The company provides the education necessary to use the product safely and effectively. This innovation offers great promise for both health care providers and consumers.

ETHICAL ISSUES ASSOCIATED WITH TECHNOLOGICAL DEVELOPMENTS

The rapid developments in health care technology have raised numerous complex social policy issues. Some of the most perplexing issues fall under the general heading of ethics. One such issue (Annas, 1991) is presented as illustrative of the larger array of concerns. Euthanasia advocate Dr. Jack Kevorkian has developed a "suicide" or "killing machine." It consists of three hanging bottles connected to intravenous tubing. Once the intravenous needle is inserted, a saline solution is delivered. The patient can switch the saline to a second bottle containing a sedative. The third bottle containing the fatal drug is activated automatically by a timer. This technology enables a person to commit suicide. Although society has become familiar with situations in which a decision is made to discontinue technology (i.e., "pulling the plug"), society is not at all comfortable with creating technology that facilitates suicide. Society is debating at least two questions embedded in the Kevorkian "suicide machine." Is the machine bad and should it be allowed in our society? Secondly, should physicians be allowed to use the technology; if so, under what conditions/controls?

In recent years people across the world have become aware of the ability to create technology to do what previous generations thought was impossible (e.g., test tube babies, heart-lung transplants). But, at least in the United States, society is far behind in developing consensus on how to use these new advances for the common good. Some health care leaders have called for a ban on all new technology being developed or used until society has resolved the ethical dilemmas specific to that technology. Without clear ethical guidelines, the technological imperative rules—We can, therefore we must (Fuchs, 1968)! And with that rule come all the unresolved ethical concerns.

Of equal concern is that the proliferation of sophisticated technologies has had a dramatic impact on the cost of health care (Fitzgerald, 1989). For example, magnetic resonance imaging (MRI) can reveal parts of the body never seen before. But the machines sell at prices ranging from $1 to 2.5 million and require $640,000 in annual operating costs.

The computed tomography (CT) scanner was the first device to provide cross-sectional views of the body. It was first marketed in London at a cost of $300,000. Four years later it was being marketed in the United States and sold at the rate of 40 per month at a purchase cost of as much as $1 million and an annual operating cost of $350,000. Although there are no hard data on the portion of health care costs attributable to technology, it is seen as a major culprit for the high costs of health care.

If there was a strong positive correlation between the use of sophisticated technology and health outcomes, the public might be less concerned about technology and rising health care costs. The fact of the matter is that there is no such strong, positive correlation. For example, the lithotripter (a device that shatters kidney stones by directing electromechanical shock waves at them from outside the body rather than removing them by invasive surgery) costs $2 million. One year after stone shattering by a lithotripter, 48 percent of those treated have stone fragments visible on x-ray. One year after stone removal by surgery, 15 percent of those patients treated have recurrence of stones. The lithotripter has recently been used to treat gallstones. It is estimated that for the majority of patients, the lithotripter treatment is more expensive and does not result in better outcomes.

The points of contention are:

- the unresolved ethical issues associated with specific technology
- the concern over the rising costs of health care, which are decreasing access for more and more people
- inadequate assurances that high technology brings better health outcomes

TECHNOLOGY AND NURSING PRACTICE

There are two generalizations regarding technology and nursing practice:

- Technology provides the tools and environment for nursing practice.
- Technology influences the nature and scope of nursing practice.

Within nursing, probably the first generalization is better understood than the second. It is only in recent years with the very rapid development of health care technologies in the fields of information and robotics that the second generalization is evident (McClure, 1995; Meierhoffer, 1995).

Technology and the Tools of Nursing Practice

CHANGES IN NURSING TECHNOLOGY

The nursing folklore (nursing stories passed on by word of mouth) includes reference to an era when the thermometer used to determine body temperature was so new it was considered a potentially dangerous weapon and only physicians were allowed to use it in the care of the ill. The nurse used the hand placed on the patient's forehead to determine body temperature. Today that thermometer is common household technology. In the clinical setting it has been replaced with more sophisticated technology frequently used by health care workers with minimal postsecondary education.

In the 1950s, water was a major technology in treating the mentally ill. Agitated patients were wrapped mummy fashion in sheets, restrained in tubs of warm water for hours at a time, or were stood at the end of a long room and hosed with cold water. Today people with similar symptoms are treated with drugs called tranquilizers. Many are able to live at home instead of spending their lives in an institution.

Even the administration of pain medication is changing. In the 1950s, glass syringes were used and sterilized for reuse. Needles were used and reused after being sharpened and sterilized. Today disposable needles and syringes are in use across the country. Technology that allows a patient to administer his or her own pain medication is used successfully. Implants that release medication are in use but are not as effective as initially hoped. And as mentioned earlier, the needleless injection system is being used in some settings for some medications. The stereotype of the nurse entering a patient's room with a syringe and foot-long needle will be a memory of the past!

The hammer was a major component of the technology of the public health nurse of the 1940s. The nurse used it to hang quarantine signs on homes of people with a communicable disease. If there was a possibility that an individual (usually a child) had a communicable disease, the nurse would visit the home and verify a diagnosis. If it was a communicable disease, the nurse would nail a sign on the front door warning people of the disease. When the person was no longer contagious, the sign was taken down.

Individuals with more life-threatening communicable diseases such as scarlet fever or tuberculosis were sent to specialty hospitals and cared for there. The technology needed to care for them was only available in the hospital. Today the home is also the site of high-technology care. Home health nursing includes the use of ventilators, dialysis equipment, apnea monitors, chest x-ray machines, electrocardiographs, and intravenous supplies (Smith et al, 1991). The nursing home is also the site of high-technology care because patients with conditions requiring long-term care are treated there before discharge to their homes (Fields et al, 1991).

FUTURE TECHNOLOGY

As dramatic as these changes are to those practicing nursing, it is clear that in the years ahead the rate of change will be even greater and the change in the technology even more dramatic. A typical response to the onslaught of new technology is "I went into nursing to nurse patients, *not machines*." Unfortunately that is an attitude that is inconsistent with contemporary nursing practice. Today's nurse functions in a world of high technology (Fig. 5–2). The paperless hospital and HANK the robot, described in the beginning of this chapter, are just part of the technology on the horizon.

THE "DE-SKILLING" OF NURSING PRACTICE

Much nursing technology is developed in an attempt to improve performance. It has the potential to substitute for some human function, save time, measure accurately, measure physiologic variables not directly perceptible by humans, and avoid frequent patient disturbance (Ashworth, 1990). Technology developed toward these ends usually begins by reconceptualizing a complex process into a series of simpler operations, one or more of which can be implemented with a technology. For example, it has been noted that the routine recording of vital signs for a group of patients frequently involves errors. A wrong temperature or pulse is recorded. Replacing the health care worker with a monitoring machine linked to a database could eliminate those errors. Consider the critically ill patient for whom it is important to accurately measure fluid intake and output. It is not uncommon to find errors in measuring the urinary output. A bedpan has now been developed that automatically measures the urinary output along with a chemical analysis of the urine.

When only one part of a complex process is replaced by technology, it is viewed as work enhancement. The health care worker can do better work in perhaps less time because of the introduction of the technology. Over time, an entire complex process may be reduced to a set of automated techniques. The use of technology in this way results in the *de-skilling* of the process. Not only are some muscular and manual skills replaced by technology, but so are the judgment skills. With de-skilling, the assumption is that a less skilled worker can be safely assigned that process.

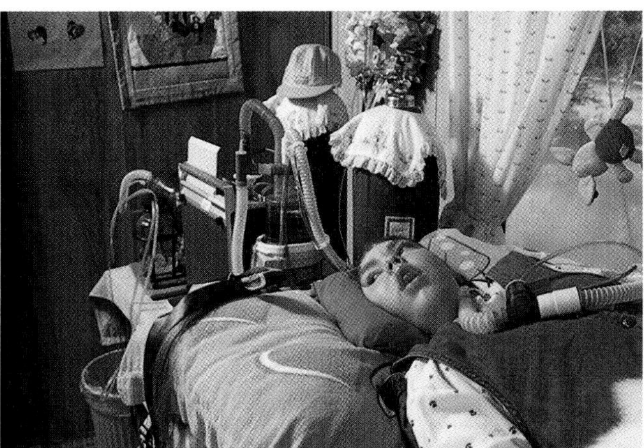

Figure 5–2. The home care setting is increasingly becoming a high-tech care setting.

Technology and the Nature and Scope of Nursing Practice

The second principle regarding technology and nursing practice is that technology influences the nature and scope of nursing practice. This principle reflects the extensive de-skilling that is taking place within health care. Specialized work such as the initial screening of a radiograph by an x-ray technician or a radiologist can now be done by a computer. This has the potential of eliminating the need for the specialist and instead placing responsibility for that work with a generalist such as a nurse case manager. Some of the personal care that nurses have protected legally as "nursing practice" is being thought of as patient care rather than nursing care. The intent is to enable less well prepared (and less well paid) health care workers to do that work. It is entirely possible that health care technology will make obsolete certain established well-defined practice acts.

GUIDELINES FOR USING TECHNOLOGY IN NURSING PRACTICE

The nurse should not use any technology until she or he has been adequately prepared and is comfortable using it.

In general, the rate of change in technology and the introduction of new technology are determined by the ability to master and use the improvements effectively. In health care this is not always the case. Nurses are often the primary link between the patient and the vast array of health care technology. Yet in many situations the decision to purchase new equipment or change technology is made by someone other than the nurse. The new technology simply appears and the old technology disappears. This situation is frustrating for

CURRENT CONTROVERSY

WILL PERSONAL CARE BE PART OF NURSING'S FUTURE?

DEBUNKING NURSING MYTHS

By Carol Lindeman

NLN Update, *August 1995, Vol. 1, No. 3*

The summer 1994 issue of *Audacity* carried a letter from the editor titled "The Power of the Myth." It begins with this statement: During the last presidential election, Ross Perot, self-described as America's pre-eminent self-made man, offered himself as the fellow uniquely qualified to sort out the mess the politicians had gotten us into. But then an embarrassing fact began to trickle out—Perot's big success had been as a governmental contractor serving the American welfare state, and the most valuable piece of property he owned, the keystone of his empire, was a computer program developed at federal expense that had somehow got stuck to his fingers. The self-made great man was in fact "the biggest welfare beneficiary in American history." The letter continues the Perot myth busting and ends "All myths seem implausible in retrospect. What takes audacity is to debunk them while they still hold us in thrall."

In an October 1994 article in the *Health Care Forum Journal,* Richard Lamm identifies eight myths and corresponding heresies regarding health care reform. It is his premise that as the old world of health care is dying and the new world is being born, it is a good time to pause to rethink many long-standing myths. He begins his list with the myth that the United States has the best health care system in the world and his list ends with the myth that medical care is the best way to improve health.

The discipline of nursing has its own myths. And we have those among us who challenge our myths; at first they are seen as heretics. One such person who was influential in the NLN curriculum revolution is Chris Tanner. Chris challenged the myths surrounding the nursing process, nursing diagnosis, and the nursing care plan. When she first proposed clinical decision making/clinical judgement as the better model of nurses' thought patterns, she was viewed as a heretic or at least her writing was viewed as heresy by many in nursing.

I am certain if you pause to think about nursing myths and heresies you will be able to identify quite a number.

In recent years, articles have appeared describing how faculty and clinicians have identified and dealt with their prized myths. For example, one nursing group met in a funeral home. Each person attending had written a myth about nursing on a card. During the meeting each person walked up to an open coffin and placed their myth into the coffin. When all had done that, the coffin lid was closed and the coffin wheeled out of the room. The group could then move on with creating something new.

A lighter version of the same idea was described to me by an NLN member. She described the sacred cow luncheon her faculty held. Each member of the faculty wrote a sacred cow about nursing practice or education on a card; during the luncheon all sacred cows were sacrificed. The curriculum could then be redesigned.

It is clear that we are now moving rapidly into a health care system that will bear little resemblance to the health care system of the 1980s. We are moving from a system where care is controlled by physicians and in some instances nurses, to a system where care is controlled by the available data/information.

We are moving from a system where conditions [are] treated through the use of surgery or chemical compounds to a system where genetic-based research will be used in the immunization and treatment of conditions. We are moving from a system where care is provided during acute periods of illness to a system where self-administered preventive care will be the norm. And we are moving from a hospital-based physician-driven system to an out-patient, home-based, provider-prescribed but self-administered system of care. It is a myth to believe that nurses are so important that no matter what the public will always need us.

As I think about the future health care system and nursing's role, I am struck by the issues that nursing, in collaboration with others, must think through. The issues include long-held beliefs about the practice of nursing. For example, a most common question about nursing practice these days relates to the role of personal care such as bathing, elimination, and nutrition. Many nurses will say it is important for nurses to provide this care for two reasons. First, it gives the nurse the opportunity to better assess the patient. Secondly, it establishes a relationship that is essential to positive outcomes of care. Many outside of nursing say it is too costly for nurses to provide personal care. Those aspects of care can be done just as well by lower paid personnel. Is it a myth that providing personal care is vital to the practice of nursing? Is personal care the essence of the nurse-patient relationship? Let me share two concrete illustrations of this issue. A nurse who was quoted recently as saying, "They tell me that others can do morning care so that I am free to do nursing care. To me personal care is nursing care." And a nurse at our university hospital, when asked to let the multi-skilled worker measure intake and output, the nurse responded. "I can't. How would I know if the patient was in congestive heart failure?"

Is it heresy to suggest that in the reformed health care system where hospitalization is rare personal care tasks CANNOT be the language we use to define nursing? Is the importance of providing personal care to the nurse-patient relationship a myth or a truth? How will we know?

CURRENT CONTROVERSY

HOW DOES DE-SKILLING AFFECT PATIENT CARE?

BE PATIENT; THEY CALL IT 'DE-SKILLING'

By Hilary Abramson

NLN Update, *March 27, 1995, p. A15*

From my hospital bed, I saw the young man as a silhouette with an edgy voice. "Didn't you notice your IV needs *changing?*"

He seized the bottle and confirmed that the drip had stopped warming its way into my veins.

In my morphine fog, I could barely respond. Less than 24 hours earlier, I had undergone a hysterectomy at what is now called California Pacific Medical Center in San Francisco.

The IV technician (or nurse's aide) had enough to say for both of us, and the questions kept coming.

Didn't I realize we were "a team?" Hadn't I been told that we have to work *together?* Hadn't I received some sort of patient orientation? *Why* wasn't *I* watching *my* IV?

During the next few days, I received a crash course in the "de-skilling" of an American hospital, where technicians and students are now assigned to what appear to be mundane chores previously performed by registered nurses. This move—recently in the news—may save hospital administrators money, but it's enough to make a patient sick. Or sicker. . . .

Was I passing the normal amount of blood? When could I move without this P-A-I-N?

"I *think* it's normal," she [a first-year nursing student] said, "I'll have to ask someone when you might be able to sit up."

Lesson Number One: Surrounded by more technicians and students than registered nurses, the patient can know as much as the caregiver.

After I insisted, a nurse finally arrived. She said that my doctor should have warned me how tough it would be for at least three days.

"There is something wrong here," I said. "I am the patient; you are the nurse. I have this feeling that you expect me to help you feel better."

She apologized, sat on the edge of the bed and began to cry. She had been working double shifts because they were so short-staffed. She feared being laid off. Her brother was dying of AIDS, and she had a stress overload.

Lesson Number Two: Nurses can be too overworked for the patient to expect comfort from them.

There was more. Having technicians do what appear to be rote tasks can be dangerous to a patient. When my neck hurt from the surgical tube and I lacked the mobility to adjust the bed, I rang for a nurse. The technician who responded barely spoke English. Instead of bringing me a pillow as I requested, he took away my pillow, lowered the upper portion of the mattress and pushed my head back against it, producing an intense episode of pain.

nurses and leads to errors in care. For example, Henney and Blatt (1984) report on errors made by patients using canister nebulizers for respiratory problems. None of the nurses involved in teaching patients how to use the nebulizers had had any formal training in nebulizer use, and only 39 percent had an opportunity to read material regarding the correct use of the nebulizer. Hutchinson et al (1987) cited nurses' confusion of nasogastric tubes and tracheostomy cuff tubing as cause of a patient's death. Furthermore, nurses who are inadequately prepared to use medical devices are likely to fear the equipment and thus experience greater stress (Malila, 1987; McConnell and Murphy, 1987; Steel et al, 1981).

Certainly the health care agency has a responsibility to provide the necessary on-the-job training for new technology. But the individual nurse also has the responsibility to provide safe care. Therefore it is important for the nurse to request training if it is not provided. Many companies offer routine training in new technology at no cost to an agency or individual. In addition, one should routinely read the reports from technology assessment agencies mentioned earlier. Patients may also be a good source of information if it is technology that involves them. For example, women in labor have very definite views on the use of fetal monitors.

If you are not familiar with a technology and have been asked to use it, first talk to your supervisor and explain the situation. Ask for direct assistance from someone who is familiar with the equipment or procedure.

The nurse should evaluate the safety and effectiveness of every technology with every patient. Just because a drug or device is in use, it should not be assumed to be safe and effective.

As noted earlier, it is possible for technology to be introduced and adopted with only minimal evaluation. It is also possible for technology developed and introduced for one purpose to be used for a new purpose without further evaluation. The data cited earlier suggest that the majority of health care technology in use has had inadequate evaluation (Jacox, 1990).

Safe nursing practice therefore requires the nurse to continue the process of evaluation in terms of the individual patient with whom it is being used. The nurse must collect data to answer questions such as "Is the technology producing the desired effect?" "Is the patient experiencing any negative outcomes?" "What is the error rate?" "Is the time required to use the equipment greater than obtaining the results another way?" and "What is the patient's response to the technology?" Negative answers to any of these questions should lead the nurse to confer with the physician or case manager.

The nurse should always educate the patient and/or family about the technology used in care.

TABLE 5-1 Ethical Issues Associated with Specific Emerging Technologies

Emerging Technologies	Ethical Issues
Artifical intelligence (computer modeling and expert systems that think)	Who will **control** the use of these systems? Will these systems allow for **choice** or will they mandate a single rule?
Diagnostic imaging (imaging that will pinpoint pathology in the disease process)	Will costly treatments be **rationed?** Will the best contrast agents be used even if **expensive?**
Genetic engineering (the use of genetic markers in early diagnosis and treatment)	Will gene therapy increase **legal** issues regarding selection of treatment? Will the public, out of fear of misuse, refuse to **fund** genetic research? Will genetic information be used to **refuse insurance** to someone?
Home health/Self diagnostics (the ability to be cared for at home and to monitor one's own progress)	Where will the **homeless** receive care? Will insurance companies fund the **social support** system needed to make home care effective?
Health care automation (integrated health care computer systems)	How will privacy be maintained? How will people be **protected** from electronically snooping?
New-wave surgery (the use of laser surgery)	Will small rural and public hospitals be able to **afford** these tools? Will the availability of these tools increase **competition** among health care providers?
Super-drugs (chemicals that are used instead of invasive procedures, e.g., a drug that dissolves plaque and is used instead of bypass surgery)	Who should **pay** the high costs of research and development? Who should have access to **experimental** drugs? Who should be used as **research subjects?**
Transplants and implants (the replacement of organs, joints, lenses, etc.)	Will **age** guidelines be used to refuse transplants? Will insurance companies refuse to **pay** for these high-cost procedures?

Based on information in Coile, R.C. [1990]. Technology and ethics: Three scenarios for the 1990s. *Quality Review Bulletin, 16,* 202-208.

There are several reasons why this is an important guideline. The first is that the patient and/or family is likely to use the technology when a nurse is not present. This could be in a hospital setting as well as a home setting. For the patient and family to use the technology, they too must be adequately prepared and feel comfortable. Education is a key to successful use of technology by patients and family.

A second reason is that the patient is likely to feel less stress and alienation if he or she can understand the technology as an extension of the nurse's practice. When the nurse helps the patient see technology in this way, the patient experiences the "high touch" that must accompany the "high tech."

A third reason why this guideline is important is that by teaching others, one also learns. When the nurse facilitates a patient learning some aspect of their care, the nurse has to rethink his or her own knowledge base as well as think through the questions raised by the patient. The end result is that the nurse will come away from the interaction better prepared to assist the next patient. We learn by teaching others.

The nurse needs to think through the legal and ethical issues associated with a specific technology and be prepared to discuss these issues with the health care team and the patient and/or family.

The technological imperative "I can, therefore I must" is no longer an acceptable approach to care. Over the last several years the public has taken actions to give individuals more authority over health care decisions—particularly at the end of life (see Chapter 8). Remember that although technology is neutral, technology-practice is not. The nurse is involved in technology-practice and therefore must be aware of the issues. Yet it is not the nurse who makes the final decision about the ethics in a specific technology-practice situation. It is the patient and/or family. The nurse must have the knowledge and clinical reasoning skills to facilitate their decision making (see Chapter 12).

Table 5–1 summarizes emerging technologies and ethical issues specific to that technology.

CHAPTER HIGHLIGHTS

- High technology is only as good as those that use it. When used by knowledgeable clinicians, it can save time and improve the outcomes of care. It may also save money. When used by inadequately prepared or inattentive clinicians, technology can waste time, detract from positive outcomes of care, and cost money.
- Contemporary nursing practice requires the nurse to have a positive attitude toward technology, to use it appropriately, and to find ways to offer the high touch that must accompany the high tech. Technology need not detract from high-quality, caring nursing practice. The key is the nurse—not the machine.

REFERENCES

Abele, J.E. (1991). Objective assessment of new technology. *Catheterization and Cardiovascular Diagnosis, 23,* 268–269.

Annas, G.J. (1991). Killing machines. *Hastings Center Report,* March-April, 33–35.

Armstrong, S.E. (1991). The cost of needle-stick injuries: The impact of safer medical devices. *Nursing Economics, 9,* 426–430, 433.

Ashworth, P. (1990). High technology and humanity for intensive care. *Intensive Care Nursing, 6,* 150–160.

Baer, C.L., Bennett, W.M., Folwick, D.A., Erickson, R.S. (1996). Effectiveness of a jet injection system in administering morphine and heparin to healthy adults. *American Journal of Critical Care, 5, 42–48.*

Coile, R.C. (1990). Technology and ethics: Three scenarios for the 1990s. *Quality Review Bulletin, 16,* 202–208.

Constans, L. (1991). Jet injection. *The (Oregon) Times,* April 18–24, 1B.

deCarteret, J.C. (1987). Needlestick injuries: An occupational health hazard for nurses. *AAOHN Journal, 35* (3), 119–123.

Fields, A.I., Rosenblatt, A., Pollack, M.M., Kaufman, J. (1991). Home care cost-effectiveness for respiratory technology-dependent children. *American Journal of Diseases of Children, 145,* 729–733.

Fitzgerald, K. (1989). Technology in medicine: Too much too soon? *IEEE SPECTRUM,* December, 24–29.

Fuchs, V.R. (1968). The growing demand for medical care. *New England Journal of Medicine, 279,* 192.

Goode, C.J., Titler, M., Rakel, B., et al (1991). A meta-analysis of effects of heparin flush and saline flush: Quality and cost implications. *Nursing Research, 40,* 324–330.

Greenberg, R.S., Maxwell, L.G., Zahruak, M., Yaster, M. (October 1994). *Preinduction of Anesthesia in Children with Midazolam using the Bioject Jet Injector.* Poster session presented as the annual meeting of the American Society of Anesthesiologists.

Health Technology Reviews. (1994). *Research Activities, 172,* January/February, 9–10.

Henney, H.R., Blatt, R.S. (1984). Knowledge of nurses and respiratory therapists about using canister nebulizers. *American Journal of Hospital Pharmacy, 41,* 2403–2404.

Holding, R., Carlsen, W. (1998). Epidemic Ravages Caregivers. *San Francisco Chronicle,* April 13, pp. A1, A6–A8.

Hutchinson, M., Himes, T.M., Davis, L.E. (1987). Preventing multiple body tubes mix-ups. *Nursing 87,* 17, 57.

Jacox, A. (1990). Technology assessment in reducing costs and improving care. *Nursing Economics, 8,* 116–119.

Luce, B.R. (1993). Medical technology and its assessment. In S.J. Williams and P.R. Torrens (eds.): *Introduction to Health Services,* 4th ed. Albany, NY: Delmar, pp. 245–268.

Malila, F.M. (1987). Caring in a technological age: Education for adaptation. *Focus on Critical Care, 14* (3), 21–26.

McClure, M.L. (1995). Tomorrow's workplace. *Dean's Notes, 17,* September, 1–2.

McConnell, E.A., Murphy, E.K. (1990). Nurses' use of technology: An international concern. *International Nursing Review, 37,* 331–334.

McKinlay, J.B. (1981). From "promising report" to "standard procedure": Seven stages in the career of a medical innovation. *Milbank Memorial Fund Quarterly/Health and Society, 59,* 374–411.

Meierhoffer, L.L. (1995). 'High-touch' versus 'high-tech.' *The American Nurse, 27,* September, 1, 12.

Nelson, V. (1997). How would health care look in a perfect world? *Nurse Week, 10* (13), 1, 6, 7.

Nursing's Agenda for Health Care Reform. (1991). Available from the National League for Nursing, 350 Hudson St., New York, NY 10014.

Office of Technology Assessment. (1986). *Nurse Practitioners, Physician Assistants, and Certified Nurse-Midwives: A Policy Analysis.* (Health Technology Case Study 37, OTA-HCS-37.) Washington, D.C.: U.S. Government Printing Office.

Pacey, A. (1984). *The culture of technology.* Cambridge, MA: The MIT Press.

Smith, C.E., Mayer, L.S., Parkhurst, C., et al (1991). Adaptation in families with a member requiring mechanical ventilation at home. *Heart and Lung, 20,* 349–356.

Steel, K., Gertman, P.M., Crescenzi, B.S., Anderson, J. (1981). Iantrogenic illness on a general medical service at a university hospital. *New England Journal of Medicine, 304,* 638–642.

6 Determinants of Health and Illness

Carol Lindeman

With contributions by Sheila Kodadek, RN, PhD, Professor, School of Nursing, Oregon Health Sciences University; Laura J. Armstrong, EdD, MPH, RN, Chief Community Health Nursing Division, Hawaii Department of Health; June Shibuya, RN, MSN, NP Malama Project Coordinator, Hawaii Department of Health

OBJECTIVES

After studying this chapter, students will have learned to:

- **incorporate nonbiologic factors associated with health and illness into clinical decision making**
- **use epidemiologic data in evaluating and planning prevention and intervention strategies**
- **contrast individual patient data with aggregate data as a basis for planning and evaluating care**
- **contrast data from a population subgroup with aggregate data as a basis for evaluating and planning care**

Health is more than the absence of disease. It is a response to the biophysical, socioeconomic, and interpersonal dimensions of a person's environment experienced in the context of living (Milio, 1981). According to the World Health Organization (Constitution of the WHO, 1964), health is a state of complete physical, mental, and social well-being. For many, health is equated with the ability to go about daily activities without restriction (Milio, 1981).

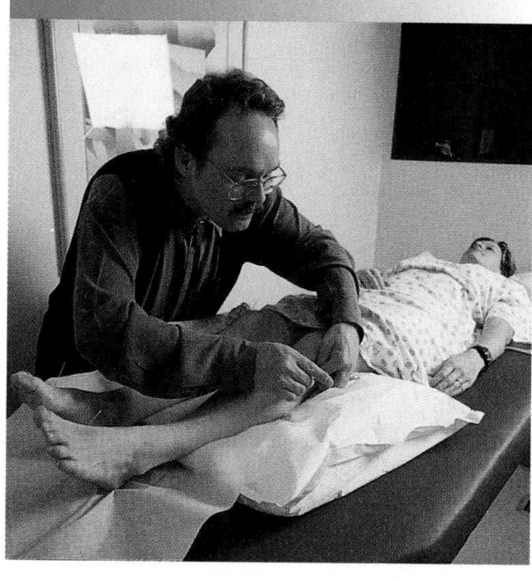

Illness is an individual's reaction to a biologic alteration. It is defined differently by different people according to their state of mind and cultural beliefs. For many, illness is something that keeps one from pursuing the usual activities of life (Milio, 1981). It is a person's **perception** of loss of functional capacity, i.e., the person feels or believes that he or she has lost the capacity to do some usual activity. For example, one person has a cold and *feels* he cannot go to work because he is ill. Another person has a cold and goes to work because the person does not *feel* ill.

Whereas *illness* refers to a lay experience of either or both a physical and psychosocial state, the word *disease* is a professional construct. A disease has a specific definition and is used to inform the patient and others about specific pathology, to decide a course of treatment, and to compare the results of therapy.

A person may feel ill but not have a diagnosable disease, e.g., a person who feels chronic severe fatigue but whose health care provider cannot identify a known disease. Similarly, a person may have a disease and not feel ill, as commonly occurs in the early stages of some cancers when the disease is picked up on routine examination. It is illness, and not disease, that causes a person to seek help.

Health and illness can be understood only in the context of a specific individual, family, or community. Neither health nor illness occurs in a vacuum. Neither can be fully explained by exposure to bacteria, viruses, or toxic agents. Environmental factors such as pollutants in the air or pesticides and lead in the work place contribute to health and illness. Likewise, patterns of personal behavior such as nutrition, alcohol and drug use, cigarette use, and exposure to stress also affect health and illness.

It is important for nurses to remember that less than healthful lifestyles are not always a matter of "free" choice but rather the result of opportunities available to people (Milio, 1981). People living at poverty level may simply not be able to afford healthy meals or safe housing. A child with parents who must hold several jobs to support the family may not have routine immunizations because the parents do not have the time available to take the child to the doctor's office. A person who cannot read may never learn about germ theory and the importance of washing hands.

Clearly, nursing practice is influenced by the nature of health and illness. It is also influenced by the demographics of the population and the nature of the leading causes of illness and death. For instance, as the population ages, nurses are learning how to support the caregivers of the frail elderly living at home. As the population becomes ethnically more diverse, nurses are learning interventions that are effective with different population groups. A little more than a decade ago, acquired immunodeficiency syndrome (AIDS) was virtually unknown in the United States. Today, nurses are well aware of AIDS and the precautions necessary in caring for affected individuals.

Nurses must consider the broad array of nonbiologic factors as well as the biologic factors that influence health, illness, and nursing practice in their clinical decision making. Culture, race, ethnicity, families, age, gender, socioeconomic status, and religion are factors influencing health and illness discussed in this chapter. The natural history of a disease is discussed using an epidemiology perspective. The following scenarios illustrate clinical decision making that considers these factors.

- Nurse A works in an integrated health care system associated with a capitated insurance program (CIP). Her focus is women's health. As she compares data about the women cared for in CIP with national data, she notes that the rate of late-stage breast tumors is higher for the CIP women. Nurse A sets a goal of bringing her group to national norms within a 2-year time frame. What factors are associated with routine screening for breast cancer?
- Nurse B works in a school-based clinic. He is very concerned about the rate of young teen pregnancies. His sex education program has not decreased the rate of pregnancies. What factors are associated with decreased rates of teen pregnancies?
- Nurse C works in a low-cost housing project. She is concerned that the elderly have no access to exercise facilities. The people with whom she has shared her concern tell her exercise facilities are a luxury and not a necessity. Are they right?
- Nurse D works in a county health department with a large population of immigrants. He notes that many of the immigrants come for initial assessment but rarely return for treatment. As he pursues this with his patients they tell him they do not trust physical or chemical interventions. They prefer alternative therapies such as herbs, acupuncture, and meditation. Should Nurse D attempt to make these alternative therapies available?

EPIDEMIOLOGY

Epidemiology is the study of how disease is distributed in the population and of the factors that influence or determine this distribution (Gordis, 1996). Epidemiologists are interested in identifying risk factors that might be altered in a population to prevent or delay disease or death (classical epidemiology). They are also interested in improving the diagnosis and treatment of people who are ill (clinical epidemiology).

Impact

The changing health problems of a community are evidence of the success of epidemiology. Table 6–1 contrasts the leading causes of death in the United States in 1900 and in 1990. In the early 1900s the leading causes of death were infectious diseases. Today, the leading causes of death are noncommunicable chronic diseases. Understanding the nature of an illness and implementing corrective actions can eliminate or minimize the incidence of that illness.

The Natural History of a Disease

The natural history of a disease can be described in terms of four factors: the host, the agent, the environment, and the vector. According to this epidemiologic perspective, disease is

TABLE 6–1 Leading Causes of Death in the United States, 1900 and 1990

Leading Causes of Death, 1900	Leading Causes of Death, 1990
1. Pneumonia	1. Heart disease
2. Tuberculosis	2. Cancer
3. Diarrhea and enteritis	3. Stroke
4. Heart disease	4. Unintentional injury
5. Chronic nephritis	5. Lung disease
6. Unintentional injury	6. Pneumonia and influenza
7. Stroke	7. Diabetes
8. Diseases of early infancy	8. Suicide
9. Cancer	9. Liver disease
10. Diphtheria	10. Human immunodeficiency virus/acquired immunodeficiency syndrome (HIV/AIDS)

Data from Gordis, L. (1996). *Epidemiology.* Philadelphia: W. B. Saunders, p. 4.

the result of an interaction of a human host, an infectious or other type of agent, the environment that promotes the exposure, and in some instances a vector than transmits the agent (Fig. 6–1).

HOST

For disease to occur, the human host must be susceptible. Susceptibility or resistance is influenced by a person's genotype (genetic inheritance), nutritional status, immune system, and social behavior (Jekel et al, 1996). A growing body of research highlights the importance of heredity in the incidence of certain types of cancers. Genetic inheritance is also linked with diseases such as hemochromatosis, in which the body's ability to restrict the amount of iron in the blood is impaired. General resistance is influenced by nutrition, as evidenced by the fact that measles is seldom fatal in well-nourished children but can be fatal in malnourished children (Jekel et al, 1996). The immune status of a person is influenced by heredity, previous exposure to an agent, and immunization. Social behavior such as personal hygiene has been linked to dysentery. Likewise social behaviors such as sexual activity and drug administration with used needles have been linked with AIDS.

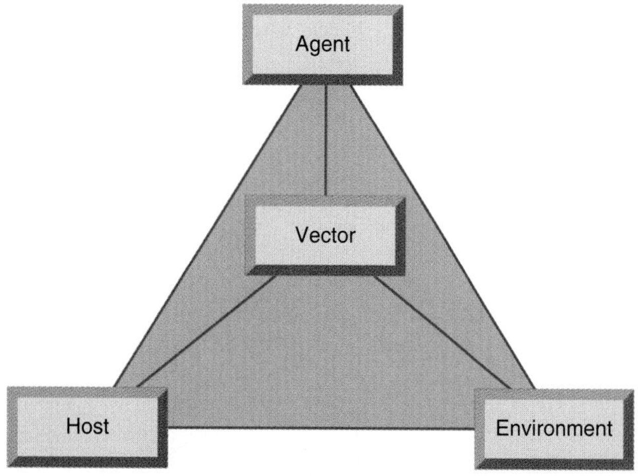

Figure 6–1. Factors involved in the natural history of a disease.

AGENT

Four categories of agents can produce serious disease in humans: biologic, chemical, physical, and social and psychological stressors. Bacteria, viruses, and allergens are examples of biologic agents. Lead, dust, and insecticides are examples of chemical agents. Bullets and automobile accidents are examples of physical agents. Loss or a job, change in residence, and death of a child are examples of social or psychological stressors.

ENVIRONMENT

The environment influences the probability and circumstances of interaction between a host and an agent. Examples include:

- People living in crowded neighborhoods have increased exposure to violence.
- People living in inner cities have increased exposure to pollutants.
- People living with poor sanitation have increased exposure to dysentery.
- People working on farms have increased exposure to injury from heavy equipment.
- Nurses have increased exposure to injury from lifting.

VECTOR

A vector is the transmitter of the disease. To be effective, the vector must have a specific relationship to the host, agent, and environment. For example, in malaria the *Anopheles* mosquito is the vector. Without that mosquito, the disease cannot be transmitted. Insects, animals, humans, and objects may all be vectors.

Disease Prevention

Jekel et al (1996) have coined the acronym BEINGS as a way to remember the categories of preventable causes of disease (Box 6–1). These factors are an important framework for nurses to use in work with individuals, families, and communities. For instance, a nurse working with an AIDS prevention and detection program would need to think through each of the seven categories of factors before an effective program could be established. The BEINGS model can be used in health promotion and disease prevention as well as when treating disease.

BOX 6-1
THE BEINGS MODEL: AN ACRONYM FOR REMEMBERING THE CATEGORIES OF PREVENTABLE CAUSES OF DISEASE

- **B**iologic factors and **B**ehavioral factors
- **E**nvironmental factors
- **I**mmunologic factors
- **N**utritional factors
- **G**enetic factors
- **S**ervices, **S**ocial factors, and **S**piritual factors

From Jekel, J.F., Elmore, J.G., Katz, D.L. (1996). *Epidemiology, Biostatistics, and Preventive Medicines.* Philadelphia: W.B. Saunders, p. 4.

BEHAVIORAL FACTORS

Human behavior is a major factor determining health and illness. Cigarette smoking contributes to a number of diseases, including lung cancer, heart disease, and chronic obstructive pulmonary disease. Intravenous drug abuse is associated with AIDS. Excessive intake of alcohol, abuse of illegal drugs, and driving while intoxicated are all associated with premature death. Changes in behavior could prevent these negative outcomes.

ENVIRONMENTAL FACTORS

Environmental factors have been discussed earlier. In terms of disease prevention, it is important to note the relationships between the prevalence and patterns of disease and environment. In recent years this approach to prevention was evident with the disease known as legionnaires' disease. In 1976, a number of people attending an American Legion convention became ill, and some died from a fatal pneumonia. The discovery was made that the disease was caused by a small bacterium that thrived in air-conditioning cooling towers and in warm water systems. By treating the water in air conditioning systems, the disease can be prevented.

IMMUNOLOGIC FACTORS

Disease can be prevented through immunization. The spread of disease can also be curtailed by immunizing large numbers of people. The possibility exists that disease can even be eradicated through worldwide immunization programs. An immune system deficiency can be created by disease (e.g., AIDS), genetic abnormalities, or other factors such as live measles vaccine.

NUTRITIONAL FACTORS

Nutrition is more important in determining health and illness than most people realize. Certainly nutritional status influences susceptibility to disease. It also influences incidence of disease. For example, diseases such as appendicitis, breast cancer, colon cancer, and coronary heart disease are very rare in the indigenous populations of tropical Africa (Jekel et al, 1996). This difference in incidence of disease is not genetically based because African-Americans have these diseases at about the same rate as other groups in the United States. Persons of Japanese descent living in Hawaii and in California have a higher rate of myocardial infarctions than those of similar age and sex living in Japan. Investigators believe that dietary differences are the single most important factor in the different disease incidences.

GENETIC FACTORS

Genetic inheritance interacts with diet and the environment to promote or protect against a variety of diseases. Cancer and heart disease are two such diseases. As genetic research increases, new insights into the links between genetics and disease will occur. It is also likely that the research will enable early detection and treatment of some diseases.

HEALTH CARE SERVICES, SOCIAL FACTORS, AND SPIRITUAL FACTORS

Health care services can be a source of illness. For example, a nurse who makes a medication error or implements a procedure incorrectly can cause a health problem for the patient. Health care providers who do not take precautions such as washing their hands between caring for patients can transmit disease. Approximately 1 out of every 20 hospitalized patients develops a nosocomial infection, i.e., an infection not associated with the reason for admission.

Although social and spiritual factors have been studied less intensely than other factors, there is growing evidence of their importance. Social factors are discussed in more detail in Chapter 29. Research shows that members of religious groups such as the Mormons and Seventh-Day Adventists have lower than average death rates for many diseases including heart disease. The differences cannot be fully accounted for by diet. It appears that personal beliefs about the meaning and purpose of life influence health and illness (Jekel et al, 1996). Recent research on prayer shows it to have a positive influence on recovery.

Epidemiologic Measurements

SOURCES OF DATA

Most countries collect vital statistics and census data. Vital statistics include data on births, deaths, causes of death, fetal deaths, marriages, and divorces. Most countries report their data to the United Nations, which then publishes compendia of national statistics.

There are many sources of morbidity and mortality statistics. The most important ongoing national databases include:

- **The U.S. Vital Statistics System,** a database that includes data on all vital statistics collected by local and state representatives.

- **U.S. Disease Reporting System,** a database that includes data on specific reportable communicable diseases, such as AIDS, and some noncommunicable reportable conditions, such as lead poisoning.
- **National Center for Health Statistics Studies,** a database that includes data from repeated surveys such as the National Health Interview Survey and National Nursing Home Survey, as well as data from specific surveys such as the population's use of preventive measures.
- **Behavioral Risk Factor Surveillance System,** a database that includes data collected from most states on prevalence of behaviors such as smoking, obesity, alcohol consumption, use of automobile seat belts, and exercise.

MEASURES OF MORBIDITY

There are two measures of morbidity: incidence and prevalence. The *incidence* of a disease is the number of new cases of a disease that occurs during a specified time period in a population at risk for developing the disease. It is usually expressed as the number per 1000 population (Box 6–2). For example, if there are 500 new cases of diabetes in a population of 5000, the incidence would be 500 divided by 5000 multiplied by 1000, or an incidence rate of 100 per 1000 population. Incidence is considered a measure of risk.

Prevalence is the number of affected persons in the population at a specified period of time divided by the number of persons in that population at the specified time. It too is usually expressed as the number per 1000 population (see Box 6–2). If there was a total of 2000 people with diabetes in a population of 5000, the prevalence is 2000 divided by 5000 multiplied by 1000, or 400 per 1000 population. Prevalence is considered a measure of the burden of disease in a community.

Four nursing practice scenarios were presented earlier. In those scenarios, Nurse A and Nurse B were using incidence data to make decisions about nursing actions.

MEASURES OF MORTALITY

There are three commonly used measures of mortality: mortality rates, case-fatality rates, and proportionate mortality. *Mortality rate* is the number of occurrences divided by the number in the population expressed (usually) in terms of 1000 population. In calculating the annual mortality rate for all causes of death, the total number of deaths would be divided by the total number of persons in the population and multiplied by 1000. If there were 3000 total deaths and 300,000 persons in the population, the mortality rate would be 10 per 1000 people. Mortality rates can be calculated for specific age groups, by sex, or by race. They can also be calculated for specific diseases or causes.

Case-fatality rates show what percent of people diagnosed as having a certain disease die within a certain time frame. The case-fatality rate is calculated by dividing the number of persons dying from the disease within a certain time frame after diagnosis by the number of people with the disease. It is expressed as a percent. For example if there were 300 persons with the disease and in 1 year after diagnosis 100 of them died from the disease, then the case-fatality rate for the disease would be 33 percent. This statistic describes the chance of dying from the disease.

Proportionate mortality describes the proportion of deaths due to a specific disease or cause. It too can be calculated for specific age groups, by sex or by race. For example, if there were 50 deaths from cancer in children under age 15 and 50,000 deaths in children under age 15, then the proportionate mortality for cancer in children under 15 years of age is 5 divided by 50,000 multiplied by 100 (to express the statistic as a percentage), or 0.1 percent. This statistic is useful for providing a quick look at the major causes of death.

Integrated health care systems use morbidity and mortality statistics to judge the cost-effectiveness of care. Data are compiled on the individuals enrolled in the specific system and compared with national data. Nurses are expected to use such data in developing plans of care for both individuals and groups of patients.

BOX 6–2
FORMULAS FOR CALCULATING INCIDENCE AND PREVALENCE OF A DISEASE

Incidence: $\frac{\text{number of new cases of a disease}}{\text{total population at risk}} \times 1000$

Prevalence:

$$\frac{\text{number of people with the disease}}{\text{total number of people in the population}} \times 1000$$

DETERMINANTS OF HEALTH

Historical Perspective

Life expectancy (i.e., the average number of years one is expected to live) is considered a measure of the health of a population. The fact that relatively poor countries such as Cuba and Costa Rica have essentially the same expectation of life as the United States highlights the complex nature of the determinants of health and illness (Terris, 1992). Clearly, neither the amount of money spent on health care nor the sophistication of the health care system is the major influence on life expectancy.

Across the world, health has improved because people become ill less often (McKeown, 1997). In particular, life expectancy has improved because of the reduction in deaths from infectious diseases. McKeown summarizes the improvements in health as follows:

> The death rate from infectious diseases fell because an increase in food supplies led to better nutrition. From the second half of

the 19th century this advance was strongly supported by improved hygiene and safer food (including pasteurized milk) and water, which reduced exposure to infection. With the exception of smallpox vaccination, which played a small part in the total decline of mortality, medical procedures such as immunization and therapy had little impact on human health until the 20th century (McKeown, 1997).

Today's health problems are primarily noncommunicable diseases, such as cancer, heart disease, and arthritis, and diseases associated with lifestyle, such as substance abuse and exposure to stress. The hope is that these diseases can also be prevented by identifying the conditions that lead to them. Genetic research may provide answers for diseases determined at the moment of conception. Other research must continue to identify the personal, social, and environmental factors associated with these conditions and the behavioral changes necessary to prevent them.

Word of Caution

Factors such as culture, age, and religion do influence an individual's health, illness, and response to disease and death. General statements regarding these factors can be made. Yet the manner in which individuals implement their health behaviors varies even among people within the same group. As with all factors influencing health and illness, the nurse must avoid stereotyping individuals because of their age, race, religion, etc. Effective nursing care requires the nurse to attend to individual differences.

Culture, Race, and Ethnicity

Terms such as culture, race, and ethnicity are often used interchangeably when reporting health and illness data. However, each factor may contribute differently to one's health status.

CULTURE

Culture is a learned set of shared perceptions about beliefs, values, and norms that affect the behaviors of a relatively large group of people (Lustig and Koester, 1993). Culture exists in the minds of people and affects behavior. Definitions of health and illness are part of a culture. Response to illness is a part of culture. Preferred treatments for illness are part of a culture. The differences in caring behaviors across cultures are discussed in Chapter 11.

RACE

Race refers to a genetic or biologically based similarity among people, which is distinguishable and unique and functions to mark or separate people from one another (Lustig and Koester, 1993). It is a more encompassing term than either culture or ethnicity. Although race may initially separate people into categories, culture is a more powerful factor in creating more homogeneous groups. For example, people from Germany, Great Britain, Norway, and the United States may all be members of the white race. Yet their cultures are distinctly different. The same is true for people from Africa, South America, and the Caribbean. They may all be members of the black race, yet their cultures are different and are their primary source of identification.

Race influences health and illness from a genetic standpoint. Sickle cell anemia is often cited as a genetic factor among blacks (Miller, 1990).

The incidence of other diseases also varies by race. However, it is very difficult to separate the impact of cultural, economic, social factors, and access to health services from the impact of genetics.

The higher mortality rates from cancer for African-Americans illustrate this difficulty (Powe, 1996). African-Americans are 1.3 times more likely to die of cancer when compared with the general population. Cancer is a disease in which mortality rates can be decreased through the use of health-promoting behaviors such as routine screening for tumors (mammography and Pap smear) and avoiding smoking. African-Americans tend not to participate in cancer screening programs. Research links poverty, poor access to care, undereducation, and a lack of knowledge about cancer to failure to participate in cancer screening programs. However, even when these factors are accounted for, African-Americans are still less likely to participate in cancer screening programs. Why? One potential answer is the presence of cancer fatalism. *Cancer fatalism* is defined as the belief that death is inevitable when cancer is present. It is thought to be the result of cultural, historical, and socioeconomic factors that have influenced the lived experiences of African-Americans. Over time people experience hopelessness, powerlessness, and social isolation to the point that they believe there is no way out of the cycle of cancer and death.

For the nurse to intervene effectively, attention must be given to all the factors that influence health and illness and to how they interact with each other to further influence health and illness. For example, if cancer fatalism is a factor in the high incidence of cancer deaths among African-Americans, nurses will need to address that belief in addition to offering screening programs or health education programs.

ETHNICITY

Ethnicity is a term used to refer to a wide variety of groups who might share a language, historical origins, religion, identification with a common nation-state, or cultural system (Lustig and Koester, 1993). In the United States many people still identify with the ethnic background of their ancestors. A person may give a self-description of being Norwegian or Swedish when in fact the person is really part of the Euroamerican culture in the United States. The wars in Bosnia have made us all aware of the three major ethnic groups (Slovaks, Croatians, and Serbians), each with a distinct culture, that live in the area once called Yugoslavia.

Ethnicity can affect health and illness in the same way that culture does. To the extent that ethnic identification exists in one's mind, it influences behavior, including behavior associated with health and illness. For example, ethnic identity may include religious beliefs identifying illness as a punishment from *God*. The individual may avoid medical treatment, believing that *God* will cure the illness when he or she has been adequately punished.

Health Outcomes and Culture, Race, and Ethnicity

Race, culture, and ethnicity influence health outcomes in complex, interactive ways. The challenge to health care providers is using this knowledge to improve health outcomes for minority groups within the population. The challenge becomes more intense when viewed in terms of the changing demographics and health status trends.

HEALTH OUTCOMES

The following statistics are reported in *Health, United States, 1996–97* (Public Health Service Centers for Disease Control and Prevention and National Center for Health Statistics, 1997):

- During the period 1990 through 1995 the infant mortality rate for black infants was 2.4 times the rate for white infants.
- In 1995 life expectancy at birth was 8.2 years longer for white males than for black males and 5.7 years longer for white females than black females.
- Death rates for American Indian males age 25 to 34 was about 60 percent higher than for white males and for American Indian females was 85 percent higher than for white females.
- Overall mortality for Hispanic Americans was about 20 percent lower than for non-Hispanic white Americans.
- Compared with white Americans, heart disease mortality was 41 percent lower for Asian Americans and 49 percent higher for black Americans in 1995.

THE CHANGING POPULATION PROFILE

The demographic contrasts between 1990 and 2000 will be dramatic. The Hispanic and Asian and Pacific Islander populations in the United States have been increasing more rapidly than the total U.S. population. Between 1980 and 1992, the Hispanic population increased by 65 percent to 24.2 million persons, and the Asian and Pacific Islander population more than doubled to 8.4 million persons. Between 1980 and 1992, the total U.S. population grew by 13 percent to 255 million persons (Public Health Service Centers for Disease Control and Prevention and National Center for Health Statistics, 1995).

By the year 2000, the racial and ethnic composition of the American population will form a different pattern. Whites, not including Hispanic-Americans, will represent a smaller proportion of the total, declining from 76 to 72 percent of the population. One particularly fast-growing population group will be Hispanics. Some estimates forecast a rise from 8 to 11.3 percent, to more than 31 million Hispanic people by 2000. Blacks will increase their proportion from 12.4 to 13.1 percent. Other racial groups, including American Indians and Alaska Natives and Asians and Pacific Islanders, will increase from 3.5 to 4.3 percent of the total (U.S. Department of Health and Human Services, 1991).

- Currently, Hawaii is the only state where non-Hispanic whites are in the minority. In the near future, this will be the case for New Mexico, Texas, and California as well.

Culturally Based Health Beliefs

It is important to remember that health practices and beliefs vary within a given culture just as they vary from culture to culture. A nurse can never assume health beliefs and practices from a person's race, culture, or ethnic identification. The nurse must be sensitive to and value the unique health beliefs of every individual. The nurse should never base clinical decisions on stereotypes.

Furthermore, in the United States there is the tendency to view Western medicine as superior to other approaches. The nurse must understand that the belief in Western medicine held by many Americans is similar to the belief in other theories of health and illness held by people of other cultures.

THE LATINO/CHICANO PERSPECTIVE

The material that follows describes the perceptions of illness for a diverse group of people known nationally as Latinos. This group is sometimes referred to as Hispanics, Spanish-Americans, Latin-Americans, Mexican Americans, Chicanos, or Boriqua. There are similarities and differences in perceptions of illness among these groups. The example provided in Box 6–3 refers to a Chicano folk health practice. It was selected because the Chicanos are the largest group of Spanish-speaking people in the United States and they have had a large influence on the culture in the Southwestern United States.

The basis for the folk health beliefs and practices of the Latino/Chicano family is the concept of equilibrium—a balance between humana and nature. A person is seen as a being whose health and welfare are guided by the maintenance of a balance between the natural and supernatural worlds. A loss of this balance or equilibrium is considered to be the basis for illness (Dorsey and Jackson, 1976).

Mal Ojo is one such disease. It results from the influence of someone outside the family, or extended family, on a person (Dorsey and Jackson, 1976). This influence is seen in terms of a desire, or envy of the victim, or another similar imbalance of the relationship between the victim and the intruder. Most often, as a consequence of unspoken emotions, there exists a mystical or psychological interplay in this condition. Children

BOX 6–3
ILLUSTRATION OF MAL OJO—A DISEASE CAUSED BY A DISRUPTION IN THE BALANCE BETWEEN A PERSON AND NATURE

It was a cool summer evening when baby Adrian suddenly became restless, feverish, and refused to eat at all. Similar symptoms were present the following day, and his parents began to trace activities of the week.

One incident that stuck out in their minds was a situation that occurred while purchasing their new car. Adrian's parents noticed that an older Anglo couple had been admiring the child. They further recalled that although the couple talked about him and smiled at him, they never touched him. With the fear that he might have been given ojo, the family took Adrian to his grandmother; she would know. Sra. H. visited her grandchild, and the diagnosis was confirmed.

That evening family members were called together as she prayed over Adrian. They were involved in the healing by their prayers and their presence. She then took an egg, and, as she prayed, she passed it over his body three times, stopping at his forehead and lips to make the sign of the cross. More prayers were recited and responses given. Sra. H. then lifted her grandson and passed him over a candle that lay on the floor, three times in circular motions. At the same time she prayed in inaudible words.

One hour later, the egg was cracked into a bowl of water, and the bowl was placed under a crib. The child was massaged and laid in the crib to sleep.

In the morning, his mother went to the crib and checked her child. Though he was restless and weak, his fever had broken. Beneath the crib, in the bowl, was a semi-poached egg that had taken the form of an eye. Sra. H. was called back to remove the egg and the diagnosis was confirmed. Her explanation to the authors was that, by some process, the fever was drawn into the water and cooked the egg.

are most frequently affected. An example of Mal Ojo is presented in Box 6–3.

CHINESE SYSTEM OF MEDICINE

Chinese medicine includes the following (in their order of importance): philosophy, meditation, nutrition, martial arts, herbology, acumassage, acupressure, moxibustion, acupuncture, and even spiritual healing (Chow, 1976). The Chinese emphasize prevention, in contrast to Western medicine, which emphasizes crisis intervention.

The theoretical and philosophical base of Chinese medicine is derived from the Taoist religion (the Right Way), with its concept that nature maintains a balance in all things. The human is seen as a microcosm within a macrocosm; the energy in humans interrelates with the energy of the universe. Chi (energy) and Jing (sexual energy) are both vital life energies. They are kept in balance by the dual polarities of Yin and Yang. Yin is described as negative, dark, cold, and feminine, and Yang is positive, light, warm, and masculine. Whatever the terminology, there must be a balance of both positive and negative polarities. This balance is illustrated in a Western context by the following example. A woman primarily produces female sex hormones, but a small proportion of male sex hormones are also produced within her system. The reverse applies to men. This delicate balance of Yin and Yang results in health; the imbalance or disturbance of this energy balance may result in disease (dis-ease). Likewise, if the hormones are in perfect balance, the person is normal, but if there is a disturbance in this hormonal balance, dis-ease or dys-function occurs.

The theory of energy balance in Chinese medicine may also be compared with the theories of immunologic competency or incompetence in Western medicine. According to Chinese medicine, most conditions are caused by an imbalance in energy resulting from a wrong diet or strong emotional feelings; therefore, bodily functions may be brought back into harmony through the application of self-restraint and through the use of certain organisms that can be controlled; the person uses them to maintain a balanced state, thus countering forces that result from immoderation. The balance of energy Chi (Yin and Yang) means that the immunity of the body is in a healthy condition. If there is an imbalance of the Yin and Yang, then the immunity of the body is disturbed, and the body is likely to be susceptible to disease or bacteria.

A further concept of Chinese medicine is that the universe and humana are susceptible to the laws of the five elements: fire, earth, metal, water, and wood. Body and mind are integrated: They are never separated. The five elements are reflected in different organs and parts of the body. Every organ of the body encompasses the properties of taste, emotion, sound, odor, season, climate, power, and fortification of other structures of the body. This cycle is a destructive as well as a constructive one, with each element having some effect on the others (Chow, 1976).

ANOTHER PERSPECTIVE

Box 6–4 details the partnership of the state of Hawaii Department of Health's Community Health Nursing Division and ethnic/cultural healers and scholars.

Clinical Decision Making

Do race and ethnicity influence perceptions of health care providers? How do practitioners construct and utilize race and ethnicity? Should the practice of racial and ethnic identification in patient care situations be discontinued?

These and related questions were addressed in a research study that included survey and interview data from 169 nurse practitioners and health care professionals (Moscou, 1995). The findings from that study are presented in the Current Controversy box.

BOX 6-4

ETHNIC HEALERS AND SCHOLARS

Laura J. Armstrong, EdD, MPH, RN
Chief Community Health Nursing Division
Hawaii Department of Health
June Shibuya, RN, MSN, NP
Malama Project Coordinator

As professional nurses approach the millennium, our values in the practice of nursing must shift to accommodate new models of care delivery, and we must recognize that we are guests in communities that we work in. We are not the experts. Public Health Nurses have long stated that the individuals, families, and communities are our clients. This is passe!! Our communities, individuals, and families are our experts, because they know what their wants and needs are. Our role in working with families and communities is to work hand in hand in partnership with them to strengthen their capacity for self-sufficiency and to support their efforts to create healthy choices for healthy outcomes. We as nurses must be humble and demonstrate humility as we work with families and communities. There is a time to exchange expertise between the professionals, our families, and communities. Respect must be given to both.

The State of Hawaii Department of Health's Community Health Nursing Division strongly fosters changes in the health care delivery system that affords all people and communities access to care that involves choices, is culturally appropriate, and is coordinated with and responsive to the needs of the community. Hawaii's Malama Na Wahine Hapai Project designated "Caring for Pregnant Women," Research Project (R18NR02678), was designed to evaluate innovative interventions for providing effective prenatal care service in the rural area of Hilo-Puna on the island of Hawaii during 1990 through 1995. We learned that partnerships with ethnic healers and scholars are a vital part of care delivery, along with the community outreach women, who knew their community, provided their wisdom and expertise, and reinforced the cultural beliefs and values held by the pregnant women and their families. Other true partnerships with local businesses (e.g., KTA Super Stores) and service organizations (e.g., Kiwanis International, Exchange Club, Jr. Jaycees) and with Hawaiian organizations also led to positive outcome measures and fostered community ownership of prenatal care.

Communities recognize that ethnic/cultural healers and scholars are designated to be the guardians of knowledge regarding health and illness. They are seen as the gatekeepers of traditional values, beliefs, customs, and practices in today's world, they promote positive awareness in their people's life and heritage, and they provide the wisdom and the "spiritual" way for many families to be able to cope with illnesses or disease, especially when families lose confidence in or are confused by the health care system.

The following stories illustrate the findings of the Malama Na Wahine Hapai Project. The first story was related to the Malama Project Coordinator by Bishop Okimura, a Buddhist Priest (Odaisan) in Honomu, a rural community on the island of Hawaii.

Delivery of the first child of a third-generation Japanese-American couple was imminent. The wife was having a difficult labor and the husband sensed that the medical staff were concerned. The husband felt very helpless as he observed his wife's difficulty. Because of fear for his wife, he turned to the most basic part of his being . . . "spirituality," the core of his culture, because he felt that there was nowhere else to go. He remembered his parents and grandparents carrying amulets (omamori) to ward off bad spirits. In desperation, he called his mother for advice and she suggested visiting the Odiasan for assistance, which he quickly did.

The Odaisan prayed for the child's birth through a formal ritual and gave the husband an omamori, which is similar to the Catholic St. Christopher medallion. The Odaisan instructed the man to give the omamori to his wife and tell her that it was blessed with unending, infinite strength of the universe and that this would be her source of strength. The Odaisan also instructed the husband to tell her that when she was instructed to push by the doctor, she was to crush the omamori in her hand and yell as loudly as possible because this would help in "sliding the baby out like a baby in slippery oil sliding out." The Odaisan gave permission for the man to have his wife yell out, which is not part of what Japanese people are comfortable in doing, especially in public. The Odaisan provided a cognitive rehearsal for this couple, using metaphors that the wife could visualize and quickly master. These instructions were followed because the woman believed in the Odaisan and his authority, and that the omamori was blessed with special powers. The husband said that when he placed the omamori in his wife's hand, her contractions became regular and strong, so that when it was time to push, she did so without instructions from the medical team because it was her body and she knew how to respond. A healthy baby was delivered.

This Japanese couple gained mastery over the birth of the baby through the Odaisan's guided imagery, the use of a metaphor, and the belief that this was the last resort. They were very grateful to the Odaisan, whom they credit for bringing their sense of self and self-esteem to a higher level. When the infant was 33 days old, the baby was allowed to leave the house (rites of passage) and be within the community. This Japanese family took their baby for a special Buddhist baby blessing. They believed that this would safeguard the baby for at least the first year in life.

The second story is told by Debbie Fujimoto, Executive Secretary with the KTA Super Stores in Hawaii, who is also a Malama client as well as Neighborhood Woman with the Malama Project on the island of Hawaii.

My second child, Deena, was five months old. Up until now, she had been a very easy baby. We felt comfort-

continued on next page

BOX 6-4 (cont'd)
ETHNIC HEALERS AND SCHOLARS

continued from previous page

able taking her everywhere, including our son's t-ball practices and games.

One day, at t-ball practice, I noticed that about one hour after she had her bottle of breast milk, she started screaming in pain. It was a different kind of crying, one that I hadn't heard from Deena before. The cycle continued throughout the night—drink from the bottle, wait an hour, and the crying would begin. She cried for about 10 to 15 minutes each time, then settled down. The next day, I called the pediatrician's office and made an appointment. The only time that he had available was after lunch. I explained the situation to my babysitter, and she said it sounded like "huli stomach." At lunch, my girlfriend asked how Deena was doing so I told her what the sitter said. She shared that she also took her two sons to Aunty Mary Fragas, a Native Hawaiian healer, when they had "huli stomach." She insisted that I take Deena to see her.

I left for the doctor's office and while I was there, my girlfriend called telling me to go straight to Aunty Mary's after the doctor's office. The doctor looked at Deena, couldn't find anything wrong with her, stuck a bag on her to catch her urine, and told me to go to the hospital to get blood tests. Instead of going to the hospital, I went to Aunty Mary's. I felt so helpless and I didn't want to have my daughter poked and prodded.

When we got to Aunty Mary's, Deena was screaming again. Aunty Mary gently massaged her tummy and asked if we flew on an airplane or took long, bumpy rides with Deena. I explained that I had given birth in Honolulu and after two weeks brought Deena home to Hilo. Both baby and I commute at least for 1 hour a day from home to the sitters, to work and back. Aunty Mary explained that Deena had "huli stomach," a condition in which a baby's intestines get tangled and the food cannot pass. She explained that bumps, whether air pockets or potholes, feel much bigger to babies. The babies gasp and jerk, which tends to tangle the intestines. To prevent this, we should therefore bind the baby with a soft cloth like a diaper. Aunty Mary massaged, or provided "lomi lomi," to Deena. Deena let out a sigh of relief and fell asleep. She slept the entire way home. I knew that Deena was relaxed and felt much better. In the early evening, she took her bottle and didn't cry. Later, the cycle started again, but this was not as severe as before.

The doctor's office called me the next day to find out if we went to get the blood tests. I told her that I didn't and that I took Deena to Aunty Mary. I heard a disappointing sigh from the doctor. She asked how Deena was and I told her she was resting. The doctor said that if Deena starts up again to call her and bring her in. I took Deena back to Aunty Mary again the next day because the binding came loose and she started the painful crying again. Aunty Mary massaged Deena and she once again sighed and fell asleep. This "huli stomach" has not occurred since that time.

I take my three children to get their immunizations and check-ups with the doctor and when they come down with colds. However, I know that there are times when modern medicine cannot be the answer to all health problems.

Aunty Mary also helped my husband David with a twisted shoulder that the doctors treated with pain killers instead of finding out the cause. Aunty Mary is a gifted healer!

As nurses, we need to know that cultural scholars are in all communities and are sought for their healing regardless of the provision of western medicine. Nurses must recognize that our clinical training must be augmented by the incorporation of traditional religious and cultural beliefs of families if we are to be partners as they maximize their well being.

Alternative Medicine

Many options are available in today's health care system. Western medicine can now be complemented or replaced with new choices of therapies learned from other cultures. Many of the alternative therapies reflect Eastern thought with the notion of health as a matter of living in harmony and balance in all areas of life. Three such options are presented as illustrative of those available.

CHINESE MEDICINE

The philosophy of Chinese medicine has already been described. The following therapies are used:

- **Herbs**, any natural material of a plant, animal, or mineral origin, or any traditional or modern preparation of natural materials short of preparing an isolated chemical (Collinge, 1996). Herbs are used to introduce certain qualities or influences into the body to balance or harmonize its dynamics.
- **Acupuncture**, the insertion of thin, sterile, stainless steel needles into points on the surface of the body to a depth just below the surface of the skin (Collinge, 1996). The diagnosis and goals of treatment determine the points used.
- **Acupressure and Shiatsu**, variations of massage technique in which a similar geography of points and meridians is used to guide the application of finger pressure rather than the insertion of needles (Collinge, 1996).
- **Chi Kung**, a form of martial arts that emphasizes meditation, relaxation, visualization, movement, postures, and breathing exercises (Collinge, 1996). These practices are designed to strengthen and direct the flow of *Chi* through the body.

CURRENT CONTROVERSY

DO RACE AND ETHNICITY INFLUENCE PERCEPTIONS OF HEALTH CARE PRACTITIONERS?

Susan Elizabeth Moscou, master's thesis, submitted to the Faculty, Yale University School of Nursing, May 1995

The study's findings suggest:

- Health care practitioners often construct race and ethnicity within a **social** context rather than a **scientific** framework which is the commonly stated reason for inclusion.
- Race and ethnicity serve as "social" markers for class, health beliefs, culture, religion, compliance, risk behaviors, and risk factors.
- Racial and ethnic identification largely rests on subjective and arbitrary indicators such as skin color, appearance, hair texture, the patient's spoken language or accent, and general assumptions based upon last names, family members, and other health care practitioner's assessments.
- Race and ethnicity do influence perceptions of health care practitioners and that race and ethnicity impact health care strategies, patient care, treatment regimens, and professional relationships.

On the basis of the data collected, the researcher raises this question.

The blurring of scientific knowledge with perceptions of class, patient behavior, risk factors, and culture make it difficult to presume that health care practitioners always have the objectivity needed to make a clinical diagnosis without some prejudicial thinking. **If race and ethnicity lead one to consider a relatively narrow set of choices, how many diagnoses and treatment options are immediately ruled out because the practitioner holds existing beliefs about the patient's race or ethnicity (p. 135)?**

The researcher challenges us to question common assumptions/stereotypes.

Several health care professionals maintained that race and ethnicity are inconsequential variables in the clinical decision making process and actually are often detrimental because race and ethnicity come with their own set of assumptions. These preformed notions, more often than not, reduce the decision-making focus to "cookbook" health care, a methodology that often fails the patient and the health care provider. **Additionally, practicing medicine or nursing in this manner enables conceptions about race and ethnicity to operate without an analysis of societal or institutional racism as the potential root cause of disease prevalence in specific racial and ethnic groups. The failure to consider the role of racism and its impact on morbidity and mortality statistics permits health care practitioners to comfortably accept genetic explanations as the cause of their patients' disease (p. 141).**

AYURVEDA

One of the four main branches of knowledge comprising the Hindu philosophical and spiritual texts called the *Vedas* is Ayurveda. Ayurveda is the science that deals with physical healing, diet, herbs, and massage or bodyworks. It may well be the oldest system of natural healing and the common root of many more modern medical traditions. Its methods are noninvasive, nontoxic, and dependent on the willingness to participate in a healthier lifestyle (Collinge, 1996).

Ayurveda is built on the concept of vital energy called *prana,* a primal energy that enlivens the body and mind. A second key principle is the belief that all of existence comprises five basic elements: earth, air, fire, water, and ether. At conception, these five elements are organized within us in patterns that last a lifetime. The organization is called a person's *prakriti.* The elements are organized into three doshas: ether and air *(vata),* fire and water *(pitta),* and earth and water *(kapha).*

Health is a state of balance of forces within the person and between the person and the environment.

Health requires persons to live in accord with their prakriti. Treatment procedures include:

- **Dietary guidance,** a diet tailored to the person's constitutional type or to pacify a dosha.
- **Rasayanas,** a herbal regimen to help balance the doshas or a behavioral regimen with specific lifestyle changes. In the latter category are yoga, meditation, and breathing exercises.
- **Massage,** the use of touch and oils at specific points on the body.
- **Panchakarma,** an intensive detoxification process that includes massage with special herbs.
- **Chronotherapy,** bringing one's daily activity pattern into line with one's natural body rhythms and cycles.

NATUROPATHIC MEDICINE

The unifying philosophy of naturopathy is contained in the following six principles:

1. Use the healing power of nature.
2. Treat the whole person.
3. First do no harm.
4. Identify and treat the cause.
5. The best cure is prevention.
6. The doctor must be a teacher (Collinge, 1996).

The training of naturopathic physicians is similar to that of allopathic (conventional) physicians. The two differ in philosophy of health and illness and types of treatments used.

Naturopathic treatment modalities include:

- clinical nutrition
- physical medicine, including therapeutic manipulation of the muscles, bones, and spine; massage therapy; ultrasound; hydrotherapy; and diathermy
- homeopathy, natural substances used to strengthen the body's vital force
- botanical medicine, the medicinal use of herbs
- natural childbirth
- Chinese medicine
- Ayurveda
- psychological counseling and therapy
- environmental medicine, detoxification, and immune restoration
- minor surgery with local anesthetic

Families

Nursing practice is as appropriately directed toward families as it is toward individuals. Individuals cannot be defined by using "one-size-fits-all" labels; they come with personal meanings, dreams, beliefs, values, attitudes, and behaviors, most of which were learned first in their families of origin and which continue to be influenced profoundly by both their past and present families. Individuals come with affective bonds to persons they define as family, and who are in relationship to them in enduring ways. At a minimum, beliefs and attitudes about what constitutes physical, emotional, and psychological health, and behaviors that impact on health, including nutrition, exercise, and stress management, are learned and reinforced in families. The power of families and the transgenerational patterns transmitted through families are substantial; family influence, past and present, can significantly enhance or inhibit healthy life changes, regardless of how urgently they may be needed (Doherty and McCubbin, 1985; Pratt, 1976).

In addition, families play significant and substantive roles in health and illness care decision making and delivery (Doherty, 1985; Doherty and Campbell, 1988). In fact, families provide the vast majority of all health and illness care delivered to individuals. Although in some cases this responsibility is perceived as a burden by families, in far more instances family involvement is the choice of both the individual and his or her family.

Families impact the experience of individual family members, but the family unit also is affected when a member has a health problem (Gilliss, 1993). A change in one family member affects all members, sometimes in ways that change the family unit forever. A diagnosis of a life-threatening disease in a member or a profound life change to a more healthy way of living can cause significant reverberations throughout family systems (Brown and Powell-Cope, 1991; Clarke-Steffen, 1993; Deatrick et al, 1988; Mishel and Murdaugh, 1987).

It is important to emphasize that family roles in health and illness are not limited to caring for seriously ill family members. Much of what safeguards and promotes health is related to nutrition, exercise, and stress management. It follows that the family that supplies food, supports patterns of daily activity, and provides emotional sustenance for family members can be a major force for health (Bomar, 1990; Gilliss, 1989; Turk and Kerns, 1985).

Historically, family roles in health and illness care have been overlooked or minimized in the United States, where medical management and hospitalization have been used liberally and with little or no appreciation for individual and family preferences. However, this picture has been changing over the last 40 years, beginning with lay advocacy efforts. First, parents of young children demanded to stay overnight with their children during hospitalizations. Then pregnant women insisted that fathers and other significant persons had a right to be present in delivery rooms. Persons who were dying began to seek out hospice programs that allowed them to stay at home with their family members, who would continue to be their primary caregivers. And today it is even possible to find articles in medical and nursing journals debating whether families should be present during resuscitation (Redley and Hood, 1996).

Attention to family involvement in care has accelerated with the advent of managed care and other cost management programs. Attention to cost control has shifted illness care from hospitals and emergency rooms to lower cost primary care settings and to homes. Family members who once were ignored or even looked down upon now are depended on for medical and nursing management in the home, from triage-type decision making when some child falls and is injured while rollerblading, to provision of highly technical and complex care in the home.

Some would say it has never been acceptable to ignore or minimize families in health care, and the best of clinicians never did. In today's health care arena, at a minimum it would be inappropriate to exclude families, without compelling legitimate reasons.

FAMILY DEFINITIONS

Definition of what constitutes a family can be controversial and even dangerous. Definitions of families set boundaries of who is included and who is excluded. Legal definitions usually focus on recognized ties of blood, marriage, and adoption. For example, in 1953 Burgess and Locke wrote that "The family is a group of persons united by ties of marriage, blood, or adoption, constituting a single household; interacting and communicating with each other in their respective social roles of husband and wife, mother and father, son and daughter, brother and sister; and creating and maintaining a common culture (pp. 7–8)." Even in 1953 many families did not fit that definition, and today there is considerably more diversity in family structures, including single-parent families, blended families, multi-adult households, communal groups with children, and cohabitating partners, both heterosexual and homosexual.

In 1985, the Department of Family Nursing, Oregon Health Sciences University School of Nursing, recognized this diversity across families. The departmental faculty adopted the following definition of family for use in their teaching, research, and practice activities: "The family is a social system composed of two or more persons who coexist within the context of some expectations of reciprocal affection, mutual responsibility, and temporal duration. The family is characterized by commitment, mutual decision making and shared goals." This definition emphasized emotional commitment, rather than legal ties, and gave latitude for families in which expectations did not match reality.

In practice, nurses who have a family perspective tend to use whatever definition of family is given by an individual client. In effect then, an individual's family is whoever he or she says it is. Although this is both pragmatic and appropriate in many, if not most, situations, in some practice arenas it is inadequate. For example, a state's legal definition of family may be evoked when child custody is in contest, when end-of-life decision making is needed, or when permission to treat a minor or an incapacitated adult is sought.

Every nurse has a personal definition of family, which he or she has internalized. It is important to know that definition, to understand what it means in relationship to practice, and to appreciate how it can impact practice. The issue here is not whether the personal definition is "right" or "good." The issue is how that definition may come into play in practice settings in ways that can influence care and healing. For example, if a nurse has a strong belief in the importance of marriage to create a family, he or she may find practice in a birth setting serving a high percentage of unmarried women to be stressful. A nurse who values equal partnerships in committed adult relationships may find himself or herself feeling anger toward a woman who refuses to enroll in a much needed health promotion program because she doesn't want to inconvenience her partner. Examining one's personal definitions and the values they represent is a necessary step in family nursing practice.

PURPOSE OF THE FAMILY

The purpose of the family has changed over time. Traditionally the purpose of the family was to provide its members with economic survival, values and religion, education, social status, and protection from extrinsic threats. Today, in the United States and much of the Western world, these functions are no longer based in the family for much of the population. Research has found that the primary purpose of families today is to meet the relational needs of individual family members, including love, intimacy, self-acceptance, nurturance, caring, and individuation, and needs to give and be given to, to share the joys of posterity, and to have support through adversity (Curran, 1983, 1985). Terkelson (1980) wrote that the purpose of the family is to create a nurturing environment to assure physical survival and personal development for all members. Given the high expectations this purpose evokes, he added that a "good enough family" was one who met most of the needs of most of its members most of the time, putting the goal in reach of many families.

Acceptance of the importance of relational needs and of individual development over the collective needs of the family is pervasive in the predominant culture. The emotional health of individuals is tied closely to the perceived healthy functioning of their families. It follows then that nurses who are concerned with holistic health must be aware of the pervasive and persistent interactions between individuals and their families.

FAMILY TRANSITIONS

Transitions or times of significant change in an individual's life are impacted by and impact family life. Normative transitions, or developmental transitions, occur in a majority of families, and include birth of a child, end of childhood, marriage, and retirement. Because these transitions are considered to be "normal," the fact that they are not necessarily easy to navigate often is ignored or minimized. In fact, assisting families to anticipate and cope with normative transitions can be a significant health promotion activity. Prenatal education programs and transition to parenting courses are examples of how health promotion for families has been integrated into health programming.

Situational transitions are those transitions that occur frequently, but not universally, across families. Examples include miscarriages; marital or couple separation and divorce, whether legal or emotional; significant changes in socioeconomic status; and extrinsic catastrophes, such as floods, war, and fires, which often result in dislocation of the family unit. Illness, death, and disability may also fit here, depending on factors such as the timing and meaning of the event. For example, a family may not experience as the same both the long expected death of a 93-year-old grandfather and the sudden, unexpected death, a week later, of his 5-year-old great-grandson.

Nursing of families requires knowledge of transitions and their impact on individuals and families. Such knowledge, provided to families with sensitivity to content, timing, and mode of delivery, can help families make healthy choices in how they move through the transition.

Nurse researchers have focused attention on family transitions around illness. The three examples that follow illustrate the differences and commonalities across stages of family life.

Clarke-Steffen (1993a, 1993b) studied the experience of families during the period immediately preceding and following the diagnosis of cancer in a child. She found that "waiting and not knowing" was the most distressing aspect for family members during this transition, and that this experience was characterized by uncertainty, worry and preoccupation, and feelings of vulnerability and helplessness (1993a). She developed a model of family transition to living with childhood cancer (1993b) that demonstrated how a diagnosis of childhood cancer affected both each family member and structure and functioning of the family as a whole. Her study findings suggested that nursing care should include attention directed not only toward the child and parent, but also to all family members, both individually and as a unit. And, when possible, information about what is happening and what will happen should be shared to help decrease ambiguity and uncertainty.

In a second example, Brown and Powell-Cope (1991) examined AIDS family caregiving and had similar findings about the roles uncertainty played in the difficulties family members experienced as caregivers. Based on their findings, the nurse researchers defined uncertainty as "the caregiver's inability to predict future events and outcomes and the lack of confidence in making day-to-day decisions about the ill person's care" (p. 340). Again, attention to family members' needs, especially information needs, was indicated.

A third example is Mishel and Murdaugh's study (1987) that examined family adjustment to heart transplantation. They found that family members developed strategies, including modifying attitudes and beliefs, to learn to live with the continual unpredictability that came with a new heart. They needed considerable support to make the internal changes necessary.

FAMILY NEEDS

Families want and need health-related information about their family members and about family health. They want accurate, complete information about health issues, management options, care delivery, and expected trajectories. They want to know what to do to help, both now and in the future. They want expert information, research-based, and they want it in ways they can use it (Brown and Powell-Cope, 1991; Chesla, 1996; Clarke-Steffen, 1993a).

Families also want and need support in their roles as family members and their experiences related to health and illness of members. They need their experiences and their own healing capacities recognized and validated (Chesla, 1996).

NURSING AND FAMILIES

Nursing of families, or family nursing, may occur (1) when the individual is the focus of care, (2) when the family is the focus of care, or (3) when both the family and individual are the focus of care. When individuals are the focus of practice, families are the context for family nursing (Wright and Leahey, 1993). The nurse acknowledges the roles of families, whether or not family members are physically present or acknowledged by an individual during a clinical encounter.

For example, a nurse working with a new mother who is learning to breast-feed her infant may focus only on skill acquisition. However, research suggests that family members, particularly the father of the infant and the maternal grandmother, can be significant in the mother's ability to feel and be successful. A family nursing intervention probes for how family members are responding to the new mother's effort, and suggests ways to enhance that support or mitigate negative effects.

When families are the focus of care, the nurse attends to the experience of family members when another member has health needs. For example, a 75-year-old man has had a heart attack in the grocery store and is hospitalized in a cardiac critical care unit at the local hospital. His wife of 50 years hurries to the hospital to see him; the last time she saw him was when he was getting into the car to go to the store; he has never been hospitalized. Now she sees him in a bed with rails keeping her from him, with tubes and monitors and sounds that further separate them. A family nursing intervention might be to walk with the woman to her husband's side, provide a chair next to the bed, lower the bed, take his hand out from under the sheet, and place her hand over his. All the while the nurse might be speaking reassuringly about what is happening, what his wife might expect, what she might do to make contact. What the nurse is doing is recognizing and reinforcing the wife's preeminent position in her husband's world, providing perspective for the wife about what is happening, and showing her how she can be emotionally and physically present for her husband. The nurse's attention to the wife is grounded in an understanding that the wife can play a significant role in her husband's healing and that role must be recognized and supported (Chesla, 1996).

When both the individual and the family are foci of nursing, attention is paid to interactions between and among the family members. Nursing interventions then focus on supporting healthy interactions and encouraging connection when appropriate.

Expert nursing practice is characterized by an emphasis on all three ways of doing family nursing, with the context of the nurse-client-family interaction determining what is in the foreground of practice and what is in the background in any given instance.

LEVELS OF FAMILY-CENTERED CARE

Doherty and Baird (1986) identified five levels in family-centered medical care. Gilliss and colleagues (1989) modified their work to make it applicable for nursing. In this conception of family care, the first level is characterized by a minimal emphasis on the family. Some family-oriented nurses joke that in this level families are seen and heard—rarely, and are tolerated—barely. Families are perceived to get in the way of "real" nursing care, they "upset" the patient and staff, and their only value is to assure compliance of the patient with a medical regimen when the patient is not in a health care setting. Families are not recognized as part of the nurse's responsibility in level one care. All a nurse would need is some common sense to manage family members; it doesn't take much to keep them quiet and out of the way.

Clinical example: Laura Green and Sarah, her 12-year-old daughter, rush to a large teaching hospital in the Midwest after being called with the news that their 45-year-old husband and father, Joseph, has had a heart attack. When Mrs. Green and Sarah reach the cardiac care unit, they are greeted by a nurse who says, in a manner that suggests this is a speech she has given many times: "You just missed the visiting period; you'll have to wait an hour to see the patient. By they way, children are not allowed in the unit. You can wait in the family waiting room over there; I'll page the doctor and he can answer your questions."

The second level of family care is the provision of ongoing medical information and advice. At this level it is assumed that families have a right to information and assistance as they relate to the patient's needs. To practice at this level, the nurse needs to have sufficient medical and nursing knowledge to provide families with accurate and appropriate information and advice. A minimal requirement here is that the nurse have an openness to engage patients and families in a collaborative way.

A half hour later, a nurse comes into the waiting room and sits next to Mrs. Green and Sarah. "I am Mr. Green's CCU nurse and I have been with him since he came into the unit. I thought you would like to know how he is doing." The nurse explains briefly what is happening medically, and asks if either Mrs. Green or Sarah has any questions. She listens carefully to their questions and concerns, and, in answer, explains what the next day or so will look like, if things continue as they have been going.

The third level of family care focuses on the nurse's ability to recognize family feelings around health issues and to provide appropriate support. The nurse practicing at this level needs to have knowledge of normal family development and family reactions to stress. He or she engages family members in a discussion of their feelings and reactions, and encourages them in their coping efforts. Level three family care also requires the nurse to be aware of his or her own feelings around the patient and family, so that the nurse's feelings do not inhibit therapeutic interventions.

After talking with the cardiologist and seeing her husband for a brief visit, Mrs. Green is sitting with Sarah in the waiting room. Both are crying. The hospital's cardiac care clinical nurse specialist comes in and introduces herself. She sits quietly with them for a few minutes, and then begins to ask questions designed to elicit their feelings and concerns about what has happened, along with clues to guide how she might help this particular family cope with the sudden change in their life. She learns that Mr. Green's mother lives in a nearby suburb. He is her only child; she is very frail and will be deeply distressed by what has happened. Mrs. Green doesn't know how to tell her. The clinical nurse specialist offers some suggestions tailored to the data she has received about and from this family. She also offers to call Mr. Green's mother after she is told, to see if his mother has questions.

The fourth level of family care focuses on systematic assessment and planned intervention around family issues. Knowledge of family systems and awareness of one's own participation in systems are critical to function at this level. The nurse meets with the family to plan for the health of all members, emphasizing their ability to collaborate for the health and well-being of all members.

Mr. Green steadily improves and nears discharge. He will need to make significant changes in his life if he is to continue to recover and prevent further cardiovascular problems. The clinical nurse specialist arranges to meet with the family, including Mr. Green's mother if they wish, to talk about the changes that will be required and how they will impact each member of the family. She is prepared with suggestions to maximize their success.

The fifth level of family care is family therapy. The focus in level five is on dysfunctional family systems; knowledge and skills are those associated with family therapy. This level is a specialized form of family care, for families in which interactions have become seriously problematic.

Six months after Mr. Green's discharge, he calls the clinical nurse specialist to discuss problems he is having with his mother. Her needs have increased and she seems not to recognize that he can no longer meet them himself, although he can and does arrange for her care. The tension is spilling over into his relationship with his wife, and both are worried about the ongoing stress impacting their daughter. The clinical nurse specialist suggests that they talk with a psychiatric/mental health nurse practitioner who is knowledgeable in helping families deal directly with situations like theirs, and she offers to make a referral that day.

FAMILIES AND DYSFUNCTION

Because families are critical to the health and well-being of their members, it follows that they are in the position to do great good, or great harm. Family violence, incest, eating disorders, alcohol and drug abuse, and attachment disorders are significant health problems in the United States (Humphreys and Campbell, 1989). Their effects can be seen in statistical increases in teenage suicide, depression, child abuse and neglect, spousal abuse, elder abuse, teenage runaways, teenage pregnancy, and dissolution of families by divorce, separation, and abandonment.

Nurses today need to be proficient in identifying family dysfunction, from inappropriate communication patterns to significant histories of abuse, neglect, and addiction. They need to know the statistical profiles of dysfunctional behaviors in their communities, and they need to be alert for sociocultural differences that may mask dysfunction or mislead health care providers. For example, spousal abuse is missed in middle and upper income families because of a pervasive and mistaken belief that spousal abuse is tied to lower socioeconomic settings. On the other hand, culturally appropriate remedies may leave marks on a child that are mistaken for abuse, and a loving family is falsely accused. Knowledge and appropriate consultation are the most effective ways of improving assessment and clinical identification skills (Campbell and Campbell, 1993; Sheridan, 1995).

Nurses today also need to know the laws of their state regarding reporting of suspected abuse and neglect, and they need to understand their own legal responsibilities. They also need to be skilled at referral, including being prepared with names and telephone numbers of individuals and agencies prepared to help families. The more nurses know and understand the families who are in their practice community, the better able they will be to make effective referrals.

Age

Age affects health and illness in several ways. Different age groups are exposed to different environmental hazards, thereby increasing the risk of a particular health problem, for example, work place accidents. Age can also be associated with exposure to organisms resulting in the disease, or over time, protection against the disease, e.g., infectious disease such as mumps and tuberculosis. Age can also be associated with physiologic changes and chronic illness such as arthritis or diabetes.

MYTHS ABOUT AGING

Elderly people are frequently stereotyped and the objects of discrimination. In health care this takes the form of attributing health problems to "old age" with the implication that the problems are untreatable. A health care provider may say to an elderly person, "Of course you are short of breath. After all, you are 80 years old." In fact, the shortness of breath may not be age related but related to an inactive lifestyle or another treatable cause.

Common myths about the elderly include the following (Butler, 1990):

- **The myth of aging.** Chronological age is an imprecise indicator of health status. There are "young" 80-year-olds and "old" 80-year-olds. In fact, in terms of physiologic health indicators, the elderly are more diverse than any other segment of the population (Fig. 6–2).
- **The myth of unproductivity.** In the absence of disease and social adversities, elderly people tend to remain productive and actively involved in life. There are numerous examples of older people beginning new, productive careers; for example, Grandma Moses, who became a world-renowned artist very late in life. Others have made their greatest contributions to society later in life, such as Golda Meir as the Prime Minister of Israel. Still others have continued highly successful careers into their 80s, such as the artist Georgia O'Keeffe. The corporate world has numerous chief executive officers over age 65. More elderly would work if jobs were available to them.
- **The myth of disengagement.** The generalization that people disengage from life as they age is not supported by evidence. Older people do not necessarily choose to disengage from life, to live alone, or to withdraw into themselves. The political strength of the American Association of Retired Persons (AARP) is a clear example that elderly people do care about society and remain involved.
- **The myth of inflexibility.** The ability to change and adapt has less to do with age and more to do with character. Change is the hallmark of living. The thought that people become less responsive to innovation and change because of age is not supported by scientific studies of healthy older people living in the community or by everyday observations and clinical psychiatric experience.
- **The myth of "senility."** The symptoms of senility (forgetfulness, confusion, and reduced attention span) are associated with irreversible brain damage diseases such as cerebral arteriosclerosis. Old people are not automatically senile. For those that do show symptoms of senility, the cause may be prescribed medications, the interaction of various prescribed medications, malnutrition, or unrecognized physical illness. The symptoms of senility deserve assessment and intervention; they should not be taken as automatic with age.
- **The myth of serenity.** Almost in contrast to other myths, this one assumes that old age is a type of adult fairyland where there are no worries or cares. Older people have nothing to do but relax and enjoy the fruits of their labors. Although this is a pleasant picture of old age, it is not true. Older persons experience more stresses than any other age group. For example, there may be stress associated with living on a fixed retirement income in the event of increasing housing and food prices. There is stress associated with the loss of a spouse and the resulting change in living patterns. There is stress associated with one's friends dying one after the other. The ability of the elderly to endure crises is remarkable.

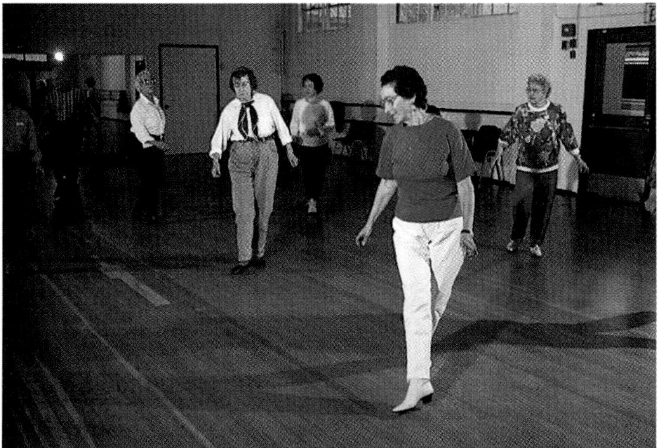

Figure 6–2. Active elderly persons such as these dispel common myths about aging.

MYTHS ABOUT CHILDREN

Children are frequently viewed as living in a carefree world. Yet children experience pressures in terms of group acceptance, sexuality, and substance abuse, to name just a few pressures.

The World Health Organization publication *Nursing Beyond the Year 2000* (1994) identifies children as one of four vulnerable groups in terms of health concerns. The data offered to support this position include:

- One third of the developing world's children suffer from malnutrition.
- The diarrheal diseases together kill approximately 4 million young children each year.
- Every year, vitamin A deficiency results in a third of a million children going blind, and 60 percent of these children die within a short time of losing their sight.

Although age is a determinant of health and illness status, like culture, race, and ethnicity, its impact is complex. The only generalization that can be made is that there is great diversity in health status in every age group. Health care providers must consider the age of the individual or community but cannot draw conclusions without considering other factors associated with health and illness.

HEALTH OUTCOMES AND AGE

The following data from *Health, United States, 1996–97* illustrate relationships between age and health and illness:

- Death rates for motor vehicle accidents are highest for those 85 years and over, second highest for those age 15 to 24 years, third highest for those 75 to 84 years, and fourth highest for those 25 to 34 years (Table 6–2).
- As shown in Table 6–3, death rates from suicide are highest for those age 85 and older, second highest for those age 75 to 84 years, third highest for those age 65 to 74 years, and fourth highest for those age 25 to 34 years.
- As shown in Table 6–4, the death rate for AIDS is highest for those age 35 to 44 years, second highest for those age 25 to 34 years, and third highest for those age 45 to 54 years.

CHANGING DEMOGRAPHICS

Healthy People 2000 (U.S. Department of Health and Human Services, 1991) provides the following picture of the American people:

- By the year 2000, the overall population of the United States will have grown to nearly 270 million people, with the slowest rate of growth in the nation's history projected between 1995 and 2000. Average household size is expected to decline from 2.69 in 1985 to 2.48 in 2000, with husband-wife households decreasing from 58 to 53 percent of all households.
- By the year 2000, the American population will be older, continuing the aging trend of the present century, with a median age of more than 36 years, compared with 29 years in 1975. The number of children under age 5 will actually decline from more than 18 million to fewer than 17 million between 1990 and 2000. By 2000, the 35 million people over age 65 will represent about 13 percent of the population, in contrast to 8 percent in 1950. The population of the

TABLE 6–2 Death Rates Per 100,000 Resident Population for Motor Vehicle Crashes According to Age: United States, 1995

Age	Deaths per 100,000
Under 1 year	4.7
1–4	5.2
5–14	5.4
15–24	29.5
25–34	19.8
35–44	15.4
45–54	13.9
55–64	14.6
65–74	17.6
75–84	28.6
85 and over	31.4

From Public Health Service Centers for Disease Control and Prevention and National Center for Health Statistics (1997). *Health, United States, 1996-97.* Washington, D.C.: U.S. Government Printing Office, Table 46, p. 151.

TABLE 6–3 Death Rates per 100,000 Population for Suicide According to Age: Unites States, Selected Years

Age	1950	1960	1970	1980	1995
Under 1 year					
1–4					
5–14	0.2	0.3	0.3	0.4	0.9
15–24	4.5	5.2	8.8	12.3	13.3
25–34	9.1	10.0	14.1	16.0	15.3
35–44	14.3	14.2	16.9	15.4	15.2
45–54	20.9	20.7	20.0	15.9	14.5
55–64	27.0	23.7	21.4	15.9	13.8
65–74	29.3	23.0	20.8	16.9	15.8
75–84	31.1	27.9	21.2	19.1	21.4
85 and older	28.8	26.0	19.0	19.2	22.5

From Public Health Service Centers for Disease Control and Prevention and National Center for Health Statistics (1997). *Health, United States, 1996-97.* Washington, D.C.: U.S. Government Printing Office, Table 48, p. 158.

TABLE 6–4 Death Rates Per 100,000 Resident Population for Human Immunodeficiency Virus (HIV) Infection, According to Age: United States, 1987, 1992, and 1995

Age	1987	1992	1995
Under 1 year	2.3	2.5	2.0
1–4	0.7	1.0	1.3
5–14	0.1	0.3	0.5
15–24	1.3	1.6	1.7
25–34	11.7	24.6	28.5
35–44	14.0	35.6	42.5
45–54	8.0	20.3	24.9
55–64	3.5	8.5	10.1
65–74	1.3	2.8	3.2
75–84	0.8	0.8	0.8
85 and older			0.4

From Public Health Service Centers for Disease Control and Prevention and National Center for Health Statistics (1997). *Health, United States, 1996-97.* Washington, D.C.: U.S. Government Printing Office, Table 44, p. 148.

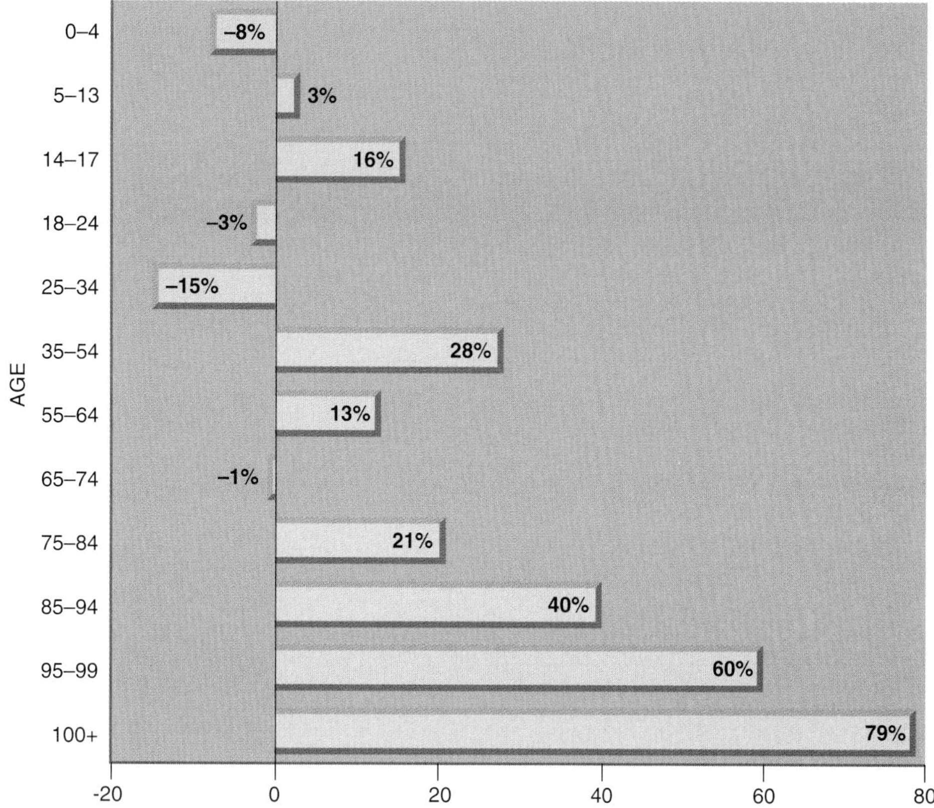

Figure 6–3. Percent change in U.S. population by age group, 1990–2000. (Source: U.S. Bureau of the Census, 1989.)

"oldest old"—those over age 85—will have increased by about 30 percent to a total of 4.6 million by 2000.

Figure 6–3 shows the projected percent of change in the population from 1990 to 2000. Of note is the growth of the elderly population.

Gender

Because the relationship between gender and health and illness is discussed in detail in Chapter 33, it is addressed only briefly in this chapter.

The World Health Organization's Report *Nursing Beyond the Year 2000* (1994) identifies women as one of four groups vulnerable in terms of health needs. The report states (p. 5) "Women are disproportionately vulnerable to disease. In comparison with men they fare less well in terms of disease prevalence, utilization of services and allocation of resources within the family. Such gender differences are found throughout the world from birth onwards."

Data comparing the leading causes of death in 1992 for white men and white women are shown in Table 6–5 and for black men and black women are shown in Table 6–6.

Research has documented gender differences in response to illness. The research report by Vallerand (1995) summarized research on gender differences in response to pain (Box 6–5).

TABLE 6–5 Leading Causes of Death for White Men and White Women, 1995

Leading Causes of Death for White Men	Leading Causes of Death for White Women
1. Diseases of the heart	1. Diseases of the heart
2. Malignant neoplasms	2. Malignant neoplams
3. Cerebrovascular disease	3. Cerebrovascular disease
4. Unintentional injuries	4. Chronic obstructive pulmonary disease
5. Chronic obstructive pulmonary disease	5. Pneumonia and influenza
6. Pneumonia and influenza	6. Unintentional injuries
7. Suicide	7. Diabetes mellitus
8. Human immunodeficiency virus disease	8. Alzheimer's disease
9. Diabetes mellitus	9. Nephritis, nephrotic syndrome, and nephrosis
10. Chronic liver disease and cirrhosis	10. Septicemia

From Public Health Service Centers for Disease Control and Prevention and National Center for Health Statistics (1997). *Health, United States, 1996–97.* Washington, D.C.: U.S. Government Printing Office, Table 33, pp. 118–119.

TABLE 6-6 Leading Causes of Death for Black Men and Black Women, 1995

Leading Causes of Death for Black Men	Leading Causes of Death for Black Women
1. Diseases of the heart	1. Diseases of the heart
2. Malignant neoplasms	2. Malignant neoplasms
3. Homicide and legal intervention	3. Cerebrovascular disease
4. Human immunodeficiency virus infection	4. Diabetes mellitus
5. Unintentional injuries	5. Human immunodeficiency virus infection
6. Cerebrovascular diseases	6. Unintentional injuries
7. Pneumonia and influenza	7. Pneumonia and influenza
8. Chronic obstructive pulmonary diseases	8. Chronic obstructive pulmonary diseases
9. Certain conditions originating in the perinatal period	9. Nephritis, nephrotic syndrome and nephrosis
10. Diabetes mellitus	10. Certain conditions originating in the perinatal period

From Public Health Service Centers for Disease Control and Prevention and National Center for Health Statistics (1997). *Health, United States, 1996-97.* Washington, D.C.: U.S. Government Printing Office, Table 33, pp. 118-119.

Socioeconomic Status

It is clear from a number of studies that the more advantaged social groups, whether determined by income, education, social class, or ethnicity, tend to have better health than other groups of their societies (Blane, 1995). This distribution of mortality and morbidity by social group is striking and consistent. Each change in level of advantage (or disadvantage) is associated with a change in health. The differences cannot be accounted for by biologic processes or access to health services. It seems that the psychosocial consequences of belonging to a particular social class are important determiners of health and illness.

HEALTH OUTCOMES AND VARIABLES ASSOCIATED WITH ECONOMIC STATUS

The following highlights are included in *Health, United States, 1996–97* (1997):

- Health status is strongly associated with family income. In 1994 the age-adjusted percent of persons with low family income (less than $14,000) who reported fair or poor health was 5.0 times that for persons with a high income of $50,000 or more. Similarly, the age-adjusted percent of low income persons who were unable to carry on their major activity due to a chronic health condition was 3 times the level for high income persons.
- Cigarette smoking is strongly associated with educational attainment. In 1994 the age-adjusted prevalence of current cigarette smoking among persons 25 years of age and over ranged from 12 percent for college graduates to 38 percent for persons with less than a high school education.

The following highlights are included in *Health, United States, 1994* (1995):

- In 1991 to 1993 nonpoor children received more ambulatory care than poor or near poor children. The mean number of physician contacts per year for nonpoor children was 23 to 26 percent greater than for poor or near poor children.
- Despite their worse health status, persons with low income are more likely to have gone without a recent physician contact than persons with high income. In 1993, the age-adjusted percent of persons without a physician contact in the previous two years was more than 50 percent greater for those with family incomes

BOX 6-5
GENDER DIFFERENCES IN PAIN

April Hazard Vallerand
Image: Journal of Nursing Scolarship, 27(3), 235–237

Celento, Linet, and Stewart (1990) suggested that women suffer less social disapproval for admitting to emotional distress than men and that physicians are more likely to recognize symptoms of distress in women than in men. Because pain is a subjective phenomenon that can be assessed most reliably from the patient's self report (AHCPR, 1992), the ability to communicate the discomfort of pain to a healthcare provider should be an advantage. However, much of the pain literature is based on male responses. When a comparison is made between responses of men and women, women's ability to verbalize their emotions causes their responses to be viewed as being psychologically based, and thus treated accordingly. Despite findings that identify either no differences in the experience of pain between men and women, or an increased sensitivity to pain in women, women's responses to pain are viewed with suspicion and treated less aggressively. A recent study by Cleeland and colleagues (1994) found that even in a population of patients with metastatic cancer, being female was a significant predictor of inadequate pain management. Patients in the Cleeland study reported that inadequate analgesia resulted in less and shorter pain relief and greater pain-related impairment of function. Of the 1308 patients in the study, 475 (36%) had severe function-impairing pain despite the fact that most were receiving some treatment for pain.

Agency for Health Care Policy and Research (AHCPR) (1992). *Acute Pain Management in Adults: Operative Procedures.* (AHCPR Publication No. 92-0019). Rockville, MD: Agency for Health Care Policy and Research, Public Health Service, U.S. Department of Health and Human Services.

Celentano, D.D., Linet, M.S., Stewart, W.F. (1990). Gender differences in the experience of headache. *Social Science Medicine, 30,* 1289–1295.

Cleeland, C.S., Gonin, R., Hatfield, A.K., et al (1994). Pain and its treatment in outpatients with metastatic cancer. *New Engl J Med, 330,* 592–596.

of less than $14,000 than for those with high incomes of $50,000 or more.
- Persons with low income use more inpatient hospital care than persons with high income.
- In 1993 levels of recent mammography were 35 percent lower among women with less than 12 years of education and 17 percent lower among women with a high school education, compared with women of higher educational attainment.

These statistics point out differences in behaviors associated with health and illness according to socioeconomic status. The statistics do not provide insight into why socioeconomic status plays such an important role in health and illness. For example, we know that people with more education (and therefore a higher socioeconomic status) are less likely to smoke. But we do not know why. Research that provides insights into the why is needed.

Religion

Religious practices do influence an individual's health, illness, and response to disease and death. General statements regarding the definition of a religion, its view on birth control and abortion, and attitude toward medical treatment can be made. Yet the manner in which individuals implement religious practices varies even among people within the same religious group. Effective nursing care requires the nurse to attend to individual differences and not make assumptions based on stereotypes or generalizations.

Major religions in the United States are described. Brief descriptions of agnostics and atheists are provided. As the U.S. population diversifies, nurses will need to be familiar with other worldwide religions such as Confucianism, Taoism, and Islam.

BAPTIST (LIPPHARD AND SHARP, 1975)

There is a great deal of diversity among people who identify themselves as Baptists. Baptists are dedicated to a high degree of personal independence and to the right of the individual to interpret the New Testament for himself or herself in terms of faith and practice. There is an insistence on purity, on personal responsibility, and on freedom of belief and worship. The Scripture, rather than the church or its hierarchy, is supreme.

VIEWS ON ABORTION AND BIRTH CONTROL

The Baptist Church has not taken an official stand on either abortion or birth control. Every Baptist is free to make up his or her own mind.

VIEWS ON MEDICAL SERVICES

The Baptist Church does not restrict its members from using any health care services.

CATHOLIC (HENDRICKS, 1975)

The Catholic Church has four distinctive beliefs:
- *One*—in doctrine, authority, and worship.
- *Holy*—Perfect adherence to its teachings leads to sanctity.
- *Catholic*—It is unchanging in its essential teachings and preaches the same gospel and administers the same sacraments to men of all times and in all places.
- *Apostolic*—It traces its ancestry back to the apostles and carries the message of Christ to all.

The Catholic Church considers itself the divinely appointed custodian of the Bible with the final word on what any passage means. Within the Catholic Church there is a specially ordained priesthood. The Pope is preserved by God from leading the Church into doctrinal error.

VIEWS ON BIRTH CONTROL AND ABORTION

The Catholic Church encourages responsible family planning using morally acceptable means such as the calendar rhythm method or abstinence. Artificial contraception and sterilization are considered immoral methods.

Because the Church believes that human life begins at the moment of conception, abortion is seen as killing an individual, unique human being.

VIEWS ON MEDICAL SERVICES

Other than for immoral birth control methods, abortion, and physician-assisted suicide, the Church does not preclude its members from using any medical services.

CHRISTIAN SCIENTIST (STOKES, 1975)

The Church of Christ, Scientist, is designed to commemorate the word and works of Jesus Christ, including the element of healing. A Christian Scientist accepts and practices the teachings of the church as found in the Bible and the Christian Science textbook, *Science and Health with Key to the Scriptures*. The discoverer and founder of Christian Science is Mary Baker Eddy (1821–1910).

VIEWS ON BIRTH CONTROL AND ABORTION

The Church of Christ, Scientist, allows married couples freedom to decide the number of children they will have. Abortion is left to individual judgment, but methods that involve operations or drugs are against the religion.

VIEWS ON MEDICAL SERVICES

Health is a spiritual reality and not a physical condition. Disease is a delusion of the carnal mind and can be destroyed by prayer and spiritual understanding. Assistance can be obtained from a Christian Science practitioner. To be a practitioner requires study, prayer, consecration, instruction under an authorized teacher and satisfactory evidence of successful healing. The practitioner applies spiritual understanding to the destruction of human ills and discords.

Ordinarily, Christian Scientists do not seek hospitalization. Christian Science sanitariums and nurses exist when expert care is needed. A non–Christian Scientist practitioner may be used at the time of childbirth and for the setting of broken bones.

EPISCOPALIAN (PITTENGER, 1975)

In the United States, Episcopalians are members of the Protestant Episcopal Church, which is one of the self-governing national churches within the Anglican Communion. They are called Anglican because the Church of England is in some way the mother of them all. The beliefs of Episcopalians are expressed in the Apostles' Creed.

VIEWS ON BIRTH CONTROL AND ABORTION

The Church believes that the responsibility for making decisions about the number and frequency of children falls upon the conscience of the parents. They are expected to consider the resources of their family as well as to consider the needs of populations, society, and future generations.

The Church has urged that methods other than abortion be made available to all women and men. It has also supported efforts to repeal all laws regarding abortion that deny women the free and responsible use of their conscience.

VIEWS ON MEDICAL SERVICES

The Church has no statements that would restrict use of any medical services.

GREEK ORTHODOX (DOUROPULOS, 1975)

The Greek Orthodox Church is defined by three key words:

- *Holy,* because its founder Jesus Christ is holy.
- *Catholic,* because the whole world is its province and it is universal in time and place.
- *Apostolic,* because it was established on earth by the apostles of Christ.

For over 1,000 years this Church and the Roman Catholic church were united. In A.D. 1054 the Church of Christ divided into Eastern and Western segments. The Western segment became known as the Roman Catholic Church. The Eastern segment became known as the Greek or Eastern Orthodox church.

VIEWS ON BIRTH CONTROL AND ABORTION

Birth control is disapproved and the Church is strictly opposed to abortion unless the mother's life is in danger.

VIEWS ON MEDICAL SERVICES

The Church has no statements that would restrict use of any medical services other than birth control and abortion.

JEHOVAH'S WITNESSES (HENSCHEL, 1975)

The Witnesses follow the Bible in every aspect of their lives. They believe it is practical for everyday living. Their beliefs include:

- Jehovah is the only true God.
- Satan challenged God's sovereignty putting the integrity of all men to the test.
- God's primary purpose is the vindication of His sovereignty.
- The beginning of the end for Satan came in 1914 when God threw Satan out of heaven.
- Since 1914, God has been destroying the wicked system and eventually the Devil himself will be put out of action.
- Following Jehovah's vindication, there will be the thousand-year reign of Christ.

A Jehovah's Witness is expected to maintain integrity to Jehovah, announce the King's reign, and help neighbors find the way to godly service and everlasting life.

VIEWS ON BIRTH CONTROL AND ABORTION

Birth control is considered a personal matter. Abortion is considered as taking away life and thus contrary to the Bible.

VIEWS ON MEDICAL SERVICES

Jehovah's Witnesses are opposed to blood transfusions, citing passages from both the Old and New Testaments of the Bible. They believe that by having a blood transfusion they would invoke the wrath of God. Other than blood transfusions and abortions, there are no restrictions on medical services.

JUDAISM (KERTZER, 1975)

Judaism is a way of life. Being a Jew may be a matter of belonging (accepting the faith of Judaism), believing (without religious affiliation accepts the teaching of Judaism), or behaving (is considered Jewish because the person claims to be).

The Jewish prayer book identifies three basic principles of faith:

1. The love of learning.
2. The worship of God.
3. The obligation of good deeds.

The Jews value the timeless truths and values of the Old Testament. They do not accept the divinity of Jesus.

The Orthodox Jew maintains the traditions established over 3000 years ago including strict observance of the Sabbath and dietary laws. Reform Jews accept as binding only the moral laws of the Old Testament. Conservative Jews follow the traditions but do believe Judaism is an evolving religion.

VIEWS ON BIRTH CONTROL AND ABORTION

Orthodox Jews allow abortion to save the mental health or life of the mother. Reform and Conservative Jews allow abortion if it is undertaken for unselfish reasons.

VIEWS ON MEDICAL SERVICES

When hospitalized, a Jewish patient may require special meals to meet the requirements of the dietary laws. Beyond that, the religion places no restrictions on the use of medical services.

LUTHERAN (RUFF AND STAUDERMAN, 1975)

The Lutheran Church is based on the doctrines of the New Testament summarized in the Apostles' Creed. Faith in Christ is an essential part of the religion. Lutherans think of the Christian life as a grateful response to a loving father rather than strict obedience to a stern monarch. Members of the Lutheran Church are urged to achieve a high ethical life without emphasis on rules and regulations. At the same time the church emphasizes thorough study of the Lutheran Catechism.

VIEWS ON BIRTH CONTROL AND ABORTION

Although the Church has made official statements on both birth control and abortion, the wording is guarded. The Church is not seen as a law-making entity but rather a vehicle through which the Holy Spirit can shape and direct Christian lives. Medical advice and spiritual counsel are recommended.

VIEWS ON MEDICAL SERVICES

The Lutheran Church places no restrictions on the use of medical services.

METHODIST (SOCKMAN, 1975)

Methodism began as a movement within the Protestant church and not as a new religion. Its founder, John Wesley, described a Methodist as one who has the love of God in his heart planted by the Holy Spirit and who loves the Lord his God with all his soul, mind, and strength. The Methodist Church emphasizes the behavior of people rather than their beliefs or creed.

VIEWS ON BIRTH CONTROL AND ABORTION

The Methodist Church believes in the sanctity of the unborn child and is therefore hesitant to approve of abortion. A Methodist would be expected to give thorough and thoughtful consideration to an abortion and first seek medical and pastoral counseling.

VIEWS ON MEDICAL SERVICES

The Methodist Church has no restrictions on the use of medical services.

MORMON (EVANS, 1975)

Mormons are members of the Church of Jesus Christ of Latter-day Saints. They believe that the Gospel of Jesus Christ was proclaimed in the heavens before the world was created; that it was known to Adam and others; that mankind has repeatedly departed from it; and that it has had to be restored through various people and means such as Abraham and Moses. They believe that the last restoration was in the early nineteenth century through Joseph Smith. The Mormons accept the Bible as well as *The Book of Mormon*. The latter is accepted as complementary scripture.

The Church has a code on health and conduct that disapproves of the use of tobacco, alcohol, and drinks such as coffee and tea. The spirit of the "Word of Wisdom" mandates abstinence from all injurious substances and urges enjoyment of wholesome things. This code may account for the positive health status of members of this religion.

VIEWS ON BIRTH CONTROL AND ABORTION

The Church has urged the rearing of large families, and birth control is contrary to its teachings. It is also opposed to all forms of abortion except where the mother's life is in jeopardy.

VIEWS ON MEDICAL SERVICES

The Church does not restrict use of medical services.

PRESBYTERIAN (BONNELL, 1975)

The word Presbyterian does not refer to a specific doctrine but rather to a particular form of church governance. The Presbyterian Church is governed by teaching elders and ruling elders. Most Presbyterians accept the Westminister Confession of Faith and the Nicene and Apostles' Creeds. They accept the Old and New Testaments as the Word of God written by inspired people. Although they see the Bible as containing the truths by which one should live, they do not emphasize the traditions contained in the Bible.

VIEWS ON BIRTH CONTROL AND ABORTION

The Presbyterian Church does not legislate on personal moral issues. Nothing in its teaching would forbid intelligent, conservative, and unselfish use of birth control. The Church advocates that women should have full freedom of personal choice concerning completion or termination of a pregnancy.

VIEWS ON MEDICAL SERVICES

The Church does not restrict use of medical services.

QUAKER (MILLER AND TUCKER, 1975)

A Quaker is a member of the Religious Society of Friends. They believe that the worship of God is the primary purpose of the religious life, in fact of life itself; their group worship is a fellowship of the spirit based on silent communion. Quakers believe that God speaks to all mankind through the still small inner voice and that His revelation is continuous. For the Quaker, truth is found in the Bible and therefore they are serious students of the Bible. Many but not all Quakers hold that nonviolent forms of peacemaking are the only ways to settle strife.

VIEWS ON BIRTH CONTROL AND ABORTION

Birth control is considered a matter for the individual conscience. Many Quakers feel the woman should have control over what happens to her own body. The nature of the Religious Society of Friends makes it unlikely it will take formal positions on such issues.

VIEWS ON MEDICAL SERVICES

The Church places no restrictions on the use of medical services.

SEVENTH-DAY ADVENTIST (MAXWELL, 1975)

A Seventh-Day Adventist:

- accepts Christ as a personal Savior.
- walks in humble obedience to the will of God.
- seeks to pattern his life according to the teaching of the Bible.
- looks for the imminent return of the Lord.
- believes it is his duty to warn mankind that the end of the world is at hand.

Saturday is considered the seventh day of the week and therefore the day observed as the Sabbath day. The Bible is accepted literally. The return of Christ is an important aspect of their beliefs. That return will mark the end of the world as we know it today.

Seventh-Day Adventists are expected to refrain from alcohol and tobacco. They are to refrain from all harmful indulgences.

VIEWS ON BIRTH CONTROL AND ABORTION

The Church has taken no formal stand on birth control and abortion. In terms of the latter it has urged its physicians and medical institutions to perform abortions when the life of the mother is in question; the child would be born with serious deformities; and when the pregnancy is the result of rape or incest.

VIEWS ON MEDICAL SERVICES

The Church does not restrict the use of any medical services. In fact, it has maintained many hospitals across the United States.

UNITARIAN UNIVERSALIST (CHWOROWSKY AND RAIBLE, 1975)

Members of this religious group are organized as free religious communities in which they unite for the celebration of life, for sharing values, for service, and for comfort—without being required to accept a dogmatic creed. They honor the ethical leadership of Jesus but do not consider him a final religious authority. All people are seen as having value. Working toward a just and peaceful social order is considered a responsibility. They believe in the principles of freedom.

Members of their churches may be agnostics, humanists, atheists, nature worshipers, and those who accept Jesus as Lord.

VIEWS ON BIRTH CONTROL AND ABORTION

Unitarian Universalists have pioneered to eliminate restrictive laws regarding birth control and abortion.

VIEWS ON MEDICAL SERVICES

The Church does not restrict any medical services.

AGNOSTICS AND ATHEISTS

An atheist is an individual who holds that humans can determine whether a God exists or not, and on serious thought decides there is no God. An agnostic is an individual who holds that there is insufficient information to determine whether or not there is a God and therefore suspends judgment.

Both agnostics and atheists look to an authority other than "God's law" as a guide to conduct. An individual may look to his or her own conscience, to the potential for punishment, or to logic as a guide to conduct.

Agnostics and atheists would accept or reject medical services based on their personal rationale.

BUDDHISM (SMITH, 1991)

Buddhism has its roots in a man, Siddhartha Gautama of the Sakyas, born about 563 B.C. in the area now known as Nepal. In his twenties he experienced a profound discontent, leading him to break with his worldly estate. His experiences taught him the unlikelihood of finding fulfillment on the physical plane. At one point he felt that he was about to experience a breakthrough in his understanding of fulfillment. He sat down under a tree now called the Bo Tree (short for bodhi or enlightenment) with the intent of staying until enlightenment was his. He experienced severe temptations as he meditated. He was able to persevere until he experienced the Great Awakening and was transformed into the Buddha.

Important teaching relevant to health and illness include the Four Noble Truths and The Eightfold Path. The first Noble Truth is that life is suffering. All will experience the trauma of birth, the pathology of sickness, the morbidity associated with old age, the fear of death, to be tied to what one dislikes, and to be separated from what one loves. The Second Noble Truth is that the cause of life's dislocations is selfish craving. The Third Noble Truth is that release from this torment is accomplished by identification with the vast expanse of universal life. The Fouth Noble Truth is that this is accomplished through the Eightfold Path.

The Eightfold Path consists of eight rights: right views, right intent, right speech, right conduct, right livelihood, right effort, right mindfulness, and right concentration.

As with other religions, Buddhism has schools of thought and it continues to evolve its philosophy.

HINDUISM (SMITH, 1991)

Hinduism has a vast literature, complicated rituals, and sprawling folkways. One recurring theme is that people are different. Therefore people take different paths toward life's fulfillment and move through life's stages in different ways and with different time tables.

The Hindu first travels the Path of Desire and then the Path of Renunciation. The Path of Desire is characterized by drives for power, position, and possessions. The guiding principle is not to turn from desire until desire turns from you. The Path of Desire could take several lifetimes. Following pleasure and success, the third great aim of the Hindu life is duty, particularly duty to the community, which is greater than one's self.

But duty too is of limited satisfaction and the time comes when the question "Is this all there is to life?" is raised. This is a key point for Hinduism. For the Hindu, life does hold other possibilities in the direction of what humans really want and want infinitely: to be, to know, and to feel joy. This is accomplished by uniting the human spirit with the Brahman (God) who lies within its deepest recesses.

Hinduism identifies four paths for coming to and remaining in touch with Brahman, for identifying with Brahman, and becoming divine while living on earth. Each path is designed for a specific personality type. One path is not superior to another. A distinct yoga is detailed for each path and is designed to capitalize on the personality associated with that path. The four paths are knowledge, love, work, and psychophysical exercises (experiments).

Hinduism emphasizes that people are different even as they travel through life toward the ultimate goal of reaching Brahman. Therefore it is even more difficult to draw generalizations about Hinduism and views on health and illness. The challenge to the nurse is first to understand where the individual is in life's journey and then to determine the implications for care.

Implications for Nursing Practice

The complex relationship between culture, race, and ethnicity and health outcomes and the rapidly changing population demographics will put a strain on the current health care system. Nurses and other health care providers will be challenged to:

- develop better understandings of the relationship between race, culture, and ethnicity and health status
- practice from a holistic framework that includes environmental factors

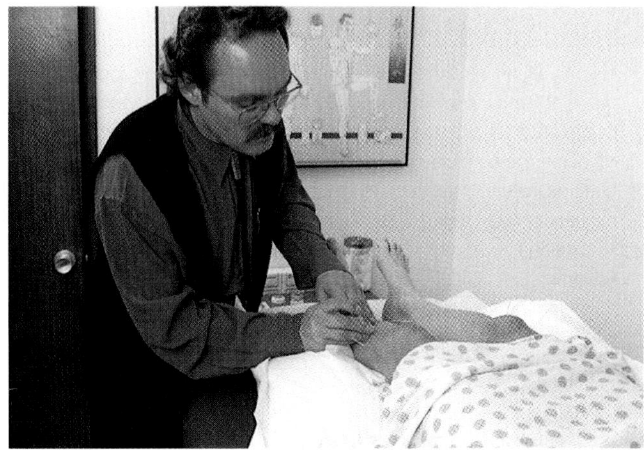

Figure 6–4. Acupuncture, a traditional Chinese treatment, has gained many proponents in the West as well.

- incorporate therapies complementary to a range of cultural beliefs about health and illness (Fig. 6–4)
- communicate effectively with people from different races, cultures, and ethnic identifications
- eliminate the discrepancies in health outcomes for people of color

The relationship between age and health status poses many challenges for health care providers:

- Because different age groups are at risk for different health problems, prevention strategies must be developed for specific age groups. Immunizations may be a first priority for very young children whereas suicide prevention may be a high priority for the frail elderly.
- Quality of life is of concern to those who are increasingly likely to live to age 90 or 100 or beyond. Prevention of chronic illnesses and depression are essential. Preparing children to assume responsibility for their health is as important as preparing the elderly for self-care and management of their symptoms.
- Health care providers have not been eager to develop careers in caring for the elderly. The country needs more nurses interested in long-term care settings and nurse practitioners and physicians interested in gerontology.

Poverty has a profound effect on health status. It reaches far beyond the issue of access to services. Nurses can mitigate the negatives of effects of poverty on health by:

- identifying effective health promotion strategies for low socioeconomic families
- using every nurse-patient encounter to empower the patient and family
- appreciating the relationship between economic status and health and illness
- serving as an advocate for economically deprived people at the health policy making level

CHAPTER HIGHLIGHTS

- Health is more than the absence of disease and disease is more than susceptibility to certain organisms. Many factors contribute to a sense of health or illness and to the presence or absence of disease.
- Unfortunately, health care practices reflect an array of biases or stereotypes regarding race, culture, ethnicity, age, gender, socioeconomic status, choice of medical philosophy, and religion.
- Each nurse must strive to understand the factors that influence health and illness for the population as a whole as well as for the individual.
- Each nurse must be reflective about preformed ideas and provide care without bias.

REFERENCES

Bender, P. (1992). Deceptive distress in the elderly. *AJN, 92* (10), 29–32.

Blane, D. (1995). Editorial: Social determinents of health—Socioeconomic status, social class and ethnicity. *American Journal of Public Health, 85,* 903–904.

Bomar, P. (1990). Perspectives on family health promotion. *Family & Community Health, 12* (4), 1–11.

Bonnell, J.S. (1975). What is a Presbyterian? In L. Rosten (ed.): *Religions of America.* New York: Simon & Schuster, pp. 200–212.

Brown, M.A., Powell-Cope, G.M. (1991). AIDS family caregiving: Transitions through uncertainty. *Nursing Research, 40,* 338–345.

Burgess, E.W., Locke, H.J. (1953). *The Family: From Institution to Companionship.* New York: American Book.

Butler, R.N. (1990). The tragedy of old age in America. In P.R. Lee and C.L. Estes (eds.): *The Nation's Health,* 3rd ed. Boston: Jones and Bartlett, pp. 363–373.

Campbell, D., Campbell, J. (1993). Nursing care of families using violence. In J. Campbell and J. Humphreys (eds.): *Nursing Care of Survivors of Family Violence.* St. Louis: Mosby, pp. 290–317.

Chesla, C.A. (1996). Reconciling technologic and family care in critical-care nursing. *Image; Journal of Nursing Scholarship, 28,* 199–203.

Chow, E. (1976). Cultural health traditions: Asian perspectives. In M.F. Branch and P.P. Paxton (eds.): *Providing Safe Nursing Care for Ethnic People of Color.* New York: Appleton-Century-Crofts, pp. 99–114.

Chworowsky, K.M., Raible, C.G. (1975). What is a Unitarian Universalist? In L. Rosten (ed.): *Religions of America.* New York: Simon & Schuster, pp. 263–276.

Clarke-Steffen, L. (1993a). Waiting and now knowing: The diagnosis of cancer in a child. *Journal of Pediatric Oncology, 10,* 146–153.

Clarke-Steffen, L. (1993b). A model of the family transition to living with childhood cancer. *Cancer Practice, 1,* 285–292.

Collinge, W. (1996). *Alternative Medicine.* Warner Books, New York. Constitution of the World Health Organization, 1948 (1964). In *Basic Documents,* 15th ed. Geneva: WHO.

Craig, J.E., Friedly, R.L. (1975). Who are the Disciples of Christ? In L. Rosten (ed.): *Religions of America.* New York: Simon & Schuster, pp. 83–95.

Curran, D. (1983). *Traits of a Healthy Family.* Minneapolis, Winston Press.

Curran, D. (1985). *Stress and the Healthy Family.* Minneapolis, Winston Press.

Deatrick, J.A., Knafl, K.A, Walsh, M. (1988). The process of parenting a child with a disability: Normalization through accommodations. *Journal of Advanced Nursing, 13,* 15–21.

Department of Family Nursing, Oregon Health Sciences University (1985). *Department of Family Nursing: Philosophy, Conceptual Framework, Objectives and Definitions.* Unpublished manuscript. Portland, OR: Oregon Health Sciences University School of Nursing.

Doherty, W. (1985). Family intervention in health care. *Family Relations, 34,* 129–137.

Doherty, W., Campbell, T. (1988). *Families and Health.* Newbury Park, CA: Sage.

Doherty, W.J., Baird, M.A. (1986). Developmental levels in family-centered medical care. *Family Medicine, 18, 153–156.*

Doherty, W.J., McCubbin, H.I. (1985). Families and health care: An emerging arena of theory, research and clinical intervention. *Family Relations, 34,* 5–11.

Dorsey, P.R., Jackson, H.Q. (1976). Cultural health traditions: The latino/chicano perspective. In M.F. Branch and P.P. Paxton (eds.): *Providing Safe Nursing Care for Ethnic People of Color.* New York: Appleton-Century-Crofts, pp. 41–80.

Douropulos, A. (1975). What is Greek Orthodox? In L. Rosten (ed.): *Religions of America.* New York: Simon & Schuster, pp. 112–131.

Evans, R. (1975). What is a Mormon? In L. Rosten (ed.): *Religions of America.* New York: Simon & Schuster, pp. 186–189.

Gilliss, C.L. (1989). Why family health care? In C.L. Gillis, B.L. Highley, B.M. Roberts, I.M. Martinson (eds.): *Toward a Science of Family Nursing.* Menlo Park, CA: Addison-Wesley, pp. 3–8.

Gilliss, C.L. (1993). Family nursing research, theory and practice. In G.D. Wegner and R.J. Alexander (eds.): *Readings in Family Nursing.* Philadelphia: Lippincott, pp. 34–42.

Gilliss, C.L., Roberts, B.M., Highley, B.L., Martinson, I.M. (1989). What is family nursing? In C.L. Gillis, B.L. Highley, B.M. Roberts, I.M. Martinson (eds.): *Toward a Science of Family Nursing.* Menlo Park, CA: Addison-Wesley, pp. 64–73.

Gordis, L. (1996). *Epidemiology.* Philadelphia: W.B. Saunders.

Hendricks, D. (1975). What is a Catholic? In L. Rosten (ed.): *Religions of America.* New York: Simon & Schuster, pp. 39–67.

Henschel, M. (1975). Who are Jehovah's Witnesses? In L. Rosten (ed.): *Religions of America.* New York: Simon & Schuster, pp. 132–141.

Humphreys, J., Campbell, J.C. (1989). Abusive behavior in families. In C.L. Gillis, B.L. Highley, B.M. Roberts, I.M. Martinson (eds.): *Toward a Science of Family Nursing.* Menlo Park, CA: Addison-Wesley, pp. 394–417.

Jekel, J.F., Elmore, J.G., Katz, D.L. (1996). *Epidemiology, Biostatistics, and Preventive Medicine.* Philadelphia: W.B. Saunders.

Kertzer, M.N. (1975). What is a Jew? In L. Rosten (ed.): *Religions of America.* New York: Simon & Schuster, pp. 142–155.

Lipphard, W.B., Sharp, F.A. (1975). What is a Baptist? In L. Rosten (ed.): *Religions of America.* New York: Simon & Schuster, pp. 25–38.

Lustig, M.W., Koester, J. (1993). *Intercultural Competence: Interpersonal Communication Across Cultures.* New York: HarperCollins College.

Maxwell, A.S. (1975). What is a Seventh-Day Adventist? In L. Rosten (ed.): *Religions of America.* New York: Simon & Schuster, pp. 244–454.

McKeown, T. (1997). Determinants of health. In P.R. Lee and C.L. Estes (eds.): *The Nation's Health,* 5th ed. Boston: Jones and Bartlett, pp. 3–17.

Milio, N. (1981). *Promoting Health Through Public Policy.* Philadelphia: F.A. Davis.

Miller, R.P., Tucker, R.W. (1975). What is a Quaker? In L. Rosten (ed.): *Religions of America.* New York: Simon & Schuster, pp. 213–243.

Miller, S.M. (1990). Race in the health of america. In P.R. Lee and C.L. Estes (eds.): *The Nation's Health,* 3rd ed. Boston: Jones and Bartlett, pp. 54–71.

Mishel, M.H., Murdaugh, C.L. (1987). Family adjustment to heart transplantation: Redesigning the dream. *Nursing Research, 36,* 332–338.

Pittenger, W.N (1975). What is an Episcopalian? In L. Rosten (ed.): *Religions of America.* New York: Simon & Schuster, pp. 96–111.

Powe, B.D. (1996). Cancer fatalism among African-Americans: A review of the literature. *Nursing Outlook, 44* (1), 18–21.

Pratt, L. (1977). *Family Structure and Effective Health Behavior: The Energized Family.* Boston: Houghton Mifflin.

Public Health Service Centers for Disease Control and Prevention and National Center for Health Statistics (1997). *Health, United States, 1996–97.* Washington, D.C.: U.S. Government Printing Office.

Public Health Service Centers for Disease Control and Prevention and National Center for Health Statistics (1995). *Health, United States, 1994.* Washington, D.C.: U.S. Government Printing Office.

Redley, B., Hood, K. (1996). Staff attitudes towards family presence during resuscitation. *Accident & Emergency Nursing, 4,* 145–151.

Ruff, G.E., Stauderman, A.P. (1975). What is a Lutheran? In L. Rosten (ed.): *Religions of America.* New York: Simon & Schuster, pp. 156–169.

Sheridan, D.J. (1995). Family violence. In S. Kitt, J. Selfridge-Thomas, J.A. Proehl, J. Kaiser (eds.): *Emergency Nursing: A Physiologic and Clinical Perspective.* Philadelphia: W.B. Saunders, pp. 482–494.

Smith, H. (1991). *The World Religions.* New York: HarperCollins.

Sockman R.W., Washburn, P.A. (1975). What is a Methodist? In L. Rosten (ed.): *Religions of America.* New York: Simon & Schuster, pp. 170–185.

Stokes, J.B. (1975). What is a Christian Scientist? In L. Rosten (ed.): *Religions of America.* New York: Simon & Schuster, pp. 69–81.

Terkelsen, K.G. (1980). Toward a theory of the family life cycle. In E.A. Carter, M. McGoldrick (eds.): *The Family Life Cycle: A Framework for Family Therapy.* New York: Gardner, pp. 21–52.

Terris, M. (1992). The health situation in the Americas. In *International Health: A North-South Debate.* pp. 71–85. Washington D.C. Human Resources Bureau Developmental Series No. 95.

Turk, D.C., Kerns, R.D. (1985). The family in health and illness. In D.C. Turk, R.D. Kerns (eds.): *Health, Illness and Families.* New York: Wiley, pp. 1–22.

U.S. Department of Health and Human Services. (1991). Healthy People 2000 (DHHS Publication No. PHS 91-50212). Washington, D.C.: U.S. Government Printing Office.

Vallerand, A. (1995). Gender differences in pain. *Image: Journal of Nursing Scholarship, 27* (3), 235–243.

WHO Study Group on Nursing beyond the Year 2000. (1994). *Nursing Beyond the Year 2000: Report of a WHO Study Group* (WHO technical report series; 842). Switzerland: World Health Organization.

Wright, L.M., Leahey, M. (1993). Trends in nursing of families. In G.D. Wegner, R.J. Alexander (eds.): *Readings in Family Nursing.* Philadelphia: Lippincott, pp. 23–33.

7 Leadership, Management, Change, and Innovation

Marylou McAthie

OBJECTIVES

After studying this chapter, students will:

- **understand the various meanings of the terms *leadership, management, change, innovation,* and *creativity***
- **be familiar with the theories of leadership and management**
- **understand concepts of change, innovation, and creativity**
- **be able to apply the theories of change**
- **recognize the importance of fostering innovation and creativity**
- **recognize the importance of using management and leadership principles in nursing practice**
- **understand the implications of change as it applies to the nursing profession and nursing practice**

Regardless of the clinical area in which nursing care is administered, nurses generally practice in organized institutional settings. These include acute care and long-term care facilities, home care agencies, community health organizations, schools, industries, military and veteran institutions, insurance companies, and others. Major changes within the health care industry have drastically affected the delivery, financing, and organizational structuring of health care institutions. As discussed in Chapter 3, the development of managed care and health maintenance organizations has fostered unprecedented change. Nursing practice and the delivery of nursing care has been affected.

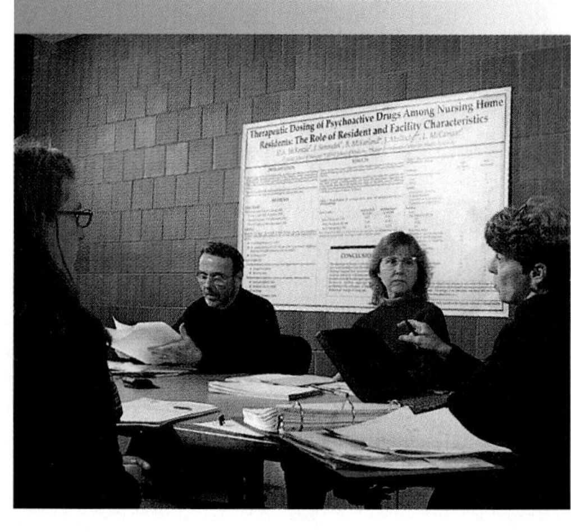

A common denominator in all institutions is the existence of some type of administrative or organizational structure. An organization is "a social system deliberately established to carry out some definite purpose. The purpose, or goal, is carried out efficiently and effectively using both human and nonhuman resources." (Kast and Rosenzweig, 1985, p. 108.) Nursing practice is affected by the organization's philosophy, mission, organizational patterns and systems, and human and material resources. To function effectively within organizations, nurses need to understand the principles of management and leadership, the relevance of innovation and change, and the interlinking of these concepts.

Nurses assume broad responsibilities. In addition to providing direct nursing care, nurses coordinate and manage groups of patients and supervise other nursing personnel. They need to be innovative and involved in the increasingly rapid changes occurring in the health care industry. Nurses manage and lead and are part of the institutional organizational team. Management and leadership principles are used in planning and implementing nursing care and in managerial positions. Nurses are caregivers and care managers (Huber, 1996). McCloskey (1995) makes the same point:

Management is the speciality of some nurses, but all nurses have a management role. Nursing is a unique discipline because of the interaction of two roles; provider of patient care and manager of the care environment (p. 307).

All nurses are in leadership positions. Leadership is exercised in various ways. Nurses assume responsibility for the care of patients and thus are held accountable for their welfare. In the latter case, the nurse guides and leads the patient and family in setting and accomplishing goals that result in desired outcomes. However, nursing is broader than taking care of a select number of patients; most nursing care is given in bureaucratic institutions and it is important that nurses be involved in leadership and management processes (Huber, 1996). Nurses participate in nursing group and team assignments, and in overseeing and coordinating nursing care administered by licensed and unlicensed subordinate staff. Professional nursing management and leadership are also demonstrated through participation in the institutions' organizational teams and in such activities as committees and educational programs. It is through these endeavors that organizational missions and personal goals are accomplished.

Every organization is different; the services provided are all unique. The challenge to those in management and leadership positions is to discover the best methods to use to accomplish the desired organizational goals.

The concepts of managing and leading are closely related. Although the processes are similar, the term *manager* is generally reserved for the individual who occupies a position within a hierarchical organization. The person assigned to a managerial position has been given decision-making authority and has the power to enforce the decisions. Leaders exercise leadership through their influence over others. Bennis (1993, p. 104) states that "management is getting people to do what needs to be done; leadership is getting people to want to do what needs to be done."

BASIC CONCEPTS: MANAGEMENT, LEADERSHIP, CHANGE, AND INNOVATION DEFINED

Management and leadership are closely related and intertwined concepts (Tappen, 1995). Various researchers and academicians have proposed different theories, approaches, and strategies of management and leadership. As a result there are many different definitions of management and leadership.

Management

Management has been defined by different individuals over the years. A few of the many definitions are presented:

- Koontz (1981) identified the following aspects of management: getting things done through and with people in formally organized groups, creating an environment in an organized group where people can perform as individuals yet cooperate to attain group goals, removing blocks to performance, and optimizing efficiency in effectively reaching goals.
- Drucker in 1967 defined management as a process of influencing others with the intention that they perform effectively and contribute to meeting the organization's goals.
- Follett in 1978 indicated that management is the art of getting things done through people.
- Swansburg (1990) viewed management as:

  The manager creates and maintains an internal environment in an enterprise in which individuals work together as a group. Managing is the art of doing. Management is the body of organized knowledge underlying the art (p. 2).

The statements represent definitions developed over a 30-year span by persons who represent a variety of different approaches to management. As can be seen, there is a common theme carried throughout, which is that people in institutions must work together.

Leadership

Leadership is also defined by many different individuals. There does not seem to be much agreement as to what the essence of leadership is (Swansburg, 1990).

- Yura and colleagues (1980) define leadership as the process of influencing the behavior of other persons in their efforts toward goal setting and achievement. Nursing leadership is a process whereby a person who is a nurse affects the actions of others in goal determination and achievement.
- Gardner (1986) indicates that leadership is the process of persuasion and example by which an individual (or leadership team) induces a group to take action that is in accord with the leader's purposes or the shared purposes of all.
- Kouzes and Posner (1995) state that leadership is a process used by all people to bring forth the best from their own and from others' efforts. They define leadership as the art of mobilizing others to want to struggle for shared aspirations.
- Grohar-Murray and DiCroce (1997) state leadership is:

  A collective function in the sense that it is the integrated synergized expression of a group's efforts; it is not the sum of individual dominance and contributions, it is their interrelationships. Ultimate authority and true sanction for leadership, where it is exercised, resides not

> in the individual, however dominant, but in the total situation and in the demands of the situation. It is the situation that creates the imperative, whereas the leader is able to make others aware of it, is able to make them willing to serve it, and is able to release collective capacities and emotional attitudes that may be related fruitfully to the solution of the group's problems; to that extent one is exercising leadership (p. 23).

The processes described in these definitions allow all staff to participate, be motivated, and involved in the ever-changing operations of the organization. The participatory process stimulates innovation and creativity. All leaders and managers are faced with the challenge of functioning in a constantly changing environment that demands the exercise of innovation and creativity.

Change, Innovation, and Creativity

CHANGE

Change is a part of daily life. Change is becoming more and more rapid. Consider that a person born in the early part of the twentieth century has experienced the advent or general use of automobiles, telephones, airplanes, nuclear power, television, radio, and computers. In addition to electronic and technological changes, change has also occurred in other fields such as medicine and in social, political, and economic areas. According to Bennis, Parikh, Lessem (1994):

> As the business world becomes more complex and more uncertain, more changeable, and more conflict ridden, so the requirements of managers proliferate. We are called upon, simultaneously, to manage complexity and uncertainty, change and conflict in ever larger doses (p. 1).

They state that the term *change* "tells us that nothing is static and that everything is moving in the stream of time."

The most effective approach to provide for positive change is to plan and influence the change. If change is not planned, it is possible that chaotic, negative circumstances will result. Bennis et al in 1976 defined *planned change* as "a conscious, deliberate, collaborative effort to improve the operation of human systems through the use of valid knowledge, . . . a goal directed process" (p. 4).

INNOVATION AND CREATIVITY

The terms *innovate* and *innovation* and *create* and *creativity* are used interchangeably in many publications. The *Random House Webster's College Dictionary* (1996, p. 319) defines *create* as "to cause to come into being, as something unique," and *creativity* as "the ability to create meaningful new forms, interpretations, . . . originality." *Innovate* (*Random House Webster's College Dictionary,* 1996, p. 695) is defined as "to introduce something new, make changes" and *innovation* as "something new or different is introduced." A creative, innovative person is one who displays productive originality.

Being creative and innovative is essential in nursing activities where change is constantly occurring. Improvements in nursing practice depend on the emerging of new ideas and strategies to meet the changing demands at all levels of health care.

LEADERSHIP AND MANAGEMENT IN NURSING PRACTICE

Managing and leading are basic components of nursing practice. All aspects of providing care for patients require application of the basic principles of management. Inherent in the process of leading is the need for the nurse to be aware of and responsive to the changes and innovations occurring in the patient care setting, in health care, and in the practice of nursing.

Understanding Management and Leadership Concepts

Rapid changes in health care have altered the activities of nursing staff and have increasingly thrust professional nurses into management and leadership roles. Nurses need to understand and practice the concepts of management and leadership because they are expected to know how to lead and manage. The nurse not only assists and helps patients who are dependent on someone "doing for" them but also is responsible for "watching over" other nursing staff members in their performance of nursing tasks. Nurses are "trustees" expected to take care of increasing numbers of patients and to manage the nursing staff who also provide direct hands-on care (Hersey and Duldt, 1989).

Another important function of the nurse is to coordinate the activities within the nursing staff and with other health professionals who interact with patients. Services are provided by laboratories, pharmacies, x-ray departments, rehabilitation and physical therapy units, and a wide variety of other departments. The nurse, as a caregiver or case manager, assumes responsibility for ensuring that services are safely and adequately provided.

Accomplishing the goals of safe, effective care is facilitated when all staff in an organization have an appreciation of fellow workers and can work well together. Several research studies indicate that accomplishment of tasks suffers when people do not respect each other or get along (Hersey and Duldt, 1989). The leaders and managers of groups need to understand the principles underlying leadership and management processes to better utilize the talents of all members of the team.

Theories of Management

The study of management in organizations has been of interest to a variety of different scientists, engineers, and institutional managers and administrators for many years. The desire to increase the productive output of organizations led to the development of different methods of organizing work and the workforce. As different ways of organizing work were devised, a variety of different theories evolved to explain the phenomena. As explained in Chapter 2, the word *theory* has multiple meanings and connotations. In science the word *theory* means the carefully formulated analysis of a set of facts or concepts in their relation to one another. A set of complex concepts known as organization theory describes how people work together to meet organizational goals (Grohar-Murray and DiCroce, 1997). Understanding the development of organizational and leadership theories provides insight as to how organizations evolve.

THE TRADITIONAL OR CLASSICAL SCHOOL OF MANAGEMENT

Engineer Frederick Winslow Taylor conducted studies and formulated management principles in the 1890s and early 1900s. He became known as the "father of scientific measurement." His concept was "knowing exactly what you want men to do, and then seeing that they do it in the best and cheapest way" (Taylor, 1910, p. 21). Taylor, a factory manager, attempted to determine how much work could reasonably be expected from one individual in a given job in a set period of time. His goal was to establish a standard of performance for a specific job. Using a stopwatch, he observed workers performing jobs or did the task himself. His work led to the beginnings of time-and-motion studies and job analysis. He tried to find the one best way of doing a job. He developed the concepts that led to mass producing of automobiles, which was introduced by Henry Ford. Application of his theories allowed the Ford Company to reduce the man-hours required to produce an automobile from 14 hours to 2 (Torrington and Weightman, 1994).

As a result of the studies conducted by Taylor, managers in other organizations began studying workers' job activities. Taylor's work led to organizational approaches that incorporated specialization, division of labor, sequence of work activities, planning, and evaluation techniques. The systems developed in many of these factories were unsatisfactory and led to employee dissatisfaction when high production standards could not be met and bottlenecks occurred on the production lines (Stevens, 1978).

Taylor's concepts were expanded by other scientists, including Henry L. Gnatt, and Frank and Lillian Gilbreth, who continued to establish standards based on the length of time it took to do a task. Workers were paid on the basis of the hours of work needed to complete an assignment. Other contemporary scientists conducted motion analysis of specific factory jobs. The focus was on the way to do a task best instead of how long the job took (Stevens, 1978).

Another major contributor to the early development of management studies was Henri Fayol, who changed the focus of his studies to review the administrative management side by devising a broader approach to management. Fayol, a French engineer, conducted a study in 1916, published in 1949, entitled *General and Industrial Management.* He concluded that there was a set of management principles that could be used in any organization in a variety of management situations. Fayol's writings are considered classic and form the basis for many of today's theories. Fayol identified the functions of management as:

- planning
- coordinating
- controlling
- organizing
- commanding

He stated that the principles of management were flexible and were dependent on individual conditions and specifications.

The approach taken by these pioneers in management studies was to provide a rational basis for management. The movement was directed to establish a scientific foundation and has been labeled the *Traditional School of Management.* Its concepts and theories have been analyzed and expanded. The traditional school continues to be refined by academicians and practitioners (Stevens, 1978).

The basic components of scientific management can be summarized as:

- analysis and synthesis of the elements of operation
- selection of the worker based on ability to meet production standards
- training of the worker
- proper tools and equipment
- proper incentives (Tappen, 1995, p. 87)

The principles and concepts devised by the Traditionalists have had a profound impact on health care agency management. Many of the present-day studies of nursing staff functions are based on an engineering approach. The results of time-and-motion studies have served as the basis for the assignment of nursing tasks to nurses with different levels of educational preparation.

At present there are efforts to restructure or reengineer nursing services. The move is based on the concept that relieving the professional nurse of nonnursing activities by assigning certain nursing tasks to less prepared individuals (described as unlicensed assistive personnel [UAP]) will reduce the costs of patient care and perhaps allow nurses more time for more advanced nursing practices (see Current Controversy in Chapter 5 on "deskilling" of nursing procedures). The assumption is that nursing procedures can be compartmentalized and anyone, regardless of limited educational preparation, can assume certain tasks. For example, multipurpose workers with on-the-job training participate in dietary activities such as delivering food to patients and then are assigned to direct nursing care tasks such as taking the patient's blood pressure and vital signs. The question arises as to whether the quality of nursing care is jeopardized by using these engineering techniques. Further research needs to be undertaken to determine the effect of these changes.

Although modern managers continue to use the ideas generated by the Traditional approach, there are drawbacks. Expectations that improved job productivity would result from analyzing tasks and setting performance standards did not always materialize. The focus was on the workers' performance only and not on the manager's performance (Stevens, 1978). Studies of the effectiveness of the manager's performance also had to be done to provide for more complete theory development. The theory base of the Traditional school seemed unfinished.

BEHAVIORAL SCHOOL OF MANAGEMENT

The failure of the Traditionalists to consider the behavior of humans in an organization led to the development of behavioral theories (also referred to as Human Relations theories). The theories evolved from the studies in the 1930s of Elton Mayo and J. F. Roethlisberger. Along with other colleagues they conducted research at the Hawthorne plant of Western Electric Company in Chicago, Illinois. A series of studies were conducted and are among the most famous reported in management literature (Roethlisberger and Dickson, 1958).

One of the studies dealt with introducing rest periods into the plant workers' schedule. The study was expected to show that controlling one variable, the rest period, would result in increased productivity. Initial results demonstrated that productivity did increase. However, when the rest periods were discontinued, productivity continued to climb. Rest periods were reintroduced and productivity further elevated. The conclusion reached was that the human factor had not been controlled. The extra attention given to the employees by including and consulting with them, and merely not the rest period, appeared to be the cause of increased productivity. This phenomenon has been labeled the "Hawthorne effect" by researchers and is always a factor to be controlled when conducting any research study (Stevens, 1978; Tappen, 1995).

Other results indicated that employee attitudes, fears, desires, sensitivity to status, and response to being treated fairly had an impact on how they performed and related to management (Tappen, 1995). Managers recognized that the way in which employees were treated greatly influenced productivity. For example, members of a health care team will respond more positively toward a leader who treats all members fairly and does not show favoritism to certain staff members.

Another contributor to the Behavioral School was Chester Barnard, who in 1938 used a sociologic approach to try to understand the concept of **cooperation.** The studies identified an institution as a social organism. His theory was based on the desire of individuals to control their own environment through cooperation with others (Stevens, 1978).

Other well-known figures associated with the Behavioral School included:

- Kurt Lewin (1951), a social psychologist, proposed that behavior is influenced by interactions between the worker's personality, structure of work groups, and the social and technical climate of the work place. He defined the steps involved in the process of change (discussed later in this chapter) (Gillies, 1989).
- Douglas McGregor (1957) developed Theory X and Y (Box 7–1). McGregor thought that employee effectiveness would be greatly improved if organizations would subscribe to Theory Y. If institutions using Theory X approaches moved to endorse Theory Y principles, major changes in management styles would have to

BOX 7-1
McGREGOR'S MANAGEMENT THEORIES: THEORY X AND THEORY Y

THEORY X

McGregor identified the conventional approaches to using human beings to meet organizational goals:

1. Management is responsible for organizing the money, materials, equipment, and people in an economical way.
2. Employees are to be directed, motivated, controlled, and assisted in modifying their behavior to fit organizational needs.
3. Without the active intervention of management, workers would be passive, perhaps even resistant to organizational needs.

McGregor indicated that inherent in the propositions were several additional beliefs:

1. The average man is indolent and works as little as possible.
2. He lacks ambition, dislikes responsibility, and prefers to be led.
3. He is inherently self-centered, indifferent to organizational needs, and resistant to change.
4. He is gullible and not very bright.

Underlying this approach is the concept that employees will be punished if the rules are not followed.

McGregor did not fully agree with the conventional assumptions and thought the approach to be inadequate. He proposed Theory Y as being more adequate for the management of people.

THEORY Y

1. Management is responsible for organizing the elements of money, materials, equipment, and people in an economical way.
2. People, by nature, are not passive, or resistant to organizational needs. They become so because of the experiences within the organization.
3. The motivation, potential for development, capacity to assume responsibility, and readiness to direct behavior toward organizational goals are present in people. Management is responsible to recognize and develop these characteristics.
4. The task of management is to arrange the organizational conditions so that people can achieve their goals and direct their own activities to meet organizational needs. They become so because of the experiences within the organization.

The basis of Theory Y is that if employees do fail it is because of poor management and leadership (McGregor, 1957).

occur so that workers were viewed and treated differently (McGregor, 1957). Theory Y proposes that work is satisfying, motivating, and rewarding. People can be enthusiastic and willing to support the organization if properly respected and treated.

- Herzberg further developed McGregor's theories. Employees were asked in a series of research studies what made them feel good or especially bad. The results were divided into hygiene factors, those factors that met an individual's need to avoid pain and discomfort (salary, appropriate supervision, good interpersonal relationships, and safe working conditions), and motivation factors such as growing personally and psychologically (satisfying work, opportunity to advance, responsibility, and recognition) (Tappen, 1995).
- Rensis Likert developed an approach in which supervisors focused on building work groups that are effective, that support the goals of the organization, and that have favorable attitudes toward the organization and coworkers. Likert developed the "system 4" approach to facilitate interaction among work groups in which supervisors and employees mutually influence and trust one another. An important component in this approach is that decisions are made at every level of the organization and not just by the top administrators. Democratic principles of governing are used. Training is provided to develop the potential of every employee (Gillies, 1989).
- Research studies by Chris Argyris found that, as individuals mature, they move toward greater independence, longer time perspectives, and increased self-control. He concluded that the rigid structure and harsh rules of the typical bureaucracy block employee growth potential and diminish job satisfaction. Employees tend to become passive and dependent (Gillies, 1989).

The **Z Theory** is an expansion of the Theory Y proposed by McGregor. Ouchi (1981) developed Theory Z as an outcome of studies conducted in well-managed Japanese industries. The theory has a humanistic viewpoint and is focused on developing improved ways to motivate people. The underlying principle of Theory Z is that motivated employees have increased job satisfaction and increased productivity (Tappen, 1995). A major component of the theory is collective decision making. Everyone affected by a decision is included in the making of that decision. For example, in a nursing team, all members of a team would be consulted about a decision; if a major change is made in the proposed agreed-upon solution, all members are again informed and participate in making another decision. The team is called a "quality circle" and all members of the circle are encouraged to assist in problem solutions. The leadership is democratic and decentralized.

Many individual social scientists contributed to the theories of the Behavioral School. These theories recognized that employees' perceptions of the work place are important and should be included when implementing any changes. The theorists also demonstrated the importance of considering the impact of formal and informal groups in the work setting because groups serve as social support systems and assist employees in either accepting or rejecting company policies (Tappen, 1995). Behavioral theorists continue to study and explore organizational behavior. Early scientists attempted to develop one theory to explain management; it is now known that organizations are too complex and the human factor too complicated to be explained by one theory.

Many health care institutions have tended to have hierarchical and bureaucratic organizational structures. In a hierarchy, power is concentrated at the top, with little authority at the bottom. Rank is determined by the individual's job description. Nurses employed in higher level managerial positions have greater authority to make decisions than do nurses working in staff positions.

In other health care institutions behavioral science studies have influenced nursing management activities. Participatory management practices have been introduced in clinical nursing settings. Decision making is being shared within all levels of nursing staff. Those in many organized nursing services within health care institutions have devised systems of shared governance in which participation and idea sharing are promoted within all levels of staff. The use of nursing teams that utilize team conferences provides for participation of all members of the team.

The Behavioral School stressed that the organization is a system of individuals working toward a common goal. Some managers and theorists did not subscribe to these theories and viewed the concepts as an extension of and a partnership with traditionalists. Behavioral scientists will continue to study and develop organizational theories; however, other ways to explain how organizations operate are being devised. One such approach is the Management Science School.

MANAGEMENT SCIENCE SCHOOL

The focus of management science, also referred to as operations research, is on the application of the scientific method of research and mathematical models to resolve tactical (operational) and strategic (long-term) problems in order to give management quantitative data as the basis for making decisions. (See Chapter 2 for a discussion of the scientific research method.) Developments within management science were greatly advanced with the increasing use of computers.

Management science is defined as the art and science of decision making. It originated in the economics field and is based on using a rational approach to make management decisions. It uses quantitative methods and mathematical models and processes. Solutions to problems are formulated by using statistical models and advanced data analysis methods (Dienemann, 1990).

In management science, models are defined as mathematical or structural descriptions of an activity. Constructing a model requires judgment and technical expertise. The development of the model requires the abstraction or simplifying of complex characteristics or systems that exist within an organization. It uses mathematical techniques to build models to solve problems and improve management practices. Different characteristics can be added or subtracted, allowing the data to be manipulated. For example, the design of a system of staffing for the operation of a nursing service organization (such as a home care program) can be developed into a mathematical model. The model is constructed by nurse managers and is based on their collective knowledge of the variables that affect the numbers of nursing staff needed to care for patients. The data produced provide managers with the information necessary to make informed decisions on staff allocation. Another example of nursing involvement in management science or operations research is participation in designing space requirements for patients, particularly in intensive care units and in planning for new facility space development. The success of management science or operations research is based on the ability of the participants conducting the research to clearly define the problem (Clark and Shea, 1979).

The use of the mathematical decision-making models has brought modern technology into organizations and allows for the use of sophisticated management tools. Managers have the opportunity to extend their knowledge base and make decisions on the basis of data rather than hunches. The use of such models requires decision makers to define problems and identify all of the elements that must be considered to make effective decisions. The use of the model in health care agencies has presented problems because of the complex nature of health institutions.

Quantitative methods are used in all aspects of operations in modern organizations. Mathematical models in health services were introduced in the United States in the early 1950s and even earlier in Great Britain. Early mathematical models included programs for scheduling outpatient services, planning menus, controlling the inventory for linens and drugs, and analyzing how inpatient services were being utilized. The approach is widely used. For example, the federal government's development of health care policy is based on the management science approach (Clark and Shea, 1979).

Quantitative methods are also used in nursing services budgetary programs. For example, the use of budgetary accounting principles and cost accounting (reports of how much it costs to provide specific services) has been incorporated into nursing management processes. Changes in reimbursement practices have created a new approach to how nurses practice nursing. The previous focus of doing all things for all patients regardless of the costs has disappeared. Measures of productivity have been introduced into most health care institutions.

An example of the use of accounting principles in patient care is the introduction of Diagnostic Related Groups (DRGs). Facilities participating in Medicare programs receive payment based on DRGs. The diagnostic groups are based on a formula in which diagnoses are divided into groups and the costs of each group averaged so that the average cost per patient per day is calculated. Reimbursement to the health care agency is based on the cost and number of patients in each group. A second accounting approach is based on patient classification systems in which nursing care hours are used as the basis for determining average costs (see Chapter 12 for discussion of patient classification systems) (Hoffman, 1988).

There are advantages and disadvantages to the management science approach. Supporters indicate that the choices for making decisions are based on objective, rational data rather than tradition or politics. Critics state that too much faith is placed in quantitative data even when the data are incomplete. The management science approach may also lead to centralized decision making rather than a decentralized system in which many individuals participate. There is agreement that three conditions need to be present to successfully use the approach:

- The goals to be reached are agreed upon.
- Only a limited number of characteristics or elements are included.
- The elements included must be amenable to quantification.

CURRENT MANAGEMENT APPROACHES

Establishing a single theory, as presented by Fayol, to explain all of the complex elements inherent in management is not possible. Different advocates have designed different theories to explain specific aspects of management processes. As already identified, traditionalists defined what managers do, behavioralists studied employees' involvement, and management scientists dealt with the quantitative processes used by managers. Theories based on previously devised concepts have been further developed and explored. There has been a logical and orderly extension of past perspectives and approaches.

The Human Resources Model. The concepts presented by McGregor in Theory X (i.e., workers are lazy, dull, and unwilling to accept responsibility) still persist in many institutions. Enlightened modern managers consider that people react to conditions around them and are promoters and utilizers of Theory Y (i.e., there are no intrinsic reasons why employees cannot be encouraged to take positive actions and to be self-motivated).

Behavioral Science. Institutions have become proficient and increasingly sophisticated in understanding human behavior. Progress in fields such as psychology, sociology, and other related sciences has affected operations in health care agencies. Studies in psychology have contributed information about learning, perception, and motivation. Social psychology and sociology have added to the knowledge base to increase understanding of group processes, leadership, cooperation, and communication. Nurses have contributed to the development of the body of knowledge in these fields through participation in and conducting of nursing research studies.

Contingency Approach. There are no simple answers or best style to communicating, leading, decision making, or structuring in any organization. The most successful managers and leaders are those that recognize that the method, style, or approach to managing and leading varies from situation to situation. Managing is more complex under these circumstances and requires greater sophistication to adapt to the use of different styles and communication patterns.

The main concept of this approach is that processes within an organization are interactive and cannot be isolated. For example, nursing activities within an agency are interactive with every other department in that agency. A change initiated in one component will affect other components (Baron, 1983).

DIFFERENCES BETWEEN MANAGERS AND LEADERS

As stated earlier, managers get work done through others and leaders serve as catalysts who, by persuasion and example, induce individuals or groups to take action. There is a difference in the power base between the manager and the leader. The manager is in a hierarchical position given authority by virtue of position, while leaders attempt to direct and influence the behavior of others to accomplish specific mutually agreed-upon goals (Gillies, 1989). Box 7–2, Leadership and Management Behaviors, displays these differences.

Roseanne Spitzer-Lehmann, a well-known nursing manager, indicates that it is difficult to distinguish between leadership and management because the "core components . . . are circular, dynamic, and interrelated." She states that the management role is to manage and ensure that the right process is being managed; the leadership role is to ensure that the right problem is being solved while focusing on the outcomes. She further explains that leadership is the vision, passion, and planning whereas management is the execution of the plan (Huber, 1996). The manager's primary aim is to accomplish organizational goals; the leader's aim may be to attain a goal associated with patient care.

Leaders in an organization are often placed in managerial positions. The most successful leaders/managers are those who are able to combine and bring vision, passion, and planning to a managerial position and exhibit the best characteristics of both. Managers who rely strictly on the authority of a hierarchical position will not be effective and will fail in meeting organizational and personal goals. As previously noted, employees tend to become passive and dependent when their talents are not used or appreciated.

BOX 7-2
LEADERSHIP AND MANAGEMENT BEHAVIORS

LEADERSHIP BEHAVIOR	MANAGEMENT BEHAVIOR	OVERLAP AREAS
Influences people to accomplish goals	Coordinates resources, integrates the use of resources	Plans for goal accomplishment
Inspires confidence	Plans Organizes	Motivates and directs follower
Envisions the future	Directs Controls	
Motivates followers	Accomplishes specific institutional goals and objectives	
Guides or leads the way		

From Huber, D. (1996). *Leadership and Nursing Care Management.* Philadelphia: W. B. Saunders.

Theories of Leadership

There are many different approaches to leadership. As with concepts of management, many theories have been developed and expanded, while some theories have been abandoned along the way. There is great interest in the area of leadership. Many researchers and authors continue to pursue different conceptual avenues to explain what leadership is.

It seems that when a group forms, a solitary person emerges as being "in charge." The person who takes over becomes either the designated or undesignated or informal leader. The leader is the person who has the most influence within a group. As stated previously in the definition by Kouzes and Posner (1995), leadership is the process used by all people to bring forth the best from their own efforts and those of others. They further state that leadership is the art of mobilizing others to want to struggle for shared aspirations.

Leadership has been traced from the time that human beings started to organize themselves into family groups, clans, or tribes. Political and governmental systems evolved. Early records from Egypt, China, Greece, and the Romans chronicle the history of this evolution.

As with management theories, efforts to determine what leadership is started in the early 1900s. Major approaches to investigating leadership have been organized into trait theories, behavioral theories, and situational theories.

TRAIT THEORIES

Trait theories, which emerged in the 1940s and 1950s, are based on the idea that "leaders are born, not made." It is assumed that certain innate abilities, or personality factors, are present within an individual that make for a great leader. The acceptance of such a theory leads to the conclusion that some people could not become leaders. Some theorists studied the biographies of people in leadership positions to determine if a single trait could explain the successful leader.

The Great Man Theory

The basic premise of the Great Man theory is that the influence of a great man changed the course of history. The individuals possessed innate characteristics that made them great leaders. Historical figures such as Hitler, Caesar, Joan of Arc, and Mao Tse Tung have been studied. The theory can be summarized as:

- Leaders differ from followers in the number of key traits possessed, and
- Traits remain unchanged across time.

Had such a theory been realized, it would be easy to select leaders; all that is needed is to identify persons with the desirable trait and appoint them to the leadership position. Obviously, the theory does not work; researchers could not identify traits that distinguished leaders from nonleaders (Baron, 1983; Tappen, 1995).

Personal Trait Theory

The pursuit of trait theories continued despite the rejection of the great man theory. Researchers were not able to identify specific traits that could be used to predict who would be an effective leader. However, there were some characteristics that were identified as significant in most of the studies (Box 7–3). Of the identified characteristics, the most frequently cited were intelligence and initiative.

Trait theories are limited because they focus only on the leader. They do not take into consideration all of the other components involved in the management-leadership situation, e.g., the employee, the work being performed, or the environment. The leader is evaluated only on his or her capacities as a leader and not on the actual job done. The characteristics demonstrated may stem from other factors such as motivation rather than on the innate capacities of the leader (Tappen, 1995).

BEHAVIORAL THEORIES

Initiated in the 1950s, behavioral theories continued to focus on the leader. Behavioral theories, also referred to as attitudinal approaches, are concerned with *how* effective the leader is and *what* the leader does rather than *who* the leader is. Management theories and leadership theories evolved at the same time. For example, McGregor's Theory of X and Y,

BOX 7-3
SIGNIFICANT PERSONAL TRAITS OF LEADERS

- Intelligence and skill
- Initiative
- Assertiveness and persistence
- Ability to relate to other people
- A strong sense of self
- Ability to tolerate stress and take the consequences of a decision
- Originality (creativeness)
- Status within a group

From Tappen, R. M. (1995). *Nursing Leadership and Management: Concepts and Practice,* 3rd ed. Philadelphia: F. A. Davis.

and Rensis Likert's concepts and studies relating to participative management are also considered as research in leadership.

Other behavioral theorists include Blake and Mouton, who developed a managerial styles grid in which two factors are considered: concern for production, and concern for people (Fig. 7–1). A scale to determine whether a leader has high or low concern for production and for people is devised. It is anticipated that both factors will be considered by managers and leaders because the concerns are interdependent. The grids are used by groups to objectively look at the attitudes and personal behavior of members (Blake and Mouton, 1967).

The scales have been used by nursing managers and leaders in clinical settings to assist in reviewing the effectiveness of management teams. The ratings assist nursing staff in strengthening staff cohesion and group interworking (Swansburg, 1990).

Major research studies on organizational behavior were undertaken at the Ohio State University and the University of Michigan. The studies at the Ohio State University were conducted to investigate leader behavior and the effects of leadership style on the work group. The University of Michigan studies were designed to identify styles of leadership that resulted in increased work-group performance and satisfaction.

In the Ohio studies, leaders, subordinates, peers, and supervisors were surveyed in an attempt to determine the best leadership style. Two different questionnaires were used. One measured the style of leadership as **perceived by the leader** and the other measured the style of leadership of the leader as **perceived by the subordinates.** Two independent leadership styles were identified:

- Task-oriented leadership style: The degree to which the leader organized and defined the tasks, assigned the work to be done, established communications and networks, and evaluated work-group performance.
- Employee-oriented leadership style: The degree to which the leader developed trust, mutual respect, friendship, support, and concern for the welfare of the employee.

The findings indicated that the organizational structure of the institution and the behavior of the leader combined to determine the style used, but the style adopted also depended on how the leader reacted as individual situations were encountered.

The University of Michigan researchers conducted a number of studies in a variety of different industries. In one setting training programs were provided to supervisors. Two groups received information to make supervisors more participative (employee-centered behavior); in two other groups the use of rules, regulations, and procedures was emphasized (job-centered behavior). Production was measured weekly and employee attitudes were measured before and after the study. The results indicated that, in using either job-centered or em-

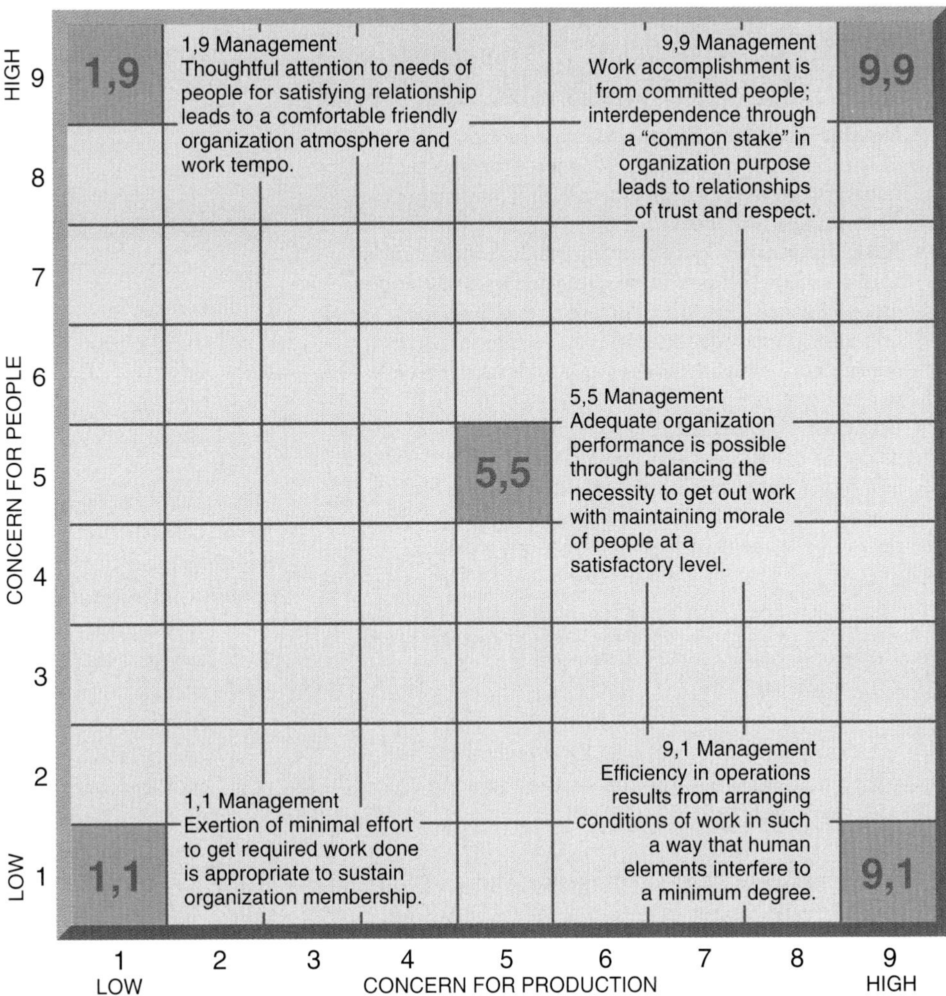

Figure 7-1. Blake and Moulton's managerial styles grid. (From Blake, R.P., Mouton, J.S. [1967]. Organization excellence through effective management behavior. *Management. 20*:42–47.)

ployee-centered leadership styles, productivity increased. However, job-centered behavior created tension and stress that resulted in lower job satisfaction and increased turnover and absenteeism (Szilagyi and Wallace, 1980).

The results of the various behavioral studies indicated that effective leadership is determined by situational factors and not by any specific leadership behavior. This led to exploring new approaches to studying leadership.

SITUATIONAL THEORIES

The late 1960s saw a move toward a more system-wide, humanistic thinking about organizations. The approach avoids the narrow perspective of earlier leadership methods by considering all of the situational factors existing within an institution.

Investigators started to focus their efforts on situational leadership studies. The trait and behavioral theorists provided a solid foundation of research on which to base a new approach. Situational leadership combines the elements of:

- Manager or leader: The personal characteristics, needs and motives, and past experiences will affect the behavior of the leader/manager.
- Employee: Employees will also have personality characteristics, needs, motives, and past experiences that will affect attitudes and behavior.
- Structure of the group and nature of the work: (1) Groups have specific characteristics and structure that may or may not support the leader/manager; (2) The nature of the task of the group will affect the leader's behavior. For example, a group assigned to routine types of tasks may require more motivation than a group assigned to experimental tasks in which changes occur frequently.
- Factors within the organization: (1) The power base of the leader will affect the influence the leader wields within the group; (2) The rules, procedures, standards, policies and routines within an organization may dictate the type of leadership exercised.
- Professionalism: Organizations in which staff are highly qualified and educated (such as nurses) may limit the leader's/manager's ability to influence the staff.
- Timing: Problems requiring quick decisions can lead to stress and tension within a group. Careful planning

BOX 7-4
FIEDLER'S CONTINGENCY MODEL OF LEADERSHIP

- **Leader-Member Relationships:** Leaders presumably have more power and influence if they have good relationships with their members than if they have poor relationships with them.
- **Task Structure:** Tasks or assignments that are highly structured, spelled out, or programmed give the leader more influence than tasks that are vague, nebulous, and unstructured. For example, it is easier to develop nursing care plans according to a set format than it is to chair a meeting.
- **Position Power:** Leaders will have more power and influence if their position is vested with such activities as hiring and firing, and being able to discipline and reprimand. Position power is determined by how much power the leader has over his or her subordinates.

Data from Fiedler, E. E. (1972). How do you make leaders more effective? New answers to an old puzzle. In K. Davis: *Organizational Behavior: A Book of Readings,* 5th ed. New York: McGraw-Hill.

may avoid situations in which staff members feel they have not had input into the decision-making process (Szilagyi and Wallace, 1980).

A situational theory, the **Contingency Theory** or **Model,** was proposed by Fiedler in the mid 1960s (Box 7–4). The model is complex and three-dimensional. The model purports to predict the most effective leadership style through an analysis of three components: leader-member relationships, task structure, and the leader's position of power. The theory demonstrates that effective leadership style depends on the interaction of many different factors, primarily within the job assigned and related to the power of the leader. For example, if a nurse leader is well-liked and has an ambiguous task to assign to a staff member, a considerate, friendly approach can be used; if the nurse leader is not well liked, a direct impersonal leadership style would be most appropriate (Grohar-Murray and DiCroce, 1997).

Another situational theory, the **Path-Goal Theory,** was suggested by R. J. House (1971). The theory considers a different set of factors including the extent of the tasks to be done, role ambiguity, employees' expectations, and the ways in which the leader can influence a group. The results of House's work indicated that a leader will have less influence if an individual has many and varied tasks to perform and enjoys the work. He also determined that employees need recognition and consideration from their leaders. The characteristics of the staff and the situational demands with which they are faced will affect the leader's need to increase employee motivation (Tappen, 1995).

Other theories have been suggested and explored. Most of these theories are based on the previous studies proposed by other situational, behavioral, and trait theorists. Many of the research studies that led to the development of specific theories identified various managerial and leadership styles. An understanding of the significant styles and leadership behaviors is important to nurses because participating in nursing care activities involves working in groups.

Leadership Styles

Studies in which the traits of leaders were examined failed to differentiate successful leaders from unsuccessful leaders. A different approach was devised in which the behavior of the leader or the style of leadership was investigated. The studying of behavior is easier because behavior can be observed and various styles of leadership could be identified.

Leadership style is defined by Huber (1996, p. 60) as "different combinations of task and relationship behaviors used to influence others to accomplish goals." Task behavior and relationship behavior are further defined:

- *Task behavior* is the way in which leaders define roles and organize the tasks to accomplish the work to be done.
- *Relationship behavior* is the way in which leaders maintain personal relationships, communicate, and support staff members (Hersey and Blanchard, 1993)

The results of the studies by Tannenbaum and Schmidt (1958, 1973) indicated that three major categories of leadership styles emerged:

- **Authoritarian Leadership**

  This style of leadership is exemplified by the person who is directive and maintains control over all situations. All decisions are made by the leader, and subordinate staff are expected to carry out orders. The stereotypical image of the "hard as nails" nurse manager on a clinical unit issuing orders to cowering staff members typifies the worst features of an authoritarian leader.

  A disadvantage of the authoritarian style is that it dampens employee creativity and leads to staff dissatisfaction. An advantage is that the style can be effective during emergencies and in crisis situations.
- **Democratic Leadership**

  Shared decision making is a central component of democratic leadership style. The leader supports participation by staff and fosters staff involvement. Teamwork and positive intrapersonal relationships are encouraged. The focus is on human relationships. Some studies indicate that absenteeism is lessened, job satisfaction is increased, and feelings of anxiety and hostility are diminished.

  There are disadvantages to the use of a democratic leadership model. Reaching group consensus in decision making takes longer. If an immediate decision must be made, all personnel may not be included in the decision, which could lead to difficulties with staff feelings. There also may be some staff members who are not interested in being involved and only want to be left alone to do their assigned task.

On the other hand, there are many advantages to using a democratic, participative leadership style. Employees are usually more satisfied and realize greater self-actualization.

- **Laissez-Faire Leadership**

  Leaders who choose to adopt a laissez-faire type of leadership behavior generally have abdicated all control of the group. The leader does not influence anyone. Although personnel may initially like the freedom, frequently members become hostile and tense because they do not have a sense of direction. This style may be advantageous if the members of a specific group work independently of each other, e.g., a group of nursing researchers working on separate aspects of a project. The group members may report only to each other rather than to a single member (Huber, 1996).

As discussed, there are advantages and disadvantages to each of the leadership styles. A leader may find that one style is exercised in one set of circumstances and other style under different conditions. Nurses generally prefer to work in a democratic work environment. As well-qualified professionals, nurses possess a body of knowledge that allows for independent decision making and working in collegial groups.

CHANGE, INNOVATION, AND CREATIVITY

Change, Innovation, and Creativity in Nursing Practice

Present within all work environments is the constant pressure to adopt, adapt, and change. Nurses, as an integral part of health care, are being placed in managerial and leadership positions in which they are expected to improve productivity with reduced budgets, fewer numbers, and less well prepared staff. New creative and innovative ideas have to be formulated to meet this challenge.

It is not possible to discuss leadership and management without considering the concept of change. Change is an everyday part of both work and personal life. Maya Angelou, author and poet, says:

> Circumstances alter cases. One never really makes a change unless one has to; difficulties cause change. But if we participate in that change, there may be the grand chance that we can direct it. If we don't participate it's going to take place anyway (Brown, 1996, pp. 4–5).

To contemplate making a change may be a pleasurable experience, or, depending on the circumstances, frightening and filled with uncertainty. The challenge nurses face in the turbulent, often chaotic, ever-changing situation existing in health care today is enormous. There are no longer choices as to whether one will participate in proposed changes, inasmuch as change is constantly occurring, but individuals have an option as to how they will participate. The shift from nonprofit to profit-making health care is increasing attention on reducing costs and increasing shareholder profits. Nurses are caring for more patients with less available material and human resources. For example, reductions in the numbers of professional nurses and increases in unlicensed assistive personnel have required nurses to be responsible and care for many more patients and oversee the work of less well-prepared staff.

Nurses are working to become proactive and have a voice in the changes happening around and to them, while at the same time reacting to those changes that have already been made. Change can be viewed positively or negatively. It can be a growth, survival, or retrenchment experience (Sample, 1994). Understanding the dynamics of the change process and the theoretical basis assists in making the response to change growth-producing and serves as a stimulus to innovative and creative behavior.

Theories of Change

As previously stated, nurses are involved in changes every day. New patients are admitted, new medications are ordered, new staff are assigned to the unit or program, and new or improved equipment is placed into service. Participating in the decisions about the way in which changes are made assists staff members in accepting and guiding the change process. It is important that nurses understand the processes and theories of change to become effective leaders and managers (Manion, 1995).

Change theory is derived from behavioral sciences, learning theory, communications theory, systems theory, and interpersonal theory. The phases of the change process proposed by Kurt Lewin have served as a foundation for the development of change theory. It is one of the most widely known theories and underlies the work of many other theorists.

FORCE FIELD ANALYSIS

Lewin proposes that, in situations in which changes are to be made, there is a dynamic balance of forces working against each other. The **driving forces** move toward the proposed change and the **restraining forces** move away from the proposed change. Lewin's theory of change, force field analysis, is based on maintaining equilibrium in systems. The change process is initiated by analyzing the whole system to determine the forces that are for and against change. There are three phases of the change process (Box 7–5):

- Unfreezing
- Freezing
- Refreezing

BOX 7-5
LEWIN'S PHASES OF THE CHANGE PROCESS

➡ ➡ ➡ **UNFREEZING** ➡ ➡ ➡ **MOVING** ➡ ➡ ➡ **REFREEZING** ➡ ➡ ➡ ➡ ➡ ➡ ➡ ➡ ➡ ➡ ➡ ➡ ➡ ➡ ➡
⬅ ⬅ ⬅ ⬅ ⬅ ⬅ ⬅ ⬅ ⬅

- **Unfreezing**
  The problem is identified and a possible solution is devised. The next step is to prepare individuals in the system to accept the change and create an environment to motivate staff toward change. If patterns of behavior are well established, it may be necessary to create uncomfortable situations so that individuals will respond and participate. Disequilibrium is created by introducing the idea that the old methods did not work. People may resist, try to ignore the problem, or become defensive.
  Guilt and anxiety may be introduced to raise the tension level of the group. The level of unease must be monitored and staff need to be assured that they are secure in their job (psychological security).
  The unfreezing stage is completed when the change is accepted by the group.
- **Moving/Changing**
  The system becomes unfrozen and movement toward change is initiated. The innovation is refined. Planning and implementing the change is undertaken. The process of unfreezing can lead to confusion and resistance to change. Efforts must be directed to overcoming the resistance.
- **Refreezing**
  The change is stabilized and integrated into the ongoing activities. An evaluation process is undertaken to determine the effectiveness of the change and make necessary adjustments in the implementation procedures.

The process of change may flow back and forth between the various phases. It is not linear and the stages may be revisited at any time.

From Huber, D. (1996). *Leadership and Nursing Care Management*. Philadelphia: W. B. Saunders.

Some forces will be at work to assist the change and others to restrain the process from occurring. The process may move quickly or may become static and remain at one phase. The goal of Lewin's model is to plan, control, and evaluate change (Huber, 1996) (see discussion of research utilization of Lewin's theory in chapter 2).

ROGERS' THEORY OF CHANGE

In 1962, Everett Rogers expanded on Lewin's theory by indicating that the background of the person instituting the change (change agent) and the environment in which the change is being introduced are antecedents to the change. Five factors are needed to ensure the success of the change:

- The change must have the advantage of being better than the existing methods.
- The change must be compatible with existing values (compatibility).
- Complex ideas will persist even if simple ones are implemented (complexity).
- Change is to be introduced on a small scale (divisibility)
- The easier it is to describe the change, the more likely it will be successful (communicability) (Swansburg, 1990).

Rogers identifies five phases to the change process:

Phase 1. Awareness: Knowledge of the need for the change to occur.
Phase 2. Interest: Commitment to the need for the change and support of the process defined to initiate the change.
Phase 3. Evaluation: Methods developed to determine the success or failure of the change.
Phase 4. Trial: Trials of the proposed change conducted.
Phase 5. Adoption: Successful programs instituted (Huber, 1996).

According to Rogers, people involved need to be interested in the innovation and be committed to making the change. There are two outcomes: the change is accepted or rejected (Huber, 1996).

LIPPITT'S THEORY OF CHANGE

Lippitt expanded on Lewin's theory and proposed an approach utilizing seven phases. The theory is specific in defining the steps necessary to plan for change.

Phase 1: Define the problem:
The person(s) recognizing the need for change initiates a process (such as group meetings) to identify the problem.

Phase 2. Assess the motivation for and capacity for making the change:
Decide on certain solutions and determine the possibility for each solution to be successful. The persons involved in the change should have a part in the decision-making process. Included in the decision-making process are considerations as to the interest of group members in making the change, cost in terms of human and material resources, and who is to make the final decision for the change to take place.

Phase 3. Assess the change agent's motivation and resources:
The individual(s) involved in promoting the change (the change agent) should be committed to improving the situation, knowledgeable about the approaches needed to institute the change, and objective and flexible in promoting the change.

Phase 4. Select the objectives necessary to accomplish the change:
A final decision is made on initiating a change. A detailed plan is developed that incorporates specific

objectives, time tables, responsibilities, and deadlines to complete the change. The change is implemented and evaluated.

Phase 5. Determine the role of the change agent:

The change agent plays an active role in facilitating the implementation of the change. Conflicts about the change are handled by the change agent.

Phase 6. Maintain the change:

The change is evaluated, with constant feedback given on any problems encountered during the implementation process. Revisions in the plan are made as necessary.

Phase 7. Change agent's role reduced and terminated:

Written policies and procedures are completed. The staff assumes responsibility for continuing the new process and monitoring additional changes that may need to be made (Swansburg, 1990).

The change theories described are similar to the problem-solving process and to the nursing process.

Types of Change

Change can be accidental or planned (as previously discussed). Accidental change or reactive change happens in response to an outside force causing an imbalance in the organization. The systems operating within the organization try to adjust to the outside force by changing. Torrington and Weightman (1994) distinguish between four broad types of change:

- **Imposition:** The initiative comes from exterior sources. Alteration in ways in which things are done is necessary to comply with the external forces. The only route open is to respond to the parameters set by someone else. Examples of this type of imposed change would include new laws, new policies mandated by an institution, or changes in nursing work schedules.
- **Adaptation:** Changes in attitudes, values, or behavior are required because of forces external to the person. For example, an institution changes its policy regarding abortions and requires that nurses assist in the abortion procedure. The nurse who does not believe in abortion may be faced with changing personal values if he or she agrees to assist or may decide to seek employment elsewhere.
- **Growth:** Individuals are allowed to make decisions and personal talents are permitted to evolve in an atmosphere in which individuals can develop more confidence and are allowed to achieve. For example, staff are encouraged to express their ideas on how procedures or policies may be improved and are recognized for their contributions.
- **Creativity:** Staff members instigate and control the way in which changes are planned and made. For example, a team of nurses representing all levels of nursing staff was assigned the responsibility of designing a new system of delivering nursing care. They were also held accountable for implementing the plan. The members received support from coworkers and administrators in their efforts to use new and different approaches in the design.

Change has far-reaching effects and can have unforeseen and potentially unexpected and undesirable outcomes. If changes are enforced from outside or from internal pressures that do not allow staff participation, greater anxiety and less success may result. Under the best of circumstances, a small change can have a ripple effect on an entire agency (Gillies, 1989).

The change agent and those involved take risks when change is instituted. There is usually some resistance to the change that should be recognized and dealt with when it happens. The greater the support of the persons involved, the greater the chance for successfully making the change. Change needs to occur and leaders should be the movers behind making the change rather than waiting for forces outside of the immediate work situation to mandate change.

Change involves being innovative and creative. According to Drucker (1985), change offers opportunities for new things and different processes. Huber (1996, p. 515) states "a purposeful and organized search for change is the basis for systematic innovation." Innovativeness and creativity are usually more evident in an environment in which individuals are supported by supra- and subordinate staff when trying new approaches and new ways of doing things.

Innovation and Creativity

Innovation and creativity, defined as the introduction of something new by a person who displays originality, are concepts basic to leadership and change processes. Solving problems requires new ways of looking at and analyzing the problem, environment, and circumstances surrounding the problem. Bennis (1989, pp. 29–30) indicates that:

> It is not the articulation of a profession or organizational goals that creates new practices but rather the imagery that creates the understanding, the compelling moral necessity for the new way.
>
> How do we identify and develop such innovators? Innovators, like all creative people, see things differently, think in fresh and original ways.
>
> The true leader not only is him- or herself an innovator but makes every effort to locate and use other innovators in the organization.

Change, and innovation and creativity are companion terms but can also be differentiated. Change occurs when the system is disrupted; innovation uses change to create new and different approaches to resolve an issue and develop new products or procedures (Huber, 1996). Systematic innovation, according to Drucker (1992) requires a willingness to look on change as an opportunity. Innovation does not create change. Successful innovations are accomplished by exploiting change not forcing it.

The innovative person will look for occasions to be creative and bring new solutions to old problems. Seven sources for innovative ideas have been identified by Drucker (1992). Four sources found internally within the institution are:

- **Unexpected opportunities:** Situations present themselves that require different methods to be adopted. Knowing what is happening in an institution allows an individual to prepare for impending changes.
- **Incongruous circumstances:** Disruptions occur that require changes to be made. Discrepancies exist between reality as it is and reality as it is assumed to be.
- **Innovation based on process needs:** Procedures and policies need to be altered to respond to new regulations, policies, or laws.
- **Changes in structure:** Organizational changes require changes in methods of operations.

Three sources are outside of the institution:

- **Changes in demographics:** Alterations in community statistics such as age and income levels affect organizational operations.
- **New information or knowledge:** New technological knowledge requires changes in practices.
- **Changes in perceptions, taste, and meanings:** Shifts in demographics, technology, and social needs create different ways of looking at situations.

Drucker (1992) further identified the skills that a leader needs to be an effective innovator:

- Looks beyond the immediate situation into the broad world for data on what is happening in other similar arenas.
- Finds out what information is needed to be an effective leader in a specific work situation; assumes responsibility for finding information for own needs; uses a variety of different data sources.
- Focuses energies and attention on the need for changes and innovations.
- Maintains learning as a lifelong process; incorporates ways to maintain current and up-to-date knowledge.

There are many opportunities for innovation. The unexpected will happen but no one knows when or how. It is important to be aware of what is going on and recognize the opportunities to be innovative.

Innovations are generally more acceptable if compatible with the values and norms of the group or organization involved. The institutional climate and culture influence how innovative-creative individuals perform because organizations seem to emphasize a particular organizational culture. For example, it is not uncommon in health care agencies to be told that "this is the right way," or "this is the way we do things on this unit." The type of uniform or dress required by an organization also reflects the culture. Creativity may be fostered or stifled, depending on the organizational climate.

Nurse leaders are responsible for helping create and support an organizational culture that is adaptable, innovative, and positive. The leader can incorporate change and innovation as a positive norm so that knowing, understanding, and accepting change become part of the nursing environment (Kawamoto, 1994). Psychologists have tried to identify the characteristics of individuals with high levels of creativity. The characteristics are summarized by Steiner (1965) (Box 7–6).

BOX 7-6
STEINER'S CHARACTERISTICS OF CREATIVE INDIVIDUALS

- **Conceptual Fluency**
  The ability to generate a large number of ideas rapidly.
- **Conceptual Flexibility**
  The ability to discard one frame of reference for another.
- **Originality**
  The tendency to give unusual or atypical answers.
- **Preference for complexity over simplicity**
  Looking for the new challenge of knotty problems.
- **Independence of judgement**
  Being different from peers and seeing superiors as conventional or arbitrary.

Data from Torrington, D., Weightman, J. (1994). *Effective Management: A Systems Approach: People and Organizations,* 2nd ed. Englewood Cliffs, NJ: Prentice-Hall.

Nurses who provide care in a creative and innovative way are highly valued by patients. Nurses who are creative give nursing care in a way that is individualized, unique, and in tune with the circumstances surrounding the patient's problems (Ferguson, 1992). Creativity is also discussed in Chapter 12.

Innovation and creativity are essential components in modern-day nursing and in the operation of any health care organization. An institution that maintains the status quo will not continue to be productive nor will it survive in the current health care marketplace. Health care institutions that support a climate of innovation and creativity will have a greater chance of continuing success.

IMPLICATIONS FOR NURSING PRACTICE

Using Management and Leadership Theory in Nursing Practice

Nursing management and leadership utilize the concepts and principles developed in the fields of psychology, sociology, anthropology, economics, social psychology, and applied fields such as business administration, accounting, computer technology, and others. Although there are no generally accepted theories of nursing management or leadership, a few theories and models have been proposed. Results of a variety of studies indicate that there is an integration of clinical nursing concepts with nursing administration knowledge, and that nursing and management knowledge is integrated. One important finding indicated that little attention was paid by nursing researchers to determining the importance of leadership in nursing practice (Huber, 1996).

Nurses realize that motivating, seeking staff participation in decision making, communicating, recognizing the contributions made by individuals, and allowing for interactive group processes will enhance employee satisfaction and lead to improved job performance. Efforts to develop new management and leadership theories in the behavioral and management sciences need to be enhanced. Nursing will continue to draw on management and leadership theories and to study and develop nursing management theories.

Nurse managers will be faced with increasing use of management science technology. The emergence of managed care systems or health maintenance organizations will force all nursing managers to utilize data gathering and data analysis techniques to accommodate the increasing focus on cost-effective care. Use of computers in health care facilities will further expand and require a high degree of literacy in the use of a computer and utilizing of data.

Using Change Theory in Nursing Practice

Nursing is in the process of redesigning its role in the health care system. The changes that are occurring in health care agency restructuring have required the nursing profession to make changes in the systems used to deliver nursing care.

Roles and responsibilities of nurses are being drastically altered. Changes demand a new frame of reference for all nursing personnel in all health care agencies. Included in these changes is the increasing need for nurses to understand and practice nursing management and leadership theories and principles. Nursing students are thrust into organizational settings from their first day of clinical practice. It is essential to have knowledge about the organizational structure and systems operating within the agency where one is practicing. Organizational structures provide a road map that portrays the decision-making process within an agency. In a hierarchy, the higher the position level in the organizational structure, the greater the authority and the greater the decision-making power.

It is expected in clinical agencies that all nurses will have management and leadership skills. Having a theoretical base provides the nurse with the tools to analyze and solve management and leadership problems. For example, understanding McGregor's X and Y Theory provides the nurse with information as to how employees may be responding to management policies and procedures. The nurse may also review personal feelings about role expectations and how personal attitudes affect his or her job performance.

Nurses can make use of leadership theories in everyday decision-making situations. A decision-making or problem-solving process is used to plan and implement change. An important element in planning for and implementing any change is the understanding that evaluating and constant monitoring are essential. The initiation of the change process is circular, and each phase or stage may be revisited several times to assess outcomes and make adaptations.

An example of how nursing uses the planning process to initiate change:

> The possible purchase of a new piece of equipment requires the development of a plan on how to introduce the changes that will be required to use the equipment in nursing practice. A staff person assumes the responsibility for being the change agent and introduces the product to the group that will utilize the instrument. Details on what changes are required and how the plan is to be formulated are made during a meeting of the group. Cost factors and resources needed (such as who is to use the equipment) are determined. Conflicts within the group are discussed and handled by the change agent and group members (Lewin's Unfreezing Phase; Roger's Phases 1 and 2; Lippitt's Phases 1, 2 and 3).
>
> A final decision is made on the basis of the desirable results that would occur as a result of the purchase and use of the equipment and the commitment of the staff to support the change. Assuming the decision is positive, a specific plan is formulated. The plan includes the objectives to be accomplished, steps to be taken to introduce the instrument to and train the staff, procedures and policies needed to ensure availability of adequate information for the staff, evaluation process, and a timetable to accomplish the change (Lewin's Moving/Changing; Roger's Phases 2 and 3; Lippitt's Phases 4 and 5).
>
> The nurse responsible for overseeing the activities associated with the implementation and evaluation of the change continues to be available for assistance in any alterations needed in the plan. For example, if problems arise with the functioning of the equipment, additional training sessions in its proper use may be held.
>
> The agent ensures that the procedures and policies are in writing and available to the staff (Lewin's Refreezing; Roger's Phase 5; Lippitt's Phases 6 and 7).

Once the implementation is completed, the involved staff assume the responsibility for continuing monitoring. A process is built in to provide for evaluating beneficial or non-beneficial effects of using the procedure and equipment. Based on the evaluation, further changes may have to be made.

Another approach for instituting change was used by a health care organization to restructure nursing care on an inpatient acute care hospital unit (Scott and Rantz, 1994). The Lewin's Phases of the Change Process model (see Box 7–5) was used as a theoretical framework. Following is a discussion of initiating change using Lewin's Phases of the Change Process.

THE SETTING

REASONS TO INITIATE CHANGE

The nursing staff of an acute care hospital was informed that budgets for personnel and material resources (i.e., equipment and supplies) were being reduced. The changes imposed by the reductions forced the nursing staff to review the way in which nursing care was being delivered. Time, money, and effort had already been expended on making changes without a great deal of success. It was decided that the best method to accomplish a significant change would be to restructure and invent new ways to provide care. A literature review was undertaken to find information on how to make the change. The Lewin model (see Box 7–5) was selected as being the clearest and providing the needed direction to plan and implement the project. A driving force was the maintenance of a patient care focus. The patient was to receive care that was coordinated and supportive.

The nursing administrative group decided that there was great value in having the staff participate in the restructuring. A task force consisting of staff nurses, assistant nurse managers, a nurse clinician, nurse specialist, and a representative from nursing administration was appointed. The three-step process proposed by Lewin was initiated.

THE PROCESS USED

UNFREEZING

The task force studied all of the facets of change for more than 2 months. Methods to promote creativity were used. That change frequently causes confusion and uncomfortableness was discussed. Change was not to be made until the staff felt an urgency to change. During this period of time the patients presented more complex problems, lengths of stay of patients decreased, and lack of coordination of patient care was creating frustration for the staff. Task-oriented behaviors rather than patient-oriented behaviors had been rewarded in the past. Rewards needed to be given to those that served the patient.

A vision of the future organization emerged, and a model for a new structure was created. The new model was designed after several weeks of discussion and a staff retreat that focused on challenging traditions and transforming roles. After reviewing the model the role of the nurse was revised to include a closer relationship between the nurse and patient. The nursing role was envisioned to include greater influence, guidance, and a continuous relationship with the patient. The care coordinator role was defined.

A team-oriented approach to making the changes had been initiated and was continued. Administrative support was evident. A climate supporting change existed. A foundation for making the change was in place. Meetings to communicate the plan for the proposed changes were held with different groups in the organization.

MOVING/CHANGING

The first unit indicating readiness to initiate the change was determined. Staff meetings were held and volunteers were recruited to make up a task force on restructuring. Orientation meetings were conducted with the intent of increasing trust and developing communication skills among the members of the group.

The roles of the various levels of nursing staff were explored. The lines between the levels of nursing aide, licensed practical nurse (LPN), and registered nurse (RN) had blurred. It became evident during the discussions that providing total patient care by RNs would not be possible. The first role developed was a patient care technician. The technician would be well prepared to provide supportive care. The next level was the LPN. The discussions were delayed until a later time because of difficulties in defining the specific role. The care coordinator role of the RN was defined. Next the staff nurse role was determined. Job descriptions for each level, except the LPN, were written.

The LPN role emerged as technical and supportive in a partnership with other team members. The LPN was also seen as a possible multicompetent worker who could be cross-trained for a variety of different jobs. The number of staff and the mix of staff to be assigned to each shift were decided. Budgetary issues were resolved.

REFREEZING

The hiring and training of staff were the first steps in the refreezing stage. The plan was implemented. Some staff, such as the care coordinator, had difficulty changing old habits and allowing other staff to provide direct patient care. Training in delegating tasks had to also be conducted for staff nurses.

Other problems were encountered such as depending on a task-driven system rather than on a total plan of care for the patient. The focus was to be placed on patient outcomes. The LPN role also had to be further defined and retraining provided. All of the staff required support during this phase.

THE RESULTS

The evaluation is ongoing and alterations are made as necessary. The commitment to support the change process continued.

The example of the use of the Lewin's Phases of Change Theory in a clinical setting can be replicated in any health care site. Not only is the Lewin model useful but also the application of other theoretical models provides a solid foundation for designing and implementing changes which are based on creative innovations.

Creativity and Innovation in Nursing Practice

Change is inevitable. The individual who looks upon change as an opportunity to be creative and innovative is to be envied. Having the ability to visualize beyond the immediate situation and envision the future is the basis for new and innovative approaches to giving nursing care. Nursing, as in all professions, is in need of individuals who have the ability to develop new ways and methods to care for patients. Creative nurses seize the opportunities when presented to try different approaches to resolve old problems.

Flexibility, curiosity, tenacity, and the commitment to try new ways of practicing nursing are but a few of the characteristics that students need to develop to foster creativity and innovation. Practicing in situations where these traits are valued allows these talents to be fostered and nourished. The nursing profession should emphasize the importance of recognizing and rewarding the creative individual.

Possessing information about leadership, management, change, and innovations allows the nurse to understand what is occurring in the clinical area. The knowledgeable nurse will be able to participate and contribute at a higher level of performance.

CURRENT CONTROVERSY
HOW CAN NURSES FEEL EMPOWERED TODAY?

EMPOWERMENT IN NURSING

A shift in organizational structure in some health care agen-cies is resulting in the decentralization of nursing services. Top level management positions are being eliminated and decision-making authority is being given to nonnursing managers. Nurses employed in these organizations are concerned that nursing input into the decision-making process is being diluted. Also, nursing priorities concerning the maintaining of quality of nursing care are being overlooked. In addition, most nurses are employed in organizations with bureaucratic structures that give them limited opportunities for input into decision-making processes.

Many nurses in these situations develop feelings of anger, abandonment, and powerlessness. Heavy work assignments and pressures from different sources lead to a high degree of tension and frustration because the nurses have little control over what is happening to and around them. Is it possible to create circumstances in which nurses can feel empowered? Nurse managers and leaders must face this challenge.

Empowerment is defined by Huber (1996) as developing a structure and environment in which people have a strong sense of self and are motivated to excel. Empowering workers means giving them the respect and trust they need to believe they are a vital part of the organization.

It has been assumed by managers that it is the manager's delegation of influence, authority, and control that empowers nurses. Surprisingly, results of a study conducted by Genevieve Chandler (Winslow, 1994) at the University of Massachusetts found otherwise.

A study was conducted in which 56 nurses at two community hospitals and three medical centers were asked to describe scenarios of empowerment and powerlessness. The greatest number of respondents (57 percent) described nurse/patient interactions as a major source of empowerment. Nurse/physician interactions ranked second at 23 percent. Nurses felt empowered when physicians asked for their advice, gave praise, and allowed nurses to collaborate in patient-care decision making. Compliments by nurse managers were recognized only 7 percent of the time. Empowerment gained from working well within a nursing team accounted for only 7 percent. Only 6 percent of the respondents indicated that they felt good about themselves.

A high degree of powerlessness (52 percent) was reported when nurses had negative interactions with physicians. A feeling of powerlessness was also reported (12 percent) when a patient died, and 11 percent when the patient or family did not appreciate the nursing care given by the nursing staff.

The results of the study point up serious problems for nursing leaders and managers. It would appear that the managerial and leadership skills used by nurses in clinical settings do little to empower nurses. The uses of authority, control, delegation, and influence have long been considered as major forces in empowering staff and increasing employees' job satisfaction. Some of the issues identified by this study that need to be further explored include the following:

- Why do nurses have such a low feeling of empowerment while working in a team relationship with other staff members?
- What can be done to produce a more positive response?
- What needs to be done to improve the organizational climate to enhance the sense of empowerment in the work place?
- What do nurse managers and leaders need to do to increase their influence and promote a sense of empowerment in the nursing staff?

It is essential that leaders and managers promote a sense of empowerment. Leaders who empower others ensure a strong and committed staff. Resolving the current controversy, in light of the findings of the Chandler research study, will require the development of new and innovative strategies to promote a sense of empowerment within the nursing staff. The path to empowerment follows three basic steps:

- Sharing information with employees: A sense of ownership in the agency is fostered.
- Creating autonomy through boundaries and guidelines: Knowing what job responsibilities are increases sense of security and confidence.
- Replacing hierarchy with self-directed teams: Self-direction fosters personal growth and allows for creativity and innovation (Kokmen, 1996).

CHAPTER HIGHLIGHTS

- Nurses generally practice in organized institutional settings. Major changes are occurring in health care institutions as a result of the development of managed care and health maintenance organizations.
- All institutions have some type of organizational structure. Nursing practice is affected by the organization's philosophy, mission, goals, organizational patterns, and systems. Nurses need to understand the principles of management and leadership, relevance of innovation and change, and the interlinking of these concepts.
- Nurses manage and lead. All nurses are involved in leadership positions. Management and leadership are intertwined and related concepts. A common theme in defining management is that people in institutions must work together. Leadership focuses on fostering participation by all levels of the nursing staff.

- Change is a part of everyday life and is becoming more and more rapid. Nursing practice includes the process of planning for change.
- A creative and innovative person is one who displays productive originality. Nursing practice is enhanced through creative and innovative approaches. An institution that maintains the status quo will not survive in the current health care marketplace.
- Managing and leading are basic components of nursing practice. Accomplishing the goals of safe, effective care is facilitated when all staff in an organization have an appreciation of fellow staff members and can work well together.

REFERENCES

Baron, R.A. (1983). *Behavior in Organizations.* Boston: Allyn and Bacon.

Bennis, W. (1989). *Why Leaders Can't Lead.* San Francisco: Jossey-Bass.

Bennis, W. (1993). *An Invented Life: Reflections on Leadership and Change.* Reading, MA: Addison Wesley.

Bennis, W., Benne, K.D., Chin, R., Corey, K. (1976). *The Planning of Change,* 3rd ed. New York: Holt, Rinehart, and Winston.

Bennis, W., Parikh, J., Lessem, R. (1994). *Beyond Leadership, Balancing Economics, Ethics, and Ecology.* Cambridge, MA: Blackwell Ltd.

Blake, R.P., Mouton, J.S. (1967). Organizational excellence through effective management behavior. *Management, 20* (2), 42–47.

Brown, J. (1996). Poems and circumstances, *Get Up and Go.* Emeryville, CA: Age Way, Inc.

Clark, C.C., Shea, C. (1979). *Management in Organizations: A Vital Link in the Health Care System.* New York: McGraw-Hill.

Dienemann, J. (1990). Strategic perspectives and application. In *Nursing Administration.* Stamford, CT: Appleton-Lange.

Drucker, P. (1985). *Innovation and Entrepreneurship: Practice and Principles.* New York: Harper & Row.

Drucker, P. (1992). *Managing for the Future: The 1990s and Beyond.* New York: Truman Talley Books/Dutton.

Drucker, P.F. (1967). *The Effective Executive.* New York: Harper-Row.

Fayol, H. (1949). *General and Industrial Management,* translated by C. Storrs. London: Pittman and Sons.

Ferguson, L.M. (1992). Teaching for creativity. *Nurse Educator, 17* (1), January-February, 16.

Fiedler, E.E. (1972). How do you make leaders more effective? New answers to an old puzzle. In K. Davis: *Organizational Behavior: A Book of Readings,* 5th ed. New York: McGraw-Hill.

Follett, M.P. (1978). In J.F. Stoner: *Management.* Englewood Cliffs, NJ: Prentice-Hall.

Gardner, J.W. (1986). *The Nature of Leadership: Introductory Considerations.* Washington, D.C.: Independent Sector.

Gillies, D.A. (1989). *Nursing Management: A Systems Approach.* Philadelphia: W.B. Saunders.

Grohar-Murray, M.E., DiCroce, H.R. (1997). *Leadership and Management in Nursing,* 2nd ed. Stamford, CT: Appleton-Lange.

Hersey, P., Blanchard, K. (1993). *Management of Organizational Behavior: Utilizing Human Resources,* 6th ed. Englewood Cliffs, NJ: Prentice-Hall.

Hersey, P., Duldt, B.W. (1989). *Situational Leadership in Nursing.* Norwalk, CT: Appleton-Lange.

Hoffman, F. (1988). *Nursing Productivity Assessment and Costing Out Nursing Services.* Philadelphia: J.B. Lippincott.

House, R.J. (1971). A path goal theory of leader effectiveness. *Administrative Science Quarterly, 16* (3), 321.

Huber, D. (1996). *Leadership and Nursing Care Management.* Philadelphia: W.B. Saunders.

Kast, F., Rozenzweig, J.E. (1985). *Organization and Management: A System Approach,* 4th ed. New York: McGraw-Hill.

Kawamoto, K. (1994). Nursing leadership: To thrive in a world of change. *Nursing Administration Quarterly, 18* (3), Spring, 5.

Kokmen, L. (1996). Out with managers, in with empowerment. *The Press-Democrat,* March 25, p. D19.

Koontz, H. (1981). The management theory jungle. *Academy of Management Journal,* December, 174–188.

Kouzes, J.H., Posner, B.Z. (1995). *The Leadership Challenge.* San Francisco: Jossey-Bass.

Manion, J. (1995). The seven stages of change. *American Journal of Nursing, 95* (4), April, 41.

McCloskey, J. (1995). Recognizing the managing role of all nurses. *Nursing and Health Care: Perspectives on Community, 16,* (6), November-December, 307.

McGregor, D. (1957) The human side of enterprise. In K. Davis (1979): *Organizational Behavior: A Book of Readings,* 5th. ed. New York: McGraw-Hill.

Ouchi, W.G. (1981). *Theory Z: How American Business Can Meet the Japanese Challenge.* Reading, MA: Addison-Wesley.

Random House Webster's College Dictionary (1996). New York: Random House.

Rogers, E. (1962). *Diffusion of Innovations.* New York: Free Press.

Roethlisberger, F.J., Dickson, W.J. (1958). Management and the worker. In H. Landsberger (ed.): *Hawthorne Revisited: Management and the Worker, Its Critics and Developments in Human Relations in Industry.* New York: Cornell University Press, pp. 14–15.

Sample, S. (1994). Guest Editorial, *Nursing Administration Quarterly, 18* (3), Spring, vii.

Scott, J., Rantz, M. (1994). Change champions at the grass-roots level: Practice innovation using team process. *Nursing Administration Quarterly, 18* (3), Spring, 7–17.

Stevens, W.F. (1978). *Management and Leadership in Nursing.* New York: McGraw-Hill.

Steiner, G.A. (1965) *The Creative Organization.* Chicago: University of Chicago Press.

Swansburg, R. (1990). *Management and Leadership for Nurse Managers.* Boston: Jones and Barlett.

Szilagyi, A.D., Wallace, M.J. (1980). *Organizational Behavior and Performance.* Santa Monica: Goodyear Publishing.

Tannenbaum, R., Schmidt, W. (1958). How to Choose a Leadership Pattern. *Harvard Business Review, 36,* 95–101.

Tannenbaum, R., Schmidt, W. (1973). How to Choose a Leadership Pattern. *Harvard Business Review,* 51 (3), 162–180.

Tappen, R.M. (1995). *Nursing Leadership and Management: Concepts and Practice,* 3rd ed. Philadelphia: F.A. Davis.

Taylor, F.W. (1910). *Shop Management.* New York: Harper.

Torrington, D., Weightman, J. (1994). *Effective Management: A Systems Approach: People and Organizations,* 2nd ed. Englewood Cliffs, NJ: Prentice-Hall.

Winslow, E. (1994). Research for practice: Who empowers nurses. *American Journal of Nursing, 94* (3), 19.

Yura, H., Ozimer, D., Walsh, M.B. (1980). Nursing leadership processes. *Nursing Leadership: Theory and Process,* 2nd ed. New York: Appleton-Crofts.

8 Legal Issues in Nursing Practice

Marylou McAthie

OBJECTIVES

After studying this chapter, students will have learned to:

- **recognize how the present system of law originated**
- **understand why knowledge of laws, types of laws, and the court system in the United States is important**
- **be familiar with statutory laws and nursing practice acts**
- **understand torts, unintentional and intentional, and how they apply to nursing practice**
- **apply legal principles in the documentation of nursing care**
- **understand advanced directives and the importance of implementing the Patient Self-Determination Act**
- **be familiar with the Good Samaritan Act and its implications in nursing**
- **understand reporting requirements in child abuse**
- **recognize the liability laws that affect students while practicing nursing**

From its earliest days nursing has been involved with the law. Patient safety and nursing competence are addressed in the laws, rules, and regulations of each state and territory of the United States and in many other countries in the world. Nursing practice is controlled by legislative bodies and the laws passed under their aegis. Laws are defined as "principles and regulations established by government or other authority and applicable to a people, whether by legislation or by custom enforced by judicial decision" (*Random House Webster's College Dictionary,* 1996.)

The legal issues facing the nursing profession increasingly become complicated. The complexity of technological advances; the litigious attitude of many U.S. citizens; the increasing body of common laws, rules, and regulations from state and federal legislative acts; and the actions of the U.S. Supreme Court provide a constantly changing health care legal environment. Nurses will have to be ever alert to the changes and alter nursing practices accordingly.

The chapter explores the legal parameters of nursing practice by reviewing the historical aspects of nursing and the law, purposes of laws, types of laws, and the United States Constitution and the court system. Nurse practice acts, standards of care, and torts as they apply to nursing are addressed.

HISTORICAL PERSPECTIVES

The legal system in the United States of America is based on the jurisprudence system that originated in England. In the early ages laws were the pronouncements of kings based on the concept that kings and rulers had "divine rights." The Magna Carta signed in 1215 by King John of England established that rights of human beings superseded the rights of kings; however, the Magna Carta primarily protected the rights of noblemen and not common men. The American and French Revolutions in the eighteenth century determined that the common man also had inherent rights that superseded the rights of kings and governments. Bodies such as the British Parliament and the U.S. Congress were formed to provide laws that would balance the power between the people and the government. The U.S. Constitution and its amendments provide a system of checks and balances between the legislative, executive, and judicial branches of the U.S. government.

Nursing leaders became involved in the legislative process early in the twentieth century. It became obvious that the profession was developing with little internal or external control over the quality of the proliferating educational programs and the increasing numbers of practicing nurses. Many poorly prepared individuals were involved in giving nursing care, putting patients at risk of suffering serious harm.

By the early 1900s, nursing leaders had become increasingly concerned and determined that there should be greater protection for the safety of the public. The leaders decided that the major focus of the emerging nursing organizations would be centered on securing legal protection for nurses and developing standards for nursing practice and nursing educational programs. Whereas other occupations and professions had attained such protection, nursing met with opposition from groups with financial interests in controlling nursing, such as physicians and hospital administrators. Legislative bodies in most states were negatively influenced by these groups, and nursing leaders had to expend great efforts to overcome the opposition. Also, there was a need to provide nursing input into the administration of the laws by ensuring nurse representation on the examining boards and ensuring that nurses would be largely responsible for setting the standards of nursing practice and education (Dock and Stewart, 1938). The fledgling nursing organizations responded to this need by forming state societies. The well-organized groups pressured the legislative bodies, and states gradually responded by passing laws that defined nursing practice and set standards for schools of nursing. The legislation was not the same in each state or territory, which led to a variety of different approaches in defining practice and in the requirements for educational programs. The first licensing laws were passed in March 1903 in North Carolina and in April 1903 in New Jersey. Two other states, New York and Virginia, also passed nursing legislation in 1903. The laws were very different. The New Jersey law omitted a board of nursing; North Carolina allowed a nurse to be licensed without attending an educational program if vouched for by a physician. In North Carolina the board had representation from physicians and nurses. Although the language and specifications varied, three provisions were included in most legislative acts:

1. Denied the use of the title Registered Nurse to untrained nurses;
2. Established a mechanism for examining training school graduates; and
3. Established a grandfathering mechanism (a time period that allowed qualified trained nurses to acquire registration without examination) (American Nurses' Association, 1984).

By 1952 all states and territories had passed nursing laws. Many of the laws were permissive, which allowed nonaccredited schools to continue to prepare nurses. The graduates of nonaccredited programs were not allowed to take licensing examinations or to use the term *Registered Nurse*. By 1980 all states had laws that mandated or required licensure for Registered Nurses.

PURPOSES OF LAWS

Nearly every known society operates under rules and regulations developed and promoted by society. A society that operates without laws would be ruled by anarchy, and no successful society has based its system of laws or politics on anarchy. Laws function to maintain society. The purposes of laws are:

- to define relationships among the members of a society;
- to define which activities are permitted and which are not;
- to allocate authority and determine who may exercise physical coercion as a recognized privilege-right;
- to dispose of troubled cases as they arise; and
- to define relationships between individuals and groups as they arise (Hoebel, 1954).

Laws have two functions: to confirm the rights and privileges for all people and to provide a framework for government. The English and American legal systems are based on the building of case-by-case decisions known as *common law* or *judge-made law*, and on laws referred to as *statutory laws*. Statutory laws are those passed by the legislative bodies at the federal, state, and local levels.

Laws define relationships and regulate behavior. Laws are general rules of conduct that are enforced by the government. Laws impose penalties when laws are violated (Pozgar, 1990). Laws may encourage and benefit society or inhibit it. Acts viewed as destructive will be prohibited; constructive acts will be encouraged. For example, acts such as the deliberate taking of the life of or inflicting harm on another person are considered as destructive and are forbidden; acts such as those passed to protect the environment are encouraged. Not all laws passed may be wise, and it is possible that some legislation that was thought to be helpful is in reality harmful. For example, in England in the 1700s the death penalty was imposed for petty theft and other minor crimes. The penalty was so severe that juries refused to convict criminals and thieves were not punished. The crime rate increased instead of decreasing (Murchison and Nichols, 1970).

Laws are not static; they change with time and circumstances. Different cultures will have different laws that vary with time. Laws that were appropriate a century ago may not be applicable to society's needs today. Consider that 100 years ago there were few automobiles, and laws governing the use of cars were virtually nonexistent.

TYPES OF LAWS

The system of law is divided into the laws that govern the relationships between individuals and society as a whole and the laws governing relationships among individual members of a society. The laws between individuals and society as a whole are "criminal" laws and between individual members are "civil" laws. Criminal laws protect all members of society from harm; civil laws regulate disputes between individuals. In some cases both criminal and civil laws may apply, for example, if a person were injured during a robbery, the injured person may sue the criminal (civil law) at the same time the state is prosecuting for the crime (criminal law).

Another way of dividing the laws is through "statutory" laws and "common" laws. The laws passed by the Congress of the United States, state legislatures, and other governmental entities are statutory laws. Common laws are those made by judges.

Criminal Law

Criminal laws are used to force people to obey the tenets of the law. Enforcement is through governmental agencies such as local, state, and federal police. Being convicted of committing a crime may result in incarceration or, in the extreme, the taking of the criminal's life. Criminal law has four functions:

- Deter violation through inducement of fear that sanctions will be imposed.
- The sanctions imposed will restrain members of society who seem unable to comply.
- Penal systems should be rehabilitative and enable the criminal to return as a useful member of society.
- The penalty imposed provides a sense of gratification to the injured person that justice has been served (Murchison and Nichols, 1970).

Civil Law

Civil laws deal with disagreements between two parties who are unable or unwilling to resolve the problems themselves. For example, if one party fails to adhere to the terms of a contract, the case may be tried in the courts. Civil matters are handled exclusively by the parties involved and are not subject to governmental policing action. Civil laws serve the purposes of settling disputes peacefully, providing decisions that are just, and ensuring that the court's decisions are honored. In the last instance, there is the possibility that if the court's decree is not followed, the coercive powers of the state could be exercised and the wrongdoer's property seized.

Statutory Law

Statutory laws are passed by legislative bodies at all levels of government. They include such areas as "criminal statutes," where sanctions and penalties are defined, and "regulatory statutes," where policy and budgetary decisions are enacted.

The U.S. Constitution with its Amendments is the highest statutory law in the United States. An article in the Constitution states that the Constitution is the "supreme law of the land." The implication is that federal laws take precedence over state statutes. Statutory laws may be amended, repealed, or expanded. Statutory laws may also be declared void by the courts if they fail to comply with a state or the federal constitution.

Regulatory statutes establish agencies at all levels of government. State regulatory statutes enable state governments to establish state boards of nursing and other licensing boards. Statutes are used to regulate many types of businesses and industries. The statutes have a great impact on individuals, organizations, and society as a whole.

Common Law

Common law is the accumulation of thousands upon thousands of legal decisions handed down through all the years that laws have existed. The accumulated decisions have led to the development of rules that provide for impartiality and equity in guiding the courts in handing down new decisions. Judges will respond to the precedence established in decisions made in similar cases. If there is a case in which there has not been a decision made previously, a new legal principle or precedent is established when a decision is made.

Common law is not the same in each state. After the American Revolution each state developed its own system of common law, so no national system of common law exists. Cases are tried on common law in each state unless a federal or state statute exists. Precedents or legal principles set forth in one state do not apply in another state. For example, if a physician is licensed in two states and licensure is rescinded in one state, the physician will be able to continue to practice in the state in which a valid license is still held. Common laws are not static and change over time. If a precedent established at a given time is no longer applicable because of technical, cultural, or social changes, the legal principle may be modified or overturned and new precedents developed. For example, technological advances, such as the development of the artificial heart, have had a great impact on establishing new legal principles involving medical and nursing care. The advances have, in some instances, led to more lawsuits and new legal precedents. As a result of the increasing number of lawsuits, almost all health care providers are covered by malpractice insurance.

THE COURT SYSTEMS

There are two main divisions of the court system: the courts created by the states and the courts created by the United States Congress. State legislators determine the system within the state, which usually consists of criminal courts and civil courts. There may also be municipal, juvenile, small claims, probate, and others. The next level of this court system is the appellate or appeals court, which reviews the decisions of lower courts.

The federal courts administer the laws passed by the United States Congress. Federal courts become involved in disputes at the state level only if a federal law is also an issue. Overlapping between the two systems may occur if there is a dispute that affects individuals from different states.

Federal courts are concerned about violations of criminal statutes. If a crime is committed that violates both state and federal law the criminal(s) may be prosecuted in either court. Crimes that concern narcotics violations are frequently prosecuted in the federal courts if the crime involved more than one state. The next level of the federal court is the Court of Appeals. There are also special courts, for example, the Court of Claims, that hear such cases as breaches of contracts with the U.S. government, or Tax Courts.

The Supreme Court of the United States has jurisdiction over both federal and state matters. The decisions made determine whether or not violations of the Constitution occurred. The Supreme Court ordinarily does not review issues that are specific to an individual state. The Supreme Court has great discretion in the cases it decides to hear. Usually only those cases that have significance to the entire country will be considered. It is the court of last resort; the Supreme Court opinions cannot be appealed to any other court and can only be changed by Congress passing new laws.

Each citizen of the United States is affected by the decisions made by the Supreme Court. For example, medical and nursing practitioners have particularly been affected by the decisions made by the Court and Congress on the abortion issue. Who has the right to make the decision as to whether a woman has an abortion: the federal government, the state, or the woman who is pregnant? What are the legal constraints placed against those who protest at clinics and other health facilities where abortions are performed? Even though the Court has stated that women have the right to seek abortions, there continue to be unresolved major problems in the application of the law from state to state and at the federal level.

STATUTORY LAWS AND NURSING: NURSING PRACTICE ACTS

Legislation to control nursing practice has existed in the United States since the turn of the century. The profession of nursing and legislative bodies in individual states have a mutual responsibility to develop the laws affecting nursing to protect the safety and welfare of the public. The legal boundaries established in each state and territory provide the framework for and define the scope of nursing practice in each legislative entity.

Nurse Practice Acts

Legislation to control nursing practice, known as nurse practice acts, has existed in the United States for over 90 years. State legislative bodies are granted the power to regulate practice through licensing laws as a result of Article X of the U.S. Constitution. The Constitution delegates police powers to individual states. Police powers provide the authority to designated individuals and groups to protect the health and welfare of the public (American Nurses' Association, 1984).

As previously stated, the profession of nursing and state legislative bodies share responsibility to develop nursing legislation. Nursing laws provide the framework for and define nursing practice in each state or territory. Standards for licensure are developed to ensure that nurses who acquire a license have the necessary knowledge base and are competent to practice, and to ensure that incompetent and inadequately prepared nurses are barred from or removed from practice.

Provisions in the nurse practice acts establish a regulatory authority that is delegated the responsibility to administer the legislation. The regulatory bodies are usually designated as boards of nursing. Although nurse practice acts vary from state to state, all share similar characteristics. The acts include provisions for establishing a board or commission and define the powers delegated by the state to the board. Table 8–1 lists typical components included in nurse practice acts.

All sections of the nurse practice acts are important. Every nurse should be aware of the components and be especially cognizant of the definitions of the practice of nursing, the scope of nursing practice, and statements relating to standards. The differences in nurse practice acts can be illustrated by reviewing the definitions from two states, Oregon and California. An example of a definition of nursing is included in the Nurse Practice Act from the state of Oregon:

> "Practice of Nursing" means diagnosing and treating human responses to actual or potential health problems through such services as identification thereof, health teaching, health counseling, and providing care supportive to or restorative of life and well-being and including the performance of such additional services requiring education and training which are recognized by nursing as proper to be performed by nurses licensed under Oregon Revised Statutes and are recognized by rules of the board (Board of Nursing, 1998, p. 3).

TABLE 8-1 Components Included in Nurse Practice Acts

- Purposes of nurse practice acts stated
- Terms used in legislation defined
- Requirements to practice mandated
- Licensing responsibilities defined:
  - Qualifications of applicants
  - Examining of applicants
  - Disciplinary procedures
- State board functions include:
  - Terms of office and appointment of members
  - Supervision of nursing practice
  - Standards setting for nursing practice and curriculum requirements for nursing education programs
  - Accreditation of nursing education program
  - Denial or revocation of Accreditation of Nursing Education programs
  - Examine, license, and renew license of qualified applicants
  - Prescribe standards for delegation of duties to other levels of nursing personnel
  - Determine scope of nursing practice
- Regulate advanced nursing practice (not included in all state nurse practice acts)

The practice of Registered Nursing is further described in the Oregon Nurse Practice Act as:

> "Practice of Registered Nursing" means the application of knowledge drawn from broad in-depth education in the social and physical sciences in assessing, planning, ordering, giving, delegating, teaching, and supervising care which promotes the person's optimum health and independence (Board of Nursing, 1998, p. 3).

The California Nurse Practice Act defines the "Scope of Regulation" (comparable to the scope of nursing practice) as:

> The practice of nursing within the meaning of this chapter means those functions including basic health care, which help people cope with difficulties in daily living which are associated with their actual or potential health or illness problems or the treatment thereof which require a substantial amount of scientific knowledge or technical skill and includes all of the following:
>
> (a) Direct and indirect patient care services that insure the safety, comfort, personal hygiene, and protection of patients; and the performance of disease prevention, and restorative measures.
>
> (b) Direct and indirect patient care services, including, but not limited to, the administration of medications and therapeutic agents, necessary to implement a treatment, disease prevention, or rehabilitative regimen ordered by and within the scope of licensure of a physician, dentist, podiatrist, or clinical psychologist, as defined by the Section 1316.5 of the Health and Safety Code.
>
> (c) The performance of skin tests, immunization techniques, and the withdrawal of human blood from veins and arteries.
>
> (d) Observation of signs and symptoms of illness, reactions to treatment, general behavior, or general physical condition, and (a) determination of whether such signs, symptoms, reactions, behavior, or general appearance exhibit abnormal characteristics; and (b) implementation, based on observed abnormalities, or appropriate reporting, or referral, or standardized procedures, or changes in treatment regimen in accordance with standardized procedures, or the initiation of emergency procedures. (California Business and Professions Code, 1997, pp. 3–4.)

As can be perceived in the definitions, the nurse functions independently except, for example, in Oregon, for the "executing of medical orders as prescribed by a physician or dentist." The language of the Oregon law clearly distinguishes between the independent and dependent functions of nursing. The definition is broad and allows for wide interpretation of the nursing role. The California legislation is more restrictive but also specifies the functions that are under the purview of nurses and indicates where the nursing and other health care professional practice overlap. Both Acts emphasize the need for the nurse to have a sound scientific knowledge base.

The Oregon Act also addresses the scope of nursing practice in a separate section that states the Nurse Practice Act "board shall determine the scope of practice as delineated by the knowledge acquired through approved courses of education or experience." (Board of Nursing, 1998, pp. 5–9.) The California law defines *standardized procedures* as policies and protocols developed in a health facility, or through collaboration between nurses, health care facility administrators, and physicians. The policies and protocols are usually developed in areas in which legal precedent has not been established or there are overlapping functions between nurses and physicians.

The wording of the definitions is extremely important. The definitions need to be specific enough to define the scope of practice, explicit enough to clarify the areas to be excluded, and flexible enough to allow for future changes. For example, the California Board of Nursing specifies in the Nurse Practice Act that "the legislature recognizes that nursing is a dynamic field, the practice of which is continually evolving to include more sophisticated patient care activities [and to] provide clear legal authority for functions and procedures which have common acceptance and usage" (California Nurse Practice Act, 1997, p. 3).

The scope of practice defines the framework for the practice of nursing. The scope should be broad and allow for changes in the nursing role. For example, early nurse practice acts were very restrictive and confined nurses to performing personal hygiene functions. Physicians took the patient's blood pressure and administered other technical treatments such as dressing changes. Today taking a blood pressure is delegated to nursing personnel. In the past, other advanced technical procedures such as intravenous therapy were also solely within the scope of physician practice. Today nurses are the primary administrators of intravenous therapy. Many states now allow nurse practitioners with advanced preparation to diagnose, treat, and write prescriptions within their area of specialization.

The enabling acts specify the powers of the administrative boards and the functions to be conducted by the boards. The board is charged with implementing the provision in the law. The membership on the boards usually consists of nurses and

TABLE 8-2 Reasons for Disciplinary Action Against Nurses by State Boards of Nursing

- Unprofessional conduct, which includes incompetence or gross negligence in carrying out nursing activities
- Practicing medicine without a license
- Obtaining a license by fraud, misrepresentation, or mistake
- Giving false information in applying for a license
- Conviction of a felony related to the qualifications, functions and duties of a registered nurse
- Impersonating an applicant or acting for an applicant in any examination needed to acquire a license
- Impersonating another licensed nurse, or permitting someone to use a license
- Holding oneself out to be a nurse practitioner when the necessary education has not been acquired
- Revocation of a license in another state or territory
- Failing to protect patients

public members. The nursing membership assumes the responsibility for ensuring that the scope and standards are continually updated to reflect the changes in nursing education and practice.

The boards also exercise control over violations of the law. The board will conduct investigations into complaints received. The basic question asked is whether the practice of the nurse being investigated is safe or unsafe. If evidence indicates that actions need to be instituted against the nurse, the complaint will be pursued, usually through a hearing. If the nurse is found guilty, his or her license could be suspended or revoked, or the nurse could be placed on probation, depending on the seriousness of the offense. State nurse practice acts specify reasons for disciplinary action. Table 8–2 lists some reasons for disciplinary actions.

Other activities of the boards include accrediting/approving of schools of nursing and determining and supervising the nursing licensure examination. Standards are developed for administering nursing educational programs including curricula and overseeing the operation of the school. All states participate in the National Council of State Boards Licensing Examination, which allows a graduate of a state-accredited program to procure a Registered Nurse license in another state without the need to repeat the examination.

TORTS

A tort is a wrong committed by one person that inflicts injury on another or others. The wrong may be against either person or property. The law provides relief by permitting the injured to institute legal action to collect for the damages sustained. Tort law deals with civil law and not criminal law. A general rule of law is that every person is liable for the torts he or she commits. A fundamental duty of all people imposed by the law of torts is the duty to behave reasonably and to act in ways that do not cause harm to others.

Tort lawsuits are usually adversarial because one person has accused another of inflicting harm. Tort law is designed to promote acceptable and responsible behavior by penalizing the wrongdoer. Torts are based on the fault principle that if through one's own fault an injury is caused to another, the person at fault will bear the loss.

There are unintentional and intentional torts. Unintentional torts are accidents that cause injury to another person or property; intentional torts are deliberate actions in which the intent is to cause injury to a person or property. The difference between the unintentional torts and intentional torts is a matter of degree of intent.

Unintentional Torts

The primary example of an unintentional tort is when an accident happens. The accident may be due to negligence or an act of nature. When injury occurs to a second party as a result of an negligent accident, e.g., an automobile accident in which one person carelessly loses control of a vehicle and causes serious physical injury to another; the person causing the accident will be held liable and will be penalized, usually by having to pay all costs.

Not all accidents are caused by negligence. There are those that result from the forces of nature and those that occur regardless of the care taken to avoid the accident. These are called inevitable or unavoidable accidents. For example, in the first instance, if a power failure results during a surgical procedure and an inaccurate sponge count occurs and a sponge is left in the abdomen, the surgical nurse would not be held accountable. In the second instance, if a nurse correctly administers the right medication to the right patient but the patient experiences an adverse effect, the nurse is not held liable.

ACCIDENTS, NEGLIGENCE, AND MALPRACTICE

Nurses can be involved in negligent acts. For example, if by accident a nurse administers a wrong medication to a patient and the patient sustains injury, the nurse can be held responsible. The injury is not intentional but is brought about by the failure of the nurse to act in a responsible manner (an act of commission). The committing of the irresponsible act is considered negligent behavior. Negligence is the basis for health care professionals being charged with malpractice.

The term *negligence* refers to the doing or not doing of an act that a reasonable person in the same circumstance would or would not do; and the doing or not doing causes harm to a person or to property. Negligence is behavior that does not conform to the standards that society expects. *Malpractice* refers to those negligent acts committed by practitioners in skilled and technical professions, for example, physicians, nurses, and dentists. An example of nursing malpractice is the failure of the nurse to properly administer a procedure, such as the starting of an intravenous infusion wherein a needle or catheter is improperly inserted resulting in permanent damage to the patient's extremity. Another example of malpractice is seen in Box 8–1.

BOX 8-1
A CASE OF NEGLIGENCE

A cardinal safety rule known to all nurses is to read the label of a medication three times: when removing the medication from the shelf, preparing the medication for administration, and after replacing on the shelf.

The Court discussed the standard in the Habuda v. Trustees of Rex Hospital, Inc.:

> An order was written for a hospitalized patient to be given a cathartic. Instead she received a surgical soap; the two bottles were in the same area in the medicine storage cabinet. The patient attempted to prove that the hospital was negligent in not carrying out proper procedures for storing medications.
>
> Evidence established that the procedure requires that the nurse read the label of the medication three times. Therefore both the nurse who breached this duty and the hospital were held liable.

From Fiesta, J. (1988). *The Law and Liability: A Guide for Nurses*, 2nd ed. Albany, NY: Delmar, p. 65.

Negligence may be an act of commission or omission. An act of commission occurs when an action results in injury to the patient; an act of omission happens when the nurse fails to carry out the proper action and the patient is harmed. An example of an act of commission, as previously stated, is the administering of a wrong medication to a patient; an act of omission would occur if the nurse failed to give the medication ordered for a patient.

NEGLIGENCE, MALPRACTICE, AND STANDARDS OF CARE

Society expects that nurses will perform nursing functions in a safe and effective manner. This implies that a standard will be used to determine whether the care given by a nurse was administered in a reasonable and prudent way and was comparable to how other nurses would have performed in similar circumstances.

The concept of reasonable and prudent behavior applies in every aspect of an individual's life. The ordinary person is expected to act prudently while driving an automobile, in caring for a family, and in all other activities of living. However, the nurse in the caregiver role is held to an even higher standard of reasonable and prudent behavior than an average person because a nurse is expected to exercise expert knowledge and skills while giving care. The use of advanced technology has added complicated new treatments and procedures to medical and nursing care, requiring practicing nurses to maintain an increasingly higher level of competency and skill. Boundaries of reasonable conduct are rapidly expanding. The performance and behavior of the nurse, as with other health care practitioners, must meet the level expected of other practitioners in the same field. It is the nurse's conduct, related to the nurse's practice, and the reasonableness of the conduct in terms of the standards of the profession, that determines whether it is prudent behavior.

TABLE 8-3 Elements Needed Before Malpractice Liability Can Be Charged

1. The nurse has a duty to care for the patient.
2. A breach of duty based upon violations of the standards of care occurred.
3. There is a cause and effect connection between the breach of duty and the harm or damage done to the patient.
4. Harm or damages were actually suffered by the patient.

Adapted from Aiken T.D. with Catalano J.T. (1994). *Legal, Ethical, and Political Issues in Nursing*. Philadelphia, F.A. Davis, pp. 8–9

Negligence and, therefore, malpractice acts are judged by the activities performed and the conditions existing at the time. There must be a close and reasonable causal relationship between the negligent conduct and the damages suffered by the injured party. The standards required in any given situation will depend not only upon the facts in that situation, but also whether or not a specific law exists that prescribes and constitutes the standard of care. Determining reasonable behavior will depend on all the facts and circumstances surrounding the person who acted negligently. Some of the factors considered include experience and educational preparation. If an individual is charged with negligence or malpractice and if there is not a statute that addresses the specific charge, a jury may decide whether the nurse is or is not to be held liable. Table 8–3 summarizes the four elements that must be present before malpractice can be charged against a nurse.

Whether or not a malpractice act occurred is also based on the standards of care existing in a community. A community may be defined as a city, a region in a state, or in less populated areas, an entire state. If the practitioner does not meet or adhere to acceptable standards, the practitioner could be found guilty of malpractice. There may be instances in which community standards are below standards existing in other communities. If the standards are deemed to be below acceptable standards existing in other communities, it is expected that regulatory bodies would review and recommend changes. Regardless of poor standards being practiced in a community, nurses must adhere to the higher standards established by the profession or face the possibility of being charged with malpractice.

Standards are set by individual institutions through policies and procedures, local and regional health care practices, state nursing boards through the nurse practice acts, private accrediting agencies such as the Joint Commission on the Accrediting of Health Care Organizations, and at the federal level through the Department of Health and Human Services, various units such as the Centers for Disease Control, and the Occupational Safety and Health Administration.

BREACH OF DUTY

A large portion of the law deals with legal duties. Legal duties exist because of contracts entered into with others. Examples of such contracts are obeying crime and traffic laws and paying debts. The fundamental duty imposed on all people is the duty to behave in a reasonable way so as to not hurt others. If one engages in conduct leading to harm, the law considers that a breach of duty has occurred. For a person to be guilty of a breach of duty, an injury must have happened as a result of the breach. For example, a breach of duty occurs if a fire exit in a health care clinic is blocked and staff and patients are injured because of not being able to exit during the fire. The law imposes an obligation or duty on health professionals to behave in a reasonable way and to avoid any harm to patients. If the nurse exercises unreasonable conduct that results in injury to a patient, a legal breach of duty results. For example, if a nurse takes a patient's blood pressure and finds it extremely elevated, it is expected that procedures would immediately be instituted to report the problem to the proper individual and initiate treatment. A breach of duty results if the nurse fails to report the elevated blood pressure and the patient suffers.

Intentional Torts

Intentional torts are deliberate actions in which the intent is to cause injury to a person or property. To be defined as intentional, the act must be carried out for a specific reason to cause a specific result. What determines whether an act is intentional or results from unintentional negligence is not entirely clear. The determination is made when one considers the intent of the person carrying out the act. For example, if a driver accidentally swerves and hits a pedestrian it may be considered as negligence and failure to drive safely; if a driver, however, purposely swerves and hits a pedestrian it is considered an intentional act. The difference between the two, negligence and intentional harm, is a matter of degree. Guido (1988, p. 50) defines the difference between negligence (unintentional) and an intentional tort as:

1. Intent is necessary in proving intentional torts.
2. The action must be a conscious action against the person.
3. Damages are not an issue with intentional torts, that is, the injured party need not show that damages were incurred. Whether the patient encounters out-of-pocket expenses or not, the patient could still show that an intentional tort had occurred.

Nurses need to be aware of the types of intentional torts that affect nursing practice.

ASSAULT

Assault is a threat or an attempt, with the ability to carry out the threat, to bodily contact another person without the consent of the person. Assault can be an action that causes a person to become fearful and apprehensive about being touched in a way that may be considered offensive, threatening, or physically injurious. The person does not have to actually be touched by another; a menacing act is sufficient to create reasonable apprehension. The action must be overt and the intended victim alert and aware that the act has occurred. Words are not enough to constitute assault; the possibility of causing harm must be present. For example, if a patient has refused an injection but the nurse insists on giving the injection, the nurse is guilty of assault. The nurse is equally guilty of assault if in any way the patient after refusing the injection *thinks* the nurse is going to administer it.

BATTERY

Battery is an executed assault. It is the inflicting of physical harm or the unlawful touching of another person. Battery is the most frequent intentional tort occurring within the practice of physicians and nurses. Factors involved in defining battery:

- A single touch is sufficient for battery to have occurred.
- The patient does not have to have experienced pain, be harmed or injured, to be considered as battered.
- The patient does not have to be aware that the battery occurred. Touching a sleeping patient could constitute battery.
- Indirect contact with the patient is also considered battery—for example, dropping an object on the patient.
- Unwanted touching of a patient's personal objects may be battery. Anything connected to the patient is considered an extension of the patient. For example, touching a patient's shoes, clothes, or jewelry could be construed as battery (Guido, 1988, p. 51).

Most of the lawsuits involving battery are associated with the process of consenting to medical, surgical, and nursing procedures. Any procedure performed without the patient's consent can be deemed battery. To be considered legally effective, consent must be considered as "informed consent." The patient must be given adequate factual information as to the expected outcome of the procedure to be performed. See Chapter 14, Documentation, for more information on the process for "obtaining the patient's consent." The competent adult has the right to decide whether or not a prescribed procedure or treatment will be completed.

A second area in which battery lawsuits may occur is in restraining of patients. Restraining of patients by physical or mechanical means can be considered as battery. The practice of using restraints is not recommended; however, there may be circumstances in which the patient could suffer self-inflicted injury such as falling from a bed or wheelchair if not restrained. In all cases, agency guidelines, policies, and procedures must be followed to avoid incurring a charge of battering the patient. Under all circumstances, the restraints need to be applied in such a manner to preserve the dignity of the patient and prevent injury from the use of the restraint.

FALSE IMPRISONMENT

False imprisonment is the unlawful confinement of a person within defined boundaries without a legal warrant. The confined area may be the patient's room, bed, or chair within the room. False imprisonment can also be charged if the nurse refuses to give a patient personal objects such as clothes, keys, or luggage. Refusal to allow family members to visit a patient can also be construed as false imprisonment.

A patient who voluntarily enters a health care facility and then decides to leave against medical advice can claim to have been falsely imprisoned if not allowed to leave. Frail, elderly, competent individuals in nursing home facilities cannot be kept against their will even if vulnerable to injury.

There are circumstances that do allow for restricting the patient. Detainment is acceptable in the case of mentally ill, confused, disoriented, or intoxicated patients. To protect the public, patients with communicable diseases may also be confined against their will. In certain cases such as the mentally ill, strict state laws control the confinement.

INVASION OF PRIVACY

Invasion of privacy is defined as the right to be left alone. Any intrusion of the person or the property of the person is considered an invasion of privacy. Creighton (1986) states that there are four elements to the right of privacy:

- Unauthorized use of the person's personality for commercial purposes, e.g., using a photograph of an individual without the person's approval. This is applicable to the medical field, e.g., in the case of a person undergoing facial plastic surgery. If a picture were taken without the patient's approval that clearly identified the patient and subsequently was used by the physician to show others, the physician would be committing an intentional tort.
- Intrusions into the person's seclusion. Examples of this element include phone tapping, listening in on a personal phone call, and spying on an individual without the person's knowledge.
- Placing a person in an embarrassing or false position. Examples include signing another person's name to a document or misrepresenting another individual's views.
- Disclosing private information that may be harmful to the patient. Information concerning the patient is confidential and is not to be disclosed unless permission has been obtained from the patient or is allowed by policies established by the agency. Release of information about births and deaths does not usually violate the individual rights of patients. Each agency should have a policy that describes how information is to be provided to the media.

DEFAMATION

Defamation is different from the tort of invasion of privacy. Invading of privacy does not require actual harm but can injure the person's feelings regardless of effect on property or reputation. Defamation causes harm to the character or reputation of the person.

Defamation may be in written or oral form. It is an intentional tort defined as an act that diminishes the reputation or character of another person. When the act is oral, it is considered slander; when in written form, it is called libel. The defamatory material must be either published or communicated to a third party who understands that the material is libel or slander.

Defamation may also involve an institution or corporation. Statements made that are derogatory about an institution, e.g., a hospital or home health agency, may be considered slander if the reputation or business activities of that organization are harmed. In libel cases, the libeled individual does not have to prove that actual damages occurred, but, generally, in slander cases there must be proof that damages were incurred. There are exceptions in some slander cases, e.g., in cases of immoral behavior or venereal diseases. If a person were to spread a rumor that a food handler was infected with a venereal disease and the food handler lost his job, the person spreading the rumor could be held for slander and be sued with no further proof other than the testimony of those that heard the rumor.

Guido (1988, p. 56) lists four conditions necessary to prove defamation:

- defamatory language that would negatively affect ones reputation
- defamatory language about or concerning a living person
- writing the accusation to a third party or several persons
- damages to the person's reputation

Caution must be exercised in recording on the patient record. Charting anything derogatory about a patient could be interpreted as defamatory. For example, recording such a statement as the patient is "crazy" could lead to a lawsuit. Only the actual behavior observed, without drawing generalized conclusions, should be stated.

There are defenses against a charge of defamation: the truth, and absolute or qualified privilege granted as a result of being protected as a health care professional. The use of truth as a defense requires that all statements made about the third party can be proven to be true. If only part of the charge is true, the person making the derogatory statements can be charged with defamation.

In the use of privilege as a defense, the law acknowledges that under certain circumstances, i.e., when records are subpoenaed by the courts, the information included in the records is not subject to charges of defamation even if false information is included. For example, reporting of information on certain diseases such as tuberculosis or venereal diseases is required by law. If there are lawsuits concerning any individual found to have such a disease, the medical record can be subpoenaed by the court. Defamation cannot be charged, even if the medical records contained false and defamatory statements about the patient. Qualified privilege exempts statements made in good faith and without malice. Many states have laws that specify how qualified privileges are applied.

Defamation can be both written and oral; the written record referred to at various times as the medical record or patient chart is a key element in defamatory lawsuits. The nurse should have a clear understanding of the legal significance of the record to avoid being included in any legal action involving defamation.

SPECIFIC LEGAL ISSUES IN NURSING PRACTICE

Documentation of Patient Records

Keeping accurate and comprehensive records is essential in any health care facility. The medical record is not only a compilation of the services provided to the patient but also a legal and business document.

Compiling of medical records and storing of the record in a medical library are mandated by governmental and nongovernmental agencies. Standards for the content and maintenance of the records originate from a variety of sources including the federal and state governments, the Joint Commission on Accreditation of Healthcare Organizations (JCAHO), and professional organizations. Standards are also established by individual health care agencies and are available to agency staff through policy and procedure manuals. The standards need to be reasonable and understandable to all who record.

Regardless of the format used to record data, the notations need to be based on fact—concise, accurate, and timely. The legal and ethical issue of veracity is also an important aspect in recording; honesty in making entries in the chart is a necessity. The confidentiality of the record must be maintained at all times. Table 8–4 lists the major purposes of maintaining medical records.

TABLE 8–4 Major Purposes for Maintaining Medical Records

- Provide a tool for planning patient care.
- Record the patient's treatment, progress, and changes in the patient's condition.
- Provide a tool for communication between practitioners and other health professionals responsible for the patient's care.
- Assist in protecting the legal interests of the patient, health care agency, and the practitioner.
- Provide a base for data used in statistical reports, research, and other legally required activities.
- Provide data for billing and reimbursement activities.

Adapted from Pozgar, G.P. (1990). *Legal Aspects of Health Care Administration*, 2nd ed. Gaithersburg, MD: Aspen Systems Publications.

NURSING NOTES OR PATIENT PROGRESS NOTES

The records documenting nursing care are considered as legal records and therefore should be carefully completed. As previously indicated, the information is to be accurate, concise, and recorded in a timely manner. They should clearly describe the care given and include any observations that reflect the patient's responses. The data need to include what is heard, seen, and believed about the patient's condition. Complete honesty is necessary in charting. The nurse's notes are usually the first document reviewed by attorneys if a lawsuit is being pursued by a patient. Alterations should not be made in the record. If mistakes are made on paper records, the material is to be crossed out, not obliterated, left in the chart, and the accurate information recorded.

Increasingly, computers are being used to record patient progress. A major legal problem in computer charting is maintaining the confidentiality of patient records. Procedures need to be in place to ensure that access to the computerized record is available only to those approved to enter the system. If computerized records are being used, it is essential that methods to access the information by staff, e.g., a password, not be shared with any other staff member.

One method of recording on nursing records is a procedure referred to as "charting by exception." The overall aim of the method is to reduce the time spent on documentation. The process requires that the institution have in place clearly defined standards of practice and established nursing assessments and interventions. The recording of routine nursing care is eliminated and the only notations made are those explaining unusual occurrences or deviations from normal responses.

Documentation of nursing notes and other nursing forms is an involved process and is discussed in further detail in Chapter 14.

INCIDENT, VARIANCE, OR OCCURRENCE REPORT

Incident, variance, and occurrence reports are used internally by an organization to report when something unusual happens to a patient, visitor, or in some instances staff. For example, a report of this type would be completed if a visitor fell and sustained injury while visiting a patient, or if a member of the nursing staff were to accidentally sustain a puncture from a needle that had been used to give an injection to a patient. These reports do not become part of the patient record. The reports are used to augment quality of care assessment activities, to alert agency administrators to potential problem areas, and to reduce the possibility of further problems from similar happenings. The report is not used to discipline staff (Lilley, 1994).

The incident report has been considered to be confidential and not available to attorneys participating in a lawsuit against the health care agency; however, in several cases, judges have allowed use of the reports in court. Reports should be written as if they were to be presented in a legal action. Language should be used in a manner that does not make a determination as to who was at fault or liable. To ensure confidentiality, only one copy of the report should be completed. Refer to Chapter 14 for further information on completing the incident reports.

PATIENT RECORDS AND ASSESSING QUALITY OF NURSING CARE

Another important reason for keeping patient care records is to provide a basis for assessing the quality of care given by a health care organization. Lawsuits can be minimized in health care agencies that provide programs to reduce the possibility of injury to patients. Quality assurance programs assess the type and level of patient care that is given by the health agency staff. Patterns and recurring incidents are reviewed to determine whether changes in policies and procedures will improve the level of care. Another quality assessment program, risk management, is a technique used to reduce or prevent financial losses before they occur. Risk management uses a process that includes analyzing problem areas to reveal the underlying causes of the problems before serious injuries to patients, staff, or visitors occur. The processes used include reviewing incident reports, conducting surveys, and assessing conditions existing in specific problem areas. Retraining of staff may be necessary to reduce incidents that lead to patient injury.

Another quality assessment program is known as Continuous Quality Improvement (CQI). Aiken and Catalano (1994) state that CQI is a more complex process than other quality assurance programs and uses work groups composed of experts to monitor the quality of care, identify problems, and propose solutions. Information collected from patients' records is utilized to identify and analyze problems. Data are collected over periods of time and are reviewed to determine that standards of care are met. Nurses involved in administering patient care are active participants in the procedure. An overall objective is to provide information to improve nursing practice. (See Chapter 12 for an illustration of this process.)

INFORMED PATIENT CONSENT

The necessity for informed consent is addressed in state laws that vary from state to state. In addition private health care professional and accrediting agencies have developed policies and procedures to guide agencies in implementing the process. The JCAHO has issued accreditation standards for hospitals and other health care agencies. The standards state:

> The patient has the right to reasonable informed participation in decisions involving his health care. To the degree possible this should be based on a clear, concise explanation of his condition and of all proposed technical procedures including the possibilities of any risk of mortality or serious side effects, problems related to recuperation, and probability of success. The patient should not be subjected to any procedure without his voluntary, competent, and understanding consent or that of his legally authorized representative. Where medically significant alternatives for care or treatment exist, the patient shall be so informed.
>
> The patient has the right to know who is responsible for authorizing and performing the procedures or treatment. The patient shall be informed if the hospital proposes to engage in or perform human experimentation or other research/educational projects affecting high quality care or treatment, and the patient has the right to refuse to participate in any such activity.

TABLE 8-5 Types of Informed Consent

Expressed consent: consent given by direct words. The form may be either written or oral.
Implied consent: consent inferred by the patient's demeanor or behavior or is presumed in emergency situations.
Oral consent: consent verbally given by the patient.
Written consent: consent signed by the patient or authorized representative.
Partial consent: consent given for only a portion of a treatment.
Complete consent: consent that is given for the performance of the entire procedure.

Consent may be obtained in different ways: by expression or implication, written or oral, and either complete or partial. Table 8–5 lists the types of informed consent.

The primary responsibility for obtaining the patient's consent rests with the physician or primary care practitioner. The health care agency takes responsibility for procuring the patient's approval if the physician or practitioner is an employee of the agency or if the institution is aware that the consent has not been obtained. Consent for major medical and surgical procedures requires the signature of the patient and must be witnessed. A written explanation of what was explained to the patient about the procedure to be performed also must be provided in the record.

Patients have the right to refuse medical treatment. Refusal is often based upon the religious preferences of the individual. For example, the Jehovah's Witnesses may not allow blood transfusions to be administered to their members and Christian Scientists usually refuse medical or surgical interventions. The right to refuse is based on the right to freely participate in religious practices and the right of privacy. In the latter case, patients may refuse treatment even if their life is in danger. For example, a patient may decide to not have a leg amputated even if the patient could die as a result of the refusal. The courts may interfere and order the treatment to be administered if it is determined that the patient is a minor and the parent's decision to refuse treatment may result in the death of the child or that the patient's condition is curable if treatment is instituted. In other instances, if a communicable disease is present, the court may order that treatment be initiated (Rhodes and Miller, 1984). Nurses become involved in the informed consent process in several ways. Consent must be obtained for all procedures and treatments, including those performed by nurses. Most nursing interventions are covered under the general consent form signed when a patient enters a health care agency. Implied or oral consent usually can be inferred through a patient's verbal statements or by actions and behavior. Specific policies and procedures regarding nursing's role in informed consent should be available in agency policy and procedure manuals.

In 1972, the American Hospital Association published the Patient's Bill of Rights. The Bill of Rights embodies the concepts of informed consent. The bill came about as a result of the actions of health consumers who wanted to have a voice and participate in decisions about their personal health care.

The bill is posted in many health care facilities and in some agencies a copy is provided to each patient. The bill is included in Box 8–2.

There are special circumstances in which the informed consent procedure includes orders initiated by the patient and the physician to not use any procedures to continue the life of the patient. The *Do Not Resuscitate* (DNR) or *No Code* order states that treatment for respiratory, cardiac, or circulatory failure is not to be started because the patient is in a terminal stage of illness. Every health care facility should have its own DNR policies. The nurse needs to be totally familiar with the policies and procedures. The orders for DNR must be in writing and should be periodically updated.

Do not resuscitate and no code orders are used if the patient does not have an advance directive such as a Living Will or durable power of attorney for health care. The Living Will or durable power of attorney expresses the patient's wishes regarding continued treatment if he or she becomes terminally ill. The do not resuscitate or no code order is a medical prescription reflecting the decision to not resuscitate in case of cardiopulmonary failure (Idemoto et al, 1993).

Refer to Chapter 14 for further information on procedures to implement the informed consent procedure. Another important facet to consider in understanding all aspects of informed consent is the area of advance directives or the right of patients to determine their own fate.

ADVANCE DIRECTIVES

The Patient Self-Determination Act (PSDA) was passed by Congress in 1991. The law requires health care agencies receiving federal monies through Medicare and Medicaid programs to inform recipients in writing of their right under state law to make decisions about health care. Included is the right

BOX 8–2
A PATIENT'S BILL OF RIGHTS

1. The patient has a right to considerate and respectful care.
2. The patient has a right to obtain from his physician complete correct information concerning his diagnosis, treatment, and prognosis in terms the patient can be reasonably expected to understand. When it is not medically advisable to give such information to the patient, the information should be made available to an appropriate person in his behalf. He has the right to know, by name, the physician responsible for coordinating his care.
3. The patient has the right to receive from his physician information necessary to give informed consent prior to the start of any procedure and/or treatment. Except in emergencies, such information for informed consent should include but not necessarily be limited to the specific procedure and/or treatment, the medically significant risks involved, and the probable duration of incapacitation. Where medically significant alternatives for care or treatment exist, or when the patient requests information concerning medical alternatives, the patient has the right to such information. The patient also has the right to know the name of the person responsible for the procedures and/or treatment.
4. The patient has the right to refuse treatment to the extent permitted by law and to be informed of the medical consequences of his actions.
5. The patient has the right to every consideration of his privacy concerning his own medical care program. Case discussion, consultation, examination, and treatment are confidential and should be conducted discreetly. Those not directly involved in his care must have the permission of the patient to be present.
6. The patient has the right to expect that all communications and records pertaining to his care should be treated confidentially.
7. The patient has the right to expect that within its capacity a hospital must make reasonable response to the request of a patient for services. The hospital must provide evaluation, service, and/or referral as indicated by the urgency of the case. When medically permissible, a patient may be transferred to another facility after he has received complete information and explanation concerning the needs for and alternatives to such a transfer. The institution to which the patient is to be transferred must first have accepted the patient for transfer.
8. The patient has the right to obtain information as to any relationship of his hospital to other health care and educational institutions insofar as his care is concerned. The patient has the right to obtain information as to the existence of professional relationships among individuals, by name, who are treating him.
9. The patient has the right to be advised if the hospital proposes to engage in or perform human experimentation affecting his care or treatment. The patient has the right to refuse to participate in such research projects.
10. The patient has the right to expect reasonable continuity of care. He has the right to know in advance what appointment times and physicians are available and where. The patient has the right to expect that the hospital will provide a mechanism whereby he is informed by his physician or a delegate of the physician of the patient's continuing health care requirements following discharge.
11. The patient has the right to examine and receive an explanation of his bill, regardless of source of payment.
12. The patient has a right to know what hospital rules and regulations apply to his conduct as a patient.

From American Hospital Association (1972). *A Patient's Bill of Rights.* Chicago: AHA.

TABLE 8–6 Essentials of the Patient Self-Determination Act

To encourage patients to complete advance directives, Congress enacted the Patient Self-Determination Act. The law requires hospitals, nursing homes, and hospices to:

- advise patients on admission of their right to accept or refuse medical care;
- advise patients of their right to execute an advance directive;
- document whether a patient has an advance directive;
- implement advance directive policies;
- educate staff and communities about advance directives; and
- in managed care organizations and home health care agencies, provide the same information to each member enrolled.

From Berrio, M., Levesque, M. (1996). Advance directives: Most patients don't have one. Do yours? *American Journal of Nursing, 96,* 8, 25–28.

to refuse medical or surgical treatments and the right to initiate "advance directives." The PSDA was passed by Congress after the Supreme Court, in 1990, issued a decision recognizing that every competent individual has a constitutional right to be free from unwanted treatment. Table 8–6 lists the essentials required by the PSDA.

An advance directive is a written statement completed in advance of a serious illness by an individual about how medical and financial decisions are to be made about his or her care. The two common forms of advance directives are *living wills* and *durable power of attorney for health care* or *health care proxy.* The advance directive allows a person to select someone to make choices when the individual is unable to make the decision (Mezey et al, 1994).

Almost every state has enacted laws that permit advance directives. States have developed their own unique requirements for the elements to be included in an advance directive. There are certain features common in all states (Table 8–7).

Durable Power of Attorney is a written designation by a competent adult for a proxy or surrogate to be appointed to make civil affairs and financial decisions if the appointor becomes incompetent and unable to do so. The preparation of the durable power of attorney requires the same process as any will. The form is signed, dated, witnessed and names the person designated as the proxy.

A *Living Will* sets forth advance treatment choices or instructions to be followed by caregivers in the event that the initiator becomes incapable of making health care decisions and also defines the future health care desired. This will is called a *Living Will* because it is in effect while the person is alive.

The advance directives are binding on health care providers. In some states only one of the directives is allowed, in others both may be implemented. Family members and the primary care provider should be aware that an advance directive has been completed. Copies should be provided to the patient's physician and available to family members.

Nurses play an integral role in assisting patients in making informed decisions about their care. The American Nurses' Association Position Statement on Nursing and the Patient Self-Determination Act (1992) suggests that questions about advance directives be included in the nursing admission assessment. Health care agencies are required to have policies and procedures regarding advance directives. Some agencies may define the role of the nurse in implementing the directive(s). The nurse should be aware of the policies and procedures at both the state and health care agency level. According to the Patient Self-Determination Act, the patient must be informed about living wills and the durable power of attorney for health care. The nurse may be in a position to assess and reinforce the knowledge base and assist in clarifying with the patient the patient's future health care needs. All discussions of treatment preferences need to be fully documented in the patient's record. The information also should be conveyed to other health care professionals. Patients have the right to change the living will or durable power of attorney for health care at any time (Schwarz, 1992).

GOOD SAMARITAN LAWS

Almost all of the states and territories have passed legislation protecting health care professionals that provide assistance in emergency situations. The laws do not require that the nurse or physician must participate but do provide protection if the help is needed and is given in an acceptable, appropriate, and prudent manner. For example, if there is a highway accident and it is obvious that the automobile occupants are injured, the nurse or physician may provide aid without fear of being sued. In these circumstances, it is not necessary to obtain the consent of the injured persons prior to administering treatment. The Good Samaritan Law does not apply to emergencies in health care institutions.

The decision to assist in Good Samaritan emergency situations involves both legal and ethical issues. The health care

TABLE 8–7 Common Features of Advance Directives in All States

Living Wills

- The individual is incapacitated and unable to make or communicate medical wishes before the advance directive can be initiated.
- A physician, and frequently a second physician, must certify that the patient's condition is not expected to improve.
- Instructions are explicit on the use or withdrawal of artificial life support in end of life situations.

Durable Power of Attorney

- An agent is appointed to make decisions regarding financial or property matters during periods of incapacity.
- An agent may be appointed to make health care decisions according to the patient's wishes, if known, or in the patient's best interest if unknown. The scope of the agent's authority is broader than in a living will and is not restricted to ending life support systems.
- The agent may be involved in health care management decisions such as access to medical records and employment of health care personnel caring for the patient.

Adapted from Fade, A. (1994). End of life decisions affect health care providers. *American Nurse* (January), 28–29.

professional will be faced with the decision to either participate or ignore the plight of the injured. Is there an ethical responsibility to give assistance? The professional will have to make the decision based upon his or her own value system.

REPORTING ABUSE

There are three forms of family violence or abuse: sexual, emotional, and physical. They are manifested in different ways: child abuse, elder abuse, and domestic violence. Child abuse is classified as a form of family violence that results in maltreatment of children. It is physical injury caused by nonaccidental acts or it is emotional injury, sexual abuse, or physical or emotional neglect, or exploitation of a child by another person (Campbell and Humphreys, 1993).

Elder abuse, also a form of family violence, is an act of omission by the one providing care, having custody, or responsibility for an elderly person that results in harm or threatened harm to the elderly person. Elder abuse includes physical, emotional, or sexual abuse; neglect, and other violations of rights (Weiner, 1991).

Domestic violence is a form of family violence. It is also known as spousal or partner abuse and refers to all types of abuse between partners, e.g., physical injury (battery), sexual assault, and emotional injury. Battering of women is of particular concern because the incidence of this type of abuse has increased (Campbell and Landenburger, 1996).

Nurses are considered mandated reporters for child abuse and elder abuse. As mandated reporters they must become knowledgeable about the detailed requirements set forth in the Penal Codes in their respective states. In California, for example, when the victim is a child (a person under the age of 18), the nurse as a legally mandated reporter must report if he or she "has the knowledge of or observes a child in his or her professional capacity, or within the scope of his or her employment whom he or she knows or reasonably suspects has been the victim" (California Penal Code 11166 [a]). The report is made to a state child protective agency. Failure of the nurse to report suspected abuse could result in a fine or jail sentence.

All states and territories have laws requiring the reporting of abuse. Many states also include legislation to protect the mentally impaired.

Health care agencies should have specific policies and procedures regarding methods used to complete the necessary reports. Emergency department, outpatient, and home care personnel should be especially aware of the possibility that the physical or psychological symptoms presented by an individual were caused by abuse. Some health care institutions require every patient admitted to the emergency room be assessed for signs of abuse. Immunity is granted to those who report abuse if the report made was made in good faith.

Nurses serve as advocates for any vulnerable group to protect their safety and well-being. Reporting of abuse in all situations is essential, including abuse by any member of the health care staff. Nurses are in a pivotal position to intervene at primary, secondary, and tertiary levels of prevention. The nurse must be alert to potential as well as actual incidents of abuse and take the necessary action, whether it be to refer the abused person to a shelter, to the police, to a family service center, or to community-based nursing organizations.

LIABILITY AND NURSING STUDENTS

All laws affecting registered nurses apply to nursing students. An act performed by a student that causes harm to a patient will be considered negligence. The courts have stated that anyone who administers nursing care usually performed by professional nurses is held to the same standards of care as that given by professional nurses.

Students have a responsibility to be prepared to safely provide patient care. They also have the responsibility to refuse to give care if unprepared or unsure of the level of their proficiency. The student should discuss any potential problem with the clinical instructor or agency nursing staff and, when necessary, to ask for assistance.

The teacher representing the educational agency will be held accountable for the supervision of the nursing student's activities. The teacher could be held equally accountable if the student commits a negligent or other illegal act. Teachers will also be liable if students are assigned to nursing functions for which they are unprepared or if they fail to exercise adequate supervision over the students.

Malpractice Insurance

It is prudent for students and professional nurses to participate in a malpractice insurance program because nurses are increasingly named as defendants in malpractice lawsuits. Insurance policies usually are available through nursing educational programs, selected insurance agencies, or professional nursing organizations such as the American Nurses' Association. The insurance will assist in providing financial assistance in the event the nurse is sued. It is important for nurses to have coverage because in some instances the employing institution may not cover all aspects included in a suit or may not cover instances of supposed malpractice that occur outside of the employing agency.

RELATIONSHIP OF ETHICAL AND LEGAL ISSUES

There is a close relationship between legal and ethical issues. It is important to recognize the differences between the two issues. Legal rights must be accorded to the patient. In most instances, there are no laws that control ethical nursing practice. Laws are made by humans to guide and regulate; ethics deals with the rightness and wrongness of human behavior. Ethical guidelines are not subject to enforcement. Nurses who are aware of both the law and ethics will be well-prepared practitioners.

CHAPTER HIGHLIGHTS

- The system of laws existing in the United States is based on the jurisprudence system that originated in England.
- All societies operate under some type of legal system. The absence of a legal system leads to anarchy.
- Laws have two functions: to provide rights and privileges for all people and to provide a framework for government. Laws provide rules of conduct and regulate behavior.
- Laws either govern the relationships between individuals and society or govern relationships among individual members of sociey. Laws are defined as statutory laws or common laws.
- There are two divisions to the court system: courts created by the states, and courts created by the federal government. The highest court in the country is the United States Supreme Court.
- The practice of nursing is controlled by laws in each state and territory of the United States. The laws are called nurse practice acts. The acts vary from state to state. Practicing nurses should be familiar with the nurse practice act in the state in which they are employed.
- A tort is a wrong committed by one person that inflicts injury on another person. Torts may be unintentional or intentional. Unintentional torts include accidents, negligence, and malpractice. Intentional torts include assault, battery, false imprisonment, invasion of privacy, and defamation.
- Standards of nursing care are established by institutions and reflect practices existing in a community.
- Accurate and comprehensive patient care records are essential in any health care agency. Nurses assume responsibility for ensuring that records are accurate, concise, and recorded in a timely manner.
- Untoward incidents are to be reported to the proper authority. The reports are called incident, variance, or occurrence reports. These reports are included in agency programs that assess quality of care.
- Patients have the right to be informed of and participate in any decisions relating to their health care. Nurses become involved in obtaining informed consents. Nursing activities are subject to patient consent.
- The Patient Self-Determination Act requires that recipients of federal health care dollars have the right to make decisions about their health care. The administration of the law provides for advance directives and living wills.
- Good Samaritan laws have been passed in most states. The laws protect health care professionals who give assistance in emergencies.
- Nurses are responsible for reporting acts of abuse of a patient. Nurses serving in emergency rooms, clinics, homes, schools, or other sites where evidence of abuse may be present are required to report the abuse to the proper authorities.
- Student nurses are held to the same standards of practice as professional nurses and should consider carrying malpractice insurance.
- There is relationship between legal and ethical issues. Both involve behavior; laws regulate behavior, ethics guide behavior.

REFERENCES

Aiken, T.D. with Catalano, J.T. (1994). *Legal, Ethical, and Political Issues in Nursing.* Philadelphia: F.A. Davis, pp. 8–9.

American Nurses' Association (1984). *Issues in Professional Nursing Practice 1. Nursing: Legal Authority for Practice.* Kansas City, MO: American Nurses' Association, p. 2.

American Nurses' Association (1990). *Nursing Practice Acts: Suggested State Legislation.* Kansas City, MO: American Nurses' Association, pp. 7–9.

American Nurses' Association (1992). *Position Statement on Nursing and the Patient's Self Determination Act.* Washington, D.C.: American Nurses' Association.

Berrio, M., Levesque, M. (1996). Advance directives: Most patients don't have one. Do yours? *American Journal of Nursing 96,* 8, 25–28.

Board of Nursing (1998). Nurse Practice Act. *Oregon Administrative Rules.* Portland, OR: Board of Nursing, Chapter 851, pp. 5–9, 52–53.

California Business and Professions Code (1997). Nurse Practice Act. Chapter 6, Nursing, pp. 3–4.

Campbell, J.C., Humphreys, J. (1993). *Nursing Care of Survivors of Family Violence.* St. Louis: Mosby.

Campbell, J., Landenburger, K. (1996). Violence and human abuse. In M. Stanhope and J. Lancaster: *Community Health Nursing: Promoting Health of Aggregates, Families, and Individuals,* 4th ed. St. Louis: Mosby.

Creighton, H. (1986). *Law Every Nurse Should Know,* 5th ed. Philadelphia: W.B. Saunders.

Dock, L.D., Stewart, I.M. (1938). *A Short History of Nursing,* 4th ed. New York: G.P. Putnam, pp. 168–169.

Edwards, B.S. (1994). When a Living Will is ignored. *American Journal of Nursing, 94* (7), 64–65.

Fade, A. (1994). End of life decisions affect health care providers. *American Nurse,* January, 28–29.

Fiesta, J. (1988). *The Law and Liability: A Guide for Nurses,* 2nd ed. Albany, NY: Delmar, p. 65.

Green, A., Crimson, C., Waddil, L., Fitzpatrick, O. (1995). Are you at risk for disciplinary action? *American Journal of Nursing, 95* (7) (July), 36–42.

Guido, G.W. (1988). *Legal Issues in Nursing: A Source Book for Practice.* Norwalk, CT: Appleton-Lange.

Hoebel, E.A. (1954). *The Law of Primitive Man.* Cambridge: Harvard University, 275–276.

Idemoto, B., Daly, B.J., Eger, D., et al (1993). Implementing the Patient Self-Determination Act. *American Journal of Nursing, 93* (1) (January), 20–25.

Joint Commission on the Accreditation of Healthcare Organizations (1990). *Accreditation Manual for Hospitals.* Chicago: JCAHO, p. XV.

Lilley, L. (1994). Now what? After an error. *American Journal of Nursing, 94* (11) (November), 18.

Lippman, H. (1994). Legally speaking: Legal risks of computer charting. *RN.* Reprint 1994, 6–8.

Medicare Omnibus Budget Reconciliation Act of 1990, Public Law No. 101–508 (4206, 4751). Nov. 5, 1990. *The Patient Self Determination Act.*

Mezey, M., Evans, L.K., Golub, Z.D., et al (1994). The Patient Self Determination Act; Sources of concern for nurses. *Nursing Outlook, 42* (7), 30–38.

Meyer, C. (1992). Beside computer charting; Inching toward tomorrow. *American Journal of Nursing, 92* (4) (April), 38–44.

Murchison, I., Nichols, T.S. (1970). *Legal Foundations of Nursing Practice.* New York: Macmillan.

Murchison, I., Nichols, T.S., Hanson, R. (1982). *Legal Accountability in the Nursing Process,* 2nd ed. London: Collier MacMillian Limited, p. 3.

Murphy, J., Burke, L.J., (1990). Charting by exception: A more efficient way to document. *Nursing, 90* (5) (May), 65–69.

National Council of State Board of Nursing (1994). *Profiles of Member Boards.* Chicago.

Pozgar, G.P. (1990). *Legal Aspects of Health Care Administration,* 2nd ed. Gaithersburg, MD: Aspen Systems Publications.

Rhodes, A.M., Miller, R. (1984). *Nursing and the Law,* 4th ed. Rockville, MD: Aspen Systems Publications, p. 201.

Schwarz, J.K. (1992). Living Wills and Health Care Proxies: Nurse practice implications. *Nursing and Health Care, 92* (13) (February), 92–96.

Supples, J.M. (1993). Self regulation in the nursing profession: Response to substandard practice. *Nursing Outlook, 41* (1) (Jan/Feb), 20–24.

Switzer, K.H., (1995). Informed consent for inserting a central venous catheter. *American Journal of Nursing, 95* (6) (June), 66–68.

Viles, S.M. (1980). Liability for the negligence of hospital nursing personnel. *Nursing Administration Quarterly, 80* (5) (Fall), 83–93.

Random House Webster's College Dictionary (1996). New York: Random House, pp. 767–768.

Weiner, A. (1991). A community based education model for identification and prevention of elder abuse. *Journal of Gerontological Social Work, 16* (3–4), 107–119.

Ethical Issues in Nursing Practice

Marylou McAthie

All people have value systems that guide their relationships with others. Everyone has morals, values, and ethical principles shaped by the total of life experiences. It is essential that persons entering the nursing profession be aware of their personal biases, ethical principles, and value systems. Nurses in their everyday activities are faced with situations in which they make ethical decisions regarding those entrusted to their care. It is expected that the decisions will be based on the highest moral and ethical principles because ethical behavior is an integral component in all nursing activities. This chapter will address the issues relating to the application of ethical principles in nursing practice.

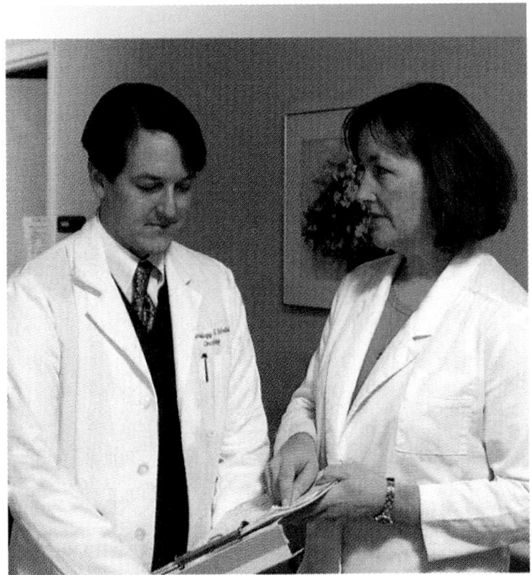

OBJECTIVES

After studying this chapter, students will be able to:

- **use the terminology associated with ethics and understand the meaning of ethics**
- **recognize various ethical theories**
- **apply the levels of the ethical decision-making process**
- **be familiar with the primary principles of ethics and their application to nursing practice**
- **understand the secondary principles of ethics and their effect on professional-patient relationships**
- **understand and apply professional codes of ethics in nursing practice**

THE MEANING OF ETHICS

Why is having an understanding of ethics important? Why do we need to study ethical principles? These questions can be answered by considering the complexity and depth of the relationships that professional nurses have with patients, physicians, other nurses, health care agencies, and society as a whole. The nurse is responsible for making decisions about the patient's welfare while participating in the therapeutic plan of care with the physician and other health care workers. Many nursing actions, referred to as independent functions, require decisions that relate solely to the individual nurse's actions and not to the actions of other health professionals. Many of these decisions are of an ethical nature.

Nurses also are held accountable for upholding the policies of employing agencies and to practice within the confines of the laws of the state or territory in which they live. Codes of ethics created by nursing professional organizations should also be observed. Conflicts of an ethical or moral nature as to the best course of action can occur as decisions are made. An understanding of ethical principles serves to guide the nurse to attain the highest standards of professional conduct and assist in resolving ethical conflicts or dilemmas.

Ethics is based in the field of moral philosophy. The term originates from the Greek word *ethos* and means conduct, customs, and character. The word *morals* is from the Latin word *mores,* which refers to habits and customs. Today, these terms are often used interchangeably.

Understanding the terms associated with the study of ethics serves as a framework for understanding ethics and ethical decision making. Box 9–1 provides definitions of these key terms.

In reviewing the definitions, it is obvious that there is overlap between the various terms, and as stated previously, many are used interchangeably. Knowing the definitions assists the nurse in gaining an understanding of the principles of ethics.

BOX 9–1
DEFINING ETHICAL TERMS

- Ethics: A system or set of moral principles; the rules of conduct recognized in respect to a particular class of human actions or governing a particular group or culture; the branch of philosophy dealing with values relating to human conduct with the respect to rightness or wrongness of actions; and the goodness or badness of motives and ends (*Random House Webster's College Dictionary,* 1996, p. 459).
- Ethical Codes: Guides to actions for professionals; acceptance of responsibility and trust that society has invested in the professions. The requirements of the code may exceed the law but not be less than that required by the law.
- Ethical Dilemma: A difficult problem seemingly impossible of being resolved.
- Principles: An accepted or professional rule of action or conduct; a fundamental law, axiom, or doctrine.
- Principle: A general law or rule that provides a guide for action.(Cooper, 1990, p. 10).
- Professional Oaths: A guide to professional action.
- Standard: Something considered by an authority or by general consent as a basis for comparison; a rule or principle that is used as a basis for judgment.
- Standards: The morals, ethics, customs, etc., regarded generally or by an individual as acceptable. Another term used in place of standards is *criterion.* Criterion refers to the basis for making a judgment or a pattern for guidance for comparing excellence or correctness.
- Moral: Pertaining to or concerned with the principles of right conduct or the distinction between right and wrong.
- Morals: Principles, standards, or habits with respect to right or wrong conduct.
- Values: The abstract concepts of what is right, worthwhile, or desirable; principles or standards.
- Value Systems: Individual values that are interrelated.
- Value Judgments: Judgments of appraisal; the forming of an opinion, decision, or conclusion about values.

APPROACHES TO ETHICS AND ETHICAL THEORIES

The practicing nurse is often faced with situations in which ethical choices must be made. Sometimes the choices are made with the patient or physician or other health care professional; at other times the nurse makes the decision alone. Often there are no clear-cut good options; the choices may be equally "bad" with no "good" alternatives. It is also possible that a nurse will be faced with choices that violate his or her personal value system. It is at this point that the nurse is confronted with an ethical dilemma. For example, the nurse who is personally opposed to abortion may be asked to participate in a surgical procedure that will result in the aborting of a fetus. To refuse will result in violating the agency's policies and possibly in the loss of employment, or could be considered as abandonment of the patient. To agree to assist in the surgical intervention will violate the nurse's own feelings of what is right and what is wrong. There is a need for some type of systematized approach to resolving these conflicts.

Historically, two ethical theories or approaches have been used to analyze ethical dilemmas: deontology and utilitarianism. Unfortunately, these theories may not provide specific answers to the nurse in clinical practice. They offer only general approaches and serve to guide the critical thinking process as one decides a moral course of action.

Deontology

Deontology makes "right" or "wrong" the central core of ethics (Husted and Husted, 1995b). The name is derived from the Greek word *deon,* which means duty, and *logos,* which is defined as discourse. In the deontologic, or formalist, approach, the rightness or wrongness of actions depends on the nature or form of the actions in terms of their moral significance. Duties and obligations are decided by moral principles and rules, e.g., always telling the truth or always keeping promises. In all deontologic approaches a *rule* establishes the right or wrong without regard to the situation, time, or circumstances.

The approach is based on the work of German philosopher Immanuel Kant (1734–1804). Kant wrote that it is *duty* that determines the moral worth of an action. Ethical action consists of doing one's duty; to shirk one's duty is wrong. A person is born knowing that he or she must do his or her duty. To be ethical one must do what is right and refrain from doing what is wrong (Husted and Husted, 1995b). Kant believed that reason ultimately is the foundation of right judgment (Veatch and Fry, 1987). He also believed that the duty to keep promises is unconditional.

Deontology has appealed to some in the health care field because medical institutions operate on systems of rules, regulations, and procedures. Czerwinski (1990) states that deontology focuses on rights and duties; a nurse has a duty to do something, based on binding principles and rules that classify acts as right, wrong, obligatory, or prohibitive. She indicates that another term for the deontologic framework is the *duty-oriented approach*. She defines the approach as "actions based

BOX 9-2
THE DEONTOLOGIC FRAMEWORK IN ACTION

An Ethical Dilemma. The duty-oriented or deontologic framework was applied by Czerwinski to an ethical dilemma that occurred in an intensive care clinical unit:

Joan Silver was a staff nurse on the Intensive Care Unit of an acute care hospital. She had been employed on the unit for a period of 3 years and was assigned to the evening shift. She was fully aware of the policies and procedures of the unit and the hospital.

During Miss Silver's tour of duty she noticed that the condition of one of her patients was deteriorating. She notified the patient's primary physician and described the symptoms. The physician told her to write an order for a "No Code" and then hung up. The hospital policy indicated that phone orders should only be accepted for emergency situations and the physician had to countersign the order within 24 hours. Silver did not consider the patient's condition serious enough to warrant emergency orders and did not want to accept the responsibility of writing an order she considered wrong for the patient.

Miss Silver considered the following:

- How would the patient react if aware of the order?
- Who would tell the family who were waiting in the hospital waiting room?
- Who would tell other health care team members of the order?
- Is not the purpose of the Intensive Care Unit to save lives?
- Why did the primary care physician order a "No Code"?

Exploring the Dilemma. The options:

- Follow the orders of the physician by recording the "No Code" order in the patient's medical record.
- Ignore the order and if the patient had a cardiac arrest, initiate the cardiac team and resuscitate the patient.
- Inform the family of the problem and turn the problem over to them to recontact the primary care physician.
- Discuss the problem with the nursing manager on duty during the evening shift.

Selecting the Appropriate Course of Action. Miss Silver's primary ethical responsibility (duty) was to do what was right for the patient by following the rule of "doing no harm." She felt the physician's order was wrong and violated the rights of the patient and family, and policies of the unit and hospital. Silver selected the fourth option as the best path to follow.

Silver determined that the dilemma needed to be resolved on two levels: the policy level and the nursing practice level. At the patient care level, she felt that the right approach was to seek care for the patient because the patient's condition continued to deteriorate. At the policy level, she decided that it was necessary (right) to follow the chain of command within the hospital by notifying her immediate nursing manager of the incident.

To select the first three options could be wrong and harmful to the patient. However, by not following the physician's order, she could be accused of failure to perform her duty and be fired. She could also have faced legal action from the patient or patient's family for failing to provide adequate care. There was no ideal solution to the dilemma; the course of action best for the safeguarding patient needed to be selected.

Resolving the Dilemma. Joan Silver talked with the on-duty nurse manager and a decision was made to contact the hospital physician-in-residence and review the problem. Miss Silver's decision to not follow the order for the "No Code" was agreed to by the supervisor and the physician. Silver obtained the necessary orders to care for the patient. She was commended for carrying out her duty to the patient and the hospital. The physician reported the problem to the chief of the medical staff. Policies and procedures were changed to prevent the problem from recurring.

Had the supervisor and resident physician not agreed with Miss Silver, she could have contacted the administrator of nursing services, the hospital administrator, or chief of the medical staff to further explore the issue. If they did not agree with her decision, she would be faced with writing the order on the patient's record and carrying out the order or refusing and be held to be insubordinate.

Adapted from Czerwinski, B.S. (1990). An autopsy of a dilemma. *Journal of Nursing Administration, 20* (6), 25–29.

on rules or principles rather than actions based on means or outcomes" and "in other words, the consequences of actions do not always determine the rightness or wrongness of the actions." (Czerwinski, 1990, p. 26). Box 9–2 presents an example of an ethical dilemma to which the deontologic framework was applied.

There are pitfalls to this approach. Deontology demands that action be taken regardless of the outcomes of the actions. It is almost impossible for nurses to be in a situation in which the results of an action are not considered.

Think of the nurse who makes a promise to a patient to control the patient's pain after a surgical procedure only to be confronted postsurgically with circumstances that do not allow pain medications to be administered. If one adhered to deontologic principles, it would be imperative to keep the promise and give the medication regardless of the harm to the patient.

Utilitarianism

The utility approach considers the "good" and the "right." "Good" includes pleasure and happiness and "right" if it leads to the greatest amount of good and the least amount of harm. John Stewart Mill in his book *Utilitarianism* (1861, p. 10) proposed the principle of utility: "Actions are right in proportion as they tend to promote happiness, wrong as they tend to produce the reverse of happiness, i.e., pleasure or absence of pain." A second principle of utilitarianism is that most people have a basic desire for unity and harmony with their fellow human beings.

Utilitarianism has also been applied to acts and rules. The *act utilitarian* asks: "What good or evil will result directly from this action in these circumstances" (Beauchamp and Childress, 1994, p. 50). Utility is grounded in the specific act, not in general circumstances. "Rules of thumb" apply that can be altered to fit the situation. For example, if it harms the patient to tell the truth about his or her condition, the nurse may alter the truth and not inform the patient of the facts. *Rule utilitarians* believe that rules cannot be compromised. The rules are considered firm and protective of individuals and society. Rules are not abandoned under any circumstances. To the rule utilitarian the truth must always be told to a patient regardless of the results.

Conflicts between rules can occur, which results in the development of a dilemma. When this happens, one rule will take precedence over another. The choice may not be easy. For example, one of the ethical principles states that health professionals shall not cause harm to a patient (as stated in the Florence Nightingale pledge for nurses and in the Hippocratic oath for physicians), but what if a nurse working in a critical care unit of a hospital develops a serious respiratory infection? Should the nurse stay on the unit and expose vulnerable patients or go home? The nurse is aware that no other qualified staff members are available and that the unit would be left with nonlicensed nursing personnel. Which action will cause the least harm? Another example would be if a health care team is faced with the problem of whether to save the life of the mother or her unborn child when both cannot be saved. Whose right to life is to be violated, the mother or the child? Either the mother or the fetus will be harmed. Is there a good answer? Seroka (1994) states that both deontologic and utilitarian theories represent appropriate frameworks for ethical decision making; however, it is imperative that nurses identify the framework in which they believe.

FOUNDATIONS OF ETHICAL DECISION MAKING

As previously stated, it is important to be aware of the theoretical discussions regarding ethical principles, but direct application of the theories to specific situations in nursing practice is complicated. It is also important to understand the arguments and approaches being postulated by various ethicists.

Ethical issues arise in many different circumstances and seem to always present difficult choices. Ethics is an active process that evolves when circumstances force individuals to deal with tension and conflict. Making ethical decisions over time tends to assist the nurse in developing an operational ethic or ethical identity. Skill in resolving ethical issues can be developed (Cooper, 1990).

Levels of Ethical Decision Making

Ethical decision making involves the development of a systematic approach to examine the values used by individuals in selecting ethical courses of actions. A framework for understanding the process, which is described as being fluid and lacking rigidity, was developed by Henry David Aiken in 1962 and is described by Cooper (1990). The process is one of ordering values and making decisions about ethical dilemmas. Aiken defines ethics as having to do with concepts of "good," "right," and "ought." He states that in everyday life the meanings of concepts are dealt with at various levels of seriousness and reflection. The level may be a response about:

- what one ought to do
- that something is good, or
- reflecting on one's world view

Four distinct levels of ethical decisions are presented:

- expressive level
- level of moral rule
- level of ethical analysis
- postethical level

THE EXPRESSIVE LEVEL

The spontaneous expression of emotion, such as venting of one's feelings, is a common form of value judgment. It is manifested in such statements as "That was a stupid thing you did" or "That clerk is completely incompetent." There is neither a description to explain the statement nor an overt attempt to influence others to agree. The words may have influence depending on who uttered the statement. If said by someone in a position of authority, the effect may have more impact than intended.

THE LEVEL OF MORAL RULES

At this level, more serious questions are raised. Moral guides acquired through socialization from family, friends, colleagues, religious institutions, education, and life experiences are brought to conscious thought. The moral guides are considered "rules of thumb" and are used to appraise a situation and decide what responses or courses of action might be undertaken. Problems of proper conduct and assessment of alternatives and consequences are considered. Answers to the questions are based on an in-depth review of courses of actions and the outcomes resulting from the actions. Moral guides in the form of rules, proverbs, and maxims (including the "golden rule") demonstrate some of the moral stances that may lead to consequences from the action:

- "Loyalty to your patient comes first."
- "Do unto others as you would have them do unto you."
- "Honesty is the best policy."
- "Love thy neighbor as thyself."
- "Truth will win out."
- "A promise made is a promise kept."
- "Never tell a lie."

What happens to the moral guide when situations occur that force the nurse to violate the rules? Consider the following:

> Joan Wright, a registered nurse, was assigned to care for Mrs. Murphy, a terminally ill patient. Mrs. Murphy was in a great deal of pain. She had never been told that she was dying. Mrs. Murphy pleaded with Miss Wright to tell her what was wrong with her and why she was having so much discomfort. Miss Wright knew that the physician and the patient's family did not want her to know that she was terminally ill. The family had decided that Mrs. Murphy would respond very negatively to the news of her impending death. Miss Wright felt that she was being untruthful by not telling Mrs. Murphy about her condition. She felt that if she knew what was happening she would be less anxious and under reduced stress, which might lessen the pain.

Miss Wright was faced with the dilemma of either not following the orders of the physician and the desires of the family or violating her own principles or moral rules. Miss Wright could search for some alternate ways of handling the situation whereby she could follow the rule that loyalty to the patient and to her own sense of honesty comes first. One course of action could lead her to discuss her feelings with the physician and to explain how she feels about the patient's lack of information; a second way to seek a solution is to ask for a conference with the family to discuss her point of view and suggest possible measures that might assist Mrs. Murphy in becoming less stressed and more comfortable. Another course of action is to ignore the problem, which in and of itself is a decision; however, Miss Wright would not have resolved her dilemma.

At this level of ethical decision making, the problem is usually resolved. The ethical problems are not long term and ad hoc decisions are usually made. To summarize, at the level of moral rules, the ethical problem is identified, alternative solutions based on moral guides are reviewed, a course of action is pursued, and the problem is resolved. The next level requires greater dimensions of reflection and thought.

THE LEVEL OF ETHICAL ANALYSIS

The ethical issues are complex, profound, and unique at this level. The moral guides or rules are ineffective and require greater review of the ethical principles involved. The definition of an ethical principle can be expanded to say that it is a statement concerning the conduct or state of being that is required for the fulfillment of a value: it explicitly links a value with a general mode of action (Cooper, 1990, p. 10). The profoundness of an ethical problem may require an in-depth review of the values that are in conflict and the principles that underlie the values. Values tend to be too vague to have great meaning in analyzing an ethical problem. For example, to say that an individual values justice or freedom or honesty conveys only a generalized meaning. Principles that identify the true meaning of the term can be formulated. The principles should clearly describe conditions and qualifications for the range of conduct implied. For example, Davis (1991) cites respect for individuals as a value inherent in nursing. The principle requires that each individual be treated as unique and as equal to every other individual and that justification is required for interference in the individual's own purposes and goals (Davis, 1991). A general principle is devised that may then be used to develop more specific statements and courses of actions. To return to the earlier scenario:

> The situation between Miss Wright and Mrs. Murphy has not been resolved. The physician refused to discuss the case with Miss Wright and the family ignored the request for a conference. Mrs. Murphy's anxiety and pain intensified. Miss Wright would need to analyze the information she had gathered and decide if Mrs. Murphy's rights as an individual were being disregarded. The situation had changed; the nurse's moral rules and patient's welfare were being adversely affected. Miss Wright was left with the task of reviewing her values and sorting out the underlying principles, then deciding on a course of action based on the principles.

Clarifying the distinction between values and principles can become an exercise that may help the nurse to understand how personal values affect the decision-making process. A list of personal values can be devised. Principles can then be formulated from each value. The process allows the nurse to objectively review how personal feeling affects the decision-making process.

THE POSTETHICAL LEVEL

The fourth level of ethical decision making involves a basic introspective review of one's fundamental beliefs. In the presence of deeply disturbing circumstances, a person may question personally held views and values. Problems and issues relating to integrity, loyalty, or justice may emerge, leading to the need to examine one's fundamental philosophy or the meaning of life.

It is unusual to engage in this level of reflection. The circumstances would be profound—for example, being placed in a situation in which one questions the meaning of one's religious beliefs or cultural traditions. Resolutions to ethical problems of this nature require a thorough examination of the person's basic world view or, in some instances, a reassessment of religious or cultural values (Cooper, 1990).

As with most processes, linear thinking is not feasible. Movement between the levels is continuous as different alternatives are explored. New information and changing circumstances create a situation of alternating between feelings and reflection. The process may or may not be at the conscious thinking level. As the situation becomes more complex, greater conscious reflective thought is given. The more that ethical or moral issues are brought into conscious thought, the more responsive the nurse will be in making sound ethical decisions.

The circumstances and environment of the nurse's practice will have an effect on the quality of the ethical decisions made. If staff members are operating at different emotional or reflective levels, conflicts may occur in deciding the best course of action to follow. Recognition of the various approaches taken by colleagues will facilitate making the best ethical decisions (Cooper, 1990).

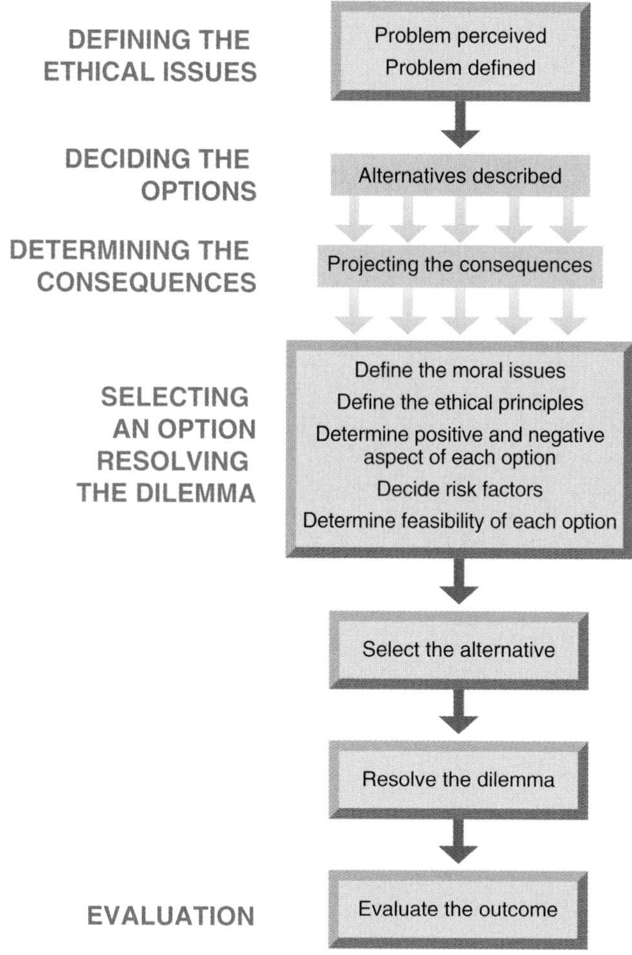

Figure 9–1. An example of an ethical decision-making model.

An Ethical Decision-Making Model

Ethical decision making requires having the most relevant objective data available. It is important to be able to describe the specific circumstances or situation. It is also essential to be able to prescribe steps to be taken and have a guide to resolve the dilemma. This section describes a typical decision-making model; this model is illustrated in Figure 9–1.

CLARIFYING THE ETHICAL DILEMMA

The first step in the decision-making process is to determine whether or not a patient care situation presents ethical concerns or questions that need to be resolved. The circumstances to be explored involve conflicts of values, obligations, interests, or disagreements between health care members, patient, family, or about the use of therapies that may be aggressive or expensive. Values that conflict may relate to respect for the patient's choices, respect for the integrity of the care providers, and reducing the patient's suffering or not causing harm to the patient (Aroskar, 1994).

When an ethical dilemma occurs, it may be presented in a disorganized, disjointed manner. It is important to systematically collect all relevant information, review the circumstances surrounding the situation, and determine the crucial elements. The following questions may be asked:

- Who should be involved in the decision-making process? Who should make the final decision? Why?
- What criteria should be used—for example, physiologic or economic conditions only; legal, social, or family considerations, or psychological status?
- What risks are involved?
- What, if any, consent should be or should have been obtained from the patient?
- What, if any, moral principles are validated or negated by the proposed choices of action? For example, truth telling, justice, respect for individuals, or self-determination (Davis and Aroskar, 1991, pp. 229–230)?

In addition to determining what and who is involved, it is essential to know the viewpoints of the key players, and, in addition, it is important to know the sequence of events.

The decision-making ability of the patient should be assessed to determine if the patient has the capacity to either make a decision or participate in the process (Aroskar, 1994).

DEFINING THE ETHICAL ISSUES

The difficult process of analyzing and defining underlying ethical problems is undertaken. After the objective data have been collected, the next step is to organize and analyze the information, and then identify the specific problem as clearly as possible. The process involves looking for patterns and clues.

While undertaking defining and analyzing the problem, many long-held personal beliefs and values may be questioned. Problems are frequently analyzed in practical terms that lead to solutions that may be expedient but not ethical. For example, rather than report a colleague for improperly performing a treatment, a nurse ignores the action, not wanting to create a problem for a coworker. This nurse saved a friend from possibly being removed from the job but violated the right of the patient to be free from harm.

DECIDING THE OPTIONS; DETERMINING THE CONSEQUENCES

All of the possible solutions or courses of actions should be explored. It is rare that there would be only one path or one "good" answer to the dilemma. Conscious critical thinking processes are used to develop alternative courses of action. Writing out possibilities or brainstorming with other individuals may assist in bringing about the most acceptable answers. Alternative choices should be explored from the perspective of how they affect ethical principles such as respect for individual autonomy, and avoiding of harm to the patient (Aroskar, 1994).

The positive and negative consequences of each proposed solution should be ascertained. Assuming that a course of action is followed, what are the events that will take place once the solution is implemented? Cooper (1990, p. 22), quoting John Dewey, calls this process one of "deliberation" in which a "dramatic rehearsal" in one's mind happens and "various competing lines of action" are imagined. The more that imagination is exercised, the more the ethical decision-making process may be improved.

SELECTING OPTIONS AND RESOLVING THE DILEMMA

Reviewing the alternative courses of action can help identify the solutions that have the greatest potential to resolve the dilemma. The moral values inherent in each option need to be determined. The positive and negative, risks, cost, feasibility, and acceptability of each option should be determined. The next step in the process is to select the specific alternative that is to be considered. The moral rules and ethical principles involved in the solution should be identified and explored in depth. The process is not linear and requires moving back and forth between the various alternatives to decide which may be the best.

The nurse must ask if the option selected can be defended to other health care professionals and the community at large. The legal implications should also be reviewed. The option must fit the accepted ethical norms of the institution in which the nurse practices, within the nursing profession, and with society as a whole. If the option cannot be defended, then it is clear that the solution is not acceptable. The option should also feel right, be consistently used, and be reflected in the values and actions of the nurse.

EVALUATING THE OUTCOMES

The course of action selected represents the end result of gathering objective data, analyzing the data, selecting options, and determining the best course of action. The final process undertaken is to decide whether the option or options selected effectively resolved the dilemma. A series of questions may be posed to decide the impact of the option(s) selected:

- Did the action reflect the values of the person or persons involved?
- Did the action achieve the desired results?
- What feedback was received from others?
- Was the option selected defensible to others?
- Did the option selected uphold the standards of the employing agency and the nursing profession?

The process is completed when the nurse involved is satisfied that sound ethical principles were used to arrive at a solution and the evaluation indicates that the results of the decisions made were acceptable. The use of the model allows for systematic ethical decision making. The model is not used to resolve every ethical problem but will be helpful when problems of the third and fourth level are encountered. To reiterate, the process is not linear; the various steps within the model are frequently revisited as new information is obtained or additional solutions are proposed.

The use of the model may provide the nurse with increased sensitivity and a greater understanding of personal values. Because of the need to respect and protect patients, it is important to have a clear perception of the specific principles or concepts which health care professionals use to respond to ethical dilemmas.

PRINCIPLES OF ETHICS

The term *principle* has been defined as "an accepted or professed rule of action or conduct" (*Random House Webster's College Dictionary*, 1996, p. 1073). Principles direct ethical behavior. Applying ethical principles to specific situations helps to clarify the ethical problem. Principles are guides and leave room for judgments in specific cases. Principles are broadly stated; therefore, it is important to ensure that principles are defined and carefully applied according to the specific situation and problem. For example, the term *truth* may start with a general principle such as "Always tell the truth" but will need greater definition if carrying out such an action would cause harm to the persons involved.

Major moral and ethical principles affect practicing nurses and other health care professionals. The principles include:

- autonomy–respect for the individual
- nonmaleficence–the obligation to not inflict harm intentionally
- beneficence–the need to contribute to the welfare of others
- justice–the provision of fair, equitable, and appropriate treatment to others

Autonomy

Autonomy is derived from the Greek *autos* meaning self and *nomos* referring to rule or law. Beauchamp and Childress (1994, p. 121) define "personal autonomy: personal rule of the self that is free from both controlling interferences by others and from personal limitations that prevent meaningful choice." According to Husted and Husted (1995a, p. 72), autonomy "describes every person's experience of being himself." They further state that autonomy "relates a nurse—the actual person she is—to the actual person her patient is" and "every ethical agent is, by nature, the ethical equal of every other."

Respect for the individual implies that every person is equal to every other person. To interfere with another person's privacy or behavior requires justification. Under all circumstances, the desires, values, and goals of the patient are to be considered and given high priority in any decision affecting the patient's welfare and care. Individuals act for themselves to the level of their abilities.

Nurses, as coordinators and managers of patient care, are in a position to ensure that the patient's wishes and interests are included in any treatment plan. A mentally competent patient who refuses treatment is not to be coerced even if the results of the refusal create a negative response for the patient's mental or physical condition. Other alternatives such as changing the treatment regimen or asking the patient's family for assistance can be pursued in an attempt to resolve the problem. The only action left for the nurse may be to comfort the patient and support his or her decision, especially if the patient's refusal could result in his or her death. The nurse must also be aware of his or her own value system and not try to impose decisions on the patient that are contrary to the patient's desires.

There is a caveat in considering the use of the principle of autonomy. The rights of the individual are to be respected as long as the actions do not harm other persons. The scope of the rights of each person involved must be defined.

All patients are to be made fully aware of the procedures and treatments ordered for their care. The patient is to be provided with adequate, reasonable information to enable an informed decision. Frequently the severity of the treatment, as in the case of an invasive procedure, may require the patient to indicate agreement by signing a consent form. The requirement for a signed informed consent protects the autonomy of the patient.

Unconscious patients, infants, and mentally incompetent patients cannot participate in the informed consent process. There is an assumption made by health care workers that patients will want to be cared for and treated. Family members may be consulted or the patient may have planned ahead and prepared documentation to explain their wishes. In some instances a legal solution may be sought and a court order specifying the treatment may be obtained.

The Patient Self-Determination Act was passed by the United States Congress and became law in 1991. (See Chapter 8 for further information about the Act.) The law requires that persons receiving Medicare and Medicaid benefits be given written information about their rights by the institution in which they are receiving care. The laws of the state in which the patient resides are used as guidelines to make decisions about medical care, including the right to refuse care. Information is also to be provided about living wills (a document listing the medical treatments the patient wishes to refuse if unable to speak for him- or herself) and the durable power of attorney (a document appointing a friend or relative to make medical decisions on the patient's behalf when the patient can no longer make decisions about health care). The wishes of the patient are to be documented in the patient's record and periodically reconfirmed with the patient. The living will and durable power of attorney are discussed in more detail in Chapter 8.

As also discussed in Chapter 8, the American Hospital Association adopted and distributed a Patient's Bill of Rights in 1972. The expectation is that patients have a right to expect respectful and competent care in any hospital in the United States. The Bill includes a detailed list of the rights of the individual patient, including participating in decisions regarding care and the right to refuse care. It is anticipated that all hospitals will adhere to the contents of the Bill.

Beneficence and Nonmaleficence

Beneficence and nonmaleficence are considered as a single principle by some ethicists; others make a distinction between the two by defining *beneficence* as the obligation to help others and *nonmaleficence* as the obligation to not cause harm to others. The two principles can be distinguished in the following way:

- Nonmaleficence: One ought not to inflict evil or harm.
- Beneficence: One ought to prevent evil or harm, remove evil or harm, and to do or promote good.

Beneficence requires helping actions or promoting good; nonmaleficence requires intentionally not causing harm (Beauchamp and Childress, 1994).

The principle of nonmaleficence (the duty to do no harm) is implied in the Hippocratic oath that serves as the basis for medical ethics. The Hippocratic oath states: "I will use treatment to help the sick according to my ability and judgment, but I will never use it to injure or wrong them." The Nightingale Pledge states: "I will abstain from whatever is deleterious and mischievous." The concept is also reflected in nursing ethical codes, which will be discussed later.

Nonmaleficence prohibits intentionally causing harm to an individual unless there are special circumstances. For example, administering a treatment, such as probing an infected incision, may cause pain to a patient, but the potential benefits accruing from the treatment outweigh the harm. The circumstances require that the risks be balanced against the benefits to be gained. There are many types of harm; therefore, the principle of nonmaleficence involves moral rules such as "do not kill" and "do not cause pain or suffering to others."

When there is a possibility of causing harm to the patient, the *Standard of Due Care* is used (Beauchamp and Childress, 1994). The standard requires that the outcomes sought justify the risks that must be taken to achieve the desired results. The taking of serious risks requires exacting justification. The failure to adequately follow the standard of care results in *negligence* when risks are intentionally imposed, are unreasonable, and cause harm to the patient. Professional malpractice (i.e., harmful or unhelpful medical or nursing therapy) is an example of negligence. Health care professionals are obligated to uphold the legal and moral standards of due care. The standard requires that health professionals have proper training, be skilled, and show competence (Beauchamp and Childress, 1994).

The principle of beneficence requires more than the principle of nonmaleficence because there is an obligation to provide positive benefits to others. The acts of mercy, charity, kindness, and altruism are beneficent actions. The concept of the "Good Samaritan" or showing compassion for another human being is an example of this principle. The providing of preventive health care programs is another example of the principle. Moral rules of beneficence include:

- Protect and defend the rights of others.
- Prevent harm from occurring to others.
- Remove conditions that will cause harm to others.
- Help persons with disabilities.
- Rescue persons in danger (Beauchamp and Childress, 1994, p. 262).

Nurses are morally required to take part in the decisions regarding the potential harms or benefits that result from the therapeutic decisions made about patient care. The nurse also reviews the plan of nursing care to determine what risks, potential harm, or positive benefits are being imposed on the patient. Under all circumstances, nurses are obliged to follow the standards of due care.

The principles of beneficence and nonmaleficence require balancing of the risks taken when harm is inflicted and the benefits gained from inflicting the harm. For instance, the nurse who is about to treat a child with an injectable medication knows that the child will feel pain but also knows that the beneficial effects of the medication outweigh the momentary pain felt. Practicing nurses encounter many situations in which decisions of this nature must be made.

Justice

Justice, as defined by Beauchamp and Childress (1994), is the fair, equitable, and appropriate treatment of all people in light of what is due or owed to them. Those who have valid claims based on justice have rights and therefore are due something. An injustice involves a wrongful act that denies benefits to those entitled to them.

The idea of justice is basic to the structure of society. Distributive justice refers to fair, equitable, and reasonable distribution of benefits and burdens, and having rights and assuming responsibilities in society. Public and private institutions, including the government, are included. The health care system is involved in maintaining and participating in upholding the principle of justice.

Problems in distributive justice arise when scarcities or competition occurs. For example, basic human need involves having access to a safe water supply; however, many people in the United States are exposed to polluted water because of industrial waste products. Should the government limit the amount of pollutants and create a problem whereby the industry causing the pollution would lay off employees? Unemployment in the community could cause serious problems for the workers and their families. Do the health concerns outweigh the economic concerns? Where does fairness and equality enter the picture? Weighing such alternatives is typical of the difficulties encountered in distributive justice. The risks, costs, and benefits of the alternatives have to be determined.

One major consideration for nurses is the fairness and equality by which health care, medical care, and nursing care is distributed. Meeting the fundamental needs of all persons implies that the individuals will be harmed if needs are not met. For example, all humans have needs for adequate nutrition, protection from bodily harm, safe water and air, and so on. The following have been proposed as valid principles of distributive justice:

- To each person an equal share.
- To each person according to his or her need.
- To each person according to his or her effort.
- To each person according to his or her contribution.
- To each person according to his or her merit.
- To each person according to free-market exchanges (Beauchamp and Childress, 1994, p.330).

Application of all principles may be impossible for health care workers. For instance, providing equal access for all individuals to the health care system is questionable when one considers the number of uninsured people in the United States. The emergence of managed care may also be considered as a way to ration medical and nursing care, which raises

CURRENT CONTROVERSY
HOW CAN NURSING DEAL WITH HEALTH CARE RATIONING?

HEALTH CARE RATIONING

Nurses are confronted with a dilemma and a clash of values because they are faced with participating in decisions that result in rationing health care to their patients. Nursing has traditionally valued and believed that all patients should receive the care they need. Professional nursing's Agenda for Health Care Reform (1991, p. 8) states:

All citizens and residents of the United States must have equitable access to essential health care services (a core of care).

Nurses are not alone in their concerns about the rationing of care. Providing for health care and access to health care in the United States are issues for all citizens. Everyone is worried about the crises and for good reason. The nation spends billions of dollars on health care, yet few Americans are receiving improved care. Many people are not insured or are underinsured (Davis, 1991).

Further, the President's Commission for the Study of Ethical Problems in Medicine and Biomedical Research (1983) concluded that society has an ethical obligation to ensure equal access to health for all. Efforts to reduce health care costs should not focus on limiting health care to the most vulnerable population groups such as the aged and the poor. In the United States, indicators of health care status such as infant mortality rate and life expectancy are poorer than in other advanced countries, yet health care costs are among the highest in the world.

In an effort to reduce escalating costs, health care providers and insurance companies are reducing services to their enrollees. Less care is available and certain medical procedures are not covered. As a result, major changes in the delivery of health are being initiated. Nurses are being forced to alter nursing delivery systems to reduce costs, often at the expense of providing adequate patient care. For example, in some health care institutions the re-engineering now taking place has reduced the number of licensed nursing personnel and increased the work of those remaining. As a result, patients may be placed at risk because poorly trained staff are being hired to assume registered nurse functions. Patients are being sent home from hospitals on the basis of how much insurance companies will pay rather than on the medical condition of the patient. These changes have caused major ethical concerns for nurses because they may be participating in changes that will cause harm to the patient.

Rationing of health care and health care resources is occurring. The double-edged problem of providing equitable access and adequate care while reducing costs has created an ethical dilemma for nurses. The nursing profession has become acutely aware of the problem of rationing of health care resources. A survey conducted by *The American Nurse* (Health care rationing tops list of pressing ethical issues, 1994, p.11) asked nurses which of the ethical issues they believed were most critical during the 1990s. The results of the survey indicated their greatest concerns:

- Health care rationing 56%
- End-of-life decision making 42%

When asked if age should be a criterion in rationing of limited health care resources, the majority of the respondents (56%) said no.

A system of rationing scarce medical resources hinges on two questions (Davis, 1991, p. 9): (1) What should the criterion of selection be? and (2) Who should make the selection? How will and how should nurses participate in making these decisions? What avenues do nursing organizations need to pursue to influence the development of a just system of health care for all? Many barriers exist to achieving access to adequate health care. For millions of people who encounter the barriers, a just system is a distant ideal (Beauchamp and Childress, 1994). For nurses the clash of values will be reduced when adequate access and care are available to all citizens.

a question in applying the concept that each person receives care "according to his need." Will basic needs of the patient be met? (See Current Controversy box.)

The individual needs of patients are of primary concern to practicing nurses. The basic need to provide a safe and therapeutic environment is necessary under all circumstances.

Scarcity of nursing services may require prioritizing needs beyond those considered basic. For example, the first priority for care may be given to patients facing life-threatening situations such as in emergency settings, and in acute and critical care sites. Other nursing care activities will be provided as determined by the policies of the nursing, medical, and administrative staff of the facility where the nurse is employed. It is essential that nurses participate in the decisions regarding the distribution of services to ensure that the principle of justice is upheld. It seems obvious that when resources are limited, inequality may occur. Sufficient services are not always available to meet every need of every person. A basic level of service for all should be determined and implemented.

PROFESSIONAL-PATIENT ETHICAL RELATIONSHIPS

Professional-patient ethical relationships involve problems of veracity, privacy, fidelity, and confidentiality. These terms may be defined as follows:

- veracity: from the Latin word *veritas;* to tell the truth

- privacy: a right of limited physical or informational inaccessibility
- fidelity: faithfulness of one human being to another, or the duty to keep promises
- confidentiality: the duty to safeguard privileged information

These principles may be considered as secondary principles that are frequently interrelated and involved with the primary principles of autonomy, beneficence and nonmaleficence, and justice.

Veracity

The question of truth-telling is inherent in all of the other principles. Truth-telling is an essential element in informed consent and in confidentiality. The nurse must be honest in all actions involving the patient.

The obligation for veracity is based on the respect owed to others. The obligation also is closely connected to fidelity and keeping promises. There is an implicit promise that, when speaking, the truth will be told and that listeners will not be deceived. When a patient agrees to a treatment, it is anticipated that the patient will be told the truth about the treatment and that promises made about the results will be kept, or explanations will be given as to why the promises could not be honored. Veracity implies a trusting relationship between the patient and the health care professional. Confidence is developed when veracity is present (Beauchamp and Childress, 1994).

The question of withholding information presents a difficult problem for the nurse, as was evident in the example when Miss Wright was told not to explain to Mrs. Murphy the reason for her pain. Practices of withholding information vary from institution to institution and from situation to situation. The tendency in most circumstances is that information is not withheld from patients so that they can make informed decisions.

Right to Privacy

The right to privacy is implied in the Bill of Rights of the United States Constitution and has been addressed by the United States Supreme Court. The right of privacy is not clearly articulated in the law and tends to be interpreted in different ways depending on the legal situation. The right to privacy and the principle of autonomy are related. The ethical issues confronting the nurse require that the patient's right to privacy be respected and protected.

Health care professionals are obligated to protect the patient's privacy and confidentiality. The World Health Organization, the American Medical Association, the Canadian Nurses' Association, the American Nurses' Association, and other international and national health professional groups include the concept of confidentiality in their codes of ethics.

Fidelity

Whenever there is an agreement, there must be fidelity. An agreement that is not honored is a contradiction in terms (Husted and Husted, 1995b). They further state:

> The evolution and traditions of nursing have produced certain cultural expectations concerning the nature of nursing. These also form a bridge of expectations between nurse and patient. When a patient enters the health care system, these expectations form an implicit agreement between them. The terms of the agreement are precisely those expectations as each is aware of them.
>
> A nurse in relating to her patient tacitly promises to live up to her patient's reasonable expectations. Behind this act of making a promise is an implicit commitment to keep it. Thus fidelity is fundamental to the nurse-patient agreement (Husted and Husted, 1995b, p. 65).

Confidentiality

The concept of confidentiality is present when one person discloses information to another, is both private and voluntary, and is told in trust and confidence. The information is not to be given to any other individual unless the originating person providing the information gives permission for it to be released and defines under which circumstances. The rule prohibits disclosures of information to a third party unless permission is specifically given. There are some exceptions in which laws exist that require reporting, as in cases such as a person entering an emergency room with a gunshot wound, in cases of venereal diseases and in child abuse (in some states), and in certain infectious diseases.

It is not uncommon for several of the principles to be involved in any ethical problem. The nurse can utilize the ethical decision-making model to assist in analyzing and resolving the problem.

PROFESSIONAL BEHAVIOR AND CODES OF PROFESSIONAL ETHICS

The values of the person participating in a nursing program have been well developed prior to entering the profession. As stated previously, values are acquired through the socialization process and life experiences. The values gained through earlier life experiences serve as the basis for the values developed in nursing. The development of professional values is essential if the nurse is to exercise ethical behavior in practice. There is an interrelationship between personal and professional values. The values of an individual become a part of the individual's identity and guide his or her conduct. According to Seroka (1994, p. 9) values are "actualized as a way of life through one's behaviors." She further states:

> A belief, which is a proposition based on information that we gather, combined with a value gained from our life experiences,

results in an attitude, which in turn shapes our behavior. Following is an example of this concept:

- Belief—All street people are lazy.
- Value—Laziness is bad.
- Attitude—Therefore, all street people are bad.

This example assists in recognizing the influence values have on behaviors, feelings, actions, and conduct. This is why one must identify and clarify one's own value system (Seroka, 1994, pp. 9–10).

The nursing profession has developed standards of conduct to guide members in their everyday behaviors. The codes of ethics have been developed and approved by members of the nursing profession. The principles of justice, beneficence and nonmaleficence, autonomy, veracity, privacy, confidentiality, and fidelity are incorporated in the codes.

The American Nurses' Association's Code for Nurses (see Box 9–3) serves as the profession's guidelines for individual and collective responsibility in response to society's need for trustworthy, competent, and accountable practitioners. The Code is a statement of belief expressing the moral concerns, values, and goals of nursing. It:

- demonstrates to society that nurses are expected to understand and accept trust and responsibility invested in them by the public
- provides guidelines for professional conduct and relationships as the basis for ethical practice
- defines the nurse's relationship to the client as one of patient advocate
- provides a means of self-regulation (Bandman and Bandman, 1995, p. 28)

Codes from other nursing organizations also have been developed for the same purposes (see Box 9–4, Canadian Nurses' Association Code of Ethics; and Box 9–5, International Council for Nurses Code for Nurses).

BOX 9–3

AMERICAN NURSES' ASSOCIATION CODE OF ETHICS

- The nurse provides services with respect for human dignity and the uniqueness of the client, unrestricted by considerations of social or economic status, personal attributes, or the nature of health problems.
- The nurse safeguards the client's right to privacy by judiciously protecting information of a confidential nature.
- The nurse acts to safeguard the client and the public when health care and safety are affected by the incompetent, unethical, or illegal practice of any person.
- The nurse assumes responsibility and accountability for individual nursing judgments and actions.
- The nurse maintains competence in nursing.
- The nurse exercises informed judgment and uses individual competence and qualifications as criteria in seeking consultation, accepting responsibilities, and delegating nursing activities to others.
- The nurse participates in activities that contribute to the ongoing development of the profession's body of knowledge.
- The nurse participates in the profession's efforts to implement and improve standards of nursing.
- The nurse participates in the profession's efforts to establish and maintain conditions of employment conducive to high-quality nursing care.
- The nurse participates in the profession's effort to protect the public from misinformation and misrepresentation and to maintain the integrity of nursing.
- The nurse collaborates with members of the health professions and other citizens in promoting community and national efforts to meet the health needs of the public.

American Nurses' Association (1985). *Code for Nurses with Interpretive Statements*. Washington, D.C.: American Nurses' Association.

BOX 9–4

CANADIAN NURSES' ASSOCIATION CODE OF ETHICS FOR NURSING CLIENTS

- The nurse treats clients with respect for their individual needs and values.
- Based on respect for clients and regard for their right to control their own care, nursing care reflects respect for the right of choice held by clients.
- The nurse holds confidential all information about a client learned in the health care setting.
- The nurse is guided by consideration for the dignity of clients.
- The nurse provides competent care to clients.
- The nurse maintains trust in nurses and nursing.
- The nurse recognizes the contribution and experience of colleagues from nursing and other disciplines as essential to excellent health care.
- The nurse takes steps to ensure that the client receives competent and ethical care.
- Conditions of employment should contribute in a positive way to client care and the professional satisfaction of nurses.
- Job action by nurses is directed toward securing conditions of employment that enable safe and appropriate care for clients and contribute to the professional satisfaction of nurses.
- The nurse advocates the interests of clients.
- The nurse represents the values and ethics of nursing before colleagues and others.
- Professional nurses' organizations are responsible for clarifying, securing, and sustaining ethical nursing conduct. The fulfillment of these tasks requires that professional nurses' organizations remain responsive to the rights, needs, and legitimate interests of clients and nurses.

Canadian Nurses' Association (1991). *Code of Ethics for Nursing Clients*. Ottawa, Canada (represents values only, obligations under value are also included in full code).

BOX 9-5
INTERNATIONAL COUNCIL FOR NURSES CODE FOR NURSES

- The fundamental responsibility of the nurse is fourfold: to promote health, to prevent illness, to restore health, and to alleviate suffering.
- The need for nursing is universal. Inherent in nursing is respect for life, dignity, and rights of man. It is unrestricted by considerations of nationality, race, creed, color, age, sex, politics, or social status.
- Nurses render health services to the individual, the family, and the community and coordinate their services with those of related groups.

NURSES AND PEOPLE

The nurse's primary responsibility is to those people who require nursing care.

- The nurse, in providing care, promotes an environment in which the values, customs, and spiritual beliefs of the individual are respected.
- The nurse holds in confidence personal information and uses judgment in sharing this information.

NURSES AND PRACTICE

- The nurse carries personal responsibility for nursing practice and for maintaining competence by continuing learning. The nurse maintains the highest standards of nursing care possible within the reality of a specific situation.
- The nurse uses judgment in relation to individual competence when accepting and delegating responsibilities.
- The nurse when acting in a professional capacity should at all times maintain standards of personal conduct which reflect credit upon the profession.

NURSES AND SOCIETY

- The nurse shares with other citizens the responsibility for initiating and supporting action to meet the health and social needs of the public.

NURSES AND CO-WORKERS

- The nurse sustains a cooperative with co-workers in nursing and other fields. The nurse takes appropriate action to safeguard the individual when his or her care is endangered by a co-worker or any other person.

NURSES AND THE PROFESSION

- The nurse plays the major role in determining and implementing desirable standards of nursing practice and nursing education.
- The nurse is active in developing a core of professional knowledge.
- The nurse, acting through the professional organization, participates in establishing and maintaining equitable social and economic working conditions in nursing.

International Council for Nurses (1973). *Code for Nurses: Ethical Concepts applied to Nursing*. Geneva, Switzerland: International Council for Nurses.

BOX 9-6
HEALTH PROFESSIONS COVENANT

As a health care professional dedicated to enhancing the well-being of individuals and communities, I am committed to achieving and sustaining the highest level of professional competence, to fulfilling my responsibilities with compassion for patients' suffering, and to helping patients make their own informed choices about health care whenever possible.

Recognizing that effective health promotion, disease prevention, and curative and long-term care are products of the combination of teams of health professionals, I pledge collaboration with all of my colleagues similarly committed to meeting the health care needs of individuals and their communities. Further, I will work within my profession to encourage placement of the patient's and the public interests above the self-interests of my individual profession.

Association of Academic Health Centers (1994). *Health Professionals Covenant*. Washington, D.C.: Association of Academic Health Centers.

Other health professional organizations have also developed codes for members of their groups. Codes of ethics for the medical profession guide the actions of the physician. The Association of Academic Health Centers has adopted a code to be used by all health professionals. The *Health Professions Covenant* promises interdisciplinary collaboration and a dedication to a common commitment to the health care needs of individuals and communities (Box 9–6). The Covenant has been endorsed by the National League for Nursing.

ORGANIZATIONAL POSITION STATEMENTS; ETHICS COMMITTEES

It becomes apparent as one reviews the issues and dilemmas that in many circumstances it is not possible to determine a solution to an ethical problem. The conflicts may be moral issues, ethical dilemmas, or ethical-legal problems. Health professional organizations have attempted to solve the problem by developing "position statements." Usually the statements are developed by groups of nurses, or nurses and physicians, or nurses and other health care workers. In some health care facilities, ethics committees may formulate position statements.

The position statement is an agreement reached between participating individuals that defines the parameters of ethical behaviors in specific ethical situations. Usually the statements are devised to provide guidance to nurses and other health care workers in circumstances when there are no clear-cut solutions to an ethical dilemma. For example, position statements have been developed by the American Nurses' Association on assisting in a suicide, actively participating in euthanasia, and caring for an anencephalic neonate.

Ethics committees operate in many health care facilities. The committees have been formed in response to the complex problems that have originated from legal, social, technological, and ethical questions regarding care and protection of patients. The committees develop guidelines and formulate policies relating to ethical problems. The committees also review research protocols to ensure that patient safety is assured in any research study being undertaken in the facility. The committee may also be called on to review and attempt to resolve ethical problems that develop when administering patient care.

It is important that nurses participate in the development of position statements and on ethical committees. In addition to nursing, the committees usually have representation from the legal profession, administrative staff, physicians, social workers, spiritual advisors, and community lay members. The nurse needs to be an active member of the group. Many of the decisions made will affect the practice of the nurse.

There is a close relationship between the resolving of ethical dilemmas and the legal aspects of nursing care. Many of the issues discussed as ethical problems will also emerge as legal problems. Chapter 8 provides added insight into ethical problems.

CHAPTER HIGHLIGHTS

- Everyone has morals, values, and ethical principles that are shaped by the total of life experiences. Nurses must be aware of their own personal biases, ethical principles, and values systems and how they affect their nursing practice.
- Many nursing actions require decisions that relate solely to the individual nurse's actions. Many of these decisions are of an ethical nature.
- Nurses are frequently faced with situations involving ethical decisions that require choices to be made. Sometimes there are no "good" alternatives.
- Two ethical theories have been used to analyze ethical dilemmas: utilitarianism and deontology.
- Ethics is an active process that evolves when circumstances force individuals to deal with conflict and tension.
- Ethical decision making involves a systematic approach to examine the value system of individuals. There are four levels of ethical decisions: expressive level, level of moral rule, level of ethical analysis, and postethical level.
- Ethical dilemmas can be analyzed through the use of a decision-making model.
- There are specific principles of ethics: autonomy, nonmaleficence, beneficence, and justice.
- Nurse-patient ethical relations involve problems of veracity, privacy, fidelity, and confidentiality.
- The nursing profession has developed standards of conduct to guide members in their everyday behaviors and in their nursing practice. The standards are included in codes of ethics.

REFERENCES

American Nurses' Association (1985). *Code for Nurses with Interpretive Statements.* Washington, D.C.: American Nurses' Association.

American Nurses' Association (1985). *Nursing: A Social Policy Statement.* Washington, D.C.: American Nurses' Association.

American Nurses' Association (1991). *Standards of Clinical Nursing Practice.* Washington, D.C.: American Nurses' Association.

Aroskar, M. (1994). Ethical decision making in patient care. *The American Nurse, 26,* March, 10.

Association of Academic Health Centers (1994). *Health Professions Covenant.* Washington, D.C.: Association of Academic Health Centers.

Bandman, E., Bandman, B. (1995). *Nursing Ethics Through the Life Span,* 3rd ed. Norwalk, CT: Appleton-Lange.

Beauchamp, T.L., Childress, J.F. (1994). *Principles of Bioethical Ethics.* New York: Oxford University Press.

Canadian Nurses' Association (1991). *Code of Ethics for Nursing Clients.* Ottawa, Canada: Canadian Nurses' Association.

Cooper, T.L. (1990). *The Responsible Administrator,* 3rd ed. San Francisco: Jossey-Bass.

Czerwinski, B.S. (1990). An autopsy of a dilemma. *Journal of Nursing Administration, 20,* (6) 25–29.

Davis, A. (1991). Ethical questions on health care rationing and the elderly. *California Nurse,* March, 8.

Davis, A.J., Aroskar, M.A. (1991). *Ethical Dilemmas and Nursing Practice.* Norwalk, CT: Appleton and Lange.

Health care rationing tops list of pressing ethical issues (1994). *The American Nurse, 26* (3), March, 11.

Husted, G.L., Husted, J.H. (1995a). Bioethical standards: The analysis of dilemmas through the analysis of persons. In J. O'Malley (ed.): *Advanced Practice Nursing Quarterly, 1* (2), 69–76.

Husted, G.L., Husted, J.H. (1995b). *Ethical Decision Making in Nursing.* St. Louis: Mosby.

International Council For Nurses (1973). *Code for Nurses.* Geneva, Switzerland: International Council for Nurses.

Mill, J.S. (1861). *Utilitarianism.* The Library of Liberal Arts. 1957, p. 10.

Nursing's Agenda for Health Care Reform (1991). Available from the National League for Nursing, 350 Hudson St. NY. 10014.

President's Commission for the Study of Ethical Problems in Medicine and Biomedical and Behavior Research (1983). Securing Access to Health Care Report, 1, 4.

Random House Webster's College Dictionary (1996). New York: Random House.

Seroka, A. (1994). Values clarification and ethical decision making. *Seminar for Nurse Managers, 2* (1), 9–10.

Veatch, R.M., Fry, S.T. (1987). *Case Studies in Nursing Ethics.* Philadelphia: Lippincott.

UNIT II

The Process of Nursing Practice

Nursing practice, at its best, is an unbroken spectrum of thought and action, a process involving cognitive and psychomotor skills. The process does not exist in a vacuum; neither does it involve randomly selected actions. "Thought-full doing" is one apt description of this process. Although both the context and content (specific nursing actions) for nursing practice will change over time, core elements of the nursing process will remain. The five chapters in this unit address the essence of the practice of nursing—the heart of professional nursing practice. They emphasize the therapeutic potential of the nurse-patient relationship, the importance of informed caring, the range of skills required for critical thinking and clinical judgment, the importance of patient and family education for empowerment, and the need for careful documentation and communication. These are the elements of practice that patients describe when they characterize quality care.

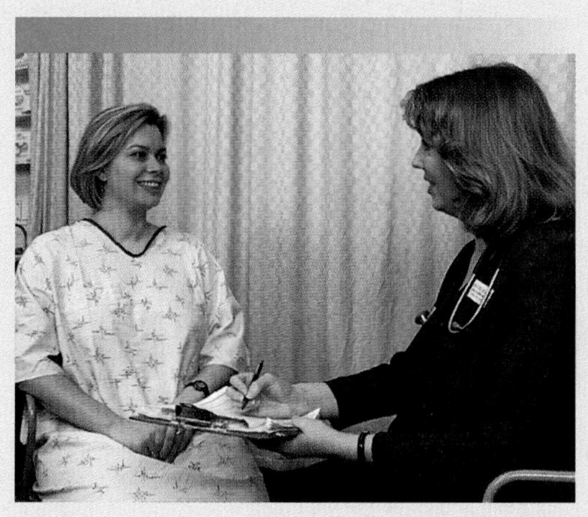

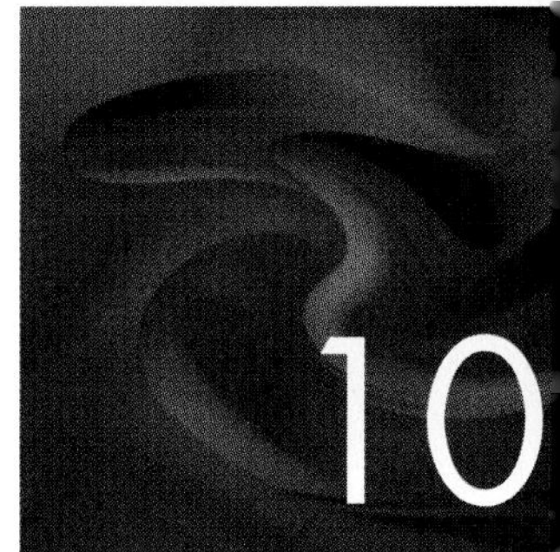

The Nurse-Patient Relationship

Carol Lindeman

Think about your relationships with your family and friends. Can you identify a relationship that was growth promoting? Can you think of one that made you feel valued and respected? Can you recall one that caused pain? Relationships are very powerful forces in our lives. The relationship between a patient and a nurse is an equally powerful force. In fact, that relationship has as much or more power as nursing procedures to facilitate health (Tresolini, C.P., et al, 1994).

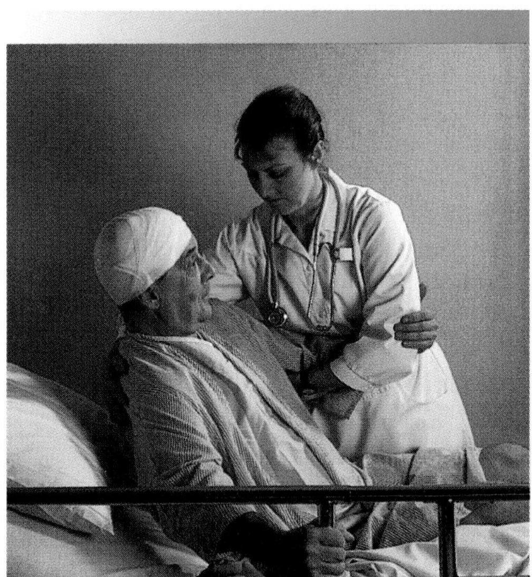

OBJECTIVES

After studying this chapter, students will:

- **understand the importance of the nurse-patient relationship**
- **know the communication and interpersonal skills involved in developing a helping relationship**
- **be ready to use those skills in their nursing practice**

RELATIONSHIP-CENTERED CARE

Models of Care

BIOMEDICAL MODEL OF CARE

To appreciate the current emphasis on the nurse-patient relationship, it is necessary to reflect on our changing understanding of health and illness. For most of this century, health care has been based on the biomedical model. Significant features of this model are as follows:

- Health is viewed as the absence of disease/illness.
- Diseases have a specific etiology (cause) with one cause sought for each disease.
- Disease is analyzed at the molecular, cellular, or chemical level.
- The body is seen as a mechanism that can be reduced to its component parts.
- The body can be treated without attention to the person's mental status, life events, and environmental conditions.
- It is assumed that it is the medical intervention that cures (Pew-Fetzer, 1994).

This view of health and illness works well with acute, curable illnesses and with infectious diseases. For example, in the 1950s polio was a dreaded disease. Its cause and cure or prevention were not understood. Through biomedical research, the cause was identified and a means of immunization developed. Today, in the United States, polio is rare.

The biomedical model of care worked so well with the diseases that were prevalent in the first part of the twentieth century that people thought the model would work for all illnesses. However, the model has been unsuccessful in treating diseases such as hypertension, cancer, and diabetes. It has had very limited success for conditions related to lifestyle such as substance abuse.

BIOPSYCHOSOCIAL MODEL OF CARE

For several decades nursing has objected to the biomedical model, believing that the mind cannot be separated from the body. One cannot treat a disease without treating the person who has the disease. Nursing has promoted a bio**psychosocial** view of health and illness that calls for consideration of the psychological and sociological aspects of illness. It is an additive approach, i.e., adding **care** for the **person** (psychosocial) to the **cure** of the **disease** (biomedical) (Pew-Fetzer, 1994).

The use of the biopsychosocial model of care is evident in the nursing history taken at the first contact a nurse has with a patient. The nurse will ask questions regarding the individual's habits, family, lifestyle, and the like, in addition to questions regarding the illness per se. This information about the person is then used by the nurse in planning and implementing care and in preparing the person for discharge and self-care.

RELATIONSHIP-CENTERED CARE

The biomedical and biopsychosocial models of care have driven the curricula for health professionals and have also directed the funding and conduct of health care research for most of the twentieth century. Yet neither of these models is adequate for contemporary practice with its focus on people with **chronic** illnesses, health problems that are the result of people living with people (violence, substance abuse, depression), health promotion and disease prevention, and the changing demographics of the population. Both of these models are reductionist in their approach to illness and disease. Both are linked to an interventionist approach to care and cure, i.e., a belief that it is the medical or nursing intervention that is important. Both are linked to Western medicine.

A recent publication from a task force supported by both the Pew and Fetzer Foundations describes a new model of care. In that model of care **health** is viewed as more than the absence of illness. Health is considered a **process by which people maintain their ability to function in the face of changes within themselves, their relationships, and their environment.** In that model, illness is not just a malfunction in the mechanism. The person's **experience** is at the center of what it means to be ill.

In this emerging model the health care provider is not an **objective** professional standing apart from the patient. Instead the provider seeks to understand the patient's experience and help those for whom there is no cure per se. The foundation of care is the **relationship between the provider and the patient** and not the interventions the provider offers. The provider-patient relationship is a medium for the exchange of all forms of information, feelings, and concerns; a factor in the success of therapeutic regimens; and an essential ingredient in the satisfaction of both patient and provider.

The Pew-Fetzer task force calls this model Relationship-Centered Care. Their monograph describing this model includes strong justification for its use (Tresolini, C.P., et al, 1994).

The Placebo Effect

The importance of the provider-patient relationship is demonstrated in research related to the **placebo effect.**

What is a placebo? The word *placebo* is Latin; the English literal translation is "I will please." An 1811 edition of one medical dictionary identified it as a label given to any medicine adapted more **to please** than **to benefit** the patient (Weil, 1988, p. 206). Indeed, most people today still think of a placebo as a sugar pill disguised to look like the real one. They think of it as an inert (nonactive) substance with no therapeutic or healing power. Many physicians and nurses schooled in the biomedical and biopsychosocial models of illness also hold this view of placebo.

However, clinicians and more recently researchers have not been able to explain instances of healing (and dying) on the basis of this narrow definition of placebo. For example, Weil

(1988) provides example after example of curious and miraculous cures of cutaneous warts. He cites the use of being touched by the neighborhood wart healer who "wishes" the wart away, rubbing a plant on the wart, rubbing a cut potato on the wart and then burying the potato under a specific tree at a specific phase of the moon, selling the wart to a sibling, and handling some kind of animal. Although there is nothing common to these procedures, the result is the same. A person will follow "the procedure" in the afternoon or evening and then go to bed. The next day the wart falls off when touched and there is clean pink skin underneath. And the wart does not regrow.

In contrast, the scientific approach is to cut warts off, burn them with sparks, freeze them with a chemical, or etch them off with an acid. These methods tend to be ineffective and at least half of the time the wart grows back even larger.

Weil believes the wart cure stories are examples of **mind-mediated healing.** He suggests that the same mechanism may underlie placebo effects. The placebo response, which originates in the mind but is based on the interworking of the mind and body, may be the key to activating true healing.

As health care clinicians and researchers tried to understand the placebo response, they created new, broader definitions of placebo. One example is the following definition (Shapiro, 1961, p. 73):

> Any therapeutic procedure (or that component of any procedure) which is given deliberately to have an effect, or unknowingly has an effect on a patient, symptom, syndrome, or disease, but which is objectively without specific activity for the condition being treated. The therapeutic procedure may be given with or without conscious knowledge that the procedure is a placebo, may be an active or inactive procedure, and includes, therefore, all medical procedures no matter how specific—oral and parenteral medication, topical preparations, inhalants, and mechanical, surgical and psychotherapeutic procedures. The placebo must be differentiated from the placebo effect, which may or may not occur and which may be favorable or unfavorable.

The narrow definition of placebo as a sugar pill or inactive substance may continue as a basis for some research, particularly studies of new drugs. However, as researchers struggle with understanding the **outcomes** of care, the broader definition of placebo is used.

"The Importance of Placebo Effects in Pain Treatment and Research" (Turner et al, 1994) illustrates current research trying to understand the placebo effect and outcomes of care. The researchers state that two questions are of interest to clinicians:

- Under what conditions and for what patients will a treatment improve outcomes of care?
- What is the mechanism that makes a treatment effective?

They list three general reasons for clinical improvement:

- Natural history and regression to the mean. (Most acute and some chronic pain problems resolve on their own. Extreme symptoms tend to move toward a more typical state on their own.)
- Specific effects of treatment reflecting the content of the intervention.
- Nonspecific effects of treatment attributable to factors other than specific active components. (This category includes factors such as physician attention, interest, and concern; patient and physician expectations of treatment; the reputation of the treatment; and characteristics of the setting. The term *nonspecific effect* is used synonymously with *placebo effect.*)

The researchers analyzed data from published studies designed to assess the outcomes of "sham" treatments. The researchers concluded:

> Placebo effects influence patient outcomes after any treatment, including surgery, that the clinician and patient believe is effective. Placebo effects plus disease natural history and regression to the mean can result in high rates of good outcomes, which may be misattributed to specific treatment effects.

Specifically, they found that:

- Patients' expectations of treatment effects clearly influence their responses.
- The provider's warmth, friendliness, interest, sympathy, empathy, prestige, and positive attitude toward the patient and toward the treatment are associated with positive effects of placebos as well as of active treatments.

Research such as the study just summarized highlights the importance of relationship-centered care. The relationship between the nurse and the patient has a powerful effect on the outcomes of care. Communication skills are crucial to establishing that relationship.

COMMUNICATION SKILLS

Communication skills are essential for effective nursing practice. Communication skills enable the nurse to know the patient, understand the patient's view of his or her health and illness, plan care, monitor the patient's progress, prepare the patient for discharge, empower the patient for self-care, and share relevant information with others. Communication skills enable the nurse to establish the type of relationship with a patient that influences the outcomes of care.

Professional communication is a process affected by many factors. The nurse must remember the importance of this process and never take it or skill level for granted. Effective communicators are not born that way. People become effective communicators through practice and study. Each communication between a patient and nurse can be used by the nurse to further develop communication skills.

Social Versus Professional Communications

Obviously, the nurse uses communication skills in situations that are not associated with the professional role. These are usually thought of as **social** communication skills. They differ from the use of communication skills in the professional role. In the professional role, the use of communication skills focuses on the patient and family and meeting their needs. In social situations, communication usually occurs to meet the needs of all the people involved. For example, in social communication, friends may discuss a recent political event. They share thoughts and feelings with the intent of developing greater insight into the event. The conversation meets both of their needs for greater insight and for a feeling of being personally connected (affiliation).

The Communication Process

Communication occurs when a message is produced by one person with the intent of stimulating meaning in another. It is a dynamic process. There is neither **a beginning** nor **an ending.** Every communication situation is unique in some respects; yet there are common elements to the process. The ten components of the communication process are shown in Figure 10–1.

The definition of each component of the communication process is presented in Table 10–1.

TABLE 10-1 The Ten Components of the Communication Process

Component	Explanation
Source	The person with the idea and the desire to communicate
Encoding	Putting ideas into symbols such as words, gestures, art
Message	The encoded thought
Channel	The means by which the encoded message is transmitted
Noise	Anything that distorts the message the source encodes
Receiver	The person who attends to the message
Decoding	Assigning meaning to the symbols received
Receiver response	Anything the receiver does after having attended to and decoded the message
Feedback	That portion of the receiver response of which the source has knowledge and to which the source attends and assigns meaning
Context	The environment in which the communication process takes place and which helps to define the communication

From Jandt, F.E. (1995). *Intercultural Communication.* Thousand Oaks, CA: Sage.

SOURCE (SENDER)/RECEIVER

In the nurse-patient relationship, the source may be the nurse or the patient. The source is the person who initiates the communication. When doing so, the source should have a purpose and a receiver in mind. In the process of communicating, the source and receiver are interdependent, i.e., they affect each other in the process. The nurse affects the patient and the patient affects the nurse.

Consider the following example. The nurse gives a pain-reducing medication to a patient and returns a little later to determine the effect of the medication. The nurse initiates the communication with the question "Has the medication reduced your pain?" The patient responds "A little bit." The communication continues until the nurse has collected enough information to determine the appropriate next steps so that the patient achieves the desired level of comfort. The nurse had a purpose in mind and a receiver in mind. The communication continued until the purpose was met for the specific patient.

In the process of communicating, the communication of the nurse produced a response in the patient. Likewise, the response of the patient produced a response in the nurse. The process of communication required the nurse and the patient to

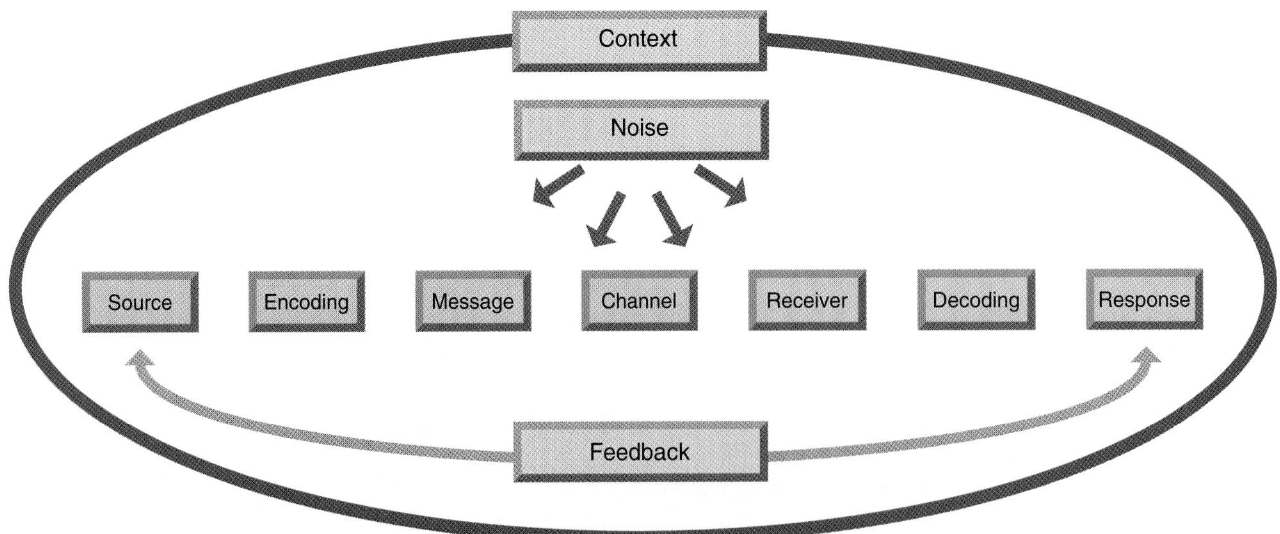

Figure 10–1. Ten components of communication.

be interdependent. If the nurse is not affected by the response of the patient (or the patient is not affected by the response of the nurse), real communication will not have taken place.

MESSAGE

The message will vary from situation to situation. The message could be information regarding nutrition. The message could be reassurance about recovery. The message could be an expression of caring. Just as the sender determines a message, so does the receiver determine a message. The patient may initiate a communication asking the nurse for information regarding his or her progress. The patient may say, "Will I have much pain after the surgery?" The nurse may respond "Don't worry. Everything will be fine." The nurse sent a clear message back to the patient—but not the message the patient wanted to hear. A better response would have been to ask the patient what he or she knew about the surgery, pursuing the topic until reassurance specific to the individual patient could be given.

COMMUNICATION CHANNEL

The majority of the nurse-patient communications will use sound waves as the communication channel. The nurse and the patient will communicate by talking to each other. However, it is important that the nurse consider other communication channels such as pictures, pamphlets, video tapes, books, and even the computer for specific situations. For example, when teaching a diabetic about diet, a pamphlet containing the information is essential. The patient cannot be expected to remember all the details about which foods fit into which category. The old adage that "one picture is worth a thousand words" is true when trying to communicate complex ideas or new information. Video or audio tapes can be used to reinforce previous instruction or to allow patients to learn at their own pace and time. Computers are rapidly growing as a medium for communication between a patient and nurse. For example, software exists to help a person understand medications and symptoms. For patients who have difficulty speaking, the nurse might use the channel of paper and pencil. When patients are in a stressful situation, it is unlikely they will remember everything that was told to them. In those situations, it is important that written information be used as a backup for the verbal information.

Factors Affecting Communication

Six major categories of factors affect the quality or outcomes of communication:

- verbal communication skills
- nonverbal communication skills
- attitudes
- knowledge level
- position
- feedback (Berlo, 1960)

VERBAL COMMUNICATION SKILLS

The first category of factors affecting the outcome of communication is the verbal skills of the sender and receiver, i.e., the nurse and the patient. Verbal communication skills include having an adequate vocabulary, using clear sentence structure, and being able to articulate the intended message. These three skills affect the clarity of the message.

The vocabulary must be appropriate to the intended receiver. Nurses quickly forget that the general public is not familiar with nursing jargon and many of the terms used by health care providers. For example, the chief nurse on a patient unit introduced herself to a patient as the "head nurse." The patient took her quite literally, thinking she was a nurse who specialized in head problems. As his problem was with his feet he continued to wait for the "foot nurse" to visit him.

Sentence structure is also important. In general, the shorter the sentence the better. Lengthy sentences may contain too much information for the listener to absorb.

It is also helpful to anticipate how to articulate key ideas so that they are clear to the intended receiver. This may require knowing interests, hobbies, education, or work background of the patient. Examples and analogies meaningful to the patient are powerful tools for influencing learning. A patient who has a skin graft and is a gardener would understand the principles surrounding a skin graft as the same as those regarding a tree graft.

There is a story in the nursing folklore about a nurse who taught a diabetic patient how to inject insulin. In teaching the patient, the nurse used insulin, an insulin syringe and needle, and an orange. An orange was used because the skin has the same resistance as the skin of a human. Therefore, sticking an orange is similar to inserting a needle into human skin. After several tries the patient was able to do the procedure correctly. The patient was discharged home but a few days later appeared in the emergency room. It turns out that the patient did at home just what he was taught in the hospital. He injected the insulin into the orange . . . and then ate the orange. The nurse never communicated the need to inject the insulin into his tissue. The intended message was never received by the patient.

COMMUNICATION FACILITATORS

In addition to the general issues of vocabulary, sentence structure, and articulateness, these techniques facilitate effective communication:

- organization
- questions
- clarification of content
- clarification of feelings
- sharing observations
- silence

Organization. Many nurse-patient communications involve the nurse giving information to the patient. To facilitate

RESEARCH HIGHLIGHT

COMPARISON OF TWO TYPES OF COMMUNICATION METHODS USED AFTER CARDIAC SURGERY WITH PATIENTS WITH ENDOTRACHEAL TUBES

Betsy Stovsky, Ellen Rudy, and Peggy Dragonette, Heart and Lung, *17 (3), 281–289, 1988*

Communication is particularly difficult for the patient in the period immediately after cardiac surgery because of the presence of the endotracheal tube. The nurse is challenged by the difficulty in interpreting patients' behavior and clinical symptoms without the benefit of oral communication.

Our purpose was to compare two types of communication methods (planned and unplanned) for effectiveness in communication in the early postoperative intubation period with patients who have had cardiac surgery. Unplanned spontaneous communication was defined as communication that is unplanned and is not carried out by a specific method. The nurse's creativity, judgment, and spontaneity determine the method used. Methods identified in the literature and in use in the surgical ICU of this study included:

1. Having the patient write.
2. Having the patient use hand gestures, such as pointing.
3. Lip-reading.
4. Asking the patient "yes" or "no" questions.
5. Trying to interpret nonverbal cues.

Planned communication consisted of use of a picture board with words, which was termed a picture board. Considering the limitations imposed by the endotracheal tube, intravenous and arterial lines, and sedated state of the patient, we chose a picture board because of its minimal prerequisites for use: "seeing, understanding, and doing."

Forty-eight patients and 22 nurses participated in the study. Four instruments were used for data collection: an open-ended patient interview, a nurse bedside assessment tool, a patient and nurse satisfaction questionnaire, and a visual analog scale on satisfaction with communication.

On the basis of this study, we (the investigators) recommend:

1. Patients who will undergo mechanical ventilation after surgery be instructed on specific communication techniques before surgery.
2. The communication techniques taught before surgery be available to all patients who have endotracheal tubes after surgery.
3. A communication board be considered as a supplement to other methods of communication presently being used.
4. Nurses identify the communication methods most useful for individual patients and integrate them into the written plan of care.
5. Nurses facilitate communication by providing the patient's eyeglasses, removing any opthalmic ointment or petroleum jelly from the patient's eyes after surgery, and, when using a communication board, placing the board in an optimal position for the patient to see.

learning, the content must be organized in a way that is helpful to the patient. Organizing information from the most simple to the most complex is one example. It is helpful to have a scheme in mind that can be shared with the patient and one that the patient can use to recall the information later. For example, the nurse might discuss nutrition by first focusing on breakfast, then lunch, and finally dinner. This may be easier for the patient to remember rather than talking about total daily requirements. Chapter 13 includes further suggestions for organizing different types of information (teaching skills, concepts, etc.).

Questions. Many nurse-patient communications involve the nurse obtaining information from the patient. This is frequently done by asking questions. One common example is the admission history. The nurse obtains information from the patient that is relevant to his or her care. This involves the use of closed-ended, open-ended, and focused questions. A closed-ended question is one that can be answered with a yes or no. For example, "Have you ever had measles?" is a closed-ended question. Open-ended questions are designed to obtain more than a simple yes or no. For example, "How did you feel when you heard you had cancer?" is an open-ended question. It is designed to elicit in-depth information. Questions must be focused or the patient will have difficulty responding. Focus may require the inclusion of a time frame, a setting, or a context to enable the patient to answer accurately. For example, "How has your chest been feeling in the last 4 hours?"

The nurse does not have the right to ask questions that are not directly relevant to the purpose of the communication. Every question, open-ended or closed-ended, must be a valid question in terms of the purpose of the communication. For example, asking the patient about political affiliation or income should not be done unless it is relevant to the patient's care. The patient also has the right to refuse to answer any question.

Clarification of Content. Within a communication it may be necessary for the nurse to respond in a way that clarifies the patient's message. There are several techniques for doing this. Three commonly used techniques are **paraphrasing, seeking clarification,** and **summarization.** In **paraphrasing,** nurses repeat back to the patient in different words what they heard the patient say. Nurses repeat it back to see if they understand what the patient said. The patient says, "When I eat spicy foods I have trouble sleeping." The nurse paraphrases it back: "Eating spicy foods keeps you awake at night?" When

RESEARCH HIGHLIGHT

HELPFUL AND UNHELPFUL COMMUNICATION IN CANCER CARE: THE PATIENT PERSPECTIVE

Sally E. Thorne, Oncology Nursing Forum, 15 (2), 167–172, 1988

It has often been noted that the emotional anguish associated with cancer can be far harder on the patient than the physical manifestations. Despite this, serious scholarly attention to the psychosocial distress associated with having cancer has lagged behind concern for the physical aspects of the disease. While communication is believed to play a significant role in the psychosocial cancer experience, its impact rarely has been investigated systematically.

The study used a descriptive design to address the following questions:

- What factors distinguish cancer patients who recall helpful communications from those who recall unhelpful communications?
- What factors distinguish the different types of communications?

Helpful communications were those perceived by the patient to be constructive, encouraging or supportive beyond what seemed necessary under the circumstances. *Unhelpful* communications were those perceived by the patient as frustrating, impeding or demoralizing beyond what seemed necessary under the circumstances.

One hundred and fifty-eight communication instances were extracted from the available data (data previously collected by the investigator and data from published autobiographical accounts).

Distinction between patients who recalled helpful communication and those who recalled unhelpful communication was not possible.

Most (77.2%) of the recalled communication occurred when the patient's expectation of the outcome of the cancer was uncertain. Helpful instances were proportionately more frequent for patients who were expecting cure than for those who were uncertain or who expected to die of cancer.

A breakdown of the contexts in which the communication instances occurred revealed that the majority of the instances took place in the context of **information-giving** (39.9%) and **advice** (39.9%). Most of the advice (90.5%) and information (65.1%) was perceived as unhelpful, while support and social exchange were usually recalled as helpful (75%).

In only a minority of instances (37.3%) did patients perceive that health care professionals expressed concern for the patients, and most (92.5%) of the unhelpful instances were associated with a communication style characterized by lack of concern.

Cancer care obviously requires special skills and special qualities from health care providers. From the patient's perspective, communication as health care professionals plays an important role in shaping the illness experience.

seeking clarification, the nurse asks the patient to further describe or elaborate on a given point. He or she may say, "I am not clear about that last statement. Could you give me another example?" In **summarization,** the nurse highlights the main themes or issues contained in the patient's message. The nurse may say, "These are the health problems that concern you. . . . Is that correct?" The point of all three techniques is to verify the message. All three techniques are used when the nurse is focused on the content of the message.

An example of where no clarification of content occurred is reported by Krupat (1986). A middle-aged man noticed a dark mole on his shoulder. He was concerned that it could be serious and made an appointment to see his physician. At the beginning of the appointment, he and the physician engaged in "small talk" during which the man mentioned his arthritis. The doctor picked up on this complaint, wrote a prescription to relieve arthritis pain, and ushered the man out the door. The patient had been shut out of the conversation and left feeling frustrated, upset, and still worried about the mole.

Clarification of Feelings. When the nurse is focused on **feelings** within the patient's message, other techniques are useful. **Reflection** is repeating or echoing part of what the patient said. The patient might have been describing his angry response to hearing that he had cancer. He then stops talking. The nurse responds "You felt angry . . . " as a way to keep the patient talking about the subject. Another technique to focus on feelings and obtain additional information is **acknowledgment.** Acknowledgment is a stated recognition of the patient's feelings. In contrast to reflection where the nurse leaves the sentence unfinished, in acknowledgment the nurse makes a statement. "You felt angry" is a response that acknowledges the feelings. This technique allows the patient to confirm or deny that the feeling was identified correctly. It also serves as an encouragement to continue discussing his angry feelings.

Sharing of Observations. This technique calls for the nurse to label an observation in a manner that allows the patient to respond to its accuracy. For example, the nurse may say "You sounded angry when you made that statement." The patient can then confirm, deny, or clarify the observation.

Silence. Silence is a very important technique in the nurse-patient relationship. It allows the patient time to think or gather courage to continue. Once the nurse and patient get beyond superficial exchange, silences will occur. **The nurse must not talk when the patient requires silence. (The perceptive nurse will infer this requirement from the nonverbal behavior.) The nurse must use silence to make certain the communication is being understood.** Silence is a normal part of every meaningful communication. Personal

RESEARCH HIGHLIGHT

BLOOD PRESSURE, HEART RATE, AND HEART RHYTHM CHANGES IN PATIENTS WITH HEART DISEASE DURING TALKING

Carolyn D. Freed, Sue A. Thomas, James J. Lynch, Richard Stein, and *Erika Friedmann,* Heart and Lung, *18,* 17–22, 1989

Blood pressure and heart rate were recorded in 37 patients with cardiac disease while they were resting quietly and talking. Heart rate, systolic blood pressure, and diastolic blood pressure were all significantly greater while the patients were speaking than while they were resting silently. In addition, ventricular and atrial arrhythmias were more frequent while they were talking than while they were quiet. Higher resting systolic blood pressure levels also were associated with larger blood pressure increases while the patients were speaking. Older patients exhibited significantly greater systolic pressure increases while talking than younger patients. Therapeutic doses of antihypertensive medications, including β-blockers, calcium channel blockers, and diuretics did not block the heart rate and blood pressure increases while the patients were talking. These findings suggest that more attention needs to be paid to the hemodynamic consequences of communication in patients with coronary heart disease. Coupled with previous research findings, these data also suggest that clinicians need to attend to verbal communications during routine diagnostic procedures for evaluating cardiovascular function.

uncomfortableness with silence must be overcome to allow silence to be used effectively. One way to overcome uncomfortableness with silence is to reflect on what the patient has just said or simply to consciously direct your energy toward the patient.

COMMUNICATION BLOCKERS

Just as there are techniques that facilitate communication between the nurse and the patient, there are responses that block the process. It is important that the nurse eliminate these types of responses from his or her professional communications:

- evaluative comments
- superficiality
- "why" questions

Evaluative Comments. Perhaps the major blocker occurs when the nurse steps out of a neutral role of attending to feelings and obtaining or giving information and becomes evaluative, i.e., passes judgment. The patient may describe his diet and the nurse responds "How could you eat those greasy hamburgers!!" This show of disapproval is likely to keep the patient from revealing other sensitive information. Another blocker occurs when the nurse gives personal advice when the patient did not ask for it. The patient may be describing taking a certain drug for joint pain and the nurse says "Oh, I don't use 'X', it gives me an upset stomach. I always use 'Y'." This type of response detracts the patient from his message and therefore is a blocker. Becoming defensive is another blocker. The patient may say "I do not want to be here. Hospitals are where people die." The nurse, instead of responding to the thought that the patient may fear she is dying, responds defensively, saying "That is not true. The majority of people admitted to the hospital leave feeling better than when they were admitted."

Superficiality. A second set of blockers is related to the nurse responding at a superficial level. Instead of being invested in the communication, the nurse responds with clichés, trite reassurances, or changes the subject. "Don't worry. Everything will be O.K." is such a response.

"Why" Questions. One final blocker that the nurse must be aware of is the tendency to ask **"why"** questions. These are the most difficult questions to answer. Frequently a person does not know why. It makes a person feel defensive when she or he must justify behavior or explain feelings. If the nurse makes the patient feel defensive, effective communication will stop.

Reflect on some of your own experiences. When someone asks you "Why did you think that?"; "Why did you do that?"; or "Why would you feel that way?" you are asked to defend yourself when you may not have a rationale for your thoughts, actions, or feelings. In social communication it is possible to handle this situation in a variety of ways. You might say "Forget it!!" or "Leave it be!" or just walk away. In the nurse-patient situation, the patient usually responds by withdrawing from meaningful communication. The nurse must avoid using "why" questions.

NONVERBAL COMMUNICATION SKILLS

Communication often involves more than a verbal message. Messages sent without words are called nonverbal messages. Table 10–2 displays the range of codes used for nonverbal communication.

Nonverbal communication skills are as important as verbal skills in the nurse-patient communication process. It is essential that the nurse look at and concentrate on the patient (eye and facial code). The nurse must sit or stand close to the patient, yet not so close that the patient feels his or her personal space has been invaded (proxemics). Hall's (1959, 1966) work suggests that there are four distances that have meaning in communication in the U.S. culture. The intimate zone is from physical contact to 18 inches. The casual personal zone is from 18 inches to 4 feet. The socioconsultative zone spans from 4 feet to 10 feet. The public zone is from 10

TABLE 10–2 Nonverbal Message Codes

Codes	Examples
Kinesics, e.g., bodily movements or "body language"	
Emblems, e.g., movements that are clearly symbolic and are used without words	Waving good-bye
Illustrators, e.g., gestures used in conjunction with words to assist in understanding	Holding the hand at a certain height with the words "It was this high!"
Affect displays, e.g., body movements that express emotion	A teacher putting on a happy face to encourage learning
Regulators, e.g., movements used to regulate or control the interaction	Making a statement and walking away
Adaptors, e.g., behaviors that once served a physical need but have been adapted to serve other needs	Scratching the head
Eye and facial behavior, e.g., eye movements and pupil dilation	Tension on the eyelids, partially closing them with a hard look
Vocalics, e.g., the use of the voice to convey emotion	Using a very rapid, excited tone
Physical appearance, e.g., clothing and artifacts, grooming	Wearing one's best clothes to make a good impression
Proxemics, e.g., the use of space to communicate	
Territoriality, e.g., claiming rights to an area	Use of a fence to keep people out
Personal space, e.g., the zones of space that surround us	Sitting next to a person while taking his or her history
Touch, e.g., stimulating meaning through physical contact	Placing a hand on another's shoulder while expressing sympathy

feet to as far away as one can still be seen and heard. Initially the nurse may give the patient about 4 feet of personal space but as the relationship develops move closer. The intimate space should not be entered unless the patient signals the nurse to be closer.

If the exchange is likely to be lengthy, the nurse should sit to convey that expectation (time). Being at eye level with the patient facilitates communication and avoids the impression of intimidation and authority associated with towering over a patient (kinesics) (Fig. 10–2). The nurse should urge the patient to assume a comfortable position, one in which he or she feels like a person, not just a patient.

The nurse must be aware of every facial expression and body movement and control them so they do not detract from the communication (kinesics). At the same time the nurse must be a careful observer of the nonverbal behavior of the patient because this provides insight into the communication.

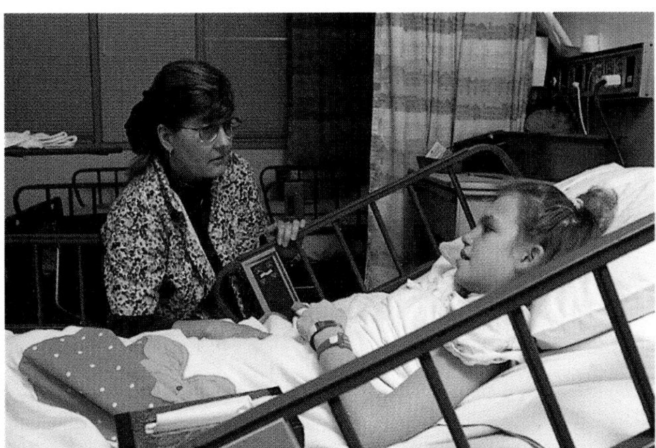

Figure 10–2. This nurse is communicating with the patient in "a posture of involvement," sitting at the patient's level to enable good eye contact. This posture indicates active listening.

Touch is an important nonverbal communication code. Chapter 32 presents this topic in depth.

ATTITUDES

The third category of factors to influence the outcomes of communication is the attitudes of the nurse. Attitude toward self, toward the content of the message, and toward the patient all influence the outcomes of the communication. Attitudes are communicated in what we say, how we say it, and by our nonverbal behavior. Toward the patient, the nurse must communicate an attitude of nonjudgmental interest. Listening to the patient's message, allowing the patient to control the flow of the communication, avoiding trite or stereotyped responses, and remaining focused are ways that positive attitudes are communicated to a patient. The opposite verbal and nonverbal behaviors, e.g., inattention, yawning, and looking at one's watch, communicate a negative attitude toward the patient.

The nurse must appear interested in the content of the message and convey an attitude that shows the importance of the material.

For example, even though there is more open discussion of sexual matters today in comparison with 20 years ago, a female nurse may feel embarrassed obtaining a sexual history on a male patient. The nurse's attitude toward that content may be conveyed to the patient. If it is, it will negatively affect the outcomes of the communication.

The attitude of the nurse toward self and nursing will also influence the outcome of the communication. A nurse who feels ineffectual either personally or professionally will send that message to the patient through his or her verbal and nonverbal behavior. For example, a student doing an aspect of patient care for the first time might feel anxious. The patient may sense that anxiety and mistake it for a negative attitude toward the patient. In such a situation the student should

CURRENT CONTROVERSY

HOW DO THE NURSE'S OWN UNMET NEEDS INFLUENCE THE NURSE PATIENT RELATIONSHIP? HOW CAN THE NURSE GAIN SELF-AWARENESS INTO THESE MOTIVATORS?

Angela M. Jerome and Adelina R. Ferraro-McDuffie, Pediatric Nursing, 18(2) 153–156

NURSE SELF-AWARENESS IN THERAPEUTIC RELATIONSHIPS

Situation 1: A ventilator-dependent child on the unit was to appear on the local television station. The nurse dressed and carefully prepared the little girl's hair, despite knowing the mother was coming to do these things and was running a little late. Often the mother stated she will visit on a particular day and did not show up, so the nurse doubted mother's ability to follow through on her word. Also, the mother did not visit as much as the staff felt was appropriate for the child's needs. When the mother arrived, she became angry because the child was already dressed and hair completely fixed. The mother changed the child's clothes and hairstyle, making the hairstyle different than what the child normally wears. The nurse was very angry at the mother because she knew the child's normal hairstyle and care. A therapeutic relationship was not maintained in this instance because the goals of parental control and independence were not the priority. What were the underlying reasons why the nurse became angry at the mother? Could there be unresolved issues that the nurse was struggling with in her personal life that could have led her to react with anger?

Situation 2: The child life specialist asked the mother to purchase a specific toy that the child developmentally needed. The mother was unable to afford it so the nurse asked the mother if the mother would mind if she bought the toy since the child "really needed it." The mother stated "yes" but later shared with the social worker that she did not feel she could say "no." She continued to say that she felt inadequate because someone else could provide for her child better than she could. The nurse's "intentions" were good when she purchased the toy. But whose needs were met by purchasing the toy?

INTERVENTIONS FOR SELF-AWARENESS

Being aware of one's own intentions is the first step to understanding difficulties one experiences in relationships with families. Interventions that can promote self-awareness when evaluating one's own intentions include:

1. Identify at least one "safe" person at work who will provide sensitive and caring feedback regarding the nurse's behaviors with families. This person should be available for the nurse to consult when questions or difficulties arise. The nurse may best relate to a person who has nursing experience dealing with difficult family situations and can fully appreciate stressors of bedside nursing, such as a psychiatric/mental health clinical nurse specialist. It may be advantageous if this person had only indirect impact on the nurse's performance appraisal. Otherwise, the nurse may perceive that asking for help or having difficulties with families could influence their annual evaluations, hindering open and honest communication.
2. Have scheduled meetings for groups of nurses to meet regarding therapeutic relationship issues. A group leader may be able to facilitate discussion regarding difficult experiences on their unit. Role-playing and scenarios often provide a nonthreatening way to examine one's motives and needs when trying to provide help. This group may be able to generate institutional guidelines, such as those developed at Children's Hospital of Philadelphia (Barnsteiner and Gillis-Donovan, 1990).
3. Use a self-awareness tool such as the one used at Children's Hospital of The King's Daughters (see Table 1), which allows the nurse to systematically evaluate the decision to provide help when one is unsure of self motives in a situation. The nurse writes: (a) the intervention to be done, (b) the underlying intentions for wanting to do this, (c) what a "safe" coworker says about the nurse doing this intervention, and (d) what interventions could be done to allow the family to complete this on their own. The nurse then lists possible negative and positive outcomes that may occur with this intervention. By weighing the possible consequences, the nurse has concrete information to decide then whether or not to follow through with the Intervention.
4. Develop an environment that promotes positive peer pressure to enforce consistent professional behaviors in coworkers. The nurse should be helped to develop skills in providing sensitive and caring feedback to coworkers regarding behaviors considered to be therapeutic or nontherapeutic within the group. It can be beneficial to develop a "buddy" system in which each nurse chooses another nurse to provide honest feedback to each other about issues of overinvolvement, overstepping family boundaries, etc.
5. Develop a library on the unit for books and audiotapes for nurses to use to help them become more aware of issues that could impact the therapeutic relationship.
6. Seek professional assistance. It can be a wonderful (and sometimes painful) journey of self-discovery that can explore one's own boundaries and family-of-origin

continued on next page

CURRENT CONTROVERSY (cont'd)
HOW DO THE NURSE'S OWN UNMET NEEDS INFLUENCE THE NURSE PATIENT RELATIONSHIP? HOW CAN THE NURSE GAIN SELF-AWARENESS INTO THESE MOTIVATORS?

continued from previous page

issues with the assistance of a skilled therapist. It does not mean that one is "unsuccessful" or "cannot handle" therapeutic relationships at work. Nor does seeking assistance need to have a stigma attached. Rather, it is a sign of maturity to seek assistance for self-growth and understanding.

Therapeutic relationships are often challenging in the best of circumstances. By developing an awareness of one's own boundaries issues, and a need for positive self-esteem, control, and a sense of belonging, nurses can begin to separate family issues and needs versus their own. Each nurse can then choose helping practices that promote independence and self-control in the child and family.

Table 1. Self-Inventory Tool
(© Children's Hospital of The King's Daughters, 1991)

WOULD MY INTERVENTION HELP?

Complete the questions below when having trouble deciding if something you would like to do for a family would be in their best interest. There are no right or wrong answers. This tool will help you to see both the possible positive and negative outcomes. After you have finished, you will need to "weigh" the outcomes to decide whether or not you will, indeed, complete the helpful task. Please consult other resources if you feel you need assistance.

1. I would like to ______________________________

______________________________ to help this family and/or child.

2. Do I think this will be a one-time event/request? ______________

3. What are my intentions? A) ______________

B) ______________

C) ______________

4. How does a trusted coworker perceive my intentions? ______________

____

____

5. Assuming they were able, what could I do to help the family do this without me? A) ______________

____

B) ______________

____

Possible positive outcomes for the child and/or family	Possible negative outcomes for the child and/or family

_______ Yes, I have decided that it would be helpful to the family to do this task.
_______ No, I have decided that it would not be helpful to the family to do this task.

practice in a non–anxiety producing environment first or have an instructor present to reassure the patient.

The self-confidence of the nurse will also be tested when a patient refuses to do something the nurse has requested. The nurse needs the self-confidence to understand the refusal from the perspective of the patient and not see it as personal rejection.

KNOWLEDGE LEVEL

The knowledge base of the nurse is the fourth category of factors influencing the outcomes of communication.

- The knowledge base includes knowledge about communication—knowledge about communication does influence communication behavior.
- The knowledge base includes information about the subject matter—one cannot communicate what one does not know.
- The knowledge base includes knowledge about the patient—the better we know the patient, the more effective we are in communicating with that person. The population in the United States is changing dramatically. In terms of age, culture, ethnic background, and values, the United States is a country of great diversity. The nurse must appreciate this diversity and develop a knowledge base that incorporates understanding these cultural differences.

POSITION

The word **position** is used to refer to the relative position of the nurse and the patient within the health care system. Nurses and patients have different roles/positions. The behaviors associated with these roles/positions influence communication. In the classroom a student will communicate differently with the teacher than when at home with a child. The patient will communicate differently with the nurse than with a spouse.

The relative position of the patient and the nurse has frequently made the patient feel powerless and dependent. The hospitalized patient in particular was placed in a position that was emotionally traumatic. **Having** to be hospitalized makes a person feel afraid and helpless. The person/patient is placed in strange surroundings under the watch of strangers. Finally the patient finds that others take care of all physical needs and make all the decisions, e.g., when to eat, what to eat, when to sleep, and so forth. The consequence of these actions is a patient who may look like an adult but who feels like a child (or a child who regresses to earlier behaviors such as bedwetting). The patient is in an uncomfortable position of **dependency.**

The experience of feeling dependent in interactions with health care professionals occurs in settings other than the hospital. In long-term care settings, many residents feel they lose their autonomy and sense of self once admitted. One resident wrote recently (Tulloch, 1995) about her experiences and described nursing care plans as tools of terror. She noted that once the nurse had developed a care plan it became a tool for **evaluating the resident.** A good resident did what was called for on the care plan. Not doing something such as sitting in the lounge from 10 A.M. to 11 A.M. quickly labeled the resident as "bad." The fear of being a "bad" resident leads to communication breakdown.

The feeling of dependency may not be as significant in home care and care provided in community-controlled settings such as high-rise apartments. However, even in these settings, patients do comment on the imbalance of power due to position. For example, elderly people receiving home care may be reluctant to ask for what they need out of fear they will lose their care and be forced into a nursing home. Parents of children dependent on ventilators may be overwhelmed by the care issues and feel helpless and dependent on the nurse. Their feelings may be expressed in appropriate or inappropriate ways. Because they feel dependent, they may try to please the nurse rather than express their needs.

As was mentioned earlier, effective communication requires interdependence. The nurse must be affected by the patient and the patient by the nurse. The nurse must do everything possible to maintain the patient's sense of control and feelings of respect. Common courtesy such as asking the patient when he or she would feel ready to provide an admission history is helpful in giving the patient a sense of control. (This might seem impractical, but at times in some settings it can be done.) Addressing an adult by his last name (Mr. Smith) rather than by his first name (Bob) or a familiar term (Grandpa) helps maintain the person's sense of worth. Using words that are meaningful to the general public is equally important. Simply being sensitive to how the patient feels is also a first step in keeping the patient from feeling dependent.

Communication is affected by perceived positions in the health care system. The patient who feels dependent and like a "room number" or medical diagnosis is not likely to communicate well with the nurse. Likewise, the patient who feels in control and respected as an individual will tend to communicate better with the nurse.

FEEDBACK

The sixth and final set of factors that influence communication is feedback processes. Feedback is simply that—a reaction or understanding that is fed back to the patient to confirm or modify. Feedback is essential because it provides the nurse with information concerning the success in meeting the goals for the communication.

On pp. 163-164 several techniques are listed for obtaining feedback during communication. These same techniques can be used after the communication has ended and the nurse has ascribed meaning to the information. For example, the nurse has completed an information session in which a patient was instructed about the diet that should be followed after discharge from the hospital. As the nurse reviews his actions and those of the patient, he concludes that the patient needs more time to discuss living with the new diet. **The nurse is giving meaning to the communication.** Before planning another session for the patient to talk about his feelings, the nurse needs to give the patient feedback and see if that interpretation is correct.

The nurse can do this by asking the patient to clarify a statement; by sharing the observation and asking for verification; or by offering the patient a summary and asking for response.

Feedback is essential in that it influences all further communication. It influences the content of future communications because one communication builds on the previous one. It also influences how the patient responds in further communication. If the patient feels misunderstood, further communication will be guarded.

GROUP COMMUNICATION

The nurse will frequently lead meetings with small groups of patients (or healthy individuals) for educational or support goals. All of the points about communication skills relate to small groups as well as individuals. In small groups the nurse must be alert to the personality and task issues and be prepared to intervene if conflict develops.

Intercultural Communication

Human beings are more alike than unalike, and what is true anywhere is true everywhere, yet I encourage travel to as many destinations as possible. . . . Perhaps travel cannot prevent bigotry, but by demonstrating that all peoples laugh, cry, eat, worry, and die, it can introduce the idea that if we try to understand each other, we may even become friends (Angelou, 1993).

Intercultural communication calls attention to the significant impact of culture on communication. Every culture, subculture, and subgroup has rules and norms that govern behavior including communication. Knowledge of these rules and norms can help avoid communication mistakes. The following examples demonstrate that point (Jandt, 1995, p. 4):

- In Germany, a *Berliner* is a jelly doughnut. In his speech at the Berlin Wall, President Kennedy when he said, "Ich bin ein Berliner," actually said, "I am a jelly doughnut!"
- Chevrolet attempted unsuccessfully to market its Nova compact car in Latin American countries. In Spanish, *no va* means "does not go" or "it doesn't run."
- Braniff Airlines promoted rendezvous lounges on its planes flying Brazilian routes. In Portuguese, *rendezvous* is "a place to have sex."
- In Australia, President Bush flashed a backhanded peace sign in motorcades. To many, that gesture is interpreted as obscene.

Effective intercultural communication requires people from different cultures and therefore with different rules and norms regarding communication to create shared meanings.

INTERCULTURAL COMMUNICATION COMPETENCE

It is impossible for one individual to know all the rules and norms of communication for all cultures, subcultures, and subgroups. Even if it were possible, that knowledge would not account for the differences among individuals within any specific group. What is possible and effective is developing the following skills (Jandt, 1995):

- Personality strength, i.e., self-concept (view of self), self-disclosure (willingness to openly and appropriately reveal information about self), self-monitoring (using social comparison information to control and modify self), and social relaxation (reveal little anxiety in communication).
- Communication skills, i.e., message skills (understand and use the language and feedback), behavioral flexibility (select appropriate behavior in diverse contexts), interaction management (attentiveness, responsiveness, ability to initiate and end a conversation), and social skills (empathy and identity maintenance).
- Psychological adjustment, i.e., acclimate to new settings and handle "culture shock."
- Cultural awareness, i.e., understand social customs and how people think and behave.

The Behavioral Assessment Scale for Intercultural Competence (BASIC) lists these eight categories of communication behavior, each of which contributes to the achievement of intercultural competence (Lustig and Koester, 1993):

- Display of Respect demonstrated through both verbal and nonverbal symbols. Within every culture there are specific ways to show respect and specific expectations about those to whom respect should be shown.
- Orientation to Knowledge demonstrated by actions showing all experiences and interpretations are personal rather than universally shared. For example, stating "New Yorkers are rude and unfriendly!" suggests all people share that view. A personal orientation to knowledge would result in this type of statement "Many of the people I interacted with when visiting New York were not friendly or courteous to me."
- Empathy demonstrated by communicating an awareness of another person's thoughts, feelings, and experiences. Empathetic behaviors include verbal statements and nonverbal codes that are complementary to the moods and thoughts of others.
- Interaction Management demonstrated by the ability to start and end interactions as well as taking turns maintaining a discussion.
- Task Role Behavior demonstrated by contributions to a group's problem-solving activities. Tasks are accomplished by cultures in many ways. For example, in the United States it is acceptable to conduct work over lunch or dinner. In another culture this may well be inappropriate.
- Relational Role Behavior demonstrated by the ability to build or maintain personal relationships within a group by verbal and nonverbal indication of support.
- Tolerance for Ambiguity demonstrated by viewing new situations as a challenge and quickly adapting to the demands of changing environments.
- Interaction Posture demonstrated by responses to others that are descriptive, nonevaluative, and non-

judgmental. Statements based on absolute judgments of rights and wrongs indicate a closed framework of attitudes, beliefs, and values. This is seen as evaluative.

This set of BASIC skills can be used to assess general communication skills as well as those related to intercultural competence.

BARRIERS TO INTERCULTURAL COMMUNICATION

There are five common barriers to intercultural communication (Jandt, 1995). The first barrier is **anxiety.** Anxiety tends to make a person focus on his or her own feelings; the person is therefore not fully engaged in the communication transaction.

The second barrier is assuming that all cultures are the same rather than being open to differences. It is better to assume differences and ask about the customs rather than make errors.

The third barrier is ethnocentrism, i.e., negatively judging aspects of another culture by the rules and norms of one's own culture. An ethnocentric person believes his or her culture is superior to all other cultures.

The fourth barrier is stereotyping, i.e., making negative or positive judgments about an individual based on observable or assumed group membership.

The fifth barrier is prejudice, i.e., irrational suspicion or hatred of a particular group, race, religion, or sexual orientation.

Issues

PERSONAL QUESTIONS

There are some aspects of social communication that initially may be troublesome in professional communication. One commonly occurring situation is a patient asking the nurse for personal information. The patient may say, "You remind me of my daughter. How old are you?" When possible, the nurse should avoid giving personal information about herself to the patient. Doing so turns the communication into a more social rather than professional one. In some instances, it may not be possible to avoid giving the patient personal information. Then it is essential to give the briefest answer and continue the goal-directed communication. If the patient asks again for personal information the nurse may need to respond (pleasantly) in a way that refocuses the communication back on the patient. In doing this, the nurse is establishing boundaries for the communication. This must be done in words and tones that do not embarrass the patient and do not make the patient feel rejected. It is also important for the nurse to understand **why** the patient asked the questions. Knowing that will enable the nurse to respond without needing to provide personal information.

SENSITIVE INFORMATION

Another common situation is when the patient asks the nurse for information that the nurse does not feel free to provide. The patient may ask "Is my physician good?" or "How do you rate this hospital?" The nurse may feel comfortable responding to some direct questions but not to others. In either case a more helpful response is first finding out what the patient's underlying concerns are. The patient may have been referred to a new physician and is therefore asking for information. If this were the case, the better response would be to arrange time for the patient and physician to develop their relationship. A question about the hospital may actually stem from the fear of dying or knowing someone who died in the hospital. Rather than responding to the direct question, a better response is to deal with the underlying fear. In general, the nurse can respond to a direct question by asking questions back until the underlying issue has been identified. One word of caution—when engaged in this process, avoid using "why" questions. Asking the patient why he is asking the question seldom produces valid responses.

HUMOR

The use of humor and side comments is common in social communication. In fact, in social communication we seek out people with a sense of humor or wit. In professional communications, humor and side comments should be used cautiously. People who feel in a vulnerable position are likely to misinterpret humor and side comments. They do not see anything funny about the situation. Even if the patient uses humor, the nurse must be cautious in making a response. Humor is personal. It has limited use in nurse-patient communications. Yet when it is appropriate, humor can be a powerful technique for relieving tension and other feelings. For example, cancer patients receiving chemotherapy who lose their hair often wear comical gear. The nurse, who in most instances has a long-time association with the patient, may be able to tease about the selection of cap or turban and make the patient feel noticed and understood.

TITLES

In social situations we usually call people by their first name or some nickname. This should be avoided in professional communications. The nurse and the patient are not communicating because they are friends but because the patient has need of the nurse's services. This purpose can be forgotten if the communication resembles social communication. The nurse also must remember that the terms used when addressing the patient reflect her attitude toward the patient. If the nurse calls the patient "Granny" instead of by her full name, the nurse has communicated that she sees the patient as just one more older person. She has responded to the patient as a stereotype rather than as an individual. The consequence is that the patient senses the lack of respect and feels depersonalized. The terms used when addressing someone communicate much more than a name. With adults the nurse should always address the person by the full given name—Mr. Jones or Mrs. Smith or Ms. Green—until such time as the patient indicates otherwise. With children the nurse should determine (from either the child or parents) what name to use.

The nurse should also expect to be addressed by his last name. He should introduce himself that way to the patient and expect the patient to address him that way. As the relationship develops between the patient and the nurse, the nurse may want the patient to use a first name. In some institutions the practice is to call nurses by their first name. In that situation the nurse would not insist on being called by a last name.

PERSONAL PREFERENCES

In social situations we can avoid people or interact with people based on our own likes and dislikes. In professional situations, the nurse must have a nonjudgmental, neutral attitude toward all individuals. For example, personally a nurse may feel that alcoholism is the result of a weak character; with willpower, a person could stop drinking. Yet when the nurse is communicating with the person who is an alcoholic, the nurse is not free to let that attitude influence the interaction. The nurse must focus on the goal of the communication and use all her knowledge and skills to help the person. It may be difficult to set aside our personal biases, but it can and must be done. The best approach is to focus on the person (not the problem) and on the goal of the communication.

Preparation for Effective Communication

The preceding material focused on the communication process. This is obviously important. Preparing for the interaction is also important. Preparation is frequently overlooked in the hustle and bustle of patient care settings.

SETTING

The nurse must consider the setting in which the communication takes place. The setting needs to be conducive to the goal of the communication. It should be well lighted, comfortable, and free of distractions. It should allow the nurse and patient to have eye contact without one having to look up and the other down. It should allow the nurse to be physically present but not invading the patient's private space. (For example, the nurse should not have to sit on the patient's bed.) The nurse may ask the patient to go to another setting if the patient's room is not suitable to the communication. Quite often patients are asked to reveal personal information in a setting where there is another patient or where relatives or distractions are present. The lack of privacy can detract from the communication.

TIME

The nurse should try to ensure enough time to accomplish the purpose of the communication. The nurse's time schedule as well as the patient's needs to be considered. If there is not enough time, the nurse needs to state this at the beginning of the communication and arrange for the additional time that is required. A sense of being rushed detracts from effective communication.

REVIEW OF INFORMATION

To the extent possible, the nurse also needs to review all the information that is known about the patient before beginning the communication. The nurse should review the patient's current chart and any previous records. The nurse needs to communicate what is known and what is not known. A major complaint of patients is that they are asked to give the same information over and over again. Even asking a simple question like "Why are you here?" produces a concerned response from the patient. In the minds of patients, you should know why they are in the hospital or clinic. It is better to say, "I understand that you are scheduled for surgery tomorrow. However, I would appreciate hearing about your health problems in your own words. That information will help us plan your care more effectively."

RECALL

Finally, the nurse should be prepared to take notes during the communication. The nurse may have an excellent memory but having notes enables the nurse to reflect on the communication and develop greater understanding. It is wise to tell the patient that notes will be taken and how the notes will be used. Do not take notes to the extent that that process detracts from the communication process.

THE HELPING RELATIONSHIP

This chapter started with a discussion of the importance of the nurse-patient relationship. Emphasis was given to the fact that the relationship is a vehicle for health and healing and is as powerful as any nursing procedure. Patients often distinguish relationships that **helped** from those that simply occurred. Communication skills essential to establishing a positive nurse-patient relationship were discussed.

Contribution of Carl Rogers

In the 1950s a well-known psychologist, Carl Rogers (1958), studied the therapeutic relationship to determine the characteristics of those relationships that do help (promote growth). His work is still used today and is considered classic. Rogers concluded that **attitudes** were more important than **techniques.** Of greatest importance is the characteristic of **genuineness.**

The patient must sense that the nurse is genuine, that words match behavior and internal feelings. A nurse who is thinking of something else while talking to the patient will not be perceived as genuine. A nurse who is bored with the practice of nursing will not be seen as genuine. A nurse who does not look at the patient or **who looks without seeing** will not be seen as genuine. **Genuineness is expressed by seeing the patient as a person and focusing energy and attention toward understanding that person** (Fig. 10–3). If the nurse withholds herself as a person and therefore deals with the patient as an object, the relationship will not be a helping one. The patient must sense genuineness to the point that he or she will trust the nurse.

In addition to being genuine in interactions with the patient, there are specific behaviors that promote a helping relationship.

- Be dependable. Do what you say you are going to do when you say you will do it.
- Be consistent in the way in which you interact with the patient.
- Respect and maintain the confidential nature of the patient's disclosures.
- Be real; be a person.
- Communicate clearly. Check with the patient to make certain the intended message was the one received.
- Allow yourself to experience positive feelings toward the patient. One can be professional without having to be impersonal.
- Understand how the patient feels. Respond with a sensitivity based on that understanding.
- Create opportunities outside of the clinical setting to grow and mature. **See yourself as in the process of becoming.**

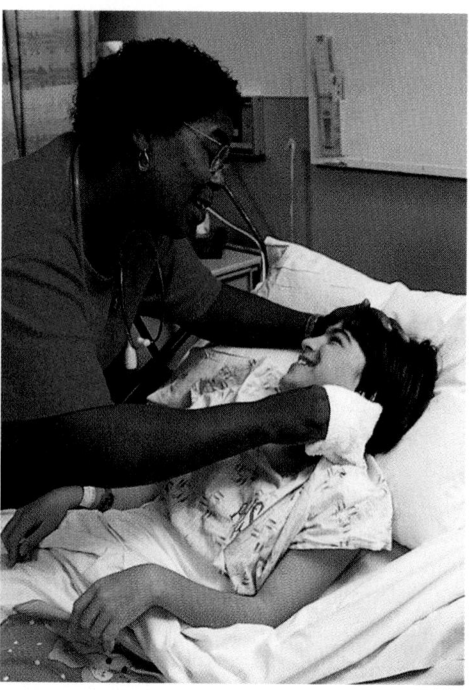

Figure 10–3. The nurse who conveys a sense of genuineness when providing care will foster a helping nurse-patient relationship.

Contributions from Nursing Research

COMMUNICATION SKILLS

Most nurses would agree that

- the nurse-patient relationship is the essence of nursing
- the nurse-patient relationship is developed through interaction
- the interaction is made possible through communication, and
- meaning is created through the communication process

Despite agreement regarding the importance of the nurse-patient relationship and communication to nursing practice, nursing research in this area has lagged. Two generalizations are warranted from the existing nursing research base (Garvin and Kennedy, 1990):

- Regardless of technique, the nurse's intention to focus on the patient resulted in desirable outcomes.
- A nurse's being available is the most supportive behavior.

TRUST

Trust has been identified as an important aspect of the nurse-patient relationship. However, within the nursing literature the term lacks clear definition and conceptual clarity. Johns (1996) subjected existing nursing and nonnursing literature relevant to the concept of trust to concept analysis. The analysis resulted in a process/outcome model of the concept of trust (Fig. 10–4). As process, it is a sequential step model with feedback. As outcome, it is a condition of the process captured at a moment in time.

The model depicts four stages associated with the concept of trust:

- **Assimilation of information** about the person or thing trusted and about the relevant situation. Elements of information include the perception of risks and benefits of entering into a trusting relationship, characteristics of the person or thing to be trusted, and past experience.
- **Decision making** based on the information. The person or thing may be trusted or may not.
- **A trusting relationship** follows if the person is found to be trustworthy. As process, this relationship includes elements of being vulnerable and relying on someone else. It is dynamic and goes through developmental stages.
- **Consequences of trusting** then occur. These can vary from being very specific such as trusting the nurse when told an injection will have little pain to quite general such as experiencing greater benefits than expected from the relationship (the nurse helped me see my life in a new way). Feedback from this stage is information that enters and influences the process.

Although this model does require empirical testing, it does have face validity as it is based on existing literature. It can serve as a useful guide for the beginning nursing student by

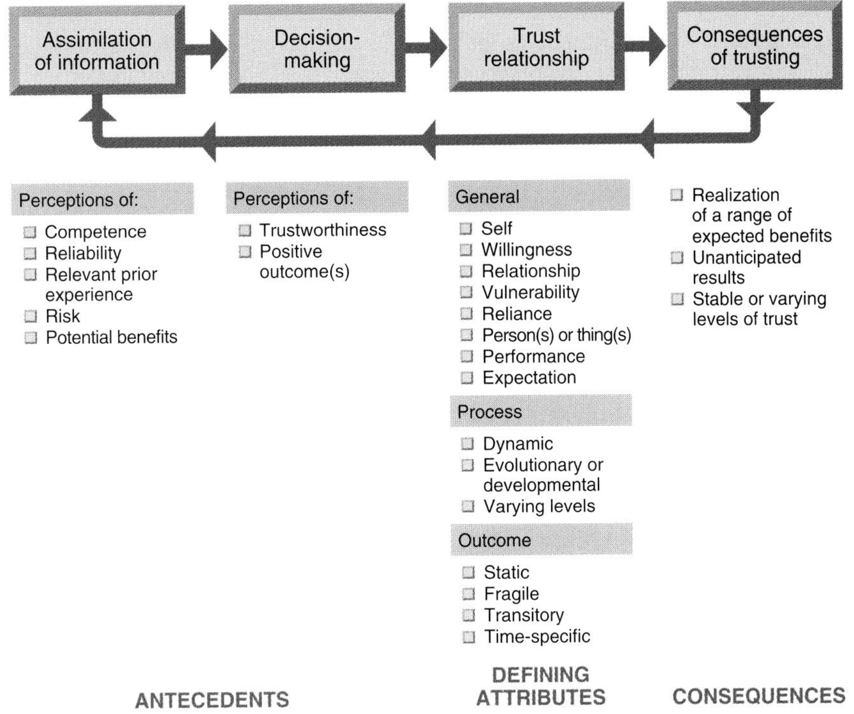

Figure 10–4. Johns' process/outcome model of a core concept of trust.

providing structure for establishing and evaluating the concept of trust within a helping relationship.

EMPOWERMENT

Using a similar methodology, Rodwell (1996) analyzed the concept of empowerment. Empowerment is a popular conept in today's world and is used frequently in the nursing literature. Empowerment has four defining attributes:

- a helping process
- a partnership that values self and others
- mutual decision making using resources, opportunities, and authority
- freedom to make choices and accept responsibility

> Empowerment, in a helping relationship, is the process of enabling people to choose to take control over and make decisions about their own lives. It is a process that values all involved (p. 309).

The antecedents to the empowerment process are mutual trust and respect; education and support; and participation and commitment. The consequences are positive self-esteem; ability to set and reach goals; a sense of control over life and change processes; and a sense of hope for the future.

The goal of empowerment is applicable for all nursing care situations. Rodwell's critical analysis of the literature clarifies the concept and provides structure for nurses attempting to implement this concept in practice.

CHAPTER HIGHLIGHTS

- Relationship-centered care has therapeutic value apart from the interventions the nurse administers.
- Communication is affected by the verbal skills, nonverbal skills, attitudes, knowledge, position, culture, and feedback of the people involved.
- Genuineness as expressed by seeing the patient as a person and focusing energy and attention toward understanding that person is key to a helping relationship.
- Communication skills are developed through practice.

REFERENCES

Angelou, M. (1993). *Won't Take Nothing for My Journey Now.* New York: Random House, pp. 11, 12.

Barker, L.L., Wahlers, K.J., Watson, K.W. (1995). *Groups in Process,* 5th ed. Boston: Allyn and Bacon.

Berlo, D. (1960). *The Process of Communication.* Chicago: Holt, Rinehart and Winston.

Bulger, R. (1991). *The Demise of the Placebo Effect in the Practice of Scientific Medicine.* Association of Academic Health Centers, Washington, D.C.

Cravener, P. (1992). Establishing therapeutic alliance across cultural barriers. *Journal of Psychosocial Nursing, 30* (12), 10–14.

Garvin, B.J., Kennedy, C.W. (1990). Interpersonal communication between nurses and patients. In J.J. Fitzpatrick, R.L. Taunton, and J.Q. Benoliel (eds.): *Annual Review of Nursing Research, 1990.* New York: Springer, pp. 213–234.

Hall, E.T. (1959). *The Silent Language.* Greenwich, CT: Fawcett.

Hall, E.T. (1966). *The Hidden Dimension.* Garden City, NJ: Doubleday.

Hollinger, L.M. (1986). Communicating with the elderly. *J Gerontol Nurs, 12* (3):8–13.

Infante, D.A., Rancer, A.S., Womack, D.F. (1993). *Building Communication Theory,* 2nd ed. Prospect Heights, IL: Waveland.

Jandt, F.E. (1995). *Intercultural Communication.* Thousand Oaks, CA: Sage.

Jerome, A., McDuffie, A. (1992). Nurse self-awareness in therapeutic relationships. *Pediatric Nursing,* 18 (2), 153–156.

Johns, J.L. (1996). A concept analysis of trust. *Journal of Advanced Nursing, 24, 76–83.*

Krupat, E. (1986). A delicate imbalance. *Psychology Today,* November, 22–26.

Lustig, M.W., Koester, J. (1993). *Intercultural Competence: Interpersonal Communications Across Cultures.* New York: Harper Collins College.

Peplau, H. (1964). *Basic Principles of Patient Counseling,* 2nd ed. Philadelphia: Smith Kline and French Laboratories.

Pike A. (1990). On the nature and place of empathy in clinical nursing practice. *Journal of Professional Nursing,* 6 (4), 235–241.

Rodwell, C.M. (1996). An analysis of the concept of empowerment. *Journal of Advanced Nursing, 23,* 305–313.

Rogers, C. (1958). The characteristics of a helping relationship. *Personnel and Guidance, 37,* 6–16.

Shapiro, A.K. (1961). Factors contributing to the placebo effect: Their implications for psychotherapy. *Am J Psychotherapy, 18, 73–88.*

Stovsky, B., Rudy, E., Dragonette, P. (1988). Comparison of two types of communication methods used after cardiac surgery with patients with endotracheal tubes. *Heart and Lung, 17* (3), 281–289.

Therapeutic Communication Teacher's Guide. (1990). Athens, Ohio: Fuld Institute for Technology in Nursing Education.

Thorne, S.E. (1988). Helpful and unhelpful communications in cancer care: The patient perspective. *Oncology Nursing Forum, 15* (2), 167–172.

Tresolini, C.P., Pew-Fetzer Task Force. (1994). *Health Professions Education and Relationship-centered Care.* San Francisco, CA: Pew Health Professions Commission.

Tulloch, G.J. (1995). A resident's view of autonomy. In L.M. Gamroth et al (eds.): *Enhancing Autonomy in Long-Term Care.* New York: Springer, pp. 109–120.

Turner, J.A., Deyo, R.A., Loeser, J.D. et al. (1994). The importance of placebo effects in pain treatment and research. *Journal of the American Medical Association, 271* (20), 1609–1614.

Weil, A. (1988). *Health and Healing,* 2nd ed. Boston: Houghton Mifflin.

The Phenomena of Caring 11

Carol Lindeman

Hello, David
David—my name is Dusty, I'm your night nurse. I will stay with you.
I will check your vitals
every 15 minutes.
I will document in-
evitability.
I will hang more blood
And give you something
for your pain.
I will stay with you and
I will touch your face.
Yes, of course, I will
write your mother and
tell her you were brave.
I will write your mother
and tell her how much you loved her.
I will write your mother and tell her to give your bratty kid sister a big kiss and hug.
What I will not tell her is that you were wasted.
I will stay with you and hold your hand.
I will stay with you and watch your life flow through my fingers into my soul.
I will stay with you until you stay with me.
Goodbye, David—my name is Dusty.
I am the last person you will see.
I am the last person you will touch.
I am the last person who will love you.
So long, David—my name is Dusty.
David, who will give me something for my pain?
(Styles and Moccia, *1993, pp. 166–167)*

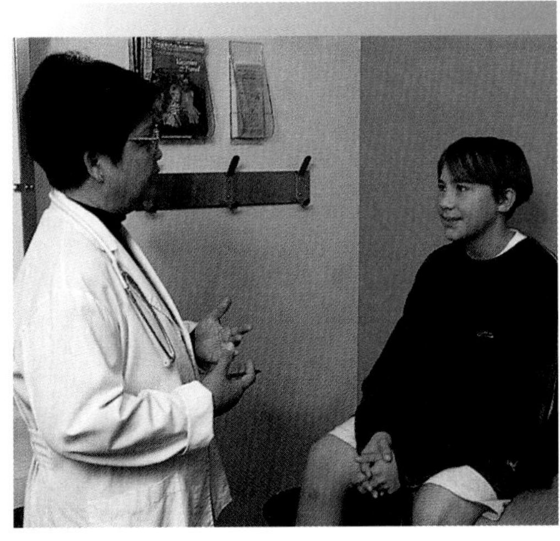

OBJECTIVES
After studying this chapter, students will be able to:
- **formulate a personal conception of care and caring based on the existing theory and research**
- **thoughtfully implement and evaluate that conception in practice**

This anonymous poem provides a vivid description of a nurse **caring.** In the quest to describe the nature and significance of nursing, no terms have been used so consistently as *care* and *caring* (Styles and Moccia, 1993). **Caring** is frequently mentioned as the core or essence of nursing (Leininger, 1984; Watson, 1988). The connection between nursing and caring can be easily verified by asking classmates why they went into nursing. When asked, nursing students are likely to say they wanted to care for people. The word is also evident in the language used by nurses. They talk about nursing **care,** the **care** given to a certain patient, or how they felt when they gave **care.**

Despite the frequent use of the word **care** in the nursing language and literature and the assumption that **caring** is a significant part of nursing practice, the concepts of care and caring are not fully understood. The concepts remain the focus of study for many nurse researchers, theorists, and ethicists.

THE NATURE OF CARING FROM A PHILOSOPHICAL PERSPECTIVE

Mayeroff (1971) refers to caring as "helping the other grow by seeing the other as an extension of one's self and yet as separate from self." He states:

> The meaning of caring I want to suggest is not to be confused with such meanings as wishing well, liking, comforting and maintaining, or simply having an interest in what happens to another. Also, it is not an isolated feeling or a momentary relationship, nor is it simply a matter of wanting to care for some person. Caring, as helping another grow and actualize himself, is a process, a way of relating to someone that involves development, in the same way that friendship can only emerge in time through mutual trust and a deepening and qualitative transformation of the relationship. Whatever the important differences are among a parent caring for his child, a teacher caring for his pupil, a psychotherapist caring for his patient, or a husband caring for his wife, I would like to show that they all exhibit a common pattern (p. 2).

The basic pattern of caring according to Mayeroff is this personal experience:

- I experience the other as an extension of myself and also as independent and with the need to grow.
- I experience the other's development as bound up with my own sense of well-being and I feel needed by it for that growth.
- I respond affirmatively and with devotion to the other's need guided by the direction of its growth (pp. 11–12).

Mayeroff identifies nine major ingredients of caring:

- **Knowledge.** To care for someone requires knowing many things. You must know who the other is; what his powers and limitations are; what his needs are; and what responses would be acceptable. You must know general information (such as the nature of the illness) as well as specific information (what this illness means to this person). In the caring process you will know some things from direct encounters and other things through information from others. Some of what you know you will be able to state explicitly while other knowledge you will feel as intuition.
- **Alternating Rhythms.** The same approach or perspective may work one time and not a second time. It is important to learn from a situation and try something new. It is also important to look at the situation as a one-time incident and also to see if there is a pattern.
- **Patience.** People grow in their own time and way. They will need space, which can be provided by patiently listening. Patience requires active involvement and tolerance.
- **Honesty.** You must be genuine in caring. What you feel and what you say must be in agreement. What you say and how you behave must be consistent.
- **Trust.** Trust is shown in caring by allowing the other to be independent. It is shown by allowing mistakes to be made and lessons learned. Forcing someone into a mold or not allowing them to make their own choices demonstrates **no** trust.
- **Humility.** Humility in caring is shown by learning from the other, by knowing one's limits and strengths, by overcoming the arrogance that exaggerates one's own power, and by knowing there is always something more to learn.
- **Hope.** In caring, hope is an expression of a *present* alive with possibilities. It is not just focused on the future. It is not just a passive waiting for something to happen.
- **Courage.** Following the lead of another may well take you into the unknown. You may find yourself in new territory without familiar landmarks. But courage is not blind, as it is informed by past experiences and is open and sensitive to the present.

Caring requires (1) a focus on the **other,** (2) a focus on the **process** and the eight ingredients just listed, and (3) actively maintaining the **ability** to care for and to be cared for.

Mayeroff's insights into caring are directly applicable to the practice of nursing. Individuals enter the discipline of nursing at different points in their personal development of the components of caring. Each situation with a patient, family and colleague can contribute to the further development and refinement of the ability to care. It is through caring and helping others grow that we grow too.

NURSING THEORY REGARDING THE PHENOMENA OF CARING

Leininger's Theory of Culture Care

DESCRIPTION

Madeline Leininger, a nurse anthropologist, is one of the most frequently quoted nurse scholars regarding the phenomena of caring. Her theory is especially important in today's diverse world as it emphasizes similarities and differences across cultures. An assumption crucial to understanding her theory is that the capacity for human cultures to develop and survive through time, and among a great variety of precarious world environments, has largely been related to the ability of the human species to **care** for itself and for others with a moral sense of responsibility and human accountability (Leininger, 1990). She believes that in the history of humankind, a caring ethos and action mode must have been vital to the survival of the human race and its environments.

According to Leininger (1991, p. 39), "culturally derived nursing care based on transcultural human care knowledge will maintain client health and well being or help clients face death in culturally appropriate ways." Nursing's focus is human **care**; it centers on providing human care to people in a way that is meaningful, congruent, and respectful of cultural values and lifestyles (Fig. 11–1).

KEY POINTS

From her field research in many cultures, Leininger (1990) identified the following tenets of a culture care theory:

1. Care is essential for development, growth, and survival of human beings. (Without human care people will not survive.)
2. Generic and professional care meanings, expressions, patterns, and action modes vary transculturally, with some culturally universal and diverse features. (In many cultures nurses are expected to help relieve pain. In the United States a nurse is expected to relieve pain through a variety of means including drugs. In Samoa a nurse is expected to protect patients from breaking cultural and social rules in order to prevent further harm and illness.)
3. Care is the essence of nursing and the distinctive feature explaining nursing. (Care is the key to outcomes and therefore the core of nursing.)
4. A culture's care meanings and action patterns are largely embedded in its world view, social structure, cultural values, language, and environment. (For example, in Turkey and Israel, nurses related their caring functions to restorative care due to frequent war activities. In New Guinea, nursing care activities were linked to religious and kinship ties. In the United States, nursing actions were associated with medical and technological structures.)
5. The use of generic and professional care knowledge is a powerful means of promoting health, well-being, and recovery from illness or disability, or of helping clients and families during the dying process. (Generic care is equated with folk, indigenous or naturalist care—the oldest form of care. Professional nursing care is what is learned in nursing educational programs. Professional care is a natural derivation from generic care. The two knowledges, generic and professional, need to be brought together.)
6. Ethical-moral care values and practices have differences and similarities in Western and non-Western cultures. (Across cultures there are some similar care behaviors and some that are distinctly different. All cultures may care for the infant. The nature of that care differs.)
7. Emic (from inside the culture) and etic (professional perspective) care knowledge are important differential aspects of care in determining and providing culturally congruent care to clients. (People of each culture know and define the ways in which they experience and perceive their nursing care world and can relate these experiences and perceptions to their general health beliefs and practices. Nursing care is derived and developed from the cultural context in which it is to be provided.)
8. Human beings may exist without curing, but not without caring. (Caring is essential to curing. There can be no cure without care.)
9. Cultural, social, and physical environmental contexts give meaning and structure to assessing and guiding professional care practices and policies. (How people live, what they value, and where they live influence the norms they set for the practice of health care.)
10. The goal of professional care is to provide culturally congruent care to people of diverse cultures. (We are

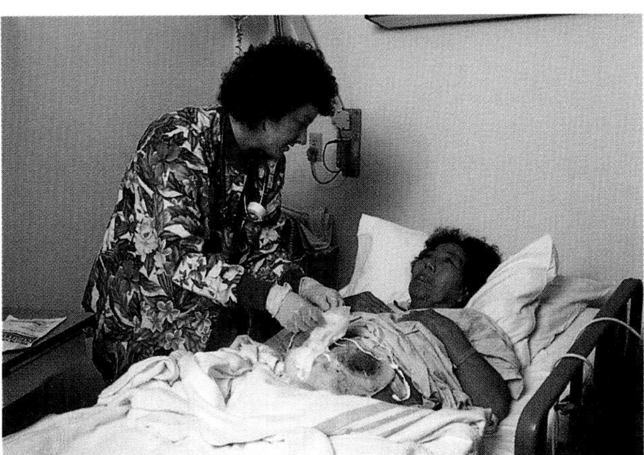

Figure 11–1. Effective nursing care transcends all ethnic and cultural barriers to focus on human care.

one world but many cultures. Only **culturally congruent care** promotes healing and health.)

ILLUSTRATION FROM RESEARCH

Leininger (1991) offers the following example of different cultural care meanings and actions. The statements were derived from research with two cultures in the United States, the Anglo-American middle class and African-Americans. The Anglo-American participants identified the following care means and their related action modes:

1. To provide *stress alleviation* measures, largely through physical and psychosocial means.
2. To provide *personalized acts* such as doing special things and giving attention to individuals.
3. To rely on *self-care* modes rather than care by others, in order to become independent and self-reliant.
4. To obtain from health personnel *health instruction and medical facts* that allow expanded self-care.

The African-American participants identified the following care means and their related action modes:

1. To show *concern for* "my brothers and sisters" at all times.
2. To demonstrate ways to *be involved with* family members.
3. To give *physical presence* when someone is ill or "under the weather."
4. To give *family support* and maintain family "get-togethers."
5. To use *touching* appropriately and frequently, when well or sick.
6. To rely on *folk home remedies* to communicate caring and to restore health.
7. To rely on *"Jesus to save us,"* especially through the use of prayers and songs.

The italicized words are the guides to nurses' thinking and actions. There was cultural variability in both groups but these are dominant themes as reported by Leininger.

CONCEPTS TO GUIDE NURSING ACTIONS

Through her research with 54 cultures, Leininger has identified some 172 care constructs. These constructs provide a focus for nursing actions and can guide nursing decisions. Examples of caring constructs are:

- comfort
- compassion
- empathy
- involvement
- presence
- sharing
- support
- surveillance
- tenderness
- touching
- trust

SUMMARY

In summary, in the theory of cultural care:

- Care is essential for survival of humankind.
- Professional care is a derivative of folk/lay care.
- Care is the essence of nursing.
- For care to be effective it must be culturally congruent.
- Nurses must learn the values, beliefs, and practices of a culture because these form the patterns, conditions, and actions associated with human care.

Watson's Theory of Human Care

DESCRIPTION

Watson sees nursing as a caring-healing art and science. The theory focuses on the transforming, healing power of the human spirit. Caring is a **way of being** for the nurse. The nurse uses self to engage in a genuine, unique transpersonal relationship with another experiencing human being (Morris, 1996). The goal of the relationship is to assist the person to obtain greater harmony among the mind, body, and spirit. This greater harmony will (according to the theory) produce self-knowledge, self-reverence, self-healing, and self-care (Watson, 1988). The goal of nursing actions is "to protect, enhance, and preserve humanity by helping the person find meaning in illness, suffering, pain, and existence and to help another gain self-knowledge, control, and self-healing wherein inner harmony is restored regardless of the external circumstance" (Watson, 1985, p. 54).

KEY ASSUMPTIONS

Watson sees caring as the most valuable attribute nursing has to offer. There are seven assumptions basic to the theory:

1. Caring can be effectively demonstrated and practiced interpersonally.
2. Caring consists of "carative" factors that result in the satisfaction of certain human needs.
3. Effective caring promotes health and individual or family growth.
4. Caring responses accept a person not only as he or she is now but as what he or she may become.
5. A caring environment is one that offers the development of potential while allowing the person to choose the best action for himself or herself at a given point in time.
6. Caring is more "healthogenic" than is curing. The practice of caring integrates biophysical knowledge with knowledge of human behaviors to generate or promote health and to provide ministrations to those who are ill. A science of caring is therefore complementary to the science of curing.

7. The practice of caring is central to nursing (Watson, 1979, pp. 8–9).

CONCEPTS TO GUIDE NURSING ACTIONS

The structure for the science of caring is built on 10 carative factors:

1. **Formation of humanistic-altruistic value system.** This is a developmental process mediated by life experiences. The nurse's own maturation promotes altruistic behavior toward others.
2. **Instillation of faith and hope.** Nurses need to recognize alternatives to Western medicine. They can then provide a sense of well-being through those beliefs that are meaningful to the individual.
3. **Cultivation of sensitivity to self and others.** Through development of and sensitivity to one's own feelings one can genuinely and sensitively interact with others.
4. **Development of helping-trust relationship.** This is accomplished through communication that reflects genuineness, empathy, and warmth.
5. **Promotion and acceptance of the expression of positive and negative feelings.** Feelings influence behavior and are therefore important to express. Listening to the feelings of a person will help understand that person's behavior.
6. **Utilization of scientific problem-solving methods for decision making.** Without the use of these processes, effective practice is accidental at best and haphazard or harmful at worst. Also, science does not always have to be neutral and objective.
7. **Promotion of interpersonal teaching-learning.** This provides people with control over their own health by giving them information and alternatives.
8. **Provision of supportive, protective, and/or corrective mental, physical, sociocultural, and spiritual environment.** The nurse must attend to both external variables such as safety and physical needs as well as internal variables such as mental and spiritual activities.
9. **Assistance with human need gratification.** Needs are hierarchical but the person must still be viewed holistically. Biophysical needs such as food and fluid and psychophysical needs such as activity and sexuality are lower order needs. Psychosocial needs such as achievement and intrapersonal-interpersonal needs such as self-actualization are higher order needs.
10. **Allowance for existential-phenomenological forces.** The nurse must understand the person from the way things appear to that person. This includes understanding the meaning the person finds in life and difficult life events. The nurse must face these questions before being able to assist others. (Watson, 1979, pp. 9–10).

The first three factors are the philosophical foundation for the science of human caring. The remaining seven are the tools for implementing the caring relationship.

USE OF WATSON'S THEORY IN PRACTICE

The Denver Nursing Project in Human Caring (DNPHC) is an outpatient, nurse-directed health care facility for clients with human immunodeficiency virus/acquired immunodeficiency syndrome (HIV/AIDS). Since its inception in 1988 programs and services have been based on Watson's philosophy and science of human caring (Astorino et al, 1994). The DNPHC mission statement is presented in Box 11–1.

DNPHC staff learned to work together in a way that nurtured their ability to care. Key factors in that process were:

- **Valuing spirituality.** Caring is not a set of behaviors. It is a way of being in the world that corresponds to a way of being in the workplace.
- **Team support.** One must care for oneself, and people must support one another.
- **Focus on healing.** Healing occurs in a relationship. In that relationship nurses grow and change *with* their clients.
- **Homelike and nurturing environment.** The environment must support and facilitate healing.
- **Interrelationships.** Understanding that we are all connected and inseparable from our environment.
- **Sense of community.** Creating a nonhierarchical organization that emphasizes cooperation rather than competition.
- **Authentic communication.** Speaking up and saying what you think and feel strengthens ties rather than severs them.
- **Self-scheduling.** Staff have the responsibility to organize themselves so that the work gets done.
- **Commitment to growth.** Team process is a day-to-day experience and not something one goes to an in-service meeting to learn. Personal and professional growth occur as a result of teamwork.
- **Valuing intuition.** It is important to listen and attend to the "wise old person within."

Key characteristics of the model of nursing care, Nursing Care Partnership, are:

- A mutually accepted, reciprocal agreement that both partners openly acknowledge and identify needs as the relationship evolves.
- An avenue for the nurse to foster client independence in his or her own health care by helping the client identify internal and external resources and offering information about how to negotiate health care systems.
- The nursing care partner is a person to help problem solve and is an advocate during crisis.
- The goals of the Nursing care Partnership are empowerment of the individuals and agencies involved.

BOX 11-1
DENVER NURSING PROJECT IN HUMAN CARING MISSION STATEMENT

THE CARING CENTER

The Denver Nursing Project in Human Caring (Caring Center) is a nurse-directed outpatient community health center offering a broad range of programs and services for persons affected by HIV/AIDS.

Mission Statement

The first mission and top priority of The Denver Nursing Project in Human Caring is facilitation of high quality health care of HIV-positive clients and their lovers, friends, families, and designated others who make up their support systems. Such health care is based on respect for each person and belief that health and well being are multidimensional—including physical, emotional, mental, spiritual, and the social components. Every person is unique and has the right and responsibility to make informed choices concerning health. Each also possesses inner resources and strengths to meet health challenges. Through establishment of authentic caring relationships, the DNPHC staff and clients encourage self-acceptance, self-love, and self-empowerment. The staff belief is that the healing process is fostered by the understanding, love, and concern of those who care.

Education is the second mission of the DNPHC. Education is the foundation for competent care of others as well as care of oneself. Clients and staff continue to share openly their knowledge and experience as greater understanding develops about the spectrum of HIV-induced health changes. DNPHC staff and clients also serve as resource persons for various education programs in the community. In addition to client and family education, training and observational programs for students and professionals from nursing and other health-related disciplines are provided at the Center.

The third mission of the DNPHC is to foster professional health care practices based on research findings. This includes staying abreast of the professional literature, participating in research conferences, initiating nursing research, and cooperating with other disciplines and agencies as appropriate in the conduct of research. DNPHC is also committed to demonstrating and disseminating information regarding the cost-effectiveness of the nursing center model.

Nursing practices carried out at the DNPHC are based on Jean Watson's theory of Human Care Nursing. This provides opportunity for ongoing validation of the theory as well as basis for research questions.

Expected client outcomes from the partnership are:

- The client will feel better able to identify needs and utilize appropriate resources.
- The client will have better decision-making and negotiating skills.
- The client will feel better able to care for himself or herself.
- The client will feel that his or her quality of life has improved.

The partnership process involves the following steps:

- An initial interview is held with a nurse who provides information about the center.
- The client is encouraged to "get to know" the DNPHC and its staff and then *to choose* whom he or she would like to have as a care partner.
- The client and nurse mutually establish a freely chosen relationship.
- The client and nurse negotiate their roles in the partnership with the understanding that these roles are flexible and variable depending on the situation (Astorino et al, 1994, pp. 23–24).

Education is an integral aspect of nursing care. In addition a variety of nontraditional healing options (meditation, art therapy, massage, reflexology, etc.) are available.

Charting is designed to reflect the individual as well as the complex nature of the disease. Each entry has a present and future focus (FF). The FF refers to issues the nurse and client are working on or concerns that the nurse has that need follow-up. The carative factors (CF) from Watson's theory are also used in charting. A note is made in the page margin noting which CF was implemented.

Since using Watson's theory, the DNPHC staff have created an eleventh carative factor—medically supportive nursing—to reflect the technical treatment requirements.

The DNPHC has demonstrated its success through client satisfaction, a continued increase in use of the program, and research showing its cost-effectiveness. It has also received six separate awards for excellence in services to the HIV/AIDS community.

SUMMARY

The Theory of Human Caring represents Watson's view of nursing as a caring-healing art and science. Its focus is the transforming, healing power of the human spirit. Through transpersonal caring, the goals of nursing are achieved.

RESEARCH ON CARING

Patients' Views on Caring

CANCER PATIENTS

Larson (1987) believes that caring is the essential and universal concept underlying nursing practice. She also believes that caring requires *mutual perception*—that is, the patient and the nurse must agree on the behaviors that demonstrate caring. She designed a study to examine whether patients and nurses differ in their rankings of nurse caring behaviors. Larson selected hospitalized cancer patients and hospital-based registered nurses giving care to cancer patients as subjects for the study. She selected this population because cancer patients require extensive nursing care and therefore should be good judges of caring behaviors.

Patients and nurses were asked to rank 50 specific nurse caring behaviors using a seven-point rating scale ranging from most important to least important. The behaviors represented the following six categories of caring behaviors:

- is accessible
- explains and facilitates
- comforts
- fosters a trusting relationship
- anticipates
- monitors and follows through

The **patients** identified the following as the ten most important caring behaviors:

1. Knows how to give shots, start IVs, manage equipment.
2. Knows when to call physician.
3. *Gives good physical care to patient.*
4. Gives patient's treatments and medications on time.
5. Checks on patient frequently.
6. Is well organized.
7. *Listens to patient.*
8. *Talks to patient.*
9. *Gives quick response to patient's call.*
10. *Puts patient first, no matter what else happens.*

Only five of these items appear in the top ten behaviors identified by **nurses.** Items 3, 7, 8, 9, and 10 (the italicized items) are on that list.

Nurses listed these five items that patients did not list among their top ten:

1. Allows expression of feelings.
2. Gets to know the patient as an individual.
3. Realizes that patients know themselves best.
4. Touches patient when he or she needs comforting.
5. Is perceptive of patient's needs.

Larson concludes from her data that nurses cannot assume that patients will interpret their behavior as caring. Whereas nurses perceived that a comforting and trusting relationship was indicative of caring, patients perceived nurse behaviors that demonstrated accessibility, monitoring, and following through as most caring.

REHABILITATION PATIENTS

A similar study was conducted with rehabilitation patients as subjects (Keane and Chastain, 1987). These patients were chosen because they too have a long and close contact with nurses. The researchers held two assumptions:

- Satisfaction with nursing care depends on how well patients and nurses agree on which needs are most important.
- Self-care and coping are improved when patients feel that their needs are understood.

The study was designed to identify areas of agreement and disagreement between patient and nurse perceptions of important nurse caring behaviors. The researchers used the same 50 caring behavior items and research method used by Larson (1987).

The data from this study support the conclusion that for patients, the most important caring behaviors are monitoring and following through associated with the skill competency of the nurse. Patients consistently placed expert physical care higher in importance than emotionally supportive care. The researchers emphasize that the greatest implication for practice is the fact that nurses cannot assume patients see their behavior as caring. Nurses must validate the effects of their caring behaviors with patients. Validation can be done through asking the patient what is important or by asking the patient if there is something that could be done to make the care better.

PATIENTS WITH SEVERE MYOCARDIAL INFARCTION

Cronin and Harrison (1988) used a slightly different research approach to study the relative importance of nurse caring behaviors to patients experiencing severe myocardial infarction. The researchers collected data using open-ended questions and a questionnaire. The items on the questionnaire represented seven categories of caring behavior based on Watson's Theory of Human Caring.

The most important nurse caring behaviors identified by these patients are as follows:

1. Know what they are doing.
2. Make me feel someone is there if I need them.
3. Know how to give shots, IVs, etc.
4. Know how to handle equipment (e.g., monitors).
5. Know when it is necessary to call the doctor.
6. Do what they say they will do.
7. Answer my questions clearly.
8. Are kind and considerate.
9. Teach me about my illness.

Despite the use of a different tool to collect patients' perceptions of nurse caring behaviors, the results are similar to those of Larson (1984) and Keane and Chastain (1987). Nurse behaviors most indicative of caring are monitoring the patient's condition and the demonstration of professional competence. It is also important to note that these researchers found no significant differences in perceptions of caring behaviors based on age, sex, educational level, or length of hospital stay.

PATIENTS IN AN ACUTE CARE HOSPITAL

When asked to comment on the quality of nursing care, a satisfied patient will make a statement similar to "The nurses really *care about* me." Paternoster (1988) interviewed patients in an acute care hospital to determine the nursing behaviors associated with the phrase *care about.* Five nurse caring behaviors were identified from interview data:

- **solicitude.** Showing concern, being careful and attentive. The nurse who is solicitous actively seeks out the patient and offers assistance.
- **dependability.** Patients defined this behavior with phrases such as: "They are there when you need something," "She follows through," and "She says 'I'll be back' and she means it."
- awareness of and **attention to the patient's comfort needs.** Patients cited things such as straightening the bed as indicative of this behavior.
- **affect.** Patients placed importance on the nonverbal affective behaviors of the nurse such as being friendly, smiling, and being cheerful.
- willing **acceptance of the responsibilities** of the caring relationship. Patients described this behavior with phrases such as: "She gives a little extra," "I realize that she is doing her job but she goes one step beyond," and "Those nurses who don't care about you. . . . (they) just do the job."

Paternoster concludes that "this study has shown that patients know when nurses care about them and they value caring. One woman, when asked if she thought that feeling cared about was important to getting well, said "Positively! Ninety percent of getting well is nursing care . . . When you are ill you need a human touch." (p. 21).

PATIENTS IN GENERAL

Warren (1988) published a critique and synthesis of results from nine research studies designed to determine what care is and what it means to patients. Table 11–1 presents her synthesis of those aspects of caring mentioned as important by patients, nurses, and the general population.

TABLE 11–1 Aspects of Caring Mentioned as Important by Patients, Nurses, and the Public

Aspects of Caring	Mentioned by: Patients	Nurses	The Public
does extra things	X	X	X
is accessible	X		X
knows procedures	X	X	X
knows when to call MD	X	X	X
responds quickly	X		
gives good physical care	X	X	X
gives care on time	X		
gives care gently	X		
gives care carefully	X		
checks patient often	X		
does assessments	X	X	
listens	X	X	X
talks	X	X	
shares	X		X
is well organized	X		
does health teaching	X	X	
is an advocate	X		
shows concern	X	X	X
expresses hope	X	X	
touches	X	X	X
uses humor, laughter	X	X	
has good relationship with patient	X	X	
builds self-esteem	X	X	
is considerate	X		
is understanding	X		
recognizes, uses patient's knowledge	X		
supports individuality, independence	X		
assists with pain	X	X	
supplies resources (teaching, referrals, etc)		X	
plans for the future		X	
aware of safety		X	
collaborates		X	
counsels		X	
conforms to preconceived role expectations			X

Modified from Warren, L.D. (1988). Review and synthesis of 9 nursing studies on care and caring. Journal of the New York State Nurses Association, December 19(4), 10–16.

It is clear from the studies presented that patients have clear, consistent perceptions of nurse caring behavior. Patients want nurses to demonstrate professional competence and attend to their physical care needs with a positive, genuine affect. When it comes to caring behaviors, patients seem to agree that "actions speak louder than words."

Caring from the Nurse's Perspective

THEMES FROM NURSING PRACTICE

Kahn and Steeves (1988) conducted open-ended interviews with 25 nurses entering a graduate program. Three questions guided the analysis of the transcripts from the interviews:

- What is the meaning of caring?
- What conditions elicit caring?
- What conditions limit caring?

Four themes emerged from the analysis, each containing categories of items as to what caring is and what it is not.

One theme from the interviews related to the background or context of caring. Over half of those interviewed expressed the notion that caring is essential to the *identity* of the nurse. From this perspective, nurses said that caring:

- underlies professional identity
- requires seeing persons as unique individuals
- requires compassion and empathy
- involves relationships that are therapeutic

They also noted that caring is limited by the need to maintain objectivity.

The second theme to emerge from the interviews was the relationship between *liking* and caring. From this perspective, nurses said that caring:

- is characterized by "fitting with" someone
- is evaluated in terms of liking someone
- includes friendship
- is reciprocated through personal recognition

The nurses noted that the absence of caring is characterized by a mutual inability to get along or by animosity.

A third theme that emerged concerned the actual practices of nurses. Nurses said that caring includes:

- physical nursing interventions
- nonphysical nursing actions
- insisting on patient independence
- actions that improve conditions for patients
- nursing actions related to communication
- being an advocate and liaison

The nurses noted that the absence of caring is indicated by performing in a routine way.

The fourth theme that was elicited from the interviews was the attributions for caring, i.e., the reasons nurses were able or unable to establish caring relationships. Caring is elicited when:

- patients are in dire circumstances
- patients have multiple psychosocial problems
- patients rely on the nurse
- patients are alert and personable
- the nurse can make a temporal investment

Caring is limited by:

- temporal circumstances
- factors that are the nurse's responsibility (a nurse cannot care with the same intensity for every person)
- patients' actions that cause problems
- patients' unwillingness to communicate
- patients' poor self-image

All of this information is helpful in understanding the dimensions of caring from the perspective of experienced nurses. However, the fourth theme regarding attributions for caring warrants emphasis. Nurses found it "easier" to care for patients who were very dependent or were outgoing and personable. Patients who were seen as demanding, constantly calling, dirty, and as having other negative qualities were found difficult to like.

Another study (Baer and Lowery, 1987) conducted with nursing students produced similar results. Students were asked to describe a patient they liked caring for and one they did not like caring for. Ninety-eight percent of the students could identify a patient they liked caring for, and 80 percent could describe a patient they did not like caring for. Liking to care for was not associated with physical attractiveness or any demographic characteristic (age, sex, and so on) of the patient. Students liked to care for patients who were cheerful, communicative, responsive to care, and required significant amounts of care (incontinent, in pain, or depressed). They disliked caring for patients who did not want them around, treated them as servants, or who shouted or yelled at them. Patient responsiveness to care seemed to be the crucial factor in a student liking or not liking to care for a patient. It is important to note that students did not indicate they did not like the patient; the focus was on "caring for."

If caring is the essence of nursing as identified in the first theme, then is it not important to care irrespective of the traits of the patient? This discrepancy between the ideal (caring is the essence of nursing) and the real (nurses care for some patients but not all patients) is a significant part of the difficulty in applying the concept of caring within the practice of nursing.

THE DIFFICULT PATIENT

Probably every nurse has had an experience similar to the one described in these reflections (Masson, 1996, p. 33):

> Not so many years ago in the glare of a modern hospital room, I stood by a bed with an egg in my hand, ordered by an implacable patient to take it back to the kitchen and inform the chef he'd cooked it too long. Boiling inside I wanted to ask if he thought the dietary staff should be bothered with minutiae and what did he take me for—a maid? Keeping my wits, I went off with the egg, came back with another, and placed it next to the toast and bagged Lipton's tea on the plastic breakfast tray.

Imagine me nursing the ill-tempered invalid mindfully, and with grace in the face of injured professional pride.

By focusing on what the patient felt he needed, this nurse was able to continue to care for him even though there were characteristics of the patient she did not like. Many nurses handle patients who are difficult to care for in this same way.

CONTROVERSIES ABOUT CARING

WHAT ARE THE DIFFERING PERSPECTIVES ON CARING IN NURSING PRACTICE?

Despite significant research and theory development, the concept of care and its role in the practice of nursing remains elusive. Analysis of the nursing literature produced five perspectives on the nature of caring (Morse et al, 1990):

- **Caring as a human trait influenced by experiences and learning.** In this perspective caring is seen as an innate human trait, a part of human nature, and essential to all human existence.
- **Caring as a moral imperative or ideal.** In this perspective caring is seen as a fundamental value or moral ideal. It is not a set of behaviors such as providing support. It is adherence to the commitment to maintain the individual's dignity and integrity.
- **Caring as an effect.** In this perspective caring is seen as an empathetic feeling for the patient experience.
- **Caring as the nurse-patient interpersonal relationship.** In this perspective caring is seen as the interaction between the nurse and the patient.
- **Caring as a therapeutic intervention.** In this perspective caring is seen as the implementation of specific nursing actions or even as all nursing actions.

Clearly, nurses are expected **to care.** However, the nurse in the clinical setting is caught between conflicting views on what that means and how to do it. Of particular concern is the

CURRENT CONTROVERSY
DOES COMMUNITY-BASED NURSING REQUIRE A DIFFERENT CONCEPTION OF CARING?

Nurses must, of course, "care" in community-based practice, but the focus and nature of that care cannot be limited to those one knows personally or those "with whom one has established some 'close' or intimate relationship."

. . . the focus of community-based nursing is building and developing the health of *communities.* As such, nurses must care about what happens to groups of citizens, as well as particular clients. A more suitable ethical paradigm for practice in this setting is one that is not solely dependent on particular relationships or "engrossment" in the life and circumstances of particular others.

Nurses can work on problems of distribution of health and related services such as housing, protection from violence, nutrition, and public assistance programs. Nurses can be spokespersons and advocates. They can bring to the attention of local-, county-, and state-level policy makers the need for essential services by those either locked out of, or invisible to, the system. Nurses can help both elected officials and the electorate understand and value the public health agenda. Working through community organizations and more directly with local government and voluntary agencies, nurses can help empower communities to address distribution problems. They can identify aggregates in the community (elderly, youth, minority groups) and involve them in planning and problem solving to increase the distribution of resources where the resources are most needed. Nurses can collect and analyze data and advocate or negotiate with policy makers for needed resources on behalf of groups that are unable to negotiate for themselves. There is need, for instance, for nurses to talk with policy makers about the necessity in their community for services to address protective and mental health needs of children, or clinics to serve minority women in neighborhoods where they have support systems, or immunization clinics to target children at highest risk.

Nurses can activate communities to be concerned about problems that affect the community as a whole. They can form partnerships with special interest groups and coalitions in the community to ensure clean air, water, soil, and food; improve emergency services; reduce occupational hazards; provide shelter for the homeless; assist the elderly; improve nutritional services; reduce violence; and increase awareness of racism and xenophobia. Nurses can lend these groups the benefits of their knowledge of community assessment and health interventions and their experience working with high-risk groups. In short, nurses can work in partnership with the community to empower and teach communities to be healthy.

Nurses can work not only to improve the just distribution of common resources, but to reduce barriers to access as well. Often, clients are unable to access services because of isolation, lack of transportation, and lack of awareness of what is available. Nurses can improve access to care within existing programs and program budgets by using and teaching others to use caring interventions. Attention to the special needs of individuals, families, and communities in ways that reduce barriers to access is an important ethical component of community-based practice.

Chafey, K. (1996). "Caring" is not enough: Ethical paradigms for community-based care. *Nursing and Health Care 17*(1), 10–15.

conflict between the view that caring is an interaction process and the view that caring is the actions/interventions of the nurse. This conceptual muddle surrounding caring needs to be sorted out quickly so that nurses can have the guides to practice that they need.

HOW WILL CHANGES IN THE HEALTH CARE SYSTEM AFFECT CARING IN NURSING PRACTICE?

Most of the nursing literature regarding caring assumes a one-on-one nurse-patient relationship. With the restructuring of the health care system toward community-based care, less and less care will be delivered one on one (one provider caring for one patient) and more care will be focused on groups and communities. Does community-based nursing practice require a different conception of caring? At least one nurse leader thinks so (see Current Controversy).

GIVEN INCREASING CONSTRAINTS ON THEIR TIME WITH PATIENTS, CAN NURSES FIND THE TIME TO CARE?

Nurses are told to care—but are they given *time* to care? Reverby (1987) has written about the dilemma of caring from this perspective. In the introduction to her book, she states:

> Although much has been written about caring from the perspective of individual nurse-patient relationships, its historical consequences for nursing as a whole have rarely been studied. This book examines the failure of our society to create the conditions under which the desire to care can be valued. Nurses, whatever else can be charged against them, continuously try to meet their obligations to care. Nurses have, however, confronted a series of limitations—of imagination, of cultural ideology, of economics, and ultimately of political power—in their efforts to care.

Reverby's position is that nurses have been instructed to care and want to care but have found the clinical setting lacking in support for caring. Hospital staffing formulas are based on tasks excluding or minimizing the importance of time to express caring. Home health care visits are analyzed in terms of reimbursable interventions—caring is not a reimbursable intervention. Clinic visits are timed on the basis of an expectation of seeing a new client every 10 to 12 minutes. There is no time to focus on caring.

In a health care system driven by the economic "bottom line," nurses must be prepared to argue the case for time to care. The first step in preparing the argument is documenting the relationship between time to care and health outcomes for the patient.

FORMULATING A PERSONAL PERSPECTIVE

Much has been written about the nature of caring and its importance to the practice of nursing. Yet there is no prescription for how a nurse cares. Within the practice of nursing caring may be an attitude, a process, a behavior, an ethical or moral perspective, or an intervention. It may be all of the above. The research literature suggests three guides:

- It is the **behavior** of the nurse that makes the patient sense caring or the lack of it.
- The nurse cannot assume that the patient senses caring without **validating** that with the patient.
- Caring always needs to be combined with clinical knowledge (Box 11–2).

These three guides apply in any setting where a nurse and patient interact—home, school, work site, or hospital. The specific behaviors that make a patient feel caring are likely to be different in different settings. In the hospital the patient is very dependent on the nurse. In that setting caring may take the form of excellent physical care and attentive monitoring. In their own home, a person may not feel that same dependency and therefore caring may be demonstrated with different behaviors. It may take the form of active listening or creative problem solving. When the patient is not acutely ill, caring may take the form of educating the patient for self-care.

In addition to understanding the nature of caring within the context of nursing practice, the nurse must be willing to care. As Gaut (1993, p.170) states:

> We can transform the present and future by reawakening to the potential within us for caring. One by one, we can choose to awaken to a universal source of all caring. Awakening brings its own assignments, unique to each of us. Whatever you may think about yourself, and however long you may have thought it, you are not just you. You are a seed—a silent promise . . . Our own thoughts and actions determine how deeply caring is experienced and how widely it is shared. We become the means of caring and peace when we become living representatives of what we study, practice, and research.

This chapter has provided a framework of caring to be used, evaluated, and modified as part of the process of practicing nursing. Caring is a set of behaviors, an attitude, specific interventions, a process, and a moral directive. It is what is done and how it is done. It is the essence of nursing, and yet nursing is more than caring. Others can help understand the concept of caring, yet the individual nurse is the only one who can commit to caring. It is important that as one practices nursing, there is continuous reflection on the concept of care and the courage to develop one's own way of caring.

BOX 11-2

BLENDING EXPERT KNOWLEDGE AND CARING

Donna Allen, RN, and Debra Lee Swett, RN.
Mercy Hospital, Portland, Oregon

Historically, postanesthesia nursing practice has focused on insuring the patient's safe and complete recovery from the effects of anesthesia and surgery. Although the fundamentals of this practice have not changed, a more sophisticated understanding about the patient's vulnerability and dependency during anesthesia emergence has evolved.

Expert postanesthesia nurses provide a sense of situation for patients and facilitate understanding of the rapidly changing postoperative course.[1] At a time when the presence of family and friends is limited, the nurse sustains patients through the confrontation of existential issues precipitated by a surgical experience. These issues are centered around fear of the unknown, loss of control, and fear of dying.

Patients emerging from the effects of anesthesia are not in a position to negotiate their own care. They cannot express the personal and particular aspects of their situations that call forth the nurse's response. Expert postanesthesia care nurses understand that patients' coping abilities will be determined by the meaning they assign to the experience. Therefore, the relationship out of which this information comes must be established in the preoperative period. The following exemplar regarding a patient undergoing maxillofacial surgery illustrates this point.

I could sense the tension when I walked into the room. Laura was sitting in the corner chair in street clothes. Her mother and husband were with her. Laura's hands were clenched tightly, her chin was quivering, and her head was bent down. I introduced myself, but she did not respond. Her family seemed equally anxious. Laura's husband was walking around the room and her mother was crying. Her mother asked several questions about the surgical procedure and the recovery room. Laura started to sob. Her husband asked her to "stop whining." Clearly, Laura needed more support. Her fear was so real that she could not hear what I was saying.

I called the operating room (OR) and requested that Laura's physician come and talk with her and the family. The physician came promptly, bypassed Laura, and talked with her mother and husband. Laura had lost control of any decision making. I directed myself toward her needs. I explained that I would be present when she awoke, I would be with her in the postanesthesia care unit (PACU) and that she would go through the procedures with my assistance and support, emphasizing that there would be no surprises. She finally spoke. "Please don't leave me alone. I need your help."

Laura's family left the room while she changed into an OR gown and she seemed calmer. I accompanied Laura to the OR and remained with her through intubation. She was frightened by the noises and sights in the OR.

Three hours later the OR called. Laura was coming into the PACU intubated. I had worked around my earlier assignments to ensure my availability as Laura's primary nurse.

Laura had an uneventful anesthetic and emergence. She recognized my voice and squeezed my hand. Her jaws were wired shut. She had a moderate amount of bloody oral drainage and moderate facial swelling. The first two hours went well. Laura remained relaxed without sedation. I knew if she were oversedated, extubation would be difficult.

I started to prepare Laura for extubation. By this time, she was pushing secretions to the front of her mouth and was free of pain and, most importantly, nausea. Writing was her form of communication. She explained that she did not want to be extubated. She feared choking and maybe death. Her eyes expressed much fear. I had a natural concern about her airway and her anxiety increased my fear. If she panicked after extubation, she could clamp down her airway and become hypoxic or take a quick breath and aspirate. However, if I did not extubate her, she would rely on the safety of the endotube and not progress. I chose to extubate her using positive pressure, forcing a cough on extubation, and moving residual secretions out with the tube.

Immediately, I began teaching Laura to suction herself. It took a while to master oral suctioning around braces and a wired jaw. She still required intensive nursing care. Occasionally, she would begin to panic, but her SAO_2 remained at 96 per cent. She needed to learn how to assess her airway, when to suction, and how to shift reliance from me to herself. I kept her 3 to 4 hours longer until she became comfortable.

My next concern was the family's reaction to Laura's edematous face. I called the nursing unit and suggested they stay in the waiting room until Laura was settled in bed. This gave me an opportunity to explain Laura's appearance and try to set a calm tone for their visit. This would be essential to Laura's response. It worked.

Vulnerability and increased dependency are common issues for patients having surgery and anesthesia. Postanesthesia nurses understand the essence of their practice as establishing trust, creating a safe environment, and blending expert clinical knowledge with caring practices when patients are unable to speak and act for themselves.

Reference

1. Benner P, Wrubel J: The Primacy of Caring. Menlo Park, CA, Addison-Wesley, 1989.

(From *Journal of Professional Nursing*, Vol 6, No 4 (July–August), 1990: p 195.)

CHAPTER HIGHLIGHTS

- Patients and nurses agree that informed caring is a core element of nursing practice.
- Leininger's Theory of Culture Care and Watson's Theory of Human Care are widely used in nursing practice.
- Research on caring has helped identify behaviors that communicate caring to the patient. Such behaviors include giving skillful physical care on time, checking the patient's condition frequently, listening to the patient, talking to the patient, being well organized, and putting the patient first.
- Patients and nurses evaluate caring behaviors differently.
- Despite significant research and theory development, the concept of care and its role in nursing practice has multiple meanings and perspectives.

REFERENCES

Astorino, G., Hecomovich, K., Jacobs, T., et al (1994). The Denver Nursing Project in Human Caring. In J. Watson (ed.): *Applying the Art and Science of Human Caring.* New York: National League for Nursing Press, pp. 19–38.

Baer, E.D., Lowery, B.J. (1987). Patient and situational factors that affect nursing students' like or dislike of caring for patients. *Nursing Research, 36* (5), 298–302.

Cameron, C., Luna, L. (1996). Leininger's transcultural nursing model. In J. J. Fitzpatrick and A. L. Whall (eds.): *Conceptual Models of Nursing,* 3rd ed. Stamford, CT: Appleton & Lange, pp. 183–198.

Cronin, S.N., Harrison, B. (1988). Importance of nurse caring behaviors as perceived by patients after myocardial infarction. *Heart and Lung, 17* (4), 374–380.

Gaut, D.A. (1993). Caring: a vision of wholeness for nursing. *Journal of Holistic Nursing, 11* (2), 164–171.

George, J.B. (1995). Madeline M. Leininger. In J.B. George (ed.): *Nursing Theories,* 4th ed. Norwalk, CT: Appleton & Lange, pp. 373–390.

Kahn, D.L., Steeves, R.H. (1988). Caring and practice: construction of the nurse's world. *Scholarly Inquiry for Nursing Practice, 2* (3), 201–221.

Keane, S., Chastain, B. (1987). Caring: Nurse-patient perceptions. *Rehabilitation Nursing, 12* (4), 182–184.

Larson, P.J. (1987). Comparison of cancer patients' and professional nurses' perceptions of important nurse caring behaviors. *Heart and Lung, 16* (2), 187–193.

Leininger, M. (1990). Historic and epistemologic dimensions of care and caring with future directions. In *Knowledge About Care and Caring.* Washington, DC: American Academy of Nursing, pp. 19–32.

Leininger, M.M. (Ed.). (1991). *Culture care diversity and universality: A Theory of nursing.* New York: National League for Nursing Press.

Leininger, M. (1993). Culture Care Theory: The Comparative Global Theory to Advance Human Care Nursing Knowledge and Practice. In D.A. Gaut (ed.): *A Global Agenda for Caring.* New York: National League for Nursing, pp. 3–18.

Leininger, M.M. (1984). *Care: The Essence of Nursing and Health.* Thorofare, NJ: Slack.

Masson, V. (1996). Art in practice: The attentive nurse. *Nursing in Health Care, 17* (1), 32–33.

Mayeroff, M. (1971). *On Caring.* New York: Harper & Row.

Morris, D.L. (1996). Watson's theory of caring. In J.J. Fitzpatrick and A.L. Whall (eds.): *Conceptual Models of Nursing,* 3rd ed. Stamford, CT: Appleton & Lange, pp. 289–304.

Morse, J.M., Solberg, S.M., Neander, W.L., et al (1990). Concepts of caring and caring as a concept. *Adv Nurs Sci, 13* (1), 1–14.

Paternoster, J. (1988). How patients know that nurses care about them. *Journal of the New York State Nurses Association, 19* (4), 17–21.

Reverby, S. M. (1987). *Ordered to Care: The Dilemma of American Nursing, 1850–1945.* Cambridge: Cambridge University Press.

Styles, M.M., Moccia, P. (1993). *On Nursing: A Literary Celebration.* New York: National League for Nursing.

Talento, B. (1995). Jean Watson. In J.B. George (ed.): *Nursing Theories.* 4th ed. Norwalk, CT: Appleton and Lange, pp. 317–334.

Warren, L.D. (1988). Review and synthesis of nine nursing studies on care and caring. *Journal of the New York State Nurses Association, 19* (4), 10–16.

Watson, J. (1979). *Nursing: The Philosophy and Science of Care.* Boston: Little Brown.

Watson, J. (1985). *Nursing: Human Science and Human Care: A Theory of Nursing.* Norwalk, CT: Appleton-Century-Crofts.

Watson, J. (1988). *Nursing: Human Science and Human Care: A Theory of Nursing.* New York: National League for Nursing.

12 Clinical Decision Making

Carol Lindeman

OBJECTIVES

After studying this chapter, students will:

- **have practiced the "thinking" skills involved in clinical decision making**
- **be prepared to use the major systems for classifying patients' problems, nursing interventions, and patients' outcomes in the clinical decision-making process**
- **be able to participate in developing critical pathways and total quality management processes as aids to clinical decision making**
- **be ready to apply this information and further develop clinical decision-making skills in the clinical setting**

Nursing practice is "thoughtful doing." The *thoughtful* part of the process is called *clinical decision making.* Clinical decision making involves decisions regarding what care to provide, how to provide that care, where care should be given, and what outcomes to use to evaluate the care. The process requires a range of thinking skills such as inductive and deductive reasoning, critical thinking, and creativity. The clinical decision-making abilities of the nurse, more than any other factor, determine the quality of care. Although this has always been true, it is more evident in today's cost-conscious health care environment.

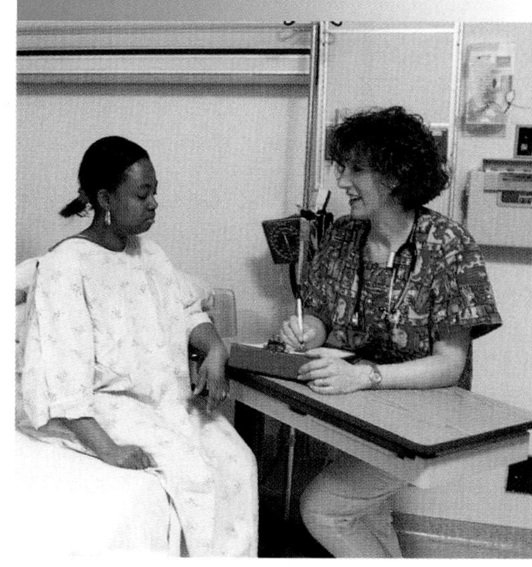

In the health care system of the twenty-first century, nurses will use clinical decision-making skills as they:

- take the lead role in developing clinical pathways and protocols to ensure cost-efficient management of patients across settings
- serve as care coordinators with a variety of lesser-trained caregivers
- case manage to reduce costs and integrate the care of other health professionals
- provide primary care to and manage the care of the chronically ill
- implement community-based initiatives in health promotion and disease prevention
- provide, monitor, and evaluate care using high technology for the high-risk, acutely ill patient
- create partnerships with patients to develop appropriate plans of care
- balance what is good for the individual patient with what is good for the greatest number of people

Because of the importance of clinical decision-making skills within nursing practice, each chapter in Unit IV begins with a case study illustrating nursing practice specific to the knowledge base presented in that chapter. Also, each chapter includes a clinical decision-making scenario to highlight the thought surrounding application of that knowledge.

Contemporary nursing practice is *not*:

- a random set of activities directed toward a vague outcome
- a set of rules and procedures applied to an individual without thought

HISTORICAL PERSPECTIVE

The Era of Linear Thinking

To fully appreciate the nature of clinical decision making for the health care system of the twenty-first century, it must be considered in the larger social context. For most of the second half of the twentieth century people viewed social systems as stable and predictable. It was assumed that through objective analysis (i.e., the scientific method), systems, including the human system, could be understood and even controlled. A linear mechanistic framework was used to describe and discuss the problems encountered in both professional and personal worlds. For example, organizations (and people) were to run like "well-oiled machines." If there was a problem, the organization (or person) would be reduced to a set of parts, the problem located and fixed. It was assumed that if one fixed a part, the whole would be fine.

In health care this linear mechanistic framework led health care providers to think of people as the "broken hip" in room 317 or the "head injury" in bed 3. A symptom or disease rather than the person was the focus of care. If a treatment did not work, only the "broken part" was studied for insight. Medical research reduced people to molecular levels seeking cause and effect with the expectation that clinicians could apply that research directly to the whole person.

The Nursing Process

Nursing practice also incorporated a linear mechanistic view of people (Kobert and Folan, 1990). From the mid 1960s through the early 1990s "the nursing process" served as the framework for nursing practice. Initially the process consisted of four phases: assessment, planning, implementation, and evaluation. In the mid 1970s, a fifth step, diagnosis, was added. The phases/steps became: assessment, diagnosis, planning, implementation, and evaluation. This stepwise linear approach served to guide and document nurses' thought processes. Because this nursing process is still used in some nursing settings, it is summarized in this text.

OVERVIEW

In the first step of the nursing process, *assessment,* the nurse collects information regarding the patient and the patient's family and environment. This is done in a systematic manner using the nursing history, physical examination, laboratory results, and other sources of information such as previous medical records. The purpose of assessment is to identify the patient's needs and problems.

In the second step, *diagnosis,* the nurse critically analyzes and interprets the information gathered during the assessment. The conclusions made regarding the patient's needs and problems are translated into *nursing diagnoses.* These diagnoses serve as the basis for the plan of care.

The third step involves *planning* nursing care. In this step, the nurse determines appropriate nursing actions for each of the identified nursing diagnoses. Depending on the number of diagnoses, the nurse may have to establish priorities among them. As the nurse determines the appropriate nursing actions, the outcomes of that action are also made explicit. This step ends with a written plan of care. The plan of care includes the nursing diagnoses, the nursing actions or interventions, and the desired patient outcomes.

The fourth step in the nursing process is *implementation* of the plan of care. The nurse shares the plan with the patient and family if appropriate and with other members of the nursing staff. The nurse is accountable for implementation but may delegate aspects of the plan to others, including the patient. This step also involves (1) collecting information regarding changes in the patient's condition, (2) documenting the care that has been given, and (3) documenting the patient's response to the care.

The fifth step is *evaluation.* The nurse is accountable for evaluating the outcomes of the care and making changes as necessary. This step continues for as long as the patient is in the care of the nurse.

ILLUSTRATION

Picture a nurse admitting a resident to a long-term care facility. The nurse notes that the resident (1) is very thin with prominent elbow bones, (2) wants to stay in bed, and (3) has very dry skin. This information leads the nurse to the diagnosis "High Risk for Impaired Skin Integrity." The plan of care lists this diagnosis along with the proposed nursing actions:

- Encourage resident to move in bed and spend time out of bed.
- Encourage resident to drink water—at least 7 glasses a day.
- Check daily for signs of skin breakdown.

The care plan contains the notation that the goal is to prevent skin breakdown.

The nurse informs all members of the nursing staff about the plan of care and delegates to the staff providing personal care the responsibility to encourage the resident to spend time out of bed and to ensure the resident drinks water frequently. The nurse will continue to monitor the skin and the plan of care to prevent skin breakdown. The nurse records observations and outcomes of care in the patient record.

CRITIQUE

The nursing process served a useful purpose for nursing. When nursing practice was simply implementing the orders written by physicians, there was no need for a framework for organizing nursing care. When nursing practice included actions independent of physicians' orders, a framework for identifying and communicating those decisions was needed. The nursing process became that framework.

Although many found the nursing process a useful framework, it has been the subject of considerable criticism within the discipline. For example, Virginia Henderson, recognized throughout the world for her contributions to nursing, stated (1982, p. 109):

> Use of the term nursing process, as I have known it, is traced from the 1950s, when I heard it discussed as a way of describing client-nurse communication conducive to mutual understanding, until the present when it is used to mean problem-solving by the nurse for the benefit of the patient. As usually interpreted, the term involves a nursing history, a nursing diagnosis of physical, but particularly psychosocial, problems, a plan for nursing intervention and evaluation of its effect. These steps seem to be taken independently of comparable activities by other health professionals, most notably physicians, with the nurse in an independent rather than an interdependent relationship with other health care providers.
>
> While the nursing process recognizes the purpose of the problem-solving aspects of the nurses' work, a habit of inquiry and the use of the investigative techniques in developing the scientific basis for nursing, **it ignores the subjective or intuitive aspect of nursing and the role of experience, logic and expert opinion as bases for nursing practice. In stressing a dominant and independent function for the nurse, it fails to stress the value of collaboration of health professionals and particularly the importance of developing the self-reliance of clients.**

The nursing process has also been criticized for its reductionist approach to patient care (Kobert and Folan, 1990). By conducting the patient through a series of steps, the nurse is forced to think in terms of components of the body rather than of the whole human being. Holism, a concept strongly supported by nursing, is philosophically in opposition to an approach that creates a hierarchy of steps. To proponents of holism, the nursing process is considered incompatible with health-promoting nursing practice (Lindsey and Hartrick, 1996). Table 12–1 compares and contrasts the nursing process and health-promoting nursing practice.

Lindsey and Hartrick (1996) offer a case study to illustrate the outcomes of the two processes. A man with gradually deteriorating spina bifida experienced frequent urinary tract infections requiring hospitalization. While in the hospital, the man felt as though he lost control of his own health and healing practices. In the hospital, the nurse assessed his physical condition, reached an appropriate diagnosis, determined appropriate treatment, and evaluated the treatment's success in terms of the medical problem.

However, even though the urinary tract infection was cured, the man felt "sicker." He attributed his decline in health experience and the interruption in healing to a loss of control in his own decision making. He was physically weakened by the experience of expending energy having to be insistent and assertive about his health needs.

TABLE 12-1 The Characteristics Underlying the Nursing Process Versus the Characteristics Underlying Health-Promoting Nursing Practice

Nursing Process	Health-Promoting Nursing Practice
Medical, behavioral	Socio-environmental
Problem-focused	Health-focused
Problem-solving	Health promotion
Structure that requires conformity	Structure that supports and allows for openness, fluidity
Nurse as expert	Nurse as facilitator
Health professional prediction and control	Client-centered control
Client as participant	Client as expert
Clinical judgment	Enhancing understanding
Cyclical process	Synergistic, expansionist process
Providing professional opinion/advice	Fostering reflection, drawing forth the client's resources
Control	Empowerment
Problem identification	Recognition of patterns and themes
Assessment and diagnosis, collecting data, seeking information	Engagement, active listening, telling narrative, participatory dialogue
Planning	Co-creating meaning, envisioning, reimagining
Intervening	Critical questioning, reflection, action
Evaluating	Reflecting on action, critical questioning and making changes (praxis)

From Lindsey, E., et al (1996). Health-promoting nursing practice: The demise of the nursing process? *Journal of Advanced Nursing, 23,* 106–112. Reprinted with permission.

Lindsey and Hartrick suggest that if a health-promotion process had instead been followed for this patient, the nurses would have used a participatory process beginning with active listening. The nurses would have found out how the patient cared for himself at home. Critical questions would have been raised by both the nurses and the patient to determine what care was needed and how best it could be provided. The patient would have felt empowered rather than powerless. Through critical reflection on the illness and health experiences, common themes would have been identified to serve as the basis for future care. The patient would not feel "sicker" after his infection was cured; rather, he would be better educated and feel more empowered to care for himself.

Tanner (1996) is critical of the nursing process because it does not resemble the thought processes used by skilled clinicians. Based on years of research, she states (1996, p. 1):

> The clinical judgment of experienced nurses resembles much more the engaged, practical reasoning first described by Aristotle than the disengaged, scientific or theoretical reasoning represented in the nursing process. Experienced nurses reach an understanding of a person's experience with an illness, and hence their responses to it, not through abstract labeling such as nursing diagnosis, but rather through knowing the particular patient, his typical pattern of responses, his story and the way

in which illness has constituted his story, and through advanced clinical knowledge, which is gained from experience with many persons in similar situations, and which sensitizes the nurse to possible issues and concerns in this particular situation.

The steps of the nursing process may be helpful to the beginning student, but it is an inadequate framework for contemporary nursing practice.

The Shift to Nonlinear Thought Processes

Today many disciplines including nursing are replacing the linear mechanistic framework with a dynamic nonlinear view of systems including the human system. In a dynamic system (Allen, 1990):

- Things do not progress in a linear predictable way. Instead of a single linear line between cause and effect, there is mutual shaping or interconnectedness. **In nursing practice one would not expect every patient or community to progress the same way. Instead one would expect the patient's or community's context to influence progress. The nurse is part of that context.**
- What appears random on the surface actually has an underlying order and rhythm. It is important to look for patterns and themes. **In nursing practice, expert nurses have been able to save lives because of pattern recognition. By understanding the importance of patterns and being alert to them, they attend to cues that others do not.**
- The whole is more than the sum of its parts. **The human body is more than its physical parts. Emotions, spirit and intelligence are important ingredients in the human being. The result is a human system that is complex and constantly changing. The nurse must consider the whole person or the whole community.**
- Patients and communities are very sensitive to initial conditions. **In nursing practice it is very important to understand the starting point for the patient or community. A community that has had a negative experience with a health care provider will react very differently than one that has not.**
- Problems are not drawn to scale. Little problems may take more time than larger ones. **A patient may be more concerned about a family member than their own health. A patient may be more worried about paying for health care than recovering from an illness.**

Comparison of Linear and Nonlinear Thinking

Linear and nonlinear thinking differ in significant ways, as described in Table 12–2. Contemporary nursing practice requires a nonlinear framework.

TABLE 12–2 Linear Thinking Versus Nonlinear Thinking

Linear Thinking	Nonlinear Thinking
Problems are separate	Problems are connected, solving one will frequently trigger new problems that are related to the old one.
Every problem has a solution	Problems do not always have solution and often return in a different form to be solved again.
Decisions are separate	Decisions are not single events but become a stream of decisions as they respond to constantly changing conditions.
Events are separate	Life is made up of streams of events; events are connected.
How to—product focus	Ways to—process focus

From Allen, KE. (1990). Making Sense Out of Chaos: Leading and Living in Dynamic Systems. *Campus Activities Programming,* May, 54.

CLINICAL DECISION MAKING

The nonlinear framework for nursing practice is **clinical decision making.** In the nursing literature there is no unequivocal definition of clinical decision making (Hamers et al, 1994). The terms clinical decision making, clinical judgment, and clinical inference are used with similar meanings by different authors (Tanner, 1993). As research in this area continues, it is anticipated that the concepts will be clarified and precise definitions developed.

In this text, the phrase **clinical decision making refers to an interactive (nonlinear) complex process of thought and action through which the nurse in partnership with the patient maximize health outcomes by ensuring the delivery of cost-effective services. It requires a range of thinking skills, knowledge, experience, and self-awareness.**

Why Is Clinical Decision Making Complex?

Health and illness are complex human experiences. If one asked classmates or friends to define "health," there would be a range of ideas such as "the absence of illness" or "feeling full of energy." Likewise, if one asked for a definition of illness, there would be varying responses. The appreciation of the importance of the **personal** definition of health and illness is a crucial component of clinical decision making. No two people respond in exactly the same way to any situation involving their health or illness. The personal nature of health and illness is one factor making clinical decision making complex.

Furthermore, maintaining health and recovering from illness is not a simple cause and effect situation. The notion that health and illness can be treated in biomolecular terms—one disease, one gene, one enzyme, one protein, one precise cure—has proven false (Bulger, 1990). There is no precise cure for most of the diseases known to mankind. The health care provider must be able to identify the most appropriate intervention for the individual. The complex nature of the disease process makes clinical decision making complex.

The role of the nurse in today's health care system has changed. Contemporary nursing practice requires the nurse to be a **care manager,** not just a care provider. As a care manager the nurse must be able to (1) implement the most appropriate intervention, (2) at the right time, (3) in the right setting, and (4) with the least cost. Accomplishing the "four rights" of care management requires knowledge and thought processes that are different from those required by the person who only provides care. Practicing nursing in today's cost-sensitive environment has made clinical decision making more complex.

Features of Clinical Decision Making

From narratives of expert clinicians, Tanner (1993) identified six features of clinical decision making:

1. **The role of context and the situation.** The nurse must understand the particulars of the specific patient situation. This occurs through being actively involved with the patient and family. Expert clinicians want to know all they can about the immediate situation as well as obtain the bigger picture.
2. **The role of narrative.** Understanding the situation from the patient's and family's perspective allows the nurse to direct attention not only to the disease but to the human world of meanings, values, and concerns.
3. **The importance of knowing the patient.** There are two components to knowing the patient: (1) knowing the patient's typical pattern of responses; and (2) knowing the patient as a person. Expert clinicians know the patient by being open to that individual's uniqueness.
4. **The role of emotion.** Expert clinicians allow themselves to feel emotions triggered by the patient. They have learned how to avoid overinvolvement, i.e., feeling the pain and suffering of the patient to the point they become ineffective. Instead expert clinicians use their feelings as part of clinical decision making. When they feel the clinical encounter with a patient is not right in some way, they use that feeling to guide their nursing actions.
5. **The role of intuition and reason.** In some situations, expert clinicians will believe something to be true but not be able to provide a rationale. This type of intuition may be related to pattern recognition developed through experience.
6. **The interplay of theoretical knowledge and practical know-how.** Expert clinicians use theory but they use it in a way that complements the knowledge of the particular situation. Theory is a guide not a rule.

Tanner's Model of Clinical Decision Making

Figure 12–1 displays the major components of Tanner's model, which she calls "Interactive Processes of Clinical Judgment in the Context of a Caring Relationship." A first glance at the model underscores the complexity of clinical decision making. Tanner identifies four categories of factors in the model:

- background for practice
- developing an understanding
- responding to the situation
- reflection and evaluation

Having done that, she emphasizes through the use of arrows the interactions among the four categories. For example, reflection is not the fourth step in the process. It must occur throughout the entire process. Evaluation interacts with the background the clinician brings to the situation. The model also highlights the balance between analytic thinking and holistic understanding. The nurse may have a piece of data such as the patient's vital signs. If those data are not put into a holistic context, the nurse may not understand the true significance of the data. The model also highlights that developing an understanding is more than collecting data. There is also intuition and the clinician's emotional responses. Furthermore, all data must still be interpreted and given meaning. Data by themselves are simply data.

This model is a useful guide for the novice clinical decision maker. Assume you are assigned to a particular patient. Think through the points in the model regarding "clinician's background" in terms of yourself and the patient. What practical knowledge do you have that might be important in this case? For example, if the person is older, you may have cared for an elderly relative that gave you practical knowledge. What assumptions do you have about the patient? Again, assume the patient is older. Do you have assumptions about older people that could affect your clinical decision making?

Consider the context for care. Is it in the hospital, the home, the clinic? What constraints might you experience in terms of financial and human resources?

After you have interacted with the patient and reached some understanding of the situation, try to diagram your thought processes. Identify the data that seemed most significant and why. Did you experience any intuitive hunches? If so, how did you respond? What meaning did you give to the data/information you obtained?

What was your response to the situation? Were you satisfied with your conclusions or did you verify them with the patient? Did you explore and negotiate with the patient? How did the patient respond to that process? How did *you* respond to that process? When the encounter was over, what thoughts kept coming back to you? Did you find yourself ruminating over some aspect of the encounter? If so, what troubled you? What would you have done differently? How did this encounter change you in terms of the next patient you care for?

This process of self-critique is essential to the development of clinical decision-making skills.

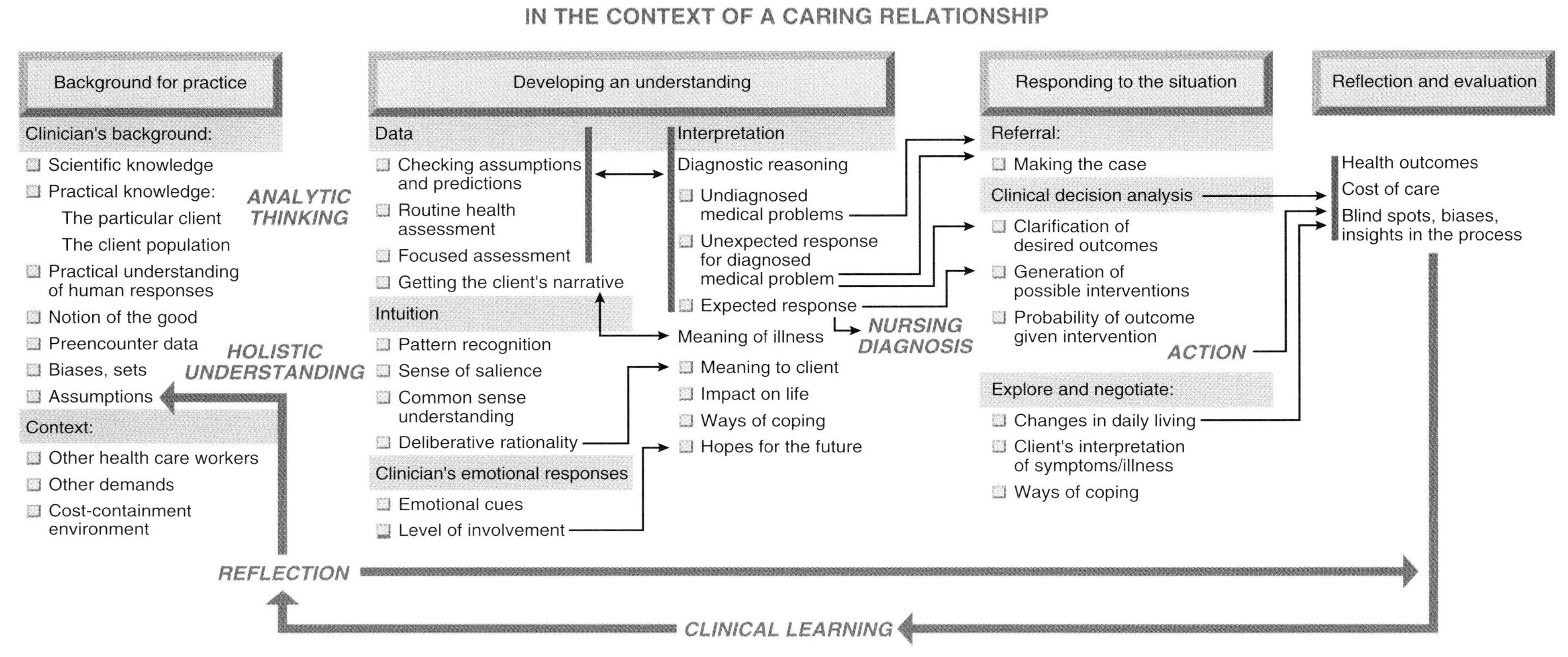

Figure 12-1. Tanner's clinical decision making model.

Descriptors of the Clinical Decision-Making Process

Additional descriptors of the clinical decision-making process are:

- It is a continuous process of conceptualizing and reconceptualizing what is known about a specific patient situation. Every patient and family encounter is used to verify or modify previous clinical decisions.
- It is a continuous process of thought and action. Thinking guides doing and doing guides thinking. Theory informs practice and practice informs theory.
- It empowers the patient and family as partners in the process of care. The nurse listens to how the patient names and frames health and illness concerns. The nurse acknowledges the meaning and significance the patient ascribes to the health situation.
- It is a process driven by **inquiry**, not rules. The process uncovers what is best for a particular patient at a specific point in time.
- Knowledge, experience, intuition, and subjective feelings are used to ascribe meaning and determine action.

Examples of Clinical Decision Making

Because experience is an important component of clinical decision making, the skill of the expert clinician will be significantly different from the skill of the beginning student. In addition to experience, expert clinicians have the self-confidence to trust their subjective feelings and intuition. Beginning students will develop self-confidence with time. However, the beginning student needs to learn to pay attention to subjective feelings and intuitions as an important part of clinical decision making. Box 12–1 presents an example of clinical decision making by a beginning nursing student; Box 12–2, an example by an expert nurse.

Comparison of the Nursing Process and Tanner's Clinical Decision Making Model

Table 12–3 presents a comparison of significant features of the linear nursing process and Tanner's nonlinear clinical decision-making process. Both processes involve assessment, diagnosis, planning, implementation, and evaluation. The differences are in how and when these actions are implemented.

The following points emphasize the differences shown in Table 12–3:

- Nonlinear clinical decision making accepts complexity as necessary to sound decision making. The nursing process eliminates complexity by reducing people to systems or problems.
- Clinical decision making acknowledges the significance of the human, financial, and environmental context of care. The nursing process does not include context as a major factor.
- Clinical decision making requires a range of thinking skills such as reasoning, creativity, and intuition. The nursing process is essentially an inductive reasoning process.
- Clinical decision making calls for ascribing personal meaning to data and the situation. The nursing process calls for the **nurse's** diagnosis.

TABLE 12–3 Nursing Process Versus Clinical Decision Making

Nursing Process	Clinical Decision Making
Reduces person to systems or problems	Maintains a holistic focus
Discipline-specific	Interdisciplinary
Individual as focus	Applicable to family and community Allows balancing what is best for the individual with what is best for the population
Needs-based	Resource-based
Episodic focus	Longitudinal focus
Process focus	Outcome focus
Nursing diagnosis	**Meaning** determined by the patient and situation
Inductive reasoning	Range of thinking skills
Nursing care plan product	Critical pathway, total quality management, or nursing care plan as product

Using a Clinical Decision-Making Process

Over time, a nurse will use the clinical decision-making process with individuals, families, and communities. It will be used when the goal is health promotion as well as when there is an acute illness. Although the process is not a set of unalterable steps, the beginning student can use the following guides:

- Begin the process by focusing on the individual (family or community) and the specific situation. Be aware of personal biases and preconceived ideas that might affect one's ability to see and hear the situation from the patient's perspective.
- Use all sources of information available—assessment data, the patient's or community's narrative, past experience, theoretical knowledge, intuition, subjective feelings.
- Use a range of thinking skills (detailed in the next section of this chapter) and maintain a holistic perspective.
- When possible, let the patient (family or community) take the lead in determining an acceptable plan of care.
- Take time to reflect on the whole situation, allowing its unique features to become clear. Discuss one's

BOX 12-1
MOST CHALLENGING DECISION

C.C. is an 81-year-old man. He is soft-spoken and looks directly at you when he speaks. I met him while taking vital signs of a series of patients. I asked if he would like to chat for awhile, and he replied that he would "be delighted to have someone to talk to." He has been in the V.A. hospital for 10 weeks due to a fractured right hip, which occurred when he slipped and fell while doing laundry. His fall was not caused by dizziness, and he was generally healthy prior to this injury. He says his son is visiting from California. I did not gather more psychosocial data (something I would do next time), but he never mentioned a wife and he lives alone and so I think that he might have a limited support network. He did not seem depressed when I was visiting with him.

The situation that challenged me involves an intervention that I chose not to do. Specifically, I allowed this man to remain in denial about moving to a rest home instead of back to his apartment. Between taking his vital signs and returning for a bedside chat, I had read C.C.'s chart and spoken with his nurse. I was told that he had been extremely upset a few hours ago upon learning that he would not be returning to his downtown apartment, his home for 30 years, as it has a flight of stairs which he now would be unable to negotiate. With this knowledge in mind, I returned to visit with him. Our conversation was general at first. We spoke of the hospital experience and how he disliked the food. He told me about his hip and about an old war injury to his back. I said that I had heard that he would be leaving the following morning, and he said "Yes! Let me tell you about my apartment." I was fairly certain that he was not cognitively impaired. He had been lucid all along, and as far as I could determine, he had no problems recalling short- or long-term memories. He described the living room and his favorite sofa. He told me how it had been his home for 30 years and even said there was a flight of stairs and that he "would manage them somehow." He complained that the only thing he disliked was that the building was old and therefore had "one of those doorbells for people to ring when they want to come up and visit, and it never works and then I don't know they are there . . ." (This is evidence of a support network of friends, and if I could repeat the situation, I would find out more.) I was very sad while he was speaking. I did not know what to do in the moment. I did not want to be the cause of any further unhappiness for him, and my mind kept trying to rationalize this by saying "You are not his nurse. You do not have to force reality on him. Let him enjoy the moment." At the same time, another internal voice was saying to me "Be strong. Don't be a chicken. He needs to confront reality by tomorrow morning, so you might as well try to help him do so now. This is what a nurse's job is."

The actual "in the moment" decision process was an internal struggle for me, and in the end I simply allowed him to continue speaking as though he would be returning to his apartment the next morning. I asked my classmates for their opinion during the evening debriefing session in the hospital conference room. People thought that I had made an appropriate and kind choice, but they were not certain either that it was correct. In the week since this conversation, I have come to the conclusion that every patient presents a somewhat unique situation, but that in general I should most often take the difficult path of helping the patient to confront reality. This is a difficult situation that is faced by many elderly people in our Western culture. However it is framed, it is a sad situation to be forced to leave one's home and go to a care facility. I see some ways that I might have helped this kindly old gentleman to face this situation. By careful use of therapeutic language, I could have encouraged him to explore what he is feeling—is he denying reality because he feels powerless, or is he afraid of being all alone? I might have led him to explore this by saying "Most patients that I know feel a loss of control over their lives when they come to a hospital and find that they cannot return to living life in the same independent way that they are used to. It's a normal reaction to be sad and frustrated and even angry. I wonder if you aren't feeling frustrated, Mr. C." I am not certain how I could help him to find some meaning, hope, or control over his situation, but using open-ended questions to allow him the opportunity to open up and share what he is feeling would be a way to begin. If he had neighbors who could visit, I could remind him of this. If there were activities he has always liked, I could remind him that he can still do those, even though he won't be living at home. (For example, reading and television are always available, as is talking on the telephone.) I would need to know more details of his life before I could find the specific items to use to encourage him.

A most important lesson that I have been reminded of by this experience is that I must continue to explore my own biases—the "context" that I bring into each nursing situation because of my upbringing. I do have an elderly father, and I am sad when I think that he is lonely sometimes. I know that I need to not transfer these feelings to the patient, who is not my father. I will become better at therapeutic communication and at setting boundaries as I go through my training to become a professional nurse, but I believe that serving the elderly population is not where my best strengths and abilities lie. Unless I find some really hidden emotional strength, I think that I will be best at working with a younger patient population with a different set of emotional challenges, although I will look for the learning and growth and giving opportunities that each patient I encounter provides.

BOX 12-2
EXCERPT FROM AN EXPERT REPORTING ON A CLINICAL SITUATION

We had a patient who had been in the operating room having heart surgery. I'd gotten word that he had been hospitalized before, had a very poor heart, and had had multiple infarctions. As I was coming to work that evening, I had also gotten word that his family was sitting and waiting in the waiting room. The patient wasn't back from surgery yet, so I thought I'd go out and meet them, which I try to do when it works out that way. They were stressed to the max; the minute I walked out they jumped off their chairs. They knew I was coming to talk with them. I introduced myself, explained that we really don't hear much until the patient actually gets up to the unit and just talked about what to expect, e.g., that they could come in after an hour or so. They proceeded to tell me this whole story about what this poor man had gone through and how it was so rough on him, and so on.

So the patient returned from surgery, and sure enough, was sick as everything, on every drip known to man, ballooned, had had a real hard time coming off bypass, the whole thing. As I listened to report and went into the room and looked at him, it was clear that it's going to be a miracle if this man leaves the hospital alive. *That was the sense I had. So, I got settled. I went out and had the family come and just tried to give them a sense of what to expect . . . And we just hit it off or something. They needed—it was like they were just looking for this release valve and I gave it to them. At that point we just kind of clicked.*

A few days went by and the patient was really sick, but eventually, amazingly, he kind of turned the corner and we were able to start weaning drips. We were all astonished that this man was alive. . . . he was extubated, he was lucid, and he was talking to me. His grandson came in and visited, and his grandson was his pride and joy. The two of them were going at it. He told me how he got his nickname, what he did with his grandson, went to this ballgame, to that ballgame. *But it was still obvious, even though he looked better, it was really obvious that he was very, very fragile and any little thing was going to tip him over the edge. And another day or so went by . . . it came time to pull his chest tubes and unfortunately he got a pneumothorax and that was all he needed. I knew that any little thing was just going to be his demise, and sure enough he ended up having to get reintubated, chest tubes put back in.*

(Tanner, 1993, pp. 24–25)

thoughts and actions with others as a means to improve care to the patient and the skills of the staff.
- Use the written plan of care as guide—not as a rigid set of rules or procedures.
- The product of clinical decision making may be the creation of an **interdisciplinary critical pathway** (described later) or a nursing care plan (see Chapter 14, Documentation).
- Concerns arising as care is evaluated may be referred for Total Quality Management analysis (described later in this chapter).

An illustration of the nursing process was presented earlier in this chapter. In that situation the nurse made an assessment, diagnosed a problem, created a plan of care, and determined implementation and evaluation. What would have been different if a clinical decision-making process had been used?

First, the nurse would have taken time to understand the person and to hear that individual's narrative. In doing this the nurse would maintain a holistic view of the situation. The nurse would attend to **why** the person wanted to stay in bed, **why** the skin was dry, and **why** the person was thin. The nurse would want to understand how the resident felt about the nursing home. The nurse would want to know more about the individual's typical patterns.

Next, the nurse would engage in interactions with the resident to make that individual feel empowered, in control, and able to participate in self-care. The nurse would not make decisions about the resident or for the resident but rather would become a partner with the resident in determining care.

In addition, the nurse would use thinking processes other than the inductive reasoning of the nursing process. Before creating a plan of care there would be time for creative thinking. If the resident needs to spend less time in bed, how might that be done other than simply "encouraging the resident to move in bed and spend time out of bed"? Could the resident be asked to water the flowers in the day room? What are the resident's usual patterns? Is there any meaningful activity in the nursing home that resembles those? If so, could the resident be asked to do that activity? The nurse might challenge herself to list 20 ways to encourage a person to move in bed and then, in terms of this resident, identify one or two that are most promising.

Furthermore, the nurse would attend to her own feelings. What did her intuition tell her about this resident? Did the resident seem depressed even though there were no obvious signs of depression? Or did the resident seem interested in living? The nurse would use all those feelings and insights as the plan of care was constructed.

The nurse would tell the resident about concerns regarding skin breakdown and educate the resident as the first line of defense against that possibility. The resident would be prepared to assess her own skin.

Finally, the resident and the nurse would agree on outcomes for care. In this instance the outcomes will be more than preventing skin breakdown; they will have a holistic focus. For example, one outcome might be that the resident views the nursing home as her "home away from home." Reaching that outcome might be more powerful in preventing skin breakdown than any other nursing intervention.

With the clinical decision-making process, the plan of care could include:

- Will water flowers in the day room daily.
- Will meet with the nurse daily to share in the assessment of skin.
- Will ask family to bring her favorite chair to the nursing home.
- Will weigh herself weekly and talk with dietitian about eating habits.

At some early point in the clinical decision-making process all members of the interdisciplinary team would meet with the resident and as a team to further develop a single plan of care.

In contrast to the traditional nursing process, clinical decision making emphasizes:

- **the role of the patient's narrative.** Building on that is key to identifying effective interventions.
- **the use of creative thinking along with inductive and deductive reasoning.** There is no one right solution. Many possible ideas should be considered and tried.
- **the use of intuition and emotion.** Important aspects of a situation are not articulated during an interaction with a patient. The nurse's intuition and emotion are the only ways that these aspects can be built into the plan of care.
- **the holistic approach.** The individual is more than the sum of his or her illness needs. Focusing on the total person helps set priorities and outcomes that are of value to the individual.

THINKING SKILLS

The importance of thinking skills in nursing practice cannot be overstated. It is the critical thinking of the nurse that will determine the quality of care (Wolf et al, 1994). In today's health care system, quality nursing care is:

- dependent on the critical thinking skills of the nurse
- focused on the unique needs of each patient
- coupled with creative approaches for meeting those needs

Thus, the thinking skills used in nursing practice must include:

- inductive reasoning
- deductive reasoning
- creativity
- intuition
- critical thinking

Thinking Styles

People think about things in very different ways. Inherited tendencies and early life experiences mold us to favor certain ways of relating to the world, making sense out of it and solving problems. For example, when reading a textbook, one student may first focus on the quality of writing, another student may focus on the table of contents, while yet another student will immediately start reading looking for the main points. Research has identified five distinct styles of thinking, although most people use a mixture of styles (Schwabbauer et al, 1985).

An increasing amount of nursing practice involves the use of interdisciplinary teams and working with groups of patients. Thus, it is important for nurses to understand their own thinking style as well as appreciate differences in styles. The following exercise can help foster this understanding.

EXERCISE 1

Table 12–4 summarizes various styles of thinking (Schwabbauer et al, 1985). Review the chart and determine which style is most like yours. Identify people who fall into the other categories. Which styles are you most comfortable with? Under what circumstances does a particular style trouble you? How will you deal with your discomfort when it occurs within a patient care situation?

These are important understandings and influence your ability to think in collaboration with patients and other health care providers.

Inductive Reasoning

Inductive reasoning moves from observation of specifics to statement of general principles. The nursing process is an inductive reasoning process. In the illustration of the nursing process earlier in the chapter, the nurse noticed specific characteristics of the patient and reached the conclusion the patient was at high risk for skin breakdown.

Inductive reasoning is common in daily living. For example, a friend does not look at you when you enter the room. When you approach her, she turns away. When you speak to her, she answers in an abrupt manner. You conclude she is angry with you. Your observation of specifics led you to a general conclusion.

Inductive reasoning can lead to the acceptance and application of health care technology. Consider the mother who notes that none of her friend's children who were immunized against chickenpox developed the disease. She decides to have her children immunized. A physician notes that breathing equipment designed to produce deep diaphragmatic breathing prevents respiratory complications in surgical patients. He decides to use that same equipment with frail elderly patients with respiratory problems who are bedridden.

These examples may suggest that inductive reasoning is easy and requires little training. That conclusion would be inaccurate and in fact would highlight a concern in inductive reasoning. Without careful attention to certain steps in the

TABLE 12-4 Styles of Thinking

	Synthesist	Idealist	Pragmatist	Analyst	Realist
Orientation					
Characteristics	Integrative view. Seeks conflict and synthesis. Interested in change. Speculative.	Holistic view. Seeks ideal solutions. Interested in values. Receptive.	Eclectic view. Seeks shortest route to payoff. Interested in innovation. Adaptive.	Deductive view. Seeks "one best way." Interested in "scientific solutions." Perceptive.	Empirical view. Seeks solutions that meet current needs. Interested in concrete results. Corrective.
Strengths	Focus on underlying assumptions. Points out abstract conceptual aspects. Good at preventing over-agreement. Best in controversial situations. Provides debate and creativity.	Focus on process and relationships. Points out values and aspirations. Good at articulating goals. Best in value-laden situations. Provides broad view, goals, standards.	Focus on payoff. Points out tactics and strategies. Good at identifying impacts. Best in complex situations. Provides experiment and innovation.	Focus on method and plan. Points out data and details. Good at model building and planning. Best in structured situations. Provides stability and structure.	Focus on facts and results. Points out realities and resources. Good at simplifying, "cutting through." Best in well-defined situations. Provides drive and momentum.
Liabilities	May screen out agreement. May seek conflict unnecessarily. May try too hard for change, newness. May theorize excessively. Can appear uncommitted.	May screen out "hard" data. May delay from too many choices. May try too hard for "perfect solutions." May overlook details. Can appear overly sentimental.	May screen out long-range aspects. May rush too quickly to payoff. May try too hard for expediency. May rely too much on what "sells." Can appear over-compromising.	May screen out values. May over-plan, over-analyze. May try too hard for predictability. May be inflexible, overly cautious. Can appear "tunnel visioned."	May screen out disagreement. May rush to over-simplified solutions. May try too hard for consensus. May over-emphasize perceived "facts." Can appear to be too results-oriented.

From Harrison, AF, Bramson, RM: Styles of thinking. In Schwabbauer M et al (1985). Medical Technologist thinking styles. *Journal of Medical Technology*, 2(8), 517–520.

process, incorrect reasoning is likely to occur, because of the following factors:

- Inductive reasoning requires precise use of language. Terms must be clearly defined and associated with observable phenomena.
- Inductive reasoning requires adequate unbiased data collection. Unfortunately, with complex human beings it is difficult to know when enough data have been collected.
- Facts must not be confused with generalizations. For example, a research report on a new drug states that all the rabbits to whom the drug was given died. That is a statement of fact. To then state that the drug is poisonous for rabbits is a generalization arrived at through induction. The second statement is no longer a statement of fact. It is a generalization and as a generalization it may be shown to be true or false.
- Logic is of little help in induction as the process is based on inference. One must continually pause and review the specifics and identify all other possible explanations or generalizations.

EXERCISE 2

Option 1. Form a work group of five students from your class. Have every student write a paragraph describing the nature of nursing practice. Distribute the material so that every student has a copy of all five statements. Then, working independently, use inductive reasoning to create a generalization about the nature of nursing practice. Have every student share his or her generalization. In what ways are they similar? How are they dissimilar? What errors were made in the process of moving from specifics to generalizations? What unfounded assumptions did people make?

Option 2. Instead of writing a paragraph describing the nature of nursing, use the data in Table 12–5. Have every member of the group develop generalizations about patients' needs from the data. Analyze the generalizations using the questions listed under Option 1.

Deductive Reasoning

In deductive reasoning, one moves from the theory or generalization to the particular. For example, research has demon-

TABLE 12-4 Styles of Thinking *Continued*

	Synthesist	Idealist	Pragmatist	Analyst	Realist
Behavioral Cues					
Apt to Appear	Challenging, skeptical, amused.	Attentive, receptive, supportive.	Open, sociable, humorous.	Cool, studious, hard to read.	Direct, forceful; quick nonverbal expression.
Apt to Say	On the other hand . . . No, not necessarily . . .	It seems to me . . . Don't you think . . .	I'll buy that . . . That's one sure way . . .	It stands to reason . . . Logically . . .	It's obvious to me . . . Everybody knows that . . .
Apt to Express	Concepts, opposite points of view.	Feelings, ideas about values, what's good.	Non-complex ideas, personal anecdotes.	General rules; supporting data.	Opinions, factual anecdotes.
Tone	May sound argumentative, sardonic.	May sound tentative, hopeful, resentful.	May sound insincere, enthusiastic.	May sound stubborn, careful, dry.	May sound dogmatic, forthright, positive.
Enjoys	Intellectual, philosophical arguments.	Feeling-level discussions.	Brainstorming, lively give-and-take.	Rational examination of issues.	Short, direct factual discussions.
Apt to Use	Parenthetical expressions, qualifying phrases, adjectives.	Indirect questions, aids to agreement.	Case examples, illustrations, popular opinions.	Long, discursive, well-formulated sentences.	Direct, pithy, descriptive statements.
Dislikes	Talk that seems simplistic, superficial, mundane.	Talk that seems too factual, too conflictive, dehumanizing.	Talk that seems dry, dull, humorless, "nit-picking."	Talk that seems irrational, aimless, "far-out."	Talk that seems too theoretical, sentimental, impractical.
Under Stress	Pokes fun.	Looks hurt.	Looks bored.	Withdraws.	Becomes agitated.

strated the value of preoperative teaching of deep breathing and coughing skills. You are assigned to care for a patient scheduled for surgery. You therefore include teaching deep breathing and coughing skills in your plan of care.

Nurse scholars have generated research and theories for clinicians to use in practice. Research and theory from other disciplines may also be applicable.

Deductive reasoning requires attention to the definition of terms and to other alternative interpretations. For example, from inductive reasoning, the head nurse has concluded that patients who recover successfully from an operation get out of bed and walk in their room within 12 hours of the surgery. You are assigned to take care of a patient scheduled for surgery. In your care plan you note that the patient should get out of bed and walk in the room within 12 hours after surgery. Is this a sound use of deductive reasoning? Not yet. First you must ask about those patients who had an unsuccessful recovery from surgery. How were they similar? How did they differ? Were they different in terms of ambulating?

In deductive reasoning it cannot be assumed that if you have A (ambulating in 12 hours) and then B (successful recovery) that B (successful recovery) is always associated with A (ambulating in 12 hours). The probability of it occurring in the context of other factors must be considered in the deductive reasoning process.

Another error made in deductive reasoning is the assumption that if A, then B, then also *not* A leads to *not* B. In the illustration of the surgical patient the assumption would be that without ambulating in 12 hours the patient would not have a successful recovery. This is shown in the reasoning embedded in the poem "To His Coy Mistress" by Andrew Marvell (Anderson, 1980, pp. 101–102):

Had we but world enough, and time,
This coyness, Lady, were no crime. . . .
But at my back I always hear
Time's winged chariot hurrying near. . . .
Now therefore, while the youthful hue
Sits on thy skin like morning dew,
And while thy willing soul transpires
At every pore with instant fires,
Now let us sport us while we may.

TABLE 12-5 Hospitalized Patients' Rank Ordering of Needs

Introduction

The nursing literature contains many statements of what is important to the hospitalized person. Many of these statements are the result of educated guesses or generalizations from one or two encounters.

The following data are the result of a card sort survey of hospitalized persons. The card sort survey consisted of 33 items representing the following broad categories of factors: physical care, physical and social environment, and information and assurance. Each item was stated as an incomplete statement and was typed on a 3 × 5 card. The patient was instructed to sort the items as very important, important, less important, and not important. There were no restrictions on the number of items that could be placed into any category. The response categories were scored as follows: very important = 5; important = 4; less important = 3; and not important = 1.

The data were first analyzed for the 45 patients that participated. The data were then analyzed by gender, then by age.

Assignment

Review the rank ordering of needs for patients as a total group as well as by gender and age. Based on your analysis of the data, develop generalizations regarding the relative importance of patients' needs. **Remember, the lower the rank, the more important the need. For example, item number 1 (rank 33) is less important than item number 6 (rank 5).**

Data

	Total Group	Female				Male		
		Age 20–35	*Age 36–60*	*Age 60+*	*Total Females*	*Age 25–60*	*Age 60+*	*Total Males*
Statement of Need	**N = 45**	**N = 8**	**N = 14**	**N = 14**	**N = 36**	**N = 5**	**N = 4**	**N = 9**
1. To be permitted to smoke.	33	25	31.5	33	33	32.5	33	33
2. To have the room or ward quiet.	19.5	18	16	17.5	18.5	26.5	19	24
3. To have the nurse rub my back often enough.	27	29.5	26	26	26.5	26.5	24.5	27
4. To have the nurses look in on me when I'm sleeping.	24.5	33	24	29	26.5	19.5	30	24
5. To have the nurses take enough time to talk with me.	23	25	27	23	24.5	23	13	21
6. To be able to get up and go to the bathroom instead of using the bedpan.	5	13.5	7	3.5	4.5	8	5	6.5
7. To have patients talk with me.	28	31.5	31.5	21	29	26.5	24.5	27
8. To have the nurse do something about it when I'm uncomfortable.	9	7	9	9.5	8.5	16	19	16.5
9. To see my family or friends often enough.	19.5	13.5	20.5	21	20	8	28	16.5
10. To have nurses use my name when they are talking with me.	24.5	18	22.5	26	23	30.5	31.5	32
11. To be able to sleep.	6.5	7	10	5.5	8.5	12	2	6.5
12. To have patients who are very ill moved somewhere else.	16	25	14	15	18.5	12	8.5	9.5
13. To be served a food tray that makes me feel like eating.	13	13.5	16	15	16	1.5	8.5	4.5
14. To have the nurses talk about things which interest me.	31	31.5	33	26	31	23	28	27

15. To have the doctors tell me the truth about my illness.	1	2	1	1.5	1	1.5	2	2
16. To have my bed screened or the door closed when I am getting a bath or the doctors are examining me.	8	4.5	3.5	12	4.5	12	19	13.5
17. To have nurses who are friendly.	3.5	7	7	1.5	3	4.5	5	4.5
18. To permit someone of my family or a special friend to stay after visiting hours if I really want them.	21	13.5	22.5	24	21	19.5	19	18.5
19. To be permitted to sleep as long as I want to in the morning.	32	28	28.5	32	32	29	31.5	30.5
20. To feel that the people here are interested in my getting well.	6.5	20.5	5	3.5	6.5	4.5	13	8
21. To have the minister, priest, or rabbi visit me.	22	29.5	20.5	19	22	26.5	8.5	21
22. To have the nurse come promptly when I call.	15	13.5	18	12	14.5	19.5	8.5	13.5
23. To have something to do to occupy my time.	29	25	28.5	31	30	23	24.5	24
24. To get my medicines on time.	17	13.5	12.5	21	17	19.5	19	18.5
25. To understand what the doctors and nurses are talking about when they try to explain my case to me.	2	1	2	8	2	4.5	2	3
26. To have doctors and nurses listen to what I have to say.	13	10	11	15	12.5	12	13	11
27. To be free of worry about bills piling up when I'm sick.	18	25	7	17.5	14.5	16	28	21
28. Not used in study.								
29. To know that the nurse will come if I need her.	3.5	18	3.5	5.5	6.5	4.5	5	1
30. To have someone explain all tests which are new to me.	10	4.5	12.5	7	10	16	13	13.5
31. To understand why I'm getting my medicines.	13	9	16	9.5	11	12	19	13.5
32. To have the nurses finish what they are doing and not run in and out.	26	20.5	25	29	24.5	30.5	19	29
33. To know which nurse is assigned to take care of me.	30	22	30	29	28	32.5	24.5	30.5
34. To know how long I will be in the hospital.	11	3	19	12	12.5	8	13	9.5

EXERCISE 3

Reread the poem. Then using the framework "if A, then B, then *not* A leads to *not* B," write out the argument of the poem. Why is it faulty?

Creativity

Creative thinking is characterized as *divergent* in that it produces elaboration, expansion, and variety of ideas. In contrast, reasoning is considered convergent thinking as it involves reduction, abstraction, and extraction of ideas.

Creativity requires three inner conditions: openness to experience, an internal locus of evaluation, and the ability to toy with elements and concepts (Rogers, 1959). Creative thinkers must be willing to be seen as nonconformist and to take risks (Egan, 1986). True creativity also requires the thinking to be original, adaptive to reality, and consistent with the original insight (MacKinnon, 1962).

Creative thinkers (Brookfield, 1987, pp. 115–116):

- Reject standardized formats for problem solving.
- Have interests in a wide range of related and divergent fields.
- Can take multiple perspectives on a problem.
- View the world as relative and contextual rather than universal and absolute.
- Frequently use trial and error methods in their experimentation with alternative approaches.
- Have a future orientation and embrace change optimistically.
- Have self-confidence and trust in their own judgment.

Creativity can be developed by creating an environment in which it is rewarded. In the classroom, students can be asked to create new methods for accomplishing an outcome. In the clinical setting where patients present unique characteristics, creative thinking can result in more effective interventions.

For example, a patient was admitted to the hospital because she had severe pain radiating down her leg. It required several days of diagnostic work to determine the origin of the problem and agree on treatment. In the meantime, the patient was on modified bed rest, meaning she was to remain in bed except to shower and use the bathroom. Inevitably while showering the patient (who continued to experience severe pain) would drop the bar of soap. To bend down and pick it up aggravated the pain. The patient shared this problem with the nurse, who came up with the idea of "soap on a rope" (a bar of soap with a rope attached to it that can hang around your neck). That creative solution enabled the patient to shower without increased pain.

EXERCISE 4

You are assigned to take care of a 5-year-old boy who is scheduled for surgery. He has never been in the hospital and his parents are also unfamiliar with hospital care. You have decided that it is necessary to educate the parents and the child about surgery in general and the surgical procedure specifically. Free yourself of preconceived ideas about patient teaching. How would you teach these parents and their son? List as many teaching strategies as you can. *Direct your thoughts to the situation, hold your attention there, allow your subconscious mind to throw up ideas, and consciously allow your imagination to wander. Have fun thinking.*

Intuition

Intuition, an understanding without a rationale, has five key aspects (Benner and Tanner, 1987):

- *Pattern recognition,* the ability to see relationships not limited to those specified in some abstract listing. For example, a nurse may decide a patient is a suicide risk based on a pattern of behaviors unique to this patient.
- *Similarity recognition,* the ability to see similarities and dissimilarities between this patient and others even when the resemblances are not clearly understood or are fuzzy. For example, the nurse working in the emergency room may treat a person with head trauma in a certain way because of a sense of similarity between this person and previous people with head trauma.
- *Common sense understanding,* a deep grasp of the culture and language so that flexible understanding in diverse situations is possible. For example, a nurse was assigned to take care of a patient just admitted with a severe heart attack. The nurse learned that the patient's daughter had just died. She used her understanding of the impact of a daughter dying as she assessed the patient and determined care. Her thought was that the death of her daughter followed by her own heart attack would leave this woman feeling vulnerable and frightened.
- *Skilled know-how, knowledge, and skills* that are so well understood, they have become part of the person of the nurse. For example, when inserting an intravenous catheter the skilled nurse can probe with the catheter tip as extension of her finger and not an unwieldy foreign object.
- *Sense of salience,* to see the world as meaningful with events as more or less important, complete with nuances. For example, when asked how a patient was doing, the nurse responded by describing sleep patterns, purposeful body movements, and physical strength. The points she commented on reflected her sense of the important factors for this individual. The factors did not come from a checklist but from in-depth knowledge of the patient.

Clinical *intuition* is accepted by practitioners as an important aspect of clinical decision making (Young, 1987). It is defined as a process whereby the nurse knows something about a patient that cannot be verbalized, that is verbalized with difficulty, or for which the source of knowledge cannot be determined. During clinical decision making, intuition functions as both a *process* and a *product*. As a process, cues, images, feelings, and recollections of past and present experiences become integrated with the current situation. As a product, the nurse knows or does something because of the processed information.

Experience will increase both one's amount of intuitive thinking and one's confidence in that intuition. The clinical experiences of the nurse will provide rich data to use in future clinical situations. The lived experiences of the nurse-person also provide rich material from which intuition may spring. Critical to experience aiding intuitive thinking is the attention the nurse must pay to intuition. When did it occur? What thoughts and feelings were associated with the intuition? Was the intuition well founded?

Intuition is a part of nursing practice. It produces useful information that could also be helpful to others. For example, when caring for patients in their home, the intuition of family members is very helpful information for the nurse.

EXERCISE 5

Picture yourself as a hospice nurse working with people who have chosen to die in their homes. You visit one of your patients and although there is no change in his physical condition, your intuition tells you he is going to die very soon, perhaps within the next 24 hours. How would you respond? Would you disregard your feeling? What process would you use to reflect on your intuition before you took action? Think of situations in which your intuition was correct. Think of situations in which your intuition was incorrect. (For example, was your intuition correct about the grades you received last term?) By analyzing these situations you may develop insight into your own intuitiveness and be willing to use intuition in your nursing practice.

Critical Thinking

Critical thinking is a rational response to questions that cannot be answered definitively and for which all the relevant information may not be available (Kurfiss, 1988). It is an act of inquiry whose purpose is to explore a situation, phenomenon, or problem to arrive at a hypothesis or conclusion about it that integrates all available information and that can be convincingly justified (Kurfiss, 1988). Discovery and justification are components of critical thinking.

Critical thinking is characterized by these nine themes (Brookfield, 1987):

1. **Critical thinking is a productive and positive activity.** Critical thinkers see themselves as able to create and recreate aspects of a situation. They see the world as open and malleable, value diversity, and are innovative.
2. **Critical thinking is a process, not an outcome.** Critical thinking involves continuous inquiry. There is no thought of universal truth or total certainty. Conclusions are seen as temporary pauses in an ongoing process.
3. **Manifestations of critical thinking vary according to the context in which it occurs.** The critical thinking process of a nurse and a mathematician will differ. Sometimes the process is internal to the individual; other times it is external and done in the context of a group.
4. **Critical thinking is triggered by positive as well as negative events.** Any event that causes questioning of previously held assumptions can lead to critical thinking. The key factor is the decision to explore new possibilities. In nursing, every patient encounter is an opportunity for critical thinking.
5. **Critical thinking is emotive as well as rational.** It is exciting to develop new insights and feel the ability to change aspects of a situation. The nurse who sees an aspect of patient care in a new way and is therefore able to facilitate a patient's return to health is going to **feel** a pleasing sense of self-confidence. Critical thinkers enjoy their feelings and use them in the process.
6. **Identifying and challenging assumptions is central to critical thinking.** Health care delivery is changing so rapidly that yesterday's assumptions and beliefs are not likely to work today and certainly will not work tomorrow. The nurse needs to constantly challenge assumptions about nursing care and patient outcomes. New assumptions that fit the current context are needed. The move to provide more care in the home and less in the hospital is a challenge to assumptions held in the 1980s. The move to provide alternatives to Western medicine also challenges assumptions by the U.S. medical establishment.
7. **Attending to the importance of context is crucial to critical thinking.** Practices, structures, and actions are never context-free. Critical thinkers are aware of this and factor it into their thinking. In the hospital patients may be very willing to do everything the nurse says. In their home, those same people may challenge everything the nurse says. The difference is the context and its impact on the individual's sense of control.
8. **Critical thinkers try to imagine and explore alternatives.** Although it is important to respect "the way things have always been done," it is equally important to imagine and explore alternate ways of doing something. For many years nurses were expected to practice by the rules of the procedure manual. Today nurses are expected to create new interventions or methods for implementing patient care. In a hospital in Wisconsin, nurses on one nursing unit challenged the idea of keeping the patients' charts in a central location (the nursing station). They decided to hang the chart on the wall right outside the patient's room. They also decided that anybody could chart—aides, patients, and family. It was a great innovation, but nurses on other units felt so threatened that they avoided any contact with the staff that challenged the assumptions.

9. **Imagining and exploring alternatives leads to reflective skepticism.** Critical thinkers are skeptical of universal truths and absolute answers. They use existing knowledge and experience as a springboard into exploring new possibilities.

Critical thinking involves the ability to:

- identify possibilities/innovations
- formulate and analyze arguments
- construct meaning
- use knowledge as context
- negotiate
- critically reflect on one's thoughts and actions

Identifying possibilities/innovations is the creative aspect of critical thinking and involves the thinking described earlier in this chapter under the heading "creative thinking."

Formulating and analyzing arguments can be thought of as the ability to make the reasoning process explicit. It is a skill used frequently in patient care. For example, the doctor thinks a patient is ready for discharge from the hospital to home. The nurse who has been caring for the patient disagrees. The nurse's ability to convince the doctor that the patient should not be discharged will, in part, depend on the nurse's ability to construct and defend that position. The **quality** of the nurse's reasoning is an essential factor. In this situation the nurse might use data about the home situation, the patient's feelings about discharge, and the nurse's perception about the ability of the patient to manage at home. The nurse must formulate feelings, knowledge, and perceptions into well-stated positions that can be defended. Defending them well requires not only understanding one's position but the position of the other person. Knowledge of the particular situation and theoretical knowledge are both important in formulating arguments.

The following errors in reasoning are common in the process of critical thinking (Kurfiss, 1988):

- *Provincialism,* the tendency to accept or reject ideas on the basis of experience in one's own group. For example, the idea of room service in a hospital setting might be rejected because that is not the practice in today's hospitals.
- *Ad hominem,* an attack on the person rather than on the ideas. For example, an idea may be rejected because a **new** employee presented it rather than because others saw major flaws in the idea.
- *False dilemma,* erroneously reducing the number of alternatives. For example, a nurse may think that the only alternative for a patient experiencing pain is drug A or drug B when, in fact, there are many other methods of alleviating pain.
- *Hasty conclusion or generalization,* drawing conclusions with too little evidence. For example, a nurse may decide a patient is ready for discharge based only on data regarding the physical aspect of recovery. If the nurse had considered the patient's mental status (level of anxiety and other factors), a different decision might have been made.
- *Begging the question*—reasoning in circles. When the conclusion is supported by itself with the words changed, it is begging the question or reasoning in circles. For example, a nurse believes that a patient who wants to recover will do everything the nurse says. Patient X does not do everything the nurse says. The nurse concludes that patient X does not really want to recover. How does the nurse "prove" that the patient does not want to recover? By restating the conclusion that patients who want to recover do everything the nurse tells them to do. If the nurse could state specific reasons why not following the dictates of the nurse is linked with a desire not to recover, it would not be reasoning in circles. Here is another example of circular reasoning: Requiring all women to have a yearly mammogram is wasteful. Therefore, passing legislation requiring health plans to provide that service would result in a great deal of harm. Because the legislation would be so harmful, it is obviously wasteful. *It is wasteful because it is wasteful!*

A third skill in critical thinking is **constructing meaning.** An event such as a surgical procedure does not have the same meaning for every person having surgery. That sounds like common sense, yet it is frequently forgotten. Automatic responses based on assumptions can occur without awareness by the health care provider. To construct meaning to an event requires the nurse to understand the event from the patient's perspective. It requires paying attention to those factors that the patient feels are important. It requires a holistic view of the situation. It means having enough knowledge of self that preconceived ideas and assumptions can be isolated and not influence the process of constructing meaning. It requires accepting the reality that the meaning the patient ascribes to an event may have more influence in determining the outcomes of the event than anything else. **Meaning** is created by the people in the situation—it is not a given. **Meaning** is a powerful force in determining the outcome of an event. The skill of constructing meaning is a major component of critical thinking.

One example of the importance of ascribing meaning comes from nursing home residents. The nursing care plan is seen by nurses as a useful tool to provide continuity of care across shifts and among nursing personnel. To the nursing home resident it may be seen as a "tool of terror" as it forces the resident into a rigid pattern of behavior not typical of life outside the institution. Furthermore, if the resident objects to something stated on the care plan, e.g., attending occupational therapy, the resident runs the risk of being labeled uncooperative. The nurse must understand the care plan from the eyes of the resident and learn to use it accordingly.

A second example of ascribing meaning comes from elderly people recovering from a broken hip. To the health care provider the broken hip is typically seen as a physical health problem to be fixed. To individuals with a broken hip the problem is more likely to be seen in terms of their self-image. The nurse may focus on rehabilitation and strengthening muscles. Patients are focused on their self-image and whether or not they will be "the same person" after the hip heals. People who have defined self in terms of gardening and independence in activities of daily living will be thinking about their broken hip and how it affects that image of self. The meaning ascribed to the broken hip is not the physical injury but how it affects self-image.

A fourth skill in critical thinking is **using knowledge as a guide.** This is in contrast to the use of knowledge as **truth.** When knowledge is viewed as just one component of the context for practice, it becomes a guide to action. When knowledge is viewed as truth, it determines the action. When knowledge is viewed as a guide, it is used in consideration with everything else that is known through other means such as intuition and experience. The nurse first considers the applicability of existing knowledge to the present situation.

Existing knowledge and beliefs can be so powerful they can inhibit seeing the situation as it really exists and learning new information.

Furthermore, when knowledge is viewed as a component of the patient care context there is the awareness that knowledge exists within the situation itself. The nurse brings knowledge to the situation. The nurse must also learn from the situation. Both sources of knowledge are used in critical thinking.

For example, the nurse is assigned to care for an elderly patient who is confused. The nurse knows that admitting an elderly person to a strange hospital setting with different stimuli in the environment can produce confusion. If the nurse assumes this is the case for this patient without further assessment, he or she will be using knowledge as though it were truth. If the nurse considers other options such as medications, health status, and the patient's own perspective, the nurse will be using knowledge as a guide.

A fifth skill in critical thinking is **negotiation.** Negotiation requires a deep understanding of the person's experience with health and illness, what the experience means to the person, ways in which the person has learned to cope with the illness, and what the person hopes for in the future. Negotiation with the patient is the process of combining this local specific understanding of the patient's interpretations, issues, concerns and ways of coping with more general practical and scientific knowledge. Respecting and supporting the client's autonomy for health care decision making is part of negotiation.

Negotiation with other health care providers frequently involves this same in-depth understanding of the patient, coupled with the capacity to make assumptions, arguments, and rationale explicit.

The sixth skill in critical thinking is **critical reflection.** Reflective thinking is an active, persistent, and careful consideration of an experience or belief in light of other experiences and beliefs that support or conflict with it. Frequently reflection occurs as a response to a perplexing situation, e.g., when the current situation does not match previous experiences or when the nurse feels uneasy about some aspect of the situation. It differs from the analysis of inductive and deductive reasoning in that it is unstructured and has an iterative component.

As has already been stated, critical thinking is more than applying predetermined theoretical knowledge to a particular situation. It involves observation, interaction, thoughts, feelings, and interpretation all done as a process of inquiry and with the active involvement of the patient. It is a process through which new knowledge is created and tested. It is this aspect of critical thinking that requires reflective thought. It is through reflection that the nurse is able to understand the rationale for an action. It is through reflection that the nurse is able to address the validity of the knowledge created. It is through reflection that the nurse determines the generalizability of the knowledge and experience.

Ford and Profetto-McGrath (1994) describe critical reflection as going beneath the surface structure of the situation to reveal the underlying assumptions that constrain open discourse and responsible action. They identify two moments of critical reflection: the critical examination of one's own practice and an understanding of the situation and the way the situation works. They state, "Critical self-reflection permits an understanding of one's perception of the situation, as well as an examination of the assumptions that guide one's practice."

Consider the following situation. The nurse has been caring for Patient A for several days. The patient is recovering from a major heart attack. He has been recovering well and is pleased with his care. The nurse enters the patient's room to check vital signs (blood pressure, temperature, pulse and respiration). They are all normal. The nurse leaves the room to chart that information. As she charts the information she reflects on the specific data collected and the interaction with the patient. She becomes aware that the nonverbal behavior of the patient did not match the verbal behavior. She decides to return to the patient's room to verify her observations. She does . . . and finds the patient crying. Something guided the nurse to return to the room—to take the right action. What was that something? In this situation it was reflecting on the situation and realizing the conflict between the data that suggested health and the nonverbal responses that suggested a problem. Only through reflective thought can that knowledge be made conscious and helpful.

Consider another situation. Several years ago a group of experienced nurses was given authority for the care of chronically ill residents in a long-term care facility. Several of the patients were fed by tubes passed through their nose into their stomach. Some had been fed this way for years. The nurses decided to remove the tubes and teach these residents how to swallow food once again. Every patient for whom the nurses removed the tube learned to swallow and was able to eat regular food once again. What cues led the nurses to know which residents could learn to swallow once again? Only through reflective thought about their practice were the nurses able to answer that question.

Reflective thought is important in critical thinking and clinical decision making because knowledge is tested and created as the process is used. The knowledge that is created is important in caring for that individual; it is equally important to consider its validity and generalizability for other patients.

EXERCISE 6

Create a study group of five students. Ask each student to individually prioritize five tasks of medication administration for two cases: a patient just admitted to the emergency room with two broken legs and an adult with chronic back pain. The five tasks are:

- assess vital signs (i.e., pulse, respiration, and blood pressure)
- identify cost
- administer pain medication
- check allergies
- evaluate pain

Have each student present his or her prioritized list and the rationale. Ascribe different roles to the others such as physician, family, and nursing supervisor. Evaluate the "critical thinking" in terms of the five skills of critical thinking. Offer comments to each student that can be used to improve their critical thinking abilities.

In summary, clinical decision making is a complex process involving a range of thinking skills, knowledge, experience, and self-confidence. In the clinical setting it is replacing discipline-specific linear processes such as the nursing process. Skill in clinical decision making evolves over time and must be considered part of lifetime professional development.

CLASSIFICATION SYSTEMS

Most care is designed and delivered by a team of health care providers. Clinical decisions need to be clearly communicated to all members of that team. To facilitate communication and clinical decision making, classification systems have been developed. These systems range from some that are in use across the world to some that are in use only by nurses in the United States. To be an effective member of a health care team, the nurse needs to be able to use the range of classification systems in use in the health care system.

Figure 12–1 shows the identification of a nursing diagnosis as a component of clinical judgment. When the nurse is part of an interdisciplinary team, the nursing diagnosis is only one of the classification systems used.

International Classification of Diseases

Classification systems evolved as health care became more and more complex and there was increasing need to be able to compare knowledge, results, and experiences within and across disciplines and within and across countries. One of the earliest national classification efforts was the standard nomenclature of diseases and operations. This classification system has been replaced by the World Health Organization (WHO) international system for reporting vital statistics including mortality data.

The classification system currently used in the United States is the International Classification of Diseases, Ninth Revision, Clinical Modifications (ICD-9-CM). This system is compatible with the WHO system. It is used primarily for statistical reporting but is also used by insurance companies and the federal government when determining payment.

The ICD-9-CM is a classification of diseases and injuries. The diseases and injuries are grouped into chapters, sections, categories, subcategories, and fifth-digit subclassifications. The classification must be so precise that there is only one place to classify each disease or injury. Each category and subcategory must be mutually exclusive. The classification system is revised as new diseases are discovered.

Box 12–3 presents an example from the ICD-9-CM. Diseases are categorized into chapters; e.g., Chapter 1 is Infectious and Parasitic Diseases. This chapter includes diseases generally recognized as communicable or transmissible as well as a few diseases of unknown but possibly infectious origin. It does not include acute respiratory infections, certain localized infections, or influenza. What a chapter includes and excludes is stated at the beginning of the chapter.

Chapters are divided into sections. For example, one section in the chapter on infectious diseases is titled Intestinal Infectious Diseases. In that section is a coded listing of all known infections of that type. For example, Salmonella food poisoning is coded 003 and then divided further in terms of type of infection. A localized Salmonella infection is thus coded 003.2. Because there are various localized sites, the classification continues with, for example, Salmonella arthritis coded 003.23. As mentioned, this detailed coding system requires precision to the point that any given disease or injury can be coded in only one place.

This system may seem extremely detailed to the average health care provider. Yet specialists find the detail inadequate for their reporting, research, and educational purposes. Specialists have moved from discussing diseased organs to discussing intracellular elements such as genes and proteins. The level of specification in the ICD-9-CM is inadequate to their needs. Therefore, for example, an ICD-O (O for Oncology/Cancer) has been developed as a companion to Chapter 2 of the ICD-9-CM. It is an expansion of that chapter/code book.

Diagnostic and Statistical Manual

The American Psychiatric Association has developed its Diagnostic and Statistical Manual, the most recent version of which is the fourth edition, known as the DSM-IV. Again this classification of mental disorders was initially developed because of the inadequacy of the ICD. Mental illness was not well understood until after World War II. For example, in 1840 the only mental illness diagnosis was idiocy/insanity. By 1880 there were seven categories: mania, melancholia, monomania, paresis, dementia, dipsomania, and epilepsy. It is not important to understand these conditions but rather to note

BOX 12-3
AN EXAMPLE OF A LISTING FROM *ICD-9-CM*, Vol. 1

1. INFECTIOUS AND PARASITIC DISEASES (001-139)

Note: Categories for "late effects" of infectious and parasitic diseases are to be found at 137–139.

Includes: diseases generally recognized as communicable or transmissible as well as a few diseases of unknown but possibly infectious origin

Excludes: *acute respiratory infections (460–466)*
carrier or suspected carrier of infectious organism (V02.0–V02.9)
certain localized infections
influenza (487.0–487.8)

INTESTINAL INFECTIOUS DISEASES (001–009)

Excludes: *helminithiases (120.0–129)*

001 Cholera

001.0 Due to Vibrio cholerae

001.1 Due to Vibrio cholerae el tor

001.9 Cholera, unspecified

002 Typhoid and paratyphoid fevers

002.0 Typhoid fever
Typhoid (fever) (infection) [any site]

002.1 Paratyphoid fever A

002.2 Paratyphoid fever B

002.3 Paratyphoid fever C

002.9 Paratyphoid fever, unspecified

003 Other salmonella infections
Includes: infection or food poisoning by Salmonella [any serotype]

003.0 Salmonella gastroenteritis
Salmonellosis

003.1 Salmonella septicemia

003.2 Localized salmonella infections

003.20 Localized salmonella infection, unspecified

003.21 Salmonella meningitis

003.22 Salmonella pneumonia

003.23 Salmonella arthritis

003.24 Salmonella osteomyelitis

003.29 Other

003.8 Other specified salmonella infections

003.9 Salmonella infection, unspecified

004 Shigellosis
Includes: bacillary dysentery

004.0 Shigella dysenteriae
Infection by group B Shigella (Schmitz) (Shiga)

004.1 Shigella flexneri
Infection by group B Shigella

004.2 Shigella boydii
Infection by group C Shigella

the limited number of diagnoses and of course the inclusion of epilepsy. After World War II, the U.S. Army found itself having to treat many soldiers for mental problems that were related to serving in the war. This led to new diagnoses and the first serious attempt to develop a classification system.

The authors of DSM-IV acknowledge the difficulty of separating mind from body when describing illness and injury. They also acknowledge that the concept "mental illness" lacks a precise definition that covers all situations. They do not claim that the categories listed are completely discrete entities with clear boundaries dividing one from another. The system includes 16 major diagnostic categories and one section for "other conditions." The system includes cross-reference to ICD codes, diagnostic criteria, and descriptive text. The DSM has proven very helpful to physicians, nurses, psychologists, and social workers. It will continue to undergo revision, expansion, and clarification as it is used.

As interdisciplinary approaches to health care are implemented, it is important for nurses to be familiar with these widely used classification systems. At a minimum, nurses must know what ICD-9-CM and DSM-IV refer to and how these systems are used.

Nursing Classification Systems

As the discipline of nursing continued to evolve and nursing practice included more independent functions (see Chapter 1 for the differentiation between dependent and independent functions), the need for a classification of nursing phenomena became evident. The same issues of communication and reporting that led to the development of the ICD, the ICD-O, and the DSM led nursing to begin developing its own classification system. As there is not national consensus on a classification system that describes the commonly accepted components of nursing practice, an overview of several widely used systems is presented.

NORTH AMERICAN NURSING DIAGNOSIS ASSOCIATION TAXONOMY

The classification system most widely used by nursing was developed by the North American Nursing Diagnosis Association (NANDA). As the name implies, this is a classification of nursing diagnoses. The phrase nursing diagnosis refers to those problems, states, or human responses that can be treated by nursing interventions (in contrast to those problems and conditions that are treated by medical interventions). This system has evolved into a taxonomy—that is, a classification system with an explicit basis for structuring/relating the groups within the system.

Developing the NANDA taxonomy involved four distinct steps. The initial NANDA listing of nursing diagnoses was developed by induction based on the health conditions nurses said they treated. The second step was reaching agreement about a consistent nomenclature that could be used to describe the health conditions identified in the first step. The third step was to group identified diagnoses into classes and subclasses according to patterns and relationships among them. NANDA made the decision that diagnoses would be listed in alphabetical order (there was no agreement on any other way to list them) and to list the basic concept of the diagnosis first followed by modifiers. The nurse caring for a patient who was constipated would record this nursing diagnosis "Bowel Elimination, Alteration in: Constipation."

The NANDA taxonomy uses the following nine patterns of human response: exchanging, moving, communicating, perceiving, relating, knowing, valuing, feeling, and choosing. An alphabetized list of approved diagnostic labels is presented in the appendix.

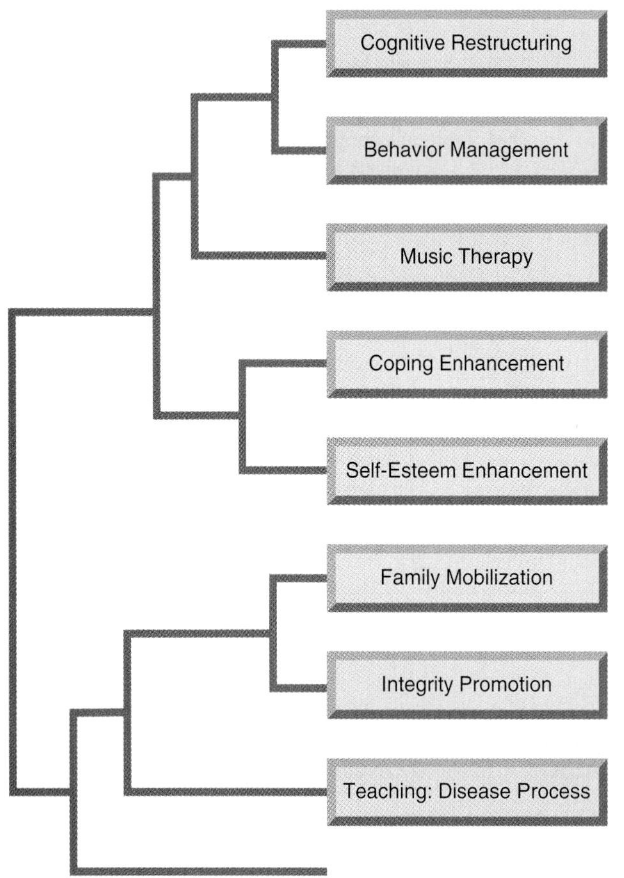

Figure 12-2. Nursing Intervention Classification (NIC) taxonomy structure.

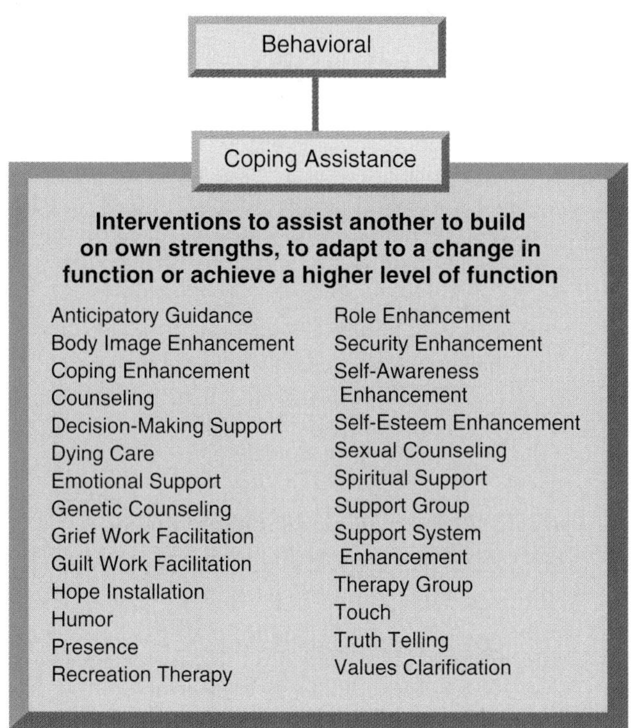

Figure 12-3. An example of a Nursing Intervention Classification (NIC) class.

TAXONOMY OF NURSING INTERVENTIONS

The focus of the Nursing Interventions Classification (NIC) is nurse behavior: those activities that nurses do to move patients toward desired health outcomes. The NIC developed under the leadership of Joanne McCloskey, RN, PhD, and Gloria Bulechek, RN, PhD. They define a nursing intervention as "any direct care treatment that a nurse performs on behalf of a client. These treatments include nurse-initiated treatments resulting from nursing diagnoses, physician-initiated treatments resulting from medical diagnoses, and performance of the daily essential functions for the client who cannot do these" (Bulechek and McCloskey 1992, p. 6). Each intervention comprises a label, a definition, a set of activities that a nurse does to carry out the intervention, and a short list of background readings.

The research that led to the NICs involved two phases. Phase one included the generation of an initial list of interventions and then the refinement of that list and defining activities. Phase two was the creation of the taxonomy and the validation of the intervention labels, defining activities, and taxonomy. Phase one produced approximately 340 intervention labels (each with a definition and a set of related activities that describes the behavior of the nurse). The NIC taxonomy produced by phase two has six domains representing the highest level of conceptualizing nursing interventions, and 26 classes representing the next level of conceptualization. Figure 12–2 shows the NIC taxonomy; Figure 12–3 presents an example of one class from the taxonomy; and Box 12–4 presents an intervention, including appropriate activities and

BOX 12-4
EXAMPLE OF A NURSING INTERVENTIONS CLASSIFICATION (NIC) INTERVENTION

HOPE INSTILLATION

DEFINITION: Facilitation of the development of a positive outlook in a given situation.

ACTIVITIES:

Assist patient/family to identify areas of hope in life

Inform the patient if the current situation is a temporary state

Demonstrate hope by recognizing the patient's intrinsic worth and viewing the patient's illness as only one facet of the individual

Expand the patient's repertoire of coping mechanisms

Teach reality recognition by surveying the situation and making contingency plans

Assist the patient to devise and revise goals related to the hope object

Help the patient expand spiritual self

Avoid masking the truth

Facilitate the patient incorporating a personal loss into his/her body image

Facilitate the patient/family reliving and savoring past achievements and experiences

Emphasize sustaining relationships, such as mentioning the names of loved ones to the unresponsive patient

Employ guided life review and/or reminiscence as appropriate

Involve the patient actively in his/her own care

Develop a plan of care that involves degree of goal attainment, moving from simple to more complex goals

Encourage therapeutic relationships with significant others

Teach family about the positive aspects of hope (e.g., develop meaningful conversational themes that reflect love and need for the patient)

Provide patient/family opportunity to be involved with support groups

Create an environment that facilitates patient practicing his/her religion as appropriate

BACKGROUND READINGS:

Brown, P. (1989). The concept of hope: Implications for care of the critically ill. Critical Care Nurse, 9(5), 97–105.
Parse, R. R. (1990). Parse's research methodology with an illustration of the lived experience of hope. Nursing Science Quarterly, 3(1), 9–17.
Snyder, M. (1988). Nursing management strategies: An overview. In P.H. Mitchell, L.C. Hodges, M. MuWasews, & C. Nalleck (Eds.), AANN's Neuroscience Nursing, Phenomena and Practice. Norwalk, CT: Appleton & Lange.

From McCloskey, J.C., Bulechek, G.M. (eds.). (1996). *Nursing Interventions Classification* (NIC), 2nd ed. St. Louis: Mosby-Year Book, p. 321.

references. These features show the movement from the general to the concrete that is an essential component of the taxonomy.

The researchers involved in the development of NICs were also committed to developing a classification of patient outcomes sensitive to nursing interventions, known as nursing outcomes classifications (NOCs). This work, which started in late 1993 and continued through late 1997, was funded by the National Institute of Nursing Research. The research aimed to (1) identify, label, validate, and classify nursing-sensitive patient outcomes and indicators and (2) evaluate the validity and usefulness of the classification in clinical field testing.

Each NOC has five levels. The first level is broad outcome categories; the other levels include classes of outcomes, labels of outcomes, indicators of outcomes, and measurement activities.

With the current emphasis by health care systems on outcomes of care rather than on the process of care, it is this latter classification system that may prove to be the most important for the discipline of nursing. This does not negate the importance of the NANDA and NIC taxonomies for documentation, communication, research, and education. It is simply a comment on the current value system within health care. When providers were paid for what they did, a NIC taxonomy was very important. When providers are valued in terms of health outcomes (recall the discussions of outcomes in Chapter 3), a NOC taxonomy may be more important.

THE OMAHA SYSTEM

The rapidly changing nature of community health care provided the stimulus for the development of the Omaha System. The narrative-type client record in use in community health nursing at the time the system was developed was not desirable for the following reasons:

- Nurses were spending too much time documenting care in a lengthy, rambling manner.
- Primary nurses and supervisors were not able to evaluate client progress by reviewing records.
- Health care professionals were not reading entries into the record because of their length and the difficulty in interpreting the narrative.
- Supervisors and administrators could not obtain aggregate clinical data from the records to produce meaningful information about services or future trends.

The Omaha System consists of three separate but related parts: the problem classification scheme, the intervention scheme, and the problem rating scale for outcomes. Martin and Scheet describe the Omaha System as follows (1992, pp. 19–20):

> The *Problem Classification Scheme* is a taxonomy of nursing diagnoses that provides consistent language for collecting, sorting, classifying, documenting, and analyzing data about client concerns. The *Intervention Scheme* is a taxonomy of community health nursing actions or activities that offers a method of describing services provided to clients. The *Problem Rating Scale for Outcomes* is an evaluation tool designed to measure client progress in relation to specific problems or nursing diagnoses. The three components of the Omaha System represent a structured, comprehensive approach to community health practice, documentation, and data management. Therefore, the System offers the following six capabilities and characteristics for community health nursing: (1) advances the scientific practice of nursing; (2) offers capabilities to quantify community health nursing; (3) is practical for general community application; (4) is congruent with the nursing process; (5) minimizes redundancy in the client record; and (6) limits documentation time.

The *Problem Classification Scheme* consists of four distinct hierarchical levels: domain, problem, modifiers, and signs/symptoms. The scheme has four domains: Environmental, Psychosocial, Physiological, and Health Related Behaviors. It includes 40 nursing diagnoses, two sets of modifiers, and a varying number of signs and symptoms. Box 12–5 presents one problem from the environmental domain; Box 12–6, one problem from the physiological domain. These are provided to illustrate the scheme.

The intervention scheme is organized into three levels to accommodate the needs of direct care delivery staff, supervisors, and administrators. The three hierarchical levels are: categories, targets, and client-specific information. Box 12–7 gives the entire scheme. Definitions have been developed for the four categories and 63 targets.

The *Problem Rating Scale for Outcomes* is based on the assumption that the interactions of a community health nurse and a client in relation to a problem affect what the client knows (knowledge), does (behavior), and is (status). The scale depicts the most positive to the most negative client state **in relation to a specific problem.** The three outcomes are considered to be of equal importance. Figure 12–4 shows the actual outcomes scale.

At the Visiting Nurse Association (VNA) of Omaha, the Omaha System is used in a variety of ways including (1) orientation, (2) communication, (3) practice, and (4) record audit (Martin and Scheet, 1988). All new nurses and other health care professionals attend an orientation session during which the three schema of the Omaha System are presented followed by an opportunity to apply the system.

Agency personnel use the concepts and terms of the Omaha System in their formal and informal communications.

BOX 12-5
A PROBLEM FROM THE OMAHA SYSTEM'S ENVIRONMENTAL DOMAIN

ENVIRONMENTAL DOMAIN

The Environmental Domain of the Problem Classification Scheme is defined as the material resources, physical surroundings, and substances both internal and external to the client, home, neighborhood, and broader community. The four problems included in this domain focus on critical factors that affect the health status, health behavior, and lifestyle of the client. A cluster of problem-specific signs/symptoms provide the diagnostic clues to problem identification. Signs and symptoms of problems in the Environmental Domain, as well as the other three domains, must be considered in relation to all other client data.

PROBLEM 02.

Sanitation. Environmental conditions pertaining to or affecting health with reference to cleanliness, precautions against infection or disease, and promotion of health

MODIFIER

Health Promotion	Family
Potential Deficit	Individual
Deficit	

SIGNS/SYMPTOMS

01. soiled living area
02. inadequate food storage/disposal
03. insects/rodents
04. foul odor

From Martin, K. S., Scheet, N. J. (1992). *The Omaha System: Applications for Community Health Nursing*. Philadelphia: W. B. Saunders, p. 67.

BOX 12-6
A PROBLEM FROM THE OMAHA SYSTEM'S PHYSIOLOGICAL DOMAIN

PHYSIOLOGICAL DOMAIN

The Physiological Domain is defined as functional status of processes that maintain life. The 15 problems focus on physical health status. Therefore, problems in this domain are usually associated with the client as an individual rather than as a family unit. Signs and symptoms of this domain may be observed, identified, or elicited through the practice skills of community health nurses.

PROBLEM 19.

Hearing. The perception of sound by the ears

MODIFIER

Health Promotion	Family
Potential Impairment	Individual
Impairment	

SIGNS/SYMPTOMS

01. difficulty hearing normal speech tones
02. absent/abnormal response to sound
03. abnormal results of hearing screening test
04. other

From Martin, K. S., Scheet, N. J. (1992). *The Omaha System: Applications for Community Health Nursing*. Philadelphia: W. B. Saunders, p. 70.

BOX 12-7
OMAHA SYSTEM: INTERVENTION SCHEME

CATEGORIES

I. Health Teaching, Guidance, and Counseling
II. Treatments and Procedures
III. Case Management
IV. Surveillance

TARGETS

01. Anatomy/physiology
02. Behavior modification
03. Bladder care
04. Bonding
05. Bowel care
06. Bronchial hygiene
07. Cardiac care
08. Caretaking/parenting skills
09. Cast care
10. Communication
11. Coping skills
12. Day care/respite
13. Discipline
14. Dressing change/wound care
15. Durable medical equipment
16. Education
17. Employment
18. Environment
19. Exercises
20. Family planning
21. Feeding procedures
22. Finances
23. Food
24. Gait training
25. Growth/development
26. Homemaking
27. Housing
28. Interaction
29. Lab findings
30. Legal system
31. Medical/dental care
32. Medication action/side effects
33. Medication administration
34. Medication set-up
35. Mobility/transfers
36. Nursing care, supplementary
37. Nutrition
38. Nutritionist
39. Ostomy care
40. Other community resource
41. Personal care
42. Positioning
43. Rehabilitation
44. Relaxation/breathing techniques
45. Rest/sleep
46. Safety
47. Screening
48. Sickness/injury care
49. Signs/symptoms—mental/emotional
50. Signs/symptoms—physical
51. Skin care
52. Social work/counseling
53. Specimen collection
54. Spiritual care
55. Stimulation/nurturance
56. Stress management
57. Substance use
58. Supplies
59. Support group
60. Support system
61. Transportation
62. Wellness
63. Other

CLIENT-SPECIFIC INFORMATION

Generated and individualized by health care provider

CATEGORY DEFINITIONS

I. Health Teaching, Guidance, and Counseling

Health teaching, guidance, and counseling are nursing activities that range from giving information, anticipating client problems, encouraging client action and responsibility for self-care and coping, to assisting with decision-making and problem-solving. The overlapping concepts occur on a continuum with the variation due to the client's self-direction capabilities.

II. Treatments and Procedures

Treatments and procedures are technical nursing activities directed toward preventing signs and symptoms, identifying risk factors and early signs and symptoms, and decreasing or alleviating signs and symptoms.

III. Case Management

Case management includes nursing activities of coordination, advocacy, and referral. These activities involve facilitating service delivery on behalf of the client, communicating with health and human service providers, promoting assertive client communication, and guiding the client toward use of appropriate community resources.

IV. Surveillance

Surveillance includes nursing activities of detection, measurement, critical analysis, and monitoring to indicate client status in relation to a given condition or phenomenon.

Box continued on following page

BOX 12-7
OMAHA SYSTEM: INTERVENTION SCHEME *Continued*

TARGET DEFINITIONS

01. **Anatomy/physiology:** Structure and function of the human body.
02. **Behavior modification:** Activities designed to promote a change of habits.
03. **Bladder care:** Activities directed toward maintenance of urinary bladder function, including bladder retraining, catheter change, and catheter irrigation.
04. **Bonding:** Unique emotional, synchronized parent-child relationship.
05. **Bowel care:** Activities directed toward maintenance of bowel function, including enema, bowel training, diet, and medication.
06. **Bronchial hygiene:** Activities directed toward maintenance of respiratory or pulmonary function, including inhalation therapy, percussion, and cannula insertion.
07. **Cardiac care:** Activities directed toward maintenance of cardiac or circulatory function, including diet, medication, vital signs, and relief of edema.
08. **Caretaking/parenting skills:** Abilities necessary to maintain a dependent child or adult, including feeding, bathing, discipline, nurturing, and stimulation.
09. **Cast care:** Activities directed toward maintenance of an immobilized body part, including relief of pain, pressure, or constriction of circulation.
10. **Communication:** The exchange of verbal or nonverbal information.
11. **Coping skills:** Ability to deal with or gain control of existing problems, including family tasks, illness, and employment.
12. **Day-care/respite:** Individual or institution providing child or adult supervision or care in the absence of the parent or caregiver.
13. **Discipline:** Activities designed to promote appropriate behavior, conduct, or action, including time out, limits, and controls.
14. **Dressing change/wound care:** Observing, cleansing, irrigating, or covering a wound, lesion, or incision.
15. **Durable medical equipment:** Nonexpendable articles primarily used for medical purposes in the presence of illness or injury, including hospital beds, respirators, walkers, and apnea monitors.
16. **Education:** Programs for development of special and general abilities, including Headstart, individualized study, GED, and vocational rehabilitation.
17. **Employment:** Occupation that provides income.
18. **Environment:** Aggregate of surrounding conditions or influences, including housing, community, and family.
19. **Exercises:** Therapeutic physical exertion, including active/passive range of motion, isometrics, and strengthening exercises.
20. **Family planning:** Practice of birth control measures within the context of family values, attitudes, and beliefs, including oral contraceptive, diaphragm, condom, and natural family planning.
21. **Feeding procedures:** Method of giving food or fluid, including breast, formula, intravenous, or tube.
22. **Finances:** Management of available economic resources in relation to family needs, including credit counseling, Assistance to Families with Dependent Children (AFDC), and Medicaid.
23. **Food:** Nourishing substance that is eaten or otherwise taken into the body to sustain life, provide energy, or promote growth.
24. **Gait training:** Systematic activities designed to promote walking with or without assistive devices.
25. **Growth/development:** Progressive physical, mental, emotional, and social maturation in relation to age, including developmental milestones and Erikson's developmental stages.
26. **Homemaking:** Management of the home, including cooking, cleaning, and laundry.
27. **Housing:** Place or type of residence.
28. **Interaction:** Reciprocal actions or influences among people, including mother-child, husband-wife, client-nurse, and parent-teacher.
29. **Lab findings:** Results of physiologic tests, including urinalysis and blood work.
30. **Legal system:** Connected with law or its administration, including legal aid, attorney, court, or Child Protective Services (CPS).
31. **Medical/dental care:** Diagnosis and treatment by a physician or dentist.
32. **Medication action/side effects:** Information regarding the purposes and positive or negative consequences of therapeutic drugs.
33. **Medication administration:** Applying, dispensing, or giving of drugs or medicines as prescribed by a physician.
34. **Medication set-up:** Organizing or arranging medicines for self-administration, including a Mediset.
35. **Mobility/transfers:** Movement of body or body parts, including activities of walking, swimming, and moving from one position or location to another.

BOX 12-7
OMAHA SYSTEM: INTERVENTION SCHEME *Continued*

36. **Nursing care, supplementary:** Therapeutic activities in addition to intermittent service, including private duty nursing and home health aide.
37. **Nutrition:** Nourishment of body with balanced food and fluid capable of providing energy, maintenance, and growth.
38. **Nutritionist:** A person who utilizes the science of nutrition to help individuals improve their health.
39. **Ostomy care:** Management of elimination through artificial openings, including colostomy and ileostomy.
40. **Other community resource:** An agency or group that offers goods or services not specifically identified in other targets, including day care/respite and education.
41. **Personal care:** Management of hygiene, including bathing, shampooing, shaving, nail trimming, and dressing.
42. **Positioning:** Placing the body into a particular position/alignment for a specified activity or response.
43. **Rehabilitation:** Process of restoring the ability to live and work as normally as possible after a disabling injury or illness, including physical, speech, and occupational therapy.
44. **Relaxation/breathing techniques:** Activities that relieve muscle tension, induce a quieting body response, and rebuild energy resources, including deep breathing exercises, imagery, and meditation.
45. **Rest/sleep:** Period of inactivity, repose, or mental calm with or without suspension of sensory activity.
46. **Safety:** A state of freedom from the risk or occurrence of injury or loss.
47. **Screening:** Individual or group testing procedures, including vision, hearing, height-weight, developmental, scoliosis, and blood pressure.
48. **Sickness/injury care:** Appropriate responses to illness or accidents, including first aid, taking temperature, and seeking medical care.
49. **Signs/symptoms—mental/emotional:** Objective or subjective evidence of a mental/emotional health problem, including depression, confusion, agitation, and suicidal threats.
50. **Signs/symptoms—physical:** Objective or subjective evidence of a physical health problem, including elevated temperature, failure to thrive, and statement of pain.
51. **Skin care:** Activities directed toward maintaining integrity of integument, including decubitus care and massage.
52. **Social work/counseling:** Plan designed by a social worker or counselor to promote the welfare of individual/ families.
53. **Specimen collection:** Obtaining samples of body fluids, secretions, or excreta, including blood, urine, feces, sputum, or drainage.
54. **Spiritual care:** Activities directed toward management of religious concerns.
55. **Stimulation/nurturance:** Activities that promote healthy physical and emotional development.
56. **Stress management:** Physical and emotional activities that immunize the body from known stressors.
57. **Substance use:** Consumption of medicines, drugs, or other materials, including prescription drugs, over-the-counter or street drugs, alcohol, and tobacco.
58. **Supplies:** Articles necessary to the management of personal care or the treatment plan, including dressings, syringes, lotions, or baby bottles.
59. **Support group:** Regular planned gatherings designed to accomplish some compatible goal, including Alcoholics Anonymous, I Can Cope, or Pilot Parents.
60. **Support system:** The circle of friends, family, and associates that provide love, care, and need gratification, including church, school, and workplace.
61. **Transportation:** Method of travel, including car, bus, and taxi.
62. **Wellness:** Practices that promote health, including immunization, exercise, nutrition, and birth control.
63. **Other:** Nursing action not identified in this list.

From Martin, K. S., & Scheet, N. J. (1992). *The Omaha System: Applications for Community Health Nursing*. Philadelphia: W. B. Saunders, pp. 82–83.

For example, the staff nurse-supervisor conferences use the Omaha System as the framework to discuss client problems and progress. The staff nurse describes the client's problems and progress based on the Problem Classification Scheme and the Problem Rating Scale for Outcomes. The Intervention Scheme terminology is used to describe nursing activities. Using this framework, the staff nurse and supervisor make decisions about the extent and frequency of continuing care. They also use the framework to determine communication with the client, family, and other health care providers, and for reimbursement.

The use of the Omaha System in practice is structured as follows (Martin and Scheet, 1988, p. 26):

> During initial and ongoing client visits, the staff member is responsible for considering and collecting client data from the Environmental, Psychosocial, Physiological, and Health-related behaviors domains. These domains provide a nursing-based data-collection model complementary to referral data, medical diagnoses, and hospitalization details. These data and the Problem Classification System are then used to identify client problems or nursing diagnoses. The Problem Rating Scale for Outcomes enables the staff member to identify client status at

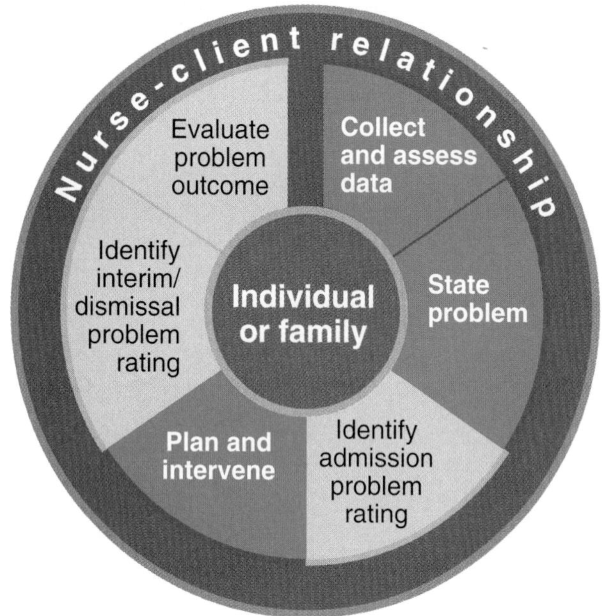

Figure 12-4. The Omaha System problem rating scale for outcomes.

admission to service, at 2-month intervals, and at dismissal. These multiple ratings can be compared by the staff nurse to evaluate client progress. The staff member is expected to use the concepts and terminology of the Intervention Scheme to develop plans and document services provided during home visits.

The VNA staff use a formal peer review process to audit records. Records are reviewed for completeness and adherence to agency documentation policies. Attention is given to consistent use of the Omaha System. The staff currently use process standards but are developing outcome standards based on the Problem Rating Scale for Outcomes.

BENEFITS OF CLASSIFICATION SYSTEMS

Classification systems serve many purposes. They enable health care providers to compare knowledge, results, and experiences within and across classification categories. For example, using the ICD, a nurse might evaluate nursing actions and outcomes for insulin-dependent diabetics to determine the most promising actions in terms of desirable outcomes. Without a means of classifying patients it would be difficult if not impossible to do the evaluation of care.

Once the nurse has reached a nursing diagnosis it becomes a clear, concise way to communicate complex clinical decision making. For example, the nurse may have spent hours with a patient understanding the health and illness problems from the standpoint of the patient. Using one of the nursing classification schemes, the nurse arrives at a set of terms/diagnoses that best summarize the situation. In communication with others, the nurse can use the language of the system rather than provide all the details of the hours spent with the patient.

In a fee-for-service health care financing system, classification schemes are used to determine reimbursement. In a capitated financing system, classification systems are used to create databases that are then used to identify critical care paths (described in the next section) and eliminate unnecessary health care activities, i.e., those that do not appear to influence outcomes.

EMERGING CARE MANAGEMENT PROCESSES

The development of classification systems is an effort to improve the planning of care and the communication of care. Those systems are obviously important. Yet, as clinical settings move to emphasize the role of the nurse in cost-effective management of care, other systems also become important in clinical decision making. Two such systems are presented in this chapter.

Critical Paths

In a managed care approach to health care, there is great emphasis on strategic management of cost and quality outcomes by the clinicians providing care. One strategic management tool used by the clinicians is called *critical path* or *care map.* Critical paths are developed for different groups of patients thought of as a "case type." A case type consists of patients that you anticipate will experience the same clinical symptoms and will therefore require the same services and resources. Examples of case types are depression, myocardial infarction (heart attack), kidney transplant, etc. The critical path includes a listing of anticipated problems with outcomes and the critical path of effects to get from the problems to the outcomes. The critical path is interdisciplinary and specifies on a day-by-day basis what should occur with and for the patient. The path covers the full episode of care. Figures 12–5 and 12–6 illustrate examples of critical paths.

Anecdotal information and the nursing literature support the position that the nurse is usually the person responsible for monitoring patient progress according to the critical path. As part of that responsibility the nurse must note any deviation from the plan and take appropriate action. That action could involve asking another member of the interdisciplinary team to do or not to do something. It could involve exercising judgment regarding individual differences that may affect progress. Whatever the situation, the nurse has the authority along with the responsibility to intervene as necessary. This makes the nurse a very powerful member of the health care team.

Total Quality Management

In recent years many health care institutions have instituted a management philosophy that emphasizes the satisfaction of the consumer. Consumer input is used to assess the value and quality of the outputs. Stated another way, patient evaluations of care guide the health care staff in making changes in care.

Patient ____________________
MD ____________________
Case Manager ____________________
Date Critical Path ____________________
Reviewed by MD ____________________
Date

Case Type Myocardial Infarction
DRG 122
Expected LOS 7 Days

MYOCARDIAL INFARCTION
CRITICAL PATH

	Day 1	Day 2	Day 3	Day 4	Day 5	Day 6	Day 7
ICU	———	———	———	65	———	———	———
Consults		Cardiac Rehab. Dietitian				Copy of Low Chol. No Added Salt Diet	
Tests	EKG	EKG ETT if nec. for Day 6 Echo, Muga, if nec	EKG Receive MBs R/I or R/O MI Holter if nec on Day 5		Holter ETT Cath. if nec		
Activity	BRP w/ Commode		OOB Chair		Amb in Rm/Hall w/Asst	Up Ad ⟶ Lib Stairs	
Treatments	O_2 ⟶			⟶ D/C O_2			
	Cardiac Monitor ⟶				⟶	D/C Monitor p. negative Holter	
	I & O qd ⟶				⟶	D/C I & O qd wt, unless CHF	
	IV ⟶	Heparin Lock ⟶				⟶	D/C Heparin Lock
Diet	No Added Salt, Low Chol. Diet ⟶						⟶
Discharge Planning			VNA		Check w/ Attending RE:D/C Date	Discharge Orders	Discharge before 12 Noon
Teaching	Angina, MI PN, Med, Teaching Plan in Chart	Begin MI Teaching Plan	3 discharge classes Formal Med tx				Amb Classes Re:Risk Factors Diet & smoking

Admission Date ________ Discharge Date ________ Discharge Time ________
Days in ICU ________ Stress test date ________ Cardiac cath. date ________
Days in Routine bed ________ Thalium ________
Routine ________
Holter date ________

	VARIATION	CAUSE	ACTION TAKEN
DATE			

Figure 12-5. Critical path for a patient with myocardial infarction. (From Zander, K. [1988]. Nursing case management: Strategic management of cost and quality outcomes. *Journal of Nursing Administration, 18,* [5], 26.)

Patient problems	Day 1 Admission–Operation	Day 2 Postoperative day 1	Day 3–13	Day 14 Post-operative day 13
Date				
1. Fear related to uncertainty of transplant outcome	Verbalizes concerns about transplant outcome	Verbalizes concern about transplant outcome Comprehends and is informed about kidney function and tests	→	Verbalizes concerns about long-term outcome and management
2. Potential for infection related to immuno-suppression	No evidence of pre-existing infection as indicated by no fever, chest clear No prior history of infection	Incision and central line shows no evidence of infection at Day 1	→	Mucous membrane shows no evidence of infection: fungal or viral
3. Pain related to surgical intervention		Pain controlled as evidenced by non-verbal indicators	→	Analgesics no longer required for pain relief
4. Potential for alteration in fluid balance (excess–deficit) related to impaired regulatory mechanisms	Pre-operative weight within 3% of dry weight Clear chest X-ray No elevation of jugular venous pressure	Post-operative weight within 3% of dry weight Chest clear on X-ray auscultation Central venous pressure of 8–12	→	Patient is euvolemic as evidenced by within 0–5 to 1 kg of dry weight, free of edema, chest clear
5. Knowledge deficit of self-management related to kidney transplant				No knowledge deficit
6. Potential for rejection related to immunological response				No evidence of rejection as indicated by good output, weight stable, no edema, no pain, blood pressure stable, afebrile
Signature Nights				
Days				
Evenings				

Note: Days 3–13 are not provided in this example.

Figure 12–6. Critical path for a patient undergoing renal transplant. (From Petryshen, P. R., Petryshen, P. M. [1992]. The case management model: An innovative approach to the delivery of patient care. *Journal of Advanced Nursing, 17,* 1190.)

The philosophy and process used is called Total Quality Management (TQM) or Total Quality Improvement (TQI). The exact process may vary slightly from institution to institution, but the philosophy behind the process is the same.

TQM is a philosophy about work. The belief is that work involves processes that can continually be improved. In addition, there is the belief that the customer or the recipient of care is the best judge of quality. If the customer is not satisfied,

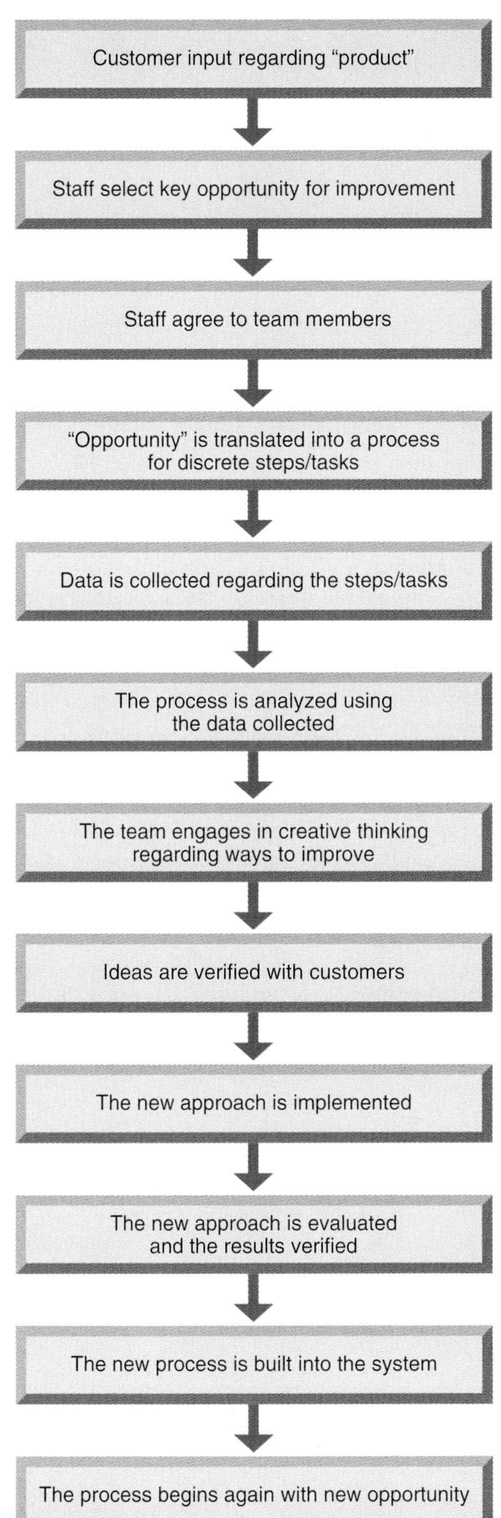

Figure 12-7. Total quality improvement (TQI) process.

quality is lacking. Other key points about the philosophy are as follows:

- Some 85 percent of quality problems are due to the process; only 15 percent are people problems.
- Change needs to be identified by teams of employees, not by the administrators.
- Change must be based on data, not on intuition.
- Teams must be free to think creatively and identify new solutions to quality issues.
- Consensus must be developed before change is initiated.
- The new process must be evaluated before it becomes routine.

As mentioned, institutions have developed a TQM/TQI process that works best in their institution. Yet they are all

BOX 12-8
USING TQI: AN EXAMPLE (EASTES, 1993)

The trauma coordinators at the Oregon Health Sciences University Hospital noted a periodic problem with the notification of trauma patients' families. When patients were unable to contact their families themselves, staff sometimes failed to notify them. The nurses on the units where the patients were sent following care in the emergency room were frustrated by the failure to notify families. Families were angry and had a negative view of the Hospital.

The trauma coordinators decided to use a TQI approach to resolve this problem. The department directors from all nursing units as well as ancillary departments met to decide the composition of the team. The team included a social worker, emergency department staff nurse, trauma surgeon, patient advocate, quality management department representative, emergency department admitting specialist, Intensive Care Unit nurse, and a trauma coordinator as team leader.

The first step was to map the present process for family notification. As soon as the team did this they saw major weaknesses in the system. The team then brainstormed all the possible causes of the problem. The causes were grouped under the headings "procedures," "patients," "provisions," and "people." The team then developed consensus about the root causes.

The team was now ready to collect data. Data were collected retrospectively. The data indicated: (1) most problems with notifying patients' families took place on the evening shift; (2) in more than half of the cases where families were not notified, the patients were either confused or intoxicated and were not carrying identification; (3) social workers usually notified the family but no policy for their doing that existed; and (4) the nursing staff consistently failed to chart family notification efforts.

The team then met to construct solutions, assign accountability for implementation, determine a time frame for implementation, and agree on evaluation criteria.

Problems with notification of families decreased from two per month to two in ten months. The staff recognized that their plan needed modification to include periodic update training for all staff and opportunity for those unhappy with the new process to give input.

The staff believe TQI is a very effective way to change problematic processes within any patient care system.

BOX 12-9
BARRIERS TO EFFECTIVE CRITICAL THINKING

CRITICAL THINKING ENEMY #1: LOGICAL FALLACIES

Non sequitur: Occurs when one statement is not logically connected to another.

Ad hominem: Occurs when the writer (or speaker) personally attacks his or her opponents instead of finding fault with their argument.

Straw man: Occurs when the writer directs the argument against a claim that nobody actually holds or that everyone agrees is weak; often involves misrepresentation or distortion of the opposing argument.

Red herring: Occurs when a writer raises an irrelevant issue to draw attention away from the central issue.

Post hoc, ergo propter hoc: Occurs when the writer implies that because one event follows another, the first caused the second. Chronology is not the same as causality.

Sequential fallacy: Occurs when the writer implies that two simultaneous events are causally related.

Begging the question: Occurs when the believability of the support itself depends upon the believability of the claim. Another name for this kind of fallacy is circular reasoning.

Failing to accept the burden of proof: Occurs when the writer asserts a claim but provides no support for it.

Hasty generalization: Occurs when the writer asserts a claim on the basis of an isolated example.

Sweeping generalizations: Occurs when the writer fails to qualify the applicability of the claim and asserts that it applies to "all" instances instead of to "some" instances.

Overgeneralizations: Occurs when the writer fails to qualify the claim and asserts that it is "certainly true" rather than that it "may be true."

Slippery slope: Occurs when the writer argues that taking one step will lead inevitably to a next step, one that is undesirable.

Equivocation: Occurs when a writer uses the same term in two different senses in an argument.

Oversimplification: Occurs when an argument obscures or denies the complexity of the issue.

Either-or reasoning or false division: Occurs when the writer reduces the issue to only two alternatives that are polar opposites.

Double standard: Occurs when two or more comparable things are judged according to different standards; often involves holding the opposing argument to a higher standard than the one to which the writer holds his or her own argument.

Reification: Occurs when the writer portrays the symbol as the actual thing and therefore misplaces his or her response to the thing onto the symbol.

Ambiguous words or phrases: Occurs when the writer uses words or phrases that have unclear, unspecific or many different meanings without clarifying his or her specific meaning. These are often used to evoke a purely emotional response.

Emotional appeal: Occurs when the writer tries to excite or appeal to only the reader's emotions.

similar in many respects. The flowchart in Figure 12–7 illustrates the general TQM/TQI process. A case study highlighting the use of TQI is presented in Box 12–8.

In summary, it is the clinical decision-making skills of the nurse that are the key to quality in contemporary nursing practice. The nurse will use clinical guidelines in some situations and clinical paths in other situations. For some patients neither will be available. In all situations, the nurse must still determine what care the patient requires and how best to provide that care.

Tools such as classification schemes are available to assist in making clinical decisions. It is important to remember that these are only tools to assist. No tool can replace the clinical judgment of the nurse. It should also be noted that tools will change over time. At one point in time a particular nursing process (assess, plan, intervene, evaluate) was the most commonly used tool. Today that particular nursing process has been replaced by the concept of clinical decision making that emphasizes the individual differences of patients and care management. In time clinical decision making will be replaced by another tool to help nurses provide high-quality care. Tools will change. What will never change is the relationship between the thinking skills of the nurse and quality care.

LIFELONG LEARNING

The only way to improve clinical decision-making skills is to make a conscious effort to do so. One way to improve these skills was discussed earlier in the chapter in terms of Tanner's clinical decision-making model. Using that model to analyze clinical experiences will help one develop insight into areas of strength and areas that need improvement.

Exercises to improve various thinking skills were included in this chapter. Clinical decision making requires the use of those skills. With thoughtful practice, the nurse will become more proficient in the use of those skills in the clinical setting. The novice should compare his or her clinical decision making with nurse experts. This can be done by asking for critique of one's own decisions or through interaction with the expert. It is

BOX 12-9
BARRIERS TO EFFECTIVE CRITICAL THINKING *Continued*

Ethical appeal: Occurs when the writer tries to convince readers to accept an argument on the basis of his or her moral credentials.

Appeal to tradition: Occurs when the writer's grounds rest solely on the "goodness" of what has been done in the past.

Appeal to ignorance: Occurs when the writer argues that something is valid because it is not known to be false.

Add to these signs of shoddy and deceptive research, such as unacceptable violations of scientific methods and statistical assumptions.

CRITICAL THINKING ENEMY #2: PSYCHO-LOGICAL FALLACIES

Assimilation: Occurs when a person distorts his or her perception and/or memory of an object, event or person to fit into his or her existing beliefs or attitudes.

Denial: Occurs when a person refuses to acknowledge certain impulses or emotions in himself or herself. Typically, he or she also becomes insensitive to or critical of similar impulses or emotions in others.

Displacement: Occurs when a person transfers an emotion from its original focus to another object, person or event.

Externalization: Occurs when a person's unresolved inner conflicts or emotions distort his or her perception of another person, event or issue.

Projection: Occurs when a person ascribes to others his or her own attitudes, emotions, beliefs or thoughts.

Rationalization: Occurs when a person attributes his or her opinions or behavior to causes that seem valid but are not the true, possibly unconscious causes.

Regression: Occurs when a person reverts to a developmentally earlier or less adapted pattern of feeling or behavior.

Repression: Occurs when a person rejects consciousness of painful or disagreeable impulses, emotions, thoughts or memories.

Resistance: Occurs when a person opposes an attempt to bring repressed impulses, emotions, thoughts or memories to consciousness.

Selective Perception/Recall: Occurs when a person fails to perceive/recall what threatens his or her existing beliefs or attitudes.

Sublimation: Occurs when a person diverts the energy of a biological impulse from its immediate goal to a higher social, moral or aesthetic goal.

Suppression: Occurs when a person consciously inhibits an impulse, emotion, thought or memory.

Transference: Occurs when a person shifts emotions (especially those experienced in childhood) from one person or object to another (especially the transfer of feelings about a parent to a therapist).

Withdrawal: Occurs when a person removes his or her energy or consciousness from situation that is currently threatening or painful.

(Courtesy of Linda B. Nilson, Vanderbilt University, Nashville, TN.)

helpful to ask the expert nurse to talk out loud when making a decision or to share after the fact the critical parts of the process.

Skill in clinical decision making depends on the extent and organization of one's knowledge base. That knowledge base includes the knowledge gained from experience. The organization of one's knowledge base requires thought. The nurse must reflect on information and experience and make associations that can be stored in memory. This mental review increases the likelihood that knowledge will be recalled. It also allows the nurse the opportunity to store it in memory with related information and experience.

Practicing asking the right question (Browne and Keeley, 1994) is another method for improving clinical decision-making skills. Asking the right question involves the ability to analyze an argument in terms of the following:

- What is the real issue?
- What is the conclusion you are asked to accept?
- What rationale is offered to support the conclusion?
- What beliefs or biases confound the rationale?
- Do you accept the definitions of key terms?
- How good is the evidence used to support the rationale?
- Are there fallacies in the reasoning? (see Box 12–9)
- What rival conclusions can be put forward?
- Was significant information omitted?

The next time you listen to a politician's campaign speech, take notes on the issue(s)/conclusion(s)/rationale(s). Use the questions to analyze the statements. Do so with someone who has a different political bent than yours. Compare the similarities and differences in your analysis and conclusions.

In addition to improving your skills through your own reflection and experience, you must continue to study what experts write about thinking and decision making. Whatever is known today about thinking and decision making will be less than what is known tomorrow. Because critical thinking and clinical decision making are understood as important to the advancement of civilization, they are the subject of considerable research and analysis. Become a lifelong student of these skills.

CHAPTER HIGHLIGHTS

- Critical thinking/clinical decision making/clinical judgment (terms used interchangeably in the nursing literature) is considered the key to quality nursing practice.
- The practice of nursing is moving from the use of a linear thought process to nonlinear interactive thought processes.
- The nursing process defined as a linear reasoning process remains one of the thought processes used in the practice of nursing.
- Thinking processes/skills used in the practice of nursing include inductive reasoning, deductive reasoning, creativity, intuition, and critical thinking per se.
- Classification systems are used to assist in clinical decision making as well as in communicating decisions to members of the health care team.
- Critical thinking skills are also involved in implementing two care management processes: critical paths/care maps and total quality management (TQM).

REFERENCES

Allen, K. E. (1990). *Making Sense out of Chaos: Leading and Living in Dynamic Systems. Campus Activities Programming,* May, 54ff.

American Psychiatric Association (1994). *Diagnostic and Statistical Manual of Mental Disorders,* 4th ed. Washington, D.C.: American Psychiatric Association.

Anderson, B. F. (1980). *The Complete Thinker.* Englewood Cliffs, NJ: Prentice-Hall.

Benner, P., Tanner, C. (1987). Clinical judgment: How expert nurses use intuition. *American Journal of Nursing, 87,* 23–31.

Brookfield, S. D. (1987). *Developing Critical Thinkers.* San Francisco: Jossey-Bass.

Brown, F. (1991). *ICD-9-CM: Coding handbook, without answers, 1991 revised edition.* (DHHS Pub. No. [PHS] 89-1260). Bethesda, MD: U.S. Department of Health and Human Services, Public Health Service, Health Care Financing Administration.

Browne, M. N., Keeley, S. M. (1994). *Asking the right questions,* 4th ed. Englewood Cliffs, NJ: Prentice-Hall.

Bulechek, G. M., McCloskey, J. C. (guest eds.) (1992). *The Nursing Clinics of North America: Nursing Interventions* (Vol. 27, No. 2). Philadelphia: W. B. Saunders.

Bulechek, G. M., McCloskey, J. C. (1992). *Nursing Interventions: Essential Nursing Treatments,* 2nd ed. Philadelphia: W. B. Saunders.

Bulger, R. J. (1990). The demise of the placebo effect in the practice of scientific medicine—a natural progression or an undesirable abberation? *Trans Am Clin Climatol Assoc,* 102, 285–292.

Eastes, L. (1993). Trauma system problems: Using the tools of quality improvement to find solutions. *Journal of Emergency Nursing, 19* (2), 163–166.

Egan, G. (1986). *The Skilled Helper: A Systematic Approach to Effective Helping,* 3rd ed. Monterey, CA: Brooks/Cole.

Ford, J. S., Profetto-McGrath, J. (1994). A model for critical thinking within the context of curriculum as praxis. *Journal of Nursing Education, 33* (8), 341–344.

Hamers, J. P. H., Huijer Abu-Saad, H., Halfens, R. J. G. (1994). Diagnostic process and decision making in nursing: A literature review. *Journal of Professional Nursing, 10* (3), 154–163.

Henderson, V. (1982). The nursing process—is the title right? *Journal of Advanced Nursing, 7,* 103–109.

Iowa Intervention Project (1993). The NIC taxonomy structure. *Image: Journal of Nursing Scholarship, 25* (3), 187–192.

Kobert, L., Folan, M. (1990). Coming of age in rethinking the philosophies behind holism and nursing process. *Nursing and Health Care, 11* (6), 308–312.

Kurfiss, J. G. (1988). *Critical thinking* (Report No. 2). Washington, D.C.: ASHE-ERIC Higher Education.

Lindsey, E., Hartrick, G. (1996). Health-promoting nursing practice: The demise of the nursing process? *Journal of Advanced Nursing,* 23, 106–112.

MacKinnon, D. (1962). The nature and nurture of creative talent. *American Psychologist, 17,* 484–495.

Martin, K. S., Scheet, N. J. (1988). The Omaha System: Providing a framework for assuring quality of home care. *Home Healthcare Nurse, 6* (3), 24–28.

Martin, K. S., Scheet, N. J. (1992). *The Omaha System: Applications for Community Health Nursing.* Philadelphia: W. B. Saunders, pp. 66–96.

Mason, G., Webb, C. (1993). Nursing diagnosis: A review of the literature. *Journal of Clinical Nursing, 2, 67–74.*

McCloskey, J. C., Bulechek, G.M. (eds.). (1996). Nursing Interventions Classification (NIC), 2nd ed. St Louis: Mosby-Year Book, p. 296.

Moorhead, S. A., McCloskey, J. C., Bulechek, G. M. (1993). Nursing interventions classification: A comparison with the Omaha System and the home healthcare classification. *Journal of Nursing Administration, 23* (10), 23–29.

Schwabbauer, M., Parlette, G. N., Weinholtz, D., Branson, R. M. (1985). Medical technologist thinking styles. *Journal of Medical Technology,* 2(8), 517–520.

Percy, C., Van Holten, V., Muir, C. (eds.) (1990). *International Classification of Diseases for Oncology,* 2nd ed. Geneva: World Health Organization.

Petryshen, P. R., Petryshen, P. M. (1992). The case management model: An innovative approach to the delivery of patient care. *Journal of Advanced Nursing, 17,* 1188–1194.

Pinkley, C. L. (1991). Exploring NANDA's definition of nursing diagnosis: Linking diagnostic judgments with the selection of outcomes and interventions. *Nursing Diagnosis, 2* (1), 26–32.

Rogers, C. (1959). Toward a theory of creativity. In H. Anderson (ed.): *Creativity and Its Cultivation.* New York: Harper.

Tanner, C. (1993). Rethinking clinical judgment. In N. Diekelmann and M. Rather (eds.): *Transforming RN Education.* New York: National League for Nursing, pp. 15–41.

Tanner, C. (1996). Clinical judgment. In P. Benner, C. Tanner, and C. Chesla (eds.): *Expertise in Nursing Practice: Caring, Clinical Judgment and Ethics.* New York: Springer.

Saba, V. K., O'Hare, P. A., Zuckerman, A. E., et al (1991). A nursing intervention taxonomy for home health care. *Nursing and Health Care, 12* (6), 296–299.

Warren, J. J., Hoskins, L. M. (1990). The development of NANDA's nursing diagnosis taxonomy. *Nursing Diagnosis, 1* (4), 168–196.

Wolf, G. A., Boland, S., Aukerman, M. (1994). A transformational model for the practice of nursing. *Journal of Nursing Administration, 24* (4), 51–57.

Young, C. E. (1987). Intuition and nursing process. *Holistic Nursing Practice, 1* (3), 52–62.

Zander, K. (1988). Nursing case management: Strategic management of cost and quality outcomes. *Journal of Nursing Administration, 18* (5), 23–30.

13 Patient and Family Education

Carol Lindeman

OBJECTIVES

After studying this chapter, students will be able to:

- **design, implement, and evaluate educational interventions as a component of nursing practice**

Patient education is a very powerful nursing intervention. It has the potential to enable patients and families to care for themselves, manage symptoms, improve the quality of life, promote health and prevent illness, and reduce the costs of health care. No other single intervention has the same potential.

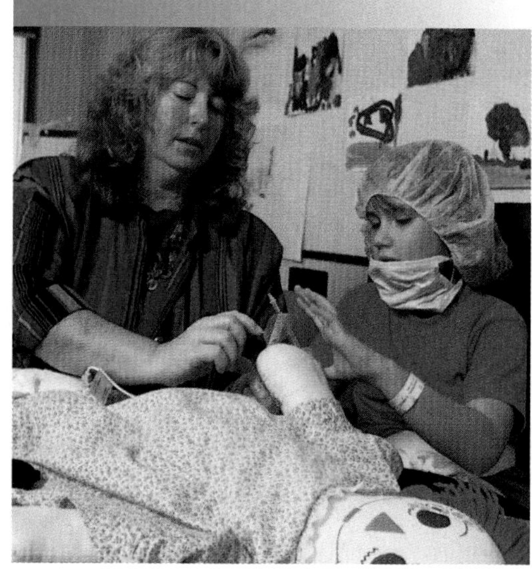

The importance of patient education is evident from an excerpt from this newspaper article (Painter, 1992):

> Instances of sudden infant death syndrome (SIDS) dropped 12% in six months after a 1992 national advisory that infants not be allowed to sleep face down, researchers said Monday.
>
> And in King County, WA, SIDS cases dropped **52%** in the first eight months after the change was urged in a single 1991 newspaper article. Research from Great Britain and New Zealand shows substantial, sustained drops in sudden infant deaths after major education campaigns.

Just imagine how many SIDS deaths could be prevented if nurses assumed the responsibility to educate every parent of every newborn to place their child on its back or side for sleep.

The importance of patient education is also clearly stated in the national goals for health promotion and disease prevention (Healthy People 2000, 1991, p. 251):

> In a democratic society, health education is particularly important to assure that individuals have the information and skills they need to protect and enhance their own health, the health of the families for which they are responsible, and the health of the communities in which they live. Effective health education enables individuals to make informed choices about behaviors that will affect their health; and enables populations to collectively make informed decisions about the allocation of resources, implementation of health programs and services, and enactment of legislation to protect the health of populations.

Educational and community-based health promotion and disease prevention interventions are important in reducing preventable disease, injury, disability, and premature death **and have the potential to increase years of healthy life from 62 to 65** (Healthy People 2000, 1991).

Based on data from the Centers for Disease Control showing that patient education programs for diabetes, asthma, and other conditions are valued by patients and can help to improve the efficiency and effectiveness of care, and patient education programs may reduce length of hospital stay, prevent hospital readmissions, and reduce emergency room visits, Healthy People 2000 calls for 90 percent of the country's hospitals, health maintenance organizations, and large group practices to provide patient education programs. In 1987 only 66 percent of the hospitals offered such programs.

In addition, the Report calls for significant increases in health educational programs in schools, work sites, and community settings. The key to good health is responsible and enlightened behavior that can only occur through education.

Education of the patient and family is a key element of contemporary nursing practice. Its importance has increased over this last decade for reasons including:

- increasing demands for knowledge from patients
- legal pressures
- earlier hospital discharges
- higher incidence of chronic diseases
- research evidence supporting the benefits of patient education
- increased self-care and care provided by family (Luker and Caress, 1989; Redman and Thomas, 1992)

In the past most patient education focused on teaching compliance with the medical regimen. Today it is primarily focused on self-care skills and enabling patients and families to make informed choices such as:

- self-management of asthma
- choice among options for surgery for breast cancer
- self-care skills in the management of diabetes including blood glucose monitoring
- cognitive control by family members of their experiences in dealing with a loved one with cancer (Redman and Thomas, 1992)

This change in focus requires teaching problem-solving and performance skills in addition to knowledge.

Patient teaching is an intervention (nursing activity) linked to a specific outcome; an interactive process that includes assessment, an educational encounter, supportive activity, directed practice, evaluation and reinforcement; broad in scope including facilitating acquiring new knowledge, skills, attitudes, problem-solving abilities, and feelings of being able to care for oneself.

NURSING RESEARCH BASE

The nursing literature contains literally hundreds of studies regarding patient education. For the purposes of this chapter, the research is summarized in terms of questions relevant to practice.

What Do We Know About the Relationship Between Characteristics of the Patient and Learning Outcomes?

PSYCHOLOGICAL CHARACTERISTICS

Psychological characteristics of the patient have been studied in relationship to learning outcomes. For example, a study was conducted to explore the relationships between locus of control (whether you believe you control your fate or that it is controlled by external forces), social support, and success in a weight loss program (Gierszewski, 1983). Neither locus of control nor social support influenced weight loss outcomes. Another example is the study conducted to see if preoperative fear and anxiety influenced the effectiveness of preoperative teaching (Kinney, 1977). Fear and anxiety did not influence effectiveness.

Studies have also been conducted to determine the relationship between patient characteristics, teaching strategy, and learning outcomes. One such study (Mills et al, 1985) analyzed the relationship between compliance and a patient's sociodemographic variables (age, education, and so on), intelligence, problem-solving ability, motivation, and knowledge. Of all these factors, motivation was most highly correlated with compliance.

To date the research base supports the following generalization. **Psychological characteristics by themselves are not strong predictors of learning outcomes. They do seem to interact with teaching strategies and thus influence outcomes. In particular, the nurse needs to consider the patient's motivation to learn** (Lindeman, 1988).

READING LEVEL

Common sense suggests that if a patient cannot read or comprehend educational material, there is little likelihood of any benefit. Yet for decades patient education materials have been developed at levels beyond the reading ability of many patients.

An early study (Mohammed, 1964) reported that in one large clinic, written educational materials were primarily at the **eighth grade level** and **only 22 percent** of the clinic population could comprehend the material. Studies conducted since then confirm: (1) the relationship between reading ability and learning outcomes, and (2) written patient education materials are beyond the comprehension of a significant number of patients (Taylor et al, 1982; Estey et al, 1991; Meade et al, 1992). Nurses and others developing patient education materials tend to forget that approximately 38 percent of American adults have no high school diploma, 20 percent of the population is functionally illiterate, and a high school diploma is no guarantee that the person can read (Dixon and Park, 1990).

To date the research literature supports the following generalization: **Reading ability does influence ability to learn and comprehend. Patient educational materials should be**

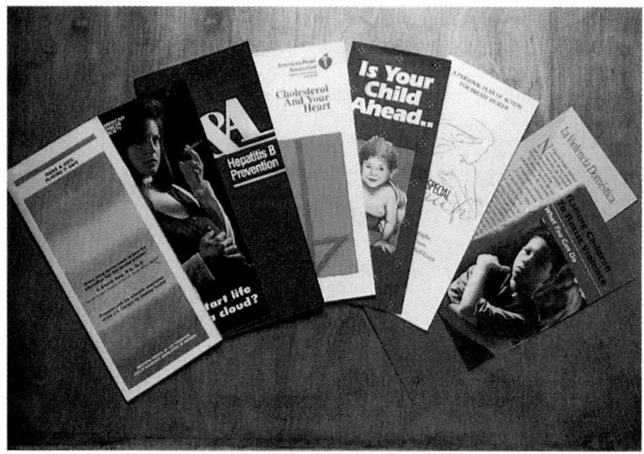

Figure 13–1. Printed patient education materials must be appropriate to the individual patient's reading ability.

at the sixth to eighth grade level (Dixon and Park, 1990) (Fig. 13–1). **The nurse needs to verify the appropriateness of the reading level of words and sentence structure used in verbal presentations and written materials. The nurse should not assume the patient can comprehend the material.** Box 13–1 presents a method that the nurse can use to rate the appropriateness of written patient education materials for a particular patient and family.

What Do We Know About Various Patient Populations and Learning Outcomes?

In general, studies in this category involve the design of a particular patient education program based on the researcher's clinical experience with the patient population. For example, a nurse experienced with home care of patients recovering from a severe heart attack might design and evaluate a patient education program regarding diet, exercise, smoking, stress, and sex offered to patients in the last few days of their hospital stay. These topics reflect the questions patients asked the nurse after they returned to their homes. The assumption of the nurse is that if patients have this information before they go home they will avoid problems and experience less stress. The nurse would offer the program to some patients and not to others. Change in knowledge due to the program would be used to determine the effectiveness of the program.

The nursing research literature is filled with studies assessing learning outcomes for various categories of patients. There is, for example, a substantial literature documenting the benefits of prenatal instruction (Orstead et al, 1985; Timm, 1979; Henderson, 1983; Cohen, 1980).

Diabetic and other chronically ill, surgical, and cardiac patients clearly benefit from patient education programs (Brown, 1990; Cupples, 1991; Devine, 1992; Dodd, 1983; Funnell et al, 1992; Milazzo, 1980; Mullen et al, 1992).

Most of the studies in this category evaluate the accuracy of the content learned and recalled at a later point in time. Very few studies actually evaluated the patient's **use** of the knowledge.

The following generalization can be made regarding patient populations and learning outcomes: **Virtually all patient populations learn when taught. Patients tend to retain the knowledge acquired in patient education programs.**

What Do We Know About the Relationship Between Teaching Strategies and Learning?

Nurses have designed and tested the use of many different teaching strategies. Examples include:

- Programmed instruction to enhance self-care following pulmonary surgery (Goodwin, 1979)
- Individualized learning activity packet for hip replacement patients (Wong and Wong, 1985)
- Contracting with hypertensive patients (Swain and Steckel, 1981)
- Self-instructional booklet designed to teach facts about heart attacks (Gregor, 1981)
- A game for diabetic children (Heston and Lazar, 1980)

Self-help diaries, computer-assisted instruction (Fig. 13–2), programmed instruction, and audio and videotapes are all effective teaching strategies for a range of patient populations (Beresford et al, 1992; Brown et al, 1992; Lindsay et al, 1991; Peterson, 1991; Vargo, 1991).

Nurses have also explored group and individual teaching (Choi-Loa, 1976; Falkiewicz, 1980; Lindeman, 1972). These studies compared the effect of using the same teaching strategy in group and individual situations.

The timing of teaching is another common research question. Nurses have explored questions such as teaching the presurgical patient several days prior to admission versus the night before surgery (Levesque et al, 1984). A similar question—when to teach maternity patients postpartum information—has also been explored (Petrowski, 1981).

Structured versus unstructured teaching has been a frequent research question (Billie, 1977; Garvey and Kramer, 1983; Lindeman and Van Aernam, 1971; Milazzo, 1980); see

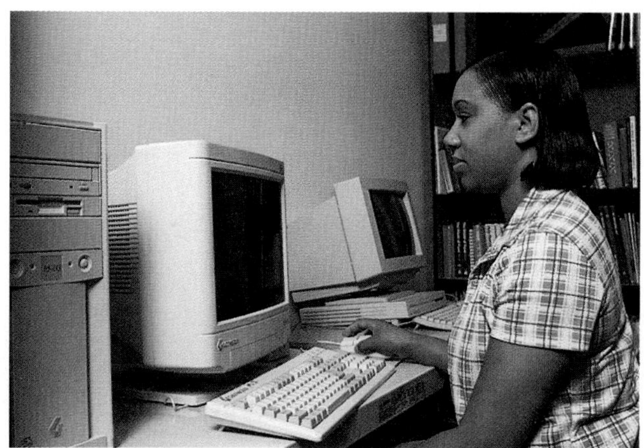

Figure 13–2. More and more patients are able to use computer-assisted instruction for self-teaching.

BOX 13-1
BERNIER INSTRUCTIONAL DESIGN SCALE 2 (BIDS - 2)(1997)

The BIDS-2 is a checklist for rating the presence (or absence) of instructional design and learning principles contained in printed education materials (PEMs) for use with patients and families.

1. Begin the rating procedure by reading each principle on the BIDS-2.
2. Next, read the PEM to be evaluated.
3. Use the Rating Scale listed below to record the level of instructional design and learning principles contained in the PEM.
4. Re-read the PEM as many times as you need to complete the rating.

Rating Scale

0 = NOT MET
1 = PARTIALLY MET
2 = MET
NA = NOT APPLICABLE

EXAMPLE: Principle #1 states, "The font or print size can be easily read by the target group."

A PEM that is written in a print size as small as this (9 point font) would not be appropriate for a general target audience since the readers would be of many age groups and some would have difficulty reading this print size.

The appropriate rating for a PEM written in the 9 point font would be 0 = NOT MET if the PEM is intended for a general audience which would include elderly persons. You would place a check mark in the column labeled 0 for principle #1.

Principle:	Scale: 0	1	2	NA
1. The font or print size can be easily read by the target group. This is a 14 point font recommended for the elderly; this is a 12 point font recommended for general audience and this is a 10 point font.	—	—	—	—
2. The vocabulary of the PEM reflects words commonly used by the target group.	—	—	—	—
3. The learning objectives & educational content of the PEM relate to one another.	—	—	—	—
4. The learning objectives relate to the intended learning outcome.	—	—	—	—
5. The information presented in the PEM is accurate.	—	—	—	—
6. The information is presented using concrete terms rather than abstract ideas.	—	—	—	—
7. The educational content is presented in a way that relates and integrates the new information to what is already known and understood by the target group.	—	—	—	—

continued on next page

8. Examples are used to bridge the gap between what the target group already knows and the new information that is presented in the PEM. — — — —

9. The information load of the material is appropriate to the target group. Information load = amount + obscurity/novelty of information. Content that is unfamiliar represents a larger information load than content that is familiar to the target group. — — — —

10. The information presented in the PEM focuses on what the target group should *do* as well as *know.* — — — —

11. The information presented in the PEM is current and up to date. — — — —

12. Important information is repeated as reinforcement throughout the PEM. — — — —

13. Accurate and coherent summaries of the informational content are included in the PEM. — — — —

14. The PEM is written at a reading level that is appropriate to the target group. Material intended for the general public should be written at the 6th to 8th grade level. — — — —

Directions for applying the SMOG Readability Formula (Doak, Doak, and Root, 1985) follow:

SMOG Formula for Determining Reading Grade Level

1. A total of 30 sentences are examined with the SMOG:
   10 consecutive sentences are selected from the beginning of the PEM.
   10 consecutive sentences are selected from the middle of the PEM.
   10 consecutive sentences are selected near the end of the PEM.

2. Count the number of syllables for each word in the 30 sentences. For example, the word cough contains one syllable; the word mucus contains two syllables (mu/cus); the word polio contains three syllables (po/li/o); and pneumonectomy contains five syllables (pneu/mon/ect/o/my)

3. Count the number of words containing three or more syllables in the 30 sentences, including words that are repetitions.

4. Determine the nearest perfect square root of the total number of words with three or more syllables in the 30 sentences selected and the number "3" (a constant in the formula) is added to the square root to obtain the grade level.

EXAMPLE: A PEM having 53 words with three or more syllables in the 30 selected sentences would have a square root of 7 since $7 \times 7 = 49$. By adding the constant number 3, the reading level is determined to be at the 10th grade since 7 (the nearest perfect square root for 53) + 3 (constant in the formula) is equal to 10.

RESEARCH HIGHLIGHT

EXCERPTS FROM EDUCATING PARENTS WITH LIMITED LITERACY SKILLS: THE EFFECTIVENESS OF PRINTED AND VIDEOTAPED MATERIALS ABOUT COLON CANCER

by Cathy D. Meade, PhD, RN, W. Paul McKinney, MD, and Gary P. Barnes, MD, American Journal of Public Health, 84, 119–121, 1994

Colon cancer, the second most common malignancy among men and women in the United States, results in over 61,000 deaths each year. Efforts to reduce colon cancer mortality and morbidity focus primarily on early detection and treatment, given the high survival rates in early stages of the disease. Printed materials are commonly used to communicate screening guidelines and detection practices, yet they are often produced at reading levels above that of the intended reader. For those with low reading skills, videotapes may offer a significant advantage over printed materials because of their visual appeal. Videotaped instruction has been demonstrated to be as effective as other instructional methods and often more effective than printed material alone. . . . We believe this is the first study to compare the effect of printed vs. videotaped colon cancer information on enhancing knowledge among individuals with limited reading skills.

Booklet. The booklet was written in medium size type, at the 5–6 grade reading level, and had five sections: facts about colon cancer, facts about the colon and rectum, signs and symptoms of colon cancer, early detection of colon cancer, and a summary.

Videotape. The videotape contained the same information as the booklet and used the same headings. It showed patients participating in desired screening behaviors.

Pretest/posttest. To evaluate colon cancer knowledge and recall, 24 questions written at grade 5–6 were developed.

Subjects (1100) were randomly assigned to one of three groups: control, booklet, or videotape. All subjects were given the pretest before the intervention and the posttest following it. Pretest scores were subtracted from posttest scores and analyzed for differences.

The investigators found that the subjects receiving either the booklet or videotape instruction had scores significantly higher than the control group. There were no significant differences in scores for the booklet and videotape groups.

The investigators conclude that appropriately designed educational materials are effective with patients with limited literacy skills.

Research Highlight. Structured teaching refers to using a planned formal teaching approach. Unstructured teaching refers to an informal approach determined by the individual nurse at the time the teaching is done.

This very extensive literature supports the following generalizations:

- All teaching strategies have the potential to produce effective outcomes. Nurses can use methods they are comfortable with and that seem appropriate to the individual patient.
- Patients learn as well in groups as when they are taught individually. Group teaching is more cost-effective and may also lead to other benefits such as higher patient satisfaction.
- The timing of teaching does not seem to be an important factor. Patients learn whenever they are taught—assuming it is an appropriate time. None of the research used times that were inappropriate such as teaching a presurgical patient on the way to surgery.
- Structured teaching is clearly superior to unstructured teaching. Nurses need to take time to develop effective teaching plans and materials.

What Do We Know About the Relationship Between the Setting and Learning Outcomes?

There are few studies comparing learning outcomes across different settings. The studies that have been conducted have typically compared teaching patients in their home with teaching done in the hospital or clinical setting (Dalzell, 1965; Lowe, 1970). These studies have not produced evidence that one setting is better than another.

Certainly the research literature contains studies where patient education was offered in different settings. The home, hospital, and clinic are all popular settings for conducting patient teaching research. Patients seem to be able to learn in a variety of settings.

The research literature supports the generalization that **the setting in which the teaching takes place is *not* a critical factor in determining learning outcomes.** Again, it is important to note that none of the research explored teaching in inappropriate settings such as a street corner. A nurse can select a setting appropriate to the individual or family and feel confident that effective teaching can occur.

What Do We Know About the Relationship Between Specific Content Areas and Learning Outcomes?

Nurses have questioned the value of specific content for a variety of patient populations. Three areas have been studied intensively: relaxation techniques, psychoeducation, and parenting behavior and skill.

Progressive muscle relaxation has intrigued nurses as a means of reducing nausea and vomiting in cancer patients and for pain reduction with surgical patients (Cotanch, 1983; Flaherty and Fitzpatrick, 1978; Holden-Lund, 1988; Warner et al, 1992). Although the investigators called the intervention by the same name, the specific content and number of educational sessions differed across investigators. In the majority of

RESEARCH HIGHLIGHT

EXCERPTS FROM EFFECTS OF EDUCATIONAL INTERVENTIONS IN DIABETES CARE: A META-ANALYSIS OF FINDINGS

by Sharon A. Brown, Nursing Research, 37, 223–230, 1988

Meta-analysis, a group of quantitative procedures useful for synthesizing a body of research in a given area, was used to integrate the results of studies conducted on patient education in diabetes. The following research questions were explored:

1. What is the magnitude of the effect of patient teaching in diabetic adults?
2. What outcomes of patient teaching of diabetic adults have been documented with regard to patient knowledge about diabetes, its management, self-care behaviors, and degree of metabolic control?

FINDINGS

Research Question 1: To determine the magnitude of the effect of patient teaching in diabetic adults, effect sizes across all 47 studies included in the analysis were pooled.

Regardless of the manner in which the mean effect size is determined, **patient teaching does appear to enhance patient outcomes in diabetes management.**

Research Question 2: To answer the second question 14 analyses were done to find the best conceptual fit of the many outcome measures.

In this study patient teaching was found to have a positive moderate effect on each of the outcome variables: **knowledge, self-care behaviors (skill performance and compliance), and metabolic control. Diabetes patient teaching appears to enhance these patient outcomes.**

METHODOLOGIC CONSIDERATIONS

While conducting this study, it became clear that the use of meta-analysis has proceeded faster than the development of the statistical theory needed as a basis for meta-analytic procedures. Certainly, it is apparent that quantitative procedures for synthesizing a body of research are needed.

In spite of the methodologic problems, some important relationships have been identified. Trends in the data are more important than any individual statistical result, and the trend of the data from this study suggests that **patient teaching in diabetes care is effective in producing positive outcomes.**

studies progressive muscle relaxation made patients feel more comfortable and in control.

For three decades nurses have investigated the effects of an intervention, primarily psychological and secondarily educational in nature, designed to reduce the negative effects of hospitalization. The research is based on the assumption that patients see the hospital experience as a threatening event.

Typical of this category of studies is the work by Johnson (1974; 1975; 1978; 1985). The psychoeducational intervention consisted of sensory description information and behavioral information. The patient received specific information about what would be done (in a given procedure) and exactly what sensations would be experienced during that time. The patient also received specific information about what to do to reduce the negative sensations. In some research the nurse assisted the patient determine those actions the patient believed would be effective.

This psychoeducational intervention was tested with adults having painful diagnostic procedures, adults having surgery, and children having casts removed. The data support this as an effective intervention.

A third area of investigation is parenting behavior and skill. Nurses interested in this topic assume a relationship between effective parenting and the immediate and future health and well-being of the infant. A variety of educational interventions have been tested, including having fathers attend classes (Bowen and Miller, 1980), educating mothers in the home after childbirth (Hall, 1980), and a variety of programs designed to help parents understand the unique characteristics of the child (Perry, 1983). This educational content has a positive effect on parenting behavior. The research does not support the effectiveness of one program over another.

In areas where there is substantial experimental research, investigators can combine data from the separate studies and apply a statistical procedure called *meta-analysis.* This enables drawing statistically supported conclusions rather than basing conclusions on inferences. An example of a meta-analysis is presented in the Research Highlight box. Meta-analyses have been performed on research related to diabetic education, presurgical education, and cardiac patient education, to name just a few.

The research supports the generalization that **teaching patients specific content relative to self-care or symptom management activities is an effective intervention. Patients are able to use such knowledge and skills to their benefit.**

Summary

The research literature makes explicit the importance of patient education as a nursing intervention. It supports the following generalizations:

- Motivation to learn and reading ability are important determinants of learning outcomes.

- All patient populations respond positively to the opportunity to learn.
- All teaching strategies have the potential to facilitate effective learning.
- Well-planned and -implemented programs (structured) are associated with positive outcomes.
- Patients are responsive to opportunities to learn knowledge and skills useful in self-care and symptom management.

LEARNING OUTCOMES AND TEACHING PRINCIPLES

Facts and Concepts

Most patient/family teaching is designed to facilitate learning of facts and concepts. For example, prior to discharge the nurse will instruct the patient on how to take medications correctly, how to change a dressing (Fig. 13–3), or how to recognize negative signs and symptoms. The nurse may facilitate a family learning good parenting behaviors or understanding what it means to live with a chronic disease such as hypertension (high blood pressure). A fact is a piece of information having objective reality. The name of a medication is a fact. A concept is a thought or abstract idea developed and generalized from specific instances. Developing an understanding of the concept of discipline is an important aspect of parenting.

PRINCIPLES FOR TEACHING FACTS

There are five important principles to keep in mind when teaching facts.

- **Organize the material in a manner appropriate to the individual.** For example, if the patient is able to concentrate only for short periods, develop the materials into brief modules. If the patient is familiar with some of the material but not all of it, arrange for a quick review and then introduce the new material. Ask the patient's preference to read material before or after you discuss it.
- **Relate the new material to knowledge the person already has.** This moves new material into a meaningful form that will facilitate learning. For example, if the patient enjoys working on automobiles, you could link facts about good health habits to preventive maintenance on an automobile.
- **Sequence material in a manner that makes sense to the patient.** One way to do this is to ask the patient to tell you his or her major questions about the drug (or whatever you are teaching) and then use the questions as the basis for sequencing the content.
- **Arrange for appropriate practice.** Recall facilitates learning and retention of material. Interact with the patient, asking him or her to repeat parts of the material presented (Fig. 13–4).
- **Develop the patient's ability to evaluate his or her own knowledge.** This could be done by asking the patient to teach you (or a family member) what you just taught the patient. Having the patient answer a set of questions is another method.

PRINCIPLES FOR TEACHING CONCEPTS

There are six principles basic to teaching concepts. By definition, a concept is learned through repeated experience with positive and negative illustrations of the concept. The principles reflect that notion.

- **Emphasize the unique features of the concept—what it is and what it is not.** Using the example of effective discipline as one parenting concept, the first instructional step is to identify the features of effective discipline and contrast that with less effective discipline.

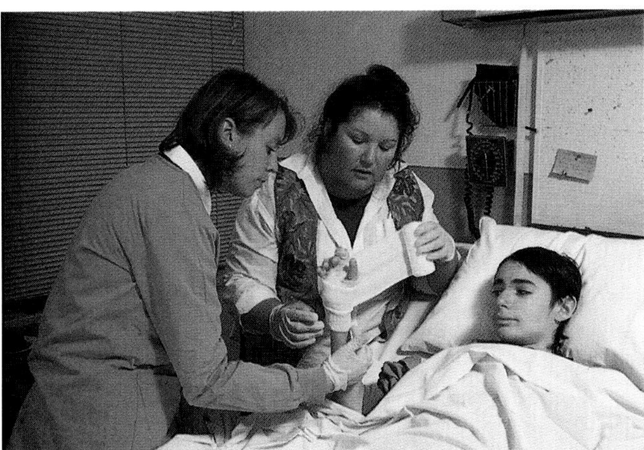

Figure 13–3. Whenever possible, family members should be included in teaching sessions.

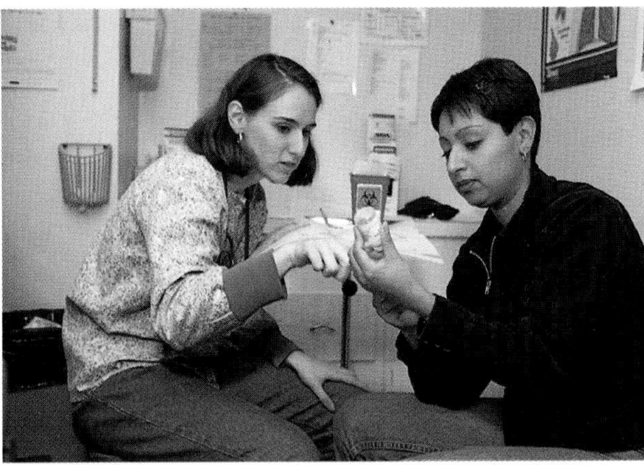

Figure 13–4. One-on-one, "hands on" teaching is often effective. Here, the nurse shows the patient how to draw up insulin and self-administer an injection.

- **Help the patient develop the correct language for the concept.** This is more important than it may at first seem. Being able to label a behavior or feeling correctly is part of being able to understand, communicate, and improve that behavior. Because the concepts being taught may be new to the individuals, you must help them acquire the correct language to use that concept.
- **Provide for experience with the concept.** Positive illustrations are better learning examples than negative illustrations and should be arranged first. With discipline, video tapes might be used to show parent-child interactions involving discipline. A field trip to a child care facility might be used. The parent could be asked to role play situations involving discipline.
- **Urge the patient to engage in self-discovery.** With the example being used, ask the individual to think back to childhood and identify discipline situations. Or ask the person to maintain a diary recording observations of situations involving discipline.
- **Encourage application in the real world.** Once the individual understands the concept, it should be tested in everyday living.
- **Develop a means for self-evaluation.** This principle was discussed for teaching facts.

EXAMPLE

An example of a patient-teaching program for teaching facts and concepts is presented in the Patient Teaching Box.

Psychomotor Skills

Nurses teach many psychomotor skills to patients and their families. A psychomotor skill is a set of physical actions by which a task is done. Illustrations of psychomotor skills are a diabetic patient learning to self-administer an insulin injection, a mother learning to instill ear drops in her child's ear, and a father learning to suction a ventilator-dependent child. With increasingly short hospital stays and more home care, the need for teaching these types of psychomotor skills has escalated.

PRINCIPLES FOR TEACHING PSYCHOMOTOR SKILLS

There are six principles basic to effective teaching of psychomotor skills. The six principles were used in developing the structured preoperative teaching program described in Chapter 2.

- **Analyze the skill from the learner's perspective.** This is critical. Once a person is proficient in a skill, it is easy to take for granted some aspects of the skill. The expert is likely to think the novice knows more than he or she does. Each step of a skill must be detailed in terms of the person who knows nothing about the task. In teaching deep breathing, the skill was analyzed in terms of the novice. As nurses designed that program they had to think through questions such as: Should you breathe through your nose or mouth? What position should you be in when doing deep breathing?
- **Demonstrate the skill correctly.** Observation and imitation help a person learn a skill. Just hearing how to do something is inadequate. The individual needs to see the skill performed correctly. In teaching deep breathing, patients viewed a set of slides that demonstrated the skill of deep breathing. The nursing staff was also prepared to demonstrate the skill.
- **Guide the initial responses verbally, and if appropriate, physically.** Talk the person through the process of implementing the skill. If helpful, put your hand on the patient to guide movements. In the example of deep breathing, the nurse used verbal commands to guide the patient. The nurse said, "Put your hand on your belly. Breathe in. As you inhale your hand should move out." If the patient had difficulty, the nurse guided the patient by placing her or his hand on the patient. It is important to prevent the patient from learning incorrect behaviors.
- **Arrange for practice.** Skills can only be acquired through practice. Some of the practice can be mental, i.e., the person can review the steps in his or her mind. However, practice must also include the actual doing of the skill to gain confidence and effectiveness.
- **Provide information about what was done correctly and incorrectly.** If errors in implementing a skill are not eliminated, they are acquired as part of the skill and are difficult to change. Anyone who has tried to correct a bad golf swing knows the problem.
- **Help the patient develop a way of evaluating his or her performance of the skill.** As with teaching other content, this is essential. In teaching deep breathing, patients were told, "If your hand moves out as you breathe in, and in as you breathe out, you will know that you are doing the skill correctly."

EXAMPLE

The Patient Teaching Box presents an example of teaching a patient about a psychomotor skill—in this case, exercises to promote hip function.

Problem-Solving Skills

Patients and families are becoming more involved in self-care and symptom management as the health care system moves toward managed care. Their ability to do that well depends on knowledge about the disease and problem-solving skills. Problem solving requires an individual to think critically and propose effective solutions for an identified problem.

Common examples of situations requiring problem-solving skills are as follows:

- A diabetic patient develops the flu and vomits everything eaten. Should he or she still take the regular dose of insulin?

PATIENT TEACHING
TEACHING FACTS AND CONCEPTS: A PATIENT WITH LOW BACK PAIN

BASIC INFORMATION

Description

Pain in the lower back usually caused by muscle strain. It is often accompanied by sciatica (pain that radiates from the back to the buttock and down into the leg). Onset of pain may be immediate or occur some hours after exertion or an injury. The symptoms get into a cycle, starting with a muscle spasm, the spasm then causes pain and the pain results in additional muscle spasm.

Frequent Signs and Symptoms

Pain. It may be continuous, or only occur when you are in a certain position. The pain may be aggravated by coughing or sneezing, bending or twisting.

- Stiffness.

Causes

- Exertion or lifting.
- Severe blow or fall.
- Back disorders.
- Infections.
- Ruptured lumbar disk.
- Nerve dysfunction.
- Osteoporosis.
- Tumors
- Spondylosis (hardening and stiffening of the spinal column).
- Congenital problem.
- Childbirth.
- Often there is no obvious cause.

Risk Increases with

- Biomechanical risk factors.
- Sedentary occupations.
- Gardening and other yard work.
- Sports and exercise participation, especially if infrequent.
- Obesity.

Preventive Measures

- Exercises to strengthen lower back muscles.
- Learn how to lift heavy objects.
- Sit properly.
- Back support in bed.
- Lose weight, if obese.
- Choose proper footwear.
- Wear special back support devices.

Expected Outcome

Gradual recovery, but backaches tend to recur.

Possible Complications

Chronic low back pain.

TREATMENT

General Measures

- Diagnostic tests may include laboratory blood studies to determine if there is an underlying disorder, X-rays of the spine, CT or MRI scan.
- Bed rest for first 24 hours. Additional bed rest will be determined by severity of the problem. Recent medical studies indicate that staying more active is better for back disorders than prolonged bed rest.
- Use a firm mattress (place a bed board under the mattress if needed).
- Ice pack or cold massage or heat applied to affected area with heating pad or hot water bottle.
- Physical therapy.
- Massage may help. Be sure person is well-trained or massage could cause more harm than help.
- Wear a special back support device.
- Other options are available depending on degree of injury, such as surgery (if disc damaged), electrical nerve stimulation, acupuncture, special shoes, etc.
- Stress reduction techniques, if needed.

Medication

- Mild pain medications such as aspirin or acetaminophen.
- Stronger pain medicine or a muscle relaxant may be prescribed.
- Note: Medications do not hasten healing. They only help to reduce symptoms.

Activity

- Try to continue with daily work or school schedules to the extent possible. Use care in resuming normal activities.
- Avoid strenuous activity for 6 weeks.
- After healing, an exercise program will help prevent reinjury.

Diet

No special diet. A weight reduction is recommended if obesity is a problem.

NOTIFY OUR OFFICE IF

- You or a family member has mild, low back pain that persists 3 or 4 days after self-treatment.
- Back pain is severe or recurrent.
- New or unexplained symptoms appear. Medications used in treatment may cause side effects.

From Griffith, H.W. (1994). Instructions for Patients, 5th ed. Philadelphia: W.B. Saunders.

- The mother of a 3-year-old checks her child's temperature. It is 102°F. Should she call the doctor?
- A middle-aged man with hypertension finds that taking the medication at the times determined by the doctor interferes with his sleep patterns. Can he take the medications at other times?
- A community is concerned over the increase in suicides among high school age children. What actions can they take to reduce that rate?

Every person living with a chronic illness, caring for someone else or caring for one's own health will have to

PATIENT TEACHING
TEACHING PSYCHOMOTOR SKILLS: HIP JOINT MUSCLE EXERCISES

EXERCISE 1

Lie face down on a firm surface and forcibly contract the gluteal (buttock) muscles to raise the extended leg. Hold for a count of 10, then slowly lower the leg (Step 1). After the muscles improve in strength, the exercise should be performed against increasing resistance by adding weight to the leg (Step 2).

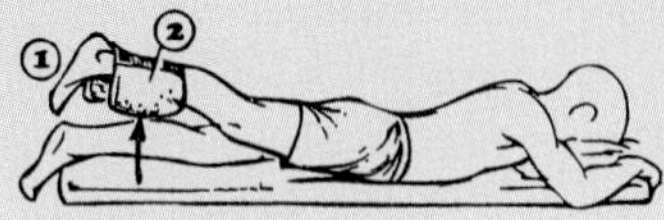

EXERCISE 2

Lie flat on your side with the affected leg upward. Lift the leg to the maximum level, without bending the knee, and hold it there for a count of 10; then lower it slowly (Step 3). Repeat 5 times.

Later the same exercise should be performed against increasing loads by adding weight to the leg (Step 4).

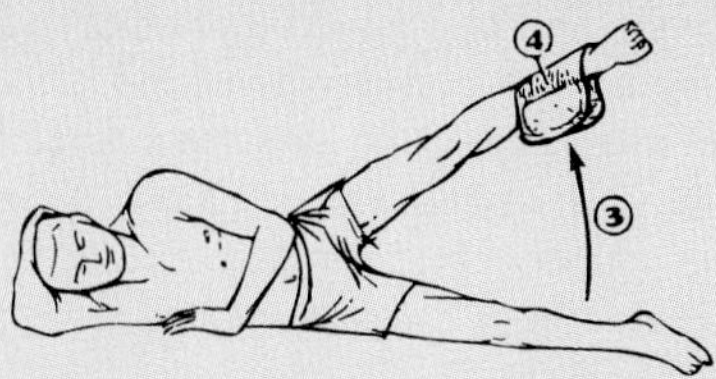

Note: Exercises for the quadriceps muscle (large muscle in the front of the thigh) may be added to this program; a powerful quadriceps adds to the hip joint stability.

From Griffith, H.W. (1994). Instructions for Patients, 5th ed. Philadelphia: W.B. Saunders.

engage in problem solving. Some people will be able to do this without assistance. Others will need help in learning these skills.

PRINCIPLES FOR TEACHING PROBLEM-SOLVING SKILLS

There are six principles for teaching problem-solving skills:

- **Activate solvable problems.** A patient might not know the problems that are likely to occur in living with an illness or recovering from a disease. Sharing a list of problems encountered by others is one way to implement this principle. Another way would be to create a group situation in which people with the disease could share experiences with each other.
- **Assist the patient in stating and delineating problems.** Problems cannot be solved if they are not made explicit. Patients could be asked to think about their style of living and identify problems that they might anticipate. The nurse needs to listen carefully to the patient's narrative and assist in clear naming and framing of the problem(s).
- **Assist the patient in finding information.** Most patients do not know where to find literature that could help them solve problems. Although an increasing number of hospitals have added reading rooms for patients and their families, many patients remain uninformed. The nurse needs to inform the patient about resources and access to them. For example, a woman having a breast removed (mastectomy) should be told about the Reach For Recovery program—a support and educational group for women who have had a mastectomy. A family that is thinking about a hospice program needs to know how to find information about such programs and also how to evaluate one.
- **Help the patient process the information.** The patient will need to think through the information and apply it to his or her situation. The nurse can ask the patient to "think out loud" as a means of determining the patient's critical thinking ability. The nurse can offer suggestions and model how to use the information.
- **Encourage stating and testing of hypotheses.** Ask the patient to identify the most likely solution to the problem. The nurse could also consider asking the patient to identify several hypotheses (potential solutions to the problem). Once they were identified, the patient could rank them from best to poorest and give the rationale. This would enable the nurse to further evaluate the patient's ability to think critically and use information.
- **Encourage independent discovery and evaluation.** As with every other learning outcome, practice and self-evaluation are essential to effective learning. Over time, patients could be asked to practice solving more and more complex problems. At the same time they could be asked to evaluate their problem-solving skills. The nurse would be available for guidance, support, and reinforcement.

EXAMPLE

Many diabetics worry about selecting food from a restaurant menu. Preparing the diabetic for this situation requires the development of problem-solving skills. After discussion of the problem and reviewing available information, the diabetic could go through the hospital cafeteria and select what might be appropriate food and servings. The nurse and patient could role play waiter and customer and the patient could test out what questions to ask about food preparation. And lastly, the patient might be given menus from local restaurants and select appropriate items. These exercises are all ways to explore problem-solving skills in situations where helpful feedback can be given.

THE TEACHING-LEARNING PROCESS

Patient Assessment

MOTIVATION AND READING ABILITY

Patient teaching is a complex process involving interactions between a patient (family or community) and a nurse. The characteristics of the patient are the most important factors influencing learning outcomes. Therefore the process always begins with an assessment of the patient. The research base identified two factors to assess: **motivation and reading ability.** Motivation can be inferred from the patient's response to the suggestion of learning the necessary knowledge or skills. It can also be inferred from the patient's communications and whether a desire to learn is mentioned. Reading ability can be inferred from the nursing history, which usually includes information about educational level. In addition, the nurse can infer that ability from the patient's language skills and reading material.

ADDITIONAL FACTORS

Additional factors that are logical to consider are:

- **The health status of the patient.** If the patient is too ill to concentrate or to remember, an educational intervention is not likely to be effective.
- **The emotional status of the patient.** If the patient is extremely anxious or depressed, an educational intervention is not likely to be effective.
- **Specific abilities prerequisite to the learning goals.** For example, is the patient's vision adequate for reading markings on a syringe (in the case of a diabetic learning to withdraw insulin from a vial)? For a hemiplegic to learn to move from bed to wheelchair, the person must first be able to (1) balance in a sitting position, (2) turn over and push up in bed, (3) follow simple instructions about movement of the unaffected side, (4) bear a goodly portion of the body weight on the arm, and (5) pay attention to a series of actions and commands for the span of a few minutes (Redman, 1980).
- **What the patient already knows.** The patient is likely to have some knowledge relevant to the situation. The nurse needs to determine what the patient knows as well as what misconceptions are held.

Structure

The patient teaching research base supports the effectiveness of structured educational programs. As initially defined by Lindeman and Van Aernam (1971), structured teaching is following a lesson plan previously developed and approved for content, method, and teaching aids. The lesson plan is a guide, not a rule. It must be adapted to the unique requirements of the individual, family, or community.

CONTENT

The nurse in partnership with the patient needs to determine goals for the educational intervention. Once the goals are determined, specific content can be identified. One goal for a presurgical patient is to prevent respiratory and circulatory complications in the postoperative period. One goal for a diabetic patient is self-care, including administration of insulin and monitoring blood glucose levels. A goal for a cardiac patient is to prevent a second heart attack. If several goals are identified, they should be put in priority order and addressed one at a time.

Once the goal is agreed to, the nurse must decide what the patient needs to **know and be able to do** to meet that goal. The clearer the nurse can be about these outcomes, the more effective and efficient the educational intervention will be. These statements, frequently called **objectives,** should be written and shared with the patient.

In the example of a diabetic patient, likely outcomes are:

- Be able to describe the action of different types of insulin.
- Be able to withdraw insulin without contamination.
- Be able to correctly identify sites for insulin injection.

In the example of a presurgical patient, likely outcomes are:

- Be able to do diaphragmatic breathing.
- Be able to clear airway by coughing.
- Be able to do leg and foot exercises.

There may be different opinions on what content is most accurate and therefore what should be taught to the patient. Clinical agencies have different approval processes. Students should use the content approved by the agency in which their clinical experiences occur. If the student believes the content is not accurate, it is necessary to use the procedures of that agency to get it changed.

The Patient Teaching Box presents the content that one hospital determined to be most pertinent and accurate for teaching patients deep-breathing and coughing techniques.

SELECTING TEACHING PRINCIPLES

There are three principles that apply to all situations:

- **Actively involve** the patient in the process. Avoid long lectures that keep the patient passive.

PATIENT TEACHING
DEEP BREATHING AND COUGH EXERCISE FOR POSTSURGICAL PATIENTS

1. Instruct and supervise patient preoperatively.
2. Patient may assume one of the following positions:
   a. Flat in bed.
   b. Back rest elevated to 45-degree angle (having the patient's head resting on two pillows will usually bring the head well forward).
   c. Sitting on the edge of bed.

   The patient should be as comfortable and relaxed as possible. Unless contraindicated, one or two pillows may be used to support the head.
3. During the exercise, the patient should place one hand on his abdomen (umbilical area) to exert a counterpressure during inhalation and use his other hand to support the area around the incision. If the patient is unable to provide support, the nurse should do this.
4. The deep breathing is effective only if the abdomen and rib cage expand on inspiration.
5. Inspiration and expiration may be done through either the nose or mouth.
6. Inspiration and expiration should be done *slowly, deliberately,* and *deeply.* Expiration should immediately follow inspiration.
7. This should be repeated three times.
8. Following the deep breathing exercise, the patient should perform the cough exercise.
9. During the exercise, the patient should place one hand on his abdomen (umbilical area) to exert a counterpressure during cough and use his other hand to support the area around the incision. If the patient is unable to provide support, the nurse should do this.
10. Patient should inhale slowly, deeply and deliberately.
11. Immediately after inspiration is completed, he should cough.
12. The patient should cough three or four times on the one expiration. The sequence is to inhale, cough, cough, cough, cough.
13. This should be repeated twice.
14. It is recommended that the entire procedure should be done every 2 hours for the first 24 hours following surgery and every 4 hours when awake for the next 48 hours. If the patient is unable to perform the procedure successfully, it should be repeated more often.
15. Depending on the nature of the surgery and the patient's condition, the nurse should use her judgment in implementing the above procedures.

From Lindeman C., Van Aernam, B. (1971). Nursing intervention with the presurgical patient—the effects of structured and unstructured preoperative teaching. *Nursing Research,* 20, 319–332.

- Create a **context** in which the patient can identify **personally.** Avoid examples that are not directly relevant to the individual.
- **Individualize** the process as people learn best in different ways.

Based on the objectives, the nurse selects the appropriate set of teaching principles. If the patient is to learn a skill such as insulin injection, the nurse would use the principles for teaching a psychomotor skill. If the patient is to learn about a medication, the nurse would use the principles for teaching facts. It is likely that several sets of principles will be used for complex teaching programs such as a diabetic educational program.

PLANNING THE EDUCATIONAL INTERVENTION

At this point, the nurse and patient have agreed on the goal(s) of the educational intervention. The nurse has assessed the patient and identified specific objectives, content, and teaching principles. The next step is to do the detailed planning.

Based on knowledge of the individual patient and of the content, the nurse thinks through each step of the process. For example, if the patient knew nothing about insulin injection, what and how would you teach him or her about holding a syringe? If the patient had arthritic hands, how would the patient hold the syringe? **A key to an effective educational intervention is thinking through the skill or knowledge from the perspective of the novice.**

The Patient Teaching Box presents a teaching plan for a presurgical patient involving the use of a slide program. The second box presents excerpts from the narrative accompanying the slide program.

DEVELOPING TEACHING AIDS

Using teaching materials that require different sense organs increases the effectiveness of an educational intervention. Hearing, seeing, feeling, tasting and smelling are all vehicles for learning. Furthermore, each sense organ can be stimulated in a variety of ways. Hearing can occur in a one-on-one situation or in a group. It can occur in a face-to-face situation or through audio tapes. Seeing can be through video tape, books, pamphlets, models (Fig. 13–5), or the computer. Developing aids to teaching is one place where creativity is important.

Teaching aids are important for initial learning and also for later recall to enhance retention. An increasing number of clinical agencies are using video tapes for use after discharge.

When developing aids to learning, keep in mind:

- the reading and comprehension level of the intended audience (Fig. 13–6)
- the perspective of the novice
- that "one picture is worth a thousand words"

PATIENT TEACHING

INFORMATION AND INSTRUCTIONS FOR PRE-OP TEACHING OF STIR-UP REGIMEN

I. PREOPERATIVE TEACHING
   A. All patients receiving general anesthesia should be taught.
   B. You may teach patients in a group or individually—use the method of choice considering the individual patient and time factors.
   C. If possible, use the 3M Sound-on-Slide Program for the initial teaching.
      If the patient will not do the complete stir-up routine (deep breathing, coughing, and bed exercises) postoperatively, remove the unnecessary slides from the slide tray.
   D. Distribute Patient Teaching Pamphlet.
   E. The patient should practice the deep breathing and coughing exercises and perform them correctly under the supervision of a Registered Nurse.
   F. A second return demonstration should be done later—again under the supervision of a Registered Nurse.

II. RECORDING
   A. On care plan under "Patient Teaching"
      1. Stir-up regimen
      2. Return demonstration—if this is to be done in A.M., note this on care plan and have ward secretary make out a white card as a reminder.
   B. On patient's chart
      1. "Stir-up" regimen, previously taught with return demonstration and note how well patient was able to do procedure.
      2. Follow-up return demonstration of stir-up regimen and how well patient did.

III. SUGGESTED TEACHING PLAN
   A. It is important that all teaching covers each point and that all patients are taught the same way.
   B. Begin with an explanation of why the stir-up regimen, previously is being taught.
      Example: For a better recovery after your surgery, I am going to describe and demonstrate some exercises that you will be asked to do.
      One is how to deep breathe and cough. The second is how to change positions, and the third is how to improve circulation in your legs.
      It is important that all of these be done frequently following surgery (at first every 2 hours) until you are up and around, and then at least four times a day.
      I will show you some slides on the correct method. After the slides you will be asked to do the exercises. Feel free to ask questions if you do not understand.
      Because of the nature of your particular operation, your doctor may order additional or different exercises. The nurses will tell you exactly which exercises you are to do.
   C. Show slides.
   D. Demonstrate deep breathing.
   E. Have patients return demonstration—instructing as necessary.
   F. Demonstrate the cough.
   G. Have patient return demonstration.
   H. Review change of position. If in bed, have patient demonstrate—if not, instruct him to practice turning before surgery.
   I. Demonstrate or explain leg exercises.
   J. Instruct patient to practice in bed (if in chair he would be able to feel muscles tighten when toes were pulled forward or pushed away and also could do foot rotating).

For patients (example: gynecologic surgery) who should do pelvic tilting—this should be taught at the time of second return demonstration.

When pamphlets are available, they would be given to patients at the start of teaching.

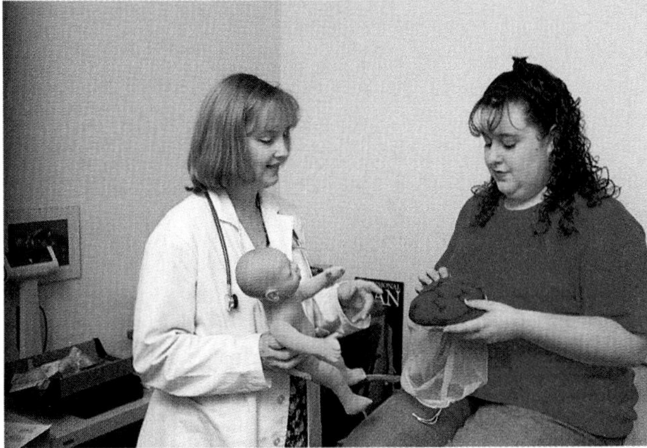

Figure 13-5. Visual aids can be effective teaching tools. Here a nurse uses a model of a neonate and placenta to teach about childbirth.

- the most important points should be highlighted in some way (e.g., bold type, repetition, or a border/box)
- the importance of maintaining interest from beginning to end

IMPLEMENTING THE PLAN

The educational intervention should be implemented in a place and at a time that is conducive to learning. Throughout the session, the nurse should attend to the patient's response to the intervention as well as overall health status. If the patient is not learning or is showing signs of health problems, the nurse should end the session and reschedule it for a time when the patient is in a better health status.

An educational intervention should be part of the written plan of care and once implemented, it should be charted.

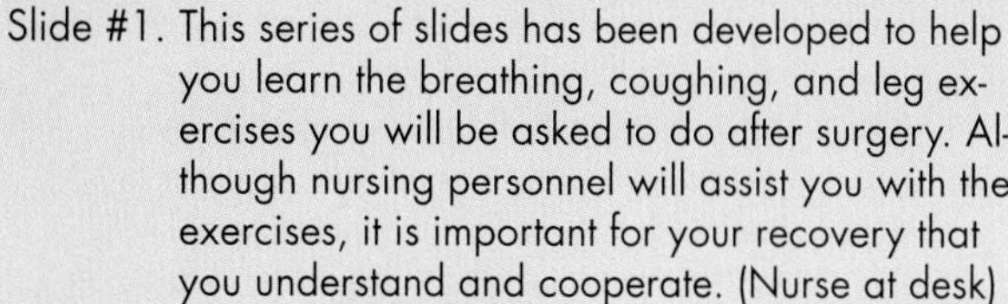

PATIENT TEACHING

EXCERPTS FROM THE NARRATION FROM SOUND-ON-SLIDE PREOPERATIVE TEACHING PROGRAM

Slide #1. This series of slides has been developed to help you learn the breathing, coughing, and leg exercises you will be asked to do after surgery. Although nursing personnel will assist you with the exercises, it is important for your recovery that you understand and cooperate. (Nurse at desk)

Slide #2. These exercises are commonly called the stir-up regimen, previously because their purpose is to stir up the circulation and breathing. This is necessary because the medicines and anesthetic you receive for surgery tend to slow down your circulation and breathing. (Stir-up Regimen printed on blackboard)

Slide #4. When deep breathing is done correctly, your lower rib area and your upper abdomen, the area you sometimes call your belly, expand or swell on inspiration and contract or sink together when you exhale. Your upper ribs and shoulders should not move or move very little when you are doing the deep breathing. (Schematic drawing of lungs)

Slide #5. Begin by getting into a comfortable position, one that will allow you to breathe easily and fully. You may sit in a chair or on the side of the bed or in bed with the back rest elevated. If necessary, because of the nature of your surgery, you may remain flat on your back. It is important that you are as comfortable and relaxed as possible.

Slide #6. Next, place either one or both hands over your incision if your surgery was abdominal. This will support the muscles and prevent pain. If your surgery was not abdominal, place one hand on your upper abdomen. If your hand moves in and out as you breathe, you will know you are doing the deep breathing correctly. (Patient with hand supporting incision)

Slide #10. Now you try to do it. And don't be too bashful to try. Remember to concentrate on making your belly and lower rib cage swell and then sink. Put your hand on your abdomen as a check on yourself. Relax your shoulders and chest. Now—inhale slowly and swell—then exhale—slowly—then sink together. (Patient exhaling)

Usually the nursing action and patient response are both noted in the record.

Implementing an educational intervention will highlight the fact that it is a nonlinear process. Objectives may change as the teaching progresses. Methods that initially seemed appropriate may be changed. An initial assessment of level of motivation or reading ability may prove inaccurate. None of these occurrences should detract from the process. **The nurse can plan an intervention but cannot control learning.**

Figure 13-6. Patient teaching materials should always be age-appropriate, as this doll used to teach a child about injections.

CHRONIC ILLNESS, EDUCATION, AND HEALTH OUTCOMES

As of 1995, 38 percent of Americans were living with a chronic condition, accounting for 76 percent of medical care costs. When looked at by age categories, the statistics show that in 1987, 25 percent of children age 17 years and younger, 35 percent of young adults, 68 percent of middle-aged adults, and 88 percent of adults age 65 years and older had a chronic condition (The toll of chronic illness, 1996).

People 60 years of age and older average slightly over two chronic diseases; the most common are hypertension, arthritis, cardiovascular disease, and lung disease (Clark et al, 1991). Overall, the morbidity and disability associated with chronic conditions have increased dramatically since the 1960s (Rothenberg and Koplan, 1990).

Learning to live with a chronic illness is an important health behavior. Educational programs that enable self-management have the potential to improve quality of life and reduce health care costs. For example, research (Breslow and Somers, 1988; Omenn, 1990) has shown that prevention programs can prolong the period of optimal physical functioning, maintain mental functioning and social activity, minimize disability and discomfort, and support people with a terminal illness.

The Chronic Disease Self-Management Program (CDSMP) is an example of an effective educational program. This program represents a collaborative research study conducted by the Stanford University School of Medicine and the Kaiser Permanente Medical Care Program, Northern California (Lorig et al, 1996).

The program was based on prior experience in working with health education programs for people with arthritis, the literature, and focus group discussions with people with chronic conditions. These three sources of information led to the following impressions:

- Different chronic diseases often cause similar problems in living with the disease.
- Many older people are willing and able to better self-manage their chronic illness when given appropriate instruction.
- Self-management tasks common across chronic conditions include symptom management, administration of medication, management of acute episodes of the disease, maintaining good nutrition and adequate exercise, avoiding health risk behaviors such as smoking, using relaxation and stress management techniques, communication with health care providers and significant others, obtaining information and using community resources, adapting work and other role functions, and managing the negative emotions and psychological responses to the illness.
- Coping with the daily challenges associated with living with a chronic condition requires knowledge and skills and a belief in one's ability to use those skills in realistic contexts and a belief that the use of those skills will produce desired outcomes. (Self-efficacy

TABLE 13-1 Examples of Outcomes Measures by Category of Outcome

	Measure	*Definition*
Self-Management Behaviors		
	Aerobic exercise	Time in past week spent walking for exercise, swimming or aquatic exercise, bicycling or stationary bike, aerobic exercise equipment, other aerobic exercise
	Communication with physician	When visiting physician, frequency of preparing list of questions, asking questions about things one doesn't know/understand, discussing personal problems related to illness
Self-Efficacy (SE) to Perform Self-Management Behaviors		
	SE get information about disease	Confidence that one can get information about disease from community resources
	SE communicate with physician	Confidence that one can ask doctor about things of concern, discuss openly any personal problems related to illness, work out differences if any
SE to Manage Disease in General		
	SE manage disease in general	Confidence that one can manage condition on a regular basis, judge when changes mean should visit a doctor, do tasks needed to manage condition so as to reduce need to see doctor, reduce emotional distress caused by condition, and do things other than take medications to reduce effect of illness on everyday life
SE to Achieve Outcomes		
	SE do chores	Confidence that one can complete household chores, get errands done, get shopping done despite health problems
	SE control/manage depression	Confidence that one can keep from feeling sad, discouraged, lonely and can do something to feel better when feeling sad, discouraged, lonely
Health Status		
	Disability	Difficulty in past 4 weeks with dressing and grooming, arising, eating, walking, hygiene, reaching, gripping, and activities
	Pain and physical discomfort	Pain and physical discomfort intensity, frequency, duration over past 4 weeks
Health Care Utilization		
	Number of hospital stays	Number of times that one stayed in the hospital overnight or longer in past 6 months
	Visits to emergency department	Number of visits to emergency rooms in past 6 months

CURRENT CONTROVERSY

WHAT ACCESS SHOULD PATIENTS HAVE TO THEIR OWN RECORDS?

MEDICAL CARE

by Steve Aylward, Portland Downtowner, *May 3, 1993*

At the heart of Planetree* is the idea that technology-driven medicine has lost sight of a fundamental in healing—the relationship between body and mind. The approach demands that patients be empowered, hospitals be humanized and health care demystified.

Under the Planetree program not only is the patient given access to the chart and other information, but is also encouraged to ask questions and express views.

"Part of the values of Planetree are really radical, that you're absolutely bone-honest about providing access to information" he (the hospital CEO) says.

"This means that the medical record is open to patients, that they have the right to read and understand it, a right to do their own progress notes if they want. It means that we provide fact sheets on every procedure, every treatment, every medication."

*Planetree is the kind of tree Hippocrates would sit beneath while teaching. The word is used to describe a hospital that emphasizes patient education and empowerment. It also refers to a non-profit consumer organization committed to changing health care.

theory is discussed in Chapter 36, Health Promotion and Self-Care.)

The CDSMP is a 7-week program of 2.5 hours per week. Between 10 and 15 people with chronic illness and their partners attend. Pairs of trained lay leaders teach the program. Sessions are held in community centers such as senior centers or libraries. The content includes how to develop an exercise program, symptom management, breathing exercises, problem solving, communication skills, use of medication, and dealing with the emotions of chronic illness (i.e., anger and depression).

The sessions are highly interactive using techniques associated with self-efficacy such as skills mastery and modeling. Skills mastery involves weekly contracting for specific skill development and feedback. Modeling involves the use of lay leaders with chronic illnesses and problem solving within the group process.

The program uses a comprehensive evaluation of outcomes. Examples are shown in Table 13–1.

TRENDS AND ISSUES IN PATIENT TEACHING

Some hospitals are experimenting with a new approach to health care. It is called the Planetree program and emphasizes the relationship between the mind and the body. These hospitals emphasize patient education and open communication. The Current Controversy Box presents excerpts from an article describing one Planetree hospital.

The importance of patient education is evident. Yet many programs are inadequate. The results of one survey addressing this dilemma are presented in the second Current Controversy Box.

Nurses must continue to develop **structured** teaching programs based on sound educational principles and clinical knowledge. Too often patient education is done in a hurried, spontaneous fashion with little actual learning occurring.

CURRENT CONTROVERSY

WHAT ARE THE BARRIERS TO PATIENT EDUCATION?

WHAT IS WRONG WITH PATIENT EDUCATION PROGRAMS?

by Marcia J. Lipetz, Margaret N. Bussigel, Julia Bannerman, and Betty Risley, in Nursing Outlook *38 (4), 184–189*

Full time faculty of the colleges of nursing and medicine at a major midwestern medical center were asked to respond anonymously to a mailed questionnaire concerning patient education.

The questionnaire suggested a number of possible impediments to patient education in hospital settings:

- structural barriers,
- the utility of patient education,
- perceptions of patients.

The data analysis showed:

- 75% of the nurses and 51% of the physicians identified other care-related tasks as a structural barrier
- 81% of the nurses and 39% of the physicians felt the length of hospital stay was a structural barrier
- 66% of the nurses and 35% of the physicians saw the lack of third party reimbursement as a structural barrier
- 46% of the nurses and 68% of the physicians saw the lack of effectiveness of patient education as a barrier
- Over 92% of both nurses and physicians saw the lack of interest in changing behavior on the part of patient as a barrier
- About 75% of both nurses and doctors saw the lack of patient interest in learning about their disease as a barrier
- About 74% of the nurses and 81% of the doctors saw the lack of patient interest in learning self-care skills as a barrier
- About 44% of the nurses and 54% of the physicians saw the patient as unable to learn self-care skills

Emerging technologies such as Internet and the World Wide Web increase opportunities for nurses to influence the health and well-being of individuals and communities.

Also, nurses need to remember that a patient may be the best person to educate another patient. Even though patient education is considered a nursing intervention, the nurse does not have to be the educator. At times the nurse may simply facilitate a group of patients teaching each other.

Finally, as health care moves into community settings, more patient education will be done with groups and in noninstitutional settings. The content of this chapter is equally applicable in those settings.

CHAPTER HIGHLIGHTS

- Patient education is a very powerful nursing intervention. Research has demonstrated its effects on health outcomes.
- Motivation to learn and reading ability are important determinants of learning outcomes.
- All patient populations respond positively to the opportunity to learn.
- All teaching strategies have the potential to facilitate effective learning.
- Well planned and implemented programs (structured) are associated with positive outcomes.
- Patients are responsive to opportunities to acquire knowledge and skills useful in self-care and symptom management.
- Effective teaching requires using teaching principles appropriate to the material—e.g., facts, concepts, skills.
- The growing elderly population, increasing incidence of chronic illnesses, shorter hospital stays, and emphasis on self-care and home care make patient education an essential component of contemporary nursing practice.

REFERENCES

Beresford, S. A., Farmer, E. M., Feingold, L., et al (1992). Evaluation of a self-help dietary intervention in a primary care setting. *American Journal of Public Health, 82,* 79–84.

Billie, D. (1977). A study of patients' knowledge in relation to teaching format and compliance. *Supervisor Nurse, 8,* (3) 55–57, 60–62.

Bowen, S., Miller, B. (1980). Paternal attachment behavior as related to presence at delivery and preparenthood classes: A pilot study. *Nursing Research, 29,* 307–311.

Breslow, L., Somers, A. (1988). The periodic health examination, and updates. *Canadian Medical Asociation Journal, 4,* 617–626.

Brown, S. A., (1990). Studies of educational interventions and outcomes in diabetic adults: A meta-analysis revisited. *Patient Education and Counseling, 16,* 189–215.

Brown, S. A., Duchin, P. P., Villagomez, E. T. (1992). Diabetes education in a Mexican-American population: Pilot testing of a research-based videotape. *Diabetes Educator, 18,* 47–51.

Choi-Lao, A. (1976). A preliminary study designed to explore the difference in effectiveness of group and individual teaching in self-medication. *Nursing Papers, 8,* 22–29.

Clark, N. M., Becker, M. H., Janz, N. K., et al (1991). Self-management of chronic disease by older adults. *Journal of Aging and Health, 3,* 3–27.

Cohen, S. (1980). Postpartum teaching and the subsequent use of milk supplements. *Birth and the Family Journal, 7,* 163–167.

Cotanch, P. (1983). Relaxation training for control of nausea and vomiting in patients receiving chemotherapy. *Cancer Nursing, 6,* 277–283.

Cupples, S. A. (1991). Effects of timing and reinforcement of preoperative education on knowledge and recovery of patients having coronary artery bypass graft surgery. *Heart & Lung, 20,* 654–660.

Dalzell, I. (1965). Evaluation of prenatal teaching program. *Nursing Research, 14,* 160–163.

Devine, E. C. (1992). Effects of psychoeducational care for adult surgical patients: A meta-analysis of 191 studies. *Patient Education and Counseling, 19,* 143–162.

Dixon, E., Park, R. (1990). Do patients understand written health information? *Nursing Outlook, 38,* 278–281.

Doak L.G., Doak C., Root, J. (1985) Teaching patients with low literacy skills. Philadelphia: JB Lippincott.

Dodd, M. (1983). Self-care for side effects in cancer chemotherapy: An assessment of nursing interventions—part II. *Cancer Nursing, 6,* 63–67.

Estey, A., Musseau, A., Keehn, L. (1991). Comprehension levels of patients reading health information. *Patient Education and Counseling, 18,* 165–169.

Falkiewicz, J. (1980). Are group classes helpful in teaching cardiac patients? *American Journal of Nursing, 80,* 444.

Flaherty, G., Fitzpatrick, J. (1978). Relaxation technique to increase comfort level of postoperative patients: A preliminary study. *Nursing Research, 27,* 352–355.

Funnell, M. M., Donnelly, M. B., Anderson, R. M., et al (1992). Perceived effectiveness, cost, and availability of patient education methods and materials. *Diabetes Educator, 18,* 139–145.

Garvey, E., Kramer, R. (1983). Improving cancer patients' adjustment to infusion chemotherapy: Evaluation of a patient education program. *Cancer Nursing, 6,* 373–378.

Gierszewski, S. (1983). The relationship of weight loss, locus of control, and social support. *Nursing Research, 32,* 43–47.

Goodwin, J. (1979). Programmed instruction of self-care following pulmonary surgery. *International Journal of Nursing Studies, 16,* 29–40.

Gregor, F. (1981). Teaching the patient with ischemic heart disease: A systematic approach to instructional design. *Patient Counseling and Health Education, 3,* 57–61.

Hall, L. (1980). Effect of teaching on primiparas' perceptions of their newborn. *Nursing Research, 29,* 317–322.

Healthy people 2000: National health promotion and disease prevention objectives. (1991). DHHS publication No. (PHS) 91-50212. U.S. Government Printing Office, Washington, DC 20402.

Henderson, J. (1983). Effects of prenatal teaching program on postpartum regeneration of the pubococcygeal muscle. *Journal of Obstetric, Gynecologic, and Neonatal Nursing, 12,* 403–408.

Heston, J., Lazar, S. (1980). Evaluating a learning device for juvenile diabetic children. *Diabetes Care, 3,* 668–671.

Holden-Lund, C. (1988). Effects of relaxation with guided imagery on surgical stress and wound healing. *Research in Nursing and Health, 11,* 235–244.

Johnson, J., Christman, N., Stitt, C. (1985). Personal control interventions: Short and long term effects on surgical patients. *Research in Nursing and Health, 8,* 131–145.

Johnson, J., Kirchhoff, K. T., Endress, M. (1975). Altering children's distress behavior during orthopedic cast removal. *Nursing Research, 24,* 404–410.

Johnson, J., Leventhal, H. (1974). Effects of accurate expectations and behavioral instructions on reactions during a noxious medical examination. *Journal of Personality and Social Psychology, 29,* 710–718.

Johnson, J., Rice, V., Fuller, S., Endress, M. (1978). Sensory information, instruction in a coping strategy, and recovery from surgery. *Research in Nursing and Health, 1,* 4–17.

Kinney, M. R. (1977). Effects of preoperative teaching upon patients with differing modes of response to threatening stimuli. *International Journal of Nursing Studies, 14,* 49–59.

Klausmeier, H. J., Goodwin, W. (1966). *Learning and Human Abilities,* 2nd ed. New York: Harper & Row.

Levesque, L., Grenier, R., Kerouac, S., Reidy, M. (1984). Evaluation of a presurgical group program given at two different times. *Research in Nursing and Health, 7,* 227–236.

Lindeman, C. (1972). Nursing intervention with the presurgical patient. *Nursing Research, 21,* 196–209.

Lindeman, C. A. (1988). Patient education. *Annual Review of Nursing Research, 6,* 29–60.

Lindeman, C. A. (1989). Patient education part II. *Annual Review of Nursing Research, 7,* 199–212.

Lindeman, C. (1995). Patient education. In S. G. Funk, E. M. Tornquist, M. T. Champagne, and R. A. Wiese (eds.): *Key aspects of caring for the acutely ill.* New York: Springer, pp. 8–22.

Lindeman, C., Van Aernam, B. (1971). Nursing intervention with the presurgical patient—the effects of structured and unstructured preoperative teaching. *Nursing Research, 20,* 319–332.

Lindsay, C., Jennrich, J. A., Biemolt, M. (1991). Programmed instruction booklet for cardiac rehabilitation teaching. *Heart & Lung, 20,* 648–653.

Lorig, K., Stewart, A., Ritter, P., et al (1996). *Outcome Measures for Health Education and Other Health Care Interventions.* Thousand Oaks: Sage.

Lowe, M. (1970). Effectiveness of teaching as measured by compliance with medical recommendations. *Nursing Research, 19,* 59–63.

Luker, K., Caress, A. (1989). Rethinking patient education. *Journal of Advanced Nursing, 14,* 711–718.

Meade, C. D., Diekmann, J., Thornhill, D. G. (1992). Readability of American Cancer Society patient education literature. *Oncology Nursing Forum, 19,* 51–55.

Milazzo, V. (1980). A study of the difference in health knowledge gained through formal and informal teaching. *Heart & Lung, 9,* 1079–1082.

Mills, G., Barnes, R., Rodell, D., Terry, L. (1985). An evaluation of an inpatient cardiac patient/family education program. *Heart & Lung, 14,* 400–406.

Mohammed, M. (1964). Patients' understanding of written health information. *Nursing Research, 13,* 100–108.

Mullen, P. D., Mains, D. A., Velez, R. (1992). A meta-analysis of controlled trials of cardiac patient education. *Patient Education and Counseling, 19,* 143–162.

Omenn, G. S. (1990, Summer). Prevention and the elderly: Appropriate policies. *Health Affairs, 9,* 80–93.

Orstead, C., Arrington, D., Kamath, S., et al (1985). Efficacy of prenatal counseling: Weight gain, infant birth weight and cost-effectiveness. *Journal of the American Dietetic Association, 85,* 40–45.

Painter, K. (1992). Fewer infants die after education blitz. *USA Today,* January 30, 1992, p 6A.

Perry, S. (1983). Parents' perceptions of their newborn following structured interactions. *Nursing Research, 32,* 208–212.

Peterson, M. (1991). Patient anxiety before cardiac catheterization: An intervention study. *Heart & Lung, 20,* 643– 647.

Petrowski, D. (1981). Effectiveness of prenatal and postnatal instruction in postpartum care. *Journal of Obstetric, Gynecologic, and Neonatal Nursing, 10,* 386–389.

Redman, B. K. (1980). *The Process of Patient Teaching in Nursing,* 4th ed. St. Louis: Mosby.

Redman, B. K., and Thomas, S. A. (1992). Patient teaching. In G. M. Bulechek and J. C. McCloskey (eds.): *Nursing Interventions: Essential Nursing Treatments,* 2nd ed. Philadelphia: W. B. Saunders.

Rothenberg, R. B., and Koplan, J. P. (1990). Chronic disease in the 1990's. *Annual Review of Public Health, 11,* 267–296.

Swain, M. A., Steckel, S. (1981). Influencing adherence among hypertensives. *Research in Nursing & Health, 4,* 213–222.

Taylor, A., Skelton, J., Czajkowski, R. (1982). Do patients understand patient education brochures? *Nursing and Health care, 3,* 305–310.

The toll of chronic illness. (1996, November 25). *U.S. News & World Report,* p. 24.

Timm, M. (1979). Prenatal education evaluation. *Nursing Research, 28,* 338–341.

Vargo, G. (1991). Computer assisted patient education in the ambulatory care setting. *Computers in Nursing, 9,* 168–169.

Warner, C. D., Peebles, B. U., Miller, J., et al (1992). The effectiveness of teaching a relaxation technique to patients undergoing elective cardiac catheterization. *Journal of Cardiovascular Nursing, 6*(2), 66–75.

Wong, J., Wong, S. (1985). A randomized controlled trial of a new approach to preoperative teaching and patient compliance. *International Journal of Nursing Studies, 22,* 105–115.

Documentation 14

Mary Lush and Christine Lush

Documentation is one of the most important functions performed by the nurse. It is also an activity that is subject to change as professional, regulatory, institutional, technological, and electrical advances alter reporting and recording requirements. As much as one third of the time spent in the delivery and support of patient care is spent charting in the patient record. This is because documentation is the recording of all pertinent care provided to and for the patient, the results of that care, and the patient's response to that care. No matter how comprehensive the documentation, it does not capture all that was done (McCloskey and Bulechek, 1994). Instead, documentation of patient care is defined by what the culture dictates should be in the legal record and in institutional reports.

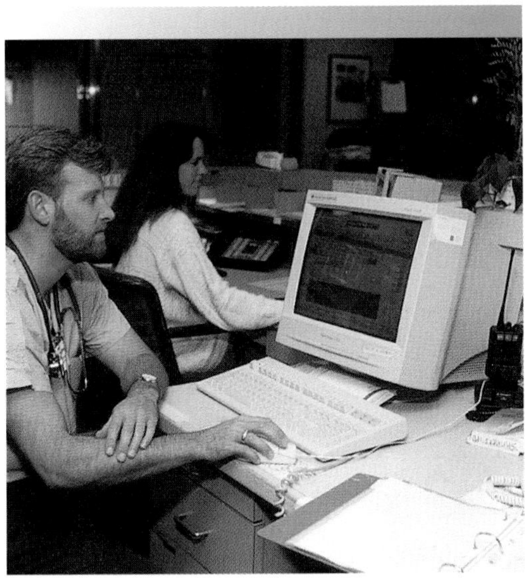

OBJECTIVES

After studying this chapter, students will be able to:

- **concisely and accurately record the pertinent observations and communications made during the course of patient care**
- **select appropriate formats for documenting the various processes of patient care**
- **document patient care in a manner consistent with the needs of the patient, the organization, and the nursing profession**

Documentation has evolved from the simple, narrative recording of the care delivered to the patient. Methods of documentation have moved from the simple use of blank pages through a complex array of structured forms to the transition of those forms to computer-based systems. However, the foundational skills through which documentation is accomplished remain the same. They are:

- observational
- intellectual
- physical/technical
- interpersonal

This chapter focuses on the importance of documentation. The uses of documentation in today's health care environment are explored. The importance of observing, recording, reporting, and communicating as elements of documentation is emphasized. Finally, an examination of the tools and methods of documenting nursing activities is considered for a variety of care settings.

THE IMPORTANCE OF DOCUMENTATION

Nursing's use of documentation to support the delivery of quality patient care dates back to the work of Florence Nightingale during the Crimean War (Nightingale, 1863). Nightingale used documentation and statistics to quantify the effects of hygiene on reducing mortality. However, issues relating to the availability of data defining the process of care that frustrated Nightingale over 100 years ago still face the profession today. It is amazing to realize that the work of Florence Nightingale still applies in today's electronic age. In 1863 Nightingale wrote:

> In attempting to arrive at the truth, I have applied everywhere for information, but in scarcely an instance have I been able to obtain hospital records fit for any purpose of comparison. If they could be obtained they would enable us to decide many other questions besides the one alluded to. They would show the subscribers how their money was being spent, what good was really being done with it, or whether the money was not doing mischief rather than good (Nightingale, 1863, pp. 175–176).

Documentation includes the process of communication. Within health care, communication is the continuous sharing and refinement of data and information for the purpose of achieving quality patient care. The process is both written (recording) and oral (reporting) and is essential to the coordination of the complex process of care. Patient care documentation is a 24-hour, seven-day-a-week process involving the patient, family, and multiple providers (medical, nursing, therapists, and social workers, among others) in a variety of settings.

In health care today, documentation is used to:

- ensure continuity and quality of care (across settings and time) through communication
- furnish legal evidence of the process and outcomes of care
- support the evaluation of the quality, efficiency, and effectiveness of patient care delivered by providers and institutions
- provide the database infrastructure supporting research and the development of nursing knowledge

Continuity of Care

Documentation includes the written summary of the ongoing and continuous communication that occurs in the support of patient care. Once recorded, events are available for review by others for multiple purposes, including the continuity of care. Patient care takes place over a period of time, in a variety of settings and with multiple providers. An elderly patient requiring surgery to replace a hip joint may:

- be provided prehospitalization assessments by physicians, physical therapists, nurses, and social workers
- have preoperative lab work and procedures completed at the hospital and/or outpatient sites
- participate in preoperative education by physical therapists and nurses
- undergo total joint replacement surgery in the hospital
- receive physician, nursing, and physical therapist care for several weeks or months in the skilled nursing facility, home, and medical offices, following discharge from the hospital

All of these activities form a part of the patient event "total hip replacement" (THR). Patient outcomes associated with THRs are a result of all facets of the care, from the initial diagnoses to the final office visit. Negative outcomes are often linked to a lapse in communication or coordination somewhere in the continuum of care for the THR event. Today, health care institutions are implementing standards of care and standardized paths of care. These multidisciplinary standards and care paths detail the normal care requirements and progression of care for a given population over time and across the settings of care. Use of care paths increases the likelihood that quality care will be provided for the patient. However, although a single path of care may well predict how the average patient can and will move through the care process, a single path of care cannot predict the unique needs of each individual patient. The nurse plays a crucial role in the assessment and documentation of the need to individualize paths of care in order to best meet the patient's needs.

Legal Record

One of the key reasons documentation is so complex is the use of the medical record as a legal document. The court refers to the record for evidence of a patient's condition, for the quality and competence of care provided, the patient's reaction to the care and to the ultimate outcome of the care provided. The medical record is the property of the health care agency. Information cannot be released without the expressed consent of the patient or the presentation of a subpoena and/or court order. All forms used for charting that are included in the medical record must go through an approval process involving a multidisciplinary medical records committee. Because of the importance of the patient record as a legal document, there are strict institutional policies and procedures surrounding its content, confidentiality, and access.

Evaluation and Accreditation Requirements

The medical record is used by regulatory and accreditation agencies to assess the quality of care provided by the institution as well the use of the record by third-party payers as a validation source for care provided for billing purposes. Regulatory agencies and insurers routinely audit charts to verify the appropriateness of admissions, discharges, interventions, and the length of stay. These audits frequently focus on nursing forms for the clearest understanding of the patient's status. Accreditation agencies such as the Joint Commission for the Accreditation of Healthcare Organizations (JCAHO) also include chart audits as a major criteria for determining the safety, effectiveness, and quality of care routinely provided by the health care facility. The simile to the legal dictum, "If it wasn't charted, it wasn't done" is the insurer's dictum, "If it wasn't charted, it wasn't used!" Chart audit for evidence of treatments implemented and supplies used is being performed by insurers and third-party payers to ensure accurate reimbursement for services provided (Box 14–1).

Chart audits of documentation have become the foundation for:

- meeting peer review requirements by JCAHO
- supporting the evaluation of care
- facilitating the efforts of professional standards review organizations to review the quality of care in federally funded programs.

Initial chart audits demonstrated the inconsistency and varying quality in the practice of documentation. As a result, forms were developed to prompt the writer to provide crucial data for process steps such as admission and discharge assessments, transfers, patient education, and the plan of care.

BOX 14-1

THE CHART AUDIT PROCESS

Goal: To assess the quality of a particular aspect of the health care system. Priority is given to issues considered high volume (occur frequently) and/or high risk to the patient or institution. Chart audits focus on the accuracy and adequacy of chart documentation. As a provider central to the care delivery process, the nurse will routinely be participating in chart audits.

Process:

- Depending on the focus of the audit, a discipline-specific or a multidisciplinary team meets to select the criteria to be studied.
- Each criterion is defined so that it can be reliably observed or measured.
- Method of data collection is determined, i.e., concurrent or retrospective review of the medical record, patient interview or direct observation of practice.
- The minimum sample size is defined, time frames established, and forms developed to gather the data.
- Data collection is normally completed by the same discipline(s) involved in the audit: particularly where judgment or interpretation of observed actions may be required.
- Results are reviewed and follow-up determined. Examples of follow-up may be an educational program for staff followed by re-audit, the decision to make changes in the standards of care, or agreement that level of quality is adequate and a schedule of maintenance audits developed.

Research

To remain cost effective, health care is rapidly shifting to less costly settings and to less costly caregivers. Research designed to evaluate the effectiveness and efficiency of new care delivery models relies heavily on data obtained during the delivery of care to understand the outcomes of that care. For example, research at Beth Israel Hospital was conducted to determine the best single predictor of in-hospital mortality in patients with pneumonia or cerebrovascular disease. In this case, the nurse's documentation that a patient required total assistance for bathing was determined to be the best predictor of mortality, even better than the patient's clinical laboratory values (Davis et al, 1995). In this case, use of admission bathing status as a predictor of outcomes will allow the early identification of high-risk patients and the implementation of a more aggressive path of care.

The documentation of care is also core to evolving research into the impact of nursing care on patient outcomes. Nursing documentation of the patient's functional status, knowledge, and engagement in care and psychosocial well-being will be used to evaluate models of patient care (Crawford et al, 1996). Data gathered in the hospital are linked with assessments in the skilled nursing facilities, the home, and in the physician offices. The objective is to return patients to their best achievable health status in the shortest time frame, and at the lowest cost.

Documentation continues to undergo significant changes in order to support these research efforts. One change is the development of common terms to describe patient care. There is little consistency in the words used by nurses to describe their actions. The language of the nurse used during oral communication differs significantly from that used in written documentation (Henry et al, 1994). Clark (1994) reports that a natural language project being conducted in the United Kingdom has identified over 40,000 terms used by nurses to document patient care. In contrast, the Nursing Intervention Classification is said to define all that nurses do for patients in all health care settings with only 433 defined intervention terms (Iowa Intervention Project, 1996)! The future nationwide reporting on the quality of patient care provided by individual health care systems and institutions will depend on the consistent, comparable documentation of patient care across all settings of care. Graduating nurses will need to link their own language to that required by the institution.

Quality

There is an evolving quality agenda in health care that has had significant implications on the requirements for documentation (Box 14–2). The introduction of Medicare and Medicaid has resulted in the development of utilization review programs for the monitoring of the cost and quality of the services provided. The JCAHO also initiated their approach to the evaluation of health care quality by focusing on structure as well as standards for process and outcome. Prior to these changes, charting was relatively straightforward with a minimum number of specialized forms.

BOX 14-2
THE EVOLVING QUALITY AGENDA

The term *evolving quality agenda* refers to the priority efforts being placed on the definition, measurement, management, and control of the quality of care. All major participants in the health care arena are involved in emphasis on quality including health care organizations, professional groups, insurers, third-party payers, employers, purchasers, and the public. It is an evolving agenda because the focus on quality has been and continues to be a learning process for all health care participants. Examples of the increasing sophistication and expansion of efforts to deal with phenomenon of quality include:

- The focus of quality assessment has shifted from the structure and the ability to provide quality care, to the study of linkages between the processes and the outcomes of care.
- The government has become a predominant third-party payer for health and has used this position to focus attention of providers on the control of the utilization of services and the assessment of the quality of care provided.
- Standards of care and practice guidelines developed by professional organizations are being developed to increase the accountability of the provider to control the costs and quality of care.
- The focus of quality has shifted from its retrospective measurement to its development into a phenomenon requiring assessment, control, management, and continuous improvement.
- The emphasis on outcome definition has shifted from traditional measures of mortality and morbidity to a focus more challenging: patient-focused concepts such as health, quality of life, goal attainment, and psychosocial well-being.
- The shift from organization-specific definitions of quality to the development of "report cards" for comparing the performance of all like organizations on common criteria.

Data from Ball, M.J. Quality assurance: Its origins, transformations, and prospects. In C.G. Meisenheimer (ed.): Quality Assurance: A Complete Guide to Effective Programs, Rockville, MD: Aspen; and Henry, S.B. (1995). Informatics: Essential infrastructure for quality assessment and improvement in nursing. *Journal of the American Medical Informatics Association,* 2(3), 169–182.

OBSERVATION, RECORDING, REPORTING: KEY COMPONENTS OF DOCUMENTATION

The documentation of patient care occurs in the medical record. The content of the medical record is used for multiple and diverse purposes. The record is accessed prior to, during, and following the delivery of care. For medical record documentation to meet the diverse needs of its users, the nurse must develop observational, recording, and reporting skills. This section of the chapter provides a basic overview of management of the medical record by the institution. In addition, foundational documentation skills of observing, recording, and reporting are reviewed.

Medical Records Committees

Because of its importance as a legal document, each agency will have strict policies and standards relating to the content, methods of documentation, and the use of abbreviations in the medical record. In addition, agency-specific policies will define the use of corrections and alterations as well as the storage, access, tracking, and confidentiality of the record.

In most institutions, the medical records committee is charged with the responsibility of defining the content, use, and maintenance of the medical record. Members of the committee typically reflect the departments and disciplines that contribute to the record. All forms used in the medical record must be reviewed and approved by the committee—even those undergoing minor changes or revisions. Elements included in the review include the necessity for the information to be collected, the clarity of the document, legal aspects associated with the form's content, and the adequacy of instructions for completion. For example, most states require that suspected child abuse be reported to a specific governmental agency. A form may be approved by the committee detailing the pertinent history; assessment data; photographs; the date, time, and name of the agency that the individual contacted; and the signatures of the providers completing the form. Institutions are mounting major efforts to reduce the amount of paperwork, to reduce costs, and to simplify data collection procedures. In addition, major efforts are being focused on the use of computer technology to reduce the staff time and costs associated with documentation.

Although the institutional medical records committee defines the content of the medical record, the nursing profession has recommended a minimum set of information that should be collected and included in the record. Identified as the Nursing Minimum Data Set (NMDS), the set includes those data needed to represent the nurse-patient interaction (Werley and Lang, 1985). Additional information on the NMDS can be found in Box 14–3.

Observation

Traditionally, observation refers to the physical assessment skills of inspection, palpation, percussion, and auscultation. In inspection sight is used to observe the appearance of specific features in contrast to auscultation, in which hearing is used, usually via a stethoscope, to listen to body sounds. Palpation gathers information through touching of the body part as opposed to percussion, in which the hands are used to tap or strike the body.

For the purposes of this discussion, the objective of observation is to gather information about the status and care needs of the patient. It is a learned skill requiring tools (i.e., thermometers, laboratory reports, monitors), techniques (i.e., physical assessment, measurement, chart review), and the ability to problem-solve and communicate effectively.

BOX 14-3
NURSING MINIMUM DATA SET

A minimum set of essential data has been identified for the purposes of supporting quality of care and patient outcome research (Werley and Lang, 1985). Called the "Nursing Minimum Data Set" (NMDS), the required elements encompass those needed to describe or understand the nurse-patient relationship including: client characteristics; nursing diagnoses; nursing objectives; nursing interventions; and outcomes of nursing care. Data for the NMDS data are collected from the documentation of the nurse completed during the course of care. This means ultimately that charting, so often seen as drudgery and left for last, will provide the foundation for:

- analyzing nursing care requirements
- evaluating outcomes of practice
- support for changes in nursing practice
- a research base to support the expansion of the knowledge base of nursing
- linking nursing care to quality patient outcomes
- linking nursing care to cost-effective health care

Observations may focus on the physiologic, psychosocial, knowledge, or safety needs of the patient. Observations of the family, the environment, and even the health care delivery system may also be required in order to effectively identify and meet patient needs. The purpose and timing of the observations will drive the frequency and detail required. For instance, observations made during the admission assessment into a nursing service will be more complete and detailed. This provides for a comprehensive baseline for future assessment as well as the basis for defining the priorities of the patient's plan of care. Once complete, limited interval observations will be based on the plan of care and any additional data provided by the patient.

The nurse must also be able to observe and interpret interactions involving and surrounding the patient. These may include the family, physician, other health care providers, and the patient's immediate (i.e., hospital, the home) and extended environments (i.e., social support, community). Observations in these areas provide critical information relating to the patient's psychosocial well-being and ability to cope. A single parent being discharged after mastectomy may be going home to young children and invalid parents requiring care. In the absence of a strong social support system, this patient will require substantial assistance in the home if recovery with a minimum risk of complication is to be expected.

The role of the nurse is changing over time. Now, as the coordinator of care, the nurse does not have the opportunity to directly gather all of the relevant data needed to monitor the progress of the patient. The nurse must "observe" these data through other persons and other sources. Instead of measuring the patient's vital signs, the nurse observes them on the graphic form. The nurse observes evidence of the patient's fluid balance on the intake and output record. The laboratory forms allow the nurse to observe whether clinical laboratory values are within expected values and to report those that are not. Communication skills are needed by the nurse to help support staff provide clear, complete descriptions of the patient's condition. Unfortunately, the nurse often finds that the tools needed to "observe" pertinent data are not readily available. Documentation or reports may be incomplete or missing. Problem-solving skills are needed to first find the relevant data and then to determine where communication or procedural protocols may have broken down.

Reporting

The accurate reporting of observations is essential to the safe ongoing care of the patient. Several categories of information require not just documentation but also the reporting or sharing with appropriate individuals or groups (Fig. 14–1). Examples include:

- facts collected that have impact on the care to be provided to the patient by other departments and providers
- facts about the current plan of care that require follow-up during the next shifts
- patient symptoms, responses, and reactions to treatment that require changes in the plan of care
- the occurrence of unusual incidents and the occurrence of errors of omission or commission
- Signs, symptoms, factors, and circumstances that the patient or family should report to the nurse and/or physician

There is much information that must be reported to other departments and providers. Collecting data on patient allergies but failing to accurately report them to pertinent departments (e.g., dietary, pharmacy, radiology) is a severe threat to patient safety. The patient's functional status may affect the method of transport for procedures. Scheduled radiology procedures may require medications from pharmacy and changes in diet in order to prepare the patient. Certain laboratory procedures (e.g., drug levels, coagulation times) require the reporting of

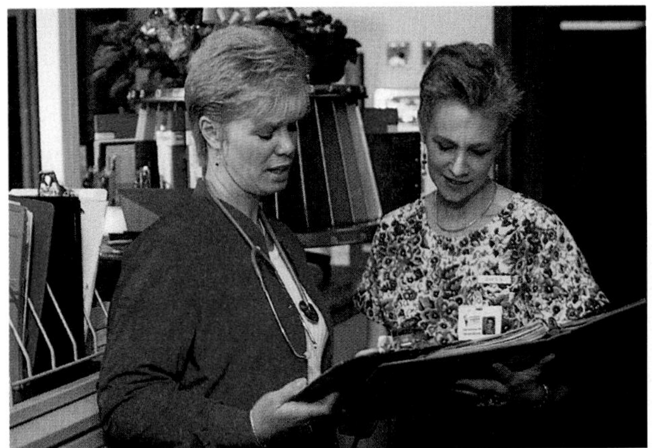

Figure 14–1. Two nurses sharing patient records. Such sharing and reporting is vital to safe, effective patient care.

scheduled medication times so that samples are collected at the appropriate time and intervals.

The change in shift report, reports of transfer of the patient to other units in the facility, and reports to providers of postdischarge care require careful thought. The key facts needed to provide immediate care must be included. For instance, sharing the information that Mrs. Jones's intravenous solution requires changing in 30 minutes and that the urgent blood transfusion for Mr. Silcox is now ready in the laboratory will assist the oncoming shift in setting care priorities. The need to report the results of upcoming laboratory work and tests to the patient's physician is also important to share. The nurse can then make sure the sample was drawn and arrange with the unit assistant to bring the results immediately to the nurse for review. Calling the admitting department and letting them know that Mr. Jones is allergic to smoke and flowers and prefers a bed close to the bathroom will help the receiving skilled nursing facility to assign an appropriate bed to the patient.

Consideration must also be given to the timing and content of reports to physicians. Some information must be reported immediately (transfusion reactions, significant changes in patient conditions), whereas other data may wait until the next time the physician makes rounds (normal lab work). New nurses often find their first professional positions on night shift. Knowing when to call physicians at night is another learned skill; one should be sure to check the plan of care for covering orders. The physician may have already ordered doses of potassium for administration when laboratory results indicated hypokalemia. If the laboratory results fall within the prescribed parameters, the potassium can be administered and the physician notified in the morning. Conversely, if the result indicates an extreme hypokalemia beyond the prescribed parameters and the patient has developed an irregular heart rate, the physician should be notified immediately. When one calls the physician at night to report on a patient's condition, one should know in advance the expected response. One needs to make sure the physician is in fact awake and has clearly in mind the correct patient and the importance of the information being reported. Nurses with many years of night shift experience will have their stories about errors they prevented on the basis of their assessment of the physician's alertness and the appropriateness of the orders received.

Another responsibility of the nurse is to report the occurrence of errors or other unusual incidents. Examples include medication errors, allergic reactions, nosocomial infections, falls, the development of decubitus ulcers, and a patient's refusal to accept treatment. One should refer to the organization's policies and procedures for details of how these situations should be handled. To provide an example, consider a patient's report of an unwitnessed fall. The nurse will obtain information from the patient regarding the circumstances of the fall. Vital signs are taken and the patient is assessed for possible injury. The environment is checked for factors that might have contributed to the fall (e.g., rails up/down, call light available, liquid on the floor). An assessment is also made of current orders that may have contributed to the fall (i.e., recent administration of medications both for pain and for sleep). The physician is notified of the fall and the patient's condition. The plan of care may be altered based on the circumstances of the fall. Nurse's notes are limited to the simple reporting of the patient's statements, the patient's status, the notification of the physician, and any changes made to the care plan. The date and time of each event should be recorded. The reporting of the incident to the quality assurance committee will be done via a "notification" or "documentation" form. These forms are used to report the event as well as circumstances that may have contributed to its occurrence.

Whether receiving direct care or being discharged to their home environment, the patient and family need to know when to communicate with their nurse or physician. The patient and family should be informed of the anticipated course of recovery and nursing and physician orders to follow at home. In addition, the patient and family need to know the signs, symptoms, factors, and circumstances that could appear during recovery. Instructions will also include when these should be reported to the physician or nurse.

Recording

Observing and reporting result in essential information that can be lost over time unless recorded. What to record, how, where, and at what level of detail are learned skills. Complete and timely charting will prevent duplication of services and treatments. Rather than miss the recording of a key observation or event, the new nurse may tend to document more than is necessary. However, it is not feasible or necessary to record every detail of the observations made, reports completed, and care provided to and for the patient. In fact, skillful, competent charting can be characterized as:

- clear and concise
- accurately capturing the essential events making up the care of the patient
- presenting a clear understanding of the patient's condition and response to the care
- providing the information needed to support continuity of care after discharge
- meeting the requirements of regulatory agencies
- reflecting the philosophy of care of the organization

Many forms make up the medical record. These forms evolved over time to increase the quality of charting while reducing the time needed for documentation. The next section reviews the forms typically used to organize and document the process of patient care.

TOOLS FOR DOCUMENTING NURSING ACTIVITIES

A well-organized medical record is essential to the coordination and monitoring of patient care. Over time, a variety of tools have been developed to facilitate the documentation process. Each organization selects the types of forms and individualizes the content to meet its needs. Forms that can be found in most paper-based and computer-based medical records include:

- consent for treatment
- patient data/admission
- patient progress notes
- laboratory, radiology, pathology, and other support services
- graphics
- medication and intravenous fluids records
- patient care flow sheets
- Kardex
- discharge and transfer forms
- plan of care
- care paths
- intake and output records

Although the detail of each form may be unique to the institution, there are common factors found in each.

Consent for Treatment

The consent for treatment on admission to the hospital typically includes information such as the medical record number, primary physician, diagnoses, important family telephone numbers, and insurance coverage. In most facilities, the consent for treatment is completed by admitting personnel. As facilities move to "patient-focused care" models, personnel on the nursing units may assume this task. It is important to verify information on the consent form with the patient or family early in the admission. In a crisis situation it may be necessary to reach family members. Finding that the phone numbers on the front sheet are incorrect can delay essential communication and care.

Prior to signing the consent for treatment, the patient will be asked to indicate if there are known aspects of care that the patient will refuse. Examples include blood transfusions and cardiopulmonary resuscitation. It is essential that these patient decisions be clearly documented on all pertinent forms (i.e., the medication record, Kardex, plan of care, the outside of the chart) and communicated to appropriate departments.

Most admission consent for treatment forms address the issue of confidentiality. Patients are asked to indicate whether information can be released regarding their presence at the institution, diagnoses, current status, and other information pertinent to their condition. It is essential for the nurse to check for any special "confidentiality tags" for patients on the unit. In these situations, the nurse needs to be absolutely clear regarding who may or may not have access to the patient record or to information about the patient. If the patient or family member does not give approval for the release of information, it is important to explicitly follow written policy on such issues as communication with the press and others seeking information on the patient's condition.

Patient Data/Admission

The patient data/admission form is typically two pages long and documents the patient's condition on admission to the facility (Fig. 14–2). It also focuses the nursing assessment of the patient, which will provide the basis for the plan of care. The first part of a patient admission form provides space for basic data such as the date and time of admission, height and weight, and the patient's chief complaint. Information on patient allergies and history of cigarette, alcohol, and illicit substance use are documented. The disposition of valuables and medications, orientation to the immediate environment, and the language spoken by the patient and family are also recorded.

The next major part of most admission forms is designed to capture the nurse's assessment of the physical and functional status of the patient. The psychosocial well-being of the patient, family, and caregiver are also documented. Knowledge deficits are identified as well as the ability of the patient to provide self-care. The risk for skin breakdown and injury is also recorded. Information from the admission form is transcribed to the Kardex and to the plan of care. Data needed by other departments is shared as needed (i.e., diet and food allergies).

Patient Progress Notes

The patient progress notes are that section of the chart in which the recording of the activities of patient care occurs. Activities include observations, interventions, the patient's response to care, and rationale for changes to the plan of care. Patient progress notes are usually organized in one of two ways. In most facilities, each provider group has a set of progress notes in its section of the medical record. Other facilities have all providers documenting the patient's progress on the same set of forms. Procedures and styles for documenting in patient progress notes are reviewed in the chapter section "Methods Used in Documenting Patient Care on Patient Progress Notes."

Laboratory, Radiology, and Other Support Services

A section of the chart is usually set aside for each of the major support services. Reports are entered chronologically by type of test or exam. The nurse must routinely review the results of laboratory tests and other examinations for abnormal results. The date and time that the physician is notified of abnormal results may be written on the laboratory work itself or in the progress notes. Orders for changes to the plan of care must also be recorded. The timeliness and adequacy of response to abnormal results has often been the basis of legal proceedings in the presence of negative patient outcomes.

Graphics

Transcription of vital signs and weights on the graphics form increases the value of the data because trends can be easily identified. Because the graphics form is used by so many providers to observe for major trends or patterns over time, it

NURSING ADMISSION ASSESSMENT - DATA BASE

SECTION A

DATE	TIME	ROOM #	TRANSPORT MODE
4/2/96	18:30	496 B	guerney
ADMITTED FROM	IDENTA-BAND	HEIGHT	WEIGHT
ER	☐ Yes ☐ No	5'6"	136.4 bed scale
TPR	BP	(SIGNATURE LINE)	
98⁴-80-18	116/78	M. White [signature] — If NA does Sections A & B, sign above.	

IMPRINT AREA

SECTION B

PT/FAMILY ORIENTATION TO NURSING UNIT

- ☑ Call light
- ☑ Bed Controls/Lights
- ☑ Console/TV
- ☐ Smoking Policy
- ☑ Siderails Policy
- ☑ Telephone
- ☑ Meals
- ☑ Visiting Hours
- ☑ Valuables — ☑ Home ☐ Safe

PROSTHESIS ☐ Limb ☐ Other: ____
☑ Glasses ☑ Dentures ☐ Disposition if applicable: ____
☐ Hearing Aid ☐ Eye

ALLERGIES	SYMPTOMS/REACTIONS
FOOD: milk products	sour stomach
MEDICINE: Erythromycin	upset stomach
OTHER	

SECTION C

MEDS TAKEN AT HOME	USUAL TIMES	LAST TIME TAKEN	REASONS FOR TAKING
Multiple Vitamins	qd	today	health
Ibuprofen 400mg	at night	last night	aches
"Water Pill"	0900	today	swelling in feet

DISPOSITION OF MEDS: ☐ Pharmacy ☑ Home ☑ With: husband

Smoking History: ☑ No ☐ Yes
If yes, how much? ______ For how long? ______

Drinking History: ☐ No ☑ Yes
Comments: glass wine with dinner

Substance Use: ☑ No ☐ Yes
Comments: ______

REASON FOR CURRENT ADMISSION: Dizziness, shortness of breath

PERTINENT HOSPITALIZATIONS/ILLNESSES: Feb, 1996 for CHF

INTERVAL NOTE: Patient transfered to bed. Bedscale weight obtained. Complains of increased shortness of breath when flat. Positioned in semi-fowlers.

Time and signature: 18:40 M. White

SYSTEMS REVIEW

SECTION D NURSING ADMISSION ASSESSMENT (CHECK OR DESCRIBE THOSE THAT APPLY) — NURSING DIAGNOSIS

CARDIOVASCULAR ☐ See Critical Care Flowsheet

- Cardiac Rhythm: ☑ regular ☐ irregular ☐ pacemaker
- Color: ☐ pink ☑ pale ☐ flushed ☐ mottled ☐ jaundiced
- Edema: ☐ none ☑ feet ☑ hands ☐ face ☐ eyelids ☐ sacral ☐ generalized
- Comments: Wants to know what else to do about ~~self~~ her swelling

Nursing diagnosis: ☐ No problem identified ☑ Fluid volume alteration ☑ Tissue perfusion alteration ☑ Knowledge deficit ☐ Other: ____

VENTILATION ☐ See Critical Care Flowsheet

- Respirations: ☑ regular ☐ irregular ☐ labored ☑ shallow
- Breath sounds: ☐ clear ☑ moist ☐ wheezing ☑ equal
- ☐ unequal-diminished (state location): ____
- Cough: ☐ none ☑ productive (describe): white
- Activity tolerance: ☐ no problem ☑ SOB at rest ☑ SOB with exertion
- Comments: Not sure when she should have called doctor

Nursing diagnosis: ☐ No problem identified ☐ Ineffective airway clearance ☐ Impaired breathing pattern ☑ Impaired gas exchange ☑ Knowledge deficit ☐ Other: ____

NEUROLOGICAL (SENSORY) ☐ See Critical Care Flowsheet

- Altered mental status: ☐ LOC ☐ orientation ☐ affect ☐ emotion
- Deficit in: ☐ vision ☐ hearing ☐ memory
- Pain – describe location, duration, precipitating factors, how controlled at home:
- Pain scale score (0-10) ______ "Comfort zone" ______ (for surgical patients)
- Comments: uses Ibuprofen for aches and pains at night - generalized.

Nursing diagnosis: ☐ No problem identified ☐ Altered sensory function ☑ Altered comfort/pain ☐ Altered orientation ☐ Alteration in thought ☐ Memory deficit process ☐ Knowledge deficit ☐ Other: ____

01263-4 (REV. 9-95) (OVER)

Figure 14–2. Patient data/admission assessment form.

NURSING ADMISSION ASSESSMENT (check or describe all those that apply) — NURSING DIAGNOSIS

BRADEN SCALE FOR PREDICITNG PRESSURE SORE RISK. If score is 16 or less, implement the Skin Integrity Protocol.

Total Score 16

ACTIVITY:
- ☑ 1 Bedfast
- ☐ 2 Chairfast
- ☐ 3 Walks occasionally
- ☐ 4 Walks frequently

MOBILITY:
- ☐ 1 Completely immobile
- ☑ 2 Very limited (requires assist)
- ☐ 3 Slight limited movement (no assist)
- ☐ 4 No limitations

FRICTION AND SHEAR:
- ☐ 1 Actual problem (mod to max assist)
- ☑ 2 Potential problem (min assist)
- ☐ 3 No apparent problem

NUTRITION:
- ☐ 1 Very poor (< 30%)
- ☐ 2 Probably inadequate (30-50%)
- ☑ 3 Adequate (50-80%)
- ☐ 4 Excellent (90-100%)

MOISTURE/INCONTINENCE:
- ☐ 1 Constantly moist
- ☐ 2 Moist (linen change q shift)
- ☐ 3 Occasionally moist (linen change x2/day)
- ☑ 4 Rarely moist (linen change x1 day)

SENSORY PERCEPTION/LOC:
- ☐ 1 Completely limited/unresponsive
- ☐ 2 Very limited/responds to painful stimuli
- ☐ 3 Slightly limited/slow to respond
- ☑ 4 No impairment

COMMENTS (Describe any skin alterations): ∅

Nursing diagnosis:
- ☐ No problem
- ☑ Skin integrity impairment/actual/potential **(call Dietitian, x4787)**
- ☐ Other

ELIMINATION/NUTRITION: ☐ See Critical Care Flowsheet

ELIMINATION:

Bowel Sounds:	☐ absent	☐ hyperactive	☑ normal
Bowel Habits:	☐ diarrhea	☐ constipation	☐ ostomy
Abdomen:	☐ distended	☐ obese	☑ flat
Last BM:	4/2		
Urination:	☐ retention	☑ frequency with water pill	☐ incontinent

NUTRITION: normal diet: Soft

(CIRCLE ONE)

YES (NO)	loss of appetite
YES (NO)	N/V diarhea x3d
YES (NO)	recent weight change
YES (NO)	dysphagia
YES (NO)	difficulty chewing

Any "YES" - call Dietitian x4787

Nursing diagnosis:
- ☑ **No problem identified**
- ☐ Alteration in nutrition
- ☐ Self care deficit: feed/toilet
- ☐ Altered bowel elimination
- ☐ Altered urinary elimination
- ☐ Knowledge deficit
- ☐ Other

PSYCHOSOCIAL ☐ See Critical Care Flowsheet

- ☐ language barrier
- ☐ unable to speak
- ☐ withdrawn
- ☑ fear/anxiety
- ☐ signs of abuse or neglect
- ☐ special cultural/religious preferences (describe):
- ☑ support system (describe): husband helps with care

COMMENTS: Is concerned about second time in hospital in 2 months. wants to know more re self care

MUST CHECK ONE
- ☐ Impaired communication
- ☐ Ineffective coping
- ☑ Fear, anxiety, anger, frustration
- ☑ Knowledge deficit
- ☐ Other

ACTIVITY (REST, MOBILITY) ☐ See Critical Care Flowsheet

Mobility: ☑ independent ☐ pain ☐ dependent (describe):

Activity Level: ☑ sedentary when SOB ☐ active ☐ very active

Rest: ☐ normal sleep pattern ☑ difficulty sleeping if no ibuprofen for aches

Safety: **Note: A patient who is found to reflect two of the criteria in this category or is over age 65 is identified as being at risk for falls.**

- ☐ history of falls prior to admission
- ☐ requires assistance with ambulation
- ☐ inability to follow/understand directions
- ☐ no falls risk identified

COMMENTS:

Nursing diagnosis:
- ☐ **No problem identified**
- ☐ Impaired mobility
- ☐ Potential for injury
- ☑ Activity intolerance
- ☐ Sleep pattern disturbance
- ☐ Knowledge deficit
- ☐ Other

SECTION E — DISCHARGE PLANNING NEEDS

1.	Is patient 75 years of age or greater and living alone?	Yes	(No)	(Circle One)
2.	Does patient have a severe chronic process (for example, COPD or diabetes mellitus)?	(Yes)	No	(Circle One)
3.	Is patient demented?	Yes	(No)	(Circle One)
4.	Is patient terminally ill?	Yes	(No)	(Circle One)
5.	Does patient have special emotional support needs (for example, domestic violence, trauma)?	Yes	(No)	(Circle One)
6.	Will patient require a caregiver upon discharge?	Yes	(No)	(Circle One)
7.	Has patient been under care of home health?	Yes	(No)	(Circle One)
8.	Will patient need help with his/her ADL's when discharged?	Yes	(No)	(Circle One)
9.	Is patient from any out-of-home placements (for example, board/care, SNF)?	Yes	(No)	(Circle One)

If you answered "Yes" to ***any*** *of the above questions, please refer this patient to the PCC/SWS referral line - 7337.*

Referral made: (Yes) No (Circle One)

10. INFORMATION OBTAINED FROM: ☑ patient ☐ family

☐ other (specify):

COMPLETED BY: M White, R.N. DATE 4/2/96 TIME ☐ A.M. ☑ P.M. 20:30

01263-4 (REV. 9-95) REVERSE

Figure 14–2. *Continued*

is important to incorporate vital sign data collected "between" the normal times if they provide information significantly different from the established pattern. In other words, a graphics form may have columns for every 4-hour vital signs on an 12–4–8 schedule. If the vital signs taken during the regular times are normal but the patient spikes a temperature of 102 degrees at 2 P.M. each day, this essential pattern will be lost unless the abnormal value is "squeezed in" or inserted on the line between the 12 P.M. and 4 P.M. results (Fig. 14–3).

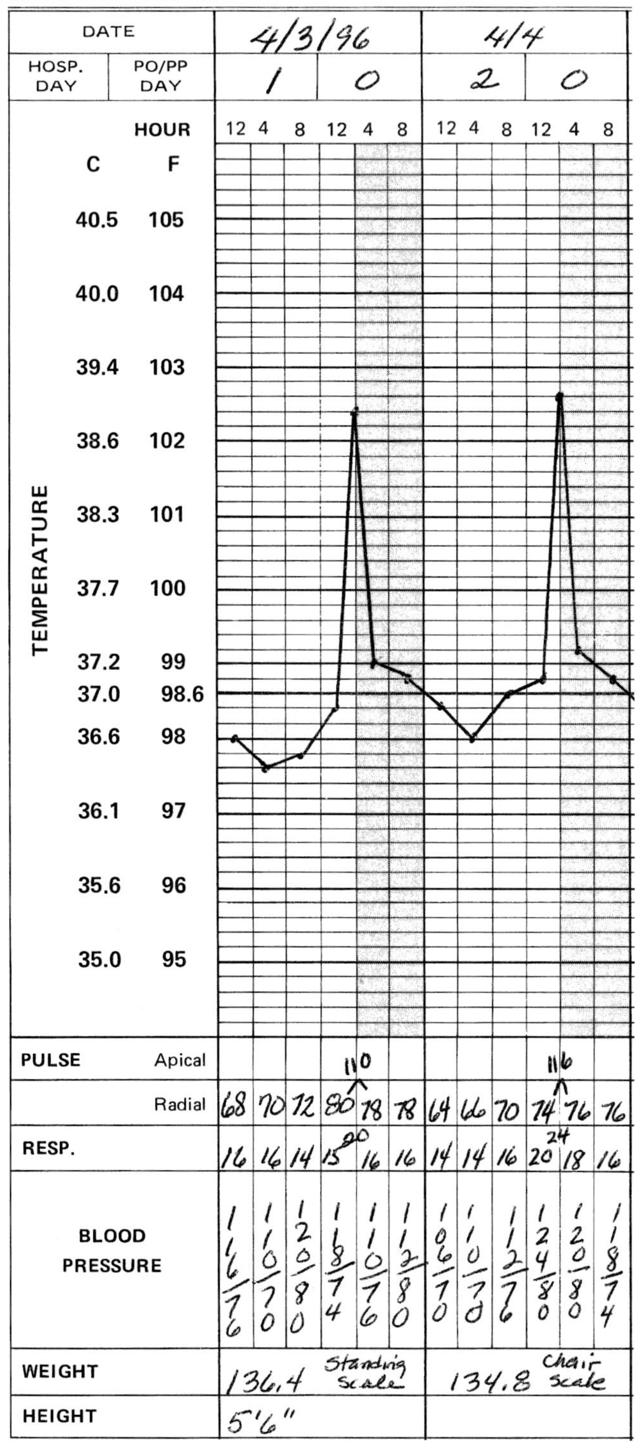

GRAPHIC RECORD

DATE		4/3/96						4/4					
HOSP. DAY	PO/PP DAY	1			0			2			0		
	HOUR	12	4	8	12	4	8	12	4	8	12	4	8
TEMPERATURE	C / F: 40.5 105; 40.0 104; 39.4 103; 38.6 102; 38.3 101; 37.7 100; 37.2 99; 37.0 98.6; 36.6 98; 36.1 97; 35.6 96; 35.0 95												
PULSE	Apical					110						116	
	Radial	68	70	72	80	78	78	64	66	70	74	76	76
RESP.		16	16	14	15	20 / 16	16	14	14	16	20	24 / 18	16
BLOOD PRESSURE		116/76	110/70	120/80	118/74	110/76	112/80	106/70	110/70	112/76	124/80	120/80	118/74
WEIGHT		136.4 Standing Scale						134.8 Chair Scale					
HEIGHT		5'6"											

Figure 14–3. Section from a typical graphics record.

It is also important to note trends in weight. If more than one scale is available on the unit, the nurse should note on the care plan the type of scale to be used. There can be significant differences between standing scales, chair scales, and bed scales. If the scale used must vary, document the scale used on the graphics form each day. Again, when weight is being closely monitored one should document what the patient should be wearing when being weighed. Robes can be very heavy and provide a false indication that the patient gained weight. This information should be placed on the Kardex, plan of care, or the graphics form—depending on the standards of the organization.

Medication and Intravenous Fluids Records

These records contain all active medication and intravenous fluids (IV) orders (Fig. 14–4). Each medication and IV order is recorded in its own space. Each time a medication is administered, the dose, route, site, date, and time of administration are recorded. Likewise, as each IV is hung, the date, time, content, volume, and site are recorded. The amount of fluid still hanging at the change of shift is often written on the IV record. The volume of IV fluids received by the patient is recorded on the intake and output record (Fig. 14–5). Patient responses to medication and IV administration are normally recorded in the patient progress notes. The nurse should pay special attention to start and stop dates for the medications.

Patient Care Flow Sheets

Flow sheets were created to ease the burden of documenting the extensive amount of information routinely gathered during patient assessments while improving its quality and the ease of data retrieval. Flow sheets are typically for a single day and have a series of duplicate columns that can be timed at the top (Fig. 14–6). This format makes possible the rapid documentation of detailed assessments and interventions.

Kardex

While not formally a part of the medical record, the Kardex is one of the most important tools used by the nurse. The Kardex is the quick reference document for the care plan and the medical record (Fig. 14–7). It summarizes all current orders of the patient care team (physicians, nurses, nutritional services, physical therapy). The Kardex reflects the range of orders of a multidiscipline team. Because the care provided for the postpartum mother differs significantly from care provided to the neurosurgical patient, the Kardexes from these units will be different. As the Kardex is a dynamic document,

MEDICATION ADMINISTRATION RECORD

SITE CODE			ALLERGIES:
	A - RIGHT UPPER QUADRANT B - LEFT UPPER QUADRANT C - RIGHT DELTOID D - LEFT DELTOID E - RIGHT ANTERIOR THIGH F - LEFT ANTERIOR THIGH G - RIGHT LATERAL THIGH	H - LEFT LATERAL THIGH I - RIGHT ABDOMEN J - LEFT ABDOMEN K - RIGHT ILIAC CREST L - LEFT ILIAC CREST M - RIGHT VENTRO-GLUTEAL AREA N - LEFT VENTRO-GLUTEAL AREA	Erythromycin Milk - sour stomach

		DATE		4/15/96	4/16	4/17
START 4/15 STOP	IV D5.45NS	TIMES 100cc/hr	N		#2 0600 (200) TBA fn	
			D	#2 12:00 MW 14:00 (800) TBA	#3↑ 0800 MW, 1400 (400) TBA	
			E	#2 22:00 KH (1000) TBA	#4↑ 1800 KH KH 22:00 (600) TBA	
START 4/15 STOP	Maalox 30cc po pc+hs	TIMES 09 13 19 22	N			
			D	0900 MW 1300 MW	09 MW (1300) MW Held for procedure	
			E	1900 KH 2200 KH	1900 KH 2200 KH	
START 4/15 STOP 4/20	Gentamicin 60mg IM q8°	TIMES 02 10 18	N	02 (A) TL	0200 fn (N)	
			D	10 (B) MW	10 (A) KH	
			E	1800 (M) KH	1800 (B) KH	
START 4/16 STOP 4/16	Demerol 50mg IM Diazepam 10mg IM 1x only pre procedure	TIMES 11:00	N	/		/
			D		11:00 Demerol (C) Diazepam (D) KH	
			E			
START STOP		TIMES	N			
			D			
			E			
START STOP		TIMES	N			
			D			
			E			

Do not forget to chart injection sites. For insulin, use diabetes flowsheet. For heparin, use anticoagulant flowsheet.	INITIAL / SIGNATURE	MW / M. White RN KH / Ken Handy RN TL / T. Lewis RN	fn / F. Welborn RN / /	/ / /

Figure 14–4. Some organizations maintain separate sheets for routine, p.r.n. (as needed), and intravenous fluids. This medication administration record is an example of a routine medication sheet.

24 HOUR NURSING CARE RECORD

IMPRINT AREA

Date	4/3/96	INTAKE						OUTPUT				
TIME	IV SOLUTION/DRUGS	IV FLUIDS	TPN	BLOOD PRODUCTS	OTHER	ORAL FLUIDS	TUBE FEEDING	URINE	NG	STOOL	OTHER	INITIAL
0100	D5/.45NS 1000	150										ML
0200	Gentamicin 60mg	100						350				ML
0600	Cefazolin 500 mg	100				120		325				ML
0600	D5/.45NS 1000	500										ML
0600	DAY SHIFT TOTALS	850	ø	ø	ø	120	ø	675	ø	ø	ø	ML
0830						340						CH
1000	Gentamicin 60mg	100						350		÷		CH
1100	D5/.45 NS 1000	500										JA
1200						240						JA
1400	Cefazolin 500mg	100				160		320				CH
1400	D5.45NS	300										CH
1400	PM SHIFT TOTALS	1000	ø	ø	ø	740	ø	670		÷	ø	CH
1600						180						JW
1800	Gentamicin 60mg	100				360		420				JW
1800	D5/.45NS	650										JW
2200	Cefazolin 500mg	100				110		370				JW
2200	D5.45NS	400										
2200	NIGHT SHIFT TOTALS	1250	—	—	—	650	ø	790	ø	ø	ø	JW
2200	**24 HOUR TOTALS**	3100	ø	ø	ø	1510	ø	2135	ø	÷	ø	JW

Figure 14–5. Although intravenous medication orders may be written on the medication sheet (Fig. 14–4), the fluid intake from IV fluids is normally recorded on the intake and output record.

it is written in pencil. The type of information typically found on a Kardex includes:

- patient information such as name, age, language, religion, allergies
- medical and nursing diagnoses
- current orders—medical and nursing orders for medications, treatments, diet, activity, laboratory work, education, therapies, procedures, and tests
- activated protocols and care paths (i.e., care of patient undergoing total hip replacement, patient at high risk for fall, and knowledge deficit)
- orders impacting activities of daily living (ambulate 20 minutes twice daily), safety precautions, use of assistive devices, functional limitations

The Kardex is used to focus the change of shift report, is used by the oncoming nurse to plan care for the shift and to make assignments, and is used to coordinate communications with family and other health care personnel. For this reason, it is imperative that the Kardex be current and accurate. Many an error in the provision of care can be traced back to a mistake in documentation on or communication from the Kardex. In

MEDICAL-SURGICAL NURSING CARE RECORD

DATE

IMPRINT AREA

	ASSESSMENT	N	D	E
NUTRITION	Abd: Soft / Tender / Firm / Distended	✓ (Soft)	✓ (Soft)	✓ (Soft)
	Bowel sounds / flatus	✓ / ✓	✓ / ✓	✓ / ✓
	Nausea			
	Vomitus (describe)			
	Tube: type			
	Describe drainage			
	Tube: type			
	Describe drainage			
	Other			
VITAL FUNCTIONS	Heart rhythm	Regular	Regular	0-1 PVC/min
	Other			
	Pulses: Popliteal L/R			
	Pulses: Pedal L/R			
	Edema	+	++	+
	Site	ankles	ankles	ankles
	Other			
	Respirations	Regular	Regular	Regular
	Lung Sounds: Right	clear	clear	clear
	Left	clear	clear	clear
	Cough: Prod/Non-Prod	Prod	Prod	Prod
	Describe sputum	clear/white	white	white
	Skin color *nailbeds*	pink	pink	pink
	Other			
ELIMINATION	Stool/describe		÷ large firm	
	Ostomy			
	Voiding	✓	✓	✓
	Rack urine			
	Color			
	Clarity			
	Incontinent: Urine / Stool			

NURSING CARE	N	D	E
Diet: Type *Soft*		B/ ✓ L/ ✓	D/ ✓ HS ✓
Amt: % taken		B/ 80 L/ 100	D/ 75 HS/ 100
Feeds: self/assist.	✓	✓	✓
Tube feeding: Type			
Amount / Hour	cc/hr	cc/hr	cc/hr
Placement: ck q shift			
Tolerance/residual			
Irrigation			
Amt/frequency			
Fluids: Restrict / Encourage			
Cardiac monitor	✓	✓	✓
Anti-emb. Stockings:	✓	✓	✓
☑ Knee ☐ Thigh			
Time off	0200	1000	2000
Elevate limb *legs*	✓	✓	✓
Incent. Spiro / Cough	✓ / ✓	✓ / ✓	✓ / ✓
O_2@ LPM	2	2	2
Aerosol mist			
Suction: Type			
Frequency			
Results			
Chest tube:			
Clamps @ bedside			
Air Leak			
Suction/pressure	cm	cm	cm
Tracheostomy Care			
Endotracheal Tube			
Spec to lab: Type / Time			
Enema: Type / Results			
Rectal tube			
Ostomy bag change			
Urinary cath: Type			
Care: Catheter / Perineal			
Irrigation/type			

02487-3 (REV. 8-88)

Figure 14–6. On this patient care flow sheet, items are checked if present and left blank if not applicable.

Illustration continued on following page

	ASSESSMENT	N	D	E
ACTIVITY / HYGIENE / SAFETY	Up ad lib			
	Bedrest/turn			
	Special position			
	Dangle			
	Out of bed ☑ Chair ☐ Commode		✓	✓
	BRP	✓	✓	✓
	Ambulation			
	Assistive device			
	Activity tolerance	well	some S.O.B.	well
	Isolation			
	Sleep	well		well
SENSORY FUNCTION	Speech	clear	clear	clear
	Aphasic			
	Numbness			
	Oriented To: Time/place/person	✓ ✓ ✓	✓ ✓ ✓	✓ ✓ ✓
	Follows directions	✓	✓	✓
	Responds to stimulation: (Verbal) Pain (describe)	✓	✓	✓
	Confused/combative			
SKIN INTEGRITY	Moisture: dry/mst/wet	dry	dry	dry
	Temperature	cool	warm	warm
	Color	pale	normal	normal
	Rash: site/descrip.			
	See Pressure Sore Flow Flowsheet			
	Incis/wound – location			
	Odor/drainage			
	Edema/redness			
	Drains			

NURSING CARE	N	D	E
Bath/linen change		✓ ✓	
Oral care/frequency	✓ x 1	✓ x 2	✓ x 2
Siderails/call light	up ✓	down ✓	up ✓
Bed in low position	✓	✓	✓
Range of motion			
CPM speed/ext/flex			
Time/tolerance			
Trapeze			
Traction: Type / Wt.			
Restraints:. Type / CMS q2h			
Seizure precautions			
Bed exer. as ordered			
Pain: ☐ See MAR			
Reoriented To: Time/place/person	✓ ✓ ✓	✓ ✓ ✓	✓ ✓ ✓
☐ See NEURO RECORD			
Pressure sore protocol			
Special pad: bed / chair			
Sheepskin/cradle			
Protectors: heel / elbow			
K-pad/location			
Dressing: condition / location			
Time changed			

Signature / title of caregiver:

N	B. White RN	N	
D	Janet Watson RN	D	
E	John Lewis RN	E	

02487-3 (REV. 8-88) REVERSE

Figure 14-6. *Continued*

some facilities, the Kardex is included with the medical record at discharge. In these circumstances, the Kardex is usually completed in ink.

Discharge and Transfer

These forms provide the format for recording the patient's status and the follow-up plan of care at the time of discharge or transfer. Hospital lengths of stay are decreasing rapidly. As a result, health care institutions are increasingly at risk of being held accountable for postdischarge complications or injury that can be linked to the premature discharge of a patient. An accurate recording of the patient's discharge status and all activities preparing for discharge is essential. For this reason, discharge and transfer forms are lengthy and require substantial time to complete. Space is provided to record the patient's physical, functional, and psychosocial status. Education provided to the patient is documented, as well as the patient's understanding of the postdischarge plan of care, medications prescribed, and follow-up appointments (Fig. 14–8).

The continuity of care for the patient also relies heavily on the information collected on the forms. The level of success of the patient in attaining each goal on the plan of care is recorded. Goals that were not achieved and that require follow-up after discharge must be clearly identified. Discharge information must be shared with the patient, family, caregivers, providers, and other facilities providing posttransfer or postdischarge care. To ensure the accurate sharing of information, discharge/transfer forms are increasingly made of paper that self-generates a number of copies. For this reason, the nurse will need to press hard while writing so all copies will be legible.

Front of Kardex

MEDICAL SURGICAL KARDEX		
Date	Physician and Nursing Orders	Interventions
	TEACHING/COPING: Planned Teaching (enter start date) □ ADLs ________ □ Trach Care ________ □ Cardiac Rehab ________ □ Wound/Decubitus Care ________ □ Diabetic ________ □ Other (specify) ________ □ Home IV Infusion ________ □ Other (specify) ________ □ Planned emotional reassurance ________ Reason/Plan/Date	□ Planned Teaching Patient □ Planned Teaching Family □ Routine/Reinforcement/Teaching/Emotional Support □ Planned Emotional Reinforcement
	MOBILITY □ Bedrest □ Total Hip/Knee Protocol ________ ________ Date D/C Date □ Out of Bed/Chair (frequency) ________ □ Ambulate (frequency) ________ □ Physical Therapy ________ ________ Date TRANSFERS: □ Independent □ Needs Assitive Device ________ □ Pivot □ Hoyer Lift □ Requires Caregiver assist (I or 2) ________	□ Up in chair/walk/dangle □ Up with moderate assist qd/bid/tid/qid □ Up with maximum assist (chair or Hoyer lift) □ Hoyer lift □ Turn q 2/3/4 hrs □ Special positioning □ CPM machine □ Simple traction □ Splints/Braces/Wraps □ TEDS □ Compression Stockings
	HYGIENE □ Use Special Skin Care Products - NO SOAP □ Aloe Vesta Fungal Cream □ Triple Care Cleanser □ Skin Protocol ________ ________ □ Uniderm Moisturizer Date D/C Date	□ Bathes Self □ Bathes with Assistance □ Bathed by Personnel □ Frequent Oral Care □ Sitz Bath
	ELIMINATION □ Incontinent ________ Last B.M. ________ Device used Date □ I&O □ Ostomy Protocol ________ □ Foley/Condom Date Started □ Other: ________ Appliance Type ________ □ Ostomy: □ New □ Old Size of Opening ________	□ BRP/Commode/Bedpan - Min/Mod/Max Assist □ Peri-Care TID □ Foley/Condom/Suprapubic Care □ CBI □ Straight cath p.r.n. distention □ Bowel Care
Patient has: □ Glasses □ Dentures: upper/lower □ Belongings □ Hearing Aid □ Prosthesis: right/left □ Valuables in Safe		
(from back) Medical Diagnosis History Surgery & Dates Allergies Room Name Age Sex Physician Admit Date Medical Record No.		

Figure 14–7. A Kardex is made of heavy-duty paper that is folded horizontally. Patient information is found on the front and on the inside of the Kardex when opened. The front (top) is normally a little shorter than the back. This allows the demographic information at the bottom of the back part to be visible whether the Kardex is open or closed. This is an example of the type of information found on a Kardex.

Illustration continued on following page

Inside of Kardex

Date	Physician and Nursing Orders	Interventions
	VITAL SIGNS/MONITORING ☐ VS q 8 hrs/routine ☐ Telemetry Protocol ____________ Date ☐ VS q 2/4/6 hrs ☐ Weights ☐ CSM Checks ☐ Neuro Checks ☐ Pulse Oximeter: ☐ Intermittent ☐ Continuous	☐ Orthostatic Checks ☐ CSM Checks ☐ Neuro Checks q 1/2/4 hrs ☐ Telemetry Monitoring ☐ Fetal Heart Tones/NST ☐ Respiratory S/P Epidural ☐ Weights Scale: standing/chair/bed
	NUTRITION Diet: ____________________ ☐ Assistance Needed (specify): ____________________ ☐ Force/Limit Fluids to _____ cc's/24 hr Days: ___ PMs: ___ Nocs: ___	☐ Feed with Assist: Partial/Full ☐ Total Feed with Dysphagia ☐ Tube Feeding
	RESPIRATORY/SUCTION ☐ O_2 at ______ liters/minute ☐ prn ☐ continuous ☐ mode______________ ☐ Nebulizer ☐ Ventilator/BIPSP continuous ☐ Trach Protocol: ______________ Date ☐ Ventilator/BIPAP at night only ☐ Trach: Type/Size ____________ ☐ Chest Tube Protocol: _______/_______ Date / Date DC ☐ Chest Tube(s) ______________ ☐ NG Tube ☐ Incisional Drain(s) ____________________	☐ Tracheostomy ☐ Naso/Oral/ET/Trach Suction ☐ Trach Suction/Dressing Change ☐ Inspirometer/Cough/Deep Breathe ☐ Vent Care and maintenance ☐ NG/OG Sump maintenance and care
	MEDICATIONS ☐Parenteral Fluids: ____________________ ____________________ ____________________ ☐ TPN/PPN Orders: ____________________ ____________________ ☐ PCA Drug: ______________ ☐ IV Protocol __________ Date __________ D/C Date BR _______ TD/hr _________ PCA Dose _____ Delay Time ____ ☐ CVC Protocol ________ Date _________ D/C Date Syringe Change ____________ D/C BR @ ______________ ☐ Pain Management Protocol _____ Date _____ Date/DC ☐ PCA Protocol _____ Date _______ Date D/C ☐ Blood Infusion Protocol _______ Date _____ Date D/C ☐ Blood Reinfusion Device Protocol _____ Date _____ Date D/C	☐ Site/Tubing Change Due ____________ Date Due ☐ Central Line Dressing Change _______ Date Due ☐ Fragile veins, monitor frequently
	OTHER DIRECT NURSING CARE ☐ Dressing Change: See below ☐ Timed Specimens: ☐ Specimen Collection: __________ Type: ______________ ____________________ Start:: ________ End: ________ ____________________ ☐ Diabetic Protocol _______ Date _______ D/C Date ☐ Guaiac: ______________ ☐ Blood Sugar Monitoring: _______ ☐ Protective Device Protocol ☐ Protective Device (type) ______________ _______ Date _______ Date D/C	

Date Treatments/Dressing Changes Times	Call MD If:
____________________ ____________________ ____________________	
Labwork ordered Date Call MD If: ____________________ ____________________ ____________________ ____________________	Date Radiology Prep ____________________ ____________________ ____________________ ____________________

Pertinent Patient Information

Medical Diagnosis			History		Surgery & Dates	Allergies
Room	Name	Age	Sex	Physician	Admit Date	Medical Record No.

Figure 14–7. *Continued*

GENERAL INFORMATION				
Date/Time	Diet Restrictions	Special Instructions	Medications	Return Appointments
To ______	Fluid Restrictions	Symptoms to Report	Purpose	Date/Time
Transportation	Activity Restrictions	Self-care Instructions	Frequency	With ______
With	Weight Bearing Status	Yes/No Change Dressing	What to Report	Purpose
	Equipment Needs	Phone Questions to ____	New/From Home	
HOME HEALTH/SNF/ACUTE CARE TRANSFERS				
Demographic Information	Medical Record No.	Hospital Information	Patient Status	Orders
Name/Date of Birth	Coverage/Group	Admit Date	Vital Signs	Direct Care
Home Address/Phone	Medicare H.I.C. No.	Discharge Date/Time	Weight	Teaching
Sex/Marital Status	Medicaid No.	Primary Diagnosis	Last B.M.	Assessment
Religion	Receiving Facility	Secondary Diagnosis	Skin Integrity	Code Status
Responsible Person	Receiving Provider	Prognosis	Status at D/C	Stable Yes/No
NURSING SUMMARY				
General Condition	Wound Care/Treatments	Referrals	Objectives Met	
Physical Status	Drug/Food Interactions	Patient Education	Objectives Not Met/Status	
Mental Status	Caregiver/Family Needs	Family Education	Outstanding Problems	
Psychosocial Status	Meds/Next Scheduled	Self-care Deficits		
PATIENT/CAREGIVER ACKNOWLEDGEMENTS				
Instructions Explained	Questions Answered	Instructions/Answers Understood	Signature(s)	
PROVIDER SIGNATURES				
Authorizing Transfer/Discharge	Writing Orders	Completing Forms	Provider Accepting Patient	

Figure 14–8. Discharge and transfer forms are designed to assure the safety of the patient and to minimize the legal risk to the organization. This is done by clearly documenting the status of the patient, providing clear instructions for follow-up care, and including instructions (with telephone numbers) for when to call the physician. To meet these needs, discharge and transfer forms are now three and four pages long. This example shows the type of information that can be found on these forms.

Plan of Care

The patient care plan can be used in any setting and by any provider of care. Although each discipline could maintain its own plan of care, regulatory and accreditation agencies strongly encourage the development of a single plan of care for each patient. The potential benefit of a single multidisciplinary plan of care for enhancing the communication and coordination of care is obvious. Despite this, the plan of care in many organizations is written and maintained primarily by nursing personnel.

It is important to document the identification of significant patient problems that may affect the patient's ability to respond as anticipated to the plan of care. For each identified problem, the planned interventions and anticipated outcomes are written (Fig. 14–9). It was once practice to write both short- and long-term goals for each identified problem on the plan. With shortened hospital lengths of stay, there is a need to focus on the most crucial problems to facilitate the patient's early response to care. For this reason, acute care plans of care define the short-term goals that can be achieved and measured during the length of stay. Problems may occur if the patient's need for care extends beyond the time hospitalized. Long-term problems should be documented in the plan of care and must be communicated to those responsible for follow-up with the patient once discharged from the acute care setting.

Care Paths

Care paths (also called *critical paths* and *plans of care*) are found with increasing frequency in health care institutions. Care paths are templates developed by a multidisciplinary team to guide and direct the care for a specific patient population (Fig. 14–10). Each path or template lists the patient problems normally seen or anticipated in the population along with the normal interventions and anticipated outcomes of care. The more sophisticated care paths coordinate the episode of care across settings of care (medical offices, hospital, skilled nursing facility, and the home). These care paths will indicate, by setting of care and day of stay, the progress the patient is expected to make each day during the episode of care.

A care path for a scheduled surgery may include preoperative education and skills training for the patient and caregiver. This education may occur in the physician's offices or in the

CARE PLAN		Patient Name:	Diagnosis: Severe dehydration - status post CVA					
Initiated		PATIENT PROBLEM	PATIENT OUTCOMES	Evaluated		NURSING INTERVENTIONS	Resolved	
Date	RN			Date	RN		Date	RN
4/15	MW	Potential impairment of skin integrity due to prolonged bedrest	Skin integrity maintained	4/18	JB	Implement Skin Integrity Protocol		
4/15	MW	Fluid volume deficit related to poor fluid intake	Patient oral intake to equal 1800 cc's per day	4/18	JB	1. Determine fluid preferences 2. Consult with dietary re plan 3. Offer 300/hr from 06:00 to 14:00 to reduce BR trips at noc.		
4/15	MW	Bowel elimination alteration (constipation) related to poor fluid intake and immobility	The patient will have at least one soft formed stool per day	4/18	JB	1. Dietary consult for high fiber diet and prune juice a.m. 2. Instruct in bed exercises 3. Offer bedpan following a.m. activities and exercises		
4/15	MW	Potential knowledge deficit for self care	Patient will perform self care as identified in CVA teaching protocol	4/17	TH	1. Determine understanding of patient and family re CVA pathology, symptomatology, activity/diet, medication regimens 2. Implement CVA teaching protocol. 3. Record patient/family response as directed	4/18	JB

Figure 14–9. Traditional nursing care plan.

home. The course of care during hospitalization is included as well as plans for discharge to skilled nursing, home health, and/or follow-up provider care. Criteria for moving from one stage to the another are made explicit (i.e., patient able to walk 100 feet with walker). Reasons for a patient's failure to move forward on the path of care as planned are documented and the care path revised accordingly.

Care paths have gained in widespread use as they have expedited the patient's movement through the care process and significantly reduced lengths of stay. The consistency, coordination, and communication facilitated by the care path have also improved the quality of care. The nurse is the provider most frequently in the role of monitoring patient progress along the care path. This is done by assessing the patient's readiness to move forward through the plan of care or determining that the plan of care requires alteration to meet the needs of the specific patient. It is essential to document the rationale for each decision made to maintain or alter the prescribed path of care for the patient.

Intake and Output Records

Intake and output (I&O) records provide visual access to trends regarding fluid balance (see Fig. 14–5). This information, in combination with daily weights, can provide crucial data regarding the fluid balance and fluid tolerance of many sensitive patient populations. Institutions have varying definitions of which food items constitute fluids. Examples might include hot cereals, custards, and puddings. The nurse will need to learn the policies of the institution.

The I&O record seems to be one of those problematic forms inasmuch as it is frequently found to be incomplete. Use of the I&O data as part of the assessment of the patient's response to treatment by each nurse will help ensure the completion of the record.

METHODS USED IN DOCUMENTING PATIENT CARE ON PATIENT PROGRESS NOTES

Perhaps the area in which institutions vary the most in their documentation standards is in methods by which the patient's progress is recorded. Examples of charting methods the nurse may find include:

- narrative charting
- source-oriented charting
- mnemonics to focus charting
- problem-oriented charting
- standards of care and protocols
- charting by exception

INTERDISCIPLINARY CLINICAL PATHWAY FOR TOTAL HIP REPLACEMENT

Note: The Care Plan will be adapted to reflect the chronological age, physical capabilities or limitations, psychoemotional and spiritual needs of the patient.

Expected Length of Stay: 4 Days.

Discharge Criteria: Independent ambulation with assistive devices & understanding of Total Hip Precautions

	PATIENT CARE PROBLEMS	
	Knowledge deficit related to hospitalization, potential risks and impaired mobility	Alteration in comfort related to surgical intervention
	PATIENT OUTCOMES	
	Verbalize and demonstrate Total Hip Precautions and use of abduction splints. If achieved, initial here. Initial: __________ Date: _________ If not achieved, a focus note must be written.	Pain is controlled at a comfortable level on P.O. meds as evidenced by ability to rest and participate in prescribed activities. If achieved, initial here. Initial: _______ Date: ________ If not achieved, a focus note must be written.
DAY	INTERVENTIONS	
DOS	Attend Pre-op class. □ Yes □ No Abductor pillow, bed exercises, TCDB and incentive spirometer. 11-7 7-3 3-11 I/C □ □ □ N/C □ □ □	Explain use of PCA or epidural. Manage pain on PCA/Epidural/IM 11-7 7-3 3-11 I/C □ □ □ N/C □ □ □
PO #1	Review Total Hip Precaution, use of abductor splint, repositioning q 2° and bed exercises. THP and picture guide on wall. 11-7 7-3 3-11 I/C □ □ □ N/C □ □ □	Manage pain on PCA/IM/Epidural. Explain use of PCA, IM and pain management. 11-7 7-3 3-11 I/C □ □ □ N/C □ □ □
PO #2	Continue Total Hip Precaution education & use of splints. Bed exercises on own. 11-7 7-3 3-11 I/C □ □ □ N/C □ □ □	Same as PO #1 11-7 7-3 3-11 I/C □ □ □ N/C □ □ □
PO #3	Patient to verbalize and demonstrate THP. Lovanox administration instruction. Staff to instruct patient. 11-7 7-3 3-11 I/C □ □ □ N/C □ □ □	Oral analgesic and supplemental parenteral/IV. 11-7 7-3 3-11 I/C □ □ □ N/C □ □ □
PO #4	Patient to demonstrate Total Hip Precautions, heparin injections and discharge instructions. If RSTC not available, staff to instruct patient. 11-7 7-3 3-11 I/C □ □ □ N/C □ □ □	Oral analgesic. Patient reveals understanding of pain management at home. 11-7 7-3 3-11 I/C □ □ □ N/C □ □ □

Figure 14–10. Multidisciplinary plan of care. This is an example of an abbreviated plan of care for a patient undergoing total hip replacement.

Narrative Charting

Narrative charting, a method of documentation used to record the patient's condition in the medical record from the beginning of patient care, is still used today. It is the chronological, free-form documentation of the patient's status, events, treatments, and response to care (see Fig. 14–11). Even in those facilities making extensive use of protocols, standards of care, and flow sheets, some amount of narrative charting is used. Certain events and aspects of care unique to

Narrative Nurse's Notes

Date	Time	
7/11/95	08:25	Patient c/o incision pain and unwilling to ambulate or
		use spirometer. Abd soft, bowel sounds present,
		incision clean and dry. Medicated patient M White RN
	10:00	Patient ~~ambult~~ ambulated in hall for ten minutes and
		used incentive spirometer. Will med for pain at
		12:30. Patient to ambulate and use spirometer q 2hrs.
		——————————— M Lewis RN

Problem-Oriented Patient Progress Notes Using a Charting Mnemonic

Date	Time	Problem Name	Progress Notes
4/11/96	10:00	Skin integrity	I: Dressing changed. Wound red, hot, weeping
		(L) thigh	pink fluid. Redressed wound with four
			4×4 dsgs.
			EP: Drainage unchanged. Labwork shows
			culture sensitive to current antibiotic.
			Continue with current plan
		Knowledge Deficit	S: I don't know how to do this when I
		Dsg Changes	get home.
			O: Patient scheduled for discharge in 2days.
			Responsible for self care.
			I: Explained process to patient during dsg change.
			P: Add knowledge deficit to care plan. Initiate
			teaching protocol. Arrange home health visit
			——————————— M White RN

S: Subjective O: Objective A: Assessment P: Plan I: Interventions E: Evaluation R: Revision

Figure 14–11. Examples of narrative nurse's notes and problem-oriented charting. In the example of problem-oriented charting, note that a mnemonic (SOAPIER) is used to organize the documentation. However, it is not necessary to document each "letter" of the mnemonic each time. Rather, date and time the note, and indicate the letters of the care process to which you are charting.

the patient do not fit into the structured chart forms provided for the medical record. Some circumstances that occur are not easily captured using a select set of words or descriptive phrases. It would be impossible to create a form that had every possible option available to the nurse. The use of narrative charting in these situations saves both time and space.

The lack of structure in narrative charting, however, makes it difficult for personnel to review the notes to find information on a specific area of concern. It is also difficult to retrieve information from the medical record for the purpose of communication, the coordination of care, and for chart audits. In the absence of the charting reminders that come with flow sheets, problem-oriented charting, and standards of care, it falls to the nurse to carefully consider what should be included in the note.

When facilities have moved to the use of flow sheets and other documentation supports, a limited amount of space is provided for narrative charting.

Source-Oriented Charting

Medical records compiled in this format have a separate documentation area for each discipline (source). Typically, sections are set aside for physicians, nurses, physical and respiratory therapy, and nutritional services. Source-oriented charting makes it easier to review and follow through on patient care issues pertinent to the discipline. When source-oriented charting is used, the nurse coordinating the patient's care must remember to review the progress notes of the other disciplines. Each discipline could elect to use a different method for recording (narrative, problem-oriented, etc.) in its section.

Mnemonics to Focus Charting

A mnemonic is a memory aid. The use of mnemonics such as SOAP and SOAPIER evolved from the need to improve the quality of documentation. SOAP stands for: (S) subjective data; (O) objective data; (A) assessment; and (P) plan. SOAPIER helps the nurse to fully document the patient care process by adding: (I) interventions; (E) evaluation; and (R) revision. The use of SOAP and SOAPIER charting is more fully described in Box 14–4.

BOX 14-4
MNEMONICS TO FOCUS CHARTING

The use of mnemonics such as SOAP and SOAPIER evolved from the need to improve the quality of documentation. SOAP stands for: S) subjective data; O) objective data; A) assessment; and P) plan. Subjective data are those contributed by the patient or the family, with the assumption being that the information came from the patient unless otherwise stated. In the absence of subjective data (e.g., patient unable to respond) the "S" is written and the space on the line left blank. Objective data include all information collected by nurses relevant to the entry. Examples would include results of a physical assessment, lab or radiology results, vital signs, and dietary intake. Objective data also include interventions and teaching completed by the nurse. Record only those data that are pertinent to the entry being written. The "P" refers to your plan for the patient based on the S, O, and A. The plan should include sufficient detail about the planned follow-up so that others can follow through appropriately.

SOAPIER helps nurses to fully document the complete process of their critical thinking by adding: I) interventions; E) evaluation; and R) revision (see Fig. 14–11). Specifying the interventions makes it easier for others to determine which interventions have been successful and which have been tried unsuccessfully. Detail is again important. Stating "will begin teaching about diabetes" does not let the readers know which specific aspects of the subject will be covered and which topic areas remain. Evaluating the response of the patient to your intervention, be it positive or negative, is essential for the planning of any follow-up. Revision provides evidence of how the plan was adjusted based on the patient's response to care.

Problem-Oriented Charting

As with mnemonic focused charting, problem-oriented charting was developed as a methodology to improve the structure of charting, improve its quality, and improve its ease of use by others to track essential elements of care. Each problem on the patient's care plan is named, numbered, and maintained as long as the patient's condition warrants. When no longer relevant, the problem is "inactivated." With each dated and timed chart entry, the problem and its number is first identified. Typically, some form of structured SOAP-like method is used for documentation, but the method selected may simply be a narrative note. Part of each note should indicate the status of the problem—whether it is active, its progress toward planned outcomes, and at what point the problem can be considered no longer active. An advantage of problem-oriented charting is the ease in tracking a problem throughout the documentation (Fig. 14–11).

Standards of Care and Protocols

Standards of care define the minimum level of care that will be provided for a patient population. Standards of care for the critically ill patient will typically include the frequency and extent of physical assessments, routine safety measures, requirements for a patient-specific plan of care, the extent of physiologic monitoring, and attention to the psychosocial needs of the patient. In contrast, protocols define the specific actions expected to be performed to manage a specific procedure, problem, or stage of care. An example would be a "falls protocol," which might be activated by the nurse based on the patient meeting defined high-risk criteria. The nurse must chart the data collected that justified the implementation of the protocol (e.g., patient disoriented, unstable when transferring or walking, postural hypotension). Each shift, the nurse determines whether the expected care was provided and whether the patient's assessed condition came within defined norm. Care that comes within the norm is indicated by a checkmark or a signature in the designated location. Exceptions are carefully noted in the patient's progress notes. The date and time of the activation and deactivation of standards and protocols must also be documented.

The plan of care must clearly delineate the standards and protocols that are active for the patient. Standards and protocols commonly implemented on a unit are often preprinted on flow sheets as a reminder to the nurse and to ease the

PROTOCOLS IMPLEMENTED		
☒ IV	☐ Shock	Standards Implemented
☒ Monitoring	☐ Arterial Line Management	☒ CCD Patient Care Standard
☒ Pulse Oximetry	☐ PAP Monitoring	☐ Rule Out MI
☒ Falls	☐ CVP Monitoring	☐ GI Bleed
☒ Age Specific	☐ Central Venous Lines	☐ Surgical Patient: Vascular
☐ Post-op Patient	☐ Blood Products	☐ Surgical Patient: Lobectomy
☐ Pain Acute/Chronic	☐ Anticoagulation	
☐ Epidural Analgesia	☐ Insulin	☐ Skin Assessment
☐ PCA	☐ Lidocaine	
☐ Chest Pain, Acute	☐ Urinary Catheter	
☐ TPA	☐ TPN	
☐ CHF	☐	
☐ Airway Management	☐	

Figure 14–12. A list of typical protocols for a critical care unit. Some are "pre-marked" on the flow sheet as they apply to all patients. Other protocols are marked to meet the specific needs of the patient.

process of documentation. Examples of standards and protocols commonly implemented in a critical care unit are shown in Figure 14–12. The nurse completing the admission assessment will activate the initial standards and protocols based on the patient's condition, the nurse's assessment, and physician orders. Most institutions require that a copy of each implemented standard or protocol be included in the patient's permanent record. This is for legal purposes and for ease of reference for third parties needing to document the care provided and the supplies used in that care.

Charting by Exception

In this charting method, the nurse documents only those findings that differ from defined standards or norms. The basic premise is that all care was provided and all patient assessments fell within defined norms unless otherwise charted. Charting by exception became a viable option with the implementation of standards and protocols for patient care. This eliminates a large amount of repetitive charting associated with activities such as positioning the patient, circulation checks, and hourly assessments of the patient's tolerance of continuous passive motion devices. Flow sheets are used to document physical assessments, treatments, procedures, and other interventions completed for the patient. Narrative notes are used to document where the patient response to treatment fell out of the expected normal range (Fig. 14–13).

THE PROCESS OF DOCUMENTATION

During an individual's orientation to an organization, the forms used for documentation will be presented. In addition, the policies and procedures of the organization relating to the documentation of care will be reviewed. What is not discussed is how to organize the process of documentation. Ideally, all documentation is done at the point of contact (bedside, treatment room) and at the time observation is made. The time will then be accurate, and essential observations are not as likely to be missed because of faulty memory. How close one can come to the ideal (point of

Narrative Nurse's Notes

Date	Time	
12/19/95	14:00	Care path day 3. Patient unable to ambulate due to
		dizziness. V/S and Hct stable. Will use Nelson bed to
		increase tolerance to standing position. J Henkins RN
12/19/95	19:30	IV site Ⓡ arm red and hard. IV catheter removed
		intact. IV started Ⓛ anterior arm without difficulty.
		Warm compresses applied to Ⓡ arm S Mellows RN —

Figure 14–13. Example of charting by exception.

contact charting) depends on the documentation systems of the organization, and the situation with the patient.

Some facilities have charting and mini nursing stations outside of each patient room. In these facilities, it is possible to document most observations, treatments, and procedures as they are completed. Exceptions to this situation will occur if another provider is using the medical record or if the medical record is with the patient in another part of the facility. In these situations, the nurse will want to make brief notes so that he or she can chart the information when the medical record is again available.

Nurses use a variety of means for making notes. Report sheets, paper towels, clipboards, pocket notebooks, and even bed linen (in an emergency) are all used. Notes typically include the exact time of the observation, the exact value of measured observations, and a few key words as reminders of important information.

In facilities where medical records are kept centrally in the nursing station, timely charting is more problematic. The nurse may be responsible for as many as 10 or more patients during a shift of care. It would not be practical to carry 10 charts around while providing the care. Nor is it practical to run back and forth to the nursing station each time a task is completed or an observation made. Again, the nurse will want to take notes until time is available to document.

When it is time to document, the nurse should take time to organize thoughts while considering what is essential to document. Box 14–5 identifies the sections of the medical record where observations and the process of care are normally recorded. Nurses usually start by completing flow sheets, graphics, and intake and output records. This organizes observations and allows identification of trends. The next step is to complete the progress notes in chronological order, referring to notes taken during the course of care to make sure this documentation is complete. Visualizing the situation makes it easier to make sure all pertinent observations are recorded.

At the end of each shift, one should:

- Review all documentation forms for completeness and then review crucial parts of the medical record
- Check the physician orders to be sure all orders have been transcribed.
- Check the medication record, intravenous fluid sheet, Kardex, and plan of care to ensure all scheduled care has been provided.

BOX 14-5
ESSENTIAL ELEMENTS OF DOCUMENTATION

Nursing Process Element →	Observation Sources →	Where to Document
Assessment of: >Physiologic Status >Functional Status >Knowledge >Psychosocial Well-being >Family >Safety	Patient/Family Interview Physical Exam History and Physical Lab and Radiology Results Medication Records The Environment	Admission Sheets Discharge/Transfer Forms Progress Notes Flow Sheets
Diagnosis	Nursing Judgment	Patient Care Plan Multidisciplinary Care Path Protocols Progress Notes Patient Problem Lists
Planning Care Outcome Definition Defining Care Priorities Defining Intervention Strategy	Patient Care Plan Multidisciplinary Care Path Projected Length of Stay Standards of Care Admission Assessment Data	Patient Care Plan Multidisciplinary Care Path Protocols Progress Notes Patient Problem Lists
Activation of Care Plan Interventions	Staff Reports Progress Notes Patient Rounds Direct Patient Care	Progress Notes Multidisciplinary Care Path Protocols
Evaluation	Patient/Family Interview Physical Assessment Staff Reports Progress Notes Diagnostic Test Results Flow Sheets	Patient Care Plan Multidisciplinary Care Plan Progress Notes Protocols Patient Problem Lists

- Review the current information in each section of the medical record.
- Verify that reports with abnormal results have been communicated to the appropriate provider.
- Compare the patient's progress for that day with the plan of care.

When the patient is progressing as expected, and additional actual or potential problems are not identified, the nurse charts that the plan should be continued as written. When changes to the plan of care are needed, one should be sure the observations leading to those decisions are charted and that the changes are communicated to the next shift.

THE IMPACT OF SETTING ON DOCUMENTATION

One of the wonders of nursing practice is its incredible diversity. Nursing participates in the delivery of patient care in many diverse settings including the hospital, skilled nursing facilities, rehabilitation centers, the home, the community, in medical offices, and in nursing clinics. In all settings, nursing documentation is driven by the process used to plan, implement, and evaluate patient care. However, what one documents and how it will be documented will vary according to the patient population, patient status, and setting. Box 14–6 provides an overview of the essential elements of documentation, which cross patient populations and settings of care. The sources of data available to the nurse and the tools available for documentation will be setting- and organization-specific. Some of the impacts of setting are discussed in this section.

Acute Care

The need to manage care across the continuum has influenced documentation in the hospital setting. Multidisciplinary, multi-setting care paths are being implemented to manage care across settings and over time. Shortened lengths of stay mean that only the highest priority problems can be addressed during the hospital stay. Discharge forms have become lengthy and complex. These forms document the patient's status on discharge, the patient's achievement of outcomes, deferred patient problems requiring follow-up, and the posthospital plan of care.

Skilled and Long-Term Nursing Facilities

Governmental oversight has had a strong impact on documentation in skilled and long-term care facilities. The content of admission and periodic assessments for all residents in nursing facilities has been defined by the Minimum Data Set (MDS) for Resident Assessment and Care Screening (Morris, et al., 1990). The MDS was created in response to the 1987 Omnibus Reconciliation Act mandate to the Health Care Financing Administration. The MDS was designed to reflect the quality of care in long-term resident nursing facilities. MDS standards define the content for the baseline assessment in addition to the timing and content of subsequent periodic assessments throughout the term of the resident's stay. There are defined triggers for

BOX 14–6
THE BASICS OF DOCUMENTATION

There are certain basic rules that cross all methods of documentation.

- Be sure you are documenting on the correct patient's record.
- Date and time each entry.
- Sign each entry with legal signature.
- If using initials on a flow sheet, be sure to link initial with signature in the appropriate location.
- When using a computer to document care, your logon and password are your legal signature. When leaving the computer always sign-off so others will not chart under your electronic signature.
- Never give your logon and password to another individual or chart for others under their logon and password.
- Entries should be legible, concise, and accurate.
- If an error is made, cross out with a single line and initial.
- Avoid language subject to interpretation, i.e., large or small. Instead use statements like "the 6 mm by 8 mm abrasion. . . ."
- Use only those abbreviations approved by the institution.
- Although units may have standards like "medication must be given within 30 minutes of the time scheduled," it is important to document the exact time the patient actually received the medication. This is important for understanding the presence of unusual symptoms should they occur.
- Record adverse reactions to medications or treatments.
- The care plan needs to indicate the potential problems you are observing for as well as seeking to prevent.
- Do not leave spaces in your documentation. If a nurse on a prior shift forgets to chart, that nurse will need to use the next available space and indicate that a late entry is being made to the medical record.
- Be sure all active protocols for safety and care are referred to in the documentation.
- In an emergency, patient care comes first. Whenever possible, chart key assessments, observations, and interventions as they occur on flow sheets. If you are restricted to narrative charting, take notes on critical observations, vital signs, events, and interventions. Chart completely once the patient has stabilized or you have been relieved.
- Remember it is just as important to document the absence of change as it is to document the presence of change in the patient's condition.

BOX 14–7
CONTENT AREAS OF THE NATIONAL RESIDENT ASSESSMENT AND CARE SCREENING INSTRUMENT

Assessment Areas for all Residents	Triggers for Protocol Implementation and Increased Assessment/Follow-up
Cognitive Patterns	Delirium
Communication/Hearing Patterns	Cognitive Loss/Dementia
Vision Patterns	Visual Function
Physical Functioning and Structural Problems	Communication
Continence in Last 14 Days	Activities of Daily Living Function/Rehabilitation Potential
Psychosocial Well-Being	Urinary Incontinence/Indwelling Catheter
Mood and Behavior Patterns	Psychosocial Well-Being
Activity Pursuit Patterns	Mood
Disease Diagnoses	Behavior
Health Conditions	Activities
Oral/Nutritional Status	Falls
Oral/Dental Status	Nutrition
Skin Condition	Feeding Tubes
Medication Use	Dehydration/Fluid Maintenance
Special Treatment and Procedures	Dental Care
Customary Routine	Pressure Ulcers
	Psychotropic Drug Use
	Physical Restraints

more frequent and more detailed assessments. The comprehensiveness of the assessment and follow-ups required by the MDS are illustrated in Box 14–7.

Home Health

The role of home health nurse is rapidly increasing in importance as lengths of stay shorten in the acute care settings, and as the adult children of our aging population seek to maximize the amount of time their parents can remain at home. The shortened lengths of stay mean that more acute treatments (i.e., intravenous therapy, complex open wound dressing changes) are occurring in the home. The care plan developed by the home health nurse for a discharged patient must be a continuation of the care plan from the hospital. Objectives not met during hospitalization must be monitored. In addition, actual or potential problems identified but deferred during the acute stage must be reevaluated and prioritized. In the hospital, the patient adapts to the acute care environment. When care is delivered in the home, the nurse must adapt to the patient's environment. It is therefore important for the nurse to document environmental and family factors that drive the decision-making process.

Because the patient has had less time to stabilize, the home health nurse must carefully document the patient's status and response to treatment. Changes in the patient's condition requiring alterations in the medical plan of care must be documented and reported to the physician. As always, the timing, accuracy, and completeness of the documentation are essential. These notes are often referred to when medical records are being audited for premature discharge from the acute care facility.

As care is rapidly shifting to the home, there is greater attention being paid to the cost of that care. Invoices for home care reimbursement are often derived directly from the nursing documentation of care delivered. Computers are finding increasing use in the home health area to support billing and quality processes. The Department of Health and Human Service's Health Care Financing Agency is sponsoring the development and testing of a standard dataset for documenting the status, interventions, and outcomes of health care delivered in the home. This dataset will be used as a basis for a required outcomes-based quality improvement program.

Community Health Nursing

Community health nurses work in the community, in schools, in industry (occupational health), and in community mental health agencies. Health care teams work together to deal with the complexities of care of community groups and populations. As the number of health care workers grows, effective documentation keeps the lines of communication between all the providers open and clear. Problem-oriented record keeping is the most common kind of documentation used in this field.

Data gathering for the purposes of analysis and application to other situations is an important function of community nursing. Communication to the public health department occurs to curb the spread of disease within a community. The Centers for Disease Control and Prevention in Atlanta, Georgia, conduct key research into the prevention of communicable disease. This work relies on the accurate recording and reporting by nurses and other health care personnel.

THE MEDICAL RECORD AS A LEGAL DOCUMENT

Any discussion of documentation must address the medical record as an important legal document. As a legal document, the record must accurately reflect the care provided to the patient. Clear, legible, unambiguous information is essential. Nursing documentation is always reviewed in detail in any legal case because it provides an ongoing, 24-hour-per-day picture of the patient's status. In addition, because nursing has a primary role in the coordination of care, nursing documentation provides evidence of the timeliness of communications between departments and providers.

The first way nurses protect themselves legally is to follow the basic principles of documentation (see Box 14–6). Next, it is important to follow the standards for documentation established by the organization. Nursing management, quality assurance departments, and medical records committees work together to ensure that approved forms for charting meet the requirements of outside agencies. Federal, state, and local agencies each have documentation and reporting requirements. These might include reporting births and deaths, reporting suspected child abuse, and reporting the occurrence of infectious diseases. Professional organizations such as JCAHO, the American Nurses' Association (ANA), and the American Association of Critical Care Nurses have published standards for care and documentation. During legal proceedings, documentation provides the evidence that standards of care were or were not followed.

Organization charting forms and standards will also require documentation directed at reducing the liability of the organization. For instance, information on the status of valuables on admission, during transfer between units, and on discharge is usually required. Instruction to the patient and family regarding the use, or the restriction of the use of electrical equipment brought from home enhances patient safety. Documentation of the orientation of the patient to the environment, the availability of the call light, and the status of the bed rails is all relevant to safety and, therefore, to reducing the liability of the nurse and the organization.

You will note that phrases like "complete and accurate documentation" are frequently used. And yet, the documentation of every task and element of care provided for the patient is not possible. Principles of documentation that provide legal protection to the nurse and his or her institution fall in the following areas.

- Document all identified actual or potential problems of the patient. Include pertinent observations, communications, actions, and changes to the plan of care implemented to address the problems.
- Record patient responses to treatment and to the plan of care.
- Document the standards of care and protocols of the organization.
- Chart all incidents or occurrences (e.g., falls, allergic reactions, medication errors, refusal of treatment) whether or not the patient appears to be injured. Attention should be paid to assessing and recording the patient's status and response to the incident. Documentation should be accurate, objective, complete, and include the exact time of the occurrence, all communications, and each intervention.
- Never falsify a record by omitting to note an incident, or by changing the facts about an incident. To do so brings into question the integrity of all documentation under your signature.
- Objective recording means clear, concise descriptions of the facts. Do not include judgments or assignment of fault (e.g., ". . . the unit was short staffed and so the dressing wasn't changed").
- Use only those abbreviations approved by the organization's medical records committee. The use of abbreviations when charting can be problematic. Does "VH" refer to vaginal hysterectomy or to ventricular hypertrophy? Are "BS" breath sounds or bowel sounds? Box 14–8 provides a sample of the hundreds of abbreviations that might be approved by a medical records committee.

COMPUTER DOCUMENTATION

Computers are rapidly being integrated into the operations of health care organizations for a variety of reasons. As efforts increase to control costs and to streamline processes of care, organizations are realizing that effective decision making must be data driven. Regulatory agencies are moving toward the mandatory electronic transmission of patient and billing information. Purchasers of health care are demanding evidence of the quality of care through the use of comparative report cards. The Health Plan Employer Data and Information Set (HEDIS) provides a standard way for health plans to specify, calculate, and report information in five performance categories: quality; enrollees' access and satisfaction; utilization; and financial data (Appleby, 1995). The ANA has recommended the development of a national report card that nurses, consumers, payers, and government agencies can use to assess the quality of hospital nursing care (ANA, 1995). Indicators in the second phase of the national report card will include nosocomial infections, decubitus ulcers, medication errors, patient injury rate, and patient satisfaction. Nursing leaders are calling for the development of an outcomes database structure through which nursing knowledge can be developed (Henry, 1995). Finally, as managed care organizations increase in number and size, the ability to track the patient across the continuum of care (hospital, skilled nursing facility, home, physician offices) has become essential for controlling the costs of care.

The meeting of these diverse needs requires the extraction of patient data from the medical record. It is extremely labor intensive to manually extract data from a paper record for

BOX 14–8
APPROVED ABBREVIATIONS

This is a selection from a 20-page list of approved abbreviations for use in a health maintenance organization. These abbreviations are used in the medical centers, the medical offices, and in home care. Because the complete abbreviation list is used across sites of care, the names of facilities and major services are also included in the complete list.

Term	Abbreviation
Abdominal	ABD
Appointment	APPT
Cancer	CA
Complains of	C/O
Diagnosis	DX
Follow-up	F/U
Fracture or broken bone	FX
Gastrointestinal	GI
History	HX
Infection	INF
Medication	MED
Message	MESS
Months	MO
Nausea & vomiting	N/V
No known allergies	NKA
No known drug allergies	NKDA
Patient	PT
Physical exam (any age)	PE
Pounds	LBS
Pregnant	PREG
Prescription	RX
Reception	RECP
Regarding	RE:
Regular	REG
Request	REQ
Return to work	RTW
Sore throat	ST
Symptoms	SX
Throat culture	TC
Treatment	TX
Unknown	?
Urinalysis	UA
Urinary tract infection	UTI
Vaginal	VAG
Weight	WT
With	W/
Years	YR
Left	LT
Right	RT
Morning	AM
Afternoon or Evening	PM
Night	NOC
Acute Care	ACC
Emergency Dept	ER
Family Practice	FPR
Medicine	MED
OB/GYN	OB
Ophthalmology	OPH
Optometry	OPT
Pediatrics	PED
Psychiatry	PSY
Teen Clinic	TCL
Physical Therapy	PTD
Antioch	ANT
Martinez	MTZ
Vallejo	VAL
Walnut Creek	WCR
Aspirin	ASA
Every day	QD
Injection/shot	INJ
Milligrams	MG
Penicillin	PCN
Suspension/liquid med	SUSP
Three times a day	TID
Twice a day	BID

entry into a computer. Each reduction in the number of hands required to handle a piece of data can significantly reduce the cost of the infrastructure supporting health care.

For the nurse, this environment increases the likelihood that some form of technology will be required in the documentation process. Computers can be found at the bedside, in the nursing station, and even in lounges and dressing rooms (Fig. 14–14). Voice-activated technology is being tested as well as hand-held and pen-based computing devices. With the implementation of this new technology comes the expectation that the process of documentation will change. For instance, it is common practice for the nurse to write vital signs and other observations on pieces of paper as reminders for when it is time to chart. With computing devices at each point of care, the nurse is expected to chart directly into the computer. Many nurses have found it very difficult to give up their "paper towel" reminders of care.

Issues with Computer Documentation

Computerized documentation systems are frequently called *clinical information systems* (CISs). In addition to documentation modules, CISs include order entry and transcription functions, linkages to laboratory and pharmacy systems, and linkages to administrative databases (admission/discharge/transfer, health information coding).

The basic principles that apply to charting in the paper record also apply to the computer record (see Box 14–6). However, the nurse will find that the process of documenta-

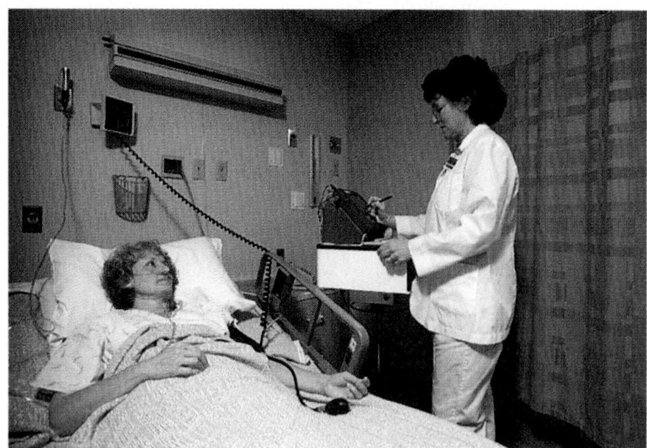

Figure 14–14. Nurse using a bedside computer for documentation.

tion on computers is different from that on paper. In addition, nurses will find that each documentation program they use will have different characteristics and approaches to recording care. It is important that thorough orientation and training be provided to personnel accessing each system. During this training, several issues are normally addressed including:

- accessibility
- security
- moving through the program
- quality edits
- responsibility for reviewing transferred data
- language and restricted choices

ACCESSIBILITY

Day shift on a busy unit can be a challenging time to try to document in the paper record. The chart might be with the physician, the therapist, the unit assistant, or even with the patient in radiology. At a computer station, nurses can have access to all of their patients at any time. Depending on the facility, however, the number and location of computer stations may be limited. Patient care personnel can document on several patients at the same computer. During this time, the same computer station cannot be used by others. Most facilities have learned the importance of having plenty of computer stations located in convenient places (e.g., lounges and outside patient rooms). Nurses may resort to assigning "computer" time throughout the day in those facilities faced with limited space or resources for additional stations.

SECURITY AND CONFIDENTIALITY

Each time CISs are accessed, a "logon" procedure is required (Fig. 14–15). Typically, the nurse types in his or her name followed by a password. Passwords are changed on a routine basis, as often as every 30 days. A specific level of security and

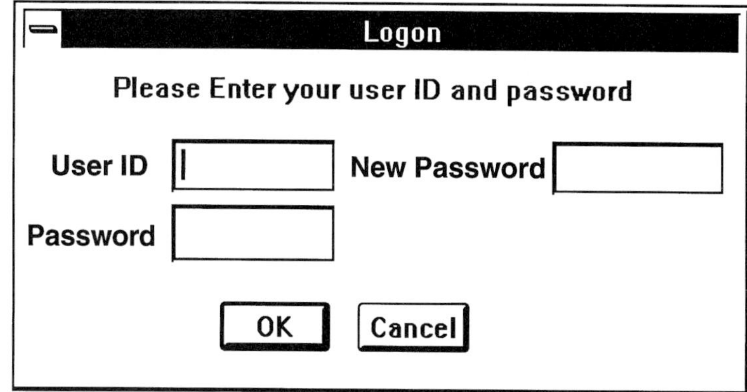

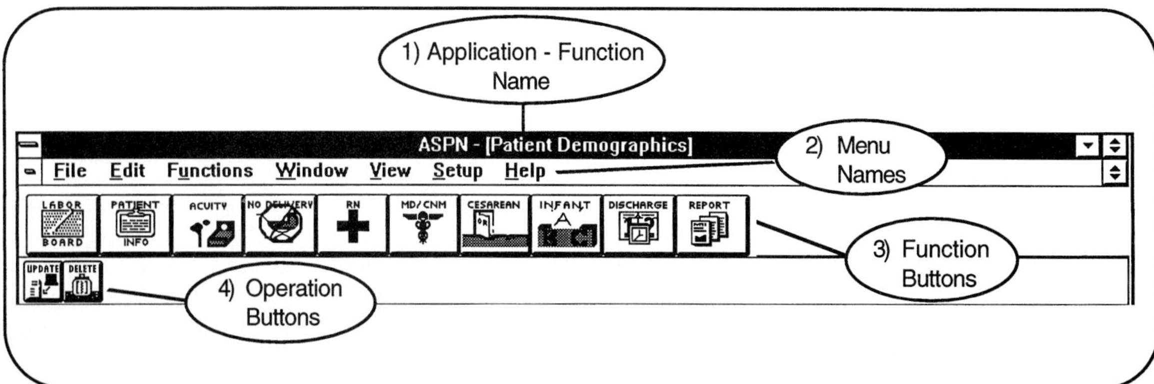

Figure 14–15. Logging on to the system is the first step in computer documentation. When in doubt, read the screen. You can usually find out where you are in the system, where you move to in the system, and how to get help.

access is associated with an individual's logon. This security gives access to certain patients and certain parts of the CIS. For instance, a physician may be able to enter and document in the medical history and physical part of the program. Nurses may be able to enter the history and physical module but be restricted to "read only" access. This means that they cannot chart or change information in the module. Registered nurses are typically given access to the orders generation part of the information system because they accept telephone orders from physicians. In contrast, nursing assistants would not be able to enter this module.

Patient confidentiality is the responsibility of every employee of the health care institution. Most institutions require all employees to sign statements holding the employee accountable for following all standards and policies on confidentiality. It is natural for individuals to be curious about the status or care of others. In the absence of strict logon procedures, access to the computer can make it especially easy to obtain information on patients, staff members, or other individuals for whom you are not providing care. Clinical information systems are establishing audit trails documenting all personnel who have accessed an electronic record in order to improve the management of confidentiality.

However, any computer security system is of little value if personnel do not take access rules seriously. Unless Nurse A is conscientious about signing off the system prior to leaving the computer, others can use his or her security access to view information for other patients, and even to chart under his or her electronic signature. The nurse should never share a logon and password with anyone. If individuals have forgotten their logon and password, refer them to their supervisor or to the information systems department. Each facility has rules providing for the emergency assignment of new logons and passwords.

MOVING THROUGH THE PROGRAM

Once the nurse has completed the logon procedure for the CIS, he or she will typically enter the system either through the medical record number of a single patient or through the patient list for a given unit. One then selects the module in which to work. Any CIS can seem overwhelming at first. Nurses find that they rapidly learn how to navigate through the system. Users who find themselves stuck in a program and are not sure how to progress can always look at the screen for clues. They will most likely find an answer somewhere on that screen (see Fig. 14–15).

Figure 14–15 is an example of a patient information screen from a labor and delivery documentation system. At the top of the screen, the "Patient Info" module was selected. Below the title of the module is a row of icons. Icons are "pictures" representing different aspects of the program. From the patient information module, one can move to any of the areas shown in the icon row. Note the "logoff" icon. This allows one to

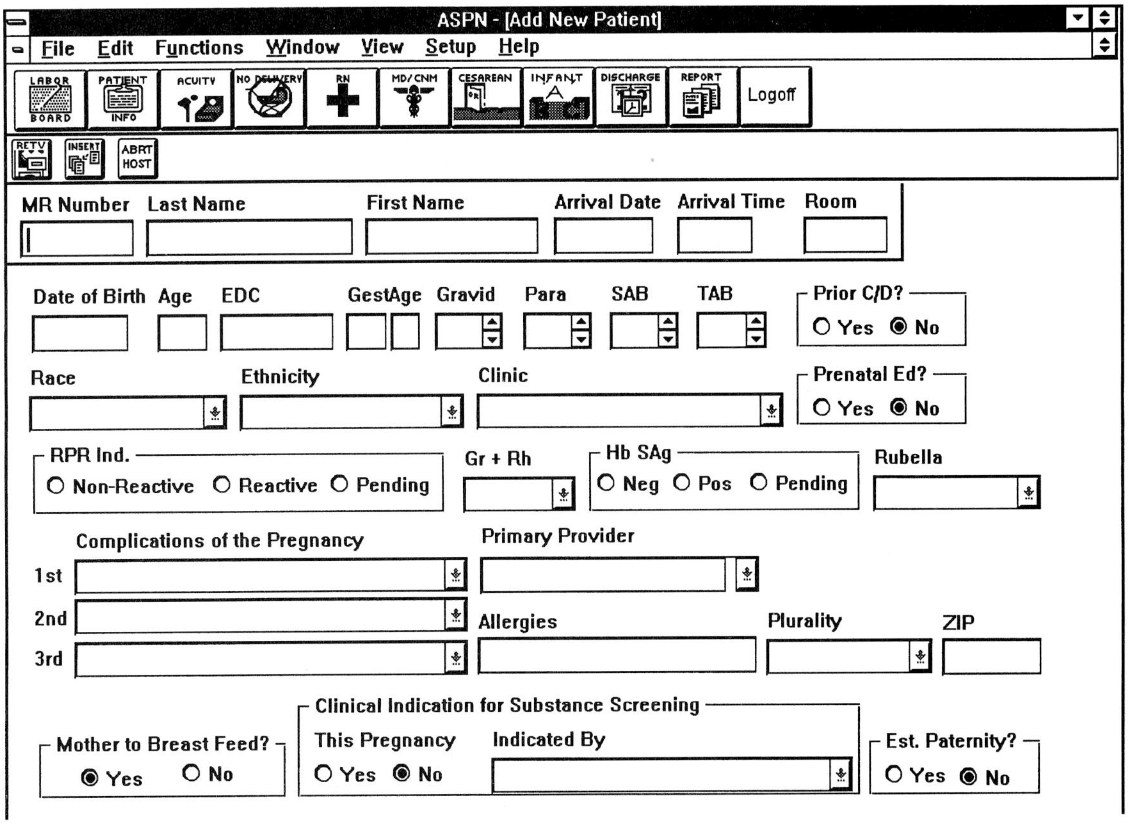

Figure 14–16. An example of a computer screen for documenting patient care in the labor and delivery department.

rapidly logoff the system in an emergency. This prevents others from charting under one's electronic signature.

REVIEWING TRANSFERRED DATA

Technology has advanced to the point that data from electronic monitors (heart, vital signs, hemodynamic) are transferred directly to the CIS. Lab and radiology results are also electronically linked. This process greatly reduces the amount of time spent in recording data. However, it does not eliminate the responsibility of the nurse to review the data, identify trends, and notify the physician of abnormal results.

LANGUAGE AND RESTRICTED CHOICES

In CISs designed to support the development of clinical databases, "free form" or traditional charting is severely limited. For information to be of value in a database, it must be able to be pulled from the medical record. In most cases, this means the computer is looking for an exact match. To make this happen, the CIS will allow limited options for each field. A "field" is where a particular piece of data is entered. In Figure 14–16, MR Number, Last Name, First Name, Arrival Date, Arrival Time, and Room each are fields. The computer will normally include some logic edits. For instance, the computer will question an age of 200. An extra "0" was probably entered. Notice there is an arrow in a small box at the end of the "Race" field. Data entry in this field is limited to a specific set of choices. Each organization has an established format for tracking data on race. The nurse "clicks" on the arrow. Clicking on the arrow opens up a small screen listing the data options. The nurse can then click on the desired option and it will appear in the field. As nurses learn the options, they have the option of typing the information directly in the field.

Just as computers are being used increasingly to support the delivery and documentation of patient care, computers are being used to increase knowledge within nursing. A discussion of nursing informatics may seem out-of-place in a chapter on documentation. However, it is through documentation and the advances in informatics that the speed in which nursing knowledge can be derived from practice will be greatly enhanced.

THE EMERGING FIELD OF NURSING INFORMATICS

Nursing informatics is a rapidly evolving field. Definitions of nursing informatics vary from "where caring and technology meet" (Ball et al, 1988) to "a combination of computer science, information science, and nursing science designed to assist in the management and processing of nursing data, information and knowledge to support the practice of nursing and the delivery of nursing care" (Graves and Corcoran, 1989). Of essential importance to nursing are the CISs being developed to support nursing in its many activities. CISs are typically made up of several software programs needed to manage the planning, delivery, assessment, and documentation of patient care. Typical programs include order entry and transcription, laboratory results reporting, libraries of standards and protocols, and patient care documentation systems. Newer CISs are incorporating knowledge-based programs.

CISs support the documentation process, reduce the time required to chart, and enhance the quality of documentation. One key time saver is the elimination of duplicate charting and reporting. For example, patient allergies can be collected once during the admission and entered into the CIS. The CIS then automatically provides this data to nutritional services, pharmacy, the operating room, and so on. The quality of documentation is supported by providing consistent prompts to the nurse and by requiring certain information prior to exiting a function. For instance, when documenting a medication, the system will check for an existing order and require that the dose, route of administration, site of injection, and reason for administration be documented prior to exiting the function (screen). If a medication requires special concentrations for administration and titration, the system will request the pertinent data and perform the calculations for the nurse.

CISs support the documentation of the nursing process and enhance the problem-solving ability of the nurse through knowledge-based programs. The nurse enters patient information

BOX 14–9
NURMETRICS: AN EVOLVING NURSING SCIENCE

The term *nurmetrics* originates from the work of Meintz at the University of Nevada, Las Vegas (Meintz, 1994). The evolving quality agenda requires the use of massive interagency, national, and international clinical and administrative databases to support the ongoing monitoring and analysis of patient care. The use of these databases requires new approaches to data quality and analysis. The high-performance computing and communication environment of supercomputers makes possible quality analysis projects of this magnitude.

Nurmetrics is the application of supercomputer technology to the nursing profession. Nurmetrics supports the growth of nursing knowledge by applying principles of mathematics and statistical techniques to the testing, estimation, and quantifying of nursing theories and solutions of nursing problems. Nurmetrics is made up of computational nursing and nursing informatics.

Computational Nursing uses models from mathematics and computer science together with simulation techniques to apply existing theory and methods to new solutions for nursing problems or for the design of new methods and techniques.

Nursing Informatics is the application of principles from computer science and informatics to understand the interplay between information form and function for the purpose of solving problems in nursing administration, nursing education, nursing practice, and nursing research.

(e.g., diagnoses, assessments, laboratory values) into the system for analysis. The system then presents to the nurse likely nursing diagnoses, protocols, actions, and treatments for consideration. These systems are designed to support and not replace the decision-making process of the nurse.

Potentially of greatest importance to nursing is the use of CISs to produce clinical, practice-based databases. Nursing produces an incredible amount of data about the patient, the care provided, and the results of that care. In fact clinical nursing databases can be so massive that research is currently being conducted to examine the use of supercomputers to support the process of data analysis (Meintz, 1994). The project team on the supercomputer project has identified a new science for development in nursing called **nurmetrics.** The focus of nurmetrics is the use of advanced statistical analysis techniques to analyze data collected by nursing for the purposes of evaluating patient care (Box 14–9).

THE FUTURE

Health care technology is changing so rapidly that anything in print can almost be considered out of date. Major trends include research into knowledge and decision support, the standardization and linkage of nursing language, and the use of clinical data to define the quality and outcomes of nursing care. One of the great challenges is the creation of an electronic clinical information system that will track patients over time, through health care events, and across settings of care. It is essential that staff nurses participate and contribute their expertise in each of these major projects. Screen designs need to reflect both the process of care and the thought process of the nurse. Different disciplines, and even individual providers within the discipline, process information in different ways and so require data presentation in different ways to support the process and documentation of care. Developers of CISs are increasingly striving to provide this kind of flexibility in their products. Nursing participation in the development of CISs will assure their effectiveness in supporting and documenting the decision-making process of the nurse, the process of care, and the analysis of its outcomes.

REFERENCES

American Nurses' Association (1995). *Nursing Report Card for Acute Care.* Washington, D.C.: American Nurses' Publishing.

Appleby, C. (1995). HEDIS: Managed care's emerging gold standard. *Managed Care,* Feb., 1995.

Ball, M.J., Hannah, K.J., Gerdin Jelger, U., Peterson, H. (1988). *Nursing Informatics: Where Caring and Technology Meet.* New York: Springer-Verlag.

Ball, M.J. (1985). Quality assurance: Its origins, transformations, and prospects. In C.G. Meisenheimer (ed.): *Quality Assurance: A Complete Guide to Effective Programs.* Rockville, MD: Aspen.

Clark, J. (1994). *An International Classification for Nursing Practice.* From paper prepared for: Informatics: The infrastructure for quality assessment and improvement in nursing. University of Austin, Texas, June, 1994.

Crawford, B.L., Taylor, L.S., Seipert, B.S., Lush, M. (1996). The imperative of outcomes analysis: An integration of traditional and nontraditional outcomes of care. *Journal of Nursing Care Quality, 10* (2), 33–40.

Davis, R.B., Iezzoni, L.I., Phillips, R.S., et al (1995). Predicting in-hospital mortality: The importance of functional status information. *Medical Care, 33* (9), 906–921.

Graves, J.R., Corcoran, S. (1989). The study of nursing informatics. *Image, 21,* 227–231.

Henry, S.B. (1995). Informatics: Essential infrastructure for quality assessment and improvement in nursing. *Journal of the American Medical Informatics Association, 2* (3), 169–182.

Henry, S.B., Holzemer, W.L., Reilly, C., Campbell, K. (1994). Terms used by nurses to describe patient problems. Can SNOMED III represent nursing concepts in the patient record? *Journal of the American Medical Informatics Association,* 1 (1), 61–74.

Iowa Intervention Project (1996). *Nursing Interventions Classification (NIC),* 2nd ed. J. McCloskey & B. Bulechek (eds.). St. Louis: Mosby-Year Book.

McCloskey, J., Bulechek, G., Iowa Intervention Project (1994). Toward data standards for clinical nursing information. *Journal of the American Medical Informatics Association, 1* (6), 469–470.

Meintz, S.L. (1994). High performance computing in nursing research. In S.J. Grobe and E.S.P. Pluyter-Wenting (eds.): *Nursing Informatics: An International Overview for Nursing in a Technological Era.* Amsterdam: Elsevier Science B. V.

Morris, J.N., Hawes, C., Fries, B.E., et al (1990). Designing the national resident assessment instrument for nursing homes. *The Gerontologist, 30* (3), 293–307.

Nightingale, F. (1863). *Notes on Hospitals.* London: Longman, Green, Longman, Roberts, & Green.

Werley, H.H., Lang, N.M. (1985). *Identification of the Nursing Minimum Data Set.* New York: Springer Publishing Company.

UNIT III

Special Considerations Basic to Nursing Practice

If asked to describe the settings in which nurses work, the average person would name hospitals, nursing homes, and doctors' offices. The description would likely focus on the technology, personnel, and quality of care. Few would offer a description of the setting as dangerous for the nurse and other health care workers. Yet health care workers are more likely than even police officers to die of job-related injuries. One million health care workers annually suffer a needle-stick injury; the total number of work-related injuries by health care workers obviously is much higher. Many of these injuries and/or consequences of working in high-stress situations can be prevented. The six chapters in this unit focus on clinical content common across all nursing situations and the prevention of injury and unhealthy reactions to stress on the part of the nurse. As appropriate, prevention of injury to the patient is also addressed.

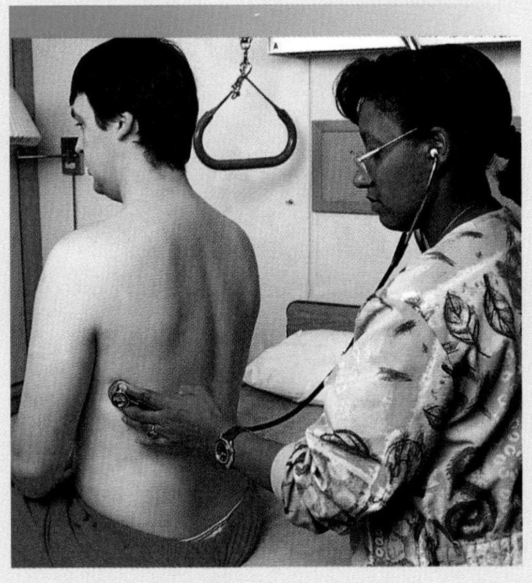

The unit begins with a chapter on assessment, the starting point for all nursing practice. The next chapter covers pharmacology and medication administration, with emphasis on safe and effective medication administration. Chapters on infection control, personal safety, the health of the nurse (and student nurse), and biomechanics and mobility complete this unit.

Patient Assessment

Pamela Hellings

Five members of the Johnson family have arrived for a clinic appointment. Mr. Johnson, age 35, has a history of high blood pressure and has been out of work after an industrial accident in which he hurt his back. Mrs. Johnson, age 28, is 3 weeks post-cesarean section from the birth of baby Audrey and has a history of obesity and anemia. They are bringing in Jeremy, age 4 years, because he has been complaining of pain in his right ear. They do not come in for regular checkups. Mrs. Johnson did receive prenatal care, but Mr. Johnson has not been in for more than 18 months. Audrey has not had her first checkup since discharge from the hospital, and Jeremy was last seen 1 year ago for an ear infection. Mr. Johnson's mother, Alma Peterson, who lives with the family, accompanies them. She is 65 years old, has diabetes, and is legally blind.

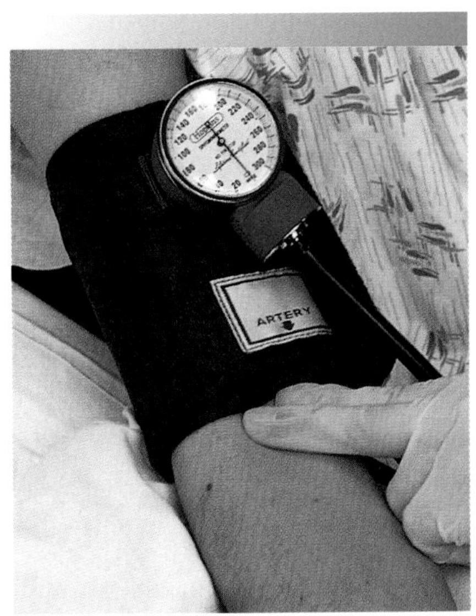

OBJECTIVES

After studying this chapter, students will be able to:

- **discriminate between subjective and objective findings while conducting a patient assessment**
- **complete a beginning-level patient assessment using a systematic and organized approach**
- **consider individual and setting differences in completing the assessment**
- **select among various types of the health history**
- **list the six components of the health history**
- **identify positive and negative findings for each body system**
- **demonstrate an awareness of privacy and confidentiality issues**
- **correctly document subjective and objective data collected during a patient assessment**

SCOPE OF NURSING PRACTICE

Assessment is part of every nurse-patient interaction. Its importance is reflected in the American Nurses' Association's (ANA, 1991; currently under revision) *Standards of Clinical Nursing Practice.* Those standards (authoritative statements by which the nursing profession describes the responsibilities for which its practitioners are held accountable) apply to all nurses in all clinical settings. The first standard of care is *assessment*: "The nurse collects client health data." Five measurement criteria accompany this standard:

- The priority of data collection is determined by the client's immediate condition or needs.
- Pertinent data are collected using appropriate assessment techniques.
- Data collection involves the client, significant others, and health care providers when appropriate.
- The data collection process is systematic and ongoing.
- Relevant data are documented in a retrievable form.

The importance of assessment as a component of nursing practice is also evident in state level nurse practice acts. For example, California's *Nurse Practice Act Rules and Regulations* (California Board of Registered Nursing, 1997) lists as one of four nursing functions "observation of signs and symptoms of illness, reactions to treatment, general behavior, or general physical condition, and (A) determination of whether the signs, symptoms, reactions, behavior, or general appearance exhibit abnormal characteristics; and (B) implementation, based on observed abnormalities, of appropriate reporting, or referral, or standardized procedures, or the initiation of emergency procedures."

In the ANA's 1995 *Nursing's Social Policy Statement,* one of the four essential features of contemporary nursing practice is "integration of objective data with knowledge gained from an understanding of the patient's or group's subjective experience."

Assessment is clearly a significant component of nursing practice. It is the framework from which the nurse determines the "what" and "how" of care. It provides the "why" of care. Assessment is an iterative process, not a single event, because

- The patient and the patient's situation is dynamic (i.e., in a state of change).
- The reliability of the assessment data must be verified.

A survey of registered nurses (Sony, 1992) supports the importance of physical assessment skills within contemporary nursing practice. The following 10 skills were used most frequently:

- Assessment of skin
- Auscultation of abdomen
- Palpation of peripheral pulses
- Palpation of abdomen
- Assessment of muscular strength
- Auscultation of thorax
- Assessment of pupillary response
- Auscultation of mitral area
- Inspection of neck
- Assessment for Homans's sign (pain in the calf when the foot is passively dorsiflexed).

When done in the context of a caring relationship, the assessment process provides the patient an opportunity to disclose private, personal health concerns to the nurse. It is a key time for establishing trust.

Developing skill in assessment requires knowledge and experience because it is an art as well as a science. Treating every patient encounter as a learning experience is one way to improve assessment skills.

ASSESSMENT PROCESS

Patient assessment provides the information base on which to build a plan of nursing care and ultimately to evaluate that plan. Thus, accurate, complete assessment is critical to the development of a realistic plan of action.

Assessment requires an organized and logical approach to data collection. The data collected are closely examined by the nurse to evaluate the contents and their meaning, thereby ensuring the completeness and accuracy of any conclusions.

Objective and Subjective Data

During assessment, data of both a subjective and an objective nature are collected. To obtain subjective data, the nurse asks the patient what he or she thinks or feels about what is happening. The patient is asked to report his or her experience of an event and to interpret the meaning of that event. The patient is questioned about past experiences (health history) and current health problems. These reports provide the basis of the subjective assessment. Current Controversy: An Interviewing Style for Nursing Assessment discusses possible forms of the subjective assessment.

Objective data, information that can be seen or measured by the nurse, are also collected. Findings from a physical examination or laboratory results from a blood test are examples of this type of data.

On the basis of connotations of the terms *objective* and *subjective,* the nurse may be led to consider the objective data accurate and reliable while viewing the subjective data with a great deal more caution. However, the potential for error and misrepresentation exists in the collection and interpretation of both kinds of data. Thus, the nurse needs to check and recheck both subjective data and objective data with the patient and other sources to ensure accuracy and reliability.

Keep in mind that assessment is an ongoing activity. New data must be collected at every patient contact. The events and the interpretation of these events are not static. New problems arise and must be included in the assessment. New information about old problems may become available. A

CURRENT CONTROVERSY

AN INTERVIEW STYLE FOR NURSING ASSESSMENT

(Brown, 1995)

In Western medicine, obtaining a health history takes the form of an interview. The health care provider is authorized to control what is discussed by asking a series of questions. The patient is expected to participate by answering the questions. The patient is not expected to initiate questions or new topics for discussion. Research on care provider-patient communication patterns supports this approach to the health history.

Research has also shown that a conversational style of interviewing, one that more closely represents normal conversation patterns, is more efficacious than traditional interviewing. Three studies of nurses revealed the use of more conversational, client-centered approaches.

"At this point, we cannot be sure whether conducting interviews in a conversational, client-centered manner will enhance or detract from the quality of the assistance rendered to clients. Advocates of humanistic caring may assert that the provider who deeply understands the client will form more meaningful human connections, will form more valid interpretations of the client's situation, and will therefore be able to formulate nursing plans of care that are more tailored to the individual client. Those clinicians who are more rational or cognitive in their view of nursing may say that re-centering clinical discourse on the client's story will result in less well founded diagnostic conclusions because the nurse will be distracted in his/her clinical reasoning. The question of the effects of client-centered, conversational interviewing on clinical decision making awaits further research."

change in a physical finding must be documented. Thus, the assessment process continues throughout the entire duration of the nurse-patient relationship.

Art and Science of Assessment

There is both an art and a science to assessment. The science base may be a little easier to teach because it has been codified over years of research. For example, the process of assessment includes basic techniques such as heart auscultation that may be practiced and evaluated in terms of known science. There are concrete data such as laboratory urine or blood values to be considered. There are anatomic landmarks that can be identified.

The scientific knowledge base for assessment requires constant reevaluation to incorporate new techniques and technology and new understandings of the meaning of clinical data. The knowledge base in the science of assessment is not static, even though it is more concrete and definable than the art of assessment.

The art of patient assessment is more difficult to translate into quantifiable terms. The feeling the nurse gets that drives her or him to pursue a topic, the look on a patient's face that suggests that a question from the nurse is not clear, a catch in the patient's voice that needs clarification, the tenseness of the muscles when the nurse touches the person, the smell in the room that has not been acknowledged relate to the art of assessment. All of the senses contribute to the development of the art of assessment. These skills are difficult to teach and evaluate. Yet they are critical skills in assessment and may be the determining factor in the adequacy of the assessment process.

Priorities for Assessment

One additional consideration in the assessment process is the need to set priorities. Time pressures, crucial health problems, and an appreciation of how much can be accomplished in a single contact often lead to the necessity of determining what will be done first and what may not be done at all during this encounter. An assessment based on past information and on an update of the current situation will provide the guidance to determine those priorities in the planning stage of nursing care.

In the case presentation at the beginning of the chapter, the Johnson family presents with many health care needs that require assessment. During the initial visit, at the very minimum, Mr. Johnson needs to have his blood pressure checked while Mrs. Johnson should be queried about her postpartum care. If she has not been seen since discharge and plans to resume care at this clinic, information about her delivery should be obtained and her surgical incision inspected for healing. Jeremy needs to be seen for the pain in his ear, and his immunization status needs to be evaluated. The baby, Audrey, needs to have a record established in her own name and her initial history obtained. In addition, if she has not been seen since discharge from the hospital, she is overdue for her first checkup. Questions about medication use and the cause for Mrs. Peterson's blindness need to be pursued.

Clearly, plans for follow-up or coordination with other clinics or the hospital need to be developed. Priorities must be established to deal with problems that may be identified, such as ongoing hypertension for Mr. Johnson, an ear infection for Jeremy, and the impact of diabetes on Mrs. Peterson's health status. Mrs. Johnson's decisions or questions about family planning need to be discussed. Finally, all family members' needs for ongoing health care must be included in the follow-up recommendations. The problems and concerns identified for management of acute and chronic illness, for implementation of health maintenance, and for follow-up of care provided at another facility require the full measure of the art and science of patient assessment to develop a workable plan with the Johnson family.

Several visits may be required to accomplish all of the goals set; if so, appointments need to be made for follow-up. It would be extremely difficult for one nurse to accomplish all of these assessments in one visit with the family. However, because this family has a history of irregular health care, a plan to accomplish as much as possible at the initial visit is important.

Subjective Data

The basis of a thorough patient assessment is the solicitation of an accurate and complete description of the patient's current and past health status. The process used to collect this data is the *health history*. Historical data are labeled subjective because of the nature of the information obtained. Subjective data include the patient's experiences as he or she perceives and reports them. The events and experiences have been interpreted by the informant (patient) and to some degree by the nurse taking or reviewing the history. The nurse cannot, for instance, objectively touch a patient's concern or see a patient's pain, but must rely on the patient's subjective report at this point in the assessment. However, the nurse has the freedom to ask questions, follow up on comments, or clarify remarks to help ensure that the subjective data are as accurate and complete as possible.

TYPES OF HISTORIES

Frequently, the history is obtained by the nurse sitting with the patient and asking a series of questions (Fig. 15–1). The discussion that ensues provides the basis for determining the subjective information. There are identified components of the history to be completed, and notes should be taken for transcription or dictation into the patient's record or chart.

Sometimes, however, the patient is asked to complete a written form, which is then reviewed and clarified with the patient. Such a form may be used to collect standard information such as immunization history. It may also be used to gather time-consuming information such as background health history on a new patient. In this situation, the nurse and patient can use their time together to delve into areas of concern rather than simply collecting data. These self-administered questionnaires must be clear and written at a reading level appropriate for the patient, because they will be reviewed only by the clinician, who likely will also expect the patient to seek clarification if he or she does not understand a particular question or word.

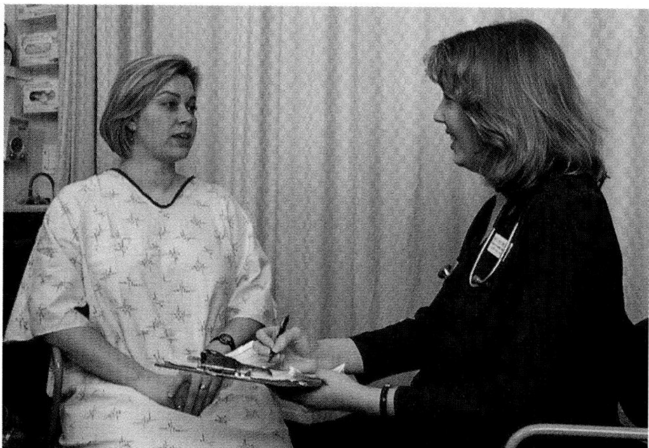

Figure 15–1. The face-to-face patient interview is the usual format for the health history.

In some cases, patients are not able to answer for themselves or to provide the necessary data. This is often the situation with young children and with those who are cognitively impaired. In this situation, a parent or other family member is asked to be the informant, or the one who provides the data. In the case presentation, Mr. or Mrs. Johnson would be the most likely informants for Audrey and Jeremy.

So far, the complete history has been noted as the norm. However, each patient does not need to provide a complete history on every encounter with the nurse. If a complete history has been obtained, it should be a part of the patient's record and available for review. An interim history is then appropriate. New problems or new information about old problems need to be explored. Mr. Johnson should have an interim history of his symptoms of hypertension and any other health concerns obtained, and his current blood pressure should be determined.

COMPONENTS OF THE HEALTH HISTORY

The health history contains six basic components:

- Chief complaint
- History of the present illness or problem
- Medical history
- Personal and social history
- Family history
- Review of systems

These six components provide the organizational framework for the history, but they serve only as a guideline. Flexibility in following the patient's lead or exploring relevant issues at the time they arise is imperative.

CHIEF COMPLAINT

The *chief complaint* is a brief phrase or statement from the patient or other informant characterizing the reason for the appointment or visit with the nurse. In the patient's record, the abbreviation *CC* is used to denote chief complaint. Often quotation marks may be used to record the patient's or informant's exact words. Examples of common chief complaints are "My head hurts"; "I have an infection in my toe"; "I brought my baby for his shots." Although it is important to note the reason the patient gives for the visit, it is also appropriate to listen for clues of other concerns or problems. Are there other reasons for the visit that have not yet been stated? Is the patient behaving in a way to suggest that he or she would like to talk in more depth about a particular issue?

Examples of clues that additional concerns have not yet been identified include vague or misleading answers to probing questions about the concerns expressed and a long delay in response to clarifying questions. Skill in the art of assessment and experience in collecting historical data assist the nurse in identifying these clues.

HISTORY OF THE PRESENT ILLNESS OR PROBLEM

In this aspect of the health history, a complete delineation of the chief complaint is obtained. In the patient's record, the abbreviation *HPI* may be used to denote this aspect of the assessment. Clarifying questions, including variations of "how," "what," "when," "where," and "why," are asked to promote a full understanding of the situation. For instance, questions such as "When did the headaches begin?" "Where does it hurt?" or "How did the baby respond to his last immunizations?" provide additional detail about the patient's concern or reason for the appointment. At the completion of this section of the history, the nurse should feel that she or he has a thorough understanding of the patient's concerns and the events surrounding those concerns.

MEDICAL HISTORY

In the medical history, the nurse has the opportunity to develop knowledge about the patient's past health problems and issues. This is also an opportunity to gain insight into the patient's general well-being. Many areas can be covered in this phase of the health history, and modifications in the process often need to be made based on the individual situation. In some cases, the birth history may be extremely relevant and may need to be documented in detail, whereas in others it may be more important to explore the patient's self-management of a chronic illness. For instance, a detailed description of the events leading up to Audrey's cesarean birth is of importance to assist in the identification of potential health problems for her, whereas it is more important to determine what medications Mr. Johnson currently uses on a regular basis. Box 15–1 lists the elements of a medical history.

PERSONAL AND SOCIAL HISTORY

The personal and social history provides data on the relevant events that may impact the patient's health status and provides information about his or her unique characteristics. Box 15–2 lists topics to cover in a personal and social history. Included are suggestions for areas to be explored.

FAMILY HISTORY

In the section for the family history, a good way to start is by diagramming the "family tree" or genogram (Fig. 15–2). The patient and family members, including parents, spouses, siblings, and children, should be recorded when appropriate. Health status, current age, cause of death, and age at time of death of various family members should be included. Attention should be paid to identifying hereditary conditions such as hemophilia and Huntington's disease as well as familial risk factors for chronic illnesses such as cancer, high blood pressure, heart disease, diabetes, and allergies. These data will provide a framework for making decisions about the necessity for and timing of screening activities such as blood glucose and cholesterol levels as well as health promotion strategies such as diet and exercise programs.

BOX 15–1
ELEMENTS OF A PAST MEDICAL HISTORY

General Health
How the patient describes his current health status in general terms such as "very healthy" or "having many problems"; as the patient describes his health status, the nurse may obtain insight into issues to probe during the remainder of the health history

Birth History
Prematurity; birth trauma; congenital anomalies; birth order; early growth and development milestones

Growth and Development
Patterns of weight gain and loss; later developmental milestones; school performance and grade completion

Previous Accidents, Major Illnesses, Hospitalizations
Broken bones; surgery; communicable diseases including the childhood illnesses such as measles, mumps, and rubella; chronic illnesses; and disabilities

Medication Use
Current prescription, over-the-counter, and home remedy drugs and medications. An increasing number of people are using medicinal plants and herbs, which needs to be probed

Immunizations
Regular childhood immunizations including the tuberculin skin test results as well as flu shots and other vaccinations

Allergies
Allergies to foods, medications, animals, and environmental agents

REVIEW OF SYSTEMS

Although health issues have been touched on in several of the body systems before the review of systems (ROS) is reached, it is still important to complete a review of systems. In the patient's record the abbreviation *ROS* may be used to denote this section of the assessment. The nurse can acknowledge what has already been heard and continue on if an area has already been covered. A thorough review of each system may not be needed; instead, the nurse may focus on just those areas relevant to the chief complaint. The focus is on present and past concerns and symptoms in each of the systems.

Box 15–3 presents elements of the review of systems. For each of the systems listed, some avenues for questions are suggested. The list is not complete, and specific questions that

BOX 15-2
ELEMENTS OF A PERSONAL/SOCIAL HISTORY

Cultural Background
Country of birth; language preference in the home; cultural beliefs about health and illness

Occupation
Usual work; job issues of safety, exposure, stress; previous/current military service

Habits
Drug use: prescribed, over-the-counter, and illicit; smoking; alcohol; exercise; leisure; sleep; travel

Religion
Religious preference; beliefs affecting health care (e.g., use of blood products)

Nutrition
Vitamins; daily diet; nutritional problems such as anorexia

Socioeconomic Status
Housing; health insurance; schooling; financial security

Sexuality
Preference; compatibility with partner; presently sexually active or not; protection from AIDS and other sexually transmitted diseases

may be related to the patient's concerns must be considered when relevant. Information about any history of disease or diagnoses in each specific system should be solicited and noted.

VARIATIONS IN THE SUBJECTIVE DATA COLLECTION PROCESS

The process used to collect subjective data must be adapted to account for individual and setting differences. The nurse must be thorough and systematic in the assessment process, yet must be able to modify that process to accommodate differences.

INDIVIDUAL DIFFERENCES

Individual differences that need to be taken into account during the collection of the subjective data and that may alter the process include the patient's age and developmental level, cultural background, and comfort with the subject matter.

Age and Developmental Level. An infant obviously cannot provide subjective data, and the presence of a knowledgeable adult or family member is imperative to ensure an accurate history. A toddler or a preschool-age child can answer certain basic questions, such as what he or she likes to eat or play with. Young children should be included in the process to maintain their interest and cooperation as well as to

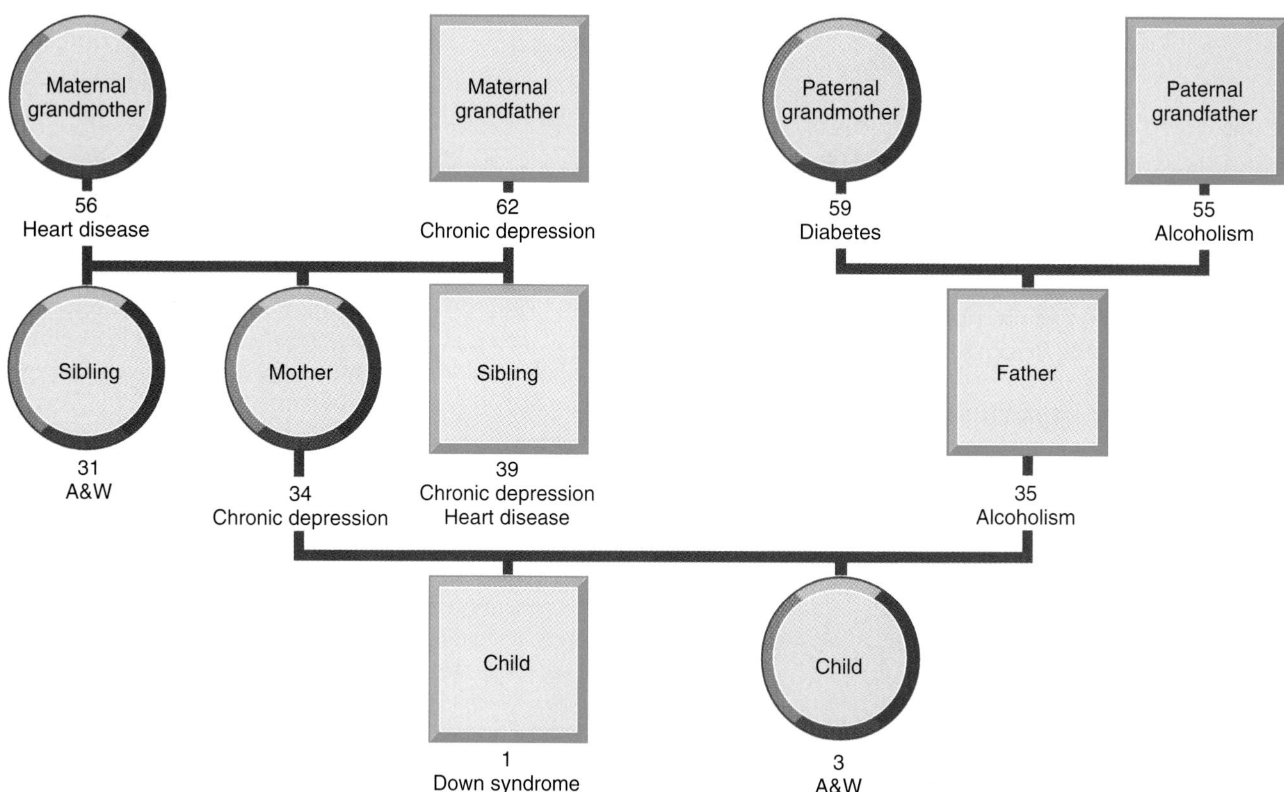

Figure 15-2. Family genogram of disease patterns. Circles represent females; squares, males. A & W indicates alive and well. (Adapted from Betz, C.L., Hunshayer, M.M., Wright, S. (eds.). (1994). *Family-Centered Nursing Care of Children,* 2nd ed. Philadelphia: W.B. Saunders, p. 46.)

BOX 15-3
ELEMENTS OF THE REVIEW OF SYSTEMS

General Symptoms
Fever; night sweats; excessive tiredness, unexplained weight loss or gain

Skin
Rash; itching; any changes in skin texture or color

Skeletal
Bony growth or deformity; pain or loss of range of motion; swelling or redness of joint or along a bone

Head
General: headaches, fainting, dizziness
Eyes: glasses or contact lenses, nearsightedness or farsightedness, eye diseases such as glaucoma or infections
Ears: loss of hearing, hearing aids, pain or ringing in ears
Nose: nosebleeds, discharge, sense of smell
Throat: frequent sore throats, changes in voice, difficulty swallowing, tongue pain or sores
Teeth and gums: cavities, swelling or bleeding from the gums, taste, regularity of dental care

Endocrine
General: thyroid enlargement, diabetes
Females: menstrual history including onset, flow, pain, menopause; last Pap smear or mammogram; pregnancy history including live births, miscarriages, abortions; use of birth control pills or other hormones; contraceptive method used
Males: onset of puberty, testicular pain or swelling, infertility

Respiratory
Difficulty breathing, wheezing or coughing, production of sputum

Cardiac
Chest pain, high blood pressure, cholesterol level

Hematologic
Past transfusions, anemia, easy bruising or bleeding

Lymphatic
Painful or enlarged lymph nodes

Gastrointestinal
Diarrhea or constipation, vomiting or nausea, hemorrhoids or polyps, change in stool frequency or color

Genitourinary
Frequent or painful urination, urine smell and color, dribbling

Neurologic
Seizures, fainting, memory loss, headaches

Psychiatric/Emotional
Mood swings, irritability, depression or mania, difficulty concentrating or sleeping, nightmares

provide an opportunity to interact with them and increase trust. School-age children and adolescents often have their own perspective, which may differ from that of their parents, and their input should be included in the subjective process. They can be particularly helpful in the current concerns and issues, but their knowledge of past events such a developmental milestone may be more limited.

Individuals of any age with cognitive impairments that affect memory or understanding of events will also need the help of a friend or family member to relay their history. For instance, the patient may not remember important details of the past event such as an allergic reaction to a medication or description of the symptoms that prompted treatment that are needed to clarify previous care and to assist in determination of a plan for the current concerns.

Age is also a variable in the type of data or the detail required. For instance, the birth history for an infant or toddler will be a great deal more detailed as the nurse pursues birth weight, details of the birth such as location, Apgar scores, and length of labor. In addition, a high level of detail sought for the growth and development milestones is more appropriate for a child than for an adult. In the case of the subjective data for an older individual, one must allow time to secure the information about lifelong experiences and symptoms. In addition, ability to care for oneself, including activities of daily living and getting to and from important locations such as the grocery store or the clinic for health care, must be included in the database. Also data about the ability to follow a treatment plan such as taking prescribed medications must be noted. For example, Alma Peterson will certainly require her family's assistance to obtain and take her medications on a consistent basis.

Cultural Background. Cultural background must also be considered. Cultural attitudes may lead to a different explanation for a particular health event such as an illness being caused by "bad behavior" rather than a virus. It is important to consider the patient's explanation or concern as it relates to their own experience of health. As a part of cultural awareness, it is important to determine the language that the patient normally speaks. Even if that language is English, it may be the patient's second language, and his or her skill or experience with medical terminology may be limited. In addition, multiple names for the same body part can add to the potential for misunderstanding (see Current Controversy: Anatomy of a Problem: Naming Body Parts). An understanding of the patient's cultural background will also be helpful in determining the plan for treatment.

Comfort with Subject Matter. Some patients may provide unclear or evasive answers to health history questions because of their lack of comfort with certain topics such as sexuality or

CURRENT CONTROVERSY

ANATOMY OF A PROBLEM: NAMING BODY PARTS (LEHMAN, 1997)

Since 1985, anatomists have been striving for a universal language for the 6000 terms used to describe the human body. The lack of a universal language has created confusion and inhibited communication among anatomists worldwide. For example, depending on where the anatomist was educated and worked, the end of the small intestine could be called Varolius, Tulp, Rondelet, or Posthius valve.

For the last 8 years, a panel of 20 scientists from 16 countries have been working to create a common language. Some of the proposed terms are already in common usage; about 1000 represent new terms. The new terms will be published in Latin and English. The panel hopes that anatomists in all countries will adopt this proposed universal language.

In the proposed lexicon, the end of the small intestine is papilla ileal and represents a move away from naming body parts after the scientist that first discovered it. The fingers are now named thumb, index, middle, ring, and little.

Will anatomists and health care providers in the United States adopt this universal language? If so, how long will it take to change practice?

bodily functions (e.g., urination or defecation). There may be a reluctance for a male patient to discuss certain topics with a female nurse. Alternatively, a young person may be hesitant to acknowledge an embarrassing problem. Care must be taken to approach these difficult topics in a manner that elicits the necessary detail for a full assessment.

SETTING DIFFERENCES

The setting in which the assessment is conducted may alter the quality and quantity of the data obtained. Subjective data may be gathered in a clinical setting such as an ambulatory center or a hospital, in the patient's home, and even over the telephone.

The patient may feel uncomfortable in an unfamiliar institutional setting. Every attempt must be made to ensure the patient's comfort and privacy. A room where the door may be closed or, at the very least, a curtain drawn helps provide a sense of privacy. Pleasant surroundings and comfortable seating also contribute to a feeling of openness. The patient's home provides an alternative in some situations, although the presence of other family members may inhibit the patient's willingness to discuss certain issues. Again, privacy must be maintained to encourage open communication during the subjective phase of the assessment. In addition, the home may provide other challenges such as competition from the television, radio, or other household activities during the collection of subjective health history data. The nurse should always provide strategies to minimize the distractions such as turning off the television or asking that the vacuuming be delayed.

In some cases, the nurse may obtain data for an interval history (between face-to-face meetings) or a prehospitalization history from the patient via a telephone conversation. Because of the length and complexity of a thorough initial history, data collection via the telephone is not practical. However, when an update is desirable, the telephone may be used. Without face-to-face contact, the telephone creates unique challenges in the accurate assessment of the patient's responses and questions. The nurse needs to be very careful to pay attention to pauses in the conversation and other clues that there are unresolved issues or questions that have not been addressed. The nurse should not hesitate to make comments like "I have a feeling you want to ask me something else" or to remind the patient that "you can always call me back if there is something else you want to add."

DOCUMENTATION OF SUBJECTIVE ASSESSMENT DATA

The nurse should take notes during each aspect of the subjective data collection process. The framework provided by the six components (CC, HPI, medical history, personal and social history, family history, and ROS) provides an organizational structure for recording of findings. Every detail need not be noted, only those that will be transferred to the medical record. Sometimes these notes will also serve to remind the nurse about items on which to follow up during the objective phase of assessment. In some cases, notes may be taken directly on the form that will go into the medical record. The form may include places to check "yes" or "no" to certain questions. If notes are taken on nonchart forms, they must then be transcribed or dictated into the medical record. The chart notes will serve as the communication link for the next visit or appointment for the patient. Care must be taken to record all pertinent findings.

Objective Data

The nurse collects objective data using the various senses to see, touch, smell, taste, and hear. Although these findings are labeled objective, a degree of subjectivity is involved. How red is red? What is firm versus hard? Experience and discussion with other clinicians improve this skill and contribute to improving the reliability and validity of the objective notations. An overview of environmental preparation for the objective assessment (also called the physical examination or physical assessment) is given in Procedure 15–1.

TECHNIQUES FOR PHYSICAL ASSESSMENT

Four techniques are routinely used in the collection of objective data:

- Inspection
- Palpation
- Percussion
- Auscultation

INSPECTION

Observation provides the framework for inspection. The nurse starts inspecting as soon as interaction with the patient begins. Does Mr. Johnson limp as he enters the exam room? Does Mrs. Johnson's voice soften as she begins to describe a symptom? Is Mrs. Peterson breathing comfortably? Does baby Audrey have a rash on her face? During the formal physical examination, the nurse observes each system carefully and notes any unusual or unexpected (positive) findings, such as crossed eyes, difficulty breathing, blue nail beds, curved spine, webbing of the fingers or toes, tics, and surgical scars, to list just a few.

Accurate inspection requires an adequate view of the area to be observed. Good lighting is imperative, and each system must be available for inspection. Thus, clothing and other coverings such as large jewelry or long hair must be moved or removed. Embarrassment on the part of the patient or the clinician must not prevent adequate exposure of the area to be inspected. Provision of privacy and sensitivity to the patient's feelings go a long way in increasing both the patient's and nurse's comfort with the process. Recognition by both the patient and nurse of the importance of a complete evaluation also contribute to a willingness to overcome feelings of discomfort. A thorough explanation of each part of the inspection provides the patient with an understanding of the process and a distraction to the actual activities.

The findings of the inspection are not immediately labeled "normal" or "abnormal" because they may require further investigation to determine the normality of them. For instance, blue nail beds may be a sign of congenital heart disease or may simply indicate that the patient is cold, perhaps from a long walk to the clinic in cold temperatures. A description of a positive finding is not a judgment as to its significance but rather a description of what is observed. Mrs. Johnson may be moving very slowly and carefully as she accompanies the nurse to the exam room, and Mr. Johnson may be breathing heavily as he enters the front door. Mrs. Johnson may be moving slowly because of continuing pain from her surgery, or she may have twisted her ankle in a recent fall. Mr. Johnson may suffer from chronic shortness of breath or may have run in from the parking lot after parking his car. The meaning of an observation requires further investigation.

It is often also important to note any findings that are usual or expected (negative) or that do not necessarily support the subjective assessment data. For instance, in the Johnson family, Jeremy may be playing and running around the room and his temperature may be normal despite his complaints of ear pain and his family's concern that he may have an ear infection. His behavior does not support the concern that he may be ill with an ear infection. However, his behavior should not be taken to mean that he does not have an ear infection, but rather that he does not appear to be feeling badly.

Thus, the record of a thorough inspection includes a description of relevant positive and negative findings. Keep in mind that inspection continues throughout entire course of the nurse-patient interaction. A change in the patient's appearance from the beginning of the encounter to the end may signal a new level of comfort or may provide evidence of tiring. A skillful observer maintains constant vigilance and adds to the database throughout the interaction.

Thoughtful and thorough observation is a vital assessment skill that must be practiced. Comparing observations with a skilled clinician is one way to sharpen skills. Also, remaining alert and processing what one's eyes, ears, and nose are noting will increase the quantity and the quality of the observations.

PALPATION

Palpation involves using touch to gather information. Light touch may be used to appreciate a fine rash (Fig. 15–3); deep palpation may be needed to find the liver's edge. Bimanual (both hands) palpation may be needed to assess adequately organs such as the kidneys or uterus (Fig. 15–4). Light palpation should always be done before deep palpation is attempted. Deep palpation may cause pain or may move tissue or fluid that should be lightly palpated first without discomfort or in the original configuration. Warm hands, a gentle touch, and short fingernails are much appreciated by patients and demonstrate respect for their personal comfort.

PERCUSSION

The nurse uses percussion to elicit sound from various body tissues to assist in the description of the density of the tissue. The more dense the tissue, the duller is the sound; the more air present in the tissue, the more resonant is the sound. Percussion

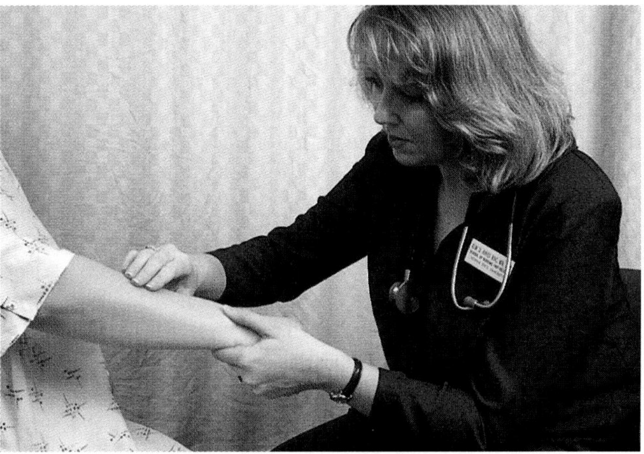

Figure 15–3. Light palpation technique.

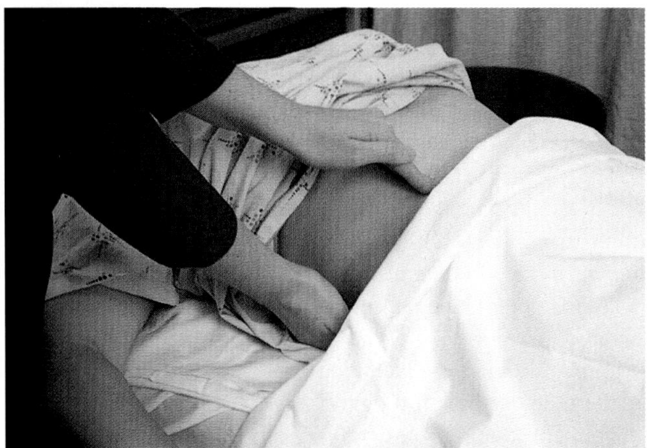

Figure 15-4. Bimanual palpation technique.

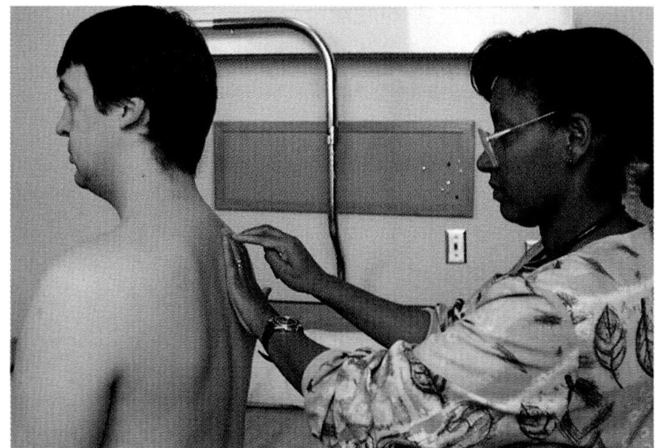

Figure 15-5. Percussion technique.

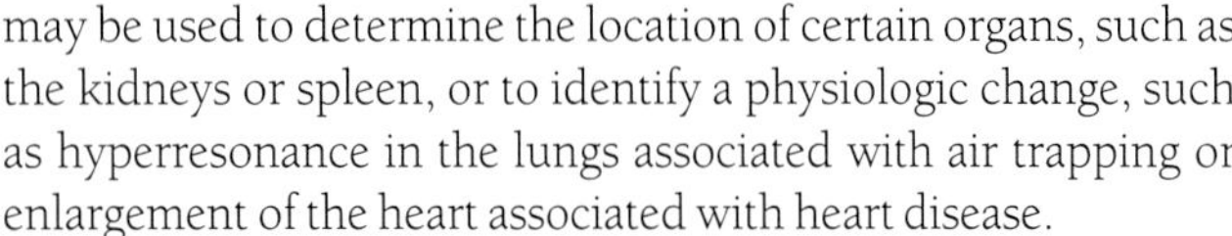

may be used to determine the location of certain organs, such as the kidneys or spleen, or to identify a physiologic change, such as hyperresonance in the lungs associated with air trapping or enlargement of the heart associated with heart disease.

The fingers are usually used for percussing, although the fist may be used. The finger of one hand (often the middle finger) is placed firmly on the location to be percussed, while the middle finger of the other hand is used in hammer-like fashion to strike the stationary finger (Fig. 15–5). The resulting sound is described in terms from flat to tympanic. Terms such as dull, resonant, and hyperresonant are used to describe the sounds between the extremes from flatness to tympany (Table 15–1). Dull and flat sounds are heard over solid areas such as the liver and muscle tissue. Resonance is characterized by a hollow, low-pitched sound; tympany, by high-pitched, drumlike sounds.

It is easier to appreciate the changes in sound when going from resonant sounds to dull sounds. Thus, percussion should proceed from normally resonant areas, such as over the lungs, to more dull areas, such as over the liver.

AUSCULTATION

Auscultation involves listening to the sounds of the body, such as heart, bowel, and respiratory sounds. Some sounds may be appreciated with the naked ear; others require the assistance of devices such as a stethoscope.

Some body sounds are rhythmic in nature and occur at regular intervals; others are heard less regularly or frequently. For example, breath sounds occur regularly and predictably, whereas bowel sounds may require more diligence to hear.

A quiet environment aids the ability to hear and describe the differences in body sounds. Sometimes, closing one's eyes to concentrate on the listening process can help focus the sense of hearing. Characteristics of sounds, such as rhythm (regular vs. irregular), pitch (high vs. low), duration (short to long), quality (e.g., harsh, musical, twanging, or machinery-like), and intensity (soft to loud) should be described.

Each sound needs to be separated from the others that may be present in the area, such as the presence of breath and heart sounds over the anterior chest. Also, the origin of sounds that are associated with the respiratory cycle need to be identified. Sounds originating in the nose that may be heard without a stethoscope may be heard even more distinctly when the stethoscope is over the lungs. One way to clarify the source is to place the stethoscope about 1 inch away from the nose and then move it down over the lungs. This technique usually helps determine whether the sound is actually coming from the lungs.

Auscultation generally should be completed as the last step in the examination of each system. Then, the information that is compiled from the both the subjective and objective assessments can be evaluated as to significance and meaning.

EQUIPMENT FOR PHYSICAL ASSESSMENT

To complete the physical assessment, some basic equipment is needed. Figures 15–6A–C show some of the equipment used in physical assessment.

TABLE 15-1 Percussion Sounds

Sound	Intensity	Pitch	Quality	Where Heard
Resonance	Loud	Low	Hollow	Healthy lungs
Hyperresonance	Very loud	Low	Booming	Emphysematous lungs
Tympany	Loud	High	Drumlike	Gastric bubble
Dull	Soft to moderate	Moderate to high	Solid	Over liver
Flat	Soft	High	Very dull	Over muscle

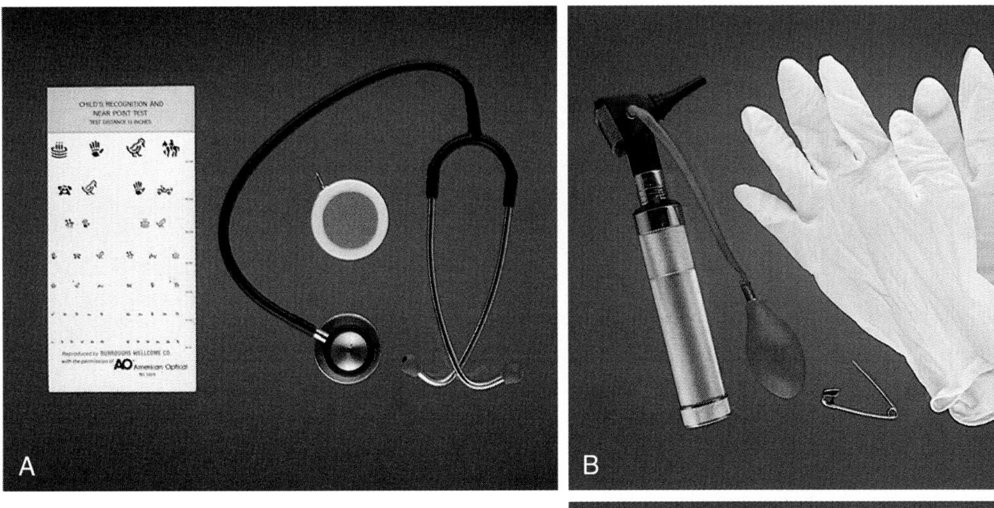

Figure 15–6. Some of the basic equipment used during physical assessment. *A*, Stethoscope and eye chart; *B*, otoscope, gloves, and pin; *C*, reflex hammer, tongue blade, and sphygmomanometer.

MEASURING TAPE

A measuring tape is used to determine head and chest circumference during the assessment of growth-related factors. It may also be used to measure findings such as the size of a skin lesion or mass. A cloth measuring tape covered with a light vinyl coating or a disposable paper tape that does not stretch should be used. Measurement in both inches and centimeters should be possible.

THERMOMETER

Thermometers for oral, rectal, and axillary measurements should be available and ready for use. The thermometer is used during the assessment of vital signs.

SPHYGMOMANOMETER

A blood pressure device and several sizes of cuffs for infants through adults are needed to determine blood pressure during the assessment of vital signs. Make sure that the sphygmomanometer has been appropriately maintained so that it is providing an accurate reading. The sphygmomanometer includes a cuff and a pressure valve. The cuffs come in a variety of sizes, and one of appropriate size should be selected for each patient. For adults, the width of the cuff should be about one third to one half the circumference of the arm or leg being used. In children, the cuff should cover approximately one half to two thirds of the upper arm or thigh.

OTOSCOPE

An otoscope with fresh batteries to provide a strong light and several sizes of specula are required for examining the ears and nose. The otoscope set also may include an ophthalmoscopic head for examination of the eye.

REFLEX HAMMER

A hammer with a flat side and a pointed side is required for the assessment of tendon reflexes during the neurologic examination.

STETHOSCOPE

A stethoscope with a bell and diaphragm should be available for use during assessment of the heart and lungs. The bell side is useful for picking up low-frequency sounds such as certain heart murmurs; the diaphragm side allows better transmission of higher pitched sounds such as those originating in the lungs. The ear pieces of the stethoscope should fit comfortably in the ear and be large enough to block out nonbody sounds.

SNELLEN VISUAL ACUITY CHART

Charts with appropriate symbols such as letters of the alphabet, the letter E turned to the sides and up and down, or nonletter figures of decreasing size from the top of the chart to the bottom are used to assess distance visual acuity. The patient is placed 20 feet from the chart in a well-lighted area.

NEAR-VISION CHARTS

A preprinted, specially designed card or even a page from a magazine may be used to assess near vision.

SHARP AND DULL IMPLEMENTS

A safety pin that can be opened to test sharp touch and closed to test dull touch should be included in the equipment list.

TONGUE BLADES

Wood tongue blades that are individually packaged or stored in a clean, covered container are need for examining the mouth or eliciting the gag reflex.

GLOVES

Gloves made of latex or other material in the event of latex allergy should be available for examination of the areas in which there might be contact with body fluids such as in the mouth and genital area.

VITAL SIGN ASSESSMENT

The basic signs of life—temperature, pulse, respiration, and blood pressure—are collectively termed *vital* (or *cardinal*) signs. Because of their value in evaluating health status, vital signs are assessed more routinely than any other single measure. For example, vital signs are usually assessed when the patient is admitted to a health care facility (hospital, office, clinic, nursing home). Some institutions have policies regarding routine monitoring of vital signs, requiring that they be taken at 8 A.M. and 6 P.M., whereas others depend on physician's and nurse's judgment about when vital signs should be monitored. Vital signs are always assessed before and after invasive procedures such as surgery and any intervention that could affect vital signs.

In today's increasingly cost-conscious health care environment, more and more guidelines and critical pathways will be written specifying when vital signs should be checked. Likewise, many patients (such as people with high blood pressure) will be expected to assess their own vital signs in between visits with their health care provider. The nurse must still exercise clinical judgment in determining when to assess vital signs more than the minimum required by guidelines. The nurse must always reflect on the significance of the data obtained or reported.

TEMPERATURE

Temperature is the degree of heat of a living body. It is controlled by balancing heat production and heat loss.

Physiology (Ganong, 1995; Guyton & Hall, 1996). Body temperature is regulated by the thermoregulatory center of the hypothalamus. Neurons in the hypothalamus function like a thermostat, sending out impulses to either conserve body heat or increase heat loss. Inputs to the neurons are provided by peripheral thermal receptors located in the skin and certain mucous membranes and central thermal receptors located in selected internal structures, such as the spinal cord and abdominal organs. As impulses affecting body temperature are received by the hypothalamus, control or thermostatic regulation processes begin.

Body heat is produced by

- Basic metabolic processes
- Specific dynamic action of food intake
- Muscular activity

Body heat is lost by

- Radiation (heat exchange between objects or substances that are not in contact)
- Conduction (heat exchange between objects or substances that are in contact)
- Vaporization of sweat
- Respiration
- Urination and defecation

Measurement. In most situations, nurses will be concerned with measurement of the surface or skin temperature. In healthy individuals, surface temperature rises and falls in relation to variables that affect heat production and loss. These variables include metabolism rate, age, sex, environment, and time of day. Daily fluctuations in temperature in a healthy person may be 1 to 2°F.

Using the traditional mercury-in-glass thermometer, surface body temperature can be measured:

- Orally by placing a thermometer under the patient's tongue with lips closed for 3 minutes. Oral temperature is usually 97.5 to 99.5°F.
- Via the axilla by placing the thermometer in the apex of the axilla with the arm pressed closely to the side of the body. When obtained this way, the temperature reading is usually 0.5 to 1°F below an oral measurement.
- Rectally by placing the thermometer into the anal canal to the depth of at least 1½ inches for 3 to 5 minutes. When obtained this way, the temperature reading is usually 0.5 to 1°F above an oral measurement.

Temperature can also be measured using one of the newer devices such as heat-sensitive tape or a tympanic thermometer; see Procedure 15–2.

In some situations, nurses will monitor core body temperature, the body's temperature in deep or internal structures. Core temperature is very stable and in health individuals usually does not vary by more than 1°F. It can be measured with a body temperature probe.

Technology. New devices for measuring temperature are replacing the mercury-in-glass thermometers. These new devices have the potential to reduce the amount of time required to obtain an accurate temperature reading, provide maximum patient comfort, and increase the reliability of the data obtained. Two such devices are the infrared ear thermometer and the chemical dot thermometer. Before using any new technology for measuring body temperature, the nurse must become familiar with the manufacturer's description of when and how to use the device.

Relevant Research. Early research on measuring body temperature compared the correlations among temperature recordings at oral, rectal, and axillary sites using mercury-in-glass thermometers. Research also focused on factors (such as drinking ice water) influencing oral temperature measurements. That research focus has been replaced by studies comparing the accuracy of different devices for measuring temperature (Brennan et al, 1995; Erickson et al, 1996; Erickson & Woo, 1994; Erickson & Yount, 1991; Flo & Brown, 1995; Hasel & Erickson, 1995; Yeo et al, 1995). When either core body temperature or the mercury-in-glass thermometer is used as the standard, tympanic thermometry and chemical dot thermometers produce valid data in some situations. For example, they work well for patients during the perioperative period but are not recommended for detection and management of fever in children.

Research beyond the studies conducted by manufacturers of these new devices is necessary to assist nurses in using them correctly. (See Chapter 5, Technology and Nursing Practice, for more details.)

Clinical Considerations. A body temperature above normal is called a *fever* or *pyrexia*. A temperature below normal is called *hypothermia*. The clinical significance of body temperature is shown graphically in Figure 15–7.

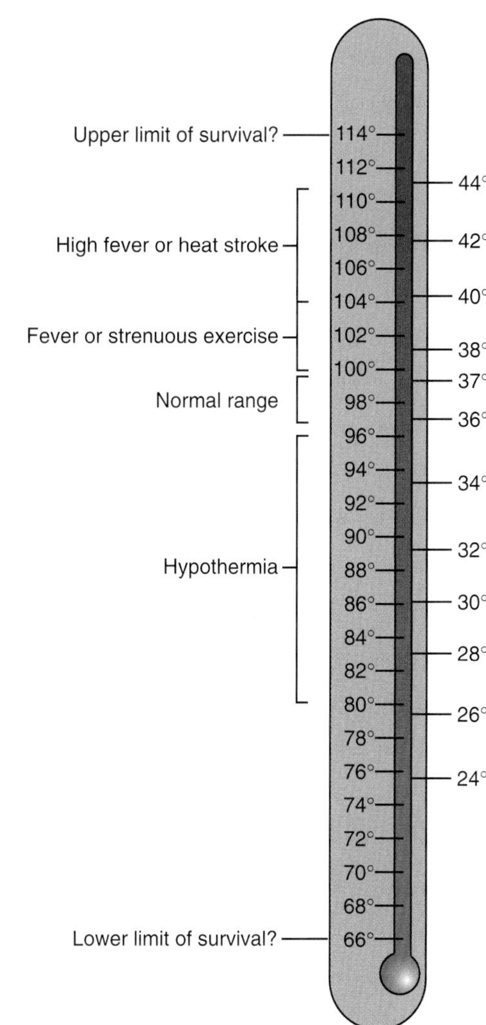

Figure 15–7. Clinical significance of changes in body temperature.

PULSE

Pulse is the throbbing caused by the alternate expansion and contraction of the artery as the fluid wave of blood rushes through it as a result of each heartbeat.

Physiology (Alcamo, 1996). As a result of the contraction and relaxation of the left ventricle of the heart, blood is pushed through the arteries, creating the pulse. The pulse is stronger near the heart and weaker further from the heart. The pulse is the same as the heart rate and averages 70 to 75 beats/minute in adults.

Measurement. The pulse rate is measured by palpating one of the body's pulse points (Fig. 15–8) and counting the total number of beats in 60 seconds. Common sites for assessing pulse include the radial artery of the wrist, carotid artery, and popliteal artery. Pulse rate can also be determined by counting the actual heart beats for 60 seconds during auscultation of the heart. Procedure 15–3 outlines the steps in assessing the pulse. The rate may be compared with that expected for various age groups, but it should be noted that the pulse rate decreases with age. Thus, a rate of 100 may be within normal limits for 2-month-old infant but not for a 30-year-old adult (Table 15–2).

Technology. In most circumstances, the nurse assesses the pulse without the aid of technology. Under some circumstances, a patient's pulse and other vital signs may be monitored with technology.

Relevant Research. Guidelines for heart rate measurement have been inadequately validated with supporting research. In one nursing study, Jones (1970) concluded that there was no advantage with normal and rapid pulse rates to counting for longer than 15 seconds. In fact, that investigator found that

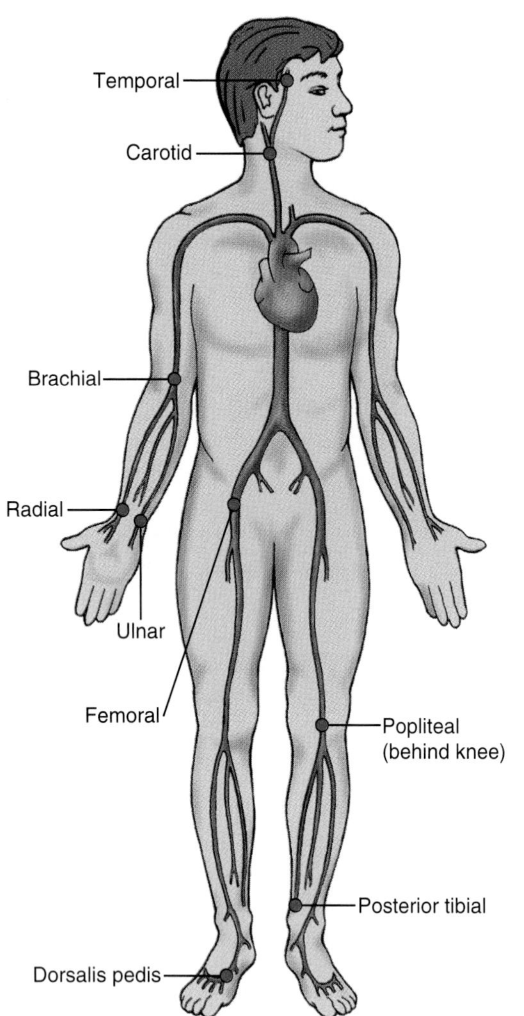

Figure 15-8. Peripheral pulses. (From Monahan, F.D., Neighbors, M. (1998). *Medical-Surgical Nursing: Foundations for Clinical Practice,* 2nd ed. Philadelphia: W.B. Saunders.)

counting for longer time periods (30 and 60 seconds) resulted in measurement errors. In a more recent study using recommendations from the earlier study, Hollerbach and Sneed (1990) concluded that the 30-second interval was the most accurate and efficient to use in counting the radial pulse. Furthermore, they recommend against using a 15-second interval for pulse rates faster than 100 beats/minute. Of note is another recommendation that the count begin with 0 rather than 1, particularly if a 15-second counting interval is used. Clearly, additional research is required before this aspect of practice can be based on standards generated from research.

Clinical Considerations. The nurse notes the rate, regularity, and strength of the pulse. A very rapid rate is called *tachycardia.* A slow rate is called *bradycardia.* The pulse may be regular or irregular and weak, normal, or strong. A weak pulse is associated with shock and is called *thready.* A strong pulse may be the result of exercise or emotion and be described as a pounding heart or heart palpations. A very strong pulse is associated with coronary disease such as aortic insufficiency.

Pulse rate is influenced by a range of factors. If the nurse notes that a patient's rate is either above or below normal for his or her age and sex, consideration should be given to the following:

- Exercise: the pulse rate usually increases during exercise
- Emotional response: emotions such as fear, anxiety, and stress tend to increase pulse rate
- Medications: specific medications may increase or decrease pulse rate
- Fever: the pulse rate increases during fever
- Hemorrhage: the pulse rate usually increases if there is hemorrhage

The assessment of a pulse rate outside the normal range is not complete until contributing factors are also assessed.

RESPIRATION

Respiration is the act of inhaling and exhaling, providing the lungs with oxygen and removing carbon dioxide.

Physiology (Alcamo, 1996). Breathing is the result of contractions of the respiratory muscles controlled by nerve stimulations. Respiratory control centers in the brain stem indirectly monitor carbon dioxide (a waste product from cell

TABLE 15-2 Age Group Norms for Pulse, Respiration, and Blood Pressure

Age	Pulse (beats/minute)	Respiration (breaths/minute)	Blood Pressure (mm Hg) Systolic*	Blood Pressure (mm Hg) Diastolic*
Newborn	120–170	30–80	66–72	55
1 year	80–160	20–40	90	56
3 years	80–120	20–30	92	56
6 years	75–115	16–22	95	56
10 years	70–110	16–20	100	62
18 and older	60–90	12–20	<130	<85
Elderly	60–90	16–20	<130	May increase

*50th percentile.

metabolism) levels in the blood. As the level increases in the arterial blood, the gas diffuses into the cerebrospinal fluid. The carbon dioxide gas causes a corresponding increase in the hydrogen ions in the fluid. The high level of hydrogen ions in the cerebrospinal fluid surrounding the respiratory centers results in activation of the center, sending impulses to the respiratory muscles. Those impulses increase the rate and depth of breathing. As carbon dioxide is released through the lungs, the hydrogen ion levels of the cerebrospinal fluid are reduced and the respiratory center is not activated.

Receptors for the respiratory system are located in other parts of the body as well. For example, chemical receptors located in the carotid artery and the arch of the aorta measure the dissolved oxygen content of the blood. When the oxygen level is low, signals are sent to the respiratory control center, again increasing the rate and depth of breathing.

The processes just described are involuntary mechanisms of respiration. These mechanisms can be partially overridden by nerve impulses originating in the cerebral cortex and passing to the respiratory control center. This voluntary control mechanism allows for holding one's breath while swimming under water, for example. With the build-up of hydrogen ions, however, this voluntary control mechanism can be overridden by the involuntary controls forcing one to breathe.

Measurement. Respirations are usually measured by direct observation of breathing for 60 seconds. The rate is the number of inhalation-exhalation cycles in 1 minute. Procedure 15–4 details the steps involved in assessing respiration.

Technology. Monitoring equipment can provide the nurse with data regarding respiratory rate.

Clinical Considerations. The nurse notes the rate, rhythm, and any other signs and symptoms (e.g., pain) associated with the patient's breathing. Various factors can influence breathing, such as exertion and emotion. Therefore, the nurse must assess a patient's breathing within this broader context.

Whether true or false, there is a widely held belief that directly watching a patient breathe will alter the rate of respiration. To count respirations in a less obvious way, the nurse may first take the radial pulse and then, while still maintaining fingers on the patient's wrist, count respirations. However, the most important outcome is that an accurate assessment of respirations is done. This may require the nurse to place a hand on the chest or abdomen.

BLOOD PRESSURE

Blood pressure is the tension exerted by blood against the arterial walls.

Physiology (Guyton & Hall, 1996; Thomas, 1997). The pressure in the vascular system rises and falls during each heartbeat cycle. It reaches its highest level when the heart pumps blood from the left ventricle; this pressure is called the *systolic pressure.* It reaches its lowest level when the heart muscle relaxes; this pressure is called the *diastolic pressure.* The actual blood pressure is determined by ventricular contraction, arteriolar and capillary resistance, elasticity of the arterial walls, and blood volume and viscosity.

The blood pressure reaches its highest level in the left ventricle during systole and then decreases in the arterial system as the distance from the heart increases. It is lower in capillaries than in arteries.

One's blood pressure varies over the course of the day, rising with activity or excitement and falling during sleep.

Measurement. Blood pressure is almost always measured in millimeters of mercury because of the long-standing acceptance of mercury manometer as the standard reference for measuring blood pressure.

Blood pressure can be measured directly or indirectly. Direct measurement is done by placing a sterile needle or small catheter inside an artery. The blood pressure is transmitted through that system to a recorder. Indirect (external) measurement is done by either auscultation or palpation. The most common method is auscultation using a sphygmomanometer and a stethoscope (see Procedure 15–5. The palpation method allows for determination of the systolic pressure only. It is determined by inflating the arm cuff (using all the same precautions as with the auscultation method), letting the pressure fall, and noting the pressure at which the radial pulse first becomes palpable. Measures obtained this way are usually 2 to 5 mm Hg lower than those obtained through auscultation.

The resulting measurement can then be compared with standard measurements of blood pressure by age.

Guidelines from the Fourth International Consensus Conference on Ambulatory Blood Pressure Monitoring include (Staessen et al, 1995) the following:

- Cuff size relative to arm circumference is an important determinant of the accuracy of noninvasive pressure measurements. The inflatable part of the blood pressure cuff, the bladder, should completely encircle the arm. If that is not possible, at least 80% of the arm should be encircled. This means that larger cuffs should be used for people with fatter arms and smaller cuffs used with children.
- The position of the arm in relation to the heart when the blood pressure is taken influences the pressure. Patients should be asked to keep their arm parallel to their trunk when the cuff is inflated.
- Short-term blood pressure variability is difficult to estimate. Noninvasive intermittent monitoring makes an accurate determination of blood pressure possible.

Technology. The technology for measuring blood pressure has changed very little. Measurements still are taken most frequently with the use of a sphygmomanometer and stethoscope.

Relevant Research. The effect of social factors on blood pressure has been investigated by researchers in fields other than nursing. The data produced show a relationship between race and hypertension. For example, severe hypertension is five to seven times more prevalent in blacks than whites in the

United States (Saunders, 1991). Hypotheses related to physiologic differences, sociologic differences, and reactivity to stress have been advanced to explain this relationship (Thomas and DeKeyser, 1996).

Social status has also been shown to affect blood pressure (Thomas and DeKeyser, 1996). For example, army recruits had higher blood pressures when they were taken by a captain versus a private (Reiser et al, 1958). It is possible that the well-documented "white coat hypertension"—higher blood pressures when measured by a physician in comparison to a nurse or technician—is a reflection of the effect of perceived authority status.

The methodology of blood pressure measurement has been the focus of several studies. In general, research supports the traditional site of measurement (upper arm), use of the bell as opposed to the diaphragm portion of the stethoscope, and differences in readings in the right and left arms (Norman et al, 1991; Thomas and DeKeyser, 1996). However, depending on the exact design of the study, different conclusions may be reached. One study using critical care patients, for example, found that using the diaphragm of the stethoscope over the brachial artery in the upper arm produced the most accurate readings (Byra-Cook et al, 1990).

Research on the effect of patient position on blood pressure has shown no significant differences between lying and sitting positions but significant differences between sitting and standing (Thomas and DeKeyser, 1996).

Clinical Considerations. A person cannot be diagnosed as hypertensive after a single blood pressure recording. The nurse must also assess various factors influencing blood pressure, including age, sex, altitude, muscular development, and mental and physical stress and fatigue. For example, when blood pressure is recorded during the first interaction or clinic visit, the patient's blood pressure may be temporarily elevated from anxiety. This is common enough that it is labeled "white coat effect" in reference to the white lab coat worn by health care providers. Also, talking while a recording is taken or drinking coffee or smoking a cigarette just before a recording is likely to raise the blood pressure. Taking the blood pressure after vigorous exercise may give a lower than usual reading. If the patient's blood pressure is abnormal for either the individual or in terms of established norms, the nurse should recheck the blood pressure after a suitable period of time.

GROWTH-RELATED ASSESSMENTS

The assessment of growth (also known as anthropometric measurement) occurs routinely throughout life but even more frequently during childhood and adolescence

HEIGHT

During the years before puberty, height or length is generally measured at regular intervals or at least every year. After growth is complete, measurements of height are not repeated on a regular basis unless there is a growth concern. Assessment of linear growth is particularly important in childhood and especially in infancy as an indicator of nutrition and health. Infant length is usually determined at least every 2 months in the first year of life and more often if there are growth concerns.

Standing height is measured in all those who are able to stand up and stand still at the measuring device, held in place firmly at a wall or other permanent location for a degree of reliability. In addition, many scales for the measurement of weight include a rod for measuring height. The headpiece should rest firmly on the top of the head in this case, or a firm tool such as a book or ruler should be used to rest on the top of the head to assist in the accurate measurement (Fig. 15–9).

For those who are unable to stand, a recumbent length may be used. Again, it is important to make sure that the head is held firmly in place while the legs are gently extended to determine full length.

Measurements determined to the nearest .25 inch or .5 cm should be recorded. For infants and children, this measurement should also be plotted on a growth grid to provide a comparison with other children of the same age and to evaluate growth patterns (Fig. 15–10).

WEIGHT

Measurement of weight is routine throughout the lifespan. In childhood, weight and height determinations should be made on the same schedule and on every visit in the first 2 years of life. In adulthood, weight is more likely to change than height and should be measured routinely at least every year.

A standard, recumbent scale that measures in pounds and ounces or in grams should be used for infants and should be

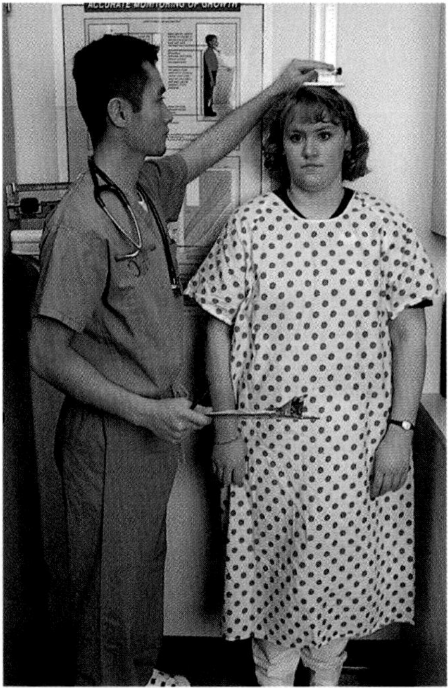

Figure 15–9. Measuring a patient's height.

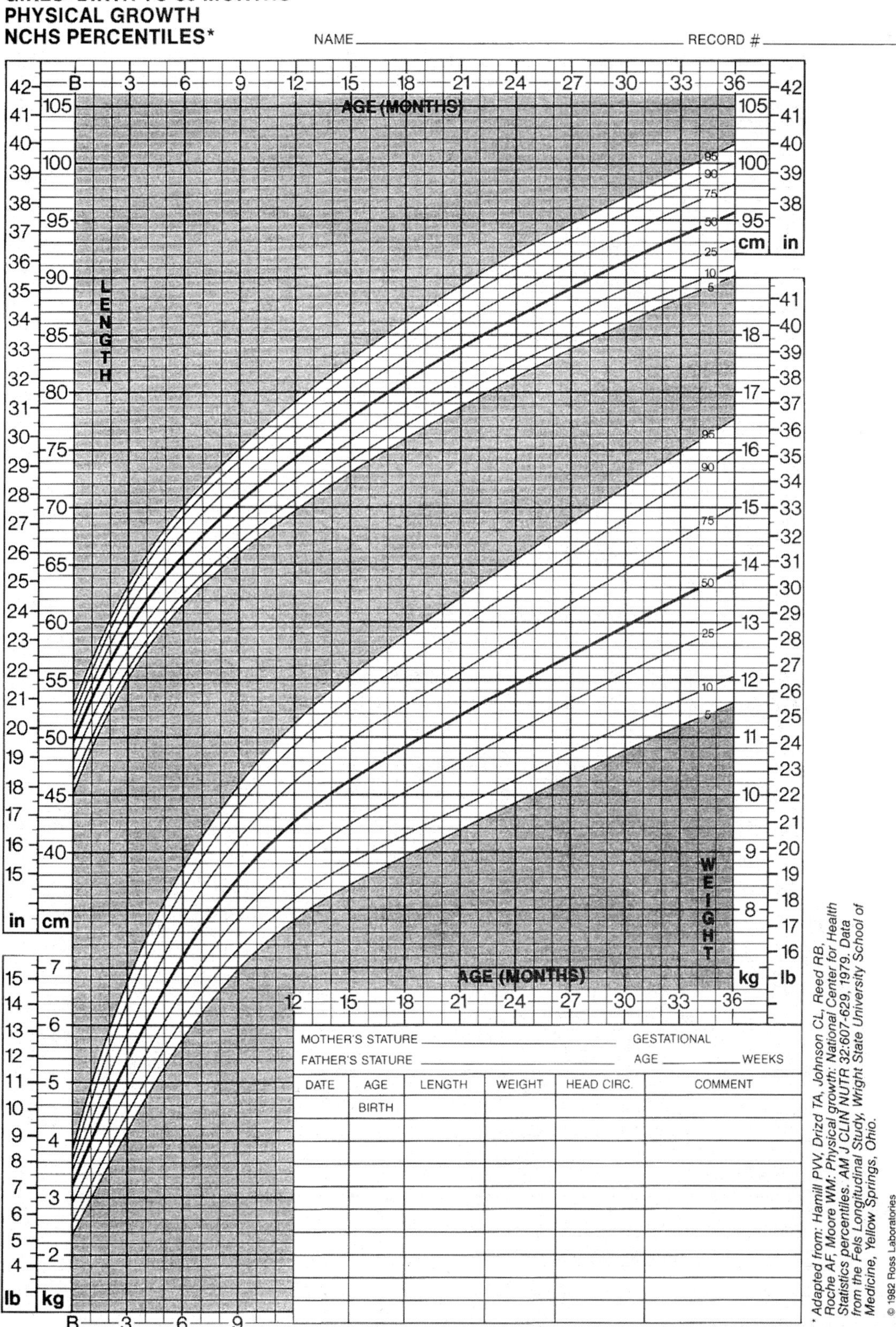

Figure 15-10. Sample pediatric height-weight chart. (Courtesy of Ross Laboratories.)

balanced daily or after heavy use. A standing scale in pounds or kilograms is sufficient for weight measurement in older children and adults. Procedure 15–6 details the steps to follow in weighing a patient.

Weights for children and adolescents younger than 18 years should be recorded on a standard growth grid for comparison with other children of the same age for visualization of growth trends and comparison of weight and height percentiles (see Fig. 15–17). Data for weight norms for adults of different heights and body types are available and should be used for comparison.

HEAD CIRCUMFERENCE

Head circumference measurements should be completed at every visit for the infant younger than 2 years. A measuring tape is used to take the measurement over the area of greatest circumference, from the occipital prominence to the bony ridge over the eyes (Fig. 15–11).

The measurement should be recorded to the nearest .125 inch or .25 cm and plotted on a growth grid. Comparison of the percentiles for the head circumference, height, and weight should be made to determine that the infant is growing appropriately and in a manner consistent with the determined norms.

OTHER GROWTH-RELATED MEASUREMENTS

Other growth-related measures that may be used in clinical practice, but less routinely, are not covered in this chapter. These measures include skinfold thickness measurement using specially calibrated calipers, assessment of gestational age in infants, and evaluation of sexual maturation using Tanner's stages. A standard textbook on physical assessment may be consulted if more information on these topics is desired.

BODY SYSTEM ASSESSMENT

The general approach to the complete physical exam or to a single system assessment should be calm, quiet, thorough, and organized. All of the equipment needed should be readily available, and the area should be free of distractions for both the patient and the nurse.

The patient should have no clothing to interfere with a thorough evaluation, but his or her modesty must be protected. Other methods to ensure comfort should be used as well, such as encouraging a young child to sit on a parent's lap during the examination.

A thorough explanation should be provided as the examination proceeds to help the patient understand what is being done. The nurse warns the patient of any anticipated pain or discomfort and verbally acknowledges normal findings.

Finally, the nurse should remain alert and keep the observational skills finely tuned. Any change in the patient's facial expression or movement that indicates worry, pain, or a question should be noted. Such observations should be followed up by asking pertinent questions and acknowledging awareness of a potential concern.

This section provides a brief overview of the process of objective assessment of each system. A complete physical evaluation is very complex and beyond the scope of this chapter. A textbook on anatomy and another dedicated to patient assessment are useful to the clinician performing thorough patient assessments routinely in the clinical setting.

The order in which the systems are reviewed or the order of the presentation of evaluation techniques within the system is not meant to convey a process for completion of the assessment. The nurse must remain flexible but always with a plan to ensure a thorough system assessment. For instance, the patient should not need to remove and replace the gown frequently. Completion of the portions of the assessment requiring removal of the covering from a particular area should be accomplished even if several different systems are evaluated. If the patient appears to be uncomfortable, the nurse should slow down and determine the cause of the discomfort before proceeding, perhaps to a less threatening part of the exam. Later, the nurse can return to complete the more troublesome areas for the patient.

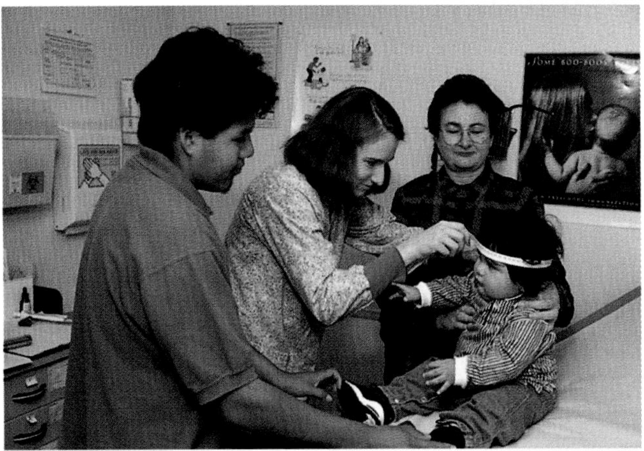

Figure 15-11. Measuring infant's head circumference.

SKIN

The skin provides a sensitive coating for the body and assists in temperature regulation, maintenance of body fluid balance, and protection from disease and injury. Techniques used in assessing the skin include inspection and palpation. First, the skin should be thoroughly inspected for color, consistency, cleanliness, and any lesions. Normal skin tones vary greatly from pale white to dark brown. A uniformity of color should be expected except in areas where darkening from sun exposure is common. Scars, stretch marks, dry patches, areas of hyperpigmentation or hypopigmentation, and skin lesions should be noted.

Palpation may be used to assess skin turgor, moistness, temperature, and texture. The presence of fluid or the height or depth of a lesion and the sensation in an area, such as pain or numbness, may also be determined by palpation. Normally,

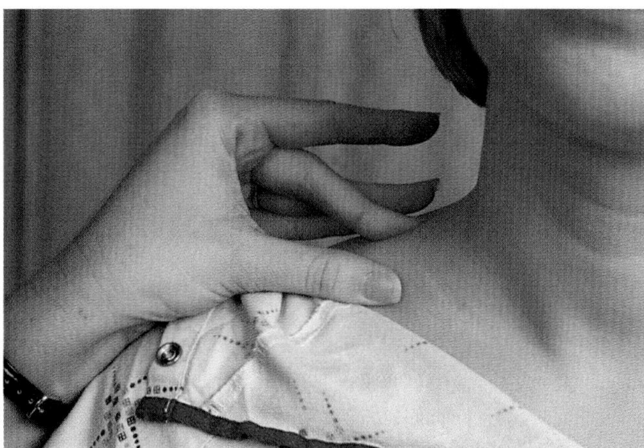

Figure 15-12. Assessing skin turgor.

the skin should feel smooth, cool to warm in temperature, and dry without much perspiration or oiliness. Turgor is assessed by pinching a small area of skin between the thumb and forefinger and then releasing (Fig. 15–12). Normally, the skin returns to normal position as soon as the skinfold is released. Abnormal turgor is present with edema or dehydration.

Finally, any lesions must be described by size (measured with a small tape), shape (e.g., round, oval, irregular) color, location, and distribution. Any pattern to the distribution, such as groups or lines of lesions, should also be noted.

HAIR AND NAILS

The techniques of inspection and palpation are also used in the assessment of the hair and nails. Inspection will reveal the color of the nails, nail beds, and hair. In addition, the texture of the nails should be noted. The smoothness of the nail edges and cuticles as well as the cleanliness are indications of individual hygiene. The uniformity of the shape and color should also be noted. The nail is normally smooth, rounded, and even in appearance.

The distribution of body hair varies greatly in the areas of the head, face, back, chest, arms, legs, and groin. Hair distribution as well as hair loss or damage should be noted. The texture and quantity of scalp hair may be evaluated by palpation, and the skin of the scalp may be revealed for closer inspection. Normally, a fine layer of hair covers the body with a thicker distribution of hair on the head and in the axilla and pubic area after puberty.

HEAD AND NECK

Assessment of the head and neck, including the eyes, ears, nose, mouth, and throat, provides an opportunity to evaluate the cranial nerves and the sensory nerves associated with vision, hearing, taste, and smell as well as an overview of this important area that provides protection for the brain. Assessment of the cranial nerves is discussed in other sections in which the particular function is found, such as the eyes or ears.

Facial symmetry should be noted during the inspection of the head. The patient's head should be held in an upright position, and the patient should be facing straight ahead to make this assessment easier and more accurate. In infants without head control, this exam is completed with the infant lying on his or her back.

The nurse observes the height and size of the eyes, position of the nose and cheeks, and movement of the mouth to check for asymmetry. Any change in the overall appearance of the face, such as puffiness around the eyes or lack of movement on one side of the mouth, is noted.

Asking the patient to swallow is an aspect of inspection of the neck. Any difficulties in swallowing or any change in posturing are noted. Also significant is any swelling, asymmetry, or webbing of the neck. The nurse asks the patient to move the head from right to left, bring the chin forward to touch the chest, tip the head back, and look from one side to the other to assess range of motion. Any pain or difficulty associated with these movements is noted.

Palpation of the head and neck includes feeling the scalp for asymmetries and noting hair loss or tenderness. In infants, the suture lines and fontanelles need to be identified. In particular, the anterior and posterior fontanelles should be measured from front to back and side to side. The measurements should be recorded until each has closed (i.e., the posterior at about 2 months and the anterior at approximately 24 months). Any bulging or depression of the fontanelles is also noted.

The position of the trachea is noted by palpating the neck. It should be felt in the midline of the neck and is easiest to feel in the lower one third of the neck. The thumbs may be brought from each side to "catch" the trachea between the fingers (Fig. 15–13).

The size and shape of the thyroid gland should also be determined. Standing behind or in front of the patient, the nurse palpates the neck for the thyroid (Fig. 15–14). Normally, the thyroid feels small, firm, and smooth and moves up with swallowing. An enlarged or painful thyroid gland requires further evaluation.

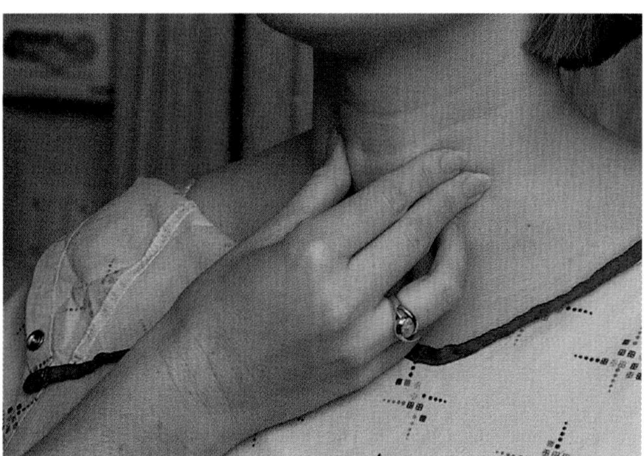

Figure 15-13. "Catching" the trachea.

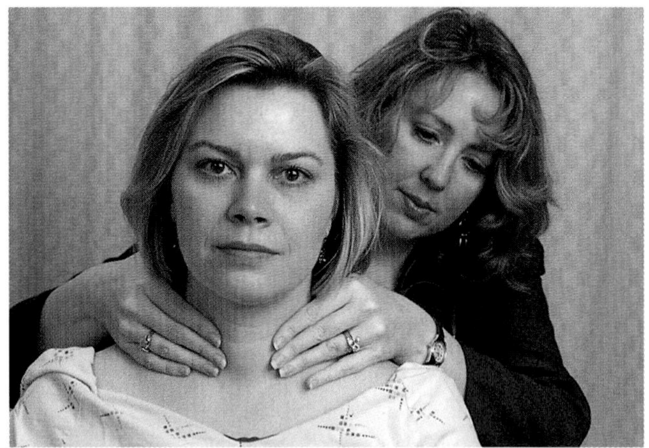

Figure 15–14. Technique for palpating the thyroid.

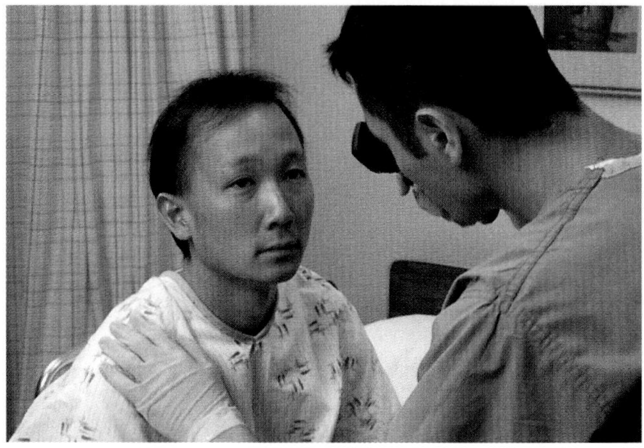

Figure 15–15. Using an ophthalmoscope to assess pupil position.

Eyes and Vision. An important aspect of assessing the eye includes screening for vision difficulties. Potential visual problems may be recognized not only by acuity testing but also by evaluating the performance of the muscles associated with eye movement. Initially, the eyes are inspected for symmetry in size, shape, and position. The patient is asked to open the eyes wide and then shut them tight. Any puffiness, eyelid drooping, excessive tearing, or impaired ability to open and close the eyes is noted. The lower lid is gently pulled down to reveal the palpebral (inside of the lower lid) conjunctiva, which is normally pink. Pale conjunctivae are associated with anemia.

The eyeball is inspected, and the color and shape of the iris and pupils are noted. The irides are normally the same color and the pupils the same size. A light is shined from the side of the patient's face across the eye to determine clarity of the cornea. The sclera is inspected and its color noted.

The pupils should be tested for response to light. The room is darkened so that the pupils will dilate to assist with this assessment. When a light is shined into one eye, both that pupil and the one in the other eye will constrict. This is called *direct* and *consensual pupillary response to light.* The pupils should also constrict in response to accommodation (the pupil becomes smaller as an object is brought from a distant point in the room to one closer). Completion of the exam of the pupil often results in the notation on the record of PERRLA (pupils equal, round, react to light and accommodation).

Next, the nurse instructs the patient to follow an object (the nurse's finger or a small toy for a child) from side to side, up and down, and in a crosswise pattern. The nurse observes for range of motion and symmetry of movement while testing the third (oculomotor), fourth (trochlear), and sixth (abducens) cranial nerves. Any jerky movements or lack of ability to sustain a certain gaze pattern is noted.

In addition to observing motion of the eyes, it is important to note the symmetry of the position of the pupil in the midline gaze. To do this, the nurse holds a light about 12 inches away from the patient's eye and directs it at the nasal bridge (Fig. 15–15). The light should be reflected from the same position on the pupil. In addition, the red light reflex should be observed. An apparent red light will shine through the pupillary opening in response to the light bouncing off of the retina. This is the same light often seen in the eyes of subjects in photographs. If the nurse does not see the red light or it is not round and symmetric, it may indicate an obstruction in front of the retina such as a cataract.

Equipment needed for the screening of vision (second cranial nerve, optic) for near and distance has been mentioned in the section on equipment. The patient is asked to look at a particular line on the appropriate chart and either read the letters or identify the symbols. If the patient cannot correctly identify at least half of the characters on the line, the nurse asks the patient to read the next line of larger figures. All persons older than 8 years should have distance vision of 20/20.

A thorough examination of the eye also includes an ophthalmoscopic evaluation. This examination requires a great deal of practice and is extremely tiring for the patient. The techniques to complete this exam are beyond the scope of this introduction to patient assessment.

The eyes should also be palpated for any swelling or lumps in the eyelids (both upper and lower) or extreme firmness of the eye itself. Gentle pressure on the eye should be able to be applied without causing pain and should result in slight movement of the globe into the orbital opening.

Ears and Hearing. The auditory system is important for both hearing and balance. Evaluation of these functions provides assessment of the seventh cranial nerve (acoustic nerve). Inspection begins with observing the external ear (auricle) for size, shape, and symmetry. Also, skin tags, deformities, and changes in color should be observed and recorded. The auricle should be about the same color as the rest of the facial skin. In addition, the placement of the attachment of the top portion of the auricle to the head should be noted to determine whether the ears are low-set. To make this determination, an imaginary line is drawn from one corner of the eye

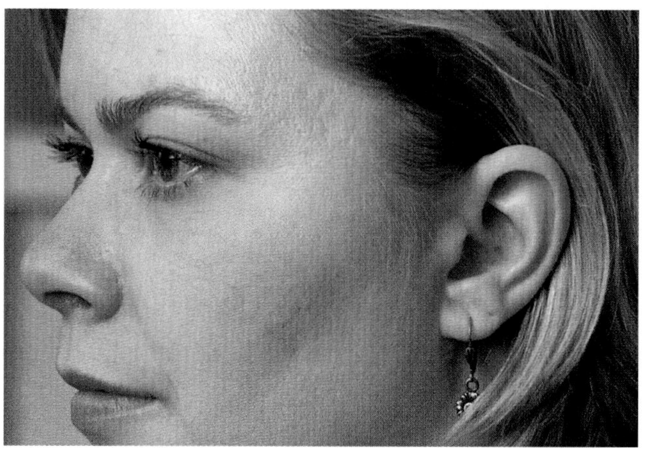

Figure 15-16. Normal ear position: aligned with an imaginary line extending from the corner of the eye to the occiput, and positioned within 10° of vertical.

through the other and continues on around to the auricular attachment. The attachment point should rest at or above the imaginary line (Fig. 15–16).

The auricles are palpated for any nodules or tenderness. The nurse also gently pulls up and out on the helix to check for discomfort.

Further inspection of the ear involves using the otoscope to assess the external auditory canal and middle ear (Fig. 15–17). The otoscope speculum comes in various sizes. The nurse selects the largest one that will fit comfortably in the patient's ear. The speculum helps provide adequate visualization of the tympanic membrane and canal; it is not intended to fit down into the auditory canal. A stream of light should be directed onto the tympanic membrane. Improper direction of the light results in an unclear image and the sensation that light is bouncing back at the nurse instead of providing a well-lighted surface.

Evaluation of hearing begins with listening to the patient speak and respond during the subjective interview. The patient should answer questions appropriately, follow directions, and not require frequent repetition of statements. Also, speech lacking in clarity or variation in tone may indicate hearing loss.

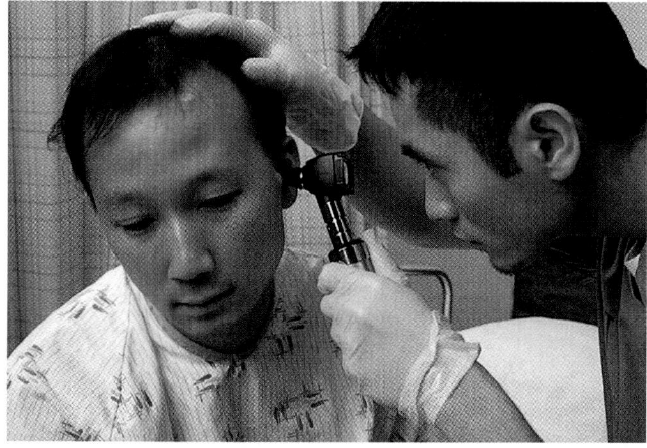

Figure 15-17. Otoscopic examination of the ear.

Further screening of hearing may be completed by using the whisper test and the ticking watch test. The whisper test may be administered by first having the patient put a finger in one ear and then having the nurse stand approximately 12 to 24 inches to the other side of the patient and whisper short words of one to two syllables. The patient is asked to repeat the words. The ticking watch test is administered by having the patient occlude hearing in one ear as in the whisper test. The nurse then holds a ticking watch approximately 6 inches from the nonoccluded ear. The watch is then slowly moved toward the ear, and the patient is asked to indicate when he or she hears the tick.

These somewhat crude screening maneuvers should be followed by a full audiometric evaluation using an audiometer to determine specific frequency (pitch) or intensity (loudness) changes if there is any concern during the screening or if the patient has a history of frequent ear infections, exposure to environmental hazards (from loud rock music to airplane engines), or hearing loss with aging.

Nose. Examination of the nose includes assessing the sense of smell (first cranial nerve, olfactory nerve) as well as the patency for breathing. The nose is inspected for any alterations in size, shape, or color. The nares should be somewhat oval and symmetric in shape. Any nasal discharge is noted and described (e.g., bloody, mucous, watery, clear). The patient is instructed to breathe in and out through one nostril at a time. Breathing should be easy and quiet.

Inspection of the nasal cavity may be completed by having the patient tip the head back lightly and by shining a light in. The nasal mucosa should appear pink and shiny. The nasal septum should be in the middle and straight from front to back.

Mouth. Evaluation of the mouth provides an opportunity to assess function related to chewing, swallowing, and taste. The patient's lips are inspected with the mouth closed in a comfortable position. Symmetry, color, and texture of the lips are observed. The lip surface should be smooth and pink.

The nurse then asks the patient to open the mouth and inspects the oral mucosa for any lesions or change in texture. Opening and clenching of the jaw are two motor functions of the fifth cranial nerve (trigeminal). The mucosa should be pinkish red, moist, and smooth. The gums are slightly more irregular in color and texture. However, the color is still pinkish except in dark-skinned patients, in whom patches of darker pigmentation may be seen. Any swelling or thickening of the gums is noted. The palate should be rounded and intact without clefts or other defects.

The receptors for taste lie in the tongue. Testing for taste by using standard sweet, sour, bitter, and salty solutions provide an assessment of some of the sensory aspects of the seventh and eighth cranial nerves (facial and glossopharyngeal nerves) but are not a routine part of the assessment. The tongue, which is normally moist and a dull pink color, is inspected for surface texture (smooth normally), asymmetry, and color changes. Palpation will reveal any nodules or lumps.

The patient's mouth is inspected for dental caries, tooth discoloration, and missing teeth. The teeth are counted, and their placement is noted. Infants begin tooth eruption by age 4 to 6 months, and for the first 2 years of life are expected to have approximately their age in months minus six teeth. Thus, a 2-year-old should have approximately 18 teeth. Shortly after the 2-year landmark, a toddler will have all 20 deciduous (baby) teeth. At maturity, a person is expected to have 28 to 32 permanent teeth depending on the eruption of the wisdom teeth. The gums below the teeth should be smooth, tight, and without inflammation or nodules. If the patient wears dentures, their fit is assessed by checking the bite and looking for a loose fit.

Throat. Inspection of the throat begins by noting placement of the uvula, which hangs down in the midline from the soft palate. The pink, shiny soft palate and the whitish, firm hard palate form the roof of the mouth. The soft palate should rise, and the uvula should remain in the midline as the patient vocalizes an "ah" sound. These maneuvers also test some functions of the ninth and tenth cranial nerves (glossopharyngeal and vagus).

The tonsils should be observed. The tonsils grow during early childhood (the preschool years) and then begin to involute (diminish in size after function has been fulfilled) when there is no infection or other problems. The tonsils should be about the same color as the rest of the pharynx and free from redness or white patches associated with infection. Even at their full size, the tonsils should not interfere with swallowing.

CHEST AND LUNGS

The chest and lung evaluation provides an opportunity to assess respiratory function. Inspection of the chest begins by having the patient expose the entire chest area. Anatomic landmarks should be used to guide the assessment process and notation of findings. These landmarks include the suprasternal notch, manubriosternal junction, clavicles, sternum, nipples, and xyphoid process (Fig. 15–18). In addition, the midclavicular line, midsternal line, scapular line, and vertebral line provide location clues to assist in describing findings (Fig. 15–19).

Chest shape and symmetry are evaluated from the front, the back, and the side. The distance from the front to the back is usually about half of the distance from one side to the other. The sternum should not protrude or recede into the chest. Observation of the chest as the patient breathes provides an opportunity to note any asymmetry of movement or difficulty breathing.

Palpation is used to note any tenderness or unusual movement as the patient breathes. During respiration, chest movement should be smooth and symmetric.

Percussion may be used to assess for any differences in sounds over the lungs. Two forms of percussion may be used: direct and indirect. With direct percussion, the fist is used. With indirect percussion, the technique involves striking one finger with another (see section on percussion). The lungs are normally resonant; any change, such as hyperresonance or dullness, may be suggestive of lung disease.

Auscultation of the lungs adds to the assessment database. With the patient sitting upright, the nurse places the diaphragm side of the stethoscope firmly on the skin over the area to be examined. There are listening areas over the posterior thorax (back), the anterior thorax (chest), and both lateral thoraces (sides). The patient is instructed to breathe in and out slowly through the mouth. The nurse moves the stethoscope from side to side to compare sounds from top to bottom as breath sounds are auscultated over each of the five lobes of the lungs. Procedure 15–7 details the steps involved in auscultating breath sounds.

Normal breath sounds are soft and smooth and are characterized as vesicular, bronchovesicular, or bronchial-tracheal. Vesicular sounds (low intensity and low pitched) are heard over most of the lung listening areas in healthy lungs. Bronchovesicular sounds (medium pitched and medium intensity) are heard over the main bronchi, whereas bronchial-tracheal sounds (high pitch and high intensity) are heard over the trachea.

By asking the patient to say common words such as names or numbers during auscultation, the nurse can assess the transmission of sound through the lungs (vocal resonance). Normally, these sounds are not distinct but may be increased or even decreased with lung conditions such as consolidation of the lungs or blockage of the respiratory tree.

Possible abnormal sounds originating in the lungs include crackles (caused by interruptions in the passage of air through small airways) that sound dry rather than moist. Crackles are usually heard during inspiration and are of short duration in each respiratory cycle. Wheezes may also be heard. They are continuous, high-pitched sounds heard during inspiration and expiration and are caused by rapid air movement through a limited airway.

HEART

With the patient lying supine, the nurse observes the chest for visible pulsations and looks for the apical pulse. In adults, it is often found at the fifth intercostal space along the left midclavicular line (an imaginary line drawn from the middle of the left clavicle down the chest). The apical pulse may not be visible in an obese or a heavily muscled patient. In a female patient, the breasts may also interfere with visualization.

The apical pulse should be located. In children, the apical pulse is usually easy to locate. In adults, it may be more difficult to find because of the thickness of the chest wall. The location at which the apical pulse is felt is called the *point of maximum intensity* (PMI).

Percussion may be practiced by locating the heart borders, although this technique is of limited assessment value. To practice this technique, one begins by percussing in the axilla and moving along the intercostal spaces toward the sternum.

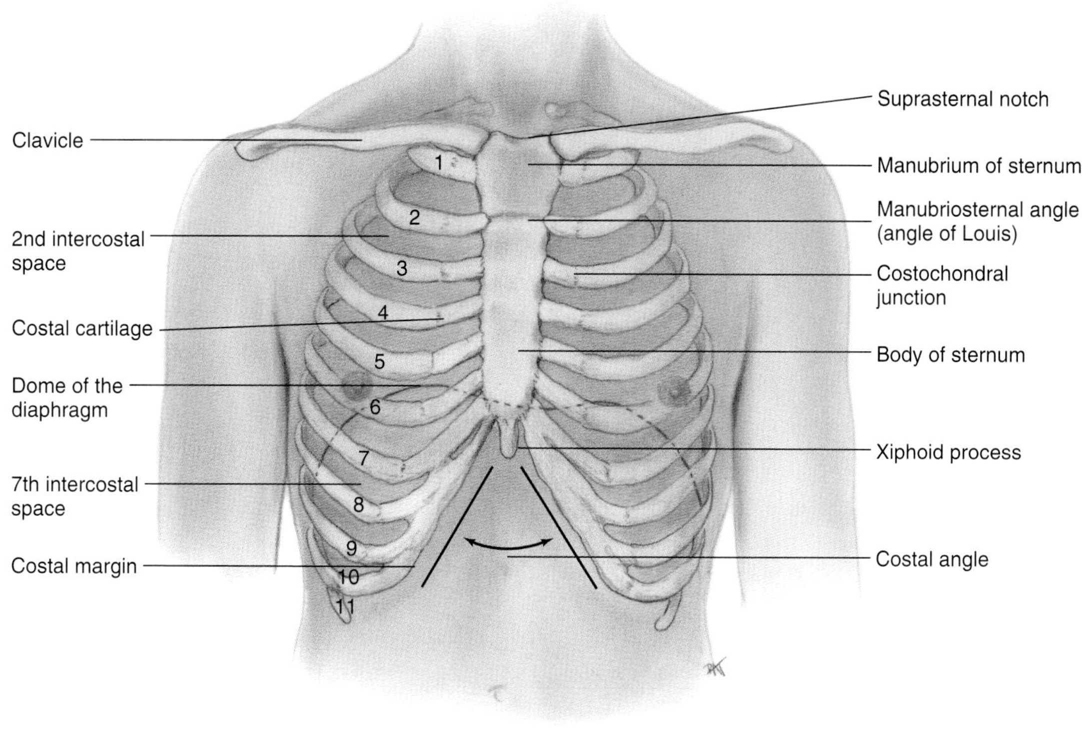

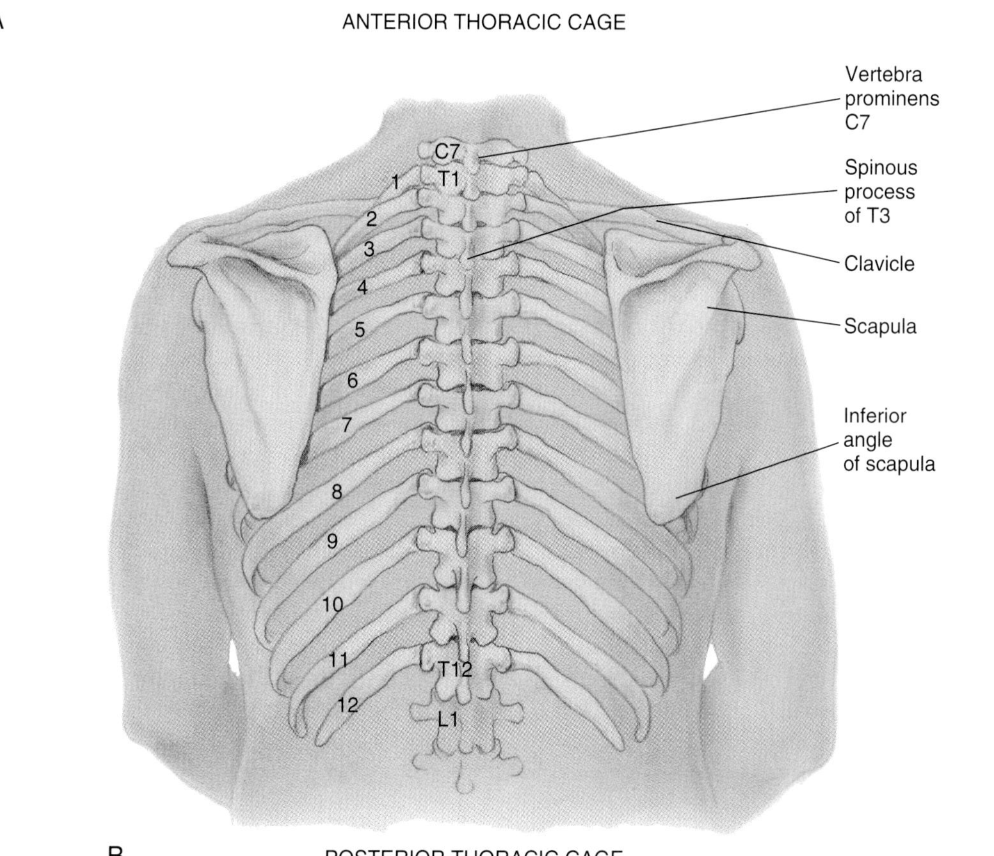

Figure 15-18. Thoracic landmarks. *A*, anterior; *B*, posterior. (From Jarvis, C. (1996). *Physical Examination and Health Assessment*, 2nd ed. Philadelphia: W.B. Saunders.)

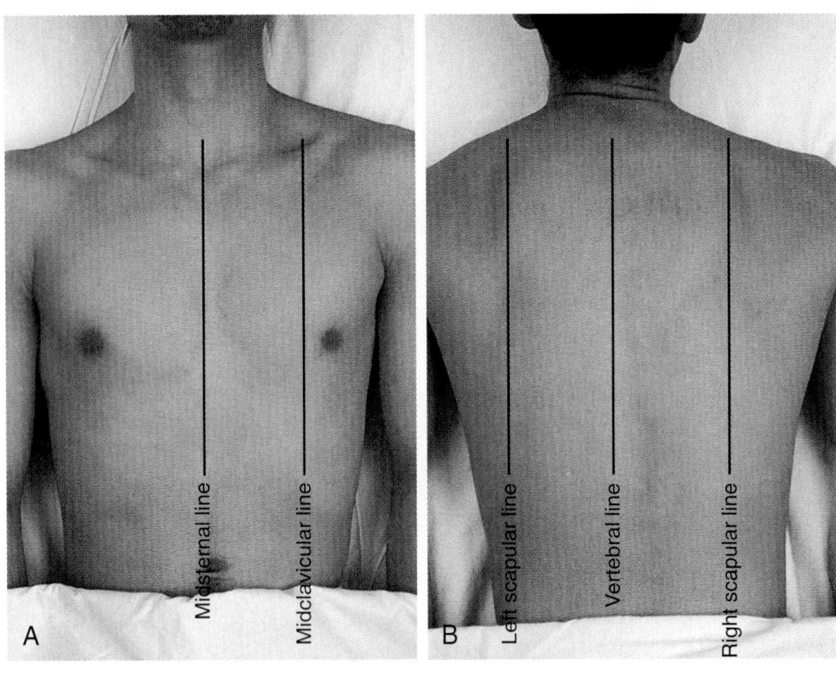

Figure 15-19. Thoracic reference lines. *A*, anterior; *B*, posterior.

On the right side, the first change in sound from resonance to dullness is usually not heard until the right sternal border. On the left side, the change is usually noted at the PMI.

Auscultation of the heart requires a quiet environment and an attentive examiner. The patient should be examined in both the lying and sitting positions. Five areas of the heart are auscultated:

- Aortic valve area at the right sternal border, second right intercostal space
- Pulmonic valve area at the left sternal border, second left intercostal space
- Second pulmonic area at the left sternal border, third left intercostal space
- Tricuspid area at the lower left sternal border, fourth left intercostal space
- Mitral area at the midclavicular line, fifth left intercostal space

The nurse auscultates each area, listening for heart rate and rhythm (Procedure 15–8). Heart rhythm should be regular and even, except in children, in whom a sinus arrhythmia is frequently heard. This normal finding, called a *sinus arrhythmia,* is heard as an increased heart rate with inspiration and a decreased rate with expiration. At any other time, an irregular heart rate or rhythm is not a normal finding. While auscultating the heart, the nurse must listen carefully and not rush. Developing a regular pattern for cardiac auscultation will help ensure thorough, accurate assessment.

Systole is the active phase of the heart cycle in which blood is pushed out of the left ventricle into the aorta and out of the right ventricle into the pulmonary artery. During diastole, the ventricles relax and receive blood from the contracting atria. The action of valve closure of the mitral and tricuspid valves at the beginning of systole and closure of the aortic and pulmonic valves at the end of systole are heard during auscultation as the "lub-dub" or S1 and S2 of the cardiac cycle. The relative loudness of the two sounds varies according to the area of auscultation (Table 15–3).

During auscultation, heart murmurs may be heard as extra sounds during systole or diastole. Murmurs are associated with abnormal flow of blood, valve abnormalities, or narrowing of the blood vessels. Murmurs should be described by their timing in the cardiac cycle (early, late, mid); their pitch (low, medium, high); their pattern (getting louder or softer or staying the same); their quality (musical, harsh, machinery like); the location where they are heard best; and finally the intensity or loudness. The intensity of murmurs are classified into six grades (Table 15–4).

The arterial pulses should also be palpated. The pulses routinely assessed from head to toe are the carotid, apical, brachial, radial, femoral, popliteal, dorsalis pedis, and posterior tibial (see Fig. 15–9). The other two—the dorsalis pedis

TABLE 15-3 Heart Sounds by Auscultation Area

Variable	Aortic	Pulmonic	Second Pulmonic	Mitral	Tricuspid
Intensity	$S_1 < S_2$	$S_1 < S_2$	$S_1 < S_2$	$S_1 > S_2$	$S_1 > S_2$
Duration	$S_1 > S_2$	$S_1 > S_2$	$S_1 > S_2$	$S_1 > S_2$	$S_1 > S_2$

TABLE 15-4 Heart Murmur Intensity: Grading System

Grade	Description
I	Barely discernible; change or disappear with change in position or exercise
II	Quiet but discernible in all positions and with exercise
III	Moderately loud; easily heard
IV	Loud, thrill present
V	Very loud may be heard with one edge of stethoscope off chest; thrill easily palpable
VI	Very loud, may be heard with stethoscope off chest, thrill palpable and visible

on the dorsal surface of the foot and the posterior tibial on the ankle by the medial malleolus—are not routinely assessed for rate but are assessed for presence and strength. The nurse uses the tips of the fingers (not the thumb) with gentle pressure to avoid occluding the pulse. Also the carotid pulse should be palpated on one side at a time only. Palpating both carotid pulses at the same time may cause the heart rate to slow (bradycardia), particularly in a patient with cardiovascular problems.

BREASTS

Breast tissue includes ligaments, muscle, subcutaneous fat, and blood vessels as well as mammary tissue, which is particularly important in the female reproductive cycle by providing optimum nutrition for infants. Inspection of the breasts in both men and women begins with the patient sitting in a relaxed position. The breasts are observed for symmetry, size, color, and any lesions. In men, breasts usually remain flat against the chest, although they may be fuller in obese males. The female breast is usually convex in shape, with one breast slightly larger than the other. The two nipples normally are about the same size and surrounded by pink to brown areolae, depending on skin color. There should be no nipple discharge unless the patient is lactating.

Assessment of the female breasts involves looking for supernumerary nipples along the embryonic ridge (an imaginary line running from the axilla through the nipple down to the groin). These are normal and may be accompanied by some mammary tissue. The areolae may not be smooth as a result of Montgomery tubercles, the remnants from the glands producing a lubricant and antibacterial solution during lactation. The nipples may be protuberant, flat, or inverted. A history of inverted nipples since childhood or adolescence supports this as a normal finding. However, a recent change in a nipple to inversion deserves further evaluation because it may be associated with internal changes in the breast tissue. It is important to note the type of nipple in prenatal care, because there are implications for breast-feeding that necessitate follow-up.

A thorough breast examination includes palpation. All quadrants of the breast should be checked for lumps or thickening. Light pressure followed by firmer pressure provide a basis for a thorough assessment. Any masses should be described, including size, shape, and consistency, and the patient referred for appropriate follow-up. It is possible for males to develop breast lesions and cancer; thus, any changes or lumps in the male breast should not be overlooked.

The female breast changes considerably throughout the life cycle. Before adolescence, the breast tissue does not appear particularly different from the surrounding tissue. Breast development begins as an early pubertal sign with the appearance of the breast bud and is considered complete when the areola recedes to a flat extension of the breast contour. The breasts undergo considerable changes associated with pregnancy and lactation to support the production of breast milk. Finally, there are changes in the menopausal years associated with the atrophy of some of the glandular tissue.

ABDOMEN

The abdominal examination provides an opportunity to assess vital organs associated with the digestive process. To promote thorough, systematic examination, the abdomen is typically divided into four regions (Fig. 15–20). The umbilicus is the central point through which the side-to-side and up and down imaginary line is drawn, one from the sternum to the pubis and the other across the abdomen.

Abdominal inspection begins by observing for any waves or tremors across the abdominal surface. Smooth movement should occur with each breath. Any lesions or scars and the color of the skin should also be noted. Normally, the skin of the abdomen is the same color as the rest of the body, but it may be paler if not exposed to sun on a regular basis. Note the placement of the umbilicus and whether it is slightly everted or inverted.

Auscultation of the abdomen is usually completed next to hear the bowel sounds before they might be changed by percussion. Using the diaphragm of the stethoscope, the nurse auscultates in the epigastric region (below the sternum and rib border) and in each of the four quadrants. Normal bowel sounds are irregular in occurrence (5–30 per minute) and sound like gurgling. The nurse must listen for at least 5 minutes before being able to determine that bowel sounds are absent. Increased bowel sounds are associated with hunger and gastrointestinal illness and decreased bowel sounds with paralytic ileus. Procedure 15–9 outlines the procedure for auscultating bowel sounds.

Percussion may be helpful in determining the size and density of the abdominal organs as well as in locating fluid, air, and masses. The nurse percusses all four quadrants and then percusses the liver, spleen, and stomach. The dull sounds heard on percussion over these organs helps determine their size and placement. Percussion, however, provides only an estimate of organ size.

Finally, palpation is completed. The nurse begins with light palpation in all four quadrants and progresses to medium and deep palpation. Any masses detected are described in terms of

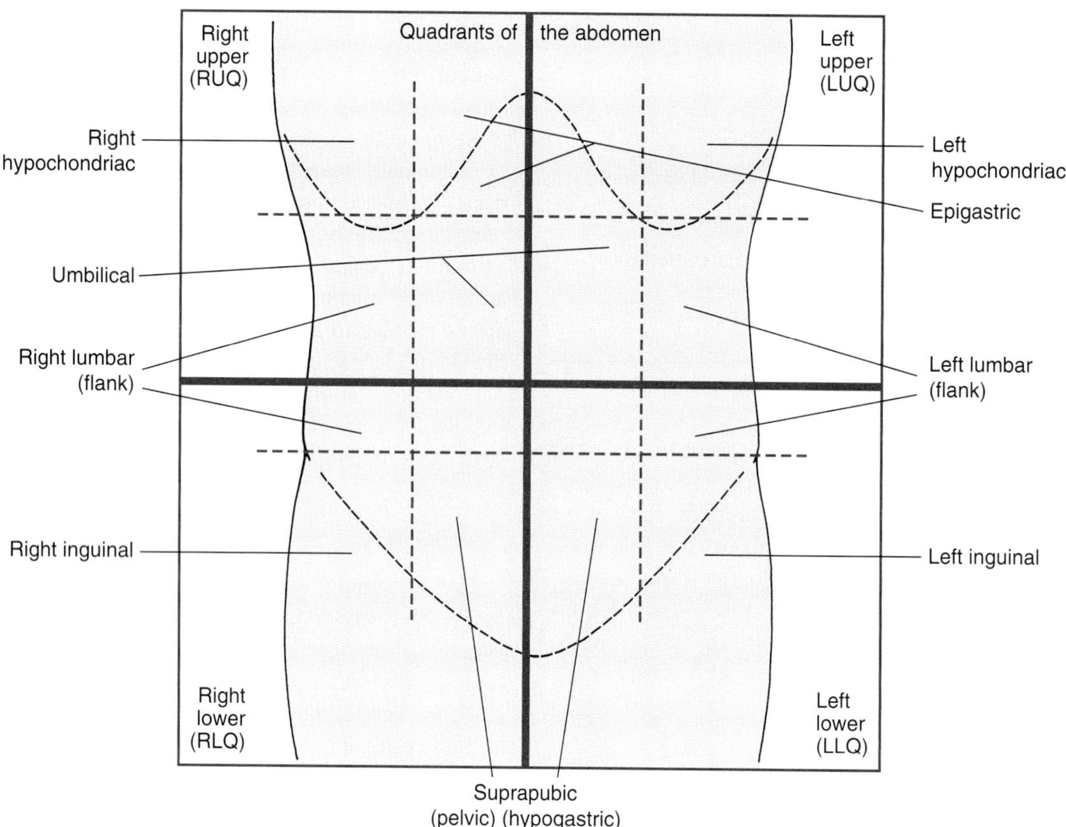

Figure 15-20. Abdominal quadrants. (From Black, J.M., Matassarin-Jacobs, E. (1997). *Medical-Surgical Nursing: Clinical Management for Continuity of Care,* 5th ed. Philadelphia: W.B. Saunders.)

their location, size, consistency, shape, and tenderness. The nurse also palpates around the umbilicus and notes whether the umbilical ring is closed. The ring is normally open in a child until 18 to 24 months of age and usually closes without any intervention. Nonclosure at any age increases the risk for an umbilical hernia.

The liver's edge may be identified at the right costal margin. However, it is usually only palpable in children or very thin adults. If it is felt, it should feel smooth, nontender, and firm. At the left costal margin, the nurse may palpate for the spleen. It should not be palpable, except in the newborn. Gentle palpation below the left costal margin is important so that an enlarged spleen is not overlooked. More information on examination of the spleen is included in the section on lymphatics.

GENITALIA

This very personal part of the assessment needs to be approached with concern for the patient's feelings. However, a thorough, but not time-consuming, exam is included as part of a routine examination. Gloves should be worn for both the male and female genitalia examinations.

Male. The patient may either lie down or stand for this exam. Inspection of the genitals begins with observation of the pubic hair. The hair is usually coarser and darker than that of the scalp and is distributed heavily in the pubic region. The hair then extends in a triangular pattern up to the umbilicus. The penis and scrotum are usually free of hair, although there may be a little hair on the scrotum.

The penis is inspected next. If the patient is not circumcised, the foreskin is gently retracted to reveal the glans. In a preschool-age child, the foreskin should never be forcibly retracted because it may tear the glans from the prepuce. Later, adhesions may result from this tearing.

The meatal opening of the urethra is inspected. It normally appears as a slit rather than a round opening. To visualize the opening, the nurse gently squeezes the head of the penis. The opening normally appears pink and shiny. The shaft of the penis is palpated for any discomfort, and any discharge is noted.

Inspection of the scrotum should reveal rough, slightly darker skin. The scrotum is normally asymmetric; the left testis hangs lower than the right one.

Palpation for a hernia should be completed. The patient should stand and bear down as if having a bowel movement. After inspection of the groin is completed, the patient should be instructed to relax and then once again bear down. The nurse should insert the index finger into the inguinal ring. If a hernia is present, a bulging against the finger is felt when the patient is asked to cough. Both sides should be examined because bilateral hernias are quite possible.

The testes are palpated to detect any tenderness or abnormal asymmetry. The testes are normally smooth and nontender to gentle palpation.

Female. For the purposes of this chapter, only the external examination of the female genitalia is discussed, because the vaginal examination and use of the speculum are beyond the knowledge base for a beginning student nurse. The nurse instructs the patient to lie supine and bring her knees up and then spread her legs. The patient should assume this position on her own; her legs should never be forced into any position.

Inspection begins by observing the distribution of pubic hair. It is usually coarser than other body hair. The mons pubis and the labia majora are then inspected. The skin should be smooth and free of redness or signs of irritation. The nurse then gently spreads the labia majora apart and inspects the labia minora, clitoris, urethral opening, and vaginal opening. These areas should be free of rashes, irritation, and swelling.

These area should be gently palpated for any lesions, swelling, or discomfort. The Bartholin glands may be palpated by placing the gloved index finger into the vaginal opening in the posterolateral area of labia majora and gently compressing between the thumb and index finger. While the finger is inserted, the patient should be asked to tighten the vaginal opening by bearing down. Patients who have not given birth can usually squeeze tightly without any loss of urine. Women who have given birth may not be able to produce as tight a response. Loss of urine or bulging of the anterior vaginal wall are associated with a cystocele and should be noted.

RECTUM AND ANUS

Examination of the gastrointestinal system includes assessment of the anus and rectum. Acknowledgment that this part of the examination is often embarrassing and even uncomfortable needs to be expressed to the patient. To visualize the area, the exam is usually performed with the patient lying on his or her back with the hips and knees flexed. Gloves should be worn throughout the assessment.

Inspection of the anal opening for fissures, skin tags, and signs of bleeding is routine. Additional light such as from a flashlight or penlight may be required to visualize the area. The nurse should ask the patient to bear down to make fissures or hemorrhoids more apparent.

In addition, a rectal examination may be performed on adults but not routinely on children. A rectal examination is performed in children when there is a history of a congenital abnormality or symptoms of rectal bleeding. To perform the rectal examination, the nurse should insert a gloved finger lubricated with a water-soluble lubricant into the anal opening. The patient should be prepared for the feeling of having a bowel movement and be reassured that is not going to happen. Ask the patient to bear down. The anal sphincter should tighten evenly around the finger. The examining finger can be inserted up to 2 to 4 inches into the rectum for palpation of the rectal walls.

The rectal exam may assist in the palpation of the cervix in females and the prostate in males. The prostate may be palpated on the anterior wall of the rectum and is about 1 to 2 inches in diameter. It should feel smooth and slightly movable. In females, the retroverted cervix may be palpated through the anterior wall of the rectum.

At the end of the rectal examination, the finger should be withdrawn slowly and any stool inspected for color and consistency. The stool should be brown and soft without any signs of blood or other secretions.

LYMPHATICS

The lymphatic system includes the lymph nodes, tonsils and adenoids, thymus, and spleen. Generally, the examination of the lymphatic system is completed as other relevant body systems in that area are assessed. For instance, the lymph nodes of the head and neck are inspected and palpated during that examination.

Lymph nodes may be palpable in the groin, axilla, and the entire region of the head and neck, including at the base of the occiput, in front of and behind the ears, at the jaw, and down the neck along the path of the sternocleidomastoid muscle, to mention just a few (Fig. 15–21). After inspecting each area for any noticeable swelling or redness, the areas should be palpated. In healthy adults, lymph nodes are usually not easily palpable. However, in children it is not uncommon to be able to palpate nodes associated with ear infections, sore throats, and even cuts of the extremities. Any palpable nodes should be described in terms of their size, mobility, tenderness, and consistency.

Lymph nodes that have not been found to be within normal limits are usually small (less than .25 inch), firm, and movable. When larger, fixed, or painful nodes are encountered, the area should be further evaluated for signs of infection or malignancy. For instance, Jeremy is likely to have enlarged lymph nodes in the area of the posterior auricular chain (behind the ear) associated with his ear infection, a normal and expected finding.

The spleen is examined as part of the abdominal assessment. The spleen is usually not palpable in adults; therefore, a palpable spleen is most likely enlarged. In infants younger than a few weeks, it may be possible to palpate the spleen just below the left costal margin. During the later months of infancy and the preschool years, the tip of the spleen may remain palpable in healthy children.

The tonsils and adenoids are assessed during the examination of the throat. Frequent infections in children often result in enlarged tonsils and adenoids, which are not a major problem unless the swelling interferes with swallowing or breathing. In adults, the tonsils may be difficult to visualize because they commonly have involuted.

MUSCULOSKELETAL

The musculoskeletal system consists of the bones, joints, muscles, tendons, ligaments, and cartilage. A thorough assessment of this system begins by watching the patient as he or she enters and moves around the room. Movements such as walking, sitting, gesturing, and bending provide clues as to the patient's musculoskeletal status. Keep in mind, however,

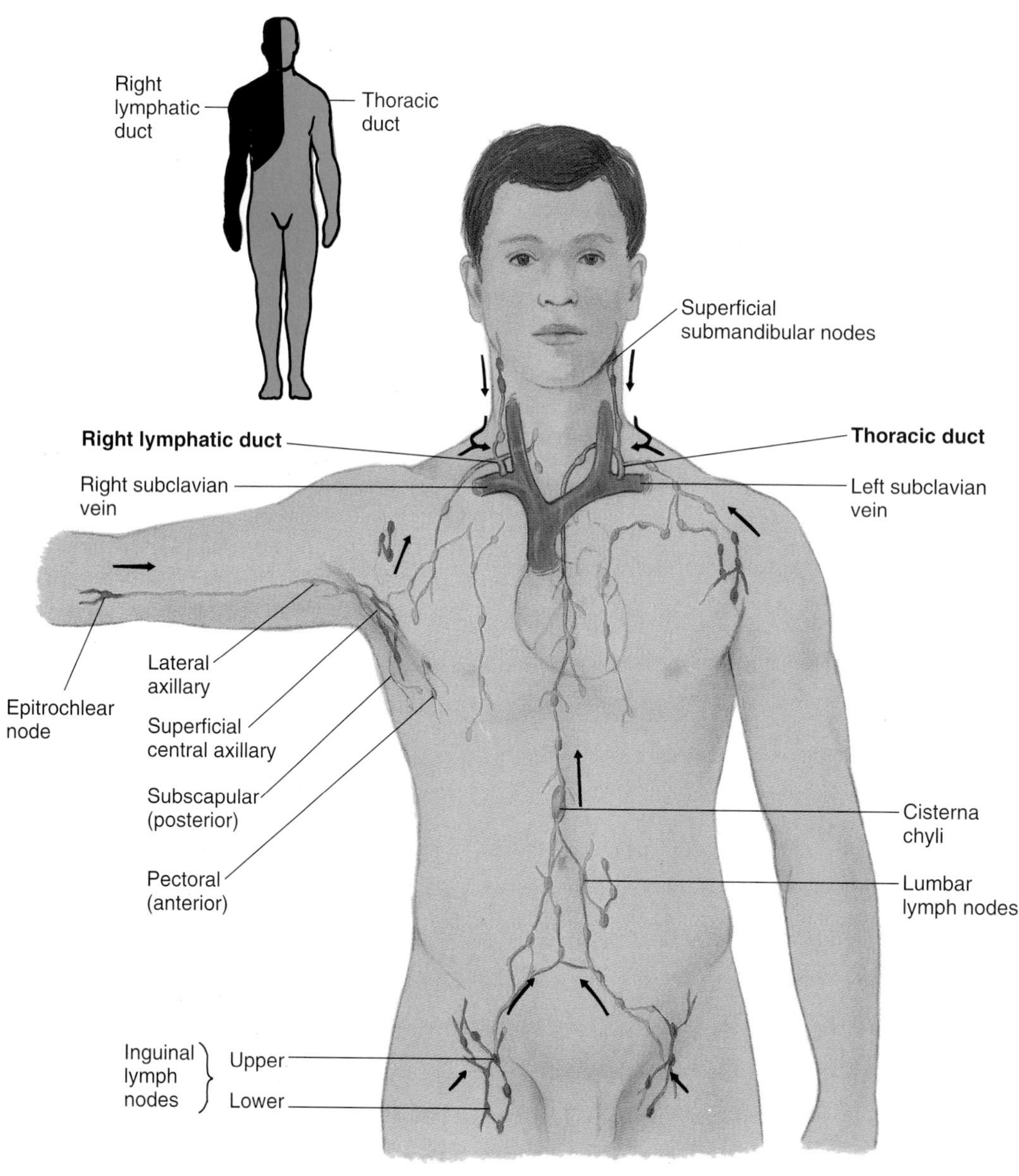

Figure 15–21. The lymphatic system. (From Jarvis, C. (1996). *Physical Examination and Health Assessment,* 2nd ed. Philadelphia: W.B. Saunders.)

that many neurologic problems also present with apparent musculoskeletal disruptions. For instance, a patient may limp as a result of a strain or sprain or the limp may be associated with nerve injury.

Inspection of the system includes noting any swelling or color changes in the areas overlying the bones and joints. Any differences in size or mobility of one side of the body versus the other should be noted. Symmetry in size, shape, and movement is expected. Inspection of the spine includes having the patient bend forward to touch the floor so that the straightness of the spine may be assessed (Fig. 15–22). Any asymmetry of the ribs or a lateral curvature of the spine is suggestive of scoliosis or lateral curvature of the spine.

The bones, muscles, and joints may be palpated for tenderness, warmth, swelling, or resistance to movement. Each joint should be moved through its range of motion and any asymmetry or pain noted. (See Chapter 20, Biomechanics and Mobility, for details on assessing range of motion.)

Muscle strength is assessed by having the patient flex a particular muscle, especially the larger muscles of the arms and legs. Then the nurse instructs the patient to resist the pull that is exerted in the opposite direction. Muscle strength is graded on a scale ranging from of 0 to 5, with 0 representing no resistance and 5 representing full resistance (Table 15–5). Normal muscle resistance should be equal from one side to the other and with full resistance.

When one suspects a difference in the length of an extremity or in the circumference of a part of it, the nurse should measure the area. Leg length is measured from the anterior iliac crest at the hip to the medial malleolus of the

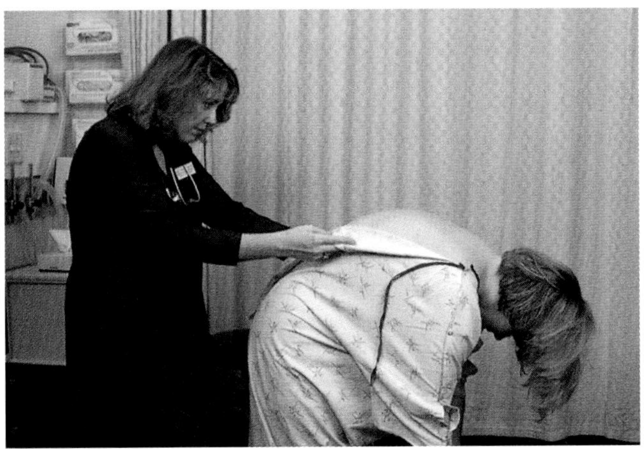

Figure 15-22. Assessing spinal curvature in the forward-bending position.

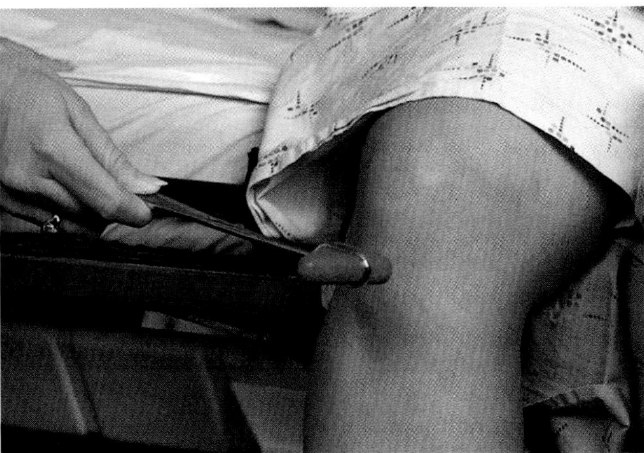

Figure 15-23. Assessing the patellar reflex.

ankle. Leg length measurements should be within .5 inch of one another.

Examination of the musculoskeletal system in infancy is particularly important to detect any congenital abnormalities such as extra digits or congenital dislocation of the hip. Screening for hip dislocation is performed by first inspecting the gluteal folds, flexing the hip and knees to 90°, and then abducting the hips as fully as possible. Normally, the gluteal folds should be equal in location and number, each hip should abduct to 80 to 90°, and the abduction should be equal from one side to the other.

NEUROLOGIC SYSTEM

Assessment of the neurologic system provides information on the system that controls all of the body's vital functions. This complex assessment includes activities to evaluate cognitive, sensory, motor, autonomic, and behavioral function.

Evaluation of the 12 cranial nerves is one aspect of the neurologic assessment. In previous sections, aspects of testing some of the functions of the cranial nerves have been mentioned. Table 15–6 reviews sensory and motor functions of all 12 cranial nerves.

Superficial and deep tendon reflexes may be elicited. Superficial reflexes are often evaluated, such as the abdominal (the umbilicus moves slightly in the direction of the abdominal quadrant stroked), cremasteric (the testicle and scrotum rise on the same side as the inner thigh that is stroked), plantar (plantar flexion of the big toe after the sole of the foot is stroked), and deep tendon reflexes, including the biceps, triceps, patellar, and Achilles. The special techniques required for each of the deep tendon reflexes are beyond the scope of a beginning nursing student. The technique for the patellar reflex is presented as an example of this part of the examination. The patient sits on the edge of the examining table with the legs dangling loosely at a 90° angle. Using the pointed end of a reflex hammer, the nurse strikes the patient's knee just below the patella (Fig. 15–23). A positive response is the extension (kicking out) of the lower leg.

Reflexes are graded on a system ranging from 0 (no response) to 4 (hyperactive or exaggerated response). The normally active response is graded as a 2 (Table 15–7).

Sensory functions are tested by having the patient respond to various stimuli, such as touch, pain, temperature, and vibration. The nurse notes any differences from one side to the other and the patient's ability to correctly interpret the stimulus and its location (Fig. 15–24).

Certain reflexes are present only in infancy. Reflexes such as the grasp (hand tightening on an object placed on the palm), Moro (startle), and stepping (a walking-like movement when

TABLE 15-5 Grading Muscle Strength

Grade	Level of Muscle Activity
0	No muscle activity
1	Slight muscle activity, no movement
2	Full passive range of motion
3	Full range of motion against gravity
4	Full range of motion with some resistance
5	Full range of motion with full resistance

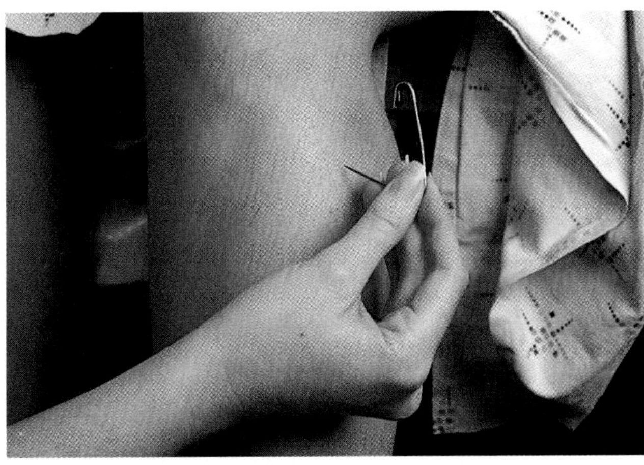

Figure 15-24. Assessing skin sensation with a pin.

TABLE 15-6 Cranial Nerves

Number	Name	Function
I	Olfactory	Sense of smell
II	Optic	Vision: acuity and visual fields
III	Oculomotor	Raise eyelids; eye movement of the inferior oblique
IV	Trochlear	Eye movements of the superior oblique muscles
V	Trigeminal	Jaw opening and tightening; chewing; sensation to the iris, cornea, eyelids, forehead, nose, tongue and
VI	Abducens	Eye movements of the lateral rectus muscles
VII	Facial	Facial expressions; taste in anterior two thirds of tongue
VIII	Acoustic	Sense of hearing and equilibrium
IX	Glossopharyngeal	Swallowing; sensation of gag, taste in posterior one third of tongue; secretion of salivary glands
X	Vagus	Voluntary muscles of phonation and swallowing
XI	Spinal accessory	Turn head; shrug shoulders
XII	Hypoglossal	Tongue movements for some speech sounds

the soles of an upright infant's feet touch a firm surface) are usually present at birth and disappear in the first 6 months of life. Presence of these primitive reflexes later in life is abnormal.

Coordination and fine motor skills are tested by instructing the patient to perform a series of activities. The nurse may instruct the patient to make rapid alternating movements such as patting the knees first with the palms and then with the back of the hand. The movements should be smooth and rhythmic. Other tests include having the patient walk by putting one foot directly in front of the other (heel to toe) and touch one finger of each hand to the nose with eyes closed. The nurse may also test balance by having the patient stand first on one foot and then the other with the arms held out straight in front of the body (Fig. 15–25).

MENTAL STATUS

Assessing a patient's mental status requires an awareness of the patient's cognitive abilities and emotional status. Thus, mental status evaluation occurs throughout the assessment process. The patient's responses to questions and his or her facial expressions provide insight into his or her awareness of the surroundings. The patient should be able to answer questions clearly and logically and should be able to talk about past and current events.

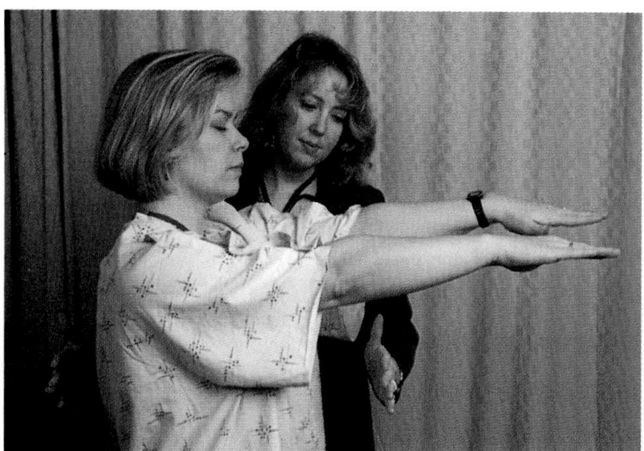

Figure 15-25. Assessing balance.

Specific areas that may be evaluated to assess cognitive abilities include level of consciousness, abstract reasoning, memory, and skills in mathematics and writing. Orientation to time and place are included in the assessment of level of consciousness. The patient should not demonstrate confusion or drowsiness. To test abstract reasoning, the nurse should ask the patient to explain a proverb or metaphor such as "a penny saved is a penny earned." Skills in math and reading may be tested by asking the patient to read a few lines from a book or magazine and to complete a problem involving addition or subtraction. Finally, short-term memory may be evaluated by asking the patient to repeat a series of 5 to 10 numbers after the nurse has said them. Long-term memory of events from the past have frequently been tested during the history-taking process.

Emotional stability may be assessed by noting the patient's mood, thought processes, and perception of events. Questions such as "How are you feeling?" or "What do you think caused this problem?" or comments by the patient regarding unrealistic fears provide evidence for assessment of these areas.

DEVELOPMENTAL ASSESSMENT

Development across the lifespan includes physical, cognitive, and psychosocial changes. Theorists such as Jean Piaget,

TABLE 15-7 Grading Deep Tendon Reflexes

Grade	Response
0	None
1+	Slow or diminished
2+	Normal response
3+	Brisk, slightly hyperactive
4+	Brisk, hyperactive; clonus may be present part of the time

Erik Erikson, Sigmund Freud, and Albert Bandura have addressed various aspects of development with theoretical perspectives that include cognitive, psychoanalytic, and psychosocial approaches.

In infancy and childhood, routine screening of development includes administering standard measures of development such as the Denver Developmental Screening Test (DDST) (Frankenburg et al, 1990) (Fig. 15–26). Areas of de-

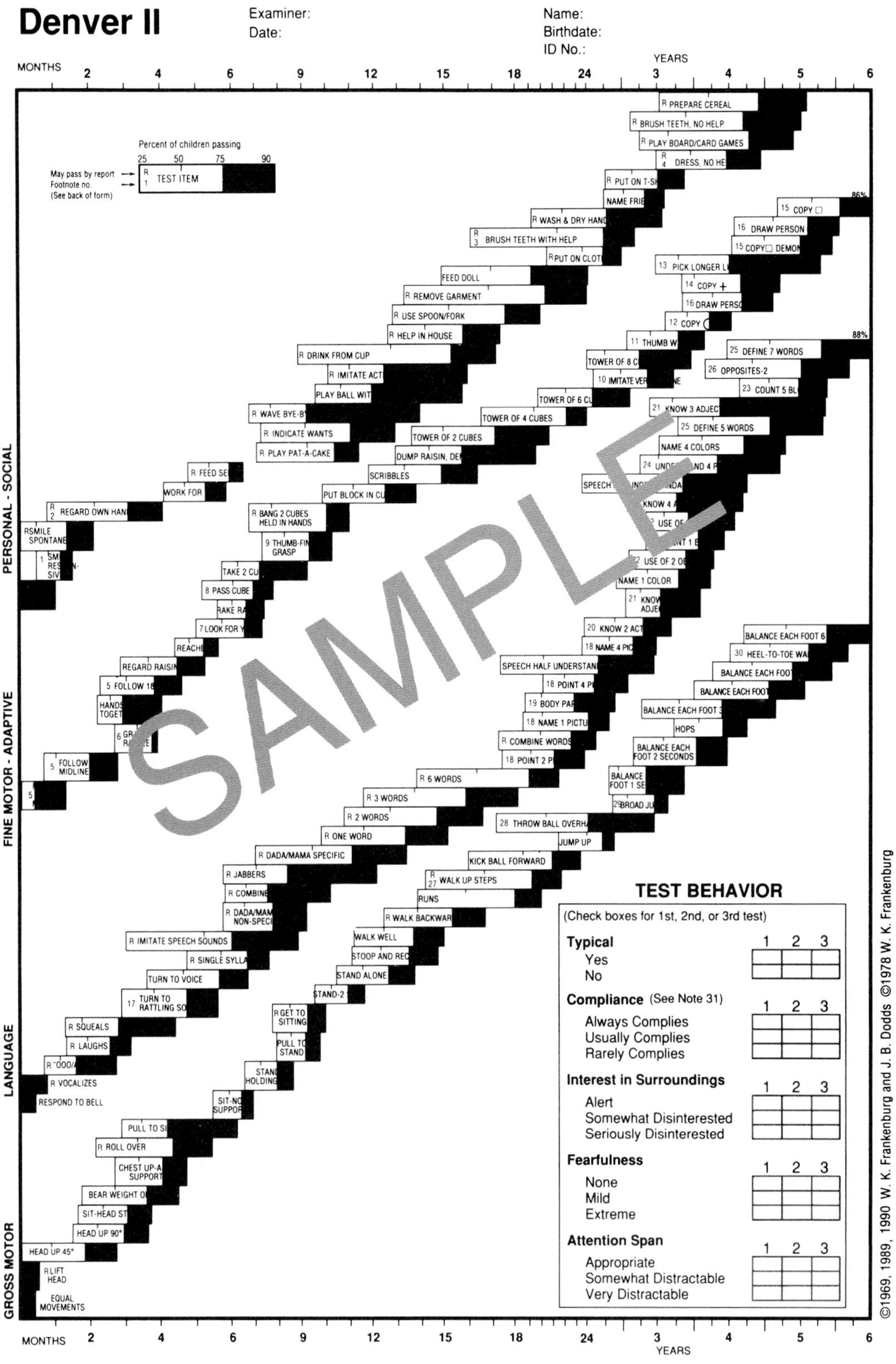

Figure 15–26. Denver Developmental Screening Test II score sheet. (Courtesy of W.K. Frankenburg.)

velopment that are frequently assessed include fine motor, gross motor, speech and language, and personal-social skills. Routine screening provides an opportunity for early detection and referral for developmental delays.

Few formal tools for developmental screening are available for adulthood. Nevertheless, developmental milestones should be evaluated in any complete assessment. Questions about finding a life partner, satisfaction in employment, success in parenting, relationships with friends and family, and ability to provide for oneself financially provide insight into the adult developmental progress.

VARIATIONS IN THE OBJECTIVE DATA COLLECTION PROCESS

INDIVIDUAL DIFFERENCES

Many differences based on age, gender, and race may be found in the objective assessment. Some of these have been noted in the sections on system assessment and measurements of vital signs. It is very important to keep these differences in mind to avoid an incorrect interpretation of findings. Infants have reflexes, such as Babinski's reflex, that are normally present, whereas such a finding in an adult would definitely not be normal. Infants with dark skin often have blue or black pigmented areas on the back or sacral area that may resemble bruising (mongolian spots) but are perfectly normal. The breast tissue of the adult female from puberty to lactation to involution changes markedly with age. The heart rate of preschool-age children may be characterized by an irregularity—sinus arrhythmia—that is not normally found in adolescence or adulthood. Changes occur in the skin with aging and may be noted to appear more transparent and dry with a less smooth texture and appearance. Visual acuity changes over the lifetime, from hyperopia (near-sighted) of the infant to presbyopia (loss of accommodation ability or increase in the distance to the near point of vision) in the aging adult. The body shape and distribution of fat varies with gender as well as age. All of these considerations must be included in a thoughtful approach to the objective assessment and determination of the significance of findings.

SETTING DIFFERENCES

Different settings provide a challenge to maintain privacy and modesty. Even in a private examination room, care must be taken to avoid the entrance of other staff or family members at an uncomfortable time. In a busy hospital room, the curtains need to be carefully drawn to maintain patient privacy. Permission of the patient should be sought before including others in the objective assessment process. Now the issue is not lack of willingness to talk as during the subjective process but may be lack of willingness to cooperate with parts of the examination during the objective process.

In the home the patient may be more comfortable, but a location with enough light and a comfortable place for both sitting and lying must be identified. The organization of the examination may be varied to take advantage of certain positions before moving the patient again.

The location of the exam within the setting is also important. For instance, infants or young children may be more cooperative if the exam is completed on a parent's lap, whereas older individuals may prefer that their spouse or significant other not be present during the examination or that at least they be on the other side of a curtain or screen.

DOCUMENTATION OF OBJECTIVE ASSESSMENT DATA

The findings from the objective assessment must be documented in the patient's record. The nurse should note both pertinent negative as well as positive findings and record all of the routine measurements that are performed. In some cases, these measurements need to be transferred to other forms (such as growth grids) to complete this aspect of documentation. Forms that address each area of the assessment may be available as authorized chart forms. If not, the nurse may need to write down each of the systems and keep notes for later transfer (in writing or by dictation) into the medical record. In either case, the form used may provide a reminder for the objective assessment so that no area is overlooked. Forms that allow a simple "examined" or "not examined" response to each system do not provide adequate documentation of the findings. There should always be room for additional notes, and the space should routinely be used to note findings specific to the individual patient. Common abbreviations are used in this process, and with experience the nurse will become familiar with these abbreviations and use them in documentation.

ETHICAL ISSUES IN PATIENT ASSESSMENT

Privacy

Patients have a right to privacy. The first priority for privacy is to ensure a quiet and not easily interrupted location for the assessment. The patient needs to feel confident that no one will walk in at an awkward or embarrassing moment. They need reassurance that what they say will not be overheard by other patients or health care workers.

The second aspect of privacy is to ensure that there is no opportunity for others to learn or overhear aspects of the patient's history or physical exam if it is not relevant to them. Although some findings from the assessment may be discussed with others on the health care team, it must be done in a private location. Conversations in a public hallway or on the elevators are not appropriate.

Finally, any written information needs to be processed and stored in such a way as to prevent noninvolved individuals from reviewing it. Charts and progress notes as well as records of assessment findings need to be kept out of public view and handled with a concern for the rights of privacy.

Confidentiality

Frequently, a patient may discuss very private and personal thoughts and behaviors. In addition, some of the findings from the assessment may reveal conditions that are potentially embarrassing to the patient. The patient may request that this information not be shared with anyone. If the information is not relevant to the patient's health and well-being, there generally is no reason to make note of it in the written and verbal notations. However, if the findings do have a bearing on the patient's care, some of the information most likely will be shared with other relevant members of the health care team. The necessity for communicating relevant findings must be explained to the patient. False reassurances must not be given. At the same time, however, a recognition of the patient's rights to a degree of confidentiality must be maintained. It is appropriate to solicit consent from the patient to discuss the matter with family members or consultants who have not previously been involved in the patient's care. With the increasing use of computer records or files in multiple locations, including the job or school site, the need to pay increased attention to patient's rights of confidentiality must be addressed.

FUTURE DEVELOPMENTS

In the immediate future, assessment practices will be influenced by two major change drivers: technology development and computer-assisted diagnosis. One example of technology development is the *palpometer* (Bendtsen et al, 1994). Manual palpation is an important method for evaluating tender myofascial tissues. Yet the method lacks reliability because palpation pressure is quite subjective. What one nurse considers mild pressure may be considered strong by another. The palpometer allows measurement of pressure exerted during palpation. It is a thin pressure-sensitive plastic device attached to the palpating finger with a scale recording the pressure exerted. This enables quantification of the pressure and the ability to replicate the examination to determine reliability of findings.

Another illustration of the influence of technology on assessment is the availability of self-diagnostic kits. Probably the most commonly advertised is the self-diagnostic pregnancy test. The health care futurists predict self-diagnostic technologies will become a routine part of the health care system. It has proven to be an excellent market for investors.

The computer is being used as an adjunct to clinical decision making and diagnosis. One example is the use of the computer to assist in the diagnosis of acute appendicitis in patients older than 50 years (Eskelinen et al, 1995). Clinicians have found it is difficult to correctly diagnosis acute appendicitis in people in this age group because of the influence of age and the presence of other diseases. Only one third of those with acute appendicitis have the typical history of initial pain. Using clinical data and mathematical techniques, researchers have been able to develop a computer-based diagnostic scoring system that works well in comparison to clinical judgment alone. This diagnostic system as well as others like it need further development and testing to determine their ultimate value in the assessment process.

Telemedicine, using computer-assisted technologies, is another rapidly developing field. A health care provider hundreds of miles away can visualize assessment data and assist with diagnosis and treatment plans.

However assessment is done today, tomorrow it will be performed using even greater technology.

PROCEDURE 15-1

Preparing the Environment for Objective Assessment

Objective

Prepare environment to facilitate patient comfort and safety during assessment process.

Terminology

- **Inspection:** visual examination of qualities or indicators that can be seen by the eye
- **Palpation:** examination of the body using the fingers or hand to detect physical characteristics of tissues or organs
- **Percussion:** tapping of body parts with the fingers to determine size, position, and density of underlying organs
- **Auscultation:** listening to sounds produced within the body by various organs

Critical Elements

Physical assessment is usually performed using a head-to-toe methodology but may vary in relationship to the patient's condition, age, and time elements.

A thorough explanation should be given to the patient before a physical examination, including the primary techniques of inspection, palpation, percussion, and auscultation.

continued on next page

PROCEDURE 15-1 (cont'd)

Patient privacy is an important element to consider when performing a physical assessment and should be maintained during the entire process.

Equipment

- Paper and pen
- Sphygmomanometer with appropriate size cuff
- Stethoscope
- Watch with second hand
- Thermometer
- Scale
- Measuring tape
- Otoscope
- Reflex hammer
- Vision charts
- Safety pin
- Alcohol swabs
- Drape

Special Considerations

Equipment selection should be appropriate to the patient and the scope of the assessment.

The patient should be positioned for safety and comfort during the examination.

Nursing Interventions

Action	*Rationale*
1. Identify patient.	1. Ensures correct patient
2. Explain to patient that you will be performing a physical assessment.	2. Provides information related to length of examination and elements contained within the examination
3. Request that patient empty his or her bladder.	3. Enhances ability to perform a successful abdominal examination
4. Gather and prepare equipment.	4. Provides organized work area
5. Assess room temperature, and provide a comfortable environment.	5. Promotes patient comfort
6. Minimize noise level in room.	6. Provides for a quiet environment for percussion and auscultation
7. Provide adequate lighting.	7. Promotes visualization during examination
8. Assist patient into examining gown and provide drape.	8. Provides privacy
9. Position patient for physical assessment based on the type of assessment being performed.	9. Provides positioning that will enhance the assessment process
10. Perform the physical assessment using assessment tools and equipment.	10. Provides data for documentation and care planning
11. Assist patient to a comfortable position after the examination.	11. Promotes patient comfort
12. Return or discard equipment as necessary.	12. Promotes a clean, organized work space

Documentation

Record pertinent findings in the patient record, including all objective and subjective findings.

Elements of Patient Teaching

Explain procedure and findings to patient and family as appropriate.

PROCEDURE 15-2

Assessing Temperature

Objective

Complete an accurate assessment of patient's body temperature.

Terminology

- **Nonfebrile (afebrile):** oral temperature within the normal range of 97–99.5°F or 36–37.5°C
- **Febrile:** body temperature exceeding the normal range
- **Hypothermia:** body temperature below the normal range

Critical Elements

Observe the patient for signs of an abnormal temperature, such as increased sweating, shivering, or flushing.

Measurement of oral temperature using a mercury thermometer for young children, infants, confused or unconscious patients, mouth breathers, or patients who are seizure prone is contraindicated.

Equipment

- Thermometer (mercury glass, digital electronic, tympanic, or chemical dot)
- Disposable probe cover or sheath
- Water-soluble lubricant (for rectal temperature)
- Watch (if indicated by type of thermometer used)
- Alcohol wipe

Special Considerations

Body temperature is a measurement of the balance between heat produced and heat lost and is useful in assessing a variety of clinical problems, such as infectious processes and fluid imbalances.

The type of thermometer and route of measurement appropriate for the patient's age and condition must be selected.

Temperature should not be taken if the patient has ingested liquids or smoked during the previous 15 minutes.

Rectal temperatures are usually 1°F (0.6°C) higher than oral temperature. Axillary temperatures are usually 1–2° lower than oral temperatures.

Follow the manufacturer's instructions for temperature measurement and time requirements when using a tympanic or electronic thermometer.

Nursing Interventions

Action	*Rationale*
1. Select the desired method of temperature measurement.	1. Ensures the most accurate measurement of temperature
2. Identify the patient.	2. Provides patient safety
3. Explain the procedure to the patient.	3. Promotes patient compliance
4. Assist patient to a comfortable position.	4. Provides for a safe and comfortable measurement time

Oral: Glass Thermometer

1. Read thermometer and ensure that mercury indicator is at its lowest point. If necessary, hold thermometer and snap wrist several times to reduce mercury reading to this point.	1. Provides consistent baseline for beginning measurement
2. Place thermometer under the patient's tongue and instruct patient to close mouth. Leave thermometer in place for at least 2 minutes.	2. Ensures accurate placement and time to register
3. Remove thermometer and wipe with an alcohol wipe.	3. Provides a clear view of mercury column for reading
4. Read the thermometer at eye level.	4. Provides optimal position for viewing temperature reading
5. Wash thermometer with soap and warm water and return to appropriate storage area.	5. Provides clean and organized environment

continued on next page

PROCEDURE 15-2 (cont'd)

Oral: Electronic Thermometer

1. Remove oral metal probe from unit and insert into disposable probe cover.
   1. Protects thermometer from transmission of organisms
2. Place covered probe under the tongue in posterior sublingual pocket of patient's mouth (Fig. 15–27).
   2. Ensures accurate placement of thermometer
3. Hold thermometer in place until auditory signal indicates final reading.
   3. Assists patient with correct placement during measurement process
4. Remove thermometer, and read temperature from digital display.
   4. Provides reading for documentation
5. Discard probe cover, and replace electronic thermometer in charger.
   5. Provides clean and organized work environment

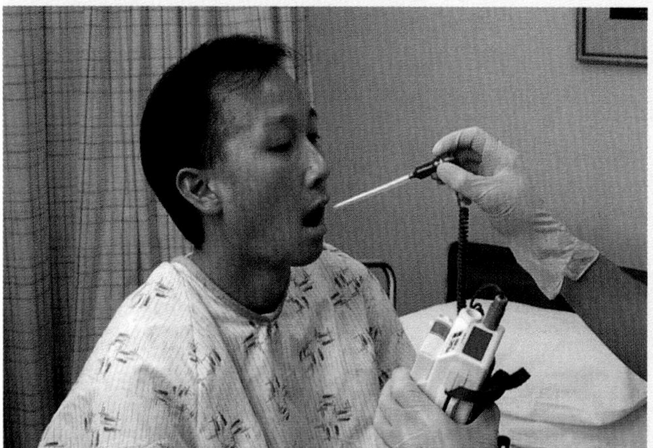

Figure 15–27. Taking temperature with a digital thermometer.

Rectal: Glass Thermometer

1. Read thermometer, and ensure that mercury indicator is at its lowest point. If necessary, hold thermometer and snap wrist several times to reduce mercury reading to this point.
   1. Provides consistent baseline for beginning measurement
2. Assist the patient into a side-lying (Sims') position.
   2. Facilitates placement of thermometer
3. Provide adequate lighting and privacy.
   3. Provides light source for thermometer insertion
4. Don gloves.
   4. Provides protection for nurse
5. Lubricate tip of thermometer.
   5. Promotes ease of insertion into the rectum
6. Raise the upper buttock.
   6. Allows for visualization of the anus
7. Insert thermometer gently into rectum 1–1½ inches.
   7. Promotes safe thermometer placement
8. Hold thermometer in place for 3 minutes.
   8. Promotes accurate temperature reading
9. Remove thermometer, and wipe with an alcohol wipe.
   9. Provides a clear view of mercury column for reading
10. Read the thermometer at eye level.
    10. Provides optimal position for viewing temperature reading
11. Wash thermometer with soap and warm water, and return to appropriate storage area.
    11. Provides clean and organized environment

PROCEDURE 15-2 (cont'd)

Rectal: Electronic Thermometer

Action	Rationale
1. Assist the patient into a side-lying (Sims') position.	1. Facilitates placement of thermometer
2. Provide adequate lighting and privacy.	2. Provides light source for thermometer insertion
3. Don gloves.	3. Provides protection for nurse
4. Remove rectal metal probe from unit and insert into disposable probe cover.	4. Protects thermometer from transmission of organisms
5. Lubricate tip of thermometer.	5. Promotes ease of insertion into the rectum
6. Raise the upper buttock.	6. Allows for visualization of the anus
7. Insert thermometer gently into rectum 1–1½ inches.	7. Promotes safe thermometer placement
8. Hold thermometer in place until auditory signal indicates final reading.	8. Assists with correct placement during measurement process
9. Remove thermometer and read temperature from digital display.	9. Provides reading for documentation
10. Discard probe cover, and replace electronic thermometer in charger.	10. Provides clean and organized work environment

Axillary: Glass Thermometer

Follow the steps for Oral: Glass Thermometer with the following exceptions:

Action	Rationale
1. Place thermometer in center of axilla with arm against chest side wall.	1. Provides maximum environment for temperature measurement
2. Hold thermometer in place for 10 minutes.	2. Promotes accurate temperature reading

Axillary: Electronic Thermometer

Follow the steps for Oral: Electronic Thermometer with the following exceptions:

Action	Rationale
1. Place thermometer in center of axilla with arm against chest side wall.	1. Provides maximum environment for temperature measurement

Documentation

Record the temperature reading and route of measurement in the patient record.

Elements of Patient Teaching

Instruct patient and family regarding the procedure and any resulting actions related to the temperature reading

PROCEDURE 15-3

Assessing Pulse

Objective

Complete an accurate assessment of patient's pulse rate, rhythm, and quality.

Terminology

- **Apical:** a point on the chest wall at approximately the midclavicular line and between the fifth and sixth ribs.
- **Radial artery:** area in forearm, wrist, and hand used for taking the pulse
- **Carotid artery:** area in neck used for taking the pulse

continued on next page

PROCEDURE 15-3 (cont'd)

- **Brachial artery:** area in antecubital space used for taking the pulse
- **Femoral artery:** area in groin used for taking the pulse
- **Popliteal artery:** area in back of knee used for taking the pulse
- **Dorsalis pedis artery:** area on the top of the foot used for taking the pulse
- **Post-tibial artery:** area in back of ankle used for taking the pulse

Critical Elements

Assess patient or review history for any influences on pulse rate such as activity level, stress, and medications taken.

Rate, rhythm, and quality should be assessed when taking a pulse. For accuracy, a pulse should be assessed for 1 minute. An apical pulse should be taken for patients who are critically ill, who have cardiovascular disease, or who are taking cardiovascular medications.

Equipment

- Watch with second indicator
- Stethoscope

Special Considerations

Report irregular, slow, or rapid heart rate to appropriate staff or physician. A variety of disease processes may cause pulse irregularities or dysrhythmias.

Nursing Interventions

Action	*Rationale*
1. Identify patient.	1. Provides patient safety
2. Explain procedure.	2. Promotes patient compliance
3. Select appropriate site, and remove clothing to expose location.	3. Ensures most accurate measurement of pulse
Radial Pulse	
1. Support patient's arm in comfortable position at heart level with wrist slightly extended.	1. Promotes patient comfort during procedure
2. Place two fingers (index and middle) over surface of wrist just inside the radius and gently palpate pulse.	2. Allows optimal access to radial groove
3. Assess for pulse and begin counting for 60 seconds, assessing rate, rhythm, and quality (Fig. 15–28).	3. Promotes accurate assessment
Apical Pulse	
1. Clean diaphragm of stethoscope with alcohol.	1. Reduces risk of transferring organisms from one patient to another
2. Assist patient to a comfortable position, and expose left side of chest using drapes.	2. Promotes patient comfort and privacy
3. Place diaphragm of stethoscope over apex of heart on left side of chest.	3. Positions stethoscope in optimal area of chest for auscultation of heartbeat
4. Auscultate and count pulse for 60 seconds assessing rate, rhythm, and quality (Fig. 15–29).	4. Promotes accurate assessment
5. Assist patient to a comfortable position.	5. Promotes patient comfort

PROCEDURE 15-3 (cont'd)

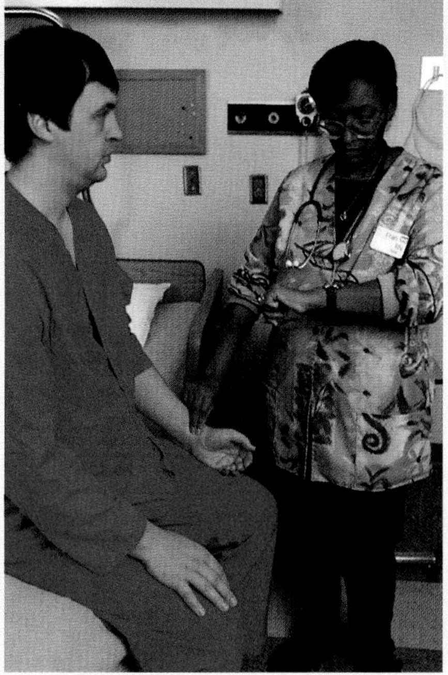

Figure 15–28. Assessing radial pulse.

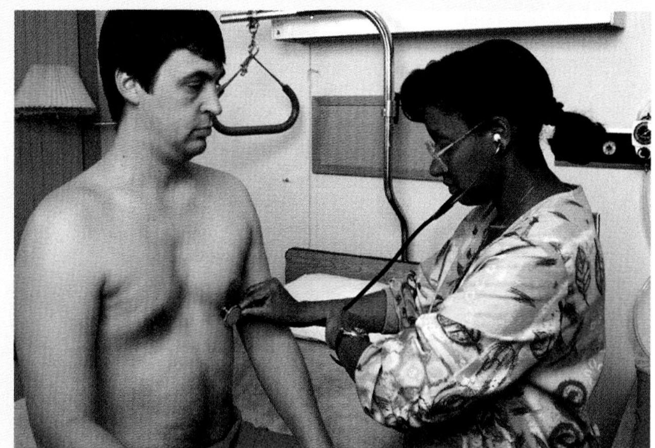

Figure 15–29. Assessing apical pulse.

Documentation

Record pulse rate, rhythm, and quality in the patient record.

Elements of Patient Teaching

Instruct patient and family regarding the procedure and any resulting actions related to the pulse assessment.

PROCEDURE 15-4

Assessing Respiration

Objective

Assess rate, rhythm, depth, and quality of patient's respirations.

Terminology

- **Normal respirations:** effortless, regular, quiet inspiration and expiration of breathing
- **Accessory muscles:** scalene, trapezius, and sternocleidomastoid muscles; often used in respiratory distress
- **Retractions:** visible inward pull on intercostal or sternal areas; seen with increased respiratory effort associated with atelectasis
- **Stertorous:** noisy respirations due to partial respiratory obstruction

Critical Elements

Place fingers on radial pulse so patient is less aware that respirations are being counted; count respirations for a full minute.

Equipment

Stethoscope and watch with second indicator are needed.

continued on next page

PROCEDURE 15-3 (cont'd)

Special Considerations

Respiratory rate may be affected by a variety of clinical conditions such as respiratory and cardiovascular disease, metabolic disorders, fluid and acid-base imbalances, trauma, medications, infection, neurologic disorders, and anxiety. Assessing respirations will frequently be done along with auscultation of breath sounds.

Nursing Interventions

Action	*Rationale*
1. Identify patient.	1. Promotes safety
2. Explain procedure.	2. Promotes cooperation
3. Wash hands.	3. Reduces risk of transmission of organisms from one patient to another
4. Count respirations just before or just after counting pulse while still holding fingers on patient's radial pulse (Fig. 15–30).	4. Allows nurse to count respirations without patient being aware

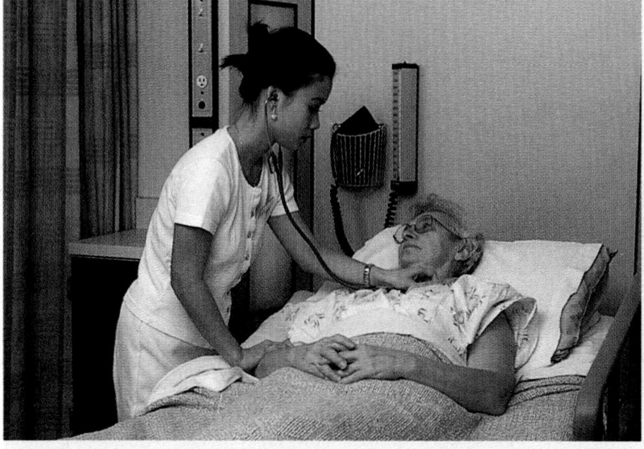

Figure 15–30. Assessing respiratory rate.

5. Assess respirations for rate, rhythm, depth, and quality; note presence of any retractions or use of accessory muscles in respiratory effort.	5. Abnormal rate, rhythm, depth, or quality indicative of possible respiratory problem
6. Note shape of chest and ribs.	6. Asymmetry may lead to respiratory problems
7. Auscultate breath sounds if indicated.	7. Abnormal finding may indicate a need for further assessment
8. Wash hands.	8. Reduces risk of transmission of organisms from one patient to another

Documentation

Document respiratory assessment on patient record; note presence of any oxygen, oxygen equipment, and position of patient in bed during assessment.

Elements of Patient Teaching

Instruct patient to notify nurse immediately if he/she experiences any difficulty breathing.

PROCEDURE 15-5

Assessing Blood Pressure

Objective

Accurate measurement of patients blood pressure

Terminology

- **Normotensive:** blood pressure in the normal range for age and gender
- **Hypertension:** blood pressure that exceeds normal range
- **Hypotension:** blood pressure below normal range
- **Korotkoff sounds:** sounds heard while taking the blood pressure

Critical Elements

Medications as well as smoking, caffeine, physical activity, stress, and environmental factors may affect blood pressure and should be considered in relation to blood pressure readings.

To promote consistent blood pressure assessment, readings should be taken on the same arm with the patient in the same position.

Blood pressure cuff size is important to accurate readings. Bladder size inside the cuff should be large enough to wrap almost entirely around the arm or leg without overlapping.

Generally, blood pressure readings should not be taken on extremities that are paralyzed or diseased, have had vascular reconstruction, or have a venous access device in place.

In most noncritical situations, a blood pressure assessment should not be repeated on the same arm for 2 minutes to reestablish normal circulation.

Equipment

- Sphygmomanometer with several size cuffs
- Stethoscope

Special Considerations

The thigh may be used for blood pressure determination using the popliteal artery behind the knee. Systolic readings are usually higher, but diastolic readings are approximately the same as using the upper arm.

There are five phases of sound changes when auscultating a blood pressure described as Korotkoff sounds, including

1. Phase 1: tapping sound, considered the systolic reading
2. Phase 2: swishing or murmur sound
3. Phase 3: crisp, intense sounds
4. Phase 4: muffling of sound, considered the first diastolic sound
5. Phase 5: absence of sound, considered the second diastolic sound

Hypertension is usually indicated by a reading greater than 140/90; hypotension is usually indicated by a reading less than 95/60, but all clinical symptoms should be considered.

When blood pressure is difficult to auscultate, the blood pressure may be obtained by palpating the brachial artery and noting where pulsations can first be felt as the cuff is deflated.

Nursing Interventions

Action	*Rationale*
1. Gather equipment, including appropriate size cuff.	1. Promotes an organized work environment
2. Identify patient.	2. Ensures correct patient
3. Explain procedure to patient.	3. Promotes patient cooperation
4. Position patient in a comfortable lying or sitting position.	4. Maintains comfort and decreases stress
5. Expose area between shoulder and elbow.	5. Removes any obstructions to the process
6. Support arm at the heart level with palm turned up.	6. Avoids tension and pressure, which artificially decrease or increase the reading
7. Wrap the deflated cuff securely around the exposed area approximately 1 inch above the antecubital space (Fig. 15–31).	7. Prevents inaccurate readings
8. Place ear pieces of stethoscope in your ears.	8. Prepares stethoscope for auscultation
9. Palpate brachial artery with middle fingers of nondominant hand (Fig. 15–32).	9. Locates artery for correct stethoscope placement and allows palpation of artery
10. Close valve on pressure bulb tightly and inflate cuff until arterial pulsations cannot be palpated. Inflate cuff 30 mm Hg above this point.	10. Provides guide for maximum inflation pressure
11. Place stethoscope over the brachial artery, making sure stethoscope is not touching the cuff.	11. Promotes optimal auscultation environment

continued on next page

PROCEDURE 15-5 (cont'd)

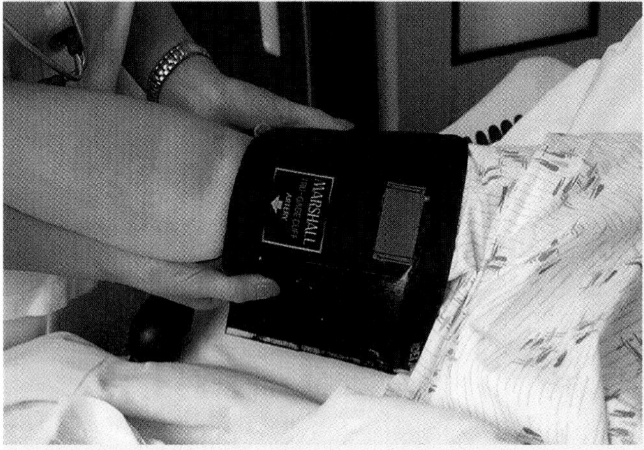

Figure 15–31. Applying the cuff.

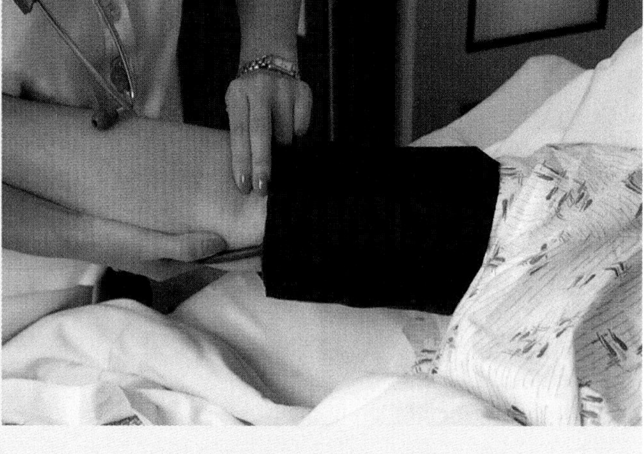

Figure 15–32. Palpating the brachial artery.

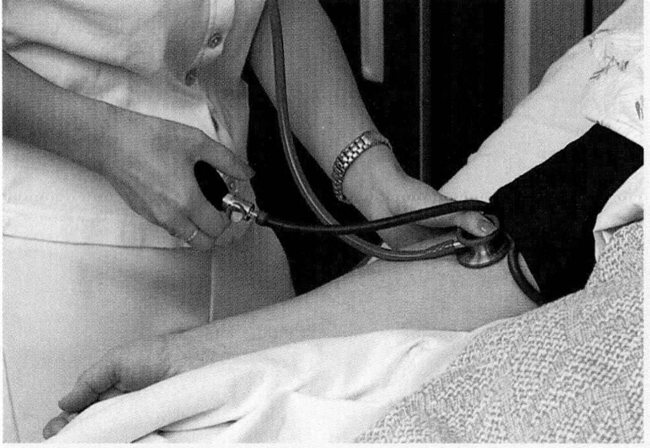

Figure 15–33. Releasing cuff pressure while auscultating over the brachial artery.

12. Slowly release pressure valve and allow gauge to drop approximately 2 mm Hg per heartbeat while auscultating sounds (Fig. 15–33).	12. Permits clear determination of points at which the sounds appear, change, and disappear
13. Note readings when the first clear sound is heard, when a muffled sound is heard, and when the sound disappears.	13. Provides information for documenting blood pressure reading
14. Allow cuff to deflate completely and remove cuff.	14. Completes measurement of blood pressure
15. Assist patient to a position of comfort.	15. Promotes patient comfort

Documentation

Record systolic and both diastolic readings, including any patient teaching.

Elements of Patient Teaching

Inform patient of the blood pressure result and provide any teaching related to medications and diet. Discuss other related lifestyle changes that may need modification. Provide blood pressure measurement teaching and a return demonstration if home monitoring is required.

PROCEDURE 15-6

Weighing a Patient

Objective

Obtain an accurate measurement of patient's weight

Terminology

- **Bed scale:** a weighing device that may be used to measure body weight of an individual who is unable to stand or sit; weight may be done with patient in horizontal position
- **Chair scale:** a weighing device that may be used to measure body weight of an individual who is unable to stand but may move out of bed and into a chair; weight is done in sitting position
- **Standing scale:** a weighing device that may be used to measure body weight of an individual who is able to stand; scale may or may not have hand rests that patient may use during weighing process

Critical Elements

Evaluate patient's condition and mobility status to choose appropriate scale. Safety is a priority.

Equipment

Bed scale, chair scale, or standing scale, paper towel or cloth towel are needed.

Special Considerations

Patient should be weighed at same time each day. Optimal time for weight is before breakfast and after voiding.

Nursing Interventions

Action	*Rationale*
1. Choose appropriate scale.	1. Ensures accurate weight assessment and maintains patient safety
2. Identify patient.	2. Promotes patient safety
3. Explain procedure.	3. Promotes cooperation
4. Assist patient in emptying bladder; if patient has an indwelling urinary catheter, empty bag before weighing.	4. Provides standardization as much as possible to avoid variances resulting from a full bladder or full indwelling urinary catheter bag
5. Balance scale at zero according to manufacturer's recommendations; balance with a cloth towel (chair scale), paper towel (standing scale), or sheet (bed scale) in place.	5. Avoids weight differences resulting from scale inaccuracies; having additional towel or linens in place helps avoid inaccuracies resulting from scale imbalance from additional objects on scale
6. Have patient remove robe and slippers (if applicable).	6. Avoids inaccuracies based on extra clothing
Standing or Chair Scale (steps 7–9)	
7. Assist patient onto standing or chair scale. Make sure patient is only touching weighing portions of scale (Fig. 15–34).	7. Ensures patient safety while getting onto scale; touching floor or any post of scale other than weighing portion may cause inaccuracies in patient weight
8. Follow any suggested manufacturer's directions for obtaining proper weight reading.	8. Facilitates weighing process
9. Assist patient back into robe and slippers and back to bed or chair as appropriate.	9. Ensures patient safety and comfort
Bed Scale (steps 10–16)	
10. If using bed scale, fan fold bed clothing down to foot of bed, leaving only a sheet over patient.	10. Avoids inaccuracies from added weight of bedding
11. With a person on each side, roll patient onto side and place bed scale sling under patient with one piece of preweighed linen between patient and sling.	11. Provides for patient safety; preweighing linen during zeroing process avoids inaccuracies based on added linen weight
12. Roll patient back onto sling; attach sling to scale frame; lift sling at least 3 inches off bed (it is important that no part of sling is touching bed) (Fig. 15–35).	12. Provides accurate position for weighing patient

continued on next page

PROCEDURE 15-6 (cont'd)

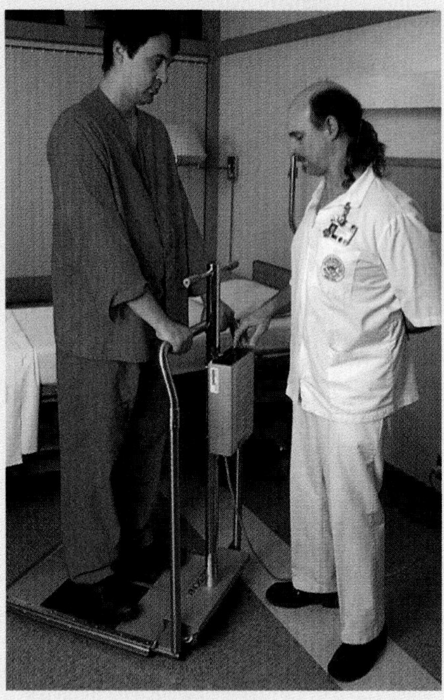

Figure 15–34. Weighing a patient on a floor scale.

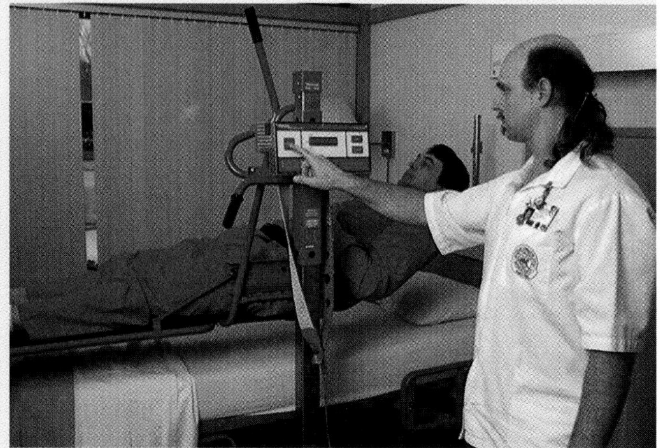

Figure 15–35. Weighing a patient on a bed scale.

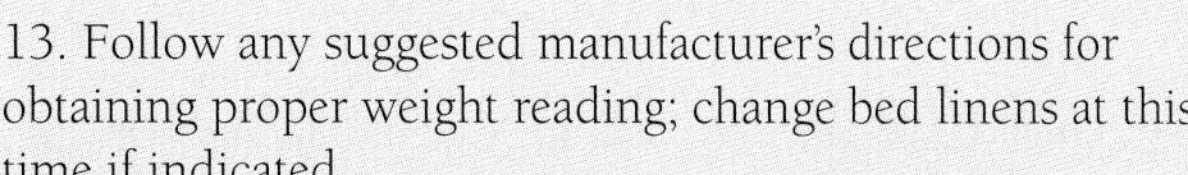

13. Follow any suggested manufacturer's directions for obtaining proper weight reading; change bed linens at this time if indicated.	13. Avoids having to roll patient again after removing sling
14. Lower sling until it is completely on bed; remove sling from scale frame; roll patient to side; remove sling from under patient.	14. Provides patient comfort and safety
15. Position patient comfortably in bed and cover with bed linens.	15. Provides patient comfort and privacy
16. Disinfect sling after use.	16. Avoids transmission of organisms from one patient to another

Documentation

Document weight in patient record.

Elements of Patient Teaching

Instruct patient regarding procedure before beginning.

PROCEDURE 15-7

Auscultating Breath Sounds

Objective

Complete an accurate assessment of breath sounds

Terminology

- **Vesicular sounds:** normal breath sound heard over lung fields; sounding like a soft whooshing sound; during inspiration
- **Bronchovesicular sounds:** normal breath sound heard over main bronchi to immediate sides of sternum just under clavicles and between scapula; a hollow, muffled sound heard during inspiration and expiration
- **Bronchial sounds:** normal breath sound heard over the manubrium; loud, tubular, and greater during expiration
- **Rales/crackles:** discontinuous sound made when air passes through fluid- or mucus-filled airways; sound like crumpling of plastic wrap; fine crackles are very high pitched and soft; coarse crackles are low pitched and bubbling or wet sounding
- **Rhonchi:** discontinuous sound heard most often on expiration; resembles snoring or a musical sound; occurs from passage of air through narrowed passages (resulting from muscle spasm, edema, or secretions)
- **Wheezes:** discontinuous sound heard during expiration caused by air passing through narrowed passages; high pitched and musical
- **Pleural friction rub:** discontinuous sound produced when irritated or inflamed pleurae rub together; sounds like rubbing leather

Critical Elements

Decreased breath sounds may indicate partial or total lung collapse, emphysema, or chronic lung disease. Louder than normal sounds may be due to consolidation; quieter than normal sounds may be due to fluid, pus, or air in pleural space.

Equipment

Stethoscope with diaphragm

Special Considerations

Provide patient with privacy before beginning assessment.

Nursing Interventions

Action	*Rationale*
1. Clean stethoscope diaphragm with alcohol.	1. Avoids transmission of organisms from one patient to another
2. Identify patient.	2. Promotes safety
3. Explain procedure.	3. Promotes cooperation
4. Turn off radio/television, and pull curtain or close door.	4. Ensures privacy and quiet to enhance ability to hear breath sounds
5. Position patient sitting upright or raise head of bed 45–90°.	5. Promotes better lung expansion
6. Remove patient's gown from chest area.	6. Prevents interference with sound transmission
7. Instruct patient to breath in through mouth and out through nose.	7. Allows for optimum airflow
8. Auscultate lungs using diaphragm of stethoscope. Auscultate the posterior chest from the apices at C7 to the bases around C10 and laterally from the axilla down to the seventh or eighth rib. Auscultate the anterior chest from the apices in the supraclavicular areas down to the sixth rib (Fig. 15–36).	8. Ensures auscultation over all of the lung fields
9. Assess for any dyspnea or pain. Report any abnormal breath sounds.	9. Any abnormal sounds may indicate respiratory problems
10. If abnormal breath sounds are heard, have patient deep breathe and cough and then listen again.	10. Promotes clearing of air passages by coughing, if abnormal air sounds are due to secretions
11. Assist patient to position of comfort.	11. Provides for patient comfort

continued on next page

PROCEDURE 15-7 (cont'd)

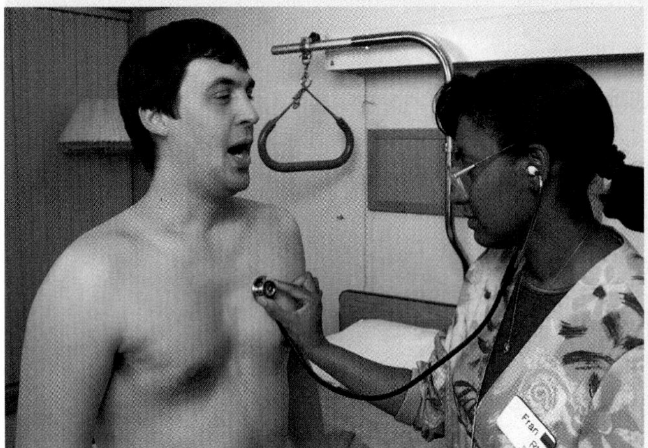

Figure 15–36. Auscultating breath sounds in the upper anterior thorax.

Documentation

Document normal and abnormal sounds in patient record.

Elements of Patient Teaching

Explain procedure to patient before beginning. Instruct patient in coughing and deep-breathing exercises.

PROCEDURE 15-8

Auscultating the Heart

Objective

Complete an accurate assessment of heart sounds.

Terminology

- S_1: sound of closing of atrioventricular valves at beginning of ventricular systole; heard over mitral and tricuspid areas; also known as "lub" sound
- S_2: sound of closing of aortic and pulmonary valves during ventricular diastole; heard over aortic and pulmonic areas during ventricular diastole; known as "dub" sound; if valves do not close together, they may be heard separately and it is thus known as a split S_2
- S_3: known as ventricular gallop; occurs right after S_2 sound at apex of heart or left lower sternal border; occurs because of early rapid filling of ventricles; is significant for cardiac decompensation in patients with heart disease; gives a "lub-DUB-dee" (or ken-TUK-y) sound
- S_4: known as atrial gallop; occurs just before S_1 as a result of increased resistance to ventricular filling after atrial contraction; heard at apex of heart or left lower sternal border; found in patients with heart disease; heard as a "DEE-lub-dub" (or TENN-ess-ee) sound
- **Heart murmurs:** sound produced by atypical or turbulent blood flow; occurs primarily during systole most of time; sound is usually faint under normal conditions

PROCEDURE 15-8 (cont'd)

Critical Elements

Sounds other than normal S_1 and S_2, or heard in other than prescribed areas are abnormal. Sounds may also be abnormal if they are not of usual quality. It is important to also note presence of any unusual rates or rhythms.

Equipment

Stethoscope with bell and diaphragm

Special Considerations

Diaphragm of stethoscope is used for detecting presence of high-pitched sounds while bell is used for detecting presence of lower pitched sounds. If any irregular rhythm, abnormal sounds, or abnormal rate is heard, listen for a full 60 seconds at that site. Report any abnormal findings.

Nursing Interventions

Action	*Rationale*
1. Clean diaphragm and bell of stethoscope with alcohol.	1. Reduces risk of passing microorganisms from one patient to another
2. Identify patient.	2. Promotes safety
3. Explain procedure.	3. Promotes cooperation
4. Pull curtain or close door.	4. Provides patient with privacy
5. Turn off television/radio.	5. Interferes with hearing heart sounds
6. Figure 15–37 indicates sites for cardiac auscultation. With the patient first supine (Fig. 15–38), then sitting upright (Fig. 15–39), use the stethoscope's diaphragm to auscultate heart sounds over the sites shown in Figure 15–30.	6. Provides landmarks for identifying S_1 and S_2 sounds

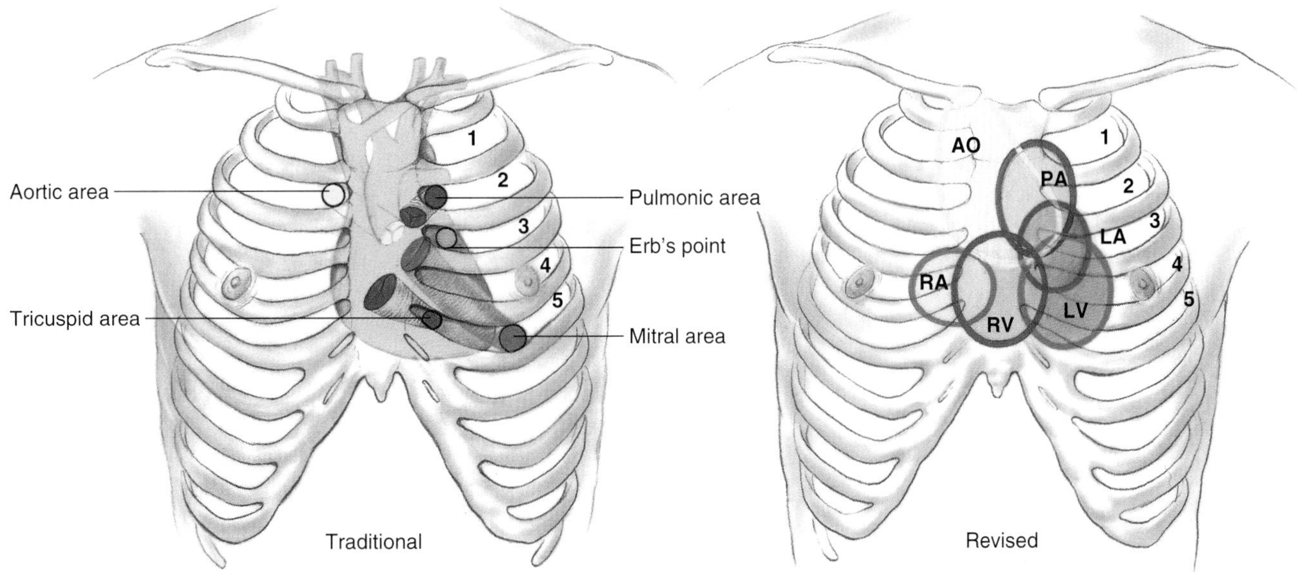

Figure 15–37. Sites for cardiac auscultation. (From Jarvis, C. (1996). Physical Examination and Health Assessment, 2nd ed. Philadelphia: W.B. Saunders.)

PROCEDURE 15-8 (cont'd)

7. Assess regularity of rhythm, rate, pitch, and intensity as well as presence of abnormal sounds.	7. Provides objective data for assessment
8. Place patient in left lateral lying position.	8. Promotes optimal position for hearing low pitched sounds
9. Repeat auscultation at the same sites as before, using the bell of stethoscope.	9. Provides mechanism for hearing
10. Assess regularity of rhythm, rate, pitch, and intensity as well as presence of abnormal sounds.	10. Provides objective data for assessment
11. Assist patient to position of comfort and safety.	11. Promotes a safe environment for patient

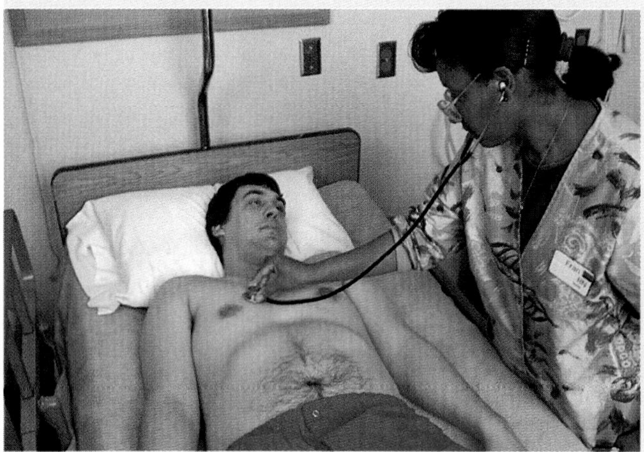

Figure 15–38. Auscultating the heart with the patient supine.

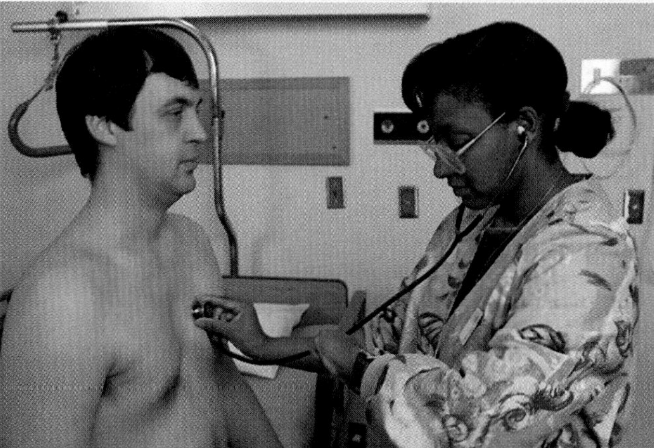

Figure 15–39. Auscultating the heart with the patient sitting upright.

Documentation

Document normal and abnormal sounds in patient record.

Elements of Patient Teaching

Explain auscultation procedure steps, including positioning and reason for auscultation.

PROCEDURE 15-9

Auscultating Bowel Sounds

Objective

Complete an accurate assessment of bowel sounds

Terminology

- **Hyperactive sounds:** increased bowel sounds, which are usually loud and high pitched; may be heard in rapid rushes, indicating increased bowel motility such as may occur with diarrhea, gastroenteritis, laxative use, and early bowel obstruction; may be heard in any quadrant
- **Hypoactive sounds:** decreased bowel sounds, which are usually quieter than normal and occurring less frequently; can be due to full colon or peritonitis; may be heard in any quadrant
- **Absent sounds:** complete absence of bowel sounds, which may be due to paralytic ileus or complete bowel obstruction
- **Tympanic sounds:** high-pitched and tinkling noises that sound as if they occur in a hollow space; result from air under tension and intestinal fluid in dilated loop of bowel

Critical Elements

Listen to all quadrants over several minutes, because bowel sounds may be intermittent, not continuous.

Equipment

Stethoscope

Special Considerations

Normal bowel sounds are fairly frequent gurgling sounds that may vary with time of day and activity directly after meals. They may be decreased or absent after surgery, recovering in 1–2 days (or 3–5 days after abdominal surgery). Review patient history of bowel elimination, laxative use, presence of pain or distention, or recent abdominal surgery. Report abnormal findings.

Nursing Interventions

Action	*Rationale*
1. Clean stethoscope diaphragm with alcohol.	1. Avoids transmission of organisms from one patient to another
2. Identify patient.	2. Promotes safety
3. Explain procedure.	3. Promotes cooperation
4. Close door or curtain.	4. Provides privacy
5. Turn off television/radio.	5. Prevents interference with hearing bowel sounds
6. Lie patient flat and expose abdomen, ensuring privacy.	6. Provides best position for listening to all four quadrants; gown or drape; may interfere with sound transmission
7. Using the diaphragm of the stethoscope, listen over each abdominal quadrant (Fig. 15–40).	7. Provides a method for locating a potential problem
8. Assist patient to position of comfort.	8. Promotes patient comfort

continued on next page

PROCEDURE 15-9 (cont'd)

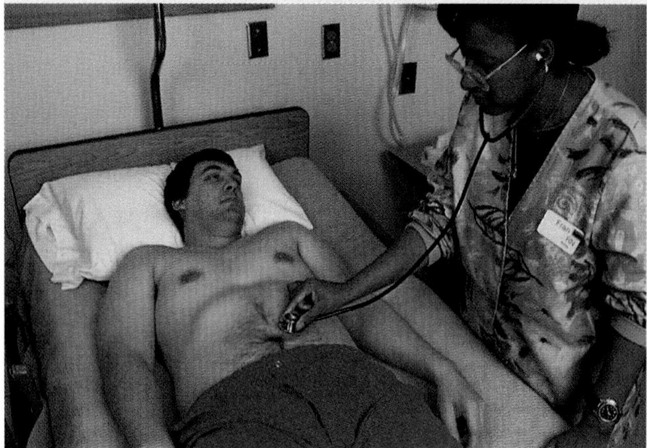

Figure 15–40. Auscultating bowel sounds with the diaphragm of the stethoscope.

Documentation

Document the bowel sounds in the patient record.

Elements of Patient Teaching

Explain procedure to the patient before beginning.

CHAPTER HIGHLIGHTS

- Assessment is a core component of nursing practice.
- There is both an art and a science component to the assessment process. They are equally important.
- The health history provides subjective data. It contains six main topics: chief complaint, history of the present problem, medical history, personal and social history, family history, and review of systems.
- The physical examination provides objective data. It requires the use of inspection, palpation, percussion, auscultation, and appropriate technology (e.g., blood pressure cuff and stethoscope).
- Each body system is assessed in a complete physical examination.
- Age and developmental status, culture, and personal comfort with the examination influence the assessment process.
- Documentation, privacy, and confidentiality are crucial components of assessment.

REFERENCES

Alcamo, I.E. (1996). *Anatomy and Physiology the Easy Way.* Hauppauge, NY: Barron's Educational Series, Inc.

American Nurses' Association (1991). *Standards of Clinical Nursing Practice.* Washington, DC: American Nurses Publishing.

American Nurses' Association (1995). *Nursing's Social Policy Statement.* Washington, DC: American Nurses Publishing.

Arnold, E., Boggs, K. (1995). *Interpersonal Relationships: Professional Communication Skills for Nurses,* 2nd ed. Philadelphia: W.B. Saunders.

Bendtsen, L., Jensen, R., Jensen, N.K., Olesen, J. (1994). Muscle palpation with controlled finger pressure: new equipment for the study of tender myofacial tissues. *Pain, 59,* 235–239.

Brennan, D.F., Falk, J.L., Rothrock, S.G., Kerr, R.B. (1995). Reliability of infrared tympanic thermometry in the detection of rectal fever in children. *Annals of Emergency Medicine, 25*(1), 21–30.

Brown, S.J. (1995). An interviewing style for nursing assessment. *Journal of Advanced Nursing, 21,* 340–343.

Byra-Cook, C.J., Dracup, K.A., Lazic, A.J. (1990). Direct and indirect blood pressure in critical care patients. *Nursing Research, 39*(5), 285–288.

California Board of Registered Nursing (1997). *Nurse Practice Act Rules and Regulations.* North Highlands, CA: Procurement Division Publications Section.

Erickson, R.S., Meyer, L.T., Woo, T.M. (1996). Accuracy of chemical dot thermometers in critically ill adults and young children. *Image: Journal of Nursing Scholarship, 28*(1), 23–28.

Erickson, R.S., Woo, T.M. (1994). Accuracy of infrared ear thermometry and traditional temperature methods in young children. *Heart & Lung, 23*(3), 181–195.

Erickson, R.S., Yount, S.T. (1991). Comparison of tympanic and oral temperatures in surgical patients. *Nursing Research, 40*(2), 90–93.

Eskelinen, M., Ikonen, J., Lipponen, P. (1995). The value of history-taking, physical examination, and computer assistance in the diagnosis of acute appendicitis in patients more than 50 years old. *Scandinavian Journal Gastroenterology, 30,* 349–355.

Flo, G., Brown, M. (1995). Comparing three methods of temperature taking: oral mercury-in-glass, oral diatek, and tympanic first temp. *Nursing Research, 44*(2), 120–122.

Frankenburg, W., Dodds, J., Archer, P., et al. (1990). *Denver II screening manual.* Denver, CO: Denver Developmental Materials, Inc.

Ganong, W.F. (1995). *Review of Medical Physiology,* 17th ed. Norwalk, CT: Appleton & Lange.

Guyton, A.C., Hall, J.E. (1996). *Textbook of Medical Physiology,* 9th ed. Philadelphia: W.B. Saunders.

Hasel, K.L., Erickson, R.S. (1995). Effect of cerumen on infrared ear temperature measurement. *Journal of Gerontological Nursing, 21*(12), 6–14.

Hollerbach, A.D., Sneed, N. (1990). Accuracy of radial pulse assessment by length of counting interval. *Heart & Lung, 19*(3), 258–264.

Jones, M.L. (1970). Accuracy of pulse rates counted for fifteen, thirty and sixty seconds. *Military Medicine, 12,* 1127–1136.

Lehman, S. (1997). Anatomy of a problem: naming body parts. *The Press Democrat,* August 29, A4.

Long, L., Higgins, P., Brady, D. (1988). *Psychosocial Assessment: A Pocket Guide for Data Collection.* Norwalk, CT: Appleton & Lange.

Norman, E., Gadaleta, D., Griffin, C.C. (1991). An evaluation of three blood pressure methods in a stabilized acute trauma population. *Nursing Research, 40*(2), 86–89.

Rieser, M.F., Reeves, R.B., Armington, J. (1958). Effect of variations in laboratory procedure and experimenter upon the ballistocardiograph, blood pressure and heart rate in healthy young men. *Psychosomatic Medicine, 17,* 185–189.

Saunders, E. (1991). Hypertension in blacks. *Primary Care, 18,* 607–621.

Seidel, H., Ball, J., Dains, J., Benedict, G. (1995). *Mosby's Guide to Physical Examination.* St. Louis, MO: C.V. Mosby.

Sony, S.D. (1992). Baccalaureate nurse graduates' perception of barriers to the use of physical assessment skills in the clinical setting. *Journal of Continuing Education, 23*(2), 83–87.

Staessen, J.A., Fagard, R., Thijs, L., Amery, A. (1995). A consensus view on the technique of ambulatory blood pressure monitoring. *Hypertension, 26,* 912–918.

Thomas, C.L. (Ed.) (1997). *Taber's Cyclopedic Medical Dictionary.* Philadelphia: F.A. Davis.

Thomas, S.A., DeKeyser, F. (1996). Blood pressure. In J.J. Fitzpatrick (ed.): *Annual Review of Nursing Research, Vol. 14.* New York: Springer, pp. 3–22.

U.S. Department of Health and Human Services (1987). *Report of the Second Task Force on Blood Pressure Control in Children.* Washington, DC: National Institutes of Health.

U.S. Department of Health and Human Services (1994). *The Fifth Report of the Joint National Committee on the Detection, Evaluation and Treatment of High Blood Pressure.* Washington, DC: National Institutes of Health.

Yeo, S., Hayashi, R.H., Wan, J.Y., Dubler, B. (1995). Tympanic versus rectal thermometry in pregnant women. *Journal of Obstetric, Gynecologic, and Neonatal Nursing, 24*(8), 719–724.

Pharmacology and Medication Administration

Part I Pharmacology

Dorie Schwertz and Mariann Piano

Part II Practical Aspects of Safe and Effective Drug Administration

Carol Lindeman

Part III Administering Medication by Intramuscular Injection

Pauline Beecroft

OBJECTIVES

After studying this chapter, the student will be able to

- **participate in decisions about drug therapy for individual patients**
- **assess patients to identify a potentially high risk for adverse drug effects**
- **administer drugs safely and effectively**

Mr. K. is a 75-year-old black patient with a history of hypertension, coronary artery disease, and chronic heart failure (HF). Mr. K. has been hypertensive for over 20 years; however, the onset of his HF was approximately 2 years ago. Within the past 2 years Mr. K. has been hospitalized four times for exacerbation of his HF. Mr. K. now presents to the heart failure clinic because of progressive swelling in his feet and lower legs and gradual weight gain of 6 lbs. over the past week. The health care management team has evaluated Mr. K. and has decided to increase his dose of diuretic. Mr. K. is required to take at least five different types of medications daily.

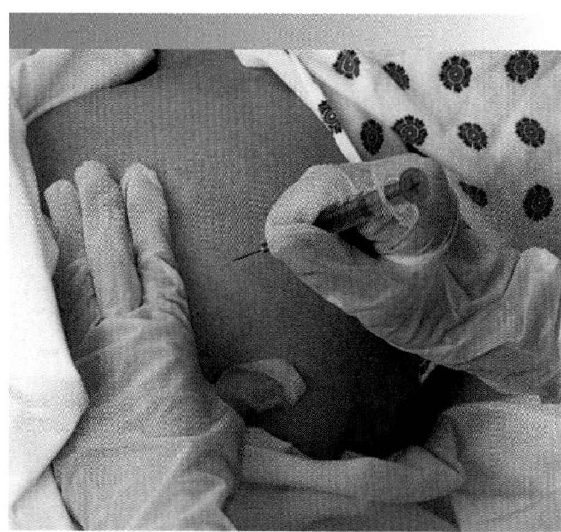

PART I: PHARMACOLOGY

SCOPE OF NURSING CARE

Pharmacotherapy—the use of drugs in the diagnosis, prevention, and treatment of disease—is a major part of health care:

- In the 1980s, outpatient prescriptions averaged over six per person per year (Manasse, 1989; Myer, 1988).
- Approximately two thirds of patient visits to a physician result in at least one prescription (Myer, 1988).
- Hospitalized patients receive an average of 15 drug administrations per day (Manasse, 1989).
- Hospitalized patients have a 3% chance of experiencing a life-threatening drug reaction, and 15% experience some adverse drug reaction (Jick, 1984).
- In the population 65 years of age and older, 20 to 25 percent of hospitalizations are due to adverse drug reactions (Shaw, 1982).
- Adverse drug reactions and toxic reactions are important factors in 8.4% of all hospital admissions (Hallas, 1996).

Managing drug regimens for patients is a responsibility of the nurse in every setting in which care is given. The scope of nursing responsibility in the administration of medications is defined by the Nurse Practice Act of each state, as well as the policies and procedures set forth by the hospital or medical institution where the nurse is employed. In 1998, there were only two states in which nurse practitioners and other advanced practice nurses had no legal prescribing authority (Pearson, 1998). First and foremost, registered nurses in all states are responsible for safe and effective drug administration.

KNOWLEDGE BASE

PHARMACOLOGIC CONCEPTS

The definition of a few key terms will help in understanding principles of pharmacology. To begin with, a *drug* is any substance that interacts with the body to produce a response. Drugs interact with the body at specific sites called *receptors*. Drugs do not produce new effects in the body but rather modify physiologic activities that are already in place. *Pharmacology* is the science of the origin, nature, chemistry, effects, and uses of drugs.

The study of pharmacology has evolved from before the scientific era, when pain and disease were associated with supernatural spirits and mysticism, to the present, when drugs are rationally conceived and designed using tools such as computer modeling. The first use of drugs came about through trial and error with natural products. For example, willow bark was used to treat pain and inflammation. As it turns out, willow bark is a source of an aspirin-like compound. *Pharmacognosy* is a division of pharmacology that involves the identification and preparation of crude drugs from natural sources. Today, the study of pharmacognosy continues to be a productive avenue for drug development.

There are at least four other divisions within the science of pharmacology that are emphasized in this chapter: pharmacokinetics, pharmacodynamics, pharmacotherapeutics, and toxicology. *Pharmacokinetics* deals with what the body does to a drug, including absorption, distribution, metabolism, and excretion. *Pharmacodynamics* is what the drug does to the body or the study of how a drug interacts with its receptor to elicit a response. *Pharmacotherapeutics* is the application of drugs to the diagnosis, prevention, and treatment of disease. Finally, *toxicology* is the study of undesirable effects of chemicals on living systems.

In this chapter we consider toxic effects of drugs. The need to determine the toxic potential or the adverse effects of new and existing therapeutic agents is illustrated by "the grey baby syndrome," in which the toxic effects of the antibiotic chloramphenicol were not fully realized until after many infant deaths had occurred. Although chloramphenicol appeared to be safe and effective in adults, it was discovered that neonates, especially premature babies, were unable to metabolize the drug. The unmetabolized drug is not excreted and therefore accumulates in the body (Weiss et al, 1960). The very high levels of chloramphenicol in neonates caused aplastic anemia, hypothermia, vasomotor collapse, and death. In other situations, the toxic effects of drugs are not always expressed immediately. For example, cancers induced by exposure to drugs or environmental pollutants are not detected until a very long time after exposure. A mother may take a drug during pregnancy, and the consequences may not be known until after the baby is born. The thalidomide tragedy, in which infants were born with distorted flipperlike limbs, is the most publicized example of this type of toxic effect.

Advances in the science of pharmacology are occurring very rapidly. A new era of pharmacologic research and development was ushered in during the 1940s and 1950s when the chemical structure of antibiotics was deciphered. In the 1960s and 1970s, the fast pace of development of chemistry and biochemistry provided a basis for understanding the relationship between drug structure and drug activity, as well as the concept of drug-receptor interactions. In the 1980s, major advances were made in understanding how a drug causes a change in cellular function after it binds to its receptor. This phenomenon is referred to as signal transduction. Today, the discipline of pharmacology is experiencing an unprecedented explosion of new discoveries based on recent advances in molecular biology and genetic engineering. For example, deoxyribonucleic acid (DNA) databases provide information that can be used to develop protein drugs (e.g., recombinant human erythropoietin), and gene transfer offers hope for new therapeutic approaches (Dykes, 1996).

The ideal drug would have a specific therapeutic effect without producing any toxic or adverse side effects. However, "ideal" drugs do not exist, and in the search for new drugs, the balance between risks and benefits must always be addressed. In some situations, nonscientific issues confound the assessment of risks and benefits. For example, the antigestation drug Mefepristone (RU486) has been shown to effectively induce abortion, as well as to have therapeutic potential for accelerating wound healing and treating other diseases (Baulieu, 1989). Studies in France have revealed no significant adverse effects. However, religious and ethical issues have delayed this drug's availability in the United States. Another sort of ethical issue arises when a highly effective drug is so expensive that economically disadvantaged populations cannot afford it.

DRUG DEVELOPMENT

The Food, Drug, and Cosmetic Act of 1906 was the first federal law enacted to protect the public from risks associated with drug consumption. The Act provided that all marketed drugs must meet standards of purity and strength as defined by the *United States Pharmacopeia and National Drug Formulary.* In 1912, the Sherley Amendment prohibited fraudulent therapeutic claims with regard to drug actions. Drug **safety** was the focus of the Food, Drug, and Cosmetic Act of 1938. This legislation established the Food and Drug Administration (FDA) as the agency responsible for enforcement of federal drug regulations. The Kefauver-Harris Amendment of 1962 mandated that pharmacologic and toxicologic testing be conducted in laboratory animals before FDA approval is sought for the marketing of a drug. The 1962 Amendment also required that all drugs be proven not just safe but also **effective** before they could be marketed.

Information gathered through animal studies is heavily relied on for initiation of clinical trials in humans. Acute and long-term toxicity studies are carried out with animals. These studies help to determine the lethal dose-50% (LD_{50}), or dose that causes death in 50 percent of a sample population of rodents. These studies also provide information regarding (1) specific organs that are adversely affected by the drug and mechanisms of toxicity, (2) the minimal effective drug dose and the therapeutic dose range, and (3) pharmacokinetic and pharmacodynamic information.

It is important to note, however, that not all adverse drug effects can be discovered during animal studies. Symptoms such as anxiety, depression, and fatigue may be difficult or impossible to measure in animals. Furthermore, the manner in which animals absorb, distribute, metabolize, eliminate, and respond to drugs may be different than those in humans in some respects. For example, the rate of drug metabolism in the liver of a rat can be 15 to 20 times faster than it is in humans (Parke, 1985).

The FDA reviews information from animal studies before determining whether a new drug should be tested in humans. Testing in humans is implemented by a three-phase process of clinical trials. Phase I clinical trials use healthy volunteers to determine pharmacokinetic and safety information. Phase II trials use a small sample of patients who have the specific pathology for which the drug is being developed to determine therapeutic effectiveness and dose range. Phase III trials use a large sample of patients from multiple sites who have the pathology for which the drug is being developed to further evaluate therapeutic effects, adverse reactions, and overall risk-to-benefit ratio. In phase II and III trials, patients are usually randomly assigned to receive the experimental drug or a placebo (an inactive substance). The trials are conducted using a double-blind research design. Neither the patient nor the clinical researcher knows whether the patient is receiving the active drug or the placebo.

The majority of drugs that enter phase I and II testing never proceed to phase III. If the drug does go through phase III and the sponsoring pharmaceutical company believes that the investigational drug is safe and effective, then the company submits the results of the studies to the FDA. The FDA reviews the data and either approves or denies the drug for marketing.

It is critical to remember that not all adverse drug effects are identified during the clinical trials. Once the drug is marketed, it will be given to a large population of patients, to special patient populations (e.g., infants, frail elderly or pregnant women), and to patients with multiple disease states who are taking many drugs. Less common adverse drug effects and effects that occur in special populations or under special conditions may be revealed during this postmarketing surveillance period (sometimes referred to as phase IV clinical trials). For example, the elderly are often excluded from phase II and phase III clinical trials even for drugs that have been developed to treat conditions most commonly seen in the elderly. In this situation, postmarketing surveillance would be especially important for evaluating efficacy and toxicity (Rochon and Gurwitz, 1995). Discovery of adverse drug reactions during the postmarketing surveillance period depends on **voluntary** reporting by the health care team. The nurse must assume accountability and responsibility to evaluate the effects of drugs in his or her patients and report adverse drug reactions to the FDA.

FACTORS INFLUENCING THE EFFECTS OF DRUGS

DOSE-RESPONSE RELATIONSHIP

In most cases, drugs cause a response by binding to a specific receptor on a target organ. Receptors are cellular macromolecules that have a high affinity for the drug. The drug fits into the receptor very much like a key fits into a lock (Fig. 16–1). Each cell in the target organ has a specific number of receptors at any given time. However, the number of receptors that a cell has can change over time. Some factors that can modify the number of drug receptors are age, genetics, disease, or prior exposure to the drug.

It may seem strange that a human cell would have receptors for drugs. Intuitively, this might make more sense if a drug were specifically developed to mimic a chemical that is naturally found in the body, like epinephrine. Epinephrine must also bind to receptors in cells to produce its effects. But why would nerve cells have receptors that are exactly the right size

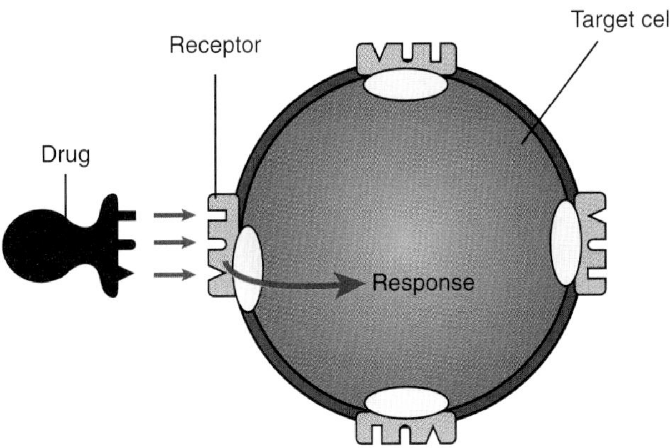

Figure 16–1. A drug binds to a receptor on a target cell to produce a response.

and shape to bind to a drug like morphine? After all, morphine is extracted from a poppy plant. Interestingly, long after the therapeutic effects of morphine and other opiates were known and after it was understood that drugs work by binding to receptors, pharmacologists discovered that there **were** natural chemicals in the body that could bind to opioid receptors. These chemicals are called endorphins.

In general, the response to a drug will increase as the concentration of a drug in the vicinity of its receptors increases until a maximal possible response is reached (Fig. 16–2). For example, diazepam (Valium) exerts its effect on receptors in the brain. The intensity of the response to Valium depends on the Valium concentration in the brain. The duration of action of Valium depends on how long the concentration of drug remains above a minimal therapeutic level in the brain. In other words, the more Valium that reaches the brain (up to a certain point), the greater the antianxiety effect. In addition, the faster Valium leaves the brain, the shorter the duration of drug action. Figure 16–2A depicts how, as the concentration of drug increases, both the amount of drug bound to receptors and the response to the drug increase. This relationship holds true until all of the receptors are occupied, at which point a maximal effect is observed. Once all of the receptors are occupied by drug, the addition of more drug will **not** produce a greater effect. This very important concept is illustrated in Figure 16–2B.

Usually the clinician does not know the concentration of drug at its receptor site; however he or she does know the drug dose and, with few exceptions, the drug dose and the concentration of drug at the receptor are directly related. In other words, the response to the drug increases as the dose of administered drug is increased, until the maximal response to a drug is reached. Using Valium as an example again, when the dose of Valium is increased, the concentration of drug at the Valium receptor sites in the brain also increases, and the antianxiety effect increases as well. This relationship between dose and response is a very important pharmacologic principle. Whereas Figure 16–2B shows the relationship among drug **concentration,** receptor occupancy, and response, the relationship between drug **dose** and response can be graphically demonstrated in the same way (Fig. 16–3). This is referred to as a dose-response curve.

STEADY-STATE PLASMA DRUG CONCENTRATIONS

It is a basic pharmacologic principle that the response to a drug is dependent on the drug concentration in the vicinity of its receptors. However, in most clinical situations, it is not possible to measure drug concentration at the receptor site. For example, measuring the concentration of Valium in the brain is impractical. Instead, the plasma concentration of a drug is measured and used as an indirect indicator of drug concentration at the receptor site.

Drugs can be given in a one-time dosage or over a period of time. Most often, when a drug is administered over time, the maintenance dose (amount of drug given each time) and dosing interval (time between doses) are designed to maintain a therapeutic steady-state plasma concentration. In other words, the drug is administered so that blood plasma concentration is maintained at a relatively constant level that will produce an optimal desired effect and minimal adverse effects (Fig. 16–4). The plasma concentration is at a "steady state" when the rate of drug absorption equals the rate of drug elimination. The steady-state plasma drug level can be manipulated by altering the maintenance dose or the dosing interval. If the maintenance dose is increased, then the steady-state plasma concentration increases. If the dosing interval is increased, then the steady-state plasma concentration decreases.

Three other major factors can modulate steady-state plasma drug concentrations (Box 16–1). One of these factors is absorption. Clearly the more of each dose of drug that is absorbed into the blood, the higher the steady-state plasma concentration. If drug absorption is decreased for some reason, such as because of an interaction with food in the gastrointestinal tract, then the steady-state plasma drug concentration falls.

A second factor that can influence steady-state plasma drug concentrations is the half-life of the drug or the time it takes

BOX 16–1
FACTORS INFLUENCING STEADY-STATE PLASMA DRUG CONCENTRATION

Factors that Increase Steady-State Plasma Drug Concentration

1. Increased absorption (increased bioavailability) **(A)**
2. Increased maintenance dose
3. Increased drug half-life **($t^1/_2$)**

Factors that Decrease Steady-State Plasma Drug Concentration

1. Increased volume of distribution **(Vd)**
2. Increased dosing interval

$$\textbf{steady-state plasma drug concentration} = \frac{\textbf{(A) (maintenance dose) } (t^1/_2)}{\textbf{(Vd) (dosing interval)}}$$

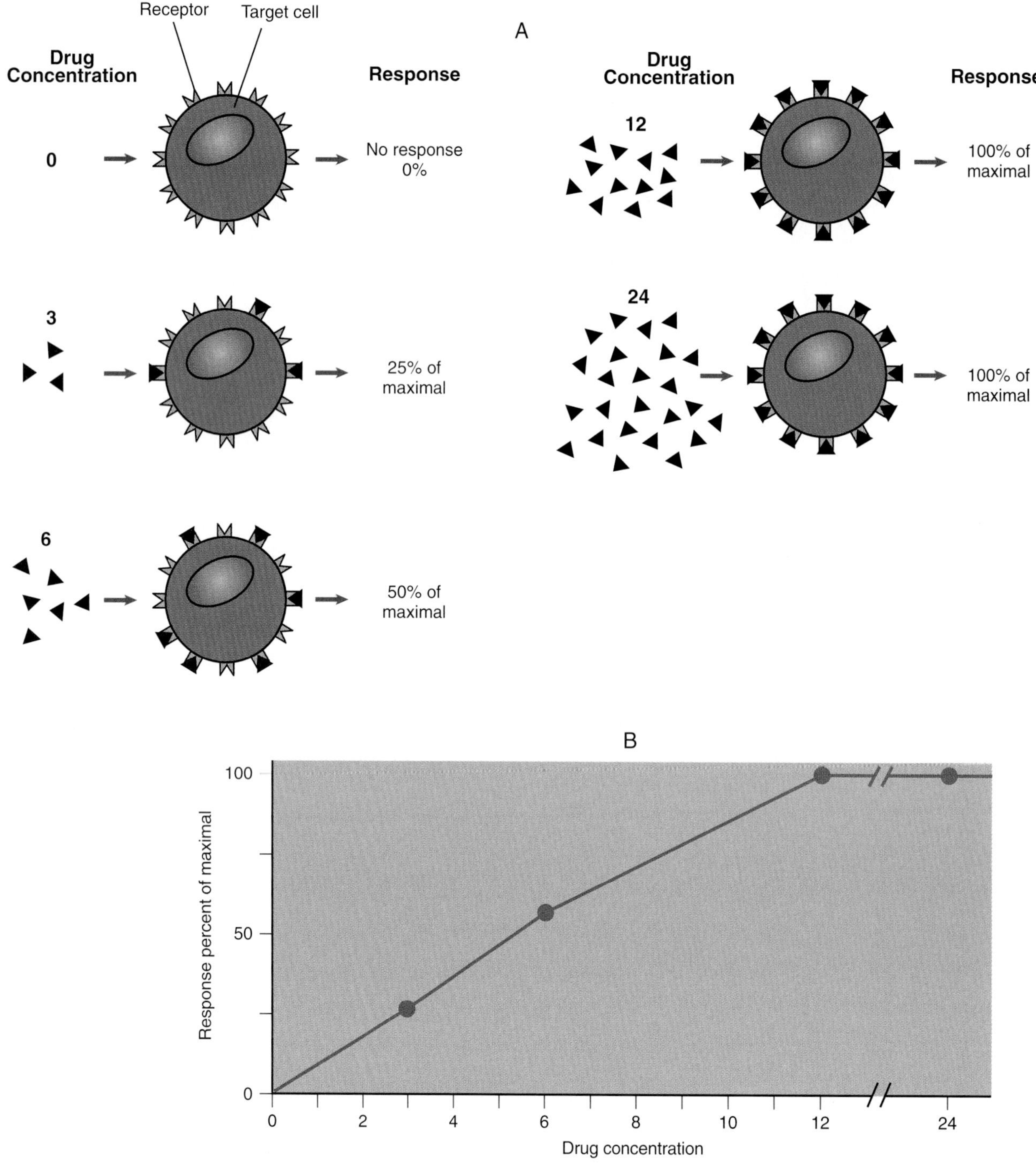

Figure 16-2. Drug concentration and response. **A**, The response to a drug increases as the concentration of the drug in the vicinity of its receptors increases. Once all of the receptors are occupied with the drug, the maximal effect is reached, and more drug will not elicit a greater effect. **B**, Graphic representation of the relationship between drug concentration and percent of maximal response.

for half of the drug to be eliminated from the body. If for some reason the half-life of a drug increases (i.e., it takes longer to eliminate half of the drug from the body), then the steady-state plasma concentration of the drug increases. The half-life of the drug is primarily dependent on metabolism and excretion. As a result, an alteration in hepatic or renal function would be likely to alter drug half-life. Specifically, if a drug is excreted by the kidneys and a patient has compromised renal function, it is likely that the half-life of the drug will increase and the plasma concentration of the drug will increase.

The third major factor that can influence steady-state plasma concentration is the volume of drug distribution. The volume of distribution essentially describes the extent to which a drug is distributed throughout the body. For

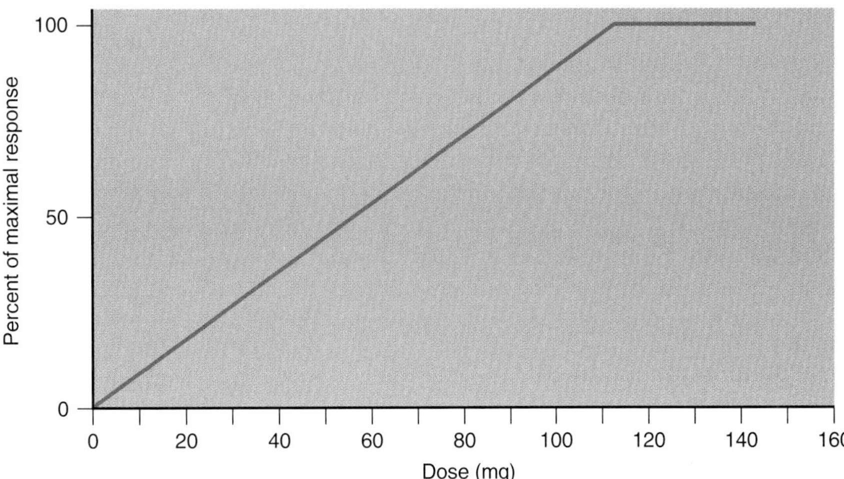

Figure 16–3. Dose-response curve. As the dose of a drug increases, the response to the drug increases until a maximal possible response is reached.

example, if a drug is given intravenously and stays in the vascular system, the drug would be narrowly distributed. On the other hand, if the drug were distributed throughout the body and taken up and stored in certain tissues, such as adipose tissue, the drug would be considered to be widely distributed. The same drug may distribute differently in different individuals. For instance, a lipid-soluble drug such as Valium has a larger volume of distribution in an obese person than in a lean person because Valium would be taken up and stored in fatty tissue. If all other factors remain constant, when the volume of distribution of a drug is increased, then the steady-state plasma level decreases. Therefore, assuming that the maintenance dose and dosing interval of a drug are the same, an obese patient has a lower steady-state plasma concentration of Valium than a lean patient. The relationship between steady-state plasma drug concentration and factors that influence it are illustrated by the equation in Box 16–1.

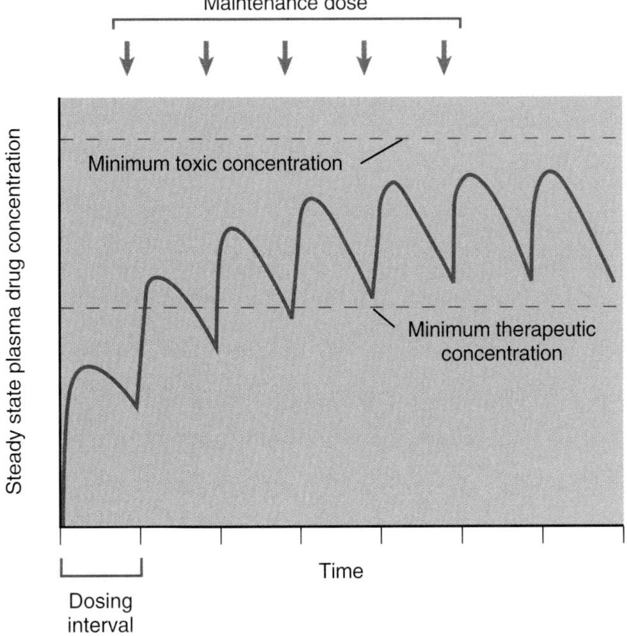

Figure 16–4. Steady-state plasma drug concentration. Drugs are administered chronically at a maintenance dose and dosing interval that will achieve a therapeutic drug level. The drug must be administered at a time interval whereby the previous dose is not completely eliminated from the body. A steady-state level is achieved after a period equal to approximately three to four times the half-life of the drug.

From this discussion it should be clear that plasma drug level is affected by many factors, including the absorption from the site of administration, how the body distributes the drug, and the rate at which the body eliminates the drug. These factors are in turn influenced by physiologic processes that regulate the pharmacokinetics of a drug; i.e., absorption, distribution, metabolism, and excretion. Physiologic processes vary among individuals. They also vary in the same individual over time because of factors such as age, disease, food consumption, and multiple drug administration. Therefore, it should be apparent that there is a substantial degree of unpredictability inherent in the outcome of drug administration.

As was mentioned earlier, *pharmacokinetics* is the study of what the body does to a drug. Pharmacokinetic factors ultimately determine the concentration of drug in the vicinity of its receptors and how rapidly the concentration of drug near the receptors changes. Because the concentration of drug near its receptor influences the intensity and duration of the drug response, it is important to know what factors can alter the pharmacokinetics of a drug.

In the following section, factors that influence pharmacokinetics are discussed. Understanding these factors helps the nurse assess the patient for factors that would alter steady-state plasma drug concentration and drug effect. Proper assessment of these factors decreases the risk of adverse drug effects and optimizes therapeutic outcome.

PHARMACOKINETICS

This section discusses the general principles involved in the regulation of drug absorption, distribution, metabolism, and excretion.

ABSORPTION

Rarely is a drug administered directly to its site of action. Instead, it must be absorbed into the systemic circulation before it can be distributed throughout the body and eventually be distributed to its receptor site. To be transported to its site of action and to exert its effect, the drug must first dissolve into biologic fluids. Unless medication is administered directly into the bloodstream (intravenously), it must diffuse around or through multiple layers of cells to reach the plasma. A drug administered orally has to diffuse through several different layers of cells, including the intestinal epithelium and the capillary endothelial wall. Because the endothelial cells that line capillaries are loosely associated, movement into and out of capillaries takes place by simple diffusion and bulk flow of fluids. However, the intestinal epithelial cells are attached by tight junctions, which necessitates the passage of the drugs through the cells.

The rate of absorption through a membrane depends on three factors:

- The difference in concentration of the drug across the membrane (i.e., the concentration gradient)
- The membrane surface area available for drug absorption
- The physicochemical properties of the drug

The greater the concentration gradient of drug across the membrane, the faster the rate of absorption. The larger the surface area, the higher the rate of absorption. The more lipid (fat)-soluble the drug, the more readily it passes through cell membranes, because the membranes themselves are composed of fatty phospholipids. In contrast, most water-soluble drugs are not able to enter cells or cross cell membranes. This is particularly important at anatomic locations such as the epithelial lining of the kidney tubules or capillaries at the blood-brain barrier, where, under normal conditions, the cells are so closely connected by tight junctions that only lipid-soluble drugs can pass through (Fig. 16–5).

The extent of ionization of a drug also affects absorption. A drug that is ionized carries a positive or negative charge and therefore cannot cross cell membranes. The degree of ionization of a drug depends on the pH of the fluid in which it is dis-

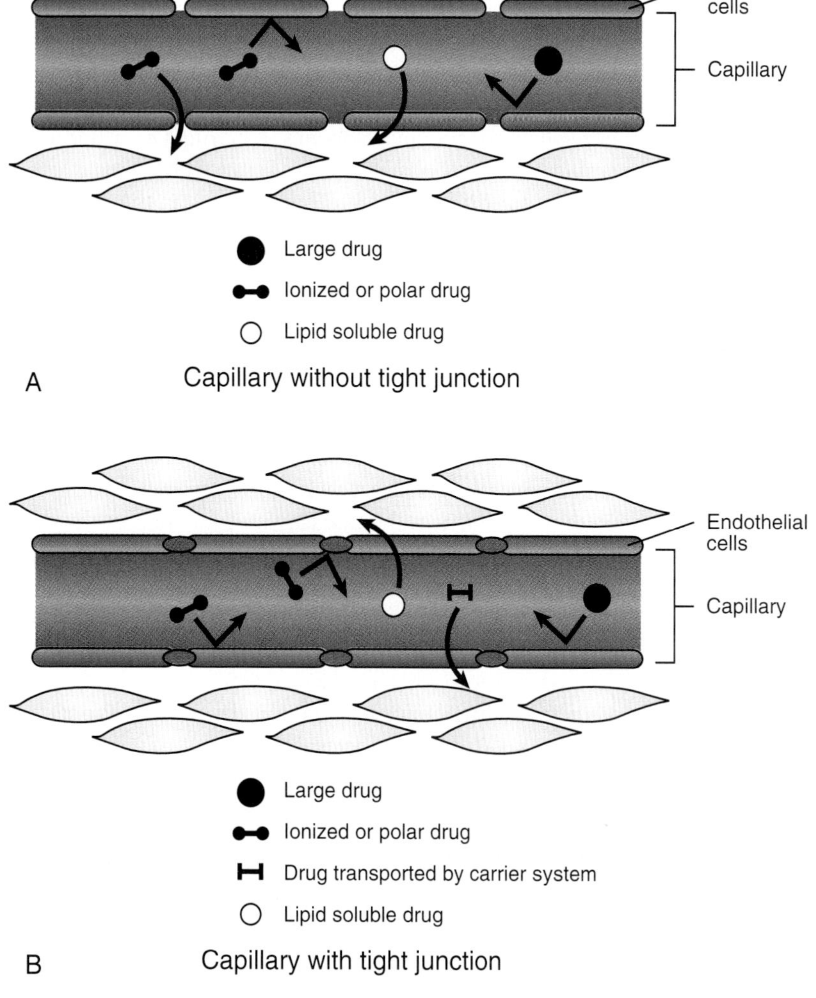

Figure 16–5. Absorption of drugs. **A**, In capillaries without tight junctions, drugs can be absorbed by passing around cells. **B**, In capillaries with tight junctions, drugs can pass out of the vasculature only if they are lipid soluble or are carried by a protein-mediated transport system.

solved. Acid drugs are more ionized in a basic environment, and basic drugs are more ionized in an acid environment. As a result, it can be predicted that altering the pH of the gut with an antacid would alter the extent of drug absorption.

A large molecule that is charged or very polar (a molecule is polar if the electronic charges are unevenly distributed throughout the structure) does not diffuse through a biologic membrane. However, some drugs that cannot diffuse through cell membranes may be shuttled across by specific protein-mediated transport systems.

In addition to the factors described here, absorption also depends on the formulation of the drug, the site of administration, and the health of the patient. For example, for drugs given orally, the rate of absorption from fastest to slowest is solutions, powders, capsules, tablets, and sustained-release preparations. Other factors such as the retention time of the drug in the gastrointestinal tract, the number of viable absorbing cells, the presence of food or other drugs, and gastric and intestinal blood flow can also affect absorption.

The rate of absorption of drugs from injection sites is affected by similar factors. A subcutaneous or intramuscular injection is affected by its formulation. A drug dissolved in oil is absorbed more slowly than if it were dissolved in water or saline. Greater blood flow at the site of injection increases rate of absorption. The muscles that are used for intramuscular injection have different degrees of blood flow, with the deltoid being highest, the quadriceps femoris next highest, and the gluteus maximus lowest. An injection mistakenly deposited in fat rather than muscle is absorbed more slowly, because fat has a lower blood supply. A medication administered subcutaneously to a patient in shock may not be absorbed at all because of decreased blood flow to the skin.

As previously described, factors that increase or decrease drug absorption increase or decrease, respectively, the steady-state plasma drug concentration. When assessing a patient in whom a drug did not produce the desired outcome or caused an unpredicted adverse reaction, the nurse should consider the possibility that drug absorption was altered and ask herself or himself the following questions:

- Has the pH of the gut been altered by disease, aging, use of antacids, or tube feedings?
- Does the patient have normal gastrointestinal retention times, or is retention time altered by vomiting or diarrhea or drugs that affect gastrointestinal motility (e.g., laxatives, opiates, or anticholinergics)?
- Has the surface area of the gut that is available for drug absorption been altered by disease or surgery?
- Has blood flow to the gastrointestinal tract or site of administration been compromised?
- Is it possible that two drugs or drugs and food are interacting in the gut, rendering a drug nonabsorbable?
- Has the drug been administered by the route that was ordered?

Changing the dose, timing, or route of drug administration could be used to correct the situation.

FIRST-PASS OR PRESYSTEMIC METABOLISM/ BIOTRANSFORMATION

A drug that has been absorbed from the gastrointestinal tract goes directly to the liver before it reaches the systemic circulation for distribution to the rest of the body. As the drug goes through the liver, an elaborate enzyme system called the mixed-function oxidase system, or P450 enzymes, causes "first-pass" metabolism. These enzymes can metabolize a portion of the drug into an inactive form before it reaches the general circulatory system for distribution to the receptor site. Obviously, for drugs that have significant first-pass metabolism to an inactive form, a greater dosage is required to produce a therapeutic effect. Though it is less common, some drugs can be converted from an inactive form to an active form by first-pass metabolism.

Liver blood flow and liver function are the major factors that determine the extent of first-pass drug metabolism. Therefore, the availability of drug for distribution after absorption can be altered by these factors. If, for example, a patient has hepatitis or alcoholic cirrhosis, the nurse should be able to predict that the plasma concentration of a drug that undergoes substantial first-pass metabolism would be altered. Thus, the nurse should question an order for the administration of a standard dose of drug to any patient with severe liver dysfunction.

PLASMA PROTEIN BINDING

In the blood, a drug is either free (in solution) or bound to plasma proteins, such as albumin. Regardless of the total plasma drug concentration, the fraction of free drug is kept constant by plasma protein binding (Fig. 16–6A). This phenomenon is very important because only the free or unbound drug can be distributed to its site of action or be metabolized and eliminated (Fig. 16–7). As a result, plasma protein binding lessens the intensity of drug action but lengthens the duration of action.

Binding of drugs to plasma proteins is reversible. A drug constantly associates and dissociates from the protein. Each drug has a different affinity for plasma proteins. For drugs that bind with high affinity, the percentage of free drug is low. For drugs that bind with low affinity, the percentage of free drug is high. Information about the percent binding of drugs to plasma proteins can be found in various sources, such as the *Hospital Formulary*, the *Physicians' Desk Reference*, and drug package inserts. It is important to note that when a plasma drug level is drawn in the clinical setting, the value for the plasma drug concentration includes both bound and free drug.

Plasma protein levels and the affinity of plasma proteins for drugs can differ among individuals. Protein binding can also differ over time in one individual. Decreased plasma protein–drug binding may be caused by extremes of age, liver disease, malnutrition, or kidney diseases that cause loss of plasma proteins in the urine. The presence of other drugs competing for the same binding site on the protein can result in decreased binding for one of the drugs, because a drug that

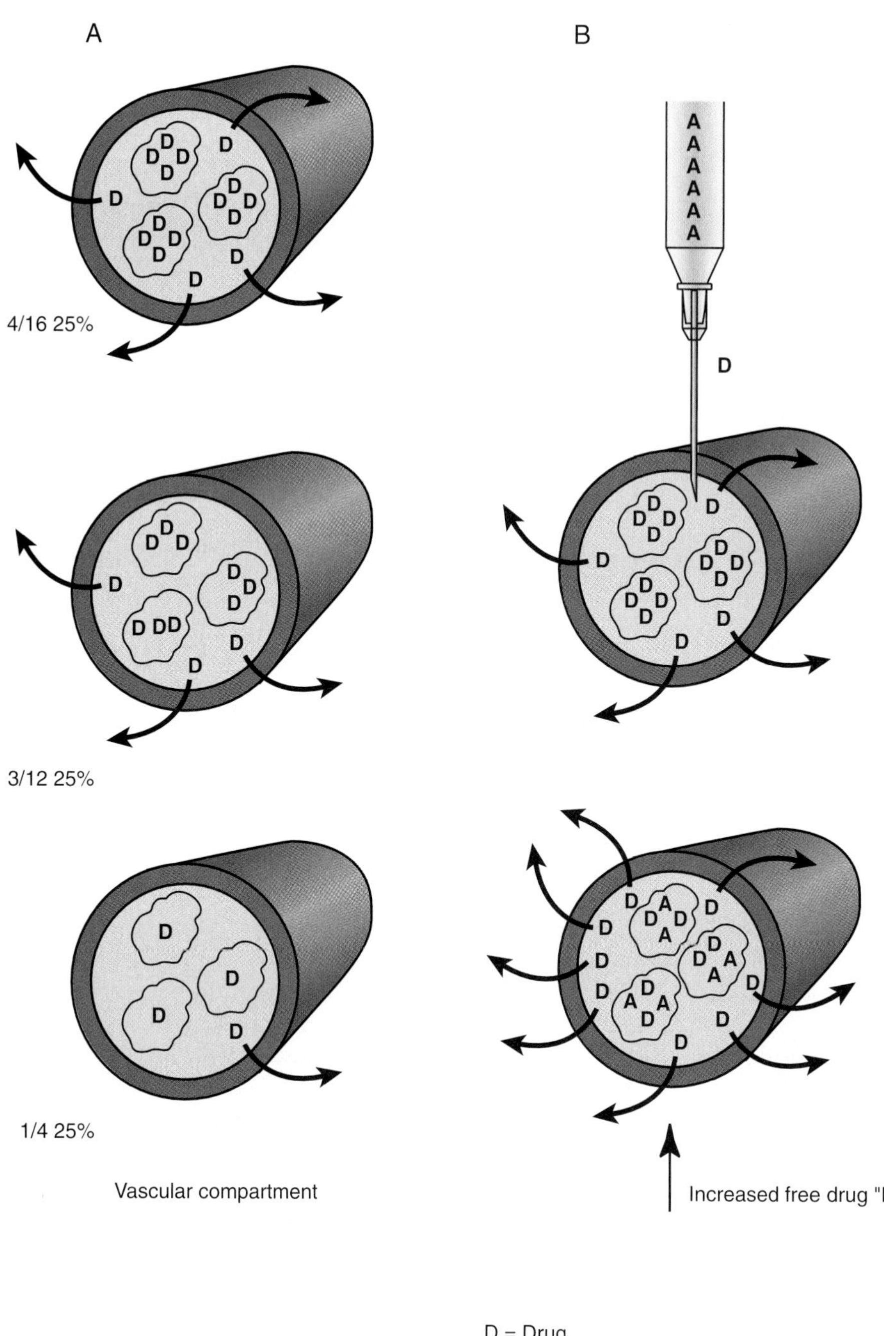

Figure 16–6. **A**, Plasma protein binding. Binding to plasma proteins decreases the intensity and prolongs the action of drugs. The ratio of bound to free drug remains constant regardless of the total amount of drug in the plasma. The ratio in the figure represents free drug/total drug. D = drug. **B**, Drug displacement. Drugs with high plasma protein binding affinity (*A*) can displace other drugs (*D*) from plasma proteins.

binds with higher affinity can displace a drug with lower affinity (see Fig. 16–6B). As previously mentioned, only free drug can be distributed to its site of action, metabolized, and excreted. Thus, because rates of distribution and elimination influence steady-state plasma drug concentration, any change in plasma protein binding could change steady-state drug levels. Moreover, any alteration that increases the fraction of unbound drug could amplify the action of a drug or increase the risk for adverse drug effect. The nurse should recognize the greater risk of adverse drug reactions when, for instance, a standard dose of drug is to be administered to a malnourished, elderly patient with liver or kidney problems who is already on multiple medications.

DISTRIBUTION

To reach a target organ and receptor site outside of the blood vessels, a drug must diffuse between cells and across cell membranes. A drug can be distributed to tissues where it has a therapeutic effect but can also be distributed to tissues where it has no effect. Factors that govern the distribution of drugs out of the plasma and into tissues are the very same

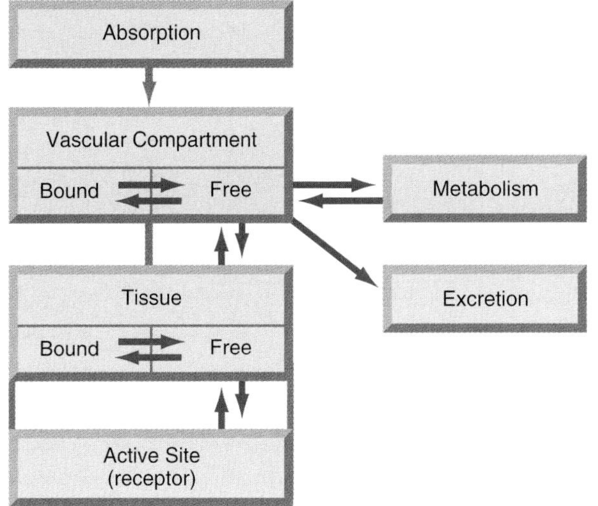

Figure 16–7. Basic pharmacokinetics. Once the drug reaches the circulation, only the fraction not bound to plasma proteins (free drug) is distributed to the active site or metabolized and excreted. At the active site, free drug elicits a response by interacting with a receptor. (From Schwertz, D.S., Buschmann, M.B. (1989). Pharmacogeriatrics. Critical Care Nursing Quarterly, 12, (1) p 28, with permission of Aspen Publishers, Inc., © 1989.)

ones that influence absorption of drugs from the site of administration. In addition, plasma protein binding influences distribution because if a drug is very tightly bound to plasma proteins, very little leaves the systemic circulation.

In general, if a single dose of drug is administered rapidly into the intravascular compartment, plasma drug concentration initially is high and then decreases over time. As shown in Figure 16–8, plasma drug concentration falls very quickly as the drug mixes in the intravascular space. Following mixing, the drug is distributed to the tissues (the alpha phase). Later, plasma drug concentration falls slowly as it is eliminated from the body (the beta phase).

Drug concentration is not the same in every tissue. Drug concentration reaches an equilibrium in some tissues more rapidly than in others. The initial phase of drug distribution primarily depends on cardiac output and regional blood flow. Assuming that a drug can diffuse across cell membranes and through other barriers rapidly, tissues having the highest blood flow rates (heart, liver, kidney, and brain) receive the greatest amount of drug first. Reasonably, therapeutic drug levels also are reached earlier in these tissues. Drugs distribute to tissues with lower blood flow rates (fat, skin, bone, and resting muscle) more slowly, and the drug concentration also comes to equilibrium in these tissues more slowly. Conversely, tissues with high rates of blood flow are cleared of a drug faster, whereas tissues with lower perfusion rates retain the drug longer.

Distribution of drug to the brain and cerebrospinal fluid is unique and warrants some discussion. The endothelial cells lining the capillaries that supply the brain have tight junctions rather than the loose junctions that are characteristic of most other capillary endothelium. These tight junctions greatly impede the diffusion of many substances, hence giving rise to the term *the blood-brain barrier.* Only drugs that are extremely small or highly lipid soluble penetrate the blood-brain barrier with relative ease. The rate of delivery of highly lipid soluble drugs to the central nervous system is limited only by cerebral blood flow. The blood-brain barrier serves to protect the brain from some compounds that may have toxic effects. On the other hand, it can limit the access of important drugs such as antibiotics. Permeability of the blood-brain barrier can be variable, with greater permeability occurring in babies, in the elderly, and during meningeal inflammation.

Some tissues act as drug reservoirs. For example, lipid-soluble drugs can be trapped in fat, and tetracycline is trapped in bone. The concentration of drug in a tissue reservoir is in equilibrium with the concentration of drug in the plasma. As a result, as the plasma concentration of a drug declines, drug "trickles out" of the reservoir, thus maintaining the plasma concentration. This may result in a prolonged drug effect. If the capacity of the reservoir is large and uptake is rapid, the drug is delivered to the reservoir first, and a large

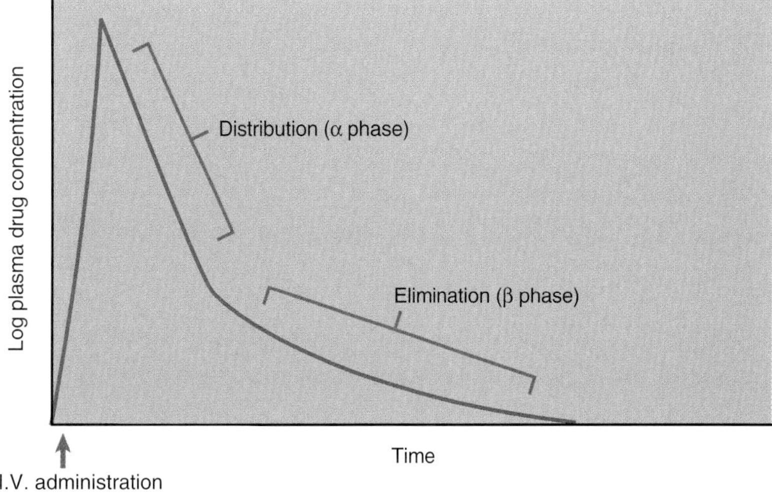

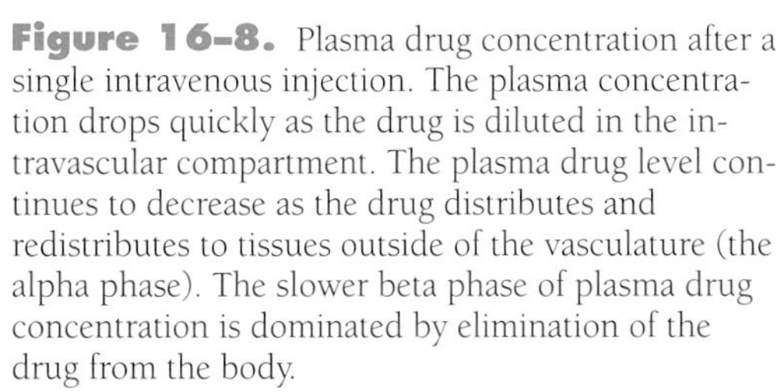

Figure 16–8. Plasma drug concentration after a single intravenous injection. The plasma concentration drops quickly as the drug is diluted in the intravascular compartment. The plasma drug level continues to decrease as the drug distributes and redistributes to tissues outside of the vasculature (the alpha phase). The slower beta phase of plasma drug concentration is dominated by elimination of the drug from the body.

dose may be needed to fill the reservoir before sufficient drug distribution to the site of action can occur. In this case, distribution of a drug into the reservoir can delay onset of drug action.

As defined previously, the term *volume of distribution* describes the extent of drug distribution throughout the body. Volume of distribution can be conceptualized as the body compartment(s) such as blood (intravascular fluid) or total body water in which a drug is apparently dissolved. A volume of distribution of 40 to 50 L indicates that the drug is distributed throughout the total body water (the total volume of body water is approximately 42 L in an adult). A volume of distribution of approximately 5 L would suggest that the drug did not leave the vascular compartment (the intravascular volume is approximately 5 L in an adult). Information about the volume of distribution of drugs can be found in such sources as the *Physicians' Desk Reference* and *Hospital Drug Formulary*. However, in these references, the volume of distribution usually is given in liters per kilogram of body weight.

Differences among patients in the apparent volume of distribution of a drug alter the steady-state plasma drug concentration and thereby alter the therapeutic or toxic response. If the maintenance dose and dose interval of a drug remain the same, the larger the volume of distribution, the lower the steady-state plasma concentration of a drug (see formula in Box 16–1). As an example, drug distribution changes across the life span. Body water is approximately 77 percent of total body mass in the infant and about 60 percent in the adult and is even lower in the elderly. Even if a drug is administered on a dose-per-body-weight ratio, the volume of distribution of the drug is different in each of these age groups. Not only does the total body water decrease with aging but, from age 20 to age 65, extracellular fluid decreases by about 40 percent (Seller, 1989).

Other changes in the elderly that influence drug distribution are a decrease in cardiac output, an increase in fat-to-total-body-weight ratio, and a drop in plasma protein concentration (Garattini, 1985; Pucino et al, 1985; Vestal and Cusack, 1990). An increase in body fat increases the volume of distribution of a lipid-soluble drug, and, conversely, a decrease in body water decreases the volume of distribution of a more water-soluble drug. These factors, as well as changes in regional blood flow, nutritional status, hydration, and specific disease states affect drug distribution.

At the other end of the age spectrum, during the first few days of life, the distribution of body water shifts radically from the extracellular to the intracellular compartment. The effect on drug distribution can be dramatic.

METABOLISM

Metabolism refers to the body's ability to change a drug from its original form to a more water-soluble and more readily excreted form. This process may also be referred to as *biotransformation.*

Elimination of drugs from the body usually requires chemical alteration of the drug by enzymatic reactions. This process usually inactivates the drug, though, more rarely, metabolism of a drug can activate it (e.g., enalapril). Metabolism can take place in the kidney, lungs, plasma, and most cells; however, the most significant biotransformation of drugs takes place in the liver.

Drug metabolism proceeds through two phases. The first phase is catalyzed by the mixed-function oxidase enzyme system (P450 enzymes) in the liver. The mixed-function oxidase enzymes either inactivate the drug or prepare it to undergo further phase 2 reactions. Phase 2 reactions are referred to as conjugation reactions. In these reactions, a chemical moiety, such as glucuronate, becomes linked to the drug. Phase 2 reactions almost always result in inactivation of a drug and an increased rate of excretion.

The half-life of a drug is the time it takes to eliminate 50 percent of the drug from the body. The half-life of a drug is directly proportional to the volume of drug distribution and inversely proportional to drug clearance. In other words, if the volume of distribution increases, then the drug half-life is longer. If the clearance of a drug increases, then the half-life is shorter (see Box 16–2).

To understand the relationship between drug half-life and clearance, the concept of drug clearance requires further clarification. Drug clearance refers to the volume of plasma that is freed (cleared) of a drug within a certain time. The greater the volume of plasma that is freed of the drug within a unit of time, the "faster" the clearance. Clearance is dependent on both metabolism and excretion. Factors that decrease the rate of metabolism decrease drug clearance, and factors that increase the rate of metabolism increase drug clearance. From the previous discussion of the apparent volume of distribution, one can instinctively see that the more extensively a drug is distributed, the longer it takes to eliminate the drug from the body.

Exposure to certain substances, such as *chronic* alcohol consumption, environmental pollutants, tobacco smoke, and certain types of drugs, increases the amount and activity of enzymes involved in phase 1 metabolizing reactions. Induction of these enzymes shortens the half-life of many drugs and thus decreases the steady-state plasma concentration. Thus, mixed-function oxidase enzyme induction should be considered in the case of an alcoholic patient when therapeutic failure occurs at the usual maintenance dose and dosing interval of a drug.

The rate of drug metabolism may be decreased by exposure to certain other drugs and by *acute* alcohol exposure. Other factors that reduce the rate of metabolism are decreased

BOX 16–2
DRUG HALF-LIFE

$$t\,½ = \frac{(c)\,(vd)}{Cl}$$

c = constant
vd = volume of distribution
Cl = clearance

hepatic blood flow or decreased hepatic function. Such changes are commonly seen in the elderly patient. A decreased rate of drug metabolism is also characteristic of newborns, in whom both phase 1 and phase 2 drug reactions are greatly reduced. Inadequate metabolism in newborns contributes to hyperbilirubinemia (jaundice caused by a decreased rate of metabolism of hemoglobin degradation products) and to an increased risk of adverse drug effects.

Another factor that has been shown to reduce the efficiency of drug inactivation through metabolism is malnutrition. Malnutrition decreases the activities of drug-metabolizing enzymes and decreases the availability of substances used in phase 2 conjugation reactions (e.g., glutathione). In elderly populations, it has been documented that malnutrition contributed to the toxicity of paracetamol and halothane (Parke, 1985).

One of the most important factors influencing the rate of drug metabolism and therefore drug clearance is genetic variability of drug metabolizing enzymes. Subgroups of patients have been identified that transform certain drugs very slowly or very rapidly compared with the normal population. A classic example involves metabolism of the muscle relaxant succinylcholine. One in 2000 Caucasians has an atypical form of the plasma enzyme cholinesterase, which is responsible for succinylcholine inactivation (Vessel, 1983). Whereas intravenous administration of succinylcholine normally produces paralysis for several minutes, a patient with the atypical enzyme may remain paralyzed for over 1 hour. If a patient has a history of abnormal metabolism of one drug, it should be suspected that there is a high risk for abnormal metabolism of other drugs and a high risk for adverse drug reactions. Taking a good drug history can uncover such potential risks.

ELIMINATION/EXCRETION

Drugs may be eliminated in bile, sweat, saliva, and breast milk, and through the lungs; however, renal excretion is by far the most important route of drug elimination. Drugs can be excreted unchanged or metabolized to compounds that are more water-soluble metabolites. The balance between elimination and absorption is reflected in the steady-state plasma drug concentration. Clearly, if elimination decreases and absorption continues, the drug accumulates and the risk for adverse effects increases.

Renal clearance of drugs takes place by glomerular filtration and active tubular secretion. In general, the rate of renal excretion of a drug depends on the degree of plasma protein binding, blood flow to the kidney, and the glomerular filtration rate. Once the drug enters the nephron by filtration from the plasma, it is either excreted in the urine or can be reabsorbed back into the plasma. The rate of passive reabsorption of drugs from renal tubules is influenced by the same factors that influence absorption of drugs (e.g., lipid solubility, pH of the urine).

Several factors such as decreased renal blood flow or loss of kidney function can influence the rate of drug elimination. For drugs that are secreted into the tubules by carrier-mediated transport, more than one drug can compete for the same transport system, thereby resulting in a decrease in the rate of excretion of one or more of the drugs. A decline in the rate of elimination causes delayed drug clearance and an increase in the half-life of a drug. If all other factors remain constant, an increase in half-life increases the steady-state plasma drug concentration. Therefore, it is important to know whether the kidneys are functioning well before administering a drug. One laboratory test that is a good indicator of renal function is creatinine clearance. The rate of clearance of this endogenous muscle protein approximates the glomerular filtration rate. A decrease in this parameter predicts that the renal clearance of most drugs will also be reduced.

Renal function is less efficient in the elderly and newborn. Renal blood flow and glomerular filtration rate are lower at birth than in the adult and decrease as much as 50% between age 30 and age 80 (Wilkinson, 1983). In the elderly, an age-dependent loss of functional nephrons also occurs (Abrams, 1985). Conditions such as dehydration or kidney disease may be superimposed on age-related changes in kidney function, thereby further compromising renal excretion of drugs. Impaired renal function should always be considered a warning sign for increased risk of adverse drug effects.

In summary, the effect of a drug is dependent on the concentration of drug at its receptor site, and in most cases this is related to the plasma concentration of the drug. Pharmacokinetic factors such as rates and extent of absorption, distribution, metabolism, and excretion influence plasma drug concentration. Clearly, there can be differences in these pharmacokinetic factors between individuals and over time in one individual. It is the responsibility of the nurse to carefully assess the patient before and during the administration of drugs to avoid therapeutic failure or the occurrence of unacceptable adverse drug effects.

Monitoring plasma drug levels is one aspect of assessment of drug effect, and observation of the patient is another. When individual differences in pharmacokinetic factors (and the pharmacodynamic factors presented next) result in unpredicted plasma drug levels or drug response, the dose or the dosing interval can be modified to achieve a target steady-state plasma drug concentration. Decreasing the maintenance dose causes the steady-state concentration to fall, and increasing the dose causes a rise in steady-state drug level. Shortening or lengthening the dose interval increases or decreases plasma drug concentration, respectively.

Increasing the dosing interval is sometimes desirable because it may improve compliance. However, this maneuver has the disadvantage of exaggerating the fluctuation in plasma drug level, which could increase the risk of adverse drug effects (see Fig. 16–4). Prolonged-release or timed-release preparations, if available, may help solve this problem. In the final analysis, each patient requires individual assessment to design a drug regimen that will provide an optimal therapeutic response.

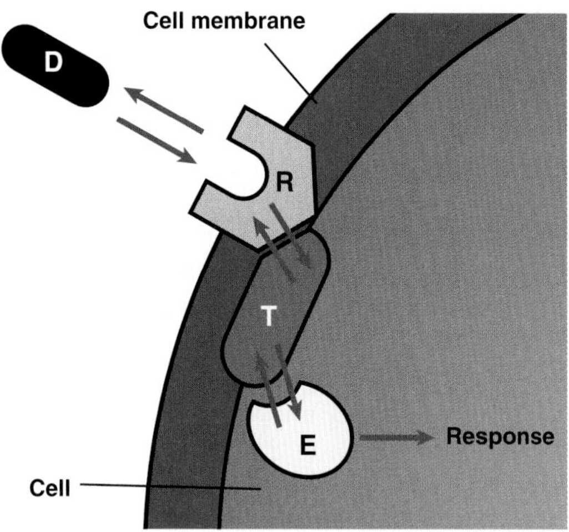

Figure 16–9. Components of a signal transduction system: D, drug; E, effector; R, receptor; T, transducer.

PHARMACODYNAMICS

Pharmacodynamics is the study of the mechanism by which a drug exerts an effect once it reaches its site of action. Usually the effect is mediated by the interaction of a drug with its receptor. However, in a few instances, drugs can exert an effect in a nonspecific manner, such as altering the cell's physical or chemical environment (e.g., an antacid changing the gastric pH). This section focuses on drug effects that are elicited by drug/receptor interactions.

DRUG RECEPTORS AND SIGNAL TRANSDUCTION

A receptor is a functional macromolecule located on the cell surface or within the cell. Binding of a drug to a receptor initiates events that lead to a cellular response. Drug-receptor interactions require a high degree of structural specificity. That is, the drug must fit its receptor exactly, in the same manner that a key fits into a lock.

A drug can be thought of as a messenger that carries a specific signal or a command to the cell. Binding of the drug to the receptor initiates a cascade of biochemical events that results in a change in cell function. This process, starting with drug-receptor binding and ending with a cellular response, is referred to as signal transduction. There are many types of signal transduction systems, but they all have three common components: a receptor, a transducer, and an effector (Fig. 16–9).

Figures 16–9 and 16–10 depict the signal transduction components for a drug that is very water soluble and binds to a cell surface receptor. The example shown in Figure 16–10 is a beta-adrenergic receptor. This receptor is associated with a transducer called a guanine nucleotide–binding protein (G protein) and an enzymatic effector system. When a drug such as isoproterenol (Isuprel) occupies the receptor, the signal is communicated through the G protein to an intracellular

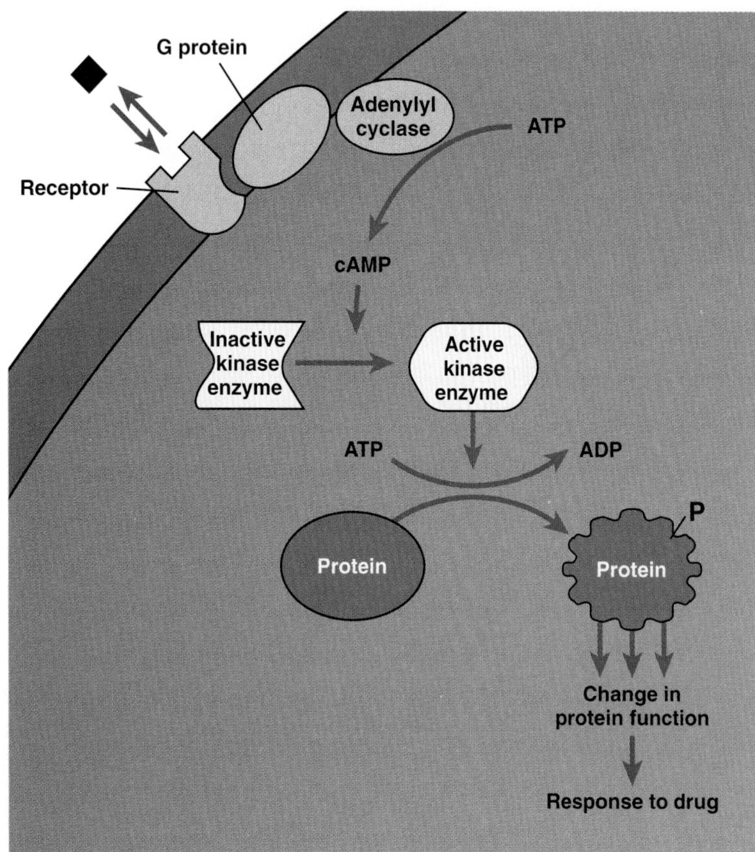

Figure 16–10. Signal transduction system at the beta-adrenergic receptor. (See text for description.) Black, drug; pink, receptor; blue, transducer; yellow, effectors.

enzyme called adenylyl cyclase. This enzyme converts adenosine triphosphate into cyclic adenosine monophosphate (cAMP). cAMP acts as a second messenger within the cell that activates another enzyme called a kinase. The kinase phosphorylates (adds a phosphate group to) proteins, which changes the protein's function and leads to a cellular response to the drug.

When the receptor is located inside the cell (and can only be reached by a drug that can cross the cell membrane), a variant of signal transduction is activated. For example, the drug dexamethasone binds to an intracellular receptor (Fig. 16–11). This drug-receptor complex, which now acts as a second messenger, moves into the nucleus and binds to specific sites in the DNA that regulate gene expression and thereby the rate of synthesis of certain cellular proteins. Thus, the information or the "signal" that is carried by the drug is translated into a cellular response.

There are many variations on the receptor/transducer/effector model of signal transduction. Currently, research on signal transduction mechanisms is one of the fastest developing areas in the biomedical sciences. Part of the importance of understanding signal transduction mechanisms lies in the role that "post-receptor" events (events that occur after a drug binds to a receptor) play in the modulation of drug response. For example, a fairly recent advance has been the understanding that extracellular signals, such as drugs, can actually tell the cell to activate or inhibit the expression of specific genes. It has also become clear that genetically defined differences in the proteins involved in signal transduction pathways can alter an individual's response to drugs. Finally, postreceptor events are involved in increasing or decreasing the number of cellular receptors. This change in receptor number can cause sensitization or desensitization to the effects of drugs.

CHARACTERISTICS OF DRUG RECEPTOR BINDING

It has already been stated that the maximal response to a drug is limited by the number of receptor sites available for drug interaction. Therefore, drug-receptor binding is saturable. Once the receptors are all occupied, a maximal therapeutic effect is elicited (refer to Fig. 16–2A). Any further increase in drug concentration at the receptor site does not produce a greater therapeutic effect but may cause an increase in toxic effects. In other words, because a prescribed amount of drug produces a good therapeutic response does not mean that more drug is better. In fact, more may be toxic. Based on this principle, it is important to teach patients that they should not take more than the prescribed dosage of drug.

With few exceptions, drug-receptor binding is reversible. Imagine that the drug is bouncing on and off the receptor instead of sticking to it permanently. The rates at which a drug associates and dissociates from the receptor are not necessarily equal. The ratio of the dissociation rate to the association rate is a measure of drug affinity for the receptor. A drug has a high affinity for its receptor when the association rate is high or the dissociation rate is low. In contrast, a drug has a low

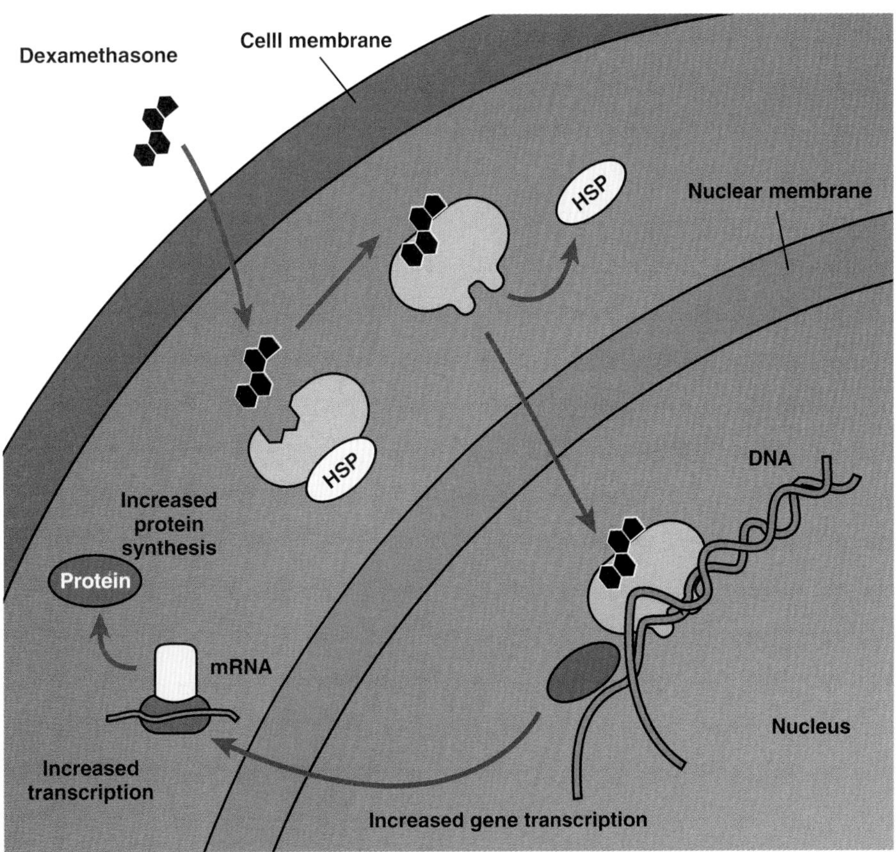

Figure 16–11. Signal transduction system for the glucocorticoid drug dexamethasone. (See text for description.) Black, drug; pink, receptor; blue, transducer; yellow, effectors.

affinity for its receptor if the association rate is low or the dissociation rate is high.

More than one drug can have affinity for the same receptor. Therefore, more than one drug can compete for binding to the same receptor. If two competing drugs are at the same concentration in the vicinity of the receptor, the one with the highest affinity occupies the most receptors. The clinical importance of these concepts of reversibility of drug binding and affinity of the drug for the receptor is clearly illustrated following a discussion of the intensity of drug effect.

INTENSITY OF DRUG EFFECT

The intensity of drug response is related to the number of receptor sites for the drug, the concentration of the drug at the receptor site, the affinity of the drug for the receptor, and another factor referred to as efficacy. *Efficacy* describes the relative ability of a drug to elicit a response once it is bound to the receptor. If two drugs bind to a receptor with the same affinity and are at the same concentration but one drug elicits a greater effect than the other, then the drug producing the greater response can be said to have greater efficacy. The concept of efficacy helps to explain the actions of agonist, antagonist, and partial agonist drugs.

Drugs that bind to a receptor and elicit a maximal possible response are called full agonists. Drugs that bind to a receptor and inhibit the action of an agonist are called antagonists. An antagonist has no ability to produce a response at the receptor by itself. In other words, while an agonist can be thought of as having an efficacy of "1", an antagonist has an efficacy of zero. Like the agonist, binding of most antagonists is reversible. When both an agonist and an antagonist are at the receptor site, they compete for receptor occupancy. The final response depends on the concentration of the agonist and the antagonist, as well as the affinities of the two drugs for the receptor.

The clinical importance of the reversibility of drug binding and differential affinities of drugs for the same receptor can be illustrated using the example of an agonist and an antagonist. The ability of the antagonist naloxone to reverse the effects of morphine is based on the reversible nature of drug-receptor binding and the fact that naloxone has a higher affinity for the opioid receptor than morphine. In the presence of an overdose of morphine, naloxone successfully competes for the opioid receptor and displaces morphine but has no efficacy of its own. Thus, the response to morphine is decreased or terminated.

A partial agonist is a drug that produces a less-than-maximal response even when it occupies all of the available receptors. Therefore, a partial agonist has an efficacy between 1 and 0. Because receptor binding is reversible, a partial agonist and a full agonist can compete for the same receptors. In the presence of a partial agonist, the response to the full agonist is reduced. The final observed response depends on the concentrations of the two drugs, the comparative affinities of the drugs for the receptor, and the efficacy of the partial agonist. Unlike the situation in which an antagonist might compete so successfully for the available receptors that the response to the agonist drops to zero, the response never drops to zero in the presence of an agonist and a partial agonist. This is because, unlike the antagonist, the partial agonist possesses at least some inherent efficacy.

The term *potency* is used to distinguish among a series of drugs that bind to the same receptor and produce the same response. The drug in the series that induces 50 percent of maximal effect at the lowest concentration would be considered the most potent, whereas the drug that requires the highest concentration to produce 50 percent of maximal effect would be the least potent. In the clinical situation, we say that one drug is more potent than another because it takes less drug to elicit the same response. Potency depends on the relative affinities and efficacies of the two drugs, as well as pharmacokinetic factors. However, the absolute potency of a drug may not be an important factor when choosing which drug to administer, because an equipotent dose (i.e., a higher dose) of the "weaker" drug could be administered. An equipotent dose of the weaker drug could be less expensive than the "stronger" drug, which could be an advantage. On the other hand, low potency would be disadvantageous if the equipotent dose of the weaker drug had more unwanted adverse effects at the therapeutic dose.

MODULATION OF RECEPTOR NUMBER

The number of cellular receptors available for drug binding is not static but varies over time. In addition, the number of certain types of receptors also differs from individual to individual. Because one of the factors that regulates intensity of drug response is receptor number, a decrease in receptor number (downregulation) would be expected to reduce the maximal effect of a drug. Conversely, an increase in receptor number (upregulation) would augment the maximal drug response. Previous exposure to a drug may change the number of receptors for that drug. Disease states, such as some forms of insulin-resistant diabetes and myasthenia gravis, have been attributed to a loss of functional receptors. The number of receptors for several neurotransmitters in the brain also has been shown to change with aging (Severson, 1984). This age-dependent pharmacodynamic alteration, as well as pharmacokinetic changes in the elderly, may account for the documented increased sensitivity to drugs that act in the central nervous system (Roberts and Turner, 1988).

A supersensitive response to an agonist may occur after a period of reduced receptor stimulation or after exposure to an antagonist. This effect is due, at least in part, to an upregulation of receptors. An example of this phenomenon is the rebound hypertension that sometimes occurs following discontinuation of a beta-adrenergic agonist (Frishman, 1983). In this case, in the presence of the antagonist, beta-adrenergic receptors become upregulated. When the antagonist is removed, endogenous agonists (such as catecholamines) bind to the receptors and produce an exaggerated response (hypertension).

Other inter- and intraindividual pharmacodynamic differences that affect drug response have been documented. For example, beta-adrenergic–mediated responses in the heart (increased heart rate and increased contractile force) are attenuated in the elderly. Evidence suggests this decreased response to beta-adrenergic agonists (isoproterenol) (Vestal et al, 1979) and antagonists (propranolol) (Kendall et al, 1982) are related to age-dependent alterations in postreceptor events (i.e., signal transduction and formation of second messengers). The adaptive desensitization response to various drugs has also been shown to be impaired in older animals (Garattini, 1985). For another example, acute and chronic alcohol consumption alter signal transduction through several pathways in many tissues (Hoek et al, 1992). Changes in these pathways in response to alcohol could theoretically influence the response to many drugs.

The Royal College of Physicians cites altered pharmacodynamics and pharmacokinetics as major factors contributing to the high rate of occurrence of adverse drug reactions in elderly patients. Inadequate clinical assessment is another factor (Abrams, 1985). Understanding the principles of pharmacokinetics and pharmacodynamics is always useful in assessing and predicting a patient's response to drugs.

HOMEOSTATIC RESERVE

A patient's response to a drug is influenced by another factor called homeostatic reserve. Homeostatic reserve refers to the sum of the body's compensatory mechanisms that act to maintain important physiologic parameters, such as temperature or blood pressure, within certain limits. When a parameter like blood pressure is outside of a specific range, feedback systems such as the baroreceptor reflex are activated to bring blood pressure back within limits.

Drugs often elicit physiologic responses that perturb homeostatic systems and activate feedback loops. If the feedback loop is intact, a cascade of compensatory mechanisms blunts the primary drug action, thus protecting the patient from experiencing a dangerously intense drug reaction. For example, if a drug induces vasodilation by relaxing vascular smooth muscle cells, blood pressure drops. As a result, the baroreceptor reflex increases cardiac output and stimulates vasoconstriction, which tends to bring the blood pressure back up and prevents the patient from experiencing severe hypotension. However, in the elderly, baroreceptor function is decreased (McGarry et al, 1975), and drugs such as direct-acting vasodilators can cause the blood pressure to drop precipitously.

Polypharmacy (the concurrent consumption of many drugs) can be associated with a decrease in homeostatic reserve. This can occur when one drug blocks the feedback loop that is recruited when another drug exerts a primary physiologic effect. For example, normally when the drug hydralazine decreases peripheral vascular resistance and blood pressure drops, the sympathetic nervous system reflexively increases heart rate and offsets the drop in blood pressure. However, if the patient is taking a beta-adrenergic antagonist, the reflex tachycardia (increased heart rate) is blocked, and the response to hydralazine is augmented. Polypharmacy is most common in the elderly and is one of the major causes of adverse drug reactions in this population (Lamy, 1986; LeSage, 1991).

This is just one example of a drug interaction that could potentially lead to an adverse drug reaction. There are many types of drug interactions, ranging from drug incompatibility within an intravenous drug line to pharmacokinetic and pharmacodynamic interactions. Thorough knowledge of potential drug interactions is extremely important. However, review of this subject is beyond the scope of this chapter. The reader is referred to LeSage (1991) and to the extensive list of references included in that publication.

THERAPEUTIC INDEX–ADVERSE DRUG REACTIONS

Dose-response curves are used to evaluate drug risks and benefits. For example, consider two pain medications, A and B. Drug A reduces pain more dramatically than drug B. However, at effective doses, drug A has severe adverse effects. On the other hand, drug B has no adverse effects at effective doses. Clearly, the risk of using drug A outweighs the benefits, and drug B is the better choice.

The relative safety of drugs can be ranked by a value called the therapeutic index (TI). *The therapeutic index is determined using laboratory animals. This index is defined as a ratio of the dose that is lethal in 50 percent of the sample of animals (e.g., mice) that are treated (LD_{50}) to the dose that is effective in 50 percent of the animal population. More practically, the therapeutic index may be calculated as ratio of* the dose at which 50 percent of patients taking a drug achieve a defined therapeutic effect (ED_{50}), to the dose at which 50 percent of the patients taking the drug experience a defined adverse or toxic effect (TD_{50}).

$$TI = LD_{50}/ED_{50} \quad TI = \frac{\text{lethal dose in 50\% of the animals}}{\text{effective dose in 50\% of the animals}}$$

$$TI = TD_{50}/ED_{50} \quad TI = \frac{\text{toxic dose in 50\% of patients}}{\text{effective dose in 50\% of patients}}$$

To determine the TI for a drug, *cumulative* dose-response curves are generated (Fig. 16–12). This is done by determining the number of persons who will respond to a drug at a given dose. These cumulative dose-response curves are done for both a defined *therapeutic* endpoint and a defined *toxic* or *adverse* endpoint. The lower the TI is, the higher the risk for an adverse drug effect. In Figure 16–12, drug X has a greater TI (5) than drug Y (1.5); therefore, drug X is considered to be safer.

Individuals vary in their response to a drug dose. Clinicians use past research and experience to order an appropriate drug dose. However, soon after the drug regimen is initiated, the patient's response should be evaluated, and the dose should be adjusted as necessary. It is important to remember that each individual can have a different response to a drug and

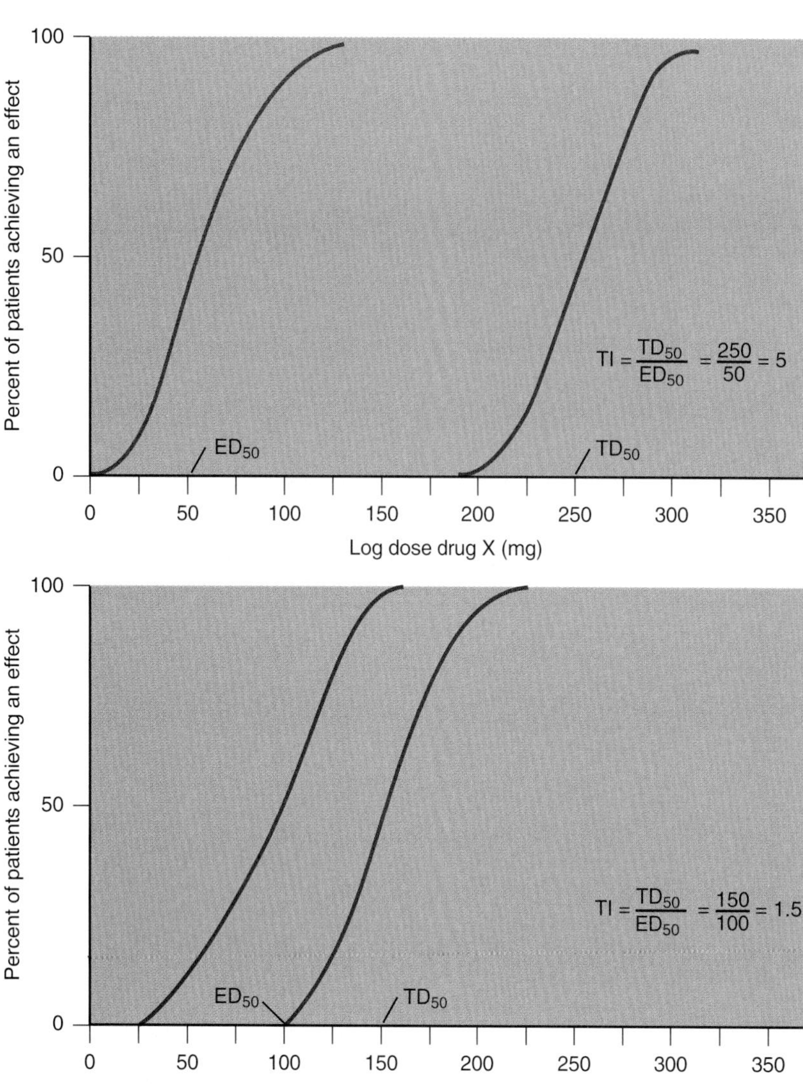

Figure 16-12. The therapeutic index, a measure of drug safety. The ED_{50} is the effective dose in 50 percent of the test population. The TD_{50} is the toxic dose in 50 percent of the test population.

that the same individual may respond differently to the same dose of a drug at different points in time or under different circumstances. The nurse should never make assumptions about how a person will respond to a drug dose.

PHARMACOTHERAPEUTICS

Pharmacotherapeutics is the use of drugs in the prevention, diagnosis, and treatment of disease. Two aspects of pharmacotherapeutics are effective drug administration and avoidance of adverse drug reactions. Nurses are responsible for safe and effective drug administration. Putting this responsibility into practice necessitates a large knowledge base that includes the usual dose of the drug; the appropriate route, techniques, and precautions for administration; indications for the use of the drug; potential adverse drug reactions; and understanding the mechanism of drug action. A large part of this knowledge base is directed toward avoiding adverse drug reactions and providing safe pharmacotherapeutics.

ADVERSE DRUG REACTIONS AND RISK ASSESSMENT

Experts define adverse drug reactions differently. Some experts include drug overdose, drug abuse, drug tolerance, drug dependence, and failure of therapeutic outcome. However, for purposes of this review, an adverse drug reaction is defined as an unintended, drug-induced noxious alteration in the patient's condition that occurs at normal dosages (Karch and Lasagna, 1975). Adverse drug reactions often require treatment, reduction of dose, or cessation of therapy.

An adverse drug reaction should be suspected when a patient's condition changes for the worse, particularly after a new medication is administered. Before administering a new medication and each time a drug is administered, the nurse should call to mind the expected drug action and the known adverse effects. Further, general pharmacokinetic and pharmacodynamic factors that are known to increase the risk for adverse drug reaction should be considered. Application of pharmacokinetic and pharmacodynamic principles can help nurses make an initial as-

BOX 16-3
PATIENT CHARACTERISTICS THAT PREDISPOSE TO INCREASED RISK FOR ADVERSE DRUG REACTIONS

- Extremes of age: the elderly, neonates, children
- Special conditions (nonpathological): pregnant women, nursing women
- Chronic illness, multiple coexisting illnesses, critical illness
- Decreased homeostatic reserve
- Hepatic dysfunction
- Renal dysfunction
- Malnutrition
- Factors that could alter absorption or bioavailability
  - Shock
  - Decreased cardiac output
  - Decreased blood flow to gut or muscle injection site
  - Decreased absorbing surface (e.g., intestinal surgery)
  - Changes in gastrointestinal retention time
  - Drug-food and drug-drug interactions
- Factors affecting distribution
  - Decreased plasma protein levels
  - Increased or decreased body fat
  - Changes in fluid balance
  - Dehydration
- Chronic alcohol consumption
- Smoking
- History of allergic disease
- History of previous adverse drug reaction
  - Known genetic differences in drug metabolism
- Psychosocial factors (compliance/noncompliance issues)
  - Dementia, confusion
  - Physical barriers to drug self-administration
  - Poor economic resources
  - Individual and cultural beliefs about drug-taking
  - Self-prescription and self-medication
  - Placebo effects

BOX 16-4
DRUG CHARACTERISTICS THAT PREDISPOSE TO INCREASED RISK FOR ADVERSE DRUG REACTIONS

- Polypharmacy
- Low therapeutic index (Wright, 1992)
  - Oral anticoagulants
  - Anticancer and immunosuppressive drugs
  - Antidysrhythmic drugs
  - Lithium carbonate
  - Oral hypoglycemic drugs
  - Anticonvulsants
  - Digoxin
  - Aminoglycosides
- Highly lipophilic drugs
- Drugs affecting the central nervous system
- Drugs that burden homeostatic systems
- Specific routes and modes of administration

sessment and prediction of risk for adverse drug reaction, even without knowledge of the specific side effects and adverse effects associated with each individual drug.

The preceding review of pharmacokinetic and pharmacodynamic principles should help the reader identify general characteristics of patients and of drugs that can increase the risk of

BOX 16-5
ASSESSMENT QUESTIONS TO HELP IDENTIFY POTENTIAL ADVERSE DRUG REACTIONS

- Is the appearance of the suspected drug reaction temporally associated with the administration of the drug? When a change in the patient's status is observed, the nurse should determine whether new drug therapy has recently been initiated. Or, does it seem that the observed alteration in the patient's condition follows every administration of a certain drug? Temporal association with drug administration may be difficult to identify in situations in which the adverse effect is delayed or occurs after cumulative doses of a drug.
- Is the suspected adverse reaction in keeping with either the therapeutic effect of the drug (e.g., vasodilation with hypotension and syncope) or in keeping with the known adverse and side effects of the drug (e.g., antihistamines with drowsiness or cholinergic antagonists with tachycardia)?
- Does the drug strongly alter a component of a physiologic feedback system, thereby causing an adverse reaction that is not obviously associated with the primary therapeutic effect of the drug? For example, autocrine regulation of renal blood flow is accomplished by a balance between the synthesis and release of vasodilating and vasoconstricting substances. When actual or effective circulating blood volume is diminished, renal synthesis of vasodilating prostaglandins normally maintains homeostatic renal blood flow. If a nonsteroidal antiinflammatory drug (e.g., aspirin) is administered, prostaglandin production is inhibited and the balance is shifted toward the synthesis of relatively more vasoconstricting substances. The result can be extreme decreases in renal perfusion (Levenson et al, 1982).
- Is it possible that the adverse effect could be explained by the patient's disease state? Or is it possible that the causal event is due to nonpharmacologic therapy?
- Has the patient had an adverse reaction to another drug from the same class of drugs or a related class?
- Does the adverse effect disappear when the drug is discontinued? Does it reappear if the drug is readministered? Does the adverse reaction reappear if a placebo is given? Interestingly, the placebo effect is more commonly thought of as a beneficial drug response that is elicited by an inert substance. However, a negative or adverse drug response may be elicited by a placebo as well. Factors such as anticipation, health beliefs, and attitudes about drug-taking can influence the patient's response to a placebo. However, taking action to test the effect of drug discontinuation or placebo effect raises difficult legal, ethical, and safety questions.

CLINICAL DECISION MAKING
PHARMACOTHERAPEUTICS

FACTORS TO CONSIDER

Refer to the case presentation at the beginning of the chapter. What information regarding Mr. K. should the nurse consider in evaluating him prior to adjusting his dose of diuretic? In the example, there are several patient variables that must be factored into the pharmacologic decision-making process, including older age, race, multiple chronic diseases, and polypharmacy. How each one of these variables affects the decision-making process and choice of pharmacotherapy is discussed here.

KNOWLEDGE BASE

Mr. K. is 75 years old; older age is associated with various physiologic changes that alter drug pharmacokinetics and pharmacodynamics. For example, aging is associated with changes in body mass, body fat, and water content, all of which affect drug distribution (Schwertz & Buschmann, 1989; Yuen, 1990). In addition, age-associated changes occur within the kidney and liver, which alter drug excretion and metabolism, respectively (Gilbert & Vaughan, 1990; Schumucker & Wang, 1980). There are also age-associated changes in the pharmacodynamic response of several drug types. Some of these pharmacodynamic changes are related to changes in the number of membrane drug receptors and/or postreceptor events (signal transduction). For example, in the aged heart, there is an attenuated (decreased) inotropic effect of beta-adrenergic drugs such as dobutamine (Scarpace, 1986). However, it is important to note that increasing the dose of a beta adrenergic drug to obtain an effect is not an option for Mr. K. because of the marked changes in renal and liver function. An alternative approach would be to choose a drug whose pharmacodynamics were not altered by aging.

Mr. K. has a history of hypertension, coronary artery disease (CAD), and heart failure. The nurse must consider how these chronic diseases have altered organ function. For example, long-standing hypertension is associated with nephrosclerosis and renal insufficiency, which in some patients progresses to renal failure. In fact, in the United States, hypertension is a leading cause of end-stage renal disease, and the highest rates occur in elderly blacks (Brown and Carter, 1994). Mr. K. has a long-standing history of hypertension and is 75 years old; more than likely, his renal function is not within normal limits. Therefore, the nurse must consider how changes in renal function will alter drug excretion. It is essential to adjust all drugs in the presence of renal insufficiency (creatinine clearance < 30 cc/min), and the drug dosage adjustment is based on the patient's glomerular filtration rate, which is estimated using creatinine clearance (Mooradian, 1988). In addition, some drugs (i.e., aminoglycosides) are nephrotoxic and are contraindicated or must be used with extreme caution in patients with renal insufficiency.

CLINICAL DECISIONS

The health care team decided to increase the amount of Mr. K.'s diuretic. The team must consider the fact that Mr. K. has a history of CAD. There are some reports that suggest that diuretic therapy (specifically, thiazide diuretic therapy) is associated with increasing cholesterol levels (Ames, 1986). This is important to consider because Mr. K. does have a CAD history. However, Mr. K. does have heart failure, and diuretic therapy is essential for reducing peripheral edema and improving several other signs and symptoms associated with this condition. Therefore, the team will increase the diuretic dose but will monitor Mr. K.'s cholesterol level every 3 months and suggest that he reduce his intake of dietary fat and cholesterol.

Mr. K. is receiving more than one type of drug (polypharmacy). The nurse must consider the multiple side effects, adverse effects, and/or interaction effects among the various drugs Mr. K. is receiving. In addition, because he is elderly, the nurse must evaluate Mr. K.'s cognitive function and mobility and how these would contribute to any problems he might have with self-administration of multiple drugs.

Mr. K. is an example of the type of patient that is very often in health care facilities today. Patients are older, have more comorbidities, and are chronically ill. Therefore, each individual must be considered unique, and health care providers must consider a multitude of variables when prescribing and administrating drug therapies.

adverse drug reactions. Boxes 16–3 and 16–4 list some of these factors but are by no means complete. Most of these predisposing risk factors are discussed throughout the chapter.

General criteria can be used to help recognize drug-induced adverse reactions. In most cases, not every one of these criteria are met. However, if several are met, the probability is greater that an unfavorable change in the patient's condition is associated with drug administration. These criteria can be put in the form of questions that can be used for patient assessment (Box 16–5).

A "user-friendly" 10-item scale has been developed for clinical determination of the probability that an adverse occurrence is, in fact, caused by an adverse drug reaction. The scale, developed by Naranjo and colleagues (1981), has been shown to have consensual, content, and concurrent validity and could be useful to nurses in patient assessment (Box 16–6).

Patient-dependent factors can affect therapeutic outcome and influence the risk of adverse drug reactions. The principal patient-dependent factor is the extent of adherence with the prescribed dose and administration protocol. Adherence with the drug regimen may be influenced by psychosocial factors such as health beliefs and economic factors. A drug may not be purchased if it is too expensive. A drug may not be taken if

BOX 16-6
ADVERSE DRUG REACTION PROBABILITY SCALE

To assess the adverse drug reaction, please answer the following questionnaire and give the pertinent score.

	YES	NO	DO NOT KNOW	SCORE
1. Are there previous **conclusive** reports on this reaction?	+1	0	0	
2. Did the adverse event appear after the suspected drug was administered?	+2	−1	0	
3. Did the adverse reaction improve when the drug was discontinued or a **specific** antagonist was administered?	+1	0	0	
4. Did the adverse reaction reappear when the drug was readministered?	+2	−1	0	
5. Are there alternative causes (other than the drug) that could on their own have caused the reaction?	−1	+2	0	
6. Did the reaction reappear when a placebo was given?	−1	+1	0	
7. Was the drug detected in the blood (or other fluids) in concentrations known to be toxic?	+1	0	0	
8. Was the reaction more severe when the dose was increased or less severe when the dose was decreased?	+1	0	0	
9. Did the patient have a similar reaction to the same or similar drugs in **any** previous exposure?	+1	0	0	
10. Was the adverse event confirmed by any objective evidence?	+1	0	0	
				Total score

From Natan JO, M.D., Busto, U., Sellers, E.M., et al (1981). A method for estimating the probability of adverse drug reactions. *Clinical Pharmacology and Therapeutics,* 30(2), 239–245.

drug-taking has strong negative connotations within a culture. A drug may not be taken correctly if the patient is simply too arthritic to open a container or too visually impaired to read the directions for administration. A higher dose may be taken if the patient believes that "if some drug is good, more drug must be better." Or, if a patient is forgetful or confused, the dosing interval may be too erratic to maintain a therapeutic steady-state plasma drug concentration.

Clearly, lack of adherence causes the steady-state drug plasma concentration to deviate from a predicted value. This

PATIENT TEACHING
ANTIHYPERTENSIVE THERAPY

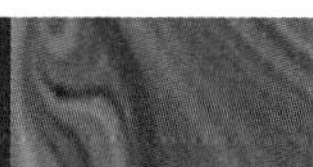

In the case study, some patient education material specific to antihypertensive therapy is discussed. However, in general there are several patient teaching tips that health care providers must incorporate and include in all patient education. These include reviewing side effects, providing the client with generic and commercial drug names, having the client orally (or in writing) repeat the names and dosing schedule, and providing the client with emergency numbers.

The major categories of antihypertensives include beta-adrenergic blockers, calcium channel blockers, vasodilators, angiotensin-converting enzyme inhibitors and diuretics. In the clinical decision making situation, the following should be considered "generic" information and taught to all patients. To begin with, a target blood pressure should be established so the patients knows what his or her desired blood pressure should be. The patient should be taught to self-monitor blood pressure by using a sphygmomanometer and that blood pressure levels cannot be determined by the way he or she feels. Patients should be advised never to discontinue therapy without consulting a health care provider, either a nurse or doctor. The health care provider needs to discuss with the patient the importance of drug compliance and adverse effects of discontinuing antihypertensive therapy. Health care providers should encourage their patients to openly discuss any side effects or symptoms. Although side effects are related to the use of specific drugs, there are some side effects that are common to many types of antihypertensives, including hypotension, which is accompanied by dizziness or lightheadedness; sexual dysfunction; and changes in cardiovascular reflexes (baroreceptor reflex). With regard to the latter side effect, some patients may experience postural hypotension or more marked changes in blood pressure with any type of change in posture.

In addition to discussing the importance of pharmacologic therapy, the nurse should also discuss the importance of risk factor reduction; for example, reducing the intake of dietary salt and fat, smoking cessation, and maintaining a routine exercise program. It needs to be emphasized that these are not to replace drug therapy but are other important ways to reduce one's blood pressure.

could result in therapeutic failure or an increased risk of adverse drug reaction. The pharmacotherapeutic team is therefore obligated to determine whether the client is following the drug regimen as prescribed. Without this information, the physician may needlessly change the prescription and increase the probability of suboptimal drug therapy.

THE NURSE'S ROLE IN PHARMACOTHERAPEUTICS

Traditionally, the nurse teaches the patient and family why it is so important to adhere to the prescribed dose and dosing interval. Because nurses spend more time than other health care workers with the patient and because of their focus on the human responses to health problems, nurses are in a key position to assess the patient for both physiologic and psychosocial factors that could affect drug therapy. They are most likely to discover whether medication is being taken inappropriately. Once the reasons for lack of adherence are understood, a plan can be formulated to improve therapy.

The nurse's role in avoiding patient injury caused by an adverse drug reaction is twofold: (1) preventing an adverse occurrence and (2) recognizing any adverse occurrence and promptly reducing or halting negative sequelae. Excellent assessment skills are invaluable in either case.

Nursing diagnosis of potential and actual alterations related to adverse drug effects may come in various forms. Some examples include

- Knowledge deficit related to insufficient instruction about gastrointestinal side effects of aspirin
- Nonadherence related to sexual dysfunction in men receiving beta-adrenergic antagonist therapy for hypertension
- Sleep pattern disturbance related to nocturnal cough caused by the angiotensin-converting enzyme inhibitor (Vasotec)
- Potential for injury related to postural hypotension caused by antihypertensive therapy.

Pharmacotherapy is a major component in the treatment of disease, disease prevention, and optimal health maintenance. Nursing's role in providing safe and effective drug administration is an extremely important element of the team approach to pharmacotherapy. The knowledge base required to adequately perform this role is large and multidisciplinary. Many areas of pharmacology that are of special interest to nurses—pharmacokinetics and pharmacodynamics in special populations (e.g., neonates, pregnant women, elderly adults), over-the-counter (nonprescription) medications and self-medication behaviors, drug abuse, drug dependence, theories related to compliant and noncompliant behaviors, and educational theory—are beyond the scope of this chapter. However, these areas and others associated with pharmacotherapeutics should not be ignored.

The goal of optimal pharmacotherapy is best achieved by a team approach. The team includes physicians, clinical pharmacists, nurses, nutritionists, and other therapists. Often, the most important members of this team are all but forgotten. These members are the patient and the patient's family or primary caregiver. One goal of pharmacotherapy should be the highest possible quality of life for the patient. Clearly, the patient should be the primary determinant of what constitutes the best quality of life to him or her (Ferrans, 1990). Therefore, there is an ethical responsibility to educate the patient with regard to the real risks and benefits of drug treatment. An additional goal of pharmacotherapy is facilitation of patient independence and self-administration of drugs.

Patient education is at the heart of these goals, and nurses are traditionally responsible for patient education. The educated patient and family can participate in an honest and mutually satisfactory therapeutic contract with the health care team. Helping the patient share the control over regulation of medications has been shown to improve compliance (Conrad, 1985).

PART II: PRACTICAL ASPECTS OF SAFE AND EFFECTIVE DRUG ADMINISTRATION

Drug administration is one of the highest-risk areas of nursing practice (Gladstone, 1995). The rate of medication error reported in the literature ranges from 5.3 to 20.6 percent, but these rates only approximate 10 to 25 percent of the administration errors actually made (Bliss-Holtz, 1994). Drug administration is a complex, multidisciplinary process. It involves

- A decision by the provider (usually a physician or nurse practitioner) to prescribe a medication
- The writing of the prescription (usually done by the person making the decision that the patient should receive a medication)
- The filling of the prescription or provision of the medication (usually done by the pharmacist)
- The preparation of the medication for administration (usually done by the registered nurse administering the medication)
- The administration of the medication (usually done by the registered nurse preparing the medication)
- The recording of the administration of the medication (usually done by the registered nurse administering the medication)

Safe and effective drug administration requires extensive knowledge from many different sources. The information in the "Knowledge Base" section of this chapter from the science of pharmacology is one source. Information about specific drugs from drug reference books is another source. In addition, the nurse needs knowledge and skill in administering drugs and knowledge about the specific patient receiving the drug. If a nurse administers a drug without full knowledge in all four of these areas, the patient may suffer adverse consequences.

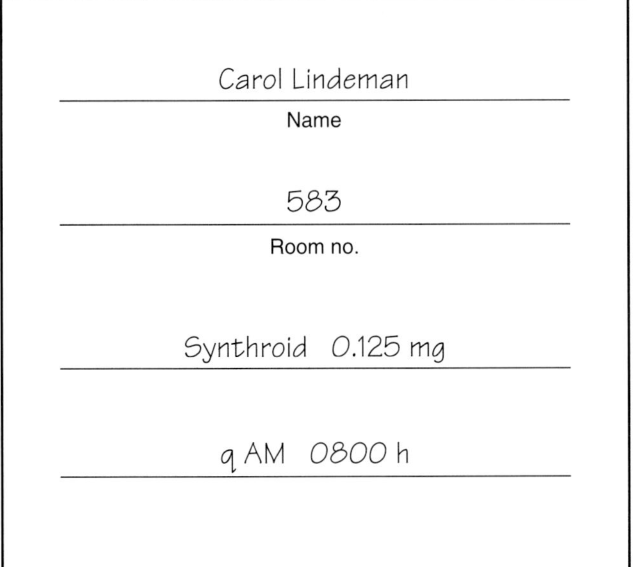

Carol Lindeman
Name

583
Room no.

Synthroid 0.125 mg

q AM 0800 h

Figure 16–13. A sample drug order.

① Name Carol Lindeman ② Date 6/6/98

Address 951 Holly Ave

Rohert Park CA

This prescription will be filled generically unless the physician signs on the line stating "Dispense as written."

③ ℞ ④ Synthroid 0.125 mg

⑤ Disp. 90

⑥ Sig. One tablet by mouth one time daily

⑦ 3 refills

Dispense as written

Jeff Thomas
⑧ Substitution permissible

Jeffrey L. Thomas, M.D.
149 Minebank Rd.
Winchester, VA 22645
540-869-5755
DEA #LDS54321

Parts of a prescription:

① Patient's name and address
② Date on which the prescription was written
③ The ℞ symbol, which means "take thou"
④ Name and strength of medication
⑤ Dispensing instructions for the pharmacist
⑥ Administration instructions for the patient
⑦ Refill and/or special labeling
⑧ Prescriber's signature

Figure 16–14. A typical prescription form.

In all situations involving the administration of drugs, a nurse needs to know

- The usual dose of the drug
- The appropriate route of administration
- The proper techniques and precautions of administration
- The approved indications for the use of the drug
- The mechanism of action of the drug
- Side effects and toxic and adverse reactions
- Drug-to-drug and drug-to-food interactions.

Remember, no drug should be administered without prior assessment of the patient and evaluation of the drug's effects.

In practice, nurses may administer a prescription drug, a nonprescription drug, or a controlled drug. A prescription drug is one that can only be taken under the supervision of a health care provider licensed to prescribe and dispense drugs according to state law. A nonprescription drug can be taken without the supervision of a health care provider. These drugs are frequently referred to as over-the-counter drugs, because they can be purchased without a prescription. A controlled drug is one whose use is controlled by state, federal, and local law because it has the potential for drug abuse or drug dependence.

Medication Orders

In institutional settings such as the hospital or nursing home, the administration of drugs is determined by the medication orders the provider writes on the order sheet in the patient's chart (Fig. 16–13). Once the order is written, it is transmitted to the pharmacy to be filled. Following that, nursing personnel administer the drug as ordered. In other settings such as the outpatient clinic, doctor's office, or home, the provider writes the drug order on a prescription pad with the expectation that the patient will have the prescription filled at a pharmacy and then take the drug as prescribed (Fig. 16–14). Whether the provider writes the order on an order sheet in the patient's chart or on a prescription pad, it must contain certain information:

- The full name of the patient
- The date the order is written
- The generic or trade name of the drug
- The dosage form and amount
- The route of administration
- The number of times per day the drug is to be taken
- Any precautions when taking the drug
- The signature of the licensed provider

Medication orders may be written with the expectation that the drug will be continued over a period of time (standard orders) or taken one time only. A one-time-only order may also be notated "stat," meaning that the drug should be given immediately. Orders may be written with the notation "p.r.n.," which means the drug should be given as needed within recommended time frames. This order is used frequently for pain medication.

Occasionally, a medication order may be given verbally, either in person or over the telephone. Verbal orders can result in miscommunication and medication error. Therefore, the nurse should avoid verbal orders whenever possible. When a verbal order must be taken, the nurse should carefully repeat the full order back to the licensed provider and arrange for the prescriber to sign the order as soon as possible. The nurse writing the order on the order page indicates it was a voice order and notes the time and date, as well as the details of the medication order itself. The licensed provider should sign the order within 24 hours.

The "Five Rights" of Drug Administration

Nursing has developed a procedure for safe drug administration known as the "five rights":

- The right drug
- The right dose
- The right patient
- The right time
- The right route

THE RIGHT DRUG

To ensure that the right drug is given, the nurse reads the label on the drug container at least four times and compares it with the order card at least two times. This becomes more and more important as the number of drugs increases and their names become more similar. The nurse first reads the medication order or medication card and compares it with the label on the medication container. Next, the nurse removes the medication from the container and while doing so again notes the name of the medication. When the medication container is returned to its storage place, the name of the drug is noted for the third time. As a final check, the nurse compares the medication order or medication card with the container returned to its storage place. When the nurse administers the medication to the patient, the name and dose of the drug should be stated for the patient. If the patient raises any question about the drug, the nurse should check for accuracy.

THE RIGHT DOSE

The second "right" is administering the right dose. If the drug is prepared in the dosage ordered, all the nurse has to do is verify the dosage ordered with the dosage printed on the container. It is always wise to check and recheck the dosage ordered against the dosage printed on the container. More and more drugs are available in the dosage ordered. However, sometimes the nurse has to create the right dosage by giving a portion of a tablet or a specific amount of liquid or by filling a syringe to the proper measurement. This may require the nurse to calculate dosage and convert from one measurement system to another. This information is provided later in the chapter. If the nurse thinks the dosage is mislabeled on the container, a drug reference book should be used or a pharmacist consulted. Many drug reference books have color pictures of drugs in which the dosage is color coded or other markings are used to verify dosage.

THE RIGHT PATIENT

Obviously, the right drug must be given to the right patient (Fig. 16–15). In an institutional setting, this is done by asking the patient to state his or her name and checking the medication order against the patient's identification band (usually worn on the wrist). In the outpatient setting, the patient may not have an identification band, requiring the nurse to depend solely on having the patient state his or her full name. In home care settings, the nurse may know the patient from previous visits but should still verify that the right person is taking the drug.

THE RIGHT TIME

In the hospital setting, there are routine times for giving drugs that have been created around the hospital's internal schedule for work. For example, a hospitalized diabetic is usually given insulin around 6:30 A.M. by the night nurse because meals are served shortly after 7 A.M. by the day shift. If a day shift worker were to give the insulin, he or she would have to delay serving the meal, as there must be a period of time between when regular insulin is given and the person eats. For efficiency, institutions create their own schedules and hope that patients can adapt to them.

The nurse must note the time or times at which the drug is to be given and administer it as closely as possible to the selected time. In institutional settings using computers to assist in

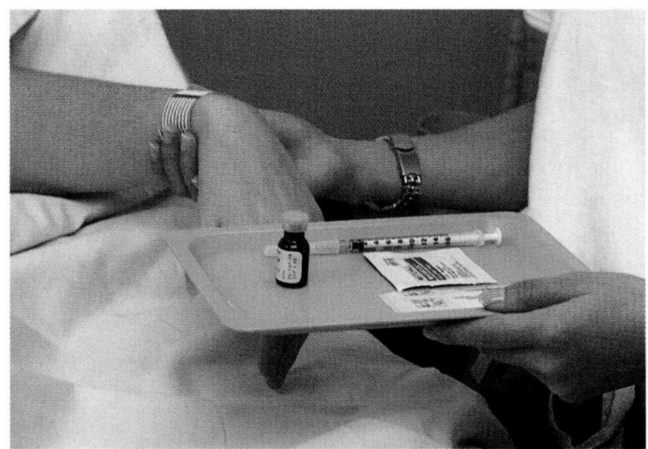

Figure 16–15. Be sure to check the patient's identification before giving any drug.

drug administration, the nurse is prompted by a computer-generated list of patients to receive drugs within the next time period (usually a 1-hour time period). Information about drug interactions may also be available from these computer systems.

In the home setting, the nurse should assist the patient in determining the best time to take medications. The nurse should determine the individual's schedule and lifestyle and then, considering the nature of the drugs, select the best schedule for the individual. In helping an individual work out a schedule for his or her drugs, the nurse should remember the information about pharmacodynamics and pharmacokinetics. The nurse should also inform the individual about the rationale for the schedule and possible modifications if the schedule does not work well.

THE RIGHT ROUTE

There are many routes for the administration of drugs (Fig. 16–16). A specific drug preparation is matched with a specific drug route when the pharmacist fills a prescription. Information about route of administration is always provided on the label or container. If the information is not provided, the nurse should check with the pharmacy before administering the drug. The nurse should never guess or make assumptions about the route of administration. Again, the route of administration is part of the order written by the licensed provider. In the institutional setting, the nurse should check the route of administration shown on the label or container with that listed on the drug order. The route used for administering a drug does influence the drug effect.

The practice of nursing requires the nurse to think about many things within a brief period. For example, the nurse may have to leave a critically ill patient to provide a drug to another patient. If the nurse continues to think about the critically ill patient while preparing a drug for the second patient, an error could easily be made. The nurse must concentrate fully on the five rights of medication administration every time a drug is administered. Adherence to the five rights is the best way to eliminate drug errors.

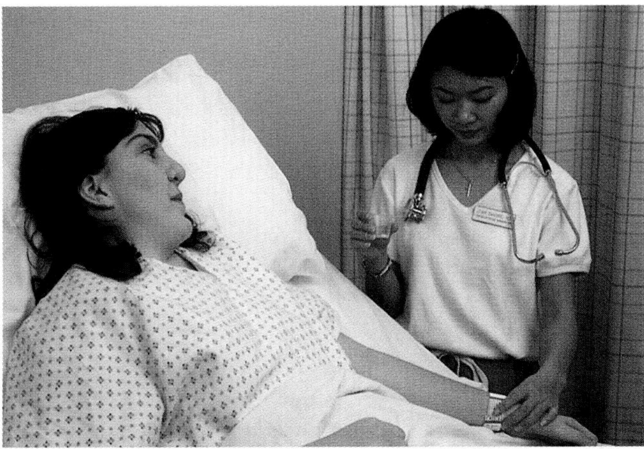

Figure 16–16. Administering oral medication.

Medication Errors

The headline read "Fatal Errors: Santa Rosa Hospitals Learn Lessons the Hard Way" (Benfell, 1997). The opening paragraphs described the deaths of two elderly women, both the results of drug errors by nurses. In both instances, the nurses used the wrong drug: undiluted potassium chloride, a chemical used to execute criminals on death row. Deaths from this drug have been so numerous that the FDA now requires distinctive black tops and inner closures, and the Institute for Safe Medication Practices has recommended that it be stored only in the hospital pharmacy. Yet some hospitals disregard these recommendations, and patient deaths from drug errors continue.

The foregoing scenario highlights the both the importance and the multidisciplinary nature of safe and effective drug administration. In 1997, concern for drug errors associated with registered nurses was so intense that the American Nurses Association set up a hotline that nurses could use to discuss drug errors.

What is a drug error? There is no universal definition. Each institution or researcher defines the phrase to match his or her particular intent. For example, the Pharmacy and Therapeutics Committee at Lutheran General Hospital (Park Ridge, IL) found that the hospital had no clear definition of drug error (Carey and Teeters, 1995). Any drug error reported on an "occurrence report" was considered an error. As the first step in improving the process of drug administration, that committee created a definition of drug error that included six categories (Box 16–7). In contrast, in a research study analyzing work-

BOX 16–7
DEFINITION OF MEDICATION ERROR AT LUTHERAN GENERAL HOSPITAL

A medication error is a discrepancy between what the physician ordered and what was actually administered, or not administered, to the patient. This includes all medications, intravenous and nonintravenous. It does not include potential errors that were caught by a check system and thus did not reach the patient.

Types of medication errors include

- Wrong medication: The medication administered to the patient was not the medication prescribed for the patient.
- Wrong route: The medication was administered by a route different than the route prescribed for the patient.
- Wrong dose: The medication dose administered was different than the dose prescribed for the patient.
- Dose omitted: One or more doses of medication were not given to the patient by the next scheduled dosing time.
- Wrong time: The dose was given 2 hours or more earlier or later than the prescribed scheduled time.
- Prescribing concern: A medication order was questioned by another health care professional (e.g., registered nurse, registered pharmacist) as to its appropriateness.

load and environmental factors associated with medication errors, Roseman and Booker (1995) defined error as any of the following occurrences:

- Omission of a scheduled medication
- Medication given at the wrong time (30 minutes before or after the prescribed time)
- Medication given to the wrong patient
- Administration of the wrong dose
- Administration of the wrong medication
- An error in transcription of the physician's order to the medication administration record
- Medication given to a patient with a known allergy to the drug
- Medication repeated without a physician's order
- Medication given by the wrong route of administration
- Medication discontinued without an authorized physician order

Numerous studies have been conducted that analyze medication errors with the intent of reducing the number of errors. One recent study (Gladstone, 1995) found 79 errors reported in a 12-month period (Table 16–1). The nurses and nurse managers in that setting identified the following reasons for why drug errors occurred:

- Drug errors occur when the nurse fails to check the patient's name band against the prescription chart.
- Drug errors occur when the doctor's writing on the prescription chart is difficult to read or illegible.
- Drug errors occur when nurses are distracted by other patients or events on the ward.
- Drug errors occur when the nurse miscalculates the dose.
- Drug errors occur when the nurse sets up or adjusts an infusion device incorrectly.

In that same study, nurses having made drug errors identified reasons that they thought contributed to the errors (Table 16–2).

TABLE 16–1 Incidence of Medication Errors in One Study

Incident Group	Incident Type (N = 79)	Number of Occurrences
Dose related	Incorrect infusion rate	14 (17.7%)
Dose related	Unprescribed/extra dose	13 (16.5%)
Dose related	Incorrect patient	10 (12.7%)
Dose related	Incorrect dose	9 (11.4%)
Drug related	Incorrect drug	6 (7.6%)
Process related	Incorrect time	6 (7.6%)
Dose related	Dose omitted	5 (6.3%)
Other	Other type of incident	5 (6.3%)
Process related	Incorrect format	4 (5.0%)
Process related	Incorrect technique	3 (3.8%)
Process related	Failure to follow protocol	3 (3.8%)
Process related	Incorrect route	1 (1.3%)

From Gladstone, J. [1995]. Drug administration errors. *Journal of Advanced Nursing, 22,* 630.

TABLE 16–2 The Factors That Nurses Thought Contributed to the Medication Errors Listed in Table 16–1

Identified Factor	Number of Comments
Workload	6
Poor skill mix	6
Interruptions	6
Loss of concentration	6
Lack of knowledge	4
Tiredness/unwell	4
Did not follow protocol	4
Poor drug chart	2
Lack of assertiveness by nurse	2
Inexperience of nurse	2
Unknown patients/unknown condition	2
Poor communication with other staff	1

From Gladstone, J. [1995]. Drug administration errors. *Journal of Advanced Nursing, 22,* 630.

When a medication error is made, it must be reported and corrective action taken to ensure patient safety. What constitutes a drug error, how it is to be reported, and who determines the corrective action are institutional policies that a nurse must know.

It is equally imperative that the nurse has the moral courage to learn from a mistake and to take action to improve the situation (Arndt, 1994). A nurse making a medication error tends to feel guilt and shame. The nurse feels devastated about the error. These feelings are intensified as the nurse considers the disciplinary action that follows a drug error.

Yet if the nurse does not report the error and reflect on the circumstances associated with the error, important changes in system factors (such as workload or methods for transcribing medication orders) will not occur. Nor will the nurse be able to grow personally and professionally.

Complex drug regimens are an increasingly important aspect of health care. Nurses must be diligent in efforts to eliminate errors from their own practice as well as attempt to identify and improve the system for drug administration.

Dosage Measurements and Calculations

There are three systems for drug administration. The primary system is the metric/international system introduced in France in 1875. The other two systems are the apothecary and household measures. The apothecary system is used only rarely. The household system is used frequently for children and for those cared for in the home.

In the metric system, the basic unit for measuring volume is the liter; that for measuring weight is the gram. This system uses prefixes to determine whether the desired amount is more or less than the basic unit. There is only one prefix to denote an amount greater than the basic unit: *kilo,* meaning 1000. A kiloliter is 1000 liters. A kilogram is 1000 grams. There are several prefixes designating amounts smaller than the basic unit. The three most commonly used are: *centi, milli,* and *micro.*

Abbreviations are used to convey the unit of measurement:

- Gram is g
- Liter is L
- Kilo is k
- Centi is c
- Milli is m
- Micro is mc

The measurement *centigram* is abbreviated cg. The measurement *microliter* is mcL. This system of abbreviations must be committed to memory. The nurse must always be alert to the ordering of these measurements from smallest to largest.

There are two rules regarding metric notations:

- The quantity is written in Arabic numbers (1, 2, etc.) and placed in front of the abbreviation with a single space between the number and the abbreviation. For example, 1 mL or 3 mcg is correct; 1mL (no space) and mcg 3 (number follows instead of precedes unit) are incorrect.
- Fractional parts of a unit are expressed as decimals, and a zero is placed in front of the decimal when it is not preceded by another whole number. For example, 0.3 mL is correct; .3 mL is incorrect.

In practice, four metric weights and two metric volumes are in common use.

The abbreviations for the apothecary and household measures systems differ from the metric system and are not based on the same simple logic for determining values. In the apothecary system, the abbreviation for the one measure of weight is *gr* for grain. There are three measures of volume. From smallest to largest, these are

- Minim, abbreviated m or min
- Dram, abbreviated ʒ or dr
- Ounce, abbreviated ℥ or oz

The household system involves three common measures:

- Tablespoon, abbreviated T or tbs
- Teaspoon, abbreviated t or tsp
- Drop, abbreviated gtt

The rules for the use of these abbreviations are the opposite of those for the metric system. For the apothecary and household notations, the quantity is placed after the unit, and it is expressed as a fraction rather than as a decimal. Roman or Arabic numbers can be used. For example, the notation would read gr ½ not 0.5 gr or gr 0.5.

Medication orders may be written using one measurement system, and the drug label, another system. Most hospital units have conversion tables available to help with calculations. The nurse working in home care or in a community setting may wish to carry a conversion table in a pocket. A student may wish to carry a conversion table until comfortable with the process.

In some situations, drugs may not be prepared or supplied in the exact quantity stated in the medication order. In that instance, the nurse must calculate the quantity of the medication the patient is to receive. Using ratio and proportion offers the most logical approach to solving dosage calculation. The nurse must also be able to add, subtract, multiply, and divide accurately. A ratio is composed of two numbers separated by a colon (1:2) or written as a fraction (½). In medication dosage, a ratio is used to express the strength of a drug. For example, 1 tab:25 mg indicates that one tablet contains 25 milligrams of the drug. An example involving a liquid is 10 units of insulin per mL (10U:1 mL). A proportion is used to show a relationship between two ratios. In drug calculations, the intent is to determine true proportions, which means that the two ratios must be equal.

Ratio and proportion can be used when one ratio is known and the second is incomplete. For example, if the medication came in 25-mg tablets and the medication order called for 75 mg, the nurse could do the following calculation:

1:25 mg = x:75 mg	(If one tablet contains 25 mg, how many tablets do I have to give to administer 75 mg of the drug?)
1/25 mg = x/75 mg	(Ratios must be written in the same sequence of measurement units.)
1/25 = x/75	(Drop the measurement units [if they are the same] and cross-multiply). [If they are not the same, convert first]
25x = 75	(Keep the unknown x on the left side of the equation.)
x = 75/25	(Divide the number on the right side of the equation by the number in front of the x on the left side of the equation.)
x = 3	(Divide the final fraction to determine the value of x.)

To give the ordered dosage, three tablets are required.

Remember to always check and recheck your calculations. Ask yourself whether your calculation makes sense. Make certain that all calculations are based on the same measurement system. In some instances it will be necessary to convert orders to the same measurement system and then do the calculations. Many experienced registered nurses use a calculator and/or have a colleague recheck medication calculations simply because they are not performed that frequently. It is always better to be safe than sorry.

PART III: ADMINISTERING MEDICATION BY INTRAMUSCULAR INJECTION

Intramuscular (IM) injections are included within the category of parenteral medication administration. Specifically, an IM injection introduces medication into the body of the muscle by needle and syringe. The IM route may be used when faster medication absorption and a more rapid response than oral route are desired. Muscles have a rich blood supply, thereby enhancing medication absorption. Also, the IM route may be an option when a patient is unable to swallow, may have a gastrointestinal illness whereby the medication is not absorbed or retained, is agitated, or is allowed nothing by mouth (NPO). Some medications may be available for IM administration only.

Administration of an IM injection requires skill and knowledge. Several important questions must be considered prior to administering a medication via the IM route. These questions include:

- What is the most appropriate *injection site* for this patient?
- What is the correct *method* for locating the injection site?
- What is the correct *angle* of injection and the correct *position* for injection?
- What is the appropriate *needle length/size* for this patient?
- How much *volume* and at what *speed* can medication be safely administered?
- Should certain *medications* be avoided for IM administration?
- Should an air bubble be used to accommodate for *dead space*?

INJECTION SITE

Traditionally, four sites are used for IM injection. These include the dorsogluteal (upper outer quadrant of the buttock), ventrogluteal (gluteus medius or hip), deltoid (upper arm), and vastus lateralis (anterior lateral thigh). Unfortunately, all of the IM injection sites except the ventrogluteal have been associated with complications such as fibrosis and contracture of skeletal muscles, abscesses, nerve injury, paralysis, and gangrene (Bergerson et al, 1982; Greenblatt and Allen, 1978; Muller-Vahl, 1983; Chung et al, 1989; Sun, 1990; Talbert et al, 1967; Napiontek and Ruszkowski, 1993; Groves and Goldner, 1974; Ling and Loong, 1962; Combes et al, 1960; Barennes et al, 1993; Zelman, 1978).

No complications from the ventrogluteal site, however, have been reported. It is unknown whether the lack of complications reported for the ventrogluteal is related to the fact that it is used less frequently than other sites (Beecroft and Redick, 1989) or whether it is indeed complication free. We do know that this site has several advantages over other injection sites. It is free of important nerves and vascular structures and is easily located from easily palpable landmarks. Furthermore, the subcutaneous (SC) fat is thinner than that of the dorsogluteal area; thus, inadvertent injection into the SC tissue is less likely than into the muscle (von Hochstetter, 1964). Therefore, the safest site for IM injection for *any* patient is the ventrogluteal.

Other factors to keep in mind when selecting the injection site are the patient's body size, age, muscle condition, skin condition, and medical diagnosis. Patients who have neuropathies or myopathies or are debilitated may have inadequate muscle mass to allow for injection without complications (Beecroft and Kongelbeck, 1994). In this case, another route for medication administration should be considered.

METHOD OF LOCATING INJECTION SITE

When locating a site for injection, it is important to identify the boundaries through anatomical landmarks. These landmarks should be palpated carefully. Next, the safe area for injection within the designated landmarks should be visualized (Beecroft and Redick, 1990). The safe areas are characterized by the bulk of the muscle mass, avoidance of injection into bony areas (as can be palpated on the ventrogluteal site), and circumventing blood vessels and nerves (at the deltoid and dorsogluteal sites) (Fig. 16–17).

ANGLE OF INJECTION AND THE CORRECT POSITION FOR INJECTION

The angle at which the needle is directed into the skin is important to make sure that the needle reaches the muscle, the medication is deposited in an area that minimizes leakage from the site of injection, and significant nerves are avoided. The angle of injection should be perpendicular (90 degrees) to the skin for all sites except the dorsogluteal. In this case the safest angle for injection is perpendicular to the surface on which the patient is lying (Johnson and Raptou, 1965). A 90-degree angle minimizes trauma to adjacent tissue and increases the likelihood that the medication will be deposited in the muscle as opposed to subcutaneous tissue.

APPROPRIATE NEEDLE LENGTH

For medication to be deposited into the muscle, the needle must be of sufficient length to penetrate the subcutaneous tissue. The thickness of subcutaneous tissue varies considerably depending on the patient's age and nutritional status. For example, subcutaneous tissue over the dorsogluteal site ranges from 9 cm (3½ inches) in the obese to 1 cm (⅜ inch) in infants, children, elderly adults, and emaciated individuals (Lachman, 1963).

Unfortunately, no reliable method exists for determining needle length for IM injection in different-sized individuals. A gross estimate can be obtained using the pinch test advocated by Lenz (1983). For the deltoid and vastus lateralis muscles, the muscle is pinched between the thumb and index finger. One-half the distance between the thumb and index finger is supposed to approximate the length of needle required to penetrate the muscle. For the ventrogluteal muscle, the layer of fat and skin above the muscle is picked up, again between the thumb and index finger. One-half of the distance between the thumb and index finger is the needle length required to reach the muscle. To penetrate the muscle, the individual practitioner must decide exactly how much length to add so the needle can reach the body of the muscle. It should be kept in mind that *no research data are available to support these recommendations.*

Pinching causes tissue compression by lifting the skin fold and cannot be considered an absolute measure of fat thickness because it represents a double fold. Also, the amount of compression varies by individuals and by skin fold site (Booth, et al, 1966; Himes et al, 1979). The pinch test is the best method currently available, but it should be used with caution.

Regardless, if the individual is obese and a needle longer than 1½ inches is needed, another administration route

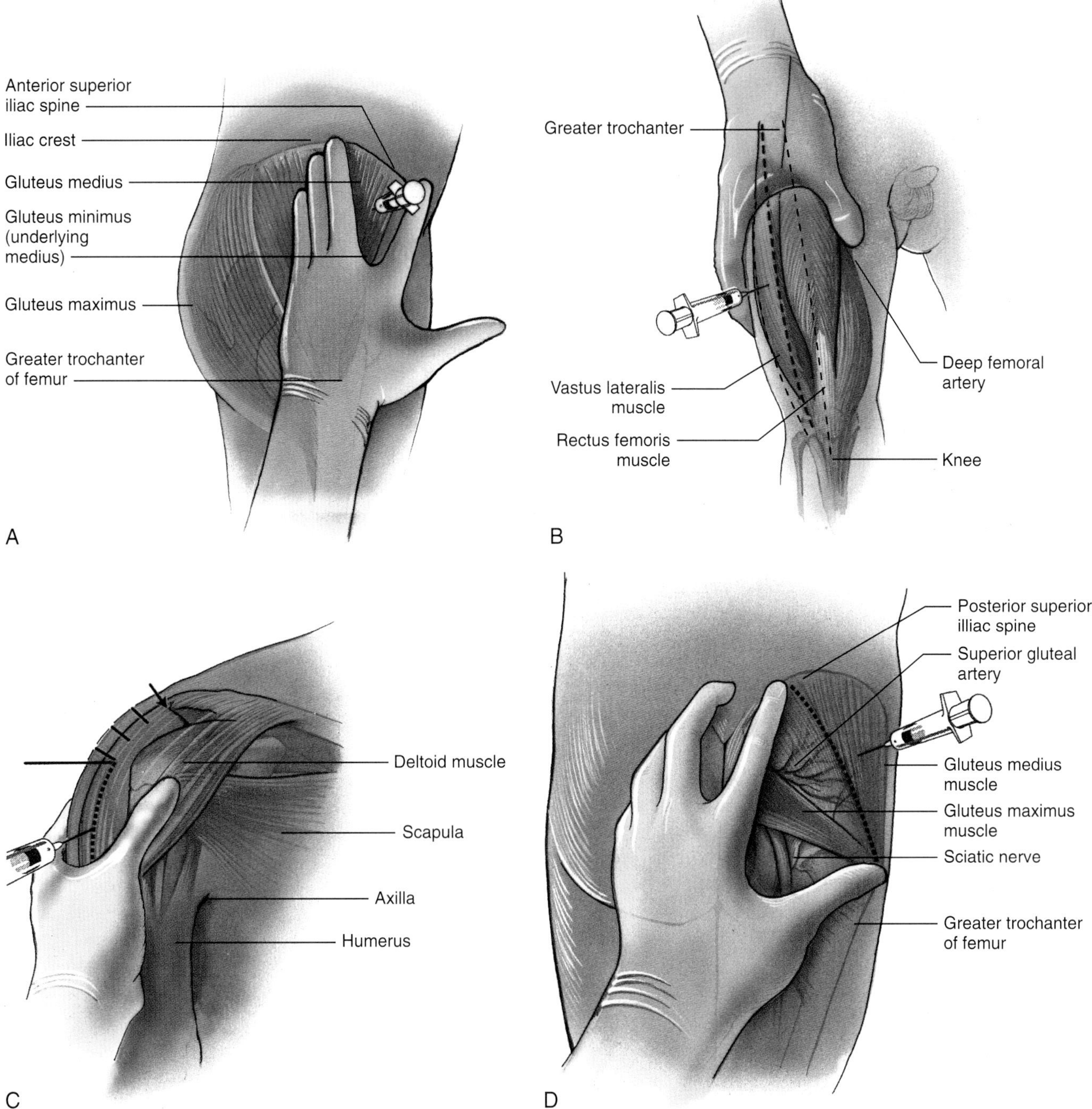

Figure 16–17. Intramuscular injection sites. **A**, Ventrogluteal; **B**, vastus lateralis; **C**, deltoid; **D**, dorsogluteal. (From Bowden, V.R., Dickey, S.B., and Greenberg, C.S. Children and Their Families: The Continuum of Care. Philadelphia: W.B. Saunders, 1998.)

should be sought. Similarly, an emaciated individual may not have sufficient muscle mass for safe injection. In all cases individual physical characteristics of the patient must be evaluated prior to IM injection.

Needle length guidelines for average-sized individuals are derived from the scant research that is available (Cockshott et al, 1989; Chugh et al, 1993; Grosswasser et al, 1997; Poland et al, 1997); see Table 16–3.

VOLUME AND SPEED OF INJECTION

Based on nurses' experience, the maximum volume of a single IM injection has been limited to 5 mL (Winfrey, 1985). This maximum may be revised to a lower limit based on individual characteristics such as age and size as well as muscle bulk. Limited research suggests that 6 mL may be safely injected into a single site without serious damage to a moderate-

TABLE 16–3 Intramuscular Injection Guidelines for an *Average* Individual

	Adult	Child/Infant
Injection Site	Ventrogluteal (first choice) Vastus Lateralis Deltoid Dorsogluteal (avoid if possible)	Ventrogluteal (first choice) Vastus Lateralis Deltoid (avoid in infants up to first year as possible) Dorsogluteal (avoid up to 5 years)
Needle Length	1½ inch	1 inch all children 4 months and older ⅝ inch (<4 months)
Needle Size	22 gauge needle	23 gauge—4 months and older 25 gauge—<4 months
Volume	3–5 mL dorsogluteal ventrogluteal 2–3 mL vastus lateralis 1–1½ mL deltoid	1 mL—infant vastus lateralis ventrogluteal ½ mL—infant deltoid 2 mL—child vastus lateralis ventrogluteal dorsogluteal 1 mL—child deltoid
Speed	Minimum of 20 seconds for 2 mL	Minimum of 20 seconds for 2 mL

sized muscle, when the injectate is nonirritating to the muscle. Similarly, speed of injection does not appear to be significant. Very slow injection (e.g., 2 mL over 20–60 seconds) may reduce local tissue damage, but only slightly. It should be kept in mind, however, that medications known to be irritating to muscles when injected rapidly or in a large volume cause more local acute discomfort than a slow injection or a minor volume (Svendsen, 1983; Chezem, 1973); see Table 16–3 for guidelines.

MEDICATIONS TO AVOID FOR IM ADMINISTRATION

Medications that cause chemical trauma, are poorly absorbed, or crystallize in the muscle should be avoided. Examples include cephalothin sodium, tetracycline hydrochloride, paraldehyde, colistimethate sodium, digoxin, and diphenylhydantin (Dilantin) (Greenblatt and Koch-Weser, 1976; Greenblatt and Allen, 1978). In addition, care should be used when injecting procaine penicillin, which is a thick solution that can clog the needle on aspiration, possibly causing inadvertent injection into an artery. To avoid this complication, aspirate for a minimum of 10 seconds and observe very carefully for signs of blood return in the penicillin solution (Weir and Fearnow, 1983).

DEAD SPACE AND USE OF AN AIR BUBBLE

Dead space is the amount of medication that is left in the needle and hub after injection (Fig 16–18). An air bubble of 0.2 cc has been used to follow the medication to clear the needle and compensate for medication that remains, as well as to avoid the tracking of the medication through the subcutaneous tissue when the needle is withdrawn. This practice can be hazardous, however, by causing inadvertent overdose of medication (Shaber and Smith, 1982; Berman et al, 1978; Chapin et al, 1985; Wong, 1982). Syringes are calibrated to deliver a specific does of medication, and manufacturers do not include the hub of the syringe in these calculations. To avoid tracking of the medication through subcutaneous tissue, the z-track injection technique is recommended (Keen, 1983).

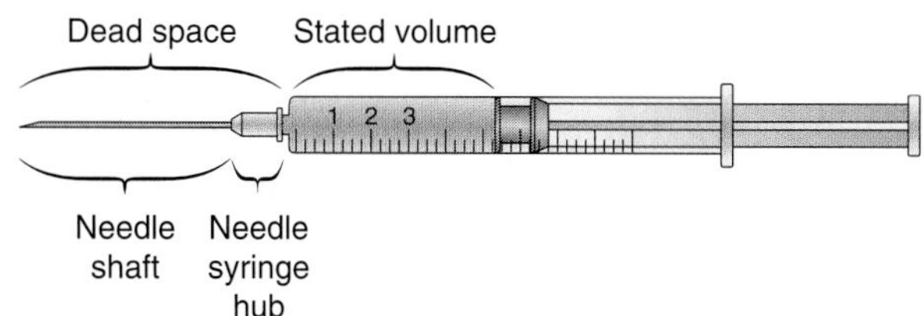

Figure 16–18. Dead space in a syringe.

The z-track technique involves pulling the skin over the injection site to one side prior to injection. After the injection, the skin is released and in effect seals medication below the subcutaneous tissue, thus preventing the leakage of medication into the subcutaneous tissue with the possibility of complications.

CONCLUSION

Administration of an IM injection requires skill and knowledge. The guidelines presented are based on the available research and case histories. Careful assessment of each patient prior to an IM injection will ensure that this procedure is performed as safely as possible.

PROCEDURES FOR DRUG ADMINISTRATION

This section presents step-by-step procedures for administering drugs via different routes. Included are

- Administering injections (Procedures 16–1 through 16–4)
- Administering oral medications (Procedure 16–5)
- Administering intravenous medications (Procedures 16–6 through 16–9)
- Administering medications via other routes (Procedure 16–10, eye medications; Procedure 16–11, ear medications; Procedure 16–12, nasal medications; Procedure 16–13, vaginal medications; and Procedure 16–14, rectal suppositories)

PROCEDURE 16-1

Preparing Medications for Parenteral Injection

Objective

Administer medication(s) as ordered by a licensed prescriber while ensuring maximum patient safety and preventing infection.

Terminology

- Ampule—a small, hermetically sealed glass flask
- Diluent—an agent that dilutes or renders fluid
- Reconstitute—to restore to a solution by adding a diluent, such as sterile water or saline
- Vial—a small bottle

Critical Elements

Use sterile equipment and sterile technique to prepare parenteral medications.

Triple-check labels:

- When removing medication from shelf, refrigerator, or drawer
- While preparing medication
- When returning medication to shelf, refrigerator, or drawer or before discarding packaging material

Medication expiration dates should always be checked and outdated medication discarded or returned to the pharmacy.

Use recommended diluent and follow instructions for reconstitution provided on the label or package insert.

Double-check all mathematical calculations. Verify calculations with another registered nurse as needed.

For reasons of cost containment and documented decreased incidence of medication errors, the pharmacies of many facilities now dispense medications by the unit dose method and mix the majority of injections and intravenous solutions. However, the nurse actually giving the medication is still responsible for all aspects of medication administration. When giving any medication, observe the five rights of medication administration:

- Right medication
- Right dosage
- Right time
- Right route
- Right patient

Prior to administering any medication, the nurse should know

- Desired therapeutic effect
- Reason for administering drug
- Usual dosage and route
- Any potential for drug or food interactions
- Potential adverse side effects

If drawing up multiple injections at one time, label syringes with patient name, medication, and dose.

Preparation of Equipment

- Sterile syringes large enough to accommodate any required diluent and final dosage (Fig. 16–19) of medication
- Alcohol swabs
- Sterile needles, with size dependent on injection type
- Correct medication
- Sterile filter needle, razor blade, or small file and paper towel if removing medication from an ampule
- Diluent for reconstitution, if applicable

Special Considerations

The correct needle size is necessary for injecting medication into the correct tissue and minimizing patient discomfort (Fig. 16–20). Viscosity of the medication must also be considered when selecting a needle. The following chart provides guidelines for which needle size to select based on the ordered route of administration:

Route	*Gauge*	*Length*
Intradermal	25–26	3/8–5/8 inches
Subcutaneous	24–27	5/8–7/8 inches
Intramuscular	19–23	1–3 inches
Intravenous	16–21	1–3 inches

Nursing Interventions

Reconstituting a Medication

Actions	*Rationale*
1. Assemble all equipment.	1. Promotes successful task completion.
2. Verify medication order, including dose, route, time, and concentration.	2. Ensures that correct medication and dose is being prepared.
3. Review and follow reconstitution instructions on label or package insert.	3. Indicates type of diluent and amount required to obtain correct concentration. CAUTION: Be sure diluent is specific for use for parenteral injection. For infants younger than 1 month, a preservative-free diluent or bacteriostatic water must be used.

continued on next page

PROCEDURE 16-1 (cont'd)

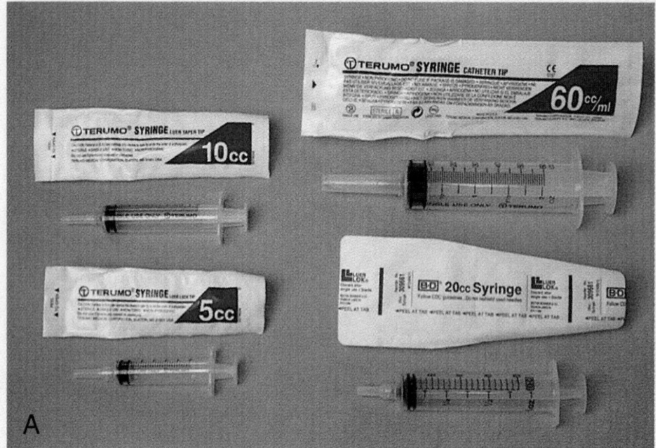

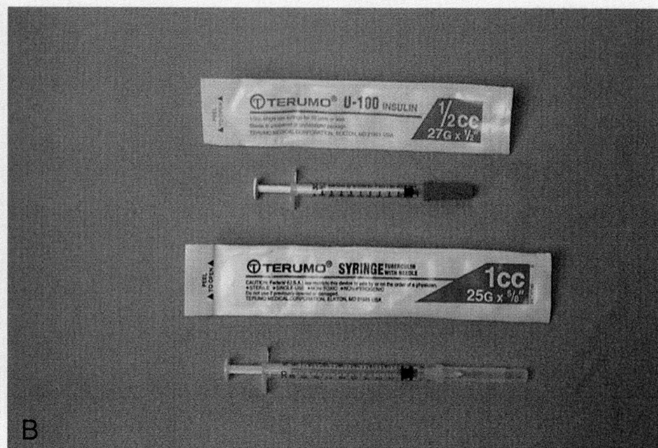

Figure 16–19. Types of syringes.

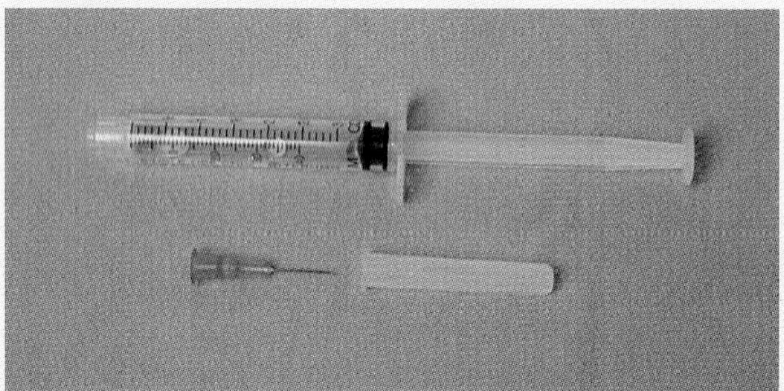

Figure 16–20. Parts of a syringe and needle.

4. Swab stopper of diluent and medication vial with alcohol and let dry.

4. Prevents contamination. Drying reduces risk of an unwanted chemical reaction.

5. Remove needle cover using aseptic technique.

5. Prevents contamination of needle.

6. Inject air equal to amount of diluent into vial.

6. Creates a positive pressure in vial, resulting in easier removal of diluent.

7. Aspirate recommended amount of diluent into syringe.

7. Ensures correct concentration of medication.

8. Inject diluent into medication bottle. Remove needle and mix well.

8. Inadequate mixing may result in wrong concentration, injection of solid particles into tissue, and decreased absorption.

9. Reinsert needle and invert vial and syringe as one. Be sure tip of needle is below fluid level. Allow syringe to fill. Gentle aspiration may be necessary to obtain ordered dose.

9. Positive pressure created with injection of diluent causes syringe to fill. Gentle aspiration minimizes turbulence, which creates air bubbles.

10. Gently tap syringe barrel to dislodge air bubbles. Expel air into vial. Continue aspirating and tapping until desired volume is obtained.

10. Ensures correct dosage.

continued on next page

PROCEDURE 16-1 (cont'd)

11. Grasp syringe barrel and remove needle from vial.	11. Prevents separation of syringe.
12. Draw air into syringe to fill dead space.	12. Assures all medication will be injected and prevents leakage into other tissue during needle withdrawal. This step is optional depending on needle angle during administration.
13. Replace needle cover using aseptic technique.	13. Prevents contamination of needle.
14. Change needle to a size appropriate for the ordered route for administration.	14. Minimizes discomfort related to improper needle size and tissue irritation caused by residue on outside of needle.
15. Label multidose vials, indicating mix date, concentration, and your initials.	15. Provides information for preparation of future doses. Check package label or insert to verify how long after reconstitution medication can be used.
16. Place disposables in proper containers. Return medication to storage if applicable.	16. Promotes a safe, clean environment and complies with universal blood and body fluid precautions.

Drawing up Medication from a Vial not Requiring Reconstitution

Actions	***Rationale***
1. Assemble all equipment.	1. Promotes successful task completion.
2. Verify medication order, including dose, route, time, and concentration.	2. Ensures that correct medication and dose is being prepared.
3. Swab stopper with alcohol and let dry.	3. Prevents contamination. Drying reduces risk of an unwanted chemical reaction.
4. Remove needle cover using aseptic technique.	4. Prevents contamination of needle.
5. Inject air equal to amount of dose into vial (Fig. 16–21).	5. Creates a positive pressure in vial, resulting in easier removal of medication.

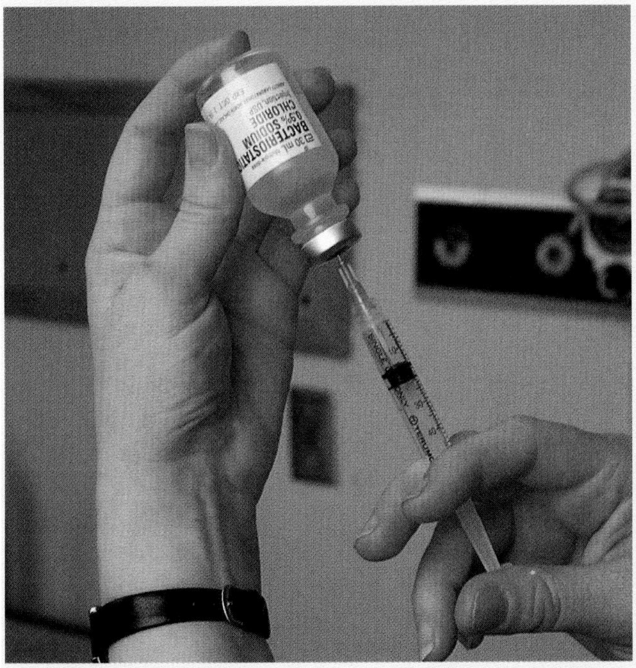

Figure 16–21. Injecting air into vial.

continued on next page

PROCEDURE 16-1 (cont'd)

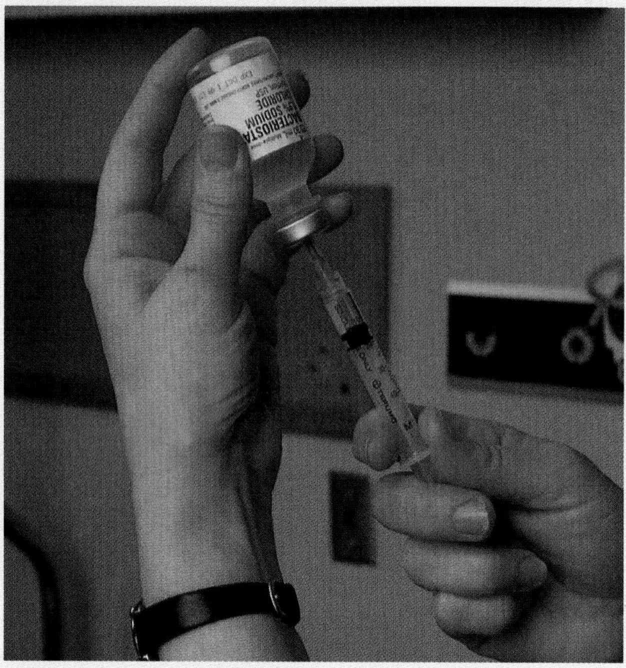

Figure 16–22. Withdrawing medication from vial.

6. Invert vial and syringe as one. Be sure tip of needle is below fluid level. Allow syringe to fill. Gentle aspiration may be necessary to obtain ordered dose (Fig. 16–22).

6. Positive pressure created with injection of air causes syringe to fill. Gentle aspiration minimizes turbulence, which creates air bubbles.

7. Gently tap syringe barrel to dislodge air bubbles. Expel air into vial. Continue aspirating and tapping until desired volume is obtained.

7. Ensures correct dosage.

8. Grasp syringe barrel and remove needle from vial.

8. Prevents separation of syringe.

9. Draw air into syringe to fill dead space.

9. Ensures that all medication will be injected and prevents leakage into other tissue during needle withdrawal. This step is optional depending on needle angle during administration.

10. Replace needle cover using aseptic technique.

10. Prevents contamination of needle

11. Change needle to a size appropriate for ordered route of administration.

11. Minimizes discomfort related to improper needle size and tissue irritation caused by residue on outside of needle.

12. Place disposables in proper containers. Return medication to storage if applicable

12. Promotes a safe, clean environment and complies with universal blood and body fluid precautions.

Drawing up Medication from a Glass Ampule

Actions

1. Assemble all equipment.
2. Verify medication order, including dose, route, time, and concentration.

Rationale

1. Promotes successful task completion.
2. Ensures correct medication and dose is being prepared.

continued on next page

PROCEDURE 16-1 (cont'd)

3. Hold ampule upright and tap gently with finger until all fluid is below neck.
3. Ensures entire contents of ampule are available for injection preparation.

4. Score top of ampule with an ampule file if not already prescored.
4. Makes opening ampule easier and prevents shattering of ampule.

5. Place ampule inside an alcohol swab and gently snap off top, maintaining aseptic technique.
5. Reduces potential for injury while maintaining aseptic technique.

6. Using a filter needle, aspirate ordered dose of medication into syringe. Do not touch ampule rim with needle.
6. Prevents glass particles that may be in medication from being drawn into syringe. Consider ampule rim to be contaminated.

7. Invert syringe and gently tap barrel to dislodge air bubbles. Expel air.
7. Ensures correct dosage.

8. Draw air into syringe to fill dead space.
8. Ensures that all medication will be injected and prevents leakage into other tissue during needle withdrawal. This step is optional depending on needle angle during administration.

9. Replace needle cover using aseptic technique.
9. Prevents contamination of needle.

10. Change needle to a size appropriate for ordered route of administration.
10. Minimizes discomfort related to improper needle size and tissue irritation caused by residue on outside of needle.

11. Place disposables in proper containers.
11. Promotes a safe, clean environment and complies with universal blood and body fluid precautions.

Preparing Medications from Prefilled Single-Dose Injection Units

Actions	***Rationale***
1. Assemble all equipment (Fig. 16–23).	1. Promotes successful task completion.
2. Verify medication order.	2. Ensures that correct medication and dose are being prepared.
3. Insert medication cartridge with attached needle into syringe-like holder and secure into place (Fig. 16–24). Follow manufacturer's instructions for assembly of unit.	3. Ensures security of syringe during medication administration.

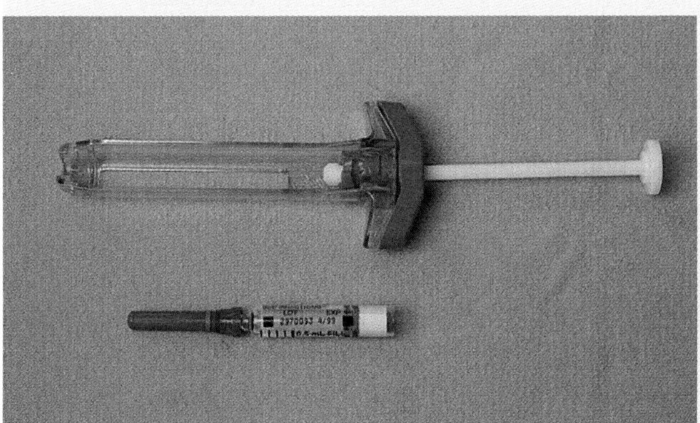

Figure 16–23. Prefilled syringe: medication cartridge and injector device.

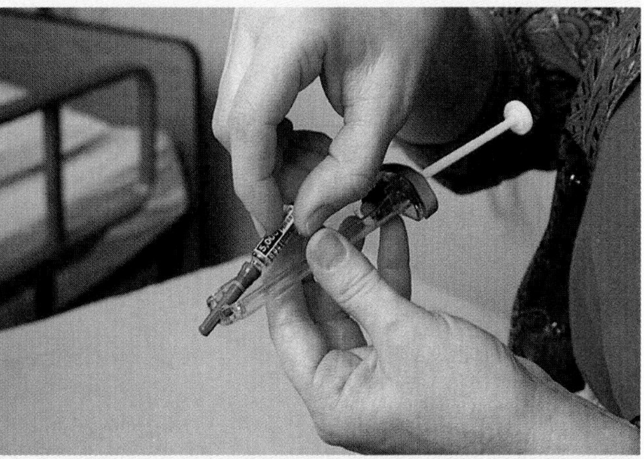

Figure 16–24. Inserting prefilled cartridge into injector device.

continued on next page

PROCEDURE 16-1 (cont'd)

4. Remove needle cover. Expel air and excess medication slowly until ordered dose remains in syringe.	4. Ensures that correct dose will be administered to patient.
5. Replace needle cover.	5. Prevents contamination of needle.

Documentation

Follow your facility's policy for tracking narcotics administration, including disposal of excess volume when utilizing prefilled injection units. All patient education should be at the assessed level of understanding.

Elements of Patient Teaching

Provide instruction to client, primary caregiver, and a back-up person. Assess their acceptance and ability to prepare and administer parenteral medication at home. Teach aseptic technique and use of equipment that may be required due to a physical limitation. Utilize demonstration/return demonstration techniques to assist in evaluating level of understanding. Instruct the patient or family about desired effects of medication, preparation schedule and how to store medication, possible untoward effects of medication, and to notify a health care professional if unusual symptoms occur.

PROCEDURE 16-2

Administering Subcutaneous Injections

Objective

Administer medication(s) as ordered by a licensed prescriber while ensuring maximum patient safety. Provide a route for administration of select medications (Fig. 16–25).

Terminology

- Injection—introduction of a fluid substance into the body, usually with a syringe or other device connected to a hollow needle
- Subcutaneous—beneath the layers of skin; accepted abbreviations include SQ and subq

Critical Elements

Assess for patient allergies prior to administering any new medication.

For reasons of cost containment and documented decreased incidence of medication errors, the pharmacies of many facilities now dispense medications by the unit dose method and mix the majority of injections and intravenous solutions. However, the nurse actually giving the medication is still responsible for all aspects of medication administration. When giving any medication, observe the five rights of medication administration:

- Right medication
- Right dosage
- Right time
- Right route
- Right patient

Prior to administering any medication, the nurse should know

- Desired therapeutic effect
- Reason for administering drug
- Usual dosage and route
- Any potential for drug/food interactions
- Potential adverse side effects

As with all procedures, handwashing is the first line of defense in infection control. The nurse may wear clean, nonsterile gloves as additional protection.

Triple-check labels:

- When removing medication from shelf, refrigerator, or drawer
- While preparing medication
- When returning medication to shelf, refrigerator, or drawer or before discarding packaging material

Medication expiration dates should always be checked, and outdated medication discarded or returned to the pharmacy.

Blood flow influences absorption of medication. Because subcutaneous tissue blood flow is minimal, the rate of absorption is usually slow. However, a few medications, such as heparin, are absorbed just as rapidly

continued on next page

PROCEDURE 16-2 (cont'd)

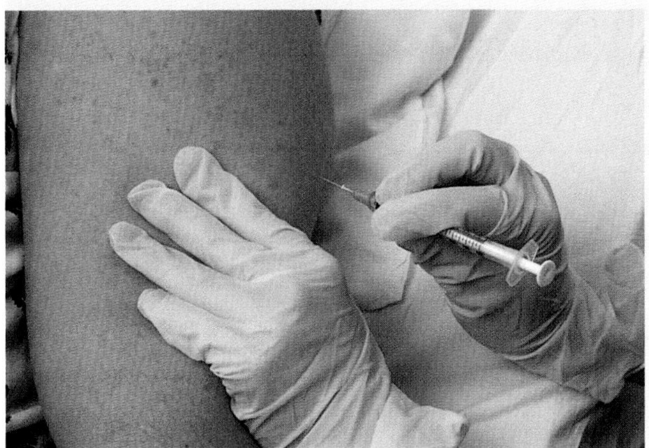

Figure 16–25. Subcutaneous injection.

when given subcutaneously as when given intramuscularly. The licensed prescriber may order a medication to be given subcutaneously if

- Subcutaneous is the preferred method of administration. The medication should be highly soluble and nonirritating. Not more than 1 cc should be injected at a time into any one site.
- The patient cannot or will not swallow or is uncooperative or unconscious.
- The patient has been ordered to have nothing by mouth.
- The effect of the medication would be destroyed by gastrointestinal secretions or would irritate the gastrointestinal tract.

Contraindications for subcutaneous administration include

- Shock
- Poor perfusion related to occlusive vascular disease
- When injection sites are grossly adipose, edematous, burned, hardened, or traumatized by previous injections or exhibit skin disease
- When subcutaneous is not a recommended route of administration for the prescribed medication

Use of heat will increase the rate of absorption of a medication and decrease pain associated with injection. However, use of heat may be contraindicated with some medications. Read the package insert or other medication references if you are unsure whether heat may or may not be used.

Preferred areas for subcutaneous injection include

- Dorsolateral aspect of arm, 3 to 5 inches above elbow
- Abdomen, avoiding area 2 inches in diameter around umbilicus and belt line
- Anterior and lateral thigh, approximately 3 inches above knee
- Scapula area

Equipment

- Antiseptic wipes
- 1-cc syringe with a ⅝-inch needle attached (tuberculin or insulin syringe)
- 25 G to 27 G needle, 0.5 inch to 1 inch in length, as needed
- Correct medication and dosage
- Clean, nonsterile gloves

Special Considerations

Appropriate needle length should be determined by placing the thumb and forefinger at the site and grasping a fold of skin. Select a needle length closest to the height of the skin fold. Generally, a 0.5-inch needle is adequate for most patients. A ⅞-inch or 1-inch needle is generally used for an overweight patient. The correct needle length ensures injecting the medication into subcutaneous tissue and minimizes discomfort associated with injection.

continued on next page

PROCEDURE 16-2 (cont'd)

Injection sites should be rotated to aid in absorption and avoid unnecessary tissue trauma. When administering heparin or insulin, use of a diagram is helpful in identifying used and unused sites to prevent excessive skin trauma and promote adequate absorption of the medication.

After drawing up the medication, air to fill dead space should be introduced into the syringe if giving the subcutaneous injection at a 90° angle. Prior to injection, position the syringe so air is located distal to the needle tip, proximal to the plunger. When the medication is injected, the bubble will force out the last amount of medication and seal it into the tissue.

When administering heparin via the subcutaneous route, follow the routine procedure, with the following exceptions:

- The abdomen is the preferred site for heparin administration. Do not inject heparin within 2 inches of the umbilicus or a scar. Avoid the area around the belt line. Be sure to rotate sites.
- Never inject heparin into an ecchymotic area. You may not be able to recognize hematoma formation resulting from the injection.
- Ice may be applied to the injection site prior to injection to reduce the possibility of hematoma formation. Some facilities require a physician's order for this; read the policy of your facility prior to using ice.
- Do not aspirate after needle placement, as this can cause tissue damage and hematoma formation.
- Never massage the site after injection.

When administering insulin via the subcutaneous route, follow routine procedure. To minimize the number of injections, regular insulin may be mixed with another type of insulin.

Draw the regular insulin dose into the syringe first, then add the second type of insulin. Be careful to withdraw the **exact** dose of the second type.

Do not discard an excess of mixed insulin into the insulin vial.

Do not administer an injection of mixed insulin that has had a portion of its contents discarded.

Actions	***Rationale***
1. Assemble all equipment and prepare medication using aseptic technique.	1. Promotes successful task completion.
2. Add air to syringe to fill dead space if giving at a 90° angle.	2. Ensures that all medication will be injected and prevents seepage from needle during withdrawal.
3. Verify medication order.	3. Ensures that correct medication is being administered.
4. Identify patient.	4. Ensures that correct patient is receiving medication.
5. Explain procedure to patient and provide privacy.	5. Promotes patient cooperation.
6. Provide adequate lighting.	6. Assists in selection of injection site.
7. Select injection site, using anatomic landmarks.	7. Lessens potential for injury.
8. Assist patient to a safe, comfortable position based on site chosen.	8. Provides clear access to injection site and placement of injection.
9. Wash hands.	9. Provides first line of defense in infection prevention.
10. Don gloves.	10. Provides protection for nurse.
11. Cleanse injection site with an antiseptic wipe, using friction, beginning at center and moving outward in a circular motion.	11. Decreases risk of infection.
12. Allow skin to dry for 30 seconds.	12. Allows antiseptic to take effect and reduces risk of introducing antiseptic into tissues, which may cause unnecessary pain.
13. Remove needle cover by pulling it straight off.	13. Prevents contamination of needle.
14. Inform patient you are ready to give injection.	14. Promotes patient cooperation.
15. Grasp a fold of skin gently but firmly, with thumb and index finger of your nondominate hand.	15. Ensures that needle will be inserted into subcutaneous tissue.

continued on next page

PROCEDURE 16-2 (cont'd)

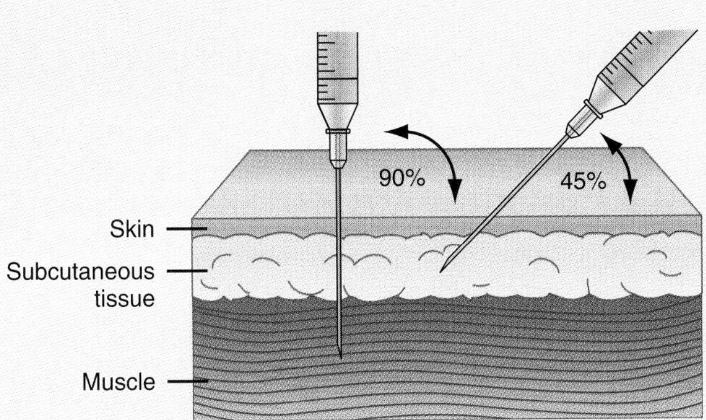

Figure 16–26. Proper angle for subcutaneous injection.

16. Insert needle to its full length at a 45 to 90° angle (Fig. 16–26) using a quick, dartlike motion. Use a 45° angle with a ⅝-inch or longer needle and a 90° angle with a 0.5-inch needle.	16. Decreases discomfort associated with needle insertion.
17. Release grasp on skin.	17. Reduces risk of irritation and discomfort associated with injections into compressed tissue.
18. Aspirate by pulling back on plunger. **Do not** move needle. If blood appears, withdraw needle and discard medication. Prepare a new injection.	18. Ensures that a blood vessel has not been entered.
19. Inject medication slowly by pushing on plunger and holding syringe steady.	19. Decreases discomfort and risk of damage to tissues.
20. Withdraw needle at same angle as inserted. Use an antiseptic swab to apply pressure at site as you withdraw.	20. Prevents discomfort related to needle withdrawal, seals punctured site, and prevents medication seepage.
21. Massage site with a circular motion.	21. Enhances absorption of medication.
22. Assess site for bleeding. Apply additional pressure if necessary.	22. Ensures patient safety after injection.
23. Assist patient to a comfortable position.	23. Promotes comfort and patient satisfaction.
24. Place disposables in proper containers.	24. Promotes a safe, clean environment and complies with universal blood and body fluid precautions.
25. Observe for adverse effects immediately following and up to 30 minutes after injection.	25. Promotes observation of medication reactions that may occur very shortly after administration.

Documentation

Document on medication record date, time, dosage, and route of medication administration, including injection site. Document in patient record patient response to procedure, postprocedure assessment, and all patient education and assessed level of understanding.

Elements of Patient Teaching

Instruct patient or family on reason for injection and type of medication, possible untoward effects of medication, administration schedule, and activity restrictions. Also instruct patient or family to notify nurse if unusual symptoms occur.

PROCEDURE 16-3

Administering Intramuscular Injections

Objective

Administer medication(s) as ordered by a licensed prescriber while ensuring maximum patient safety. Provide a route for administration of select medications (Fig. 16–27).

Terminology

- Injection—introduction of a fluid substance into the body, usually with a syringe or device connected to a hollow needle
- Intramuscular—within the muscular substance; may be abbreviated IM

Critical Elements

Assess for patient allergies prior to administering any new medication. For reasons of cost containment and documented decreased incidence of medication errors, the pharmacies in many facilities now dispense medications by the unit dose method and

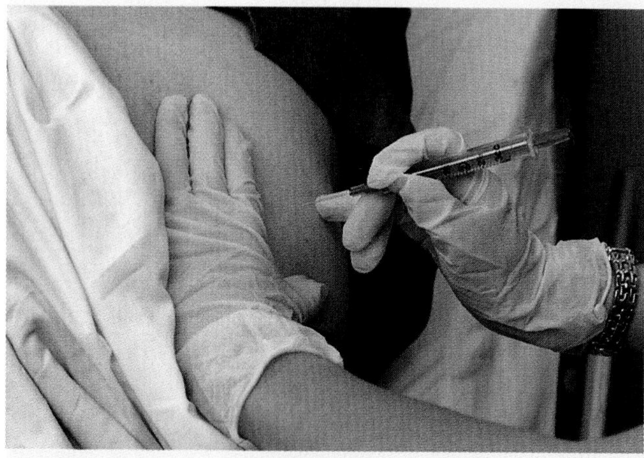

Figure 16–27. Intramuscular injection.

mix the majority of injections and intravenous solutions. However, the nurse actually giving the medication is still responsible for all aspects of medication administration. When giving any medication, observe the five rights of medication administration:

- Right medication
- Right dosage
- Right time
- Right route
- Right patient

Prior to administering any medication, the nurse should know

- Desired therapeutic effect
- Reason for administering the drug
- Usual dosage and route
- Any potential for drug or food interactions
- Potential adverse side effects

As with all procedures, handwashing is first line of defense in infection control. The nurse may wear clean, nonsterile gloves as additional protection.Triple-check labels:

- When removing medication from shelf, refrigerator, or drawer
- While preparing medication
- When returning medication to shelf, refrigerator, or drawer or before discarding packaging material.

Medication expiration dates should always be checked and outdated medication discarded or returned to the pharmacy.

Blood flow influences absorption of medication. Because muscular tissue is very vascular, the rate of absorption is usually quick. The licensed prescriber may order a medication to be given intramuscularly when

- Intramuscular is the preferred method of administration, such as with aqueous suspensions, solutions in oil, or those substances not available for oral administration.
- A rapid effect is desired.
- The patient cannot or will not swallow or is uncooperative or unconscious.
- The patient has been ordered to have nothing by mouth.
- The effect of the medication would be destroyed by gastric secretions or would irritate the gastrointestinal tract.
- Long-term absorption is desired by formation of a medication deposit.

continued on next page

PROCEDURE 16-3 (cont'd)

Use of heat increases the rate of absorption of a medication and decreases pain associated with the injection. Read the package insert or other medication references and the policy of your facility if you are unsure of whether heat may or may not be used.

Risks associated with intramuscular injections include

- Damage to blood vessels, resulting in bleeding and hematoma formation
- Inadvertent entry into a blood vessel, resulting in an intravenous injection and improper medication absorption and possible overdose
- Damage to nerves, resulting in discomfort or paralysis
- Damage to bone
- Breakage of needle

Preferred sites for intramuscular injections include

Muscle	*Location*	*Position*	*Comment*
Ventrogluteal	Hip, just below iliac crest	Back, side, or abdomen with knee and hip flexed on injection side	Can be used for all patients; site relatively free of large nerves and fat tissue
Dorsogluteal	Buttock	Prone, with toes pointed inward, arms flexed toward head, or on side with upper knee and hip flexed	Used for adults; do not use for infants and children younger than 3 years, muscle is not well developed; be careful to avoid sciatic nerve; only site that can be used for Z-track method (Fig. 16–28)
Deltoid	Upper arm	Sitting or supine with lower arm flexed and across abdomen	Seldom used, as muscle is small and only small doses can be injected; radial nerve is in close proximity

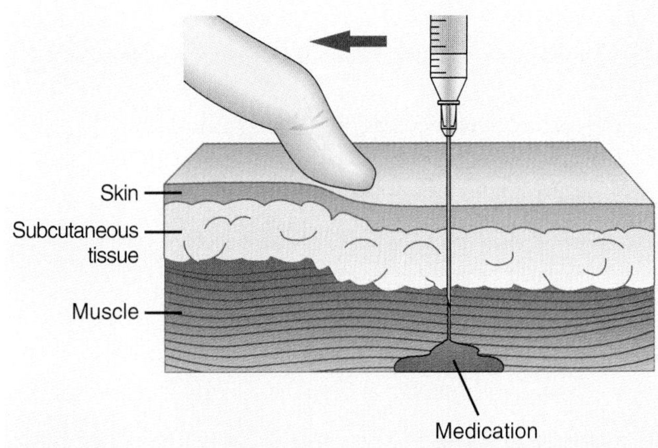

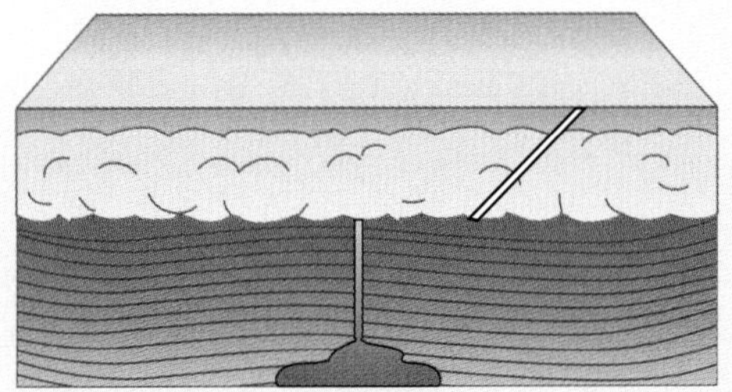

Figure 16–28. Z-track technique for intramuscular injection.

continued on next page

PROCEDURE 16-3 (cont'd)

Vastus lateralis	Lateral thigh	Supine with knee slightly flexed	Used for all patients, especially children
Rectus femoris	Anterior thigh	Sitting or supine	Most often used for self-injections because of accessibility of site

When administering intramuscular injections, give consideration to the following:

- The amount of solution given via the intramuscular route varies with the medication. In general, if the injection volume is greater than 5 cc, it should be divided and given into separate sites. Whether to divide a solution volume is also dependent on body size.
- A muscle that is painful or has hardened areas is not appropriate for an injection site.

The size of the needle and syringe vary depending on the amount and viscosity of the medication, the size of the patient, and the muscle selected for the injection. Select the smallest needle appropriate for the site and solution.

A 22-gauge, 1.5-inch needle is most commonly used for adult intramuscular injections. Rotate injection sites to aid in absorption and avoid unnecessary tissue trauma.

Equipment

- Antiseptic wipes
- Sterile needle (19 to 22 gauge, 1.5 to 3 inches)
- Sterile syringe (1 to 5 cc)
- Correct medication and dosage
- Clean, nonsterile gloves

Special Considerations

Patients receiving intramuscular injections should be placed in a position of safety and comfort, as well as one that is consistent with the condition of the patient and offers adequate exposure of the injection site.

The patient should be given a thorough explanation of the procedure prior to drug administration to reduce anxiety.

Actions	*Rationale*
1. Assemble all equipment and prepare medication using aseptic technique.	1. Promotes successful task completion.
2. Verify medication order.	2. Ensures correct medication is being administered.
3. Identify patient.	3. Ensures correct patient is receiving medication.
4. Explain procedure and provide privacy.	4. Promotes patient cooperation.
5. Provide adequate lighting.	5. Assists in selection of injection site.
6. Select injection site, using anatomic landmarks.	6. Lessens potential for injury.
7. Assist patient to a safe, comfortable position based on site chosen. Restrain if small child.	7. Provides clear access to injection site and placement of injection.
8. Wash hands.	8. Provides first line of defense in infection prevention.
9. Don gloves.	9. Complies with universal blood and body fluid precautions.
10. Cleanse injection site with an antiseptic wipe, using friction, beginning at center and moving outward in a circular motion.	10. Cleansing from inner to outer decreases risk of infection.
11. Allow skin to dry for 30 seconds.	11. Allows antiseptic to take effect and reduces risk of introducing antiseptic into tissues, which may cause unnecessary pain.
12. Remove needle cover by pulling it straight off.	12. Prevents contamination of needle.
13. Inform patient you are ready to give injection.	13. Promotes patient cooperation.
14. Draw skin taunt with thumb and index finger of your nondominant hand.	14. Displaces subcutaneous tissue and makes needle insertion easier.
15. Thrust needle quickly to its full length at a 90° angle, using a quick, dartlike motion.	15. Decreases discomfort associated with needle insertion.

continued on next page

PROCEDURE 16-3 (cont'd)

16. Aspirate by pulling back on plunger. **Do not** move needle. If blood appears, withdraw needle and discard medication. Prepare a new injection.	16. Ensures that a blood vessel has not been entered.
17. Inject medication slowly by pushing on plunger and holding syringe steady.	17. Decreases discomfort and risk of damage to tissues.
18. Rapidly withdraw needle at same angle of insertion. Use an antiseptic swab to apply pressure at site as you withdraw.	18. Pressure prevents discomfort related to needle withdrawal, seals punctured tissue, and prevents medication seepage.
19. Massage site with a circular motion.	19. Distributes medication over a greater area and enhances absorption of medication.
20. Assess site for bleeding. Apply additional pressure if necessary.	20. Ensures patient safety after injection.
21. Assist patient to a comfortable position.	21. Promotes comfort and patient satisfaction.
22. Place disposables in proper containers.	22. Promotes a safe, clean environment and complies with universal blood and body fluid precautions.
23. Observe for adverse effects immediately following and up to 30 minutes after injection.	23. Medication reactions usually occur very shortly after administration.

Documentation

Document on the medication record date, time, dosage, and route of medication administration, including injection site. Note on the patient record patient response to procedure and postprocedure assessment, as well as all patient education and assessed level of understanding.

Elements of Patient Teaching

Instruct the patient or family regarding reason for injection, type of medication, possible untoward effects of medication, administration schedule, and any activity restrictions. Also instruct to notify nurse if unusual symptoms occur.

PROCEDURE 16-4

Administering Intradermal Injections

Objective

Administer medication(s) as ordered by a licensed prescriber for diagnostic uses or local anesthesia while ensuring maximum patient safety. Provide a route for administration of select medications (Fig. 16–29).

Terminology

- Injection—introduction of a fluid substance into the body, usually with a syringe or other device connected to a hollow needle
- Intradermal—within the substance of the skin

Critical Elements

Assess for patient allergies prior to administering any new medication.

For reasons of cost containment and documented decreased incidence of medication errors, the pharmacies of many facilities now dispense medications by the unit dose method and mix the majority of injections and intravenous solutions. However, the nurse actually giving the medication is still responsible for all aspects of medication administration. When giving any medication, observe the five rights of medication administration:

- Right medication
- Right dosage
- Right time
- Right route
- Right patient

continued on next page

PROCEDURE 16-4 (cont'd)

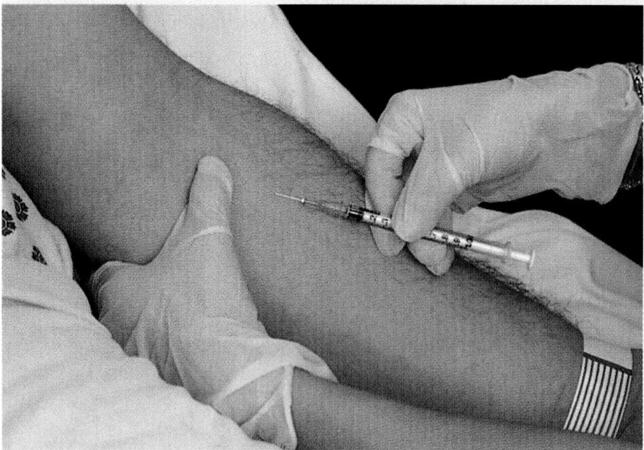

Figure 16–29. Intradermal injection.

Prior to administering any medication, the nurse should know

- Desired therapeutic effect
- Reason for administering the drug
- Usual dosage and route
- Any potential for drug/food interactions
- Potential adverse side effects

As with all procedures, handwashing is the first line of defense in infection control. The nurse may wear clean, nonsterile gloves as additional protection.

Triple-check labels:

- When removing medication from shelf, refrigerator, or drawer
- While preparing medication
- When returning medication to shelf, refrigerator, or drawer or before discarding packaging material.

Medication expiration dates should always be checked and outdated medication discarded or returned to the pharmacy.

Blood flow influences absorption of medication. Because blood flow in intradermal tissue is minimal, the rate of absorption is slow. The intradermal route is ideal for medications for which the desired action produces a local effect. Typically, the intradermal route is used for skin testing for allergies or respiratory diseases or when injecting local anesthesia.

When using the intradermal route for diagnostic purposes (skin testing), select a site that is lightly pigmented, thinly keratinized, and relatively free of hair. The preferred sites are the ventral forearms, the upper chest, or the scapula area. If administering multiple skin tests, identify each injection site with the type of test, date, and time on a diagram.

Never mix medications for intradermal injection. If a reaction occurs, you will not be able to determine which medication caused the reaction.

Equipment

- Antiseptic wipes that will not discolor skin (70 percent isopropyl alcohol preferred)
- 1-cc syringe with a 26-gauge, ⅝-inch needle attached (tuberculin or insulin syringe)
- Correct medication and dosage
- Clean, nonsterile gloves
- Diagram of injection sites if administering multiple skin tests

Special Considerations

Epinephrine should be readily available when performing allergy skin testing in the event of an anaphylactic reaction.

Therapeutic doses of medications may cause allergic reactions in patients with negative skin tests.

The injection site must be observed periodically over the ensuing 48 to 72 hours for signs of reaction. Typically, a positive reaction includes a significant area of induration **and** erythema. Strongly positive reactions may include vesiculation, ulceration, or tissue necrosis at the injection site. Review and save the package insert for the specific medication or utilize other reference material to accurately identify a positive reaction.

continued on next page

PROCEDURE 16-4 (cont'd)

Actions	*Rationale*
1. Assemble all equipment and prepare medication using aseptic technique.	1. Promotes successful task completion.
2. Verify medication order.	2. Ensures that correct medication is being administered.
3. Identify patient.	3. Ensures that correct patient is receiving medication.
4. Explain procedure to patient and provide privacy.	4. Promotes patient cooperation.
5. Provide adequate lighting.	5. Assists in selection of injection site and administration of medication.
6. Select injection site, using anatomic landmarks.	6. Lessens potential for injury.
7. Assist patient to a safe, comfortable position based on site chosen.	7. Provides clear access to injection site and placement of injection.
8. Wash hands.	8. Provides first line of defense in infection prevention.
9. Don gloves.	9. Provides protection for nurse.
10. Cleanse injection site with an antiseptic wipe, using friction, beginning at center and moving outward in a circular motion.	10. Decreases risk of infection.
11. Allow skin to dry for 30 seconds.	11. Allows antiseptic to take effect and reduces risk of introducing antiseptic into tissues, which may cause unnecessary pain.
12. Remove needle cover by pulling it straight off.	12. Prevents contamination of needle.
13. Inform patient you are ready to give injection.	13. Promotes patient cooperation.
14. Use thumb of your nondominant hand to pull skin taut over injection site.	14. Promotes easier needle insertion.
15. Position syringe so that it is parallel to and lying almost flat on skin (Fig. 16–30).	15. Ensures injection into correct tissue.

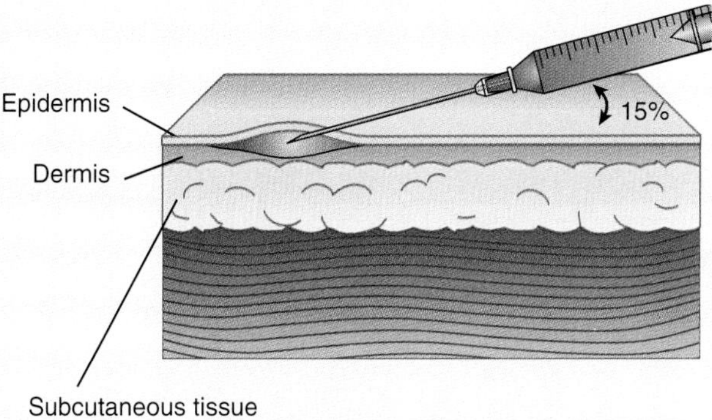

Figure 16–30. Proper angle for intradermal injection.

16. Insert needle, bevel up, approximately ⅛ inch below surface of skin. Tip and bevel of needle should be visible through skin. **Do not aspirate after needle is in position.**	16. Ensures that medication will be injected between epidermis and dermis. Prevents possible collapse of tissue at injection site.
17. Inject medication slowly by pushing on plunger and holding syringe steady. There should be some resistance. If none, withdraw needle slightly.	17. Decreases discomfort and risk of damage to tissues. No resistance indicates that needle is too deep.

continued on next page

PROCEDURE 16-4 (cont'd)

18. Watch for a bleb or bubble to form.	18. Indicates medication injected correctly.
19. Withdraw needle at same angle as inserted. Use an antiseptic swab to apply light pressure at site as you withdraw.	19. Prevents discomfort related to needle withdrawal, seals punctured site, and prevents medication seepage.
20. Do not massage site.	20. Ensures medication remains in correct tissue and accurate test results.
21. Assess site for bleeding. Apply additional pressure if necessary.	21. Ensures patient safety after injection.
22. Outline border of bleb with a non–water soluble marker.	22. Provides reference point when assessing for reaction.
23. Assist patient to a comfortable position.	23. Promotes comfort and patient satisfaction.
24. Place disposables in proper containers.	24. Promotes a safe, clean environment and complies with universal blood and body fluid precautions.
25. Observe for adverse effects immediately following and up to 30 minutes after injection.	25. Promotes observation of medication reactions that may occur very shortly after administration.

Documentation

Document in the medication record date, time, dosage, and route of medication administration including injection site. Document in the patient record response to procedure and postprocedure assessment, as well as all patient education and assessed level of understanding.

Elements of Patient Teaching

Instruct patient or family regarding reason for injection and type of medication, possible untoward effects of medication, and to notify nurse immediately if unusual or allergic symptoms occur. Instruct patient not to remove border outline until all observations are complete. Give instructions regarding indicators of a positive reaction and when to observe site for a reaction. Instruct to notify designated health care provider regarding results or schedule a follow-up appointment if in an outpatient setting.

PROCEDURE 16-4A

Administering Intramuscular Injections Using Z-Track Method

Objective

Administer medication(s) as ordered by a licensed prescriber while ensuring maximum patient safety and providing a route for administration of select medications.

Terminology

- Z-track—a method of administering intramuscular injections; the skin is grasped and pulled in such a way that the needle track is sealed off after removing the needle, minimizing subcutaneous irritation and discoloration (see Fig. 16–28).

Critical Elements

Assess for patient allergies prior to administering any new medication.

For reasons of cost containment and documented decreased incidence of medication errors, the pharmacies of many facilities now dispense medications by the unit dose method and mix the majority of injections and intravenous solutions. However, the nurse actually giving the medication is still responsible for all aspects of medication administration. When giving any medication, observe the five rights of medication administration:

- Right medication
- Right dosage

continued on next page

PROCEDURE 16-4A (cont'd)

- Right time
- Right route
- Right patient

Prior to administering any medication, the nurse should know

- Desired therapeutic effect
- Reason for administering drug
- Usual dosage and route
- Any potential for drug or food interactions
- Potential adverse side effects

As with all procedures, handwashing is the first line of defense in infection control. The nurse may wear clean, nonsterile gloves as additional protection.

Triple-check labels

- When removing medication from shelf, refrigerator, or drawer
- While preparing medication
- When returning medication to shelf, refrigerator, or drawer or before discarding packaging material

Medication expiration dates should always be checked and outdated medication discarded or returned to the pharmacy.

Risks associated with Z-track injections include

- Damage to blood vessels, resulting in bleeding and hematoma formation
- Inadvertent entry into a blood vessel, resulting in an intravenous injection and improper medication absorption and possible overdose
- Damage to nerves, resulting in discomfort or paralysis
- Damage to bone
- Breakage of needle

When administering Z-track injections, give consideration to the following:

Do not use on infants and children younger than 3 years.

Only dorsogluteal muscle (buttock) can be used.

A muscle that is painful or has hardened areas is not appropriate for an injection site.

Use a 19- to 20-gauge, 2- to 3-inch needle.

Alternate injection sites to aid in absorption and avoid unnecessary tissue trauma.

Equipment

- Antiseptic wipes
- Sterile needle (19 to 20 gauge, 2 to 3 inches)
- Sterile syringe (1 to 5 cc)
- Correct medication and dosage
- Clean, nonsterile gloves

Special Considerations

Patients receiving Z-track injections should be placed in a position of safety and comfort, as well as one that is consistent with the condition of the patient and offers adequate exposure of injection site. Preferred positions are

- Prone with toes pointed inward, arms flexed toward head
- Side, with upper knee and hip flexed

The patient should be given a thorough explanation of the procedure prior to drug administration to reduce anxiety.

Nursing Interventions

Actions	*Rationale*
1. Assemble all equipment and prepare medication using aseptic technique.	1. Promotes successful task completion.
2. Add air to syringe to fill dead space.	2. Addition of air ensures that all medication is injected and prevents seepage from needle during withdrawal.
3. Replace needle.	3. Prevents staining and irritation of subcutaneous tissue caused by residue left on original needle.
4. Verify medication order.	4. Ensures that correct medication is being administered.
5. Identify patient.	5. Ensures that the correct patient is receiving medication.
6. Explain procedure and provide privacy.	6. Promotes patient cooperation.
7. Provide adequate lighting.	7. Assists in selection of injection site.
8. Assist patient to a safe, comfortable position, exposing dorsogluteal muscle.	8. Provides clear access to injection site and placement of injection.
9. Wash hands.	9. Provides first line of defense in infection prevention.
10. Don gloves.	10. Complies with universal blood and body fluid precautions.

continued on next page

PROCEDURE 16-4A (cont'd)

11. Grasp skin with thumb and index finger of your nondominant hand. Pull skin laterally away from intended injection site.	11. Moves subcutaneous tissue from one area to another.
12. Cleanse injection site with an antiseptic wipe, using friction, beginning at center and moving outward in a circular motion.	12. Cleansing from inner to outer decreases risk of infection. Cleansing after pulling tissue away ensures preparation of intended injection site.
13. Allow skin to dry for 30 seconds.	13. Allows antiseptic to take effect and reduces risk of introducing antiseptic into tissues, which may cause unnecessary pain.
14. Remove needle cover by pulling it straight off.	14. Prevents contamination of needle.
15. Inform patient you are ready to give injection.	15. Promotes patient cooperation.
16. Thrust needle quickly to its full length at a 90° angle, using a quick, dartlike motion.	16. Decreases discomfort associated with needle insertion.
17. Aspirate by pulling back on plunger. **Do not** move needle. If blood appears, withdraw needle and discard medication. Prepare a new injection.	17. Ensures that a blood vessel has not been entered.
18. Inject medication slowly by pushing on plunger and holding syringe steady.	18. Decreases discomfort and risk of damage to tissues.
19. Wait 10 seconds, then rapidly withdraw needle at same angle of insertion.	19. Prevents medication seepage from site.
20. Apply gentle pressure to site. **Do not massage** site.	20. Massaging can force medication into subcutaneous tissue, causing irritation and discoloration.
21. Assess site for bleeding. Apply additional pressure if necessary.	21. Ensures patient safety after injection.
22. Assist patient to a comfortable position.	22. Promotes comfort and patient satisfaction.
23. Place disposables in proper containers.	23. Promotes a safe, clean environment and complies with universal blood and body fluid precautions.
24. Observe for adverse effects immediately following and up to 30 minutes after injection.	24. Medication reactions usually occur very shortly after administration.

Documentation

Document on medication record date, time, dosage, and route of medication administration, including injection site. Also document patient response to procedure and postprocedure assessment, as well as all patient education and assessed level of understanding.

Elements of Patient Teaching

Instruct the patient or family regarding the reason for injection, type of medication, possible untoward effects of medication, and administration schedule. Also instruct the patient or family to notify the nurse if unusual symptoms occur. Encourage walking or other activity to increase rate of absorption, if appropriate, and instruct the patient to avoid tight-fitting clothing, which could force medication into subcutaneous tissue.

PROCEDURE 16-5

Administering Oral Medications

Objective

Administer prescribed medication safely by oral route.

Terminology

- Mortar—a glass or ceramic dish used for pulverizing medications
- Pestle—a glass or ceramic wand with a rounded tip used to pulverize medications in a mortar
- Meniscus—upper, curved surface of a liquid that is in a container
- Pulverize—to grind into small, powderlike particles

Critical Elements

Assess for patient allergies prior to administering any new medication.

For reasons of cost containment and documented decreased incidence of medication errors, the pharmacies of many facilities now dispense medications by unit dose method and mix the majority of injections and intravenous solutions. However, the nurse actually giving medication is still responsible for all aspects of medication administration. When giving any medication, observe the five rights of medication administration:

- Right medication
- Right dosage
- Right time
- Right route
- Right patient

Prior to administering any medication, nurse should know

- Desired therapeutic effect
- Reason for administering drug
- Usual dosage and route
- Any potential for drug or food interactions
- Potential adverse side effects

As with all procedures, handwashing is the first line of defense in infection control. Nurse may wear clean, nonsterile gloves as additional protection.

Triple-check labels

- When removing medication from shelf, refrigerator, or drawer
- While preparing medication
- When returning medication to shelf, refrigerator, or drawer or before discarding packaging material

Medication expiration dates should always be checked and outdated medication discarded or returned to pharmacy.

Equipment

- Mortar and pestle (if indicated)
- Medication record
- Medication
- Medication cup
- Water, milk, juice (as indicated)

Special Considerations

Determine with the pharmacy if a drug must be crushed or a capsule opened, as this may be contraindicated because of action of the drug or altered rate of absorption. Dissolve pulverized medications if necessary for administration. Assess the patient's level of consciousness, ability to swallow, gag reflex, nausea and/or vomiting, and compliant behavior. Assess whether medication can be taken with water, milk, or juice, with meals, or on an empty stomach. Perform any dosage calculations prior to preparing medication. Have the patient sit in a high Fowler's position if not contraindicated. Measure all liquid medications at eye level to note the level of the meniscus on the measuring line.

Action	*Rationale*
1. Verify medication.	1. Ensures that correct medication being administered.
2. Obtain medication from medication storage area (medication cart or drawer, refrigerator, or cupboard).	2. Prepares supplies.
3. Identify patient and explain procedure.	3. Promotes safety and increases patient compliance.
4. Cross-check patient identification band with patient medication record form or medication card.	4. Ensures that this is the right patient.
5. Raise patient to high Fowler's or assist patient to sitting position (unless contraindicated by patient condition).	5. Facilitates swallowing and decreases chance of choking.
6. Cross-check medication with medication record and put medication into medication cup.	6. Ensures that this is the right medication, dose, time, route, and patient.
7. Give medication to patient or assist patient by putting medication in mouth if necessary—offer water to patient.	7. Assists patient in taking medication.
8. Confirm that medication is actually swallowed.	8. Patients with swallowing problems may have difficulty.

continued on next page

PROCEDURE 16-5 (cont'd)

9. Discard medication cup.	9. Provides for clean patient care area.
10. Assist patient to position of comfort.	10. Provides for patient comfort.
11. Document medication on medication record.	11. Ensures an accurate record of patient care.
12. Observe for possible adverse effects.	12. Enables patient care provider to take adverse reaction steps if indicated.

Documentation

Record medication, dose, time, route, and rate of administration, if indicated, on patient medication record. In patient record, note therapeutic effect of drug (if any); any adverse reactions, interventions, and results; and patient or family teaching done and assessed level of understanding.

Elements of Patient Teaching

Explain procedure to patient or family. Explain medication name, purpose, anticipated effects, possible untoward effects, and schedule of administration. Always instruct patient or family to notify nurse if unusual symptoms occur.

PROCEDURE 16-6

Adding Medication to Intravenous Fluid

Objective

Add medication to intravenous fluid as ordered by a licensed prescriber.

Critical Elements

When administering medication into an intravenous port, the nurse must use a needle that is long enough to allow medication to pass through the port and into the fluid.

Assess for patient allergies prior to administering any new medication.

For reasons of cost containment and documented decreased incidence of medication errors, the pharmacies of many facilities now dispense medications by the unit dose method and mix the majority of injections and intravenous solutions. However, the nurse actually giving the medication is still responsible for all aspects of medication administration.

When giving any medication, observe the five rights of medication administration:

- Right medication
- Right dosage
- Right time
- Right route
- Right patient

Prior to administering any medication, the nurse should know

- The desired therapeutic effect
- The reason for administering the drug
- The usual dosage and route
- Any potential for drug or food interactions
- Potential adverse side effects

As with all procedures, handwashing is the first line of defense in infection control. The nurse may wear clean, nonsterile gloves as additional protection.

Triple-check labels

- When removing medication from the shelf, refrigerator, or drawer
- While preparing medication
- When returning medication to the shelf, refrigerator, or drawer or before discarding the packaging material

Medication expiration dates should always be checked and outdated medication discarded or returned to the pharmacy.

Equipment

- Intravenous solution
- Medication
- Syringe
- Alcohol wipe
- Label

continued on next page

PROCEDURE 16-6 (cont'd)

Special Considerations

Closely assess the intravenous site and intravenous patency prior to starting administration. Inspect the intravenous solution to make sure there is no precipitate or clouding. Prior to adding the medication to the solution, make sure there are no incompatibilities between the solution and the medication. After the medication is added to the solution, assess to be sure the medication is completely dissolved. Whenever medication is administered by the intravenous route, the patient may experience reactions quickly; therefore, the patient must be closely observed.

Action	*Rationale*
1. Wash hands.	1. Prevents transmission of organisms from one patient to another.
2. Verify medication order.	2. Ensures that correct medication is administered.
3. Assemble equipment.	3. Promotes successful task completion.
4. Prepare medication using aseptic technique, drawing medication into syringe.	4. Prevents contamination of medication.
5. Remove cover from medication port on intravenous bag or cleanse injection port with alcohol wipe (depending on type of access provided by manufacturer).	5. Provides aseptic mode of access to the intravenous fluid.
6. Inject medication through intravenous port.	6. Provides means of introducing medication into intravenous fluid.
7. Inspect intravenous solution to verify there is no precipitate and that all medication has gone into solution.	7. Ensures that medication is safe to deliver to the patient.
8. Label intravenous solution with name of medication, amount of medication, date, time, and signature.	8. Provides information needed to correctly identify contents of intravenous solution.
9. Discard and return equipment to appropriate areas.	9. Keeps a safe and uncluttered working environment.

Documentation

Record the medication, dose, time, route, and rate (if indicated) of administration on the patient medication record. In the patient record, note the therapeutic effect of the drug (if any); any adverse reactions, interventions, and results; and patient and family teaching done, and assess level of understanding.

Elements of Patient Teaching

Explain the procedure to the patient or family, including the medication name, purpose, anticipated effects, possible untoward effects, and the schedule of administration. Always instruct patient or family to notify the nurse if unusual symptoms occur.

PROCEDURE 16-7

Administering Intravenous Medications with a Piggyback/Volume Control Set

Objective

Administering intermittent medication into venous system through an established primary line.

Terminology

- Burette—an inline chamber capable of holding and delivering a specific amount of fluid and to which medication can be added
- Piggyback—an intravenous infusion that is administered by attaching and running it through an established primary line
- Primary line—an intravenous tubing that provides direct access to venous system while delivering continuous fluid therapy
- Secondary line—an intravenous tubing that provides venous access to administer intermittent medication or fluid by infusing through primary tubing; access is established through an infusion port on primary tubing

Critical Elements

Assess for patient allergies prior to administering any new medication.

For reasons of cost containment and documented decreased incidence of medication errors, the pharmacies of many facilities now dispense medications by unit dose method and mix majority of injections and intravenous solutions. However, the nurse actually giving the medication is still responsible for all aspects of medication administration. When giving any medication, observe the five rights of medication administration:

- Right medication
- Right dosage
- Right time
- Right route
- Right patient

Prior to administering any medication, the nurse should know

- Desired therapeutic effect
- Reason for administering drug
- Usual dosage and route
- Any potential for drug or food interactions
- Potential adverse side effects

As with all procedures, handwashing is the first line of defense in infection control. The nurse may wear clean, nonsterile gloves as additional protection.

Triple-check labels

- When removing medication from shelf, refrigerator, or drawer
- While preparing medication
- When returning medication to shelf, refrigerator, or drawer or before discarding packaging material

Medication expiration dates should always be checked and outdated medication discarded or returned to the pharmacy.

Most manufacturers of intravenous products now make ports for needleless access. Ports may be covered with a sterile port cap or may need to be cleansed with an alcohol wipe. The nurse should familiarize himself or herself with the manufacturer's recommended method of use prior to using equipment.

Equipment

- Secondary tubing (for piggyback administration)
- Primary tubing
- Volume control set (for volume control administration)
- Medication/fluid piggyback (for piggyback administration)
- Medication-filled syringe (for volume-control administration)
- Alcohol wipe (if indicated)
- Sterile port cover (if indicated)

Special Considerations

Prior to any intravenous administration, assess the patency of the intravenous line. Also assess the site for possible infiltration or phlebitis. Review incompatibility of the medication to be administered with all intravenous solutions and medications already in the primary line. If an incompatibility exists and another intravenous site cannot be established, medication may be administered by stopping primary fluid, preflushing with a compatible solution, administering medication, and postflushing with a compatible solution. Always follow the manufacturer's recommendations for use of equipment. It is optimal to have intravenous solutions prepared by the pharmacy in a controlled environment. Assess the patient closely, as adverse reactions to intravenous medications can occur very rapidly.

Intravenous Piggyback Administration

Action	*Rationale*
1. Assemble equipment.	1. Aids in organization of task.
2. Verify order on medication record with physician's order.	2. Promotes safety.

continued on next page

PROCEDURE 16-7 (cont'd)

3. Wash hands; glove.	3. Provides first line of defense and protection for nurse.
4. Check intravenous piggyback for sediment or precipitates and expiration date (on premixed solutions).	4. Promotes safety by ensuring that defective or expired products are not administered.
5. Close clamp on secondary tubing.	5. Keeps solution from entering tubing until intravenous piggyback is inverted and drip chamber is filled.
6. Remove covering from spiking port and cleanse with alcohol if necessary.	6. Avoids contamination of solution from organisms on spiking port.
7. Insert spike into spiking port of bag or bottle.	7. Connects secondary tubing to solution in preparation for administration.
8. Hang intravenous solution bag and fill tubing drip chamber halfway by squeezing drip chamber.	8. Purges air from spike and keeps drip chamber only half full, so drops can be visualized during administration process.
9. Prime secondary tubing by opening clamp and purging air until solution is to end of tubing.	9. Avoids danger of air in line and also avoids wasting of medication.
10. Keep end of secondary tubing covered.	10. Avoids contamination.
11. Identify patient.	11. Promotes safety.
12. Explain procedure, including information about medication.	12. Increases patient compliance and gives patient necessary information regarding medication being given.
13. Examine intravenous site.	13. Allows nurse to determine line patency and absence of phlebitis.
14. Lower primary bottle until it is below level of secondary bottle.	14. Allows secondary bottle to run prior to primary line, because it is higher.
15. Prepare port on primary line per manufacturer's recommendations.	15. Provides safe, sterile access to primary line.
16. Insert secondary line into primary port (use port closest to intravenous site unless using infusion pump).	16. Establishes path for delivery of secondary solution through primary line.
17. Open clamp or controller completely on secondary line.	17. Allows flow adjustment through primary tubing or pump.
18. Adjust rate per controller on primary line (or adjust rate on pump if applicable.	18. Provides for delivery of medication at prescribed rate.
19. When infusion has completed, close clamp or controller on secondary line.	19. Prevents air from entering primary line.
20. Raise primary bag or bottle to original position.	20. Establishes flow of primary solution.
21. Adjust rate controller on primary bottle.	21. Administers primary solution at prescribed rate.

Volume-Control Set

1. Assemble equipment.	1. Aids in organization of task.
2. Verify order on medication record with physician's order.	2. Promotes safety.
3. Wash hands; glove.	3. Provides first line of defense and protection for nurse.
4. Remove covering from volume-control set tubing spike.	4. Keeps tubing spike sterile until time of administration.
5. Spike volume control tubing into prescribed solution bag or bottle.	5. Ensures air-tight connection.
6. Open rate controller and purge air from volume-control tubing.	6. Prevents administration of air to patient.
7. Close clamps or controllers above and below burette.	7. Prevents loss of fluid from line.

continued on next page

PROCEDURE 16-7 (cont'd)

8. Open clamp above burette and fill chamber with prescribed amount of fluid; then close clamp or controller.	8. Allows administration of small amounts of fluid or ability to dilute medication.
9. Draw up prescribed medication as listed on medication record.	9. Ensures administration of right medication.
10. Prepare port on top of burette chamber per manufacturer's recommendations.	10. Avoids contamination of medication or fluid.
11. Inject medication into port.	11. Allows method for adding medication to fluid in chamber.
12. Open clamp below burette chamber and adjust rate of flow.	12. Allows for administration of medication at prescribed rate.
13. When chamber is empty, refill and repeat procedure as necessary (if prescribed).	13. Provides means to administer multiple medication doses.

Documentation

Record medication, dose, time, route, and rate of administration, if indicated, on patient medication record. In patient record, note therapeutic effect of drug (if any); any adverse reactions, interventions, and results; and patient or family teaching done and assessed level of understanding.

Elements of Patient Teaching

Explain procedure to patient or family. Explain medication name, purpose, anticipated effects, possible untoward effects, and schedule of administration. Always instruct patient or family to notify nurse if unusual symptoms occur.

PROCEDURE 16-8

Administering Intravenous Bolus Medications

Objective

Administer medication by intravenous route for immediate effect or due to inability to give medication by another route.

Terminology

- Intravenous/heparin lock—intravenous device that provides direct access to venous system and may be used intermittently; it is filled with saline/heparin between uses
- Primary line—an intravenous tubing that provides direct access to venous system while delivering continuous fluid therapy

Critical Elements

Assess for patient allergies prior to administering any new medication.

For reasons of cost containment and documented decreased incidence of medication errors, the pharmacies of many facilities now dispense medications by unit dose method and mix the majority of injections and intravenous solutions. However, the nurse actually giving medication is still responsible for all aspects of medication administration.

When giving any medication, observe the five rights of medication administration:

- Right medication
- Right dosage
- Right time
- Right route
- Right patient

Prior to administering any medication, the nurse should know

- Desired therapeutic effect
- Reason for administering drug
- Usual dosage and route
- Any potential for drug or food interactions
- Potential adverse side effects

As with all procedures, handwashing is the first line of defense in infection control. The nurse may wear clean, nonsterile gloves as additional protection.

continued on next page

PROCEDURE 16-8 (cont'd)

Triple-check labels

- When removing medication from shelf, refrigerator, or drawer
- While preparing medication
- When returning medication to shelf, refrigerator, or drawer or before discarding packaging material

Medication expiration dates should always be checked and outdated medication discarded or returned to pharmacy.

Most manufacturers of intravenous products now make ports for needleless access. Ports may be covered with a sterile port cap or may need to be cleansed with an alcohol pad prior to use. The nurse should familiarize himself or herself with the manufacturer's recommended method of use prior to using equipment.

Equipment

- Medication filler syringe
- Alcohol wipes or sterile port cover (as indicated)
- Saline-filled syringe (3 to 5 cc)
- Watch with sweep hand

Special Considerations

Assess the intravenous line for patency. Also inspect the site for signs of phlebitis and/or infiltration. Note reports of any discomfort during or after infusion. Review compatibility of the medication with the solution in the line or lock. Follow the manufacturer's recommendations for use of ports on the primary line. Assess the patient closely for signs of adverse reaction, as the intravenous route of medication administration provides quick action and reaction to medication. Note any manufacturer's recommendation on intravenous administration of the drug to be given.

Action	*Rationale*
1. Assemble equipment.	1. Promotes successful task completion.
2. Prepare medication using aseptic technique and according to manufacturer's directions.	2. Promotes safety by reducing possible contamination of medication and possible harm to patient from giving medication in inappropriate strength or dilution.
3. Verify medication order.	3. Ensures that correct medication is being administered.
4. Research intravenous administration of medication being used and determine any possible incompatibilities with contents of primary line or lock.	4. Promotes maximum effectiveness of drug action and provides for safe administration of medication.
5. Identify patient.	5. Promotes patient safety.
6. Explain procedure.	6. Promotes patient compliance.
7. Wash hands.	7. Avoids transmission of organisms from one patient to another.
8. Glove.	8. Provides protection for nurse.

If Administering Medication Through a Primary Line

9. Cleanse port or remove protective cap (as indicated).	9. Allows access to primary line and prevents contamination from microorganisms.
10. Flush line with 3 to 5 cc saline after clamping line just above port if giving a medication that is incompatible with the solution in the line.	10. Provides protection from reactions such as crystallization or precipitation, which may occur with incompatible drugs.
11. Insert medication-filled syringe into port and clamp tubing just above port.	11. Keeps medication from backflowing into primary tubing and into solution bag.
12. Attempt to aspirate blood.	12. Checks for patency.
13. Inject medication at recommended rate, then remove syringe from port.	13. Allows for maximum effect of medication while protecting patient from adverse reactions due to administering medication too rapidly.
14. Unclamp tubing and ensure that previous flow rate is established.	14. Allows continued administration of intravenous solution at prescribed rate.

continued on next page

PROCEDURE 16-8 (cont'd)

Action	Rationale
15. Discard or return equipment to proper location.	15. Provides a safe and uncluttered working environment.
16. Observe for possible adverse effects.	16. Enables patient care provider to take steps for adverse reactions if indicated.

If Medication Is Being Delivered Through an Intravenous/Heparin Lock

Action	Rationale
16. Remove cap or cleanse lock opening according to manufacturer's instructions.	16. Prevents contamination from microorganisms.
17. Attach saline-filled syringe to lock and attempt to aspirate. Then preflush site with 3 to 5 cc saline.	17. Checks for line patency and removes any possible incompatible solution from lock.
18. Instill medication at appropriate rate, then remove syringe.	18. Allows for maximum effect of medication while protecting patient from adverse reactions due to administering medication too rapidly.
19. Attach saline-filled syringe to port and flush lock with 3 to 5 cc. Remove syringe and cap lock (if indicated).	19. Ensures that all of medication is delivered into venous system, fills lock with saline to prevent clotting, and maintains sterility of lock opening.
20. Discard or return equipment to appropriate location.	20. Keeps a safe and uncluttered working environment.
21. Observe for possible adverse effects.	21. Enables patient care provider to take steps for adverse reaction if indicated.

Documentation

Record medication, dose, time, route and rate of administration, if indicated, in patient medication record. Note therapeutic effect of drug (if any), any adverse reactions, interventions taken, and results.

Elements of Patient Teaching

Explain procedure to patient or family. Explain medication name, purpose, anticipated effects, possible side effects, and schedule of administration. Always instruct patient or family to notify nurse if unusual symptoms occur.

PROCEDURE 16-9

Introducing Medications Through Intravenous/ Heparin Lock Using Saline Push

Objective

Administer intermittent medication directly into the venous system.

Terminology

- Intravenous/heparin lock—intravenous device that provides direct access to venous system and may be used intermittently; it is filled with saline or heparin between uses

Critical Elements

Assess for patient allergies prior to administering any new medication.

For reasons of cost containment and documented decreased incidence of medication errors, the pharmacies of many facilities now dispense medications by the unit dose method and mix the majority of injections and intravenous solutions. However, the nurse actually giving the medication is still responsible for all aspects of medication administration.

continued on next page

PROCEDURE 16-9 (cont'd)

When giving any medication, observe the five rights of medication administration:

- Right medication
- Right dosage
- Right time
- Right route
- Right patient

Prior to administering any medication, the nurse should know

- Desired therapeutic effect
- Reason for administering drug
- Usual dosage and route
- Any potential for drug or food interactions
- Potential adverse side effects

As with all procedures, handwashing is the first line of defense in infection control. The nurse may wear clean, nonsterile gloves as additional protection.

Triple-check labels

- When removing medication from shelf, refrigerator, or drawer
- While preparing medication
- When returning medication to shelf, refrigerator, or drawer or before discarding packaging material

Medication expiration dates should always be checked and outdated medication discarded or returned to the pharmacy.

Most manufacturers of intravenous products now make ports for needleless access. Ports may be covered with a sterile port cap or may need to be cleansed with an alcohol pad prior to use. The nurse should familiarize himself or herself with the manufacturer's recommended method of use prior to using equipment.

Equipment

- Medication-filled syringe
- Saline-filled syringe (6 to 10 cc)
- Alcohol wipes or sterile port cover (as indicated)
- Watch with second hand

Special Considerations

Assess intravenous line for patency. Also inspect site for signs of phlebitis and/or infiltration. Note any reports of discomfort at intravenous site during or after infusion. Review compatibility of medication with solution in line or lock. Follow the manufacturer's recommendations for use of the ports on the primary line. Assess the patient closely for signs of adverse reaction, as the intravenous route of medication administration provides quick action and reaction to medication. Note any manufacturer's recommendation on intravenous administration of the drug to be given.

Action	*Rationale*
1. Assemble equipment.	1. Promotes successful task completion.
2. Prepare medication using aseptic technique.	2. Reduces risk of contaminating medication.
3. Verify medication order.	3. Ensures correct medication being administered.
4. Research intravenous administration of medication being used and determine any possible incompatibilities with contents of lock.	4. Promotes maximum effectiveness of drug action and provides for safe administration of medication.
5. Identify patient.	5. Promotes patient safety.
6. Explain procedure.	6. Promotes patient compliance.
7. Wash hands.	7. Avoids transmission of organisms from one patient to another.
8. Glove.	8. Provides protection for nurse.
9. Remove cap or cleanse lock opening, according to manufacturer's instructions.	9. Provides a sterile port into which medications may be instilled.
10. Attach saline-filled syringe to lock and attempt to aspirate. Then preflush lock with 3 to 5 cc saline.	10. Checks for line patency and removes any possible incompatible solution from lock.
11. Instill medication at recommended rate, then remove syringe.	11. Allows for maximum effect of medication while protecting patient from adverse reactions due to administering medication too rapidly.
12. Attach saline-filled syringe to port and flush lock with 3 to 5 cc. Remove syringe and cap lock (if indicated).	12. Ensures that all medication is delivered into the venous system, fills the lock with saline to prevent clotting, and maintains the sterility of the lock opening.

continued on next page

PROCEDURE 16-9 (cont'd)

13. Discard or return equipment to appropriate location.
14. Observe patient for adverse reaction.

13. Provides a safe and uncluttered working environment.
14. Enables patient care provider to take steps for adverse reaction if indicated.

Documentation

Record medication, dose, time, route, and rate of administration, if indicated, on the patient medication record. In the patient record, note the therapeutic effect of the drug (if any), any adverse reactions, interventions taken, and results.

Elements of Patient Teaching

Explain the procedure to the patient or family. Explain medication name, purpose, anticipated effects, possible side effects, and schedule of administration. Always instruct the patient or family to notify the nurse if unusual symptoms occur.

PROCEDURE 16-10

Administering Eye Medications

Objective

Administer medication(s) as ordered by a licensed prescriber while ensuring maximum patient safety. Instill medication into the eye for therapeutic effect (Fig. 16–31).

Terminology

- Conjunctival sac—mucous membrane that lines the eyes and can be visualized when pulling back the eyelid
- Cornea—anterior portion of the eye that is normally clear and transparent

Critical Elements

The cornea of the eye is very sensitive and may be easily damaged. Never instill drops or ointment directly onto the cornea but into the conjunctival sac instead. Sterile technique should be used whenever administering eye medications.

Assess for patient allergies prior to administering any new medication.

For reasons of cost containment and documented decreased incidence of medication errors, the pharmacies of many facilities now dispense med-

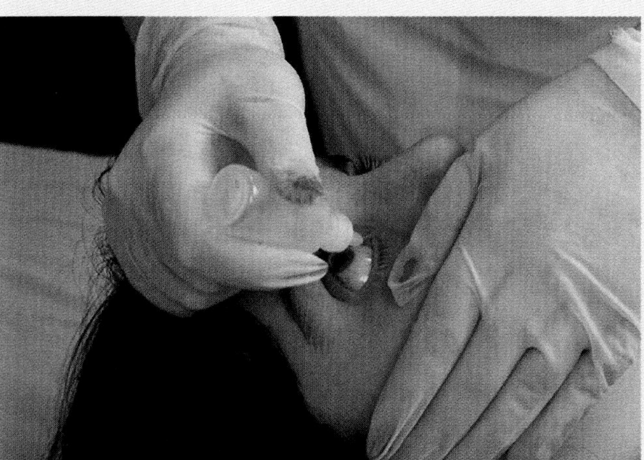

Figure 16–31. Administering eye drops.

continued on next page

PROCEDURE 16-10 (cont'd)

ications by the unit dose method and mix the majority of injections and intravenous solutions. However, the nurse actually giving the medication is still responsible for all aspects of medication administration.

When giving any medication, observe the five rights of medication administration:

- Right medication
- Right dosage
- Right time
- Right route
- Right patient

Prior to administering any medication, the nurse should know

- The desired therapeutic effect
- The reason for administering the drug
- The usual dosage and route
- Any potential for drug or food interactions
- Potential adverse side effects

As with all procedures, handwashing is the first line of defense in infection control. The nurse may wear clean, nonsterile gloves as additional protection.

Triple-check labels

- When removing medication from the shelf, refrigerator, or drawer
- While preparing medication
- When returning medication to the shelf, refrigerator, or drawer or before discarding the packaging material

Medication expiration dates should always be checked and outdated medication discarded or returned to the pharmacy.

Equipment

- Sterile 2 × 2 gauze sponges
- Sterile saline
- Eye medication prescribed
- Tissue

Special Considerations

Separate supplies should be used for each eye to avoid the transfer of organisms from one eye to another.

Action	*Rationale*
1. Verify medication order.	1. Ensures that correct medication is being administered.
2. Assemble all equipment.	2. Promotes successful task completion.
3. Identify patient.	3. Promotes patient safety.
4. Explain procedure.	4. Promotes patient compliance.
5. Emphasize to patient importance of not moving.	5. Reduces possibility of injury to eye during medication instillation process.
6. Wash hands.	6. Prevents transmission of organisms from one patient to another.
7. Position patient in sitting or supine position with head tilted back.	7. Facilitates administration of medication.
8. Wipe eyelid if secretions are present with sterile 2 × 2 dampened with saline.	8. Removes any matter that may interfere with medication administration.
9. Instruct patient to look upward.	9. Decreases chance of corneal reflex, which may cause patient to move when medication is applied.
10. Gently pull down on lower lid distal to center of lower lashes with nondominant hand.	10. Exposes conjunctival sac.
11. Rest dominant hand on patient's forehead.	11. Allows hand applying medication to move if patient's head moves, therefore avoiding possible injury.
12. Administer drops or squeeze ointment without touching eyelid.	12. Avoids possible injury to patient and possible contamination of medication container.
13. Instruct patient to close eyes and move eye back and forth under closed lid.	13. Distributes medication throughout the eye.
14. Wipe excess medication off of areas around eye.	14. Promotes patient comfort.
15. Discard or return all equipment to appropriate areas.	15. Provides for clean work area.
16. Assist patient to position of comfort.	16. Promotes patient comfort.

continued on next page

PROCEDURE 16-10 (cont'd)

Documentation

Record the medication, dose, time, and route of administration on the patient medication record. In the patient record, note the therapeutic effect of the drug (if any); any adverse reactions, interventions, and results; and patient or family teaching done and assess level of understanding. Record assessment of the eye and any observed exudate.

Elements of Patient Teaching

Explain the procedure to the patient or family, including the medication name, purpose, anticipated effects, possible untoward effects, and the schedule of administration. Explain the importance of lying or sitting still during the procedure. Always instruct the patient or family to notify the nurse if unusual symptoms occur. Instruct the patient or family to administer eyedrops if necessary.

PROCEDURE 16-11

Administering Ear Medications

Objective

Administer medication(s) as ordered by a licensed prescriber while ensuring maximum patient safety. Instill a prescribed medication into the ear for therapeutic effect (Fig. 16–32).

Terminology

- Auricle—the outer, cartilaginous portion of the ear

Critical Elements

The ear canal of the adult is in a forward and downward direction. To facilitate passage of medication into the ear canal, pull the adult auricle up and back. The ear canal of an infant is almost straight and therefore requires the ear auricle to be pulled down and back.

Assess for patient allergies prior to administering any new medication.

For reasons of cost containment and documented decreased incidence of medication errors, the pharmacies of many facilities now dispense medications by the unit dose method and mix the majority of injections and intravenous solutions. However, the nurse actually giving the medication is still responsible for all aspects of medication administration.

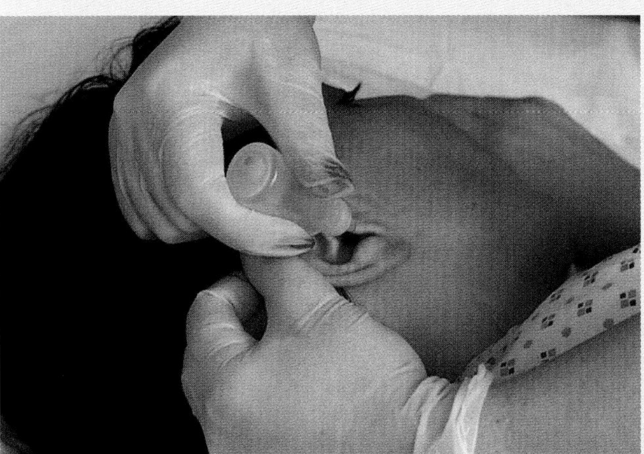

Figure 16–32. Administering ear drops.

continued on next page

PROCEDURE 16-11 (cont'd)

When giving any medication, observe the five rights of medication administration:

- Right medication
- Right dosage
- Right time
- Right route
- Right patient

Prior to administering any medication, the nurse should know

- The desired therapeutic effect
- The reason for administering the drug
- The usual dosage and route
- Any potential for drug or food interactions
- Potential adverse side effects

As with all procedures, handwashing is the first line of defense in infection control. The nurse may wear clean, nonsterile gloves as additional protection.

Triple-check labels

- When removing medication from the shelf, refrigerator, or drawer
- While preparing medication
- When returning medication to the shelf, refrigerator, or drawer or before discarding the packaging material

Medication expiration dates should always be checked and outdated medication discarded or returned to the pharmacy.

Equipment

- Medication with medicine dropper
- Cotton balls
- Normal saline

Special Considerations

Administer ear drops at body temperature for patient comfort.

Action	*Rationale*
1. Verify medication order.	1. Ensures that correct medication is being administered.
2. Assemble equipment.	2. Promotes successful task completion.
3. Identify patient.	3. Provides patient safety.
4. Explain procedure.	4. Promotes patient compliance.
5. Position patient supine with head to one side, affected ear up.	5. Provides a position conducive to medication administration.
6. Wash hands.	6. Prevents transmission of organisms from one patient to another.
7. Warm medication to body temperature.	7. Increases patient comfort.
8. Measure prescribed medication in medicine dropper.	8. Ensures that accurate dose of medication is to be given.
9. Pull auricle of ear up and back with nondominant hand.	9. Provides a means to straighten ear canal in preparation for medication administration.
10. Position hand holding dropper by resting it on side of patient's head.	10. Increases safety in case of head movement.
11. Administer prescribed medication with dropper, without touching dropper to ear.	11. Protects medication dropper from contamination.
12. Aim drops at wall of the canal, not eardrum.	12. Lessens chance of patient movement from startling.
13. Place cotton ball in outer ear loosely.	13. Absorbs excess medication.
14. Keep patient's head in turned position 10 to 15 minutes, unless otherwise ordered.	14. Allows medication to contact canal surface before running out.
15. Discard or return all equipment to appropriate areas.	15. Provides for clean work area.
16. Assist patient to position of comfort.	16. Promotes patient comfort.

Documentation

Record the medication, dose, time, and route of administration on the patient medication record. In the patient record, note the therapeutic effect of the drug (if any); any adverse reactions, interventions, and results; and patient or family teaching done and assess level of understanding.

Elements of Patient Teaching

Always instruct the patient or family to notify the nurse if unusual symptoms occur.

PROCEDURE 16-12

Administering Nasal Medications

Objective

Administer medication(s) as ordered by a licensed prescriber while ensuring maximum patient safety. Provide a means to administer prescribed medication to nasal area (Fig. 16–33).

Terminology

- Nares—openings of nasal passages located at the end of the nose

Critical Elements

Nasal medications may be used to treat infection, shrink edematous tissue, prevent or control bleeding, or provide topical anesthesia.

Aseptic technique should be observed when instilling nasal medication, because the nasal passages are in close proximity to the sinuses.

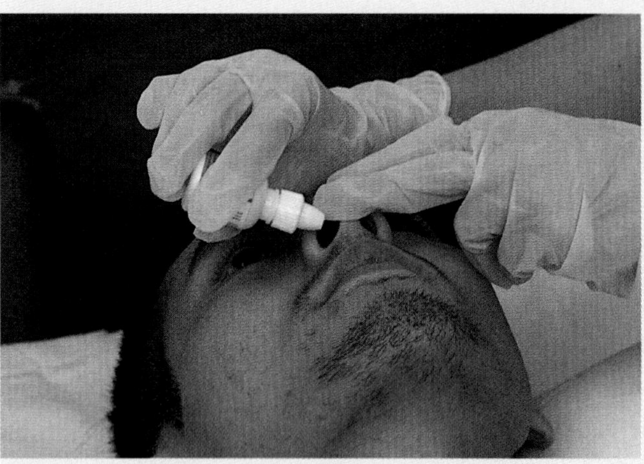

Figure 16–33. Administering nasal drops.

Avoid touching the inner surfaces of the nose with the dropper, because it may precipitate sneezing.

Assess for patient allergies prior to administering any new medication.

For reasons of cost containment and documented decreased incidence of medication errors, the pharmacies of many facilities now dispense medications by the unit dose method and mix the majority of injections and intravenous solutions. However, the nurse actually giving the medication is still responsible for all aspects of medication administration.

When giving any medication, observe the five rights of medication administration:

- Right medication
- Right dosage
- Right time
- Right route
- Right patient

Prior to administering any medication, the nurse should know

- The desired therapeutic effect
- The reason for administering the drug
- The usual dosage and route
- Any potential for drug or food interactions
- Potential adverse side effects

As with all procedures, handwashing is the first line of defense in infection control. The nurse may wear clean, nonsterile gloves as additional protection.

Triple-check labels

- When removing medication from the shelf, refrigerator, or drawer
- While preparing medication
- When returning medication to the shelf, refrigerator, or drawer or before discarding the packaging material

Medication expiration dates should always be checked, and outdated medication discarded or returned to the pharmacy.

Equipment

- Medication with medicine dropper
- Pillow
- Tissue

Special Considerations

During nasal instillation, it is best to position the patient supine with the head over a pillow. The effectiveness of the medication will be reduced if the head is only tilted backward, because the medication will run into the back of the throat, reducing its effectiveness.

continued on next page

PROCEDURE 16-12 (cont'd)

Place the patient in one of the following positions to provide medication flow to the appropriate area:

- Frontal and maxillary sinuses—flat supine with shoulders supported by a pillow and head hyperextended and turned toward affected side (Parkinson position)
- Ethmoid and sphenoid sinuses—flat supine with shoulders supported by a pillow and neck hyperextended (Proetz position)
- Eustachian tube—flat supine with head turned partially to affected side

Action	*Rationale*
1. Verify medication order.	1. Ensures that correct medication is being administered.
2. Identify patient.	2. Promotes patient safety.
3. Explain procedure.	3. Promotes patient compliance.
4. Instruct patient to blow nose gently.	4. Clears nasal passages in preparation for medication instillation.
5. Position patient supine with head back and small pillow under neck.	5. Promotes medication being delivered to nasal passages and decreases chance of its going down the throat.
6. Wash hands.	6. Avoids transmission of organisms from one patient to another.
7. Push back gently on end of nose with nondominant hand.	7. Opens nares.
8. Rest dominant hand on face.	8. Increases safety in case of head movement.
9. Instill drops just inside nare.	9. Provides for medication administration.
10. Instruct patient to stay in position 3 to 5 minutes.	10. Allows medication to be distributed through nasal passage.
11. Provide tissue to patient.	11. Promotes comfort by allowing patient to expectorate medication that goes to throat or mouth.
12. Assist patient to comfortable position.	12. Provides for patient comfort.
13. Discard or return all equipment to appropriate areas.	13. Provides for clean work area.
14. Assist patient to position of comfort.	14. Promotes patient comfort.

Documentation

Record the medication, dose, time, and route of administration on the patient medication record. In the patient record, note the therapeutic effect of the drug (if any); any adverse reactions, interventions, and results; and patient or family teaching done, and assess level of understanding. Record any nasal drainage present and assessment of nasal passages.

Elements of Patient Teaching

Explain the procedure to the patient or family, including the medication name, purpose, anticipated effects, possible untoward effects, and the schedule of administration. Always instruct the patient or family to notify the nurse if unusual symptoms occur.

PROCEDURE 16-13

Administering Vaginal Medications

Objective

Administer medication(s) as ordered by a licensed prescriber while ensuring maximum patient safety. Administer a prescribed medication via the vaginal route for therapeutic effect (Fig. 16–34).

Terminology

- Dorsal recumbent position—back-lying position in which legs are bent, with knees leaning outward; arms are bent with hands leaning outward
- Perineum—area of the pelvic outlet; external region between the vulva and anus in females

Critical Elements

Assess for patient allergies prior to administering any new medication.

For reasons of cost containment and documented decreased incidence of medication errors, the pharmacies of many facilities now dispense medications by the unit dose method and mix the majority of injections and intravenous solutions. However, the nurse actually giving the medication is still responsible for all aspects of medication administration.

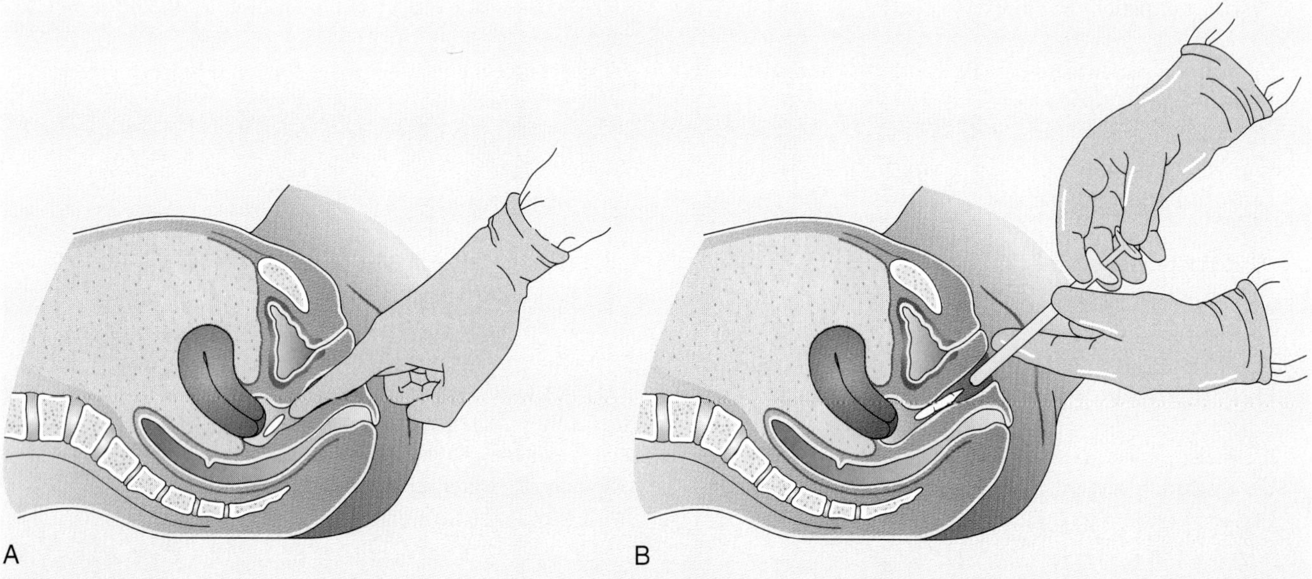

Figure 16–34. Administering vaginal medications. **A**, Inserting a suppository. **B**, Instilling ointment with an applicator.

When giving any medication, observe the five rights of medication administration:

- Right medication
- Right dosage
- Right time
- Right route
- Right patient

Prior to administering any medication, the nurse should know

- The desired therapeutic effect
- The reason for administering the drug
- The usual dosage and route
- Any potential for drug or food interactions
- Potential adverse side effects

As with all procedures, handwashing is the first line of defense in infection control. The nurse may wear clean, nonsterile gloves as additional protection.

Triple-check labels

- When removing medication from the shelf, refrigerator, or drawer
- While preparing medication
- When returning medication to the shelf, refrigerator, or drawer or before discarding the packaging material

Medication expiration dates should always be checked and outdated medication discarded or returned to the pharmacy.

Equipment

- Medication with applicator
- Clean gloves
- Bath blanket
- Cotton balls

continued on next page

PROCEDURE 16-13 (cont'd)

Special Considerations

If medication is to be administered along with a vaginal irrigation, the irrigation procedure should be completed prior to medication administration. In some facilities, patients may administer their own vaginal medications. The nurse should refer to the policies of the facility for clarification on self-administration of vaginal medications.

Action	*Rationale*
1. Verify medication order.	1. Ensures that correct medication is given.
2. Assemble equipment.	2. Promotes successful task completion.
3. Identify patient.	3. Provides patient safety.
4. Explain procedure.	4. Promotes patient compliance.
5. Position patient in dorsal recumbent position.	5. Positions patient so vaginal area may be visualized.
6. Have bath blanket cover patient's upper body and sheet pulled up over lower legs.	6. Provides privacy and comfort for patient.
7. Don gloves.	7. Provides protection for the nurse.
8. Cleanse perineum (if necessary) with soapy water on a cotton ball, wiping down only and then discarding cotton ball.	8. Removes gross contamination from perineal area.
9. Spread labia with nondominant hand.	9. Allows visualization of vaginal opening.
10. Insert medication 2 inches into vaginal opening, using a downward and backward motion.	10. Promotes medication administration, based on vaginal anatomy.
11. Instruct patient to stay in bed 30 minutes.	11. Provides time for medication to be absorbed.
12. Wipe excess medication off perineal area.	12. Provides for patient comfort and cleanliness.
13. Assist patient to position of comfort.	13. Provides patient privacy.
14. Discard and/or return equipment to appropriate areas.	14. Provides for safe and uncluttered working environment.
15. Don gloves and wash medication applicator with warm soapy water and allow to air dry (if applicable).	15. Removes gross contamination from equipment.

Documentation

Record the medication, dose, time, and route of administration on the patient medication record. In the patient record, note the therapeutic effect of the drug (if any); any adverse reactions, interventions, and results; and patient or family teaching done and assessed level of understanding. Assess any vaginal drainage and document on medical record.

Elements of Patient Teaching

Explain the procedure to the patient or family, including the medication name, purpose, anticipated effects, possible untoward effects, and the schedule of administration. Always instruct the patient or family to notify the nurse if unusual symptoms occur.

PROCEDURE 16-14

Administering Rectal Suppositories

Objective

Administer medication(s) as ordered by a licensed prescriber while ensuring maximum patient safety. Administer a prescribed medication via the rectal route for therapeutic effect (Fig. 16–35).

Terminology

- Sims position—the patient lies semiprone, on the left side, with the top leg flexed at the knee

Critical Elements

Assess the patient for any history of rectal bleeding, rectal surgery, or hemorrhoids.

Assess for patient allergies prior to administering any new medication.

For reasons of cost containment and documented decreased incidence of medication errors, the pharmacies of many facilities now dispense medications by the unit dose method and mix the majority of injections and intravenous solutions.

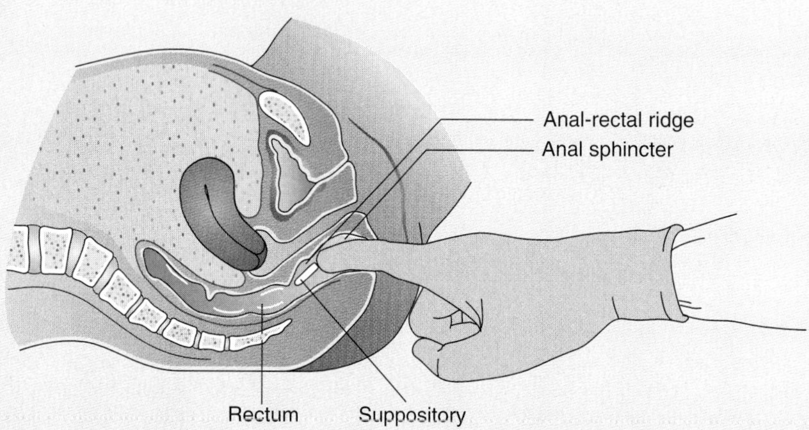

Figure 16–35. Inserting a rectal suppository.

However, the nurse actually giving the medication is still responsible for all aspects of medication administration.

When giving any medication, observe the five rights of medication administration:

- Right medication
- Right dosage
- Right time
- Right route
- Right patient

Prior to administering any medication, the nurse should know

- The desired therapeutic effect
- The reason for administering the drug
- The usual dosage and route
- Any potential for drug or food interactions
- Potential adverse side effects

As with all procedures, handwashing is the first line of defense in infection control. The nurse may wear clean, nonsterile gloves as additional protection.

Triple-check labels

- When removing medication from the shelf, refrigerator, or drawer
- While preparing medication
- When returning medication to the shelf, refrigerator, or drawer or before discarding the packaging material

Medication expiration dates should always be checked, and outdated medication discarded or returned to the pharmacy.

Equipment

- Suppository
- Gloves
- Lubricant (water soluble)
- Tissue
- Blanket

Special Considerations

The nurse should examine the patient to determine the presence of a fecal impaction. If present, it should be removed prior to instillation of medication, because the presence of fecal material may block the absorption of the drug.

continued on next page

PROCEDURE 16-14 (cont'd)

Action	*Rationale*
1. Verify medication order.	1. Ensures that correct medication is given.
2. Assemble equipment.	2. Promotes successful task completion.
3. Identify patient.	3. Provides patient safety.
4. Explain procedure.	4. Promotes patient compliance.
5. Position patient in Sims position.	5. Positions patient so that the rectal area can be visualized.
6. Cover patient with bath blanket, leaving only buttocks exposed.	6. Provides for patient comfort while allowing access to the rectal area for medication administration.
7. Don gloves.	7. Provides protection for the nurse.
8. Separate buttocks with nondominant hand.	8. Allows for visualization of anal opening.
9. Instruct patient to breathe through mouth.	9. Assists in relaxation of rectal sphincter during medication administration.
10. Insert lubricated suppository with dominant hand, advancing the suppository beyond the rectal sphincter.	10. Ensures that medication enters the rectal vault.
11. Wipe rectal area with tissue and assist patient to position of comfort.	11. Promotes patient comfort.
12. Discard and/or return equipment to appropriate areas.	12. Provides a safe, uncluttered work space.

Documentation

Record the medication, dose, time, and route of administration on the patient medication record. In the patient record, note the therapeutic effect of the drug (if any); any adverse reactions, interventions, and results; and patient or family teaching done and assessed level of understanding.

Elements of Patient Teaching

Explain the procedure to the patient or family, including the medication name, purpose, anticipated effects, possible untoward effects, and the schedule of administration. Always instruct the patient or family to notify the nurse if unusual symptoms occur. Instruct the patient to hold the medication in the rectal area for approximately 20 minutes to allow for medication absorption. If the suppository is given for laxative effect, the patient should be instructed to hold the suppository until there is a strong urge to evacuate the bowels. Also instruct the patient not to flush the toilet until the results are examined by the nurse.

CHAPTER HIGHLIGHTS

- *Pharmacotherapy* refers to the use of drugs in the diagnosis, prevention, and treatment of disease. It is a major component of health care in the United States.
- Contemporary nursing practice mandates that nurses be knowledgeable regarding pharmacokinetics (what the body does to a drug), pharmacodynamics (what the drug does to the body), pharmacotherapeutics (use of drugs in the diagnosis, prevention, and treatment of disease), and toxicology (undesirable effects of chemicals on living systems).
- Safe and effective administration of intramuscular injections requires the nurse to consider **each time an injection is given,** seven questions: What is the most appropriate site? What is the correct method for locating the site? What is the correct angle and correct position for injection? What is the appropriate needle length? How much volume and at what speed can the medication be safely administered? Should the medication be administered by this route? Should air bubbles be used to accommodate for dead space?
- Drug administration should be considered "thought-full doing" and be based on the rules and principles generated by research and practice. Each time a drug is administered, the nurse must consciously review or reflect on specific information about the drug, the individual, and the method of administration.
- Evaluation of the effects of administration of a drug is as important as administering the drug.
- The patient and family should be educated regarding the purpose of the drug, its negative side effects, and how and when to take the medication. Information should be given orally (in person) and in writing. Because it is easy to forget information or confuse drugs, it is important to schedule a time to review the material with the patient or family.

REFERENCES

Abrams, W.B. (1985). Drugs and the elderly. *Rational Drug Therapy, 19,* 1–6.

Ames, R.P. (1986). The effects of hypertensive drugs on serum lipids and lipoproteins. I. Diuretics. *Drugs, 32*(3), 260–278.

Arndt, M. (1994). Nurses' medication errors. *Journal of Advanced Nursing, 19,* 519–526.

Barennes, H., Raharinivo, S., Delorme, E. (1993). Intramuscular injections and post-injectional paralysis. *Médecine Tropicale, 53,* 373–378.

Baulieu, E.E. (1989). Contragestation and other clinical applications of RU 486, an antiprogesterone at the receptor. *Science, 245,* 1351–1356.

Beecroft, P.C., Kongelbeck, S.R. (1994). How safe are intramuscular injections? *AACN Clinical Issues, 5,* 207–215.

Beecroft, P.C., Redick, S. (1989). Possible complications of intramuscular injections on the pediatric unit. *Pediatric Nursing, 15,* 333–336.

Beecroft, P.C., Redick, S.A. (1990). Intramuscular injection practices of pediatric nurses: Site selection. *Nurse Educator, 15,* 23–28.

Benfell, C. (1997). Fatal errors: SR hospitals learn lessons the hard way. *The Press Democrat, March 23,* A1, A9–10.

Bergerson, P.S., Singer, S.A., Kaplan, A.M. (1982). Intramuscular injections in children. *Pediatrics, 70,* 944–948.

Berman, W.J., Whitman, V., Marks, K.H., et al (1978). Inadvertent overadministration of Digoxin to low birth weight infants. *Journal of Pediatrics, 92,* 1024–1025.

Bliss-Holtz, J. (1994). Discriminating types of medication calculation errors in nursing practice. *Nursing Research, 43,* 373–375.

Booth, R.A.D., Goddard, B.A., Paton, A. (1966). Measurement of fat thickness in man: A comparison of ultrasound, Harpenden calipers and electrical conductivity. *British Journal of Nutrition, 20,* 719–725.

Brown, T.E., Carter, B.L. (1994). Hypertensive and endstage renal disease. *Annals of Pharmacotherapy, 28*(3), 359–366.

Carey, R.G., Teeters, J.L. (1995). CQI case study: Reducing, medication errors. *Journal of Quality Improvement, 21,* 232–237.

Chapin, G., Shull, H., Welk, P.C. (1985). How safe is the air bubble technique for IM injections? *Nursing, 9, 59.*

Chezem, J.L. (1973). Multiple intramuscular injections: Effects of mechanical trauma on muscle tissue and clearance rates of I 131 Hippuran. *Nursing Research, 22,* 138–143.

Chugh, K., Chawla, D., Aggarwal, B.B. (1993). Optimum needle length for DPT inoculation of Indian infants. *Indian Journal of Pediatrics, 60,* 435–440.

Chung, D.C., Ko, Y.C., Pai, H. (1989). A study on the prevalence and risk factors of muscular fibrotic contracture in Jia-Dong Township, Pingtung County, Taiwan. *Kao-Hsiung-I-Hsueh-Ko-Hsueh-Ysa-Chi, 5,* 91–95.

Cockshott, W.P., Thompson, G.T., Howlett, L.J., Seeley, E.T. (1982). Intramuscular or intralipomatous injections? *New England Journal of Medicine, 307,* 356–358.

Combes, M.A., Clark, W.K., Gregory, C.F., James, J.A. (1960). Sciatic nerve injury in infants. *Journal of the American Medical Association, 173,* 1336–1339.

Conrad, P. (1985). The meaning of medications: Another look at compliance. *Social Science and Medicine, 20,* 29–37.

Dykes, C.W. (1996). Genes, disease and medicine. *Journal of Clinical Pharmacology, 42,* 883–895.

Ferrans, C.E. (1990). Quality of life: Conceptual issues. *Seminars in Oncology Nursing, 6,* 248–254.

Frishman, W.H. (1983). Pindolol: A new beta-adrenergic agonist with partial agonist activity. *New England Journal of Medicine, 308,* 940–944.

Garattini, S. (1985). Drug metabolism and actions in the aged. *Drug and Nutrient Interactions, 4,* 87–97.

Gilbert, B.R., Vaughan, E.D. (1990). Pathophysiology of the aging kidney. *Clinics in Geriatric Medicine, 6*(1), 13–30.

Gladstone, J. (1995). Drug administration errors: A study into the factors underlying the occurrence and reporting of drug errors in a district general hospital. *Journal of Advanced Nursing, 22,* 628–637.

Greenblatt, D.J., Allen, M.D. (1978). Intramuscular injection complications. *Journal of the American Medical Association, 240,* 542–544.

Greenblatt, D.J., Allen, M.D. (1978). Intramuscular injection—site complications. *Journal of the American Medical Association, 240,* 542–544.

Greenblatt, D.J., Koch-Weser, J. (1976). Drug therapy. Intramuscular injection of drugs. *New England Journal of Medicine, 295,* 542–546.

Groves, R.J., Goldner, J.L. (1974) Contracture of the deltoid muscle in the adult after intramuscular injections. *Journal of Bone & Joint Surgery, 56A,* 817–820.

Hallas, J. (1996). Drug-related hospital admissions in subspecialities of internal medicine. *Danish Medical Bulletin, 43*(2), 141–155.

Hick, J.F., Charboneau, J.W., Brakke, D.M., Goergen, B. (1989). Optimum needle length for diphtheria-tetanus-pertussis inoculation of infants. *Pediatrics, 84,* 136–137.

Himes, J.H., Roche, A.F., Siervogel, R.M. (1979). Compressibility of skinfolds and the measurement of subcutaneous fatness. *The American Journal of Clinical Nutrition, 32,* 1734–1740.

Hoek, J.B., Thomas, A.P., Rooney, T.A., et al (1992). Ethanol and signal transduction in the liver. *FASEB Journal, 6,* 2386–2396.

Jick, H. (1984). Adverse drug reactions: Magnitude of the problem. *Journal of Allergy and Clinical Immunology, 74,* 555–557.

Johnson, E.W., Raptou, A.D. (1965). A study of intragluteal injection. *Archives of Physical Medicine and Rehabilitation, February,* 167–177.

Karch, F.E., Lasagna, L. (1975). Adverse drug reactions: A critical review. *Journal of the American Medical Association, 234,* 1236–1241.

Keen, M.K. (1983). Adverse effects of frequent intramuscular injections. *Focus on Critical Care, 10,* 15–16.

Kendall, M.J., Woods, K.L., Wilkins, M.R., Worthington, D.J. (1982). Responsiveness to beta-adrenergic receptor stimulation: The effects of age are cardioselective. *British Journal of Clinical Pharmacology, 14,* 821–826.

Lachman, E. (1963). Applied anatomy of intragluteal injections. *American Surgeon, 29,* 236–241.

Lamy, P.P. (1986). The elderly and drug interactions. *Journal of the American Geriatrics Society, 34,* 586–592.

Lenz, C. (1983). Make your needle selection to the point. *Nursing '83, 13*(2), 50–51.

LeSage, J. (1991). Polypharmacy in geriatric patients. *Nursing Clinics of North America, 26,* 273–289.

Levenson, D.J., Simmons, C.E., Brenner, B.M. (1982). Arachidonate acid metabolism and the kidney. *American Journal of Medicine, 72,* 354–374.

Ling, C.M., Loong, S.C. (1962). Injection injury of the radial nerve. *Injury, 8,* 60–62.

Manasse, H.R. (1989). Medication use in an imperfect world: Drug misadventuring as an issue of public policy. *American Journal of Hospital Pharmacy, 46,* 1141–1152.

McGarry, K., Laher, M., Fitzgerald, D., et al (1975). Baroreflex function in elderly hypertensives. *Hypertension, 5,* 763–766.

Mooradian, A.D. (1988). An update of clinical pharmacokinetics, therapeutic monitoring techniques and treatment recommendations. *Clinical Pharmacokinetics, 18,* 165–173.

Muller-Vahl, H. (1983). Adverse reactions after intramuscular injections. *Lancet,* May 7; *1*(8332), 1050.

Myer, B.R. (1988). Improving medical education in therapeutics. *Annals of Internal Medicine, 108,* 145–147.

Napiontek, M., Ruszkowski, K. (1993). Paralytic foot drop and gluteal fibrosis after intramuscular injections. *Journal of Bone & Joint Surgery Br, 75B,* 83–85.

Naranjo, C.A., Busto, U., Sellers, E.M., et al. (1981). A method for estimating the probability of adverse drug reactions. *Clinical Pharmacology and Therapeutics, 30,* 234–245.

Parke, D.V. (1985). Adverse effects of drugs—Their causes and prevention. *Journal of the Royal Society of Health, 105,* 39–46.

Pearson, L.J. (1998). Annual update of how each state stands on legislation issues affecting advanced nursing practice. *Nurse Practitioner, 32*(1), 14–66.

Pucino, F., Beck, C., Seifert, R., et al (1985). Pharmacogeriatrics. *Pharmacotherapy, 5,* 314–326.

Roberts, J., Turner, N. (1988). Pharmacodynamic basis for altered drug reaction in the elderly. *Clinical Geriatric Medicine, 4,* 127–149.

Rochon, P.A., Gurwitz, J.H. (1995). Drug therapy. *Lancet,* 346, 32–36.

Roseman, C., Booker, J.M. (1995). Workload and environmental factors in hospital medication errors. *Nursing Research, 44,* 226–230.

Scarpace, P.J. (1986). Decreased beta-adrenergic responsiveness during senescence. *Federation Proceedings, 45*(1), 51–54.

Schumucker, D.L., Wang, R.K. (1980). Age-related changes in liver drug metabolism: Structure versus function. *Procedings of the Society of Experimental Biology and Medicine, 165*(2), 178–187.

Schwertz, D.S., Buschmann, M.B. (1989). Pharmacogeriatrics. *Critical Care Nursing Quarterly, 12*(1), 26–37.

Seller, E.M. (1989). Geriatric clinical pharmacology. In H. Kalant and W.H.E. Roschlau (eds.): *Principles of Medical Pharmacology,* 5th ed. Toronto: B.C. Becker, p. 699.

Severson, J.A. (1984). Neurotransmitter receptors and aging. *Journal of the American Geriatrics Society, 32,* 24–27.

Shaber, E.P., Smith, R.A. (1982). Techniques of drug administration. *Dental Clinics of North America, 26,* 35–38.

Shaw, P.G. (1982). Common pitfalls in geriatric drug prescribing. *Drugs, 23,* 324–328.

Sun, X. (1990). An investigation on injectional gluteal muscle contracture in children in Mianyang City. *Chung-Hua-Liu-Hsing-Ping-Hsueh-Tsa-Chih, 11,* 291–294.

Svendsen, O. (1983). Intramuscular injections and local muscle damage: An experimental study of the effect of injection speed. *Acta Pharmacology and Toxicology, 5,* 305–309.

Talbert, J.L., Haslam, R.H.A., Haller, J.A. (1967). Gangrene of the foot following intramuscular injection in the lateral thigh: A case report with recommendations for prevention. *Journal of Pediatrics, 70,* 110–121.

Vessel, E.S. (1983). Assessment of methods to identify sources of interindividual pharmacokinetic variations. *Clinical Pharmacokinetics, 8,* 378–409.

Vestal, R.E., Cusack, B.J. (1990). Pharmacology and aging. In E.L. Schneider and J.W. Rowe. (eds.): *Handbook of the Biology of Aging,* 3rd ed. San Diego: Academic Press.

Vestal, R.E., Wood, A.J., Shand, D.G. (1979). Reduced beta adrenoreception sensitivity in the elderly. *Clinical Pharmacology and Therapeutics, 26,* 181–186.

von Hochstetter, V.A. (1964). Über die intrglutäale injktin, ihre komplikationen und deren verhütung. *Schweizerische Medizinische Wochenschrift, 84,* 1226–1227.

Weir, M., Fearnow, R.G. (1983). Transverse myelitis and penicillin. *Pediatrics, 71,* 988.

Weiss, C.F., Glazko, A.J., Weston, J.K. (1960). Chloramphenicol in the newborn infant: A physiologic explanation of its toxicity when given in excessive doses. *New England Journal of Medicine, 262,* 787–794.

Wilkinson, G.R. (1983). Drug distribution and renal excretion in the elderly. *Journal of Chronic Diseases, 36,* 91–102.

Winfrey, A. (1985). Single-dose IM injections: How much is too much? *Nursing, July,* 38–39.

Wong, D.L. (1982). Significance of dead space in syringes. *American Journal of Nursing, 82,* 1237.

Wright, J.M. (1992). Drug Interactions. In K.L. Melmon, H.F. Morrelli, B.B. Hoffman, and D.W. Nierenberg (eds.): *Clinical Pharmacology,* 3rd ed. New York: McGraw-Hill Inc., p. 1016.

Yuen, G.J. (1990). Altered pharmacokinetics in the elderly. *Clinics in Geriatric Medicine, 6*(2), 257–267.

Zelman, S. (1978). Abscesses from parenteral injection. *Journal of the American Medical Association, 240,* 23.

Sterile Technique and Infection Control

Sandra Blake-Von Behren

OBJECTIVES

After studying this chapter, students will be able to:

- **describe the interaction of the causative agent, mode of transmission, and susceptible host in infection transmission**
- **identify scientific principles of hand washing**
- **demonstrate proper hand-washing techniques**
- **identify when to use antiseptic hand-washing soap**
- **identify the scientific principles underlying gowning, gloving, and using a mask**
- **demonstrate how to correctly don and remove gloves, gowns, and masks**
- **prepare and present a teaching plan for a patient in isolation**
- **explain principles of surgical asepsis**
- **properly apply a sterile wet-to-dry dressing**
- **describe factors that can affect isolation procedures and other aseptic techniques**

Molly Brown is a 60-year-old diabetic patient with an open, draining ulcer on her left foot. She is admitted to the hospital for debridement of the infected wound. Mrs. Brown has had multiple courses of antibiotic therapy over the previous 2 months and suffers from copious diarrhea, which her physician suspects is caused by *Clostridium difficile.*

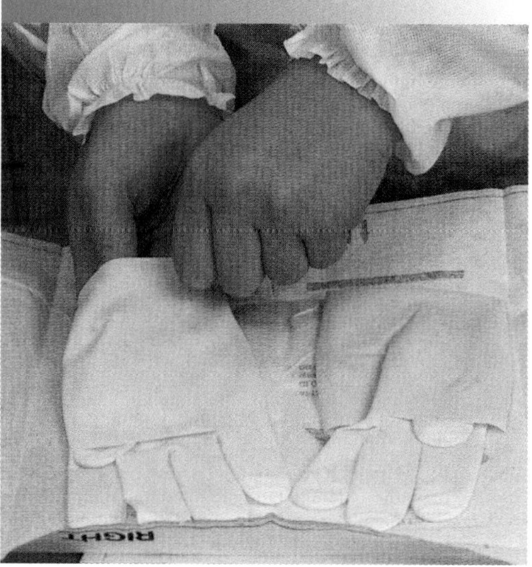

Mrs. Brown is placed on contact isolation because the drainage cannot be adequately contained in a dressing. Other patients on this unit may have open wounds or invasive devices and are susceptible to cross-infection.

Mrs. Brown has an open wound that is infected, and her wound is thus a source of microbial contamination. Because of Mrs. Brown's exposure to antibiotics, the nurse realized that the wound might be contaminated with antibiotic-resistant bacteria. Contact isolation procedures must be followed, and Mrs. Brown should be placed in a private room.

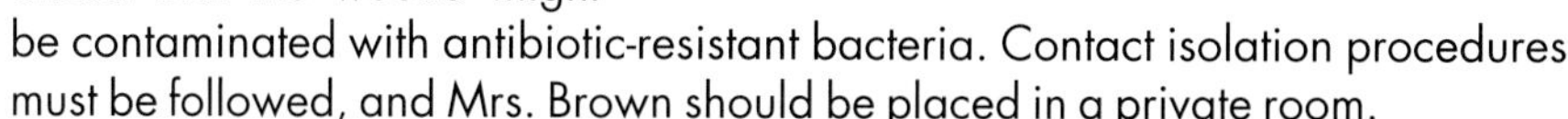
Contaminated hands of health care workers are often the means by which infections are transmitted from one patient to another. Other patients may be very susceptible to infection. Therefore, hand washing (medical asepsis) must be done before and after care of Mrs. Brown and all other patients.

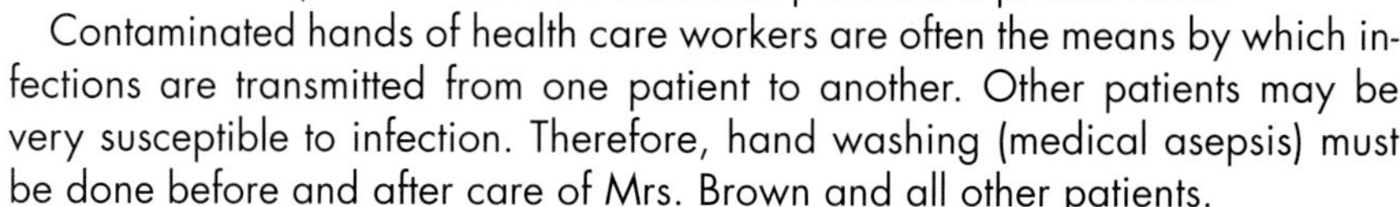
Mrs. Brown is susceptible to infection because of her impaired immune status caused by diabetes and the open skin area. Solutions used for the wet-to-dry dressings, as well as the dressings themselves, must be sterile. Meticulous aseptic technique (surgical asepsis) must be maintained in her wound care.

SCOPE OF NURSING PRACTICE

The risk of an infectious complication is always present regardless of the patient's underlying pathophysiology. Basic techniques such as hand washing and barrier precautions are vital to patient care. Only when the health care provider follows scrupulous aseptic technique can the patient be assured of receiving optimal care. Although some infections are not preventable, meticulous adherence to these techniques will minimize the patient's risk of infection and subsequent, prolonged illness, with its attendant complications and vastly increased cost.

The value of all isolation practices must be seriously reviewed in light of new diseases, such as acquired immunodeficiency syndrome (AIDS) and multiple drug-resistant tuberculosis, and the emergence of antibiotic-resistant microorganisms, such as methicillin-resistant *Staphylococcus aureus* (MRSA) and vancomycin-resistant *Enterococcus*. Studies are also needed to validate which isolation practices are effective and which ones are merely costly rituals.

Today's nurses are left to work with the procedures handed down from predecessors. As in all nursing practice, however, common sense and rational thinking are the cornerstone of sound infection control practice. The nurse must always keep in mind that the chain of infection is most effectively broken at the transmission link by good hand washing and other aseptic practices.

To practice good aseptic technique, the nurse must always keep in mind what is dirty, what is clean, what is sterile, and then keep these items and conditions strictly segregated. The conscientious nurse must also constantly search the literature to substantiate beneficial practices and disprove harmful ones.

KNOWLEDGE BASE

Infection is the entry and multiplication of an infectious agent (a microorganism) into the tissue of a host with subsequent tissue damage. A microorganism is a minute living body not perceptible to the human eye. *Apparent* infections cause disease with clinical signs and symptoms such as a fever, purulent (pus) drainage, inflammation, productive cough (one producing mucus or other secretions), diarrhea, myalgias (muscular tenderness or pain), and elevated white blood cell count. *Inapparent* infections do not cause signs or symptoms and, therefore, are not immediately apparent to the clinician. *Sepsis* is the spread of an infection through the blood stream from its initial site to vital organs. (See Box 17–1 for more definitions of infection-related terms and concepts.)

Infections may be categorized as either *community acquired* or *nosocomial*. Community-acquired infections are present or incubating at the time of admission to a health care facility and have no association with previous hospitalization. Nosocomial infections, on the other hand, are not present or incubating at the time of admission and are acquired during a hospital stay. Some nosocomial infections may be associated with admission to a hospital, having been acquired during a previous hospitalization. Figure 17–1 shows the chain of infection; Figure 17–2 illustrates common sources of nosocomial infection.

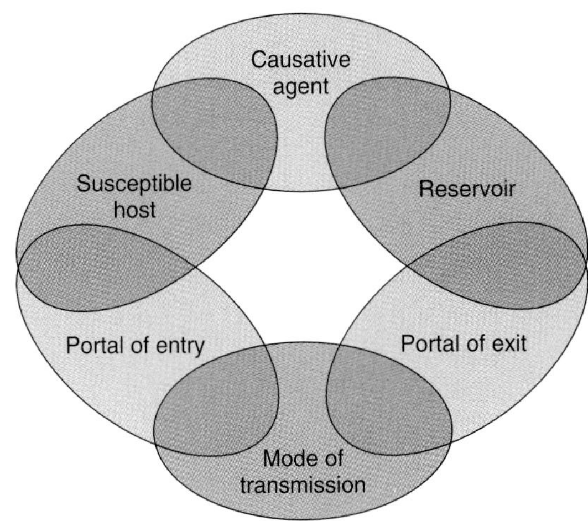

Figure 17–1. The chain of infection.

Nosocomial infections are a major cause of morbidity (disease) and mortality in hospitalized patients. The Study of the Efficacy of Nosocomial Infection Control (SENIC), a large-scale study conducted by the Centers for Disease Control (CDC) in 1975 to 1976, statistically sampled all U.S. hospitals to determine the national nosocomial infection rate. SENIC found a rate of 5.7 nosocomial infections per 100 hospital admissions, almost 6 percent of all hospitalized infections (Haley, 1985). SENIC further estimated that more than 8 million extra hospital days were required every year to care for patients with nosocomial infections, and that the estimated annual cost of this care was a staggering $4 billion nationwide. It also estimated that 20,000 deaths per year were directly attributable to, and another 60,000 attributable at least in part to, nosocomial infections (Haley, 1986).

Aseptic technique has been understood since the days of Florence Nightingale to reduce the transmission and occurrence of infection. Sufficient studies do not currently exist to validate every principle of infection control. Some clinical studies have been done to help validate aseptic techniques, but many practices are based on tradition or even ritual. Nurses and other health care professionals must, therefore, rely on the basic sciences of epidemiology, microbiology, medicine, and nursing to validate established practices.

Despite continuing advances in microbiology and pharmacology, common sense is still a major factor in preventing infection. One noted infection control researcher made the following observations about aseptic technique:

- Aseptic technique is a purposeful prevention of the transfer of infection.

BOX 17-1
INFECTION-RELATED TERMS AND CONCEPTS

Antiseptic—An agent used on the skin to inhibit or destroy microorganisms.
Apparent infection—An infection resulting in clinical signs and symptoms, such as redness, swelling, or heated skin.
Asepsis—Freedom from pathogenic organisms.
Body substance isolation (BSI)—A system of precautions designed to prevent cross-transmission of infections. BSI requires barriers for contact with any body fluid, mucous membrane, or nonintact skin.
Carrier—An individual who harbors germs of a disease and may transmit the disease to others, but has no disease symptoms.
Category-specific isolation—A system of isolation in which diseases are grouped into categories based on the route of transmission; one set of instructions applies to all diseases in a particular group.
Colonizing flora—Organisms that are part of the body's flora; does not denote infection.
Community-acquired infection—Infection present or incubating at the time of admission to a health care facility.
Contamination—Introduction of microorganisms on or in any area.
Disease-specific isolation—A system of isolation in which isolation procedures are established for each individual disease.
Disinfection—A process that eliminates many or all pathogenic organisms with the exception of bacterial spores.
Endogenous flora—Microorganisms inside the body.
Exogenous flora—Microorganisms outside the body.
Inapparent infection—An infectious process not producing clinical symptoms.
Infection—Entry and multiplication of a microorganism in the body with resulting tissue damage; clinical disease may not be present.
Microorganism—A minute living body not perceptible to the human eye.
Normal flora—Microorganisms normally present on skin and mucosal surfaces.
Nosocomial infection—Hospital-acquired infection; an infection not known to be present or incubating on admission.
Pathogen—An organism capable of causing disease.
Reservoir—A person or component of the environment (bed, table, stethoscope) harboring potentially pathogenic microorganisms.
Resident microorganisms (skin flora)—Organisms persistently isolated from the skin of most persons.
Sepsis—Spread of the infection through the bloodstream to vital organs.
Septicemia—Presence of infectious agents in the bloodstream with clinical illness (fever, chills, hypotension).
Sterile—Free from living microorganisms.
Transient microorganisms (flora)—Organisms isolated from the skin, not demonstrated to be consistently present in the majority of persons. These flora may be readily transmitted on hands of health care personnel unless removed by handwashing.
Universal precautions—CDC-recommended blood and body fluid precautions to be utilized universally in the care of all patients.

- The practice of asepsis can reduce nosocomial infections.
- Rational thinking based on common sense must remain the validation for many aseptic practices (Crow, 1989).

Basic Science

Understanding the mechanisms by which infections are transmitted is the basis for developing effective prevention and control practices. The science of epidemiology has provided the foundation for virtually all nursing practice in infection control.

EPIDEMIOLOGY

Epidemiology is the study of the occurrence, distribution, risk factors, and control of disease in a defined population. Data are collected and analyzed to determine rates of infection in the defined population, mode of transmission, and risk factors. Epidemiologic methods can be applied to the study of any disease, including infectious diseases.

Infection-control programs in hospitals and other health care facilities apply epidemiologic methods to study nosocomial infections. Surveillance is a key component of these programs. In a nursing context, surveillance is a dynamic activity that includes gathering information about individual episodes of infection, collating and analyzing these data, and summarizing the findings. These efforts help facilities identify modes of transmission, which then enables infection control practitioners to develop effective prevention and control measures. In addition, infection rates are established, which provide information on the endemic (normally occurring) incidence of infection. Then, using statistical methodology, threshold rates of infection are established. Thresholds serve as "bell ringers" and alert practitioners that infection rates have exceeded an acceptable level. Whenever infection rates significantly exceed this threshold level, the facility launches an investigation to determine whether cases are related and whether additional preventive and control measures are necessary. For example, a nursing unit may have a usual rate of two urinary tract infections (UTIs) per 1000 patient days. The threshold or maximum acceptable rate may be four UTIs per 1000 patient days. If the monthly report reveals 10 UTIs per 1000

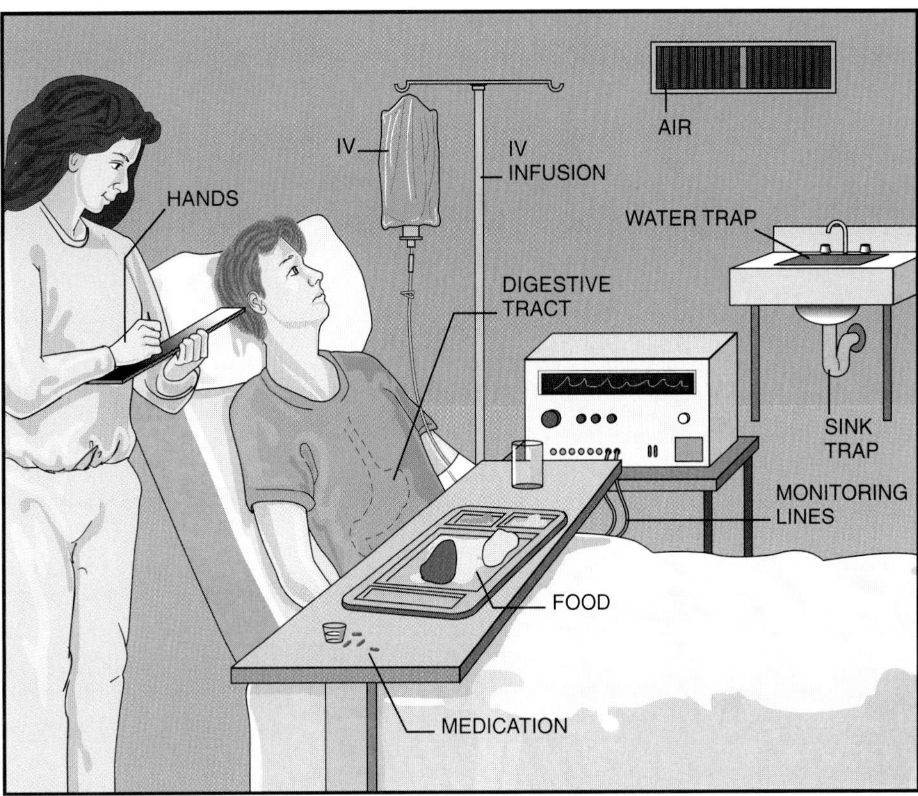

Figure 17–2. Potential sources of microbial contamination in the hospital.

patient days, a review of cases will be conducted to determine whether there are common patterns such as a common organism found, breaks in procedures such as urinary catheterizations, or excessive use of indwelling urinary catheters.

MICROBIOLOGY

Microbiology is the scientific study of microbes. Microbes are unicellular or multicellular organisms, including bacteria, fungi, protozoa, viruses, and in some instances selected algae and worms.

CHAIN OF INFECTION

The chain of infection is composed of six "links": causative agent, reservoir, portal of exit, mode of transmission, portal of entry, and susceptible host (see Fig. 17–1).

CAUSATIVE AGENT

The biologic agent or microorganism causing the infectious process is the causative agent. These agents include bacteria, viruses, fungi, protozoa, and helminths. Organisms that cause disease are often referred to as *pathogens.*

Bacteria are usually single-cell microorganisms, of which there are many variations. Under the microscope, bacteria can be partially identified by their shape (cocci, rod, or spiral) and their morphology, or structure (pairs, clusters, or chains). Different species of bacteria also have different chemical compositions with different growth requirements. Some are *aerobic* and grow only in the presence of oxygen, such as *S. aureus, Pseudomonas aeruginosa,* and *Streptococcus pyogenes.* Others are strictly *anaerobic,* growing only in the absence of oxygen, such as *Clostridium* and *Bacteroides* species.

A special staining procedure called a *Gram's stain* groups bacteria as either gram positive (retaining the stain) or gram negative (losing the stain and taking the counterstain). Gram's stain is a procedure conducted in the laboratory that identifies the type of bacteria present and provides information to determine an effective treatment. The procedure involves the preparation of a laboratory slide in which the film on the slide is stained with crystal violet and then immersed in Gram's iodine solution. The iodine solution is rinsed and counterstained with a solution of safranine or carbolfuchsin. Gram-positive bacteria retain a violet stain, whereas gram-negative bacteria adopt a red counterstain. Final identification is done by *culture.* In this procedure, the infected body secretion is transferred to a medium, where it is allowed to incubate and grow, and is then identified by various methods, including biochemical testing of the bacterial colony. *Sensitivity* tests are then done to determine which antibiotics are most effective in treating that particular species.

Viruses are the smallest known infectious agents. They are not complete cells, and they depend on host tissue to survive and multiply. Special laboratory methods, including fluorescent and electron microscopy and tissue culture, are necessary to identify viruses.

Fungi are plantlike organisms, including yeasts and molds. Fungal (mycotic) infections sometimes occur when normal flora are altered by antibiotic therapy.

Protozoa are single-celled organisms found everywhere in nature. Malaria and amebic dysentery are examples of infections caused by protozoa. *Helminths* are parasites, such as tapeworms and roundworms.

All people and virtually every facet of the environment are colonized with a multitude of microorganisms. *Normal flora* are a family of microorganisms normally present on the skin and mucous membranes that cause no infections. When these flora invade a body part where they are not "normal," however, an infection may occur. For example, when *Staphylococcus epidermidis,* bacteria that are part of the normal skin flora, invade the vascular system by way of an intravenous catheter, a serious blood stream infection can occur. This is referred to as an *endogenous* infection, meaning that the patient's own flora is the source of the infecting organism. An infection from a source outside the patient's own body (e.g., from a virus transmitted from another person) is referred to as an *exogenous* infection.

Pathogenicity refers to an organism's ability to cause disease. The severity of disease caused by an organism is a measure of that organism's *virulence.* Organisms also vary in the number of organisms necessary to cause an infection. For example, 10^2 (10 to the second power, or 10×10) colonies of *Shigella* bacteria can produce gastrointestinal symptoms, such as diarrhea, while 10^5 colonies of *Salmonella* are usually required to produce symptoms ranging from gastroenteritis to typhoid fever. *Shigella* are thus considered more virulent. Actual infections may vary considerably based on route of transmission and host susceptibility, however.

RESERVOIR

A *reservoir* is the location in which an organism is usually found. The organisms may or may not multiply in the reservoirs. Patients, health care personnel and equipment, and the environment are reservoirs associated with nosocomial infection. A *source* is the person or item from which the organism is transmitted to a host. The reservoir and the source may be the same location, such as an infected wound, or the source may be a piece of equipment that is contaminated and subsequently comes in contact with a susceptible host.

PORTAL OF EXIT

A *portal of exit* is the means by which the infectious organisms leave the host. Portals of exit from human hosts include the respiratory, gastrointestinal, and genitourinary tracts. Skin, wounds, and blood can also serve as portals of exit. In the case study, Molly Brown's wound is a reservoir for microorganisms, which, if not properly cared for, becomes an infectious portal for other patients and nurses.

MODE OF TRANSMISSION

The fourth component in the chain of infection, *transmission,* is the mechanism by which organisms transfer from the source and reservoir to a susceptible host. Microorganisms do not jump or fly to a susceptible host; rather, they must be transported. The means of transport is often the hands of health care personnel. This is why effective hand washing is so vital.

Transmission of an infectious organism to a susceptible host can occur through four routes:

- Contact
- Airborne
- Vehicle
- Vectorborne

Contact transmission, the most common route, can be divided into three types: direct, indirect, and droplet contact. *Direct contact* involves person-to-person transmission, and occurs from physical contact between the source and the susceptible person. Contact can occur continuously in daily patient care; again, health care workers are the most frequent means of transmission. Respiratory viruses, for example, are often spread from person to person. A common scenario is as follows: An infected man coughs and covers his mouth with his hands, and then does not wash his hands before touching another's hands; the second person may then contaminate his own eyes or nose with his hands and thus become infected with the respiratory virus. Another example of direct contact is an emergency room situation in which a patient with a bloodborne pathogen (such as human immunodeficiency virus [HIV]) is bleeding and a nurse applies a pressure dressing without gloves. If the nurse has cuts on her hand, the patient's pathogen may be directly transmitted to her blood via the cut.

Indirect contact involves personal contact of the susceptible host with a contaminated intermediate object. For instance, an inadequately disinfected endoscope can transfer microorganisms to a patient. In the case study, bacteria from Mrs. Brown's wound could be transferred to another patient by the nurse's contaminated hands or by a contaminated piece of equipment such as bandage scissors.

Droplet contact occurs when an infectious agent briefly passes through the air. The infected source and susceptible host are usually within a few feet of each other. This is considered contact transmission rather than airborne transmission, because droplets are usually 5 mm or greater in size and travel only a few feet. Organisms are typically dispersed when an infected person coughs, sneezes, or talks. Diseases spread by this route include meningococcal meningitis, *Haemophilus influenzae* meningitis, and pertussis (whooping cough) and influenza.

Airborne transmission occurs when infectious agents remain suspended in the air for long periods and are inhaled or deposited on the susceptible host. Organisms carried in this manner are smaller than 5 mm and can be widely dispersed by air currents. Infectious diseases spread by airborne transmission include tuberculosis, rubeola, and chickenpox.

Vehicle transmission occurs when contaminated items such as blood, blood products, food, water, contaminated solutions, or drugs transmit infections to multiple persons. An example of this type of transmission is the spread of *Salmonella* from contaminated dairy products or poultry.

Vectorborne transmission occurs when insects or other animals serve as intermediate hosts for an infectious agent. Examples are malaria, transmitted by mosquitos, and Rocky Mountain spotted fever, and Lyme disease transmitted by ticks. Vectors have not played a significant role in the transmission of nosocomial infection in the United States.

Some infectious agents are transmitted by more than one route. For example, chickenpox may be transmitted by direct contact with an infected person's lesions or by inhaling an airborne virus. *Salmonella* may be acquired by one person through eating contaminated eggs (the vehicle) and then transferred to another person by direct or indirect contact.

PORTAL OF ENTRY

The portal of entry into a susceptible host may be via the respiratory tract, genitourinary tract, gastrointestinal tract, breaks in skin or mucous membranes, parenteral routes (needle sticks), or any other body opening or orifice.

SUSCEPTIBLE HOST

The last link in the chain of infection is the *susceptible host.* For a host to become susceptible to pathogens, an elaborate defensive array designed to limit the entry of microorganisms into the human body must first break down. The skin and mucous membranes are often referred to as the body's first line of defense against microbial invasion. Very few organisms can penetrate intact skin. In the case study, Mrs. Brown is susceptible to additional infection because of the open, nonintact skin of her foot ulcer.

The mucous membranes lining the respiratory, gastrointestinal, and urinary tracts secrete substances with antimicrobial properties. The upper respiratory tract is equipped with cilia, fine, hairlike projections that are in constant wavelike motion to sweep pathogens toward the pharynx, where they may be swallowed or expectorated. In the gastrointestinal tract, the stomach's high acid content destroys microorganisms that are swallowed. Sneezing, coughing, vomiting, and diarrhea are additional mechanical defenses, body reflexes by which pathogens and their toxins are expelled. The normal microbial flora of the body also help prevent invasion of pathogenic organisms. For example, normal vaginal flora protects the vagina from invasion of disease-causing organisms. When women receive antibiotics for treatment of a pharyngeal infection, the antibiotic can also kill the normal vaginal flora and allow overgrowth with yeast, resulting in fungal vaginitis.

In addition to its mechanical defenses, the body is also equipped with a very complex immune system. The immune system comprises many components that act in harmony to combat infection. White blood cells, specifically *polymorphonuclear leukocytes* (or granulocytes), destroy microbial invaders by phagocytosis, the engulfment and digestion of foreign material.

Important underlying host factors that determine whether a person will develop an infection include age and chronic underlying disease. Newborn infants, especially those born with low birth weight, have undeveloped immune systems and thus fewer physical resources to combat infectious microorganisms. Elderly persons likewise have less efficient immune systems and thus decreased resistance to infection.

Chronic underlying diseases, such as diabetes, immune deficiency diseases, and cancers, also increase host susceptibility to infection. For example, Mrs. Brown of the case study has diabetes, which increases her susceptibility to infection. Treatment of the underlying disease also may increase susceptibility to infection by interfering with the body's normal defense mechanisms. During chemotherapy treatment for cancer, the granulocytes may decrease to such low numbers that the patient may have little ability to fight infection.

Normal microbial flora are often altered in the hospitalized patient because of antimicrobial therapy, invasive procedures, trauma, or aspiration. Invasive devices that penetrate the skin or pass through the protective area of the mucous membranes, for instance, provide a direct entry for microorganisms into normally protected internal body parts.

BREAKING THE CHAIN OF INFECTION: CONCEPTS OF INFECTION PREVENTION

Preventing the transmission of infection involves interrupting one or more of the components in the chain of infection.

CAUSATIVE AGENT

Recognizing and then containing the source or reservoir of potential pathogens represents one step in preventing the spread of infection such as localized redness, swelling (edema), and pain. The nurse must be alert to physiologic changes in a patient that may indicate infection. An elevated white blood cell count, for instance, may also indicate that the body is producing more cells to fight an infection. Pus, or exudate, is another sign of infection. As microbial cells are destroyed, exudate may accumulate at the site. Purulent discharge from a wound is supportive evidence of infection. Production of thick, tenacious sputum or cloudy urine also usually indicates infection.

As the body responds to inflammation, internal body heat increases and fever results. Body temperature exceeding 38°C (100°F) may be a sign of infection. Other conditions such as lupus, drug reactions, and neoplasms are also associated with inflammation and can produce fever. Therefore, fever must be evaluated to determine whether the origin is infectious or noninfectious. Once an infection is identified, appropriate therapy can be initiated. This therapy may include antibiotics or other antimicrobial agents. Wet-to-dry dressings may be used for infected wounds. Although this is controversial, it is still used in many settings.

The nurse must always be alert for any possible inapparent infection as well. Although a patient may have no clinical signs of disease, organisms may be shedding from previously infected, or colonized, sites. Colonized sites are contaminated with a low number of organisms but exhibit no signs of infection.

The environment or inanimate objects may be reservoirs or sources for microbial contamination. Equipment in an infected patient's immediate environment may be contaminated, and any item in the patient's bedside area must be considered contaminated. Articles soiled with blood or other body fluids are especially capable of harboring microorganisms.

TRANSMISSION

Hand washing, barrier techniques (e.g., isolation procedures), and sterile technique are practices that interrupt the transmission link in the chain of infection.

Hand Washing. Hand washing is considered the single most important procedure for preventing nosocomial infections (Garner and Favero, 1985). It should be the first step in any patient care procedure and the last step after patient care is completed.

The microbial flora of the skin consists of resident and transient microorganisms. *Resident microorganisms* survive and multiply on the skin, can be repeatedly cultured from the skin, and are not easily removed by scrubbing. These organisms rarely cause infections, except when introduced into the body through invasive procedures, such as catheterization. *Transient microorganisms* are more likely to be acquired from colonized or infected patients. These organisms generally survive on the skin for only a short time and can be removed by hand washing.

Barrier Techniques. The use of barriers in a hospital setting to interrupt the transmission of infection is referred to as isolation precautions or procedures. Isolation precautions are designed to prevent the spread of microorganisms among patients, health care personnel, and visitors. Historically, all patients with infections were totally isolated. Regardless of the infection and how it was transmitted, patients were placed in a separate room or cubicle, and all personnel wore gloves, a gown, and mask to physically isolate themselves from the infection.

As knowledge of modes of transmission has increased, isolation procedures have been modified. Most hospitals today use a *category system* of isolation in which diseases with similar modes of transmission are grouped together. A list of required procedures, such as gowning, gloving, or masking, is developed for each category.

Since 1987, hospitals have implemented a series of procedures known collectively as *Universal Precautions.* These procedures require the use of appropriate barriers whenever there is a risk of exposure to body fluids that might be contaminated with a bloodborne pathogen, such as hepatitis B or HIV. These precautions are implemented for all patients, not only those known to be infected.

Some hospitals have adopted a system called *body substance isolation* (BSI) (Lynch et al, 1987, 1990). BSI requires all health care personnel to put on clean gloves immediately before coming into contact with any body fluid, mucous membranes, or nonintact skin. All personnel may also wear aprons or other barriers, as necessary, to keep skin and clothing clean. Personnel must also be certified as immune or immunized against airborne diseases such as rubella and measles. A separate "stop sign alert" card with instructions is placed outside the rooms of patients with airborne infections. Other forms of isolation are not used with this system.

The BSI system was designed to have two benefits: decrease the transmission of nosocomial infection to patients and reduce the exposure of health care workers to viral and bacterial pathogens from patients. BSI differs from isolation systems such as the CDC's in that it is used for all patients rather than being diagnosis driven. It differs from Universal Precautions in intent: Universal Precautions are designed to protect health care workers from exposure and potential infection with bloodborne pathogens, whereas BSI aims to protect both patients and health care workers from cross-transmission of *all* infections, not just those transmitted through blood and body fluids.

CONTROL OF THE ENVIRONMENT

Sanitation, proper disinfection, and sterilization techniques greatly reduce the transfer of microorganisms by contact with surfaces or equipment. When using disinfected or sterile equipment, the nurse must maintain sterile precautions to avoid contaminating objects before use.

Careful waste management is also necessary to avoid contamination. All wet wastes, including dressings saturated with body drainage or blood, are considered potentially infectious medical wastes and must be disposed of in accordance with hospital policy. Because state and local laws vary regarding the definition of infectious medical wastes, the nurse must become familiar with hospital policy regarding waste disposal. All needles and other sharp objects used in patient care ("sharps") must be disposed of in puncture-resistant sharps boxes to decrease the risk of puncture wounds and transfer of bloodborne pathogens to other health care workers. Figure 17–3 shows the Occupational Safety and Health Administration's (OSHA) biohazard alert symbol, which is to be displayed (on a bright orange sticker) on all containers of regulated waste and on refrigerators and freezers storing blood and other potentially infectious substances.

Properly functioning ventilation systems also aid in preventing the transmission of infection, particularly by the air-

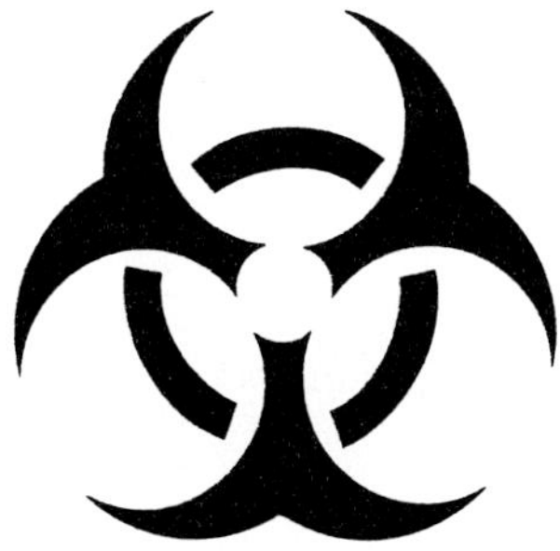

Figure 17–3. Occupational Safety and Health Administration's biohazard alert symbol.

borne route. Air exchange and exhaust systems prevent high levels of pathogenic organisms from accumulating to infective levels in these closed spaces.

HOST RESISTANCE

Although the major focus of infection prevention is aimed at the transmission link, some actions aim to increase host resistance. Vaccination is an important method of protecting elderly and chronically ill patients from influenza and pneumococcal pneumonia and protecting children from diphtheria, pertussis, tetanus, mumps, measles, rubella, *H. influenzae,* and hepatitis B. It is particularly important that children receive their scheduled vaccines. Health care workers must be current in their vaccinations, including influenza and hepatitis B. Unvaccinated health care workers put themselves, their colleagues, and their patients at risk for infection.

Relevant Research and Common Practices

It is true that scientific research is lacking to validate many infection control practices. Scientific knowledge regarding epidemiology, microbiology, and cross-contamination largely support current practices, however. Although barrier precautions have been shown to substantially reduce the risk of certain infections, such as respiratory syncytial virus (RSV), studies are still needed to determine the efficacy of the various isolation systems and barriers in preventing nosocomial transmission of infection.

HISTORICAL PERSPECTIVE

Nosocomial infection is not new. Hospital-acquired infections have occurred since the time sick people were first congregated together for care. Investigation of nosocomial infections did not occur until the mid-nineteenth century, however, spearheaded by visionaries such as Oliver Wendell Holmes, Ignaz Semmelweis, Joseph Lister, and Florence Nightingale.

Ignaz Semmelweis is regarded as the first person to demonstrate person-to-person transmission of infection and the role of hand washing as a barrier to such transmission. When Semmelweis was an obstetrician at the Lying-In Hospital in Vienna in 1847, the hospital was divided in two divisions. The first division was a teaching unit for medical students, staffed by physicians, and the second division was a normal convalescent unit staffed by midwives. Semmelweis noted that the maternal death rate was 10 percent in the first division but only 3 percent in the second division. He further noted that medical students generally entered the delivery room of the first division directly from the autopsy suite. After a colleague died of sepsis, acquired from a cut sustained during a postmortem examination, Semmelweis realized that the material causing the sepsis was being transmitted from autopsy material from women who had died of the disease.

BOX 17-2
THE SEMMELWEIS CHILDBED FEVER STUDY

Ignaz Semmelweis, a mid-nineteenth century Viennese obstetrician, noted a dramatic difference in maternal mortality rate in his hospital's two divisions. One was a teaching unit with frequent autopsy classes, the other a normal obstetric ward staffed by midwives. The teaching unit's mortality rate was almost triple that of the midwives'.

Semmelweis reasoned that the physicians and students might be carrying infectious material, particularly puerperal sepsis, or "childbed fever," as it was then known. He ordered all physicians and students to wash their hands in chlorinated lime before examining women in childbirth. The results were dramatic and form one of the foundations of infection control and sterile technique.

Mortality Rate from Childbed Fever:
Before staff hand washing with chlorinated lime: 11.4%
After staff hand washing with chlorinated lime: 3%

Semmelweis then reasoned that the hands of physicians and medical students were contaminated by cadaveric materials, and ordered everyone to scrub their hands in chlorinated lime until the cadaver smell had been removed from their hands. He subsequently documented a dramatic decline in mortality from puerperal sepsis (Box 17–2), and the mortality rate in the first division became similar to that in the second division (Semmelweis, 1861/1981).

Florence Nightingale is probably one of the first nurses to survey nosocomial infection. She and William Farr, a British health statistician, analyzed mortality data from British hospitals. In her *Notes on Nursing,* Nightingale suggested a direct relationship between the sanitary conditions of a hospital and postoperative complications. She proposed a comprehensive reporting system for all deaths in hospitals, suggesting that ward sisters (nurses) maintain these statistical records. *Notes on Nursing* also presents Farr's analysis of mortality among hospital employees, which showed that mortality from contagious disease was more common in hospital personnel than in non-health care workers (LaForce, 1987).

Despite the work of these early pioneers, however, infection control in hospitals received little subsequent attention until the 1950s, when hospitals experienced epidemic transmission of penicillin-resistant *S. aureus.* Epidemics of staphylococcal infections in surgical and pediatric patients were the main impetus for the development of modern hospital epidemiology (LaForce, 1987). Early epidemiologic efforts tended to emphasize extensive environmental culturing such as sampling of environmental surfaces and equipment. However, organisms often found did not correlate with infections in patients. Therefore, later efforts concentrated on identifying infections occurring in patients and emphasis on aseptic patient care practices.

During the 1970s, many U.S. hospitals initiated infection control programs with a designated person assigned to manage the program. Components of these infection control programs included surveillance and reporting of nosocomial infections and development of effective control and prevention techniques. Infection control practitioners were responsible for identifying and reporting all nosocomial infections. Based on their findings, standard policies and procedures were developed for the prevention and control of nosocomial infections. Many of these were based on well-established aseptic techniques.

By 1980, the average U.S. hospital had an infection control program that was 5 years old (Dixon, 1991). Increasing use of invasive devices, widespread use of antimicrobial agents, earlier discharge of hospitalized patients, and diversion of personnel and resources from infection control to other areas characterized infection control in the 1980s.

In the 1990s, the emergence and increased public awareness of bloodborne diseases has made the safety of health care workers a major infection control issue. The U.S. Public Health Service has formulated national objectives for the year 2000 that include plans for preventing and controlling nosocomial infections judged to be preventable. Along with protecting patients, these objectives include goals to reduce the risk of occupational transmission of HIV and hepatitis B virus infection to health care workers (Martone, 1991). Also, various advisory and regulatory agencies are involved in setting standards for infection control (Box 17–3).

HAND WASHING

For more than a century, hand washing has been universally accepted as reducing transmission of infection in the hospital. Little published experimental work related to hand washing followed Semmelweis' 1861 publication, however.

In 1897a physician named Galapin at the London Lying-In Hospital reported a decrease in rates of septic fevers from 40 percent in 1885 to 2.5 percent in 1890. Galapin attributed the decreased rate to the introduction of antiseptic hand washing. Likewise, in the United States in 1898, Shumaker reported a steady decline in mortality from puerperal fever. He cited the dramatic reduction as evidence of the effectiveness of antisepsis related to hand washing (Larson, 1988a).

One contemporary researcher reviewed 423 articles on hand washing published from 1879 through 1986. The collective evidence from both nonexperimental and experimental studies is consistent with the hypothesis that hand washing is causally associated with reduced risk of infection (Larson, 1988a). The evidence for hand washing's effective-

BOX 17-3
ADVISORY AND REGULATORY AGENCIES

Several regulatory and advisory groups on the federal and nursing professional levels set standards for infection control, conduct inspections, and recommend practices and procedures to protect both patient and nurse.

JCAHO

The Joint Commission on Accreditation of Healthcare Organizations (JCAHO) sets standards for infection control practice in hospitals and other health care facilities. JCAHO standards establish surveillance programs, infection control policies and procedures, and regular continuing education for all employees in infection control (JCAHO, 1998).

JCAHO also conducts on-site visits to hospitals and other facilities to evaluate compliance with their standards. Participation with the JCAHO survey process is voluntary and, in fact, hospitals pay a fee to have a JCAHO survey performed. However, because JCAHO accreditation is a prerequisite to receive Medicare reimbursement, most hospitals participate in the JCAHO accreditation process.

OSHA

The Occupational Safety and Health Administration (OSHA) is a governmental agency responsible for establishing safe working environments for all employees of all businesses, including health care. OSHA inspectors conduct unannounced visits to work sites and levy large fines for noncompliance to its published standards. OSHA has traditionally focused on industrial settings, but since 1990 it has also become concerned with safe working environments for health care personnel. OSHA has conducted many hospital inspections, some of which resulted in large fines.

APICE

The Association for Practitioners in Infection Control and Epidemiology (APICE), the national professional organization for infectious control practitioners, provides resources to its membership in various ways. Educational programs are provided locally and at the national level. APICE publishes the *American Journal of Infection Control*, distributed to its membership. APICE supports the Certification Board for Infectious Control (CBIC), which administers the certification exam for infection control practitioners. APICE also develops practice guidelines for infection control procedures, such as hand washing (Larson, 1988b, 1995) and selection and use of disinfectants (Rutala, 1990).

CDC

The Centers for Disease Control and Prevention (CDC), a branch of the United States Public Health Service, has had a major role in shaping infection surveillance and control programs in U.S. hospitals. The CDC has published many guidelines on surveillance, prevention, and control techniques, such as hand washing (Garner, 1985), isolation (Garner, 1983, 1996), and universal precautions (CDC, 1987, 1988). Guidelines from the CDC are merely recommendations for practice; the CDC is not a regulatory agency and does not inspect or issue fines.

ness is primarily anecdotal rather than empirical, however. Many hospital investigations in Larson's review readily identified the presence of the outbreak organism on the hands of hospital personnel, and subsequently noted a decrease in infections when hand washing was made mandatory.

CONTEMPORARY STUDIES

Not until the 1960s were more scientific experiments conducted in a newborn nursery to trace the airborne and direct contact spread of staphylococci and streptococci between infants and nurses. These studies confirmed the importance of hand washing. In one study, 54 percent of infants handled by a "carrier" nurse with unwashed hands became colonized with the nurse's strain of *S. aureus* (Wolinsky et al, 1960). In another study, nurses who handled a "carrier" infant and subsequently handled another infant without washing their hands had a transmission rate of 43 percent. Antiseptic hand washing reduced this rate to 14 percent (Rammelkamp et al, 1964). In another portion of the study, 92 percent of infants attended by a nurse who did not wash hands acquired the same staphylococcal strain as the "carrier" nurse and infected infants compared with 53 percent of infants handled with washed hands (Mortimer et al, 1962).

Hand washing has been shown to reduce infection spread by the fecal-oral route as well. In one outbreak of shigellosis in a newborn nursery, only 3 of 32 health care workers providing care for the infected infant acquired shigellosis. (This infant had probably acquired the infection from its mother during birth; other family members tested positive for *Shigella*.) It was believed that strict enforcement of hand-washing policies may have interrupted further spread of the infection (Beers et al, 1989).

Other studies document the interruption of transmission of RSV in newborn nurseries and pediatric units by effective hand washing (Isaacs et al, 1991; Snydman 1988). Hand washing has likewise been associated with decreased transmission of diarrheal illnesses in day care centers (Black et al, 1981; Butz et al, 1990).

NOSOCOMIAL INFECTIONS

Hand washing is an effective intervention in nosocomial infection. For example, nosocomial outbreaks of MRSA have been frequently reported in U.S. hospitals since 1980. Enforcement of hand washing along with other infection control measures has been anecdotally associated with decreased MRSA infection rates in intensive care units (Griffiths, 1988; Guiguet et al, 1990).

Although there have been many other reports of hand washing's effectiveness in curtailing nosocomial infection, many questions could still be answered through randomized clinical trials. However, these studies will probably never be performed because of the complex ethical and practical issues involved. (For example, it is not ethical to plan a clinical trial involving a control group for whom hand washing is withheld, increasing their exposure to infectious organisms.) Nonetheless, based on the studies of early investigators such as Semmelweis and continued reports of successful hand-washing interventions for infection outbreaks, hand washing is and will remain a basic infection control practice.

HAND-WASHING AGENTS

The effectiveness of various hand-washing agents has also been studied. One investigator undertook a comparative trial in a surgical intensive care unit of three hand-washing agents: a nongermicidal tissue soap, a 10 percent povidone-iodine detergent, and a 4 percent chlorhexidine solution. Each agent was used for approximately 6 weeks, and then random hand cultures were obtained from personnel and surveillance for colonization and infection of patients was performed. Nosocomial infections were reduced by nearly 50 percent from using the two antiseptic-containing hand-washing agents compared with the nongermicidal soap (Maki & Hecht, 1982).

In contrast, however, a year-long study by other investigators found no significant differences in the rates of nosocomial infections when nongermicidal hand-washing agents were used exclusively compared with alternating cycles using either 4 percent chlorhexidine or povidone-iodine solution (Massanari and Hierholzer, 1984). However, a more recent study of hand-washing agents in intensive care units demonstrated lower infection rates when chlorhexidine solution was used than when alcohol and soap were used (Doebbeling, 1991). Clearly, more studies are needed to determine which hand-washing agents are most efficacious in reducing nosocomial infections.

COMPLIANCE WITH HAND WASHING

The primary factor limiting the effectiveness of hand washing in preventing infection transmission is lack of compliance with hand-washing procedures in health care institutions. One evaluation of compliance in a neonatal intensive care unit found that a substantial number of physicians and nurses did not wash their hands either before (25 percent) or after (50 percent) patient contact (De Carvalho et al, 1989). In another study, medical-surgical nurses were observed for compliance with aseptic techniques. About 40 percent failed to wash their hands before or after a patient care procedure requiring hand washing (McLane et al, 1983). A third study monitored 1233 opportunities for hand washing and found that hands were washed 42 percent of the time when chlorhexidine was available and only 38 percent of the time when an alcohol-soap combination was available (Doebbeling et al, 1992).

Nurse surveys, observation, monitoring, educational sessions, staff feedback, and physician role models have all been used in attempts to increase compliance. In one study, investigators administered a questionnaire to nurses asking them

RESEARCH HIGHLIGHT

REDUCING THE TRANSMISSION OF MICROORGANISMS THROUGH HAND-WASHING TECHNIQUES

Hand washing is an important factor in reducing the transmission of infections. The procedure is important in any setting in which nursing care is given and in the personal life of every nurse. Preventing the spread of infectious organisms is essential in all societies and in every nation.

Numerous studies have been cited demonstrating that proper hand-washing procedures will reduce the spread of bacteria and other disease-producing organisms. However, there are also studies that indicate that there are problems with medical and nursing staff compliance with the established standards. Many nurses fail to wash their hands before or after contact with patients. Many different approaches have been used to increase compliance. One study illustrates some of the methods used.

THE STUDY: THE DUBBERT HANDWASHING COMPLIANCE STUDY (1990)

Two programs were devised in an attempt to improve nurses hand-washing standards. In *Program One* a series of three classes in hand-washing techniques was developed by infection-control nurses. Nurses involved with direct patient care were taught the proper hand-washing techniques and standards of application.

Results: There was in immediate increase in handwashing compliance, followed by a decline in compliance within 4 weeks.

In *Program Two* infection control nurses observed other nurses and tallied the number of errors committed in performing or not performing hand-washing procedures. The tally of errors committed during the previous day was reported to the involved nursing staff.

Results. The program resulted in 97% compliance rate that was sustained during the study period.

Implications for Nursing Practice

The study suggests that having basic knowledge is not sufficient to motivate individuals to properly implement hand-washing procedures. Constant attention must be provided to focus on the need to reduce infections. The daily reminders provided through feedback on the results of errors committed the previous day seemed to be a motivating factor and did increase compliance. This study demonstrates the need to devise methods to increase compliance rates. Nurses must take seriously the need to constantly and consistently apply proper hand-washing techniques. Additional studies should be conducted to determine successful methods to increase compliance rates.

to report how frequently they washed their hands in accordance with CDC criteria. A compulsory in-service session about hand washing was also held, and each nurse was given several publications promoting the importance of hand washing. This was followed by a second campaign in which buttons encouraging hand-washing practices were handed out. Despite all of these measures, overall hand-washing compliance increased only gradually, from 22 percent before the program to 29.9 percent afterward—a statistically insignificant increase (Simmons et al, 1990). Another study tried two programs—education and feedback—to increase compliance with hand washing (Dubbert, 1990); see Research Highlight: Reducing the Transmission of Microorganisms Through Hand-Washing Technique, for further details.

A further study evaluated the effects of an attending physician serving as a role model for hand-washing behavior. The investigator accompanied two medical teams on rounds: one team with an attending physician who placed little emphasis on hand washing, the other with an attending physician who emphasized its importance. The team with the role model complied with hand washing 48.1 percent of the time that hand washing was indicated; the team without a role model, only 24 percent of the time (Larson, 1983b). This study has significant implications for health care personnel who are designated leaders and who might have the capacity to influence the behavior of others. An essay by two researchers supports the concept that hospital role models could be identified to achieve desired behavior among nursing personnel, students, other staff, and attending physicians (Wenzel and Pfaller, 1991).

Significant microbial contamination can occur even with proper hand washing, however. One study reported that the subungual (beneath the fingernails) region appears to be an important reservoir of bacterial and microbial transmission (McGinley et al, 1988). The nurse must, therefore, take particular care to clean under the fingernails during hand washing. Short nails are preferred because they are easier to clean. Artificial nails have been shown to harbor higher numbers of gram-negative bacterial colonies after hand washing than natural nails (Pottinger et al, 1989). Nurses who wear artificial nails must consider them a potential carrier of gram-negative rods. The wearing of rings can also interfere with thorough hand scrubbing and has been associated with higher bacterial counts on the hands (Hoffman et al, 1985; Jacobsen et al, 1985).

ISOLATION AND BARRIER PRECAUTIONS

Isolation systems are primarily based on logic and the knowledge of disease transmission. A review of the nursing literature was conducted to evaluate the effectiveness of quarantine or isolation practices in reducing the risk of nosocomial transmission of infection (Jackson and Lynch, 1985). Recommendations were found to be usually based on opinions of individuals, not on scientific evidence related to effective interruption of disease transmission. One researcher stated that using barrier precautions to prevent cross-infection has all of the characteristics of a typical ritual, and health care workers have accepted barrier precautions without question despite very little scientific evidence of efficacy (Goldman, 1991). One study of isolation practices observed 467 subjects entering patient rooms (Pettinger and Nettleman, 1991). The study was conducted in an isolation bay of a surgical intensive care unit and was performed by a nurse on duty without the knowledge of subjects. The nurse-researcher found less than 50 percent compliance with isolation procedures; hand washing was the single most common cause of noncompliance. An additional observation was that health care workers were more compliant with isolation precautions when they were part of a group as opposed to when they were alone. This finding suggests that role models may be effective in increasing compliance. Also noted was a trend toward decreased compliance when a nurse's patient assignments increased. This observation may be especially pertinent in the current atmosphere of managed care and cost containment.

Although no formal study has compared the effectiveness of the various approaches to isolation, several reports in the literature do substantiate that barriers such as gowns, gloves, masks, and goggles are apparently effective in interrupting transmission of specific infectious diseases.

Gowns and Gloves

Compliance with gowning and gloving procedures has been reviewed by several nursing investigators. One study of compliance with isolation procedures for 52 patients on some type of isolation found that the type of isolation was appropriate 94.2 percent of the time, but personnel wore appropriate barriers only 46.1 percent of the time. The two most common errors found were failure to wear a gown when changing the dressing on contaminated or infected wounds and failure to wear gloves when handling excreta of patients on enteric precautions (Larson, 1983a).

Researchers from Children's Hospital in Boston observed isolation practices as part of an investigation of a cluster of RSV infections in infants and toddlers. Initial observation found only 39 percent compliance with the wearing of gloves and gowns for contact with patients infected with RSV (Leclair et al, 1987). Over the next few weeks, staff were made aware that they were being observed for compliance with gown and glove techniques. At the end of the monitoring time, compliance was nearly 95 percent. This compliance remained at very high levels for nearly 1½ years after the investigation. The investigators believed that the continued compliance was related to the successful curtailment of RSV transmission (Leclair et al, 1987).

In another study, patients in a pediatric intensive care unit were assigned to one of two study groups: a group receiving standard care and a group cared for by staff using disposable gowns and nonsterile latex gloves (Klein et al, 1989). The investigators found a rate of nosocomial colonization of 31 percent in the group receiving care with barrier precautions compared with 42 percent in the group receiving standard care. They also found a nosocomial infection rate of 4.4 infections per 100 patient-days in the group receiving care with barrier precautions, and a rate of 8.6 infections per 100 patient-days in the group receiving standard care. These researchers concluded that using disposable gowns and gloves in the care of high-risk children in intensive care units reduced the incidence of nosocomial infection (Klein et al, 1989).

After implementation of body substance isolation (BSI) at the Harborview Medical Center, Seattle, Washington, compliance with recommended gloving procedures increased from 61 percent to 81 percent. The investigators used certain "marker" organisms to evaluate the success of BSI in limiting transmission of nosocomial pathogens. The rate of *Serratia* isolates fell from 2.0 per 1000 patient-days to 1.0 per 1000 patient-days after implementation of BSI (Lynch et al, 1990). However, nosocomial infections were not monitored in this study, and it is uncertain whether this trend continued after the study was concluded.

Other studies have examined the efficacy of gowns and gloves in relationship to particular infections, particularly RSV. In the Children's Hospital of Boston study cited earlier (Leclair et al, 1987), the transmission of RSV was found to be 2.9 times greater during the period when gowns and gloves were not routinely used than when compliance with gown and glove usage for care with children was high. However, earlier studies had suggested that masks and gowns made no statistically significant difference in the acquisition of RSV and other respiratory viruses (Hall and Douglas, 1981; Murphy et al, 1981). Additional studies are needed to validate the effectiveness of gowns and gloves in preventing transmission of specific infections.

Masks and Goggles

Several investigators have evaluated the use of eye, nose, and mask goggle barriers for preventing RSV transmission. One study evaluated disposable eye-nose goggles to determine their usefulness in reducing nosocomial RSV infection of patients and staff members on their infant ward (Gala et al, 1986). When the eye-nose goggles were worn, 5 percent of the adult staff and 1 percent of the children acquired nosocomial infection. However, when the eye-nose goggles were not used, 34 percent of the adult staff and 43 percent of the children acquired nosocomial infection. Thus, this study suggests that using disposable eye-nose goggles can produce a significant decrease in nosocomial RSV infections.

In another small study, RSV transmission rate was compared in two groups of pediatric health care workers (Agah et al, 1987). In the mask and goggle group, 5 percent acquired RSV, whereas in the no mask and goggles group, 61 percent acquired RSV. This study did not evaluate the occurrence of nosocomial infections, but it clearly showed a reduced incidence of RSV infection associated with the use of mask and goggles.

With the advent of Universal Precautions and the implementation of BSI in some hospitals, the need for hand washing after the wearing of gloves has been questioned. One study evaluated the effectiveness of three different types of hand-washing agents in decontaminating gloved hands that were inoculated with nosocomial pathogens in a laboratory setting (Doebbeling et al, 1988). After the gloves were cleansed, they were cultured. After the gloves were removed, the wearers' hands were also cultured in a similar manner. Both gloves and hands were positive for test organisms. This study suggests that microorganisms adhere to gloves and are not easily washed off despite friction of a cleansing agent. The study demonstrates that wearing gloves does not eliminate the need for hand washing after the gloves are removed.

STERILE FIELDS

Setting up a sterile work field is based on the principles of surgical asepsis. By defining areas of sterility and contamination, infective microorganisms are not allowed to come in contact with sterile equipment or instruments. These principles are based entirely on what is known about the epidemiology and microbiology of infection transmission. These procedures have long been a part of nursing practice and have been described by some as ritualistic, because studies do not exist to validate their importance. However, it would be difficult to discontinue what is a currently accepted standard of practice to determine whether a change in sterile technique would alter the infection rate. Therefore, the principles of establishing a sterile work field must be based on an existing basic knowledge.

When preparing a sterile field, the nurse must be constantly aware of what is sterile and what is unsterile, and keep the two apart. No bacteriologic studies exist that define where sterility begins and ends. Therefore, certain "ritualistic" parameters have been established to identify what is and what is not sterile. Tables draped with sterilized material are considered sterile only on the surface and above. A person wearing sterile gloves may touch the items in the sterile field but should not lean or reach over the sterile field. A person wearing sterile gloves should always keep the hands in front of the body to avoid accidental contamination when the hands are out of sight. Talking should be kept to a minimum when working over a sterile field. Also, movement and other air currents around the sterile field should be kept to a minimum to avoid contamination.

FACTORS AFFECTING CLINICAL DECISIONS

Basic requirements for hand washing, barrier techniques, and aseptic practices are generally the same for all patients. However, each patient has unique circumstances that determine what specific infection control measures are needed. Some circumstances may affect the kind of barriers required or whether the patient should be in a private room. For example, the nurse caring for Mrs. Brown in the case study must wear a gown while performing dressing changes because of Mrs. Brown's extensive wound drainage. In contrast, a nurse caring for a patient with a small superficial wound infection may only need to wear gloves. Besides differences in patient's conditions, other differences in individual circumstances also affect nursing care of patients with infection.

Age

The patient's age may be a factor in determining what barriers are needed. For example, an adult patient with diarrhea does not normally need a private room or require health care workers to wear protective gowns. However, for an infant who wears diapers and has copious diarrhea requiring frequent diaper changes, a private room is indicated, and the nurse must wear a protective gown or apron when in direct contact with the child.

The patient's age may also be an indicator of contagiousness. For example, infants and very young children with pulmonary tuberculosis (TB) rarely cough, and their bronchial secretions contain few TB organisms. This age group thus is less likely to transmit the TB infection than older children and adults. In another example, children with acute respiratory infections require contact isolation, whereas adults do not. Children are often touched, cuddled, or held by a nurse, whose clothing may then become contaminated with respiratory secretions. The infection then may be transmitted by indirect contact to the next child whom the nurse holds. Contact isolation requires the nurse to wear a clean gown or apron for direct contact with each child.

Immune system function is also affected by age. The very young, especially preterm infants, often have underdeveloped immune systems that cannot adequately respond to infection; elderly persons may have failing immune systems. People in both of these age groups are at increased risk for infection because of impaired immune responses.

Individual and Family Values

The specific circumstances of the patient and family must be considered when implementing various infection control procedures. Previous knowledge, values, and life experiences may affect the way patients and families understand and subsequently cooperate with control measures.

EDUCATIONAL BACKGROUND

The nurse must assess a patient's level of education before teaching the patient and family about infection prevention. Some patients and their families may have little, if any, knowledge of how infections are spread, and their fear of infection may interfere with learning. The nurse may find it helpful to supplement verbal teaching with teaching aids such as brochures, illustrations, and videos. The nurse must also keep in mind that some patients may not be able to read, and special efforts may be needed to meet their needs.

Patients and families must be taught the importance of barriers and how to use them properly. This teaching should include assurance that the disease is being isolated, not the patient, to help reduce feelings of rejection. If dressing changes will be required after discharge, the patient and family must be taught proper technique. The nurse may wish to refer the patent and family to a home health agency for follow-up at home.

SOCIOECONOMIC STATUS

Hospital-acquired infections are unanticipated complications that may delay a patient's discharge and subsequent return to work. The patient's feelings of anxiety and frustration about the hospitalization may lead to anger and hostility toward hospital staff. These feelings may be intensified with the addition of barrier precautions and perceived seclusion. The patient may further be worried about family members, insurance coverage, job security, and the possibility of permanent disability. This stress, and associated depression, may actually delay recovery. Assistance from support services, such as social service or pastoral care, may be indicated.

CULTURE AND ETHNICITY

Culture and ethnicity may also impact required nursing interventions. Whenever isolation procedures are initiated, it is important that the patient and family understand why barriers are being used. For some, isolation procedures are associated with social rejection and banning. Patients raised in countries where leprosy is prevalent may associate isolation with leper colonies, for example, and resist isolation.

Language barriers may hinder nurse-patient communication. A patient who cannot speak or read English, for instance, and needs patient teaching may require an interpreter. Many hospitals provide their staff a list of persons who can interpret when these barriers emerge. These interpreters must not only educate patients about their illnesses and isolation needs, but also reassure them that they are not being banned or rejected.

The nurse must also address family needs for closeness. Family associations are vital; illness itself impacts family relationships, and use of isolation barriers may only intensify feelings of separation. Use of a mask and, especially, the use of respirators now required for TB patients prevent crucial nonverbal communication linked with facial expressions: A smile may not be seen for days.

It is almost always permissible for family members to hold the hand or pat the face of a loved one, even though isolation barriers are in place. The nurse must teach appropriate handwashing technique to these family members, however. On rare occasions, it may be necessary to isolate a mother from her newborn, such as when TB is diagnosed at admission for delivery. The infant should not have contact with the mother until the mother is treated, responding to treatment, and determined to be noninfectious. This process may require 2 weeks or longer and is a devastating experience for a new mother who longs to bond with her newborn. The nurse is faced with the challenge of providing support and encouragement to this new mother.

Patients may experience depression on isolation, which may result in decreased immunity, delaying healing. Again, the nurse must provide support to help keep the patient from feeling lonely and rejected.

Setting in Which Care Is Delivered

Patients with infections may be cared for in any setting: hospital, ambulatory care units, long-term care facilities, or home. Regardless of the setting, infection control measures include hand washing, barrier precautions, and aseptic technique. Some modifications of these measures may be necessary in different settings, however. For example, most nursing homes do not have rooms to safely house patients with TB, and some nursing homes and physician's or clinic offices have no private rooms and thus cannot accommodate a patient with an infection requiring a single room.

Most patients can be cared for effectively at home if they are well enough to be discharged and have a caretaker at home. Even patients with TB may return home, because persons in the home were already exposed to the patient for weeks or months before diagnosis. In this case, the entire household is evaluated for TB and possible treatment. A patient with airborne or severe infection must not live in the same household with a severely immunocompromised person, however.

Ethical and Legal Considerations

The nurse and all health care team members have an ethical obligation to provide the same level of care to infected patients as to patients free of infection. Unfortunately, equality of care is not always maintained. For example, health team members may avoid going into an isolation room except when absolutely essential. Thus, a patient who is already prohibited from venturing outside the room may be further isolated by poor interaction with caregivers, denying the patient human contact. Because the patient can be isolated from care, the nurse must review the patient's need for isolation in the daily assessment and discontinue isolation as soon as possible.

Confidentiality issues have intensified with the advent of AIDS. Laws exist to protect the confidentiality of the patient, and some nurses fear that these laws put them at risk of infection. In some states, written informed consent must be obtained from the patient before testing for HIV infection. If Universal Precautions are always applied, however, the health care worker is protected from known and unknown infection.

However, all patients, not just those with AIDS, are entitled to privacy. No aspect of patient care must ever be discussed in public areas, such as an elevator or cafeteria. All health care providers must be very cautious that isolation signs do not breach the patient's right to confidentiality. Isolation signs are designed to provide health care workers with the information they need to provide safe care to the patient. However, these cards are visible to family and visitors and should not provide details of a patient's illness.

Lawsuits have become more prevalent. Patients are more aware of infection standards than at any time in the past, and transmission of infection resulting from lack of compliance with established policies and procedures may result in the nurse, physician, and hospital being named in a lawsuit.

Financial Considerations

Financial concerns associated with the cost of preventing and treating infections are increasing as third-party payors move toward fixed payment of all services. Added hospital days, drugs, and supplies may not be covered expenses for the patient with nosocomial infection and may thus represent lost revenue for the hospital. Continuous application of procedures to prevent transmission of infection is also in everyone's best interest. Likewise, barriers should be used as indicated: Overuse creates unnecessary cost, which managed care organizations may refuse to reimburse.

FUTURE DEVELOPMENTS

Implementing cost-effective measures to curtail infection will become increasingly important as health care reform evolves. It will likewise be necessary to monitor the efficacy of these measures. Products, procedures, and equipment that are not efficacious will likely not be reimbursable.

Hospital building design must include provisions for patients with infections, particularly airborne infections such as TB. Patient rooms, treatment rooms, and public waiting areas, such as emergency or clinic waiting rooms, must be adequately ventilated. Air must be continuously exchanged and, in some instances, filtered or exhausted to the outside. Incoming air is also filtered and in some cases passes through a high-efficiency particulate air (HEPA) filter.

The homeless population, persons with superresistant TB, and infants with HIV infections all present special problems for the future. If transmission of infection is to be curtailed, sick people need to be provided care in environments conducive to breaking the chain of infection.

New technologies for molecular tracing of organisms such as pulse field gel electrophoresis and polymerase chain reactions allow more specific and potentially earlier identification of microorganisms. These technologies will enhance abilities to associate infective organisms with those found in the environment. This type of identification may eventually enhance research efforts to validate many of our traditional, but not research-based, practices.

Research is ongoing to develop vaccines to prevent HIV and TB, including multidrug-resistant TB. These vaccines will enhance overall public health but will be especially beneficial for health care workers. Development of vaccines to prevent nosocomial infections is also on the horizon. For example, one project is the development of a vaccine to prevent *Pseudomonas* infections in cystic fibrosis patients.

NURSING CARE ACTIONS

Principles and Practices

The implementation of nursing care to both prevent the transmission of and to treat patients with infectious diseases must be conducted with great accuracy. Nurses must be highly knowledgeable and skilled in caring for patients with diseases of any infectious nature.

HAND WASHING

Hand washing is the single most important procedure in the prevention and control of nosocomial infection. Nurses and other health care workers contaminate their hands by touching contaminated equipment and material. These transient microorganisms can then be transmitted from patient to patient. Several published guidelines (Larson, 1988b, 1995) direct when hand washing should be performed (Box 17–4). The type of hand-washing agent selected must be determined by the specific situation.

Scrubbing with detergent (plain non-antimicrobial soap) and water physically removes microbes, but antiseptic agents are needed to kill infectious organisms. The primary action of plain soap is to mechanically remove viable transient organisms. Antimicrobial soap mechanically removes and also chemically kills or inhibits both contaminating and colonizing flora (Larson, 1995).

The choice of a plain or an antiseptic soap should be based on whether it is important to reduce or maintain minimal counts of colonizing flora as well as to mechanically remove noncolonizing or contaminating flora. Situations requiring an antiseptic soap are defined in Box 17–5. In Mrs. Brown's case,

BOX 17–4
WHEN TO WASH HANDS

There are certain times when all health care workers must wash their hands. These situations have been mandated by several guidelines, including the CDC's, and encompass:

- Before and after each patient contact
- After contact with a source of microorganisms, such as body fluids, mucous membranes, nonintact skin, or any object that might be contaminated
- Before performing invasive procedures
- After removing gloves

BOX 17-5
WHEN TO USE ANTISEPTIC SOAP

Several common hospital and outpatient procedures mandate the use of antiseptic soap. These include

- During preoperative scrub
- Before performing or assisting with invasive procedures, such as inserting intravascular or urinary catheters
- When the goal is to reduce resident and transient flora
- Before and after providing wound care

the nurse should use an antiseptic agent for hand washing before and after changing her dressings.

ISOLATION

The CDC periodically updates isolation precautions. The latest was published in 1996. In 1970, the CDC published their first manual, *Isolation Techniques for Use in Hospitals.* This manual placed all diseases with similar modes of transmission into one of seven categories of isolation: Strict, Contact, Respiratory, Acid-Fast Bacteria, Enteric, Drainage and Secretion, Blood and Body Fluid. The seven isolation categories were derived by grouping diseases with similar isolation precautions. In 1983, the CDC updated these isolation procedures and published them in *Guidelines for Isolation Precautions in Hospitals.* In this update, the CDC provided two alternative isolation systems: a revised category-specific system reflecting new epidemiologic research, and a disease-specific system listing specific barrier precautions for each individual disease (Garner and Simmons, 1983). This new disease-specific isolation system considered each infectious disease individually. Specific isolation requirements and barrier precautions were determined by identifying the disease from an alphabetical table. A generic instruction card with a checklist helped nurses quickly identify required precautions. This card was then placed on the patient's door.

The CDC has published new isolation guidelines (Garner, 1996). This is a two-tiered system composed of *Standard Precautions* and *transmission-driven precautions.* Standard precautions incorporate elements of Universal Precautions and BSI (Box 17–6). Transmission-driven precautions include airborne precautions (Box 17–7), droplet precautions (Box 17–8), and contact precautions (Box 17–9). Transmission-driven precautions may be used in combination, as with chickenpox, which requires both airborne and contact precautions. Instruction cards have been designed to give concise information about appropriate precautions. These cards should be posted where they are visible to all personnel who are providing care to the patient. Cards must be designed in such a manner that the patient's right to confidentiality is maintained. The patient and family should be informed that an isolation cared has been posted.

Special care must be taken to avoid contamination during donning and removal of protective attire.

TUBERCULOSIS GUIDELINES

The rising incidence of TB in the late 1980s and early 1990s, the increase in drug-resistant strains, and outbreaks of

BOX 17-6
STANDARD PRECAUTIONS

1. Wash hands after touching blood, body fluids, secretions, excretions, mucus-contaminated items.
2. Wear gloves when touching blood, body fluids, secretions, excretions, mucous membranes, non-intact skin, and contaminated items. Remove gloves promptly after use and WASH HANDS.
3. Wear a mask and eye protection when performing procedures or patient care activities that are likely to generate sprays or splashes.
4. Wear a gown during procedures or patient care activities that may generate sprays or splashes of blood or other body fluids.
5. Disinfect or sterilize all reusable equipment between patients. Handle contaminated equipment in a manner that prevents contamination of skin, clothing, and the environment.
6. Disinfect environmental surfaces, beds, and bedside equipment.
7. Prevent injuries by safe handling of sharps (see Box 17–10).
8. Use mouthpieces, resuscitation bags, or other ventilation devices as an alternative to mouth-to-mouth resuscitation.

BOX 17-7
AIRBORNE PRECAUTIONS

Use in Addition to Standard Precautions

1. Private room that has:
   - Monitored negative air pressure
   - Discharge of air outdoors or HEPA filtration before air is recirculated.

   KEEP THE ROOM DOOR CLOSED AND THE PATIENT IN THE ROOM
2. Respiratory Protection
   - **Wear an N95 respirator mask for known or suspected tuberculosis.** Susceptible persons should not enter the room of patients with known or suspected measles (rubeola) or varicella (chickenpox) if immune caregivers are available. If susceptible persons must enter the room, a mask is required.
3. Limit the movement and transport of patients from room to essential purposes only. During transport, minimize the spread of droplet nuclei by placing a surgical mask on the patient if possible.

Illnesses Requiring Airborne Precautions

1. Measles
2. Varicella (Chickenpox and disseminated zoster).
3. Tuberculosis

BOX 17–8
DROPLET PRECAUTIONS

Use in addition to Standard Precautions

1. Place the patient in a private room. When a private room is not available, cohort with patient(s) who has active infection with the same microorganism but with no other infection. Maintain spatial separation of at least 3 feet from other patients and visitors if cohorting or private room is not available. The door may remain open. Special ventilation is not required.
2. Mask required when working within 3 feet of patient (or when entering room). Check your hospital's policy.
3. Limit the movement and transport of patients from room to essential purposes only. During transport, minimize the spread of droplets by placing a surgical mask on the patient if possible.

Illnesses Requiring Droplet Precautions

1. Invasive *Haemophilus influenzae* type b disease, including meningitis, pneumonia, epiglottitis, and sepsis.
2. Invasive *Neisseria meningitidis* disease, including meningitis, pneumonia, and sepsis.
3. Invasive multidrug-resistant *Streptococcus pneumoniae* disease, including meningitis, pneumonia, sinusitis, and otitis media.
4. Other serious bacterial respiratory infections spread by droplet transmission, including:
   a. *Diphtheria* (pharyngeal)
   b. Mycoplasma pneumonia
   c. Pertussis
   d. Pneumonic plague
   e. Streptococcal pharyngitis, pneumonia, or scarlet fever in infants and young children
5. Serious viral infections spread by droplet transmission, including
   a. Adenovirus
   b. Infuenza
   c. Mumps
   d. Parvovirus B19
   e. Rubella

TB in health care settings led to the development of specific TB control guidelines (CDC, 1990).

One of the critical components of TB control is the prompt identification and isolation of persons with TB. The nurse must be alert for patients with a chronic cough, weight loss, or night sweats. These patients must then be isolated until the TB is appropriately treated or until diagnostic tests indicate the patient does not have TB. Some patients, such as infants and young children with pulmonary TB, do not require isolation. They rarely cough, and their bronchial secretions release few organisms.

Masks are indicated for all persons entering the room of a patient with suspected or diagnosed TB. Room requirements include that the room be under negative air pressure in relation to the corridor, have six air exchanges per hour, and exhaust to the outside. In addition, respirators classified by

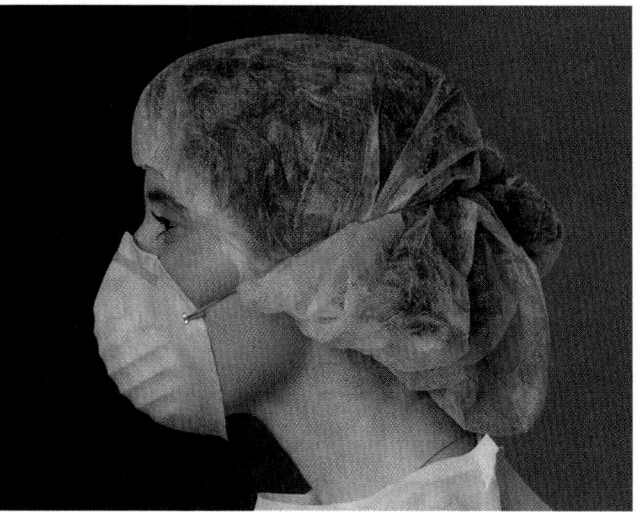

Figure 17–4. Type N95 particulate respirator.

the National Institute of Occupational Safety and Health as N95 (Fig. 17–4) or HEPA are the minimum protection required by the CDC for those providing direct care to infectious TB patients (CDC, 1994). The N95 respirator requires a special fit test before use. Every health care facility is required to have a TB control plan and to provide employees with adequate protection.

UNIVERSAL PRECAUTIONS

In August 1987, the CDC responded to increasing concerns among health care workers about minimizing the risk of infection from occupationally transmitted bloodborne diseases such as hepatitis B and AIDS. These recommendations are referred to as *universal blood and body fluid precautions,* or simply Universal Precautions (CDC, 1987, 1988). In the CDC's original publication, the precautions were applicable to blood and all body fluids, but redefined in a later publication to apply to blood and *certain* other body fluids. Universal Precautions are intended to protect health care workers from all infectious diseases, both unrecognized and recognized.

In the 1996 isolation revisions, previously reviewed Standard Precautions essentially replaced and expanded on Universal Precautions. Standard and universal precautions include the following:

- All health care workers should routinely use appropriate barriers to prevent skin and mucous membrane exposure when contact with blood or other body fluids of any patient is anticipated. Gloves should be worn for touching blood and body fluids, mucous membranes, and nonintact skin of all patients; for handling items or surfaces soiled with blood or any body fluid; and for performing venipuncture and other vascular access procedures. Masks and protective eye wear or face shields should be worn during procedures that are likely to generate droplets of blood or other body

BOX 17-9
CONTACT PRECAUTIONS

Use in Addition to Standard Precautions

1. Place the patient in a private room. When a private room is not available, cohort with patient(s) who has active infection with the same microorganism but with no other infection.
2. Wear gloves when entering room. Change gloves after contact with infective material. Remove gloves before leaving the patient's room.
3. WASH YOUR HANDS immediately with antimicrobial agent before leaving the patient's room. After glove removal and hand washing, ensure that hands do not touch potentially contaminated environmental surfaces or items in the patient's room to avoid transfer of microorganisms to other patients or environments.
4. Wear a gown if you anticipate that your clothes will have substantial contact with the patient, environmental surfaces, or items in the patient's room or if the patient has any of the following:
   - Incontinence
   - Diarrhea
   - Colostomy
   - Ileostomy
   - Wound drainage not contained in a dressing.
5. Remove gown before leaving the patient's environment.
6. Limit the movement and transport of patients from room to essential purposes only. During transport, ensure that all precautions are maintained at all times.
7. When possible, dedicate the use of noncritical patient care equipment for each patient.

Illnesses Requiring Contact Precautions

1. Gastrointestinal, respiratory, skin, or wound infections or colonization with multidrug-resistant bacteria judged by the infection control program, based on current state, regional, or national recommendations, to be of special clinical and epidemiologic significance.
2. Enteric infections with low infectious dose or prolonged environmental survival, including:
   a. *Clostridium difficile*
   b. For diapered or incontinent patients: enterohemorrhagic *Escherichia coli* O157:H7, *Shigella,* hepatitis A, or rotavirus.
3. Respiratory syncytial virus, parainfluenza virus, or enteroviral infections in infants and young children.
4. Skin infections that are highly contagious or that may occur on dry skin, including
   a. Diphtheria (cutaneous)
   b. Herpes simplex virus (neonatal or mucocutaneous)
   c. Impetigo
   d. Major (noncontained) abscesses, cellulitis, or decubitus
   e. Pediculosis
   f. Scabies
   g. Staphylococcal furunculosis in infants and young children
   h. Staphylococcal scalded skin syndrome
   i. Zoster (disseminated or in the immunocompromised host)
5. Viral/Hemorrhagic conjunctivitis
6. Viral hemorrhagic fevers (Lassa fever or Marburg virus)

Prevention of Injuries from Contaminated Needles and other Sharps

1. Never recap needles using two hands.
2. Use a one-handed "scoop" technique or a resheathing device.
3. Do not remove needles from disposable syringes.
4. Place used needles and sharps in puncture-resistant containers located as close as possible to the point of use.
5. Use needleless intravascular system components whenever possible.

CLINICAL DECISION MAKING
CARING FOR AN ILL DIABETIC WITH AN OPEN ULCER

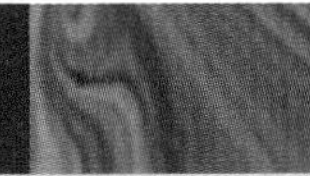

Molly Brown, a 60-year-old diabetic patient with an open draining ulcer on her left foot, is admitted to the hospital. Within eight hours of admission Ms. Brown has had five episodes of liquid stool and complains of severe abdominal cramping.

FACTORS TO CONSIDER

1. How well does Ms. Brown understand her diabetes and comply with diet and medication requirements?
2. Who has been caring for her wound?
3. What is the cause of her diarrhea?
4. Who will be caring for Ms. Brown when she is discharged?

GOAL OF CARE

Return Ms. Brown to independent living with her diarrhea resolved, her wound healing, and her diabetes controlled.

Interventions

1. Contact isolation for infected wound and diarrhea.
2. Stool specimen to lab for identification of possible infectious process.
3. Consult wound therapist for best wound care protocol.
4. Assess Ms. Brown's understanding of her illness.
5. Teach Ms. Brown and her caretaker about diabetes control measures, proper hand-washing technique, and aseptic techniques for wound care.
6. Assess Ms. Brown's ability to obtain the medications and supplies she needs.

PATIENT TEACHING
TOPICS TO DISCUSS WITH PATIENT AND FAMILY MEMBERS

PROPER TECHNIQUE FOR DRESSING CHANGES

Patients with open incisions or traumatic wounds need to be instructed in the proper technique to apply dressings to the open lesion. The main objective in surgical wound care is to reduce the possibility of sepsis caused by microorganisms. Wounds created by trauma may already be contaminated. In all instances the prevention or reduction of infection is of primary importance.

GENERAL INFORMATION

In general, the patient and family members need to understand the following factors:

- How infection is transmitted
- A demonstration of proper hand-washing techniques
- The importance of adequate nutrition and rest in reducing infections and promoting wound healing
- Hygienic measures important in maintaining general health care practices
- If appropriate, isolation procedures to protect the family and patient
- Importance of vaccinations in reducing spread of contagious disease
- Type of dressing materials and solutions used to change dressings
- Proper dressing change techniques

SPECIFIC FACTORS TO TEACH THE PATIENT AND FAMILY

The patient's physician will indicate the type of dressing, the frequency of the dressing change and any special type of solution to be used to clean the incision.

Specific steps to teach to change dressing:

- Type of supplies to use and placement of supplies on a clean, flat workspace
- Comfortable placement of patient for the dressing change
- How to remove old bandage from the patient's incision and safe disposal of dressing in a plastic bag. How to securely tie or close bag and dispose in a closed container
- Importance of when and how to wash hands
- How to cleanse wound with solution such as soap and water
- How to apply a clean dressing over the wound
- How to inspect incision for signs of infection such as purulent drainage, swelling, heat, redness, and elevated body temperature
- When to call the physician if signs of infections occur

fluids to prevent exposure of mucous membranes of the mouth, nose, and eyes. Gowns or aprons should be worn during procedures that are likely to generate splashes of blood or other body fluids.

- Hands and other skin surfaces must be washed immediately if contaminated with blood or body fluids.
- All health care workers should take precautions to prevent injuries caused by needles, scalpels, and other sharp instruments. To prevent needle-stick injuries, needles should not be recapped, purposely bent or broken by hand, removed from disposable syringes, or otherwise manipulated by hand. All sharps are to be disposed of in puncture-resistant containers located as close as possible to the area of use.
- Mouthpieces, resuscitation bags, or other ventilation devices should be available for use in areas where the need for resuscitation is predictable. This minimizes the need for mouth-to-mouth resuscitation.

The body fluids to which Universal Precautions were originally applied included blood, semen, vaginal secretions, cerebrospinal fluid, synovial fluid, pleural fluid, peritoneal fluid, pericardial fluid, and amniotic fluid. Universal Precautions did not apply to feces, nasal secretions, sputum, sweat, tears, urine, and vomitus unless they contained visible blood (CDC, 1988). Standard Precautions have the same requirements as Universal Precautions, but have been expanded to include *all* body fluids. Standard Precautions protect both the health care worker and patient from cross-infection.

Under OSHA regulations, hospitals must implement Universal Precautions in the care of all patients. If a nurse is allergic to powder or latex, the health care facility must provide alternative products for the employee. OSHA also obliges all employers of health care workers to provide hepatitis B vaccine to employees frequently exposed to blood and other potentially infectious materials, to provide postexposure evaluation and medical follow-up, to train all employees in the use of Universal Precautions, and to maintain records of training and occupational exposure (U.S. Department of Labor, 1994).

ASEPTIC TECHNIQUES

The nurse uses aseptic technique as an infection control routine in all patient care activities. *Medical asepsis,* also known as clean technique, inhibits the transmission of infection in nonsterile situations. Hand washing between caring for different patients is the key to medical asepsis. Patient care activities requiring medical asepsis include monitoring blood pressure and temperature, changing linen, and serving food.

Surgical asepsis, known as sterile technique, requires an environment free of all microorganisms. Procedures requiring surgical asepsis include care of surgical wounds, insertion of intravascular catheters, insertion of urinary catheters, and performance of operative procedures.

Sterilization is the complete elimination of all microbial life, including bacterial spores. All equipment used for sterile procedures must be sterilized. Sterilization is performed using methods such as *autoclaving* (steam pressurization at 250°F) or exposure to ethylene oxide, a highly flammable, toxic gas. Some chemicals such as glutaraldehyde and peracetic acid can also be used to achieve sterilization.

Disinfection eliminates many or all pathogenic organisms, with the exception of bacterial spores. Liquid chemicals such as glutaraldehyde, alcohol, and hydrogen peroxide are used for disinfection.

The nurse must ensure that all equipment used in patient care has been appropriately sterilized or disinfected. Whether a medical device or other item should be sterilized or disinfected between patients is determined by the degree of infection risk. There are four categories of medical devices: critical instruments or devices, semicritical instruments or devices, noncritical instruments and devices, and environmental surfaces (Favero and Bond, 1991).

Critical instruments enter the blood stream or normally sterile body areas. Examples include surgical instruments, cardiac catheters, implants, needles, and transfer forceps. Biopsy forceps that penetrate mucosal barriers also fall into this category. A substantial risk of infection exists if instruments in this category are contaminated with any microorganism. Critical instruments should be sterile.

Semicritical instruments are those that come in contact with mucous membranes or nonintact skin. These include flexible fiberoptic endoscopes, endotracheal tubes, bronchoscopes, respiratory therapy equipment, anesthesia breathing circuits, ophthalmic devices, and vaginal specula. Semicritical devices must be meticulously cleaned manually and submitted to a high-level disinfection process that eradicates all microorganisms. High-level disinfection usually requires 20 minutes of soaking in a liquid chemical labeled as a high-level disinfectant.

Noncritical instruments have contact only with nonbroken skin, including blood pressure cuffs, face masks, most neurologic and cardiac diagnostic electrodes, and bedpans. Sterility for these items is not critical. However, these items should be disinfected between patients, using chemicals such as alcohol or iodophor preparations.

Environmental surfaces include medical equipment surfaces, such as adjustment knobs on dialysis machines, ventilators, x-ray machines, and intravenous (IV) pumps as well as nonmedical equipment such as floors, walls, tabletops, and curtains. Although items in this category do not usually come into direct contact with patients, hand contact with these surfaces may lead to cross-contamination between patients. Cleaning with a detergent or hospital-grade disinfectant detergent is adequate for environmental surfaces.

ASSESSMENT

The nurse must continuously monitor the patient for signs and symptoms of infection such as elevated temperature, hypotension, redness, and drainage. Table 17–1 lists common signs and symptoms suggesting infection. (See Chapter 28, Skin Integrity, for additional information regarding wound assessment.)

TABLE 17-1 Assessing for Signs and Symptoms of Infection

A diverse group of signs and symptoms may be suggestive of infection, depending on body site. Some of the major sites, with common signs and symptoms, are listed next.

Site	Observation
General	Elevated temperature Elevated white blood cell (WBC) count Chills, rigors Hypotension
Wound	Warmth, erythema Tenderness Purulent drainage
Pulmonary	Increased respirations Cough Purulent sputum
Gastrointestinal	Diarrhea Nausea, vomiting Epigastric or abdominal pain
Urinary	Frequency, urgency, burning A WBC count of 5 or less on urinalysis
Skin	Erythema, warmth, tenderness Draining skin lesions Pustules
Neurologic	Irritability Confusion Altered level of consciousness

INFECTION CONTROL IN VARIOUS HEALTH CARE SETTINGS

HOSPITALS

U.S. hospitals have no standard approach to isolation because of the various systems available. Each hospital evaluates its patient population and personnel to determine which system of isolation best suits its needs. Various approaches were used in the past. Some hospitals simply added Universal Precautions to its existing category- or disease-specific isolation policy. Some deleted blood and body fluid precautions; others incorporated Universal Precautions but maintained a blood and body fluids category. Others deleted all isolation categories and implemented BSI with a special category for airborne-transmitted diseases. Still others developed policies that combined BSI, Universal Precautions, and Centers for Disease Control (CDC) category- or disease-specific systems.

As hospitals implement the new CDC isolation system, infection control policies among institutions should become more consistent. However, each nurse beginning practice in a hospital must become familiar with that hospital's approach to isolation. The hospital's infection control manual will be a vital resource in answering questions regarding isolation needs of each patient.

LONG-TERM CARE FACILITIES

Appropriate infection control and prevention procedures must be in place and enforced in long-term facilities such as nursing homes and hospices. Hand washing, isolation, sterilization, and disinfection are the integral components of infection prevention in these settings.

A resident health program should also be established. This program should ensure tuberculin skin testing both on admission and annually for all residents, administration of appropriate vaccines, and nursing measures to prevent aspiration and skin breakdown.

HOME CARE SETTINGS

Many infections acquired by home care patients are related to devices used in the home. Home intravenous (IV) therapy has expanded rapidly in recent years; the home care nurse must use sterile technique in the insertion and care of all IV catheters. The nurse must also teach the patient's family members to perform dressing changes using surgical asepsis. All members of the home health team—nurse, patient, and family—must be alert for the early signs and symptoms of blood stream or catheter site infection (see Table 17–1).

Patients on mechanical ventilation may also be cared for at home. Again, the nurse must use aseptic technique in caring for tracheostomies, performing suctioning, and using respiratory care equipment.

As in other settings, hand washing is the most important infection control measure in the home setting. Home health nurses may need to carry a waterless antiseptic hand rinse for use when soap and water are not available.

The home health nurse's bag is considered a clean piece of equipment. Any contaminated equipment should be either cleaned in the home or placed in an impervious (i.e., plastic) bag for removal from the home. Hand washing and strict adherence to Standard Precautions in a patient's home are effective infection control measures for the home health nurse.

Procedures

Important nursing procedures to help prevent infection transmission include

- Hand washing
- Putting on sterile gloves, gown, and mask
- Properly applying wound dressings: sterile dressings, wet-to-dry dressings, pressure bandages, transparent dressings, and elastic bandages

HAND WASHING

The effectiveness of hand washing in removing transient microbes that may transmit infection is well supported by the scientific literature. Procedure 17–1 details the steps in proper hand-washing technique.

GLOVING

Gloves protect health care workers' hands from contamination with microorganisms in body fluids, nonintact skin, and mucous membranes. Procedures 17–2 and 17–3 present the proper technique for putting on sterile gloves.

GOWNING

Gowning protects health care workers' uniforms from contamination with organisms colonizing or infecting patients. Isolation gowns also prevent soiling clothing with moist body substances. The proper technique for putting on a sterile gown is detailed in Procedure 17–4.

MASKING

Masks protect health care workers from inhaling large-particle and small-particle aerosols suspended in the air. Masks may also prevent transmission of some infections spread by direct contact with mucous membranes, because masks discourage personnel from touching mucous membranes of their eyes, nose, and mouth until they have properly washed their hands and removed the mask. Procedure 17–5 outlines the steps involved in sterile masking technique.

DRESSING AND BANDAGE CHANGES

Sterile dressings are applied to protect a patient's wound from contamination with microorganisms and possible infection. Procedure 17–6 details the steps involved in properly applying a sterile dressing.

Wet-to-dry dressings are frequently indicated for infected or draining wounds to *debride* (remove foreign, dead, or damaged tissue) the wound. As the wet dressing dries, damaged tissue clings to the dressing and is removed when the dressing is changed. Debridement removes necrotic or damaged tissue. The physician will determine the type of solution to be used for the wet dressing. Procedure 17–7 lists the steps involved in changing a wet-to-dry dressing.

Transparent dressings are nonabsorbent dressings that are impermeable to microorganisms and water, yet allow oxygen to reach the wound beneath, facilitating healing. These dressings are commonly applied to ulcerated areas and burn wounds. Procedure 17–8 describes how to apply a transparent dressing.

Elastic bandages come in various widths, usually in rolls, for easy application to body parts. They are applied to provide support, exert pressure, and sometimes to hold a wound dressing in place. Procedure 17–9 details the steps involved in applying elastic bandages.

Pressure bandages, also known as antiembolic or elastic stockings, are applied to the lower extremities to promote venous return in patients with circulatory problems in the legs and feet. Procedure 20–3 in Chapter 20 outlines the steps in applying these bandages.

PROCEDURE 17-1

Hand Washing

Objective

To prevent or minimize the spread of microorganisms by hands

Terminology

- **Superficial contact:** patient contact in which there is little chance of coming into contact with contamination, such as handing medications to the patient, taking the blood pressure, setting up food tray
- **Intense contact:** patient contact in which there is a definite chance of contamination occurring to care provider's hands, such as tasks that cause prolonged contact with the patient's body and skin surface.

Critical Elements

The single most important means of prevention of transmission of microorganisms is hand washing. Although regular soap is often sufficient for hand washing, some areas of health care provide antimicrobial soaps for the use of the care provider. Hand lotion after washing can help decrease the chance of dry, cracked skin, which increases the risk of contamination to the care provider.

When turning off water control handles, use a dry paper towel because control handles are considered contaminated.

Hand washing is not always necessary after superficial patient contact but should always be performed after intense contact.

Equipment

- Soap
- Towels

Special Considerations

Nails should be kept short to reduce the area under which microorganisms might be found. Rings and watches should be removed before washing because they may prohibit thorough cleansing of the entire skin surface. Regular soap is sufficient for hand washing in most patient care areas; however, antimicrobial agents should be used in high-risk (invasive procedures) situations.

Nursing Interventions

Action	*Rationale*
1. Turn on water and adjust temperature (Fig. 17–5).	1. Promotes comfort during procedure

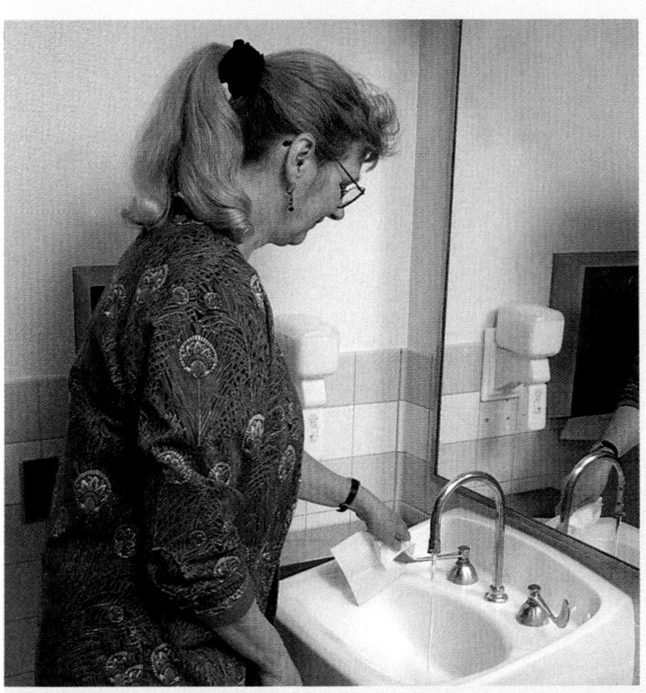

Figure 17–5. Adjust the water temperature to a comfortable level.

continued on next page

PROCEDURE 17-1 (cont'd)

2. Wet hands, and apply cleansing agent while keeping fingers pointed downward (Fig. 17–6).	2. Prevents water from running up arms to wrists and causing further contamination
3. Lather hands thoroughly, going up wrist areas, interlacing fingers, and rubbing around nail areas. Wash for 10–15 seconds (or per facility's policy) (Fig. 17–7).	3. Assists in the removal of microorganisms from the skin surface
4. Thoroughly rinse hands, allowing water to run from wrist downward off fingers.	4. Allows rinsing while keeping contaminated water from running up arms
5. Dry hands with disposable towel, and then use towel to grasp the water control handles to turn off water.	5. Keeps clean hands from contacting contaminated control handles
6. Dispose of towel in appropriate receptacle.	6. Maintains clean work area

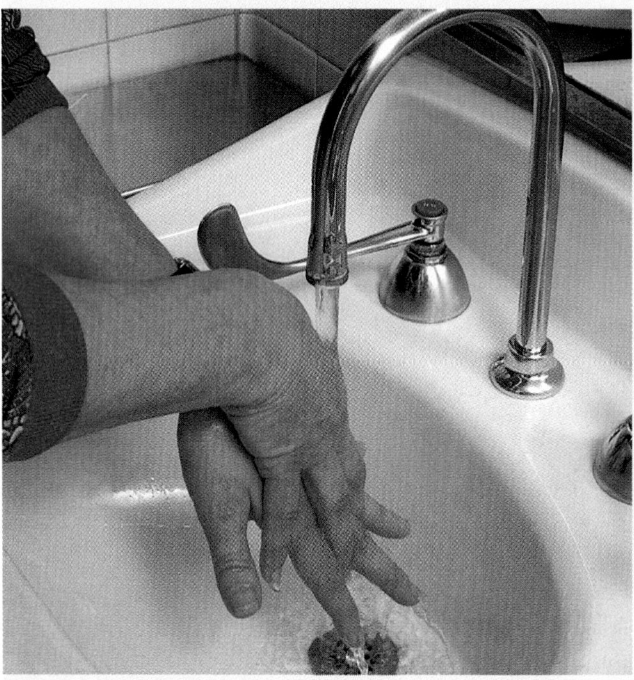

Figure 17–6. Keep fingers pointed downward when applying cleansing agent.

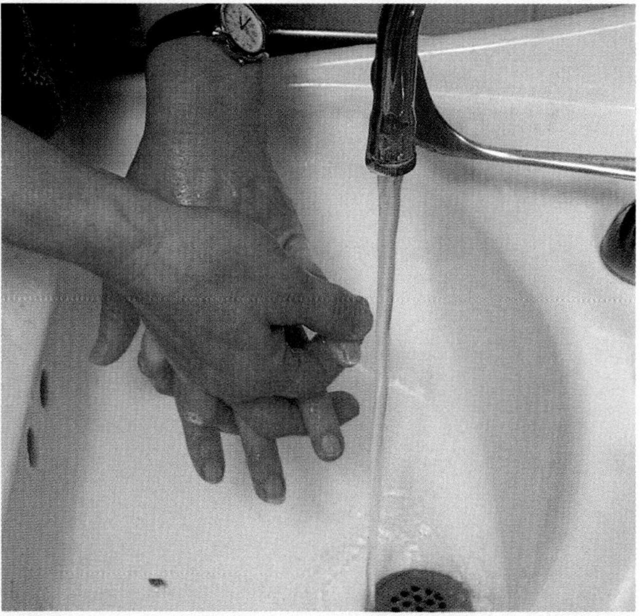

Figure 17–7. Wash extra carefully around the nails.

Documentation

Record in patient record any patient or family teaching done regarding hand washing.

Elements of Patient Teachings

Instruct patient and family on the importance of hand washing and demonstrate the appropriate hand-washing technique. Observe return demonstration after teaching.

PROCEDURE 17-2

Sterile Gloving Technique

Objective

Promotes asepsis for invasive procedures as well as providing protection for care provider

Terminology

- Asepsis: free from any form of germ/infection; sterile

Critical Elements

Wearing of gloves does not replace hand washing. Sterile gloves should be used when sterile technique is necessary for a procedure and should be used only once and discarded. When donning gloves, no part of the outside of either glove should be allowed to come into contact with any nonsterile surface.

Equipment

- Sterile gloves

Special Considerations

When sterile gloves are worn with a sterile gown, the gloves should be pulled up over the sleeve cuff of the gown. Always inspect gloves for any imperfections, because these can allow the passage of microorganisms. Latex allergies on the part of the patient care provider or patient should be noted. Nonlatex gloves must be worn under these conditions.

Nursing Interventions

Action	*Rationale*
Applying Gloves	
1. Wash and dry hands.	1. Reduced risk of transmission of organisms
2. Read manufacturer's instructions on package and open package per instruction.	2. Avoids contamination of gloves during opening procedure
3. Grasp first glove by cuff (folded edge) and insert hand into glove, pulling glove into place with folded cuff (Fig. 17–8).	3. Provides means to grasp glove while not touching outer sterile surface
4. Slip fingers of gloved hand under cuff (folded edge) of second glove, and pull glove over second hand (Fig. 17–9).	4. Provides means to apply second glove while maintaining sterility of first glove

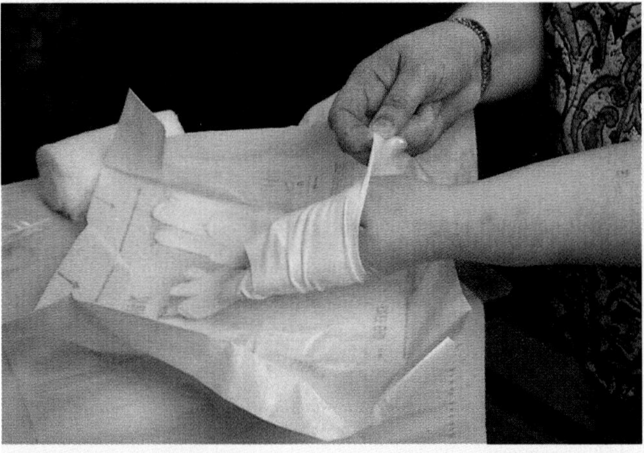

Figure 17–8. Grasp the glove by the cuff and insert other hand.

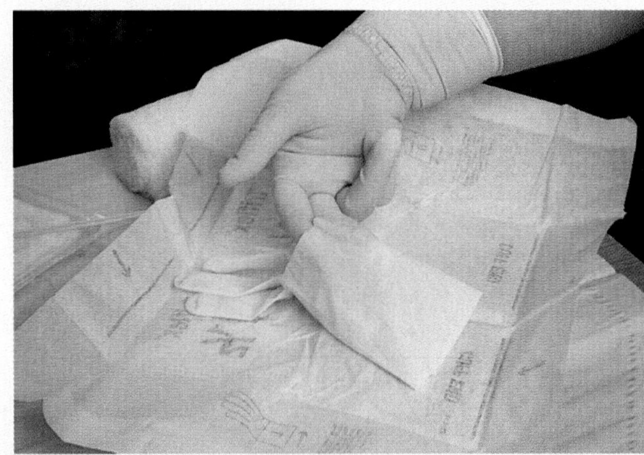

Figure 17–9. Slip gloved fingers under the cuff of the second glove.

Action	*Rationale*
Removing Gloves	
1. Remove first glove by grasping the outside surface of glove near top (but not at top edge) and pulling glove off. Hold removed glove in fingers of hand that remains gloved.	1. Provides means to remove first glove while preventing contamination of care provider with contaminated surface of gloves

continued on next page

PROCEDURE 17-2 (cont'd)

Action	Rationale
2. Slip fingers of hand that is now ungloved under the edge of remaining glove and pull glove off, enfolding glove that is being held in the fingers of hand inside glove being removed.	2. Protects care provider from contamination from surface of used gloves
3. Dispose of gloves in appropriate receptacle.	3. Maintains clean, organized work space
4. Wash hands.	4. Protects care provider and patient from potential contamination from organisms on hands

Documentation

Record procedure performed in patient record indicating sterile procedure was used.

Elements of Patient Teachings

Explain to patient and family the purpose of using sterile technique.

PROCEDURE 17-3

Gloving Technique for Isolation

Objective

Prevent cross-contamination from one patient to another. Provide personal protection for the care provider.

Terminology

- **Isolation technique:** special procedures used for patients with infectious processes to prevent transferring organisms

Critical Elements

Gloves must be worn for contact isolation or when the care provider may come into contact with blood or body fluids. Always inspect gloves for impaired integrity that may allow the entry of microorganisms.

Equipment

- Gloves

Special Considerations

Latex allergies on the part of the patient care provider or patient should be noted. Nonlatex gloves must be worn under these conditions.

Nursing Interventions

Action	*Rationale*
1. Wash hands.	1. Reduces risk of transmission of organisms from one patient to another
2. Remove gloves from dispenser and pull glove on up to wrist area; then repeat with second hand.	2. Provides coverage of hand and wrist area
3. Pull gloves over wrist cuff of isolation gown (Fig. 17–10).	3. Provides complete coverage of care provider's wrist/lower area
4. Change gloves after handling any body fluid or drainage.	4. Reduces risk of cross-contamination from one site to another
5. Remove gloves by grasping at the cuff and pulling glove off. Hold removed glove in hand that remains gloved (Fig. 17–11). Using ungloved hand, slip fingers under cuff of remaining glove, and pull glove off folding it over the first glove being held in gloved fingers.	5. Provides means for removing gloves without touching outer surface of gloves

continued on next page

PROCEDURE 17-3 (cont'd)

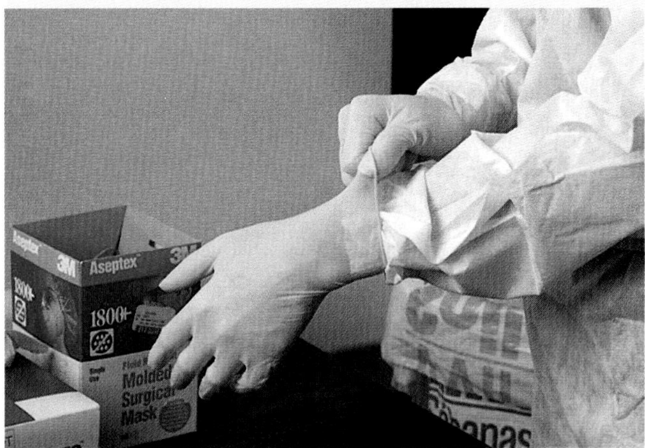

Figure 17–10. Putting on glove.

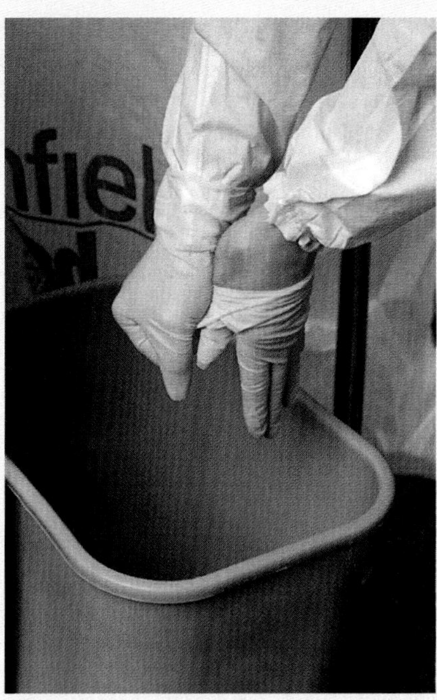

Figure 17–11. Disposing of glove.

6. Dispose of gloves in appropriate receptacle.
7. Wash hands.

6. Provides safe and clean workspace
7. Reduces risk of transmission of organisms from one patient to another

Documentation

Record in patient record the use of isolation technique.

Elements of Patient Teachings

Explain the purpose of gloving to the patient and family. Demonstrate to family and visitors how to apply and remove gloves before entering isolation. Allow family and visitors to provide a return demonstration of gloving technique.

PROCEDURE 17-4

Gowning

Objective

Provide a barrier of protection to minimize transfer of microorganisms to or from clothing

Terminology

- *Isolation technique:* special procedures used for patients with infectious processes to prevent transferring organisms

Critical Elements

A new gown is worn each time the patient care provider enters an isolation room. The gown is worn during direct contact with the patient or

continued on next page

PROCEDURE 17-4 (cont'd)

items contaminated with body secretions/fluids.

Equipment

- Gown (cloth or disposable)
- Trash/linen receptacle

Special Considerations

Long-sleeved uniforms should be rolled up from wrists before gowning.

Nursing Interventions

Action	*Rationale*
Applying Gown	
1. Wash hands.	1. Reduces risk of transmission of organisms from one patient to another
2. Select and open gown with opening facing away from you (Fig. 17–12).	2. Positions gown for application
3. Grasp inside of gown and slide arms into sleeves and cuffs (Fig. 17–13).	3. Facilitates application of gown
4. Fasten neck ties.	4. Secures upper portion of gown
5. Overlap edges of gown at waist and tie waist tie.	5. Secures gown and covers care clothing of care provider

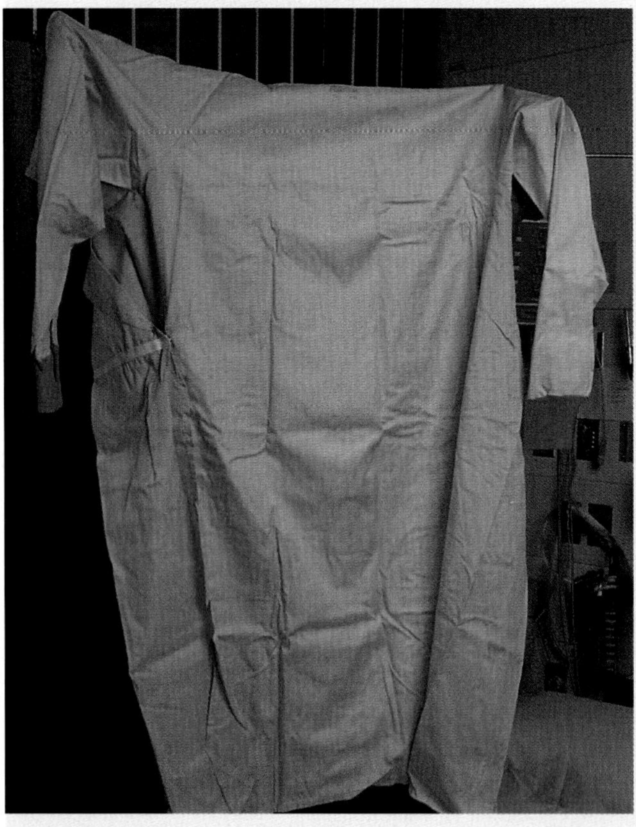

Figure 17–12. Isolation gown.

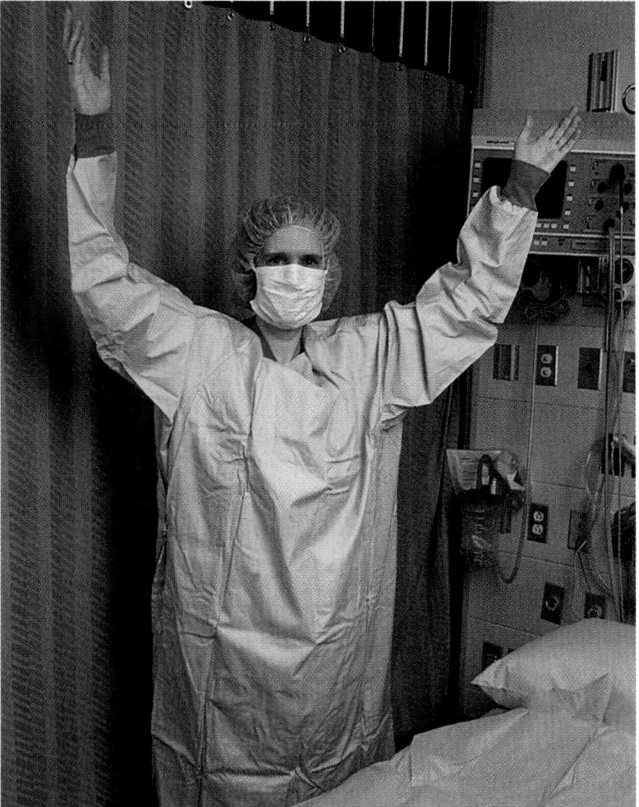

Figure 17–13. Putting on isolation gown.

continued on next page

PROCEDURE 17-4 (cont'd)

Removing Gown

1. Untie waist tie.
   1. Loosens gown in preparation for removal
2. Wash hands and then untie neck ties.
   2. Reduces risk of transmission of organisms to patient care provider from hands
3. Withdraw arms from sleeves and fold outer surface of gown away from you by grasping neck ties or inside of gown at shoulders (Fig. 17–14).
   3. Prevents contamination of care providers clothing with soiled outer surface of gown
4. Dispose of gown in appropriate receptacle.
   4. Provides clean work area
5. Wash hands.
   5. Protects care provider and patient from potential contamination from organisms on hands

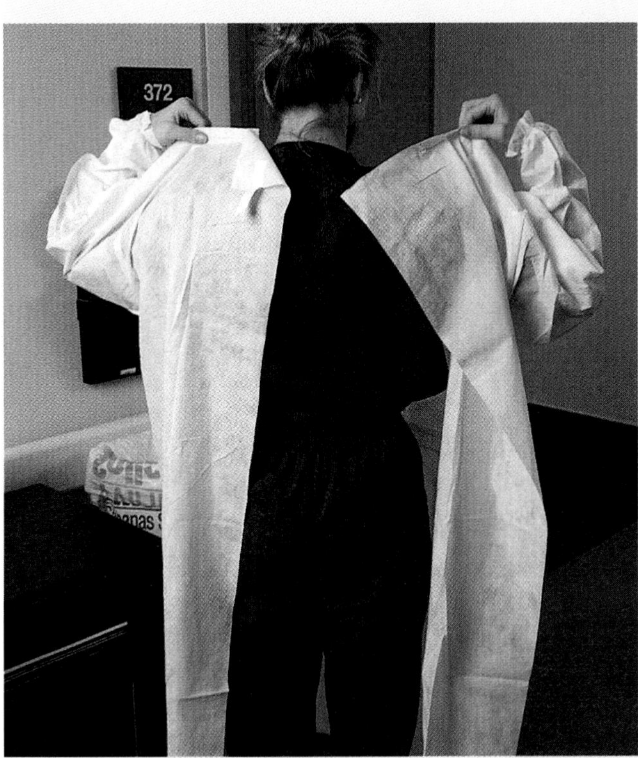

Figure 17–14. Removing gown.

Documentation

Record use of isolation technique in the patient record, including care given.

Elements of Patient Teachings

Explain to the patient and family the rationale for gowning. Instruct family and visitors in proper gowning technique. Observe family and visitors in a return demonstration of the procedure.

PROCEDURE 17-5

Masking

Objective

Prevent or reduce the transmission of microorganisms from care provider to patient or patient to care provider.

Terminology

- **Isolation technique:** special procedures used for patients with infectious processes to prevent transferring organisms

Critical Elements

Masking should be done before entering the patient's room and discarded before leaving the room. Masks should fit closely over the mouth and nose and should be worn only once and then discarded. They should not be lowered and draped around the neck. A mask should also be replaced if it becomes too moist because it may be ineffective (damp/wet materials allow the transmission of microorganisms).

Equipment

- Masks
- Trash receptacle

Special Considerations

Special respiratory masks may be needed when working with patients with tuberculosis, measles, and chickenpox. Refer to the infection control guidelines of your facility.

Nursing Interventions

Action	*Rationale*
Applying Mask	
1. Wash hands.	1. Reduces risk of transmission of organisms
2. Remove mask from container and place it so that it covers mouth and nose completely, tying strings over head or placing elastic straps behind ears (depending on the mask structure).	2. Promotes effectiveness of mask in preventing organisms from contacting oral or nasal mucosa or from allowing organisms to escape around the mask

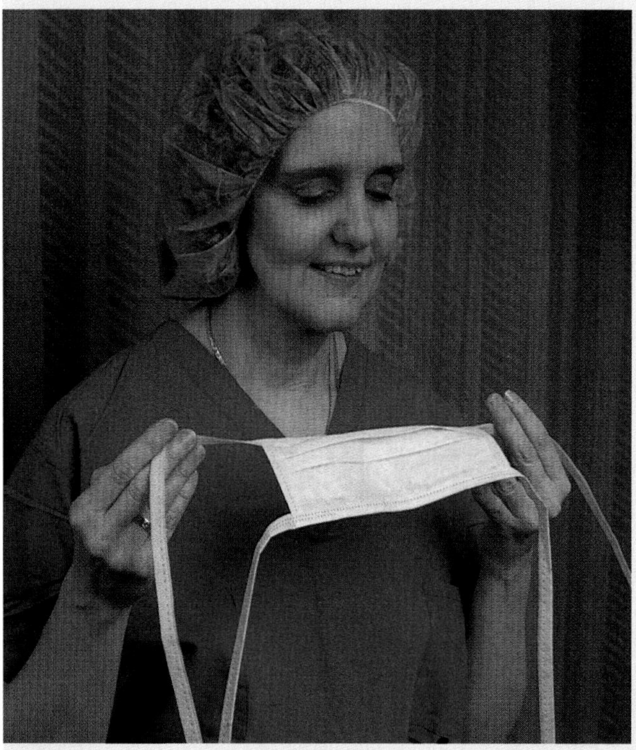

Figure 17–15. Removing face mask.

continued on next page

PROCEDURE 17-5 (cont'd)

Removing Mask

1. Wash hands.	1. Reduces risk of transmission of organisms from hands to facial area
2. Remove mask by untying strings or removing the elastic bands.	2. Prepares mask for removal
3. Remove mask by touching only strings/bands or inner surface (Fig. 17–15).	3. Reduces risk of contamination of hands with microorganisms from the outside of the mask
4. Dispose of mask in appropriate receptacle.	4. Provides safe workspace
5. Wash hands.	5. Protects care provider and patient from potential contamination from organisms on hands

Documentation

Record in patient record use of isolation technique in the care given the patient.

Elements of Patient Teachings

Instruct patient and family regarding the rationale for masking. Demonstrate and assist patient's family and visitors in the masking procedure. Observe family and visitors in a return demonstration of the masking procedure.

PROCEDURE 17-6

Changing a Sterile Dressing

Objective

Provide means to assess wound while providing a sterile cover for the wound, which helps promote healing and prevent infection.

Terminology

- **Clean gloves:** gloves that are free of pathogenic organisms
- **Sterile gloves:** gloves that are free of all living microorganisms
- **Montgomery straps:** tape straps that have cloth ties attached; the tape stays attached to the patient's skin at all times using the ties to secure and release the dressing.

Critical Elements

A physician order is required to change a dressing. The physician will often prefer to change the operative dressing for the first time and instruct nursing personnel to do subsequent dressing changes. Nurse should assess the old dressing for drainage (type and amount), redness or irritation of surrounding skin, edema, and the progression of healing. Any signs of infection should be reported to the physician. Before changing a dressing, the patient should be assessed for level of comfort and offered pain medication if indicated. The dressing change should then occur at least 20 minutes after the administration of medication. The supplies used should be based on the size, location, and amount of drainage.

Equipment

- Clean gloves
- Sterile gloves
- Sterile dressing supplies (as indicated)
- Antiseptic swabs (if ordered)
- Tape or Montgomery straps
- Waste receptacle (plastic bag may be used)

Special Considerations

Evaluate and change dressing according to the time frames indicated in the physician order. Respond promptly to any patient complaints regarding the wound. Reinforce a dressing if necessary. If there is enough drainage occurring that the dressing must be reinforced, the nurse should notify the physician of the amount of drainage. All surgical wounds should be carefully observed for the first 24 hours for signs of hemorrhage. If the dressing should adhere to the wound when it is being removed, a small amount of sterile saline (unless contraindicated) may help loosen the dressing and ease the removal of the old dressing.

continued on next page

PROCEDURE 17–6 (cont'd)

Nursing Interventions

Action	*Rationale*
1. Verify order.	1. Ensures correct procedure is done
2. Identify patient.	2. Promotes patient safety
3. Explain procedure.	3. Promotes patient compliance
4. Position and drape patient.	4. Provides patient comfort and privacy
5. Wash hands.	5. Prevents transmission of organisms from one patient to another
6. Open supplies using sterile technique.	6. Provides sterile organized workspace
7. Don clean gloves.	7. Protects care provider from contact with potential contamination while providing patient care
8. Loosen tape and remove dressing slowly while touching only outer surface of old dressing (Fig. 17–16).	8. Prevents accidental removal of drains, which can occur if dressing is removed quickly
9. Assess old dressing and then discard in appropriate receptacle.	9. Allows care provider to report and document the status of the old dressing before the disposal
10. Assess wound.	10. Allows care provider to report and document the status of the wound
11. Remove and discard gloves in appropriate receptacle.	11. Provides for proper disposal of contaminated materials.

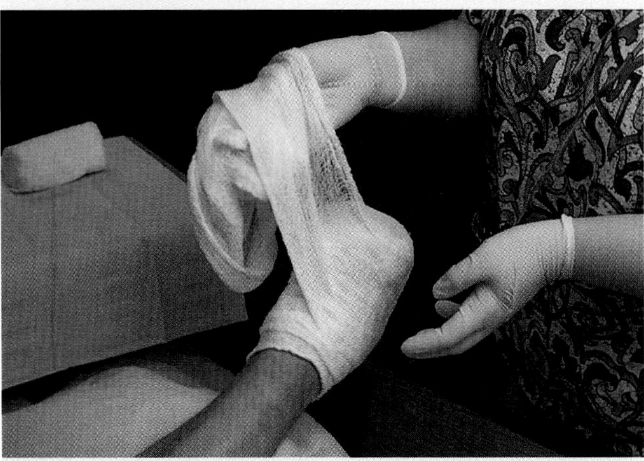

Figure 17–16. Removing dressing.

If Ordered by the Physician:

12. Cleanse the wound with antiseptic swabs.	12. Allows for physician preference in regards to use of antiseptic swabs
13. When swabbing the wound: *Incision*—Roll swab down incision line from proximal to distal, then do the same for 1 inch on either side of the incision. *Drain site*—Swab in circular motion starting immediately around the drain and progress outward in a circular manner.	13. Provides cleansing from the least to the more contaminated surfaces

continued on next page

PROCEDURE 17-6 (cont'd)

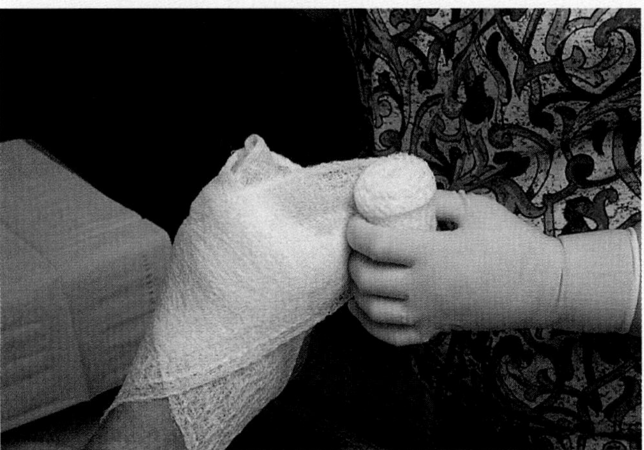

Figure 17–17. Applying dressing.

14. Don sterile gloves.	14. Allows use of aseptic technique with dressing change
15. Apply sterile dressing with aseptic technique; use split gauze around drains and put heavier pads over areas (Fig. 17–17) that may drain.	15. Protects wound and allows dressing to absorb drainage, thereby protecting surrounding skin
16. Remove and discard gloves in appropriate container.	16. Protects patient and care provider from contamination from used gloves
17. Secure dressing with tape or Montgomery straps.	17. Provides means to hold dressing in place
18. Cover patient and assist to position of comfort.	18. Promotes patient comfort
19. Discard or return equipment to appropriate place.	19. Provides clean, organized workspace
20. Wash hands.	20. Prevents transmission of organisms from one patient to another

Documentation

Record in the patient record the date and time of the dressing change as well as the appearance of the wound. Note and record in the patient record the presence of drainage, including the amount, color, consistency, and any odor. Record the patient's response to the procedure.

Elements of Patient Teachings

Explain procedure to the patient and family. Stress to the patient the importance of not moving or handling the dressing. Inform the patient of the need to notify the nurse immediately if there is an increase in drainage, odor, or pain associated with the area or the dressing. If necessary, instruct the patient and family in the dressing change procedure. Allow them to do a return demonstration.

PROCEDURE 17-7

Changing a Wet-to-Dry Dressing

Objective

Provide a means to protect the wound, promote healing, and debride the wound during dressing removal.

Terminology

- **Debridement:** removal of dead or diseased tissue or foreign material from a wound area
- **Wet-to-dry dressing:** wound cover that is applied wet and remains in place until dry to promote wound debridement when removed
- **Clean gloves:** gloves that are free of pathogenic organisms
- **Sterile gloves:** gloves that are free of all living microorganisms
- **Montgomery straps:** tape straps that have cloth ties attached; the tape stays attached to the patient's skin at all times, using the ties to secure and release the dressing.

Critical Elements

A physician order is required to change a dressing. When removing the old dressing, the wound should be assessed for drainage (type and amount), redness or irritation of surrounding skin, edema, and the progression of healing. Any signs of infection should be reported to the physician. Before changing a dressing, the patient should be assessed for level of comfort and offered pain medication if indicated. The removal of a wet-to-dry dressing can be uncomfortable for the patient; therefore, the dressing change should occur at least 20 minutes after the administration of pain medication. The supplies used should be based on the size, location, and amount of drainage.

Equipment

- Sterile dressing supplies (as indicated)
- Solution (per physician order)
- Clean gloves
- Sterile gloves
- Antiseptic swabs (as indicated)
- Sterile basin for solution
- Tape or Montgomery straps
- Sterile Q-tip or hemostat (if indicated)
- Waste receptacle (plastic bag may be used)

Special Considerations

Evaluate and change dressing according to time frames indicated in physician order. Respond promptly to any patient complaints regarding the wound. When applying the new dressing, the gauze should be only damp, allowing for drying before the next dressing change. This allows the dressing to adhere to the wound and debridement to occur during the removal process. If moistened gauze is being packed into a wound, care should be taken to place the gauze gently into the wound. Forceful packing may cause damage to the wound site.

Nursing Interventions

Action	*Rationale*
1. Verify order.	1. Ensures correct procedure is done
2. Identify patient.	2. Provides patient safety
3. Explain procedure.	3. Promotes patient compliance
4. Position patient and drape so that dressing area is exposed.	4. Provides patient comfort and as much patient privacy as possible during procedure
5. Wash hands.	5. Prevents transmission of organisms from one patient to another
6. Open supplies using aseptic technique and pour prescribed solution into sterile bowls.	6. Provides a sterile, organized work area
7. Don clean gloves.	7. Protects care provider from possible contamination from soiled dressing
8. Remove old dressing slowly and discard in appropriate receptacle.	8. Provides wound debridement during the removal process
9. Assess wound.	9. Provides means to gauge wound healing
10. Don sterile gloves.	10. Allows for use of aseptic technique during dressing change

continued on next page

PROCEDURE 17-7 (cont'd)

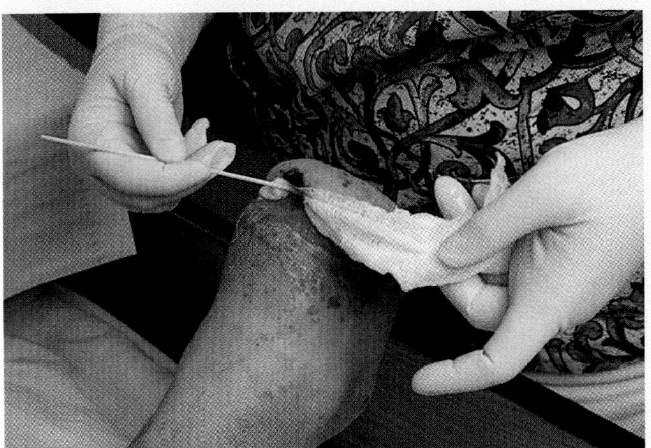

Figure 17–18. Cleansing wound with aseptic swab and gauze.

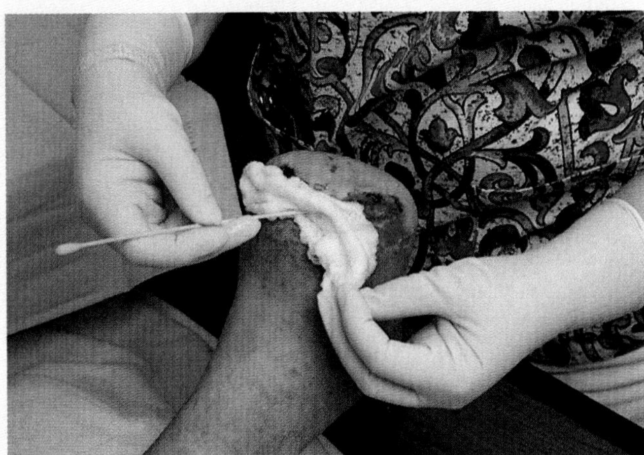

Figure 17–19. Packing wound with moistened gauze.

If Ordered by the Physician

11. Cleanse the wound with antiseptic swabs or gauze dampened with solution (Fig. 17–18).

11. Allows for physician preference in regard to use of antiseptic swabs or dampened gauze

12. When swabbing the wound:
Incision—Roll swab or dampened gauze down incision line from proximal to distal; then do the same for 1 inch on either side of the incision.
Drain site—Swab or wipe with dampened gauze in circular motion, starting immediately around the drain and progressing outward in a circular manner.

12. Provides cleansing from the least to the more contaminated surfaces.

13. Using gauze moistened with the prescribed solution, pack the wound as ordered (wring out gauze so it is only moist, not wet). (Fig. 17–19). Note: It may be necessary to use a sterile Q-tip or hemostat to pack deep wounds.

13. Provides moist gauze, which will dry before the next dressing change and adhere to the wound surface

14. Cover wound with sterile dressing.

14. Provides protection for wound site

15. Remove gloves and dispose in appropriate container.

15. Protects patient and care provider from contamination from used gloves

16. Secure dressing with tape or Montgomery straps.

16. Provides protection for the wound, keeping dampened gauze in place

17. Discard or return supplies to appropriate place.

17. Provides a clean and organized workplace

18. Wash hands.

18. Prevents transmission of organisms from one patient to another

Documentation

Record in the patient record the date and time of the dressing change as well as the appearance of the wound. Note and record in the patient record the presence of drainage, including the amount, color, consistency, and any odor. Record the patient's response to the procedure.

Elements of Patient Teachings

Explain procedure to the patient and family. Stress to the patient the importance of not moving or handling the dressing. Inform the patient of the need to notify the nurse immediately if there is an increase in drainage, odor, or pain associated with the area or the dressing. If necessary, instruct the patient and/or family in how to do the dressing change procedure. Allow them to do a return demonstration.

PROCEDURE 17-8

Applying Transparent Dressings

Objective

Provide occlusive protection while still allowing visualization of site.

Terminology

- **Asepsis:** protection against infection during a procedure by the use of sterile dressings and equipment

Critical Elements

Transparent dressings allow visualization of the site; however, they do not provide for absorption of drainage. Therefore, transparent dressings should be used on nondraining sites such as intravenous sites and small skin tears.

Equipment

- Transparent dressing
- Gloves

Special Considerations

Transparent dressings may be used to hold other dressing materials in place over wound breakdown sites.

Nursing Interventions

Action	*Rationale*
1. Assemble supplies.	1. Promotes successful task completion
2. Identify patient.	2. Provides patient safety
3. Explain procedure.	3. Promotes patient compliance
4. Expose site and inspect area.	4. Allows nurse to access site for procedure and to determine condition of site
5. Open dressing materials.	5. Promotes task organization
6. Don gloves.	6. Protects nurse from organism transmission
7. Remove protective covering from back of transparent dressing.	7. Facilitates application of dressing
8. Apply transparent dressing using aseptic technique and making sure all edges are secure.	8. Provides means for dressing to remain in place without edges peeling
9. Assist patient to position of comfort.	9. Promotes patient comfort
10. Discard and/or return equipment to appropriate area.	10. Provides clean and organized work environment

Documentation

Record in patient record date and time of application as well as location of transparent dressing. Be sure to note site location, size, appearance of site, and patient's response to procedure.

Elements of Patient Teachings

Explain the purpose of the procedure to the patient/family. Instruct the patient/family to notify the nurse if any problems or changes occur at the dressing site.

PROCEDURE 17-9

Applying Elastic Bandages

Objective

Provide immobilization and support, minimize swelling, and prevent venous stasis.

Terminology

- **Spiral wrap:** wrapping in a circular pattern around a limb
- **Figure-eight wrap:** wrapping using a crossover pattern, which looks like the figure 8

Critical Elements

When wrapping with an elastic bandage, start at the most distal part of the limb, wrapping distal to proximal. Application should be firm, not tight, because having a bandage that is too tight may compromise circulation. A baseline neurovascular assessment should be done before application. After application, the nurse should perform neurovascular assessments per facility policy during the time the wrap is in place.

Equipment

- Elastic bandages
- Fasteners and/or tape

Special Considerations

When wrapping a long cylindrical body part, a spiral wrap is usually used. When wrapping a joint the figure-eight wrap is preferable. Wrapping should be done so wraps are equidistant apart so that even pressure is applied. The size of the wrap used should be appropriate for the size of the patient and the body part to be wrapped. The bandage should be unrolled with the wrap coming off the bottom of roll.

Nursing Interventions

Action	*Rationale*
1. Verify order.	1. Ensures that correct procedure is done
2. Assemble equipment.	2. Promotes successful task completion
3. Identify patient.	3. Provides patient safety
4. Explain procedure.	4. Promotes patient compliance
For Spiral Wrap	
5. Wrap limb starting at distal end, wrapping around one time before proceeding up the limb.	5. Provides a firm anchor for bandage
6. Use spiral turns as wrap proceeds up limb overlaying previous wrap by one-half width of wrap.	6. Provides an even distribution of pressure

continued on next page

PROCEDURE 17-9 (cont'd)

For Figure-Eight Wrap

7. Wrap one time around body part distal to joint (Fig. 17–20).	7. Provides a firm anchor for bandage
8. Proceed with figure-eight wrap by going above joint and returning for one additional wrap below joint (Fig. 17–21).	8. Provides support for joint area

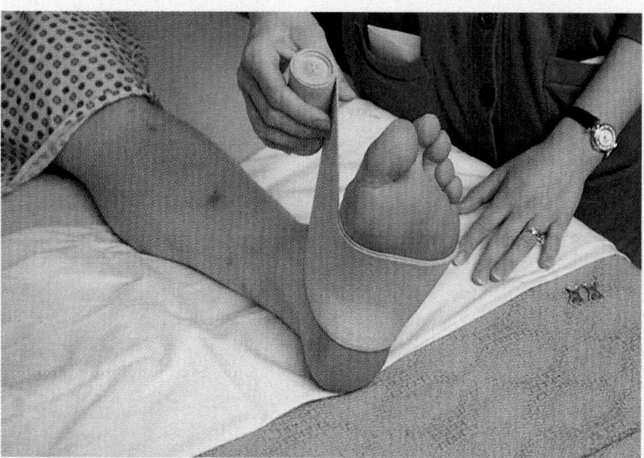

Figure 17–20. Applying Ace bandage.

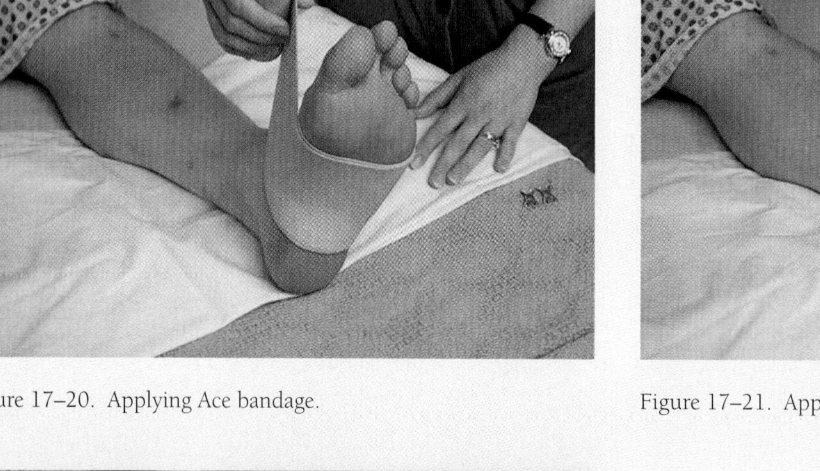

Figure 17–21. Applying Ace bandage.

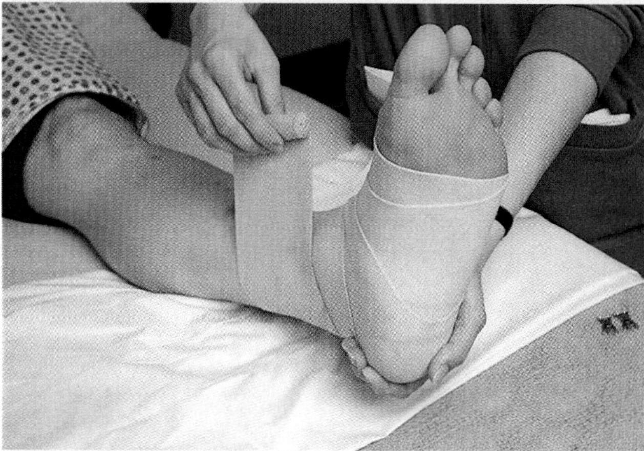

Figure 17–22. Applying Ace bandage.

9. Continue wrapping up limb as indicated (Fig. 17–22).	9. Provides even pressure along length of limb
10. Place fasteners and/or tape at end of wrap.	10. Anchors bandage so it will not come unwrapped
11. Remove elastic bandage for skin and neurovascular assessment per policy.	11. Provides opportunity for skin care and assessment

continued on next page

PROCEDURE 17-9 (cont'd)

Documentation

Record date, time, and location of elastic bandage application in patient record. Assess and record neurovascular status of limb before application of elastic bandage and after ongoing neurovascular checks. Note presence of edema or any break in skin integrity.

Elements of Patient Teachings

Explain purpose of elastic wrap to patient/family. Instruct patient/family to report immediately an increase of pain in limb as well as presence of any numbness, tingling, cyanosis, swelling, change of sensation, and temperature change.

CHAPTER HIGHLIGHTS

- Infection is the entry and multiplication of an infectious agent into the host with subsequent tissue damage.
- Infections cause signs and symptoms such as fever, purulent drainage, inflammation, productive cough, diarrhea, and myalgias.
- Nosocomial infections are a major cause of morbidity and mortality in hospitalized patients.
- Transmission and occurrences of infections are reduced by aseptic technique.
- Epidemiology is the study of the occurrence, distribution, risk factors, and control of disease in a defined population. Microbiology is the study of microbes, which include bacteria, fungi, protozoa, viruses, and in some cases algae and worms.
- The chain of infection is composed of six links: causative agent, reservoir, portal of exit, mode of transmission, portal of entry, and susceptible host. Preventing the transmission of infection involves interrupting one or more of the components in the chain of infection.
- Sanitation, proper disinfection, and sterilization techniques greatly reduce the transfer of microorganisms. Proper waste management is essential to control the spread of infection in the hospital environment.
- Hand washing has been universally accepted as an important factor in reducing the transmission of infection.
- The lack of compliance in using hand-washing techniques increases the incidence of infections in health care agencies.
- Research reports substantiate that barriers such as gowns, gloves, masks, and goggles are effective in interrupting transmission of specific infectious diseases.
- Consideration in providing nursing care is given to the age, educational level, culture, and ethnicity of the patient with an infectious disease.
- Nursing care of patients with infectious diseases is based on sound scientific principles.
- Patient and family teaching is an essential part of caring for patients with infectious diseases regardless of where the patient is housed (hospital, long-term care facility, clinic, or home).

REFERENCES

Agah, R., et al. (1987). Respiratory syncytial virus (RSV) infection rate in personnel caring for children with RSV infection. *American Journal of Diseases in Children, 141,* 695–697.

Beers, L.M., et al. (1989). Shigellosis occurring in newborn nursery staff. *Infection Control and Hospital Epidemiology, 10,* 147–149.

Black, R.E., et al. (1981). Handwashing to prevent diarrhea in day-care centers. *American Journal of Epidemiology, 113,* 445–451.

Butz, A.M., et al. (1990). Occurrence of infectious symptoms in children in day care homes. *American Journal of Infection Control, 18,* 347–353.

Centers for Disease Control (1970). *Isolation Techniques for Use in Hospitals* (DHEW publication no. [PHS] 70-2054). Washington, DC: U.S. Government Printing Office.

Centers for Disease Control (1987). Recommendations for prevention of HIV transmission in health care settings. *Morbidity and Mortality Weekly Report, 36*(2S, Suppl), 1S–16S.

Centers for Disease Control (1988). Update: universal precautions for prevention of transmission of human immunodeficiency virus, hepatitis B virus, and other bloodborne pathogens in health care settings. *Morbidity and Mortality Weekly Report, 37,* 377–388.

Centers for Disease Control (1990). Guidelines for preventing the transmission of tuberculosis in health care settings, with special focus on HIV-related issues. *Morbidity and Mortality Weekly Report, 39,* (RR-17) 1–29.

Centers for Disease Control and Prevention (1994). Guidelines for preventing the transmission of Mycobacterium tuberculosis in health care facilities. *Morbidity and Mortality Weekly Report, 43,* (RR-13) 1–132.

Crow, S. (1989). Asepsis, The Right Touch. Something Old Is Now New. Bossier City, LA: The Everett Companies.

De Carvalho, M., et al. (1989). Frequency and duration of hand-washing in a neonatal intensive care unit. *Pediatric Infectious Disease Journal, 8,* 179–180.

Dixon, R.E. (1991). Historical perspective: the landmark conference in 1980. *American Journal of Medicine, 91*(3B), 65–75.

Doebbeling, B.N., et al. (1988). Removal of nosocomial pathogens from the contaminated glove. *Annals of Internal Medicine, 109,* 394–398.

Doebbeling, B.N., et al. (1992). Comparative efficacy of alternative hand-washing agents in reducing nosocomial infections in intensive care units. *New England Journal of Medicine, 327,* 88–93.

Dubbert, P.M. (1990). Increasing ICU staff handwashing: effects of education and group feedback. *Infection Control and Hospital Epidemiology, 11,* 191–193.

Favero, M.S., Bond, W.W. (1991). Chemical disinfection of medical and surgical materials. In S.S. Block (ed.): *Disinfection, Sterilization and Preservation,* 4th ed. Philadelphia: Lea & Feibeger.

Gala, C.L., et al. (1986). The use of eye-nose goggles to control nosocomial respiratory syncytial virus infection. *Journal of the American Medical Association, 256,* 2706–2708.

Garner, J.S. (1996). Guideline for isolation precautions in hospitals. *American Journal of Infection, 7,* 53–80.

Garner, J.S., Favero, M.S. (1985). *Guideline for Handwashing and Hospital Environmental Control.* Atlanta: Centers for Disease Control.

Garner, J.S., Simmons, B.P. (1983). Guideline for isolation precautions in hospitals. *Infection Control, 4,* 245–325.

Goldman, D.A. (1991). The role of barrier precautions in infection control. *Journal of Hospital Infection, 18*(Suppl A), 515–523.

Griffiths, D. (1988). Outbreak of methicillin-resistant *Staphylococcus aureus* on a surgical service. *American Journal of Infection Control, 16,* 123–126.

Guiguet, M., et al. (1990). Effectiveness of simple measures to control an outbreak of nosocomial methicillin-resistant *Staphylococcus aureus* infections in an intensive care unit. *Infection Control and Hospital Epidemiology, 11,* 23–26.

Haley, R.W. (1986). *Managing Hospital Infection Control for Cost Effectiveness.* Chicago: American Hospital Publishing.

Haley, R.W., et al. (1985). The nationwide nosocomial infection rate: a new need for vital statistics. *American Journal of Epidemiology, 121,* 159–167.

Hall, C.B., Douglas, R.G. (1981). Nosocomial respiratory syncytial viral infections. *American Journal of Diseases in Children, 135,* 512–515.

Hoffman, P.N., et al. (1985). Micro-organisms isolated from skin under wedding rings worn by hospital staff. *British Medical Journal, 290,* 206–207.

Isaacs, D., et al. (1991). Handwashing and cohorting in prevention of hospital acquired infections with respiratory syncytial virus. *Archives of Disease in Childhood, 66,* 227–231.

Jackson, M.M., Lynch, P. (1985). Isolation practices: a historical perspective. *American Journal of Infection Control, 13,* 21–31.

Jacobsen, G., et al. (1985). Handwashing, ringwearing, and number of microorganisms. *Nursing Research, 34,* 186–188.

Joint Commission on Accreditation of Health Care Organizations (1998). *Accreditation Manual for Hospitals.* Chicago: Joint Commission on Accreditation of Healthcare Organizations.

Klein, B.S., et al. (1989). Reduction of nosocomial infection during pediatric intensive care by protective isolation. *New England Journal of Medicine, 320,* 1714–1721.

LaForce, M.F. (1987). Control of infections in hospitals, 1750 to 1950. In R.P. Wenzel (ed.): *Prevention and Control of Nosocomial Infections.* Baltimore: Williams & Wilkins.

Larson, E. (1988a). A causal link between handwashing and risk of infection: examination of the evidence. *Infection Control and Hospital Epidemiology, 9,* 28–36.

Larson, E. (1988b). APIC guideline for use of topical antimicrobial agents. *American Journal Infection Control, 16,* 253–266.

Larson, E. (1983a). Compliance with isolation technique. *American Journal of Infection Control, 11,* 221–225.

Larson, E. (1983b). Influence of a role model of handwashing behavior (abstract). *American Journal of Infection Control, 11,* 146.

Larson, E. (1995). APIC guideline for handwashing and hand antisepsis in health care settings. *American Journal of Infection Control, 23,* 251–269.

Leclair, J.M., et al. (1987). Prevention of nosocomial respiratory syncytial virus infections through compliance with gown and glove isolation precautions. *New England Journal of Medicine, 317,* 329–334.

Lynch, P., et al. (1987). Rethinking the role of isolation practices in the prevention of nosocomial infections. *Annals of Internal Medicine, 107,* 243–246.

Lynch, P., et al. (1990). Implementing and evaluating a system of generic infection precautions: body substance isolation. *American Journal of Infection Control, 18,* 1–12.

Maki, D.G., Hecht, J. (1982). Antiseptic-containing handwashing agents reduce nosocomial infection—a prospective study. In *Proceedings of the Twenty-Second Interscience Conference on Antimicrobial Agents and Chemotherapy,* Miami Beach.

Martone, W.J. (1991). Year 2000 objectives for preventing nosocomial infections: how do we get there? *American Journal of Medicine, 91*(Suppl 3B), 39S-43S.

Massanari, R.M., Hierholzer, W.J. (1984). A crossover comparison of antiseptic soaps on nosocomial infection rates in intensive care units. *American Journal of Infection Control, 12,* 247–248.

McGinley, K.J., et al. (1988). Composition and density of microflora in the subungual space of the hand. *Journal of Clinical Microbiology, 26,* 950–953.

McLane, C., et al. (1983). A nursing practice problem: failure to observe aseptic technique. *American Journal of Infection Control, 11,* 178–182.

Mortimer, E.A., et al. (1962). Transmission of staphylococci between newborns. *American Journal of Diseases in Children, 104,* 289–295.

Murphy, D., et al. (1981). The use of gowns and masks to control respiratory illness in pediatric hospital personnel. *Journal of Pediatrics, 99,* 746–750.

Pettinger, A., Nettleman, M.D. (1991). Epidemiology of isolation precautions. *Infection Control and Hospital Epidemiology, 12,* 303–307.

Pottinger, J., et al. (1989). Bacterial carriage by artificial versus natural nails. *American Journal of Infection Control, 17,* 340–344.

Rammelkamp, C.H., et al. (1964). Treatment of streptococcal and staphylococcal infections. *Annals of Internal Medicine, 60,* 753–758.

Rutala, W.A. (1990). APIC guidelines for selection and use of disinfectants. *American Journal of Infection Control, 58,* 99–117.

Semmelweiss, I.P. (1981). The Etiology of the Concept and the Prophylaxis of Childbed Fever (F.P. Murphy, trans.). Birmingham, AL: Classics of Medicine Library. (Original work published 1861)

Simmons, B., et al. (1990). The role of handwashing in prevention of endemic intensive care unit infections. *Infection Control and Hospital Epidemiology, 11,* 589–594.

Snydman, D.R., et al. (1988). Prevention of nosocomial transmission of respiratory syncytial virus in newborn nursery. *Infection Control and Hospital Epidemiology, 9*(3), 105–108.

Wenzel, R.P., Pfaller, M.A. (1991). Handwashing efficacy versus acceptance. A brief essay. *Journal of Hospital Infection, 18*(Suppl B), 65–68.

Wolinsky, E., et al. (1960). Acquisition of staphylococci by newborns: direct versus indirect transmission. *Lancet, 2,* 620– 622.

U.S. Department of Labor (1994). Occupational exposure to bloodborne pathogens. *Federal Register, 58,* 56(235): 64175–64182.

Personal Safety in Nursing Practice

Bonnie Rogers, Marguerite Jackson, Thérése Rymer, and Lisa Pompeii

Janice Johnson has been a registered nurse for 10 years. She has a bachelor of science degree in nursing and is enrolled in a master's degree program in critical care nursing. She has had experience in a variety of different services in hospitals and in home care nursing. She has taken short-term courses in caring for acquired immunodeficiency syndrome (AIDS) patients and in infection control. Miss Johnson is well aware of the precautions needed to protect herself and others from cross-contamination with body fluids such as blood, mucus, and saliva.

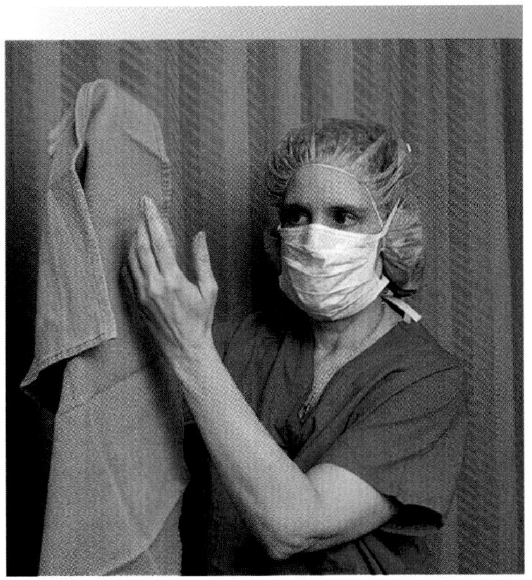

Miss Johnson was caring for James Duffy, a patient in the intensive care unit who had a positive diagnosis for the human immunodeficiency virus (HIV). Mr. Duffy had been in a car accident and was in critical condition. Intravenous fluids were ordered. The fluids being administered through a needle inserted in the patient's arm had infiltrated into the tissue. Miss Johnson was in the process of removing the needle from Mr. Duffy's arm when he raised his arm, causing the needle to puncture the skin on Miss Johnson's left arm. The needle penetrated deeply into her arm tissue. Miss Johnson was immediately aware that she was at risk of being infected with HIV.

Many questions arose in Miss Johnson's mind: Did she take all of the precautions she should have? How could she have prevented such an incident? What should she now do to care for herself? In her 10 years in the nursing profession, she had never had any type of injury.

OBJECTIVES

After studying this chapter, students will be able to:

- **describe the five major categories of health and safety hazards faced by nurses and other health care workers in the hospital setting**
- **identify specific occupational health risks associated with the various hazard categories**
- **discuss preventive strategies to reduce or mitigate occupational risks to health care workers**
- **distinguish between the various types of prevention and control strategies (engineering controls, administrative controls, work practice controls, and personal protective equipment) and give two examples of each**

SCOPE OF NURSING PRACTICE

By the year 2000, nearly 11 million workers will be employed in health services in the United States (U.S. Department of Labor, 1991). Hospitals are the largest employers of health care workers (nearly 50 percent); registered nurses, practical nurses, orderlies, and nursing assistants compose 40 percent of the total hospital work force (U.S. Department of Health and Human Services [DHHS], 1987a). Other large employers include nursing facilities, research centers, home health care agencies, medical and dental offices, schools, and emergency response units.

Nurses are committed to providing the best possible care for their patients. At the same time, they must look out for themselves in what is undoubtedly a high-risk work environment, be it a hospital, nursing home, community health clinic, or prison. The federal government reports that the incidence of nonfatal occupational injuries and illnesses among health care workers in 1993 was 11.8 per 100 full-time workers in hospitals and 17.3 per 100 full-time workers in nursing and personal care facilities. This compares with a private industry rate of 8.5 per 100 workers (U.S. Department of Labor [DOL], 1994).

Chapter 17, Sterile Technique and Infection Control, discussed the practices and procedures nurses use to protect their patients from infection. In this chapter, the focus shifts to how nurses, with their institution's help, can protect themselves and their coworkers from potential exposure to workplace hazards such as infectious diseases, toxic substances, and radiation; accidental injuries, fatigue, shift work, stress; and sometimes violent patients. Risks do not need to be accepted or tolerated; nurses must always be aware of hazards on the job and insist on safe working conditions. Using the preventive strategies discussed in this chapter, nurses and other health care workers can maintain a safer, more healthful work environment for everyone.

BOX 18–1
OCCUPATIONAL HAZARDS IN THE NURSING ENVIRONMENT

Safety and health hazards are grouped into five major categories.

1. Biologic hazards: infectious pathogens such as bacteria, viruses, fungi, and parasites, which may be transmitted via contact with infected patients or contaminated body secretions or fluids
2. Chemical hazards: various forms of chemicals that are potentially irritating to body systems, including medications, solutions, and gases
3. Environmental and mechanical hazards: factors encountered in work environments, such as poor equipment, slippery floors, or violent patients, that cause or potentiate accidents, injuries, strain, or discomfort
4. Physical hazards: agents within work environments, such as radiation, electricity, extreme temperatures, and noise, that can cause tissue trauma
5. Psychosocial hazards: factors and situations encountered or associated with the job or work environment that create or potentiate stress, such as emotional strain and substance abuse.

KNOWLEDGE BASE

Occupational health hazards are classified as biologic, chemical, environmental/mechanical, physical, and psychosocial agents (Box 18–1). Recent research in these five areas reveals the true dimensions of the health and safety problems encountered by health care workers and also points the way for corrective actions.

Basic Science

BIOLOGIC HAZARDS

Health care workers are routinely exposed to biologic agents such as bacteria, viruses, fungi, and parasites such as lice and mites. Important viral agents include human immunodeficiency virus (HIV); hepatitis A, B, C, and D; rubeola (measles); rubella (German measles); varicella (chickenpox and shingles); herpes simplex; cytomegalovirus; and influenza A and B. Important bacterial agents include *Mycobacterium tuberculosis* (TB); *Salmonella* and *Shigella,* which cause acute diarrhea; and *Staphylococcus aureus,* which causes abscesses and infections. An arthropod parasite, the scabies mite (*Sarcoptes scabiei*) is important because it causes a skin disease that is easily transmitted from patients to health care workers and from health care workers to patients. All of these biologic hazards are summarized in Table 18–1.

Biologic agents become health hazards (cause disease) only if a precise set of conditions exist to favor their growth and spread. This set of conditions is called the *chain of infection* (Jackson and Checko, 1983) and is summarized in Box 18–2. Following your institution's infection control procedures is the best way to keep this class of hazards under control. See later discussion for occupational health aspects, and consult Chapter 17, Sterile Technique and Infection Control, for more information.

CHEMICAL HAZARDS

Many chemicals are used in health care facilities to *disinfect* or *sterilize* work surfaces, medical instruments and equipment, and articles of clothing. Disinfectants kill only disease-causing organisms; chemical sterilants kill all types of organisms, and are typically more toxic than disinfectants. Both types of chemicals are useful for preparing equipment that would be damaged by the high heat required for sterilization by steam (autoclaving) or ovens.

Because they must be strong enough to destroy viruses, bacteria, and other disease organisms, these chemicals are

TABLE 18–1 Common Biologic Hazards

Biologic Hazard	Exposure Factors	Remarks
Viruses		
Human immunodeficiency virus (HIV)	Primarily needlestick injuries at initial use and subsequent disposal; splattering with blood and body secretions; breaks in skin; failure to use universal infection precautions (see Chapter 17) significantly increases risk of exposure	Destroys body's immune defenses, opening the way to many opportunistic infections; there is no cure
Hepatitis A virus (HAV) (infectious hepatitis)	Poor hygiene/hand washing; contamination of food and water; handling infected wastes; poor or inconsistent barrier precautions	Damages the liver; no specific drug therapy available
Hepatitis B virus (HBV) (serum hepatitis)	Needlestick injuries; splattering with blood and body secretions; breaks in skin; can be sexually transmitted	Damages the liver; vaccine is available and effective
Hepatitis C virus (HCV) (non-A, non-B hepatitis)	Use of contaminated needles, hemodialysis units; can be sexually transmitted	Damages the liver
Hepatitis D virus (HDV) (delta hepatitis)	Use of contaminated needles; needlestick injuries; possibly hemodialysis units	Damages the liver; only occurs with hepatitis B infection; HBV vaccination helpful
Rubeola (measles)	Direct contact with nose and throat secretions; contaminated airborne droplets	Causes rash, high temperature, severe cough; vaccine is available
Rubella (German measles)	Direct contact with nose and throat secretions; blood, urine, stools, nasopharyngeal secretions; can infect fetus and cause birth defects	Causes rash, low-grade fever, lymphadenopathy, vaccine is available
Herpesvirus (herpes simplex)	Direct contact; oropharyngeal secretions; breaks in skin, especially of fingers	Causes cold sores, fever blisters, herpetic whitlow; treatment is palliative
Varicella-zoster (chickenpox, shingles)	Direct contact; contaminated airborne droplets	Causes chickenpox and shingles; vaccine is available
Cytomegalovirus	Direct contact; poor hygiene; urine, saliva, breast milk, respiratory-cervical secretions; can cross placenta	Infection is usually mild; may cause blindness or brain damage in immunocompromised persons; birth defects in fetus
Influenza A and B	Direct contact; contaminated airborne droplets	Causes chills, fever, cough; may progress to pneumonia, other complications; vaccines available
Bacteria		
Mycobacterium tuberculosis (TB)	Contaminated airborne droplet nuclei; poor infection control technique	Damages lung tissue; requires aggressive antibiotic therapy
Salmonella	Poor hygiene/hand washing; contamination of food, water	Causes typhoid fever; food poisoning; diarrhea; requires aggressive antibiotic therapy
Shigella (bacillary dysentery)	Direct contact; poor hygiene/hand washing; contamination of food, water	Causes fever, vomiting, diarrhea; requires fluid-electrolyte replacement, possibly antibiotics
Staphylococcus aureus	Direct contact	Occurs naturally in nasal passages; common cause of many types of purulent infections, abscesses
Arthropod		
Scabies mite (*Sarcoptes scabiei*)	Direct contact	Mite lives in skin, causing itching and infection; requires treatment with lindane cream or sulfur

only used on *nonliving* tissue or objects. They are potentially toxic to health care workers unless care is taken to limit exposure through proper handling and use. Glutaraldehyde and formaldehyde are widely used as disinfectants and sterilants; ethylene oxide is a very effective sterilant.

Other potentially toxic workplace chemicals include chemotherapeutic drugs such as antineoplastic or antimicrobial agents (e.g., nitrogen mustard, ribavirin and pentamidine), and waste anesthetic gases. These are discussed as examples of toxic or potentially toxic substances. Table 18–2 provides a summary of chemical hazards.

Toxic exposures occur when excessive amounts of the chemical are inhaled, ingested, or absorbed through the skin or mucous membranes. The chemicals may cause irritation, allergic reactions, or tissue damage. Some may also cause cancer or birth defects under certain circumstances (such as chronic exposure). Prevention and control of exposures substantially reduce health risks. Whether or not an individual is

BOX 18-2
UNDERSTANDING THE CHAIN OF INFECTION

The chain of infection is composed of six "links": causative agent, reservoir, portal of exit, mode of transmission, portal of entry, and susceptible host.

Factors influencing the *causative agent's* success or failure include the number of individual organisms present (concentration); the agent's ability to invade the host's body and overcome the host's defenses (virulence); how long the agent can live outside the host; and how well it can develop resistance to drug treatments.

The *reservoir* is the place where the causative agent may survive but may or may not multiply. Reservoirs may be human, animal, or environmental. Humans may serve as a reservoir if they have an acute or subclinical (asymptomatic) infection, or they may act as carriers, harboring the causative agent without suffering any ill effects.

The *portal of exit* is the path by which the causative agent leaves the reservoir before transmission to another host. This may occur via the respiratory, genitourinary, and gastrointestinal tracts; the skin and mucous membranes; across the placenta (from the mother to the fetus); and via blood or other body fluids and secretions.

The *mode of transmission* bridges the gap from a reservoir to a susceptible host and is accomplished by *contact* (direct—touching an infected site or person—or indirect—touching an inanimate object contaminated by an infected person); by *common vehicle* (when a reservoir such as food or fluid is consumed by one of more susceptible hosts); by a *vector* (transmitted by a nonhuman carrier, such as an insect or animal); or by an *airborne contaminant* (contacting or breathing in suspended droplets from a person who sneezes).

The *portal of entry* into a *susceptible host* may follow the respiratory tract, genitourinary tract, or gastrointestinal tract; breaks in skin or mucous membranes; parenteral (percutaneous, via blood) routes; or any natural body orifice.

A *susceptible host* is at risk of becoming infected. Susceptibility is influenced by many factors, including age, sex, socioeconomic status, disease history and underlying disease, lifestyle, nutritional status, occupation, health status, medication usage, and pregnancy.

When the chain is broken at any point, the infection process is disrupted. Hand washing, use of disinfectants, and infection precautions are some effective ways to break the chain of infection and protect yourself. Vaccination when appropriate is the best way to break the chain.

at risk of exposure will depend on factors such as the type of agent, its concentration, frequency and duration of exposure, work practices, and the individual's health and susceptibility (Rogers and Travers, 1991).

ENVIRONMENTAL AND MECHANICAL HAZARDS

Major environmental and mechanical hazards in the health care setting are summarized in Table 18–3. These include repetitive patient care tasks that cause back injuries; shift work scheduling that disrupts normal sleep-wake cycles; general environmental hazards such as slippery floors, environmental scatter (materials left lying on the floor, equipment blocking thoroughfare access, and other trip and fall hazards), poorly designed or inadequate equipment and work stations, and poor ventilation and lighting (Rogers and Travers, 1991); and violent patients.

BACK INJURIES

Health care workers are at high risk for sustaining back injuries because they must lift, bend, and pull while moving and transferring patients (see Chapter 20, Biomechanics and Mobility, for more information). Musculoskeletal injuries can be caused by poor body mechanics, lifting excessive asymmetric weights, prolonged sitting, and lack or disuse of assistive devices (Jorgensen et al, 1994). Occupational back injuries are considered the most expensive workers' compensation problem today (Buckler, 1995).

SHIFT WORK

Hospitals use various staffing patterns in an attempt to balance the needs of health care workers and their patients on one hand and control costs on the other hand. Nurses often find themselves working 10- or 12-hour shifts on rotation to ensure continuous staff coverage 24 hours a day. Because shift work often involves working through the night, the night shift nurse is awake and on duty while the body, which is usually day oriented, would rather be asleep (Glazner, 1991). This disrupts the person's natural biorhythms, also called *circadian rhythms* because they recur about every 24 hours. (See Chapter 25, Rest and Sleep, for more information on circadian rhythms.) Many human biologic rhythms peak during daylight hours and are synchronized by external forces such as light and darkness, clock time, and social stimulation (Siebenaler and McGovern, 1992).

Along with other job-related stressors, disruption of biorhythms resulting from shift work contributes to physical and psychological problems, including gastrointestinal disturbances, exhaustion, depression, anxiety, interpersonal relationship difficulties, and higher accident rates (Moore-Ede and Richardson, 1985). Part-time and night-shift health care workers have the highest incidence of needlestick injuries (Neuberger et al, 1984).

VIOLENT PATIENTS

Violent behavior toward health care workers by medical, surgical, and psychiatric patients and by persons seeking care in emergency departments is common (Lavoie et al, 1988; Rix, 1987; Wasserberger, 1988). Violent incidents include verbal threats of violence, physical attacks, and destruction of property (U.S. DOL, 1991).

It is likely that societal trends toward increased violence among the general population, increased use of drugs and alcohol, and increased availability of weapons all contribute

TABLE 18-2 Common Chemical Hazards

Chemical Hazard	Exposure Factor	Remarks
Disinfectants-Sterilants		
Glutaraldehyde	Inhalation; skin contact	Irritates eyes, nose, throat, respiratory tract; provide ventilation, use personal protective equipment
Ethylene oxide	Inhalation; skin, eye contact	Has mutagenic, carcinogenic, and explosive properties; causes respiratory irritation, nausea, vomiting; provide ventilation, use personal protective equipment, environmental monitoring(?)
Formaldehyde	Inhalation; skin contact	Irritates eyes, nose, throat, respiratory tract; may be mutagenic/carcinogenic; provide ventilation, use personal protective equipment
Chemotherapy Agents		
Antineoplastics Nitrogen mustard	Inhalation; skin contact	Has mutagenic and carcinogenic properties; provide ventilation, use personal protective equipment
Antimicrobials Ribavirin Pentamidine	Inhalation (of aerosols)	Has mutagenic and carcinogenic properties; provide ventilation, use personal protective equipment
Waste Anesthetic Gases		
Nitrous oxide, cyclopropane, halothane	Inhalation	Linked to liver and kidney disorders, central nervous system, and immune dysfunction; possible abortifacient; provide ventilation, prevent leakage, use personal protective equipment

to violence in health care settings. The problem may be compounded by inadequate training, policies, and procedures regarding how to handle violent patients.

PHYSICAL HAZARDS

Physical hazards commonly encountered in the health care setting include exposure to various types of ionizing and nonionizing radiation and excessive noise levels. These phenomena generate potentially tissue-damaging forces in the form of high-energy particles or vibrations. Table 18–4 provides a summary of physical hazards.

IONIZING RADIATION

This type of radiation results when high-energy particles are emitted during the spontaneous disintegration of unstable atomic nuclei to more stable energy states (such as gamma rays from radioactive cobalt or cesium) and when other atomic particles are artificially accelerated to high energy states (such as x-rays). The resulting particles are collected and focused into a beam, or the particle source is placed directly into target tissues. The particles are powerful enough to dislodge electrons from other atoms, a phenomenon called *ionization*. When these particles collide with living tissue, they damage cellular contents, including chromosomes, thereby causing cell death, mutations, or defective cell division. Generally, cells that grow and proliferate most actively—especially cancer cells—are more sensitive to radiation than cells that grow more slowly (such as bone, muscle, and connective tissue). Hence, ionizing radiation is used to kill cancer cells and halt tumor growth. X-rays are also used for radiographic procedures (such as chest films or computed tomography [CT] scans), and radioactive elements are used in

TABLE 18-3 Common Environmental and Mechanical Hazards

Environmental Mechanical Hazard	Exposure Factor	Remarks
Back injuries	Body mechanics (poor posture or conditioning); anxiety level; lifting, transferring patients; lifting heavy equipment; availability of assistive devices; low nurse-patient ratio	Causes sprains and strains; sciatica; spinal injuries; nurse's aides at highest risk; training in body mechanics and use of assistive devices reduces problems; staffing adjustments may be required
Shift work	Shift scheduling (rotating vs. permanent); low nurse-patient ratio; other demanding job requirements	Causes biorhythm alterations; fatigue, depression, gastrointestinal disturbances, "night shift paralysis," reduced alertness, increased incidence of errors-accidents; individual training and flexible staffing patterns may be required
Demanding, violent patients	Emergency rooms, mental health facilities, medical-surgical units, pediatric units	Threats and assaults cause physical danger as well as high stress/anxiety and posttraumatic stress disorder; requires security procedures, counseling

TABLE 18–4 Common Physical Hazards

Physical Hazard	Exposure Factor	Remarks
Radiation		
Ionizing radiation x-rays, gamma rays Nuclear medicine testing Radiation implant therapy	Proximity to energy source; energy levels; duration of treatment	Causes tissue trauma (skin, deeper tissue); carcinogenic-mutagenic effects; linked to stillbirths, miscarriages; limit exposure times, use adequate shielding, monitoring devices, and personal protective equipment
Nonionizing radiation Laser therapy Ultraviolet sterilization or therapy	Proximity to energy source; energy levels; duration of treatment	Causes tissue trauma (skin); burns; eye damage; limit exposure times, use personal protective equipment
Noise		
Emergency rescue work Critical care units	Loudness-duration; proximity to source	Causes hearing loss, psychological stress; limit exposure times, use personal protective equipment

diagnostic testing (such as radioactive iodine for thyroid uptake studies).

NONIONIZING RADIATION

As the term suggests, this type of radiation does not cause chemical changes in target tissue; rather, its energy acts on the tissues in the form of heat. Nonionizing radiation sources in the health care setting include several types of lasers and ultraviolet (UV) lighting, which is sometimes used to disinfect air in operating rooms and in rooms of patients with pulmonary tuberculosis (CDC, 1990a; Iseman, 1992).

Lasers are widely used in microsurgery (especially for eye and skin conditions) and for measuring various blood elements. The term *laser* is an acronym for light amplification by stimulated emission of radiation. A laser consists of a crystal or a tube of gas or liquid lasing material enclosed in a mirrored container. This is energized until the atoms of the lasing material emit photons of light, which impact other atoms, in turn releasing more photons. The ensuing reaction is reflected and confined until all the atoms reach a high-energy level. At last, this energized light escapes from the container as a highly focused light beam. Depending on the type of gas, liquid, or crystal used as the lasing material, lasers emit light in ultraviolet, infrared, or visible frequencies of the spectrum.

Ordinary light is a mixture of different frequencies moving in various directions, whereas laser light is a single frequency and moves in the same direction with all waves in phase. Because of this, the laser beam can be precisely focused and is powerful enough to melt a hole through a metal plate. In eye surgery, the laser beam may be concentrated 100,000 times at the retina, where it instantly vaporizes diseased tissue and seals blood vessels while leaving surrounding tissues unharmed (U.S. DHHS, 1987a).

NOISE POLLUTION

Noise can cause hearing loss if decibel levels are high enough to damage the delicate sound receptors lining the inner ear. The Occupational Safety and Health Administration (OSHA) standard for occupational exposure to noise specifies a maximum permissible noise exposure level of 90 dB for a duration of 8 hours (U.S. DOL, 1991). Although most health care settings do not have noise exposures above allowable levels, occasionally the volume or duration of noise from equipment, alarms, visitors, suction equipment, ventilators, and patients' and colleagues' voices can cause sensory overload and psychological stress as well (Rogers and Travers, 1991). In some settings, such as air rescue operations, first responders, or critical care units, nurses are commonly exposed to excessive noise for short periods, which may cause fatigue, anxiety, and decreased productivity (Falk and Wood, 1973).

PSYCHOSOCIAL HAZARDS

Psychosocial hazards common to the health care setting include excessive stress and substance abuse, a high-risk reaction to stress (Table 18–5). Psychosocial stressors can lead to

TABLE 18–5 Common Psychosocial Hazards

Psychosocial Hazard	Exposure Factors	Remarks
Stress Physical Mental	Patient deaths; low nurse-patient ratio; overwork; high-stress environments (intensive care unit, burn unit); lack of control	Causes irritability, fear of mistakes, fatigue, sleep disturbances, burnout; requires training, counseling, changes in routines
Substance abuse Tobacco Alcohol Drugs	High stress-anxiety levels; poor self-esteem; burnout	Causes poor job performance, increased incidence of errors-accidents, absenteeism; requires counseling-rehabilitation

decreased morale, reduced practice effectiveness, staff conflicts, absenteeism, and increased employee turnover (Doering, 1990; Fielding and Weaver, 1994; MacNeil and Weisz, 1987; Rees and Cooper, 1992).

STRESS

Job-related stress is a given, especially in critical care nursing. Repeated exposure to death and dying, increased workload, communication problems, and other environmental factors are important contributors (Gardam, 1969; Hay and Oken, 1972; Vreeland and Ellis, 1969). Adverse effects of psychosocial stress are physical (headache, gastrointestinal problems, fatigue, substance abuse) and psychological (insomnia, depression).

SUBSTANCE ABUSE

Substance abuse among health care workers is well documented. In one study, the American Nurses' Association estimated that 7 of every 100 nurses were abusing drugs (Brice, 1990). Workers who are impaired on the job can create hazardous situations for themselves, colleagues, and patients through faulty judgment and performance. Strategies to deal with workplace stressors that contribute to substance abuse include counseling and rehabilitation programs. (See Chapter 19, Health of the Nurse, for more details.)

Relevant Research

BIOLOGIC HAZARDS

Nurses and other health care workers are exposed to biologic agents in hospitals and all other health care settings. High-risk areas in the hospital typically include emergency rooms, ambulatory care areas, and infectious disease wards. Research has pinpointed important areas where infection prevention and control can be improved. Where appropriate, this information is provided next under specific disease headings.

HUMAN IMMUNODEFICIENCY VIRUS

The discovery that HIV could be transmitted through blood and other body fluids caused immediate concern in the health care community. This retrovirus weakens the body's immune defenses by gradually destroying the important helper (CD4) T cells. Currently, antiviral therapy can add months or even years to the life of a person infected with HIV. In 1984, the first case of occupational HIV exposure, a nurse who sustained a needlestick injury, was reported in *The Lancet* (Jagger, 1994). Since then, the number of reported cases of occupational transmission of HIV has increased. However, it is important to bear in mind that the risk of exposure is less than 1 percent (CDC, 1988a; Gerberding, 1995; Marcus et al, 1991), and that *seroconversion* must occur before a person is considered HIV positive. Seroconversion means that a person who was known to be HIV negative when first exposed to blood or body fluids containing the HIV retrovirus subsequently acquires serologic evidence of HIV infection (i.e., a serologic test showing the presence of antibody to HIV).

Most HIV exposures result from skin injuries, primarily needlestick punctures. Much of the concern about needlestick injuries stems from the threat of contracting acquired immunodeficiency syndrome (AIDS). As of December 1997, the CDC had identified 54 documented and 132 possible cases of occupationally acquired HIV (CDC, 1998). Most needlestick injuries result from recapping and breaking used needles and from "downstream" injuries of housekeepers and aides who are accidentally injured by contaminated needles placed in laundry or trash (Becker, 1990; English, 1992; Willy et al., 1990). Failure to use Universal Precautions has also been cited as a significant risk factor for HIV exposure. Nurses have begun a campaign to encourage hospitals to adopt safer needle systems that are equipped with special shielding or are "needleless," using short plastic needles that connect to special diaphragm valves (see Research Highlight for more details).

HEPATITIS A VIRUS

Hepatitis A is transmitted primarily by the fecal-oral route. The incubation period (the interval between first exposure to the pathogen and the appearance of symptoms) ranges from 2 to 6 weeks, but averages 4 weeks. Hepatitis A virus (HAV) is most contagious (i.e., produces the highest number of infectious virus particles) about 2 weeks before the infected person becomes physically ill. By the time this occurs, the amount of virus in the stool has dropped sharply.

Hepatitis A exposures in health care units through fecal-oral transmission of contamination have occurred but are rare (Rosenblum et al, 1991). The source for the hepatitis A infection is not usually sought until secondary cases of hepatitis A occur in health care workers with no other identifiable risk factors for acquiring the virus.

Many persons infected with HAV have no obvious symptoms and are never diagnosed. HAV outbreaks can occur in several ways. For example, infected kitchen workers with poor hygiene habits can contaminate food while still apparently healthy. Meanwhile, the infection is not recognized until someone eats the contaminated food and becomes ill 2 to 6 weeks later (Lettau, 1992). Health care workers may also become infected by patients with HAV who have diarrhea (Drusin et al, 1987; Edgar and Campbell, 1985; Goodman et al, 1982; Krober et al, 1984). Typically, such a patient is hospitalized for other reasons during the contagious period. Workers become infected when they assist the patient with fecal hygiene but neglect to use barrier precautions (such as gloves) or good hand-washing technique. The original contact for the resulting outbreak often is not identified until the hospital epidemiology staff investigates.

HEPATITIS B VIRUS

Hepatitis B virus (HBV) is the most prevalent type of hepatitis infection in hospitals. Of the 140,000 new cases of

RESEARCH HIGHLIGHT
BLUNTING THE IMPACT OF NEEDLESTICK INJURIES

In 1983, the Centers for Disease Control and Prevention (1983b) recommended that used needles not be bent, broken, or recapped by hand and that they be discarded in a puncture-resistant disposable "sharps" container placed near the point of use. Jagger and colleagues (1988) identified characteristics of devices that caused needlestick injuries in a large teaching hospital during 1986. Of the 326 injuries studied, 12 percent were caused by disposable syringes; 7 percent were caused by winged-steel needle intravenous sets; 5 percent were caused by phlebotomy (blood drawing) needles; 2 percent were caused by stylets used with intravenous catheters; and 13 percent were caused by other devices.

Although disposable syringes caused the most injuries in this study, they had the lowest *rate* of injuries (6.9 injuries per 100,000 syringes purchased). Devices requiring disassembly, such as intravenous tubing-needle sets, had the highest rate (36.7 injuries per 100,000 devices purchased).

Recapping Increases Health Risk

One third of needlestick injuries were related to recapping. When asked why they recapped needles, health care workers said they had to disassemble a device before disposal and that it was hard to carry several uncapped needles to a distant sharps container.

In an extension of the same study, investigators found that other types of sharp objects (surgical instruments, lancets, and glass) were liable to cause injuries because of faulty implement design and work practices (Jagger et al, 1990). Concluding that needlestick injuries will not be reduced solely by emphasizing safe handling, the authors urged adopting safer designs for needled devices and eliminating all activities that do not require skin penetration.

Encouraging Use of Safer Needles

In late 1996, a Philadelphia nurses' group announced a campaign to urge hospitals to adopt safer needle systems. The group claims that safer needle designs are available now and could prevent about 80 percent of infection-causing needlestick injuries (Hilchey, 1996).

Implications for Practice

For nurses and other health care workers to carry out safe work practices, they must be knowledgeable about the various potential health hazards in their workplace. They also must incorporate proper prevention and control strategies into their daily practice. Hospital administration should be sensitive to health care workers' needs and provide adequate equipment and safety training.

HBV reported annually, about 1000 involve health care workers. Each year, about 150 persons die of HBV (CDC, 1996).

Hepatitis B is usually transmitted by needlesticks or other injuries involving sharp objects; by blood contact with mucous membranes, as occurs when blood or bloody body fluids are splashed into the eyes or mouth; and through skin breaks or "hangnails." Nonimmunized health care workers have a 6 to 30 percent risk of contracting HBV from a single needlestick injury (Marcus et al, 1991).

Hepatitis B has a longer incubation period than hepatitis A (45–160 days, averaging 120 days). The CDC estimates that 15 to 30 percent of health care workers who experience frequent blood contact are infected with HBV and that 1 to 2 percent are chronic carriers. However, health care workers whose jobs require no blood contact are no more likely to be infected with HBV than the general population (CDC, 1990b). Infection with HBV confers lifelong immunity.

HEPATITIS C VIRUS

Hepatitis C virus (HCV) is one of many viruses formerly collected under the term *non-A, non-B hepatitis.* HCV causes most cases of so-called bloodborne non-A, non-B hepatitis worldwide. Prevalence of HCV among health care workers is low, about 1 percent; however, it is high among injection drug users and persons with hemophilia (50–80 percent) and among persons who have multiple sex partners (5–15 percent) (Lettau, 1992).

In persons with acute or chronic HCV, the presence of antibodies to the hepatitis C virus (anti-HCV) appears to indicate infectivity; however, persons with antibody and no history or evidence of illness may or may not be infectious to others. More research is needed to resolve this question (Alter, 1994).

Hepatitis C infection in patients receiving hemodialysis has been studied (Jeffers et al, 1990). The investigators determined the prevalence of anti-HCV in 90 patients and 37 health care workers. Eleven of the patients (12 percent) were positive, but none of the staff demonstrated evidence of infection. The prevalence of anti-HCV was significantly higher in injection drug users and patients who were also HIV-antibody positive, but not for patients who required multiple transfusions but were neither injection drug users nor HIV positive.

HEPATITIS D VIRUS

Hepatitis D (formerly called delta hepatitis) virus (HDV) occurs only in persons who have acute or chronic hepatitis B infections. Infection with hepatitis D can be measured with a special antibody test. Transmission of hepatitis D to health care workers via needlestick injury and in dialysis units via nonparenteral exposure has been reported (Lettau et al, 1986). The best protection against hepatitis D is vaccination against the hepatitis B virus.

RUBEOLA (MEASLES)

Hospital outbreaks of rubeola were relatively uncommon during the 1970s and early 1980s, but have since become a major concern. The increase has been attributed to two major factors: inadequate immunization of susceptible children and prevention vaccine failure. On one measles outbreak in a pediatric office in 1981, the virus spread through the building's ventilation system (Bloch et al, 1985). This has implications for occupational exposure and the need for effective engineering controls to reduce infection risks. The CDC has recommended that health care workers born after 1956 provide evidence of receiving two doses of measles vaccine unless they can prove immunity by serology or physician-documented illness (CDC, 1989, 1991b). Because many health care workers are not immunized against measles (Smith et al, 1990), most health care agencies and schools of nursing now require job applicants and students to be immunized.

RUBELLA (GERMAN MEASLES)

Rubella, like rubeola, has caused outbreaks in health care facilities. One such incident, a group of 47 cases in a Boston hospital in 1979, resulted in more than $50,000 in losses as a result of lost work time, diagnostic testing, and personnel costs (Polk et al, 1980). This disorder is worrisome because it poses a serious risk to unborn children through transplacental exposure.

Overall, rubella outbreaks have decreased sharply since a vaccine became widely available in 1969. The CDC recommends immunization of all health care workers against rubella (CDC, 1984, 1991b). As with rubeola, most health care agencies and schools of nursing now require job applicants and students to be immunized against rubella.

HERPESVIRUSES

This group includes herpes simplex, varicella-zoster virus, and cytomegalovirus (CMV). Most adults have been infected with at least one form of these viruses. Herpes simplex commonly causes fever sores, cold sores, or canker sores and usually is self-limiting (requiring little if any treatment before subsiding). However, in health care workers, it can also cause herpetic whitlow and other localized infections (Stearn et al, 1959). In herpetic whitlow, unprotected fingers become infected through a skin break or hangnail if they contact herpes-contaminated oropharyngeal secretions. Nurses (particularly those in intensive care units), dentists, respiratory therapists, and anesthesiologists are at increased risk (Greaves et al, 1980; Jackson and Emerson, 1979).

Herpetic whitlow is painful and may require convalescence for 2 to 3 weeks until the lesion has healed. Like other herpes infections, it may recur. The CDC recommends that infected health care workers avoid direct contact with patients until whitlow lesions are healed, and that those who have cold sores avoid caring for newborns or patients with burns or who are otherwise immunocompromised (CDC, 1983a).

Varicella-zoster virus, which causes chickenpox, may migrate to the dorsal root ganglia of the nervous system and become dormant there after the initial infection. The virus can become active at any time, migrate down the nerve, and cause painful skin eruptions or vesicles (shingles), which contain virus particles. The incubation period can begin as much as 5 days before eruption of vesicles, although 1 to 2 days is more common (Benenson, 1995). The virus-filled vesicles are a threat to health care workers who have not had chickenpox. At least 10 hospital outbreaks of varicella-zoster virus have been reported since 1970 (Sherertz and Hampton, 1987). Varicella zoster also causes substantial morbidity and mortality in immunocompromised patients, particularly bone marrow transplant recipients (Schimpff et al, 1972).

A vaccine for varicella zoster is now available. Control strategies involve appropriate room ventilation for patients with infection and preventing susceptible health care workers from caring for patients with chickenpox or shingles (Benenson, 1995).

CMV, another in this group of herpesviruses, occurs everywhere; 45 to 79 percent of adults in the United States are believed to have had a CMV infection at some time (Sherertz and Hampton, 1987). CMV is transmitted by prolonged or multiple contact with infected body fluids and secretions (such as urine, saliva, breast milk, cervical and respiratory secretions) and by poor hygiene. Infection risk is highest among young children; patients who are immunocompromised as a result of leukemia, burns, kidney failure, or HIV infection; and patients who have had an organ transplant. Mothers who become infected during pregnancy may pass the virus to their newborns as well, increasing the risk of birth defects (Benenson, 1995).

Despite its ubiquity, the incidence of CMV among nurses and other health care workers is no higher than in the general population (Balcarek et al, 1990; Demmler et al, 1987; Gerberding et al, 1987). Use of Universal Precautions and barrier precautions for contact with any body substance is recommended, and health care workers who may be pregnant or immunocompromised may wish to obtain guidance about assignment to patients with confirmed or suspected CMV (CDC, 1992a).

INFLUENZA A AND B

Nationwide outbreaks of these common respiratory viruses occur each year; the A strain is more prevalent than the B strain. Outbreaks also have been reported in health care facilities (Sherertz and Hampton, 1987), particularly nursing homes. Control of influenza in health care facilities depends on rapid diagnosis of the organism in the community followed by prompt vaccination of susceptible workers. Amantadine, an antiviral drug, may be given with the vaccine. Because influenza viruses are highly variable, the CDC publishes new guidelines for prevention and control annually.

MYCOBACTERIUM TUBERCULOSIS

Tuberculosis (TB), a highly contagious respiratory disease spread by airborne droplet nuclei, was successfully controlled in health care settings for almost 30 years by drug therapy (Lancaster, 1991). However, incidence of TB increased sharply in the late 1980s, driven by the epidemic of HIV. Once infected with TB, persons with HIV infection often progress quickly to active pulmonary TB (Iseman, 1992). The problem is further complicated by the appearance of drug-resistant strains of TB. The CDC has published guidelines for preventing the transmission of TB in health care settings, with special focus on HIV-related issues (CDC, 1990a).

A number of studies of transmission of *M. tuberculosis* in health care settings have been reported over the years. A patient in a respiratory intensive care unit was the source for an outbreak of nosocomial tuberculosis that involved 14 of 45 (31 percent) exposed personnel (Catanzaro, 1982). The problem was recognized when a physician on the staff experienced symptoms compatible with TB.

The CDC studied outbreaks of multidrug-resistant tuberculosis that occurred in four hospitals between 1988 and 1991 (CDC, 1991a). The study identified several contributing factors:

- In all four hospitals, diagnosis of the source cases was often delayed for lack of conclusive radiologic or bacteriologic evidence.
- Infection control precautions were sometimes delayed or not maintained for a sufficient time to ensure noncommunicability.
- Health care workers reported that doors to isolation rooms were often left open, personnel and visitors often entered rooms without masks, and ventilation for isolation rooms was rarely adequate.
- In these outbreaks, eight cases of active TB were reported among health care workers; five of the eight were known to be HIV positive, and one was known to be HIV negative.

In two of the hospitals, positive tuberculin skin test reactions were reported in 19 of 51 health care workers, for a conversion rate of 37 percent.

SALMONELLA, SHIGELLA, AND *STAPHYLOCOCCUS AUREUS*

Outbreaks resulting from *Salmonella* and *Shigella* are well documented in hospitals and other health care settings. Health care workers usually are infected by ingesting the organisms from their contaminated hands. *Salmonella* outbreaks most commonly involve children who were infected while passing through the birth canal; foodborne outbreaks are relatively rare (Sherertz and Hampton, 1987). Both patients and health care workers can become chronic asymptomatic carriers of *Salmonella* and excrete the organisms in their stool for prolonged periods.

Outbreaks of *Shigella* are less commonly reported than *Salmonella,* perhaps because the chronic carrier state is rare. On the other hand, very few *Shigella* bacteria (10–100 organisms) are required to transmit the infection (Benenson, 1995). Control measures for *Salmonella* and *Shigella* begin with good hand-washing technique and use of personal protective equipment, such as gloves (Garner, 1996).

Although *S. aureus* causes numerous infections in patients and is most frequently transmitted by direct contact, the infection risk to health care workers remains unclear. This is partly because some people are persistent carriers and are always culture positive, whereas others are intermittent carriers and are culture positive and culture negative at different times (Jackson, 1992). In addition, the bacterium lives normally in nasal passages in 30 to 40 percent of the adult population.

SCABIES

Hospital outbreaks of *Sarcoptes scabiei* usually begin with an undiagnosed patient. Because the incubation period can be as long as 4 weeks, an infested patient may be identified only after several health care workers report severe itching to the employee health service. Effective control depends on prompt evaluation of skin eruptions in patients and health care workers, especially if they are accompanied by severe itching.

CHEMICAL HAZARDS

DISINFECTING AND STERILIZING AGENTS

These chemicals evaporate rapidly into the surrounding air and can irritate the skin, eyes, mucous membranes, and respiratory tract. Symptoms of exposure usually develop rapidly. However, chronic exposures can also cause delayed hypersensitivity reactions. Sometimes it is easy to match the causative agent with the irritant effect (Rutala and Hamory, 1989), but chronic exposure to low levels of some chemical agents may not become evident until after the worker has left the health care setting, making later attribution difficult.

Glutaraldehyde is used for disinfection or chemical sterilization of certain instruments, such as endoscopes with fiberoptics (e.g., those used for bronchoscopy, arthroscopy, or endoscopy), which may be damaged by steam autoclaving under pressure. Glutaraldehyde inhalation may cause respiratory tract irritation and cough and burning of the eyes, nose, or throat (Frazier et al, 1995).

Ethylene oxide (ETO) is a toxic, explosive gas widely used to sterilize heat-sensitive equipment as well as drapes, bandages, surgical packs, and clothing. It is used, for example, in operating rooms, anesthetic areas, and dental clinics. An estimated 100,000 health care workers are exposed to ETO each year (Rutala and Hamory, 1989).

Workplace exposure is primarily by inhalation; high dosages typically occur when the gas sterilizing unit is opened to remove articles. Additional exposures occur when the freshly sterilized items or packets are handled and opened, when ETO cylinders are changed without activating proper ventilation, and when ETO vessels are cleaned (Rogers and Travers, 1991). This gas is odorless except at high concentrations (700 parts per million [ppm] or greater).

Acute exposures to ETO can cause respiratory tract irritation, headache, nausea, dyspnea (shortness of breath), vomiting, drowsiness, weakness, and incoordination. Direct skin or eye contact with the liquid form can cause severe irritation, contact dermatitis, and burns (LaDou, 1990). In addition, ETO has mutagenic and carcinogenic properties. In animals, ETO has been shown to depress fertility, increase the incidence of leukemia, and cause chromosomal aberrations (Jay and Swift, 1982; Snellings et al, 1982). It also has reportedly caused spontaneous abortions among exposed health care workers (Hemminki and Mutanen, 1982).

OSHA has set airborne ETO exposure limits of 1 ppm average over an 8-hour period. Environmental monitoring of ETO in the work area, health surveillance for exposed workers, training and education of workers regarding ETO hazards, and compliance with recommended engineering controls such as installation of local exhaust ventilation at the sterilizer door should be part of the ETO control programs (U.S. DOL, 1984).

Formaldehyde is used to preserve pathology specimens, to prepare some medications, and to disinfect renal dialysis units. It is highly irritating to the skin, eyes, mucous membranes, and lungs and can cause allergic reactions and contact dermatitis (La Dou, 1990). Adequate workplace ventilation, work practice controls, and use of personal protective equipment minimize exposures.

CHEMOTHERAPEUTIC AGENTS

Toxic chemicals used in chemotherapy include antineoplastic (anticancer) agents and antimicrobial agents. Antineoplastics (such as nitrogen mustard) act by killing malignant cancer cells or slowing their growth. Nurses working in hospitals, oncology (cancer treatment) clinics, and private offices may be exposed during preparation and handling of dosage forms. The chemicals may be inhaled, absorbed through the skin, or, possibly, accidentally ingested with food or cigarette smoking. Headache, skin rash, and gastrointestinal disturbances have been reported (Rogers and Emmett, 1987), as well as evidence of birth defects, spontaneous abortions (Rogers and Emmett, 1987; Selevan et al, 1985), and chromosome damage (Falck et al, 1979; Nikula et al, 1984).

Detailed guidelines for handling antineoplastic agents have been published by OSHA (U.S. DOL, 1986) and the Oncology Nursing Society (1989).

Antimicrobial chemotherapy agents present health risks when given to patients as inhalants. For example, ribavirin (Virazole) is used to treat respiratory syncytial virus (RSV), primarily in infants and young children (Hodgson et al, 1997). The drug may be given by oxygen tent, mist mask, or ventilator, which exposes personnel to aerosol particles. A study of 19 nurses who worked with ribavirin did not find the drug in their red blood cells, plasma, or urine (Rodriguez et al, 1987). However, nurses and respiratory therapists have complained of various subjective adverse reactions from their exposure to ribavirin aerosol. These include eye, nose, and throat irritation and headaches (Arnold and Alonso, 1993). These reactions have not been conclusively linked to exposure, however (Arnold and Buchanan, 1991). Because of a lack of dose-response data in humans, adverse effects have not been conclusively documented. However, the CDC recommends against using ribavirin in pregnant patients (CDC, 1988b); thus, health care workers who are pregnant or may become pregnant should be advised of the potential health risks of exposure.

Pentamidine, another antiviral agent, is used in its aerosol form for primary and secondary prophylaxis against *Pneumocystis carinii* in persons infected with HIV (CDC, 1992c). It can be given by different types of nebulizers, thus exposing caregivers to airborne particles. Exposure can cause respiratory irritation; caregivers who have asthma should avoid working with the drug. Although reproductive risks are not yet known, caregivers who are in the first trimester of pregnancy should not handle the aerosolized agent. OSHA guidelines have not been issued for pentamidine.

Finally, some patients with HIV may also have pulmonary TB, which presents an additional exposure hazard when they cough or wheeze while receiving pentamidine or other aerosolized drugs. Without adequate ventilation, particles from the drug and the disease may remain suspended in room air long enough to infect persons who enter the patient's room after pentamidine treatment (CDC, 1988c).

WASTE ANESTHETIC GASES

Gases (such as nitrous oxide and cyclopropane) and volatile liquids (such as halothane) are used during surgery as inhalation anesthetics to relieve pain, relax muscles, and depress consciousness. They are administered with oxygen in carefully controlled mixtures. Health care workers may be exposed to unsafe concentrations of anesthetics in operating rooms, postoperative recovery units, and labor-delivery units. Gases may escape from improperly inflated endotracheal tubes, poorly fitted facial masks, improperly connected waste disposal lines, or premature or accidental gas releases. Another source of waste gas exposure is the patient who continues to exhale the gas after surgery (Rogers and Travers, 1991).

Chronic exposure to waste anesthetic gases has been implicated in liver and kidney disease as well as central nervous system and immune system dysfunction (Brodsky and Cohen, 1985; National Institute for Occupational Safety and Health [NIOSH], 1977). Nitrous oxide has been found to cause increased incidence of spontaneous abortions among wives of exposed anesthesiologists as well as among women who were directly exposed (NIOSH, 1977). However, compelling evidence directly linking these gases to toxic effects is still lacking. Engineering controls such as effective ventilation and scavenging systems and work practices related to proper disposal techniques are effective.

PHYSICAL HAZARDS

IONIZING RADIATION

The level of background radiation emitted by rocks, building materials, radon, and the human body itself totals approximately 100 to 150 millirems (mrem) per year. An average chest x-ray examination causes approximately 30 mrem of radiation exposure. In terms of occupational exposure to ionizing radiation, the Nuclear Regulatory Commission (1974) has set maximum exposure limits of 500 mrem/year or 125 mrem/quarter for nonoccupationally exposed workers such as nurses.

The amount (dosage) of external ionizing radiation depends on the duration of exposure, the distance from the source to the worker (Fig. 18–1), and the available shielding placed between the source and the worker (U.S. DHHS, 1987b). Health care workers who work with radioactive diagnostic materials as in gallium scans and thallium heart imaging procedures are at increased risk; contamination of hands, clothing, and urine of personnel has been documented (Upton, 1982). The skill level, difficulty of the procedure, and most certainly the closeness of the health care worker to the radiation source greatly influence the health risk (Nishiyama et al, 1980). In some cases even the patient's liquid and solid wastes must be handled following specific protocols to minimize unnecessary exposure.

NONIONIZING RADIATION

Laser beams can seriously damage normal eye or skin tissue by causing burns or tissue breakdown. Health care workers are at risk if the laser is not properly calibrated, maintained, or handled (Cohen, 1990; Plog et al, 1988). Use of laser safety glasses guards against accidental reflections of the beam.

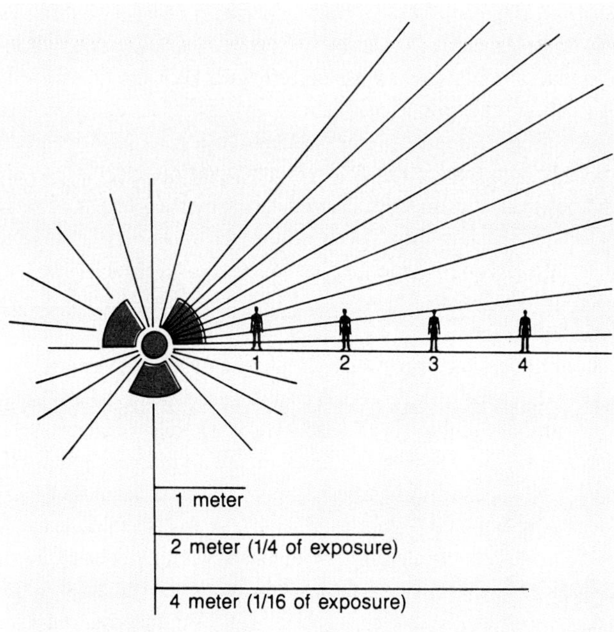

Figure 18–1. Radiation safety guidelines. The greater the distance from the radiation source, the lower is the exposure to ionizing radiation. The intensity of radiation decreases inversely to the square of the distance from the source. For example, a person standing 4 meters from a radiation source is exposed to approximately one quarter the amount of radiation than a person standing 2 meters from the source. (From Sedholm, L.N., Yann, M.I.Y. (1985). Radiation therapy and nurses' fears of radiation exposure. *Cancer Nursing, 8,* 129–134. Used with permission.)

ENVIRONMENTAL AND MECHANICAL HAZARDS

BACK INJURIES

McAbee (1988) found that the typical hospital staff nurse lifts 20 patients into bed and assists 5 to 10 patients with transfers from beds to chairs during each work shift. Another study found that assisting a patient from a toilet to a wheelchair carried the highest risk of musculoskeletal stress (Owen and Garg, 1991). The incidence of back injuries rises when the nurse-patient ratio is low, reflecting the increased workload (Larise and Fiorito, 1994). Nurses' aides appear to bear the brunt of these tasks and the resulting injuries; in the study by Owen and Garg, nurses' aides reported significantly more low back pain and sciatica severe enough to make them unable to perform daily tasks. In a study of 4000 hospital employees (including dietary and housekeeping staff, registered and practical nurses, as well as nurses' aides), nurses' aides sustained 40 percent of reported back injuries, and nearly 40 percent of these cases resulted in lost work time (Greenwood, 1986).

Although back injuries are among the most prevalent causes of workers' compensation claims, the extent of the problem may be severely underreported; in two studies of nurses experiencing back injuries, claims were reported by only 36 percent and 6 percent of sufferers, respectively (Newman and Callaghan, 1993; Owen, 1989).

SHIFT WORK

Factors that affect how well one adapts to shift work include age, physical health, gender, and attitudes about shift work (Siebenaler and McGovern, 1992). Twenty percent of workers are unable to tolerate night work (LaDou, 1982; Scott and LaDou, 1990), and health problems in shift workers usually increase with age (Akerstedt, 1984). However, workers who are in good physical condition adapt better to shift work because they are less susceptible to fatigue (Harma et al, 1986). Gender is not necessarily a factor in shift work performance, but women who are the primary child caretakers at home may find it more difficult to adapt (Levy and Wegman, 1993).

Shift work scheduling strongly influences worker effectiveness in several ways: shifts may be permanent or rotating; rotations may take place slowly (every 1–3 weeks or more) or rapidly (every 2 days); and the direction of the rotation may be clockwise ("forward") or counterclockwise ("backward"). Health care workers who work rotating shifts appear to have the lowest performance levels and highest stress levels. A study of 463 nurses at five hospitals found that those working on rotating and evening shifts rated themselves lower in job performance than did day and night shift nurses (Coffey et al, 1988). Rotating shift nurses also experienced the most job-related stress. Night shift nurses reported the least, possibly because of reduced patient and staff contact.

There is little agreement on the number of days workers should spend on each shift. One school of thought holds that slow rotation (over more than 3 weeks) is best, because it allows the person's biorhythms to adapt to the work schedule most easily. Another view is that rapid rotations (every 2 days) allow biorhythms to remain relatively day oriented (Siebenaler and McGovern, 1992).

Night shift workers do not usually get enough sleep, because sound sleeping is difficult when the body is trying to prepare for an upcoming new day. In addition, if the night shift worker does not maintain a regular schedule of sleeping during the day and working at night, the sleep-nighttime activity will tend to return to the normal nocturnal pattern (Tepas, 1982). Finally, some nurses working night shifts report experiencing episodic "night shift paralysis," with periods of temporary gross motor paralysis lasting an average of 4 minutes (Folkard et al, 1984). The nurses reported these symptoms during early morning hours while they were sitting and charting.

Personnel who must work night shifts can improve their chances of obtaining sufficient sleep during the day by sleeping in a dark, cool, sound-insulated bedroom, using ear plugs, and turning off the telephone and television. In the workplace, monitoring programs can be implemented to evaluate continuously other environmental safety problems, such as trip and fall hazards, needlestick injuries, and burns, which increase when workers are fatigued and poorly adjusted to shift work.

VIOLENT PATIENTS

Physical assaults against nurses are a continuing problem. One study of victims' reactions to such events in a psychiatric care setting found that assaults were very common (67 nurses reported 91 assaults in 1 year), and they have significant psychosocial costs (Lanza, 1983). The victims experienced anger, anxiety, helplessness, irritability, fear of other patients, self-blame, and a guilty feeling that they should have done something to prevent the assault. Some nurses experienced adverse emotional, cognitive, and social-behavioral reactions for up to a year after the incidents occurred. A study of emergency department workers at a teaching hospital revealed that one third of the 127 respondents reported being verbally threatened at least once daily. Another 18 percent noted that a threat incident involving a weapon occurred at least once a month (Lavoie et al, 1988).

In psychiatric institutions, as many as 37 to 45 percent of all patients may engage in violent behavior, and more than 50 percent of psychiatric nurses and other workers in these settings have experienced at least one assault during their career (Lipscomb and Love, 1992).

Posttraumatic stress disorder (PTSD) results from exposure to overwhelming environmental stress, such as combat or a major disaster. The victim undergoes recurrent episodes of reexperiencing the traumatic event. Perhaps not unexpectedly, PTSD also appears among health care workers. A study investigating the incidence of PTSD among hospital staff who were assaulted by patients found that 138 of 224 (62 percent) experienced a serious threat to life or physical safety or witnessed a serious injury or death, and that more than half of this group evidenced PTSD (Caldwell, 1992).

Alternatively, many assault victims report experiencing no psychological symptoms after the event, primarily because they attempt to suppress their emotional reactions. Some nurses accept that being assaulted is part of their job, and others believe that if they allowed themselves to worry about the likelihood of assault, they would not be able to function (Caldwell, 1992; Lanza, 1983). At least partly for these reasons, violent incidents in the health care setting are underreported. Some nurses cite lack of time to complete reports as well as a feeling that reporting is basically wasted effort (Mahoney, 1991). Besides staff tolerance or indifference, underreporting may also reflect lack of an institutional policy or management problems (Lipscomb and Love, 1992). Finally, other research suggests that the risk of threatening or violent patient behavior may increase if frequency of nursing staff changes (such as use of agency nurses) interferes with continuity of care (Fineberg et al, 1988).

More research is needed to define further the risks of violence toward health care workers and to identify and test preventive measures to reduce the risks. Clearly, effective protective strategies are crucial to maintaining an atmosphere of trust and safety for health care workers (Box 18–3).

BOX 18-3
PSYCHOLOGICAL DEMANDS ON THE INTENSIVE CARE UNIT NURSE

A study of intensive care unit (ICU) nurses working in six hospitals in southern California identified and ranked 16 stressful factors in the intensive care unit:

1. Workload and amount of physical work
2. Death of a patient
3. Communication problems between staff and nursing office
4. Communication problems between staff and physicians
5. Meeting the needs of the patient's family
6. Numerous pieces of equipment and their failure
7. Noise levels
8. Physical setup of the unit
9. Number of rapid decisions that must be made
10. Amount of knowledge needed to work in the ICU
11. Physical safety in the unit
12. Communication problems between staff members
13. Meeting the psychological needs of patients
14. Communication problems between staff and other departments
15. Cardiac arrest
16. Patient teaching

BOX 18-4
NURSES ACT TO CURB WORKPLACE VIOLENCE

Several nursing associations in the United States have taken proactive measures to stop violence in the workplace. For example, the state council of the California Emergency Nurses Association helped enact state legislation to address these issues:

- Educating and training of health care workers
- Establishing a reporting mechanism for violent incidents
- Conducting a security and safety assessment
- Developing a security plan to protect health care workers, patients, and visitors from violent behavior.

Nursing organizations in California have also requested assistance from California's Occupational Safety and Health Administration to develop guidelines to help managers and administrators implement safety programs to protect employees. In Mississippi and Connecticut, Emergency Nurses Association state councils helped enact legislation to make assaulting an emergency department staff member either a misdemeanor or a felony.

The Emergency Nurses Association suggests the following preventive strategies for emergency room settings:

- Increasing access control and visibility of entrances
- Using metal detectors and silent alarm systems
- Using closed-circuit television to monitor all hospital entrances
- Separating patients with minor illnesses from those who are more seriously ill
- Retaining a psychiatrist on call to assist emergency staff workers after a particularly bad shift.

TABLE 18-6 NORA Priority Research Areas

Category	Priority Research Areas
Disease and injury	Allergic and irritant dermatitis Asthma and chronic obstructive pulmonary disease Fertility and pregnancy abnormalities Hearing loss Infectious diseases Low back disorders Musculoskeletal disorders of the upper extremities Traumatic injuries
Work environment and work force	Emerging technologies Indoor environment Mixed exposures Organization of work Special populations at risk
Research tools and approaches	Cancer research methods Control technology and personal protective Equipment Exposure assessment methods Health services research Intervention effectiveness research Risk assessment methods Social and economic consequences of workplace Illness and injury Surveillance research methods

From U.S. Health and Human Services, Centers for Disease Control, National Institute of Occupational Safety and Health. 1995 *National Occupational Research Agenda*, Cincinnati, OH.

PSYCHOSOCIAL HAZARDS

STRESS

In a study of 46 intensive care unit nurses working in six hospitals in southern California, researchers identified and ranked 16 stress factors in an intensive care unit (Huckabay and Jagla, 1979) (Box 18–4). Similar findings have been reported elsewhere (Gray-Toft and Anderson, 1981; Leppanen and Olkinuora, 1987; Van Ameringen et al, 1988). Nurses in high-stress environments require support systems to help with psychosocial well-being and job satisfaction, access to grief counseling when a patient dies, and improved methods for coping with stress to enhance both professional and personal performance.

FUTURE DEVELOPMENTS

Research into and development of protective measures for occupational health hazards continues. NIOSH published its National Occupational Research Agenda (NORA) in 1996, 25 years after enaction of the Occupational Safety and Health Act. The document contains 21 priority research areas that will have research emphasis (Table 18–6). In 1996, the CDC published guidelines for post-HIV exposure management for health care workers. These guidelines include postexposure prophylaxis with zidovudine (ZDV) and other antivirals. Also in 1996, OSHA released new guidelines for workplace violence prevention that focused on programs for health care workers in institutional and community settings. In 1977, OSHA released TB and respiratory protection standards, which apply to health care workers. OSHA is currently evaluating whether or not to develop a latex guideline or standard.

Strategies for Prevention and Control

General methods for controlling occupational health hazards for health care workers include engineering and work practice controls, administrative controls, and personal protective equipment. Specific examples of these are listed in Table 18–7.

Engineering and Work Practice Controls

Engineering controls aim to reduce or prevent worker exposures by modifying the source of the exposure or reducing the level of contamination in the work environment. Examples of engineering controls include eliminating the hazard; substituting a less harmful material; changing or altering a work process to minimize exposures; and providing better and safer designs for devices such as needles (Lewy, 1991; Plog et al, 1988).

TABLE 18-7 Reviewing Control Strategies

Work Example	Control Strategies
Biologic Hazards	
Nurse examines a patient with tuberculosis, is exposed to *Mycobacterium tuberculosis* when the patient coughs: risk of infection from airborne droplet nuclei.	Engineering: provide contained ventilation system to prevent contaminated air from escaping from the patient's room to other areas. Work practice: employ scrupulous hygiene and hand-washing technique. Administrative: isolate the infected patient. PPE: use a NIOSH-approved N95 particulate respirator.
Emergency medical technician (EMT) is splattered with patient's blood while administering CPR. The patient is HIV positive: risk of infection from exposure of open wounds and mucous membranes to blood and other body fluids.	Work practice: rinse mouth thoroughly; wash face and hands with antibacterial soap. Administrative: provide training about proper use of PPE. PPE: use gloves, mask, goggles or glasses, one-way rebreather CPR mask.
Nurse sustains needlestick injury while recapping a needle used to obtain blood sample from patient who is HIV positive: risk of infection via transcutaneous route.	Engineering: place puncture-resistant containers in patient's room; label containers properly. Work practice: use one-handed technique or use puncture-resistant container to discard sharps. Administrative: provide training about proper handling and disposal of needles, sharps.
Chemical Hazards	
Hospital pharmacist or nurse prepares antineoplastic agent such as nitrogen mustard: risk of contamination through skin contact or inhalation.	Engineering: install and use exhaust hood in preparation area. Work practice: handle substances cautiously and clean work area carefully after use. Administrative: limit duration of exposures. PPE: use gloves, gown-lab coat, and mask.
Nurse anesthetist works in pediatric operating room: risk of inhaling waste anesthetic gas (such as nitrous oxide).	Engineering: install and use proper room ventilation. Design face masks and endotracheal tubes that will prevent gas leakage. Use gas-scavenging system. Work practice: use scrupulous techniques and maintain equipment properly. Administrative and PPE: adhere to NIOSH-recommended exposure level of no more than 25 ppm of nitrous oxide in an 8-hour time-weighted average.
Technician sterilizes hospital equipment using gas sterilizer: risk of inhaling ethylene oxide (ETO) sterilant gas; possible absorption through skin.	Engineering: install and use appropriate local exhaust system during sterilization. Work practice: perform all work under local exhaust ventilation. Administrative: train health care workers to limit exposure, and implement medical surveillance program for all those who work with ETO. PPE: wear gloves.
Environmental and Mechanical Hazards	
Nurse manager uses computer for scheduling and other documentation tasks: risk of tissue trauma to right hand and wrist (carpal tunnel syndrome).	Engineering: design work station to allow proper body alignment. Work practice: adjust chair height, provide padding for wrists, perform wrist exercises. Administrative: provide job breaks to reduce number of hours of keyboarding.
Housekeeper slips and falls on wet, slippery floor while mopping: risk of musculoskeletal injury.	Engineering: substitute different flooring product that is less slippery when wet or waxed. Work practice: use caution when mopping. Administrative: place signs in area warning of wet floors. PPE: wear rubber-soled shoes.
Floor nurse works rotating 12-hour shifts, experiences sleep deprivation: risk of poor work performance, accident.	Work practice: take steps to ensure adequate rest at home during the day. Administrative: implement scheduling to give workers adequate time off between shift changes; clockwise rotations; train workers about adapting to shift work.

Table continued on next page

TABLE 18-7 Reviewing Control Strategies *Continued*

Work Example	Control Strategies
Physical Hazards	
X-ray technician in early stage of pregnancy is exposed to ionizing radiation during procedures: risk of chromosome damage, birth defects.	Engineering: Configure x-ray unit controls to prevent accidental activation. Work practice: technician leaves the room while films are taken. Administrative: implement policies for female health care workers to prevent exposure to x-rays during pregnancy through job rotation or limit exposure to less than 0.05 cGy per day. PPE: use lead apron (caution about weight of lead apron on abdomen).
Nurse in intensive care unit uses portable cardiac defibrillator to resuscitate patient with congestive heart failure: risk of electrical shock.	Engineering: ensure that defibrillator has functional alarm to warn operator to stand clear of electrical pathway before discharging paddles. Work practice: follow proper defibrillation procedure to avoid shock hazard. Administrative: provide training in proper use of cardiac defibrillator.
Hospital maintenance worker performs general lawn and grounds work: risk of hearing loss from loud mowing equipment.	Engineering: repair-replace noisy machinery; maintain exhaust mufflers, acoustic housings, etc. Administrative: teach proper use of ear protection (plugs or muffs). PPE: use ear protection: plugs or muffs.
Psychosocial Hazards	
Pediatric patient dies in intensive care unit after chronic illness: distress, feelings of guilt, loss, and grief increase risk of emotional fatigue, burnout.	Work practice: recognize own feelings of loss-grief and seek counseling, if needed. Administrative: provide counseling services or support groups for employee to share feelings of grief and loss.
Implementation of new, complex technology generates fears of change, feelings of inadequacy and self-doubt.	Engineering: improve or modify equipment layout or design of work area. Work practice: attend training sessions. Administrative: provide training in how to use new and complex equipment.
Increased workload resulting from staff reductions generates psychophysiologic stress, with fear of job loss and financial insecurity: increased risk of fatigue, burnout.	Work practice: communicate with nursing manager about new work responsibilities and future position. Administrative: provide workers with avenues for career opportunities outside of company (such as a jobs fair, career counseling).

PPE, personal protective equipment; CPR, cardiopulmonary resuscitation, HIV, human immunodeficiency virus; NIOSH, National Institute of Occupational Safety and Health

Engineering controls for *biologic* hazards include using safer needles or needle-free intravascular access devices; placing sharps containers as near as possible to the point of use so that needles do not need to be recapped (one-handed method) or misplaced while other tasks are completed; providing adequate facilities for waste disposal, hand washing, and laundry; and ensuring adequate ventilation, filtration, exhaust, and air exchange rates to prevent the spread of airborne pathogens such as *M. tuberculosis.*

Engineering controls for *chemical* hazards focus on substituting less toxic chemicals, if possible, and on reducing toxic exposures. Fume hoods in clinical laboratories and pharmacies control exposures to formaldehyde, glutaraldehyde, ETO, and other volatile chemicals. Closed gas systems and scavenging units control anesthetic gases in operating rooms. Routine air sampling and sampling when a chemical exposure occurs are essential in determining levels of exposure.

Engineering controls for *physical* hazards include designating areas and rooms where ionizing and nonionizing radiation emissions are likely; placing equipment controls to avoid accidental activation, and providing adequate shielding; and muffling sound with acoustic ceilings, resilient flooring, carpets, and barriers. Complete enclosure of some machinery or placement of machinery outside of the immediate work area will also reduce noise.

Engineering controls for *environmental* and *mechanical* hazards include selection of ergonomically suitable lifting devices and patient transfer aids, computer work stations, and safety devices to reduce physical injury risks from muscle strain and repetitive motion. They also include modifications to reduce the risk of threatening and assaultive patient behavior, such as providing security windows at access points and exit options for threatened workers in the emergency department and installing metal detectors to identify patients who may be carrying weapons.

Engineering controls for *psychosocial* hazards include measures to reduce the stressors affecting nurses working in intensive care units, including equipment failures, high noise levels, and poor physical layout of the work unit.

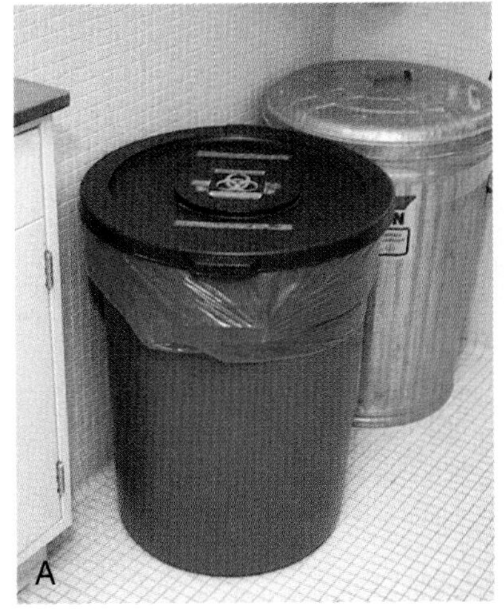

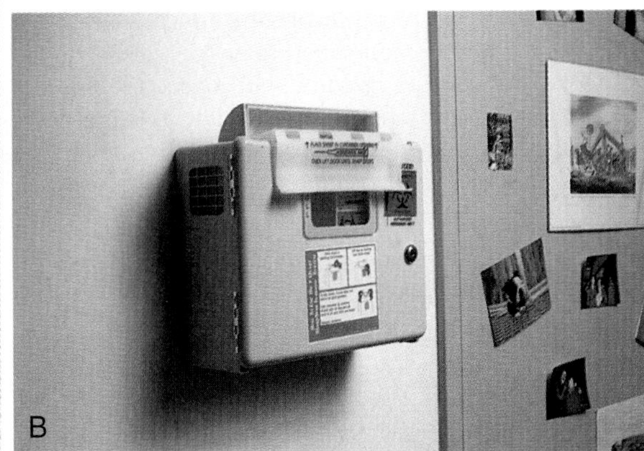

Figure 18-2. Appropriate and properly labeled and located waste (*A*) and sharps (*B*) containers are examples of good work practice controls.

Work practice controls aim to enhance appropriate work practices and modify risk-intensive practices. Examples of work practice controls include practicing good hygiene and good housekeeping, including waste disposal (Fig. 18–2).

Good work practices call for routine equipment maintenance tasks, including lubrication, adjustment, and repair of loose or worn parts, and limitations on the weight of items that must be carried through the use of small trays or handled carryalls. Other examples include use of mechanical devices to alter work practices such that items can be handled without excessive torque or lift and provision of adequate lighting to reduce risks for slips, falls, and injuries from equipment. In addition, a work practice modification for needles that must be recapped, such as needles used for some specialized procedures, is to use a one-handed recapping technique or recapping device.

Administrative Controls

Administrative controls aim to prevent or reduce hazards through institutional modifications such as flexible staffing, rotations, work assignments, and training. When hazardous situations cannot be reduced to acceptable limits through engineering and work practice controls, then administrative controls should be tried (Lewy, 1991; Plog et al, 1988). One of the most important administrative controls involves implementing vaccination programs to protect workers against vaccine-preventable diseases such as measles, rubella, HBV, influenza, and tetanus. Health maintenance, biologic-chemical exposure screening and surveillance programs, and training and education in safety, equipment monitoring and maintenance are also effective administrative controls. Accurate documentation of all procedures and hazardous conditions and substances coupled with careful incident reporting is key to the administrative control program and helps establish useful engineering controls. Agencies that have established numerous administrative guidelines for hazardous risk abatement include OSHA, NIOSH, Environmental Protection Agency, American National Standards Institute, and CDC.

Administrative controls to reduce psychosocial hazards include clearly delineating worker responsibilities and accountability; providing programs for education and counseling about job burnout and death and dying; participative management for decision making to deal with staffing patterns and work overload; communication among administrators, physicians, nurses, and other health care personnel; and implementation of counseling and support programs (Celentano and Johnson, 1987).

Personal Protective Equipment

Personal protective equipment (PPE) is the last resort for worker protection and should be relied on only when hazardous conditions cannot be eliminated through engineering, work practice, or administrative controls. The use of PPE places the burden of protection on the health care worker, who must take the initiative to use the equipment correctly. Administrative controls facilitate this process through written policies and procedures for selection, use, fit, and maintenance and through appropriate training programs and monitoring for compliance.

PPE includes gloves, goggles or other eye protection, face masks of various types, gowns, aprons, laboratory coats, head and foot coverings, lead shielding, hearing protection, and laser goggles or glasses. The CDC has developed specific recommendations for the use of PPE.

Perhaps the most important issue with the use of PPE in reducing the risk of disease transmission by bloodborne pathogens is that the strategies adopted for barrier use are intended primarily to interrupt cross-contamination between and among patients and from patients to health care workers. Strategies for isolation precautions should more strongly emphasize engineering and work practice controls, which have much to offer in dealing with bloodborne pathogens. Additional research needs to be done in this area to influence regulatory agencies to shift their positions to the most cost-effective strategies, and there is considerable room for nursing research in this area as well (Jackson and Lynch, 1995; McPherson et al, 1991).

CHAPTER HIGHLIGHTS

- Occupational hazards are classified as biological, environmental/mechanical, physical, and psychosocial agents, all of which affect the health and safety of patients and nurses.
- Among the specific hazards that nurses face are back injuries; disruptions in biorhythms while working shifts; patient violence; exposure to radiation, noise, stress, and infectious organisms, chemicals, and gases.
- Strategies for controlling occupational health hazards for health care workers include engineering and work practice controls, administrative controls, and personal protective equipment.

REFERENCES

Akerstedt, T. (1984). Work schedules and sleep. *Experientia, 40,* 417–422.

Alter, M.J. (1991). Hepatitis C: a sleeping cat? *American Journal of Medicine, 91* (Suppl 3B), 112–115.

Alter, M.J. (1994). Occupational exposure to hepatitis C virus: a dilemma. *Infection Control and Hospital Epidemiology, 15,* 742–744.

American Association of Critical Care Nurses (1989). *Handbook on Occupational Hazards.*

Arad, D., Ryan, M. (1986). The incidence and prevalence in nurses of low back pain: a definitive survey exposes the hazards. *Australian Nurse Journal, 16,* 44–48.

Arnold, S.D., Alonso, R. (1993). Ribavirin aerosol: methods for reducing employee exposure. *AAOHN, 41*(8), 382–391.

Arnold, S.D., Buchanan, R.M. (1991). Exposure to ribavirin aerosol. *Applied Occupational and Environmental Hygiene, 6*(4), 271–279.

Balcarek, K.B., Bagley, R., Cloud, G.A., Pass, R.F. (1990). Cytomegalovirus infection in employees of a children's hospital: no evidence for increased risk associated with patient care. *Journal of the American Medical Association, 263,* 840–844.

Becker, M.H., Janz, N.K., Band, J., et al. (1990). Noncompliance with universal precautions policy: why do physicians and nurses recap needles? *American Journal of Infection Control, 17*(46), 232–239.

Benenson, A.S. (ed.) (1995). *Control of Communicable Diseases in Man,* 15th ed. Washington, DC: American Public Health Association.

Bloch, A.B., Orenstein, W.A., Ewing, W.M., et al. (1985). Measles outbreak in a pediatric practice: airborne transmission in an office setting. *Pediatrics, 75,* 676–683.

Brice, J. (1990). Confronting drug abuse on the job. *Healthcare Forum Journal, 1,* 25–29.

Brodsky, J., Cohen, E. (1985). Health experiences of operating room personnel. *Anesthesiology, 68,* 461–463.

Buckler, G.F. (1995). Environmental hazards for the nurse as a worker. In A.M. Pope, M.A. Snyder, and L.H. Mood (eds.): *Nursing, Health, and the Environment.* Washington, DC: National Academy Press, pp. 134–141.

Caldwell, M.F. (1992). Incidence of PTSD among staff victims of patient violence. *Hospital and Community Psychiatry, 43*(8), 838–839.

Carmel, H., Hunter, M. (1989). Staff injuries from inpatient violence. *Hospital and Community Psychiatry, 40*(1), 41–46.

Carney, R.M. (1993). Protect your nursing athletes! *Nursing Management, 24*(3), 69–71.

Catanzaro, A. (1982). Nosocomial tuberculosis. *American Review of Respiratory Diseases, 125,* 559–562.

Celentano, D.D., Johnson, J.V. (1987). Stress in health care workers. *Occupational Medicine: State of the Art Reviews, 2*(3), 593–608.

Centers for Disease Control (1983a). Guideline for infection control in hospital personnel. *Infection Control, 4*(4), 326–349.

Centers for Disease Control (1983b). Guideline for isolation precautions in hospitals. *Infection Control, 4*(4), 245–325.

Centers for Disease Control (1984). Rubella prevention. *Morbidity and Mortality Weekly Report, 33,* 301–323.

Centers for Disease Control (1988a). Update: universal precautions for prevention of transmission of human immunodeficiency virus, hepatitis B, and other bloodborne pathogens in health-care settings. *Morbidity and Mortality Weekly Report, 37,* 378–388.

Centers for Disease Control (1988b). Assessing exposures of health-care personnel to aerosols of ribavirin—California. *Morbidity and Mortality Weekly Report, 37,* 560–563.

Centers for Disease Control (1988c). Update: acquired immunodeficiency syndrome and human immunodeficiency virus infection among health-care workers. *Morbidity and Mortality Weekly Report, 37,* 229–239.

Centers for Disease Control (1989). Measles prevention: recommendations of the Immunization Practices Advisory Committee (ACIP). *Morbidity and Mortality Weekly Report, 38,* 1–18.

Centers for Disease Control (1990a). Guidelines for preventing the transmission of tuberculosis in health-care settings, with special focus on HIV-related issues. *Morbidity and Mortality Weekly Report, 39*(RR-17), 1–29.

Centers for Disease Control (1990b). Hepatitis surveillance (report 53). Atlanta: Author, pp. 1–36.

Centers for Disease Control (1990c). Protection against viral hepatitis: recommendations of the Advisory Committee on Immunization Practices (ACIP). *Morbidity and Mortality Weekly Report, 39*(RR-2), 1–26.

Centers for Disease Control (1991a). Nosocomial transmission of multi-drug-resistant tuberculosis among HIV-infected persons—Florida and New York, 1988–1991. *Morbidity and Mortality Weekly Report, 40,* 585–591.

Centers for Disease Control (1991b). Update on adult immunizations: recommendations for the Advisory Committee on Immunization Practices (ACIP). *Morbidity and Mortality Weekly Report, 40*(RR-12), 1–94.

Centers for Disease Control (1992a). *Cytomegalovirus: Circumstances When CMV Infection Could Be a Problem.* Atlanta: Author.

Centers for Disease Control (1992b). Prevention and control of influenza: Recommendations of the Advisory Committee on

Immunization Practices (ACIP). *Morbidity and Mortality Weekly Report,* 41(RR-9), 1–17.

Centers for Disease Control (1992c). Recommendations for prophylaxis against *Pneumocystis carinii* pneumonia for adults and adolescents infected with human immunodeficiency virus. *Morbidity and Mortality Weekly Report, 41*(RR-4), 1–11.

Centers for Disease Control (1992d). The second 100,000 cases of acquired immunodeficiency syndrome—United States, June 1981–December 1991. *Morbidity and Mortality Weekly Report, 41,* 585–591.

Centers for Disease Control and Prevention (1996). *Disease Burden from Viral Hepatitis A, B, and C in the United States.* Atlanta: Author.

Centers for Disease Control and Prevention (1998). *HIV/AIDS Surveillance Report,* 9(2).

Centers for Disease Control and National Institute for Occupational Safety and Health (1988). *Guidelines for Protecting the Safety and Health of Health Care Workers* (DHHS [NIOSH] publication no. 88–119). Washington, DC: U.S. Government Printing Office.

Coffey, L.C., Skipper, J.K., Jung, F.D. (1988). Nurses and shiftwork: effects on job performance and job related stress. *Journal of Advanced Nursing, 13,* 245–254.

Cohen, B., Brady, M. (1992). Practices surrounding ribavirin administration. *Pediatrics Nursing, 18*(3), 253–257.

Cohen, R. (1990). Injuries due to physical hazards. In J. LaDou (ed.): *Occupational Medicine.* San Mateo, CA: Appleton & Lange, pp. 106–130.

Demmler, G.J., Spector, S.A., Reis, S.G., et al. (1987). Nosocomial cytomegalovirus infections within two hospitals caring for infants and children. *Journal of Infectious Diseases, 156,* 9–16.

Doering, L. (1990). Recruitment and retention: successful strategies in critical care. *Heart and Lung, 19*(3), 220–224.

Drusin, L.M., Sohmer, M., Groshen, S.L., et al. (1987). Nosocomial hepatitis A infection in a pediatric intensive care unit. *Archives of Diseases in Children, 62,* 690–695.

Edgar, W.M., Campbell, A.D. (1985). Nosocomial infection with hepatitis A. *Journal of Infections, 10,* 43–47.

English, J.F. (1992). Reported hospital needlestick injuries in relation to knowledge/skill, design, and management problems. *Infection Control and Hospital Epidemiology, 13*(5), 259–264.

Falck, K., Grohn, P., Sorsa, M., et al. (1979). Mutagenicity in urine of nurses handling cytotoxic drugs. *Lancet, June 9; 1*(8128): 1250–1251.

Falk, S.A., Wood, N.F. (1973). Hospital noise-levels and potential health hazards. *New England Journal of Medicine, 289,* 774–781.

Fielding, J., Weaver, S.M. (1984). A comparison of hospital- and community based mental health nurses: perceptions of their work environment and psychological health. *Journal of Advanced Nursing, 19*(6), 1196–1204.

Fineberg, N.A., James, D.V., Shah, A.K. (1988). Agency nurses and violence in a psychiatric ward. *Lancet, Feb. 27; 1*(8583): 474.

Folkard, S., Condon, R., Herbert, M. (1984). Night shift paralysis. *Experientia, 40,* 510–512.

Frazier, L.M., Thomann, W.R., Jackson, G.W. (1995). Occupational hazards in the hospital, doctor's office, and other health care facilities. *North Carolina Medical Journal, 56*(5), 1–7.

Gardam, J.E.D. (1969). Nursing stresses in the intensive care unit (letter). *Journal of the American Medical Association, 208*(12), 2337–2338.

Garner, J.S. (1996). Guidelines for isolation precautions in hospitals: evaluation of isolation practices. *American Journal of Infection Control, 24,* 24–52.

Gerberding, J.L. (1995). Management of occupational exposures to blood-borne viruses. *New England Journal of Medicine, 332*(7), 444–449.

Gerberding, J.L., Bryant-LeBlanc, C.E., Nelson, K., et al. (1987). Risk of transmitting the human immunodeficiency virus, cytomegalovirus, and hepatitis B virus to health care workers exposed to patients with AIDS and AIDS-related conditions. *Journal of Infectious Diseases, 156,* 1–8.

Glazner, L.K. (1991). Shiftwork and its affects on workers. *AAOHN Journal, 39,* 416–421.

Goodman, R.A., Carder, C.C., Allen, J.R., et al. (1982). Nosocomial hepatitis A transmission by an adult patient with diarrhea. *American Journal of Medicine, 72,* 220–226.

Gray-Toft, P., Anderson, J.G. (1981). Stress among hospital nursing staff: Its causes and effects. *Social Science and Medicine, 15A,* 639–647.

Greaves, W.L., Kaiser, A.B., Alford, R.H., Schaffner, W. (1980). The problem of herpetic whitlow among hospital personnel. *Infection Control, 1,* 381–385.

Greenwood, J.G. (1986). Back injuries can be reduced with worker training, reinforcement. *Occupational Health and Safety, 55*(5), 26–29.

Harber, P., Billet, E., Gutowski, M., et al. (1985). Occupational low-back pain in hospital nurses. *Journal of Occupational Medicine, 27,* 518–524.

Harma, M., et al. (1986). The effect of physical fitness intervention on adaptation to shiftwork. In M. Haider, M. Koller, and R. Cervinka (eds.): *Night and Shift Work: Long-Term Effects and Their Prevention.* Frankfurt: Peter Lang, pp. 221–228.

Harvey, B.J., Hannah, T.E. (1986). The relationship of shift work to nurses' satisfaction and perceived work performance. *Canadian Journal of Nursing Research, 18,* 5–14.

Hay, D., Oken, D. (1972). The psychological stresses of intensive care unit nursing. *Psychosomatic Medicine, 34*(2), 109–118.

Hemminki, K., Mutanen, P. (1982). Spontaneous abortions in hospital staff engaged in sterilizing instruments with chemical agents. *British Medical Journal, 285,* 1461–1463.

Hilchey, T. (1996). Nurse with HIV emphasizes safety. *New York Times,* February 28, A-15.

Hodgson, B., Kizior, R., Kingdon, R. (1997). *Nurses Drug Handbook.* Philadelphia: W.B. Saunders.

Huckabay, L., Jagla, B. (1979). Nurses' stress factors in the intensive care unit. *Journal of Nursing Administration, 1,* 21–26.

Iseman, M.D. (1992). A leap of faith: what can we do to curtail intrainstitutional transmission of tuberculosis? *Annals of Internal Medicine, 117,* 251–253.

Jackson, M.M. (1989). Implementing universal body substance precautions. *Occupational Medicine: State of the Art Reviews, 4*(Special Issue), 39–44.

Jackson, M.M. (1992). The facts about methicillin-resistant *Staphylococcus aureus. Today's OR Nurse, 14*(10), 15–21.

Jackson, M.M., Checko, P.J. (1983). Section one: epidemiology and statistics. In B.M. Soule (ed.): *The APIC Curriculum for Infection Control Practice.* Dubuque, IA: Kendall/Hunt Publishing, pp. 8–127.

Jackson, M.M., Emerson, S.C. (1979). Paronychial infections in nurses in clinical practice: a questionnaire survey. *Association for Practitioners in Infection Control Journal, 7,* 16–19.

Jackson, M.M., Lynch, P. (1995). Development of a numeric health care worker risk assessment scale to evaluate potential for blood-borne pathogen exposures. *American Journal of Infection Control, 23*(3), 13–21.

Jagger, J. (1994). A new opportunity to make the health care workplace safer. *Advances in Exposure Prevention, 1*(1), 1–2.

Jagger, J., Hunt, E.H., Brand-Elnaggar, J., Pearson, R.D. (1988). Rates of needlestick injury caused by various devices in a university hospital. *New England Journal of Medicine, 319,* 284–288.

Jagger, J., Hunt, E.H., Pearson, R.D. (1990). Sharp object injuries in the hospital: causes and strategies for prevention. *American Journal of Infection Control, 18,* 227–231.

Jay, W.M., Swift, T.R. (1982). Possible relationship of ethylene oxide exposure to cataract formation. *American Journal of Ophthalmology, 93, 727–732.*

Jeffers, L.J., Perez, G.O., deMedina, M.D., et al. (1990). Hepatitis C infection in two urban hemodialysis units. *Kidney International, 38,* 320–322.

Jensen, R.C. (1987). Disabling back injuries among nursing personnel: research needs justification. *Research in Nursing and Health, 10,* 29–38.

Jorgensen, S., Hein, H.O., Gyntelberg, F. (1994). Heavy lifting at work and risk of genital prolapse and herniated lumbar disk in assistant nurses. *Occupational Medicine, 44*(1), 47–49.

Jung, F. (1986). Shiftwork: its effect on health performance and well-being. AAOHN Journal, 34(4), 160–164.

Krober, M.S., Bass, J.W., Brown, J.D., et al. (1984). Hospital outbreak of hepatitis A: risk factors for spread. *Pediatric Infectious Diseases, 3,* 296–299.

LaDou, J. (1982). Health effects on shiftwork. *Western Journal of Medicine, 137*(6), *525–529.*

LaDou, J. (1990). *Occupational Medicine.* Norwalk, CT: Appleton & Lange.

Lancaster, E. (1991). Tuberculosis in the OR. *Today's OR Nurse, 13*(10), 31–35.

Lanza, M.L. (1983). The reactions of nursing staff to physical assault by a patient. *Hospital and Community Psychiatry, 34*(1), 44–47.

Larise, F., Fiorito, A. (1994). Musculoskeletal disorders in hospital nurses: a comparison between two hospitals. *Ergonomics, 37*(7), 1205–1211.

Lavoie, F.W., Carter, G.L., Danzl, D.F., Berg, R.L. (1988). Emergency department violence in United States teaching hospitals. *Annals of Emergency Medicine, 17,* 1227–1233.

Leppanen, R.A., Olkinuora, M.A. (1987). Psychological stress experienced by health care personnel. *Scandinavian Journal of Work and Environmental Health, 13,* 1–8.

Lettau, L.A. (1992). The A, B, C, D, and E of viral hepatitis: spelling out the risks for healthcare workers. *Infection Control and Hospital Epidemiology, 13, 77*–81.

Lettau, L.A., Alfred, H.J., Glew, R.H., et al. (1986). Nosocomial transmission of delta hepatitis. *Annals of Internal Medicine, 104,* 631–635.

Levy, B.S., Wegman, D.H. (1993). *Occupational Health: Recognizing and Preventing Work-Related Diseases,* 3rd ed. Boston: Little, Brown.

Lewy, R.M. (1991). *Employees at Risk: Protecting the Health of the Health Care Worker.* New York: Van Nostrand Reinhold.

Lipscomb, J.A., Love, C.C. (1992). Violence toward health care workers: an emerging occupational hazard. *American Association of Occupational Health Nurses Journal, 40*(5), 219–228.

Lynch, P., Cummings, M.J., Roberts, P.L., et al. (1990). Implementing and evaluating a system of generic information precautions: body substance isolation. *American Journal of Infection Control, 18,* 1–12.

MacNeil, J.M., Weisz, G.M. (1987). Critical care nursing stress: another look. *Heart and Lung, 16*(3), *274–277.*

Mahoney, B.S. (1991). The extent, nature, and response to victimization of emergency room nurses in Pennsylvania. *Journal of Emergency Nursing, 17,* 282–294.

Marchett, J.M., Weisz, G.M. (1987). Critical care nursing stress. *Orthopaedic Nursing, 4*(6), 25–29.

Marcus, R.A., Tokars, J.I., Culver, P.S., McKibben, D.M. (1991). *Zidovudine Use After Occupational Exposure to HIV-Infected Blood* (abstract 979). Presented at the 31st Interscience Conference on Antimicrobal Agents and Chemotherapy (ICAAC), Chicago.

McAbee, R. (1988). Nursing and back injuries. *AAOHN Journal, 36,* 200–209.

McPherson, D.C., Jackson, M.M., Rogers, J.C. (1991). Evaluating the cost of the body substance isolation system. *Journal of Healthcare Material Management, 6*(6), 20–28.

Monk, T.H. (1987) Shiftwork, determinants of coping ability and areas of application. In J.M. Hekkens, G.A. Kerkhof, and W.J. Rietveld (eds.): *Advances in Biosciences: Vol. 73. Trends in Chronobiology.* New York: Pergamon Press, pp. 195–207.

Moore-Ede, M.C., Richardson, G.S. (1985). Medical implications of shiftwork. *Annual Review of Medicine, 36, 607–617.*

National Council on Radiation Protection and Measurement (1987). *Ionizing Radiation Exposure of the Population of the United States.* Washington, DC: Author, p. 93.

National Council on Radiation Protection Measurement (1987). *Recommendations on Limits for Exposure to Ionization.* (NCRP Report No. 91) Bethesda MD: National Council on Radiation Protection.

National Institute for Occupational Safety and Health (1977). *Occupational Exposure to Waste Anesthetic Gases and Vapors.* Cincinnati, OH: DHEW.

National Institute for Occupational Safety and Health (1988). *Guidelines for Protecting the Safety and Health of Health Care Workers* (bulletin 2259). Washington, DC: Author.

Neuberger, J.S., Harris, J. Knudin, N.D., et al. (1984). Incidence of needlestick injuries in hospital personnel: implications for prevention. *American Journal of Infection Control, 12,* 171–176.

Newman, S., Callaghan, C. (1993). Work-related back pain. *Occupational Health, 45,* 201–205.

Nikula, E., Kivinitty, K., Leist, J. (1984). Chromosome aberrations in lymphocytes of nurses handling cytostatic agents. *Scandinavian Journal of Work and Environmental Health, 10,* 71.

Nishiyamja, H., Lukes, S.J., Feller, P.A., et al. (1980). Survey of 99mTc contamination of laboratory personnel: its degree and routes. *Radiology, 135,* 467–471.

Nuclear Regulatory Commission (1974). *Standards for Protection Against Radiation.* Washington, D.C.: Nuclear Regulatory Commission.

Owen, B.D. (1989). The magnitude of low-back problems in nursing. *Western Journal of Nursing Research, 11*(2), 234–242.

Owen, B.D., Garg, A. (1991). Reducing risk for back injury in nursing personnel. *AAOHN Journal, 39*(1), 24–33.

Plog, B.A., Benjamin, G.S., Kerwin, M.A. (1988). *Fundamentals of Industrial Hygiene,* 3rd ed. Chicago: National Safety Council.

Polk, B.F., White, J.A., DeGirolamki, P.C., Modlin, J.F. (1980). An outbreak of rubella among hospital personnel. *New England Journal of Medicine, 303,* 541–545.

Rees, D., Cooper, C.L. (1992). Occupational stress in health service workers in the UK. *Stress Medicine, 8*(2), 79–90.

Rix, G. (1987). Staff sickness and its relationship to violent incidents on a regional secure psychiatric unit. *Journal of Advanced Nursing, 12*(2), 223–228.

Rodriguez, W.J., Dang Bui, R.H., Connor, J.D., et al. (1987). Environmental exposure of primary care personnel to ribavirin aerosol when supervising treatment of infants with respiratory syncytial virus infection. *Antimicrobial Agents and Chemotherapy, 31*(7), 1143–1146.

Rogers, B. (1987). Work practices of nurses who handle antineoplastic agents. *AAOHN Journal, 35*(1), 24.

Rogers, B., Emmett, E.A. (1987a). Handling antineoplastic agents: urine mutagenicity in nurses. *Image: Journal of Nursing Scholarship, 19,* 108–113.

Rogers, B., Travers, P. (1991). Occupational hazards of critical care nursing. Overview of work-related hazards in nursing: health and safety issues. *Heart and Lung, 20*(5), 486–499.

Rosenblum, L.S., Villarino, M.E., Nainan, O.V., et al. (1991). Hepatitis A outbreak in a neonatal intensive care unit: risk factors for transmission and evidence of prolonged viral excretion among preterm infants. *Journal of Infectious Diseases, 164,* 476–482.

Rosenstock, L., Cullin, M. (1994). *Textbook of Clinical Occupational and Environmental Medicine.* Philadelphia: W.B. Saunders.

Rutala, W.A., Hamory, B.H. (1989). Expanding role of hospital epidemiology: employee health—chemical exposure in the health care setting. *Infection Control and Hospital Epidemiology, 10*(6), 261–266.

Schimpff, S., Serpick, A., Stoler, B., et al. (1972). Varicella-zoster infection in patients with cancer. *Annals of Internal Medicine, 76,* 241–254.

Scott, A.J., LaDou, J. (1990). Shiftwork: effects on sleep and health with recommendations for medical surveillance and screening. *Occupational Medicine State of the Art Reviews, 5,* 273–300.

Selevan, S.G., Lindbohlm, M.L., Hornung, R.W., Hemminki, K. (1985). A study of occupational exposure to antineoplastic drugs and fetal loss in nurses. *New England Journal of Medicine, 313*(19), 1173–1178.

Sherertz, R.J., Hampton, A.L. (1987). Infection control aspects of hospital employee health. In R.P. Wenzel (ed.): *Prevention and Control of Nosocomial Infection.* Baltimore: Williams & Wilkins, pp. 175–204.

Siebenaler, M.J., McGovern, P. (1992). Carpal tunnel syndrome priorities for prevention. *AAOHN Journal, 40*(2), 62–71.

Smith, E., Welch, W., Berhow, M., Wong, V.K. (1990). Measles susceptibility of hospital employees as determined by ELISA. *Clinical Research, 38,* 183A.

Snellings, W.M., Maronpat, R.R., Zalenak, J.P., Laffon, C.P. (1982). Teratology study in Fischer 344 rats exposed to ethylene oxide by inhalation for one generation. *Toxicology and Applied Pharmacology, 63,* 383–388.

Stearn, H., Elek, S.D., Millar, M.D., Anderson, H.F. (1959). Herpetic whitlow: a form of cross-infection in hospitals. *Lancet, 2,* 871–874.

Tepas, D.I. (1982). Work/sleep time schedules and performance. In W.B. Webb (ed.): *Biological Rhythms, Sleep and Performance.* New York: Wiley, pp. 175–200.

Upton, A.C. (1982). The biological effects of low-level ionizing radiation. *Scientific American, 246,* 41–49.

U.S. Department of Health and Human Services, Centers for Disease Control, National Institute for Occupational Safety and Health (1987a). *Guidelines for Protecting the Health and Safety of Health Care Workers* (DDHS [NIOSH] publication no. 88–119). Washington, DC: U.S. Government Printing Office.

U.S. Department of Health and Human Services, Centers for Disease Control, National Institute for Occupational Safety and Health (1987b). *A Report from the Division of Surveillance, Hazard Evaluations, and Field Study Task Force on Hospital Worker Health.* Washington, DC: U.S. Department of Health and Human Services.

U.S. Department of Labor (1984). Occupational exposure to ethylene oxide: final standard. *Federal Register, 49,* 25734–25809.

U.S. Department of Labor, Bureau of Labor Statistics (1984). *Occupational Employment in Selected Nonmanufacturing Industries.* Washington, DC: Author.

U.S. Department of Labor (1986). *Guidelines for Cytotoxic (Antineoplastic) Drugs.* Washington, D.C.: U.S. Department of Labor.

U.S. Department of Labor, Bureau of Labor Statistics (1991). *Occupational Injuries and Illnesses in the United States by Industry, 1989* (bulletin 2379). Washington, DC: Author.

U.S. Department of Labor, Bureau of Labor Statistics (1994). *Issues in Labor Statistics* (summary 94-6). Washington, DC: Author.

U.S. Department of Labor, Occupational Safety and Health Administration (1991). Final rule (29 CFR Part 1910.1030). *Federal Register, 56.*

U.S. Government Printing Office (1976). CFR. 1910.95 Noise Standard. Washington, DC: Author.

Van Ameringen, M.R., Arsenault, A., Dolan, S.L. (1988). Intrinsic job stress and diastolic blood pressure among female hospital workers. *Journal of Occupational Medicine, 30*(2), 93–97.

Vreeland, R., Ellis, G.L. (1969). Stresses on the nurse in an intensive-care unit. *Journal of the American Medical Association, 208*(2), 332–334.

Wasserberger, J., Ordog, G.J., Kolodny, M., Allen, K. (1989). Violence in a community emergency room. *Archives of Emergency Medicine, 6,* 266–269.

Willy, M.E., Dhillon, G.L., Loewen, N.L., et al. (1990). Adverse exposures and universal precautions practices among a group of highly exposed health professionals. *Infection Control and Hospital Epidemiology, 11*(7), 351–356.

Health of the Nursing Student

Sarah E. Porter and Anita Lohman

It was 1 hour before the midterm exam. Five nursing students were gathered together over coffee. "I can't look at these notes for 1 more minute. I was up until 3 A.M. cramming. I can't seem to get my life organized. After graduating from the university, I thought nursing school would be very manageable. Maybe I'm getting burned out. This is my fifth year of college." This was Sally, 22 years old and single. She lived in the residence hall.

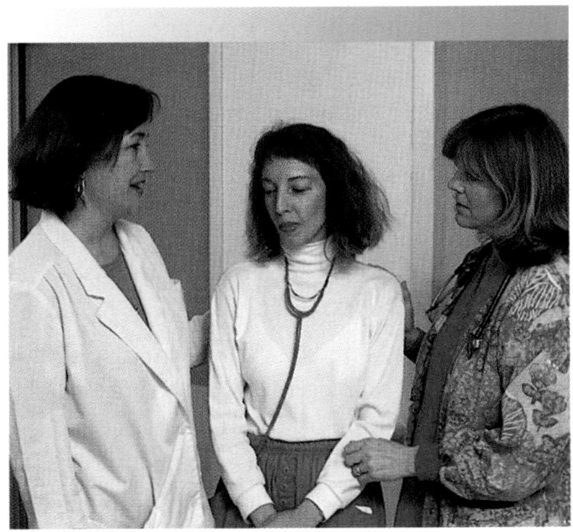

"Lucky you," said Lucy, a 36-year-old single mother. "My 18-month-old decided to get an earache last night, and I ended up in the ER trying to get some medication, again! I got some studying done because I had to wait for 2 hours. It is a good thing I dropped being manager of little league. I guess I will just have to go with what I know. It's too late now to put anything else into my poor tired brain."

"I thought I saw you last night around midnight in the ER," Robert interjected. "I had to work a full shift; they couldn't find anyone else and Sunday night is always busy. These two night shifts a week are killing me. Before I came to nursing school I thought it would be easy. Little did I know. When I was in Nam as a medic, I would stay up for 24 or 36 hours sometimes. I was 19. At 48 it is a little different. Just you wait, you'll see. I'm afraid I am going to flunk out. Ironic, isn't it? The only way I can go to school is to work, and if I work I can't make my grades."

Lisa, 28, chimed in, "I'm worried about my grades, too. My whole family—from my mom to my husband and children—really want me to be a nurse, but they don't seem to understand that I have to study, read, write papers, and practice skills. They keep asking and expecting me to do all the things I did before I came to this school, including working at my parents' restaurant. I get interrupted so many times I can't produce one coherent thought. I'm completely stressed out."

Finally, Markesha speaks. "Listen up, you guys. I can't believe what I am hearing. I thought I was the only one to have so many pushes and pulls on my time. I thought I was the only one trying to balance and juggle all the pieces of my life. I was beginning to wonder whether I made the right choice, what I've

PRACTICE OBJECTIVES

After studying this chapter, the student will be able to:

- **identify a number of stressors in your life and sort out those that are appraised as threatening, harmful, and challenging**
- **define self-care activities you are currently performing, and list additional activities that might enhance your well-being and promote your own health**
- **investigate new coping strategies by observing how peers and faculty handle situations**
- **practice ways of becoming more self-reflective**
- **gain insight into the myriad choices you have for directing your life**
- **gain a new understanding of how your own self-care enhances your nursing practice**

done to myself. Every time my instructor watches me do a new skill, I want to crawl in a hole. It is so hard."

Lucy jumps in, "I know what you mean, Markesha. I feel the same way. I was almost ready to quit, when I had the most wonderful experience with my client. She was so appreciative of my care. That experience made me reevaluate what I was doing. Now, whenever I get discouraged I think of that experience, and it keeps me going."

SCOPE OF NURSING PRACTICE

Being able to care for others, to connect with others in a meaningful way, depends fundamentally on care for one's self. (Chinn, 1994, p. 426)

Nursing students joke about not seeing the dining room table for months because it is stacked with books. They spend long evening hours preparing for the next day's clinical experience. Learning psychomotor skills in public and being closely supervised by faculty and staff nurses can create feeling of being overwhelmed and threatened (Kushner, 1986). Students may feel self-conscious about having to find a private place to cry alone after a patient dies because the topic never came up in postconference.

By definition, the student nurse's learning experience is fraught with stress and stressful events. Nursing is more challenging than ever. Today's patients are, on average, older and sicker. The threat of acquired immunodeficiency syndrome (AIDS) looms large from the pediatric clinics to the geriatric wards. Ethical dilemmas must be solved each day; the bureaucratic and financial complexities of managed care increase the turmoil and ambiguity of the health care setting. Along with the joys and sorrows of caring for patients comes the task of juggling school and family demands, finances, and personal needs, all of which arise in new and intense ways (Julian, 1990). The dual challenges of learning to be a nursing student and learning to be a nurse may leave a person wondering how to develop quickly new coping strategies that will ensure success as a student and competence as a nurse (Porter-Tibbetts, 1992).

The will to put nursing first in one's life comes very easily for most nursing students and many nurses. However, scholastic success and professional competence may come at a high price. At times, caring for another person is an invigorating and self-nurturing experience. At other times, one may feel mentally and physically drained. Instead of confidence comes self-doubt, confusion, and shame.

As a student, attempts to meet one's standards in all areas of one's life tends to generate ever-increasing mental and physical demands. These demands can be met in either of two ways. First, students and nurses may try to cope with the workload, anxiety, and stress in ways that damage their personal health through "workaholism," smoking, poor diet, or alcohol or drug abuse. Eventually, these unhealthy practices lead to physical, emotional, and mental exhaustion, or "burnout" (Fig. 19–1). Burnout is defined as physical, emotional, and mental exhaustion (Pines et al, 1981). Unless this situation is corrected, it can progress to tardiness, absenteeism, errors, vague somatic problems, staff conflicts, transfer requests, and finally exit from the profession.

Alternatively, students and nurses can learn to care for themselves as much as they care for others. A balance can be struck by providing for one's own needs. The student and the nurse can continue to give effective care to others throughout their career. This requires new and different attitudes and habits (Jarrett, 1993).

The second of these approaches, the focus of this chapter, is called *self-care*. Self-care is not to be confused with Orem's

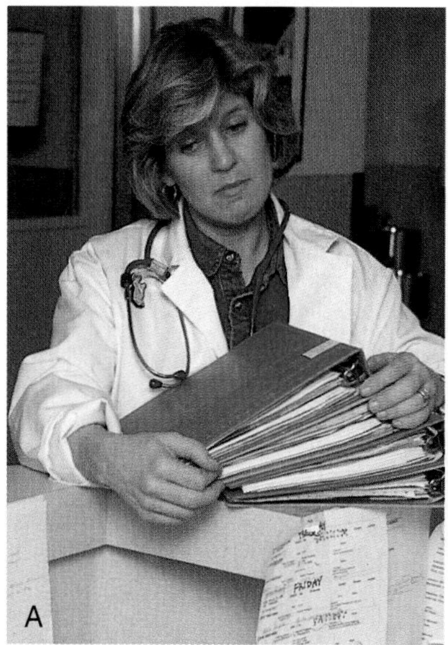

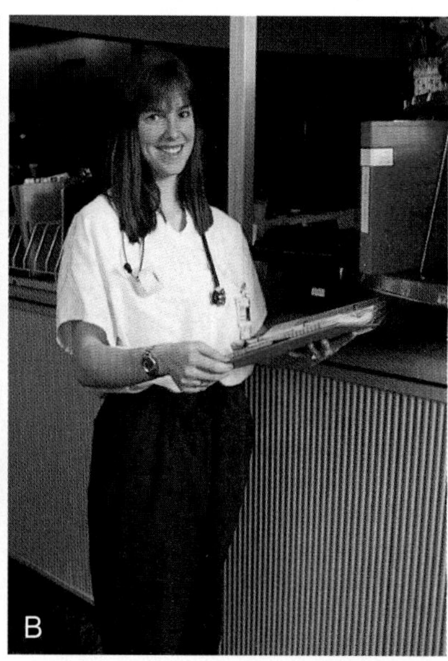

Figure 19–1. Burnout—physical, mental, and emotional exhaustion—is a serious problem in nursing (*A*). Good self-care helps keep a nurse's career on track (*B*).

(1980) definition of self-care: levels of nursing care activities performed depending on the ability of the client to provide self-care. Nursing's main interest traditionally has focused on teaching patients how to perform their own self-care (Johns, 1991). In this chapter, self-care means that caring for one's self is just as essential to the caring process as caring for the patient.

Nursing is a profession that identifies caring for others as its primary mission, yet it is only recently that self-care of the caregiver has gained attention. Self-care requires that one understand one's physical, emotional, cognitive, social, and spiritual needs. Self-care also requires that one finds functional effective ways of meeting these needs. Caring for oneself also requires love and respect for the self, together with the recognition of one's personal limits and boundaries. Caring for others and caring for oneself must be balanced so that caring for others does not come at the expense of caring for oneself. Awareness of personal vulnerabilities and strengths, together with awareness of risks, opportunities, and pressures associated with nursing school and nursing, will help nursing students recognize what steps are needed to strengthen self-care practices and coping activities while in nursing school.

Self-care is an activity influenced by one's individual differences (e.g., age, personality, gender, and cultural and linguistic background). Self-care is also influenced by the broader context of the interdependence of one's changing social setting. Self-care includes the facets of health promotion, self-knowledge, and coping.

In addition to the obvious need to take care of oneself, the practice of self-care has professional implications. Personal self-care and health practices affect a nurse's ability to serve as a model or exemplar for patients. Nurses influence their patients and students not only by what they say but also by what they do. For example, a nurse who smokes is not likely to confront a patient's smoking; nor can a nurse who overworks or neglects to diet or exercise properly hope to convince a student of the stress-reducing benefits of a balanced lifestyle, proper diet, and exercise.

It is important to understand the dynamics of self-care and its foundation composed of the related concepts of self-knowledge and coping, and their use in health promotion. All of these concepts can help the nursing student understand better how to recognize and avoid the harmful effects of stress and find healthful responses to stress.

KNOWLEDGE BASE

Basic Science

STRESS, COGNITIVE APPRAISAL, AND COPING

Traditional theories of stress were cause and effect based, sometimes referred to as "knee-jerk" or stimulus-response. Researchers discovered small events called hassles can have as much impact as a major life event such as divorce and that not everyone reacts to the same events with the same outcome (Lazarus and Folkman, 1984). In addition, outcomes to stress can be short term or long term and can in and of themselves lead to additional stress. Stress tends to be a reciprocal, circular process. (See Chapter 31, Stress and Anxiety, for more information.) Hassles are those numerous small events that are inconvenient, irritating, or demanding (e.g., waiting in traffic, waiting for an elevator, losing one's wallet, having the copy machine break down, maintaining constant vigilance to stay safe while walking, or having to redo a financial aid form). Mounting numbers of hassles can constitute a stressful event.

Current theories of stress state that between an event that looks like it could be stressful and the outcome are several *mediating forces* that can modify the impact of the event. Mediating forces can occur on three levels: social, psychological, and physical. Examples of mediating forces are social support (social), cognitive appraisal (psychological), and immune resources (physical).

Social support often buffers the impact of stressful events when they occur. For example, nurses tended to view a work situation as more of an exciting challenge when they also experienced work-related social support (Pagana, 1990).

Cognitive appraisal is a mediating force between an event that could be stressful and the actual outcome of the potentially stressful event. How one appraises the event and how one sizes up one's own resources to meet the situation play an important role in the outcome of the event. Sizing up the event and sizing up one's resources are cognitive appraisal schemes that are accessible to self-scrutiny and choice. Becoming aware of one's appraisal schemes, how they are applied, and how to change one's appraisal is pivotal in learning to manage stress.

Immune responses as mediating forces are the current focus for psychoneuroimmunology research. Immune responses like cognitive appraisal have the potential for influence by an individual's action.

Coping strategies will vary depending on the situation and the person. The classic example: in anticipating an examination, students will enact a set of coping skills such as problem solving; during the exam, they may use various methods to stay focused, and after the exam they may distract themselves until they find out the results. No one coping strategy would be appropriate for the whole process (Folkman and Lazarus, 1985). Some coping strategies are more useful in general than others. Smoking, alcohol, and over- or undereating have short-term consequences of dulling the pain, distracting, or reducing tension. The short- and long-term consequences create further hassles, requiring more effort to manage, and in the long run contribute to serious health problems.

The significance to nursing students is that it is possible to make creative choices about one's lifestyle to modify the daily hassles. It is also possible to identify, analyze, and modify one's cognitive appraisal schemas to reduce stress. A broad range of strategy options for self-care are available to nursing students.

Relevant Research

NURSING RESEARCH

The nursing literature is beginning to legitimize and value self-care among nurses (Beck, 1991; Hutchinson, 1987; Jarrett, 1993; Kairns, 1992; Leininger and Watson, 1990;

Yovanovich, 1991; Zimmerman, 1991). Even so, rigorous conceptual development is lacking. By reviewing current research and literature about the self and care related to the nurse, one can begin to construct a framework of understanding that includes nurses' own concerns.

In works such as those just cited, nurses are being urged to attend to their mental health, assess their coping strategies, pay attention to physical symptoms, be realistic in their expectations, take a break from work, exercise regularly, reward themselves, and just plain laugh at themselves. They are learning to be assertive, to establish appropriate boundaries (Seed, 1995), to share their feelings with someone they trust, and to accept their own imperfections.

SELF-CARE

As might be expected, nurses' reactions to the self-care idea range from indifference to enthusiastic action. Hutchinson (1987) described a "continuum" of self-care attitudes and practices. At one end of this continuum are nurses who are reactive rather than proactive. They respond to situations emotionally or by rote and do not engage in self-reflection or analysis. Reactive nurses do not see their on-the-job behaviors as related to self-care. In the middle range of the continuum are nurses who are younger or new to the nursing profession. They react to events without forethought; however, they later reflect on the events, analyze the appropriateness and effectiveness of their behaviors, and use the data to plan alternative approaches if confronted with similar situations. Finally, Hutchinson identified a group of nurses who consciously and deliberately plan for their self-care. They can articulate the type and nature of their stressors and have well-developed strategies for combating stress. A sample of nurses in this group actually used the words "caring for myself" and could discuss how their strategies could help to protect, maintain, and restore the self (Hutchinson, 1987, p. 193).

The concept of self-care can be summarized as a collection of actions and attitudes about and toward the self. Self-care involves

- Taking oneself seriously
- Taking actions that protect oneself
- Avoiding damage to the self
- Liking and being willing to care for oneself
- Learning to balance one's needs in a situation with the needs of others
- Being reflective and mindful as a way to enhance the care of the self
- Making the effort to maintain or restore relationships
- Finding ways to relieve one's own suffering
- Initially, one learns self-care by being cared for (Beck, 1991), and self-care behaviors are further developed to the extent that they are rewarded within one's social matrix. (Hughes, 1992).

SELF-KNOWLEDGE

Just as self-care is a prerequisite for caring for others, self-knowledge influences how one understands others. "It is not as ye judge that ye shall be judged, but as you judge yourself so shall you judge others" (Sullivan, 1947, quoted in Markus and Smith, 1981, p. 233). Self-knowledge includes awareness of one's personality traits and dynamics, how one interacts with others, how one copes with tension and stress, and how one regulates self-esteem.

Self-knowledge is a reflective process that leads to altered perceptions and understandings of oneself and others. Developing self-knowledge skills requires the ability to focus and attend to increasing levels of honesty and complexity in one's thoughts and feelings. Learning to accept things as they are, not as they should or ought to be, is central to self-knowledge. Courageous honesty about one's feelings, thoughts, and behaviors is crucial (Leininger and Watson, 1990). Self-knowledge can progress only after accepting oneself as one is. Through self-knowledge, "people can become aware of themselves as experiences, as actors, as phenomena in their own right" (Carver and Scheier, 1985, p. 305). With awareness, one takes the first steps toward autonomy or responsibility; one must be prepared to follow in whatever direction this process leads (Blattner, 1981, p.35). Box 19–1 presents a stress self-test designed to help increase self-awareness of personal stress. Self-knowledge is obtained from internal and external sources, inner thoughts, and feelings, as well as feedback from others. Self-awareness derives from one's attending to this internal and external information (Carver and Glass, 1976).

Information coming into the self from internal and external sources tends to be processed through categories one has created from childhood; a measure of maturity is how well one is able to alter or create new cognitive categories to make sense out of one's evolving experience.

Maturity is built in part on increasing self-complexity: the ability to define oneself by an increased number of roles (husband, wife, partner, friend, nurse), relationships (nurturer, colleague), peer activities (studying, writing, cooking, exercising), traits (positive, problem solver, hard working), and goals (graduation, career, vacations). Thus, appraisal of events as harmful or threatening become diluted. This self-complexity helps to buffer the individual against negative feelings leading to stress (Linville, 1987).

As self-knowledge grows, emotional awareness also gains in complexity. Lane and Schwartz (1987) found that these levels can be viewed as a progression from a diffuse subjective awareness of bodily sensations to final differentiation of the self from the other (Box 19–2). At this level, self-other differentiation has reached its peak, so that self and other are both recognized as unique as well as sharing universal characteristics (Lane and Schwartz, 1987, p. 139).

COPING

With self-knowledge comes an enhanced ability to consciously and deliberately deal with the anxiety and stress of nursing school and other life and career demands. This ability is called *coping*. Coping is generally understood as a complex of behavioral, cognitive, and physiologic responses that aim

BOX 19-1
STRESS SELF-TEST

Directions: Answer yes or no to the following questions:

Do you frequently:	YES	NO
1. Neglect your diet	____	____
2. Fail to exercise regularly	____	____
3. Ignore self examinations	____	____
4. Ignore symptoms of stress	____	____
5. Procrastinate	____	____
6. Fail to see humor in situations	____	____
7. Fail to use some time each day for relaxation	____	____
8. Try to do everything yourself	____	____
9. Set unrealistic goals	____	____
10. Look to others to make things happen for you	____	____
11. Have difficulty making decisions	____	____
12. Keep everything inside	____	____
13. Feel disorganized	____	____
14. Get too little rest	____	____
15. Race through the day	____	____
16. Make a "big deal" of everything	____	____
17. Feel your life is out of control	____	____
18. Find yourself getting angry because others are not doing what is expected	____	____
19. Find yourself worrying about the past or future	____	____
20. Say yes to everything	____	____

Score 1 for each "yes" answer. The closer your score is to 20, the higher your stress index. A score of 14 or above indicates the need for stress management strategies.

Adapted from Slaby, A. E. (1988). *60 Ways to Make Stress Work for You.* Summit, NJ: PIA Press. Used by permission.

BOX 19-2
LEVELS OF EMOTIONAL AWARENESS

Lane and Schwartz (1987) proposed five levels of emotional awareness that build toward self-knowledge. These levels progress from merely rudimentary to highly developed and discriminating, as follows:

Level 1. The subjective quality of emotional experience focuses on *bodily sensations.* There is little or no differentiation of emotion. Arousal is global and diffuse. The individual is not able to describe sensations, although the quality of the emotion can be described by an observer. Infants exhibit this level of development.

Level 2. The subjective quality of the emotional experience focuses on bodily sensations *and an urge to act.* Actions are based on a drive to maximize pleasure or minimize distress. The individual may be able to provide only a vague verbal description, such as "I feel bad." An outside observer could identify the emotional quality based on voluntary movements (running, hitting) and involuntary motor movements (flushing, sweating). Also, one can more accurately anticipate how one might feel in the future, which leads to better decision making. Self-knowledge increases one's awareness of multiple role-playing ability and emotional maturity.

Level 3. The subjective quality of the emotional experience focuses on bodily sensations (as in Levels 1 and 2) with the addition of a *psychological* experience. The range of emotion is limited and experienced as *either-or:* one is either all happy or all sad. Verbal descriptions are likewise limited and unidimensional. At this level, the individual has little or no capacity to understand that others may have separate emotions that may differ from one's own state.

Level 4. The subjective quality of the emotional experience focuses on blends of feelings. There is an awareness that emotions can change over time, can supplement or replace one another, or can be subtly differentiated. One can be happy, pleased, and grateful as well as sad and disappointed, all at once. One develops a capacity to modulate extremes of emotions and to experience an emotion such as hope in the face of what appears to be a hopeless situation. The individual has gained the ability to describe complex nuances of emotion. However, the ability to appreciate others' emotional reactions remains unidimensional and shallow.

Level 5. The subjective quality of the emotional experience in this final level is one of added complexity, of blends of feelings with varying qualities and intensities. One may describe new patterns of feelings unique to oneself and can make subtle distinction between emotions. The individual can now perceive the complexity of another's emotions without bias from one's own emotional state, even when the situation involves one's self.

to prevent or minimize unpleasant or harmful experiences (stressors) that tax one's personal resources (Lazarus and Folkman, 1984). Nursing research has found that nursing students use different coping strategies depending on the situation, one's personality style, and cultural and family backgrounds. Therefore, there is no one "correct" way to cope with a situation.

Individuals deploy their coping strengths in characteristic ways depending on whether the situation is a conflict or "business as usual" (Porter, 1973). Some nursing students will initially withdraw from an argument for the sake of harmony, but will reluctantly defend their side only if cherished values were threatened. Other students will take a stand immediately and back down only as a last resort. Nursing students tend to use emotional control and distancing (emotion-focused coping) to avoid faculty-student conflicts in the clinical setting (Parkes, 1986). A student who is normally assertive among friends may avoid speaking up if it means disagreeing with the instructor. In contrast, when students had more authority and experience, as in patient care settings, they were more likely to confront the patient or engage in more planful problem solving (behavioral coping). Similarly, nursing students tend to adjust their coping strategies to resolve a conflict between the desire to appear "in control" to their fellow students, as in not appearing ignorant by asking questions of instructors, versus the need to appear competent as nurses by speaking up and asking questions on behalf of their patients (Wilson, 1994).

Because a sense of control is central to managing stress, nursing students seek to juggle multiple demands. An extensive review of research related to nursing students and stress (Porter-Tibbetts, 1992) revealed that students coped by setting new priorities, sacrificing personal and leisure time, working harder and longer, mobilizing family assistance, and dropping nonessential activities. They also were found to redefine meaning in a situation (a passive form of coping) and to reassess their career choice (a cognitive form of coping).

At some point in their education, nursing students may begin to wonder whether they are suited to the nursing profession; in trying to reconcile their expectations with their experience, students are often surprised by how strongly the two differ. By reflecting on their values and their nursing experience, most students begin to anchor themselves in their career; they determine that it is worth the effort. They also begin to notice how their experiences are changing them.

Some researchers (e.g., Stoyva and Anderson, 1982) hypothesize that one's reaction to stressful events will oscillate between active coping (e.g., assertiveness, imagery, self-statements) and restful coping (e.g., progressive relaxation, meditation). Both of these aspects ". . . are necessary, as is a fairly frequent alternation between the two. In fact, our daily existence can be thought of as a series of shifts from one mode to the other" (p. 746).

HEALTH PROMOTION

Self-care, as discussed earlier in this chapter, starts with self-knowledge, from which one learns to sharpen one's coping skills. From enhanced coping skills comes the ability to recognize and avoid the harmful effects of stress and to respond to it in healthy ways. In practicing and benefiting from self-care in their own careers, nurses and students can serve as exemplars of health promotion to patients and colleagues alike.

Over the past two decades, the concept of health promotion has grown in importance as the health care system shifts emphasis to preventing disease rather than treating it. Thus, as nursing increasingly moves into the community, nursing practice will become more holistic, emphasizing wellness and preventive strategies (Sohier, 1992). As nurses focus more on health promotion and disease prevention, they need to be exemplars of health promotion practices. To begin this process, it will be helpful to contrast the ideal vision of health with the reality.

Health is defined broadly as well-being, congruence between one's possibilities and one's actual practices and lived meanings, and is based on caring and feeling cared for (Benner and Wrubel, 1989, p. 160). As such, there would be healthy ways to live within the limits of a situation even when the limits are severe, as in disease (Bermosk and Porter, 1979). As nursing moves into the twenty-first century, one finds increasing emphasis on wholeness and agent-environment-host interactions as opposed to the reductionist concept of agent as cause and host as victim. The traditional Eastern model of health (preserving harmony and wholeness of oneself in balance with one's environment) is becoming more accepted in nursing (Benner and Wrubel, 1989).

Descriptions of health given by undergraduate nursing students in Beck's 1991 survey augment current conceptions of health:

- *Peaceful contentedness* is a sense of satisfaction with life in areas of self, family, and friends. It includes being happy and secure in one's identity, being able to interact with others and enjoy life, feeling harmony in one's life, feeling at peace with oneself, and feeling fulfilled.
- *Optimal unfolding* means functioning at maximum potential physically and mentally; achieving personal and professional goals; and continuing to challenge oneself to grow and learn by setting new goals.
- *Perpetual vigilance* means continuing to strive for a positive lifestyle, both physically and mentally, through such acts as setting aside a portion of each day to exercise, relax, and having time for oneself; ensuring proper diet, adequate sleep and rest, and weight control; finally, avoiding unhealthy coping by abusing substances that are harmful to health such as alcohol, drugs, and tobacco.

Given this ideal concept of health care, it is instructive to examine how well nursing students and professional nurses cope and promote their own health. Studies conducted over the past 25 years reveal a wide gap between the ideal conception of health and actual practice by nursing students.

GENERAL HEALTH PRACTICES

A survey of health practices among a large group of nursing students (Dittmar et al, 1989) revealed that most students slept 6 to 8 hours nightly, exercised regularly, and had annual dental and physical examinations. However, less than half had good eating habits. Students ate between meals, skipped breakfast, and did not limit fat, salt, and sugar in their diets. Moreover, less than one third of this group performed monthly breast self-examinations, and only half had annual Papanicolaou smears.

Practicing positive health behaviors was the focus of another research study (Soeken et al, 1989). Senior nursing students responded that 20 various nutrition, safety, lifestyle behaviors and participating in medical decisions were very important. However, when students' participation in these behaviors was compared with that of a group of similar non-nursing individuals, the nursing students were significantly less compliant.

Why would a group of health-conscious nursing students not be the shining examples of health practice? The amount of effort to engage in the health behavior was very important. It did not matter whether the nursing students thought the behaviors were important: what predicted compliance was the perceived difficulty of the behavior. In addition, the participants thought their health was excellent or good. They did not feel vulnerable to poor health and, therefore, were not motivated to make the effort to change their behavior. The authors of this study also suggested that faculty as role models who only pay lip service to positive health behaviors fail to teach students by example.

A more recent study (Clement et al, 1995) of first-year undergraduate nursing students found that students' perception of self-efficacy (that one is capable and has the skills to be successful), perception of one's state of health, the influence of professors, and one's place of birth were predictive of enacting health-promoting behaviors. The importance of professors supporting students' confidence to commit to health-promoting behaviors was stressed.

Alcohol and drug abuse, smoking, and workaholism are three addictions to which nurses are vulnerable. Learning about the addictions in nursing school helps students to institute an early intervention plan for oneself if necessary.

ALCOHOL AND DRUG ABUSE

Perhaps 6 to 20% of registered nurses have a substance abuse problem (American Nurses' Association, 1984; Crosby and Bissell, 1989). The actual degree of drug and alcohol use among nurses is difficult to determine because many abusers do not respond to surveys, or they distort their self-reports. Nurses do not admit their substance abuse problems because of job repercussions and negative peer attitudes. Although nurses acknowledge that substance abuse occurs, they also have reservations about the return of recovering colleagues to the work force (Canon and Brown, 1988).

Job stressors, low self-esteem, and family problems ranked highest among student nurses as factors leading to drug addiction (Spencer-Strachan, 1990). McDonough (1989) found that 22% of graduate student nurses in anesthesiology had personality traits that predispose to drug use, such as impulsivity and sensation seeking.

Alcohol has long been relied on as a negative coping behavior related to stressors such as overwork, demanding patients, difficult schedules, and poor interpersonal relations. Students and nurses risk impaired performance and physical and mental deterioration after chronic alcohol use.

Dittmar and colleagues (1989) found that 90% of surveyed nursing students consumed alcoholic beverages, 66% consumed more than three drinks per occasion, and 25% had five or more drinks per occasion and were identified as binge drinkers. "Binge drinking is defined as consuming five or more drinks on one occasion for men and four or more drinks for women at one to two week intervals" (Wright, 1996, p. 483). Haack (1987) found that 14% of nursing students surveyed had experienced poor work and school performance because of alcohol abuse. Subjects tended to drink more as they progressed through the program, typically blamed others or external events for their failures, and lacked social-family support. They reported increased depression and increased alcohol consumption and felt more "burned out." In contrast, students who did not increase their drinking took more responsibility for their actions and had supportive friends and family.

SMOKING

The level of smoking among nurses is unacceptably high. Surveys conducted in 1959 to 1972 showed that 36% of nurses smoked. In 1976 this proportion rose to 39%, but more recent studies show that the proportion had dropped to 27.2% in 1985. Gritz and others (1989) reported that 24.6% of white nurses smoked compared with 20.7% of black nurses and 5.6% of Asian-American nurses.

Smoking among nursing students is also high. Students were found to begin smoking just before or on beginning the program and to increase the amount as they progressed through their education. Contributing factors included peer influence and entry into a stressful profession (Elkind, 1988).

Surveys of smoking behavior among nursing students revealed rates of 6 to 57% (Casey et al, 1989). Thus, health practices of both professional nurses and nursing students are not exemplary and diminish their ability to fulfill their role as health educators (Padula, 1992).

WORKAHOLISM

Nurses who work longer and longer hours in an attempt to control their workload are often given institutional and organizational rewards, which makes it difficult to maintain balance and set limits. Besides having a need for this reward stimulus, a "workaholic" is someone who has multiple addictions, high denial, and low (or overinflated) self-esteem and is externally directed and perfectionistic (Fassel, 1990). Box 19–3 lists some characteristics of workaholism.

Implementing health promotion requires more than amassing large amounts of health-related data. "Creating a belief in one's own self-care and self-healing ability takes trust, courage, and patience" (Blattner, 1981). Changing lifelong habits of mind and action is not easy. However, the effort must be made. One nurse-author (Jarrett, 1993) stated, "Let us begin to look at our bodies with love and compassion instead of disdain and disrespect. Florence Nightingale was so right when she described the human body as a temple" (p. 10). "Loving oneself begins with taking care of the body. That is basic." (p. 11).

BOX 19-3
CHARACTERISTICS OF WORK ADDICTION

- Work relieves emotional and physical discomfort.
- There is an experience of pleasure, a "rush," that can be brought about only by work.
- Work becomes the center of life, and all other activities and relationships are adjusted to accommodate it. Nothing is allowed to interfere with the pursuit of the addictive behavior.
- Addicts believe that they need only themselves and their work to be self-sufficient.
- There is denial of any problems. The addict cannot see what everyone else can see.
- If work is eliminated, there is a period of physical and emotional withdrawal characterized by anxiety and depression, which can be relieved only by work.

Adapted from Pugh, J.B., Woodward-Smith, M.A. (1997). *Nurse Manager: A Practical Guide to Better Employee Relations*, 2nd ed. Philadelphia: W.B. Saunders. Used with permission.

Relevant Theory

Relevant theory related to stress is found in Chapter 31 where four major concepts are presented: stressors, reactions, consequences, and mediators. In this section, appraisal as a mediator of stress is presented in more detail.

APPRAISAL OF STRESSFUL EVENTS

Appraisal is a cognitive activity to determine meaning and significance of an event or situation. Appraisal can be conscious or unconscious. The evaluation process is focused on the importance of the situation to one's well-being (Lazarus and Folkman, 1984). Three levels of appraisal occur in relation to stressful events. The first level is *primary appraisal.* This is one's initial thinking. The question that is implied in primary appraisal is "Am I going to be okay, am I going to be safe, am I going to be benefited now or in the future?" In other words, "Is this situation irrelevant, benign positive, or stressful?" Stress appraisals are understood as being harmful, threatening, or challenging. To the extent that the situation is viewed as containing stressful elements the next step is taken.

If stressful elements are perceived, the individual engages in *secondary appraisal.* One asks "What can I do about it?" This line of concern has two aspects: what might or can be done about the situation, that is, how to cope, and what is at stake. For example, a nursing student giving an injection for the first time to a client may appraise the situation as stressful in that failing to perform adequately could harm the client, and the faculty might express disappointment in the student's performance. The student may use the outcome of one incident as an indicator of his or her ability to be a good nurse and think that what is at stake is one's future career. To minimize this threat, the student would cope by practicing until a comfortable level of competence with the procedure is attained before giving the actual injection. In this situation, the student believes that the behavior of practice will lead to the outcome desired, or outcome expectancy, and that he or she would actually be able to practice injections to reach a comfortable level of competency with the procedure or efficacy expectation.

The student has turned what could be a threatening experience into a challenge by gaining a sense of control in the situation. Exerting substantial effort is related to feeling a sense of challenge (Lazarus and Folkman, 1984). The appraisal of coping options and recognition of what is at stake is strongly influenced by the emotions, past experiences, and habitual ways of thinking. For example, externalizing blame, avoiding the problem, and assuming that external factors will override individual efforts in problem-solving and other coping strategies of benefit to the individual. Asking for help, using resources, and examining various options and possible outcomes enhances coping.

Reappraisal is the third level. Reappraisal is the ongoing evaluation of how the coping strategies are working out, reassessing one's stake in the event, analyzing one's commitment in the situation, and adjusting one's perspective to match the reality of the situation. The more accurately one can appraise the situation and resources available, the closer one can come to reducing the stress.

FUTURE DEVELOPMENTS

Career Options

Job opportunities for registered nurses are expected to grow until at least 2005 (Abraham and Reich, 1996). Dramatic transitions in the health care delivery system, the aging population, and the aging of the nursing work force are creating ongoing and new exciting opportunities for nurses (Salmon et al, 1996).

HOSPITALS

Hospitals will continue to be a major employer of nurses (Salmon et al, 1996). Substantial changes in the nurses' role are anticipated. Expect to see a focus on *primary care* and *health promotion,* including emphasis on disease prevention and lifestyle modification. As baby boomers age, causing an expansion in the elderly population, more focus on *managing chronic conditions* will occur.

HOME CARE SETTINGS

Earlier discharge from the hospital means more nursing care required in the home. Home health care is anticipated to be the fastest growing service over the next 10 years (Abraham and Reich, 1996). The growing number of older persons with functional disabilities, complex medical problems, and consumer preference for care in the home will require a nurse who can manage the complexities of biopsychosocial dysfunctions. Instructing patients and their families in nursing care techniques is central to the home health nurse. The home health nurse must be able to work independently. Understanding families is essential.

OTHER SETTINGS

The graying of America will also impact nursing employment availability in nursing homes. Earlier release of clients from hospitals to nursing homes and growth in specialized long-term rehabilitation units for stroke and Alzheimer's disease victims will increase jobs. Physicians' offices, outpatient clinics, emergency units, ambulatory surgicenters, and health maintenance organizations (HMOs) are the sites of an increasing number of highly technical medical procedures, once the purview of hospitals. Nurses with health education and counseling skills as well as technical skill will be marketable in these areas.

As HMOs continue to develop and health care evolves into integrated health care networks, nurses may have options to float among units and geographic sites. Flexibility is the key for nurses who want the competitive edge in these settings (Abraham and Reich, 1996).

ADVANCED PRACTICE NURSING

Nurse practitioners and clinical specialists are a fast-growing career option. Currently, the family nurse practitioner is one of the more popular advanced-practice specialties. New specialties are emerging (e.g., neonatal nurse practitioner, acute care nurse practitioner). Nurse anesthetist, midwifery, women's health care, mental health, pediatric, geriatric, and adult nurse practitioner are among the more established practitioner roles. Home health, case management, administration, community health, transcultural, oncology, cardiology, emergency room, flight trauma, rehabilitation, infection control, hospice control, and school nurse are specialty areas that clinical specialists have been developing (Mundinger, 1994).

Regardless of career option chosen, the changing health care delivery system and technological developments demand that future nurses be able to:

- Manage care along a continuum
- Work as peers in interdisciplinary teams
- Integrate clinical knowledge with knowledge of community resources (Salmon et al, 1996).

Regardless of where nursing students begin their educational preparation, whether it begins with a diploma, associate degree, or baccalaureate program ongoing education that fosters:

- Critical thinking
- Adaptation to change
- Problem-solving skills
- Ability to communicate and analyze data
- A sound foundation in a broad range of basic, behavioral, social, and management sciences

will position one to stay current and relevant for the future in the fast changing health care system (Salmon et al, 1996, p. 7).

INFORMATICS AND PATIENT CARE TECHNOLOGY

INFORMATICS

Informatics refers to all aspects of the computer environment. The demand for nursing expertise in nursing informatics is strong and growing. Nurse informaticians is a new specialty recognized by the major nursing associations. The purpose of nursing informatics is to analyze information requirements; design, implement, and evaluate information systems and data structures that support nursing; and identify and apply computer technologies for nursing (Saba, 1994). For example, many clinicians want to know immediately what is significant about their client. By creating a program called Patient Event Documentation, clinicians were able to quickly sort out what was significant and make knowledgeable decisions (Goldsmith, 1996). With nursing providing sophisticated data support, communications and decision making are enhanced so that health care delivery is improved, clients have more informed choices, and the advancement of nursing science proceeds (Saba, 1994). One project using informatics that improved patient care tracked patient falls. By having access to computerized data, nursing staff discovered that most cases involve elderly women getting out of bed in the middle of the night to go to the bathroom. Staff developed protective actions for the women (McAlindon, 1994). Informatics is a fast-paced growing field in nursing completely linked to the rapid changes in technology.

PATIENT CARE TECHNOLOGIES

In an urban hospital, a 12-year-old in protective isolation to allow her bone marrow transplant to become fully functional chatted away with her classmates and teacher via the Internet and a video camera (Goldsmith, 1996, p. 11). The computer video conference, which lasted 45 minutes, was part of a therapeutic intervention of a nursing student studying the clinical problem of isolation and coping with illness. In a rural hospital, two nurse clinicians are able to view and discuss the wound of a homebound patient using a portable 5-pound still-image transmission system called Picasso. The system connects to a regular telephone line, resembles a video telephone, but transmits diagnostic quality images (Penny, 1996). Telemedicine technology, which provides highly visible data, now has "simultaneous access to the patient record as well as real-time video and remote data collection tools (e.g., digital blood pressure cuff, otoscopes)" (Caton, 1997, p. 9). Assessments, health teaching, and coordination of care are among the first nursing activities to be the subject of research using distance technology. Clearly, technological innovations can remain in the service of care, compassion, and competence for nursing (Dreher, 1996).

Trends in Self-Care and Coping

Because change is happening at a faster pace than ever before, trends in self-care must address how one copes with change itself. Lazarus and Folkman (1984) analyzed numerous research studies related to stress. They identified *situational factors* influencing whether one's appraisal of an event will be as threatening, harmful, or challenging. These factors are ever present in both change and nursing school.

AMBIGUITY

Ambiguity refers to a great lack of clarity in the areas of knowing what is going to happen, when it will happen, how long it will last, and what it means. The less one can put that pattern of information together into a meaningful whole, the more ambiguous is the situation. If a nursing student has never been inside a critical care unit and has not studied any of the patient conditions, the experience would be very ambiguous. The initial weeks of nursing school may also be ambiguous as one sorts out priorities, people, and places.

PREDICTABILITY

Predictability means knowing that an event or the environment can be known or understood in advance. When an event is predictable, the choice of coping method can also be anticipated. One has an enhanced sense of control even if the control is focused on one's attitude. There are numerous events in nursing that are unpredictable. The more experience one has with client care, the better one becomes at predicting outcomes, but for the novice nurse events are less predictable. The rapid changes in health care delivery have also decreased the ability of faculty to predict the availability of clinical placements, patient assignments, and nursing staff teaching support for students. Thus, students' clinical experiences include those added unpredictable features.

NOVELTY

Novelty is defined as situations that a person has not experienced before. Most situations are not completely new; they may resemble other situations. The meaning in the situation is usually inferred based on past experience. Hence, if the situation resembles a negative experience, the appraisal of the new situation may be one of threat or harm. Inferring meaning itself can also be threatening. There are many novel situations in nursing school and throughout one's nursing career. The more experience one gains, the easier it is to make inferential meanings that approximate the reality of the situation. When confronted with numerous novel situations, it is more difficult to match the coping skill required with the demand of the situation. Awareness of the coping skill deficit can add to the feeling of threat.

Perspectives from a new science, Chaos Theory (Wheatley, 1992), serve as a useful paradigm for a shift in attitude for being in a rapidly changing system. Rather than increased attempts to exert control over a situation, chaos theory tells us that order emerges as a process and does so with very few controls. Order emerges as partners with change. Flux and chaos are opportunities for growth and new understandings. Nursing students are introduced into ambiguous and unpredictable situations within which one's natural responses may now be inadequate. The search for gaining control, seeking predictable patterns, and making sense lead one to develop higher orders of self-complexity. What feels like fluctuations, disturbances, and imbalances are the seeds of a new self-order forming.

An important activity that guides an emerging and unfolding of a new self-order is asking questions of oneself and others. The act of asking questions calls into being the source of an answer. One cannot obtain an answer unless the question has been asked.

Failure is a great educator. The fear of making mistakes locks out learning. Use practice sessions for more attempts, quicker insight, faster solutions. This is not about being sloppy or ill prepared. Be honest, admit mistakes, and seek to recover the situation. How one recovers after a mistake and how one cleans up a situation contains the seeds for a new respect. Always ask the question: "What have I learned and what else am I to be learning from this situation?"

Work smarter. Take time to reflect and ponder. By reflecting, the ambiguity in situations is reduced. Perspectives can be reconfigured. Lessons can be learned through reconsidering the events in a new light.

PRINCIPLES AND PRACTICES

Implementing Self-Care

Awareness of personal vulnerabilities and strengths, together with awareness of the risks, opportunities, and pressures associated with a nursing career, will help the student recognize what steps to take to strengthen self-care practices, self-knowledge, and coping responses during nursing school and beyond.

There should be a balance between caring for others and caring for one's self, so that the nurse and patient benefit equally. When nurses and nursing students neglect or avoid self-care, they become candidates for burnout and poor exemplars or models for their patients and other caregivers.

What about the satisfaction that comes from serving others or, as Thomas put it (1983, pp. 64–65), "the matchless opportunity to be useful friends to great numbers of human beings in trouble?" At what point does self-care become self-absorption or selfishness? How does one know whether or not one is being selfish in a situation or taking legitimate care of oneself?

It is true that focused attention on the self, whether it be about accomplishments or about worries and concerns, is a form of self-absorption that shows a lack of interpersonal balance. Paradoxically, the more self-absorbed one becomes, the more the self feels neglected and starved for self-acceptance (Moore, 1992). Loving one's self as an object rather than as ego is love of one's deep soul. The boundaries of who one thinks one is breaks up, and a new image of self emerges. "Love of a new image of self leads to new knowledge about oneself and one's potential" (Moore, 1992, p. 63). The more one is able to accept oneself as one truly is, the less self-absorbed one becomes. It becomes easier to identify one's needs and meet one's needs in a healthy way. More energy is available to care for others based on their needs, not as an attempt to meet one's own needs.

For many women, the sense of self may be defined largely in terms of human relationships (Gilligan, 1982). A woman's self-esteem is related to her ability to nurture and care for others (Miller, 1976). A study of moral responses (Peter and Gallop, 1994) found that female nurses tended to be more concerned than male nurses with moral responses about relationships, alleviating suffering, and resolving conflicts as opposed to moral responses about enforcing rules, obligations, and standards over the situation. However, neither sex had a monopoly of unwavering moral orientation in every situation. Another study found that nursing students in general hold responsibility, honesty, and loving as their highest values (Thurston et al, 1989).

However, the very socialization that facilitates women as caregivers can handicap them when it comes to applying care to the self. Many women often feel guilty or selfish about taking time for themselves, seeing it as more virtuous to look after the needs of others. When setting priorities, they often put their needs at the bottom of the priority list. This is just the opposite of what needs to happen. An initial way to disengage from this response is to ask oneself: By doing this for another, am I keeping that person from learning something? Are there others who are not helping because I am doing it all? Would I be of more service if I took better care of myself? As one middle-aged nurse said, "I just found out I am at moderate risk for a heart attack. I was never taught to exercise. I don't have time to exercise. I have a sick husband, and I am taking care of my daughter's child and my teenagers." Then she paused and reflected, "Of course, I have even less time to die of a heart attack." Some nursing students have been amazed that their families actually learned how to take care of the house, do the shopping, and help each other with homework.

Maximizing self-care while a nursing student requires determination and perseverance; some specific strategies are as follows:

- Set aside a minimum schedule of self-care that you will engage in no matter what.
- Keep in mind that promises to yourself are as important if not more important as promises to others.
- Your own personal integrity is at the heart of developing a self-care program.
- Choose activities that you already know how to do and feel good about doing.
- Schedule time that is possible and reasonable.
- A moderate list of self-care activities that you can actually accomplish is more important than an impressive list that never happens.
- Think small and manageable.
- Itemize the innumerable small things that make you happy, that trigger good memories.
- Think of those triggers as feeding your immune system with positive neurohormones.

Hans Selye, the father of stress theory, wrote the Foreword for *Holistic Health* (Blattner, 1981). He elegantly asserted three general principles for everyday life that balance the caring efforts in one's life:

1. Find your own natural predilections and stress level. People differ with regard to the amount and kind of work they consider worth doing to meet the exigencies of daily life to assure future security and happiness. In this respect, all of us are influenced by hereditary predispositions and the expectations of our society. Only through planned self-analysis can we establish what we really want. Many people suffer all their lives because they are too conservative to risk a radical change and break with traditions.
2. Practice altruistic egoism. The selfish hoarding of the good will, respect, esteem, support, and love of our neighbor is the most efficient way to give vent to our pent-up energy and create enjoyable, beautiful, or useful things.
3. Earn your neighbor's love. This motto, unlike "love thy neighbor as thyself," is compatible with our biologic structure, and although it is based on altruistic egoism, it could hardly be attacked as unethical. Who could blame a person who wants to assure homeostasis and happiness by accumulating the treasure of other people's benevolence? Yet this makes one virtually unassailable, for people would not attack and destroy those upon whom they depend. (pp. vi, vii)

Gaining Self-Knowledge

Certain areas of self-knowledge seem especially worthwhile for the student nurse to explore. These include family of origin dynamics and personality characteristics such as locus of control hardiness and self-esteem.

FAMILY OF ORIGIN DYNAMICS

Psychodynamically oriented psychologists believe that one's early childhood experiences within the context of the family exert a formative influence on the personality in terms of values, self-esteem and self-image, relations with others in later in life, management of feelings, and coping with anxiety or stress (Briere, 1992). Through personal reflection and attention to these areas, we can become conscious of how they influence our adult behavior.

The implications for nursing students are important. In the academic setting, students are confronted with situations characterized by ambiguity, dominance, and autocratic control, intensity, and intimacy. These situations may reactivate old traumas, fears, and hurts for some students who come to nursing with a family background that included some form of substance, physical, or emotional abuse. In such dysfunctional family settings, lack of parental empathy and appropriate responses to a child's needs may leave the child with coping strategies that do not transport well into adult life.

The stress of nursing school and career can be overwhelming. The feeling of being overwhelmed may stem from the earlier family traumas. Inability to be self-assertive or provide adequate advocacy for patients, constant feelings of inadequacy and low self-esteem, unrealistically high standards and perfectionism, and poor interpersonal boundaries are examples of coping outcomes for individuals struggling to use what they have learned in dysfunctional family situations.

As you think about your own family background and your own motivations to become a nurse, you may want to identify whether or not you are vulnerable in some ways. It is also possible to obtain feedback from instructors about areas that need attention if one is to achieve professional development. Receiving feedback from an instructor about behavior patterns can be unsettling and distressing. It is important to obtain from the instructor as much detail and example about the pattern as possible. Using the phrase "Please help me understand your perception of this behavior" may help you avoid sounding defensive. Take this as an opportunity to learn more about yourself and your coping skills. Take notes, and ask for an instructor's observations in writing, if possible. Do not hesitate to ask other instructors for their perceptions of you.

Using your nursing school advisor and counseling at this point in the experience is a valuable way to exercise self-care in gaining self-knowledge. Seeking therapy (if that is what seems appropriate) to help heal past wounds is a professional way to enact self-responsibility. Other possible resources include self-help books, Adult Children of Alcoholics groups, various 12-step programs, Adults Molested as Children groups, or individual psychotherapy or group therapy.

PERSONALITY CHARACTERISTICS

Locus of control, hardiness, and self-esteem are three personality factors influencing stress. Inherent in these personality traits are styles of coping that tend to mediate the impact of stressful events. Each trait can be developed and strengthened.

LOCUS OF CONTROL

Locus of control (LOC) deals with whether an individual thinks he or she can influence events in one's life (internal LOC) or whether or not one is at the mercy of forces and events beyond one's personal control (external LOC) (Folkman et al, 1979). For the internal LOC the phrases "I am the master of my ship" or "I did it my way" fit. For the external LOC the phrase "Cast your fate to the winds" fits.

Several researchers investigated nursing students' locus of control and stress. For example, one study (Sobol, 1978) found that students who have an internal LOC (i.e., who feel they have more control over their lives and have the ability to make things happen for themselves) show less anxiety in stressful situations than students who have an external LOC (i.e., who believe that events happen to them and are beyond their control). More recent work (Parkes, 1984) showed that students with an external LOC failed to assess adequately stressful situations and thus used fewer and less adaptive coping strategies; they tended to process a situation internally before seeking help. Students who had an internal LOC used accurate situational appraisal skills and were more willing to seek additional information to help manage threatening situations.

Assertiveness, empowerment, and ability to express feelings are examples of ways in which an internal LOC can be developed.

Assertiveness. Assertiveness comes from self-confidence, in which the student compels recognition of one's rights, feelings, and values without unduly restricting those of others. Assertiveness training can help nurses learn to deal constructively and effectively with others' verbal anger, abuse, and frustrations, whether they be patients or colleagues. The importance of assertiveness skills is underscored by the American Association of Colleges of Nursing, which has listed it as a vital exit behavior for graduating nurses. The lack of assertiveness, together with low self-confidence and dependency, was found to correlate with burnout in mental health professionals (Gann, 1979). Assertiveness training has been positively correlated with performance and self-esteem (Barr, 1989).

Box 19–4 presents a self-test to help determine how assertive you are in daily life.

Another area requiring new learning and self-care involves advocating for patients, in which the student must speak up to authority figures on the behalf of the patient (Fig. 19–2). In the American nursing system, it is expected that the professional nurse will advocate with physicians or supervisors on the patient's behalf. However, for students from many cultures, this would be considered rude, particularly if one is a woman.

Speaking up for the patient may take some practice. Just remember that this is what is expected and is acceptable practice. Sometimes, too, you may have to advocate for yourself. For example, if you are assigned to a patient who requires unfamiliar and difficult treatment, you must speak up and ask for help. If you cannot hear a blood pressure or read a gauge, you must seek help on behalf of your patient's well-being. Students from cultures valuing "saving face" may need to learn the higher value of saving face by admitting ignorance or wrongdoing in the interest of preserving safe patient care. It is always more commendable to admit mistakes on behalf of the patient than to attempt to hide the mistake out of embarrassment.

Empowerment. This is the feeling that one has the power and control to effect change. One cannot act in an empowered way if self-esteem is low, and self-esteem is lost when one is

BOX 19-4
ASSERTIVENESS SELF-ASSESSMENT

In order to be an effective nurse, you must be assertive enough to represent your patients and yourself. Test your Assertiveness Quotient by completing the following questionnaire. Give each question a 1, 2, or 3 based on how comfortable you feel about each item:

1—I feel very uncomfortable
2—I feel moderately comfortable
3—I feel very comfortable

A Q TEST

Assertive Behavior

Speaking up and asking questions at a meeting _____

Commenting about being interrupted by someone the moment he or she interrupts you _____

Stating your views to an authority figure (e.g., minister, boss, teacher, parent) _____

Attempting to offer solutions and elaborating on them when others are present _____

Your Body

Entering and exiting a room where superiors are gathered _____

Speaking in front of a group _____

Maintaining eye contact, keeping your head upright, and leaning forward when in a personal conversation _____

Your Mind

Going out with a group of friends when you are the only one without a "date" _____

Being especially competent, using your authority and/or power without labeling yourself as "bitchy," impolite, bossy, aggressive, castrating, or parental _____

Requesting expected service when you haven't received it (e.g., in a restaurant or a store) _____

Apology

Being expected to apologize for something and not apologizing since you feel you are right _____

Requesting the return of borrowed items without being apologetic _____

Compliments, Criticism, and Rejection

Receiving a compliment by saying something assertive to acknowledge that you agree with the person complimenting you _____

_____ Accepting a rejection

_____ Not getting the approval of the most significant person in your life

_____ Discussing another person's criticism of you openly with that person

_____ Telling someone that she or he is doing something that is bothering you

Saying No

_____ Saying "No"—refusing to do a favor when you really don't feel like it

_____ Turning down a request for a meeting or date

Manipulation and Countermanipulation

_____ Telling a person when you think she or he is manipulating you

_____ Commenting assertively to someone who has made a patronizing remark to you

_____ Talking about your feelings of competition with another person with whom you feel competitive

Anger/Humor

_____ Expressing anger directly and honestly when you feel angry

_____ Arguing with another person

_____ Telling a joke

_____ Listening to a friend tell a story about something embarrassing, but funny, that you have done

_____ Responding with humor to someone's put-down of you

If you have mostly 3's and a few 2's, you are assertive enough to advocate for your patients and yourself. If you have a few 1's, write each one down and seek out three occasions to try more assertive behaviors in these situations. If you have five or more 1's, you need an assertiveness course and/or some real work on your part.

blocked from exerting influence and power over one's environment. Without feelings of self-worth and the ability to act in an empowered way, nurses cannot effectively cope with the stresses they encounter in their education and career practice. One way to empower one's self is to ask the question, "How can I?" instead of stating "I can't." Other keys to empowerment have to do with committing to a choice and investing the choice with effort or energy.

Ability to Express Feelings. Learning to express feelings of fear, sadness, anger, and frustration in constructive ways is

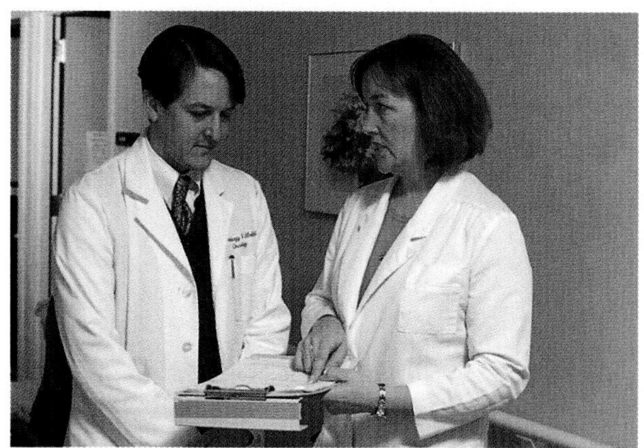

Figure 19-2. Advocating for patients is an important nursing role that helps promote assertiveness, a key attribute of an effective nurse.

now valued for stress reduction. Expression of feelings is an important coping strategy of critical care nurses, among others (Schaefer and Peterson, 1992). Use of assertiveness and problem-solving skills, along with emotional expression, can be a powerful combination to effect change. Nurses are increasingly turning to their peers and supervisors to share their feelings and draw emotional support. Nurses confront the realities of death and dying more frequently than any other group of health professionals. A study of hospice nurses found that these nurses established collaborative relationships with the dying patient and family, balancing their involvement between too much and too little (Eakes, 1988). Hospice nurses also maintained and used support systems—family members, spouses, and peers—to work through their feelings of loss.

In addition to using support and verbalizing feelings, nurses need to be able to plan and anticipate to reduce the trauma of loss (Davidhizer and Giger, 1991). Discussing the loss can increase realistic perceptions, and planning and hoping for the future can facilitate working through a separation.

HARDINESS

Hardiness is a trait that helps one cope with stress (Kabasa, et al, 1982). Key components of hardiness are *control, challenge, and commitment.* Hardy persons feel a greater sense of control over their lives like persons with an internal LOC, tend to view stressors as opportunities for change, appraise situations as challenging rather than threatening, and have a higher commitment to work and self. The hardy person has a high degree of purpose and a well-integrated sense of self. Safety, stability, and predictability are less important to hardy individuals than growth and change. Researchers have found that hardiness correlates with lower susceptibility to stress-related illness and burnout (Rich and Rich, 1987).

SELF-ESTEEM

Closely related to hardiness are one's feelings of self-esteem, which is an individual's feelings about his or her own worth, self-regard, and confidence. Individuals who feel good about themselves tend to interpret events in a more positive light and interpret events as less emotionally ladened. There is a positive relationship between personal self-esteem and professional self-esteem. Unless nurses are affirmed, valued, and emotionally supported in their relationships with other nurses and health care professionals, they will feel professionally devalued and suffer a loss in personal esteem. Student nurses look to their teachers for positive role models and positive affirmation of their abilities.

Nursing students can develop self-esteem in nursing school by attending to the skills and attitudes that increase academic success: preparing for class and developing study strategies, knowing that achievement is possible, and enhancing reading, language, and math abilities (Chacko and Huba, 1991). In addition, learn how to negotiate the system (nursing school and clinical agencies). Read the policies that govern your behavior in nursing school. Become aware of your rights and responsibilities as a nursing student. Become acquainted with your advisor early, before any potential problems develop. Students who feel they do not fit in need to focus on how to find a place for themselves in nursing school (Kornguth et al, 1994).

ADDITIONAL SELF-KNOWLEDGE TECHNIQUES

Many practices in Western and Eastern traditions can be used to increase one's ability to become more aware. These practices usually involve regularly performing a kind of single-pointed concentration or focus activity. Progressive relaxation exercises (Benson, 1975; Titlebaum, 1988) and hypnotic techniques are examples from Western traditions. Various forms of meditation (Leviton, 1995) are examples from Eastern traditions.

Journal writing is another effective way to gain awareness of your inner life (Bernard, 1991). Reflecting on a significant event of the day in writing can add new meaning and provide a reinterpretive function (Progoff, 1975). Returning again and again to the feelings associated with the events provides new insights. It is important to notice whether one has a balance in providing detailed description of the event and differentiated emotions. Sometimes individuals will be more conscious of the event and less aware of how they felt as the event unfolded. Other individuals may be more conscious of how they felt as the event unfolded and paid little attention to the details of the event. Work to enrich descriptions of both emotions and events. The more detailed information one has about the totality of the experience, the better able one is to gain a deeper meaning.

USING COPING STRATEGIES

Coping strategies can be divided into three types of activities: behavioral, cognitive, and emotion focused (Lazarus and Folkman, 1984). Behavioral coping involves modifying or eliminating a problem through direct action. Cognitive coping involves altering one's perspectives to redefine a situation when direct action is impossible or inappropriate. Emotional coping uses various methods of enhancing internal equilibrium. Table 19–1 outlines strategies associated with the three types of coping.

Behavioral Coping

Behavioral coping takes the form of modifying or eliminating the problem through direct action. Seeking advice from others about what to do or how they have handled a similar situation is useful. A common example is asking a classmate how he or she managed time during a particular clinical rotation. Gathering information about the social or political dynamics of the situations is another aspect. Students often find out about their classmates' perceptions of and experiences with an instructor or clinical experience. Negotiations to alter a situation to meet one's needs better is another direction that usually requires negotiation skills. Assertiveness is defined as behaviors that facilitate the expression of one's feelings, needs, and rights in a way that does not deny the rights or humanity of others. Standing up for oneself without putting others down and voicing a concern instead of allowing one's feeling to be ignored are part of being assertive. Confronting or facing a situation means to bravely step forward and handle a problem.

Cognitive Coping

Cognitive coping involves altering one's perspectives. Redefining the meaning of the situation is a useful coping strategy when direct action is not possible or is inappropriate. Upward comparison (Taylor, et al, 1983) or seeing that someone is managing better than oneself offers incentive and motivation: "If she can do that, then so can I." Downward comparison provides a prospective that infuses one's situation with gratefulness: "I am more lucky than I thought. At least I can do X." Selective ignoring means that certain aspects of a situation or person are overlooked. One makes the decision to not be bothered or concerned in the situation. Alternate rewards are sought when one must endure a situation. Some benefit to the situation is sought. Situation redefinition provides one with an alternative perspective. Thinking of a situation as a challenge instead of a threat changes how ones views opportunities. Looking for the lesson provides one with an alternative meaning after a situation has occurred. Asking oneself, "What is the lesson in this?" and "What is to be learned?", invites new information and enhances self-reflection.

Emotional Coping

Emotional coping provides enhanced internal equilibrium. During certain phases of dealing with a situation, one must handle emotional turmoil. Emotional discharge such as crying or laughing prepares one for the next step in coping (Fig. 19–3). At times, withdrawing emotionally from a situation is necessary. This may be used in conjunction with distracting oneself. Self-consolation takes the form of affirmations and self-talk, such as deliberately saying comforting phrases such

TABLE 19-1 Three Types of Coping Responses

Coping Response	Strategies
Behavioral coping: modifying or eliminating a problem through direct action	• Seeking advice from others about what to do or how they have handled a similar situation • Gathering information about social or political dynamics of the situation • Negotiating to alter a situation to better meet one's needs • Asserting one's feelings, needs, and rights in a way that does not deny the rights or humanity of others • Confronting or facing a situation directly.
Cognitive coping: altering one's perspective or redefining the meaning of a situation; useful when direct action is not possible or is inappropriate	• *Upward comparison:* seeing that someone is managing better than oneself offers incentive and motivation: "If she can do that, then so can I." • *Downward comparison:* provides a perspective that infuses one's situation with gratefulness: "I am luckier than I thought. At least I can do this." • *Selective ignoring:* overlooking certain aspects of a situation or person; one decides to not be bothered or concerned. • *Seeking alternate rewards:* when one must endure a situation, one searches for some benefit from it. • *Looking for the lesson:* asking oneself what can be learned from a situation invites new information and enhances self-reflection.
Emotional coping	• Emotional discharge such as crying or laughing prepares one for the next step in coping. • Emotional withdrawal from a situation may be necessary, possibly used in conjunction with self-distraction. • Self-consolation: uses affirmation and self-talk; deliberately saying comforting phrases such as "I can do it," "I'm going to be okay, this won't last forever." • Emotional control: used when any display of felt emotion would have negative repercussions. At times emotional control is the best effort one can make in a difficult situation.

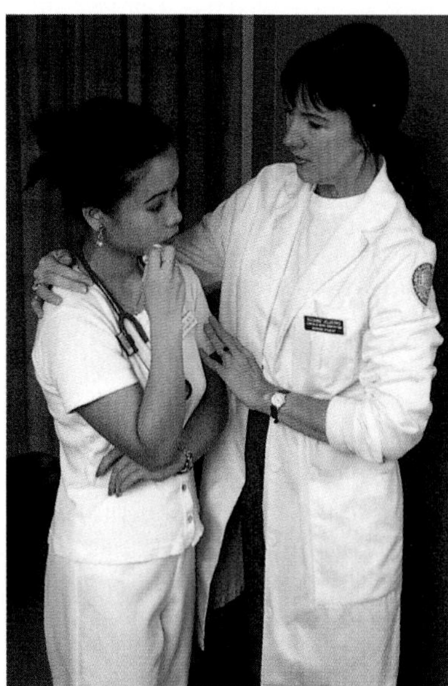

Figure 19–3. Sometimes showing one's emotions is an important step in coping with stress effectively.

as "I can do it . . . I'm going to be okay . . . this won't last forever." Emotional control is used when any display of the felt emotion would be seen to have negative repercussions. At times, emotional control is the best effort one can make in a difficult situation.

Because coping is a process (Folkman and Lazarus, 1985), one may use several coping responses within the same situation. Students may cope in one way before an exam: seek more information, for example. During the exam they may use emotional control or self-consolation. After the exam they may use alternative rewards by saying "I learned a lot even if I wasn't tested on what I knew."

Coping strategies can also be used to provide a general management of stressful events. General coping strategies focus on physiologic (e.g., biofeedback, exercise), cognitive (e.g., imagery, affirmations), and behavioral (e.g., assertiveness, negotiation) changes (Stoyva and Anderson, 1982). Individuals can practice these coping activities as a way of minimizing the impact of stressful events. Skill in general coping influences the way in which one perceives events as a challenge or a threat. The goal is to appraise an event as a challenge and an opportunity for growth and learning.

Not all coping strategies succeed in reducing stress in the long run. Although in the moment a period of denial may be useful or distracting oneself for awhile may provide the body with a rest, prolonged use of a few coping strategies to the exclusion of others can become detrimental. Using alcohol to relax rather than exercise or smoking to calm the nerves instead of using calming affirmations will in the long run become the stressors themselves.

Ensuring Health Promotion

Health promotion activities fall into two realms: active and passive. Active health promotion activities are those that individuals initiate on their own behalf, such as an exercise program or stress management. Passive health promotion activities are large-scale programs affecting whole populations, such as clean water, fluoridation, and clean air programs, in which individuals are the recipients of organized efforts.

ACTIVE HEALTH PROMOTION

For purposes of discussion, active health promotion activities are divided into three categories. The first is derived from traditional behaviors of good health and substantiated by surveys done at the University of California, Los Angeles, School of Public Health and the University of Wisconsin (Leonard, 1976). These behaviors include:

- No smoking
- Moderate drinking
- Seven to 8 hours of sleep each night
- Regular meals
- Breakfast every day
- Maintaining normal weight
- Engaging in moderate regular exercise

The second category of health promotion activities involves proactive behaviors targeted at specific situations. Such behaviors include self-breast or testicular examinations, practicing safe sex, wearing seat belts, keeping immunizations up to date, and lowering fat intake.

The third category of behaviors are the self-care practices that promote self-healing through the alignment of body, mind, and spirit. The basic underlying assumption of these practices is "the world and the body are trustworthy and capable" (Benner and Wrubel, 1989, p. 163). This model does not assume that the world or the self are badly flawed and in need of constant correction or vigilance. The assumption is that the body already has an immense amount of wisdom and healing potential. Access to this wisdom and natural healing is through self-cooperation and letting go of preconceived notions about reality. Access requires being open, centered, and trusting.

Progressive relaxation, meditation, visual imagery, and biofeedback are among the practices available to learn deeper centering skills. Self-healing is enhanced through calming and centering oneself. When one becomes more centered and the mind is calmed down, the wisdom of the body is more accessible (Williams, 1988).

PASSIVE HEALTH PROMOTION

Passive health promotion activities affecting nursing students within the nursing school and health care environment mirror the intent of active health promotion activities: the individual matters. This attitude would be reflected within the policies and procedures of nursing schools and health care agencies. These policies and procedures would be designed to maximize a supportive learning environment (Schlossberg et al, 1989). Examples of policies include:

- Adequate orientation and transition for returning students

- Reasonable work load
- Recognition of the demands on students' time outside of school
- Respect for students' working schedules
- Quiet study spaces
- Procedures to handle student grievances
- Posting of students' rights
- Voice in student-faculty governance
- Respectful relationships
- Tutoring and counseling services

Part of taking care of oneself might include an active involvement within the nursing school to create and promote those policies that support a caring environment.

Mentoring of less experienced nurses by more experienced and successful professionals can provide help with career advancement, emotional support and encouragement, and role socialization; ease the transition from school to professional work life; and affirm one's personal identity as a nurse. Mentoring can also help nurses who are switching careers or switching from one type of nursing to another (Adams-Ender, 1991). Mentoring could be used throughout nurses' educational experience to help empower them to achieve greater control over their practice and experience greater job satisfaction (Carlson-Catalano, 1992). Effective social support from clinical instructors, staff nurses, and student peers helps to buffer against job stress and prevent burnout.

INDIVIDUAL DIFFERENCES

Nursing students bring a rich diversity to their nursing school experience. Diversity is based on differences. Three common types of diversity in schools of nursing are students of color, men in nursing, and immigrant and English-as-a-second-language (ESL) students.

Although historically the white female dominated the nursing profession, this scenario is changing and in some cases has been superseded by a majority of persons of color; however, nursing as a whole continues to display an overriding Anglo-Saxon value structure. Therefore, students of color, male nurses, and students who are recent immigrants or who have limited English proficiency continue to need additional understanding. Holders of these differences usually carry with them valuable insights and strengths that benefit themselves and others as well as possible vulnerabilities to the emotional challenges in nursing school and nursing. Such life situations present nursing students with challenges in developing strong self-care patterns, which include self-knowledge, health promotion, and coping skills. How these individual differences influence nursing students' experience in nursing school is discussed in this section.

Student of Color Experience

As the United States becomes more diverse, nursing is in greater need to develop and maintain culturally competent care for all clients. Nursing students from many different cultural and ethnic backgrounds have the potential to infuse nursing education and practice with culturally sensitive care. Unfortunately, nursing students of color are and have been chronically underrepresented in nursing (Walker, 1987). Admission and retention policies have failed to overcome the dearth of students of color. Initial college experiences of alienation and loneliness for students of color often lead to dropping out of school. The educational experiences of nursing students of color and those of their Anglo peers may be very different. Anglo students at predominately white universities vastly underestimate the lack of support perceived by their ethnic minority peers (Loo and Rolison, 1986).

Coping strategies for nursing students of color aimed at retention include active participation in student government; seeking peer tutoring; social strategies to overcome social isolation; and special attempts to share one's cultural heritage and celebrate one's diversity.

Confronting racism and discrimination takes active behavioral coping strategies. A student of color may have the experience of being expected to be a spokesperson for the whole culture in an academic setting. It is important for students of color to learn to protect themselves from being singled out, pointing out to faculty or others that each culture is very complex with many variations. There is no way any one person can speak for a whole culture. One can speak of one's experience and one's background, however, making a valuable contribution to one's peers. Other stressful experiences faced by students of color are being mistaken for the cleaning staff, being spoken to as though one does not understand English, and being ignored while an Anglo student is receiving all the attention (Porter-Tibbetts, 1992). Assertiveness training is useful if one chooses to deal with discriminatory situations (Alberti and Emmons, 1986).

Students may also elect to selectively ignore racist remarks or to distance themselves emotionally from discriminatory practices found in the clinical setting. Emotional management and redefining meaning are common strategies for ethnic minority nursing students in coping with the ongoing day-to-day subtle discrimination (Porter-Tibbetts, 1992).

The diversity of America will continue to increase as we move into the twenty-first century. Nursing schools will reflect that diversity. Even now nursing students are fairly diverse. Older students, second-career students, students with learning disabilities and dyslexia, gay and lesbian students, and students with physical and emotional handicaps are part of the richness of the nursing student body. Nursing students with varied life experience bring to their clients new depth of compassion and understanding. Transforming one's adult self into a nursing professional requires much self-responsibility and care.

Men in Nursing

Men in nursing school will generally be in a minority, given that less than 10% of nurses are men. Men in nursing are in the peculiar position of being a minority within a profession that as a whole is less valued by society (Reverby, 1994). In addition, men's presence in nursing is tainted with caution and distrust by their female peers (Ryan and Porter, 1993). Within the profession men may experience discrimination by their female peers and faculty because of their gender and by the larger health care system because of their role as nurse. The male nurse is frequently asked why as a man he would want to go into nursing with the implication that he has made a mistake. "Men in nursing are not only transgressing the sex role stereotyping, they are also becoming associated with downwardly mobile female behaviors" (Smith, 1985, p. 86).

Skepticism about men's ability to nurture the right way, provide comfort care, and function adequately in labor and delivery (Cooper, 1987) are barriers that men in nursing face.

Yet several studies document the care and compassion that are part of the nursing perspective held by men in nursing. Ingle (1988) found through repeated interviews with baccalaureate-educated men in nursing that the overriding theme was the business of caring. Supporting physical, psychological, emotional, and spiritual well-being as well as providing advocacy and respect emerged as subthemes. Ingle noted that men exhibited empathy, caring, compassion, and kindness as well as assertiveness and independence (Fig. 19–4). The author encouraged nursing personnel to provide positive reinforcement for these caring behaviors.

Another area where men in nursing may experience distrust is with faculty. The feeling may occur that one must prove one's self more that women in nursing or that one just does not fit in well. Eddy (1989) found that for men in nursing the values of aesthetics and justice were significantly higher and the values of freedom and human dignity were significantly lower than the those of the nursing faculty who were predominately women. Men's values also differed significantly from those of their female peers. Older men in nursing did have values more similar to female values.

In addition, a study of noncognitive factors related to academic success of 125 baccalaureate nursing students suggested that male students were more likely to need support for their academic plans (Kornguth et al, 1994). Strategies of

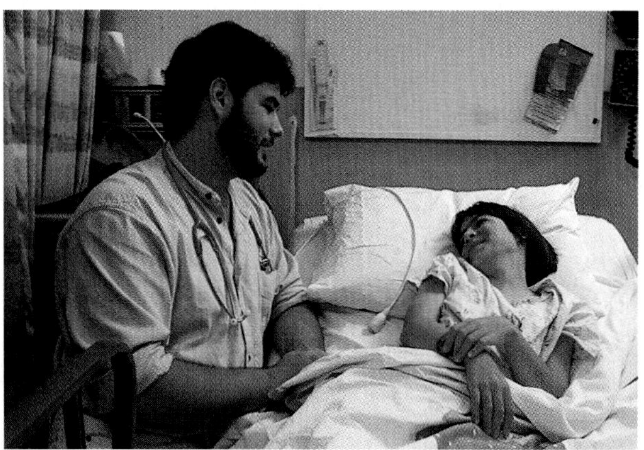

Figure 19–4. Male nurses can be just as empathic, caring, compassionate, and kind as female nurses.

negotiation, conflict resolution, and compassion are invaluable in these situations.

Men in nursing are also confronted with subtle and not so subtle homophobia. The stereotype of the male nurse as gay continues to be played out, much to the detriment of gay and straight men in nursing (Anonymous, 1983; Sharkey, 1987).

Historically, nursing has been a profession dominated by women. Although the profession as a whole has struggled with sexism within the health care system and society in general, it has been a place where women could excel and advance. Even so, men have easier access to leadership positions than their female peers (Squires, 1995). The presence of men in nursing has been welcomed as a way to provide balance and gender equality in the health care system. At the same time, there has been a great unease that men in nursing would have better access to leadership and positions of power, mirroring the sociopolitical culture and thus place more women in the one-down position once again (Ryan and Porter, 1993).

What men in nursing must cope with are the two extremes of being held up as the saviors of the profession and as the interlopers. The resentment and skepticism among women nurses are ever present (Ryan and Porter, 1993; Smith, 1985). Being aware of the broader societal forces that are played out at the individual level provides the nursing student with a broader perspective.

Immigrant and Limited-English Proficiency Experience

As the world political turmoil continues, the United States and other Western countries continue to experience an influx of immigrants. In addition, universities and colleges are reexperiencing a surge of prejudice and racism. Ethnic minority and immigrant nursing students receive their education within a climate of overt and covert ethnocentrism and racism (Bruyere, 1991). Nursing education continues to mirror the dominant culture. Strong expectations for conformity to this dominant culture are present among health care administrators, health care providers, and clients who form the Anglo majority (Amaya, 1991). Isolation, loneliness, and alienation are common experiences of minority nursing students regardless of color or language background (Wright, 1987).

Entering nursing school facilitates the acculturation process as well as provides an economic base for a newcomer to the country. It is not uncommon for the immigrant to attempt to learn nursing and English at the same time. The women and men who enter nursing school with a limited proficiency in English are courageously facing a most challenging experience.

The language of nursing is replete with the nuances of American values, which native speakers have learned from childhood. The notions of self-responsibility, autonomy, and independence are core American values not necessarily shared by cultures with stronger family-, group-, and tribal-based systems. Nursing has much to gain from learning about the family and tribal or group orientation of other cultures. It is important for ESL students to share their perceptions of the American culture and to share their own cultural heritage with their classmates.

However, it is important to know that speaking up in English is a taxing and threatening situation for many limited English proficiency (LEP) nursing students (Phillips & Hartley, 1990; Porter-Tibbetts, 1992). Nursing students with LEP are afraid of saying the wrong thing or having attention called to themselves; they are afraid of sounding different. Even when these students do speak up, they are frequently asked to repeat themselves. This too can become taxing. Students also find that faculty, nursing staff, and patients have a limited tolerance for listening to their attempts at communication. Brink (1990) noted, "How many faculty prefer not to teach foreign students for whom English is a second language because, 'they take too much time'" (p. 524). LEP students speak of being "shut off" by faculty or staff if they are not able to communicate their message quickly enough to satisfy the listener (Porter-Tibbetts, 1992). Patients may request to have a native language student take care of them.

LEP students tend to cope with the language barrier by withdrawing, speaking up only when it is absolutely necessary. Keeping silent is a common coping strategy (Porter-Tibbetts, 1992). Much is lost for students when this happens, among them the opportunity to practice English. Furthermore, native English speakers lose the opportunity to hone their listening skills. Much can be done to improve one's linguistic competency while in nursing school.

Strategies to improve linguistic competency include diligently speaking English only while at school. Make it a point to have conversations with native English speakers. Taping lectures is helpful for some students. Some schools have developed a partnership-type program in which native and nonnative speakers are paired up for the purposes of social conversation. Both speakers benefit in this activity because much cultural exchange occurs. Some cities have accent reduction programs for immigrants. These programs, although relatively new, are quite effective in targeting the phonetics of American English.

Speaking English is a high-stress activity for many newcomers, and even though Americans have a generally high tolerance for language diversity, there continues to be subtle prejudices associated with language. It may take anywhere from 4 to 8 years to develop the English fluency needed for scholastic achievement (Phillips and Hartley, 1990).

CHAPTER HIGHLIGHTS

- Personal self-care and health practices affect a nurse's ability to serve as a model or exemplar for patients. Nurses influence their patients and students not only by what they say, but also by what they do.
- The concept of self-care can be summarized as a collection of actions and attitudes about and toward the self. Self-care involves taking oneself seriously; taking actions that protect oneself; avoiding harm to oneself; liking and being willing to care for oneself; learning to balance one's needs in a situation with the needs of others; being reflective and mindful as a way to enhance the care of the self; making the effort to maintain or restore relationships; and finding ways to relieve one's own suffering.
- Self-knowledge is a reflective process that leads to altered perceptions and understandings of oneself and others. Developing self-knowledge skills requires the ability to focus and attend to increasing levels of honesty and complexity in one's thoughts and feelings.
- Coping is generally understood as a complex of behavioral, cognitive, and physiologic responses that aim to prevent or minimize unpleasant or harmful experiences that tax one's personal resources.
- Health is defined broadly as well-being, congruence between one's possibilities and one's actual practices and lived meanings, and is based on caring and feeling cared for.
- Appraisal is a cognitive activity to determine meaning or significance of an event or situation. The evaluation process is focused on the importance of the situation to one's well-being.
- The search for gaining control, seeking predictable patterns, and making sense lead one to develop higher orders of self-complexity. What feels like fluctuations, disturbances, and imbalances are the seeds of a new self-order forming.
- One way to empower one's self is to ask the question "How can I?" instead of stating "I can't."
- Self-healing is enhanced through calming and centering oneself. When one becomes more centered and the mind is calmed down, the wisdom of the body is more accessible.
- Part of taking care of oneself might include an active involvement within the nursing school to create and promote those policies that support a caring environment.

REFERENCES

Abraham, K., Reich, R. (1996). *Occupational Outlook Handbook* (1996–97 ed.). Washington DC: U.S. Bureau of Labor Statistics.

Adams-Ender, C. (1991). Taking charge. Mentoring: nurses helping nurses. *RN, 54,* 21–23.

Alberti, R., Emmons, M. (1986). *Your Perfect Right: A Guide to Assertive Living.* San Luis Obispo, CA: Impact Publishers.

Amaya, M. (1991). Official English amendment: a nurse's commentary. *Nursing Forum, 26*(3), 24–26.

American Nurses' Association (1984). *Addictions and Psychological Dysfunction in Nursing: The Profession's Response to the Problem.* Kansas City, MO: ANA.

Anonymous. (1983). Glad to be gay . . . a male nurse describes the problems he has. *Nursing Mirror, 156*(20), 33–34.

Barr, A. (1989). The effect of assertiveness training on performance of self esteem and sex role in nurses (doctoral dissertation, California School of Professional Psychology). *Dissertation Abstracts International, 50,* 4210.

Beck, C. (1991). Undergraduate nursing students' lived experience of health: a phenomenological study. *Journal of Nursing Education, 30*(8), 371–374.

Benner, P., Wrubel, J. (1989). *The Primacy of Caring: Stress and Coping in Health and Illness*. Reading, MA: Addison-Wesley.

Benson, H. (1975). *The Relaxation Response*. New York: William Morrow.

Bermosk, L., Porter, S. (1979). *Women's Health and Human Wholeness*. New York: Appleton-Century-Crofts.

Bernard, M. (ed.). (1991). *Using Rational-Emotive Therapy Effectively: A Practitioner's Guide*. New York: Plenum Press.

Blattner, B. (1981). *Holistic Nursing*. Englewood Cliffs, NJ: Prentice-Hall.

Boyd, E., Fales, A. (1983). Reflective learning: key to learning from experience. *Journal of Humanistic Psychology, 23,* 99–117.

Briere, J. (1992). *Child Abuse Trauma*. Newbury Park, CA: Sage.

Brink, P. (1990). Cultural diversity in nursing: how much can we tolerate? In J. McCloskey and H. Grace (eds.): *Current Issues in Nursing,* 3rd ed. St. Louis, MO: C.V. Mosby.

Bruyere, J. (1991). Personal growth and the minority student. *Journal of Nursing Education, 30*(6), 278–279.

Cannon, B., Brown, J. (1988). Attitudes of registered nurses towards chemically dependent peers. *Image, 20,* 96–101.

Carlson-Catalano, J. (1992). Empowering nurses for professional practice. *Nursing Outlook, 40,* 139–142.

Carver, C., Glass, D. (1976). The self-consciousness scale: a discriminant validity study. *Journal of Personality Assessment, 40,* 169–172.

Carver, C., Scheier, M. (1985). Self-consciousness, expectancies, and the coping process. In T. Field, P. McCabe, and N. Scheidman (eds.): *Stress and Coping*. Hillsdale, NJ: Erlbaum, pp. 305–330.

Casey, F., Haughey, B., Dittmar, S., et al. (1989). Smoking practices among nursing students: a comparison of two studies. *Journal of Nursing Education, 28*(9), 397–401.

Caton, K. (1997). *Technology - SoN External and Internal Data Collection*. Unpublished report, Oregon Health Sciences University, School of Nursing (SoN), Portland.

Chacko, S., Huba, M. (1991). Academic achievement among undergraduate nursing students: the development and test of a causal model. *Journal of Nursing Education, 30*(6), 267–273.

Chinn, P. (1994). Looking into the crystal ball: positioning ourselves for the year 2000. In E.C. Hein and M.J. Nicholson (eds.): *Contemporary Leadership Behavior: Selected Readings,* 4th ed. Philadelphia: J.B. Lippincott, p. 436.

Clement, M., Bouchard, L., Jankowski, L., Perreault, M. (1995). Health promotion behaviors in first-year undergraduate nursing students: a pilot study. *Canadian Journal of Nursing Research, 27*(4), 111–131.

Condon, E. (1992). Nursing and the caring metaphor: gender and political influences on an ethics of care. *Nursing Outlook, 40*(1), 14–19.

Cooper, M. (1987). A suitable job for a man? Nursed by men in obstetric wards. *Nursing Times, 83*(34), 49–50.

Crosby L., Bissell, L. (1989). *To Care Enough: Intervention with Chemically Dependent Colleagues. A Guide for Healthcare and Other Professionals.* Minneapolis, MN: Johnson Institute.

Davidhizer, R., Giger, J. (1991). When the nurse faces separation and loss. *Advances in Clinical Care, 6*(5), 19–21.

Dittmar, S., Haughey, B., O'Shea, R., Brasure, J. (1989). Health practices of nursing students: a survey. *Health Values, 13,* 24–31.

Dreher, M. (1996). Technology not technocracy. *Reflections, 22* (1), 2, 7.

Eakes, G. (1988). Grief resolution in hospice nurses. *Nursing and Health Care, 11,* 243–248.

Eddy, D. (1989). Men in nursing: comparison and contrast of values and professional behaviors of male baccalaureate students and female faculty in Ohio (doctoral dissertation, University of Akron). *Dissertation Abstracts International, 50,* 2335.

Elkind, A. (1988). Do nurses smoke because of stress? *Journal of Advanced Nursing, 13,* 733–745.

Fassel, D. (1990). *Working Ourselves to Death*. San Francisco: Harper.

Feldman, B., Richard, E. (1986). Prevalence of nurse smokers and variables associated with successful and unsuccessful smoking cessation. *Research in Nursing & Health, 9,* 131–138.

Folkman, S, Lazarus, R. (1985). If it changes it must be a process: study of emotion and coping during three stages of a college examination. *Journal of Personality and Social Psychology, 48*(1) 150–170.

Folkman, S., Schaefer, C., Lazarus, R. (1979). Cognitive processes as mediators of stress and coping. In V. Hamilton and D. Warburton (eds.) *Human Stress and Cognition*. New York: John Wiley & Sons, pp. 265–298

Gallop, R., McKeever, P., Toner, B., et al. (1995). The impact of childhood sexual abuse on the psychological well-being and practice of nurses. *Archives of Psychiatric Nursing, 9*(3), 137–145.

Gann, M. (1979). The role of personality factors and job characteristics in burnout: a study of social workers (doctoral dissertation, California School of Professional Psychology). *Dissertation Abstracts, 40,* 3366.

Gilligan, C. (1982). *In a Different Voice*. Cambridge, MA: Harvard University Press.

Goldsmith, J. (1996). A field of cyberdreams. *Reflections, 22*(2), 9.

Gritz, E., Berman, B., Marcus, A., et al. (1989). Ethnic variations in the prevalence of smoking among registered nurses. *Cancer Nursing, 12,* 16–20.

Haack, M. (1987). Alcohol use and burnout among student nurses. *Nursing & Health Care, 8,* 239–242.

Hughes, L. (1992). Faculty-student interactions and the student-perceived climate of caring. *Advances in Nursing Science, 14,* 60–71.

Hutchinson, S. (1987). Self-care and job stress. *Image: Journal of Scholarship, 19,* 192–196.

Ingle, J.R. (1988). *The Business of Caring: The Perspective of Men in Nursing*. Birmingham, AL: University of Alabama at Birmingham.

Jarrett, R. (1993). *Caring for the Caregiver*. Beaverton, OR: Happy Talk Books.

Johns, J. (1991). Self-care today: In search of an identity. In B. Spradley (ed.): *Readings in Community Health Nursing,* 4th ed. Philadelphia: J.B. Lippincott, pp. 44–50.

Julian, D. (1990). Women in transition: educational implications (doctoral dissertation, University of Oregon). *Dissertation Abstracts International, 51,* 754A.

Kairns, D. (1992). Taking charge. *RN, 55,* 19–22.

Kabasa, S., Maddi, S., Kahn, S. (1982). Hardiness and health: a prospective study. *Journal of Personality and Social Psychology, 42* (1), 168–177.

Kornguth, M., Krisch, N., Shovein, J., Williams, R. (1994). Noncognitive factors that put students at academic risk in nursing programs. *Nurse Educator, 19*(5), 24–27.

Kritsberg, W. (1988). *The Adult Children of Alcoholics Syndrome.* Bantom, NY: Health Communications.

Kushner, T. (1986). Stress and social facilitation: the effects of the presence of an instructor on student nurses' behavior. *Journal of Advanced Nursing, 11*(1), 13–19.

Lane, R., Schwartz, G. (1987). Levels of emotional awareness: a cognitive-developmental theory and its application to psychopathology. *American Journal of Psychiatry, 144*(2), 133–143.

Lazarus, R., Folkman, S. (1984). *Stress, Appraisal and Coping.* New York: Springer.

Leininger, M., Watson, J. (1990). *The Caring Imperative in Education.* Thorofare, NJ: Charles Slack.

Leonard, G. (1976). The holistic revolution. *New West, May 10,* 42.

Leviton, R. (1995). *Brain Builders.* New York: Parker.

Linville, P. (1987). Self-complexity as a cognitive buffer against stress-related illness and depression. *Journal of Personality and Social Psychology, 2,* 663–676.

Loo, C., Rolison, G. (1986). Alienation of ethnic minority students at a predominantly white university. *Journal of Higher Education, 57,* 58–77.

Markus, H., Smith, J. (1981). The influence of self-schemata on the perceptions of others. In N. Cantor and J. F. Kihlstrom (eds.): *Personality, Cognition & Social Interaction.* Hillsdale, NJ: Erlbaum, pp. 233–262.

McAlindon, M. (1994). The nurse and informatics. In M. Mundinger (ed.): *The Pfizer Guide: Nursing Career Opportunities.* New York: Merritt Communications.

McDonough, J. (1989). *Personality and Addiction Tendency: An Initial Comparison of Graduate Students of Nursing and Nurse Anesthesia.* Unpublished Master's thesis, Drake University.

Miller, J. (1976). *Toward a New Psychology of Women.* Boston: Beacon Press.

Moore, T. (1992). *Care of the Soul in Everyday Life.* New York: HarperCollins.

Morse, J., Bottorff, J., Neader, W., Solberg S. (1991). Comparative analysis of conceptualizations and theories of caring. *Image: Journal of Nursing Scholarship, 23*(2), 119–126.

Mundinger, M. (ed.). (1994). *The Pfizer Guide: Nursing Career Opportunities.* New York: Merritt Communications.

Orem, D. (1980). *Nursing: Concept of Practice.* Chevy Chase, MD: McGraw-Hill.

Padula, C. (1992). Nurses and smoking: review and implications. *Journal of Professional Nursing, 8,* 20–132.

Pagana, K. (1990). The relationship of hardiness and social support to student appraisal of stress in an initial clinical nursing situation. *Journal of Nursing Education, 29,* 255–261.

Parkes, K. (1984). Locus of control, cognitive appraisal, and coping in stressful episodes. *Journal of Personality and Social Psychology, 46*(3), 655–668.

Parkes, K. (1986). Coping in stressful episodes: The role of individual differences, environmental factors, and situational characteristics. *Journal of Personality and Social Psychology, 51*(6), 1277–1292.

Penny, N. (1996) Rural nurses retool for expanding health needs. *Reflections, 22* (2), 14–15.

Peter, E., Gallop, R. (1994). The ethic of care: a comparison of nursing and medical students. *Image: Journal of Nursing Scholarship, 26*(2), 24–51.

Phillips, S., Hartley, J. (1990). Teaching students for whom English is a second language. *Nurse Educator, 15*(5), 29–32.

Pines, A., Aronson, E., Kafry, D. (1981). *Burnout.* New York: Free Press.

Porter, E.H. (1973). On the development of relationship awareness theory: a personal note. *Group & Organization Studies, 1*(3), 302–309.

Porter-Tibbetts, S. (1992). Perceiving and coping with exclusion: the socialization experiences of ethnic minority nursing students (doctoral dissertation, Portland State University). *Dissertation Abstracts International, 53,* 4096.

Progoff, I. (1975). *In a Journal Workshop.* New York: Dialogue House Library.

Pugh, J.B., Woodward-Smith, M. (1997). *Nurse Manager: A Practical Guide to Better Employee Relations,* 2nd ed. Philadelphia: W.B. Saunders.

Reverby, S. (1994). A caring dilemma: womanhood and nursing in historical perspective, 1987. In E.C. Hein and M.J. Nicholson (eds.): *Contemporary Leadership Behavior,* 4th ed. Philadelphia: J.B. Lippincott, pp. 3–15.

Rich, V., Rich, A. (1987). Personality hardiness and burnout in female staff nurses. *Image: The Journal of Nursing Scholarship, 19,* 63–66.

Ryan, S., Porter, S. (1993). Men in nursing: A cautionary comparative critique. *Nursing Outlook, 41*(6), 262–267.

Saba, V. (1994). Informatics: an overview. In M. Mundinger (ed.): *The Pfizer Guide: Nursing Career Opportunities.* New York: Merritt Communications.

Salmon, M. (ed.). (1996). *Report to the Secretary of the Department of Health and Human Services on the Basic Registered Nurse Workforce.* Washington, DC: National Advisory Council on Nurse Education and Practice. Health Resources and Services Administration, Bureau of Health Professions, Division of Nursing.

Schaefer, K., Peterson, K. (1992). Effectiveness of coping strategies among critical care nurses. *Dimensions of Critical Care, 11,* 28–34.

Schlossberg, N., Lynch, A., and Chickering, A. (1989). *Improving higher Education Environments for Adults.* San Francisco: Jossey-Bass.

Seed, A. (1995). Crossing the boundaries: experiences of neophyte nurses. *Journal of Advanced Nursing, 21,* 1136–1143.

Sharkey, L. (1987). Nurses in the closet: is nursing open and receptive to gay and lesbian nurses? *Imprint, 34*(3), 38–39.

Smith, E. (1985). Career versus job orientation: a power dilemma in nursing and feminism. In R. Wieczorek (ed.): *Power, Politics, and Policy in Nursing.* New York: Springer.

Sobol, E. (1978). Self-actualization and the baccalaureate nursing student's response to stress. *Nursing Research, 27*(4), 238–244.

Soeken, K., Bausell, R., Winklestein, M., Carson, V. (1989). Preventive behavior: attitudes and compliance of nursing students. *Journal of Advanced Nursing, 14,* 1026–1033.

Sohier, R. (1992). Feminism and nursing knowledge: the power of the weak. *Nursing Outlook, 40,* 62–93.

Spencer-Strachan, F. (1990). Attitudes of registered nurses toward perceived substance abusing peers and education specific to substance abuse. *The ABNF Journal, 1*(2)27–32.

Squires, T.E. (1995). Men in nursing. *RN, 58,* 26–28.

Stoyva, J., Anderson, C. (1982). A coping-rest model of relaxation and stress management. In L. Goldberger and S. Breznitz (eds.): *Handbook of Stress.* New York: Free Press, pp. 745–763.

Taylor, S., Wood, J., Lichtman, R. (1983). It could be worse: selective evaluation as a response to victimization. *Journal of Social Issues, 30,* 19–40.

Thomas, L. (1983). *The Youngest Science: Notes of a Medicine-Watcher.* New York: Viking Press, pp. 64–65.

Thurston, M., Flood, M., Shupe, I., Gerald, K. (1989). Values held by nursing faculty and students in a university setting. *Journal of Professional Nursing, 5*(4), 199–207.

Titlebaum, H. (1988). Relaxation. *Holistic Nursing Practice, 2*(3),17–25.

Walker, H. (1987). Recruitment strategies for increasing minority environment in nursing and other professional schools. *Journal of Nursing Education, 26,* 169–171.

Wheatley, M. (1992). Searching for order in an orderly world. *Journal of Management Inquiry, 1*(4), 337–342.

Williams, K. (1988). World view and the facilitation of wholeness. *Holistic Nursing Practice, 2*(3), 1–8.

Wilson, M. (1994). Nursing student perspective of learning in a clinical setting. *Journal of Nursing Education, 33*(2), 81–86.

Wright, D. (1987). Minority students: developmental beginnings. In D.J. Wright (ed.): *Responding to the Needs of Today's Minority Students* (New Directions for Student Services Series No. 38). San Francisco: Jossey-Bass.

Wright, S. (1996). Alcohol abuse among college students: implications for nurse practitioners. *Journal of the American Academic of Nurse Practitioners, 8,* 433–438.

Yovanovich, L. (1991). A caregiver's guide to self-care. *Nursing, 21,* 149–150.

Zimmerman, J. (1991). Nursing and mental health: taking care of ourselves. *AARN, 47,* 8–9.

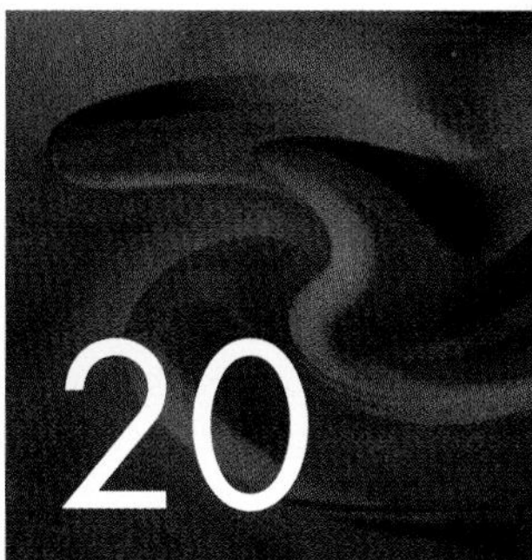

Biomechanics and Mobility

Ellen Kreighbaum

Imagine that you are a nurse on the unit of a hospital that has postoperative orthopedic patients. You have been on duty for a very busy 6 hours. Because you have been on your feet much of the time, your lower back is aching and you have a burning painful sensation at the base of your right first toe. It is time to get Mrs. Jones up for her walk. She has had a total hip replacement. You must help her out of bed and assist her with her walker as she walks down the hall. As she walks you must be ever vigilant, because she may need your assistance at any time. (Her leg and hip are not yet dependable.)

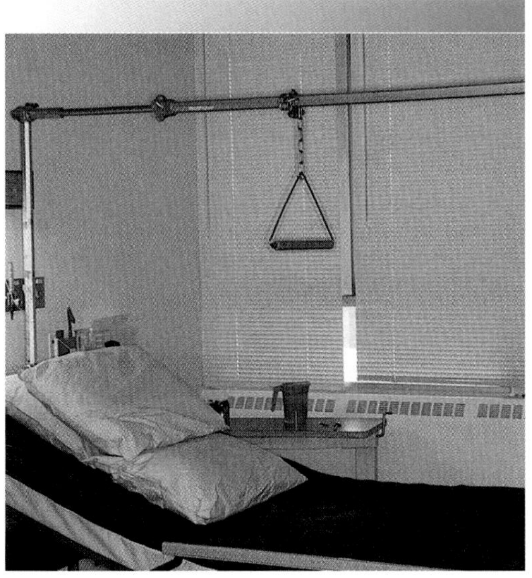

Proper application of biomechanics of the musculoskeletal system to you as a moving person may help your back and foot problems. The application of biomechanics knowledge is essential for effective movement and reduced risk of injury to you and to your patient as you assist her from bed to walker and as you guide her through her postoperative exercise protocol.

OBJECTIVES

After studying this chapter, students will be able to:

- **define and describe the biomechanical bases of movement and mobility and their applications to nursing practice**
- **describe pertinent nursing and non-nursing health-related research and discuss its application to nursing practice**
- **incorporate individual patient differences while providing nursing care**
- **recognize how injury resulting from poor body mechanics in daily living, work, and leisure affects finances**
- **demonstrate that nursing care principles related to biomechanics are the same regardless of where care is given**
- **understand the impact of new technological advances in biomechanics and nursing practice**
- **demonstrate and implement sound biomechanical principles in standing, sitting, walking, and lying down and in providing nursing care**

SCOPE OF NURSING PRACTICE

Biomechanics concepts may be applied to any human environment to make human movement more effective and more efficient and to prevent or decrease the possibility of injury. One must know the parts and movements of the musculoskeletal system, the basic mechanical concepts to which the body is subjected, and the interaction of the two to apply biomechanics to everyday situations.

Nurses and their patients are constantly moving or being moved in a gravitationally dependent world. The forces to which the body is subjected can cause the body to move, can resist the movement of an already moving body, can influence the acceleration of a body, and can produce injury in a body that misuses basic biomechanical principles and guidelines. The nurse must know the proper application of biomechanical principles so that the patient or the nurse is not injured beyond the existing condition.

Application requires knowledge of the musculoskeletal system, the bones, the articulations, and how the articulations move. Proper application also requires an understanding of forces, their magnitudes and directions, and the accelerations that those forces cause. The following sections of this chapter give the reader definitions of the biomechanical concepts and examples of the functional relationships of these concepts to human environments. Biomechanical concepts are used specifically to help the nurse in the safe accomplishment of the procedures that must be used everyday.

The environments in which a nurse must apply these concepts are varied. In a hospital environment, there are tools, machines, and other nurses and aides who may help in the safe accomplishment of tasks. In the home environment, frequently the nurse is alone with the patient and has few machines to assist in moving the patient. Understanding how the body moves, the biomechanical principles under which the body is subjected, and the principles of safety will aid the nurse in the accomplishment of tasks in whatever environment they are performed.

KNOWLEDGE BASE

Biomechanics is a relatively new and unique field of study. It is derived from knowledge of musculoskeletal and neural anatomy and mechanical physics. It forms the basis of inquiry into the most effective practices used in a variety of movement environments. In this chapter, knowledge from biomechanics is applied to the movement environment of the nurse so as to enhance the nurse's own movements and is used as a basis for developing sound fundamental practices and procedures for interaction with a variety of patients in different settings.

The knowledge from the basic sciences includes the names and locations of bones of the body; the names, movements, and ranges of motion of the joints of the body; the names of skeletal muscles of the body and the movements they affect; and the types of movements displayed and forces encountered by the body. The knowledge base is then applied to the nurse as a mover within the nursing environment and also to the patient.

Basic Science

ANATOMY AND PHYSIOLOGY

There are four anatomic subdisciplines related to human movement: *osteology,* the study of the skeletal system; *arthrology,* the study of the articulations or joints; *myology,* the study of muscles; and *neurology,* the study of the nervous system (Kreighbaum and Barthels, 1996). There are two mechanical subdisciplines related to movement: *kinematics,* the study of time and motion; and *kinetics,* the study of forces and torques that cause or change motion.

BONES

The framework of the body is made up of 206 individual bones that can be divided into the axial skeleton (the skull, thorax, pelvis, and vertebral column) and the appendicular skeleton (the bones of the upper and lower extremities). The bones of the skeletal system are shown in Figure 20–1.

These bones serve six functions (Kreighbaum and Barthels, 1996):

- Protect vital organs
- Support soft tissues
- Produce red blood cells
- Serve as a reservoir for calcium and phosphate
- Provide attachments for skeletal muscles
- Act as a system of machines to make movement possible

In biomechanics, the attachment of the skeletal muscles to the bones of the body and the resulting system of levers used to produce movement are most important.

Types of Bones

There are four types of bones, classified by shape. *Long bones* are found in the appendicular skeleton and are used to provide levers for movement. The long bones of the upper extremity are generally shorter and lighter than those found in the lower extremity, because the lower extremity must repeatedly bear weight whereas those found in the upper extremity are used for reaching and grasping. *Short bones* appear as chunks of bones, such as those found in the hands and feet. They are compact; and, in addition to providing attachments for skeletal muscles, they serve collectively to absorb shock. *Flat bones* give a protective covering to the soft tissues below them as well as have muscle attachments to allow movement. Examples of flat bones are the skull, pelvis, and scapula. *Irregular bones* such as the vertebrae have muscle attachments, protect the spinal cord, and, along with the discs between them, partially absorb the shock of landing when walking and running.

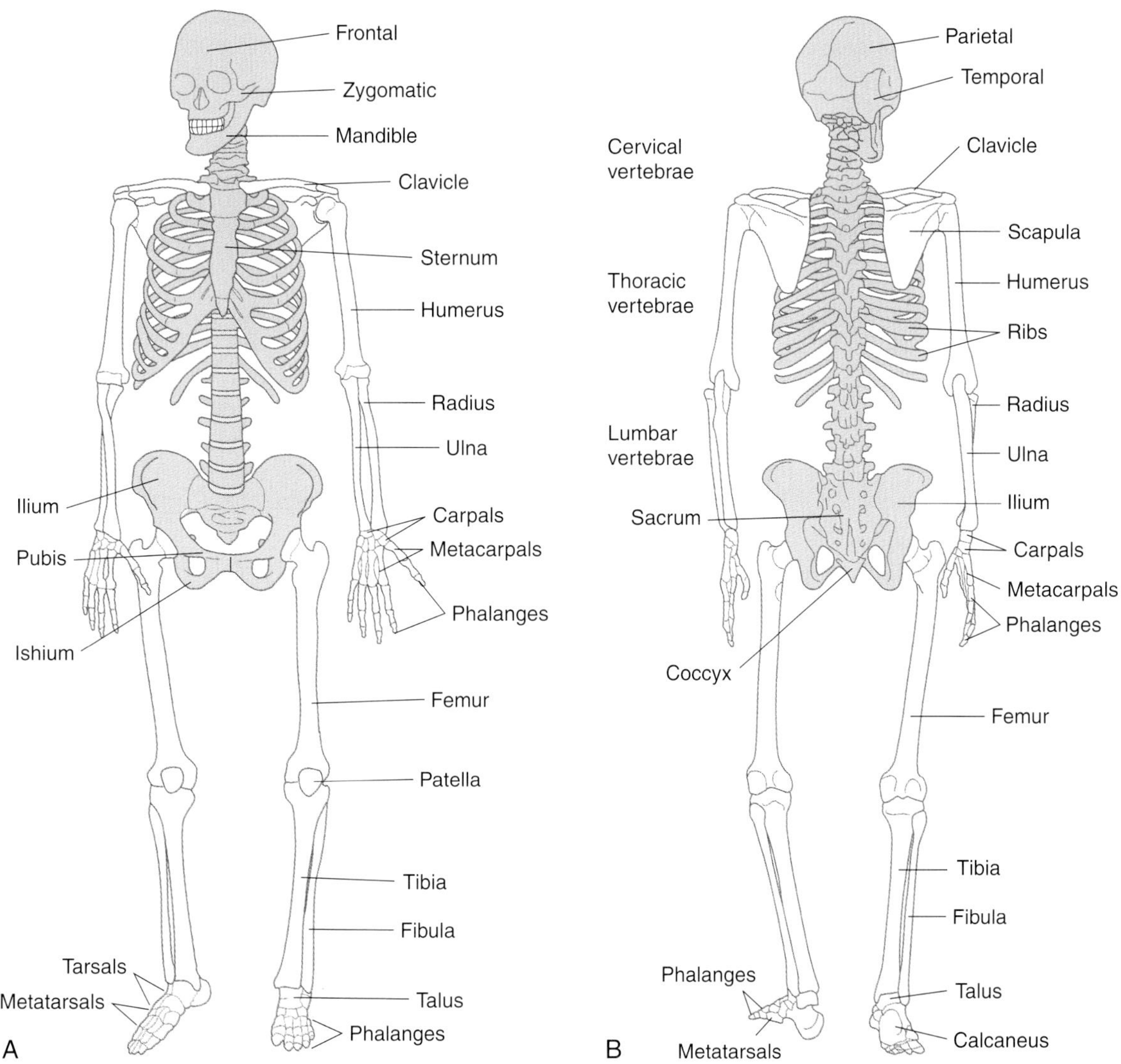

Figure 20–1. The human skeleton. The axial skeleton is indicated by the darker color: *A*, Front view; *B*, Posterior view. (Adapted from Kreighbaum, E., and Barthels, K.M. (1996). *Biomechanics: A Qualitative Approach for Studying Human Movement,* 4th ed. Boston: Allyn & Bacon.)

Structure of Bones

Growth of the long bones takes place at the ends of the bone along what is called the epiphyseal plate. The parts of a typical long bone are shown in Figure 20–2.

The shaft of the long bone is covered with an outer shell called the *cortex* and surrounds the medullary cavity. The entire shaft area of the bone is called the *diaphysis.* The *medullary cavity* contains the bone marrow where red blood cells are produced. On either end of the diaphysis is the metaphysis. The *metaphysis* is filled with spongy bone or *trabecular bone.* It is the numerous fine strands of trabeculae that align themselves in accordance with the physical stresses placed on the bone and help the bone withstand the continual forces that the bone encounters. The *epiphyseal plate* is located at the ends of the metaphysis. The *epiphysis* is located on the other side of this plate.

Bone growth takes place along the epiphyseal plate by depositing *osteoblasts* (new bone cells) there. The bone continues to grow and lengthen in this manner until maturational or nutritional signals trigger a stop. This completion of the bone's growth is called *ossification,* or the bone is said to have ossified. The ossification time varies with the particular bone, sex, and nutritional circumstances. In rare cases, a bone that is subjected to a high impact or repeated smaller stresses may be triggered into premature ossification. For the most part, physical stresses stimulate the bone to grow stronger and thicker.

The location of muscle and muscle tendon attachments often forms an *apophysis,* a raised section of bone that is separated from the cortex by an apophyseal plate. The tension or pulling of the muscle on the bone as it attempts to shorten stimulates the depositing of osteoblasts along the apophyseal plate. Thus, the continued use of the muscle encourages increased bone strength at that location. The radial tuberosity where the biceps muscle attaches to the radius is an obvious example. Changes in bone with age, sex, and hormonal changes are presented in a later section of this chapter.

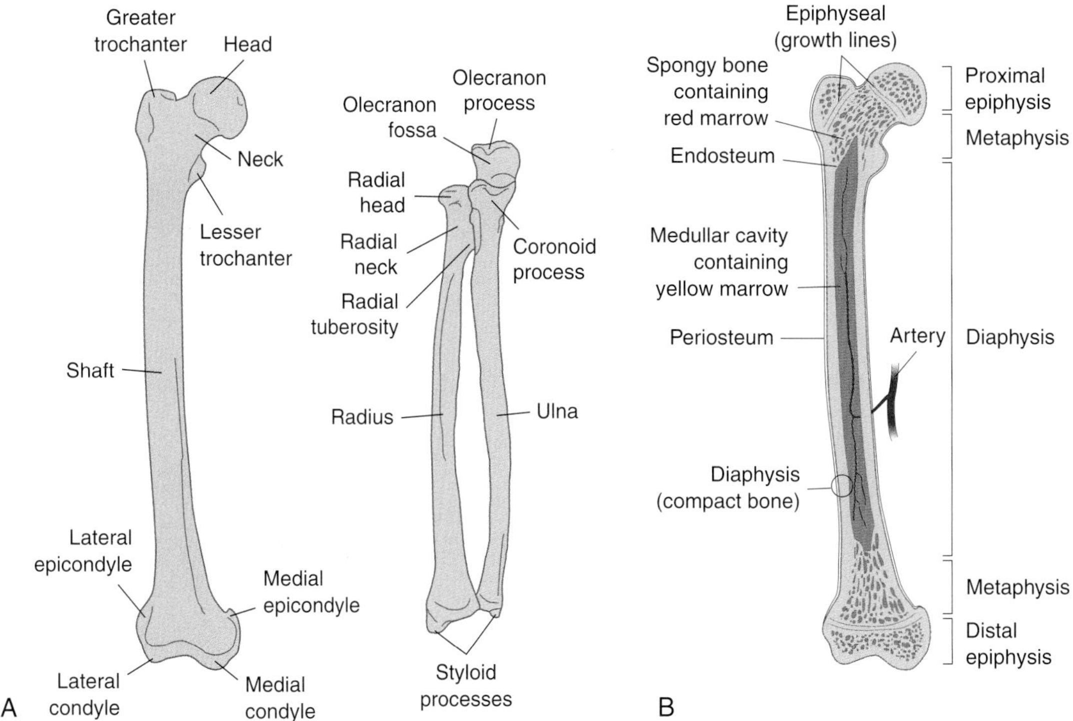

Figure 20–2. Parts of a long bone. (Adapted from Kreighbaum, E., and Barthels, K.M. (1996). *Biomechanics: A Qualitative Approach for Studying Human Movement,* 4th ed. Boston: Allyn & Bacon.)

ARTICULATIONS

The place where two or more bones come together is called an *articulation,* or joint. Depending on the shape of the ends of the bones articulating, the type of material between the two bones, if any, and the type of articulation, various movements are possible between the two segments.

Types of Articulations

Articulations may be categorized according to how much movement is allowed. *Synarthrodial articulations* are considered immovable but may display slight movement when responding to an applied force and thus help to absorb shock. An example is the sutures in the skull. *Amphiarthrodial articulations* are considered slightly movable because there is a fibrous disc, a membrane, or a ligament between the two bones that allows the bones to shift relative to each other. Hormonal changes during pregnancy, for example, can change the amount of movement possible in the symphysis pubis, a fibrocartilage between the pubic bones and the right and left pelvis. Another example is the intervertebral joints.

The most common articulation is the *diarthrodial articulation,* which is described as freely movable, although there is some restriction in the range of motion owing to the shapes of the bones and the flexibility of the ligaments and muscle tendons surrounding the articulations. A typical diarthrodial articulation is shown in Figure 20–3. Examples of this type of articulation are elbows, knees, wrists, and ankles.

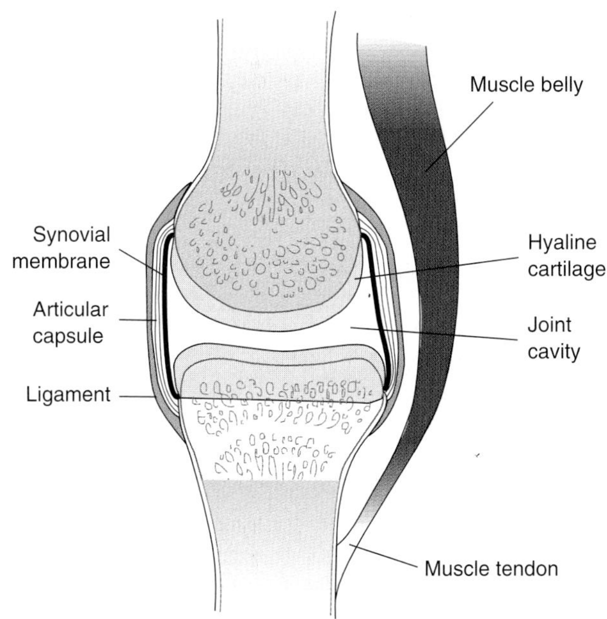

Figure 20–3. A typical diarthrodial articulation.(Adapted from Kreighbaum, E., and Barthels, K.M. (1996). *Biomechanics: A Qualitative Approach for Studying Human Movement,* 4th ed. Boston: Allyn & Bacon.)

Structure of Articulations

The *hyaline cartilage* on the ends of the bones is smooth and elastic. It absorbs shock and provides a frictionless surface over which the bones can slide. Degeneration of the hyaline cartilage can occur due to aging, or high-impact repetitive stress resulting in cracks, chips, and wear that can be painful and restrictive. Between the two bones is a cavity that houses a fluid called synovial fluid. It is the synovial fluid that lubricates the cartilage and aids in smooth movement. The fluid is encased by the *synovial membrane,* which is filled with nerve endings and is sensitive to pressure changes such as from swelling of the joint or chips of cartilage that may become lodged next to it. The *articular capsule* surrounds the articulation and aids in holding the bones together. *Ligaments* are connective tissues outside the capsule that hold one bone to the other. Examples are the anterior cruciate ligament in the knee joint and the annular ligament in the elbow. Finally, muscle *tendons* cross articulations and help to stabilize the articulation from dislocation. Tendinitis is the inflammation of a tendon associated with a muscle such as Achilles tendinitis or tendinitis in the tendons surrounding the elbow causing tennis elbow.

Axes of Rotation in Articulations

The movements possible in diarthrodial articulations take place around one, two, or three axes. Axes may be imagined as rods or dowels that pass through the articulation similar to the pins in a door hinge that allow the door to swing or rotate open or closed. The *mediolateral axis* runs from the medial (middle most) side of the articulation to the lateral (outside most) side. The *anteroposterior axis* runs from the front of the articulation to the back. The *longitudinal axis* runs along the adjoining segment from the *proximal* (near) end to the *distal* (far) end. The two-dimensional path that a body segment sweeps during its rotation around an axis is called a *plane.* When a body part rotates around the mediolateral axis, it sweeps along a frontal plane. When a body part rotates around the anteroposterior axis, it sweeps along the *sagittal plane,* and when a segment rotates around the longitudinal axis, it sweeps along a *transverse plane.* Figure 20–4 illustrates these planes and axes.

Movements of Articulations

The movements possible at the articulations are performed by the individual body segments. For example, flexion at the knee joint may be demonstrated by the lower leg moving toward the thigh as in the push-off and recovery phase of walking or by the thigh moving toward the lower leg as in sitting down. The movements of the segments of the body are illustrated in Figures 20–5 through 20–7.

Functions of Articulations

Properties of articulations include mobility and stability. *Mobility* is determined by the degree to which a segment can move before being restricted. Commonly, it is called flexibility. Mobility is measured by the range of motion of the segment or the total number of degrees a segment can move from one extreme to the other. Mobility may be restricted by any one of five factors:

- Shape of the articulating bones
- Flexibility of the ligaments surrounding and crossing the articulation
- Flexibility of the muscle tendons crossing the articulation
- Tissue bulk in the adjoining segments
- Restrictive clothing

The average range of motion for the movements of the articulations of the segments is noted in Figures 20–5 through 20–7.

Stability is determined by the degree to which the body segment and its articulation can withstand external force without injury to the articulation and surrounding tissues. Both of these functions are influenced by the shape of the bony articulating surfaces and the strength of the surrounding ligaments and muscle tendons. Frequently, it is incorrectly thought that mobility and stability are mutually exclusive functions, that is, if stability is great, mobility must be sacrificed. One needs only think of a gymnast who is certainly strong yet may have great ranges of motion (flexibility) of the joints. The strength of the surrounding ligaments and tissues is often lost with age and lack of exercise. The weakening of these tissues allows the articulation's stability to be compromised such that when the articulation is subjected to an external force as common as the body weight in some cases, tissue damage or dislocations can occur. The mobility and the stability of articulations should be maintained through an ongoing flexibility and muscle-strengthening exercise program.

MUSCLES

Mechanics of Muscle Function

Skeletal muscles are attached to two or more bones by way of direct muscle fiber attachment or by way of a tendinous attachment. Recall that a tendon is connective tissue that connects muscle fibers to the bone. When prompted by an electrochemical stimulus, muscles attempt to shorten and to pull both its ends toward the middle or belly of the muscle. Each muscle attaches to two bones that have at least one articulation between them. The two attachments are called an origin and an insertion. The *origin* is the more proximal, is usually larger and frequently fleshy, and is usually attached to the less movable segment. The *insertion* is the more distal attachment, is frequently tendinous, and is attached to the more movable segment. For example, the biceps has one of its origins on the acromion process of the scapula and its insertion on the radius. In this case there are two articulations, the shoulder and the elbow, between the origin and the insertion.

A shortening muscle will attempt to cause movement at all of the articulations that it crosses and therefore will try to move both of the bones to which it is attached. Sometimes it is not desirable to move segments at all of the articulations; therefore,

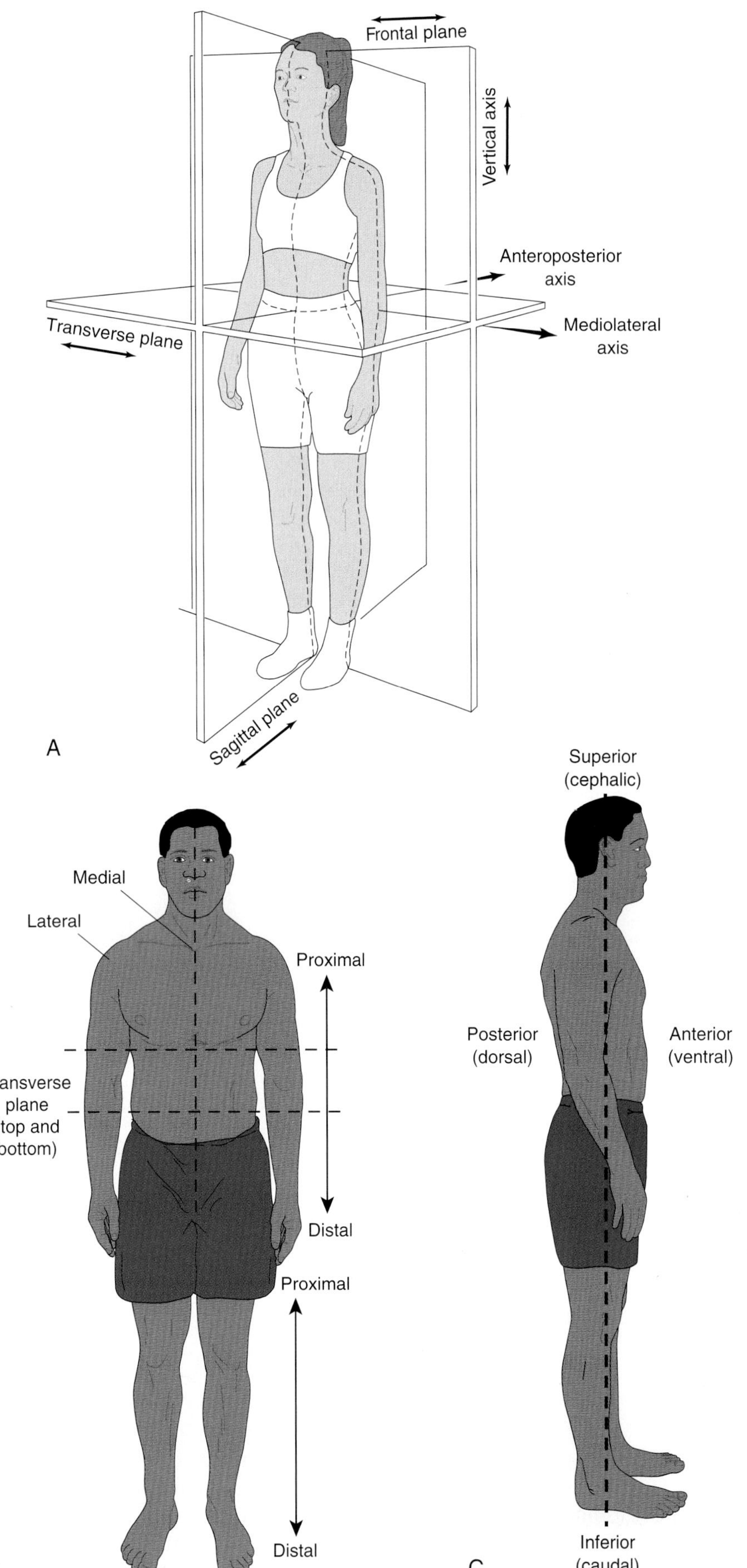

Figure 20-4. *A–C,* Planes and axes of joint movement.

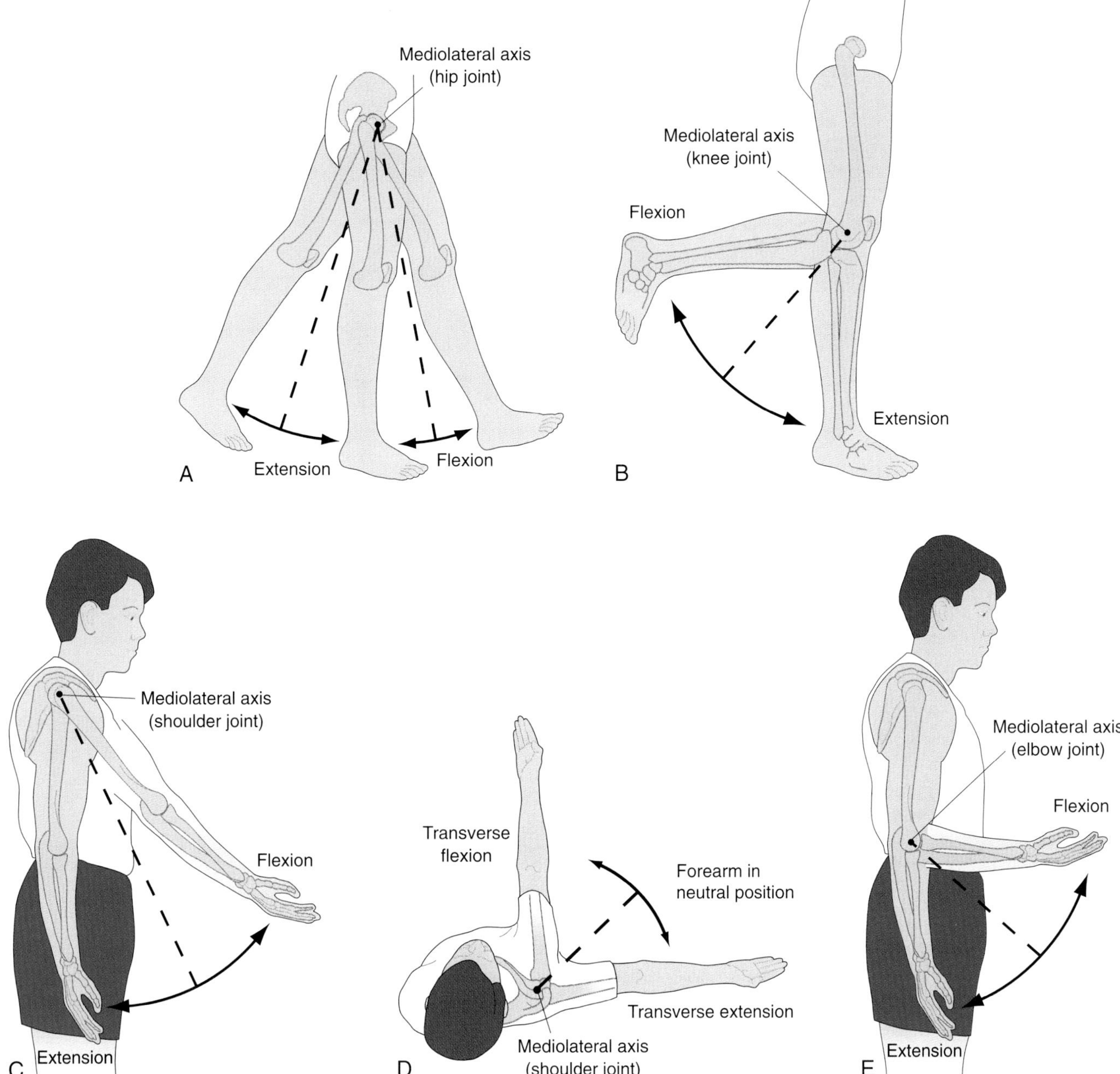

Figure 20–5. *A–H,* Segmental movements and ranges of motion in the sagittal plane. (Adapted from Kreighbaum, E., and Barthels, K.M. (1996). *Biomechanics: A Qualitative Approach for Studying Human Movement,* 4th ed. Boston: Allyn & Bacon.)

movement must be prevented by other muscles or other external forces such as a wall, table, or another person. Similarly, other outside forces besides muscles can cause segments to move. These other external forces are discussed subsequently. However, one must keep in mind that whenever a segmental movement occurs, muscular contraction may not be the cause. For example, when sitting down, gravity causes the hips, knees, and ankles to flex, not the hip, knee, and ankle flexors. Moreover, muscles can only pull bones, they cannot push them, so the direction of movement caused by muscles can always be derived if one knows the location and attachments of the muscles relative to the bones and their articulations. Figure 20–8 illustrates the action of a muscle force on a body segment.

Muscle Functioning

Muscles may be grouped into those that cause the same movement at a given articulation. Thus, there is the group called the elbow extensors that consists of all muscles that can cause the forearm or the upper arm to extend at the elbow joint. All of the muscles that can cause the same movement are part of that functional group.

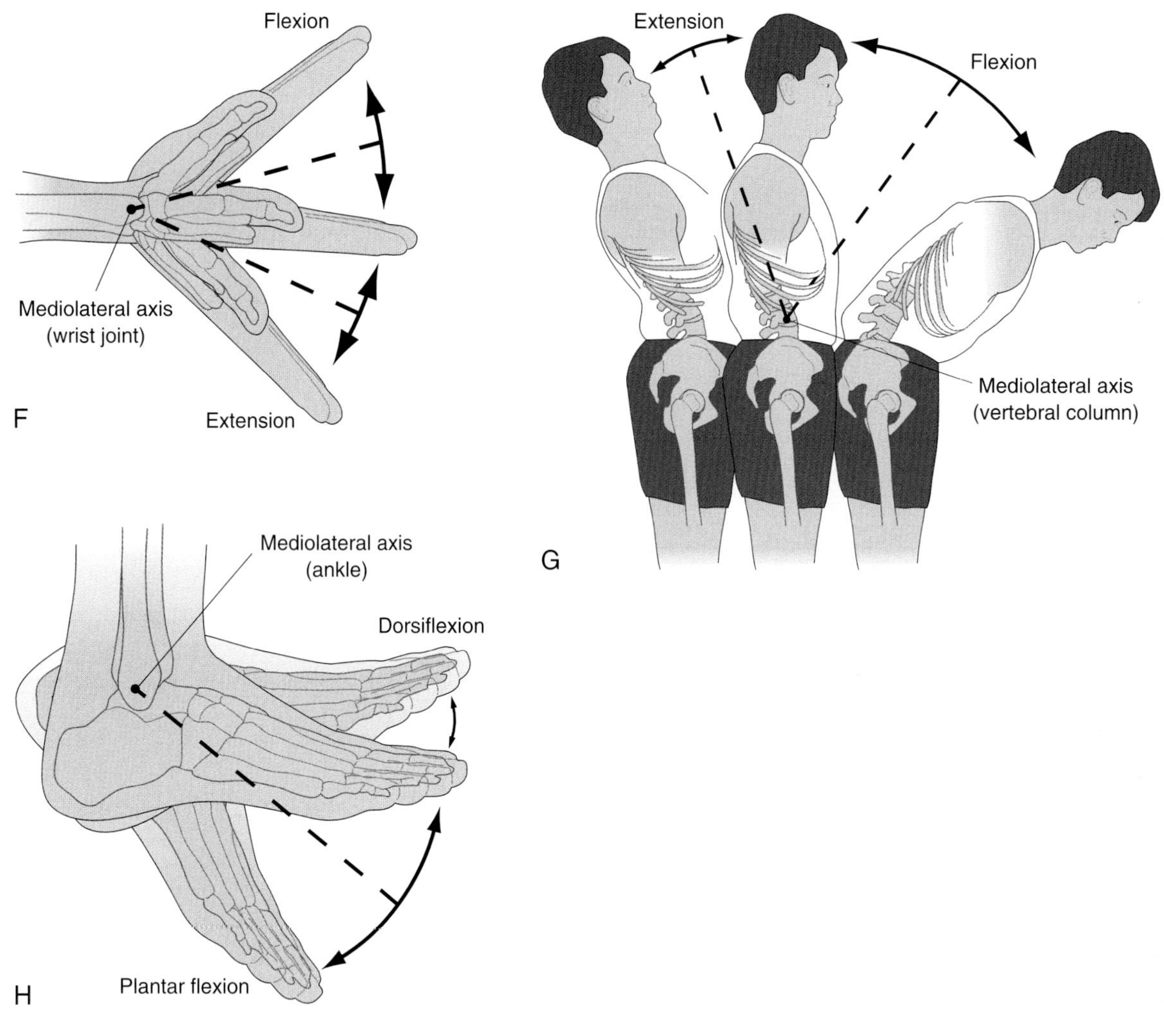

Figure 20–5. *Continued*

Muscles are called *agonists* when they are working to cause movement. The muscles that carry out the opposite function to the agonists are called *antagonists*. Antagonists relax and are lengthened passively when their agonists are shortening and causing movement.

Synergy means working together, as when two or more muscles work together to perform the same movement. Thus, the functional groups just described are synergists, all working together to produce the same movement. A second type of synergy is one in which one muscle produces movements at two joints but only the movement at one joint is desired. Because a muscle cannot "chose to" perform only one of its movements, a second muscle, an antagonist, must contract so as to prevent movement at the other joint.

A muscle that crosses one articulation is called a *uniarticulate* muscle; a muscle that crosses two articulations is called a *biarticulate* muscle; and a muscle that crosses three or more articulations is called a *multiarticulate* muscle. A muscle can only shorten a given amount. Likewise, a muscle can only be stretched a given amount without pain or injury. A biarticulate muscle that is asked to shorten over two articulations at the same time may not *be able to shorten enough* to cause full range of motion at both the articulations. This is called *active insufficiency.* For example, it is easy to fully flex your knee if your hip is not extended, but when you attempt to flex the knee fully at the same time that you are extending your hip, you will commonly get a cramp in the hamstring muscle group. These three hamstring muscles are located in a position to *cause* both of these motions but *cannot shorten enough* to cause both movements at the same time.

Conversely, when the hip is flexed the hamstring group, which is on the opposite side of the articulation, is stretched. If the knee is extended at the same time, the hamstrings are stretched over the back of the knee as well. The resulting discomfort in the hamstrings is felt when performing sit-and-reach toe touches. The muscle *cannot be stretched enough* to allow full range of antagonistic movement over both of the articulations that it crosses at the same time. This is called *passive insufficiency* (Kreighbaum and Barthels, 1996). One must keep these relationships in mind when designing flexibility or strengthening exercises or when moving patients' segments with two or more articulations between them.

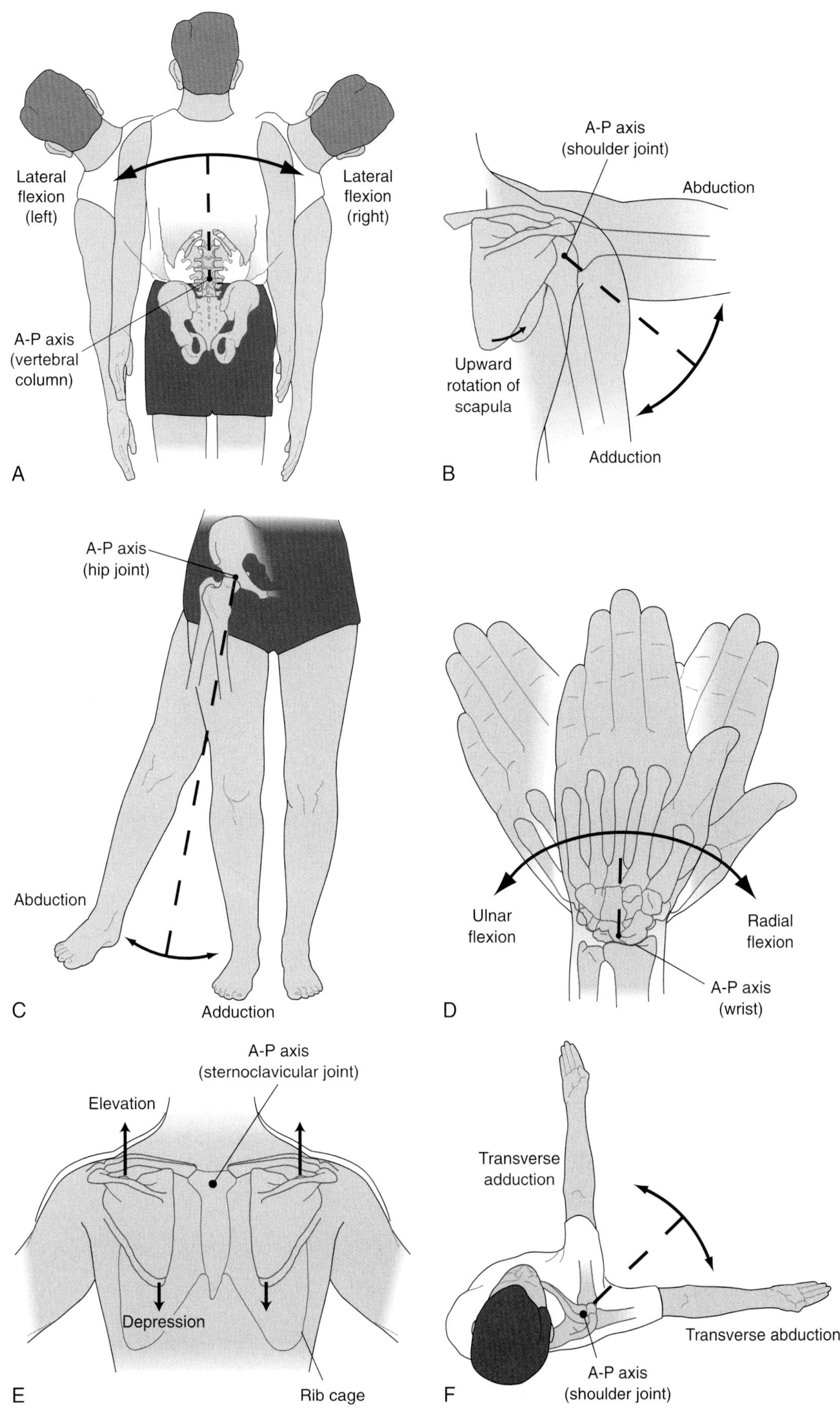

Figure 20-6. *A–F,* Articulations of the frontal plane. (Adapted from Kreighbaum, E., and Barthels, K.M. (1996). *Biomechanics: A Qualitative Approach for Studying Human Movement,* 4th ed. Boston: Allyn & Bacon.)

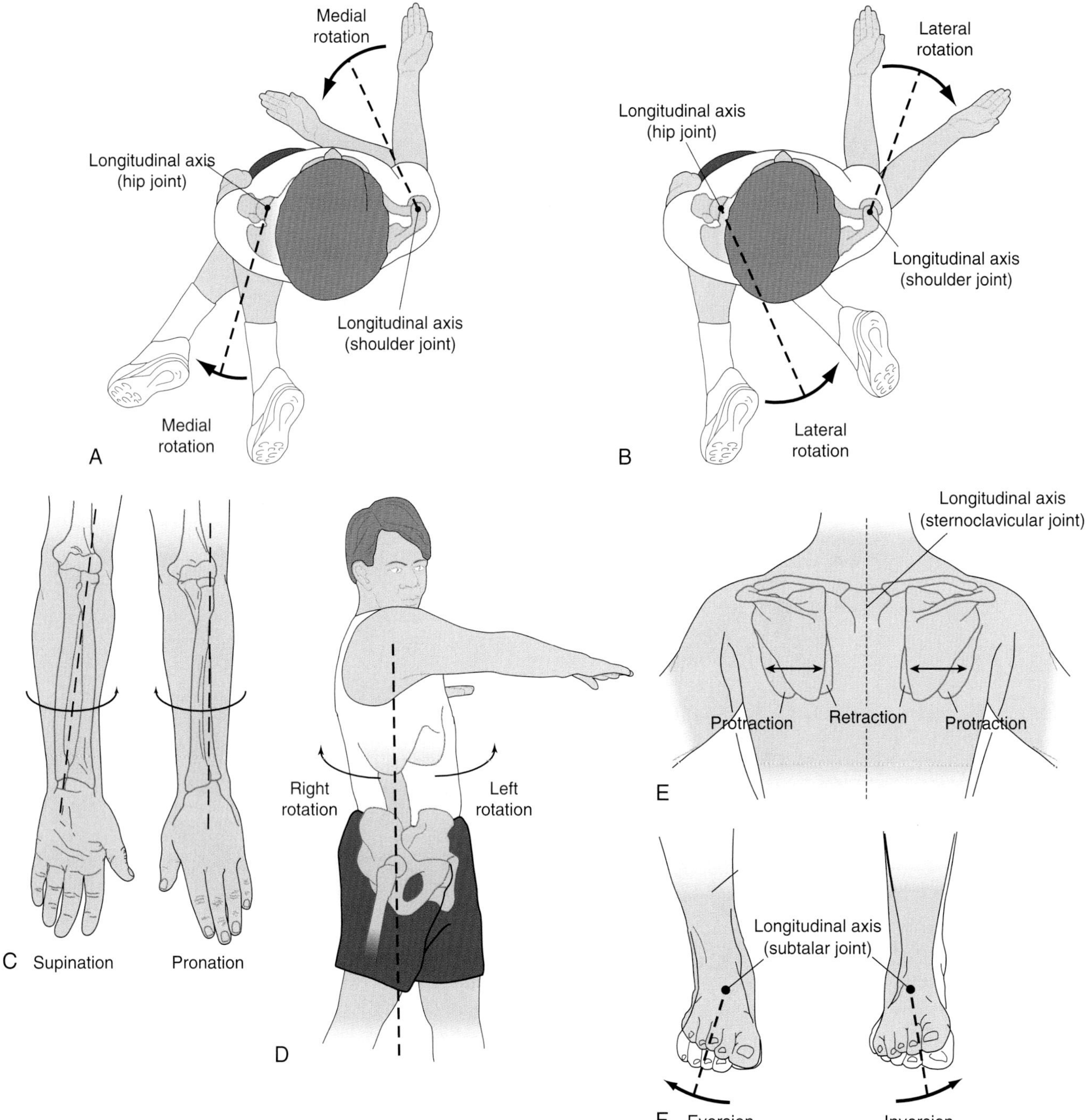

Figure 20-7. *A–F,* Articulations on the transverse plane. (Adapted from Kreighbaum, E., and Barthels, K.M. (1996). *Biomechanics: A Qualitative Approach for Studying Human Movement,* 4th ed. Boston: Allyn & Bacon.)

Functions of Muscular Tension

When skeletal muscle tissue is stimulated by the electrochemical processes of the nervous system, it responds by attempting to shorten. This response produces tension in the muscle tissue and at the ends of the muscle where it attaches to the bones. Tension is a particular type of force that when it is applied to a bone pulls on the bone. Thus, the muscle attempts to pull the two attached bones together. (Tension is discussed further under musculoskeletal mechanics.) If the bone is free to move, the muscle shortens and the segment moves. When the muscle operates in this way it is called *concentric* (toward the center) *tension* or contraction.

If another force, such as gravity, applies a greater effective force than the muscle and in the opposite direction, the body segment will move in the direction of the greater force, in this

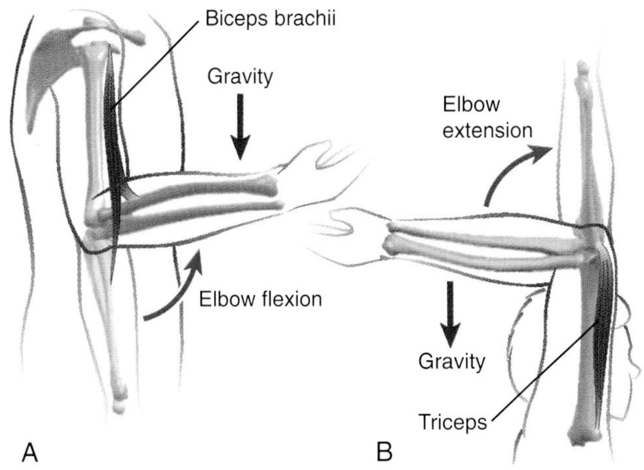

Figure 20-8. Contraction of muscle fibers. (Adapted from Kreighbaum, E., and Barthels, K.M. (1996). *Biomechanics: A Qualitative Approach for Studying Human Movement,* 4th ed. Boston: Allyn & Bacon.)

case toward the center of the earth, the direction that gravity acts. The term *effective force* is used to refer to the amount of torque that muscle force can produce, because not all of a muscle's force contributes to the movement of the bones. (Muscle torque is discussed in a subsequent section.) The oppositely directed muscle tension may still be present and serves to control the speed of the antagonistic movement. The muscle will have tension in it, also directly toward the center of the muscle, but the muscle will be lengthening, because it is losing the battle to the greater effective and oppositely directed force of gravity. This muscle tension is called *eccentric* (away from the center movement of the muscle) *tension.* An example is when a person squats: the body is moving toward the earth, but the quadriceps are tensed, not to pull the person toward the ground but to control the movement toward the ground so it is not too fast.

In some cases, the muscle will produce tension and the segment will attempt to move against an immovable object such as a wall or the muscle's antagonistic group. In this case, the tension is called *static* or *isometric* (same measure) tension. Thus, the three functional muscle tensions act to move a body part (concentric tension), to resist or control the movement of a body part caused by another force (eccentric tension), or to stabilize or fixate a body segment (static or isometric tension).

Neuromuscular Stimulation and Control

Skeletal muscle shortens when the tissue responds to electrochemical stimulation. The electrical impulse originates in the cerebral cortex of the brain and descends on motor nerve fibers that cross to the opposite side of the body before descending down the spinal cord. The crossing of the motor nerves results in the left side of the brain controlling movements of the right side of the body and the right side of the brain controlling the left side of the body.

The electrical impulse continues down the spinal cord to the "exit ramp" to the muscles being stimulated. Efferent nerve fibers carry the impulse to the muscle where chemicals called *neurotransmitters* transfer the impulse across the neuromuscular junction, causing the muscle fibers located on the other side to shorten. The *neuromuscular junction* is where the nervous system and the muscular system come together. As the individual fibers slide together, tension is created at the ends where the muscle or muscle tendon is attached to the bone. The contraction of the muscle fibers creates tension through a "pulling force" on the bone, thereby effecting movement.

Within one muscle there are numerous fibers. A relatively small portion of the fibers are grouped around one nerve, ending so as to make what is called a *motor unit.* A range from relatively few to several hundred motor units is contained within one muscle. The muscles used for fine motor skills like those required of the fingers and eye muscles have numerous motor units so that very precise movement is possible. The muscles that are used for gross motor skills, such as the leg muscles, have relatively few motor units.

ANTHROPOMETRICS

Anthropometrics is an area of study that includes the height, weight, lengths, and proportions of the body, and/or its segments. For example, whereas two people may be of the same standing height, they may be at very different eye levels when they sit down. Two individuals may have quite different sitting heights but see eye-to-eye when standing erect. In a care setting, a person's thigh length determines the chair depth needed for comfortable sitting, whereas lower-leg length determines the height of the seat. Seat dimensions are therefore important, especially to patients who have reduced knee and hip muscle strength or have knee joint and hip joint problems that impair their ability to sit or rise from a chair safely. Crutches and walkers must be adjusted for a person's total body height and for arm length as well. Reaching distance may be quite different for people of similar heights.

Body types vary widely but can be grouped into three categories for convenience. The *ectomorphic* body type is characterized by long and thin body segments. The *endomorphic* body type is characterized by a shorter and fatter body build. The *mesomorphic* body type is characterized by average body lengths and muscle builds, midway between the other types. These body types have nursing implications, because body mass distribution and center of gravity are different in each type. Patients with an ectomorphic build may have trouble with pressure sores, because they have much less surface area than either endomorphs or mesomorphs. Ectomorphs also tend to be less stable because the center of gravity lies higher in the body. People with an endomorphic build tend to have more body fat than the other two types. Consequently, they have less muscle mass and muscular strength. Although they appear to have larger proportions, they are weaker and care should be taken when they are moving. People with a mesomorph build tend to have a medium center of gravity location and have more muscle mass relative to fat. In general, mesomorphs are least susceptible to injury from biomechanical problems. It must be stressed that these body types are meant to serve as general guides to body assessment and allowances must be made for a patient's individual differences.

MECHANICS OF MOTION

Mechanics may be described in terms of the motion a body displays and in terms of the forces that cause such motion. The following section presents concepts related to the motion of bodies and the forces that are applied to them.

Mechanics of movement may be divided into *kinematics*, which is the study of the time and motion characteristics of movement, and *kinetics*, which is the study of the forces causing or influencing that motion. For the nurse, the following concepts are important for understanding movement and preventing injury: acceleration, force, mass, pressure, center of gravity, torque, and equilibrium/balance/stability.

ACCELERATION

Acceleration is the rate of change in the direction or magnitude of velocity (or speed). Whenever an object increases or decreases its speed or when an object changes its direction of movement there is acceleration (negative acceleration in the case of decreasing speed). Acceleration is seen when one begins to move from a nonmoving state, when one increases the speed or changes direction of an existing movement, or when one decreases the speed of movement or stops moving. Acceleration requires a net force. Thus, Newton stated his first law, the law of inertia: an object at rest remains at rest and an object in motion remains in motion unless acted upon by a net external force. Acceleration (negative or positive) is one of the main states that contributes to injury of the musculoskeletal system or the body's soft tissues. For example, when one hits one's skull on the floor at the end of a fall, the brain, which is encased inside the moving skull, continues to move forward after the skull is suddenly negatively accelerated (law of inertia). The brain is suddenly decelerated when it hits the negatively accelerated skull. First the floor serves as the external force to negatively accelerate the skull, and the skull serves as the external force that negatively accelerates the brain. Similarly, a fall onto a hard surface like concrete or a wooden floor produces a greater negative acceleration (or deceleration) to the body part first coming in contact with it, such as a hip or the heel of one's hand.

FORCE

There are four types of force, classified by the relationship of the force to the object to which it is applied: tension, compression, torsion, and shear. *Tension* is a force that pulls away from the object to which it is applied. The skeletal muscles apply tension to the bones when they contract. *Compression* is a force that pushes into the object to which it is applied. A compression force is applied to the hip, knee, and ankle joints during weight bearing. *Torsion* is a twisting force. Torsional forces are set up in the tissues surrounding the knee joint when the lower leg is turned laterally relative to the femur. *Shear* is a force that causes a sliding across the object. A shear force is produced when the patella slides up and down in the patellar groove of the femur. The four types of forces are illustrated in Figure 20–9.

Force is a *vector* quantity, as is acceleration, because it has direction and magnitude (bigness). Force also has a point of application, the place where the force is applied to the body, and a line of action, an imaginary line extending forever in the direction of the force.

Forces influence the direction and magnitude of the acceleration of a body. To effect acceleration, a force must be external to the body to which it is applied. An internal force, such as the pressure inside a sealed balloon, cannot cause acceleration of the balloon. Muscles, although they are internal to the skin, are external to the bones on which they are pulling and therefore can cause those bones to accelerate.

There must be a *net force*. A net force means that the sum of the forces acting in one direction is greater than the sum of the forces acting on that body in the opposite direction. For example, during a tug of war there will be no movement of either side as long as the two sides are pulling equally in opposite directions. Once one side pulls with a greater total force, there will be an acceleration in the direction of the greater force. The greater the difference between the two sum forces (net force), the greater the acceleration. The acceleration will continue until the sum of the two forces is again equalized.

Forces and the resulting accelerations are important aspects of injury. The relationship of force and acceleration is called Newton's second law of motion, the law of acceleration, and is shown in the following:

$$a = F/m$$

where a is the acceleration produced, F is the net force applied to the object, and m is the mass of the object (discussed later).

Weight

The most common force with which we deal continuously is weight, which is the force of the earth's gravitational pull on a body. Weight has magnitude and direction, always toward the center of the earth. Force causes accelerations, as in the previous example of a fall injuring the skull. The force of the body's weight caused the body to accelerate toward the center of the earth (the fall).

Ground Reaction Force

The concept of reaction force is expressed in Newton's third law of motion, the law of action–reaction: For every force

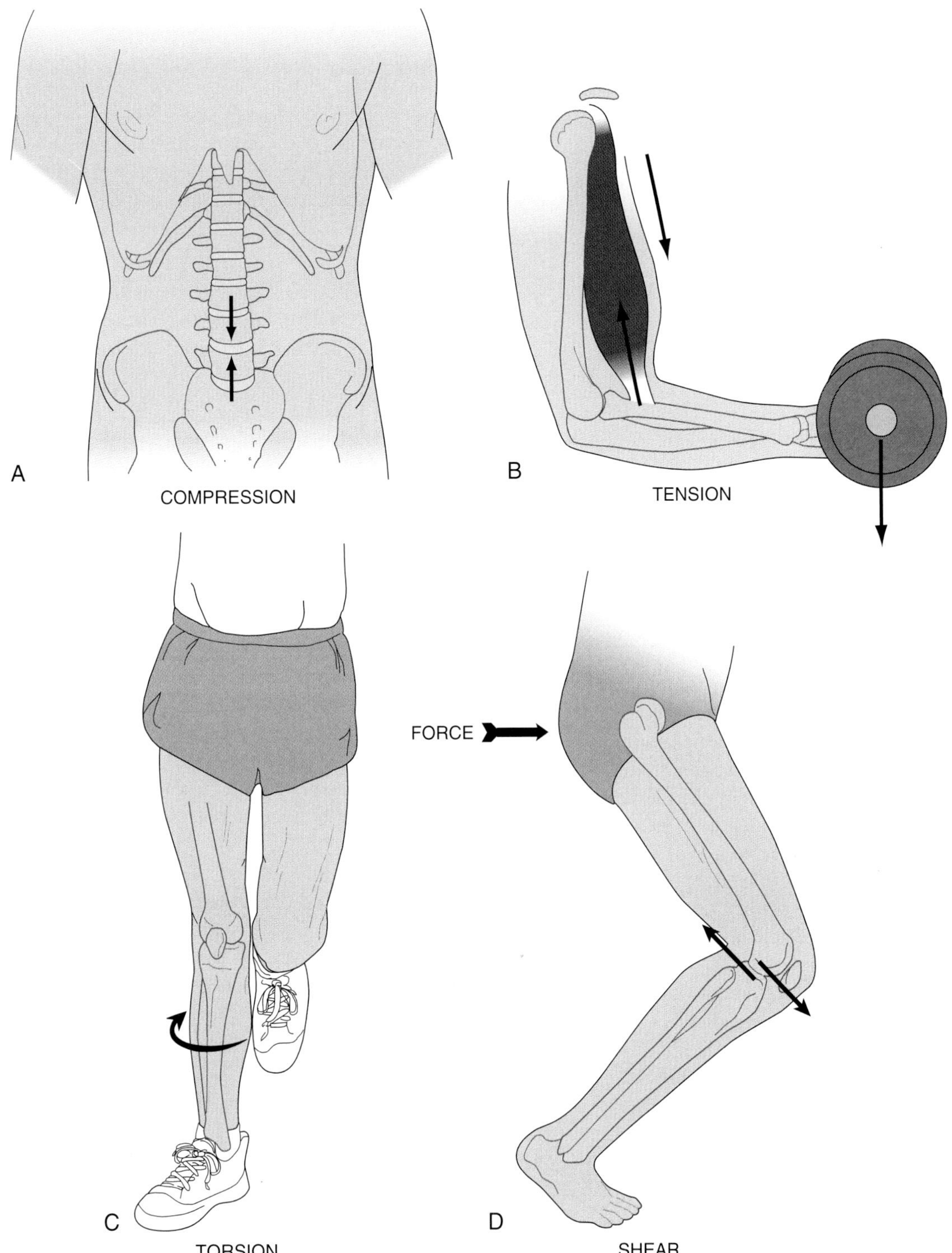

Figure 20–9. Four types of forces: *A*, compression; *B*, tension; *C*, torsion; *D*, shear. (Adapted from Kreighbaum, E., and Barthels, K.M. (1996). *Biomechanics: A Qualitative Approach for Studying Human Movement,* 4th ed. Boston: Allyn & Bacon.)

applied (action) by one body on a second, the second body applies an equal and oppositely directed force (reaction) on the first. The most common example is that of the weight of the body while standing. The force of the body's weight is directed downward and has a given magnitude. The floor pushes back on the body with a magnitude equal to the body's weight but directed upward. Thus, the forces cancel each other out and the body does not accelerate. However, if the body pushes downward with a greater magnitude than its weight, as in jumping vertically, then the ground reaction force will be greater than the body's weight, and the body will accelerate upward because of the net upward force. (By subtracting the body's weight from the upward ground reaction force, one is left with a remainder that is the net force on the system.) If one is in the unfortunate situation of standing on thin ice, one may fall through, because the thin ice is not strong enough to produce an upward reaction force equal to the downward weight force, and, thus, there is a net force downward (the difference between the weight downward and the smaller upward force that is generated).

Friction

There are three basic types of friction force: static friction, sliding friction, and rolling friction. *Static friction* is the friction generated as one pushes or pulls on an object that is resting on another so as to move one surface parallel to the contacting surface. Static friction force builds as one applies a greater pushing or pulling force until the static friction is "overcome" by the applied force.

Once sliding happens, the object begins to slip on the other surface. The objects are now generating sliding friction. *Sliding friction* is always less than static friction so once the two surfaces begin sliding past one another, friction is reduced. Any acceleration requires greater force than merely sliding the object at a constant speed.

Rolling friction is much smaller than sliding friction and is generated when one body rolls on another. Because friction is a type of reaction force, it cannot cause motion, but it can prevent motion or can negatively accelerate the bodies that are sliding. Friction force is always applied opposite in direction to the direction of the applied force, or to the motion of the sliding or rolling bodies.

The magnitude of friction is influenced by the normal force of the object and the coefficient of friction. The *coefficient of friction* is determined by the smoothness of the surfaces, the type of material that the surfaces are, and the environment (wet or dry). The *normal force* is defined as that part of the body's weight that is directed perpendicular to the surface on which it is resting. On a horizontal surface, 100 percent of the body's weight is equal to the normal force because the weight force is directed to the center of the earth. However, when the body is resting on an inclined surface, a smaller percentage of weight is directed perpendicular to the surface. The greater the incline, the less the normal force and thus the less the friction.

The smoother and drier the surfaces of the two objects, the smaller the friction. Thus, on a smooth rubber surface or on wet roads, friction is reduced considerably. Also, like surfaces generate greater friction than different surfaces. A common misconception is that apparent surface area influences the friction force. It does not. A size 12 shoe does not generate any greater coefficient of friction than a like shoe in a size 7.

In nursing practice, one should attempt to diminish friction force when moving a patient so that the move requires less force on the part of the nurse. Similarly, one should reduce the friction force on the patient's skin when sliding the patient. This may be done by lubricating the skin surface or by rolling the patient instead of sliding.

Muscle Force

As discussed in the previous section, muscles are internal to the surface of the body but external to the bones. Therefore, muscles are external forces that can cause, or influence, the movement of the bones to which they are attached. The way muscles influence movement is worth additional discussion and is covered later in this chapter.

Fluid Forces

Water and air are fluids. These fluids can apply force to the body, as is felt when holding the hand in front of an operating garden hose or standing broadside in a windstorm. Hydrotherapy (water) and air-resistant exercise machines use these fluid forces to provide beneficial effects to the users.

Other External Forces

Objects such as crutches or a walker or other people such as the patient on the nurse or the nurse on the patient apply influential forces on the body.

MASS

Mass is sometimes confused with weight, but mass is not a force. Mass is a measure of inertia. Inertia is the resistance of a body to acceleration. It is a scalar quantity; that is, it has magnitude but no direction. Forces act on masses that are the actual molecules of matter in a body. The greater the number of molecules, the greater the mass and the greater resistance to acceleration. The greater the mass of the body, the more force it takes to accelerate it. It takes more force to push a massive person in a wheelchair than it takes to push a less massive person. This is due to mass being a measure of resistance to acceleration in all directions. (There is also a greater friction force on the tires of the wheelchair owing to the patient's greater weight downward, but the two concepts of mass and weight should not be confused.) Remember, pushing is a horizontally directed force, and weight is a vertically directed force. In lifting a person, however, one must generate enough force, greater than the weight of the person, to accelerate the patient upward.

PRESSURE

Pressure is defined as force per unit area. It is measured in pounds per square inch or grams per square centimeter. The greater the force, the greater the pressure over *the same area.* The greater the area, the less the pressure with *the same force.* A larger area serves to spread the force out, so that a single square inch does not have as much force applied to it. A large-soled shoe, such as a snowshoe, to go to an extreme, applies less force per square inch on the snow cover than a regular hiking boot, even though the hiker's weight is the same. Large tires show less wear per square inch than small tires placed on the same weight car. A patient sitting on a narrow bench has more pressure on the buttocks than the same patient sitting on a chair that supports the body from the buttocks to the knees. (The area over which the weight is supported is greater, resulting in less pounds per square inch.)

CENTER OF GRAVITY

The center of gravity is the hypothetical point within the body, or in space, around which all of the body mass is equally *distributed*. Another description of the center of gravity is that point around which the body would balance in all three dimensions. Yet, a third way to think of the center of gravity is that point at which the body's mass is thought to be concentrated.

Most conveniently, the last definition can be used. When dealing with the entire body's weight force, think of the entire body's weight as being located at the body's center of gravity and, of course, always directed toward the center of the earth. When the body is standing with arms at the sides, the entire body's center of gravity is located in the pelvis, 1 to 3 inches below the navel, centered right to left and front to back. Because of the different mass distributions between males and females, a man's center of gravity is usually a centimeter or two higher than a woman's. A child's center of gravity is higher in the body than an adult's because of the unusually greater proportion of head mass relative to the extremities. A leg amputee's center of gravity (without a prosthesis) is higher and toward the supporting leg side of the body.

Each body segment has its own center of gravity. For the long bones of the body, the center of gravity is located approximately one third of the way down from the proximal articulation. This is because more mass is located toward the proximal end of long bone segments. Hands, feet, and heads have their centers of gravity approximately in the middle of the segment.

TORQUE

When a force is applied to a body, the body may display two types of motion: translation and/or rotation. If a body is free to move, that is, not restricted in any way, and the force on it is directed through its center of gravity, then the body will translate, or move in a straight line in the direction of the applied force. If a body is free to move and the applied force is not directed through the center of gravity of the body, or the body is restricted in some fashion, then the body may translate in the direction of the applied force but will also rotate or spin around its center of gravity or fixed point. This is what happens when one applies force to one end of a table with wheels—it translates and rotates.

Torque is produced when a force is directed eccentric (off center) from some fixed point in the system. The body's center of gravity, or the joint center in the case of the body segments, serves as the fixed point in the body system. Forces that do not pass through the body's center of gravity or the axis of rotation of a segment will cause the body or segment to rotate. (Recall, the axes of rotation pass through the articulation center.)

Two examples of rotation caused by an off-center (eccentric) force, or torque, are pushing a stretcher and flexing the forearm about the elbow joint. When the nurse applies an off-center force (torque) to a stretcher, the force of the push does not pass through the stretcher's center of gravity and therefore creates a torque and causes the stretcher to turn or rotate as well as move forward. Redirecting the force off center is useful when wanting to cause the stretcher to turn a corner.

In the case of all of the skeletal muscles, the tensile force created does not pass through the joint centers or axes. The muscle force thus is torque producing and causes the body segment to rotate around the axis of rotation through the joint. If muscles merely created forces through the joint centers, there would be no segmental rotations and we would not be able to move our body segments at all.

When lifting a weight with the hand, there are two weights that the muscle must manipulate: the weight of the forearm and hand and the force of the weight, which is located in the center of the weight. Both of these forces are directed vertically downward and are torque producing because they are not directed through the axis of rotation at the joint center. The segment is restricted at the elbow joint and cannot move away from this articulation unless it is dislocated. If there are no muscle torques acting, these weight torques will cause the segment to rotate around the mediolateral axis of rotation through the elbow joint. Because the forearm and hand segments are restricted from dislocation at the elbow, they will not translate but will rotate in an arc around the axis of rotation through the elbow articulation.

If a force is directed through a body's center of gravity or the segment's axis of rotation, the body will translate or move in a line. If the force is not directed through the center of gravity or the axis of rotation, then a torque is produced and, in the case of a net external torque, the body or segment will rotate (move in a circle around the center of gravity or axis of rotation). As another example, torques are produced about the hip joint by the weight torque of the upper body when leaning over and counteracted by the torque produced by the hip extensor muscles.

The magnitude of the force acting eccentric to the body's axis of rotation is as important as the distance the line of force is from the axis of rotation. The greater the force or the greater the distance from the axis, the greater the torque. Using the concept of applying a force at a greater distance is frequently called *leverage*. With leverage, one is able to apply more torque with less force by applying the force at a greater distance from the axis of rotation. Common examples are using a crowbar, a shovel, and a lift.

MACHINES OF THE MUSCULOSKELETAL SYSTEM

The musculoskeletal system is composed of classical machines. There are pulleys and wheels and axles represented in the body, but most of the bones are configured as levers. Levers consist of three parts, the lever (bone), the fulcrum (axis through the articulation), and two types of forces: the motive force, which is the force causing the lever to move, and the resistive force, the force to be moved.

Because most of the segmental movements are rotations and not translations, torques must be generated by any force that is to influence segmental movement. (Recall, torques are forces whose lines of action do not pass through the axis of rotation.) Because neither the line of action of the muscle force nor the segment weight goes through the axis of rotation, both influence the rotation of the body segment. The magnitude of the torque created is determined by the magnitude of the force and the distance that the force is from the axis of rotation. All of the skeletal muscles pass close to the axis of rotation and therefore must generate very large forces to create large torques.

External weights, held in the hand or applied to the ankle for example, are large distances from the axis of rotation. A weight held in the hand during forearm flexion or a weight on the ankle during knee extension produces a large resistive torque because of the length of the lever (the distance of the weight from the joint axis of rotation).

Moving the weight or resistance closer to the articulation will reduce the resistive torque against which the muscles must work. In all movement situations, one should attempt to keep the weight that must be lifted as close as possible to the center of the articulation around which the movement takes place.

EQUILIBRIUM, BALANCE, AND STABILITY

If there is no net external force or no external torque on a body, it is in a state of *equilibrium*. It may also be said that the body is *balanced,* that is, there are equal torques on all sides. Disequilibrium results in movement (acceleration) of some kind. An important concept for a nurse to understand is the control of equilibrium and disequilibrium so that injury will not occur to the nurse or the patient. Frequently, a nurse is required to provide a "counteractive" force or torque so that equilibrium can be maintained.

Stability is the term used to describe a body's resistance to losing equilibrium or balance (Kreighbaum and Barthels, 1996). For the nurse and the patient, stability is an important state to be achieved. Unstable bodies fall or tip over. To counteract this falling or tipping, another force or torque is needed. Once instability is reached, the force or torque needed to counteract it is hard to achieve in the small amount of time available. For example, if one begins to fall during walking, it is difficult to place the foot forward in time to prevent the fall. In the case of a patient, it is often impossible to move that fast. In the case of the nurse, who is tending to a patient's ambulation, a movement with such high acceleration may exceed the ability of the hip muscles to contract fast enough or with enough force and to do so without injury.

MECHANICAL PROPERTIES OF TISSUE

The previously mentioned mechanical concepts of acceleration, force, mass, pressure, center of gravity, torque, and equilibrium/balance/stability may be applied to musculoskeletal tissue. The tissues are bone, muscle, and muscle tendons and ligaments.

Stress, Strain, and Sprain

In biomechanical applications, *stress* denotes a force. When a force is applied to material, it causes deformation of that material. The deformation is called *strain.* In anatomic applications, strain refers to the deformation of bone or muscle tissue whereas *sprain* is commonly used to refer to an excessive deformation of ligamentous tissue.

Elasticity and Plasticity

Elasticity is the ability of a tissue to return to its original shape after being distended or deformed. *Plasticity* is the property of tissue that does not return to its original shape after being deformed. Bones and connective tissue in the body have varying degrees of elasticity and plasticity. For example, young bones (before ossification) when subjected to stress (force) may bend (display strain) but not break, whereas an adult bone under stress will initially deform very little, owing to its hardness, but will break when subjected to too much stress. The young bone has a greater elasticity and will return to its original shape after the stress has been removed. The adult bone will reach its elastic limit quickly and will break. The *elastic limit* is the level of stress or force beyond which a tissue will not return to its original shape. A bone that breaks is in a plastic state, that is, it stays in the fractured state and does not re-form unless it is reset.

Ligaments also have elastic limits. If one "turns an ankle" and the range of the deformation is not great, the ligaments of the ankle that have been stretched will return to their original lengths. If, however, the deformation is excessive and the ligament exceeds its elastic limit, the ligament will not return to its original length and will remain stretched. Sometimes, the ligaments are deformed to such an extent that they can no longer do their jobs of holding the articulation together, and a mechanical procedure is necessary to shorten the natural ligaments and reattach them, or an artificial ligament must be inserted to replace the damaged ones.

Relevant Research

NURSING AND OTHER HEALTH-RELATED RESEARCH

Physical functional status of patients may be assessed through the use of biomechanical measures of selected parameters during performance of three daily living tasks. Baseline research data are just beginning to be gathered on adults performing daily living tasks. Three daily living tasks of interest to nurses are the walk, the sit-to-stand motion, and stair ascent and descent. Initial research data assist nurses in aiding patients maintain or recapture effective daily living task performance.

WALKING GAIT, SIT TO STAND, AND STAIR ASCENT/DESCENT STUDIES

During walking, older adults may trip or slip, resulting in a fall. In a classic study, Sheldon (1960) found that the 75- to 84-year-old subjects who were likely to trip had the following in common: they did not lift their feet as high as they used to, they found it almost impossible to recover their balance, and tripping occurred most frequently when they were tired or in a hurry. These three situations suggest that muscular strength, speed of movement, and muscular endurance were functional status measures that influenced their precarious situations. In addition, Sheldon reported that the greatest percentage of falls

RESEARCH HIGHLIGHT
FALLS IN ELDERLY ADULTS

Falls are the leading cause of fatal and nonfatal injuries in people older than age 65 (Baker et al., 1984). Many elderly people injured by a fall suffer from acute morbidity, long-term loss of function, substantial risk of institutionalization, and an increased risk of death. Studies have reported a mortality rate as high as 43 percent, owing to injury suffered from a fall (Mosenthal et al., 1995). Hip fractures are the most commonly treated fall-related injury. Every year 250,000 older adults are treated for hip fractures; a fourth of them will die within 6 months (American Association of Retired Persons, 1993). Falls increase a person's chance of institutionalization; many lose their ability to live independently and perform a number of daily living activities. Half of all community-dwelling older adults who sustain an injury from a fall will move to a nursing home after hospitalization (American Association of Retired Persons, 1993). One in three people older than 65 report falling each year, and this increases to one in two of those older than 80 (Campbell et al., 1981). With the numbers of seniors growing to a projected 33 million by the year 2000, 11 million people will seek medical attention due to fall-related injury if steps for prevention are not taken (Statistical Abstract of the United States, 1995).

The number of deaths and disabilities and high costs associated with falls make them an important concern for health care professionals, policy makers, and the general public. In otherwise healthy elderly adults, fall-related costs place a tremendous financial burden on the patient, family, and society. Nearly $10 billion is spent each year treating fractures caused by falls. The medical costs are even greater when one considers the costs of institutionalization or medical care for falls that did not result in fracture. This financial burden strains people who fall, their families, and the health care system (American Association of Retired Persons, 1993). Fall prevention programs can help save millions of dollars, as well as prevent pain, disability, and in some cases even death in elderly people.

(36 percent) occurred during walking. Other situations that elicited falls were standing (14 percent), beginning to move (8 percent), and rising from sitting (8 percent). In another study, Murray and associates (1960) reported one increases the toe floor clearance distance with advancing age. Gehlsen and Whaley (1990a) did not support the finding that height of foot lift during the swing phase was significantly different for those who had a history of falls and those who did not. A serious problem of the older adult is the tendency to fall. Mobility is directly related to this problem. However, the research studies on the biomechanics of walking gait and falling are inconclusive. Discussion of the risk factors to falls in the elderly is presented under the section on the older adult. (See also Research Highlight: Falls in Elderly Adults.)

In another study relating to falls, Hogue, Studenski, and Duncan (1990) included 69 participants who were older than 50 and homebound. The purpose of the study "was to develop and test a clinical assessment tool that would be useful in identifying people at high risk for falls because of physical mobility impairments." All of the participants were involved in a Veterans Administration home care program and had a caretaker available 24 hours a day. Each subject was evaluated at home. Assessment data relating to the patient's report of being able to perform activities of daily living were collected, and a neuromuscular examination was conducted.

The results of the study indicated that 20 patients (29 percent) had repeated falls, 12 patients (17 percent) had single falls, and 37 patients (54 percent) had no falls. Analysis of the data indicated that seven mobility performance skills discriminated nonfallers from one-time and repeat fallers:

- Sitting balance
- Sitting reach
- Bending down to pick up a pencil
- Standing reach
- Rising from chair
- Gait without assistive device
- Descending stairs

The researchers indicate that the mobility scale should be useful to clinicians in screening patients and reducing the risk of falling.

Whereas standing from a seated position has been recognized as a basic function of independent living, there are relatively few recent studies on the sit-to-stand function. Ellis and associates (1979) found that morale and lifestyle of older adults were correlated with their ability to stand from a seated position without help. Some studies have collected movement and force data on young and old adults standing from a seated position; however, the descriptive nature of these studies does not lend itself to understanding the changes in the dynamics of chair sitting and standing with aging and their influences on successful and unsuccessful performance. Few studies have attempted to observe differences in standing performance before and after an exercise program or the standing function in relation to lower extremity muscle strength.

Ascending and descending stairs involves a series of single leg stances, controlled concentric and eccentric muscular contractions, and balance. Although stair climbing has been studied, there are few studies that help us understand the dynamics of stair ascent and descent and, in particular, the patterns of older adults. Evidence exists that for young women, stair climbing kinematics is dependent on the height of the climber and the patterns mirror the kinematics of an individual's walking gait (Livingston et al, 1991). There is no information available regarding changes in stair climbing kinematics with advancing age or information on stair descent with advancing age.

WORK-RELATED BACK INJURIES

Nursing personnel are at risk for serious back injuries if attention is not given to proper lifting techniques. Financial burdens are experienced by the nurse and the employing agency. A study that tracked reported back-injury cases and the cost per claim of nursing staff was completed by Coleman and Hanson in 1994. The study evaluated the efficacy and cost effectiveness of an educational program. The program was designed to (1) increase the awareness prevention of back injury, (2) decrease the cost of workers' compensation claims resulting from work-related back injury/pain, (3) decrease the amount of employee sick time taken because of back pain, (4) increase work productivity through proper ergonomics, and (5) teach staff members to take care of their backs. The study describes the process used to evaluate the program.

Another study conducted by Garrett, Singiser, and Bank (1992) indicated that female nurses in the early phases of assignment on long-term care units are at greatest risk for back injury, but risk factors that relate significantly to the severity of the injury are tour of duty (evening) and weight of the nurse (200 + pounds). Recommendation from this study include evaluation of lifting techniques and practices; orientation whenever assignments are changed; accurate assessment of nurse, patient, and situation; and regular use of an assessment tool incorporating all of these factors.

USE OF RESTRAINTS

The application of restraints in long-term care residences has served as the bases for studies by nurse researchers. In the United States the use of physical and chemical restraints escalated after the mid 1960s. A 1988 study by the Health Care Financing Administration indicated that an average of 41 percent of nursing home residents were restrained on a regular basis. Other surveys indicate that 60 percent of the nursing home patients received psychotropic medications (Evans and Strumpf, 1992). In recent years the use of restraints has been criticized particularly if used to reduce falls in the elderly.

A study by Evans and Strumpf (1992) was conducted to develop and test the effects of a structured educational program on the prevalence of use of restraints and the effects of their use on patients and staff. The research was carried out on a 62-bed unit of a long-term care facility. Ten educational sessions were designed to:

- Improve staff outcomes (burnout, beliefs about restraining efficacy and knowledge of alternative methods)
- Reduce use of restraints
- Improve resident outcomes (function, cognition, and affect)
- Maintain or decrease the number of resident injuries

Seventy-nine resident noncomatose patients participated. Thirty-three full- or part-time clinical nursing staff agreed to enroll. Only 13 staff members and 43 patients completed the entire project.

The results of the study indicate that systematic educational programs for staff in long-term care facilities can make a difference. Differences were found in attitudes, beliefs, and knowledge, but the differences did not produce change in restraint practice during a short time period. The researchers attributed part of the lack of positive results to the frequent changes in administrators made in the long-term facility during the study period. Institutional and nursing administrators did not assign staff to attend the educational sessions. Anecdotal information from various staff participants indicated that the behavior of some staff toward limiting the use of restraints did occur.

RESEARCH FROM OTHER FIELDS

Several other disciplines may be used by the nurse to solve biomechanical problems and enhance mobility in patients. *Human factors engineering* is an area of study dealing with the interactions of the person with the work environment. Examples of this research relevant to nursing practice include studies in vision, hearing, perception, fatigue, lifting weights, and, most currently, the effectiveness of lifting belts in preventing back injuries, a topic discussed later in this chapter under Biomechanical Principles of Lifting. *Ergonomics*, the study of the physiology of work, and *biomechanics*, the study of the mechanics of work, are two subcategories of human factors research that may be applied to nursing practice. In addition, the findings from human factors research can certainly be applied to the physiology and biomechanics of the patient's movements and can be applied by nurses in their practice.

Motor learning, how one learns motor skills/tasks, and motor control, how one controls ones movement, are two subdisciplines of physical education and health that provide important information to the nurse regarding neuromuscular aspects of patients and may be helpful in assessing and diagnosing conditions. Of particular concern is the patient's ability to maintain postural control and balance. One of the most serious results of balance impairment is the tendency to fall, particularly in older adults.

Unfortunately, research within the human factors or motor control areas is very limited. It is hoped that more helpful information will be brought to the nursing professional.

FACTORS AFFECTING CLINICAL DECISIONS

Age

The responses of the body to forces and torques applied to it are somewhat dependent on the age of the person. As discussed earlier, the bones of a child may bend and return to normal when an external torque is applied, whereas the same bone in an elderly person may break if subjected to the same torque. Conversely, a child's epiphyseal plate may be dislocated when subjected to a shear force, but in an adult the ossified epiphyseal plate will not be deformed. The following section describes the considerations to be given to patients and clients of different ages.

INFANTS

The infant is born with a spinal column that is C-shaped without the anteroposterior curves of the mature adult spine. It is impossible for the infant to sit or stand because of the large size and weight of the forward head, the lack of muscle strength, and the high center of gravity in the body. Moreover, if the infant could stand, the center of gravity and its line of gravity would be so far forward that it would fall outside of the base of support and the infant would topple.

As the infant encounters the forces of a gravity-dependent environment and as muscles begin to contract and apply tensile force to the bones, the musculoskeletal structure begins to strengthen. The strength of the small ligaments surrounding the articulations does not provide much stability to these joints, and they can be easily dislocated with too great a misdirected force.

TODDLERS

Eventually, the infant begins pushing up from a prone position, and the cervical and lumbar curves begin to form. The straightening of the vertebral column allows sitting up, because the center of gravity has shifted to the middle of the body. The total body center of gravity is still high in the body, and therefore balance is difficult. In response to the lack of stability, the toddler widens the base of support by walking with the feet wide apart but the steps are small from front to back.

SCHOOL-AGE CHILDREN

As a child grows, so does the strength of the bones and connective tissues. In response to stress, the trabeculae of the long bones increase and align themselves with the predominant force so as to best counteract those forces. Because the muscle tension on the apophysis stimulates the laying of osteoblasts at the site, the junction of the muscle tendons and bone strengthens with the use of the muscles. Because of the strengthening process, exercise is important during the growing years. With the lengthening of the trunk and extremities and little change in the head size, the child's center of gravity lowers in the body and balance is easier.

ADOLESCENTS

The adolescent grows very rapidly and unevenly, particularly in the extremities. It may be difficult for the adolescent to adjust to these rapid changes, and they may appear awkward. If the adolescent is in sports activities, the muscle mass and strength may be developmentally ahead of the strength of the muscle's attachment to the bone. If the adolescent participates in vigorous jumping activities, the muscle tendon or muscle fibers themselves may begin to tear away from their bony attachment. A common condition called Osgood-Schlatter syndrome is characterized by the tearing of some of the fibers of the patellar tendon away from the tibia due to the strong contraction of the quadriceps muscles. It is seen mostly in those adolescents who are in events that require forceful jumping and landing such as the long jump, high jump, basketball, volleyball, and gymnastics.

ADULTS

During the adult years, the composition of the body changes. The lean body mass decreases (the mass of the bones, muscles, connective tissues) and the body fat content increases even though the total body weight may remain the same. Because a pound of fat has a larger volume than a pound of lean body tissue, the body volume increases. Spot reducing by exercising a particular body part is not possible. For example, exercising the thigh and hip muscles, one can build muscle tissue in those areas but cannot eliminate fat deposits in the particular part of the body. Exercising adds to the muscle mass and the lean body weight. However, because the density of muscle is greater than that of fat, the volume of 5 pounds of fat is greater than that of 5 pounds of muscle. Thus, the circumference of those parts will decrease if 5 pounds of fat is taken off a given area and replaced with 5 pounds of muscle.

OLDER ADULTS

Older adults experience degenerative changes in the bones, articulations, muscle, and connective tissues. A reduction in the amount of fluid contained in the vertebral discs results in a reduction in height. Most older adults are several inches shorter than they were during their early adult years. The bones will begin to lose calcium and become brittle. The hyaline cartilage on the ends of the long bones becomes more dry and can begin to show wear by becoming rough or having chips break off and float around the joint capsule. The ligaments and muscle tendons surrounding the articulations become less flexible. The result of these joint changes is that the joints lose range of motion and movements that have been possible before become limited or impossible. The elasticity of the ligaments and muscle tendons is reduced, and this results in more frequent sprains and strains. Older adults who have participated in strength and flexibility exercises throughout their adult and older years will not experience the degenerative changes as early or as rapidly as those who do not exercise.

Degenerative changes in elderly adults put them at risk for falling and other injuries (see Research Highlight). Falls among older adults can result in dramatic change in life quality. Falls are the leading cause of fatal and nonfatal injuries in those older than age 65 (Baker et al, 1984). It is important to realize most falls can be prevented even among the frail elderly by understanding the risk factors and providing prevention education to older patients (Box 20–1).

The United States Public Health Service has joined in the campaign to prevent older adults from falling. In *Healthy*

BOX 20-1
FALL-RELATED RISK FACTORS FOR ELDERLY PATIENTS

- Sociodemographic characteristics: age, gender, living quarters
- Psychological factors: depression, cognitive impairment, fear of falling
- Sociological factors: isolation, lack of companionship, lack of public transportation
- Physiologic factors: osteoporosis, foot problems, dementia, low body weight, postural hypotension, use of sedatives, palmomental reflex, and vestibuloocular reflex

People 2000: National Health Promotion and Disease Prevention Objectives (1990), the policy makers have outlined a plan to reduce falls by the year 2000. Some of these objectives include the following:

- Reduce hospitalization for hip fractures in 85+ women by 20 percent
- Reduce deaths from falls by 5 percent in the 65- to 84-year age group
- Reduce deaths from falls by 10 percent in the 85+ age group

To meet these objectives a number of prevention strategies can be implemented, such as exercise to increase agility and strength, medication monitoring, assessment and intervention of environmental risks, and education of risk factors (Button, 1996).

As people age, they begin to suffer from physiologic and psychological changes. A number of these changes can be factors that lead to falls or put someone at risk for a fall. Some chronic problems in the senior age group include osteoporosis, decreased physical strength and mobility, impaired vision and hearing, postural hypotension, and depression. Although many of these factors are part of the aging process, steps can be taken to delay their onset and to decrease their impact on falls. Seniors can participate in exercise classes, regular physician check-ups, and risk factor education programs (Button, 1996).

A closer look at causes of falls helps us understand the importance of this kind of health promotion. Many cite a strong fear of falling. This fear is associated with decreased independence, decreased quality of life, and increased risk of falling (Arfken et al, 1994). "Fear of falling" causes severe psychological and social concerns for this age group. Individuals may become afraid to leave their homes and begin to restrict themselves from social activities. This fear can contribute to increased frailty, depression, and risk of falling.

For any fall prevention program to succeed it must be designed to eliminate the factors that contribute to falls. It must educate about various risks and empower older adults to modify these risks. A number of studies evaluate the risk factors. Some of the most commonly cited risk factors include:

- Lack of physical activity
- Use of psychoactive medications
- Impaired vision and hearing
- Environmental hazards
- Improper footwear and clothing

Lack of physical activity creates a number of added difficulties for an aging person. This deprivation can result in poor muscle strength, decreased bone mass, gait/balance disorders, and reduced flexibility. All of these factors increase one's risk of falling but can be modified with a regular exercise program.

Exercise is considered one of the best behavioral and physical intervention plans. Exercise programs that consist of strength training and exercises focusing on balance and flexibility can quickly improve one's physical health. Even in old age weight-bearing activities have dramatic effects on one's muscle tone and strength. Exercise can help one improve body mechanics, which will help the person make judgments on the environmental hurdles that might be encountered (see Patient Teaching Box: Identifying Common Environmental Hazards in the Home).

Environmental hazards have been implicated in at least a third of the falls among older adults (American Association of Retired Persons, 1993). For example, an older person may be using an unstable chair to sit in. When the person tries to rise or sit in the chair he or she is at risk. The chair may collapse or give just enough for the person to lose balance and fall. This hazard can easily be too much for the older person to compensate for, and the resulting fall can have life-threatening effects. Environmental hazards can be found in every home. They can be as apparent as a loose throw rug or as pervasive as the height of a toilet seat.

The use of psychoactive medication also puts an older person at risk for falling. Drugs can be one of the most potent risk factors, yet one of the easiest to change. Medications such as long-acting benzodiazepines and neuroleptics have been associated with increased hip fractures (Ray et al, 1989). They can reduce mental alertness, worsen gait, and decrease systolic blood pressure (American Association of Retired Persons, 1993). Older adults should be instructed to ask their physicians about the medications they are taking and they should inform all health care providers of the medications so that they might assess the interactive side effects. Sensory changes in vision and auditory abilities play a risk in falls. Thirty percent of older adults have significant hearing loss (Gray-Vickrey, 1984). Hearing loss can place people at risk when out in public and within the home, because their awareness of hazards may be lessened. For instance, they may not hear the smoke detector, making it difficult for the older person to get to safety before the fire becomes life threatening. Impaired vision, often associated with aging, can disrupt one's depth perception and peripheral vision. Both may aid in slowing down a person's reaction time and judgment of environmental hazards (Kane et al, 1984).

PATIENT TEACHING
IDENTIFYING COMMON ENVIRONMENTAL HAZARDS IN THE HOME

Most falls and other accidents occur in the home, particularly in the bathroom and the bedroom. Many of these accidents are a direct result of hazardous conditions—loose throw rugs, unstable footstools, and so on. Many existing environmental hazards can be easily modified; others may require a little work or just education on their risks. The following questionnaire can help identify potential risks in the home.

KITCHEN

- Are kitchen items stored where they can easily be reached? Do you need to bend a lot or reach up too high?
- Is there a footstool? If so, is it sturdy?
- Is the kitchen table sturdy?
- Do the chairs have armrests and are they sturdy?
- Is the floor waxed and slippery?
- Is there a rubber mat near the sink?
- Are the dials on the stove easy to read?

BATHROOM

- Does the bathtub or shower have a slippery floor?
- Does the side of the bathtub have a support or transfer rail?
- Does the toilet have a stable grab rail?
- Is the toilet seat at the proper height, neither too high nor too low?
- Is there a lock on the door? (optional)

STAIRWAYS

- What is the rise between steps?
- Are there hand rails on both sides of the stairway?
- Do the hand rails extend the full length of the stairs?
- Is the stairway long and steep?
- Are there nonskid treads on each of the stairs or carpet?
- Is the lighting adequate?
- Are any objects stored on the steps?
- Are the top and bottom steps marked with bright contrasting tape?
- Are the steps in good repair?

GENERAL HOUSEHOLD

- Is the lighting adequate throughout the house or apartment? (Does it create a glare, is it dim, or too direct?)
- Are the lights accessible on entering each room?
- Do any of the carpets need repairing?
- Are all of the rugs tacked down or have nonskid backs?
- Are hallways cluttered with furniture or other obstacles?
- Are there adequate pathways through each room?
- Are all tables stable and sturdy?
- Do the chairs have armrests and high backs?
- At what temperature is the house kept during the winter? (preferably 72° F)
- Are there any cords in the walking path?

Orthostatic hypotension is one of the many physical disorders associated with falling. Orthostatic hypotension is a fall in blood pressure occurring on standing. Dizziness, blurred vision, and faintness can result after standing. It often occurs in older adults who are malnourished, taking certain medications, or have poor vascular tone (Chipman et al, 1981). An older person with orthostatic hypotension may fall as a result of faintness while rising from a chair or when getting out of bed. Improvements in nutrition and regular medical examinations can help alleviate this risk factor (Button, 1996).

Improper clothing and footwear should also be regarded when studying the risks associated with falling. Loose garments and robes can catch on furniture. Shoes with high heels and little support may disrupt balance and gait. They may hinder the ability of an older person to react to many environmental hazards, such as icy sidewalks and steps. Sturdy leather shoes with nonskid soles provide the most effective traction (Button, 1996).

Many of the risk factors associated with falls among the elderly can be modified. To a great degree the risks involved in elderly falls are interrelated; therefore, a multiple-risk factor intervention strategy works best (Tinetti et al, 1994). The best approach to begin an assessment of an at-risk older person is to do a complete patient history and a physical examination. This allows for careful determination of the problems associated with that specific individual. Intervention programs can consist of education of risk factors, exercise programs, environment modifications, and regular physician visits (Button, 1996).

Gender

Center of gravity location is influenced somewhat by sex. In a lean-bodied adult, the center of gravity of men is an inch or two higher in the body than in women. Men generally have more massive shoulders, whereas women have more massive hips. Genetics predetermines the hierarchy of fat placement. Typically, men put on fat in the trunk and upper abdominal area whereas women put on fat in the hips and thighs. Usually, women put fat on first in the hips and thighs and last in the shoulders and arms; unfortunately, fat reduction begins in the shoulders and arms and occurs last in the hips and thighs in women.

The center of gravity in men will remain higher than in women because of the increased fat put on in a man's stomach area and in a woman's hips and thighs. Postural changes between men and women relate to the accumulation of fat. If the center of gravity shifts to the front as with men, the individual will lean backward slightly. Women, whose center of gravity shifts backward with the increased weight in the posterior, will lean forward slightly.

CLINICAL DECISION MAKING
CARE AFTER HIP REPLACEMENT SURGERY

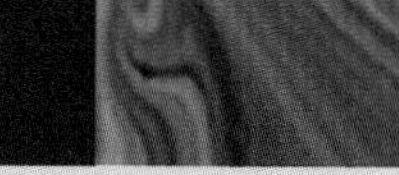

Nursing student Mary Conners was assigned to Mrs. Jones (see Case Study) to provide assistance in Mrs. Jones' completion of activities of daily living (ADLs). Mrs. Jones had a total hip replacement. Mary realized that she had to accomplish two goals: to tend to her own back problems by using proper body mechanics and to teach Mrs. Jones to use safe and appropriate techniques in ambulating. Mrs. Jones needs assistance in getting up from the bed, sitting in the chair, and walking using a mechanical device such as a walker.

Application of biomechanics is important for both the patient and the nurse. Improper movements by the nurse can lead to serious injury of the musculoskeletal system of both the nurse and the patient. The patient should be protected from falling, and the nurse should use proper biomechanical procedures.

FACTORS TO CONSIDER REGARDING MRS. JONES' HIP REPLACEMENT

Patients suffering from hip replacements may suffer from chronic diseases such as osteoporosis or arthritis.

- Assess Mrs. Jones' physical condition to determine her stamina, energy level, nutritional status, and health practices.
- Assess status of the hip replacement surgical incision and aseptic techniques required to care for the incision.
- Assess the ability of Mrs. Jones to comprehend and apply information regarding proper walking techniques and biomechanical principles. Arrange for input from the physical therapist to determine whether Mrs. Jones needs additional training.
- Assess Mrs. Jones' motivation to become independent and assume responsibility for her own care.
- Assess the potential for Mrs. Jones to be ambulatory and independent and able to care for herself.

If the potential for independence does not exist, determine, with Mrs. Jones and her family, what future living arrangements need to be made. Assist family in arranging for any mechanical devices that may be needed by Mrs. Jones.

Nursing personnel need to be aware of and apply the principles of biomechanics while aiding Mrs. Jones. Since Mary Conners is experiencing back pain, she may have already strained her musculoskeletal system. She should seek help from other staff members while assisting in lifting Mrs. Jones and helping her to ambulate.

GOALS

- To assist Mrs. Jones to return to normal daily living activities with as much independence as possible.
- To prevent any further injury to Miss Conners.

INTERVENTION IN MRS. JONES' CARE

Nursing care is conducted with other health care team members including the physician, dietitian, pharmacist, physical therapist, social worker, other nursing staff, and patient's family. Specific interventions are as follows:

- Determine the status of Mrs. Jones' knowledge about the use of biomechanics. Instruct her in proper methods to move in bed, stand at the bed side, and use a walker. Supervise her in trying out the procedures.
- Determine with other team members Mrs. Jones' future living arrangements.
- Teach the principles of body mechanics to family members who will care for Mrs. Jones after her discharge.
- Determine needs for dressing changes of Mrs. Jones' surgical incision and teach patient and family how to care for the incision.
- Assist Mrs. Jones to reduce pain while in and out of bed by using proper body positioning. Provide proper and adequate medications to keep the patient comfortable.
- Review with Mrs. Jones her nutritional and health practices and provide information that will facilitate the healing process.

With greater weight in the anterior area, older overweight men and pregnant women are susceptible to lower back injuries. The additional anterior weight creates a greater resistive torque around the mediolateral axis running through the lumbar vertebrae. This forward-tending resistive torque must be counteracted by the back extensor muscles. Recall that the muscles are placed very close to the axis of rotation and therefore must generate greater forces to equal the torque produced by the weight of the forward-leaning trunk.

Women who do not have the back extensor strength during pregnancy will be predisposed to backache. Carrying the fetus in the front of the body causes a shifting of the center of gravity forward. Stability is enhanced by widening the base of support during standing and walking.

Of particular interest to women is a potentially debilitating condition called osteoporosis. *Osteoporosis* is the increased sloughing off of calcium in the bones. During childhood and the early adult years, calcium is ingested from the high calcium foods that we eat. The hormonal system causes the calcium to be taken up by the bones so that a net loss does not result. However, changes in hormones in the late adult and older adult years prevents the system from replacing the calcium that the bones have lost, causing the bones to become brittle. Whereas both men and women experience osteoporosis, it is particularly evident in postmenopausal women. Estrogen seems to be the key to this phenomenon. With the reduction and elimination of estrogen production, calcium is not taken up in the system. If estrogen replacement therapy is not undertaken, the bones continue to deteriorate and become porous and thus are very susceptible to fracture. The deterioration of the vertebrae may be seen in older women whose stature is severely compromised. The head and upper thoracic region is carried forward, owing to the deterioration of the thoracic and cervical vertebrae.

Settings in Which Care Is Delivered

As mentioned previously, biomechanical principles apply in any setting in which nursing care is administered. In hospital, outpatient, and clinic settings other nurses or mechanical equipment can assist the nurse in performing measures that involve patient mobility. In home settings the nurse may be alone and not have access to any devices that assist in moving the patient. It is essential that regardless of the setting proper body mechanical principles be used.

The environment in which patients exist needs to be assessed for potential safety hazards. Many of the accidents that occur result from hazardous conditions found in the environment, such as unseen objects on the floor, equipment or utensils placed in the normal traffic flow, high beds, and items placed beyond reach. (See Patient Teaching Box: Identifying Common Environmental Hazards in the Home for additional information.)

Caring for patients in home care settings is more complicated than caring for patients in organized health care institutions. Generally, home settings do not have the proper facilities or equipment for patients with immobility problems. In many instances, nurses providing care under these circumstances will need to use their creative and innovative talents to provide for an adequate environment. Some patients will be able to rent or purchase mechanical aids (e.g., wheelchairs, crutches) to help in ambulation. In cases in which the family is not financially able to afford the equipment, the nurse may have to contact charitable organizations and ask for assistance in providing the necessary materials. There may be times in which improvising and using what is available in the home may be necessary, such as using a large man's belt to assist the patient in moving. Nurses need to provide guidance to the family in those instances in which families can afford to purchase equipment for use in the home. The patient and members of the family need to be taught proper use of the equipment.

In the home care setting, patients and families assisting the patient need to be taught proper body mechanics to prevent personal injury that can result from misusing the body while moving (patient and family) or lifting (family). Simple procedures such as range of motion exercises can also be taught to the family so that procedures instituted in the acute or long-term setting can be continued at home.

Ethical Considerations

A primary consideration in caring for any patient in any care setting is to protect the patient from injury. Nurses have an ethical responsibility to ensure patient safety. Many devices are available to assist in safeguarding the patient. One such group of devices are mechanical restraints used to physically impair the patient from moving. (See Procedure 20–4: Applying Restraints.) Patients may be restrained to prevent them from falling or from removing intravenous needles and catheters, urinary catheters, or other types of tubes inserted into body spaces or to prevent injury while they are comatose or delirious.

The physical restraining of patients causes ethical problems for nurses. They are acutely aware of the response of the patient to being restrained—of the loss of dignity and feeling of powerlessness. In some instances the very act of applying the restraint can cause a patient to become angry, upset, and combative.

To restrain a patient involves a violation of the ethical principle of autonomy, which affirms that individuals are to be permitted personal liberty to determine their own actions according to their own plans. Individuals (i.e., nurses) who accept the principle of autonomy will respect the individual choices of others. A dilemma is created when the patient is not capable of making an autonomous choice. There are times when the nurse is convinced that what is best for the patient is not to the patient's liking or best interest. In this case, the nurse must act for the patient. For example, if the patient is irrational and has the potential to injure himself or herself, it is essential that the nurse intercede to protect the patient. In this instance, it would be appropriate to apply physical and chemical restraints. By entering the health care system there is an implied consent that the patient has agreed to such an intervention. Husted and Husted (1995) indicate that the nurse should ask the following question before applying restraints, "What argument would you accept for someone taking control of your autonomous situation when you had not agreed to this?"

Nurses need to be constantly alert to recognize when they are faced with instances that may involve ethical problems. There are many situations encountered with patients with impaired mobility that are ethical. Understanding and practicing the principles of ethics is essential to providing safe nursing care.

Financial Considerations

Sound biomechanics when applied throughout life can result in a reduction in costly injuries. National work injury and illness trends show that whereas the percentage of some categories of injury such as skin disorders, respiratory ailments, and illness due to physical agents is staying the same or going down, the percentages are increasing in the category of musculoskeletal injuries. These injuries are mostly due to biomechanical factors and could be prevented if sound biomechanical principles were followed. The average cost for a person with carpal tunnel syndrome, for example, is $15,000, and up to $30,000 if surgery is involved. In addition, productivity is lost.

Individuals have differing dispositions to biomechanical injuries. Walking on a concrete floor all day will result in knee, back, or foot pain in some but not in others. Nurses may lift patients for 3 or 4 years and suddenly back pain develops. Equipment that the nurse must use often is not designed to prevent injury in those who are susceptible. Unfortunately, researchers do not know enough about biomechanically related problems or enough about individual differences to be able to identify who is at risk for injury and how much stress it will take to injure them. However, the nurse can take necessary precautions if he or she knows how to avoid potential problems. Frequently, employers do not concern themselves with work-related injuries, and so it is a "worker beware" environment.

Working on assembly lines without the benefit of biomechanical assessment of postural requirements may result in permanent injury. Such injuries can mean financial ruin for the worker and a loss of talent to the employer. Human factors is an area of study that, in part, applies biomechanical principles to the worker and the work place to reduce stresses on the worker and thereby increase productivity. Because few employers have the benefit of human factors specialists, many costly injuries occur in the work place.

A nurse is required to work in positions and postures that can be very injurious, sometimes resulting in the inability to work. Lower back and lower extremity aches and pains develop if biomechanical principles are not applied during the routine workday. In the case study outlined in the beginning of the chapter, the nurse was suffering from an aching back that could have been reduced or prevented by using proper lifting practices. Broadly, there are two areas of biomechanics to consider relevant to nursing practice: proper segmental body alignment when applying force and cumulative trauma disorders due to repetitive tasks. Each of these areas is discussed later in this chapter.

FUTURE DEVELOPMENTS

The field of biomechanics is undergoing change as a result of research that is being conducted in the areas of neurology, orthopedics, sports medicine, nutrition, and other related fields. For example, the increase in private and governmental funding into spinal cord injury is being sparked as a result of the efforts of a well-known celebrity, Christopher Reeve, injured in a horseback riding accident. Through his and his supporters' efforts, attention has been brought to the mobility problems of thousands of people who are suffering from total or partial paralysis. Research studies involving this group of patients will result in better treatment methods and new types of mechanical aids to assist in ambulation.

Technological advances in the development of artificial limbs are continuing to be made. Many improvements have been and are being made in this arena to assist individuals with amputations of an arm or leg to return to productive lives with the use of an artificial limb. For example, connecting the muscles remaining in the stump of an arm to a mechanical device that includes the hand has allowed for controlling finger muscle movement, enabling the mechanical hand to perform small functions. Other developments include lightweight wheelchairs and wheelchairs that can be activated through devices controlled by the patient's tongue. Research continues in these areas, with the promise of continuing improvements being made in mechanical assistive devices.

Recommendations emanating from the field of nutrition and the efforts of organizations (particularly the federal government) to provide information to improve nutritional practices and promote positive health practices will affect the field of biomechanics in the future. An adequate, well-balanced diet and exercise program assists in improving overall health and well-being. Research in these areas will lead to further information regarding how diet affects the muscular and skeletal structure of the body. Research in exercise physiology and sports medicine will provide information to assist in designing exercise regimens and rehabilitation programs for injured individuals.

NURSING CARE ACTIONS

Principles and Practices

The use of proper body mechanics for both the nurse and the patient is an essential component of safe nursing care. As previously mentioned, the nurse can sustain serious injury if the body is used improperly, for example, while lifting a patient. The patient can suffer discomfort from improper positioning and serious injury from poorly administered transferred technique, ambulating assistance, or falling.

BODY ALIGNMENT

The muscles and articulations of the lower extremities, including the feet, legs, and the cervical and lumbar areas of the vertebral column, are most susceptible to misalignment injuries, because they are the weight-bearing areas of the body. Recall that a compression force pushes two bodies together and that for every force there is an equal and opposite reaction force. Applying these two principles to a standing human body, the weight force of each segment of the body has a given magnitude and pushes downward onto the next segment below it; in turn, the segment below pushes back against the segment with an equal and opposite force.

Weight bearing results in a compression force at every articulation of the vertebral column and the lower extremities. For example, while the first cervical vertebra has only the weight of the head as a compressive force, the single ankle in one-limb weight bearing, has the entire weight of the body (minus the foot) as its compressive force.

If the body is out of alignment, muscles must contract to hold the misaligned segment in place. The needed muscle tension in a misaligned body creates a compressive component of its own and is added to the total compressive force on the articular surfaces. Thus, a person with a forward leaning head or a forward leaning trunk puts excessive compressive force on the cervical and lumbar vertebral articulations. Neck and back pain result.

Just as a column on a large building is constructed in a vertical manner without pieces out of alignment, so the lower extremities should be in vertical alignment to hold the body weight. Because fast walking, jogging, or running places additional stresses on the lower extremity articulations (up to four times more than the body weight), proper vertical alignment is critical to alleviating injury. Placing the foot with the toes pointing outward can result in pain in the knee, hip, or even back. Uneven leg length is common and can cause pain in the lower back and hips. Some leg misalignments can be corrected by proper exercises; others require the assessment of a professional such as a podiatrist, osteopath, or chiropractor. In the case presentation, the burning sensation in the first metatarsal joint that the nurse felt may be relieved by an orthotic (in shoe corrective surface), which reduces the stress on that joint and may prevent the development of painful and troublesome bunions later on.

ASSESSING BODY POSTURES

Standing

Body alignment while standing, or **posture,** should follow basic biomechanical principles. Each weight-bearing segment—the head, vertebral column, pelvis, femurs, tibias and feet—should be centered over the next vertical segment below it such that each segmental center of gravity is located in the approximate center of the next segment. The center is located in three dimensions so that the line of gravity, a plumb line hanging from the center of gravity point, falls equidistant from right to left and front to back. The center of gravity will be located from top to bottom of the segment usually closer to the proximal end.

If the segments are vertically centered, there will be very little muscular torque needed to balance the body in standing. For example, if one stands with the trunk and head leaning forward, the centers of gravity of these two segments will fall outside the base of the next vertical segment, and the extensor muscles of the vertebral column must contract to hold the segments up and prevent them from falling forward. If a person is standing for a long time in a forward leaning position, the extensor muscles tire and begin to ache. Recall also that with muscular contraction additional compression forces are applied to each articulation. In the case of the forward-leaning vertebral column, excess compression is produced at each of the multiple intervertebral articulations. For an older adult who may have degenerative changes in the hyaline cartilage or the vertebral discs, the excessive compressive force hastens the degeneration and causes pain.

Three abnormal vertebral postures have been identified: lordosis, scoliosis, and kyphosis. These postures are illustrated in Figure 20–10.

Lordosis is an exaggerated curvature of the lumbar vertebrae. Lordosis is seen normally in children of early school age but is abnormal after that age. If the abdominal muscles are weak, and there is excess weight in the anterior stomach and abdomen, lordosis will result. It is important for women to

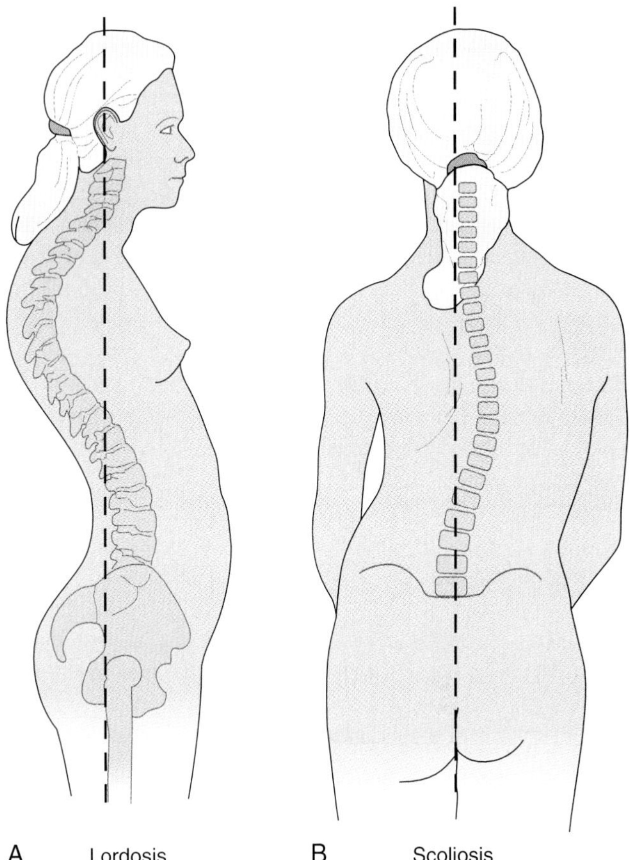

Figure 20–10. *A, B,* Lordosis and scoliosis.

have strong abdominal muscles before and during pregnancy or the weight of the fetus will pull the lumbar vertebrae forward and back pain will result. Back pain is also common in men with a large abdomen, because men put on weight in the stomach and abdomen and not the buttocks and thighs. With added weight in one anterior trunk, the center of gravity of the lumbar segments is pulled forward, and the lower back muscles must contract to counteract a forwardly displaced center of gravity.

Scoliosis is abnormal sideways curvature of the lower thoracic and lumbar areas. Sometimes the condition is genetic, but frequently it is induced by having one lower extremity shorter than the other. Surprising as it may seem, one short leg is quite common, and a difference of a quarter of an inch over time can cause a scoliotic condition of the vertebral column. The excessive side curvature causes stress on the muscles on the convex side of the vertebral column and on the lateral hip muscles (abductors) of the higher hip.

Kyphosis is the condition in which there is an excessive forward curvature of the thoracic vertebrae so that the person's shoulders, neck, and head are leaning forward. Because of the forward thoracic area, the natural curvature in the lumbar area is reduced. The forward lean requires the back extensor muscles to work constantly to hold the forward leaning segments up. The kyphotic posture is frequently seen in osteoporotic women because of a deterioration of the vertebral bodies.

Walking

The basic principles of standing should also be observed while walking. There are four phases to the gait: the plant, the stance, the push off, and the swing. Some people plant the heel first. Others are called mid-foot strikers, and their foot lands first in the mid-foot area rather than the heel. The mid-foot striker probably has better balance and is less likely to damage the tissues of the heel. During the stance phase, the weight (line of gravity) begins at the initial contact area and moves to the metatarsophalangeal area and out the second toe. People who have flat feet or are excessively pronate transfer their weight over the first metatarsophalangeal joint and toe. Eventually, this pattern can lead to medial ankle problems or bunions at the first metatarsophalangeal joint. The push-off phase may be accomplished normally by the plantarflexors of the ankle. However, people with weak calf muscles may accomplish the push-off phase with the use of the knee and hip extensors. During the swing phase, it is important for the person to "pick up the foot" by means of the dorsiflexors of the ankle. In some, the dorsiflexors of the ankle or the knee or hip flexor muscles may not be strong enough to lift the foot adequately off of the floor and the toes may catch, causing a trip or fall.

Footwear for the ambulatory person must be frictionless enough (no crepe soles) so that the person with weak flexor muscles can move forward by shuffling. The surface of the sole should not be too frictionless (smooth leather) so that a slip and fall is probable. At no time should patients be taken over wet surfaces, and inclines up or down should be avoided unless the friction of the surfaces is adequate and a handrail is used.

Sitting

Sitting for long periods of time is typical of the older adult or people with other health problems. Several problems during sitting are the leaning forward of the head, neck, and upper trunk, the sitting with the pelvis tilted backward, and inadequate surface support of the thighs.

The leaning forward of the head, neck, and trunk results in the same stress problems of the extensor muscles of the vertebral column as when standing. Excessive posterior tilt of the pelvis occurs when one slouches or slides down in the chair (Fig. 20–11). In this case, tensile stress is placed on the extensor muscles of the lumbar area and the internal organs become squeezed. Increased internal pressure makes breathing difficult.

Surface support of the thighs should be along the length of the posterior thighs. Recall that pressure is force per unit area. The greater the area of support, the smaller the pressure produced by the upper body weight. Because the ischial tuberosities protrude downward, they often get the brunt of the body weight and consequently the skin over them becomes sore. Softer chair coverings will increase the area of support and decrease the pressure. The chair must not be so soft that it encourages slouching. A chair that lacks depth results in a reduced surface area and increased pressure. A chair that is too deep for the sitter results in increased pressure behind the knees, and the sitter will sit forward of the back of the chair so that the legs fit comfortably. If the sitter is not sitting with the buttocks to the back of the chair, a leaning backward of the trunk results in posterior pelvic tilt. If the person's legs are not long enough to touch the floor, excess pressure will be produced above the knees.

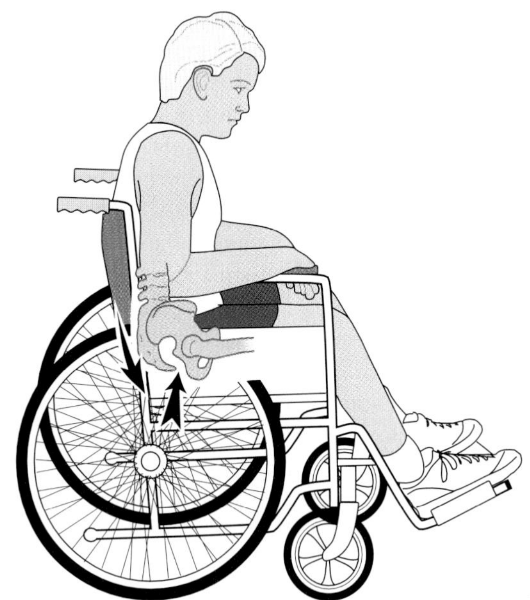

Figure 20–11. Posterior tilt of the pelvis in seated posture.

Lying Down

When lying down, a person is susceptible to misalignment of the vertebral column and pelvis and to *pressure points*, places of inordinate amounts of pressure. To give the body good support, the mattress should be firm but not hard. The more firm the mattress, the less it will "give in" to lumps and bumps of the body shape. The more firm the mattress, the less the surface area available to the body and the greater the pressure on those points of the body touching the mattress. Mattress firmness is a compromise.

Taking the example of a female, middle-aged patient, one can imagine that the posterior pelvis and the lateral pelvis are wider than the posterior upper thoracic and the lateral shoulder area, respectively. Thus, on a hard surface and lying on the back, her posterior pelvis would be pushed higher than her posterior shoulder area. Likewise, when lying on her side, her pelvis would be pushed higher than her shoulder area. Both of these situations would cause an undesirable alignment of the vertebral column. In the case of a male patient, the shoulders are usually wider than the hips and the upper back is usually more deep than the posterior hips. Thus, the back lying position should present few problems in terms of alignment but the side-lying position could result in scoliosis because of the ratio of the shoulder to the hip width.

The pressure points in side lying are the shoulders, the pelvis, the medial sides of the knees if the legs are together, and the ankles. In back lying, the pressure points are the *right* posterior pelvis and the heels for a woman and the shoulders, the pelvis (to a lesser extent than a woman), and the heels for a man.

LIFTING

Lifting an external load changes the body's center of gravity, because in biomechanics the load is considered part of the body system. Lifting a load in the front of the body will shift the body's center of gravity forward. If the load is carried at the height of the body's original center of gravity, then the center of gravity height will not change. However, if the load is carried above the middle of the pelvis, then the center of gravity will move upward while carrying it. If the load is carried below the middle of the pelvis, then the center of gravity will move downward. Recall that stability is better maintained when the center of gravity is positioned in the center of the base of support (the feet or foot in one-leg support) and is as low as possible. Thus, for balance considerations, the load is best carried lower if possible. Also, the closer to the body the load is carried, the less the center of gravity will move forward (Fig. 20–12).

The external load affects the body's biomechanics like standing with the head and trunk forward. The extensor muscles of the back must produce enough torque to counteract the forward-producing torque effects of the load. The farther forward the load, the greater the torque and the more force must be produced by the muscles. To prevent excessive forward torque, one should lift loads below the elbow level. One should move downward by flexing the knees and hips and keeping the trunk as vertical as possible. In other words, lift from the legs, the strongest muscles in the body.

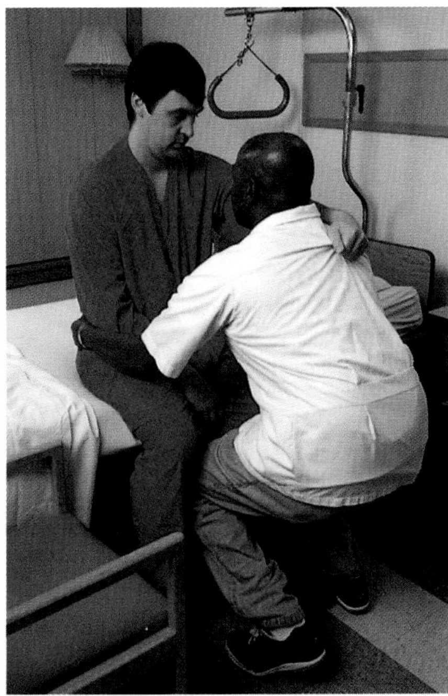

Figure 20–12. Proper body mechanics for lifting.

When lifting a load at the side, the same lifting principles should be used. Get down to the load by flexing the hips and knees and not by leaning the trunk sideways and forward. Twisting while extending the trunk results in even greater deleterious effects than leaning forward without twisting, because the muscles that rotate the trunk are even smaller than the extensors and can be injured easily.

If it is possible to divide the sideward-carried load into two loads, one to be carried on each side, all the better. Biomechanical lifting models have shown that more torque is required from the back muscles when *one* 100-pound load is carried on one side than when carrying *two* 100-pound loads, one on each side (LaVeau, 1992).

Recently, nurses have been encouraged to use a lifting belt or an ergonomically designed corset during the performance of lifting tasks. Because back injury brings high financial cost to the employer as well as the employee, not to mention the personal costs of pain and suffering, the lifting belt or corset has been an encouraging innovation to prevent such injuries. Troup (1965) reported that 40 percent of back injuries result from lifting and 33 percent are from twisting movements of the spine.

There are four factors that serve as rationales for using support devices:

- Tightly cinched belts assist in increasing the intra-abdominal pressure during a lift; this pressure supports the anterior vertebral column and helps prevent strains and/or dislocations.
- The snug corset helps prevent the lifter from lifting by flexing and extending the vertebral column; the lifter must lift by using the stronger leg muscles while keeping the "back straight."
- Some corsets are worn such that they prevent a "twisting" (vertebral rotation) during a lift that has been associated with injury.
- Wearing any device foreign to one's typical attire serves as a reminder to the lifter to remember and employ biomechanically proper lifting techniques.

Whereas initial studies have indicated some success in preventing injuries and once injured reducing pain and discomfort in workers who wear these devices, firm evidence is still out on their effectiveness. Unfortunately, workers frequently do not wear the devices or, if they must, do not tighten them securely enough because they are uncomfortable or hot to wear. In the nursing field, constant repetitive lifting is not usually performed and wearing an ergonomically designed back support should be part of the equipment assembled and used during any lifting, repositioning, or transferring procedure.

PATIENT POSITIONING, MOVING, AND TRANSFERRING

Positioning a patient must be considered from the perspective of the nurse (preventing back injuries and tissue strains) and from the perspective of the patient (preventing injury or discomfort from incorrect repositioning by the nurse or being left in a stressful position). Before moving, repositioning, or transferring a patient, the nurse should assess the patient's:

- Musculoskeletal alignment of body segments
- Mobility of the joints
- Neuromuscular system relative to proprioception (body awareness) and balance

If possible, nurses should ask the patient to assist in the moving. Even if the force the patient can produce is small, it reduces the amount of muscle torque that is required of the nurse. When the patient can assist, the nurse must be prepared to tell the patient exactly what the procedure is going to be and where and when the patient should apply force. Of course, there are situations in which the patient cannot help and in these cases the nurse must use the very best biomechanical principles to prevent injury. Finally, whenever the patient is going to be repositioned in bed, the bed should be raised to a height appropriate for each nurse, that is, as close to possible to the height of the nurse's elbow.

The objectives of these positioning procedures are to:

- Place the patient in a comfortable position in a bed or a chair
- Avoid negative effects of pressure on parts of the patient's body
- Avoid injury to the patient or the nurse when the nurse is positioning the patient in a bed or a chair

BASIC BED POSITIONS

There are five basic bed positions for patients (Fig. 20–13):

- *Prone*—the position of the body or the body's forearm segment in which the body is faced down (lying on one's front) or in which the forearm is positioned such that the palm surface is facing backward when standing or downward when lying on one's back
- *Semi-prone (Sims') position*—the position of the body in which one is midway between the side-lying and prone position in bed
- *Supine*—the position of the body or the body's forearm segment in which the body is faced upward (lying on one's back) or in which the forearm is positioned such that the palm surface is facing forward when standing or upward when lying on one's back
- *Fowler's position*—the position of the body in which one is midway between supine lying and sitting upright in bed
- *Side lying*—body turned on either right or left side

POSITIONING THE PATIENT IN BED

Prone

The prone position is one in which the patient is on the dorsal surface with the head and neck turned to one side. The true prone position will be uncomfortable for most adults, because the cervical and lumbar vertebral column will be forced into hyperextension. The limited range of motion of the cervical vertebrae will produce pain because of the resulting hyperextension. The thoracic vertebrae may not be accustomed to the extension produced by prone lying, and the lumbar area may be forced into greater hyperextension than it should be. Thus, the semiprone position is best.

If the head is turned to the right, the right shoulder is abducted and externally rotated and the forearm is pronated. The left shoulder is internally rotated and abducted and the elbow flexed so as to place the hand by the left hip. The right hip and knee are flexed, and the ankle is in neutral position. The vertebral column is in neutral position and supported by the right elbow, forearm, and hand and the right knee, leg, and foot. The left hip and knee are extended, and the left ankle is in neutral position. Thus, the support of the trunk and vertebral column is such that it remains in a neutral, non-rotated position.

For some older adults, the internal rotation of the lower arm is uncomfortable and the patient must be positioned so that the lower arm is not internally rotated. It may be placed also directly under the trunk, with the elbow flexed.

Semi-Prone (Sims' Position)

The semi-prone position is frequently more comfortable than the side-lying or full prone position, both of which may place stress on the vertebral column. The semi-prone position is easily assumed from the side-lying position.

Supine

Although the supine position seems to be the most comfortable for most people, the patient should not remain in this position for extended periods of time. The nurse should position the patient so as to reduce or prevent hyperextension of the neck and lumbar vertebrae and to reduce the pressure on the buttocks and heels.

The head and neck should be supported with a pillow. The pillow should not be so thick that the neck is hyperflexed. The lumbar vertebrae is easily forced into hyperextension when lying flat, particularly in people with large buttocks and/or weak abdominals and/or limited flexibility in the hip flexors. The limited range of motion of the hip flexors is common because most people do not do hip extension exercises to stretch them. The pelvis can be kept in a neutral posture by flexing the hips and knees about 20° and supporting this position with a pillow. The flexion of the hips and knees will reduce the pressure on the lower buttocks (coccyx area) as well. If the posterior ankles are supported with a pillow, pressure on the heel will be reduced.

Tightly tucked bedding can put undue pressure on the toes and feet. The bedding should be loosened and may be taken off of the feet entirely with the use of a footboard (Fig. 20–14). To place the feet at the proper position relative to the leg, the nurse may use a footboard to push the foot into a 140° angle (measured anteriorly) with the lower leg.

To further the comfort of the patient, one may place support pillows under the forearms, which are positioned in

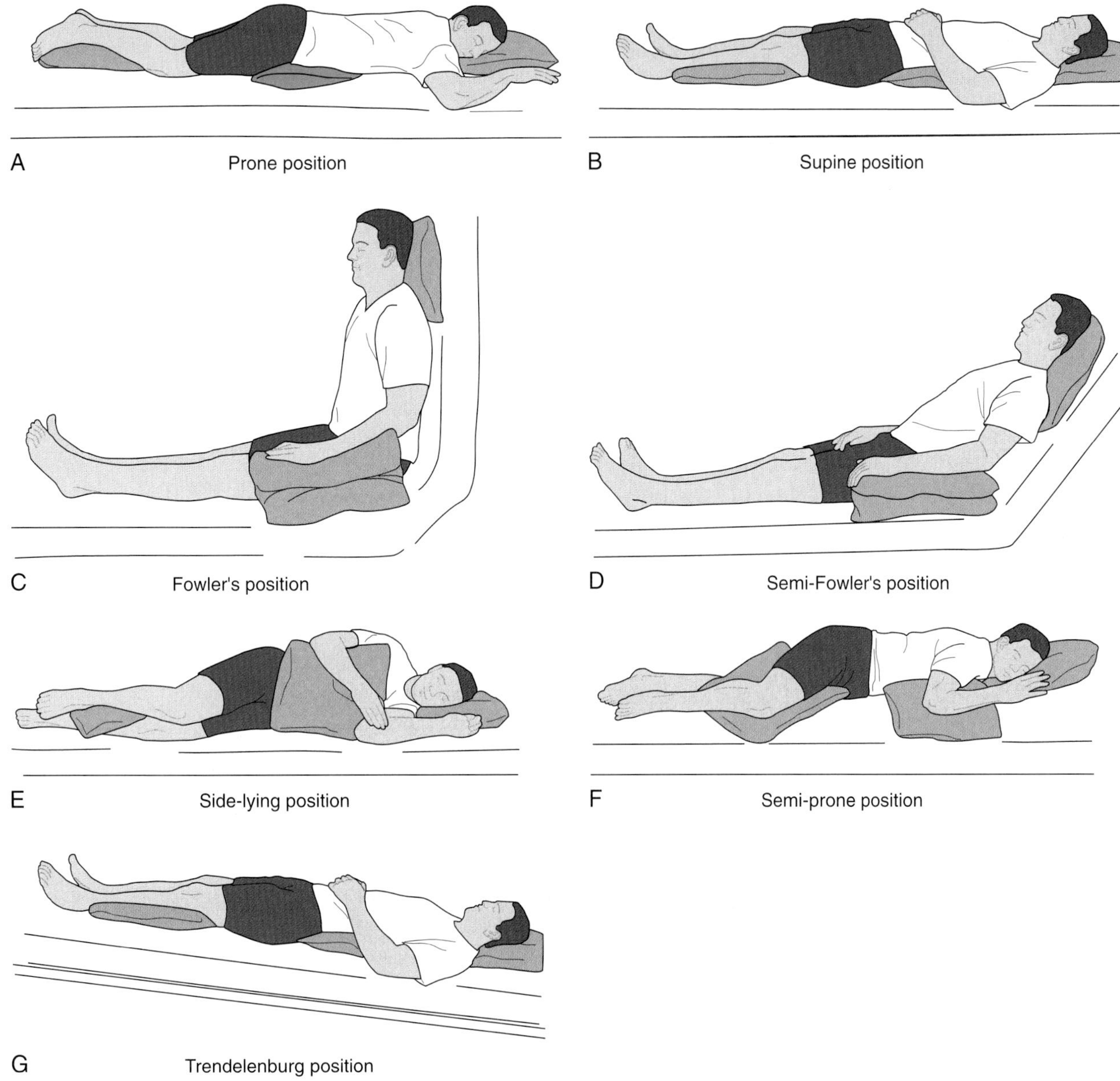

Figure 20-13. *A–G,* Basic positions for patients in bed.

pronation. This will relieve the pressure on the medial epicondyles of the humeri. In some cases, the thighs fall naturally into lateral rotation. When the patient remains in that position, stress may develop in the medial and lateral tissues surrounding the hip joint. To prevent the lateral rotation of the hip joints, towels or pillows may be rolled and tucked into the lateral interfaces of the thighs and the bed. The lateral support will prevent the unwanted outward rotation of the lower extremities.

Fowler's/Semi-Fowler's

When the patient is sitting up in bed it is called Fowler's position. The angle of the upper bed is from 45° (semi-Fowler's) to 60°. In this position, the upper body is resting on an incline and downward slippage is likely to occur. Increased pressure is assumed by the coccyx area and discomfort results. To reduce the pressure on the coccyx area, the hips and knees are flexed so that the surface area onto which the body weight rests is increased from the small coccyx area to the lower buttocks and the thighs. The body weight is the same, of course, but the pressure on any small area is reduced by the increased surface area.

The flexed knee position also reduces the pressure on the heels because the weight of the legs and feet is at an angle to the supporting surface. The nurse must always check the pillow that is placed at the head and neck area, because the same thickness of pillow used in a back-lying position will cause the head and neck to be hyperflexed when the patient is in Fowler's position. Therefore, the thickness of the support

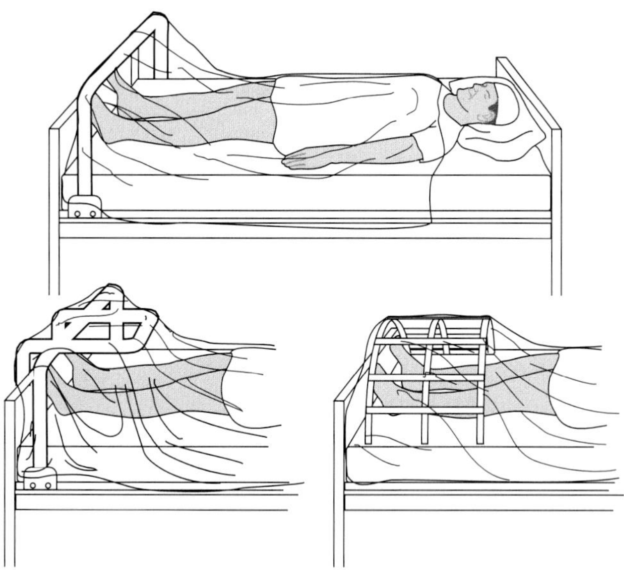

Figure 20-14. Bed cradle.

for the head and neck must be reduced in Fowler's position so that the head is not pushed forward and results in hyperflexion of the cervical vertebrae. On the other hand, the weight of the head pushing downward on the neck can produce hyperextension of the neck if adequate support is not provided so some support under the base of the skull and in the concave cervical curvature should be provided.

Side-Lying

In the side-lying position, the patient should have support at the cervical vertebrae so that the neck does not laterally flex and at the lumbar vertebrae so that the lower back does not laterally flex. The support may be provided by a small pillow or towel placed in these areas.

Pressure soreness often is induced in the shoulder, pelvis, knee, and ankle areas. Placing the support at the neck and the lumbar areas will reduce the pressure somewhat at the shoulder and hip because increased surface area will reduce the force per square inch. The pressure at the knees may be relieved by placing a pillow between the knees if the patient feels more comfortable with the legs together, but a more biomechanically appropriate position is that in which the top lower extremity is flexed at the hip and knee and a pillow support is placed beneath the upper knee and lower leg. This position eliminates the pressure point between the knees and stabilizes the upper portion of the pelvis from falling forward.

The forward displacement of the pelvis with the knees together produces a rotation or twisting of the lumbar vertebrae. Twisting or rotation of the vertebral column should be avoided when possible. A support or pillow also may be placed under the topside upper extremity so that it is not forced into adduction. The pillow placed from the elbow to the hand will increase the surface area and decrease the pressure on these segments.

Special Considerations

The safety and comfort of the patient in various positions will depend on the patient's condition. Several of these special considerations are if the patient is pregnant; is paraplegic, quadriplegic, or hemiplegic; has broken bones or recently dislocated joints; or has had surgery. Each of these conditions requires special care by the nurse to avoid further damage to the part of the body affected. The plegic patient is particularly susceptible to pressure sores because the pressure on the affected limbs cannot be felt. Usually, patients can assist the positioning and position their legs into a comfortable position. This is not true for the plegic patient, although in the case of the paraplegic and hemiplegic person, the nonaffected side may be used to assist.

The nurse should avoid excessive pushing, pulling, or tugging on any body part, but when a patient's body part is in a pathologic state, the nurse must avoid placing any stress on it. This stress can be in the form of direct lifting or pulling by the nurse or created by the movement of another body part that results in the affected part being forced against the mattress, pillows, or the rails or being squeezed between the body and the mattress.

MOVING A PATIENT HEADWARD IN BED

During positioning in which the patient is sitting at some angle in a supine position, slippage downward may occur. Thus, the nurse will be required to move the patient headward. It is difficult to move the patient up in bed without putting undue stress on one of the patient's shoulders or putting excess stress on the nurse's back. The best situation is one in which there is a second person to assist in the repositioning, either another nurse or the patient. If there is a second person, that person will perform a similar procedure on the opposite side of the bed. In case there is no extra help, and one nurse is required to move the patient up in bed alone, other procedures are necessary. Similar to the two-person move, the bed should be horizontal and, after the bed leveling, the patient's hips and knees should be flexed on both sides. A pillow should be placed under the patient's head. If it is possible for the nurse to position himself or herself at the head of the bed, the nurse's forearms should be placed under the patient's arms with the elbows resting on the end of the bed. The nurse's elbow flexors, not the nurse's back extensors, should be used to lift and move the patient headward.

If the nurse cannot position himself or herself at the head of the bed, then a two-step procedure, right and left side, must be used. On the left side of the patient, the nurse places the right hand under the patient's shoulders and the left arm under the patient's pelvis. Lift and slide the patient headward. Go to the right side of the patient and place the left hand under the patient's shoulders and the right arm under the patient's pelvis. Lift and slide the patient upward.

The procedure may have to be repeated several times, because one-sided lifting produces eccentric forces on the patient; thus, the procedure must be repeated so as to "walk the patient" upward. The friction produced due to the sliding of the patient's pelvis on the bed will counteract the intended move. Frequently with male patients, the hips will not produce as much resistant friction force as for female patients because males have less weight in the posterior pelvis area. It is difficult to assess how one may proceed because there are three basic contact areas—head, shoulders, and hips—and it is difficult to alleviate the weight of three areas with the two available arms of one nurse.

To reemphasize biomechanical principles, lift with the legs and supported arms, not the back, and lean the trunk forward as little as possible. One does not lift the patient off the bed but rather lifts so that the entire downward weight of the patient is reduced. This reduces the resistive friction force generated during the slide. The nurse should not twist at the trunk, so the sliding is best done by abducting the hips to widen the base of support in the right and left direction. Begin the force application with the nurse's center of gravity on the leg that is nearer the patient's foot end. Lift the patient upward slightly with the use of the legs while shifting one's own center of gravity horizontally toward the patient's head end.

If two nurses are lifting, the move must be coordinated and may be done also by counting to 3 before applying force. If it is possible for the patient to help in the move, coach the patient to push with the legs at the count of 3 when the nurse(s) apply force. Because the patient's feet will tend to slip on the bed sheet, the patient should attempt to help by lifting the pelvis off of the bed to reduce resistive friction force during the slide. If it is not possible for the patient to help, the nurse(s) must do this by applying additional upward force (see Procedure 20–1).

TRANSFERRING A PATIENT

Transfer techniques are those in which the nurse must assist the patient in a move from one supporting surface to another (e.g., between the bed and a chair or between the bed and a stretcher). Transfers frequently require more lifting than repositioning and should only be done with two people, either a nurse with the assistance of the patient or two nurses. One nurse should not attempt to transfer a totally dependent patient. In addition, the strength of the patient must be assessed by the nurse, because if the patient's leg strength is needed, for example, and the patient's legs give way during the transfer, injury to the patient and to the nurse may result. Also, transfers should proceed in stages, so that the patient may easily return to the previous stage if failure occurs.

Bed-to-Chair Transfer

In bed-to-chair or chair-to-bed transfers, lower extremity support by the patient is required. The transfer involves the patient sitting up on the edge of the bed or chair, a short period of standing, a 90° rotation, or pivot, of the patient's body, and a lowering of the patient into a sitting position on the receiving surface. If the chair is placed correctly, the patient should not have to take a step during lower extremity support. The height of the bed should be adjusted so that the patient's feet touch the floor completely with at least a 140° angle at the knee joint. A lesser joint angle reduces the effective torque production of the leg muscles, and the patient may not be able to support his or her entire body weight. In this position, the patient can return to the bed without extending the hips and knees and the extension required on weight bearing will be possible without undue strength of the extensor muscles.

The chair should be locked in place near the head of the bed such that the front of the chair is located just headward of the place where the patient is seated or will be seated on the bed. Of course, all obstacles should be moved well away from a 180° semicircle so that the nurse can move from behind the chair around the chair and to the opposite side of the patient without tripping or falling. The four-step procedure should be outlined to the patient so that his or her participation is clearly understood.

Transfers from chair to bed are made by following the reverse procedure of bed to chair. It should be kept in mind that the lift is made with the use of the stronger hip and knee muscles and through transferring weight from the forward to rear foot. Twisting the vertebral column is avoided by using a two-foot pivot.

Bed-to-Stretcher Transfer

If an immobilized patient is to be transferred from a bed or stretcher to another bed, the three-person carry should be employed. To maintain a proper body alignment of the patient, the three carriers should be of approximately the same height so that their forearms are on the same plane when the elbows are flexed to 90°.

The patient is carried as close to the nurses' bodies as possible to reduce the resistive torque required of the back extensor muscles. The lifting and lowering of the patient should be done by the leg muscles and not by the back extensor muscles. Because the dropped rail of the bed will hinder the flexing of the lifters' knees forward, the bed should be high enough so that the lifters do not have to flex a great amount. The stretcher or other bed to which the patient is to be transferred should be of approximately the same height so that a great deal of lifting and lowering is not required.

Two locations for the destination apparatus may be used depending on whether there is a fourth person available to move the stretcher while the three lifters support the patient. If there is a fourth person, the stretcher is located beside and at the foot end of the bed such that the near corner of the foot end of the bed is adjacent to the far corner of the head end of the stretcher when transferring from bed to stretcher. When transferring from stretcher to bed, the stretcher is wheeled adjacent and parallel to the bed and is rolled out from under the lifted patient. The procedure in this case is to lift the patient, translate the patient backward, slide the stretcher under the patient, and lower the patient onto it. When transferring a patient from the stretcher to the bed, the order is to lift the patient from the stretcher, slide the stretcher out from under the supported patient, translate the patient forward, and lower the patient to the bed.

If there are only three lifters and no fourth assistant, the bed and stretcher are positioned perpendicular to each other such that the foot end of the stretcher is adjacent to the head end of the bed. The procedure in this case is lift, translate, rotate, and lower when moving from bed to stretcher and lift, rotate, translate, and lower when moving from stretcher to bed. See Procedure 20–1 for four- and three-assistant lifts.

If the patient is being transferred from the bed to the stretcher, the order of the lift is reversed-lift, translate backward three steps, rotate 90° around the lifter at the head end of the patient, and lower the patient to the stretcher. Again, the rotation is accomplished by the middle-and-foot-end lifter moving (rotating) around the head-end lifter. The lifters at the foot end should be able to travel the greatest path in the rotation.

RANGE OF MOTION

All joints in the human body have a normal range of motion. As discussed, range of motion is the extent of the movement of which a joint is normally capable. The maintenance of the normal range of motion in body joints is important despite the age, health status, or physical impairment of the individual. The nursing care of any patient should include a plan for maintaining range of motion of the joints. There are active and passive exercises. Active exercises are performed by the patient. Passive exercises require the assistance of the nurse. It is particularly important that patients with mobility problems be assisted to perform range of motion exercises to ensure that activities of daily living can be performed (see Procedure 20–2). Activities of daily living include using the toilet, feeding oneself, bathing, urinary and bowel continence, transferring from a bed to a chair, and ambulating.

ANTIEMBOLISM OR PRESSURE STOCKINGS

Antiembolism or pressure stockings are used when patients experience edema in the lower extremities. The edema is usually associated with phlebitis or formation of a thrombus (blood clot). The elastic stockings force blood from the external veins to the deeper veins, reducing the possibility of stagnation of the blood. The stockings need to be removed from the patient during morning care and reapplied before getting out of bed (see Procedure 20–3).

RESTRAINTS

Restraints may be either physical, chemical, or pharmacologic. They are used to limit the activity of the patient. Chemical and pharmacologic restraints include sleeping medications, tranquilizers, and other drugs that reduce cognitive awareness. Physical restraints include bed rails; "soft" wrist, hand, or leg restraints made from fabric or leather; chest restraints; belts; and canvas total upper body restraints.

The increasing public and professional awareness of the effects of the use of restraints on elderly patients resulted in the passage in 1987 by Congress of the Nursing Home Reform Act (Public Law 100–203). This act, effective as of October 1990, requires reduction in the use of physical restraints. The legal and ethical issues surrounding restraints prompted the congressional action.

Restraint application may be necessary under certain circumstances, such as when a patient has intravenous therapy and there is danger of the needles or cannulas being disturbed, a patient is unconscious or delirious and pulls at tubes or dressings, or there is danger of the patient falling. Under all circumstances, the dignity of the patient is to be respected. Restraints should be used only as a last resort. Documentation as to why the restraints were applied is to be detailed.

There are dangers associated with restraint application. Patients need to be routinely checked to determine if the patient is in any jeopardy of suffocation from poorly applied restraints; contractions from restraints applied to tight, dehydrated, skin irritations; or untoward emotional responses such as irrationality, anger, or fear.

Nurses should be innovative and creative and find other methods to reduce or prevent the use of restraints. The use of restraints may cause more problems than they resolve (see Procedure 20–4).

AMBULATION WITH ASSISTANCE

Patients with impaired mobility will need assistance from the nursing staff in ambulating. There are devices available to aid the patient in walking. These include walkers, canes, and crutches. There are also some instances in which braces may be used by the patient. Usually the patient will be taught the proper techniques for use of the mechanical devices in a physical therapy or rehabilitation unit. The role of the nurse may be to teach proper procedures for using the device but under ordinary circumstances the nurse will reinforce the information learned from the physical therapist.

There are precautions to be taken while assisting the patient to ambulate. For example, the patient must be assessed to determine if there is adequate physical strength to stand to use a cane, walker, or crutches. If the patient is weak, specific exercises need to be initiated to strengthen the patient's appropriate muscles before ambulating. The patient must have the appropriate shoes so that improper footwear does not cause the patient to fall. Rubber-soled, well-fitting shoes are essential.

The mechanical devices selected for the individual patient must fit correctly. For example, walkers, crutches, and canes come in various sizes and the patient must be measured to ensure that the equipment is right.

CANES

Canes may be single tipped or three or four pronged. They may be solid wood or metal or could be adjustable. Single-tipped canes are used to provide minimal support; three- or four-pronged canes are used for patients who have difficulty maintaining balance. Handles on canes may be curved or straight. Straight-handled canes are used by patients who have impaired gripping ability (see Procedure 20–5).

WALKERS

Walkers are used to provide balance and stability to the patient. They are usually made from a lightweight metal and may be adjustable. Some walkers have two wheels to provide for greater patient mobility (see Procedure 20–5).

CRUTCHES

Crutches may be metal or wood, and some are adjustable. The different types of crutches are the forearm type and the axillary type. The physical condition and strength of the patient determine the type of crutch selected.

There are four different types of crutch gaits:

- *Swing through*—weight bearing on one foot
- *Four-point*—weight bearing on both legs
- *Three-point*—weight bearing on one foot, the second foot acts as a balance
- *Two-point*—weight bearing on two feet, a more rapid four-point gait

The selection of the specific gait depends on the physical disability of the patient.

Procedures

This section presents the following procedures:

- Patient transfers, bed positioning, and comfort measures
- Performing range-of-motion (ROM) exercises
- Applying pressue stickings
- Applying restraints
- Assisting with ambulation

PROCEDURE 20-1

Patient Transfers, Bed Positioning, and Comfort Measures

Objective

Provide a safe method for positioning and moving the patient with limited mobility while promoting comfort.

Terminology

footboard—a board that is placed at the foot of the bed and positioned so that the patient's feet gently rest against it in the correct anatomic position, therefore preventing footdrop.

Fowler's—bed position with head of bed elevated 45°.

hand roll—a small rolled cloth or premanufactured roll that is placed in the hand to maintain functional alignment of the fingers and thumb.

high Fowler's—bed position with head of bed elevated 90°.

lateral—body position in which patient is lying on side so that the weight is primarily on the hip and shoulder, which are in contact with the bed. Also known as side-lying position.

prone—body position in which patient is lying on the stomach with the head turned to one side and arms flexed at the elbows with forearms lying on bed with hands pointing to head of the bed.

semi-Fowler's—bed position with head of bed elevated 15° to 45°.

semi-prone—body position in which patient is lying on side with slight forward rotation so that the weight is on the anterior ilium of the pelvis, humerus, and clavicle, which are in contact with the bed. Also known as Sims' position.

supine—body position in which patient is lying on back with arms extended downward and legs extended toward the foot of the bed. Also known as dorsal recumbent.

trochanter roll—a rolled towel or small blanket that is placed along the trochanter region of the femur to prevent external rotation of the hip joint. Sandbags or a premanufactured roll may also be used for this purpose.

Critical Elements

Safety is the most important issue in positioning or transferring a patient. The care provider must review the physician's mobility/activity order for the patient before beginning the procedure. The care provider must assess that patient's abilities and needs before attempting to position or transfer the patient. When assessing the patient the care provider

continued on next page

PROCEDURE 20-1 (cont'd)

should take into consideration the presence of dressings, suture lines, and any equipment in use. Physical conditions that may contraindicate any exertion must also be noted. In addition, it is important to note whether the patient is physically able to assist with the positioning or transfer and whether instructions can be understood.

The care provider should have the bed at a level that prevents back strain during the procedure. The bed wheels should be locked, and the side rails should be raised on the side away from the care provider. Proper body mechanics should always be utilized to protect the care provider. The care provider should assess whether the procedure can be safely completed alone or if assistance is needed from other care providers. If the bed has been raised during the procedure, it should be returned to the low position, with side rails up before leaving the patient.

Equipment

Pillow(s)
Bath blanket or towel (if trochanter roll is needed)
Washcloths (if hand roll is needed)
Gait belt (if transferring patient to sitting at side of bed or assisting out of bed)
Footboard (if indicated)
Stretcher/wheelchair/chair (if indicated)
Slide/roller board (optional)

Special Considerations

When transferring a patient from a lying to a sitting position be sure to note the presence of dizziness. If dizziness continues or fainting occurs, vital signs should be monitored and the physician notified.

An overhead trapeze may be added to the bed frame to allow the patient to assist with bed mobility.

Before repositioning or transferring procedures, the care provider should assess the patient's pain level. Pain medication administration may be necessary to perform the procedure with maximum comfort to the patient.

Gloves should be worn if the care provider believes that contact may be made with blood or body fluids, such as with a draining wound or incontinency.

Action	*Rationale*
1. Assemble equipment.	1. Promotes task organization.
2. Identify patient.	2. Provides patient safety.
3. Explain procedure.	3. Promotes patient compliance.
4. Close door/curtain.	4. Maintains patient privacy and dignity.
5. Position bed.	5. Promotes good body mechanics.
a. For bed positioning and stretcher transfers, raise bed to comfortable working height for care provider.	
b. For bed-to-chair transfers, lower bed so patient may easily reach floor with legs when transferring.	Allows patient to secure footing during transfer process.
6. Fold top linen to foot of bed.	6. Allows access to patient for positioning procedure.
7. Lower side rail on side of bed where care provider is working and keep side rail up on other side of bed.	7. Promotes patient safety.

Supine Position

1. Position patient flat on back with arms extended at sides, legs extended toward foot of bed, and pillow under head.	1. Positions patient in supine position.
2. If indicated, place small folded towel under forearm, hand roll in hands, trochanter roll at area of greater trochanter of femur, and feet flat against footboard.	2. Provides support for arms, legs, and feet for immobile patient.
3. If indicated, place pillow under patient's lower legs so heels are not touching bed.	3. Avoids potential skin breakdown from heel pressure on bed.

continued on next page

PROCEDURE 20-1 (cont'd)

Fowler's Position

1. Position patient as in supine position and raise head of bed 15° to 45°.	1. Places head of bed in Fowler's position.
2. Raise knee gatch slightly.	2. Reduces back strain for patient in this position.
3. For comfort, if indicated, place small folded towel under forearms or place forearms in lap. Place hand rolls in hands and trochanter rolls bilaterally along both greater trochanters and femurs. Place feet gently against footboard.	3. Provides support for arms, legs, and feet for immobile patient.
4. If indicated, place pillow under lower legs so that heels are not touching bed.	4. Avoids potential skin breakdown from heel pressure on bed.

Lateral Position

1. Position patient's legs with leg farthest from care provider crossed over leg nearest care provider.	1. Prepares patient for turning to lateral position.
2. Standing close to bed, extend care provider's arm closest to patient's head under patient's farthest shoulder and care provider's other arm under patient's farthest hip.	2. Positions care provider's arms to assist patient with turn.
3. Turn patient toward care provider being sure to move patient in log rolling fashion.	3. Protects patient's back from twisting during turning procedure.
4. After patient is on side, place pillow under head so neck is in alignment with spinal cord.	4. Prevents lateral flexion of cervical vertebrae and provides comfort.
5. Flex arm on mattress at shoulder and elbow, bringing arm outward from body with forearm extending up toward pillow, rotating shoulder slightly forward.	5. Positions arm so body is not on top of arm and full weight is not on shoulder joint.
6. Flex top arm at elbow, position forearm extending outward from body and place small folded blanket or pillow under forearm.	6. Provides support for forearm.
7. Flex top leg slightly at hip and knee bringing leg slightly in front of bottom leg and place pillow under leg from thigh to foot.	7. Prevents hyperextension of leg and prevents pressure areas on bony prominences.
8. Roll pillow or blanket and place along thoracic and lumbar/sacral areas of patient's spine.	8. Provides support for back and prevents patient from rolling back into supine position.

Semi-prone Position (or Sims' Position)

1. Turn patient to lateral position as described earlier.	1. Prepares patient for placement in semi-prone position.
2. While facing patient's back, extend care provider's arms under shoulder area and slide bottom shoulder back and rotate top shoulder forward until patient is lying on front aspect of bottom shoulder. Then ease lower arm behind patient so arm is extending outward on mattress behind patient's back.	2. Positions upper body in semi-prone position.
3. While facing patient's back, extend care provider's arms under hip area and slide bottom hip back causing top hip to rotate forward until patient is lying on iliac crest area of hip closest to mattress. *Note:* Steps 2 and 3 can be done simultaneously if two care providers are working with patient.	3. Positions bottom half of body in semi-prone position.

PROCEDURE 20-1 (cont'd)

Semi-prone Position (or Sims' Position) (cont'd)

Action	Rationale
4. Position top arm extended from body at shoulder and flexed at elbow with forearm lying on bed.	4. Provides support for top arm.
5. Flex top leg slightly at hip joint and knee and place pillow under top leg from thigh to ankle.	5. Positions leg with support and prevents pressure on body prominences.

Prone Position

Action	Rationale
1. With patient in supine position, extend care provider's arms under patient's shoulder and chest and slide top part of patient's body toward side of bed. Extend care provider's arms under patient's hips and thighs and slide remainder of body toward side of bed. *Note:* If move is being done with two care providers, patient's entire body can be moved to side of bed simultaneously.	1. Prepares patient for moving to prone position.
2. While facing patient, place patient's arm closest to care provider straight along patient's side and place patient's arm farthest from care provider above patient's head. Turn head to side facing away from care provider.	2. Positions arms in preparation for turning patient.
3. Cross leg farthest from care provider over leg closest to care provider.	3. Positions legs in preparation for turning patient.
4. Grasp patient at side of chest farthest from care provider and at hip farthest from care provider and roll patient toward you.	4. Rolls patient from supine to prone position.
5. Position patient's arms extended at shoulders and flexed at elbow with forearms pointing toward head of bed.	5. Provides appropriate support for arms.
6. Position head turned to side with face directly on mattress, and place pillow under patient's lower legs and ankles so toes are not touching bed.	6. Prevents hyperextension of cervical vertebrae and avoids footdrop.

Transferring from Bed to Chair

Action	Rationale
1. Position chair at side of bed. If patient has a weaker side, make sure chair is positioned so it is next to the stronger leg.	1. Promotes patient stability by positioning chair so leg with dominant strength will bear weight during transfer procedure.
2. Place one arm on patient's shoulder farthest from care provider and one arm on hip farthest from care provider; then log-roll patient to side facing care provider.	2. Brings patient to edge of bed while avoiding straining of abdominal or back muscles.
3. Raise head of bed as much as possible.	3. Assists patient into upright position.
4. With arm closest to patient's legs, ease legs over side of bed allowing them to drop downward, while using arm closest to patient's head to slip under patient's shoulder and assist upper body to sitting position (Fig. 20–15).	4. Raises patient to sitting position.

continued on next page

PROCEDURE 20-1 (cont'd)

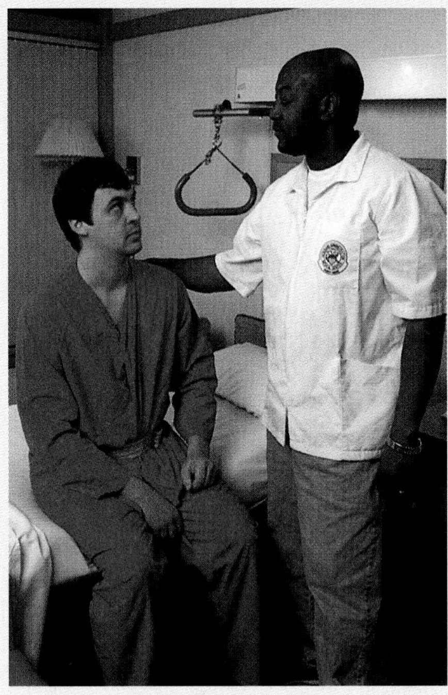

Figure 20–15. Assist patient to a sitting position on the edge of the bed.

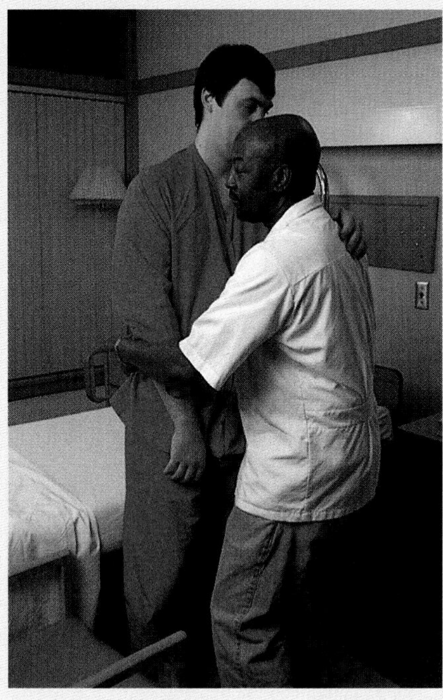

Figure 20–16. Assist patient to standing position.

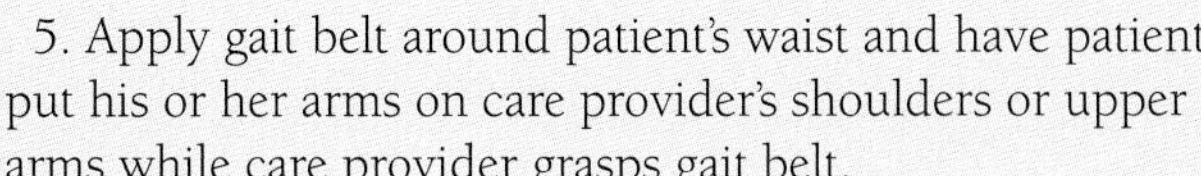

5. Apply gait belt around patient's waist and have patient put his or her arms on care provider's shoulders or upper arms while care provider grasps gait belt.	5. Promotes safety by promoting stability during transfer.
6. Place shoes or socks with nonskid bottoms on patient's feet.	6. Promotes safety and prevents sliding or slipping.
7. Stand with feet slightly apart and foot closest to chair slightly behind other foot.	7. Provides wide base of support for care provider.
8. Monitor patient for dizziness, nausea, and general level of awareness while dangling at side of bed.	8. Provides opportunity for care provider to assess patient before continuing procedure, therefore promoting safety.
9. Instruct patient to stand on your command and pivot toward chair (Fig. 20–16).	9. Prepares patient for transfer.
10. Rocking patient forward, assist patient to stand and pivot, reminding to reach back for arm of chair with hands after feeling chair on back of legs (Fig. 20–17).	10. Assists patient to stand through use of momentum.
11. Assist patient to sitting position, remove gait belt, provide lap covers as necessary, and leave call light within reach (Fig. 20–18).	11. Provides for patient comfort and safety.

continued on next page

PROCEDURE 20–1 (cont'd)

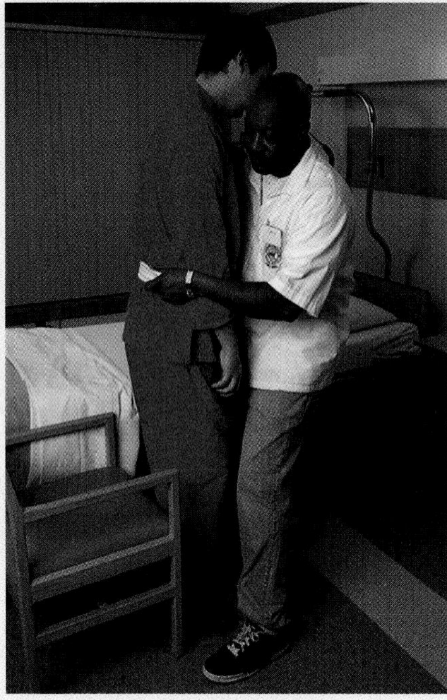

Figure 20–17. Assist patient to pivot in front of chair.

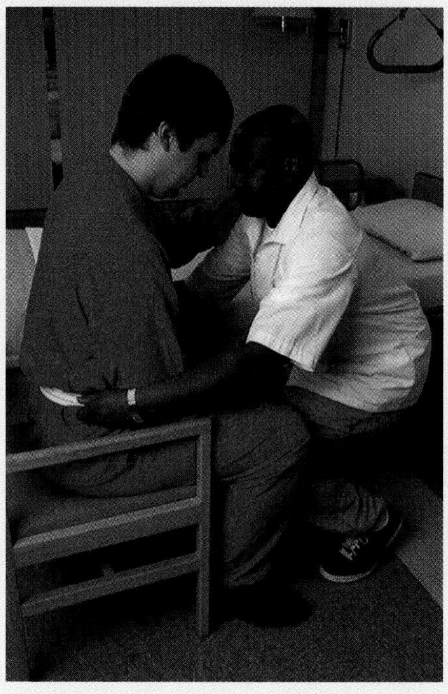

Figure 20–18. Assist patient to sitting position in chair.

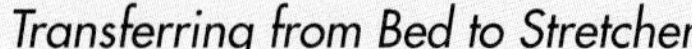

Transferring from Bed to Stretcher

Action	Rationale
1. Assess number of people needed to safely transfer patient.	1. Provides safe transfer for both patient and staff.
2. With patient in supine position, instruct patient to fold arms over chest and extend legs toward foot of bed. Move equipment as necessary and loosen top sheets (if several layers of top linens are present these may be replaced by a bath blanket to facilitate transfer).	2. Positions patient for transfer.
3. Raise bed to height of stretcher making sure both bed and stretcher wheels are locked.	3. Provides for level, safe transfer.
4. Position care providers on side of bed farthest from stretcher and on side of stretcher farthest from the bed. Have care providers grasp draw sheet, under pad, or bottom sheet edges (Fig. 20–19).	4. Reduces chance of friction or shear and helps maintain skin integrity.
5. If using slide/roller board, log-roll patient toward care providers (using sheet or pad) while other care providers at side of stretcher slip slide board under patient. Gently roll patient back to supine position so patient is lying on slide board.	5. Positions slide board for use during transfer.
6. Grasp sheet or pad and inform patient at time of move, coordinating move effort between care providers so all move at same time.	6. Allows smooth transfer of patient by coordinating all efforts.
7. Ask the patient to lift head off the mattress, or if patient is unable, make sure lift sheet is under patient's head for support.	7. Provides support for patient's head and neck during transfer procedure.

continued on next page

PROCEDURE 20-1 (cont'd)

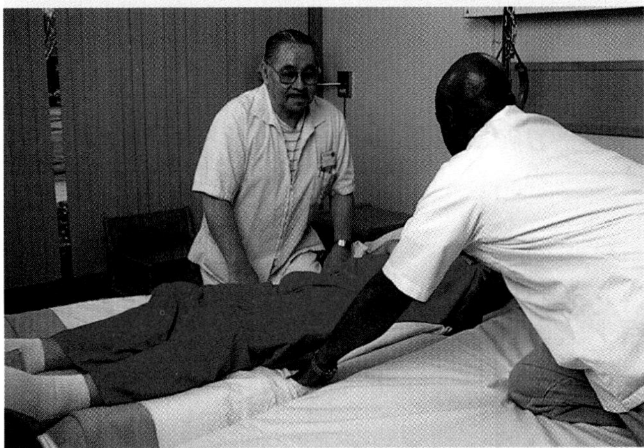

Figure 20–19. Grasp draw sheet to move patient from bed to stretcher.

8. Move patient to stretcher with all care providers lifting and moving simultaneously.

8. Provides for smooth transfer with the least jarring of patient.

9. If using slide/roller board, roll patient toward care providers at side of stretcher using sheet/pad and have care providers on side of bed slip slide/roller board out from under patient.

9. Removes slide/roller board from under patient.

10. Replace top covers (or bath blanket) and place patient in position of comfort. Raise side rails on stretcher.

10. Provides safety, comfort, and warmth, as well as maintaining dignity.

Moving the Patient Up in Bed (One Person—with Patient Assisting)

1. With patient in supine position, loosen top linens and have patient bend legs at knees, placing feet flat on the mattress. Raise bed to appropriate working height.

1. Positions patient to assist with moving procedure.

2. Stand at bedside facing patient turned slightly toward foot of bed and with feet apart and foot closest to head of bed behind other foot.

2. Positions care provider for use of appropriate body mechanics during procedure.

3. Lower side rail on side where care provider is standing.

3. Provides access to patient.

4. Instruct patient, if he or she is able, to grasp side rail with arm on side opposite care provider. If patient is able to use an overhead trapeze, instruct patient to grasp the trapeze and lift head while tucking chin to chest (Fig. 20–20).

4. Enables patient to assist with move.

5. Place care provider's arm which is closet to the head of bed under patient's shoulders, and arm closest to the foot of bed under patient's lower back.

5. Positions care provider for move.

6. When ready, inform patient so care provider's effort can be coordinated with effort from patient.

6. Maximizes potential of move effort.

continued on next page

PROCEDURE 20-1 (cont'd)

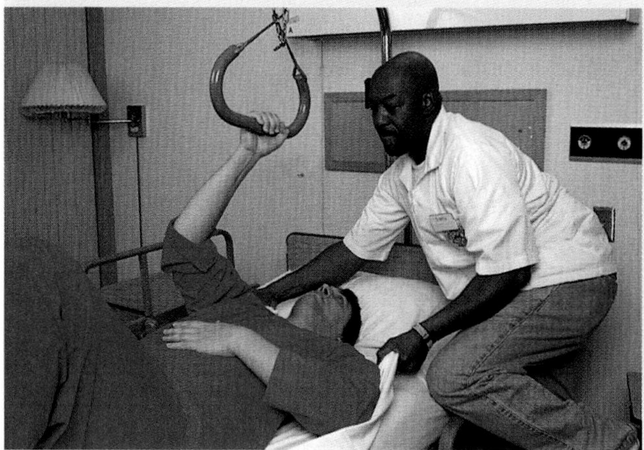

Figure 20–20. If patient able, have him grasp trapeze bar to aid moving up in bed.

Moving the Patient Up in Bed (One Person—with Patient Assisting) (cont'd)

7. Shifting weight from front foot to back foot gently move patient toward head of bed.	7. Allows shifting center of gravity in care provider's stance to assist with movement of patient.
8. Place patient in position of comfort, replace top linens, and leave patient with side rails up and bed in low position.	8. Provides for patient comfort and safety.

Moving the Patient Up in Bed (with Two People—Patient Unable to Assist)

1. With patient in supine position, cross patient's arms over chest, remove pillow, and place at top of bed. Loosen top sheets.	1. Positions patient for move procedure.
2. Place a care provider (more if indicated) on each side of the bed, facing bed with body slightly turned to head of bed and feet apart with foot closest to head of bed in front.	2. Positions care provider for move procedure.
3. If using draw sheet or underpad, grasp pad. If not using linens to assist, place arm closest to head of bed under patient's shoulders and arm closest to foot of bed under patient's thighs.	3. Positions care provider's arms to support patient during move procedure.
4. Move patient to head of bed by shifting weight from back foot to front foot as patient is moved using a coordinated effort.	4. Maximizes potential of move effort.
5. Place patient in position of comfort, replace top linens, and leave patient with side rails up and bed in low position.	5. Provides for patient safety and comfort.

continued on next page

PROCEDURE 20-1 (cont'd)

Documentation

Note the procedure performed as well as the time completed, comfort devices or equipment used, and how the patient tolerated the procedure. Note any assessment of patient during the procedure.

Elements of Patient Teaching

Instruct patient/family regarding the purpose of the procedure or comfort measures used. If family members will be transferring or positioning the patient along with providing comfort measures, instruct them in the appropriate procedure, including all safety and body mechanics principles that should be used. Allow them time to perform a return-demonstration so the care provider may assess the patient's competency level.

PROCEDURE 20-2

Performing Range-of-Motion (ROM) Exercises

Objective

Perform exercises to maintain and build muscle strength, maintain joint mobility, stimulate circulation, and prevent disuse syndrome.

Terminology

abduction—movement of a body part away from the body center.
active exercise—exercise done by the patient to maintain joint mobility, prevent contractures, and promote muscle strength.
adduction—movement of a body part toward the body center.
eversion—turning outward.
extension—straightening of joints which increase the angle between the two bones.
flexion—bending of joints that decreases the angle between the two bones.
inversion—turning inward.
passive exercise—exercise done for the patient by care provider to maintain joint mobility and prevent contractures.
pronation—turning downward.
rotation—a body part turning on its axis.
supination—turning upward.

Critical Elements

Range of motion is needed daily for immobilized patients with normal joints. Those patients who cannot move independently are most at risk. In conditions such as the flaccidity and spasticity seen after spinal cord injury the exercises may need to be modified.

ROM may be performed in conjunction with other patient care activities, such as giving a bath, making the bed, or with evening care.

ROM is contraindicated in patients with joints that are dislocated or fractured or for patients with rheumatoid arthritis during periods of inflammation.

Equipment

Bath blanket

Special Considerations

During ROM exercises, the patient should be covered with a bath blanket to maintain patient privacy and warmth. Placement of the patient in the supine position before exercises (if not contraindicated) is preferable. Elevate the bed to a comfortable level so that the patient care provider can maintain proper body mechanics.

Perform exercises on one side of the body and then on the other. If the patient complains of discomfort or if resistance is met, do not extend the movement beyond that point and report the finding to the patient's physician. During ROM exercises, always support the joint being exercised.

Action	*Rationale*
1. Identify patient.	1. Promotes safety.
2. Explain procedure.	2. Promotes cooperation.
3. Position patient in supine position.	3. Provides neutral position for body.

continued on next page

PROCEDURE 20-2 (cont'd)

ROM of Fingers

1. Grasp with nondominant hand just proximal to patient's hand. — 1. Provides support for wrist joint.
2. Hold patient's fingers with dominant hand. — 2. Provides means to hold fingers for movement.
3. Straighten fingers by gently pulling fingers away from palm with dominant hand (Fig. 20–21). — 3. Promotes extension of fingers.

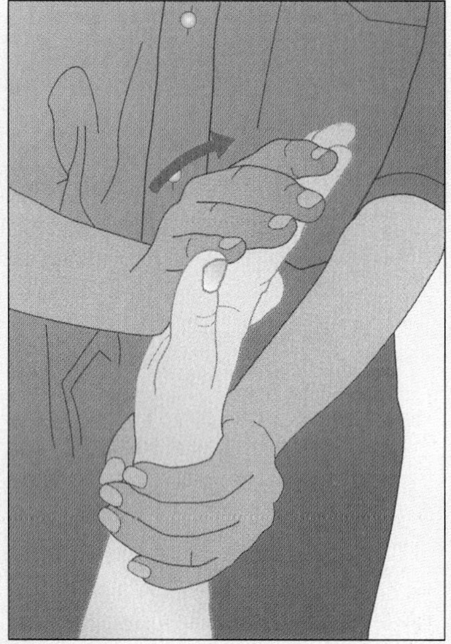

Figure 20–21. Straighten fingers.

4. Curl fingers toward palm. — 4. Promotes flexion of fingers.
5. Holding fingers straight with nondominant hand, fold thumb toward palm with dominant hand. — 5. Promotes adduction of thumb.
6. Holding fingers straight with nondominant hand, gently pull thumb away from palm with dominant hand. — 6. Promotes abduction of thumb.

ROM of Wrist/Forearm/Elbow

1. Position patient's arm out from side of body, with hand pointing up and elbow bent. — 1. Provides arm position for ROM exercises.
2. Hold patient's wrist with nondominant hand and patient's hand with dominant hand. — 2. Positions care provider's hand in appropriate manner for ROM.
3. Flex patient's hand forward (palm of hand moving toward wrist) using gentle pressure from dominant hand (Fig. 20–22). — 3. Provides flexion of wrist.
4. Using gentle pressure from dominant hand in patient's palm, extend patient's hand back toward forearm (Fig. 20–23). — 4. Provides flexion of wrist.

continued on next page

PROCEDURE 20-2 (cont'd)

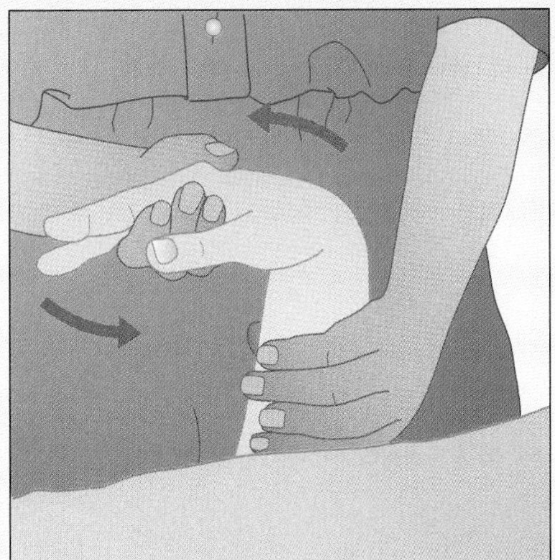

Figure 20–22. Flex wrist forward.

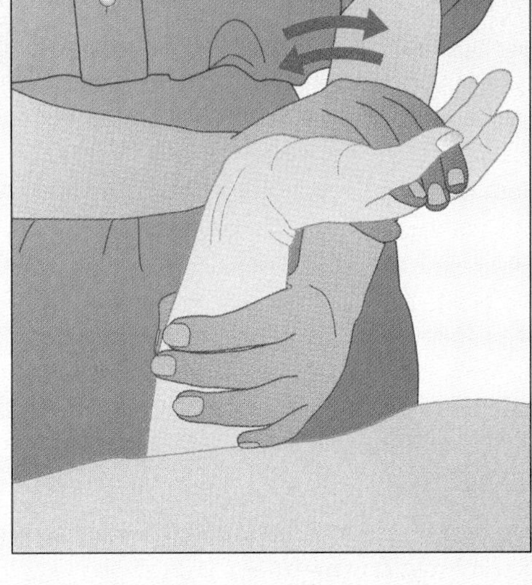

Figure 20–23. Extend wrist backward.

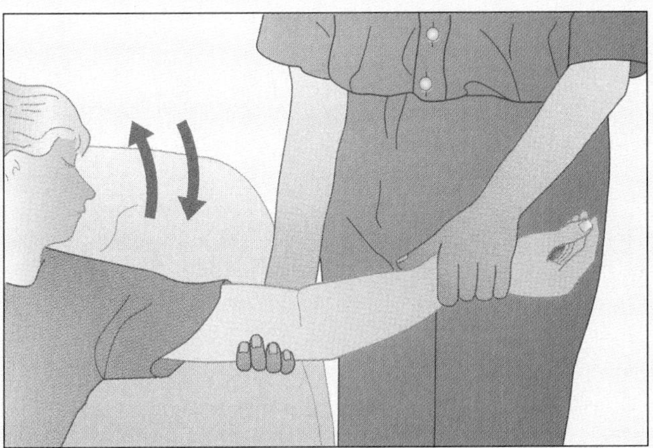

Figure 20–24. Hold arm properly.

ROM of Wrist/Forearm/Elbow (cont'd)

Action	Rationale
5. Place nondominant hand on patient's upper arm just above elbow and dominant hand holding patient's heel of hand/wrist area (Fig. 20–24).	5. Positions care provider's hand in appropriate manner for ROM.
6. Position patient's arm at side with palm down.	6. Provides pronation of forearm.
7. Run patient's hand upward.	7. Provides supination of forearm.
8. Flex patient's arm at elbow, bringing patient's hand as close as possible to shoulder.	8. Provides flexion of elbow.

continued on next page

PROCEDURE 20-2 (cont'd)

ROM of Shoulder

1. Position arm on bed, palm up, next to patient's body, while grasping patient's arm with nondominant hand just above patient's elbow with dominant hand holding patient's hand.

1. Provides position for ROM of shoulder.

2. Maintain patient's palm up while moving arm away from the body. Flex arm at the elbow and have upper arm next to patient's ear and upper forearm across top of patient's head.

2. Provides adduction, extension, and rotation of shoulder.

3. Move patient's arm back again to patient's side.

3. Provides abduction of patient's shoulder.

4. Lift arm from side-lying position until hand is pointing to ceiling.

4. Provides movement from flexion to partial extension of shoulder.

ROM of Toes/Foot

1. Grasp heel of patient's foot in nondominant hand and gently move toes downward toward the plantar surface of the foot (Fig. 20–25).

1. Provides flexion of toes.

2. Holding foot in same manner bend toes gently back toward plantar surface of the foot.

2. Provides extension of toes.

3. Place nondominant hand under knee, hold patient's heel with dominant hand and patient's foot lying along wrist of dominant hand.

3. Positions foot for ROM of ankle.

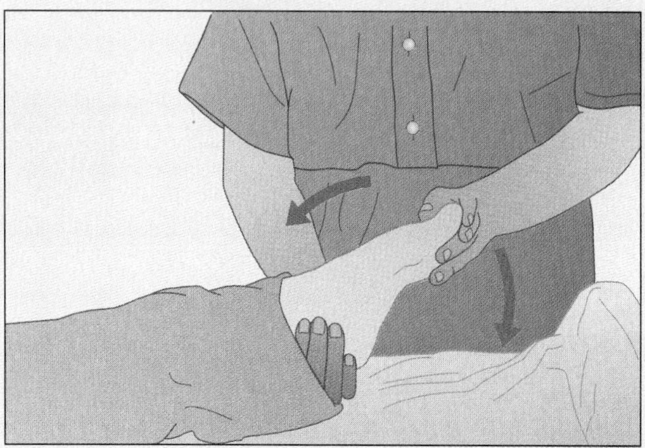

Figure 20–25. Flex toes.

4. Gently move foot toward patient's skin.

4. Provides flexion of ankle.

5. Grasp patient's heel in nondominant hand and place dominant hand on dorsal surface of foot gently moving foot down toward bed surface.

5. Provides extension of ankle joint.

6. With hands in same position turn foot inward so sole of foot faces other foot.

6. Provides inversion of foot.

7. Turn sole of foot so it faces away from other foot.

7. Provides eversion of foot.

continued on next page

PROCEDURE 20-2 (cont'd)

ROM of Knee

1. Flex patient's leg at knee by lifting heel and moving patient's leg toward the chest as far as possible (Fig. 20–26).

1. Provides flexion of knee.

2. Extend patient's leg placing nondominant hand under leg just below knee and dominant hand under patient heel. Lower leg to bed.

2. Provides extension of knee.

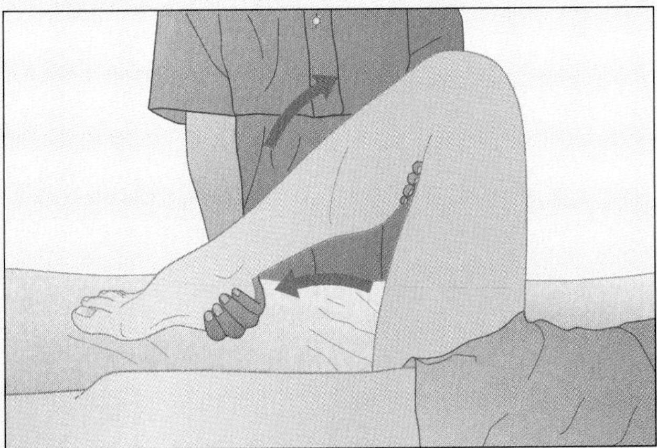

Figure 20–26. Flex knee.

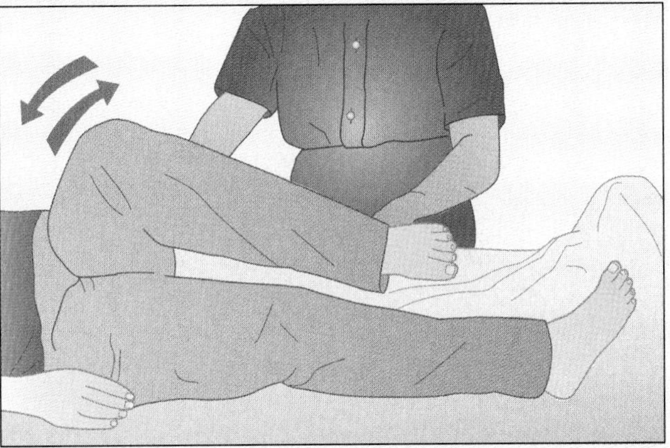

Figure 20–27. Rotate leg outward, then inward.

ROM Hip

1. Extend patient's leg straight on bed.

1. Provides extension of hip.

2. Place one hand on ankle and one on knee and rotate leg outward and then inward (Fig. 20–27).

2. Provides rotation of hip.

3. Move leg outward from body.

3. Provides abduction of hip.

4. Move leg in toward other leg.

4. Provides adduction of hip.

5. Move hands under patient's heel and knee, lifting leg upward until toes point at ceiling.

5. Provides flexion of hip.

6. Return patient to position of comfort and cover patient.

6. Provides patient comfort.

Documentation

Record ROM exercises on patient record. Indicate which joints were exercised, range of movement possible, and patient's response to exercises. Record teaching and response.

Elements of Patient Teaching

Instruct patient/family of purpose of ROM exercises. In many instances a family member can be trained to perform ROM exercises for the patient. Instruct patient and family members to inform nurse of any discomfort occurring during exercises.

PROCEDURE 20-3

Applying Pressure Stockings

Objective

Promote venous return from the lower extremities as an aid to preventing deep vein thrombosis.

Terminology

thrombosis—formation of blood clots in a blood vessel.

Critical Elements

Usually these stockings are used for patients who have limited mobility. Before ordering the stockings it is necessary to measure the patient's leg for proper fit. Measurements should be taken around the widest point of the calf (for the knee-high stocking) and around the thigh (for thigh-length stockings). In addition, the length of the leg should be measured from heel to just below the knee (for knee length) and from heel to the top of the thigh (for thigh high).

Equipment

Elastic stockings
Measuring tape
Powder/cornstarch (optional)

Special Considerations

Stocking should be applied with the patient in a supine position for ease of application. Stockings should be removed for 30 minutes twice a day (or per the policy of your facility) for skin care and assessment. The tops of the stockings should not be rolled down at any time. Having a second pair of stockings available, if possible, will allow one pair to be in use while the other is washed. Applying powder or cornstarch to the legs may facilitate the application process.

Action	*Rationale*
1. Verify order.	1. Ensures correct procedure is done.
2. Identify patient.	2. Promotes patient safety.
3. Explain procedure.	3. Promotes patient compliance.
4. Assist patient to a supine position.	4. Promotes ease of application and decreases dependent position of extremity.
5. Assess circulation in each extremity.	5. Provides baseline for continued assessment of circulation.
6. Turn stocking inside out.	6. Prepares stocking for application.
7. Grasp end of stocking and stretch over toes and foot (Fig. 20–28).	7. Allows stocking to ease over toes and foot without causing discomfort.
8. Grasp side and pull up over heel area.	8. Provides anchor for stocking while applying remaining portion of the stocking.
9. Apply stocking to remainder of leg by gently grasping sides, pulling out and moving stocking up 2 to 3 inches at a time until stocking is up to prescribed area (Fig. 20–29).	9. Protects joint from upward pushing motion while applying stocking.

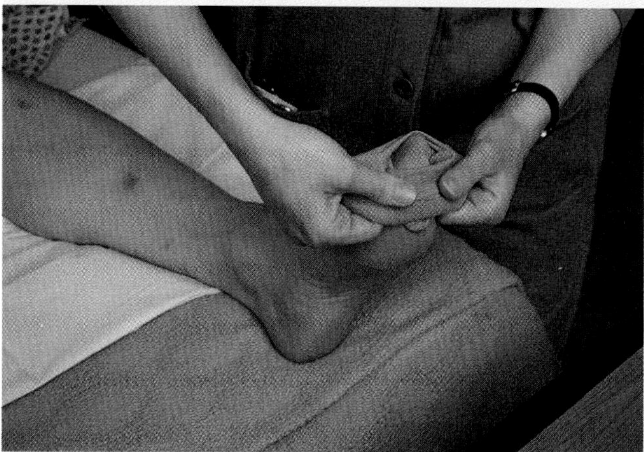

Figure 20–28. Apply stocking over toes and foot.

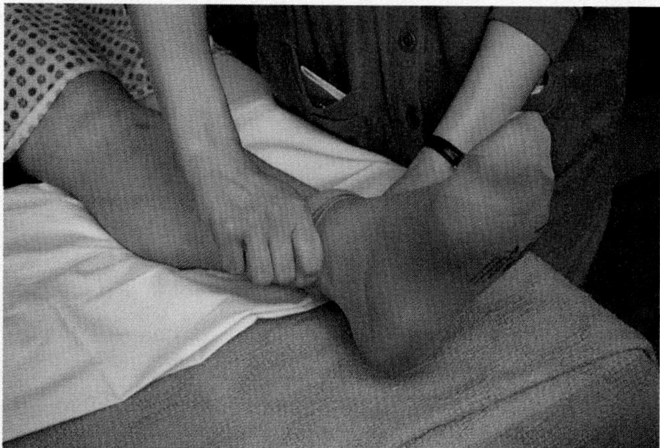

Figure 20–29. Gently pull stocking up the leg.

continued on next page

PROCEDURE 20-3 (cont'd)

10. Smooth out any wrinkles.	10. Prevents pressure sites from wrinkles.
11. Avoid any rolling of stocking at cuff.	11. Prevents stricture effect from rolling stocking.
12. Apply other stocking using same technique.	12. Provides consistency of application.
13. Assist patient to comfortable position.	13. Promotes patient comfort.

Documentation

Record in the patient record the application of the pressure stockings. Note the skin assessment including color, temperature, skin integrity, and pulses. Document the presence of any edema.

Elements of Patient Teaching

Explain to patient and family the purpose of the pressure stockings. Teach patient and/or family members how to apply stockings. Allow them to do a return-demonstration.

PROCEDURE 20-4

Applying Restraints

Objective

Prevent patient from injuring self or others or removing tubes or dressings. Remind patient to maintain limited movement of an extremity.

Terminology

leather restraints—limb restraints made of leather that usually lock in place.

restraint jacket/belt—a form of soft restraint used to restrain a patient by application to the waist/torso.

restraint mittens—glovelike apparatus used to restrain a patient's hands.

soft restraints—limb restraints made of cloth or gauze.

Critical Elements

Less prohibitive means of maintaining patient safety must always be explored before the use of restraints (i.e., use of side rails, bed alarms, frequent patient reminders, attendance in room of a family member). Restraints are often applied only by physician order. Refer to the policy of your facility before the application of any restraint.

Always use the type of restraint that employs the minimum amount of restraint possible to protect the patient and/or others.

Never attach restraints to side rails because the lowering of rails with restraints attached may result in patient injury.

When applying restraints because of patient confusion, a careful assessment should be completed focusing on medication changes, environment changes, or change in physical status.

Always read the manufacturer's recommendations before applying a restraint product.

Equipment

Restraint
Washcloth

Special Considerations

Restraints should be removed at least every 2 hours to assess skin condition and circulation status. Refer to the policy of your facility before the application of any restraint. The presence of restraints does not replace the need for careful, frequent observation of the patient. If restraining only one hand and one foot, then restrain them on opposite sides of the body. It may be necessary to pad leather restraints to protect the patient's skin.

continued on next page

PROCEDURE 20-4 (cont'd)

Action	*Rationale*
1. Verify order.	1. Ensures proper procedure is done.
2. Identify patient.	2. Provides patient safety.
3. Explain procedure.	3. Promotes patient compliance.
Waist/Belt Restraint	
1. Assist patient into waist restraint with opening at back.	1. Prevents patient from using opening as means for removing restraint.
2. Cross straps at back, adjusting size to patient and tie straps to the bed frame.	2. Provides safe anchor for straps avoiding possible injury.
Vest Restraint	
1. Assist patient into vest with cross over closure at the front.	1. Protects patient from possible choking, which may occur if higher cut back panel is placed in front inappropriately.
2. Cross straps in front and secure to bed frame.	2. Provides safe anchor for straps avoiding possible injury.
Soft Limb Restraints	
1. Apply around extremity in manner that restrains patient but still allows adequate circulation (Fig. 20–30 and Fig. 20–31).	1. Protects patient extremity from inadequate circulation and/or skin damage from restraint being applied too tightly.
2. Secure restraint ties to bed frame (Fig. 20–32).	2. Provides safe anchor for ties avoiding possible injury.

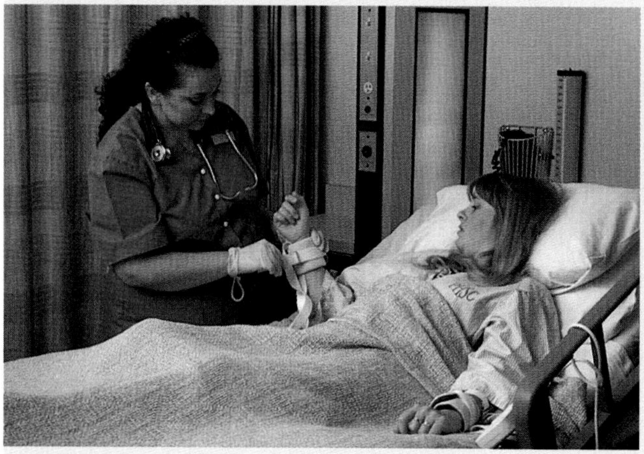

Figure 20–30. Apply limb restraints.

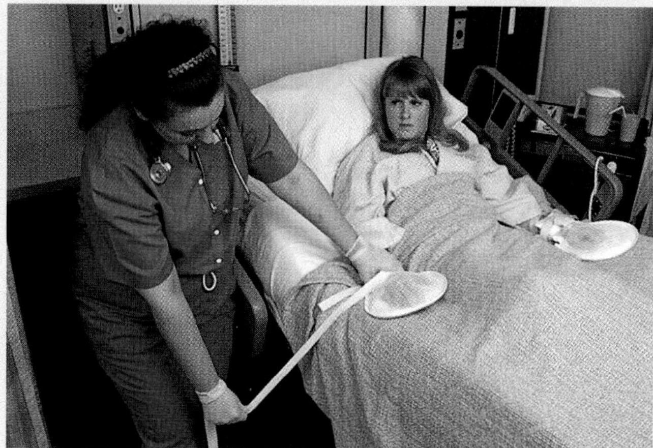

Figure 20–31. Apply hand restraints.

continued on next page

PROCEDURE 20-4 (cont'd)

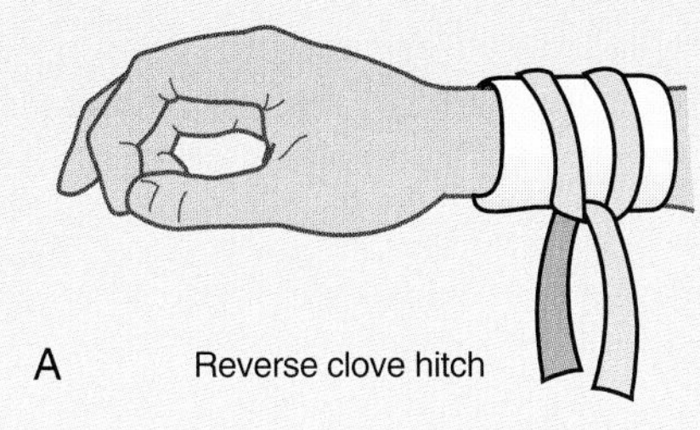

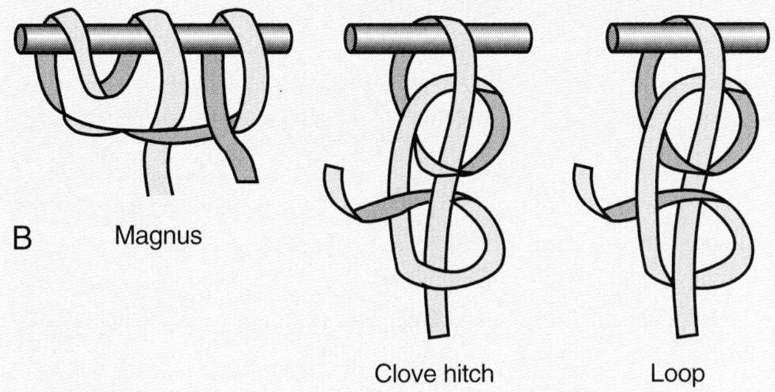

Figure 20–32. Methods for securing restraints to bed frame.

Leather Restraint

Action	Rationale
1. Refer to your facility's policy on application of leather restraints.	1. Provides patient safety by ensuring appropriate guidelines are followed.
2. Apply restraints to limb (if unpadded then may use washcloth to pad), tightening enough to secure limb without impeding circulation.	2. Protects limb while allowing adequate circulation and protecting skin integrity.
3. Secure leather straps to bed frame.	3. Provides safe anchor for straps, avoiding possible injury.

Documentation

Record in the patient record the application of the restraints, including the reason for the restraint, the type of restraint, and the patient's response. Record the circulatory assessments of the patient's extremity at the appropriate time intervals (refer to the policy of your facility). Include skin temperature, color, sensation, movement, and capillary refill.

Elements of Patient Teaching

Explain to the patient and family the need for the restraints. Encourage the family to participate in reorienting the patient, if appropriate.

PROCEDURE 20-5

Assisting with Ambulation

Objective

Promote patient mobility and assist patient in the correct use of assistive devices.

Terminology

gait belt—a belt used during ambulation or transfers that allows the patient care provider to have a secure hold on the patient.

Critical Elements

Mobility benefits all body systems, especially the cardiovascular and musculoskeletal systems. It is also important to the patient's psychological well-being. The longer the patient has been immobile, the weaker the patient may be.

All assistive devices must be the correct size for the patient to be effective and promote patient safety. The assistive device should also be inspected to make sure it is in proper working order (i.e., rubber tips, wheels, hand holds). The physician may order the frequency, duration, weight-bearing status, and assistive device to be used during ambulation, or it may be determined using a physical therapy evaluation.

Equipment

Gait belt
Walker (as indicated)
Crutches (as indicated)
Cane (as indicated)

Special Considerations

A gait belt should be applied before ambulating. This allows the patient care provider to have a secure handhold on the patient during the ambulation exercise. If the patient has a weaker side or a side to which he or she leans, the patient care provider should walk on that side.

Slippers or socks with a nonslip sole are preferable for the patient to wear. The slippers should be easy for the patient to slip into and should surround the foot (avoid a slipper with no back at the heel area).

Before ambulation, assess the patient's strength, orientation, and ability to follow directions. Also determine if the patient has previous experience using the assistive device. It may be necessary to have another person aid with ambulation. If the patient has been supine, allow him or her to sit upright for a few minutes before ambulation.

Action	*Rationale*
1. Verify order.	1. Ensures proper procedure is done.
2. Identify patient.	2. Promotes patient safety.
3. Explain procedure.	3. Promotes patient compliance.
4. Apply gait belt.	4. Provides support and safety for patient.
Ambulation with Assistance	
1. Place hand closest to patient on gait belt at patient's back and hold other hand out in front of you with patient's hand resting on this arm/hand (Fig. 20–33).	1. Positions care provider in manner to promote safe ambulation.
If two persons are assisting:	
1. Position one person on each side of patient.	1. Provides balanced support for patient.
2. Put hand closest to patient under the patient's arm while holding patient's hand with other arm (Fig. 20–34).	2. Provides a means for care provider to grasp patient and patient to hold onto care provider.
Ambulation with Crutches	
1. Adjust crutches so that tips are approximately 6 inches in front and to the side of the patient's toes and the patient's elbows are slightly flexed. Leave a 2-inch space between the axilla and the top crutch.	1. Positions crutches for safe ambulation while keeping pressure from being exerted on axilla.
2. Instruct patient never to lean on top bar of crutches.	2. Promotes safety by avoiding axilla pressure, which may cause nerve damage.
3. Hold hand to gait belt in back of patient and one hand on patient shoulder.	3. Promotes patient safety.

continued on next page

PROCEDURE 20-5 (cont'd)

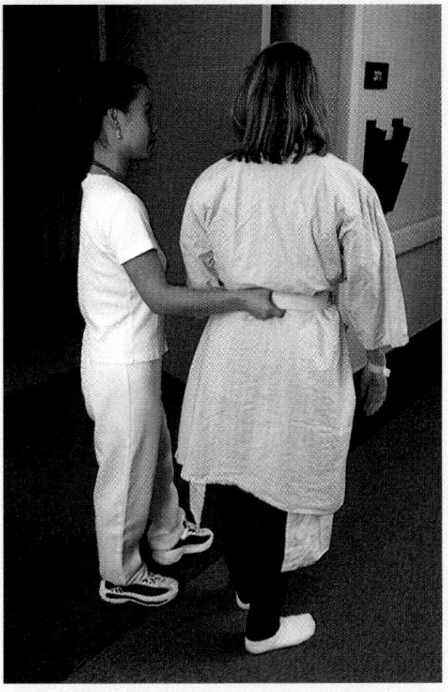

Figure 20–33. Grasp gait belt when assisting a patient with ambulation.

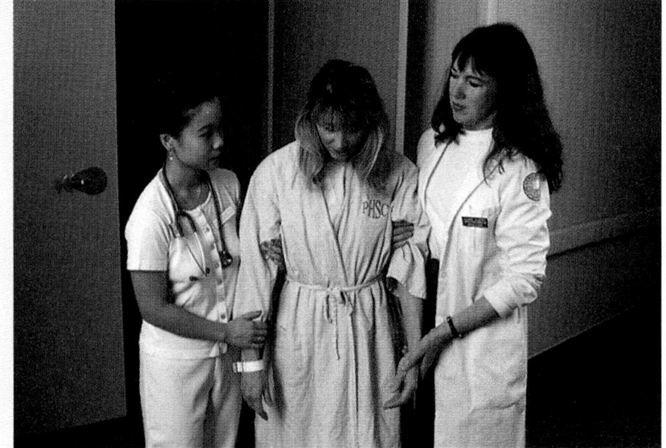

Figure 20–34. Two-person assistance.

Ambulation with Crutches (cont'd)

4. Instruct on gaits as follows: a. Four-point gait—used for partial weight bearing on both extremities. b. Three-point gait—used for no weight bearing on affected leg. c. Two-point gait—used for partial weight bearing on both extremities. d. Swing-through gait—used for paralyzed lower extremities.	4. Provides correct gait for patient condition.

Ambulation with a Walker

1. Adjust walker height so patient can rest hands on walker with arms bent 15 to 20 degrees.	1. Positions walker at optimal height for ambulation.
2. Stand on patient's affected side holding gait belt in back.	2. Provides safe position for assisting with ambulation.
3. Instruct patient to move walker and affected leg forward 6 to 8 inches. Move unaffected leg forward and parallel to affected leg (Fig. 20–35).	3. Promotes safety by keeping center of balance within range of walker.
4. Remind patient never to pull up from sitting to standing by pulling on walker.	4. Promotes patient safety by avoiding a potential fall situation.

continued on next page

PROCEDURE 20-5 (cont'd)

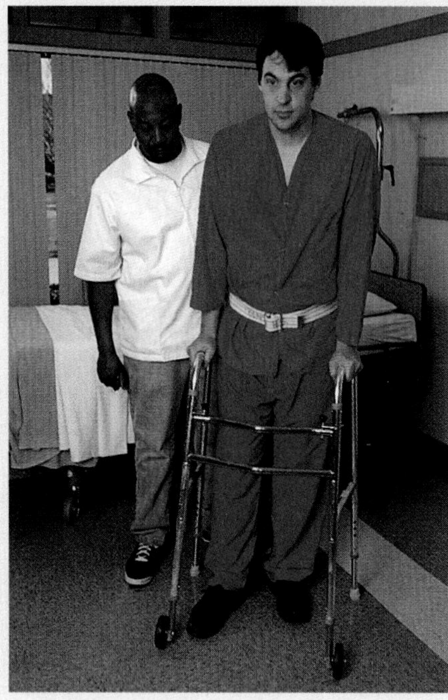

Figure 20–35. Assist patient to maintain balance when using a walker.

Ambulation with a Cane

Action	Rationale
1. Stand on patient's affected side while holding gait belt in back.	1. Promotes patient safety.
2. Instruct patient to hold on unaffected side (with arm slightly flexed) and cane tip 6 inches forward and 6 inches to the side of the foot.	2. Positions cane for optimal balance.
3. Instruct patient as follows: a. Move affected leg forward and parallel to cane. b. Move unaffected leg forward and just beyond cane. c. Move affected leg forward and even with unaffected leg. d. Move cane forward 6 inches to front and side of foot. e. Repeat.	3. Provides ambulation technique that allows assistive device to promote balance.
4. Offer support as needed.	4. Promotes patient safety.
5. Assess patient balance and endurance.	5. Provides data for ongoing therapy.
6. Assist patient back to comfortable position.	6. Promotes patient comfort.
7. Return equipment to appropriate area.	7. Maintains safe environment.

Documentation

Record ambulation exercise in patient record and results of patient/family teaching. Describe how far patient ambulated and patient's response to exercise, including any assistive devices used.

Elements of Patient Teaching

Instruct patient and family members regarding the purpose of the gait belt and any assistive devices being used. Allow patient and family members to give return-demonstration on ambulation techniques, including the use of any assistive devices.

CHAPTER HIGHLIGHTS

- Understanding and applying principles of body mechanics is essential to providing safe nursing care.
- Application of biomechanical research findings is important to continue improving nursing practice.
- Injury to the patient and the nurse is prevented when proper body mechanics are used.
- Nursing care principles are applied in the same way regardless of where the patient is located (home, clinic, long-term or acute-care facilities).
- Ethical principles are incorporated in administering procedures relating to biomechanics.
- Clinical decisions concerning the patients are based on age, gender, and financial considerations.
- Technological advances are being made in the field of biomechanics.
- Biomechanical principles are included in all procedures involving patient mobility, range of motion exercises, applying pressure stockings, and using restraints.

REFERENCES

American Association of Retired Persons (1993). *Developing Fall Prevention Programs for Older Adults: A Guide for Program Planners and Volunteer Leaders.* Washington, DC: AARP Health Advocacy Services.

Arfken, C.L., Lach, H.L., Birge, S.J., Miller, J.P. (1994). The prevalence and correlates of fear of falling in elderly persons living in the community. *American Journal of Public Health, 84,* 565–570.

Baker, S.P., O'Neill, B., Karpf, R.S. (1984). *The Injury Fact Book.* Lexington, MA: Lexington Books.

Button, S. (1996). *Evaluating the Risk Factors Associated With Falls in Older Adults.* Unpublished manuscript.

Campbell, A.J., Reinken, J., Allen, B.C., Martinez, G.S. (1981). Falls in old age: a study of frequency and related clinical factors. *Age Aging, 10,* 264–270.

Chipman, C. (1981). What does it mean when a patient falls? Part 1. Pinpointing the cause. *Geriatrics, 36,* 83–85.

Coleman, S., Hansen, S. (1994) Reducing work-related back injuries. *Nursing-Management, 25*(11), 58.

Corwin, D., Miller, C.A. (1990). Get your patient off on the right foot. *RN,* Nov; *53*(11), 44–46.

Di Fabio, R.P., Badke, M.B. (1990). Relationship of sensory organization to balance function in patients with hemiplegia. *Physical Therapy, 70*(9), 542–548.

Ellis, M., Seedholm, B.B., Amis, A.A., Wright, D. (1979). Forces in the knee jont whilst rising from normal and motorized chairs. *Mechanical Engineering, 8*(1), 33–40.

Evans, L.K., Strumpf, N.E. (1992). Reducing restraints: One nursing home's story. In S.G. Funk, E.M. Tornquist, M.T. Champagne, and R.A. Wiese (eds.): *Key Aspects of Elder Care.* New York: Springer, pp. 118–128.

Finley, F.R., Cody, K.A., Finizie, R.V. (1969). Locomotion patterns in elderly women. *Archives of Physical Medicine and Rehabilitation, 50*(3), 140–146.

Garrett, B., Singiser, D., Bank, S. (1992). Back injuries among nursing personnel: The relationship of personal characteristics, risk factors, and nursing practices. *American Association of Occupational Health Nurses, 40*(11), 510–516.

Gehlsen, G.M., Whaley, M.H. (1990a). Falls in the elderly: Part I. Gait. *Archives of Physical Medicine and Rehabilitation, 71,* (10), 739–741.

Gehlsen, G.M., Whaley, M.H. (1990b). Falls in the elderly: Part II. Balance, Strength, and Flexibility. *Archives of Physical Medicine and Rehabilitation, 71,* (10), 739–741.

Groer, M.W., Shekleton, M.E. (1989a). Musculoskeletal anthrophysiology. In: *Basic Pathophysiology: A Holistic Approach,* 3rd ed. St. Louis: C.V. Mosby, pp. 430–435, 457–462, 465–479, 483–488.

Groer, M.W., Shekleton, M.E. (1989b). Impaired physical mobility. In: *Basic Pathophysiology: A Holistic Approach,* 3rd ed. St. Louis: C.V. Mosby, pp. 490–502, 512–518.

Gray-Vickrey, M. (1984). Education to prevent falls. *Geriatric Nursing.* 5(3), 179–183.

Hasselkus, B.R., Shambes, G.M. (1975). Aging and postural sway in women. *Journal of Gerontology, 30*(6), 661–667.

Hogue, C.C., Studenski, S. Duncan, P. (1990). Assessing Mobility: The first step in preventing falls. In S. Funk, E.M. Tournquist, M.T. Champagne, L. Copp, and R. Wise, (eds.): *Key Aspects of Recovery: Improving Nutrition, Rest, and Mobility.* New York: Springer, pp. 275–280.

Husted, G.L., Husted, J.H. (1995). *Ethical Decision Making in Nursing.* 2nd ed. St. Louis: C.V. Mosby, p. 59.

Iverson, B.D., Gossman, M.R., Shaddeau, S.A., Turner, M.E., Jr. (1990). Balance performance, force production, and activity levels in noninstitutionalized men 60 to 90 years of age. *Physical Therapy, 70*(6), 348–355.

Jeng, S-F., Schenkman, M., Riley, P.O., Lin, S-J. (1990). Reliability of a clinical kinematic assessment of the sit-to-stand movement. *Physical Therapy, 70*(8), 511–520.

Johnson, V. (1989). The effect of age on the sit to stand pattern in women. Master's thesis, Microfiche. University of Oregon.

Kane, R.L., J.G. Ouslander, I.B. Abrass. (1984). *Essentials of Clinical Geriatrics.* New York: McGraw-Hill.

Kreighbaum, E., Barthels, K.M. (1996). *Biomechanics: A Qualitative Approach for Studying Human Movement,* 4th ed. Boston: Allyn and Bacon.

LaVeau, B. (1992). *Williams & Lissner's Biomechanics of Human Motion,* 3rd ed. Philadelphia: W.B. Saunders.

Lichtenstein, M.J., Shields, S.L. Shiavi, R.G., Burger, C. (1989). Exercise and balance in aged women: A pilot controlled clinical trial. *Archives of Physical Medicine and* Rehabilitation, *70,* (2), 138–143.

Livingston, L.A., Stevenson, J.M., Olney, S.J. (1991). Stair climbing kinematics on stairs of differing dimensions. *Archives of Physical Medicine and Rehabilitation, 72,* (6), 398–402.

McGill, S.M., Norman, R.W., Sharratt, M.T. (1990). The effect of an abdominal belt on trunk muscle activity and intra-abdominal pressure during squat lifts. *Ergonomics, 33*(2), 147–159.

Morton, D. (1989). Five years of fewer falls. *American Journal of Nursing, 89*(2), 204–205.

Mosenthal, A.C., Livingston, D.H., Elcavage J., et al. (1995). Falls: Epidemiology and strategies for prevention. *Journal of Trauma, 38, 753–756.*

Murray, M.P., Kory, R.C., Clarkson, B.H. (1960). Walking patterns in healthy old men. *Journal of Gerontology, 24,* 169–178.

Public Law 100–203 (1987). Omnibus Budget Reconciliation Act. Subtitle C. Nursing Home Reform. Washington, DC: U.S. Government Printing Office.

Ray, W.A., Griffin, M.R., Downey W. (1989). Benzodiazepines of long and short elimination half-life and the risk of hip fracture. *JAMA, 262,* 3303–3307.

Reuben, D.B., Laliberte, L., Hiris, J., Mor, V. (1990). A hierarchical exercise scale to measure function at the advanced activities of daily living (AADL) level. *Journal of the American Geriatrics Society, 38*(8), 855–861.

Roach, K.E., Miles, T.P. (1991). Normal hip and knee active range of motion: The relationship to age. *Physical Therapy, 71*(9), *656–665.*

Rubin, M. (1988). The physiology of bed rest. *American Journal of Nursing, 88*(1), 50–56.

Saleh, M., Murdoch, G. (1985). In defense of gait analysis. *Journal of Bone and Joint Surgery, 67*B(2), 237–241.

Schenkman, M., Berger, R.A., Riley, P.O., et al. (1990). Whole-body movements during rising to standing from sitting. *Physical Therapy, 70*(10), 638–651.

Schultz, A. B. (1992). Mobility impairment in the elderly: challenges for biomechanics research, *Journal of Biomechanics,* 25(5):519–528.

Sheldon, J.H. (1960). On the natural history of falls in old age. *British Medical Journal,* Vol. 5214, 1685–1690.

Statistical Abstract of the United States (1995). Washington, DC: U.S. Department of Commerce, Bureau of the Census.

Tinetti, M.E., Baker, D.I., McAvay, G., et al. (1994). A multifactorial intervention to reduce the risk of falling among elderly people living in the community. *New England Journal of Medicine, 331,* 821–827.

Troup, J.D.G. (1965). Relation of lumbar spine disorders to heavy manual work and lifting, *Lancet,* Vol. *7399,* April 17 857–861.

U.S. Department of Health and Human Services, Public Health Service (1990). *Healthy People 2000—The National Health Promotion and Disease Prevention Objectives.* Washington, DC: U.S. Government Printing Office.

Watkins, M.A., Riddle, D.L., Lamb, R.L., Personius, W.J. (1991). Reliability of goniometric measurements and visual estimates of knee range of motion obtained in a clinical setting. *Physical Therapy, 71(2),* 90–97.

Whittle, M. (1991). *Gait Analysis.* Oxford: Butterworth-Heinemann.

Winter, D.A., Patla, A.E., Frank, J.S., Walt, S.E. (1990). Biomechanical walking pattern changes in the fit and healthy elderly. *Physical Therapy, 70*(6), 340–347.

Woollacott, M.H., Shumway-Cook A. (1989). *Development of Posture and Gait Across the Life Span.* Columbia: University of South Carolina Press.

UNIT IV

The Content of Basic Nursing Care

The 16 chapters in this unit reflect Virginia Henderson's view of the basic components of nursing practice present in all situations and settings in which direct nursing care is given. Each chapter begins with a case to help the student visualize the particular component of nursing practice and also begin to develop a sound clinical decision-making framework. Next, the knowledge base associated with each component of nursing practice is presented, with emphasis on science and research, relevant for nursing practice. With recognition that more health care is being delivered in community and home settings, each chapter discusses variations in nursing practice related to the health care setting. Patient-related factors that influence nursing practice are also described. Referring back to the introductory case presentation, the role of these factors in the clinical decision-making process is considered. Each chapter ends with specific guidelines for nursing actions. Relevant nursing procedures are detailed in this final section.

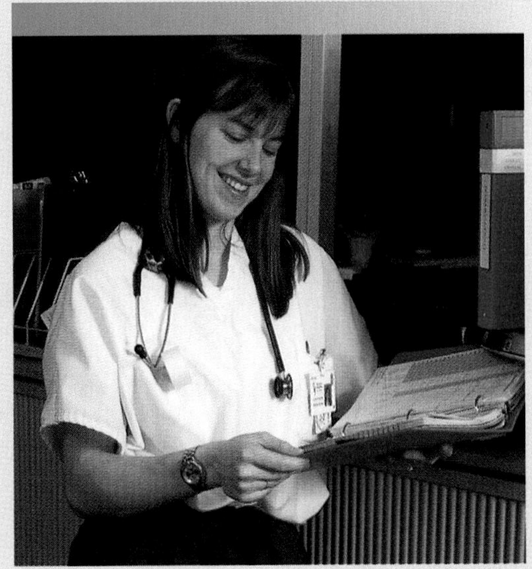

Respiration 21

May Timmons and Fay Bower

Mr. Taylor, a 70-year-old man with a history of chronic lung disease, was hospitalized yesterday with right lower lobe pneumonia. He has a hacking cough and a temperature of 103°F, measured electronically. His skin is dry and flushed, and he says he has no energy. His pulse rate is 88, his respirations are 26, and he is bracing his left side with his arm when he takes a breath. He is receiving antibiotics intravenously until his temperature reaches normal limits.

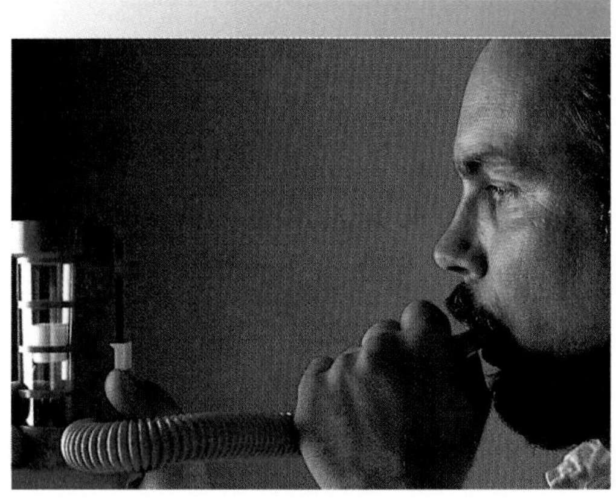

Mr. Taylor is retired and has lived alone since his wife's death 10 years ago. He has no children and spends most of his time fishing and playing poker with his buddies. When Mr. Taylor first began feeling feverish and lethargic, he stayed home and treated himself, believing he had the "flu." Three days later, when his buddy Jake stopped by to see why Mr. Taylor had not been to the club to play poker, he found his friend curled up in bed delirious. Jake dialed 911 and had Mr. Taylor taken to the hospital. In 2 days, Mr. Taylor will be dismissed, and it is unclear where he will live because he is unable to care for himself.

OBJECTIVES

After studying this chapter, students will be able to:

- **use knowledge about pathophysiology of various respiratory conditions to design nursing diagnoses, which will provide direction for nursing interventions**
- **use relevant research findings to determine appropriate nursing interventions for patients with respiratory problems**
- **apply knowledge of demographics and lifestyle to a plan of care for a patient**
- **determine which modalities and technologies are appropriate for treating specific respiratory problems**
- **include ethical and financial considerations when planning care for patients with respiratory conditions**

SCOPE OF NURSING PRACTICE

Nursing care for a patient with a respiratory problem is defined by the nurse's level of preparation and the level of decision making required by the patient's condition and where the nurse encounters the patient. For instance, most hospital-based nurses caring for people with acute respiratory conditions practice using clinical pathways or other kinds of protocols. Their scope of independent decision making is limited to the implementation of the pathway, whereas home care nurses doing follow-up care for patients with chronic respiratory conditions usually function more autonomously. Advanced practice nurses (those with master's degrees) function independently or in collaborative practice with physicians as nurse practitioners, providing primary care that includes the diagnosis and treatment of all kinds of respiratory conditions. However, whereas location and education often define the scope of practice, it varies from state to state, so nurses should check with the board of nursing in their state to determine the current scope of practice requirements.

Nurses who function as community health nurses and as primary care providers are often faced with an immediate need to make decisions because of the problems they encounter. For instance, the nurse may make a visit to a patient with bronchitis as a follow-up to a hospitalization and find that the patient is not doing well because he or she, or the family, do not fully understand the prescribed treatment regimen. The nurse will then have to devise an educational plan to help the patient and family manage the problem. There are no hospital protocols or physician's orders to follow. The nurse often has to plan, improvise, and devise on the spot. This need for independent action is also true for school nurses who encounter unexpected respiratory problems in children. The school nurse must provide immediate attention and decide where to refer the child. Occupational health nurses have a similar type of practice with much autonomy and much responsibility.

Should the nurse encounter a respiratory problem in an elderly resident in a nursing home, the usual action is to call the attending physician. The situation of that same elderly person encountered in a rural nurse practitioner's practice may result in the nurse diagnosing and prescribing the therapy for the patient.

KNOWLEDGE BASE

Anatomy and Physiology

The basic structures of the respiratory system are divided into two parts: the upper respiratory tract and the lower respiratory tract (Fig. 21–1). The upper respiratory tract, consisting of the nose with its nasal cavities and the paranasal sinuses, pharynx, and larynx, conducts air to and from the lungs. The lower respiratory tract is made up of the trachea, bronchial tree, lungs, and pleura. The lower respiratory tract conducts air to and from the upper airway and the numerous alveoli in the lungs where oxygen and carbon dioxide are exchanged.

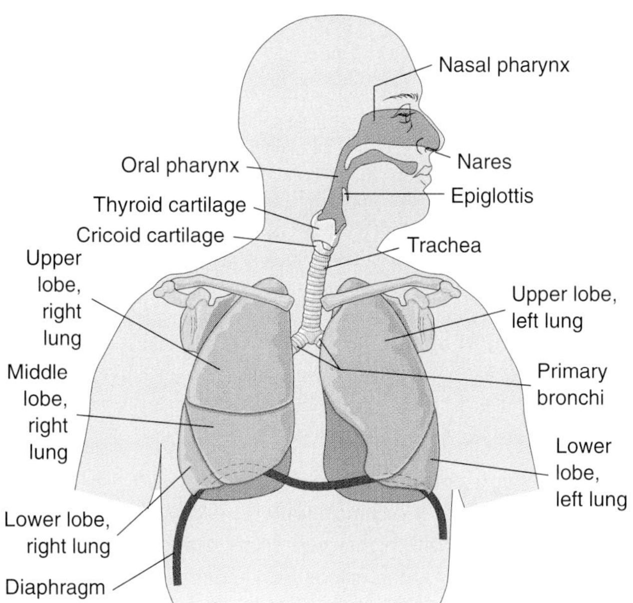

Figure 21–1. Basic anatomy of the respiratory tract.

UPPER RESPIRATORY TRACT STRUCTURES

NOSE AND PARANASAL SINUSES

The nose is the only visible external part of the respiratory system and serves the important functions of:

- Providing an airway for respiration
- Moistening and warming entering air
- Filtering inspired air and cleansing it of foreign matter
- Providing the center for olfactory receptors and providing a chamber for resonating speech

Surrounding the nasal cavity is a ring of paranasal sinuses that are located in the frontal, sphenoid, ethmoid, and maxillary bones. The sinuses lighten the skull and act as resonance chambers for speech. They also produce mucus that drains into the nasal cavities that help trap debris. Because the nasal mucosa connects to the rest of the respiratory tract, infections in the nasal cavity often spread throughout those regions as well.

PHARYNX

The pharynx, commonly called the throat, is a funnel-shaped tube that serves as a passageway for food and air. It measures about 5 inches long and extends from the base of the skull to the sixth cervical vertebra. The pharynx is divided into three parts: the nasopharynx, oropharynx, and laryngopharynx. The nasopharynx serves only as an air passageway, whereas the oropharynx services both the respiratory and digestive systems. The laryngopharynx, like the oropharynx, serves as a passageway for food and air and extends from the hyoid bone to the larynx where the respiratory and digestive pathways diverge.

LARYNX

The larynx, or voice box, is located between the laryngopharynx and the trachea and connects to both of them. The larynx serves three functions: it provides a permanent patent (unobstructed) airway, it acts as a switching mechanism to route air and food into the proper channels, and it is involved in voice production. When food is propelled through the pharynx, the inlet to the larynx is closed. When only air is needed, the inlet opens wide to let air pass through into the lower portions of the respiratory tract.

LOWER RESPIRATORY TRACT STRUCTURES

TRACHEA

The trachea, or windpipe, begins in the neck and connects to the inferior larynx. It is 4 to 5 inches long and 1 inch in diameter and can stretch and descend during inspiration and recoil during expiration. The lining of the trachea is a ciliated cellular layer containing many seromucous glands that produce a thick, mucus-containing secretion. The cilia continuously propel the mucus, loaded with dust particles and other materials, to the throat, where they are swallowed. Figure 21–2 shows structures of the lower respiratory tract.

BRONCHIAL TREE

The bronchial tree extends from the trachea and has a right and left branch. The right main stem bronchus connects to the right lung, and the left main stem bronchus connects to the left lung. The left main stem is angled more sharply than the right one; thus, aspiration into the right lung is more common. However, because the right branch is straighter, suction of the right lung is easier. The two bronchi divide into lobular branches and further into smaller bronchi, leading to the comparison of the bronchial structure to a tree.

The arrangement of bronchi in both the right and left lungs is similar, except the left bronchus divides into two lobular branches and the right bronchus divides into three lobular branches. Thus, there are three lobes in the right lung and only two in the left lung. The bronchi continue to subdivide 20 or more times into subsegmented bronchi, terminal bronchi, bronchioles, and terminal bronchioles. The terminal bronchioles are then further subdivided into the respiratory bronchioles, alveolar ducts, and alveolar sacs; together these structures make up the *terminal respiratory unit.* The respiratory bronchioles in this unit act as a conduit for the air that enters the alveolar ducts and alveolar sacs. Because the ducts and sacs are lined with alveoli, they are unable to exchange oxygen and carbon monoxide.

Two major types of epithelial cells comprise the *alveoli.* Type I cells provide structure, and type II cells secrete surfactant, a lipoprotein that coats the inner surface of the alveoli and facilitates expansion during inspiration. By lowering surface tension during expiration, surfactant keeps the alveoli from contracting or collapsing. A deficiency of surfactant is often the cause of alveolar collapse in respiratory disorders (e.g., adult and infant respiratory distress syndrome) and is also linked to problems associated with prolonged inhalation of 100 percent oxygen.

The third type of alveolar cell is the macrophage. Its chief role is to remove particles from the terminal respiratory units that settle on the alveolar surfaces. Dysfunction of this macrophage transport system can contribute to pulmonary infections.

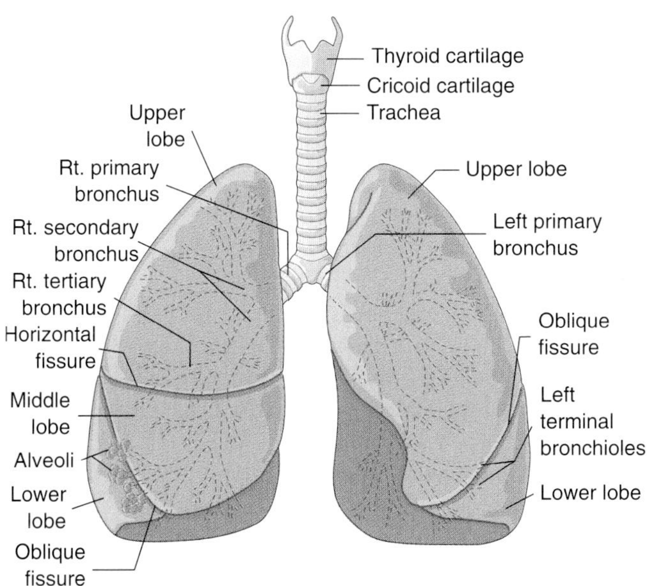

Figure 21–2. Structures of the lower respiratory tract.

LUNGS

The chief organs of respiration, the lungs are a pair of soft, spongy, cone-shaped organs located in the thoracic cavity. The two lungs are separated by the heart and the mediastinum and are supported at the bottom by the diaphragm. Each lung occupies most of the thoracic space on either side of the thoracic cage and is suspended by the bronchus and the large blood vessels. The rounded top portions of the lungs are called the apices; the concave portions of the lungs that rest on the surface of the diaphragm are known as the bases of the lungs. The spaces that divide the lobes of the lungs are called fissures. Two major fissures in the left lung separate the upper lobe from the lower one, and three major fissures separate the upper, middle and lower lobes of the right lung.

The lungs receive blood from two different types of circulation: pulmonary and bronchial. Pulmonary circulation provides the lungs with blood for gas exchange. The pulmonary artery receives venous blood from the right side of the heart and transports it into the right and left pulmonary arteries. The poorly oxygenated blood is shuttled through the smaller arteries and arterioles until it reaches the pulmonary capillaries, where gas exchange occurs. This oxygen-rich blood then leaves the lungs and drains into the left side of the heart, where it is pumped through the systemic circulation for use by the body tissues. Bronchial circulation, by contrast, provides nutrients to the conducting airways, large pulmonary vessels, and the pleura that surround the lungs. Blood from bronchial circulation that enters the pulmonary veins is oxygen depleted.

Each lung has two layers of serous membranes: the visceral and the parietal *pleura*. The pleurae give the lungs a very smooth, polished appearance. Between surfaces of these pleurae is a small amount of serous fluid that permits the pleurae to slide against each other with minimal friction during inspiration. The space between the visceral and parietal pleura is called the pleural cavity. (It is such a minimal space that the only time it is evident is when the lung collapses or fluid collects between the layers.)

The skeletal framework that encases the lungs is called the *bony thorax*. It is composed of 12 pairs of ribs and their cartilages, 12 thoracic vertebrae and intervertebral discs, and the sternum. It also includes the scapula and the clavicles, which serve as important attachments for the respiratory muscles and as landmarks for the assessment of the lungs. The movement of air in and out of the lungs is dependent on a system of open airways and the contraction and relaxation of the muscles of the thoracic cage—the diaphragm and intercostal and accessory muscles.

The main purpose of the accessory muscles is to contribute to inspiratory movements of the chest. Their action is most evident when an individual is involved in extremely strenuous physical activity or experiencing marked respiratory distress.

FUNCTION OF THE RESPIRATORY SYSTEM

Although we can go without food for several days and without water for about a day, we cannot go without oxygen for more than a few minutes. The body comprises trillions of cells that require a continuous supply of oxygen to carry out their vital functions. Furthermore, as each cell uses oxygen, it gives off carbon dioxide, a waste product that the body must discard. The term *oxygenation* refers to those processes by which oxygen is delivered to the cell and carbon dioxide is removed from the cell. Effective oxygenation requires a balance between the supply of and demand for oxygen at the cellular level. The delivery of an adequate supply of oxygen to the cells depends on the processes of ventilation, gas exchange, and perfusion.

VENTILATION

Ventilation refers to the mechanics of inspiration and expiration. Factors that govern air flow in and out of the lungs include movement of the respiratory muscles, intrapulmonary pressure changes, control by neural and chemical factors, lung volume and the compliance of the lung tissue, and airway patency and resistance.

Muscles of Respiration. The dome-shaped *diaphragm*, which performs 80 percent of the work of breathing, lies below the lungs and divides the chest cavity and abdominal cavity. During inspiration, the diaphragm contracts and flattens out while the ribs move upward and outward so the lungs can expand and fill with air. On expiration, the diaphragm relaxes, causing it to rise while the ribs descend and the lungs recoil to their normal position. At the same time, contraction of the external intercostal muscles and the anterior portion of the internal intercostal muscles causes the ribs and the thoracic cage to lift as the lungs are filled with air. In contrast, expiration during quiet breathing occurs passively as a result of the recoil of the lung. The diaphragm relaxes, which decreases the size of the thoracic cage and allows passive exhalation. (Because this is a passive process, it does not require active muscular activity.)

Pressures. Air moves in and out of the lungs by a process that involves pressures. Before inspiration or expiration, the intrapulmonary pressure (the pressure of the air in the lungs) is equal to atmospheric pressure. However, the pressure in the pleural space, called intrapleural pressure, is always less than the intrapulmonary or atmospheric pressure. It is this negative aspect of the intrapleural pressure that overcomes the elastic recoil of the lungs and prevents the lungs from collapsing. During inspiration both pressures decrease, but a greater decrease occurs in the intrapleural pressure than in the intrapulmonary pressure.

Neural and Chemical Control. Control of ventilation is also achieved by a complex network of receptors that send impulses to the brain, which in turn activates the muscles of breathing. Receptors that respond to a change in the chemical composition of the surrounding fluid are known as chemoreceptors. The two major types of chemoreceptors—central and peripheral—differ in their location, their chemical response, and their effect on the respiratory center in the brain stem.

Central chemoreceptors are located in the medulla and respond to levels of carbon dioxide in the blood. When blood carbon dioxide levels increase, the central chemoreceptors are stimulated, which triggers a compensatory mechanism—hyperventilation—in an attempt to eliminate the excess carbon dioxide from the body.

Peripheral chemoreceptors are located in the carotid bodies at the bifurcation of the common carotid arteries and in the aortic bodies above and below the aortic arch. Several receptors in the lungs, in the airways, and in the chest wall react to certain changes and trigger defensive reflexes. Peripheral chemoreceptors respond to decreased arterial oxygen levels, triggering a compensatory increase in respiratory rate.

Lung Volume and Compliance. The lung's ability to distend is determined by connective tissue (collagen and elastin) and the surface tension in the alveoli. A compliant lung distends easily when pressure is applied, whereas a noncompliant lung requires greater than normal pressure. Various devices are used to measure and graphically display lung volumes and capacity. One such device, the incentive spirometer, can measure the patient's maximum inspiratory volume. This simple device is frequently used by the nurse at the bedside to monitor and encourage an increase in inspiratory capacity to prevent respiratory complications.

Airway Resistance. Airway resistance is determined by the size of the airway through which air flows. Any process that changes the bronchial diameter will, therefore, affect airway resistance and alter the rate of air flow during respiration. Common factors that may alter airway diameter include constriction of bronchial smooth muscle; thickening of bronchial mucosa; obstruction of the airway due to mucus, tumor, or a foreign body; or loss of lung elasticity.

GAS EXCHANGE

Gas exchange refers to the diffusion of oxygen from the alveoli into the blood and subsequently into the body tissues, replacing carbon dioxide. Exchange depends on several factors:

- The integrity, thickness, and surface area of the membrane across which the exchange occurs
- The relative pressure gradients and solubility of gases on each side of the membrane
- The affinity between oxygen and hemoglobin
- The relative distribution of ventilation and perfusion at the alveolar level

Membrane Integrity. The membrane that surrounds each alveolus contains many capillaries, is thin, and has a large surface area, thus making it an ideal medium for gas exchange. As long as the membrane remains intact without inflammation due to a disease process, gas exchange occurs properly. But various disease processes can alter the membrane, which in turn severely reduces lung compliance and impairs alveolar ventilation. For instance, certain disorders alter the membrane, making it more permeable. This allows fluids, proteins, and blood cells to leak from the capillary bed into the pulmonary interstitium and alveoli, causing the lungs to become less compliant and impairing alveolar ventilation. Other disorders can cause damage to the pulmonary bed, increasing the volume of air in the alveoli and leading to air trapping in the alveoli, which can result in dyspnea, even at rest.

Pressure Gradient. The exchange of gases in the alveolar capillary membrane occurs in response to a difference in the partial pressure of the gases on either side of the membrane. This difference is known as the pressure gradient. As a rule, a gas moves from the area of higher pressure across the membrane to the area of lower pressure, until pressures are equal on both sides. The pressure gradient of oxygen and carbon dioxide determines the movement of these gases between the systemic capillary blood and tissues as well as between pulmonary capillary blood and the alveoli. This process of oxygen and carbon dioxide exchange at the alveolar capillary membrane is known as diffusion. The larger the difference between pressure gradients of these gases, the faster the diffusion of gases across the alveolar capillary membrane.

Affinity of Hemoglobin for Oxygen. Another important measure used to determine adequate gas exchange is the affinity of hemoglobin for oxygen. Oxygen is carried in the blood in two forms: dissolved oxygen and oxygen in chemical combination with hemoglobin. Oxygen delivery to the tissues depends on the amount of oxygen transported to the tissues and the ease with which hemoglobin releases oxygen once it reaches the tissues.

PERFUSION

Perfusion refers to the flow of blood that allows the transport of oxygen and carbon dioxide between the alveoli and body tissues. Perfusion depends on the strength of the pump (heart), intact blood vessels, maintenance of pressure and flow within the vessels, and the oxygen-carrying capacity of the blood.

The distribution of ventilation in the lung tissue differs by region and position. When the individual is upright, the volume of inspired air that reaches the alveolar level for gas exchange is greater at the apex than at the base. This same imbalance occurs when the patient lies on his or her abdomen, back, or side. However, the alveoli in the apex of the lung are less able to accept oxygen and give off carbon dioxide; conversely, those alveoli at the base of the lung accept oxygen more readily and empty more fully. These differences occur because the blood flow is gravity dependent (i.e., there is more blood flow in the base and in dependent areas when the position is changed) and alveolar pressures are greater in the base and in dependent areas than in the apex.

Relevant Research

A review of the current nursing and related non-nursing research provides the nurse with valid data about the efficacy of certain practices commonly used to care for patients with respiratory problems. The discussion that follows focuses on the research available about mobilizing pulmonary secretions, clearing the airway, oxygenating the system, decreasing the effort of breathing, and self-management strategies for those with chronic pulmonary diseases.

MOBILIZING PULMONARY SECRETIONS

Several studies have investigated methods for clearing mucus from the airways using postural drainage, percussion, and deep-breathing techniques and also under what conditions these techniques should be altered. After postural drainage in patients with chronic obstructive pulmonary disease (COPD), sputum mobilization increases but pulmonary function does not appear to be altered (Mazzocco et al, 1985). A combination of postural drainage and exercise has been shown to be effective in promoting sputum expectoration in hospitalized patients with cystic fibrosis (Cerney, 1989). Another study recommended that patients be moni-

RESEARCH HIGHLIGHT
SIGNIFICANT RESEARCH ABOUT PULMONARY PROBLEMS

Until very recently, most research about respiratory problems has focused on the ways that nurses can treat patients with pulmonary problems in hospitals. Newer studies, however, have focused on ways that individuals can manage their condition at home. Although controlled studies about dyspnea treatment are new and thus findings are preliminary, some offer promising directions for practice. A particularly interesting study by Dunlevy and associates (1995) demonstrated a reduction of health problems that affected the social and sexual life of patients with COPD who participated in a 10-week pulmonary comprehensive rehabilitation program (including nutrition, medication, equipment, and panic training) and three sessions of a Chairobics video exercise program each week for nine weeks. Another study by Honeyman and colleagues (1996) demonstrated the value of a wheeled walking aid for patients with chronic irreversible air flow limitations. Significant decreases in disability, breathlessness, and hypoxemia were noted in patients who used the wheeled walker. They were able to walk longer and farther with less hypoxemia and breathlessness as measured by the modified Borg Scale. Steele and Shaver (1992) propose two dimensions of dyspnea, a sensory component and an affective component; both dimensions remained to be studied and measured. Research by McCord and Cronin-Stubbs (1992) suggests that because of the multidimensional nature of dyspnea and the fact that most of the instruments available measure only one dimension, the impact of treatment on dyspnea will not be known until we can further test the validity of multidimensional instruments.

tored for oxygen saturation during postural drainage because the saturation level can be affected by the treatment (Ross et al, 1992).

Percussion enhances the speed, flow, and rate of sputum production without altering pulmonary function or oxygen saturation (Gallon, 1991). Percussion should be used in conjunction with postural drainage in patients with copious secretions that cannot be removed by other means (Zidulka et al, 1989). Coughing exercises are effective in enhancing sputum production and clearance and various parameters of lung function (Thornlow, 1995). The forced expiratory technique has also been found to be superior to coughing (Pavia, 1990).

Using an incentive spirometer to promote maximum inhalation can also help mobilize secretions. According to Thomas and McIntosh (1994), this method is very useful for mobilizing secretions and also is an excellent method for preventing *atelectasis* (a collapsed or airless state of the lung) and pneumonia, particularly for patients undergoing upper abdominal surgery.

CLEARING THE AIRWAY

Suctioning is an important procedure for preventing stasis of pulmonary secretions and maintaining a patent airway. The nurse is expected to suction patients in various situations; however, research has focused primarily on endotracheal suctioning and the potential adverse effects of its use. Much of the early research focused on hypoxemia, hypotension, increased intracranial pressure, cardiac arrhythmias, and cardiac arrest as detrimental outcomes of endotracheal suctioning. As a result of these studies, nurses were encouraged to administer oxygen-enriched breaths of air (hyperoxygenation) as well as a volume greater than the patient's resting respiration (hyperinflation) both before suctioning and 10 to 15 seconds after suctioning. However, a recent study found that endotracheal suctioning, even when augmented by the hyperoxygenation, caused adverse effects for adults with severe head injuries (Rudy et al, 1991).

In a study involving piglets, Gunderson and colleagues (1991) discovered that the reduction of heart rate during endotracheal suctioning was not related to hypoxemia but rather was the result of a vagal response (an irritation of the vagus nerve). These researchers concluded that hyperoxygenation before suctioning only prevented hypoxemia and had no effect on the decreased heart rate.

Other researchers demonstrated that the hyperinflation technique caused an increase in mean arterial pressure of the postoperative heart patient (Stone et al, 1991a). Using the same population of open-heart surgery patients, Stone and associates (1991b) found an alteration in both cardiac rate and rhythm using the hyperinflation procedure. As a result of this study, they recommended that nurses watch the cardiac monitor during the insertion of the catheter during suctioning. Another study found that using a catheter designed to allow oxygen administration simultaneously with suctioning is a valid alternative to the hyperoxygenation/hyperinflation method (Taft et al, 1991).

In yet another study researchers found that nurses were unable to meet the standard for increased volume or oxygen delivery using a manual resuscitation bag during endotracheal suctioning (Glass et al, 1993). This study led to the recommendation that nurses ensure a consistent oxygen liter flow and develop a uniform hand-to-forearm method while compressing the resuscitation bag when hyperinflating before, during, and after endotracheal suctioning.

Other studies have focused on the kinds of catheters used for endotracheal suctioning. Crimlisk and colleagues (1994) reported that nurses generally prefer a closed tracheal suction device over an open system. DePew and associates (1994) supported a change in equipment to a closed system as the result of a cost-benefit analysis.

The criteria identified by nurses and how they make decisions about suctioning were identified in a study by Copnell and Fergusson (1995). Most of the nurses in this study indicated that they rely on a deterioration in the patient's condition to indicate when suctioning is required. Based on these findings, the researchers recommended development of a suctioning policy and staff education.

Nursing care of intubated patients commonly requires the instillation of a small amount of normal saline into the tube before suctioning. The rationale for this action is to loosen secretions or stimulate a cough. Current research indicates the routine instillation of normal saline during a suctioning episode is ineffective in improving immediate suctioning outcomes (Gray et al, 1990; Ackerman, 1993; Ackerman and Guerty, 1990). In addition, the saline bolus has shown increases in the release of viable bacteria into the lower airway, which increases the risk of infection (Ackerman, 1993; Hagler and Traver, 1994). The researchers of this study recommended that the frequency of suctioning be determined on an individual basis and the practice of saline instillation be omitted as a routine part of the suctioning procedure.

OXYGENATING THE SYSTEM

Oxygen therapy is used in the management of conditions of hypoxia (lack of oxygen in the body tissues). Frequently, postoperative patients are given supplemental oxygen to prevent hypoxemia, which may result from decreased lung expansion. One study discovered that patients on continuous oxygen often received only intermittent therapy over 70 percent of the time because of mask removal due to routine tasks, such as mouth care and systematic nursing observations (Baxter et al, 1993). Another found that it is important to instruct patients to breathe through their nose when the nasal cannula is worn (Dunlevy and Tyl, 1992). During oxygen therapy, oxygen concentration received during mouth breathing is significantly lower than oxygen concentration received during nasal cannula breathing. Regardless of the delivery methods, when subjects hyperventilated the oxygen concentration was even lower.

Traditionally, it has been standard practice to humidify oxygen as it is administered. In recent years, this practice has been altered for patients receiving low-flow oxygen (1 to 4 L/min). A study comparing complications from using dry low-flow oxygenation (i.e., dry nose or throat; dry, burning eyes; headache; chest discomfort; infections of the nose, throat, and sinuses) with complications from using humidified oxygen found no evidence that humidification of low-flow oxygen affected the incidence of side effects (Estey, 1990). Furthermore, the study indicated that substantial cost savings could be realized by using dry rather than humidified oxygen.

REDUCING THE EFFORT OF BREATHING

Innovative treatment techniques to reduce the perception of respiratory effort and thus improve lung function have been studied. A breathing retraining program using biofeedback has been found to improve lung function in patients with cystic fibrosis (Delk et al, 1994). A study used the distracting power of music during exercise for patients with COPD. Results indicated that the music decreased patients' perceived symptoms of respiratory discomfort, which in turn allowed them to exercise at a greater intensity (Thornby et al, 1995). Another study found that after 4 weeks of guided imagery, subjects with chronic bronchitis and emphysema reported a significant improvement in their quality of life (Moody et al, 1993).

SELF-MANAGEMENT STRATEGIES

Exercise training in rehabilitation programs for people with chronic respiratory problems frequently includes treadmill use, upper-body weight training, and outdoor walking. Studies related to exercise training verify that patients who comply with such training demonstrate greater improvement in exercise performance (Sassi-Dambron et al, 1994). Patients' baseline measurements of exercise endurance generally improve after a 6-week rehabilitation program (Vale et al, 1993). The ideal exercise program should alternate intervals of work with rest and should continue over a period of 2 months to effectively reduce pulmonary difficulties and improve exercise tolerance (Preusser et al, 1994).

Several research studies have been conducted to determine the effect of pulmonary rehabilitation on the reduction of dyspnea (shortness of breath) for patients with COPD. Two studies found that training programs that increase the strength and endurance of arm and leg muscles reduce dyspnea and improve the quality of life in patients with COPD (Lake et al, 1990; Simpson et al, 1992). To be still more effective, the training programs should be coupled with walking exercises as well as strategies that either support the arms during activity or allow frequent rests during which the arms are lowered.

According to two other studies, participation in a pulmonary rehabilitation program can reduce exertional dyspnea during treadmill testing (Reardon et al, 1994) and participation in a muscle training program lasting over 6 months results in improved respiratory muscle endurance and dyspnea (Kim et al, 1993). However, another study demonstrated that dyspnea management coping strategies did not produce significant improvement in dyspnea (Sassi-Dambron et al, 1994).

Inhaled medication has been the cornerstone of therapy in chronic lung disease for more than a decade. The most important barrier to effective delivery of inhaled medication is the ability of the patient to use the delivery systems correctly. Several studies have demonstrated that a significant proportion of patients cannot properly use one of the oldest aerosol delivery systems available to the public: the aerosol metered-dose inhaler (MDI) (De Blaquiere et al, 1989; Hilton, 1990; Thompson et al, 1994). In older adults, the main obstacles to using MDIs properly are cognitive impairment and impaired hand-grip strength (Allen and Prior, 1986; Armitage and Williams, 1988).

Misuse of MDIs is also prevalent among health care workers (Interiano and Guntupalli, 1993). One study found that respiratory therapists were most knowledgeable (67 percent) about the use of inhaler devices, followed by physicians (48 percent) and registered nurses (39 percent). In addition, more respiratory therapists (77 percent) had received formal instruction on the use of these devices than either registered nurses (30 percent) or physicians (43 percent) (Hanania et al, 1994).

Newer inhaled medication delivery systems and add-on spacer devices have been developed in the hope of creating a more "user friendly" system that can deliver an accurate amount of medication (Kesten et al, 1994). Patients generally are better able to use the new multidose dry powder inhaler device but need periodic follow-up and reinstruction (Kesten et al, 1994). Large-volume spacer devices have advantages over MDIs for older patients in terms of patient preference and ease of inhaler use (Connolly, 1995).

According to another study (Corbett, 1992), subjects taught to use an MDI using a leaflet, video demonstration, and supervised nurse practice session significantly improved their MDI technique as compared with subjects who received only leaflet instruction or leaflet plus video demonstration. This study recommended that nursing staff should not assume that inhaler users know how to use the inhaler correctly, because skills deteriorate over time.

Relevant Theory

Although different conditions and situations affect the respiratory system in different ways, they all have one thing in common: they create a problem with breathing. This difficulty in breathing is commonly termed *dyspnea,* a multidimensional disorder that nurses and physicians see in a variety of settings.

DYSPNEA

Early definitions of dyspnea focused on objective, measurable parameters; but more recent ones focus on the condition as a subjective experience, much like pain. Accordingly, dyspnea can be defined as an uncomfortable and unpleasant feeling of the inability to breathe normally (Comroe, 1974; Gold, 1983; Killian and Jones, 1988). Based on this perspective, a theory of dyspnea has been developed that includes the concepts of antecedents, mediators, reactions, and consequences (McCord and Cronin-Stubbs, 1992) and that is used to direct nursing interventions for a wide range of respiratory disorders.

ANTECEDENTS

Although no single theory explains the causes of dyspnea, it is generally agreed that two categories of antecedent events precede dyspnea: physiologic and psychogenic (Sweer and Zwillich, 1990). Physiologic antecedents vary. The most widely accepted antecedent is the inappropriateness theory. In this theory, dyspnea results from an inappropriate relationship between the change in respiratory muscle length and the resulting muscle tension. However, other mechanisms such as changes in the intrapulmonary and central nervous system chemoreceptors, motor output, muscle tension, gas exchange, thoracic movement, metabolic load, and respiratory drive could also be antecedent events causing dyspnea (Altose, 1986; Wasserman and Casaburi, 1988).

Psychogenic antecedents develop without any physiologic alterations. For example, hyperventilation might be induced by anxiety or anger (Carrieri and Janson-Bjerklie, 1986).

MEDIATORS

Mediators are the personal and environmental factors that alter the person's response to the antecedent and the outcome. Such aspects as culture, lifestyle, environment (including changes in the temperature and pollutants), and psychological states, such as fatigue, anxiety, or fear, can mediate reactions and/or outcomes (Lowery, 1987).

REACTIONS

Reactions are an individual's immediate responses to a perceived change due to an antecedent event. Subjective reactions to a conscious awareness of breathing usually result in labored or uncomfortable breathing. Physiologic reactions are usually noted as an increased respiratory rate, change in the depth of breathing, or the use of accessory muscles (McCord and Cronin-Stubbs, 1992).

CONSEQUENCES

Consequences are the final outcomes that result from an individual's reaction to the antecedent event. Consequences of dyspnea include adaptation, resolution, or no response. Individuals with chronic dyspnea develop ways to control their symptoms, such as decreasing activity, changing jobs, obtaining assistance in dressing and grooming, or isolating themselves socially (Carrieri and Janson-Bjerklie, 1986). Transient episodes of dyspnea can usually be resolved by stopping or avoiding the activity that precipitated the breathing problem. If the person does nothing to control the problem, the dyspnea either resolves itself or becomes increasingly severe until a visit to an emergency department or a health care provider becomes necessary.

This model of dyspnea has proved enormously useful to practitioners because it explains the individual's experience of dyspnea, provides a way to assess various aspects of the experience, and pinpoints the specific area for intervention. Several measuring techniques have been developed to assess the various dimensions of dyspnea with some success. But although multidimensional instruments may provide a more thorough assessment of dyspnea, to date these types of instruments have not been widely tested (McCord and Cronin-Stubbs, 1992).

FACTORS AFFECTING CLINICAL DECISIONS

The onset, prognosis, and factors that affect the incidence, prevalence, and extent of respiratory problems vary. Age, gender, lifestyle, socioeconomic status, educational background, culture and ethnicity, spirituality and religion, the settings in which care is provided, ethical considerations, and financial considerations affect the prevention of respiratory disease and the effectiveness of therapy for those with respiratory problems. These individual differences need to be considered before any nursing intervention or plan of therapy is pursued.

Age

Very young and very old individuals are at higher risk for respiratory problems than are people of other age groups. Infants, especially premature newborns, and toddlers are at highest risk for respiratory infections because their physical immaturity makes them particularly vulnerable. Preschool and school-age children are also at high risk because of their frequent exposure to other sick children, the structural position of their ear canals, and their hygiene habits. The elderly are also a vulnerable group for respiratory problems because of the many degenerative changes that take place in the respiratory system throughout a lifetime.

INFANTS AND CHILDREN

Premature infants are at risk for pulmonary problems because of a surfactant deficiency. The surfactant-synthesizing ability of the lungs develops late in fetal development and is therefore lacking in those born before term. A condition known as hyaline membrane disease occurs in which the lungs literally stick together, unable to expand to fill with adequate air. Adequate prenatal care should be encouraged as a way to prevent prematurity and the resulting pulmonary problems that are likely to occur.

Toddlers, especially those who are teething, frequently put their fingers in their mouths, which introduces many organisms into the nasopharynx. As a result, they often develop nasal congestion, which encourages the growth of bacteria and, in turn, increases the potential for an upper respiratory tract infection. Furthermore, because the eustachian tubes, which open into the lateral walls of the nasopharynx, are at a straight angle in children, many organisms introduced into the mouth by a child make their way into the middle ear, causing ear infections (otitis media). As the child grows older, the eustachian tube develops an angle that allows the middle ear to drain into the nasopharynx, thereby reducing the potential for ear infections.

Many preschoolers are particularly susceptible to upper respiratory tract infections because of their frequent exposure to others with respiratory tract infections. At child care centers and in neighborhood play groups, invariably there is a child with a runny nose, a cold, or an ear infection. Compounding the problem is the fact that children learn about their world by touching everything and by putting much of what they see in their mouths. Although recovery from most of these infections is usually quick, frequent exposure to organisms can develop into pharyngitis, influenza, or tonsillitis. A child with a fever or one who is pulling at an ear should be referred to a physician and separated from the other children.

Some children are prone to laryngotracheal bronchitis (croup), a condition in which the larynx, trachea, and bronchi are inflamed. A characteristic "barking" cough accompanied by a fever indicates that the child has laryngotracheal bronchitis. This condition is serious in children because their bronchi are smaller and more easily obstructed. Teaching toddlers and young children to keep their fingers out of their mouths, keeping sick children away from the well ones, and seeking health care early will reduce the number and the severity of upper respiratory tract infections in young children.

Although school-age children and adolescents are exposed to many respiratory tract infections, they rarely suffer any adverse pulmonary effects. However, the adolescent who starts smoking and continues into middle age increases the risk for cardiopulmonary disease later in life. An unhealthy diet (high in fatty fast foods and/or lacking in fruits and vegetables), a lack of exercise, and excessive stress add to the adolescent's risk for respiratory problems, and teens should be encouraged to reduce these modifiable risks.

ELDERLY ADULTS

Elderly adults, like premature infants, have a higher risk for pulmonary disease, but for different reasons. The arterial system of the aged becomes less distensible, owing to atherosclerotic plaques and a concomitant rise in blood pressure. The connective tissue and the bronchial tree undergo structural changes, the lung loses elasticity, and the bronchial ducts become dilated. The alveoli often become enlarged so that ventilation and transfer of oxygen and carbon dioxide decline. Furthermore, osteoporotic changes in the thorax and kyphosis (abnormal curvature) of the vertebrae, which are normal aging processes, often keep the lungs from fully expanding, leading to lower oxygenation levels. All of these changes heighten the risk of respiratory problems, the most frequent of which is pneumonia. Because the elderly are slow to recover and subject to secondary infections, the first signs of respiratory disease should be addressed. Mr. Taylor, the 70-year-old man with pneumonia described in the introductory case study, is a good example of what can happen when early intervention is not sought.

Gender

Little has been written about gender differences in the incidence, prevalence, or severity of respiratory problems. Nonetheless, it appears that men and women may cope with respiratory disease differently. A two-part study of men and women with COPD participating in a formal pulmonary rehabilitation program (Kersten, 1990) found that men showed more improvement in total self-concept than women during the 3-week program. However, after discharge, the men's self-concept dropped more than the women's, suggesting a need for more intensive follow-up care for men. Similarly, a study of the predictors of walking distance for people with chronic bronchitis and/or emphysema suggests that men respond to respiratory problems differently than women. Compared with the women, the men in the study estimated that they would walk farther, did in fact walk farther, but overestimated the distance they would walk (Thompson, 1989). Clearly, more research needs to be done to determine whether gender makes a difference in the way people respond to respiratory problems.

Lifestyle

Of all the factors that affect respiratory function, lifestyle (habits, experiences, and preferred activities) is the most important. Smoking, nutrition, physical exercise, and use of alcohol and other drugs are clearly factors that influence the respiratory health of individuals and families and the clinical decisions made to improve or promote respiratory health.

SMOKING

Of all the lifestyle factors linked to respiratory problems, smoking is by far the most dangerous. For instance, the risk of lung cancer is 25 times greater for a person who smokes more than 20 cigarettes a day than for someone who does not smoke at all (McCance and Huether, 1994). Even passive smoking (i.e., exposure to someone else's smoke) increases the risk of cancer; it also increases susceptibility to respiratory infections by impairing mucociliary clearance. Furthermore, inhaling smoke from any source can cause chronic bronchitis and emphysema and holding smoke in the upper airway (as is done by cigar and pipe smokers) can cause gum disease, tooth deterioration, mouth ulcers, and cancer of the tongue, neck, jaw, and throat.

Research indicates that those who quit smoking can greatly reduce their risk of cancer, especially of the lungs (Chyou et al, 1992). In recent years, the incidence of lung cancer is decreasing somewhat in men; however, it is actually increasing in women, reflecting an increased incidence of smoking in women (American Cancer Society, 1996).

WEIGHT AND NUTRITION

Severe obesity affects lung expansion, both because of greater pressure against the diaphragm and because the body demands more oxygen. Conversely, the malnourished person may experience respiratory muscle wasting, which creates decreased muscle strength and respiratory excursion. Furthermore, muscle weakness decreases the ability to cough productively, putting the person at risk for the accumulation of pulmonary secretions and thus secondary infections. Finally, both obese and malnourished people are at risk for anemia, which means the cells will not be adequately supplied with oxygenated blood. Therefore, a well-balanced diet is very important both as a preventive measure for respiratory disease and as a treatment for existing respiratory problems. Planning care for someone who is obese, is malnourished, or who simply has unhealthy eating habits should be considered in light of the person's lifestyle.

EXERCISE

Physical activity increases the rate of respirations and the heart rate, enabling the individual to inhale more oxygen and expire more carbon dioxide. Compared with inactive individuals, those who exercise daily have a lower pulse rate and blood pressure, lower blood cholesterol, increased blood flow, and greater oxygen extraction by working muscles. Furthermore, a sedentary lifestyle inhibits alveolar expansion and deep breathing and makes it difficult to respond effectively to respiratory threats. Clearly, moderate exercise can be beneficial in many ways. Regularly scheduled short walks should be considered when planning care for people who are vulnerable to respiratory threats. More vigorous activity should be discussed with the patient's physician.

ALCOHOL AND OTHER DRUGS

Excessive use of alcohol and other drugs can impair tissue oxygenation in two ways. First, chronic substance abuse is associated with poor nutrition, including a low intake of iron-rich foods and a resulting decline in rate and depth of inspiration, which, in turn, decreases the amount of oxygen inhaled. These alterations in normal respirations and ventilation leave the individual vulnerable to environmental threats, which often lead to the development of frequent, then chronic, respiratory problems.

Second, excessive use of alcohol and certain other drugs depresses the respiratory center in the brain, decreasing the rate and depth of inspiration; this decreases the amount of oxygen inhaled. A lack of adequate oxygen to the rest of the body leads to multiple health problems.

ENVIRONMENTAL FACTORS

OCCUPATIONAL HAZARDS

The work place is a major source of pulmonary health problems. Thousands of pollutants in U.S. work places are occupational lung hazards, and many acute respiratory illnesses—hypersensitivity reactions, asthma, chemical pneumonia, chronic diffuse interstitial fibrosis, silicosis, coal worker's pneumoconiosis, and asbestosis—are caused by occupational conditions. Furthermore, exposure to some industrial substances increases the risk for lung cancer, especially if the individual is a cigarette smoker (Table 21–1). Planning care should include an assessment of the patient's work place so that these factors are considered.

OVERCROWDED LIVING CONDITIONS

Working or living under crowded conditions is also a major factor in the incidence and prevalence of respiratory diseases. Sneezing and coughing place droplet infections in the atmosphere, and cramped conditions increase the likelihood of exposure to these infections. Untidy, cramped quarters also tend to cause an accumulation of more potential allergens than

TABLE 21-1 Common Causes of Occupational Lung Disease

Substance	Occupation	Disease
Animal hair and urine, including insects and birds	Animal handler; e.g., farmer, veterinarian, laboratory worker	Asthma
Asbestos fiber	Asbestos miner; shipyard worker; construction worker; demolition worker; insulation worker; electrician; brake mechanic	Asbestosis; lung cancer (mesothelioma)
Coal dust	Coal miner	Coal worker's pneumoconiosis (black lung)
Cotton fiber	Textile worker	Asthma (byssinosis or brown lung)
Diisocyanates: toluene diisocyanate (TDI); diphenylmethane diisocyanate; hexamethylene diisocyanate	Automobile worker; TDI manufacturer; foundry core worker; polyurethane foam worker; painter	Asthma
Drugs: ampicillin, penicillin; glycyl-containing compounds; piperazine	Pharmacist; pharmaceutic industrial worker	Asthma
Enzymes: subtilisin; trypsin; pancreatin	Detergent manufacturer; pharmacist; pharmaceutical industrial worker	Asthma
Formaldehyde	Laboratory worker; fur, tanning, and clothing industrial workers; home insulation worker	Asthma
Grain dust and flour	Baker; miller; farmer	Asthma
Henna extract	Hairdresser	Asthma
Insoluble gases; e.g., phosgene, nitrogen oxides	Industrial worker; participants in chemical warfare (phosgene)	Chemical pneumonia; pulmonary edema
Irritant gases; e.g., chlorine, sulfur dioxide, ammonia	Industrial worker; housekeeper, maid	Upper respiratory tract symptoms; bronchitis
Metal oxides: copper, zinc, magnesium, cadmium, iron, manganese, mercury	Welder; industrial worker	Metal fume fever
Metallic salts:		Asthma
Nickel	Metal plating worker	
Chromium	Cement, tanning, and metal plating workers	
Aluminum	Aluminum fluoride and sulfate workers	
Nitrogen dioxide in filled silos, closed welding spaces, and chemical laboratories	Farmer; welder; laboratory technician	Silo filler's disease; nitrogen oxide exposure
Polyvinyl chloride; rosin (colophony); silica	Meat wrapper; electronics worker; sandblaster; foundry worker; jeweler; stonemason; pottery maker; ceramist; construction worker; miner	Asthma; silicosis (from silica)
Spores from moldy hay	Farmer	Farmer's lung
Wood dust	Carpenter; cabinet/furniture maker; wood carver; construction worker; mill worker	Asthma

well-kept, spacious places. Nonsmokers are at much greater risk of developing respiratory problems when in contact with smokers if they are in poorly ventilated or crowded rooms.

Families who live in crowded environments that are also poorly heated or cooled are doubly at risk, because they both risk more exposure to infection and must also respond to often dramatic environmental changes. In response to heat, the peripheral blood vessels dilate, thus decreasing the resistance to blood flow. In response, the heart increases output to maintain blood pressure. This increase in cardiac output requires additional oxygen, which is acquired through increased respiratory rate and depth.

In a cold environment, by contrast, the peripheral blood vessels constrict, raising the blood pressure, which in turn decreases cardiac action and thereby reduces the need for oxygen. Whereas healthy people can adjust to these body alterations, people compromised by illness and subject to crowded, polluted spaces are likely to develop more severe health problems. The nurse needs to help patients understand these environmental influences when planning care so that a realistic approach to preventing and resolving respiratory conditions can be devised.

HAZARDS IN THE HOME

Exposure to lung irritants or allergens in the home environment can be as hazardous as exposure on the job site. Some lung diseases are related to hobbies in the home, such as pottery, painting, and wood carving. In addition, pollen from blooming or cut flowers and molds that grow easily on the surface of pots or potting dirt are allergens that can cause lung disease.

Forced-air heating systems may aggravate breathing problems, especially if airborne particles are not filtered out. Humidifiers may be sources of infection if they are not cleaned regularly, with the water changed daily. High-pile carpets and throw rugs are notorious collectors of dust, animal hairs, and other allergens. Other notorious dust catchers are draperies, mini blinds, window frames, and upholstered furniture. If vacuuming or dry dusting aggravates pulmonary symptoms, wet dusting is suggested. Other potential allergens include stuffed toys, perfumes, insect sprays, tar paper, or camphor. Outdoors, shrubs, trees, grasses, and weeds are common sources of allergens. Allergies that become worse in spring are usually due to flowers, shrubs, or tree pollens. Late spring-summer allergies are usually caused by grasses, whereas late summer allergies are usually due to weeds.

Animals, especially pets, are common sources of respiratory problems. Animal hair and dander are the common precipitating factors for asthma and hay fever. Contact with pigeon excrement may lead to cryptococcosis, whereas contact with parrots may lead to psittacosis, a viral disease also called parrot fever. Among rural residents, contact with dust contaminated by sheep or cattle may lead to Q fever. Allergens responsible for pulmonary symptoms can be either eliminated completely (e.g., replacement of down pillows with synthetic ones) or controlled to tolerated levels (e.g., house cleaning to control dust accumulation). Conducting a thorough assessment with the patient to determine what lung irritants or allergens exist and how to modify them is essential so that the patient can take appropriate steps to protect his or her respiratory health.

ENVIRONMENTAL POLLUTION

In densely populated cities, air pollution from vehicles and industry has become well recognized by the public as a significant cause of pulmonary symptoms. Pollution can aggravate mucus hypersecretion along the tracheobronchial tree and cause impairment of respiratory function in smokers. In addition, hot, smoggy weather in an industrial region or urban area is a common precipitating factor for acute respiratory failure for ambulatory patients with cardiopulmonary disease.

The industries that pollute the air with sulfur oxide, nitrogen dioxide, and particulate matter include electric utilities, iron and steel producers, petroleum refineries, and chemical producers. Other sources of air pollution are motor vehicle exhaust and smoke from wood-burning stoves. While government legislation and regulations have limited the amount of pollution by these industries, in many areas pollution remains a serious respiratory threat to some individuals. If a vulnerable patient lives or works near pollutant operations, relocation may be necessary.

GEOGRAPHIC LOCATION

There are also certain areas of the United States where people are more prone to pulmonary disease. Histoplasmosis is most commonly contracted in the farming states of the Midwest, whereas coccidioidomycosis is more common in the desert southwestern states and in northern Mexico. Although tuberculosis is commonly thought to be confined to Third World countries, in fact it is frequently diagnosed in the United States, most often in areas where large numbers of immigrants from Third World countries have settled. The increased incidence of the acquired immunodeficiency syndrome and human immunodeficiency virus infection is a factor in the increased incidence of tuberculosis. Frequent screening and education are the most effective ways for nurses to help keep the incidence of tuberculosis under control.

STRESS AND ANXIETY

Many people live stressful lives, and stress creates different problems. Some become more susceptible to illness; others develop cardiovascular conditions, such as heart palpitations. A common response to stress is to develop a cold, the flu, and other respiratory problems. Being stressed seems to reduce one's resistance so that during the winter, when colds and the flu are more prevalent, those in stressful situations (such as a demanding job, an unhealthy marriage, job loss, new baby, or other life-changing event) are more prone to develop a respiratory illness. To prevent this situation, it is wise to get more rest, exercise regularly, and stay away from people with respiratory infections. It is also important to reduce the stress. (See Chapter 31, Stress and Anxiety, for more information.)

Some people have difficulty breathing (dyspnea) when they become anxious. Because of fear, the unknown, or incidences that are not expected, the individual becomes anxious and finds it hard to breathe. The usual response is to hyperventilate. The dyspnea is real and can cause serious respiratory alkalosis. The person will feel dizzy, have heart palpitations, and be diaphoretic (sweaty). If the alkalosis is severe, the person could become panicky and even have periods of apnea. Fortunately, the treatment is self-induced. The person only needs to breathe into a paper bag to rebreathe his or her own expired carbon dioxide to correct the condition. If the anxiety-induced hyperventilation occurs frequently, the individual should seek definitive therapy.

Managing stress and anxiety is important, because they both lead to respiratory problems, some that can be easily cured, such as anxiety-induced hyperventilation, and others that require more complicated treatment, such as bronchitis. Prevention is the best approach and that means managing one's life stresses so resistance is not reduced and hyperventilation induced.

Socioeconomic Status and Educational Background

Socioeconomic status often defines how a person acts when a respiratory problem occurs and whether prevention is part of the individual's considerations. For instance, patients who have adequate health insurance and are astute consumers of health care will probably focus their efforts on keeping well by having periodic checkups and adhering to a healthy lifestyle. They will faithfully get an annual flu shot and a tuberculosis screening test, avoid smoking and exposure to second-hand smoke, exercise regularly, and avoid crowded places. They do these things because they know that this will help them stay well.

On the other end of the continuum are those people who do not know what they should do to avoid respiratory problems and even if they did know would not have the resources to act appropriately. The poor and uneducated are at risk for respiratory problems because they are uninformed or so stressed by the daily need for survival that they cannot be bothered thinking about prevention and health care. These individuals often seek health care only when they are so sick that they can no longer ignore their symptoms.

Educational level and socioeconomic status tend to be coupled. The poor often are not educated, not because they are uneducable or not interested in learning but because they cannot afford the "luxury" of education. Because of family need, they often drop out of school to help support their family. They are often so focused on day-to-day survival that education seems like an option available only for others who are more fortunate.

The nurse often plays an important role in the health education of these people. During acute episodes of respiratory illness, the nurse can offer suggestions about ways to stay well. For instance, helping the patient understand the value of a balanced diet and how to plan one that is affordable will go a long way in establishing wellness. Emphasizing a balance of rest and work, the value of immunizations, the role exercise plays in keeping fit, and the importance of not smoking helps the individual learn a more healthful lifestyle. None of these suggestions costs money; they may be a new way of functioning and are excellent ways to prevent respiratory illness that is a threat to all of us during certain times of the year.

An important reason for knowing the educational level of the patient experiencing a respiratory problem is that it helps the nurse customize the care and instruction. After an assessment of the patient, the nurse is better able to plan care and instruction that is appropriate to the patient's abilities. Nothing is worse than talking down to a patient or talking about issues that the patient cannot understand. For instance, if the nurse knows the patient is a college graduate and has critical analysis capabilities, then the nurse can give the patient pamphlets to read, suggest other resources to explore, and have the patient list questions to ask during a follow-up visit. On the other hand, if the patient is a high school dropout with poor reading skills, the nurse would need to spend more time on face-to-face explanation, with pictures and models if possible to enhance learning, and rely less on printed instructional materials. We all know that behavioral change is very contingent on using an approach that is consistent with the patient's individual needs.

Teaching patients about lung problems begins when the patient is ready to learn. Rewards for correct behavior are more likely to work than threats about what might happen if change is not pursued. Behavioral therapy has been very successful for those trying to lose weight or stop smoking. The biggest task for the nurse is to realize how difficult it is to get people to change the way they live, particularly if there are no immediate visible negative outcomes associated with the high-risk behavior. Patience and keeping incentives and rewards relevant are the secret to successful behavioral change.

Culture and Ethnicity

Culture and ethnicity also affect the care planned for people with respiratory problems. For example, the nurse must be sensitive to the cultural aspects of a patient's diet when helping that patient plan a dietary regimen for preventing or resolving respiratory problems. In some cultures, obesity is considered healthy, so it is important for the nurse to be aware of such attitudes before making recommendations for change. The nurse should also be aware of differing attitudes toward alcohol use. In many cultures, alcohol is an integral part of each meal or of religious rituals, while in other cultures even moderate drinking is frowned upon. Health practices initiated and the relationships developed with health care providers also are influenced by culture and ethnicity. For example, some Hispanic families still consult the *curandero* (healer) for advice and use "old way" therapies. Black families often use remedies that have been passed from generation to generation, and, although not harmful, they may benefit from modification. Asians often use approaches to health care rooted in centuries of tradition. An awareness of such traditions and beliefs is important; otherwise, a nurse may suggest an approach only to discover much of what was recommended was contraindicated by the individual's cultural beliefs. A thorough assessment of the individual's and family's beliefs about health, nutrition, and medication will make the planning and outcome of care more effective. In many cases, the "traditional old ways" can be incorporated into the plan of care.

Spirituality and Religion

Some individuals because of their religious or spiritual beliefs do not seek care for respiratory conditions; others limit the degree to which their families and themselves get involved. For instance, Christian Scientist believers generally do not seek medical care because their desired approach is to pray for healing. They focus on preventing health problems by living a healthful lifestyle and pray during episodes of illness. Some families do not believe in prevention, so they do not want their children immunized or screened for tuberculosis.

Some spiritual groups use homeopathic ingredients for the care of their respiratory conditions. There is little evidence that these methods are not useful, so the nurse should be as knowledgeable as possible about the value or quality of those interventions that are not medically based. For instance, most of the medical community scoffed at the use of home remedies, such as poultices made of herbs for a congested chest, when in reality they worked and were found to be safe and based on sound scientific data.

Setting in Which Care Is Provided

Nurses need to know about the respiratory system and how to help people with respiratory problems, because no matter where the nurse works, patients with respiratory problems will need nursing care. For instance, people with acute respiratory problems, such as pneumonia, chest trauma, status asthmaticus (severe asthma attack), late-stage tuberculosis, and late-stage lung cancer are most often hospitalized. The nurse in the hospital setting must be prepared to provide acute care. People with chronic conditions, such as emphysema, COPD, asthma, bronchitis, or inactive tuberculosis are most often seen in clinics, physician's offices, or the home. Nurses in clinics and nursing homes and those who visit patients in the home often care for patients with chronic respiratory conditions.

Nurses in schools screen well children for tuberculosis and provide immediate care for children with colds, sore throats, earaches, and other minor ailments. Clinic nurses give immunizations to the elderly for pneumonia or the flu. Many people go to clinics for diagnostic workups where early respiratory problems are detected. Even nurses in psychiatric settings encounter patients with respiratory problems precipitated by anxiety.

Rehabilitation centers often have nursing staff who work with patients with chronic respiratory conditions and help them learn better lifestyles or how to perform prescribed breathing exercises.

Health care in rural America is different. Rural nurses often care for all kinds of patients with respiratory problems (acute, chronic, and diagnostic) because there are no clinics, diagnostic centers, or rehabilitation agencies. Nurses in these settings need to be versatile, competent, and ready to respond to a wide variety of respiratory conditions.

Ethical Considerations

The ethical aspects of helping people change their lifestyle include considerations about informed consent, confidentiality, and the right to self-determination. Individuals with chronic pulmonary problems must be informed about the adverse effects of noncompliance with the treatment plan; however, there can be no coercion or pressure to comply. Informed consent also means that the individual must be told about both the benefits and the *risks* of treatment so an informed decision can be made. *Informed choice* may be a better term, because it implies that a decision regarding lifestyle and treatment has been made only after all the pertinent information has been made available and that the individual has made the decision freely.

Confidentiality is always necessary when a patient has shared personal information and when knowledge of the patient's condition is available to other health care workers. However, when a patient has a communicable disease that is a threat to others, it is important to share the information with others who may have been exposed. For example, when a person is diagnosed with pulmonary tuberculosis, those exposed by close contact must be informed and tested so they can be treated and also so they can avoid infecting others. Even in these circumstances, confidentiality is maintained to the degree possible.

Another example of a potential ethical dilemma is when a patient who had a respiratory condition, such as lung cancer, has died and the family are not told the primary site of the disease. Why a person dies is important and should be conveyed to the family. Many families are in such grief at the time of death that they do not ask the cause or arrange for an autopsy to be performed so the site of the primary cancer can be identified. This lack of information for relatives, particularly those of direct descent, can be problematic. Some respiratory conditions are familial (found in families) and are a risk factor for those remaining. Nurses are often the people closest to the patient and the family and are in a position to encourage the family to seek this important information regardless of the cost. The possible future cost to the family members could far exceed that of an autopsy.

Self-determination also must be addressed when working with patients with chronic respiratory conditions. Because some respiratory problems can quickly escalate to a life-threatening emergency, the patient should know the options available in case he or she becomes unable to decide a course of action. There are two ways that a patient can implement rights granted by the Self-Determination Act of 1990: using the living will or using the durable power of attorney for health care. If the individual is unable to make choices because of incompetence or unconsciousness or because of other physical or mental conditions, the law allows the individual to make known his or her wishes through a previously written living will or to let another person make the choice (the durable power of attorney). (See Chapter 9, Ethics in Nursing Practice, for more information.)

Financial Considerations

The economic aspects of respiratory care depend on the extent of the illness. However, with a growing trend toward the development of more sophisticated technology, diagnostic workups, therapeutic treatment, and a growing number of medications, care has become increasingly expensive. Because even the simplest treatment plan can be costly, efforts to *prevent* disease should be emphasized. The nurse will need to give special attention to encouraging patients to live healthier lifestyles—eating a well-balanced diet, getting plenty of exercise, reducing stress, and modifying high-risk behaviors such as smoking and excessive alcohol use—as a means of avoiding expensive care. Responsibility for one's own health must be valued and practiced.

The trend toward more home care will mean that care for chronic lung diseases (emphysema, COPD, asthma, bronchitis) will increasingly be provided in the home and will involve the patient and the patient's family as integral members of the health care team. The home care nurse will coordinate the

CLINICAL DECISION MAKING
AN ELDERLY PATIENT WITH LUNG DISEASE

Mr. Taylor, as described in the case study, is a 70-year-old man with chronic lung disease. His care needs to be carefully planned to ensure that he will be able to care for himself since it is uncertain where he will go after his discharge. The goals for Mr. Taylor's care are to provide therapeutic measures to overcome his pneumonia and for discharge and posthospitalization care.

In order to formulate clinical decisions for this patient, his physical condition must be assessed to determine his energy level, health practices, living style, and nutritional status. Mr. Taylor's vital signs must be determined in order to determine how he is responding to therapy. The nurse should provide therapy to assist Mr. Taylor in coughing, deep breathing, and pain control.

His ability to become independent and assume self-care must be assessed. If potential for independent living does not exist, determine with Mr. Taylor what future living arrangements must be made.

Nursing care is a team effort involving physicians, nurses, dieticians, pharmacists, social workers, respiratory therapists, and significant others. Assess Mr. Taylor's level of knowledge about his lung condition and present pneumonia. Teach deep breathing exercises. Determine, with other staff, his possible future living arrangements. Use comfort measures and medications for chest pain. Review with him how diet and exercise affect his condition.

care provided by other health care professionals (e.g., physical therapists, occupational therapists) and ancillary workers (home health aides) as well as other support services (e.g., Meals on Wheels, transportation, home delivery of groceries and medications). A major responsibility of the home care nurse will be educating the patient and family members so they can manage the chronic condition by themselves with assistance from the nurse only when necessary and to keep the patient stable, thus avoiding expensive hospitalization.

FUTURE DEVELOPMENTS

Over the past decade, dramatic advancements have been made in knowledge about pulmonary health problems and pharmacology, as well as in diagnostic technology. We now know much more about cellular and biochemical changes in the respiratory system and about new diagnostic methods that are faster and require less effort on the part of the patient. Also, effective treatment requires less time than in the past. All of these advances help the patient recover more quickly, but they also tend to be expensive, both for the third-party payers and the patient. Cost is now the number-one issue facing health care consumers, providers, and institutions.

If these trends continue, we can expect some of the following developments:

- Diagnostic procedures will be less intrusive and more easily done in ambulatory settings in the home.
- Increasingly low-risk diagnostic technology for visualization of soft tissue (such as the lungs) will become even more sophisticated.
- Prevention of respiratory disease, particularly importance of a nutritious diet, regular exercise, and avoidance of high-risk behaviors such as smoking and excessive alcohol use will be emphasized.
- Increasing responsibility for health will be given to patients both for prevention and treatment (e.g., pulmonary toilet given at home for those with chronic emphysema; those with acute illness treated at clinics rather than expected to care for themselves at home).
- More effective symptom-specific drugs will alter or cure specific aspects of the disease process.
- The public will press for legislation to protect the environment from allergens and contaminants.
- Individuals will be better educated so they can better control their health-related behavior. Television will play a major role in this education process, as will computers as they become a part of more households and connect users to a wide range of health resources.
- The ethics of health care will continue to be debated and discussed as more issues with a moral dimension become part of health care delivery.
- The cost of care will be controlled as new ways to finance health care are devised and more emphasis is placed on health promotion and disease prevention.

NURSING CARE ACTIONS

Principles and Practices

Caring for patients with respiratory problems is best accomplished when the course of action(s) is consistent with principles related to the research available about the patient's condition and/or the response to the condition. Using nursing process, the nurse would design the plan of care based on assessment and intervention principles. For instance, if the patient has dyspnea due to pain on inspiration, the nurse would determine which principle would guide the actions.

PATIENT TEACHING
TEACHING MR. TAYLOR

The nurse needs to provide information and skills to Mr. Taylor to help him get well after his acute episode of pneumonia, as well as prevent the recurrence of catastrophic episodes.

PRE ENCOUNTER

- Before Mr. Taylor's discharge, determine what information was given to him regarding his medications, activity level, breathing exercises, and next scheduled physician(s) appointment(s).
- Ask about Mr. Taylor's ability to perform breathing exercises and upper arm–strengthening exercises.
- Review all medications, both prescribed and over-the-counter, that Mr. Taylor is currently taking.
- Prepare a summary sheet (written in lay terminology) that includes both generic and trade names of the medication(s), purpose of the medication(s), a drawing of the medication (showing form and color), dosage, time to take the medication(s), common side effect(s), special instructions for medication preparation and administration, and when to contact the physician or pharmacist.
- Observe Mr. Taylor's ability to perform activities of daily living.
- Obtain appropriate materials (e.g., audiovisuals, pamphlets) that can be used for the teaching episodes.
- Ask Mr. Taylor the best time for teaching sessions.

DURING THE ENCOUNTER

- Reinforce and supplement information given to Mr. Taylor before discharge regarding any phase of his recovery from the acute illness.
- Describe and demonstrate body position(s), upper arm–strengthening and coughing exercises, and pursed-lip and abdominal-diaphragmatic breathing exercises aimed at improving ventilation and oxygenation. Use audiovisual and written materials as appropriate. Have Mr. Taylor demonstrate these techniques to ensure that he understands how to do them properly.
- Teach walking exercises that will improve Mr. Taylor's endurance and thus improve his ventilation and oxygenation.
- Use the medication summary sheet to discuss the medications Mr. Taylor will take in a 24-hour period. Ask Mr. Taylor to keep the medication summary sheet in a convenient place and to refer to the sheet as necessary.
- Design a 24-hour medication reminder device that Mr. Taylor can use to store medications and remind him to take the medications. Observe Mr. Taylor as he prepares and takes the medications.
- Explain what signs and symptoms Mr. Taylor should report to his physician.
- Involve significant others in the teaching sessions. Have a relative, friend, or neighbor listen to the teaching with Mr. Taylor, then perform return-demonstrations along with Mr. Taylor to ensure their understanding.

POST ENCOUNTER

- Provide follow-up evaluation of teaching encounters as necessary. Ask Mr. Taylor and/or another responsible person to perform demonstrations, as necessary.
- Call Mr. Taylor or another responsible person as necessary to supplement teaching episodes and check on progress.
- Contact a physician or other consultants as necessary about Mr. Taylor's condition (e.g., to determine whether he needs a physical therapist, occupational therapist, respiratory therapist, dietitian, or social worker).

The following principle would provide direction for the nurse: reduction of pain by the administration of an analgesic and positioning that facilitates ventilation, thereby promoting full inspiration and thus better exchange of oxygen and carbon dioxide. The nurse then knows that the patient must be given an analgesic and positioned for full lung expansion, which will ease the patient's breathing and thus allow for full inspiration and a better exchange of oxygen and carbon dioxide.

This section covers several principles that guide action related to respiratory problems and the accompanying nursing actions based on the available research. For ease of understanding, the principles to be discussed have been categorized into five major areas:

- Mobilizing pulmonary secretions
- Clearing the airway
- Oxygenating the system
- Reducing the effort of breathing
- Self-management strategies for coping with chronic respiratory problems

MOBILIZING PULMONARY SECRETIONS

Sometimes the secretions in the lobes of the lungs are so copious that the patient requires assistance to remove them. Percussion should be used with postural drainage for patients with copious secretions that cannot be removed by other means (Zidulka et al, 1989). Percussion enhances the speed of flow and rate of sputum production without altering pulmonary function or oxygen saturation (Gallon, 1991). Several principles will guide the nurse's actions:

- The proper technique for removing mucus from the lobes of the lungs is based on a thorough assessment of the person with mucus accumulation.
- The risk for infection is reduced when mucus is mobilized and removed from the lung.
- Breathing is more effective and less fatiguing when the airway is clear.
- Gas exchange is more efficient when diffusion of oxygen is improved.

Clearly, these principles indicate that the lungs must be clear if proper ventilation is to occur (the exchange of oxygen and carbon dioxide) and the threat of infection is to be prevented. Two effective procedures for mobilizing and removing pulmonary secretions are chest percussion, vibration, and postural drainage (see Procedure 21–1) and incentive spirometry (see Procedure 21–2).

CLEARING THE AIRWAY

Keeping the airway clear of mucus is also an important way to ensure good respiration and ventilation. Once the mucus in the lungs is mobilized and available for coughing or suctioning there are several ways the nurse can remove the secretions from the airway. Below are principles that will guide the actions selected by the nurse:

- Removal of secretions from the airway promotes a more effective breathing pattern.
- The potential for aspiration is reduced when the airway is clear of secretions.
- The proper way to remove the secretions from the airway depends on a careful assessment of the patient's ability to cough.

People who are at risk for an accumulation of mucus in any portion of the respiratory airway (mouth, pharynx, trachea, bronchi) can be taught a deep-breathing and controlled coughing technique (Thornlow, 1995) or the superior forced expiration technique (Pavia, 1990) to help clear the airway. If that procedure cannot be done or is ineffective, suctioning may be necessary to clear secretions. Suctioning techniques include nasopharyngeal (bulb syringe) suctioning, oropharyngeal (Yankauer) suctioning, tracheobronchial suctioning, and, for intubated patients, endotracheal and tracheostomy tube suctioning.

OXYGENATING THE SYSTEM

When a patient is seriously ill and unable to obtain adequate oxygen for ventilation, oxygen is frequently administered. The following principles guide the nurse's decisions about when to administer oxygen and how to select the proper delivery mode.

- Ineffective breathing patterns will improve when hypoventilation is reversed.
- The exchange of oxygen with carbon dioxide will improve when adequate oxygen is available for exchange.
- The oxygen delivery system selected to improve ventilation depends on the cause of oxygen deprivation, the age of the patient, and the seriousness of the condition (Box 21–1).
- Frequent assessment of the patient for signs and symptoms of oxygen deprivation while receiving oxygen promotes appropriate decisions about the amount and way to administer the oxygen.

REDUCING THE EFFORT OF BREATHING

Chronic pulmonary diseases that cannot be cured are frequently treated by teaching the patient techniques for decreasing the effort expended to breathe. Abdominal-diaphragmatic breathing and pursed lip breathing are two exercises that can help patients decrease the effort of breathing. Together, these exercises lessen the effort of breathing because they increase the tidal volume, decrease the respiratory rate, increase oxygen saturation, and increase exercise tolerance, thus reducing dyspnea (Carrieri-Kohlman and Janson-Bjerklie, 1993). Three basic principles guide the nurse's actions in prescribing these exercises:

1. Fatigue from breathing is reduced when dyspnea is reduced.
2. Promoting complete exhalation improves the ability to inspire fully.
3. Improved exhalation of carbon dioxide improves the exchange of oxygen and carbon dioxide.

SELF-MANAGEMENT STRATEGIES

Self-management strategies are approaches that a patient with chronic pulmonary diseases can take to cope with and minimize dyspnea. One common strategy is to position himself or herself so as to make breathing easier. A patient with COPD may tend to lean forward when feeling short of breath. This position stabilizes the upper chest while allowing freedom of movement of the lower chest (Carrieri-Kohlman and Janson-Bjerklie, 1993). Leaning forward allows the abdominal organs to drop away from the diaphragm, decreasing accessory muscle use and permitting better diaphragmatic excursion, which may help relieve dyspnea.

Some other self-management techniques to reduce the patient's perception of excessive respiratory effort and thus improve lung function include a breathing retraining program involving biofeedback, which has been shown to improve lung function in patients with cystic fibrosis (Delk et al, 1994); a program that uses music as a distractor, decreasing patients' feelings of respiratory distress and thus allowing them to exercise at a higher intensity (Thornby et al, 1995); and guided imagery, which has been shown to improve the quality of life of patients with chronic bronchitis and emphysema (Moody et al, 1993). The nurse should consider incorporating pertinent alternative techniques in the patient's plan of care whenever possible.

A key component for the self-management of a chronic pulmonary condition is the teaching that the patient receives from nurses and other health care professionals. The basic principles that guide teaching patients strategies for self-managed care stem from learning theory and are as follows:

- Readiness to learn is promoted by the seriousness of the condition and the interest of the learner in making change.

BOX 21-1
METHODS OF OXYGEN DELIVERY

Devices commonly used for oxygen delivery include the nasal cannula, face mask, partial rebreathing mask, nonrebreathing mask, and Venturi mask.

NASAL CANNULA

This oxygen delivery system consists of plastic tubing that fits around the patient's ears and provides oxygen through nasal prongs inserted into the nostrils (Illustration A). This device allows the patient to receive oxygen while breathing through the nose; in fact, to ensure maximum oxygen delivery, the nurse should instruct the patient to breathe through the nose when the cannula is used (Dunlevy and Tyl, 1992). Nasal cannulas are inexpensive, disposable, and comfortable for most patients. They can be used for both short-term and long-term oxygen therapy.

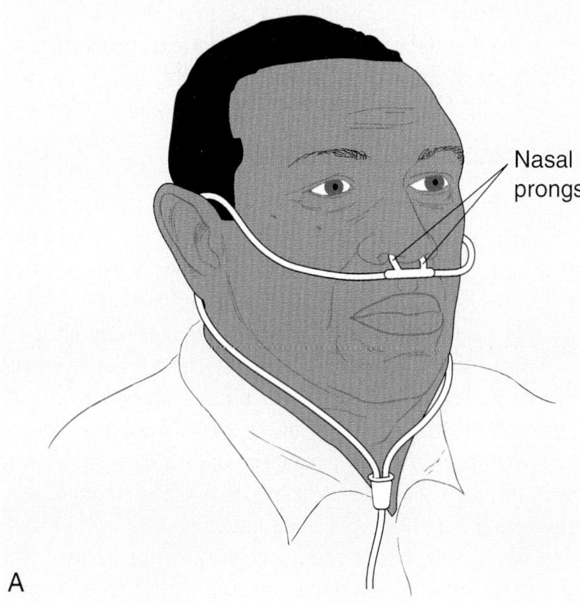

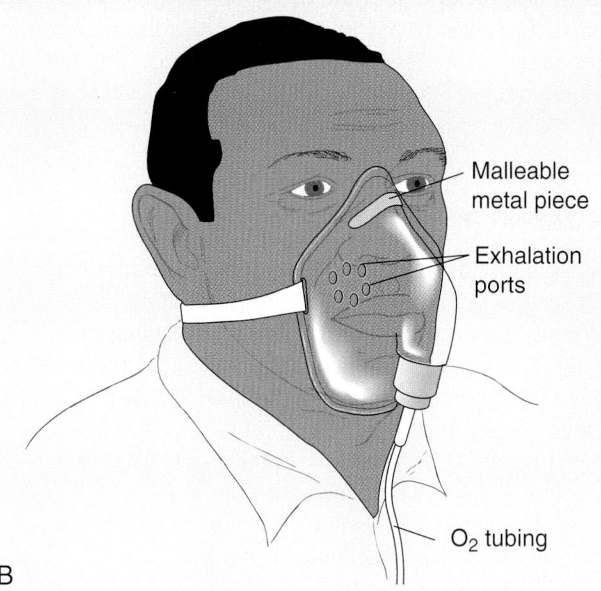

FACE MASK

This device is designed to fit snugly over the patient's mouth and nose and is secured in place with a strap over the back of the head (Illustration B). Oxygen tubing is attached to the mask for connection to the oxygen source. Exhalation ports on the sides of the mask allow outward flow of the patient's exhaled air. The face mask is used for short-term oxygen therapy for patients who do not require low-flow oxygen or precise concentrations of oxygen.

One common problem with oxygen delivery via face mask is that patients who need continuous oxygen therapy often receive only intermittent oxygen delivery because of frequent mask removal (Baxter et al, 1993). To ensure maximum effectiveness of oxygen therapy via face mask, the nurse should plan routine care to minimize the number of times the mask needs to be removed during the day; for example, provide mouth care immediately after a meal, when the mask is already off so that the patient can eat, to avoid the need to remove the mask again later.

PARTIAL NONREBREATHING MASK

This device is similar to a face mask but with a reservoir bag that provides a higher concentration of oxygen delivery (Illustration C). The bag should remain inflated at all

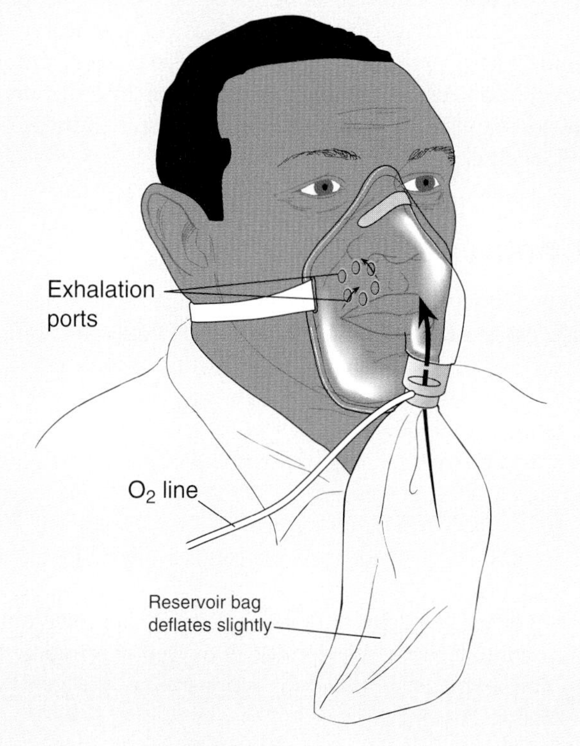

continued on next page

BOX 21-1 (cont'd)
METHODS OF OXYGEN DELIVERY

continued from previous page

times; deflation may cause the patient to breathe large amounts of exhaled carbon dioxide. Exhalation ports are frequently covered to enable the patient to draw all of the oxygen from the reservoir bag.

NONREBREATHING MASK

This device is similar to the partial nonrebreathing mask except for two features: a one-way valve between the mask and reservoir bag that prevents exhaled breath from entering the bag, and a one-way valve on the side-exhalation port that allows air to leave the mask during exhalation, while preventing room air from entering during inspiration (Illustration D). Therefore, the patient inspires pure oxygen from the reservoir bag and exhales through the exhalation port. This mask is used for short-term oxygen therapy for patients requiring high concentrations of oxygen.

VENTURI MASK

This mask has an adapter between the bottom of the mask and the gas source that permits air to mix with the oxygen, thus allowing precise delivery of oxygen (Illustration E). The Venturi mask is the most accurate device for delivering a prescribed amount of oxygen. Pure oxygen is inhaled from the flex tube and exhaled via the side exhalation port. The percentage of inspired oxygen concentration (FIO_2) is controlled by changing the size of the narrowed orifice at the base of the flex tube.

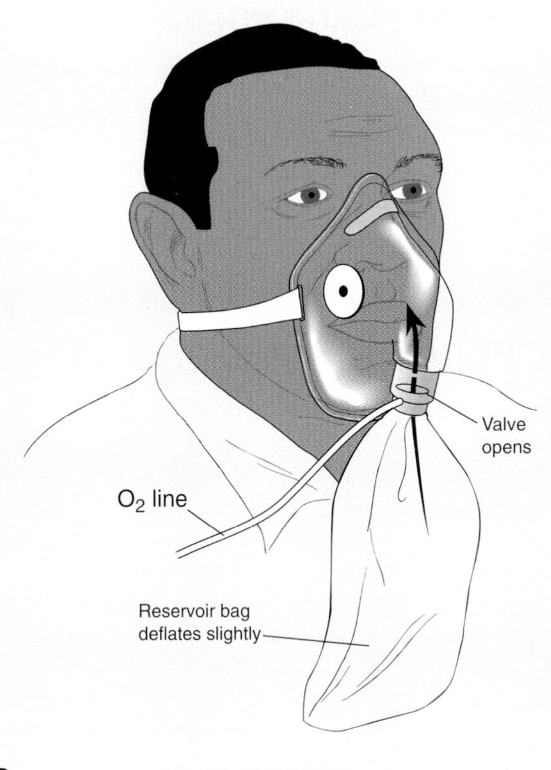

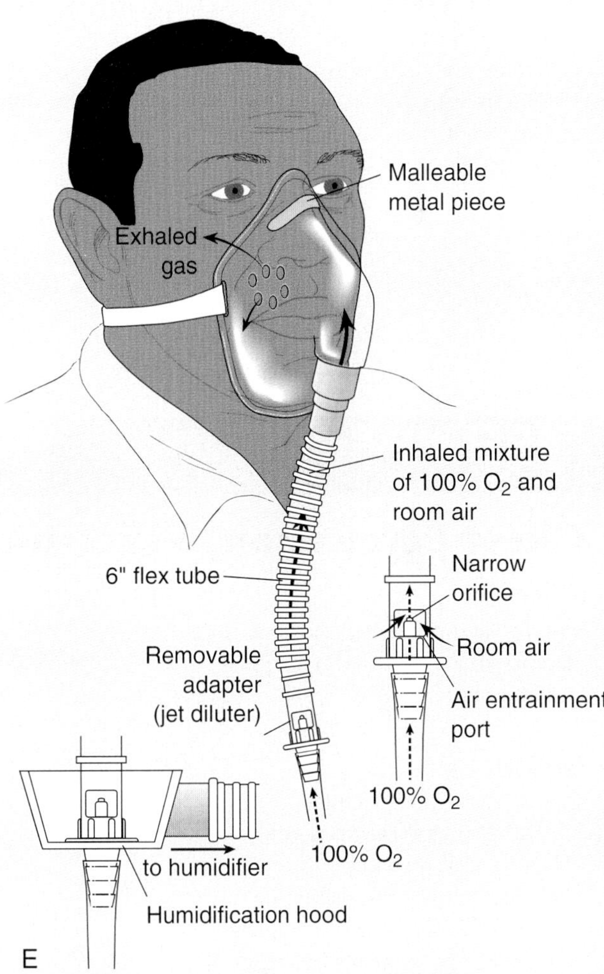

- Motivation for change is directly related to the value of the outcome.
- Active learning is more likely to be remembered and transferred to other learning experiences.
- Some learning experiences need to be reinforced so that the learner can gain maximum results. (See Chapter 13, Patient and Family Education, for more information on teaching and learning concepts.)

Pulmonary rehabilitation programs have been most successful in helping patients manage their respiratory conditions when these guidelines are followed:

- If the patient pursues an upper-body weight training program and outdoor walking to improve respiratory function, the nurse must emphasize the importance of complying with the regimen, as well as the importance of alternating exercise with rest (Sassi-Dambron et al, 1994).

- The nurse should encourage the patient to try an exercise program aimed at increasing the strength and endurance of the arm and leg muscles in an effort to reduce dyspnea. The nurse should emphasize that such exercises will be more effective if they are augmented by walking with the arms supported and the arms are rested periodically (Lake et al, 1990; Simpson et al, 1992).
- The nurse should encourage the patient to sustain an exercise program for best results. Optimum improvement of respiratory endurance and decrease in dyspnea results from muscle training programs lasting more than 6 months (Kim et al, 1993).
- A patient who uses an aerosol MDI needs repeated instruction in its use (De Blaquiere et al, 1989; Thompson et al, 1994). If the patient is elderly and/or suffering from impaired hand grip, someone in the family should be taught how to administer the inhaled medication. The most effective teaching programs combine printed instructions, a video demonstration, and supervised practice sessions (Corbett, 1992).

Procedures

MOBILIZING PULMONARY SECRETIONS

Procedure 21–1 outlines the techniques for chest percussion, vibration, and postural drainage. Procedure 21–2 discusses how to help a patient use incentive spirometry.

CLEARING THE AIRWAY

Procedure 21–3 presents guidelines for teaching a patient the deep-breathing and controlled coughing technique. Procedure 21–4 covers the forced expiration technique. Procedure 21–5 presents the steps in nasopharyngeal suctioning, oropharyngeal (Yankauer) suctioning, tracheobronchial suctioning, and endotracheal and tracheostomy tube suctioning.

OXYGENATING THE SYSTEM

Procedure 21–6 presents guidelines for the safe and effective administration of oxygen.

REDUCING THE EFFORT OF BREATHING

Procedure 21–7 presents guidelines for assisting patients with pursed-lip breathing.

PROCEDURE 21-1

Chest Percussion, Vibration, and Postural Drainage

Objective

Mobilize and facilitate removal of secretions, thereby improving ventilation and oxygenation.

Terminology

percussion—the striking of the chest wall with cupped hands using firm pressure.

postural drainage—positioning of patient to facilitate the drainage of the lung segments by means of gravity.

vibration—fine shaking pressure applied to the chest wall only during exhalation.

Critical Elements

This procedure is usually ordered by the physician. It may be performed by nursing staff, respiratory staff, or trained family members. Refer to your facility's policy before proceeding. The total time for treatment may take as long as 30 minutes.

It is often recommended that postural drainage, percussion, and vibration be performed immediately after a respiratory treatment. The medications used in these treatments will often cause bronchodilation, therefore facilitating the removal of secretions.

Before performing these respiratory treatments, a complete respiratory assessment should be done. This should include an evaluation of lung sounds, respiratory rate and effort, color, oximetry readings (if applicable), and presence of secretions. The respiratory assessment should be done again after the treatment as well as every 8 hours or whenever necessary. In addition, the care provider should assess the patient's vital signs, medications, and medical condition. The following precautions should be followed:

- The use of these treatments for some patients receiving medications affecting hemodynamic status may be contraindicated.
- Postural drainage is contraindicated for patients with increased intracranial pressure or spinal injuries.
- Chest percussion is contraindicated for patients with fractured ribs, severe osteoporosis, or bleeding disorders.
- If hemoptysis occurs, the treatment should be stopped immediately and the physician notified.

continued on next page

PROCEDURE 21-1 (cont'd)

Postural drainage is the act of positioning the patient in a variety of possible positions, depending on their respiratory assessment, to facilitate the removal of secretions using gravity. Not all positions are needed for each patient. Review of the patient's chest x-ray film or the results of lung auscultation should guide which positions to use. Postural drainage is usually used in conjunction with percussion and vibration. The patient should remain in each position used for 5 to 10 minutes. The positions used for drainage of the various lung segments include (Fig. 21–3):

- Right upper lobe, anterior segment—supine with head raised on pillows

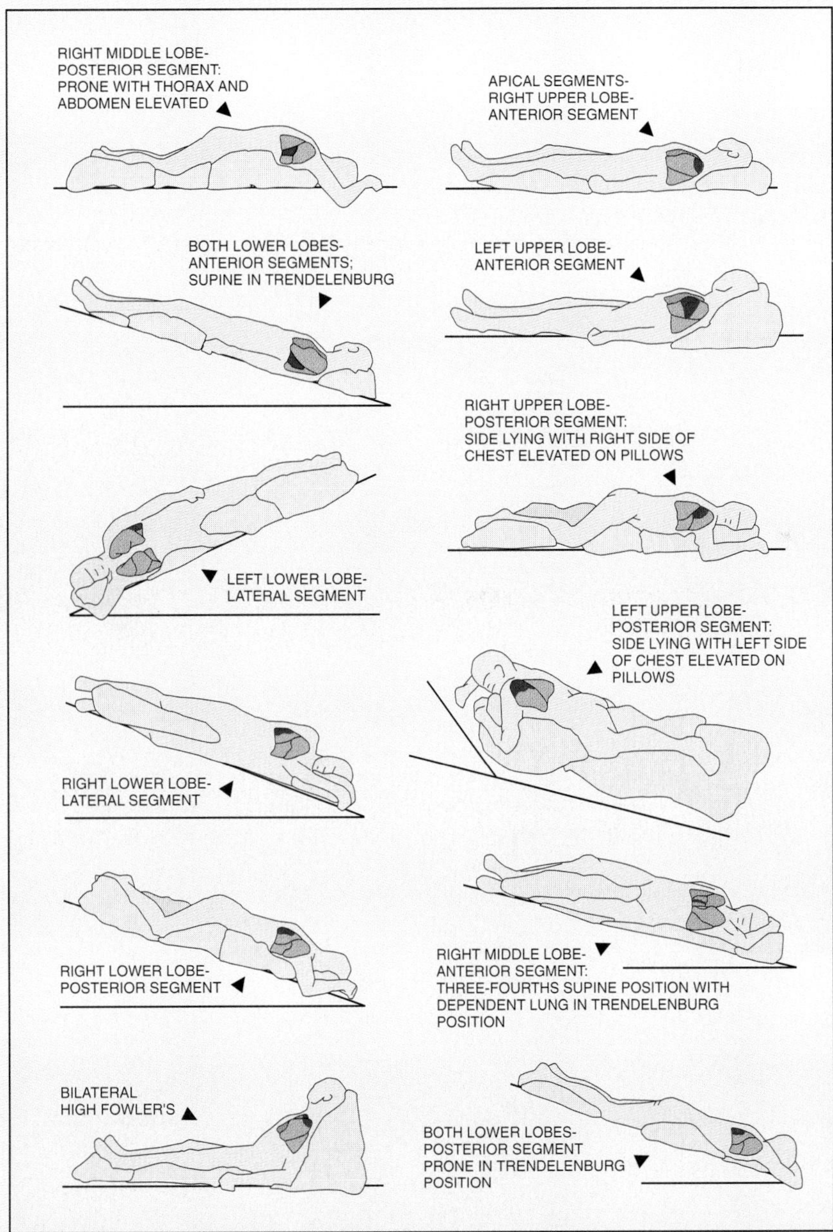

Figure 21–3. Patient positioning to drain specific bronchial segments.

continued on next page

PROCEDURE 21–1 (cont'd)

- Right upper lobe, posterior segment—left side with head elevated on pillows
- Left upper lobe, anterior segment—supine with head elevated
- Left upper lobe, posterior segment—right side with head elevated
- Right middle lobe, anterior segment—slight tilt to the left while in Trendelenburg position
- Right middle lobe, posterior segment—prone with body elevated off the bed at the waist with pillows
- Lower lobes, anterior—supine while in Trendelenburg position
- Lower lobes, posterior—prone while in Trendelenburg position
- Left lower lobe, lateral segment—right side while in Trendelenburg position
- Right lower lobe, lateral segment—left while in Trendelenburg position
- Right lower lobe, posterior segment—prone with slight tilt to left while in Trendelenburg position

Percussion is done with cupped hands. The care provider cups the hands, with finger and thumb touching the palm of hand forming the cup (Fig. 21–4). The hands alternate action and create a hollow popping sound and firmly slap the patient's chest for periods of 1 to 2 minutes. Care should be taken not to do percussion over any areas of clothing with zippers, buttons, or any other item that may cause injury.

Vibration is done with the hands placed with the palms down on the patient's chest (Fig. 21–5). As the patient exhales, the hands, using mostly the heel of the hand, vibrate downward over the lung segment.

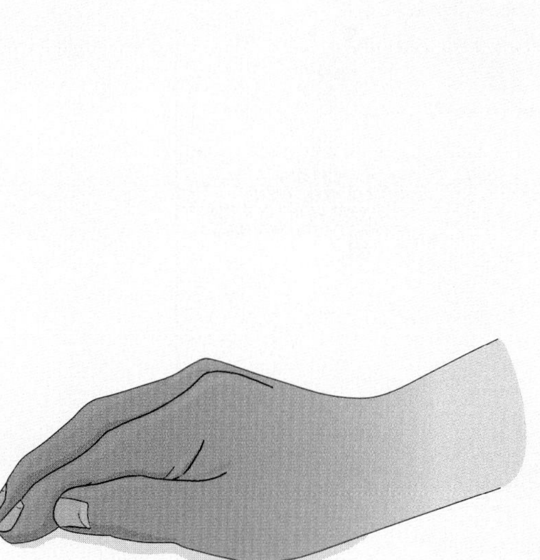

Figure 21–4. Proper cupping of hand for chest percussion.

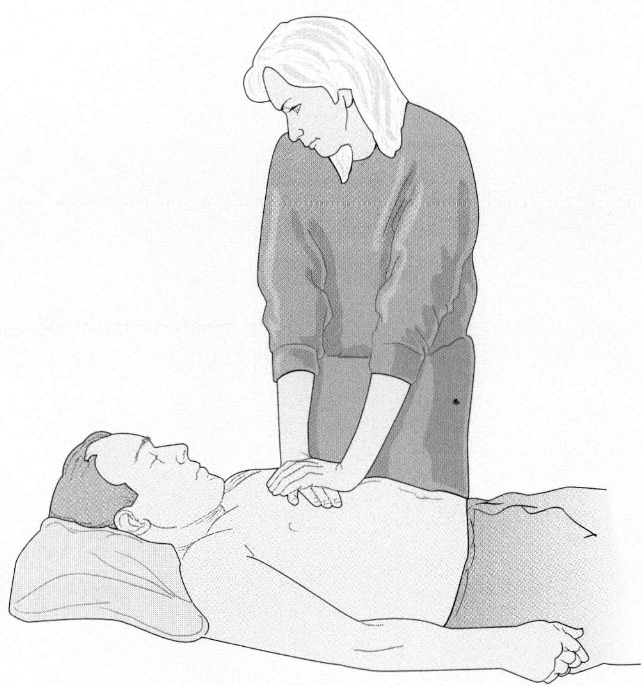

Figure 21–5. Hand positioning for chest vibration.

This procedure is done only during exhalation.

Equipment

Pillows
Bath blanket
Tissues
Emesis basin
Stethoscope
Manual percussion cup (if desired)
Mechanical hand vibrator (if desired)

Special Considerations

To protect the patient, percussion and vibration should not be done over the patient's bare skin. It should be done with one layer of clothing (such as patient gown or T-shirt) in place. These procedures should not

continued on next page

PROCEDURE 21-1 (cont'd)

be done over areas of bony prominence (such as scapula or sternum) or areas easily injured such as the breasts and kidneys.

These respiratory treatments should be scheduled before meal time or at least 2 hours after meal time. Doing them while the patient has a full stomach may cause nausea and vomiting. If the patient is receiving tube feedings, the treatment should be scheduled 2 hours after feeding.

The care provider should evaluate the patient's cognitive function before proceeding. The patient should be able to understand and follow directions to work with the care provider in the administration and successful completion of these treatments.

Action	*Rationale*
1. Verify order.	1. Ensures correct procedure is done.
2. Assemble supplies.	2. Promotes task organization.
3. Identify patient.	3. Provides for patient safety.
4. Explain procedure.	4. Promotes patient compliance.
5. Close door or pull curtain.	5. Maintains patient privacy and dignity.
6. Remove or loosen top linen and cover patient with bath blanket.	6. Allows freedom to position patient.
7. Place patient in position to drain indicated lung segments.	7. Ensures correct position is used to drain congested lung segments.
8. Perform percussion over indicated lung segment for 1 to 2 minutes (Fig. 21–6).	8. Loosens secretions.
9. Perform vibration over indicated lung segment for five exhalations.	9. Mobilizes secretions and assists with expectoration.
10. Allow patient to remain in postural drainage position for 5 to 10 minutes.	10. Facilitates drainage of secretions.
11. Change position to treat next indicated lung segment and repeat percussion, vibration, and drainage.	11. Ensures all indicated lung segments are treated.
12. Return patient to position of comfort and replace top linens.	12. Provides for patient comfort, dignity, and warmth.

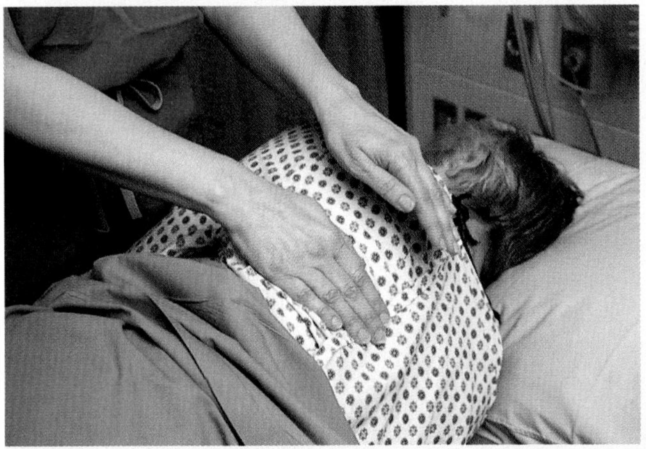

Figure 21–6. Percussion technique.

continued on next page

PROCEDURE 21-1 (cont'd)

Documentation

Record in the patient record the procedure and the patient's response. Record which lung segments were treated and the results. Include a description of the color, consistency, odor, and amount of any sputum produced. Also record the complete respiratory assessment before and after the treatment.

Elements of Patient Teaching

Instruct the patient/family regarding the purpose of the procedure. If the family will be assisting the patient with the procedure, review all safety measures, comfort measures, and contraindications involved. Also provide the family with an opportunity to perform the procedure with the care provider's supervision to assess the family's competency level.

PROCEDURES 21-2

Incentive Spirometry

Objective

Improve ventilation and oxygenation while mobilizing secretions

Terminology

atelectasis—a collapse of lung tissue that prevents exchange of oxygen and carbon dioxide.

incentive spirometer (ICS)—device for measuring the rate and volume of breathing that encourages voluntary deep breathing by providing visual feedback to users.

pulse oximetry—measures arterial blood saturation by means of a sensor usually attached to the finger.

sustained maximal inspiration—the longest length of time that the patient can inhale and hold a breath.

Critical Elements

The use of the incentive spirometer often requires a physician's order. Refer to your facility's policy before proceeding. This device may also be known as a sustained maximal inspiration device (SMI). It has proven very effective in mobilizing secretions and helping prevent atelectasis and pneumonia, particularly for postoperative patients (Thomas and McIntosh, 1994). The device is either flow oriented or volume oriented. The flow-oriented device requires less effort to raise the balls or disc in the plastic chamber and is often for single use and taken home by the patient after discharge. The volume-oriented spirometer has a preset volume and permits slower, more sustained inspirations. It can be either disposable or nondisposable.

The most effective use of the incentive spirometer for postoperative patients is to teach the use of the device before surgery. The patient and family should be instructed regarding the purpose and use of the incentive spirometer at a time when they will be able to focus on the instructions and practice with the device. The patient should be able to understand and follow the instructions regarding the use of this device.

Before using the incentive spirometer, the patient should be placed in an upright position to facilitate maximum ventilation. To use the device, the patient should be able to inspire and hold a breath for 5 seconds to achieve effective lung expansion. The patient should be encouraged to use the incentive spirometer at least ten times each hour.

The care provider should assess the patient's lung sounds, respiratory effort, color, and pulse oximetry (if applicable) before use of the incentive spirometer and every 8 hours and whenever necessary thereafter. If the patient's inspiratory capacity is known, a value of about one half to three fourths of the normal value serves as a realistic goal.

With patients who have reduced tidal volumes, it may take three to five sustained inspirations to find a maximum preset goal for each practice session. After the goal is established the patient should try to reach the goal ten times each session. Resting between attempts helps avoid fatigue and hyperventilation.

continued on next page

PROCEDURE 21-2 (cont'd)

Equipment

Incentive spirometer
Stethoscope

Special Considerations

Patients wearing dentures should have the dentures in place before using the incentive spirometer.

If the patient is unable to perform mouth breathing, the use of a nose clip may be required to successfully use the spirometer.

The care provider may need to assist if the patient is unable to hold the device in an upright position because the device will not function properly unless positioned correctly.

The mouthpiece of the incentive spirometer should be washed daily to reduce the possibility of contamination with microorganisms.

Action	*Rationale*
1. Verify order (if applicable).	1. Ensures correct procedure is done.
2. Assemble equipment.	2. Promotes task organization.
3. Identify patient.	3. Provides for patient safety.
4. Explain procedure.	4. Promotes patient compliance.
5. Position patient in upright position.	5. Promotes maximum inspiratory effort.
6. Instruct patient to exhale completely and seal lips around mouthpiece of incentive spirometer.	6. Ensures good seal for proper use of incentive spirometer.
7. Instruct patient to breathe in slowly to raise the balls or piston in the chamber. Have patient inhale until goal is reached, then hold breath for at least 3 seconds, then exhale slowly (Fig. 21–7).	7. Maintains maximum inspiration and reduces risk of progressive collapse of individual alveoli.

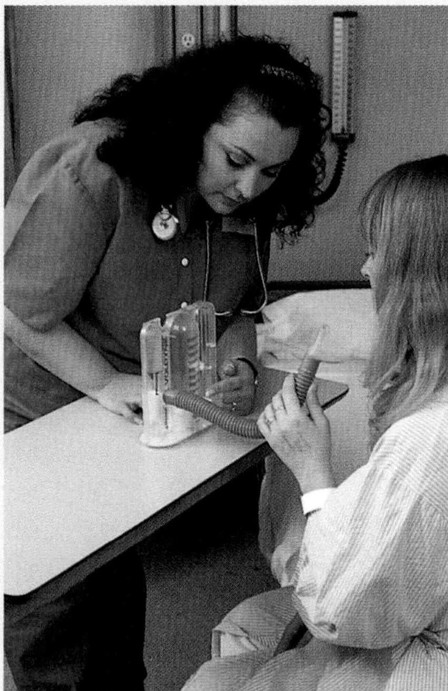

Figure 21–7. Using a disposable volume incentive spirometer.

continued on next page

PROCEDURE 21-2 (cont'd)

8. Have patient remove device from mouth and breathe normally for a short period.	8. Prevents hyperventilation.
9. After patient has reached maximum volume goal, instruct patient to repeat breathing exercise with incentive spirometer at least 10 times, with interspersed periods of normal breathing.	9. Provides for maximum inspiration while preventing hyperventilation.
10. Encourage patient to remove mouthpiece and try to cough productively.	10. Mobilizes secretions that may be present due to atelectasis.
11. Leave incentive spirometer within easy reach for patient at end of procedure. Encourage patient to repeat procedure every hour while awake.	11. Facilitates patient independence with procedure.
12. Return patient to position of comfort.	12. Provides safe, comfortable environment.

Documentation

Record in the patient record the respiratory assessment as well as the time of the procedure, maximum effort attained, and the patient's response.

Elements of Patient Teaching

Instruct the patient/family in the purpose and steps to use in the procedure. Allow the patient to do the procedure several times with the care provider to assess competency. Providing preoperative instruction with the incentive spirometer provides optimal teaching.

PROCEDURE 21-3

Deep Breathing and Controlled Coughing

Objective

Improve ventilation and oxygenation while mobilizing secretions and reducing risk of atelectasis.

Terminology

atelectasis—collapse of lung tissue that prevents exchange of oxygen and carbon dioxide.

pulse oximetry—measures arterial blood saturation by means of a sensor usually attached to the finger.

Critical Elements

Because this procedure is often used with postoperative patients, it is important to assess the patient's comfort level and administer pain medication as indicated before deep breathing and controlled coughing.

Splinting should be taught to the patient before deep breathing and controlled coughing to reduce the pain experienced during this procedure for the postoperative patient who has had abdominal or thoracic surgery. Splinting may be performed with a pillow or with a folded small blanket. The pillow or blanket is placed over the patient's surgical site and pressure is applied very gently by crossing the patient's arms over the pillow/blanket or by pressing with the hands. This prevents a rebounding effect at the site when the patient coughs, which in turn prevents additional discomfort.

The patient's lung sounds, respiratory effort, color, and pulse oximetry (if applicable) should be assessed before the procedure. Assessment of these parameters should continue at least every 4 hours and whenever necessary (for the immediate postoperative patient) and at least every 8 hours for all other patients. Any sputum produced should be assessed for color, consistency, odor, and amount.

Equipment

Tissues
Emesis basin
Small pillow or blanket (for splinting)

continued on next page

PROCEDURE 21-3 (cont'd)

Special Considerations

Deep breathing and controlled coughing are usually performed together. If no secretions are present, the controlled coughing portion may not be necessary. The presence of secretions should be reassessed frequently.

Action	*Rationale*
1. Identify patient.	1. Provides for patient safety.
2. Explain procedure.	2. Promotes patient compliance.
3. Position patient in upright position if possible. Use splinting as necessary. Provide patient with tissue or emesis basin for mucus expectoration.	3. Facilitates diaphragmatic excursion.
4. Have patient inhale slowly and deeply through the nose until the lungs are filled as much as possible.	4. Prevents hyperventilation.
5. Have patient hold breath for at least 3 seconds, then instruct patient to exhale slowly.	5. Allows air to distribute to all areas of the lungs before exhaling.
6. Repeat deep breathing two more times.	6. Improves ventilation and oxygenation.
7. As third breath is being expelled, have patient cough two or three times in succession, with mouth open, using abdomen (not throat). Repeat two or three times (Fig. 21–8).	7. Mobilizes mucus more effectively and completely than one forceful cough.

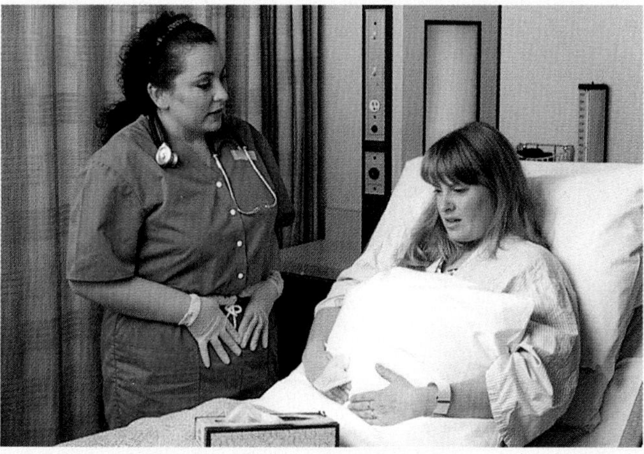

Figure 21–8. Splinting the abdomen with a pillow while coughing.

Action	*Rationale*
8. Instruct patient to rest after two or three times and to breathe normally for several minutes before repeating controlled coughing.	8. Reduces discomfort and prevents fatigue.
9. Deep breathing should be repeated 10 times every 2 hours while awake until patient ambulates unassisted. Coughing should be repeated two or three times every 2 hours while awake.	9. Prevents postoperative atelectasis.
10. Return patient to position of comfort.	10. Conserves energy.

continued on next page

PROCEDURE 21-3 (cont'd)

Documentation

Record in the patient record the procedure, the patient's response to the procedure, and results of coughing. Describe any sputum by color, consistency, odor, and amount. Also record the patient's respiratory assessment.

Elements of Patient Teaching

Instruct patient/family regarding purpose and technique of the procedure. Assist until patient is able to perform procedure independently. If family will be assisting patient, the care provider should supervise the patient and family until confirming independent competency.

PROCEDURE 21-4

Forced Exhalation Technique (Huffing)

Objective

Improve exhalation portion of ventilation cycle while mobilizing secretions.

Terminology

bronchiectasis—condition of the bronchial tree in which there is irreversible dilatation and destruction of the bronchial walls; it is characterized by a productive cough and copious sputum.

glottis—opening between vocal cords.

pulse oximetry—measures arterial blood saturation by means of a sensor usually attached to the finger.

Critical Elements

Forced exhalation technique is useful for patients with cystic fibrosis and bronchiectasis due to the copious amount of thick sputum produced in these diseases. It is also helpful to many patients with chronic obstructive pulmonary disease (COPD).

The forced exhalation technique consists of one or two forceful expiratory efforts, or "huffs," made with an open glottis at mid to low lung volume. After huffing, the patient should rest and perform abdominal breathing.

The care provider should assess the patient's lung sounds, respiratory effort, color, mucus production, and pulse oximetry (if applicable) before the forced exhalation procedure and every 8 hours and whenever necessary afterward.

Equipment

Tissues
Emesis basin

Special Considerations

Huffing can be used during postural drainage to increase the efficiency of sputum removal.

Action	*Rationale*
1. Identify patient.	1. Provides for patient safety.
2. Explain procedure.	2. Promotes patient compliance.
3. Position patient in sitting position leaning slightly forward. Provide patient with tissues and emesis basin for expectoration.	3. Promotes optimal lung expansion.
4. Instruct patient to take a deep breath and then exhale forcefully with the mouth and throat open and with firm contraction of the abdominal muscles, making a "huffing" sound.	4. Facilitates mucus drainage and expectoration because "huff" causes less airway compression than a cough.
5. Instruct patient to relax by dropping shoulders and letting arms fall limp in lap.	5. Prevents uncontrolled coughing and worsening bronchospasm.

continued on next page

PROCEDURE 21-4 (cont'd)

6. Instruct patient to take slow breaths using abdominal muscles.	6. Increases strength, coordination, and efficiency of respiratory muscles.
7. Repeat "huffing," interspersed with slow abdominal breathing.	7. Promotes mobilization of mucus.
8. Return patient to position of comfort.	8. Provides for patient comfort.

Documentation

Record in the patient record the time of the procedure and the patient's response. Record the sputum produced describing the color, consistency, odor, and amount. The care provider's assessment of lung sounds, respiratory effort, color, and pulse oximetry (if applicable) should also be recorded.

Elements of Patient Teaching

Instruct the patient/family regarding the purpose and steps for performing the procedure. Observe the patient and coach as necessary to promote competency and independent performance. The family may serve as a coach for this procedure once the care provider determines competency level.

PROCEDURE 21-5

Suctioning (Oropharyngeal, Tracheobronchial, Endotracheal, and Tracheostomy Tube)

Objective

Remove mucus from airway passages resulting in improved gas exchange and decreased risk of infection.

Terminology

cuff—an inflatable balloon-like part of the tracheostomy or endotracheal tube that is bonded to the distal end of the tube; when inflated with air, the cuff stabilizes the tube in the center of the trachea and seals the airway so that all air movement is through the tube.

endotracheal tube (ET)—plastic artificial airway that is inserted by a physician (or specially trained person) through the patient's mouth or nose past the epiglottis and vocal cords into the trachea (Fig. 21–9).

hyperoxygenation—increased oxygen delivery to the patient before and between suctioning.

oxygen flowmeter—a calibrated device that measures and controls the liter flow of oxygen to the patient.

suction catheter—plastic disposable catheter with small eyelets on one end through which secretions enter when suction is applied. Designed with a vented device on the opposite end that controls the amount of suction.

tracheostomy tube (TT)—artificial airway made of metal or plastic inserted by a physician directly into the trachea through a small incision in the patient's neck (Fig. 21–10).

Yankauer catheter—a rigid, minimally flexible plastic device with one large and several small eyelets at one end used to remove oropharyngeal secretions (Fig. 21–11).

Critical Elements

A physician's order may be necessary for this procedure. Refer to your facility's policy before beginning.

Suctioning of the tracheobronchial tree is considered a last resort in the management of tracheobronchial secretions. Every effort should be made by the care provider to ensure that the patient turns, coughs, and deep breathes so secretions do not accumulate. If secretions do accumulate, it is important to have the patient expectorate. If the patient's condition does not permit adequate self-management of secretions, suctioning must be performed.

continued on next page

PROCEDURE 21–5 (cont'd)

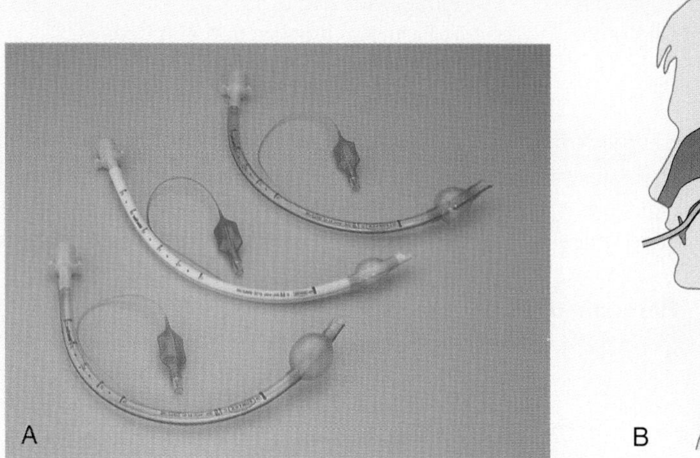

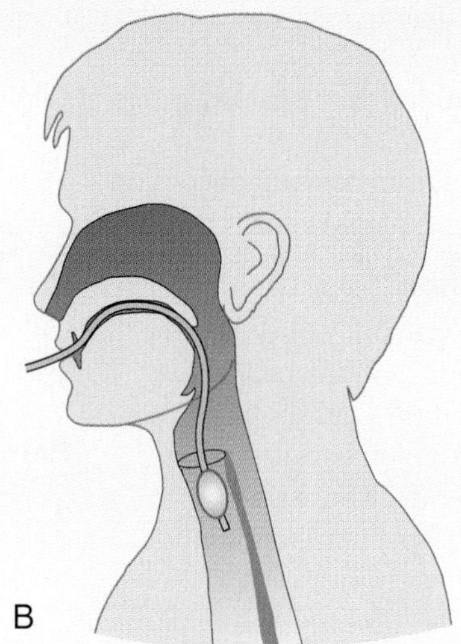

Figure 21–9. Endotracheal tube (A) and proper tube placement (B). (A, courtesy of Sims Portex, Inc.)

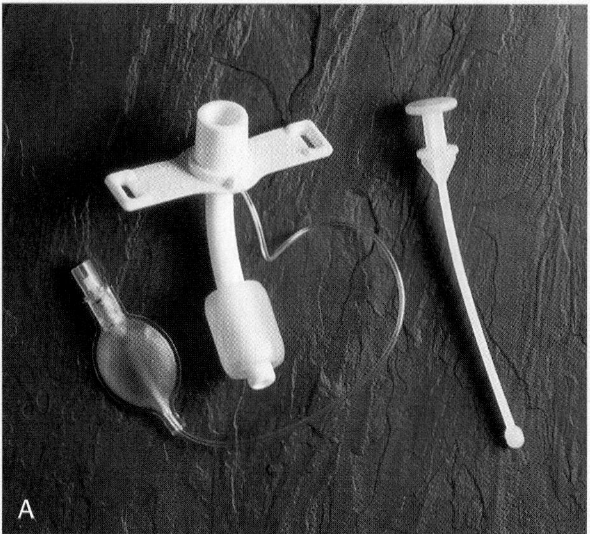

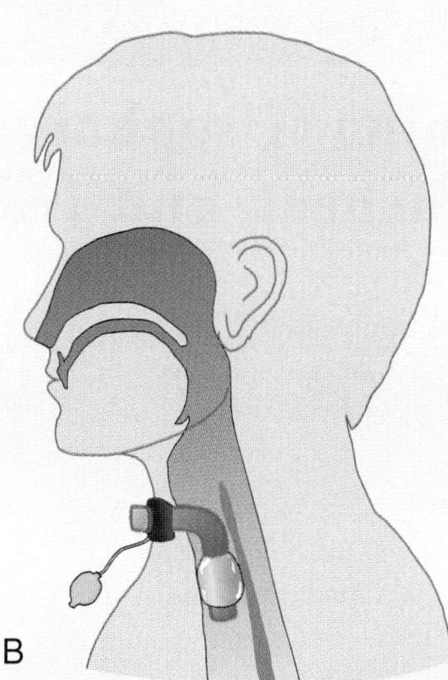

Figure 21–10. Single-lumen tracheostomy tube (A) and proper tube placement (B). (A, courtesy of Shiley Tracheostomy Products, Mallinckrodt, Inc.)

Suctioning of the pharynx through the nose or the mouth (oropharyngeal) is necessary when patients are able to cough but are not able to expectorate the secretions. Suctioning of the trachea is necessary for patients with excessive secretions who are unable to cough.

A sterile suctioning procedure is always used when the oropharynx is suctioned and a clean suctioning procedure is used for the mouth because the mouth is considered clean whereas the oropharynx is considered sterile. When suctioning both areas, always suction the oropharynx first and the mouth last.

The entire suctioning procedure should be performed quickly and should take no longer than 15 seconds. Because the air does not reach the patient during the actual suctioning procedure, the patient may become hypoxic if suctioning is performed over a longer period of time.

continued on next page

PROCEDURE 21-5 (cont'd)

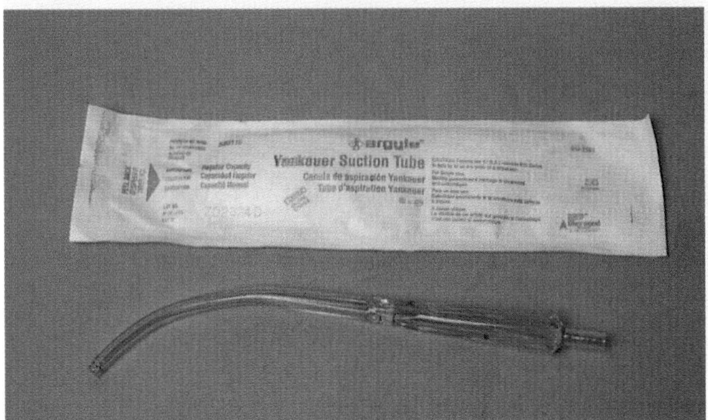

Figure 21–11. Yankauer suction catheter.

Never apply suction during the insertion process because this could damage delicate mucous membranes. Once the catheter is in place, suction can be applied and the catheter can be slowly withdrawn with a rotating motion.

A complete respiratory assessment should be done on the patient before and after suctioning. This should include vital signs, lungs sounds, respiratory rate and effort, color, oximetry readings (if applicable), and presence of secretions. The patient should be assessed at least every 4 hours and whenever necessary.

Mask and goggles are recommended for the care provider to provide protection from contact with secretions that may be expelled in droplet form or splattered by coughing during the procedure.

Equipment

Yankauer catheter (if applicable)
Suction catheter (if applicable)
Sterile or clean gloves (as indicated)
Tap water or sterile water (as indicated)
Sterile or nonsterile basin (as indicated)
Water-soluble lubricant (as indicated)
Wall or portable suction
Connecting tubing

Special Considerations

If secretions are very thick, tracheal lavage may be used. Using this method, approximately 5 ml of sterile saline is introduced into the trachea immediately before suctioning, which assists in loosening the secretions for more effective removal.

Caution should be used when suctioning patients with head injury, increased intracranial pressure, or hypertension because episodes of hypoxemia and vagal stimulation may lead to cardiac arrhythmias.

Suctioning can cause stimulation of the mucous membranes, which may in turn produce more secretions. Therefore, suction the patient only as indicated or as ordered to avoid this problem. For adults, suction pressure should not exceed 120 to 150 mm Hg to avoid unnecessary trauma to the respiratory passages.

Closed suction systems are now available. With this type of system, the care provider never touches the catheter, which is usually encased inside a thin plastic cover. The catheter may be used for up to 24 hours before being changed and is often indicated for patients with tracheostomy or endotracheal tubes who require frequent suctioning. Always read the manufacturer's instructions before use. When choosing the size of the suction catheter, it is important that the catheter does not occlude more than half of the lumen of the tracheostomy or endotracheal tube. When the cuff is inflated the only air movement is through the tracheostomy or the endotracheal tube; therefore, patency becomes critical.

If oxygen therapy is removed to suction the patient, it may be necessary to replace the oxygen between catheter insertions to help prevent

continued on next page

PROCEDURE 21-5 (cont'd)

suction-induced hypoxia. Always be sure to replace oxygen therapy at the appropriate flow rate when the suctioning procedure is completed. Patients who are ventilator dependent may need to be hyperoxygenated before suctioning. This procedure should be performed with caution if the patient has a large amount of secretions because it may cause secretions to be driven farther into the respiratory passages. Refer to your facility's policy regarding this procedure.

A Yankauer catheter may be cleansed by soaking in hydrogen peroxide. Thoroughly rinse the catheter after cleansing and before use.

Action	***Rationale***
1. Verify order.	1. Ensures correct procedure is done.
2. Assemble the equipment.	2. Promotes task organization.
3. Identify patient.	3. Provides for patient safety.
4. Explain procedure.	4. Promotes patient compliance.

Oropharyngeal (Yankauer) Suctioning

1. Don gloves.	1. Protects care provider from contact with blood and body fluids.
2. Fill nonsterile container with tap water.	2. Provides means to flush catheter.
3. Turn on suction device and set regulator to appropriate setting. Connect one end of tubing to suction setup and other end to Yankauer (Fig 21–12).	3. Reduces risk of trauma to oral mucosa from inappropriately high suction settings.

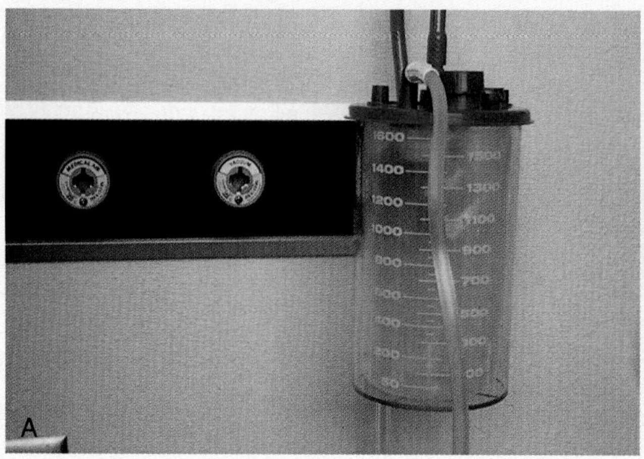

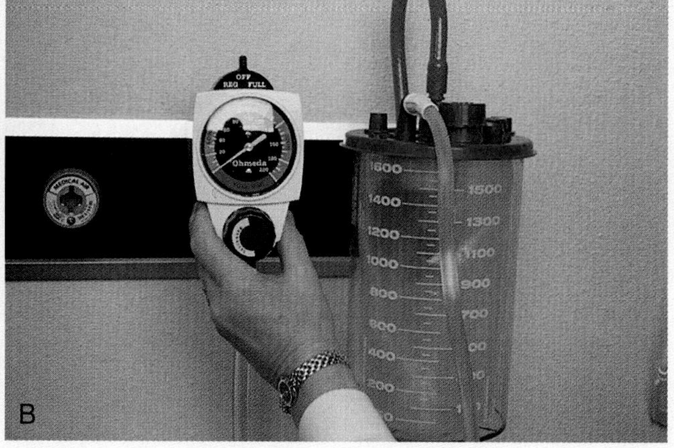

Figure 21–12. Connecting suction catheter to wall suction unit.

4. Insert Yankauer catheter into mouth between base of teeth and tongue and toward pharynx area and manipulate catheter tip around interior of mouth until secretions are removed (Fig. 21–13).	4. Removes secretions from oral cavity.
5. Encourage patient to cough between suctioning attempts.	5. Mobilizes secretions and brings them into mouth and pharynx for removal.
6. Place suction tip in water and rinse.	6. Clears secretions from inside of Yankauer catheter.
7. Discard or return equipment to appropriate place.	7. Maintains clean, organized work area.

continued on next page

PROCEDURE 21-5 (cont'd)

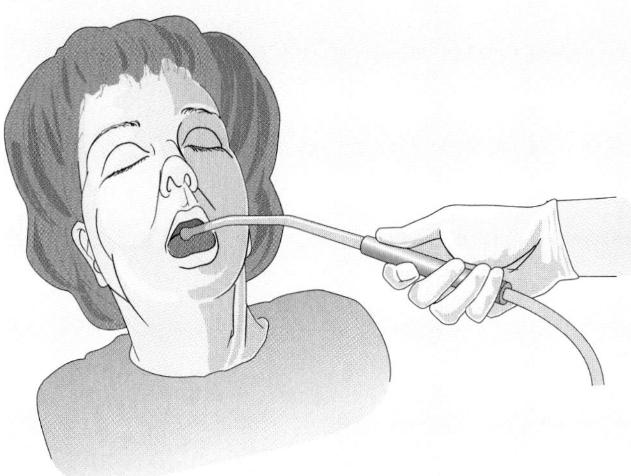

Figure 21–13. Technique for oropharyngeal suctioning.

Tracheobronchial Suctioning

1. Turn on suction device and set regulator to appropriate setting.

1. Reduces risk of trauma to trachea and bronchi from inappropriately high suction settings.

2. Before removing oxygen, hyperoxygenate if indicated.

2. Decreases chance of suction-induced hypoxia.

3. Prepare suction equipment:
   a. Set up sterile container touching only outside and add sterile water.
   b. Open suction catheter package leaving catheter inside so that it touches only sterile packaging.
   c. Squeeze lubricant onto end of catheter.
   d. Place sterile drape or clean towel across patient's chest.

3. Prepares areas for suction procedure.

4. Don sterile gloves.

Note: Dominant hand will remain sterile, and nondominant hand will function in clean capacity.

4. Protects patient's airways from contamination from microorganisms.

5. Using aseptic technique, pick up suction catheter with dominant hand and connecting tubing with nondominant hand. Connect tubing to suction catheter with nondominant hand.

5. Maintains sterility of suction catheter.

6. Assess function of suction catheter by suctioning small amount of water.

6. Ensures suction is functioning appropriately.

7. With distal end of catheter covered in water-soluble lubricant and holding catheter in dominant hand, insert catheter into patient's nare using a slight downward slant or through mouth when patient inhales. Do not apply suction during insertion process (Fig. 21–14).

7. Introduces catheter into air passages and decreases risk of hypoxia by not using suction during insertion.

8. Insert catheter approximately 16 cm for pharyngeal suctioning and another 4 to 6 cm for tracheal suction of an adult.

8. Provides access to areas where secretions have pooled for maximum airway clearance.

continued on next page

PROCEDURE 21-5 (cont'd)

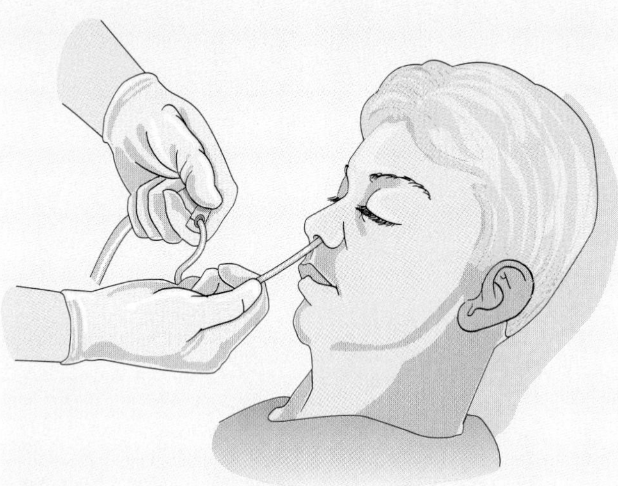

Figure 21–14. Technique for tracheobronchial suctioning.

9. Apply intermittent suction with nondominant hand while rotating and pulling catheter out slowly.	9. Protects mucosa from injury by intermittent suction and rotation.
10. Encourage patient to cough between suction attempts.	10. Mobilizes secretions for more effective removal.
11. Replace oxygen (if applicable) or allow patient rest period before suctioning again.	11. Reduces risk of suction-induced hypoxemia.
12. Place tip of catheter in sterile water and rinse by applying suction and drawing water through catheter.	12. Removes secretions from inside of suction catheter.
13. Repeat process as needed to clear secretions.	13. Removes additional secretions from respiratory passages.
14. When pharyngeal or tracheal suction is complete, suction patient's mouth.	14. Removes upper airway secretions.
15. When suctioning is complete, hold catheter in dominant hand and pull glove off with catheter inside. Remove second glove and discard both.	15. Reduces risk of transmission of microorganisms on catheter to any other surface.
16. Discard and/or return equipment to appropriate place.	16. Maintains clean, organized work area.

Endotracheal and Tracheostomy Suctioning

1. Turn on suction device and set regulator to appropriate setting.	1. Reduces risk of trauma to trachea and bronchi from inappropriately high suction settings.
2. Prepare suction equipment: a. Set up sterile container touching only outside and add sterile water. b. Open suction catheter package leaving catheter inside so that it touches only sterile packaging. c. Squeeze lubricant onto end of catheter. d. Place sterile drape or clean towel across patient's chest.	2. Prepares area for suction procedure.
3. Don sterile gloves. *Note:* Dominant hand will remain sterile and nondominant hand will function in clean capacity.	3. Protects patient's airways from contamination from microorganisms.

continued on next page

PROCEDURE 21-5 (cont'd)

4. Using aseptic technique, pick up suction catheter with dominant hand and connecting tubing with nondominant hand. Connect tubing to suction catheter with nondominant hand.

4. Maintains sterility of suction catheter.

5. Assess function of suction catheter by suctioning small amount of water.

5. Ensures suction is functioning appropriately.

6. Using nondominant hand, remove oxygen tubing or humidity device. Hyperoxygenate if indicated.

6. Reduces risk of suction-induced hypoxia.

7. With distal end of catheter covered in water-soluble lubricant and holding catheter in dominant hand, gently insert catheter until tip of catheter touches tracheal wall (this will be felt as catheter meets resistance), then pull back 1 to 2 cm (Fig. 21–15).

7. Stimulates cough reflex that assists in mobilizing secretions.

8. Apply intermittent suction with nondominant hand while rotating and pulling catheter out slowly (Fig. 21–16).

8. Protects mucosa from injury by intermittent suction and rotation.

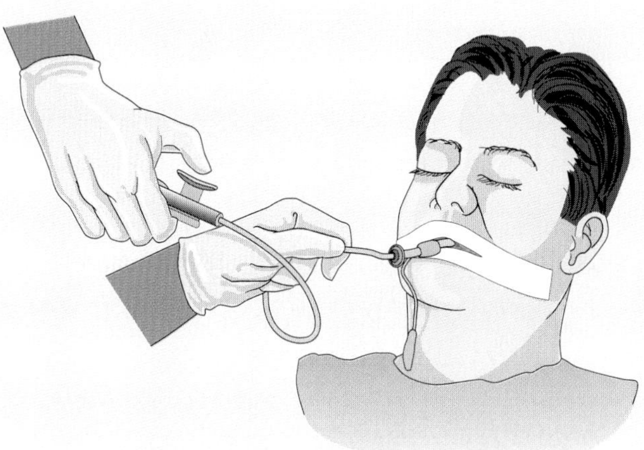

Figure 21–15. Inserting the suction catheter into the endotracheal tube.

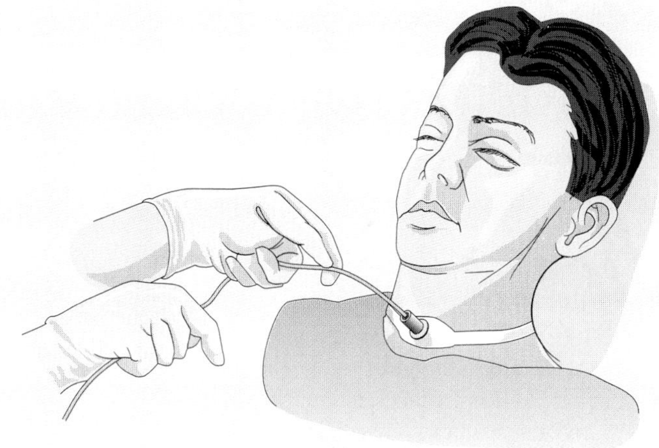

Figure 21–16. Suctioning a tracheostomy tube.

9. Encourage patient to cough between suction attempts.

9. Mobilizes secretions for more effective removal.

10. Replace oxygen (if applicable) or allow patient rest period before suctioning again.

10. Reduces risk of suction-induced hypoxemia.

11. Place tip of catheter in sterile water and rinse by applying suction and drawing water through catheter.

11. Removes secretions from inside of suction catheter.

12. Repeat process as needed to clear secretions.

12. Removes additional secretions from lower respiratory passages.

13. If indicated, suction secretions from pharyngeal and oral cavities.

13. Removes secretions from upper airways.

14. Reattach any oxygen or ventilator equipment as indicated.

14. Prevents hypoxia.

continued on next page

PROCEDURE 21-5 (cont'd)

15. Holding suction catheter in dominant hand, remove glove keeping catheter inside glove. Remove nondominant glove and discard both.	15. Reduces risk of transmission of microorganisms on catheter to any other surface.
16. Discard or return equipment to appropriate area.	16. Maintains clean, organized work area.

Documentation

Record in the patient record the procedure, the complete respiratory assessment, and the patient's response. Include a description of the color, consistency, and amount of secretions obtained.

Elements of Patient Teaching

Instruct the patient/family regarding the steps and purpose of the procedure. Reassure the patient/family about removal of any oxygen or ventilator equipment during the procedure. If Yankauer suctioning is used, and the patient is able to perform the suctioning procedure independently, supervise the procedure until the patient demonstrates competency.

PROCEDURE 21-6

Providing Oxygen Therapy

Objective

Provide adequate oxygenation for patient.

Terminology

hypoxemia—deficient oxygenation of the arterial blood.

hypoxia—diminished amount of oxygen available to the body tissues.

oxygen—a colorless, odorless gas that comprises about 20 percent of the atmosphere.

oxygen flowmeter—a calibrated device that measures and controls the liter flow of oxygen to the patient.

Critical Elements

The administration of oxygen is a procedure that must be prescribed by the physician. The physician's order will indicate the concentration, method of delivery, and liter flow per minute. Refer to your facility's policies related to oxygen and oxygen equipment. Familiarize yourself with the use of the flowmeter so that you may control the oxygen flow as ordered.

If the patient becomes short of breath while receiving oxygen, the liter flow should not be increased unless ordered by the physician. The patient may receive relief from coughing, suctioning, repositioning, or other methods. If dyspnea continues, the physician should be notified. It is especially hazardous to increase the oxygen flow on patients with chronic obstructive pulmonary disease (COPD). These patients can have their respiratory effort severely compromised by increasing the oxygen flow and therefore decreasing the carbon monoxide that has served as a stimulus to respiration.

Placing the patient in the semi-Fowler's position may help facilitate respiration. This position helps shift the abdominal contents downward, away from the diaphragm, and therefore allows easier movement of the diaphragm during respiration.

The care provider should do a complete respiratory assessment on the patient receiving oxygen at least every 8 hours and whenever necessary. This should include auscultation of lung sounds and assessment of respiratory effort, color (assessing oral mucous membranes, lips, earlobes, and fingertips), and vital signs. The care provider should also observe for signs of hypoxemia such as anxiety, apprehension, or changes in level of consciousness and/or behavior. In addition, the care provider should review all pertinent laboratory values, such as hemoglobin levels and arterial blood gas studies.

There are two main types of oxygen delivery systems:

- *Oxygen tank*—a tank filled with oxygen that has a valve and

continued on next page

PROCEDURE 21-6 (cont'd)

flowmeter attached to the top of the tank. It may also have a humidifier added if indicated. The oxygen tank should always be secured in a holder. Often these tanks are used to ambulate or transport a patient while still administering oxygen therapy.

- *Wall-mounted oxygen system*—a permanent oxygen delivery system whereby oxygen is piped directly to a wall valve in the patient's room. A flowmeter is plugged into the valve to facilitate oxygen delivery. A humidifier can be added if indicated.

Oxygen is a combustible gas and may create a fire if it comes in contact with a spark (as from a cigarette) or piece of equipment. Use of oxygen in a patient's room necessitates adherence to several safety factors, including:

- *Use of warning signs*—each room should be posted with a "NO SMOKING" or "OXYGEN IN USE" sign. The signs should be displayed over the patient's bed as well as outside the room. Many hospitals are now "smoke-free" (meaning no smoking is allowed anywhere in the facility); however, "NO SMOKING" signs should be posted when oxygen is in use.
- *Proper use of oxygen tanks*—tanks should be at least 10 feet away from any open flame (this is especially important when educating a patient who will be returning home on oxygen).
- *Prevention of sparks*—all electrical equipment used in the room should be in good working order and grounded. Refer to your facility's policy on use of patient equipment such as electric razors, blow dryers, and radios.
- *Avoiding use of oily lotions*—oily lotions, face creams, and petroleum jelly should not be used near oxygen because these substances are flammable.
- *Fire safety procedures*—each care provider should be familiar with the fire safety procedures for your facility.

Several types of oxygen delivery systems are available, including:

- *Cannula* (also called nasal cannula or nasal prongs)—the most common and the least expensive type of oxygen delivery system. It is easy to apply, having two small prongs that rest at the opening of the nares, and allows the patient freedom to talk and eat. It can adequately deliver low concentrations of oxygen (24 to 45 percent) at flow rates of 2 to 6 liters/min.
- *Simple face mask*—covers the patient's nose and mouth, usually with a metal clip that allows the mask to be adjusted to fit snugly around the patient's nose. Exhalation ports on the side of the mask allow the escape of carbon dioxide. It can deliver oxygen concentrations from 40 to 60 percent at flows of 5 to 8 liters/min.
- *Partial rebreather mask*—has an oxygen reservoir bag attached to the end of the mask that allows the patient to rebreathe a portion of exhaled air with the oxygen. The reservoir should not completely deflate during the breathing process. It can deliver oxygen concentrations of 60 to 90 percent at 6 to 10 liters/min.
- *Nonrebreather mask*—has a reservoir bag as well as a one-way valve that prevents the patient from inhaling room air or exhaled air. It can deliver concentrations as high as 95 to 100 percent at 10 to 15 liters/min.
- *Venturi mask*—a very precise method of oxygen delivery (to within 1 percent of accuracy). It is often used to obtain the precise flows necessary in the management of patients with COPD. The concentrations may be varied by the use of a variety of jet adapters that are color coded. The adapters each deliver a different flow rate that can vary oxygen concentration between 24 to 50 percent.

Equipment

Oxygen source
Cannula/mask (as ordered)
Tubing
Flowmeter
Humidifier (as indicated)
Sterile/distilled water (as indicated)

Special Considerations

If the patient is ambulating to the bathroom or getting up and about in the room, the oxygen tubing should be adequate to allow this activity without disconnecting. If the patient is mobilizing outside the room, portable oxygen must be available.

Oxygen can be drying to the mucous membranes of the nose and mouth. For this reason it is recommended that for flow rates over 4 liters/min, a humidifier be added. (*Note:* in drier climates a humidifier may be used with lower flow rates.) This will keep the mucous membranes from drying, reduce irritation, and loosen secretions. Tap water, sterile water, and distilled water have been used successfully in humidifiers; however, you should refer to your facility's policy for the type of fluid to be used.

continued on next page

PROCEDURE 21-6 (cont'd)

The care provider should remove the mask/cannula and provide skin care daily or more often if necessary. The patient should be assessed frequently to determine that the mask, cannula, or tubing is not causing pressure areas on the patient's skin.

Before discharging a patient with oxygen therapy, the care provider should instruct the patient and family regarding use of the equipment as well as safety factors.

Action	*Rationale*
1. Review order.	1. Ensures correct procedure is done.
2. Assemble equipment.	2. Promotes task organization.
3. Identify patient.	3. Provides for patient safety.
4. Explain procedure.	4. Promotes patient compliance.
5. Attach flowmeter and tubing to oxygen source and adjust liter per minute according to physician's order (Fig. 21–17).	5. Ensures equipment is ready for patient use.
6. When using cannula: Place cannula so that the prongs are at opening of nares. Adjust tubing/elastic strap so that fit is comfortable yet secure (Fig. 21–18).	6. Allows oxygen delivery to nares.

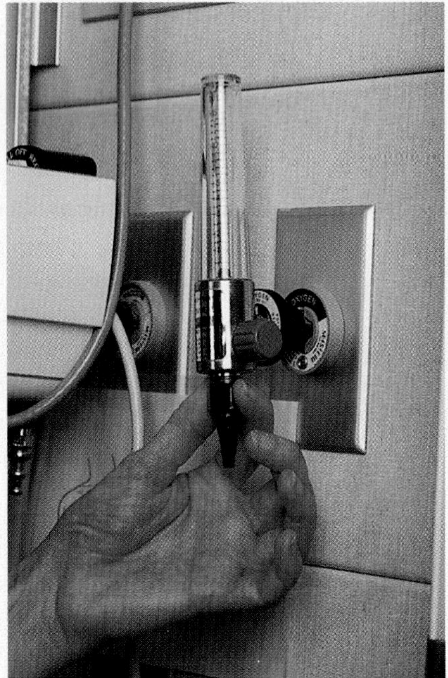

Figure 21–17. Attaching oxygen tubing to delivery device.

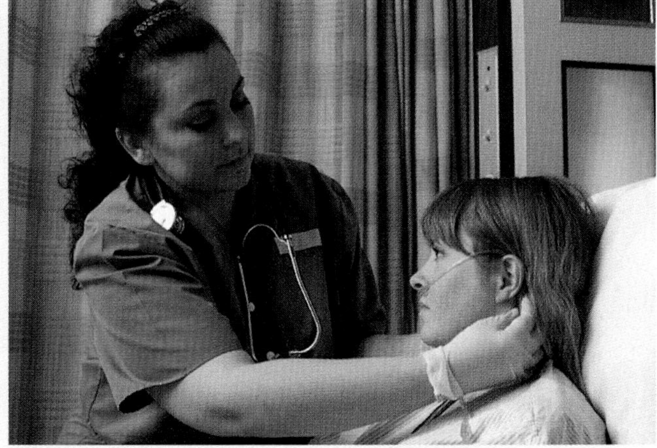

Figure 21–18. Adjusting a nasal cannula.

Action	*Rationale*
7. When using mask: Place mask over mouth and nose. Adjust straps and confirm reservoir bag is filled appropriately (when applicable) (Fig. 21–19).	7. Ensures specialized masks are functioning properly.
8. Attach bubble humidifier (Fig. 21–20).	8. Prevents drying of nasal and oral mucosa.
9. Assess patient and equipment every 4 hours and whenever necessary. Adjust oxygen flow according to any change in physician's orders.	9. Maintains prescribed flow of oxygen.

continued on next page

PROCEDURE 21-6 (cont'd)

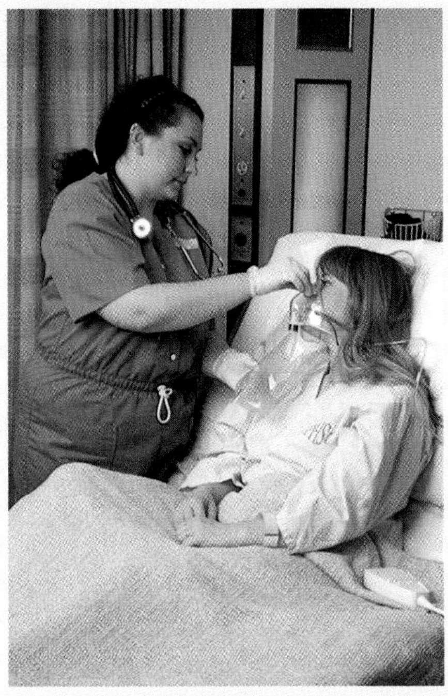

Figure 21–19. Adjusting a face mask.

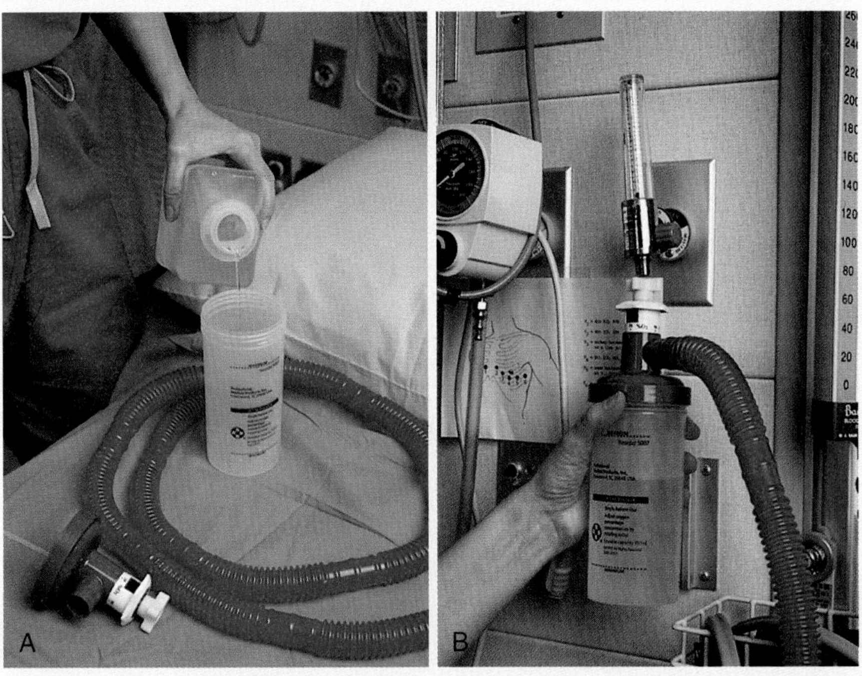

Figure 21–20. Adding a bubble humidifier to the oxygen delivery system.

continued on next page

PROCEDURE 21-6 (cont'd)

Documentation

Record in the patient record the oxygen flow rate, the delivery system in use, the complete respiratory assessment, and the patient's response to treatment.

Elements of Patient Teaching

Instruct the patient/family regarding the purpose of oxygen therapy and all safety factors involved. If family members will be assisting the patient with equipment, allow them to demonstrate the procedure so the care provider may assess their competency level.

PROCEDURE 21-7

Assisting with Pursed-Lip Breathing

Objective

Improve ventilation and oxygenation by assisting in prevention of alveolar collapse.

Terminology

alveoli—an air sac that is the terminal portion of lung tissue, where the exchange of gases takes place with the capillary

dyspnea—difficulty breathing often described as shortness of breath.

pulse oximetry—measures arterial blood saturation by means of a sensor usually attached to the finger.

tachypnea—abnormally rapid respiratory rate.

Critical Elements

This breathing technique is easily taught and may be employed by the patient in any setting. It is often used for patients who have chronic obstructive pulmonary disease (COPD). Because of a loss of lung elasticity and narrowed airways, small airways frequently collapse during exhalation in patients with COPD. Pursed lip breathing is often taught as part of a pulmonary rehabilitation program.

The patient should practice this exercise until able to do it 5 to 10 minutes, four times a day. This breathing exercise may be used after exercise and after any activity that makes the patient tachypneic or dyspneic.

Before and after this exercise, the care provider should assess the patient's respiratory rate, effort, color, and pulse oximetry (if applicable).

Equipment

Pulse oximeter (if indicated)

Special Considerations

The patient should be positioned upright with the forearms resting on a hard surface (such as the overbed table) to give maximum support during the exercise. In addition, leaning forward will position the abdominal organs away from the diaphragm and allow more freedom of respiratory movement.

If the patient wears dentures, make sure they are in place before doing pursed-lip breathing. This assists in supporting the lips during the procedure.

Action	*Rationale*
1. Verify patient.	1. Provides patient safety.
2. Explain procedure.	2. Promotes patient compliance.
3. Position patient in upright position with patient leaning slightly forward and forearms resting on hard surface.	3. Positions patient to allow freedom of chest movement and optimal diaphragmatic movement.
4. Have patient inspire through nose, with mouth closed, while counting to 2. Abdomen should rise during this inspiration.	4. Prevents hyperventilation and provides warm, humidified, filtered air to lungs.

continued on next page

PROCEDURE 21-7 (cont'd)

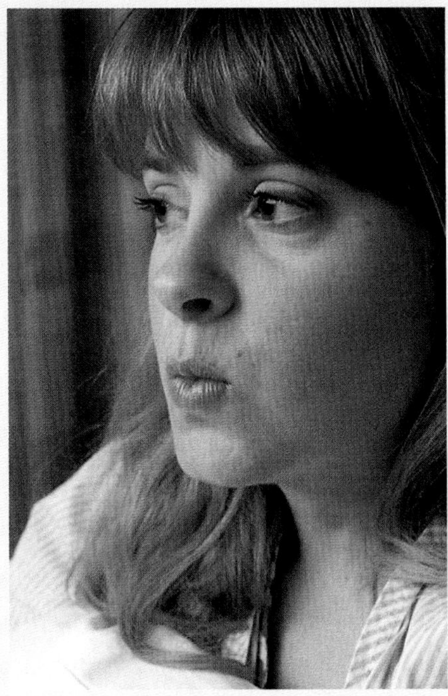

Figure 21–21. Pursed-lip breathing technique.

5. Have patient purse lips (as if attempting to whistle) and exhale slowly (without puffing out cheeks) through pursed lips while counting to 7; abdomen should fall during expiration (Fig. 21–21).	5. Creates back pressure in small airways that prevents collapse of small airways and alveoli.
6. Continue exercise until no longer short of breath.	6. Reduces feeling of dyspnea.
7. Return patient to position of comfort.	7. Provides safe, comfortable environment.

Documentation

Record on the patient record the time, duration, and patient response to the procedure. Note the care provider's assessment of the patient's respiratory status before and after the procedure.

Elements of Patient Teaching

Instruct the patient/family on the purpose of the procedure. Observe the patient to confirm that the procedure is being performed correctly. If family members are instructing or supporting the patient during this procedure, observe their performance to determine their competency.

CHAPTER HIGHLIGHTS

- A sound knowledge of the anatomy and physiology of the respiratory system is essential to provide nursing care to patients with respiratory problems.
- Research has focused on methods to clear the patient's airway, reduce efforts of difficult breathing, and increase self-management strategies for respiratory compromised patients.
- A theory relating to dyspnea has resulted in the development of a model that explains the experience of a person who has dyspnea and provides the practitioner with a way to assess the experience and propose interventions.
- Respiratory problems affect people of all ages and both genders.

- Lifestyles, cultural traditions, religious practices, and the environment affect the human respiratory system.
- People can suffer from respiratory problems in any environmental setting; at home, at work, in school, in health care settings, or out in the open air.
- Confidentiality becomes an ethical issue when patients suffer from respiratory communicable illnesses such as tuberculosis.
- To reduce health care costs, more attention will be given by health care professionals to reducing the incidence of respiratory illnesses.
- Care of patients with respiratory problems is enhanced by nurses being aware of and applying the results of relevant research findings in nursing practice.

REFERENCES

Ackerman, M.H. (1993). The effect of saline lavage prior to suctioning. *American Journal of Critical Care, 2*(4), 326–330.

Ackerman, M.H., Guerty, R. (1990). The effect of normal saline bolus instillation in artificial airways. *Journal of the Society of Otolaryngology, Head and Neck Nursing, 8*(2), 14–17.

Allen, S.C., Prior, A. (1986). What determines whether an elderly patient can use a metered dose inhaler correctly? *British Journal of Diseases of the Chest, 80,* 45–49.

Altose, M. (1986). Dyspnea. In E. Simmons (ed.): *Current Pulmonology.* Chicago: Year Book Medical.

American Cancer Society (1996). *Cancer Facts & Figures—1996.* New York: Author.

Armitage, J.M., Williams, S.J. (1988). Inhaler technique in the elderly. *Age and Aging, 17,* 275–278.

Baxter, K., Nolan, K.M., Winyard, J.A., et al. (1993). Are they getting enough? Meeting the oxygen therapy needs of post-operative patients. *Professional Nurse, 8*(5), 310–312.

Carrieri, V., Janson-Bjerklie, S. (1986). Strategies patients use to manage the sensation of dyspnea. *Western Journal of Nursing Research, 8,* 284–305.

Carrieri-Kohlman, V., Janson-Bjerklie, S. (1993). Dyspnea. In V. Carrieri-Kohlman, A.M. Lindsey, and C. West (eds.): *Pathophysiological Phenomena in Nursing: Human Responses to Illness,* 2nd ed. Philadelphia: W.B. Saunders, pp. 247–278.

Cerney, F.J. (1989). Relative effects of bronchial drainage and exercise for in-hospital care of patients with cystic fibrosis. *Physical Therapy, 69*(8), 633–639.

Chyou, P., Nomura, A., Stemmermann, G. (1992). A prospective study of the attributable risk of cancer due to cigarette smoking. *American Journal of Public Health, 82*(1), 37–40.

Comroe, J.H., Jr. (1974). *Physiology of Respiration: An Introductory Text,* 2nd ed. St Louis: Mosby–Year Book.

Connolly, M.J. (1995). Inhaler technique of elderly patients: Comparison of metered-dose inhalers and large volume spacer devices. *Age and Aging, 24,* 190–192.

Copnell, B., Fergusson, D. (1995). Endotracheal suctioning: Time-worn ritual or timely intervention? *American Journal of Critical Care, 4*(2), 100–105.

Corbett, K. (1992). An experiment to improve patient's closed-mouth metered-dose inhaler technique using a prototype spirometric training device. *Journal of Clinical Nursing, 1*(5), 289–290.

Crimlisk, J., Paris, R., McGonagle, E., et al. (1994). The closed tracheal suction system: Implications for critical care nursing. *Dimensions of Critical Care Nursing, 13*(6), 292–300.

De Blaquiere, P., Christensen, D.B., Carter, W.B., Martin, T.R. (1989). Use and misuse of metered-dose inhalers by patients with chronic lung disease. *American Review of Respiratory Disease, 140,* 910–916.

Delk, K.K., Gevirtz, R., Hicks, D.A., et al. (1994). The effects of biofeedback assisted breathing retraining on lung functions in patients with cystic fibrosis. *Chest, 105*(1), 23–28.

Depew, C.L., Moseley, M.J., Clark, E.G., Morales, C.C. (1994). Open vs. closed-system endotracheal suctioning: A cost comparison. *Critical Care Nurse, 14*(1), 94–100.

Dunlevy, C.L., Glenn, T.L., Servick, C., Baez, S. (1995). Physiological and psychological responses of patients with obstructive pulmonary disease to the Chairobics exercise program. *Canadian Journal of Respiratory Therapy, 31*(3), 109–113.

Dunlevy, C.L., Tyl, S.E. (1992). The effect of oral versus nasal breathing on oxygen concentrations received from nasal cannulas. *Respiratory Care, 37*(4), 357–360.

Estey, W. (1990). Subjective effects of dry versus humidified low flow oxygen. *Respiratory Care, 35*(12), 1265–1266.

Gallon, A. (1991). Evaluation of chest percussion in the treatment of patients with copious sputum production. *Respiratory Medicine, 85,* 45–51.

Glass, C., Grap, M.J., Corley, M.C., Wallace, D. (1993). Nurses' ability to achieve hyperinflation and hyperoxygenation with a manual resuscitation bag during endotracheal suctioning. *Heart & Lung, 22*(2), 158–165.

Gold, W. (1983). Dyspnea. In R. Blackwell (ed.): *Signs and Symptoms.* Philadelphia: J.B. Lippincott, pp. 335–348.

Gray, J.E., MacIntyre, N.R., Kronenberger, W.G. (1990). The effects of bolus normal saline instillation in conjunction with endotracheal suctioning. *Respiratory Care, 25,* 785–790.

Gunderson, L.P., Stone, K.S., Hamlin, R. (1991). Endotracheal suctioning–induced heart rate alterations. *Nursing Research, 40*(3), 139–143.

Hagler, D.A., Traver, G.A. (1994). Endotracheal saline and suction catheters: Sources of lower airway contamination. *American Journal of Critical Care, 3*(6), 444–447.

Hanania, N.A., Wittman, R., Kesten, S., Chapman, K.R. (1994). Medical personnel's knowledge of and ability to use inhaling devices: Metered-dose inhalers, spacing chambers, and breath-actuated dry powder inhalers. *Chest, 105*(1), 111–116.

Hilton, S. (1990). An audit of inhaler technique among asthma patients of 34 general practitioners. *British Journal of General Practice, 40,* 505–506.

Honeyman, P., Barr, S., Stubbing, D.E. (1996). Effect of a walking aid on disability, oxygenation, and breathlessness in patients with chronic airflow limitation. *Journal of Cardiopulmonary Rehabilitation, 16*(1), 63–67.

Interiano, B., Guntupalli, K.K. (1993). Metered-dose inhalers: Do health care providers know what to teach? *Archives of Internal Medicine, 153,* 81–85.

Kersten, L.D. (1990). Changes in self-concept during pulmonary rehabilitation, Part I. *Journal of Critical Care, 19*(5), 456–462.

Kesten, S., Elias, M., Cartier, A., Chapman, K.R. (1994). Patient handling of a multidose dry powder inhalation device for albuterol. *Chest, 105*(4), 1077–1081.

Killian, K., Jones, N. (*1988*). Respiratory muscles and dyspnea. *Clinical Chest Medicine, 9,* 237–248.

Kim, M.J., Larson, J.L., Covey, M.K., et al. (1993). Inspiratory muscle training in patients with chronic obstructive pulmonary disease. *Nursing Research, 42*(6), 356–362.

Lake, F.R., Henderson, K., Briffa, T., et al. (1990). Upper-limb and lower-limb exercise training in patients with chronic airflow obstructions. *Chest, 97,* 1077–1082.

Lowery, B. (1987). Stress research: Some theoretical and methodological issues. *Image, 19,* 42–46.

Mazzocco, M.C., Owens, F., Kirilloff, L., Rogers, R. (1985). Chest percussion and postural drainage in patients with bronchiectasis. *Chest, 88,* 360–363.

McCance, K.L., Huether, S.E. (1994). *Pathophysiology: The Biological Basis for Disease in Adults and Children,* 2nd ed. St. Louis: Mosby–Year Book.

McCord, M., Cronin-Stubbs, D. (1992). Operationalizing dyspnea: Focus on measurement. *Heart and Lung, 21,* 167.

Moody, L.E., Fraser, M., Yarandi, H. (1993). *Clinical Nursing Research, 2*(4), 478–486.

Pavia, D. (1990). The role of chest physiotherapy in mucus hypersecretion. *Lung, 168,* 614–621.

Preusser, B.A., Winningham, J.L., Clanton, T.L. (1994). High- vs low-intensity inspiratory muscle interval training in patients with COPD. *Chest, 106*(1), 111–117.

Reardon, J., Awad, E., Normandin, E., et al. (1994). The effect of comprehensive outpatient pulmonary rehabilitation on dyspnea. *Comprehensive Outpatient Pulmonary Rehabilitation, 105*(4), 1046–1052.

Rudy, E., Turner, B.S., Baun, M., et al. (1991). Endotracheal suctioning in adults with head injury. *Heart & Lung, 20*(6), 667–674.

Ross, J., Dean, E., Abboud, R. (1992). The effect of postural drainage positioning on ventilation homogeneity in healthy subjects. *Physical Therapy, 72*(11), 794–799.

Sassi-Dambron, D.E., Eakin, E.G., Ries, A.L., Kaplan, R.M. (1994). The effects of compliance with exercise training on pulmonary rehabilitation. *Rehabilitation Nursing Research, 3*(1), 3–10.

Simpson, K., Killian, K., McCartney, N., et al. (1992). Randomized controlled trial of weightlifting exercise in patients with chronic airflow limitation. *Thorax, 47,* 70–75.

Steele, B., Shaver, J. (1992). The dyspnea experience: nociceptive properties and a model for research and practice. *Advances in Nursing Science, 15*(1), 64–76.

Stone, K.S., Bell, S.D., Preusser, B.A. (1991a). The effect of repeated endotracheal suctioning on arterial blood pressure. *Applied Nursing Research, 4*(4), 152–158.

Stone, K.S., Talaganis, S., Preusser, B.A., Gonyon, D.S. (1991b). Effect of lung hyperinflation and endotracheal suctioning on heart rate and rhythm in patients after coronary artery bypass graft surgery. *Heart & Lung, 20*(5), 443–450.

Sweer, L., Zwillich, C. (1990). Dyspnea in the patient with chronic obstructive pulmonary disease: Etiologies and management. *Clinical Chest Medicine, 11,* 417–445.

Taft, A., Mishoe, S., Dennison, F., et al. (1991). A comparison of two methods of preoxygenation during endotracheal suctioning. *Respiratory Care, 36*(11), 1195–1201.

Thomas, J., McIntosh, J. (1994). Are incentive spirometry, intermittent positive pressure breathing, and deep breathing exercises effective in the prevention of postoperative pulmonary complications after upper abdominal surgery? A systematic overview and meta-analysis. *Physical Therapy, 74*(1), 3–10.

Thompson, D.L. (1989). Predictors of walking distance of people with chronic bronchitis and/or emphysema. Doctoral dissertation, Case Western Reserve University, p 89.

Thompson, J., Irvine, T., Grathwohl, K., Roth, B. (1994). Misuse of metered-dose inhalers in hospitalized patients. *Chest, 105*(3), 715–717.

Thornby, M.A., Haas, F., Axen, K. (1995). Effect of distractive auditory stimuli on exercise tolerance in patients with COPD. *Chest, 107*(5), 1213–1217.

Thornlow, D.K. (1995). Is chest physiotherapy necessary after cardiac surgery? *Critical Care Nurse, 15*(3), 39–46.

Vale, F., Reardon, J.A., ZuWallack, R.L. (1993). The long-term benefits of outpatient pulmonary rehabilitation on exercise endurance and quality of life. *Chest, 103*(1), 42–45.

Wasserman, K., Casaburi, R. (*1988*). Dyspnea: Physiological and pathophysiological mechanisms. *Annual Review of Medicine, 39,* 503–515.

Zidulka, A., Chrome, J.F., Wight, D.W., et al. (1989). Clapping or percussion causes atelectasis in dogs and influences gas exchange. *Journal of Applied Physiology, 66,* 2833–2338.

Nutrition and Fluids 22

*Marylou McAthie**

Mary Smith, age 80, a thin, frail nursing home resident, developed difficulty in swallowing as the result of a stroke. Because she could not swallow properly, her caregivers were reluctant to give her anything to drink because they feared she would choke. Over a period of a week, she developed a serum sodium level of 185 mEq/L and became markedly confused. While a high serum sodium level would normally cause severe thirst and lead to drinking, the combination of this patient's decreased awareness and inability to swallow had led to her dehydrated state.

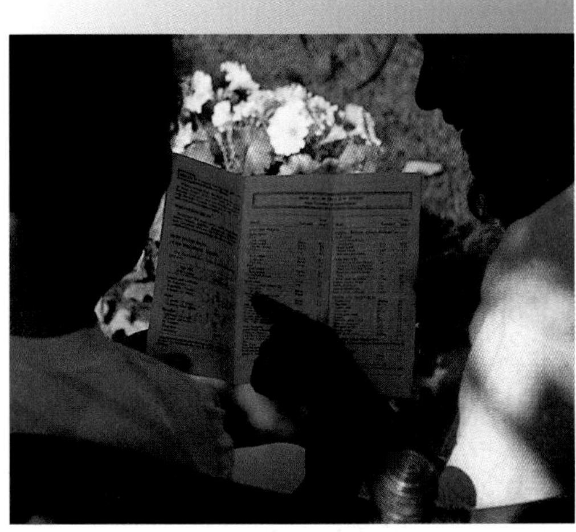

On admission to the acute care facility, she received intravenous fluids containing dextrose and small concentrations of sodium chloride (D_5 in 0.3% NaCl) until her serum sodium level returned to normal. After this, she received 2 L of D_5 in 0.45 percent sodium chloride (containing 340 calories) intravenously for 10 days. Her weight dropped from the admission weight of 109 pounds to 103 pounds, and her blood laboratory values suggested malnutrition (a serum albumin level of 2.5 g/dl). Because she was not eating and displayed obvious signs of malnutrition, a nasogastric feeding tube was inserted so that liquid nutrients and water could be continuously administered directly into her stomach; she received 1.5 L of formula each day with small water supplements every 6 hours. Because she was at risk for aspirating the tube-feeding formula into her lungs, the head of her bed was kept elevated to at least a 45° angle. Physical therapists worked with her each day to help her adapt to her decreased ability to swallow. Three weeks later she was able to eat with assistance and was returned to the nursing home.

OBJECTIVES

After studying this chapter, students will be able to:

- **describe functions of and problems involving proteins, carbohydrates, fats, and major electrolytes**
- **identify essentials of assessing fluid and electrolyte balance**
- **explain how nutritional needs vary with age, gender, culture, ethnicity, and religious practices**
- **describe essential characteristics of a nutritional screening tool**
- **discuss methods to assist patients to eat and drink**
- **explain how to insert a large-bore nasogastric tube**
- **describe how to administer NG tube feeding**
- **identify tube feeding complications and their management**
- **describe how to change an (IV)**
- **describe the procedure for calculating IV flow rates**
- **identify complications of parenteral fluid use**

*Edited from content provided by expert researchers and clinicians.

SCOPE OF NURSING PRACTICE

Nurses are responsible for the total needs of their patients. This includes ensuring that patients receive adequate nutrients and fluids to enable them to maintain or restore optimum nutritional status. Broadly defined, proper nutrition means that all the essential nutrients—carbohydrates, proteins, and fats (all of which contain calories, that is, produce food energy), vitamins, minerals (also called electrolytes), and fluids (primarily water)—are made available and utilized in sufficient, balanced quantities to enable the body to function normally.

Proper nutrition is required for normal growth, reproduction, and maintenance of basic life processes; normal organ development and function; and for the ability to resist and recover from infection, disease, and bodily injuries. Everyone needs the same nutrients and everyone needs adequate water intake, but, as in Mary Smith's case, individuals differ widely in their nutrition and fluid requirements according to such factors as age, gender, body structure and size, genetic background, and socioeconomic status.

Nutritional and dietary concerns are not new to nursing. In the mid 1800s, Florence Nightingale commented that nurses should observe patients' food intake and report findings to the physician, stating, "It is quite incalculable the good that would certainly come from such sound and close observation in this almost neglected branch of nursing . . ." (Nightingale, 1859).

A steadily growing body of knowledge developed by nurse researchers and other health care professionals is available to guide nutrition and diet therapy. Perhaps not surprisingly, much of this knowledge relates to the elderly patient population in hospitals and nursing homes. Much recent nursing research has also focused on the twin challenges of maintaining optimal feeding tube function and reducing or preventing complications related to nutrient and fluid administration (preparation and equipment) and metabolism (how the body uses nutrients and fluids).

Specific nursing skills related to nutritional status and fluid balance include performing nutritional assessment to detect signs of malnutrition and selected fluid/electrolyte problems; providing patients in a variety of settings with adequate fluids and nutrients, either enterally (by mouth or by feeding tube) or parenterally (via peripheral or central IV routes); monitoring fluid and nutrient intake; and working with other members of the health care team to correct fluid and nutrition problems.

If the patient is unable to eat but retains a functional gastrointestinal tract, the nurse may be responsible for inserting a large-diameter nasogastric tube to administer tube feedings or helping to administer IV fluids through a peripheral vein and for maintaining these devices. Although the nurse is not solely responsible for giving fluids and nutrients by the central IV route (central venous catheter), principles of safe management of this modality are also provided.

KNOWLEDGE BASE

Basic Science

Core concepts vital to an understanding of nutrition and fluid balance include the structures and processes involved in ingestion, digestion, absorption, and metabolism of nutrients and fluids; mechanisms involved in maintaining homeostasis (fluid and electrolyte balance); methods of nutrient and fluid delivery; and types of diets and enteral/parenteral nutrients and fluid formulations.

ANATOMY AND PHYSIOLOGY

THE GASTROINTESTINAL SYSTEM

Fluids and solid nutrients are usually consumed orally and then processed by the gastrointestinal system (see Fig. 22–1 for an illustration of gastrointestinal system structures and Table 22–1 for descriptions of gastrointestinal functions). This process, called digestion, takes place in a series of mechanical and chemical steps to break foods and fluids into nutrient components that can be absorbed into the circulation and carried to their final destination, the cells. Once nutrients are distributed to the cells, they are changed further for use in a complex array of processes called metabolism.

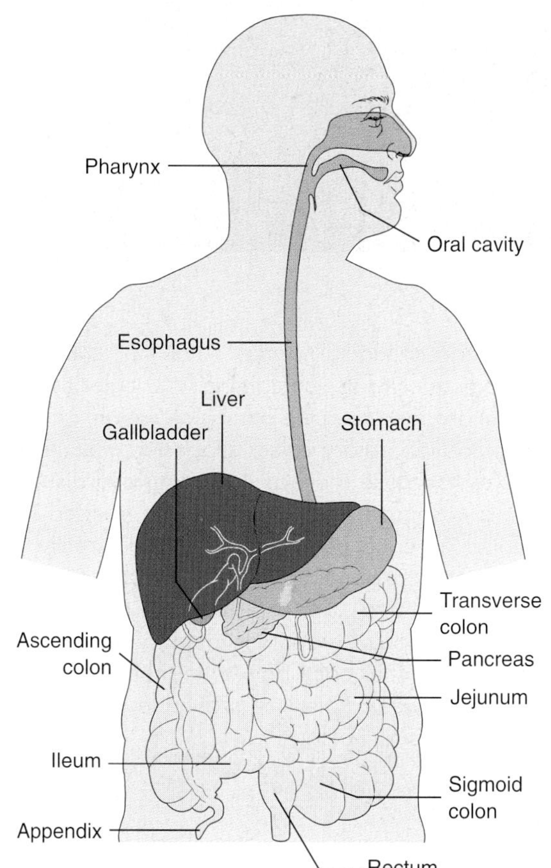

Figure 22-1. Basic anatomy of the gastrointestinal system.

TABLE 22-1 Gastrointestinal Structures and Their Functions

Structures	Description	Digestive Functions
Mouth and throat	• Beginning of digestive tract • Includes lips, cheeks, teeth, tongue, hard and soft palates, salivary glands, pharynx	• *Mechanical digestion:* food is broken up into small particles to increase its surface area for exposure to digestive enzymes. • *Chemical digestion:* food particles are mixed with saliva, which contains ptyalin, an enzyme that breaks down starches, and mucus which moistens and lubricates food. • Chewed food is formed into a bolus by tongue and cheeks, moved into pharynx by voluntary tongue movements, then moved into esophagus by involuntary swallowing reflex.
Esophagus	• Connects mouth to stomach • Hollow tube of striated and smooth muscle, lies behind trachea and heart but in front of vertebral column • Collapsed at rest, distends to accommodate fluids and solid foods	• Transports food bolus to stomach by peristaltic muscle contractions.
Stomach	• Irregularly shaped pouch, located below diaphragm in upper abdomen • Separated from esophagus by lower esophageal sphincter and from small intestine (duodenum) by pyloric sphincter • Stomach wall lined with gastric glands • Capacity varies from 1 quart to ½ gallon	• Stores food and begins digestion by mixing food with gastric secretions by churning and peristaltic action. Food bolus is converted into semiliquid called chyme. • Chyme is slowly emptied into small intestine; rate of gastric emptying varies with volume and composition of food.
Small intestine	• Consists of three sections: *duodenum, jejunum,* and *ileum;* fills most of lower abdominal cavity • Circular folds (plicae) and villi (tiny fingerlike projections from intestinal walls) vastly increase interior surface area for digestion and absorption • Intestinal glands secrete digestive hormones and enzymes.	• Serves as major site of digestion and absorption. • Food from stomach (chyme) enters duodenum, stimulating release of hormones, which in turn activate enzymes from the liver, gallbladder, pancreas, and duodenal mucosa. Enzymes break down carbohydrates, proteins, and fats into absorbable components. • Transports chyme from stomach to large intestine.
Large intestine	• Consists of five sections: *cecum, ascending colon, transverse colon, descending colon,* and *sigmoid colon* (includes rectum and anal canal)	• Continues to absorb water and electrolytes from chyme. • Transports chyme through colon to rectum and initiates urge to defecate.
Accessory Organs of Digestion		
Pancreas	• Located behind the stomach and spleen • Connects to duodenum via pancreatic duct	• Secretes pancreatic juice into duodenum; this contains enzymes that break down carbohydrates, proteins, and fats, and also contains bicarbonate ions to help neutralize pH level of chyme • Produces hormones (insulin) that regulate sugar metabolism
Liver	• Largest organ in the body located under diaphragm in upper abdominal area • Connects to common bile duct via hepatic duct • Performs many important bodily functions besides digestion	• Produces bile, which is not digestive in itself but acts on fats to allow their digestion in the small intestine • Stores glycogen, fat-soluble vitamins, and some water-soluble vitamins • Metabolizes carbohydrates, proteins, and fats
Gallbladder	• Located beneath the liver; connects to duodenum via cystic duct and common bile duct	• Stores and concentrates bile from the liver. This is released when chyme (especially if high in fat content) enters the duodenum from the stomach.

When healthy people eat, food is allowed to come into contact with enzymes in the mouth while it is being chewed and readied for swallowing. Swallowing is a complicated process that is partially voluntary and partially involuntary (Fig. 22–2). In the voluntary phase, the individual purposely initiates swallowing. From that point on, however, the process is involuntary and the food passes through the pharynx into the esophagus and then into the stomach. As food passes through the pharynx, the trachea is closed and the esophagus is opened, and a fast peristaltic wave (a muscular contraction) forces the food into the esophagus (Guyton, 1991). In certain illnesses, swallowing is impaired and food and fluids may accidentally enter the trachea rather than the esophagus. This dreaded occurrence is known as aspiration, a risk that Mrs. Smith's caregivers tried to avoid. It may be a witnessed event but more commonly occurs unnoticed (silent aspiration).

The severity of symptoms after aspiration depends on how much fluid was aspirated and its pH. Obviously, large

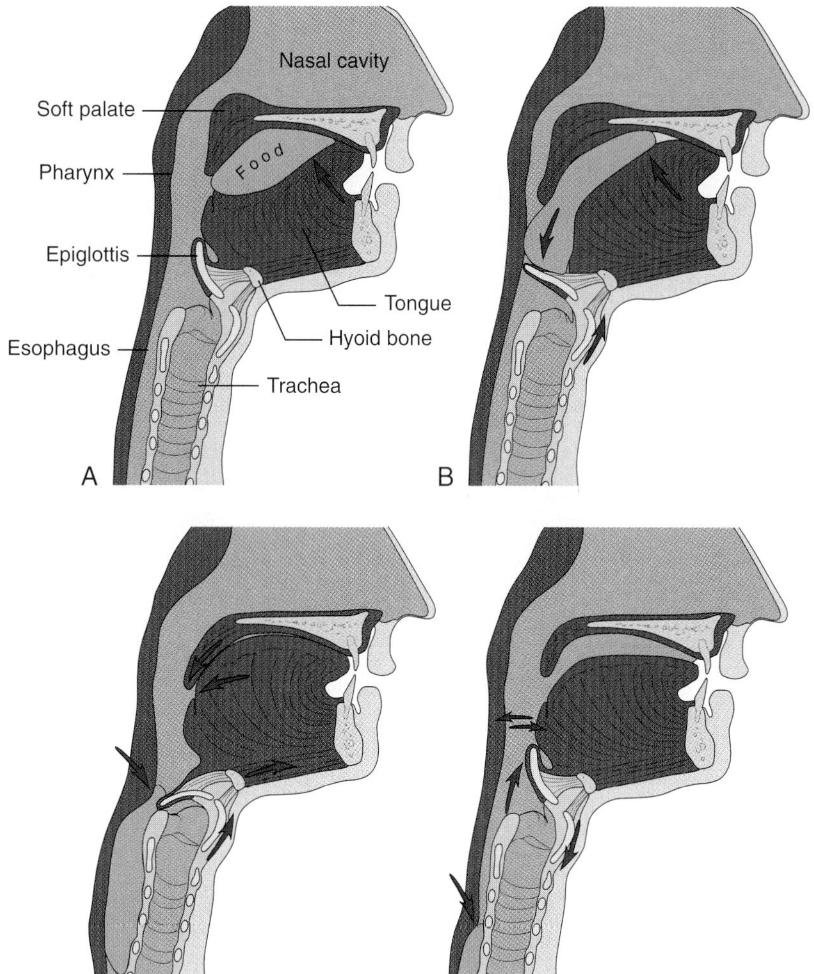

Figure 22-2. How swallowing occurs. Once food has been chewed and mixed with saliva in the mouth, it is ready to be swallowed. In step A, the tongue voluntarily pushes the food toward the back of the mouth toward the pharynx, where it stimulates sensory receptors to initiate the swallow reflex. Once a swallow begins, it continues involuntarily, as shown in steps B and C. The soft palate rises to prevent food from entering the nasal cavity, the epiglottis closes, the larynx and hyoid bone rise to prevent food from being aspirated by the trachea, the tongue rises to seal off the mouth, the upper esophageal sphincter relaxes, and the esophagus opens. Finally, in step D, a peristaltic wave begins in the upper esophagus to force the food down the esophagus.

volumes are more likely to produce serious pulmonary problems than are small volumes (such as less than 50 ml). Perhaps most crucial in determining pulmonary damage after aspiration is the fluid's pH; a highly acidic pH (less than 2.5) is especially harmful because it causes serious damage to the pulmonary tissue. After aspiration into the lung, gastric fluid is rapidly distributed to the periphery of the lung, where it produces changes that are visible on a chest x-ray film.

The esophagus transports the food to the stomach. The stomach serves as a temporary reservoir and can hold up to several liters of food and fluids. Here, food is physically churned and exposed to the action of pepsin and other digestive enzymes. The partially digested food, now in a semiliquid state known as *chyme,* is slowly emptied into the small intestine. Gastric emptying time partly depends on the nature of the food. Several hours are needed to completely empty a typical meal, and fats are emptied more slowly than other nutrients. (Slower emptying is one reason why fats produce more satiety—a feeling of fullness—than other nutrients.)

Unlike the stomach, the small intestine does not function as a reservoir. Instead, it normally propels the food bolus forward by means of frequent peristaltic waves. Thus, while relatively large quantities of fluid can enter the stomach without producing cramping, the introduction of a large bolus of food into the small intestine will likely produce cramping and diarrhea. Along the way, the food is further digested by intestinal enzymes, and the digestion products are absorbed through the intestinal walls into the blood or lymph systems, which carry the nutrients to the cells. Digestion is greatly aided by additional secretions provided by the accessory organs of digestion—the liver, pancreas, and gallbladder.

Large volumes of digestive juices secreted into the gastrointestinal tract facilitate peristaltic movement and mixing and supply adequate water to hold food particles in suspension. In the normal adult, 3 to 6 L of gastric, pancreatic, biliary, and intestinal fluids is secreted into the gastrointestinal tract every day. Counting the normal fluid intake and the body's own gastrointestinal secretions, 8 to 9 L enters the upper intestine each day. Nutrients are primarily absorbed in the jejunum and ileum of the small intestine; most of the fluid is reabsorbed in the ileum and proximal colon. This constant fluid movement is sometimes called the "gastrointestinal circulation."

After food is digested and absorbed in the small intestine, the undigested residue enters the colon, which extracts additional water and fluids and solidifies the remainder for excretion in the form of feces. In a normal adult, the resulting stools contain only 150 to 200 ml of fluid.

ALTERNATIVE NUTRITIONAL PATHWAYS

Many patients' nutritional needs can be met using special oral diets or, if necessary, enteral feeding tubes that allow liquid nutrient preparations to be delivered directly to the stomach or small intestine. (Recall that Mrs. Smith was given feedings through a nasogastric tube.) Usually the tube is threaded through a nasal passage into the esophagus until it reaches the stomach (nasogastric tube) or the upper part of the small intestine (nasoduodenal or nasojejunal tubes). In some cases, nutrients can be introduced directly into the gastrointestinal tract through a surgically or endoscopically placed tube (gastrostomy or jejunostomy). If the gastrointestinal tract must be bypassed, as when a patient is recovering from surgery or has certain disorders, nutrients and fluids are introduced parenterally, directly into the venous system. Such nutrients must be in a form that can be utilized immediately by body tissues without being acted on by the gastrointestinal tract. Parenteral feedings are usually called IV feedings because they are introduced through needles or plastic catheters threaded into one of the body's many veins. Usually peripheral veins are used rather than central veins. Enteral and parenteral feeding modalities are discussed later in this chapter.

NUTRITION

Foods provide three basic classes of essential nutrients: carbohydrates, proteins, and fats. These nutrients must be reduced by digestion into their simplest forms—sugars, amino acids, fatty acids, and glycerol—before they can be absorbed by body cells and used for energy. Three other types of nutrients—vitamins, minerals (also called electrolytes) and water—can be used by cells directly without benefit of digestion.

The process does not end with digestion and absorption by the gastrointestinal tract. Water-soluble nutrients pass from the gastrointestinal tract through the bloodstream to the liver. Fats and fat-soluble vitamins reach the liver by another pathway, the lymphatic system. The liver metabolizes some nutrients, stores some, and delivers others to cells in the rest of the body for further utilization.

Metabolism, Energy, and Calories

Metabolism comprises all the physical and chemical processes related to cellular nutrition. Metabolism can be thought of as a kind of chemical "engine." It consists of two phases, anabolism and catabolism. Anabolism builds tissues by changing simple substances into complex ones (such as those needed for growth and tissue repair), and catabolism generates energy by changing complex substances into simpler ones. Anabolic and catabolic metabolism take place simultaneously; anabolism is powered by the energy released by catabolism. The body needs food energy to perform its functions. The energy comes from metabolism of carbohydrates, proteins, and fats, with substantial help from water, minerals (electrolytes), and vitamins. The energy derived from the three nutrient groups is made available in two forms: chemical energy in the form of a complex molecule, adenosine triphosphate—the basic "fuel" used by cells throughout the body—and heat.

The energy produced by different nutrients at metabolism is measured in units of heat energy called kilocalories. Kilocalories are measured in grams. For example, 1 g of carbohydrate or protein produces approximately 4 kcal of energy and 1 g of fat produces 9 kcal of energy. Kilocalories provide a useful way to quantify food energy values and bodily energy requirements in nutrition and diet therapy.

It is helpful to review the ways in which major food sources (carbohydrates, proteins, and fats) and vitamins and minerals (electrolytes) are metabolized and utilized by the body. All of these nutrients are available for administration in enteral and parenteral forms.

Carbohydrates

Dietary carbohydrates are classified as either complex or simple sugars. Examples of simple sugars are glucose and fructose. Examples of complex carbohydrates are starch and fiber from plants. The three main dietary sources of carbohydrates are sucrose (cane sugar), lactose (milk sugar), and starches from grains and numerous other foods. Digestion reduces carbohydrates almost entirely into glucose, fructose, and galactose. If the body takes in more carbohydrates than are needed, the excess is converted to fat.

Almost all carbohydrates are transported into tissue cells as glucose. Glucose must be transported through cell membranes by facilitated diffusion, which is influenced by insulin, a hormone secreted by beta cells in the pancreas. Once glucose enters cells it can be either metabolized for release of energy or stored as glycogen. The primary purpose of glucose is to produce the energy needed to maintain cellular function. Most of the energy produced from the metabolism of carbohydrates is used to form adenosine triphosphate, which fuels all cellular metabolism and is therefore critical to nearly all body functions.

Glucose metabolism is highly responsive to the body's energy demands and is regulated by two hormones produced by the pancreas: insulin and glucagon. A rise in the plasma glucose level above normal signals the pancreas to secrete insulin, which in turn increases the rate of glucose transport through the cell membrane. In this way, insulin causes the blood glucose level to drop toward normal. Conversely, an abnormally low plasma glucose level stimulates pancreatic alpha cells to release glucagon. Glucagon acts to convert glycogen (stored in the liver) into glucose, thereby restoring the blood glucose level to normal.

Carbohydrate metabolism is also influenced by epinephrine (a hormone secreted by the medulla of the adrenal gland) and by B vitamins. Stress causes an increased release of epinephrine, which activates the breakdown of glycogen into glucose. The primary role of the B vitamins is to form active coenzymes that, in concert with enzymes, are involved in one of several of the metabolic steps needed for glucose synthesis and degradation. Vitamins specifically needed for carbohydrate metabolism include B_1 (thiamine), B_2 (riboflavin), B_3 (niacin), pantothenic acid, biotin, folic acid, and B_6 (pyridoxine).

Also needed for carbohydrate metabolism are the minerals magnesium, chromium, and zinc. Magnesium is involved with adenosine triphosphate in most reactions, whereas chromium is important in the cellular uptake of glucose. Zinc has been shown to be important in the binding of insulin to the cell surface.

Protein

Proteins are composed of amino acids, which are various combinations of carbon, hydrogen, oxygen, and nitrogen. Proteins are an important component of numerous body substances, such as muscle, enzymes, antibodies, hormones, buffers (compounds that help maintain acid-base balance), and albumin, and thus are essential for many functions.

The body constantly breaks down and builds new protein. This cycle of synthesis, degradation into amino acids, and resynthesis into new protein is referred to as "protein turnover." The nitrogen component of protein is sometimes used to evaluate a patient's protein status. When the patient is in nitrogen balance, the amount of nitrogen excreted equals the amount ingested. During growth and pregnancy, the body makes more protein than it breaks down and is in positive nitrogen balance. Conversely, in trauma, disease, or restricted food intake, the body loses more nitrogen than it makes, causing negative nitrogen balance. During fasting, some amino acids are converted to glucose.

Because proteins are not stored, it is important that the body's energy needs be met by carbohydrates and/or fats. In short-term starvation, skeletal muscle, which comprises about half of the body's total protein mass, is sacrificed. If starvation occurs in an already malnourished individual, skeletal muscle reserves will be exhausted, causing the body to sacrifice visceral proteins to obtain energy.

The body appears to be able to synthesize amino acids for critical body needs (such as liver function or wound healing) despite widespread protein degradation during starvation. For example, wound healing has been shown to occur in the presence of total negative nitrogen balance in some individuals; that is, the body loses more nitrogen than is being ingested. However, this synthesis takes place at the expense of other body tissues, such as muscle, skin, and gastrointestinal structures.

Fats

Like carbohydrates, fats are composed of carbon, hydrogen, and oxygen. However, fats (also called lipids) contain a lower ratio of oxygen to hydrogen and carbon than do carbohydrates and proteins. Therefore, fats yield a much higher caloric content (9 kcal/g) than either carbohydrate (4 kcal/g) or protein (4 kcal/g). Fats are composed of fatty acids (saturated or unsaturated), glycerides, compound lipids, and derived lipids (which include cholesterol).

An essential body constituent, fats perform numerous functions. Adipose (fat) tissue forms a major reserve energy source. It helps spare protein because its availability decreases the need to burn protein for energy. Also, adipose tissue helps protect vital organs by acting as a cushion against injury and provides insulation under the skin to help maintain constant body temperature.

All body cells (except red blood cells, central nervous system tissue, and the renal medulla) can use fatty acids to provide energy. Lipolysis (fat breakdown) and lipogenesis (fat buildup) occur continuously in the body. Adipose tissue cells can increase or decrease in size, according to caloric intake. Whereas excess caloric intake causes fat to be stored, reduced caloric intake causes adipose cells to release fat.

To reduce the risk of fat buildup in the large blood vessels (atherosclerosis), it is recommended that saturated fats be limited in the diet. Examples of saturated fats are butter, cream, and animal fat in meats. Examples of unsaturated fats are corn oil and safflower oil. It is generally recommended that the total intake of fats be limited to 30 percent or less of daily caloric intake (Alpers et al, 1995).

Water

Water is the essential solvent for all metabolic activities, such as nutrient transport in and out of cells; elimination of wastes through the kidneys, gastrointestinal tract, skin, and lungs; and regulation of body temperature by evaporation from the skin. In addition, water and electrolytes are crucial to maintaining the body's fluid balance (a subject discussed in more detail later in this chapter).

Without water, survival is possible only for a matter of days; in an extremely hot and dry environment, dehydration and death can occur within 24 hours. Infants conserve water less efficiently than adults and thus tolerate water deficit more poorly.

Depending on a person's age, gender, and body build, water makes up 50 to 70 percent of body weight. Because of this, it is possible to sustain a substantial rapid weight loss by taking diuretics (medications to cause increased urinary losses) or laxatives. Of course, the weight quickly returns when fluids are replaced. Some weight-conscious individuals occasionally take diuretics to achieve weight loss. However, this is potentially dangerous because diuretics may cause electrolyte imbalances and other metabolic disturbances.

Vitamins

Vitamins are organic compounds that occur in minute quantities in food and are necessary for normal metabolism. Although vitamins provide no calories, many are important in releasing the energy from carbohydrates, fats, and proteins.

They are usually classified as fat soluble (vitamins A, D, E, and K) or water soluble (vitamin C [ascorbic acid], thiamine, riboflavin, niacin, vitamin B_6, pantothenic acid, biotin, folacin, and vitamin B_{12}).

Water-soluble vitamins cannot be stored in the body; therefore, a daily supply must be provided for each person. Deterioration can also occur, so vitamins need to be carefully stored. Fat-soluble vitamins can be stored (although vitamin E and K have limited storage time) and do not require daily amounts to be provided. Vitamin therapy may be needed for persons unable to consume adequate vitamins through oral dietary intake.

Normal Nutritional and Dietary Recommendations

Recommendations for a prudent diet have been made in similar forms for Americans by the American Heart Association, the American Cancer Society, and the National Research Council Committee on Diet, Nutrition, and Cancer (Weinsier et al, 1989). In general, the recommendations include the following:

- Eat a wide variety of foods from the four major food groups (dairy products, cereals and grains, meat, and fruits and vegetables) to ensure an adequate intake of nutrients necessary for tissue maintenance and growth. If an entire food group must be eliminated because of intolerance or personal beliefs, other foods must be supplemented to provide the missed nutrients.
- Limit calories to achieve and maintain body weight within 20 percent of the ideal body weight.
- Eat a high carbohydrate diet (50 to 55 percent calories or more); emphasize complex carbohydrates and high-fiber foods—fresh fruits, fresh vegetables, and whole grain products.
- Limit total fat intake to less than 30 percent of calories to reduce the risk of coronary artery disease and certain cancers (such as breast and colon cancer). Limit cholesterol intake to less than 300 mg/day.
- Limit protein intake to approximately 15 percent of calories. Excess meat consumption may result in a large intake of saturated fats. Also, there is some evidence that a long-term high protein intake may have adverse effects on renal function and bone mass.
- Limit sodium intake to less than 3 g/day because reduced salt intake reduces the incidence of salt-sensitive forms of high blood pressure. The average American eats more than 4 g of sodium per day, despite the fact that daily requirements are less than 500 mg/day.

Food Groups. The United States Department of Agriculture has developed guidelines to provide ample room for foods from all food groups to be included in the American diet. Emphasis is placed on the number of servings in each group, not on the quantity consumed. The original "four" food groups devised to prevent illness and promote health have been modified (Fig. 22–3). The groups provide the quantities of nutrients needed to meet daily recommended dietary allowances (RDAs). Using the food groups provides an easy way for individuals to select a balanced diet. The food group plan emphasizes the need for breads, cereals, potatoes, pasta and rice, with limited fat intake.

Recommended Daily Food Allowances. The RDAs are defined as the daily amounts of essential nutrients as estimated by the Food and Nutrition Board. The RDAs are devised from the available scientific knowledge that determines the adequacy of physiologic needs of healthy people. The Food and Nutrition Board is part of the National Research Council of the National Academy of Sciences. Dietary standards are not consistent between countries; however, there is no difference in the RDA of iron between women residing in Canada as compared with those living in the United States.

RDAs were not developed to be used by consumers; instead they were to serve as standards for planning food supplies for population groups. The RDAs are used by the Food and Drug Administration to develop standards for food labeling and food fortification programs. For example, food labels require nutrient information to be printed on each label. For the consumer, RDAs should be averaged over several days. Health-promoting diets must consider the individual consuming the diet (Herron, 1991).

Electrolytes

Electrolytes are minerals that dissociate in solution into electrically charged particles called ions. This property allows electrolytes to conduct tiny electric currents that are needed for many chemical reactions essential to normal functioning of cells, muscles, and nerve fibers. Some electrolytes (sodium, potassium, calcium, and magnesium) have positive charges, and others (chloride, bicarbonate, and phosphate) have negative charges. Positively charged ions are called cations, and negatively charged ions are called anions. In the body, the number of cations must always equal the number of anions to achieve a chemical balance. (This topic is discussed further in the next section.) Electrolytes frequently act cooperatively in achieving body functions; yet, each has specific functions. The important functions of major electrolytes are listed in Table 22–2.

Although present only in trace amounts, elements such as chromium, cobalt, copper, iodine, iron, manganese, molybdenum, selenium, and zinc are essential to normal body functioning. For example, zinc plays a role in many physiologic functions, including bone growth, immunocompetence, and maintenance of special senses such as vision, taste, and smell.

FLUID AND ELECTROLYTE BALANCE

Fluid and Electrolyte Movement

Body fluids are the mechanism by which nutrients are transported to cells and by which waste products of metabo-

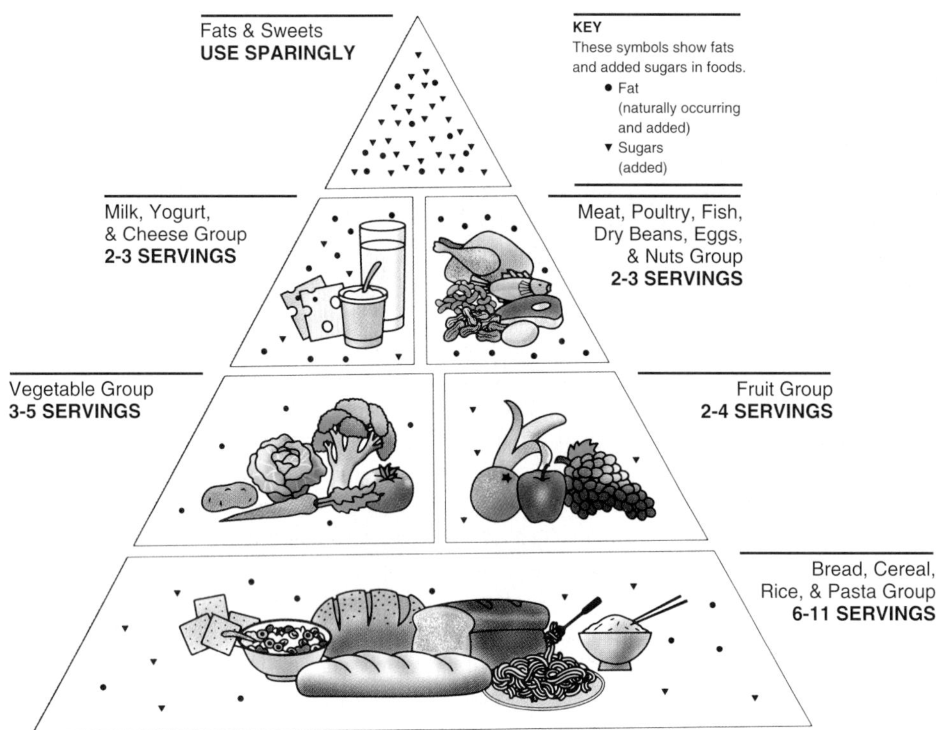

Figure 22-3. The U.S. Department of Agriculture Food Guide Pyramid.

lism are transported back to the kidneys and other organs for excretions. Body fluids are classified as either intracellular (ICF—fluid inside millions of tiny body cells) and extracellular (ECF—fluid between the cells and inside the blood vessels). The portion of ECF that bathes the cells is called interstitial fluid, whereas fluid within the bloodstream is called intravascular fluid (Figs. 22–4 and 22–5).

TABLE 22-2 Functions of Major Electrolytes

Electrolyte	Functions
Sodium (primary cation in extracellular fluid)	• Water balance • Neuromuscular function
Potassium (primary cation in intracellular fluid)	• Transmission of nerve impulses • Muscle contraction • Protein and glycogen synthesis
Calcium	• Transmission of nerve impulses • Contraction of muscle • Plays role in coagulation
Magnesium	• Plays role in carbohydrate and protein metabolism • Activator for many intracellular enzyme activities • Transmission of nerve impulses • Contraction of muscle
Phosphorus	• Critical constituent of all body tissues • Essential to intermediate metabolism of carbohydrate, proteins, and fats • Transmission of nerve impulses • Contraction of muscle
Chloride	• Maintains acid-base balance • Formation of gastric secretions

Infants have a higher body fluid content (70 to 80 percent of their body weight) than adults. In addition to having proportionately more body fluid, the infant has relatively more ECF. Because the ECF is lost more readily than cellular fluid during times of illness, infants are more vulnerable to fluid volume deficit after fluid losses, such as occur in diarrhea and vomiting. By the end of the second year of life, the total body fluid content approaches the adult percentage. At puberty, the adult body composition is attained (40 percent cellular and 20 percent extracellular). For the first time, a sex differentiation in fluid content occurs. Women have a lower percentage of body fluid than men because they have proportionately more body fat (fat cells contain little water, whereas muscle tissue is rich in water).

After absorption into capillaries of the digestive tract, nutrients are transported through the circulatory system to the cells and waste products are returned from the cells to the circulation for elimination. Body fluids are in constant motion, maintaining healthy living conditions for the cells. Remarkably, the capillary bed in the adult provides close to 6300 square meters of filtering surface! Movement of fluid through the capillary walls into the tissues depends on the force of hydrostatic pressure (equalization of pressure in liquids generated by contraction of the heart) at both the arterial and venous ends of the vessel. Conversely, the osmotic pressure (the diffusion of fluids through membranes) exerted by plasma albumin draws fluid back into the capillary. These two opposing forces determine the direction of fluid flow. At the arterial end of the capillary, hydrostatic pressure exceeds

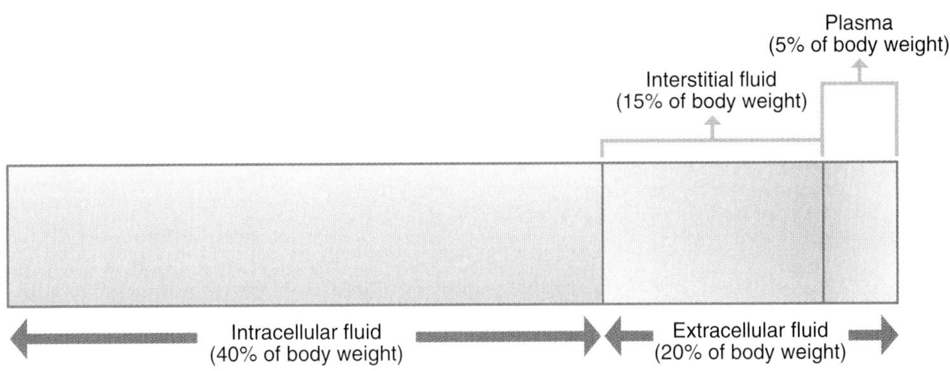

Figure 22-4. Body fluid distribution. The intracellular fluid (ICF) comprises the fluids inside the millions of body cells. The extracellular fluid (ECF) comprises the fluids outside and between the cells and includes the blood. The ECF that bathes the cells is called interstitial fluid (ISF) and that within the bloodstream (i.e., the plasma) is called intravascular fluid (IVF). This diagram shows the proportions of these fluid compartments in the normal adult.

osmotic pressure, forcing fluid out of the capillary to the cell. However, at the venous end of the capillary, osmotic pressure exceeds hydrostatic pressure, drawing fluid back into the capillary. This flow of fluids constantly provides the cells with delivery of nutrients and removal of wastes.

Homeostatic Mechanisms

The body has a remarkable ability to keep its numerous interrelated functions in balance. Some of these homeostatic mechanisms exist to keep the composition and volume of body fluids within narrow limits of normal. Organs actively involved in homeostasis include the kidneys, pituitary gland, adrenal glands, parathyroid glands, and lungs.

Kidneys. Of vital importance to normal fluid and electrolyte balance is the ability of the kidneys to excrete water, electrolytes, and organic materials and to conserve whatever amounts of these substances the body requires. They normally perform this function superbly and with ease. For example, an adult's kidneys filter 170 L of plasma every day; yet, because of their remarkable ability to return over 99 percent of the filtrate to the circulation, only 1 to 2 L is excreted as urine. The kidneys excrete the end-products of metabolism of proteins (in the form of urea), carbohydrates (in the form of water), and unneeded quantities of electrolytes and other substances to maintain normal electrolyte and acid-base (pH) balance. In addition, the kidneys can actually generate some electrolytes (such as bicarbonate) when needed to maintain pH balance.

Pituitary Gland. The hypothalamus in the brain manufactures a substance known as antidiuretic hormone, which is stored in the posterior pituitary gland and released as needed to adjust the sodium concentration in the ECF. Because antidiuretic hormone causes the body to retain water, it is sometimes referred to as the "water-conserving hormone."

Adrenal Glands. The adrenals, small glands situated on top of each kidney, are separated into two sections (the cortex and medulla). The hormone aldosterone, manufactured in the adrenal cortex, is extremely important in fluid and electrolyte homeostasis, particularly in sodium and potassium balance. It acts on the kidneys to cause sodium retention and potassium excretion. Factors that increase aldosterone activity include a drop in the plasma sodium level or a rise in plasma potassium level and a diminished blood volume. The primary stimulus is

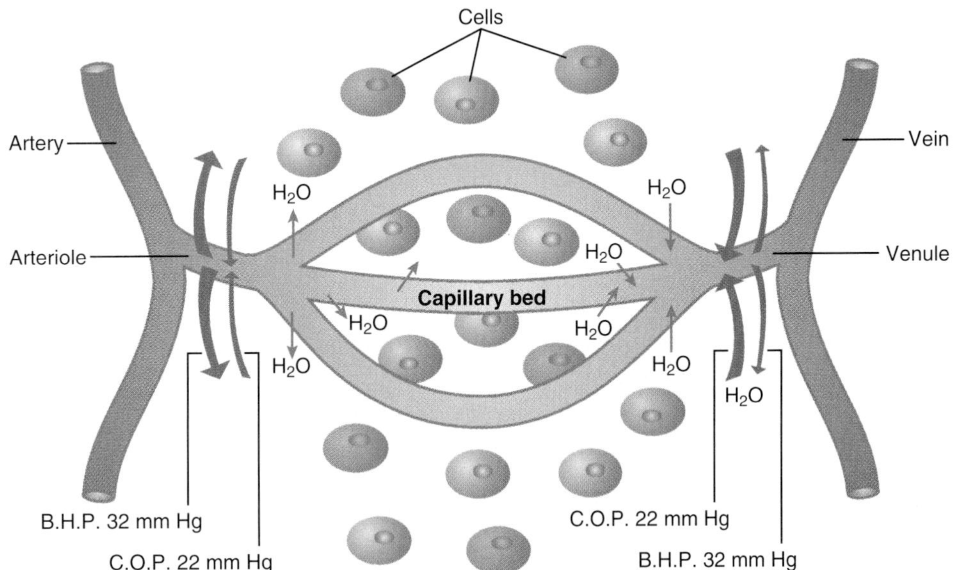

Figure 22-5. Movement of fluid and electrolytes between compartments. The relationship between hydrostatic and osmotic pressures is shown at the arteriole and venule ends of a capillary bed. (Redrawn from Lankford.)

reduced blood volume. An elevated plasma sodium level or a drop in plasma potassium level will increase aldosterone secretion. Another hormone from the adrenal cortex is cortisol; it mimics the action of aldosterone but has only a fraction of the potency.

Parathyroid Glands. The four pea-sized parathyroid glands are embedded in the corners of the thyroid gland and regulate calcium and phosphate balance by means of parathyroid hormone. This hormone can stimulate bone to release calcium into the ECF when needed to correct a fall in the blood calcium concentration (hypocalcemia). Conversely, when the extracellular calcium level is too high (hypercalcemia), parathyroid hormone secretion is depressed so that almost no bone calcium is released. Parathyroid hormone also influences the amount of calcium absorbed through the intestine and the amount eliminated through the kidneys.

Lungs. The lungs are vital in regulating acid-base (pH) balance. Their primary function in this capacity is the elimination of carbon dioxide (a potential acid) in the ECF. When the ECF pH becomes too alkaline, the lungs hypoventilate to retain carbon dioxide. Conversely, when the ECF pH becomes too acidic, the lungs hyperventilate to blow off excess carbon dioxide. The lungs also remove about 300 ml of water daily through exhalation.

APPROACHES TO NUTRITION AND DIET THERAPY

Depending on the level of physical activity, a healthy person requires 2000 to 3000 kcal/day. A person suffering from trauma, disease, or serious burns may require up to 10,000 kcal/day. A person who fails to obtain adequate fluids and nutrients becomes malnourished and without proper treatment will eventually develop serious disruptions in body functions. The most immediate problem is lack of water, which interferes with cellular activities and leads to death in a matter of days. Problems with water deprivation occur relatively early because the body lacks a fluid reservoir to draw upon in time of need. In contrast, food deprivation can be tolerated for much longer periods because the body has a ready supply of calories in various forms. For example, shortly after an individual stops eating, sugar (glycogen) stored in the liver and muscle cells is sufficient to supply energy needs for 6 to 12 hours.

Fat stores (adipose tissue) are drawn on next to help prevent destruction of vital lean body tissues. However, not all body tissues can accept fat as a fuel. For example, the central nervous system, red blood cells, and the kidneys require sugar for normal metabolism. Because fat cannot be converted to sugar, the body is forced to draw protein from lean tissues (muscle and organs) for this purpose. Thus, prolonged starvation depletes the patient of both fat and lean body mass. Whereas fat loss is easily tolerated, protein loss disrupts numerous body functions. Starvation also disrupts the function of important minerals by altering metabolic processes involved in their regulation.

Because starvation, or even partial starvation, interferes with virtually every normal body function, it must be prevented or at least minimized whenever possible by encouraging adequate fluid and nutrient intake. Fluids and nutrients can be administered enterally (by mouth or feeding tube) or parenterally (by peripheral or central IV routes).

ENTERAL ROUTES

Normal chewing and swallowing provides many benefits. The patient derives psychological rewards from being able to eat normally, especially when eating favorite foods. He or she also benefits physiologically from gradual absorption and efficient utilization of food and fluids, as well as minimal disturbance of fluid and electrolyte balances compared with tube feeding or parenteral feeding. Finally, the typical oral diet is least expensive to administer.

If the patient cannot accept foods orally but retains a functional gastrointestinal tract, enteral tube feeding should be considered. In tube feeding, liquid preparations are administered through a tube inserted into the stomach or small intestine. Usually the tube is threaded through a nasal passage and down the esophagus until it reaches the stomach (nasogastric tube) or the upper part of the small intestine (nasoduodenal or nasojejunal tubes). As a rule, tubes inserted nasally are not left in place for more than 6 weeks. If prolonged care is anticipated, nutrients can be introduced directly into the gastrointestinal tract through a surgically or endoscopically placed tube (gastrostomy or jejunostomy) (Figs. 22–6 and 22–7).

Several factors influence tube placement. For alert, ambulatory patients with normal gastrointestinal function, the gastric site is preferable because it allows intermittent feedings, which facilitates patient mobility. For patients at high risk for pulmonary aspiration of tube-feeding formula, interstitial placement in the duodenum or jejunum is preferable.

At times, tube feedings may be used for seriously ill patients who experience reduced or absent gastrointestinal motility (peristalsis), a condition sometimes called paralytic or postoperative ileus. Often, however, normal motility returns to the small intestine before it returns to the stomach and colon. Because of this, it is sometimes possible to administer feedings into the small intestine within hours of a traumatic event. This knowledge has greatly improved the ability of clinicians to nourish even critically ill patients by the enteral route.

Liquid feedings can be introduced into the stomach every few hours as boluses or continuously over 24 hours. In contrast, feedings introduced into the small intestine must be administered continuously.

Types of Oral Diets

Oral Diets for Health Maintenance. As discussed in the normal nutrition section, recommendations for a prudent diet have been made in similar forms for Americans by the American Heart Association, the American Cancer Society, and the National Research Council Committee on Diet, Nutrition, and

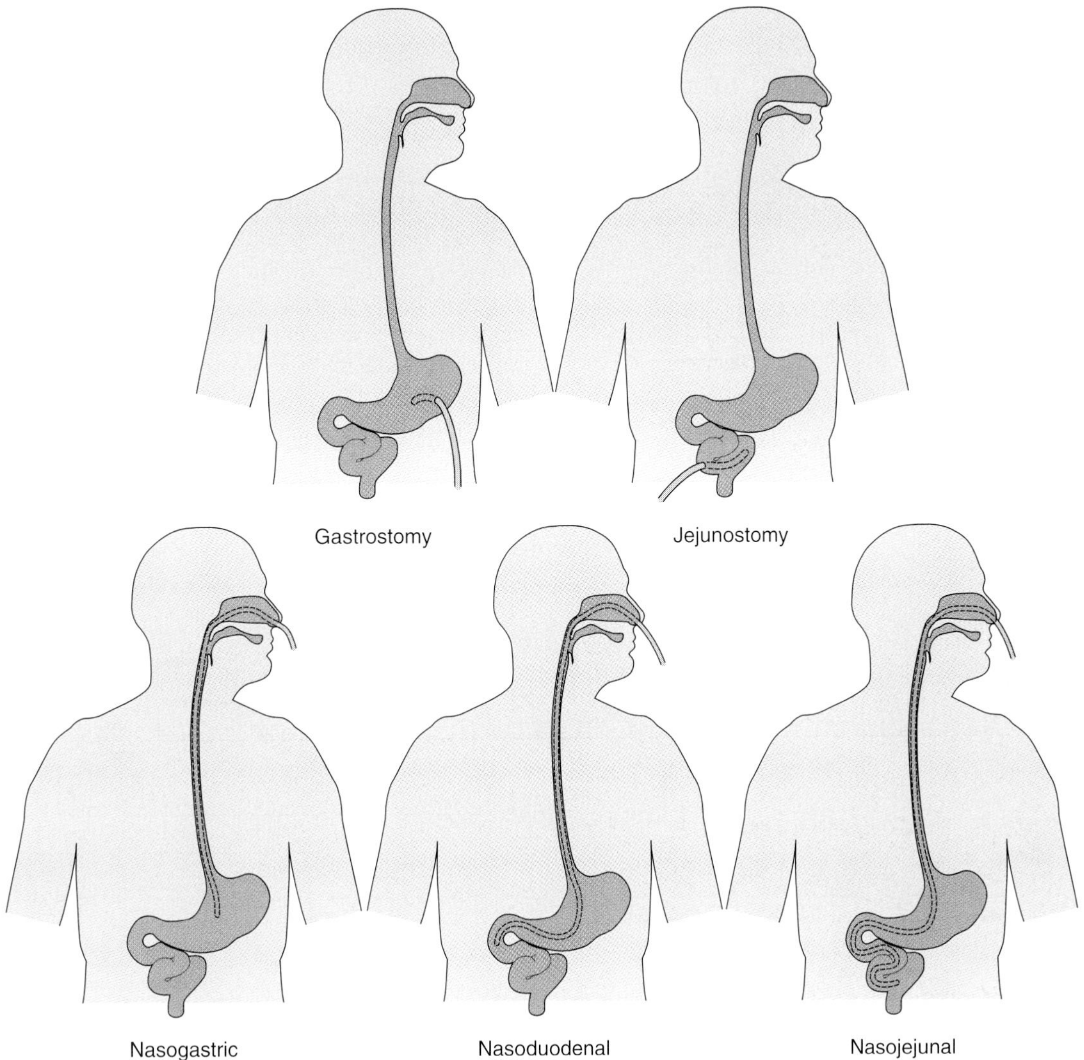

Figure 22-6. Positioning of feeding tubes.

Cancer (Weinsier et al, 1989). Recommendations are constantly under review as new research studies change requirements.

Modified Diets. Specific disease conditions often mandate severe dietary alterations. For example, individuals with lactose intolerance should avoid milk and liquid milk products. Those with hypertension should limit sodium intake. Patients with chronic hepatic or renal disease often need severely restricted protein intake.

Modified diets include clear liquid diets, full liquid diets, and soft or pureed diets. Soft and pureed diets usually supply all nutritional requirements whereas liquid hospital diets do not. Full liquid diets furnish 1000 to 1500 calories and about half of the protein contained in a regular hospital diet. Clear liquid diets are grossly inadequate and contain only about 300 calories and 10 g of protein (Pestana, 1989). If clear liquid diets must be continued for more than a few days, consideration should be given to the use of commercially prepared liquid formulas containing partially digested nutrients.

Oral Liquid Supplements. Forms of oral liquid supplements range from milkshakes to complete balanced diets packaged as individual servings (such as Ensure). Although primarily developed for tube feedings, some liquid formulas are available in flavored forms to increase palatability. Because of bad taste, not all tube-feeding formulas are suitable for this purpose. For example, monomeric (elemental) formulas, such as Vivonex, have a very unpleasant fishy taste.

Liquid balanced complete supplements are helpful in bolstering the patient's usual diet. In fact, some patients prefer these over regular foods that are more difficult to prepare and eat. Others may refuse even the flavored supplements because of unpleasant taste.

Characteristics of Enteral Formulas

A wide variety of tube-feeding formulas are commercially available. They vary in a number of important characteristics,

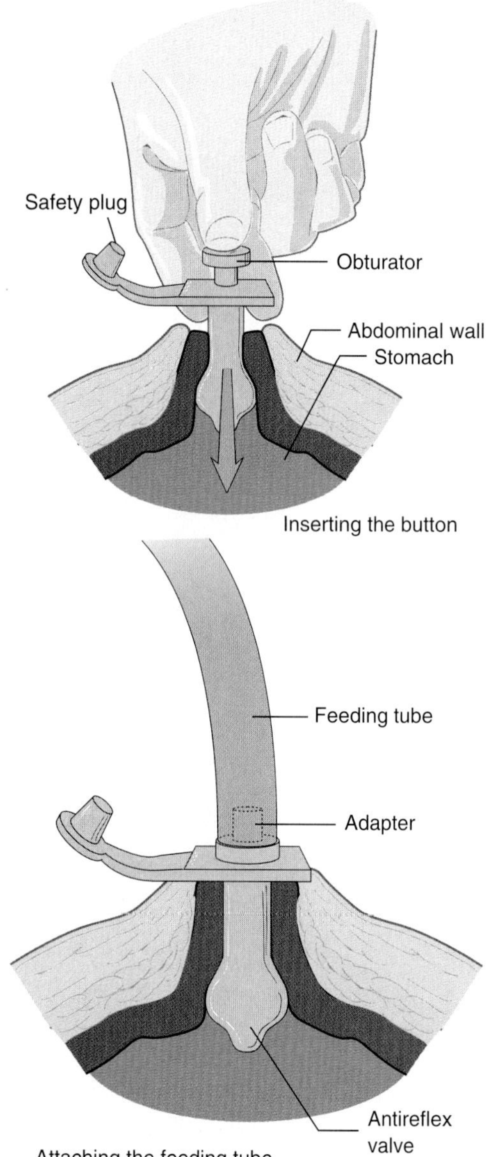

Figure 22-7. Gastrostomy feeding button. A patient receiving long-term enteral feedings may have this small plastic device implanted into a stoma in the abdominal wall. The enteral feeding tube connects to the device instead of being inserted directly into the stoma. This helps keep the feeding tube from dislodging, reduces skin irritation, and helps prevent reflux of gastric contents through the stoma.

including caloric density, nutrient content, osmolality, and electrolyte content.

Caloric density refers to the number of calories in a given volume of fluid. Most formulas range from 1.0 to 2.0 calories/ml. Tolerance for fluid is a major factor in the determination of the caloric density selected for an individual patient. For example, patients with poor fluid tolerance may require high-caloric density formulas to limit their fluid intake.

Nutrient content of liquid feeding preparations varies widely. Of the percentages and sources of protein, fat, and carbohydrate, the most important is protein. Formulas may be polymeric or monomeric. *Polymeric* formulas contain intact protein that requires digestion and absorption by the digestive tract; *monomeric* formulas contain proteins that are predigested and require only absorption. The former is suitable for patients with normal digestive abilities; the latter is needed for those with malabsorptive conditions.

Osmolality of a tube feeding is largely determined by protein, carbohydrate, and electrolyte concentrations. Osmolality is primarily a function of the number and size of molecules and ionized particles in a given volume. Plasma osmolality is approximately 300 mOsm/kg; therefore, formulas with an osmolality of approximately 300 mOsm/kg are called iso-osmotic. Those that are appreciably above 300 mOsm/kg are called hyperosmotic; those below 300 mOsm/kg, hypo-osmotic (Fig. 22–8).

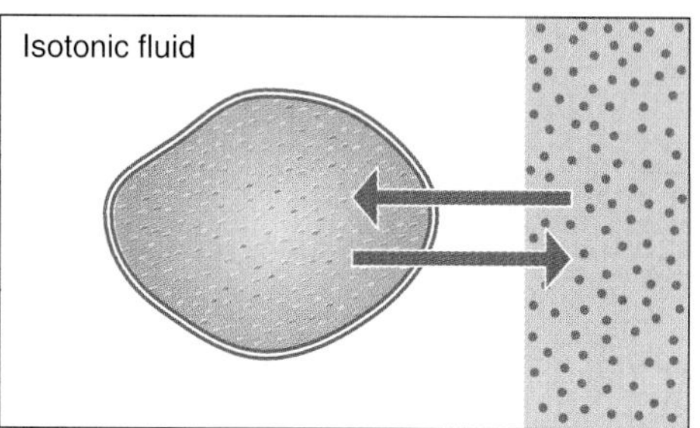

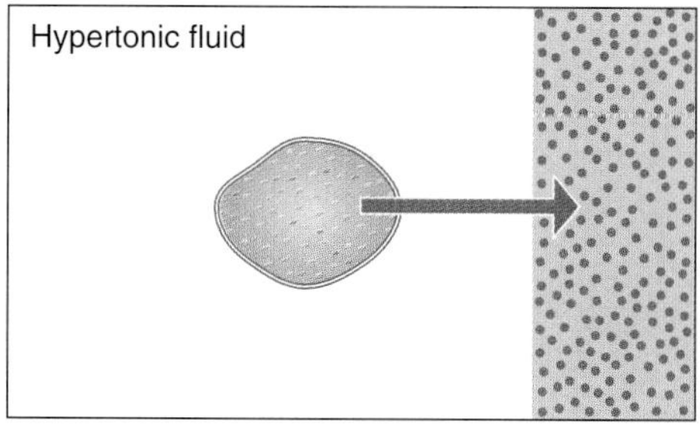

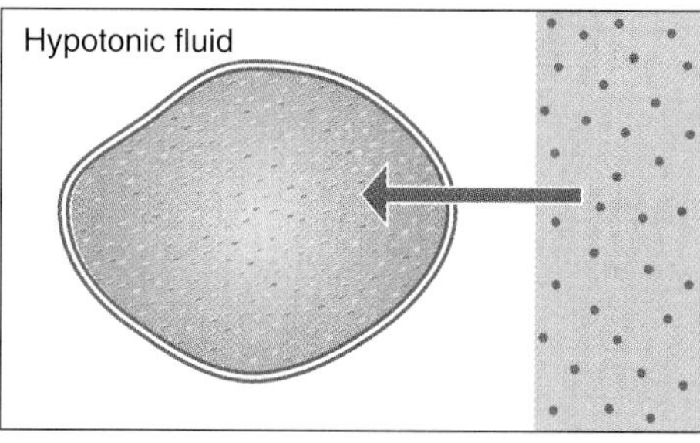

Figure 22-8. Fluid tonicity. An *isotonic* fluid (e.g., 5 percent dextrose in water, 0.9 percent sodium chloride) is equal in tonicity to intracellular fluid (ICF). An isotonic fluid entering the circulation causes no net water movement across the semipermeable cell membrane. Because osmotic pressure is the same inside and outside of the cells, cell size remains the same. A *hypertonic* fluid (e.g., 3 percent sodium chloride, 50 percent dextrose) has a greater tonicity than ICF. When infused into the circulation, hypertonic fluid moves from the cells to the area of greater concentration, causing the cells to shrink. A *hypotonic* fluid (e.g., 0.45 percent sodium chloride) has a lower tonicity than ICF. Infusion of a hypotonic fluid causes water to diffuse into the ICF, resulting in cell enlargement.

The *electrolyte content* of most formulas is based on usual requirements; however, there is variability among individual products. Thus, depending on the formula and the patient's condition, additional electrolytes may be needed or the preestablished amount may exceed the patient's tolerance.

PARENTERAL ROUTES

Patients who require more nutrition than can be provided by the gastrointestinal tract should receive supplemental feeding by the parenteral (IV) route. Some patients may receive nutrients by both enteral and parenteral routes. For others who lack gastrointestinal function, the parenteral route is the only option. Parenteral feedings are usually called IV feedings because they are introduced through needles or plastic catheters threaded into one of the body's many veins. Usually peripheral veins are used rather than central veins (Fig. 22–9).

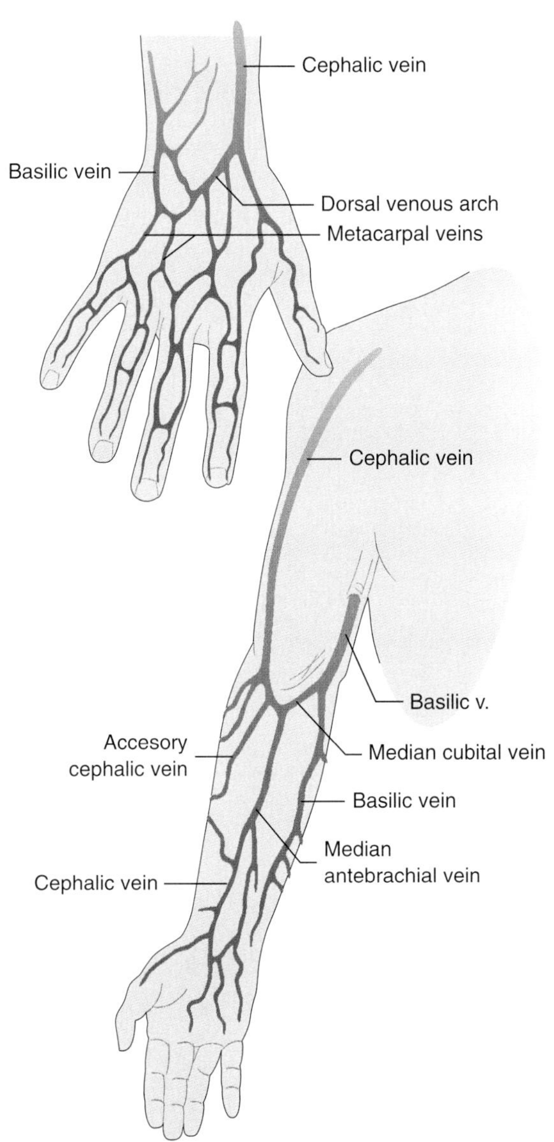

Figure 22–9. Peripheral venipuncture sites.

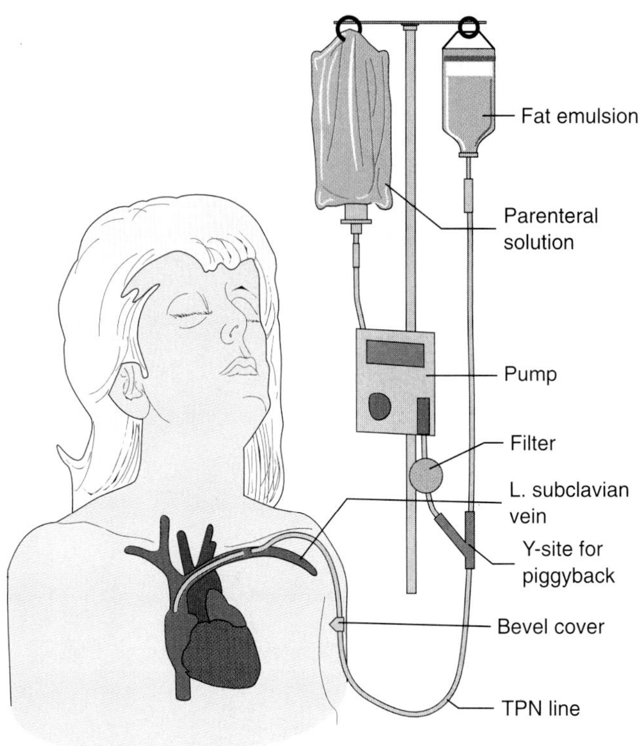

Figure 22–10. Administering parenteral nutrition through a central venous catheter.

For problems likely to last only a few days, a simple solution of glucose and water with added minerals (electrolytes) can easily be infused through a peripheral vein, usually in the lower arm or back of the hand (see Fig. 22–9). This treatment would typically be used with a patient who has just undergone surgery and is unable to consume food and fluids for 1 or 2 days because of nausea and temporarily diminished gastrointestinal motility (peristalsis) secondary to the effects of anesthesia.

If gastrointestinal dysfunction is likely to preclude nutrient intake for several days, additional nutrients should be supplied parenterally. Protein and fat (lipid) emulsions can be infused with dextrose through a needle in a forearm vein, or, if more concentrated, through a central venous catheter (Fig. 22–10).

For many years, clinicians have been able to infuse dilute solutions of dextrose, proteins, and fat emulsions through peripheral veins. However, because these solutions lack sufficient calories, peripheral vein nutrition has limited value. In the 1970s, researchers found that concentrated solutions of dextrose, proteins, and fat emulsions could be infused in large volumes through central veins and that adequate calories could be provided to fill maintenance needs and promote tissue growth, even for those with great need (Blackburn et al, 1976). These improved catheters allow patients to receive total parenteral nutrition (TPN) indefinitely, if necessary. Some catheters are surgically implanted and can be easily concealed (Fig. 22–11).

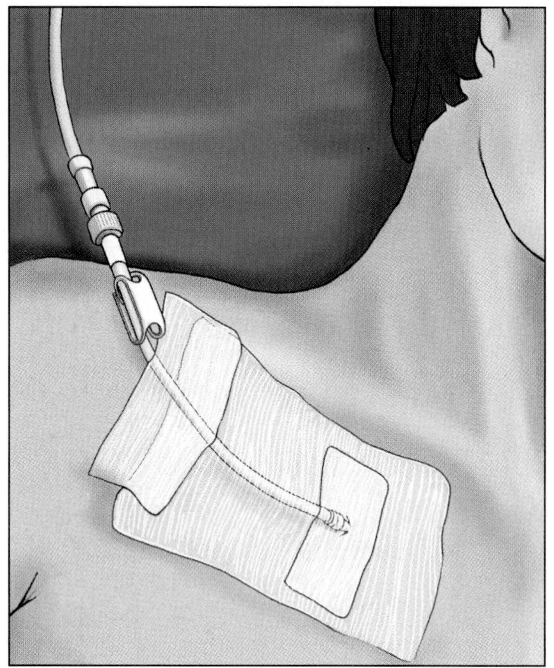

Figure 22-11. Implanted central venous catheter with dressing. (From Monahan, F.D., Neighbors, M. [1998]. Medical-Surgical Nursing: Foundations for Clinical Practice. Philadelphia: W.B. Saunders.)

Characteristics of Parenteral Fluids

Parenteral (IV) fluids range from simple solutions of water and electrolytes, or water and dextrose, to complex mixtures that supply all of the essential nutrients for TPN. As with enteral fluids, considerations of caloric density, nutrient content, osmolality, and electrolyte content are important. For patients requiring only brief periods of IV fluid therapy, simple dextrose and electrolyte solutions suffice. These include isotonic solutions of electrolyte and water, such as isotonic saline (0.9 percent sodium chloride) and lactated Ringer's solution and dextrose and water (D_5W) (Table 22–3).

Prepackaged IV fluids contain a variety of proportions of electrolytes and calorie sources. As long as the fluids are close to the osmolality of plasma (isotonic) and do not contain grossly irritating substances, they can be administered into peripheral veins.

Solutions containing only dextrose and electrolytes are inadequate for patients requiring prolonged parenteral fluid therapy. For example, a liter of D_5W contains only 170 calories and no electrolytes, and 0.9 percent sodium chloride (without added dextrose) contains no calories. Fortunately, as indicated earlier, all of the essential nutrients can be infused by the IV route, using TPN solutions. A typical TPN formulation is composed of 25 percent dextrose and 4.25 percent amino acids and has a concentration about four times that of plasma. Because of this high density, such a solution must be infused into a large central vein (such as the subclavian) to prevent trauma to venous walls. Electrolytes, trace elements, and vitamins are added according to individual needs. Fat (lipid) emulsions of soybean or safflower oil are available in 10 percent and 20 percent concentrations and are used to supply fatty acids and added calories.

Relevant Research

Research has been conducted to attempt to identify the best methods to care for patients requiring nutrition support. Health care workers most involved in this care are nurses, physicians, dietitians, and pharmacists. Some studies have been done by nurses working alone or by members of the other disciplines working alone. However, many have been conducted by members of two or more disciplines working together to solve problems shared by all health care workers who care for patients requiring nutrition support. This is a rational approach to clinical research because many patient care problems require intervention from all of these disciplines. Most nutrition- and fluid balance–related research studies conducted solely by nurses have focused on technical aspects of nutrient and fluid delivery to prevent complications. Some studies of fluid and electrolyte balance have dealt with assess-

TABLE 22-3 Electrolyte Content of Commonly Used Intravenous Fluids

Solution	Composition	Comments
0.9% NaCl (isotonic saline)	Na^+: 154 mEq/L Cl^-: 154 mEq/L	• Used primarily to expand plasma volume in hypovolemic patients. • Supplies an excess of Na and Cl; can cause hypernatremia and hyperchloremia if given in excessive volumes.
0.45% NaCl (half-strength saline)	Na^+: 77 mEq/L Cl^-: 77 mEq/L	• A hypotonic solution that provides Na, Cl, and free water.
Lactated Ringer's solution (LR)	Na^+: 130 mEq/L K^+: 4 mEq/L Ca^{++}: 3 mEq/L Lactate: 28 mEq/L (metabolized to bicarbonate) Cl^-: 109 mEq/L	• An isotonic solution that contains multiple electrolytes in roughly the same concentrations as found in plasma (contains no magnesium or phosphorus)
5% dextrose in water (D_5W)		• Furnishes free water but no electrolytes • Furnishes 170 calories

ment for specific imbalances; this is reasonable because nurses are responsible for monitoring the patient's changing health status. Nurse researchers studying nutrition and fluid balance problems have focused on technical aspects of nutrient and fluid delivery to prevent complications. Additional research has been done on improving methods of assessing patients for specific fluid and electrolyte imbalances.

ORAL INTAKE

Because nurses are primarily responsible for helping patients to drink and eat, it is understandable why they would want to learn more about how much and under what circumstances patients consume fluid and nutrients by mouth. However, this area remains underresearched; most oral administration studies have explored aspects of geriatric nutrition and the ethical problems of feeding frail or incompetent patients.

ENSURING ADEQUATE WATER INTAKE

Although elderly patients need to drink enough fluids to prevent serious problems such as confusion and constipation, administration is often difficult and time consuming, especially for institutionalized individuals, as seen in Mrs. Smith's case.

Elderly patients are more prone to develop sodium and water imbalances after periods of water deprivation than are younger adults (Phillips et al, 1984). Apparently this is because older persons lack a normal thirst response during periods of water deprivation. Recall that Mrs. Smith did not express sensations of thirst despite serious water deprivation; because of her poor water intake, her serum sodium level rose to a dangerous level (185 mEq/L).

Elderly patients in institutional settings tend to consume less fluid than those in other settings—most likely because residents commonly are offered fluids only when they receive their meals and medications (Adams, 1988). Because these patients tend to drink whatever amount of fluid is offered to them (provided that they can swallow), nurses might try offering larger volumes of fluid when providing care.

A study of nursing home patients found that patients consumed about 76 percent of the desired fluid amount (1600 ml/M^2 body surface area) and that older patients consumed less than comparatively younger patients (Gaspar, 1988). However, some patients drank slightly more than was required. It is therefore important to evaluate each patient's fluid needs individually. For example, some patients may need fluid restrictions if they have advanced congestive heart failure.

Thirst

In a study of terminally ill patients McCann and associates (1994) found that there was scant evidence that dehydration caused thirst. The study conducted in a comfort care unit of a hospital found that 62 percent of the dying patients experienced no thirst or were thirsty only during the early phases of their illness. The study supports the need to keep terminally ill patients comfortable but individual patient needs must be given consideration. Zerwekh (1997) indicates that fluids should be neither artificially forced nor withheld from dying patients.

SHOULD PATIENTS BE FORCE FED?

In some situations, patients are coaxed or actively forced to consume foods. When this occurs, it is usually because caregivers believe the patient's life should be preserved at all costs. A Swedish psychogeriatric clinic served as a site for a study of 39 health care workers (including registered nurses, practical nurses, and nurses' aides) regarding ethical concerns of force feeding patients (Akerlund and Norberg, 1985). Force feeding took the form of spoon feeding because the setting's policy was to avoid tube feedings and IV feedings. For most of the interviewed workers, force feeding was equated with holding the patient's head while forcing the spoon in the patient's mouth. Because they found this action reprehensible, most reported not participating in the activity. Those workers who did practice forced feeding of patients reported being guided by the rule "keep people alive." Some reported feeling anxious because they feared forced feeding would cause the patient to choke. A similar survey was taken of 30 nurses on an acute neurological-neurosurgical unit in an urban American hospital. Although all of the respondents overwhelmingly agreed that competent patients have the right to refuse any treatment, they were less in agreement about what should be done when an incompetent patient refuses nutritional support (Mumma, 1986). Over half (56 percent) thought that an incompetent patient should be fed by any means necessary.

TUBE FEEDING COMPLICATIONS

Tube feedings have been extensively studied by nurses because the majority of complications associated with this feeding method are primarily managed by nurses. Much of the research has centered around preventing complications such as diarrhea, tube clogging, and aspiration of fluids by the lungs. Some studies have also assessed physical and emotional distress and testing tube placement.

PHYSICAL AND EMOTIONAL DISCOMFORT

Mechanical complications vary according to the type of tube and its location. There are two types of nasally placed tubes (large-diameter firm nasogastric tubes and small-diameter soft tubes are suitable for either nasogastric or nasointestinal use). Different kinds of complications occur with each type. Large-diameter firm nasogastric tubes left in place for a prolonged period can cause irritation of the nose, throat, ears, sinuses, esophagus, and stomach. In contrast, the small-diameter soft tubes cause little mechanical irritation. The problem most commonly associated with gastrostomy and jejunostomy feeding sites is local irritation if secretions are allowed to leak onto the skin.

Although health care providers commonly consider the newer small-diameter tubes to be relatively comfortable for patients, numerous tubes are pulled out by confused patients (Eisenberg et al, 1987). Whether this action is purely a function of restless behavior or is partly related to discomfort is not known.

Although local tissue irritation problems can be quite troublesome in tube-fed patients, emotional concerns may be even greater. In an attempt to describe patients' subjective experiences with tube feedings, a team of investigators interviewed 30 hospitalized tube-fed patients, using a checklist to identify common experiences causing distress (Padilla et al, 1979). Among the factors most frequently selected by patients were thirst, sore throat, dry mouth, having a tube in the nose, breathing through the mouth, and taking nutrients through the tube instead of experiencing the satisfaction of tasting, chewing, and swallowing food. Since the time this study was conducted, the characteristics of feeding tubes have changed drastically from large-diameter rigid plastic material to small-diameter extremely pliable materials such as polyethylene or Silastic rubber. Thus, use of the newer tubes has largely eliminated the discomfort in the nose and throat associated with physical irritation by stiff, large-diameter tubes. However, despite the greater comfort associated with small-diameter tubes, deprivation of normal eating remains a major problem. Rains (1981) interviewed 10 tube-fed patients at home and found these individuals also experienced a sense of loss at being deprived of favorite foods.

GASTROINTESTINAL INTOLERANCE

Abdominal cramping, fullness, and nausea and vomiting can accompany tube feedings, especially when given too quickly. A study of the rate at which intermittent (bolus) feedings could be administered to normal subjects without causing symptomatic intolerance was conducted by a group of nurse researchers (Heitkemper et al, 1981). The investigators concluded that normal patients can tolerate bolus feedings of 250 to 750 ml when administered at a rate of 30 ml/min without distress. Because almost half the subjects experienced gastrointestinal symptoms early in the feeding, the investigators recommended that the initial intermittent feedings be given in small volumes at a slow rate. Because illness affects a patient's feeding tolerance to tube feedings (probably by altering the gastrointestinal tract), the investigators recommended that the research be repeated using ill subjects. Because the stomach acts as a reservoir, it can serve as a site for either continuous or bolus feedings; however, the small bowel can only tolerate slow, continuous feeding rates.

DIARRHEA

Diarrhea has been extensively studied because it is a common problem in tube-fed patients. Certainly diarrhea is more prevalent in severely ill individuals. Over 60 percent of the 73 mechanically ventilated tube-fed patients in one study developed diarrhea (Smith et al, 1990); high osmolality of tube-feeding formula as well as rapid infusion rates contributed to both the incidence and duration of diarrhea.

The most common cause of diarrhea in tube-fed patients is thought to be the administration of certain medications (such as antibiotics, sorbitol, and hyperosmolar agents). Another frequently cited cause is too rapid administration of concentrated formulas, especially into the small bowel. Other causes include formula contamination, lactose intolerance, and temperature of the formula. A controversial issue is whether the absence of fiber in the formula contributes to diarrhea.

Medications

In a study of 100 acutely ill tube-fed subjects, Guenter and coworkers (1991) found that antibiotic use was the most strongly associated factor with diarrhea. That is, diarrhea developed in 29 (41 percent) of the 71 patients who received antibiotics during, or within 2 weeks before, the feeding period whereas it occurred in only 1 (3 percent) of the 29 patients not receiving antibiotics. Another finding in this study was that hypoalbuminemia was statistically more prevalent in patients with diarrhea than in those without diarrhea. Hypoalbuminemia is often cited as a cause of diarrhea, presumably because of changes in the intestinal mucosa brought on by the low serum albumin level. One study indicated that a partially predigested (peptide-based) formula was less likely to produce diarrhea in hypoalbuminemic patients than was a standard formula (Brinson and Kolts, 1988).

Formula Contamination

Bacterial contamination of tube-feeding solutions has been implicated as a possible cause of diarrhea. Nurses are especially concerned with this problem because they are primarily responsible for preparing and administering feedings; it is generally during these maneuvers that formulas become contaminated. To determine the effect of sterile water versus tap water added to formulas, Perez and Brandt (1989) compared bacterial growth in six bags of formula diluted with sterile water and six diluted with tap water. Cultures of the formula found that lower levels of bacteria existed in the bags containing formula mixed with sterile water than in the bags containing formula mixed with tap water. The investigators suggested that it is prudent to use sterile water rather than tap water until further studies justify a change. Probably the most important finding in this study was that all of the feeding bags became unacceptably contaminated after 24 hours; thus, it was recommended that disposable feeding bags be changed every 24 hours.

Clinicians sometimes wonder if it is necessary to use sterile (versus clean) technique when handling enteral feedings. The effect of two methods of formula handling (aseptic versus clean) on the incidence of formula contamination and diarrhea was studied by Michschi and colleagues (1990). Cultures of formula were obtained on the first 4 days of tube feeding. Although a significantly greater incidence of contamination was found for the routine (clean) method group versus the aseptic method group, there were no significant differences in the incidence of diarrhea between the two groups. A larger study was recommended to address the pros and cons of clean versus sterile technique for handling tube-feeding formula.

It is best to handle tube-feeding formula and equipment as little as possible and only after washing one's hands carefully. In a study conducted in an intensive care nursery, both manipulated formulas (those mixed with water or other substances) and nonmanipulated formulas were tested for bacterial growth (Anderson et al, 1984). As expected, manipulated formulas contained significantly greater bacterial growth. Another important finding was that bacteria cultured from the feeding equipment were the same as those cultured from the nurses' hands.

Another factor that impacts on bacterial growth in tube-feeding formula is the length of time it has been allowed to hang in the feeding bag during administration to the patient. One group of researchers recommended that hang times not exceed 12 hours (Kohn and Keithley, 1989). Many tube-feeding formulas are now commercially available in single-use containers that do not require manipulation by the nurse; these formulas are less likely to become contaminated than those requiring pouring from containers into feeding bags.

The need to change feeding bags and tubing at 24-hour intervals is made clear by a study conducted in a community hospital (Schroeder et al, 1983). These researchers reported that five of nine feeding sets were heavily contaminated when cultured after 24 hours; however, the majority of sets showed no growth when cultured at 12 hours.

Lactose Intolerance

In the past, almost all tube-feeding formulas were milk-based and thus contained lactose. Today, relatively few contain lactose. Mostly this change in practice stemmed from research conducted by Walike and Walike in 1977. In this study, two identical diets, differing only in the presence or absence of lactose, were administered to 11 patients over a 10-day period in a clinical research unit where careful intake and output and total nitrogen balance studies were possible. Nine of the 11 patients had a significant increase in the frequency of stools while on the lactose-containing diet. These patients were found to have either a classic intolerance to lactose or a relative lactose intolerance when large quantities of lactose were administered in the tube feedings. Based on these findings, the need to avoid high-lactose tube feedings was recognized. Not only is lactose intolerance a constant problem in some well individuals (primarily black Americans), it can be a temporary problem in very ill individuals.

Fat Intolerance

The fat content of enteral formulas has been the subject of research. In one study, patients had a significantly lower incidence of diarrhea when formulas contained less than 20 g of fat per liter than when formulas contained more than this amount (Gottschlich et al, 1988).

Temperature of Formula

Temperature of tube-feeding formula has been studied as a possible cause of diarrhea in normal humans, based on the assumption that a cold formula could stimulate peristalsis (Kawaga-Busby et al, 1980). Results suggested that refrigerated tube-feeding formula is not as well tolerated as formula that is allowed to warm to room temperature before administration. Because most tube-feeding formulas in use today are packaged in ready-to-use cans or containers, the need for refrigerating formulas has largely been eliminated.

Fiber Content in Formula

Fiber content in tube-feeding formulas has been the basis of a number of studies related to the control of gastrointestinal symptoms. It has been suggested that patients may develop diarrhea when suddenly changed from a high- to low-roughage diet, such as occurs when a change is made from normal eating to ingestion of a low-fiber tube-feeding formula. Although most commercially available formulas are low in fiber, a few have recently been developed with added dietary fiber. Controversial findings exist regarding the efficacy of high-fiber formulas in reducing diarrhea. One group of researchers (Zimmaro et al, 1989) reported that a high-fiber formula is associated with a lower incidence of diarrhea than one without fiber; however, another group of researchers failed to find any significant difference in the rate of diarrhea in patients receiving and those not receiving high-fiber formulas (Guenter et al, 1991).

TUBE CLOGGING

The widespread use of small-diameter tubes is a mixed blessing. Although they are far more comfortable than their older stiff, wide-diameter counterparts, they are inclined to clog frequently. Among the common causes of clogging are formula residue adhering to the tube's lumen, inadequately crushed medications given through the tubes, and physical incompatibilities between enteral products and liquid pharmaceutical preparations.

Problems with Medication Administration

Administration of medications through small-bore tubes was identified as a common cause of tube clogging (Petrosino et al, 1989). This is especially true if tablets with a special coating (sometimes referred to as enteric coating) are crushed and given through the tube. Of course, failure to completely crush other types of pills can also lead to clogging. To avoid chemical reactions between two or more solid medications to be given at the same time, it is helpful to crush each one separately and dissolve it in several milliliters of water before administration. Five milliliters of water should be injected through the feeding tube before each medication is given. It is also helpful to inject 5 ml of water after each medication to thoroughly flush it through the tube before the next one is administered. A laboratory study of methods to prevent tube clogging found that irrigating the tube before and after administration of each medication was effective in preventing tube clogging (Scanlan and Frisch, 1992). It is recommended that medications *not* be added to the formula itself because the medications can cause the formula to curdle and also because the rate of administration is erratic, according to the flow rate of the formula.

Maintaining Tube Patency

An experimental laboratory study was conducted by a group of nurse researchers to compare the effectiveness of three commonly used irrigant fluids: cranberry juice, Coca-Cola, and tap water (Metheny et al, 1988). One hundred and eight tubes were connected to gravity-flow feeding bags containing isotonic enteral formula. Some of the tubes were composed of polyurethane, and others were made of silicone; the tubes were equally divided as to external diameters of 8, 10, and 12 French. Formula was allowed to flow through the tubes into beakers of fluid with a pH of 3. One third of the tubes were irrigated with cranberry juice, one third with Coca-Cola, and one third with water. Water and Coca-Cola were found to be consistently superior to cranberry juice as irrigants. The researchers concluded that because water and Coca-Cola were equally effective, it is logical to use water as an irrigant because it is readily available and less expensive.

The superiority of water over cranberry juice was soundly demonstrated by other researchers in a clinical setting (Wilson and Haynes-Johnson, 1987). These researchers studied patients receiving continuous tube feedings via nasointestinal tubes. Virtually all of the tubes irrigated with cranberry juice eventually clogged during use, whereas none of those irrigated with water did so.

Use of Infusion Pumps/Flow Rate of formula

There is a decided advantage to administering tube feeding by infusion pump (as opposed to gravity flow) to ensure an even delivery of formula. In a laboratory study by a group of researchers, a severe drop in formula flow was demonstrated within a few minutes of adjusting the gravity flow rate (Metheny et al, 1988). Apparently this is due to changes in configuration of the tubing while compressed by the clamp. Similar findings were reported in a study of 217 patients receiving parenteral fluids by gravity flow regulated by roller clamps; flow rates varied as much as 56 percent from desired rates (Bivins et al, 1980).

Clogged feeding tubes are a concern to all health care workers. A physician-led multidisciplinary team conducted a laboratory study to evaluate the ability of six solutions to dissolve clotted tube-feeding formula (Marcuard et al, 1989). In a laboratory setting, the investigators tested a variety of clotted enteral feeding products by attempting to dissolve them with Adolph's Meat Tenderizer, pancreatic enzyme (Viokase), Sprite, Pepsi-Cola, Coca-Cola, or Mountain Dew. It may seem strange that these substances were selected; however, these have been recommended in varying degrees by clinicians who have tried to unclog feeding tubes. The effectiveness of the agents was scored from 0 to 3, with 3 representing total dissolution and 0 representing no dissolution of the clotted material. By far the best clot dissolution was obtained with pancreatic enzyme (Viokase) adjusted to an alkaline pH; this substance had a score of 2.9. The next effective substances (in this order) were Mountain Dew (1.8), Pepsi-Cola (1.5), Classic Coca-Cola (1.4), Sprite (1.4), distilled water (0.9), Adolph's Meat Tenderizer (0.8), and plain pancreatic enzymes (not activated by an alkaline additive) (0.8). In a later clinical study, using activated pancreatic enzymes, the same investigators reported being able to restore patency in 23 of 24 instances in which formula clotting was the likely cause of tube clogging (Marcuard and Stegall, 1990).

PULMONARY ASPIRATION

Aspiration of tube-feeding formula from a distended stomach is a dreaded complication in tube-fed patients. Reports of the incidence of aspiration range from 0 to over 70 percent of tube-fed patients. Actually, the incidence varies with patient populations and the presence or absence of significant risk factors. Risk factors most likely to be associated with aspiration include decreased level of consciousness, decreased cough and gag reflexes, and slowed gastric emptying (Metheny et al, 1986). Aspiration of formula into the lungs is less likely when feedings are introduced into the small intestine because of the added protection of the pyloric sphincter. Frequently cited by authors favoring the small bowel feeding site is the work by Gustke and associates (1970). In this classic study, a group of physicians described the degree of reflux from various segments of the upper gastrointestinal tract. They reported that the likelihood of reflux (and thus of aspiration) is least likely when the tube's ports are beyond the ligament of Treitz (in the proximal jejunum). For this reason, it is considered good practice by most clinicians to feed patients at high risk for aspiration in the proximal jejunum or distal duodenum. A study of 23 patients who previously had nasogastric feedings and were switched to jejunostomy feedings indicated that the incidence of aspiration decreased from 13 episodes during gastric feedings to 5 during jejunostomy feedings (Kaplan et al, 1985).

Position of Tube

Because it is thought that high-risk patients should receive tube feedings in the proximal intestine rather than the stomach, it is important for nurses to be able to distinguish between gastric and intestinal positioning of feeding tubes. Studies have indicated that feeding tubes sometimes spontaneously dislocate upward in the gastrointestinal tract; for example, the distal end of a nasogastric tube that was once properly positioned may spontaneously move upward into the esophagus, whereas the distal end of a nasointestinal tube may spontaneously migrate upward into the stomach (Metheny et al, 1986). Risk factors include coughing, retching, tracheobronchial suctioning, and vomiting.

Position of Patient

Several studies have demonstrated that the position of the head of the bed has a strong effect on the incidence of gastroesophageal reflux and subsequent aspiration (Ibanez et al, 1992; Torres et al, 1992). Placing the patient with the head of the bed elevated to 30 to 45 degrees does not eliminate pulmonary aspiration, but it results in lessening of this complication. For example, Torres and coworkers (1992) found that the incidence of gastroesophageal reflux of formula with inhalation into the lungs increased steadily over time as the head of the bed of tube-fed patients remained in a flat position.

Emptying of Gastric Contents

Slowed gastric emptying resulting in a distended stomach increases the chance for gastroesophageal reflux and subsequent aspiration of gastric contents into the lungs. Therefore, it is recommended that gastric residual volumes be measured before each intermittent feeding and at least once a shift during continuous gastric tube feeding. Unfortunately, several studies have indicated that this procedure is performed only sporadically (Breach and Saldanha, 1988; Flynn et al, 1987). Among the reasons for this are the faulty belief that small-bore feeding tubes collapse when attempts are made to aspirate fluid from them, confusion as to what is too much residual volume, and belief that checking residual volumes will clog the feeding tube. Although it is true that it is more difficult to aspirate fluid from small-bore tubes than it is from large-bore tubes, it is indeed possible to do so with minimal effort (Metheny et al, 1993a).

Measurement of gastric residual volume is a frequently recommended nursing action to determine the patient's tolerance for tube feeding. One measures gastric residual volume with a large syringe. Immediately after the formula flow is interrupted, a large syringe (usually 60 ml) is attached to the end of the feeding tube and gastric fluid is aspirated into the syringe for measurement. While the most frequently cited volume for excessive residual fluid from the stomach is 150 ml or more, a recent clinical study indicated that a volume of 200 ml for nasogastric tubes and a volume of 100 ml for gastrostomy tubes is probably more realistic (McClave et al, 1992). These authors further state that the presence of only one excessive gastric residual volume is not sufficient to discontinue tube feedings if the patient is not experiencing signs of gastric discomfort (such as nausea, distention, and vomiting). One study reported that checking gastric residual volumes resulted in significantly more clogged feeding tubes than that observed in patients not having residual volumes checked (Powell et al, 1993). The significance of the latter study is that more care must be used when checking residual volumes from gastric tubes; this should be in the form of more frequent flushes with water, especially immediately after aspiration of fluid from the stomach to measure the gastric residual.

Gastrostomy Tubes. In the past, it was considered better to administer feedings through gastrostomy tubes than nasogastric tubes for patients at high risk for aspiration. This belief was based on the fact that nasogastric tubes interfere somewhat with closure of the lower esophageal sphincter. Because gastrostomy tubes bypass this sphincter and open directly into the stomach from the abdominal wall, it was thought that aspiration would be less likely with gastrostomies. However, several studies have demonstrated that the incidence of aspiration is essentially the same for both routes (Ciocon et al, 1988; Hassett et al, 1988). Thus, when a high-risk patient is fed through a gastrostomy tube, it is important to take the same aspiration precautions as would be taken with a nasogastric tube. These precautions include elevating the head of the bed and checking frequently for excessive gastric retention.

Continuous Versus Intermittent Feedings. The type of feeding (continuous vs. intermittent) also has implications for the development of gastroesophageal reflux and pulmonary aspiration. A group of physicians found that the lower esophageal sphincter pressure in a group of gastrostomy patients was made worse by bolus administration of 350 ml of fluid than when smaller volumes (80 ml/hr) were administered; this is important because absence of an intact lower esophageal sphincter increases the chance of fluid from the stomach refluxing into the esophagus and then the possibility of inhalation of the fluid into the lung (Coben et al, 1994).

INADVERTENT PLACEMENT OF FEEDING TUBE IN LUNG

Accidental placement of a feeding tube in the lung can cause grave damage. Reports regarding the frequency of this complication vary widely. In an attempt to identify risk factors for this complication, as well as evaluate commonly accepted methods to rule out respiratory placement, a group of researchers conducted a 2-year study of tube-fed patients (Metheny et al, 1990a). During the study, 10 cases of inadvertent respiratory placement of small-diameter feeding tubes were documented by x-ray studies. Four of the 10 misplaced tubes ended in the tracheobronchial tree, and the other 6 perforated the lung and entered the pleural space. The most frequent risk factor was decreased level of consciousness, interfering with the patient's ability to cooperate by swallowing during tube insertion. Bedside methods commonly employed by nurses and physicians failed to detect the incorrect tube placements; had x-ray films not been taken, the misplacements would have been missed in most of the patients. Catastrophic results can follow the accidental administration of tube-feeding formula into the lungs, particularly if the volume administered is large.

METABOLIC COMPLICATIONS OF TUBE FEEDINGS

The incidence of sodium imbalances in tube-fed patients depends on the patient population being studied. For example, sodium imbalances are relatively common in individuals with neurologic problems. The severity of symptoms with sodium imbalances is dependent on the magnitude of the imbalance and on how quickly the imbalance develops. It is recognized that sodium balance is difficult to maintain in some tube-fed patients and requires careful regulation of sodium and water intake. The sodium balance is difficult to maintain in some tube-fed patients (e.g., those with neurologic problems such as stroke) and requires careful regulation of sodium and water intake. The frequency of sodium imbalances in tube-fed subjects was studied by Bowman and colleagues (1989). Hyponatremia (lack of sodium in the blood plasma) was found to occur more often than hypernatremia (excess sodium in the blood plasma) (34 percent vs. 21 percent). It was concluded that hyponatremia was a more frequent imbalance because of excessive free water administration in many of the subjects, both from unnecessary dilution of isotonic formulas (to hypotonic levels) and use of D_5W as a vehicle for IV medications. Hypernatremia was more frequent among older individuals, presumably because they have relatively greater losses of free water than do their younger counterparts.

MEASURES TO TEST FEEDING TUBE POSITION

At present, most practitioners use a variety of methods to confirm that a feeding tube is in correct position before feedings are introduced through the tube. Some of these are more reliable than others. Most often recommended is the aspiration of "recognizable" gastrointestinal secretions to prove that the tube is located in the gastrointestinal tract (rather than the lung). The question then arises: "What do gastrointestinal aspirates look like?" In a study of aspirates from feeding tubes, researchers classified the fluids as having one of six colors. Gastric aspirates were most frequently cloudy and green, tan or off-white, or bloody or brown. Intestinal fluids were primarily clear and yellow to bile-colored. In the absence of blood, pleural fluid was usually pale yellow and serous and tracheobronchial secretions were usually tan or off-white mucus. However, respiratory samples often contained blood and therefore failed to have the expected characteristics of respiratory fluid. Staff nurses were shown photographs of the aspirates and asked to predict their source (stomach, small intestine, or lung). It was found that they could usually identify gastric fluid and could often identify intestinal fluid; however, they had difficulty in differentiating respiratory fluids from gastrointestinal fluids. The researchers concluded that the appearance of aspirates from feeding tubes is often helpful in distinguishing between gastric and intestinal fluid but is of little value in ruling out inadvertent respiratory placement of feeding tubes (Metheny et al, 1994).

Another study concluded that pH of aspirates from feeding tubes can be very helpful in determining tube location (Metheny et al, 1993b). It was found that approximately 85 percent of the pH meter readings from gastric fluid were between 0 and 6.0, whereas over 87 percent of the pH meter measurements performed on intestinal aspirates were greater than 6.0. Four aspirates from feeding tubes inadvertently placed in the respiratory tract (two in the pleural space and two in the tracheobronchial tree) were tested with a pH-meter; all had pH values greater than 6.5. Although pH is not a foolproof method by any means, it is the best nonradiographic method available.

Another commonly used method to test feeding nasogastric tube placement is the "auscultatory" method; this involves pushing 5 to 10 ml of air through the tube with a syringe and listening with a stethoscope over the epigastric region. Supposedly if the tube is correctly positioned a rush of air will be heard (or bubbling if fluid is present in the stomach). However, a study has indicated that air was also heard in eight subjects with tubes inadvertently positioned in the respiratory tract (Metheny et al, 1990a). Although three of these eight cases involved muffled or soft sounds, the involved clinicians assumed all but one tube was correctly placed. Furthermore, loud distinctive sounds were reported in the other five cases, causing physicians and nurses alike to feel assured the tubes were properly placed. Another study demonstrated that nurses were unable to differentiate between gastric and intestinal placement of tubes using air insufflations as the test (Metheny et al, 1990b). This could be very important if the tube were supposed to be positioned in the intestine of a patient at high-risk for aspiration. It is known that tubes originally positioned in the intestine may migrate upward into the stomach during coughing or vomiting or by accidental pulling of the portion of the tube extending from the nares (Metheny et al, 1986b).

In the past, when only large-diameter rigid tubes were used, one could assume that accidental placement in the respiratory tract would produce a series of signs, such as inability to speak (due to separation of the vocal cords), coughing, and cyanosis. However, owing to the small diameter and softness of most currently used feeding tubes, these signs are not as likely. In fact, no observable serious changes in respiratory status were noted in any of 10 cases of inadvertent respiratory placement of small-bore tubes in a report by Metheny and coworkers (1990a). At times, even large-bore feeding tubes can enter the lung without causing obvious respiratory symptoms.

Some nurses still use the "bubbling method" (placing the end of the feeding tube under water and observing for bubbling when the patient exhales). If no bubbling is present, proponents of this method assume the tube cannot be in the lung. This is an incorrect assumption because the tube's ports may merely be occluded by the respiratory mucosa.

Hanson (1979) studied the length of tubing needed to reach the stomach. Distance was measured using a well-lubricated 18-French red rubber nasogastric tube. Although the length of tube insertion remains a valid issue, one must be aware that a tube can be inserted a relatively great distance and remain coiled high in the stomach. Thus, length of insertion alone does not determine correct placement.

In summary, it is prudent to obtain radiologic confirmation of correct placement of small-bore feeding tubes, especially in high-risk patients. High-risk patients are those with decreased level of consciousness, decreased swallowing and gag reflexes, presence of tracheal tubes, recent removal of tracheal tubes, and debilitation. In fact, most facilities require radiologic confirmation of correct placement of all newly inserted small-bore nasogastric and nasointestinal feeding tubes before feedings or medications are given through the tubes.

MAINTAINING PATENCY OF PERIPHERAL INTRAVENOUS DEVICES

An IV therapy issue that has been studied rather widely by nurses concerns the type of irrigant used to keep "heparin locks" patent. A *heparin lock,* also known as an intermittent infusion device, refers to a needle in a peripheral vein that has been capped off until it is needed for an infusion of IV fluid or medications. Some authorities recommend dilute heparin solutions, and others recommend isotonic saline alone. In one study of 424 patients, no significant differences were found in rates of needle clotting or phlebitis when sites were flushed with heparin or isotonic saline (Taylor et al, 1989). Other researchers found similar results when comparing isotonic saline to heparinized saline (Ashton et al, 1990). Because isotonic saline is less potentially harmful and less expensive than heparin, it is logical to irrigate peripheral heparin locks with isotonic saline. Most hospitals have incorporated these research findings into their protocols for irrigating peripheral IV devices to maintain patency.

TOPICAL OINTMENTS AT INTRAVENOUS ENTRY SITE

Some practitioners recommend applying a topical ointment or antiseptic solution to the IV site to prevent infection of the vein (thrombophlebitis). Others do not believe this is necessary. In a trial using adult patients, nurse researchers found no difference in outcome when a topical antiseptic agent (povidone-iodine) was used and when one was not used (Thompson et al, 1989). The investigators concluded that the use of povidone-iodine antiseptic solution does not reduce the incidence of cannula-related thrombophlebitis. Despite these findings, many practitioners still advocate application of povidone-iodine ointment or solution at the insertion site. Therefore, there is wide variability in practice among institutions and even among various units within the same institution.

MONITORING FLUID BALANCE STATUS

The most frequently recommended methods for nurses to detect fluid volume disturbances include measurements of intake and output, body weight, skin turgor, changes in vein filling, and urinary specific gravity.

INTAKE AND OUTPUT MEASUREMENT

Intake and output (I & O) measurements have been studied by several nurse researchers and found to be poorly done and recorded (Bowman et al, 1989; Pflaum, 1979). This is especially true in noncritical care areas. Similarly, body weight measurements are often performed inaccurately.

Despite the widespread use of high technology in critical care areas to monitor fluid status and cardiac function, a descriptive study of factors considered by physicians when making fluid management decisions in new postoperative coronary artery bypass graft patients indicated that urine output was one of the most frequently used and trusted (Pierson and Funk, 1989).

BODY WEIGHT MEASUREMENT

A small but significant percentage of scales in clinical use were found to be inaccurate and imprecise to a clinically significant degree (Schlegal-Pratt and Heizer, 1990). The problems stemmed more from breakage and wear than from manufacturer defects. For this reason, institutions should check their scales for accuracy at regular intervals and make repairs as needed.

Errors may occur not only because of faulty scales but also because of faulty weighing techniques. A quality improvement program for staff nurses to improve the accuracy of body weight measurements was described by Savage and Wilkinson (1994). In the program, the following protocol was developed and followed:

- All patients were weighed on electronic scales unless bed scales were needed. Staff nurses were required to review the procedure for using the scale at regular intervals.
- Patients were weighed, before breakfast, by the night nurse, and the weight was recorded on the patient's medical record.
- Patients were weighed in gown or pajamas with slippers; all appliances (e.g., Foley catheter and drainage bags) were emptied before the procedure.
- A nursing assessment was required if a significant weight change ($\geq$1 kg) was found; the house officer was to be notified of significant weight changes unless the variance could be easily explained (such as a large weight loss after the administration of a diuretic).

After implementation of this protocol, the number of weights performed increased significantly, as did the accuracy of the measurements.

MEASUREMENT OF URINE SPECIFIC GRAVITY

The concentration of urine, as measured by specific gravity, is an important measure of fluid status in many situations. Nurses can obtain this measure by means of a urinometer or a refractometer. For greater accuracy, the urine should be fresh. However, because neonatal intensive-care unit nurses are not always able to test diaper urine specimens immediately, a study was conducted to compare specific gravity values at 0, 1, 2, 3 and 4 hours post urination (Stebor, 1989). A convenience sample of 20 infants was used. An open disposable diaper was placed under the infant until urination occurred. Urine was aspirated with a syringe from the diaper and tested using a refractometer. The diaper was then folded, rolled, and taped so that the urine was not exposed to light, air, or heat. Urine was tested again at hourly intervals up to 4 hours post urination. The investigator found no significant differences in the specific gravity readings. It was concluded that as long as diapers are unexposed to air, heat, or light, specific gravity readings may be performed accurately at various times up to 4 hours post urination.

INDICATORS OF FLUID VOLUME DEFICIT

The diagnostic label "Isotonic Fluid Volume Deficit" has been approved by the North American Nursing Diagnosis Association. To attempt to validate the indicators of this diagnosis, a group of researchers mailed a validation tool containing 72 proposed clinical indicators of isotonic fluid volume deficit to a national sample of critical care nurses with advanced preparation (Gershan et al, 1990). Nurses in the sample rated the clinical indicator on a scale from 1 to 5, evaluating their perceived relevancy to this diagnosis. Seventeen of the 72 factors were categorized as critical indicators. Listed as most important were negative fluid intake and output, decreased urine output, and decreased venous pressure. The latter refers to a pressure reading reflected from a catheter inserted into the central veins, near the heart (an invasive maneuver). The others, listed in order of importance, were changes in body weight, weight loss, increased urine osmolality, decreased blood pressure, postural blood pressure changes, increased heart rate, thready pulse, increased hematocrit, decreased pulse volume and pressure, decreased venous filling, dry mucous membranes, pulmonary capillary wedge pressure less than 6 mm Hg, decreased cardiac output, and poor skin turgor. This study succeeded in reporting the opinion of nurses with advanced preparation regarding the most important clinical indicators of isotonic fluid volume deficit. Because it was a sample of critical care nurses, it was assumed that nurses regularly have access to data generated from catheters placed in or near the heart. The study did not experimentally compare the effectiveness of the various indicators in actually validating the presence of isotonic fluid volume deficit.

Among the indicators of fluid volume deficit identified in a study of patients between 61 and 98 years of age were tongue dryness and increased longitudinal tongue furrows, dry oral mucous membranes, sunken eyes, confusion, and body muscle weakness (Gross et al, 1992).

Poor vein filling was a more accurate indicator of fluid volume status than were decreased body weight, postural blood pressure changes, poor skin turgor of the forehead, and decreased degree of moisture under the axilla or inner lip in a study of 36 elderly patients admitted for diagnostic studies requiring laxatives and fluid restriction (Robinson and Demuth, 1985). The investigators compressed a vein on the top of the foot by finger pressure and emptied it of its blood by stroking it proximally with another finger. They concluded that veins of well-hydrated patients filled instantly, as opposed to slow filling (over 3 seconds) in volume-depleted patients.

DETECTION OF ELECTROLYTE IMBALANCES

Because hypercalcemia is very common in cancer patients, most studies of this condition are conducted by nurses specializing in oncology. For example, in a group of eight advanced cancer patients, Mahon (1987) found that those with severe hypercalcemia displayed inappropriate behavior, slowed thinking ability, and shortened attention spans. Fortunately, these symptoms disappeared when the serum calcium levels returned to normal after treatment. One patient with a markedly elevated serum calcium level (17 mg/dl) suffered cardiac arrest, presumably secondary to the effects of hypercalcemia.

CALCIUM

Another study of hypercalcemia examined knowledge levels of signs and symptoms of hypercalcemia in cancer patients at high risk for this disorder (Coward, 1988). The investigator conducted an exploratory study to determine what patients at risk for hypercalcemia knew about this potentially lethal imbalance. The questionnaire was administered in a one-time interview with 22 hospitalized patients and 18 clinic patients. Approximately 90 percent of the subjects were unaware that hypercalcemia might be a complication of their disease. Two thirds of the subjects did not recall being told of simple measures that might prevent hypercalcemia, such as drinking 2 to 3 quarts of liquid daily and standing and walking to help keep calcium in the bones. Findings from this study are particularly disturbing because they indicate that patient teaching for this group of high-risk patients was sorely lacking. The question is raised about the same phenomenon among similar cancer patients in other settings. On the basis of findings from this study, the author designed a patient information handout on cancer-induced hypercalcemia and a guide to its use.

POTASSIUM

Potassium imbalances, particularly hypokalemia, are very common and can be life threatening if not detected and treated early. The incidence, causative factors, and symptoms of hypokalemia and hyperkalemia in 210 tube-fed patients were studied by Metheny and coworkers (1991). Of these 210 subjects, 48 developed hypokalemia and 9 developed hyperkalemia. The most frequent causative factors identified in those with hypokalemia were use of potassium-losing diuretics (primarily furosemide and thiazides), diarrhea, history of poor dietary intake before tube feedings, and administration of insulin or corticosteroids. Most frequently identified symptoms were anorexia, fatigue, muscle weakness, slowed gastrointestinal motility, and electrocardiographic changes. The researchers acknowledged that although all of these symptoms are commonly believed to accompany hypokalemia, they also could have had other origins. Of the 9 patients with hyperkalemia, 6 had end-stage renal failure (a condition commonly associated with elevated serum potassium levels). Two of the other 3 were found to have artifactual (false) readings due to clotting of the blood sample, and 1 had metabolic acidosis. Clotting of the blood sample releases cellular potassium into the serum, causing falsely elevated readings. Metabolic acidosis characteristically is associated with shifting of intracellular potassium into the ECF. Specific electrolyte disturbances are important variables related to confusion (Foreman, 1989). For example, it was found that hypernatremia, hypokalemia, hyperglycemia, and elevated blood levels of creatinine and urea nitrogen were more common in confused patients than in nonconfused elderly patients. The author concluded that it is impossible to determine whether these variables are causes, effects, or just simply correlates of confusion. Nonetheless, the study points out a relationship of some sort between hypernatremia and hypokalemia and confusion.

A condition called "pseudohyperkalemia" associated with drawing blood specimens for analysis of potassium levels has been recognized for at least four decades. (Fist clenching during phlebotomy leads to an increase in the local potassium concentration.) To study this phenomenon, a group of physicians used a patient with a history of hyperkalemia and four normal adult men who served as controls (Don et al, 1990). Blood samples were tested during periods of fist clenching and unclenching and after a period of no clenching. It was reported that fist clenching (done to make the veins more prominent for visualization during venipuncture or to pump blood into a specimen container) can increase the plasma potassium concentration by 1 to 2 mEq/L. The authors pointed out that the occurrence of potassium increase through fist clenching could mislead clinicians about the true potassium concentrations, perhaps resulting in unwarranted treatment. They concluded that it seems advisable to avoid fist clenching altogether and to rely on venous stasis from a tourniquet (if needed) to make the vein more prominent.

EFFECT OF VENIPUNCTURE SITE ON TEST RESULTS

Another laboratory study was conducted to determine where blood should be drawn for electrolyte testing during periods when the patient is receiving IV fluids (Watson et al, 1983). It was found that blood drawn from above an infusing IV line yielded faulty serum biochemical values; therefore, the researchers recommended that blood either be drawn from the arm not receiving the IV fluids or be drawn below the infusing IV site.

COMPLICATIONS OF INTRAVENOUS FLUID AND NUTRIENT ADMINISTRATION

Over 85 percent of all hospitalized patients receive IV therapy, most commonly by peripheral IV devices (Masoorli, 1996). Numerous IV therapy complications exist, and some have been studied to variable extents.

INFILTRATION OF FLUIDS AND TISSUE

The most frequently reported complication of IV therapy and the most common cause of litigation against nurses is infiltration (Masoorli, 1996). *Infiltration* is defined as inadvertent administration of solution into tissue surrounding the intended venous site of fluid delivery. This complication can occur when the IV device punctures the vein wall owing to patient activity or vein fragility. The most common symptoms associated with infiltration include swelling, coolness, and blanching at the site (Masoorli, 1996).

A study compared infiltrates intentionally made by different IV solutions (Yucha et al, 1993). Among the fluids studied were two dilute salt solutions (0.45 percent sodium chloride and lactated Ringer's solution), a dilute dextrose solution containing a small concentration of potassium chloride (10 mEq/L) and a concentrated salt solution (3 percent sodium chloride). The greatest pain was caused by the concentrated salt solution; the greatest surface area of induration was caused by the dilute sugar solution containing a small quantity of potassium chloride. It should be noted that this study used a very dilute potassium chloride concentration; in practice, concentrations of 40 mEq/L or higher are often used. In the latter case, very severe tissue necrosis can accompany infiltration of the solution.

COMPLICATIONS OF TOTAL PARENTERAL NUTRITION

A number of metabolic complications of TPN have been documented. Probably the most common electrolyte imbalance in TPN patients is hypophosphatemia. In a study of 100 TPN patients, 30 were found to have serum phosphorus levels below 2 mg/dl (Weinsier et al, 1982). Still another common complication identified in this study was hyperglycemia; that is, 47 of the 100 subjects had blood sugar levels greater than 300 mg/dl. Hypokalemia was also a common finding, occurring in 18 of the 100 subjects.

Hypoglycemia is a possible reaction to sudden discontinuation of TPN because the pancreas may temporarily continue to secrete extra insulin even after the heavy glucose load has been stopped. While several studies suggest that this is unlikely (Krzwda et al, 1993; Wagman et al, 1986), many authorities still believe that it is more prudent to taper TPN flow rates in all patients who receive 200 to 300 g or more of IV glucose per day when it is necessary to discontinue TPN (Inadomi and Kopple, 1994).

PHLEBITIS

Phlebitis (inflammation of the vein) is a common complication of peripheral IV fluid administration. There are reports that infusion-related phlebitis affects 25 to 70 percent of all hospitalized patients: approximately 60 percent of these develop indicators of phlebitis within 8 and 16 hours after the IV device is inserted (Perucca and Micek, 1993). The most frequent causes of phlebitis are chemical and mechanical irritants. Examples of chemical irritants are highly acidic or alkaline fluids, those with high concentrations, and fluids containing particulate matter. Examples of mechanical irritants are the IV device itself and frequent movement of the device against the venous wall.

AIR EMBOLISM

Another complication that has puzzled clinicians is the amount of air that is lethal when inadvertently entered into the bloodstream. Although the volume is unknown, it is likely related to the rate of entry. Ordway (1974) extrapolated data from animal studies and concluded that the lethal dose of air intravenously in humans would be between 70 and 150 ml/sec. Yeakel (1969) reported a fatal episode after the sudden intravenous administration of 100 ml of air.

PSYCHOSOCIAL PROBLEMS

Psychosocial responses to prolonged IV feedings vary according to the level of illness and length of time on TPN therapy. Manifestations observed in 59 patients receiving prolonged IV feedings (TPN) were reported by Malcolm and coworkers (1980). In acutely ill patients receiving brief TPN, the observed problems were mainly biopsychological. Improvements in mood and cognitive ability occurred within the first week of TPN. For patients who were convalescing while receiving intermediate-term TPN, psychosocial reactions began to emerge. Anxiety and apprehension related to receiving nutrients through a central vein as well as cost of therapy were more likely than in the acutely ill. Chronically ill patients receiving long-term TPN were more likely to develop concerns and even phobic behaviors based on rational or irrational fears related to their TPN therapy. Questions regarding risk for complications and financial burdens were more frequent in this group. A patient who suffered a psychotic episode related to his TPN therapy was described; this patient's delusional thinking led him to believe he was "bionic" because he no longer ate food or had bowel movements. The authors concluded that patients receiving long-term TPN need access to psychiatric support to deal with their somatopsychological reactions.

Although the preceding discussion may give the impression that most areas of nutrition and fluid/electrolyte balance have been researched, this is not the case. When sound scientific data are lacking, the next best source of knowledge is expert opinion. In fact, much of what is done in clinical practice is based on recommendations of experts with advanced knowledge through practice.

FACTORS AFFECTING CLINICAL DECISIONS

Dietary practices and nutrition therapy are influenced by a number of factors, such as age, religious beliefs, ethnic origin, family and social customs, economic status, education, and emotions. Daily mineral and fluid requirements are also affected by age and gender.

Age

Age influences nutritional needs, as well as eating ability and habits.

INFANTS AND CHILDREN

Infancy is a period of great energy needs to support the high rate of metabolism and rapid growth. Fortunately, full-term infants are born with the ability to coordinate breathing, suckling, and swallowing. Stroking of the infant's cheek will cause turning in the direction of the nipple (rooting reflex). Many authorities believe that breast feeding has decided advantages over bottle feeding. Human milk is readily available at the right temperature and is usually less costly while supplying immune factors that protect the infant from infections. However, breast feeding may be contraindicated if the mother is ill or a drug abuser, or even if she is taking certain prescription drugs. (The mother should consult with her physician about any medications that could potentially harm the infant.) The infant needs proportionately more fluid than older children and adults because of inability of the immature kidneys to conserve water and also because of the proportionately greater body surface area allowing greater insensible fluid loss.

Some solid foods can usually be given by age 3 to 4 months. At 6 months, the infant begins to sit up and responds to the offering of food with opening of the mouth. After this period, the infant progresses to a variety of fruits, vegetables, and meats. Eventually the child learns self-feeding; this process is messy at first because the child learns by feeling food and has difficulty with hand-to-mouth coordination.

Meeting the nutritional needs of a *toddler* can be a taxing endeavor. The child may refuse food as an assertive action. Making an issue of this behavior by punitive action or forced feeding is not recommended. Parents should provide foods appropriate for the child's level of development, in a nonstressful environment. Snacks are important to help maintain the child's energy level. Young children prefer bland foods with light seasoning at lukewarm rather than hot temperatures. To avoid the possibility of asphyxiation from inhalation of food into the airway, children younger than 3 years of age should not be given round pieces of food such as hot dogs, grapes, jelly beans, gum drops, popcorn, and raw carrots.

ADOLESCENTS

As the child reaches *adolescence,* a new set of problems arises. Some adolescents may indulge in a variety of fad reducing diets in an attempt to get or remain thin. A psychological problem is manifested in the form of anorexia nervosa. This condition is found predominantly in adolescent and young adult women. About 0.5 percent of young women develop anorexia, and 15 to 20 percent develop bulimia, an eating disorder involving gorging followed by self-induced vomiting (Worthington-Roberts, 1985). It seems that bulimic individuals tend to be preoccupied with eating and its control, whereas those with anorexia are preoccupied with weight and appearance. Adolescent boys tend to have voracious appetites during this period. In general, the diets of adolescent boys and girls are deficient in the recommended allowances for calcium, vitamin A, and ascorbic acid; girls often do not take in enough iron.

Emotionally, food means different things to us at different ages. Love and security are attached to food by infants, whereas toddlers are likely to view food as either a reward or a punishment. Certain foods (such as ice cream or chicken soup) are viewed as comforting to us when given during time of illness by a loving parent. Adolescents may use food as a means to attract attention or as a crutch for emotional problems. These same food associations often carry over into adulthood.

Adolescents have greater calcium needs (1200 mg/day) than those of young adults (800 mg/day); pregnant or lactating females require 1200 mg/day (Alpers et al, 1995). Maintaining body weight within normal limits during young adulthood may help prevent certain illnesses (e.g., type II diabetes, hypertension, and heart disease) in later life.

ELDERLY ADULTS

The elderly have special problems not present in earlier phases of life. With aging, there are decided physiologic changes. Body composition is altered, leading to a decrease in lean body mass. The decreased muscle mass is associated with increased adipose tissue. These changes do not generally affect organ functioning; however, older adults do not have the capacity to respond to physiologic stressors as well as their younger counterparts. Adding to their problem is a multitude of other factors. For example, gastrointestinal motility and absorption changes in the elderly can lead to intolerance for some types of foods (Chernoff, 1990). Decreased visual ability can interfere with food preparation, especially in poorly lighted rooms; hearing impairment may cause elderly persons to avoid eating with others. Senses of taste and smell are less acute in the elderly, causing them to use more salt and spices than younger adults. Decreased ability to chew is not uncommon due to dental problems. Furthermore, reduced salivary flow makes foods dry and difficult to swallow.

Faulty esophageal sphincter function is more common in the elderly and predisposes to regurgitation of fluid from the stomach. The presence of chronic conditions, such as type II diabetes mellitus and congestive heart failure, is more common in the elderly and may significantly limit the dietary choices.

Although the elderly are a substantial part of the American population, there has been little research regarding their nutritional requirements. It is generally assumed that the RDAs are the same for elderly persons as they are for younger adults (with the exception of decreased caloric intake because of lower levels of activity).

The elderly are more likely to frequent fast-food restaurants featuring high-fat foods because of the relatively low cost of meals and the close proximity to their homes. Finally, government surveys indicate that older Americans consume an imbalance of certain foods, which leads to nutritional deficiencies (Rosofsky et al, 1990). For example, overconsumption of meat and dairy products at the expense of fruits, vegetables, and cereals is common. This eating pattern promotes the excess prevalence of the three major causes of death in the United States (heart disease, cancer, and stroke).

Gender

There are some differences in nutrition requirements between men and women. Women have a lower percentage of body fluid than men because they have proportionally more body fat, and fat cells contain more water. Because of increased muscle mass, men usually require more calories and protein. Menstruation in women may lead to lower iron levels, resulting in anemia.

Individual and Family Values

An individual's food habits are greatly influenced by family environment. Throughout life, certain foods trigger a flood of childhood memories. Understandably, children learn to like foods prepared and enjoyed by their parents. Similarly, negative attitudes to food may be learned in the home as children watch parents who do not like certain foods. In some instances, children who do not have a good relationship with their parents may prefer to assume eating habits different from those of their parents.

Eating is sometimes used by children to control parents; for example, slowness in eating may be used as an attention-getting maneuver by children. Parents, in turn, may use food as a bribe or threat to obtain desired behavior from a child. For example, if a child has finished the entire meal, a dessert may be given; if the reverse is true, dessert may be withheld. It is little wonder that food habits learned as a child remain a major force throughout the life span.

Food is a symbol of sociability, warmth, and social acceptance. Indeed, most social occasions are linked closely to food and drink. Foods that one prefers are sometimes viewed as indicators of personal attributes. In some settings, meat and potatoes are viewed as masculine foods, whereas salads and souffles are thought of as feminine foods. Children are more likely to be associated with preferences for peanut butter and jelly sandwiches, and adolescents with hamburgers, pizzas, and milkshakes. If a monotonous diet is consumed on the basis of social pressure, it is possible that certain food groups will be neglected and dietary deficiencies will develop.

Early in life we learn that food is comforting, and the comfort gained from food persists throughout the life span. During times of happiness and celebration, food is used as a reward. During times of insecurity and loneliness, food is often used as an important source of solace. It is not surprising that individuals seeking to lose weight may gain psychological support from others also attempting to lose weight.

EDUCATIONAL BACKGROUND AND SOCIOECONOMIC STATUS

Well-educated individuals may eat healthier diets because they have been exposed to the importance of diet on health and longevity. Of course, other factors may override the effect of knowledge. For example, emotional cravings for sweets may cause even knowledgeable individuals to eat an excess of unhealthy foods.

Most affluent individuals may consume more balanced diets because they can afford a variety of foods. Without doubt, poverty adversely affects food habits because of inadequate income to purchase a variety of foods and limited time and facilities to prepare food in a healthy manner. Also, the poor often lack adequate information about nutrition.

CULTURE AND ETHNICITY

Food habits are deeply entrenched in many cultures and greatly influence behavior. For example, immigrants to new countries usually give up their native speech and dress before they give up their native foods. Understandably, immigrant children give up ethnic food practices more easily than their parents because they are socialized into school lunch programs and other social functions where they want to conform to social norms. By necessity, food patterns are adapted to the availability of foods in local markets. In ethnic neighborhood markets, one can usually find foods that are characteristic of that group's eating patterns.

Ethnic groups sometimes hold beliefs about categories of foods needed to maintain health. For example, many Mexicans and Puerto Ricans believe it is important to maintain a balance between "hot" and "cold" foods (with the specific foods that fall into either category differing from one group to another). Some Asians may believe nutrition is the most important force in maintaining harmony with the universe and nature; foods are classified as yin (cold) and yang (hot), and a balance of the two is thought to be necessary for health. Too much of the wrong kind of food is thought to cause illness. If proper nutrition fails to maintain health, Asians may use herbs as the next alternative. Specific herbs, brewed as tea, are thought to be protective and/or healing for specific parts of the body.

Although in modern society the eating habits of black Americans and white Americans are essentially the same, many markets serving predominant African American populations still make available "soul food," such as greens boiled in salt water with ham hocks, black-eyed peas with molasses and bacon, fried chicken, and fried fish. Because a high percentage of adult African Americans have an intolerance to lactose, they do not consume much milk. Probably this intolerance stems from a hereditary deficiency of lactase, the enzyme in intestinal juice that splits up lactose. Lactase deficiency also occurs frequently in Native Americans, Asians, and Hispanics. Whereas milk should not be excluded from the diet of children of these ethnic origins, attention should be paid to the possibility for intolerance, manifested by flatulence, abdominal cramping, and diarrhea.

SPIRITUALITY AND RELIGIOUS PRACTICES

Many religions attach symbolism to food. Some Catholics abstain from meat on fast days as a means of denial and penitence. Similarly, Muslims abstain from pork and alcoholic beverages and fast from dawn to dark for 1 month (Ramadan) each year. Buddhists are vegetarians and refuse to eat animal flesh. Seventh-day Adventists do not eat meat or consume coffee, tea, or alcoholic beverages.

Orthodox Jews take no food or drink for 24 hours during Yom Kippur (Day of Atonement). They abstain from pork and shellfish at all times and eat other meats only after they have been prepared in a certain manner referred to as koshering. Animals are slaughtered according to ritual, and the meat is soaked in water, salted to remove the blood, and then washed. No dairy foods are served at a meal with meat, and separate utensils are used for cooking meats and dairy products. Only unleavened bread is eaten during the Passover, and separate sets of dishes are used during Passover week. Conservative Jews are less stringent in observing dietary restrictions, and Reform Jews give minimal emphasis to these practices.

Although a particular religion has definite dietary practices, it must be remembered that not all members of a religion concur with all of the tenets of the religion's doctrine. Also, within a religion, various factions often exist that hold divergent views on food practices.

Whether due to religious or personal beliefs for other reasons, a small percentage of individuals in the United States are vegetarians of varying degrees. Some eliminate only meat from the diet. Others also eliminate milk, milk products, and eggs. Strict vegetarians (vegans) consume only plant foods. Reasons for adopting this type of diet range from religious and ethical beliefs to concern about the most efficient use of available land for food production. Obviously, it is more difficult to plan a nutritionally adequate diet for strict vegetarians than for those who will consume milk, milk products, and eggs.

Various ethnic and religious groups are frequently associated with having specific food habits (Table 22–4). However, it is impossible to generalize because individual preferences, experiences, economic status, and environmental considerations determine dietary intake. Other factors influencing food choice include the impact current public information campaigns have on food habits and the worldwide proliferation of fast-food outlets.

Setting in Which Care Is Delivered

Because of changes in the health care system, more very ill patients are being cared for at home. Many of these patients

TABLE 22-4 Ethnic and Religious Groups: Nutritional Concerns and Dietary Recommendations

Nutritional Concerns	Dietary Recommendations
Black	
Low milk intake (related to lactose intolerance) Excessive use of pork (high in saturated fats) Use of salty meats (ham, bacon, sausage) Vegetables cooked for a long time in a large amount of water (pot liquor) that is later eaten with corn bread Use of gravies Deep fat frying with lard (saturated fat) Excessive use of soft and fruit drinks	Use milk treated for lactose intolerance (available in stores) and use hard cheeses Use polyunsaturated fats for frying Instead of frying, boil or stew Reduce water when cooking vegetables Use leafy green vegetables Reduce use of fatty, salty meats Reduce snack foods with empty calories
Chinese	
Excessive sodium in sauces (e.g., hoisin and soy sauce) Excessive sodium intake from monosodium glutamate, smoked and dried meat, dried fish Monosaturated oil (peanut oil) used for stir-frying Low in dairy products (related to lactose intolerance) Tend to be low in meat group Deep frying used for some dishes	Reduce use of salty sauces Use polyunsaturated fats for stir-frying (safflower, sunflower, corn, or soybean oil) Instead of deep frying, boil, steam, or lightly stir fry Increase use of tofu (soy bean curd) and soy beans to increase protein and calcium intake Use milk treated for lactose intolerance (available in stores) Supplement with vitamins A and D if necessary
Greek	
Excessive salt from anchovies, feta cheese, and olives	Limit use of anchovies, feta cheese, and olives
Italian	
Excessive use of bread and pasta Low milk intake Excessive use of salt in tomato sauce, anchovies, olives, and processed meats	Use less salty cheeses, such as ricotta and mozzarella, rather than Parmesan and other hard cheeses Reduce use of salty and starchy foods
Japanese	
Excessive sodium in sauces and in dried and pickled foods Low in dairy products (related to lactose intolerance)	Reduce use of salty sauces and dried and pickled foods Use milk treated for lactose intolerance (available in stores) Increase use of tofu (bean curd) and soybeans to increase calcium and protein intake Supplement with vitamins A and D if necessary
Mexican-American	
Low in dairy products Low in meat Use of lard in cooking Excessive use of coffee	Discontinue use of lard Use polyunsaturated oils in cooking Fry less; steam tortillas instead of frying Increase use of green leafy vegetables for folacin Increase use of lean meats Increase use of dark green and yellow vegetables and fruits Continue use of corn tortillas (high in calcium as a result of soaking corn in limewater)
Puerto Rican	
Use of salt cod Use of lard High-caloric diet Lack of yellow and green vegetables	Decrease use of salt pork Soak salt cod very well and rinse well before using Substitute polyunsaturated oil for lard in cooking Increase green and yellow vegetables Use more milk and cheese Add meat to rice and beans Use margarine instead of butter
Scandinavian	
Excessive use of milk, cream, butter, and cheese	Reduce intake of high-cholesterol dairy products

Table continued on following page

TABLE 22-4 Ethnic and Religious Groups: Nutritional Concerns and Dietary Recommendations *Continued*

Nutritional Concerns	Dietary Recommendations
Central European	
Overcook vegetables, resulting in loss of vitamins	Reduce water and cooking time for vegetables
Jewish	
High in saturated fats and cholesterol	Reduce use of high-cholesterol dairy foods Substitute polyunsaturated fat for butter in cooking Reduce use of meats, especially organ meats high in cholesterol, such as liver and tongue
Catholic	
Possible excessive restriction of nutrients during Lenten season	Maintain a balanced diet and use acceptable nutritious substitutes
Seventh Day Adventist	
Exclusion of meat and fish from diet	Maintain sufficient intake of protein from dairy products and combinations of foods (see under "Protein" in text) Use meat analogs (e.g., textured vegetable protein made from soybeans may be used as a meat extender)

From Heckheimer, E.F. (1989). *Health promotion of the elderly in the community.* Philadelphia: W. B. Saunders, pp. 76–77.

require complex treatments, such as parenteral nutrition, to sustain their lives. Among the most common diagnoses of patients receiving home parenteral nutrition are acquired immunodeficiency syndrome, malignancy, and hyperemesis gravidum. Parenteral nutrition may also be given to patients who have had a bone marrow transplant and to preoperative malnourished patients with ulcerative colitis, Crohn's disease, or pancreatitis (Sanville, 1994). Although infusions can be delivered safely in home settings, special attention must be given to matching the type of venous access device to the type and duration of therapy, the patient's and caregiver's ability to care for the infusion, appropriateness of the environment to the treatment, and how financial reimbursement for the treatment will be arranged. Patients and their caregivers need to be educated to foster independence and to prevent complications as well as to respond to problems that can arise. A crucial element in determining the appropriateness of treating patients in the home is the willingness of the patient and/or caregiver to participate in the care (Sanville, 1994).

There is risk that the ability to handle advanced forms of therapy may be diminished in home settings. A regional survey of IV therapy practices in 25 health care agencies identified a lack of consistency in tube flushing and dressing change protocols and in the types of equipment used (Williams et al, 1994). The authors concluded that more emphasis on technological expertise is needed in outpatient settings as sophisticated equipment and complex forms of therapy are increasingly offered to patients in home settings.

To care for a patient in a home infusion therapy program effectively and efficiently, all of the parties involved must take part in the planning and decision-making processes (Haddad et al, 1993). This is particularly challenging because the health care workers often do not work in the same physical location.

Printed patient education materials are important in all settings, but especially so in patients receiving home IV therapy (Hur, 1994). These materials serve as resources to support the patient and family between home health nurse visits.

Ethical Considerations

Enteral and parenteral nutrition is generally considered a form of life-sustaining medical procedure, along with mechanical ventilation and potent drugs. Although some individuals seek to separate tube feedings from this category because they are usual events in everyday life, the trend is moving away from this. For example, the Consensus Report of the Ethics of Foregoing Life-Sustaining Treatments in the Critically Ill (1990) concludes that there are no intrinsic moral differences between categories of treatment. That is, ventilator support, vasopressors, antibiotics, and the provision of nutrition and fluids by artificial means are all considered life-sustaining treatments. In an earlier case tried in New Jersey, the courts acknowledged the "emotional" significance of food but insisted that tube feeding is a medical problem and a "medical procedure with inherent risks and possible side effects."

Although the technology exists to feed patients artificially for indefinite periods of time, a dilemma arises when patients or those acting on their behalf request that this treatment not be initiated or maintained. All methods for artificial feedings have drawbacks that enter into debates about whether the benefits of feedings outweigh the risks. Benefits of artificial feedings in terminally ill patients may possibly include better quality of life in the remaining time. However, risks and unpleasant factors associated with artificial feedings are numerous. Some of these are summarized next. Nasogastric and nasointestinal tubes are uncomfortable to some degree and are aesthetically unpleasant; gastrostomy and jejunostomy tubes require invasive techniques and can leak onto the abdomen, causing severe skin irritation and discomfort. Gastrointestinal tube feedings risk pulmonary aspiration and potentially lethal pneumonia, as well as a variety of other complications. Peripheral IV feedings cannot provide adequate long-term nourishment and are associated with discomfort, and central IV feedings require highly skilled staff for line placement and monitoring, are relatively expensive, and carry the risk of potential life-threatening complications. Thus, the dilemma confronting the health care team and patient/family is a major one. The question remains: "Will the benefits from feeding outweigh the associated risks?" If patients are demented, they are usually restrained to discourage them from pulling out feeding tubes or IV devices; the humanity of this practice is questioned by most health care providers. Without doubt, undertaking any method of artificial feeding requires thoughtful reflection on the part of health care providers and input from the patient and significant others.

The use of artificial feedings (most often in the form of tube feedings) in severely demented or terminally ill patients evokes passionate arguments among health care providers and others. Advocates of tube feedings contend that withholding these feedings from patients causes suffering and discomfort from thirst and hunger. Also, they feel that there is a moral responsibility to care for helpless individuals. Opponents argue that for patients near death or those in a persistent vegetative state, not eating is a natural way to let go of life. Opponents of tube feedings further argue that tube feedings cannot reverse the underlying problem and only prolong the dying process.

Probably the most important case on record regarding the withdrawal of tube feedings involved Nancy Cruzan, a young woman caught in the void between progress and the limits of modern medicine. She suffered severe anoxic brain damage in an automobile accident and was rendered in a persistent vegetative state. Shortly after injury, a feeding gastrostomy tube was placed to facilitate nutrition and hydration. Over a period of 8 years, her parents watched Nancy become transformed into a contracted, drooling, grimacing caricature of her former self. Because they wanted to end their daughter's suffering, her parents sought permission from a Missouri court to remove her feeding tube, emphasizing that their daughter would not want to be kept alive in her condition if she were able to decide. A lower court concurred with the parents' decision to remove the tube; however, on appeal, the Supreme Court of Missouri reversed this decision, citing Nancy Cruzan's "right to life." The United States Supreme Court considered the case and cited a lack of "clear and convincing evidence" of Nancy Cruzan's wishes to not be maintained in a vegetative state. Later, after an acquaintance came forward and reported a conversation with Nancy in which she made clear her desire to not be sustained by artificial means, a Missouri Probate Judge stated that clear evidence existed to indicate that Nancy Cruzan, if mentally able, would terminate her nutrition and hydration (Capron, 1991). He authorized her parents to cause removal of the gastrostomy feeding. Nancy Cruzan died 12 days later. According to those in attendance, her death was quiet and peaceful. While some of the nurses who had cared for Nancy agreed with the action, others did not and refused to be involved further with her care. Although public sentiment appeared to be largely in favor of ending Cruzan's tube feedings, a small group of opponents stood vigil during the time of her death as a means of quiet protest.

It is highly likely that many more cases of the nature of the Nancy Cruzan case will be tried in the courts in the coming years. Issues raised by patients who resist medical feeding include competency to make treatment choices, decision making on behalf of incompetent patients, and the competent patient's right of self-determination (Dresser, 1985). Legal authorities encourage individuals to write living wills stating what they want done in the event of a catastrophic event in which they would be unable to make their wishes known. In the event a living will is not acknowledged, it is often recommended that power of attorney be assigned to another individual to make appropriate decisions as necessary about life-preserving treatments.

Financial Considerations

Malnourishment increases hospitalization time and cost, as well as morbidity and mortality, as is demonstrated by a 2.5-year study conducted by the American Dietetic Association concerning the effect of malnutrition on variable costs and charges for hospitalization (Cost Effectiveness of Nutrition Support, American Dietetic Association, 1986). Data were collected from the medical records of 800 patients with diagnoses such as pneumonia, fractured hip, inflammatory bowel disease, surgical hip repair, bowel surgery, and abdominal vascular surgery. Although 55 percent of the patients in this study were at risk for malnourishment, less than 5 percent received nutrition support before developing complications. Length of hospitalization was 2 to 5 days longer for malnourished patients than for those without malnutrition. Poorly nourished patients had three times the number of major complications, and they were three times more likely to die. Even without a complication, malnourished patients cost hospitals more per patient than well-nourished patients; these increases were $5,000 and $10,000 for medical and surgical patients, respectively. It is reasonable to assume that adequate nutrition in at-risk patients can be a cost-effective measure.

It has been estimated that approximately 900,000 persons are tube fed annually in hospitals in the United States, whereas 80,000 are tube fed in nursing homes and 60,000 in home settings. In contrast, approximately 550,000 patients receive parenteral nutrition in hospitals. One reason for the prevalence of tube feedings is that enteral feedings are less expensive than TPN. In addition to being more cost effective than TPN, enteral feeding may be physiologically more beneficial as well. Lickley (1978) demonstrated that intragastrically fed laboratory animals showed greater weight gain than did intravenously fed laboratory animals given the same amount of nutrients. Of course, the enteral route is only possible if the patient has a functional gastrointestinal tract.

FUTURE DEVELOPMENTS

Home care has become a primary strategy for reducing health care costs. Managed care plans are expanding rapidly, and there are increasing concerns about how reimbursement for home therapy (including enteral and parenteral nutrition) will be affected. Home care health providers, like their hospital counterparts, are struggling with rapid changes in their work settings and the increased pressure to reduce costs while increasing productivity (Viall et al, 1995).

Increasing emphasis on standards for nutrition support are likely in the future. The 1995 standards developed by the Joint Commission on Accreditation of Health Care Organizations are in effect and focus more on interdisciplinary delivery of care, including nutrition care (Dougherty et al, 1995).

Americans are living longer than ever before. In 1990, the percentage of the population older than 50 was close to 27 percent (Taylor, 1992). People older than 50 are disproportionate users of health resources; while they represent about one fourth of the population, they consume approximately half of all health care resources (Taylor, 1992). Thus, the need to increase our understanding of health promoting nutritional behaviors in this segment of the population is obvious.

Research is ongoing to improve types of nutrient solutions available for both enteral and parenteral feedings. Experiments have led to specially formulated solutions for patients with specific conditions, such as renal and hepatic failure, or severe trauma. Manufacturers are working to improve equipment to deliver parenteral and enteral nutrients. Numerous infusion pumps exist to force fluid into the vein or gastrointestinal tract regardless of patient position or other variables problematic to gravity flow systems. Some of these are extremely precise and are quite helpful when careful control of the flow rate is essential (as in TPN via a central vein). Various types of tube-feeding formula containers are available; some are prefilled for a 24-hour period.

If advances in technology related to nutritional support made during the past two decades are paralleled in the upcoming years, the future holds dramatic promise for improving the nutrition of both sick and well individuals. With these advances, it is possible that nutritional support will be based on a firmer understanding of clinical biochemistry, allowing caregivers to provide precise nutritional requirements for individuals with all types of conditions.

More research is needed to develop nutritional assessment techniques that go beyond merely identifying high-risk patients to highlighting subgroups that are more likely to benefit from nutritional support (Twomey, 1990). Also recommended are clinical trials to demonstrate benefits from specific types of feedings, both in terms of cost-effectiveness and physiologic improvements. Although it is reasonable to believe that nutritional support improves the health of both critically and chronically ill patients, there is lack of convincing data in many situations. This could be because too little is understood at present about altered metabolism in specific types of illnesses.

Population projections indicate that by the year 2040, more than 21 percent of the population will be older than 65 years of age (Chernoff and Lipschitz, 1990). Because chronic illness increases with advancing age, it is likely that increasing numbers of patients requiring nutritional support will confront the health care system in the future. One of the most controversial issues associated with artificial feedings of elderly individuals is that of ethics. With shrinking health care dollars, it is likely that guidelines will need to be explored about circumstances under which frail, elderly long-term care patients should be fed by artificial means.

Much remains to be learned about desired methods to provide care for malnourished patients with acquired immunodeficiency syndrome. There is little information on the specific mechanism causing the altered metabolism and poor absorption of nutrients noted in these individuals.

NURSING CARE ACTIONS

Principles and Practices

Nursing activities that support the maintaining of adequate nutritional status of patients are linked to scientific principles and practices previously discussed. These activities include performing a nutritional assessment, providing patients with adequate fluids and nutrients enterally or parenterally, monitoring fluid and nutrient intake, and interacting with other health care team members to correct nutritional problems.

NUTRITION ASSESSMENT

Nutrition assessment is the first step in delivering nutrition support. It determines who requires nutrition support and which form of intervention is indicated. Furthermore, it determines for how long the support is needed; as such, it is a dynamic, ongoing process. Although assessment methods have been widely studied, no foolproof indicators for malnutrition have emerged. For this reason, the clinician usually must integrate many pieces of information to identify malnutrition and arrive at the best course of action. Specialized nutrition support should be started when the benefits outweigh the possible risks. Unfortunately, this is a difficult decision to make because there is considerable variability in recommendations and practice.

The Joint Commission for Accreditation of Health Organizations has issued standards regarding nutrition assessment (Standards of Practice, 1995). The standards require that all patients admitted to hospitals for a specified length of stay undergo nutrition screening using subjective and/or objective criteria. Screening results must be documented. Examples of screening methods include a nursing checklist, percent of weight loss, serum albumin levels, and identification of specific disease codes. The purpose of the nutrition screening is to provide a baseline and document when a more detailed nutrition assessment is indicated. In this way, nutritional problems can be detected early in the patient's course of treatment.

Complete nutritional assessment includes taking the patient's nutritional history, inspecting for signs of obvious malnutrition, performing anthropometric measurements, and evaluating results of laboratory tests.

HISTORY

In completing a history, it is necessary to compare the patient's nutrient intake and utilization to the current level of need. To describe nutrient intake, a food history or 24-hour dietary recall can be used; if a more precise measure is needed, a calorie count can be performed. This consists of recording all nutrients taken in orally, by tube feedings, or by the IV route and tallying the caloric intake. In the case study at the beginning of the chapter, the patient received only 340 calories per day during her early hospitalization when her only source of nutrients was by the IV route. This was because she received only 2 L of 5 percent dextrose in 0.45 percent sodium chloride solution (containing 340 calories and 77 mEq/L of sodium and 77 mEq/L of chloride) each day.

Another part of the history requires describing any conditions that may interfere with absorption or utilization of ingested nutrients, such as frequent nausea and vomiting, diarrhea, protein loss from wounds or gastrointestinal fistulas, proteinuria from renal disease, and disease states associated with impaired intestinal absorptive ability. One also needs to consider the effect of drug–nutrient interactions. For example, is the patient receiving medications that increase nutrient loss (e.g., renal potassium loss due to potassium-wasting diuretics, such as furosemide or hydrochlorothiazide)? Another important consideration is if any conditions are present that greatly increase metabolic rate (e.g., severe trauma, major surgery, and sepsis). Simple equations exist to allow dietitians to calculate the patient's caloric and protein needs. The most frequently used is the Harris-Benedict equation; it requires the patient's weight in kilograms, height in centimeters, and age in years.

Part of the screening process involves comparing the patient's current weight with his or her usual weight to calculate the percent of change in body weight over the past 6 months (and even the past 2 weeks). Although decreased body weight is not a specific indicator of malnutrition, it has been found to correlate well with this condition.

Examples of questions on a nutrition assessment form are:

- Is the usual body weight 20 percent above or below normal?
- Has there been recent loss or gain of 10 percent of usual body weight?
- Are there ill-fitting dentures?
- Is there any evidence that income is inadequate for food purchasing?
- Does the patient live alone and prepare his or her own meals?
- Are there any swallowing difficulties?
- Is there paralysis of the arms (making feeding of self difficult)?
- Are there any mobility problems, interfering with food preparation and eating?
- Is there any chronic illness (e.g., arthritis, chronic obstructive pulmonary disease, renal or liver disease, malabsorption)?
- Is there any recent major illness, surgery, or injury?
- Has the patient been maintained more than 10 days on "routine" IV fluids?
- Is there a history of excessive use of alcohol?
- Is there frequent use of a monotonous diet?
- Is the patient taking any medications interfering with appetite or metabolism or absorption?
- Have abnormal losses of body fluids occurred such as vomiting, loose stools, or drainage from enterostomy, colostomy, fistulas, or wounds?

CLINICAL ASSESSMENT—PHYSICAL ELEMENTS

Body Weight

Despite limitations, body weight is one of the most widely applied measures of nutritional status because of its simplicity and generally satisfactory correlation with other nutritional indices. Body weight may be compared with the patient's usual weight or to that of a healthy population (Table 22–5). A patient's weight can be calculated as a percentage of ideal body weight by dividing the actual weight by the ideal body weight and multiplying by 100 percent. Actual body weight less than 80 percent of ideal body weight is considered a significant deficit (Silberman, 1989).

Body weight is a poor indicator of nutritional status when edema and/or ascites (accumulation of fluid in the abdominal cavity) are present, because both of these mask fat and protein depletion. In overweight patients, a weight loss due to illness may not be readily apparent unless the illness weight is compared with the pre-illness weight. Therefore, a frequently asked question on a nutritional assessment is "Has there been a weight loss of greater than 10 to 20 percent in the past month?" Another potential problem with body weight measurement as an indicator of nutritional status is the difficulty in obtaining accurate readings. For example, scales frequently vary by several pounds, and other factors (such as different clothing, timing of meals and IV fluids, and timing of last voiding and defecation) affect weight readings.

In review, the following points should be kept in mind when weighing patients:

- Check accuracy of scales before weighing the patient. Try to use the same scales each time to minimize variability.

TABLE 22-5 Healthy Weight Ranges by Height

Height (without shoes)	Weight in Pounds (without clothes)	
	Ages 19–34	*Ages 35 and older*
5′0″	97–128	108–138
5′1″	101–132	111–143
5′2″	104–137	115–148
5′3″	107–141	119–152
5′4″	111–146	122–157
5′5″	114–150	126–162
5′6″	118–155	130–167
5′7″	121–160	134–172
5′8″	125–164	138–178
5′9″	129–169	142–183
5′10″	132–174	146–188
5′11″	136–179	151–194
6′0″	140–184	155–199
6′1″	144–189	159–205
6′2″	148–195	164–210
6′3″	152–200	168–216
6′4″	156–205	173–222
6′5″	160–211	177–228
6′6″	164–216	182–234

Age and height are the main factors that determine healthy weight. Within each range, higher weights generally apply to men, who tend to have more muscle and bone. Lower weights generally apply to women. Source: Derived from the National Research Council, 1989.

- Weigh patient at the same time each day (preferably in the morning before breakfast).
- Weigh the patient in same amount of clothing each time.
- Have the patient void before weighing.
- Empty drainage bags (such as Foley catheter bags) before weighing.
- Investigate any major weight change (such as ≥1 kg).
- Record the weight on the patient's record.

Body Fat and Muscle Mass

In addition to measuring body weight, nutrition screening includes visually examining the subcutaneous fat stores. This can best be done by examining the triceps region of the arms, deltoid regions of the shoulders, and the tissues in the interosseous and palmar areas of the hand (Detsky et al, 1994). Positive findings are loss of fullness in one or more areas where the skin fits too loosely over the deeper tissues (this finding may be falsely positive in some elderly patients). It is also important to assess the patient's muscle mass; this can be done by visually inspecting various muscle groups (e.g., the deltoid region and quadriceps). Severely malnourished patients have a squared-off appearance to the shoulders from loss of muscle mass.

Measures of muscle strength are important in a nutrition screening. This test may merely consist of describing the patient's ability to squeeze the examiner's hand or observing the patient's cough strength. More sophisticated measures consist of having the patient squeeze a device called a *dynamometer*; this device actually measures the amount of pressure the patient is capable of producing with a hand grip.

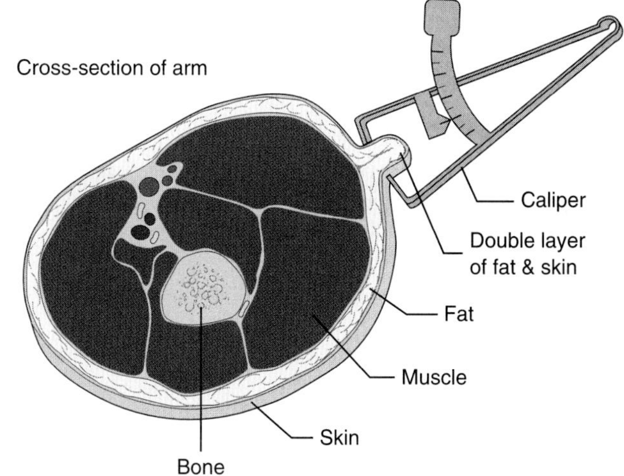

Figure 22-12. Measuring triceps skinfold thickness.

Another type of assessment for nutritional deficiencies involves measurement of the triceps skin fold thickness (Fig. 22–12) and the midarm muscle circumference (Fig. 22–13). These measures are thought to reflect fat stores and skeletal muscle mass, respectively. Although these anthropometric measurements are useful in the study of large populations, they are often of limited use in reflecting the day-to-day nutritional status of individuals. Values obtained from the same patient by different examiners may vary greatly. Also, normal

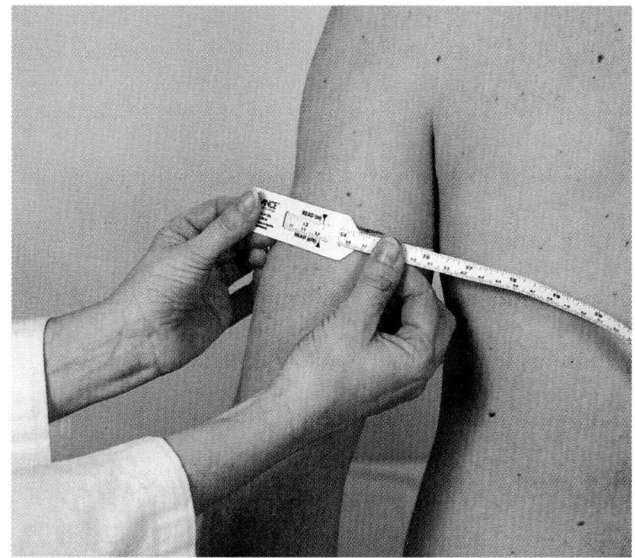

Figure 22-13. Measuring midarm circumference. (From Jarvis, C. [1996]. Physical Examination and Health Assessment, 2nd ed. Philadelphia: W.B. Saunders.)

standards for comparison with individual measurements are not well defined.

Edema is a sign of severe malnutrition and can be assessed for by inspecting the ankles and sacrum. Pressing the skin over these areas and observing for fluid moving out of the subcutaneous tissues is helpful in detecting edema; if the point of pressure stays indented for more than 5 seconds, *pitting edema* is said to be present.

The following points may be helpful in performing a physical assessment for malnutrition:

- Is the hair sparse, dry, and easily broken? Can small clumps of hair be pulled out with moderate force and no pain, especially from the side of the head? Sparse hair can indicate protein, biotin, and zinc deficiency. Similarly, hair that is easily plucked can indicate protein deficiency.
- Do nails on more than one extremity have cross-wise ridges or grooves? Transverse ridging of the nails is a sign of protein deficiency.
- Does the skin "break down" easily?
- Do wounds fail to heal normally? Poor wound healing could indicate protein, vitamin C, and zinc deficiencies.
- Do muscles have a wasted appearance? If so, this could be an indication of protein deficiency.
- Does the skin display pinpoint areas of bleeding (petechiae) or large areas of bruising (purpura)? If so, this could be an indication of vitamin C deficiency.
- Is there scaling of the skin? If so, this could be the result of deficiencies of vitamin A, zinc, and essential fatty acids.
- Are there cracked, ulcerated lips? If so, this could be a sign of deficiencies of riboflavin, pyridoxine, and niacin.
- Is there swelling and redness of the mouth and lips? A scarlet red tongue can result from vitamin (riboflavin, niacin, and pyridoxine) deficiencies. A slick tongue can signal protein, iron, or vitamin B deficiencies.
- Is edema present? If so, this could be the result of reduced albumin in the bloodstream, allowing plasma fluid to leak into the tissue spaces.

LABORATORY TESTS

Serum Albumin

Serum albumin is the most frequently used and tested laboratory measure of the body's protein status. The advantage of this laboratory test is that it is routinely obtained on admissions to hospitals and even in routine physical examinations in physicians' offices. The normal value for serum albumin is greater than or equal to 3.5 g/dl; values less than this correlate rather well with varying degrees of nutritional impairment. For example, a level less than or equal to 2.5 g/dl is thought to represent severe nutritional impairment. There are causes of low serum albumin levels other than malnutrition; among these are renal and liver disease, chronically draining wounds, and fluid volume overload. Serum albumin levels are not good indicators of a patient's response to nutritional support because it takes 20 days for any significant change to occur in measured laboratory values. Other more sensitive blood tests exist to measure protein status, such as serum transferrin and transthyretin. Advantages of these tests are that they will show changes in protein status more quickly than serum albumin levels. Unfortunately, they, too, are affected by a number of conditions other than malnutrition.

Total Lymphocyte Count

Total lymphocyte count is another laboratory test used to assess for malnutrition that theoretically helps measure the body's immune function, which is, in turn, influenced by the state of nutrition. A level greater than 1800/mm^3 is normal. An advantage of this method is that it is readily available in routine blood work; a disadvantage is that many factors other than malnutrition can cause a decreased count (among these are stress, cancer, and use of corticosteroids).

Urine Tests

Urine tests can be used to help assess the patient's protein status. This is because nitrogen (a component of protein) is largely excreted in the urine. In fact, 90 percent of daily nitrogen loss in humans is through the kidneys; about 90 percent of this loss is in the form of urea. Therefore, the 24-hour urine urea nitrogen test is a method for estimating nitrogen balance. Nitrogen (protein) balance is determined by subtracting nitrogen loss from dietary nitrogen intake. Nitrogen balance is used to estimate protein needs, assess the patient's response to therapy, and follow the metabolic status. A similar urine test is the creatinine height index. Creatinine is an index of lean muscle mass. In this test, the patient's creatinine excretion is compared with that expected of a person of similar age and height.

ASSESSING FLUID AND ELECTROLYTE BALANCE

Assessment of fluid and electrolyte balance requires review of the patient's history and laboratory data as well as careful clinical observations.

HISTORY

The history is designed to identify patients at risk for specific imbalances. Fluid and electrolyte and acid-base imbalances are indicative of many disease conditions. By using information gained from the history, it becomes easier to pinpoint problems likely to occur in specific patients. Anticipation of an imbalance makes it easier to detect and allows the nurse to focus on the most relevant observations. In addition to knowing what to look for, it is important to be aware that the symptoms of an imbalance depend on how long the imbalance has been present as well as its severity and rapidity of onset and how effectively it is compensated for by homeostatic mechanisms.

Questions to consider for a history include:

- Does the patient have a disease condition or injury state that can disrupt fluid and electrolyte balance?
- Has the patient received any medications that can disrupt fluid and electrolyte balance?
- Does the patient have abnormal routes of fluid loss?
- Have any dietary restrictions been imposed?
- Has the patient taken adequate amounts of water and other nutrients by mouth or some other route? If not, how long has the inadequacy been present?
- How does the patient's total intake of fluid compare with the total output?

CLINICAL ASSESSMENT OF FLUID AND ELECTROLYTE BALANCE

Because nurses typically spend more time with patients than do other health care team members, they are in a unique position to detect, describe, and interpret subtle changes. Assessment of fluid and electrolyte status is an ongoing process, varying with factors impacting on the patient's current status. Because fluid and electrolyte balance involves virtually every body system, the physical assessment must consider many factors. Among these are fluid intake and output, urine volume and concentration, body weight, skin and tissue changes, vital signs, and neuromuscular changes. As with nutritional assessment, changes in these factors do not necessarily indicate fluid and electrolyte problems and must be evaluated in relation to findings from the history and laboratory data. Some of the observations (e.g., the expected hourly urine volume in a particular situation) are straightforward and have relatively clear-cut values for normal and abnormal. Others, such as mild behavior changes, are more subtle.

Intake and Output Monitoring

Fluid intake and output is one of the most important measures of the patient' s fluid balance. Records of these measures should be maintained on all patients with real or potential fluid balance problems (see Procedure 22–1). Although these measurements are relatively easy to obtain, careful vigilance is necessary to ensure accuracy. A common assumption is that a procedure as "easy" as intake and output measurement cannot be as important as those involving complex technology. This could not be farther from the truth. In many instances, changes in fluid balance, either excess or deficit, show up on an accurate intake and output record. If detected early, interventions can be undertaken to remedy the situation before the imbalance becomes serious.

Urine Volume

Much can be learned about a patient's fluid balance status by assessing urine volume and concentration. As a general rule, the normal urinary output is between 0.5 and 1 ml/kg of body weight per hour. For example, a 70-kg individual would normally excrete between 35 and 70 ml of urine per hour. Another way to consider the normal urine volume is in terms of daily normal fluid intake and output. Note that the typical normal adult excretes about 1500 ml of urine per day. In times of stress, urinary volume is slightly less than usual because of the stress hormones (primarily aldosterone and antidiuretic hormone), which cause urinary retention in an attempt to maintain the body's blood volume. In stressful situations, an hourly urine volume of 30 to 50 ml is accepted as a normal adult range. An output less than 30 ml/hr, however, should be evaluated. It could be due to inadequate fluid intake or hypovolemia secondary to hemorrhage or large fluid loss from the gastrointestinal tract, skin, or lungs. In these situations, the decreased urine volume represents the kidneys' attempt to conserve fluid and maintain an effective circulating blood volume. Of course, the urine volume can also be greater than the usual range, as occurs in times of excessive fluid intake when the kidneys attempt to rid the body of unneeded fluids.

Urine Concentration

In addition to urine volume, urine concentration is an important clue to fluid balance status. A small-volume, concentrated urine indicates a healthy renal response to fluid volume deficit. More ominous is a dilute, small volume of urine, which probably indicates kidney damage. A dilute, large volume of urine probably signals fluid volume overload or a deficit of antidiuretic hormone. A large volume of urine can have a high concentration when it contains abnormal constituents (e.g., glucose, albumin, or radiocontrast dyes from diagnostic tests).

Urine concentration is usually measured in one of two ways. Specific gravity is the measure by which urine concentration is most frequently assessed. In this test, the concentration of urine is compared with the specific gravity of 1.000 of distilled water. Because urine contains electrolytes, urea, and other substances, its specific gravity exceeds 1.000. Most random urine specimens range between 1.012 and 1.025; extreme ranges are from 1.003 to 1.035. Urine specific gravity can be measured with a urinometer, a refractometer, or a dipstick that has a reagent area for specific gravity.

Another measure of urine concentration is *osmolality.* Typically, urinary osmolality ranges between 500 and 800 mOsm/kg; extreme ranges are from 50 to 1400 mOsm/kg. This measure is usually obtained in the laboratory and is definitely indicated when the urine contains substantial quantities of albumin or glucose.

Daily Weighing

The daily weighing of patients with potential or actual fluid balance problems is of great clinical importance. Rapid variations in weight, when measured correctly, reflect changes in body fluid volume. For example, a loss of 2 pounds over a day or less indicates a loss of approximately 1 L of fluid. Long-term body weight variations reflect changes in tissue mass as well as body fluid volume (Table 22–6).

TABLE 22-6 Possible Clinical Significance of Weight Changes

Weight Loss	Possible Significance
Rapid loss of 2% of total body weight	Mild fluid volume deficit
Rapid loss of 5% of total body weight	Moderate fluid volume deficit
Rapid loss of 8% or more of total body weight	Severe fluid volume deficit
Chronic weight loss	Protein deficiency
Weight Gain	
Rapid gain of 2% of total body weight	Mild fluid volume excess
Rapid gain of 5% of total body weight	Moderate fluid volume excess
Rapid gain of 8% or more of total body weight	Severe fluid volume excess

Skin Turgor

The elastic condition of skin, referred to as turgor, is partially dependent on the amount of tissue fluid supporting the skin and is therefore useful in the assessment of fluid balance. In a normal person, pinched skin will immediately fall back to its normal position when released. In a person with fluid volume deficit, the skin may remain elevated for many seconds after the pinch is released. Although the aim of the skin turgor test is to measure only the interstitial fluid volume, it measures skin elasticity as well. Because skin elasticity decreases with age, skin turgor is more difficult to assess in the elderly. The most reliable areas for testing skin turgor are the tissues over the sternum or forehead. (See Chapter 15, Patient Assessments, for details on how to assess skin turgor.)

Edema

Edema, defined as excessive accumulation of tissue (interstitial) fluid, is often an indicator of fluid volume overload. Excessive interstitial fluid that accumulates predominantly in the lower extremities of ambulatory patients and in the sacral region of bedridden patients is referred to as dependent edema. Generalized edema is spread throughout the body and is often most visible in the face and hands. Edema may be manifested in some situations by pressing one's finger into soft tissue, leaving a temporary "pit." After the pressure is removed, the pit gradually disappears. Description of peripheral edema by appearance is somewhat subjective; therefore, measurement of an extremity or body part with a millimeter tape, in the same area each day, is the most exact method.

Vital Signs

Vital signs, including temperature, pulse, respiration, and blood pressure, are measured regularly in all hospitalized patients. Changes in any or all of these measures may indicate fluid and electrolyte problems as well as a multitude of other conditions.

Fever increases body fluid loss and thus predisposes to fluid volume deficit. Metabolic wastes are formed in greater amounts in patients with fever, causing a larger urine volume to permit excretion of the metabolic wastes. In addition, the hyperpnea (deep, rapid breathing) associated with fever increases water vapor loss through the lungs. Changes in body temperature may also be symptoms of fluid and electrolyte problems. For example, hypernatremia can cause fever, presumably by decreasing the amount of water available for sweating and heat dissipation from the skin.

Pulse changes that may signal fluid and electrolyte problems are varied. A heart rate greater than 100 beats per minute (tachycardia) is an early sign of the decreased vascular volume associated with fluid volume deficit. A weak thready pulse is associated with fluid deficit, and a bounding full pulse is associated with fluid overload. Irregular pulse rates may occur with potassium and magnesium deficits.

Rapid breathing, as experienced in high-stress situations, may produce a too alkaline blood pH by blowing off large amounts of carbon dioxide (an acidic substance), or it may be the body's attempt to compensate for an acidic blood pH. Moist respiratory sounds heard with a stethoscope, in the absence of cardiopulmonary disease, signal excess fluid in the lungs (as occurs in fluid volume overload). Respiratory muscle strength is decreased in severe hypokalemia or hyperkalemia and in severe hypermagnesemia.

Blood pressure is one of the most frequently assessed variables in the identification of hypovolemia. A fall in systolic blood pressure greater than 15 mm Hg or an increase in the pulse rate greater than 15 beats per minute is suggestive of intravascular volume deficit. Conversely, an excess of intravascular fluid can cause an elevation in the systolic blood pressure. In addition to fluid volume changes, variations in plasma electrolyte concentrations can affect blood pressure. For example, hypotension can occur in patients with hypermagnesemia.

Neurologic Status

Changes in mental functioning may be the result of a number of fluid and electrolyte problems. For example, severe fluid volume deficit decreases the sensorium because of reduced blood flow to the brain. Low or high plasma sodium levels have direct effects on the brain volume and thus have profound effects on mental function. Indeed, these changes are among the most important in the clinical detection of hyponatremia or hypernatremia.

Assessment of neuromuscular irritability is frequently necessary when imbalances in calcium and magnesium are suspected. The nurse may, as necessary, check for Chvostek's sign and Trousseau's sign (Fig. 22–14); also, deep tendon reflexes may be tested to monitor neuromuscular irritability. To test Chvostek's sign, the facial nerve is tapped about an inch in front of the earlobe. A positive response shows a unilateral

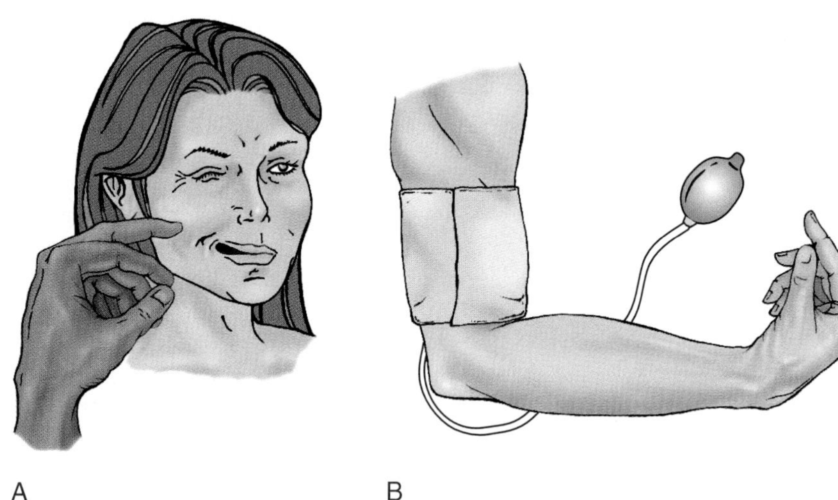

Figure 22-14. Chvostek's (*A*) and Trousseau's (*B*) signs. (From Monahan, F.D., Neighbors, M. [1998]. Medical-Surgical Nursing: Foundations for Clinical Practice. Philadelphia: W.B. Saunders.)

twitching of the face, and can indicate hypocalcemia or hypomagnesemia. To test Trousseau's sign, a blood pressure cuff is placed on the arm and inflated above systolic pressure for about 3 minutes. A positive reaction is a spasm of the hand and is likely to be present in hypocalcemia and hypomagnesemia.

A deep tendon reflex is elicited by tapping a partially stretched muscle with a percussion hammer. The extent of the reflex is graded from 0 to 4+, with 0 representing no response and 4+ indicating hypersensitivity. A 2+ response is generally described as normal.

LABORATORY TESTS

Tests performed on blood and urine are indispensable in the evaluation of patients with fluid and electrolyte disorders. In addition to serum and urinary electrolyte concentrations, tests of renal function (such as serum creatinine and blood urea nitrogen) are commonly performed (Table 22–7).

TABLE 22-7 Normal Laboratory Values for Common Tests of Fluid/Electrolyte and Nutrition Status

Test	Normal Value
Serum sodium	135–145 mEq/L
Serum potassium	3.5–5.0 mEq/L
Total serum calcium	8.9–10.3 mg/dl
Serum phosphorus	2.5–4.5 mg/dl
Serum magnesium	1.3–2.1 mEq/L
Serum bicarbonate	26 mEq/L
Blood urea nitrogen	8–25 mg/dl
Serum creatinine	0.6–1.5 mg/dl
Serum albumin	≥3.5 g/dl
Serum transthyretin	200–350 mg/dl
Total lymphocyte count	>1800 mm^3

ASSISTING PATIENTS WITH ORAL DIETARY INTAKE

Because illness may greatly decrease the desire and/or ability to eat, patients are often poor eaters. Nursing responsibilities extend beyond serving trays to helping patients overcome obstacles to eating (see Procedure 22–2). It is crucial to remember that any program of diet therapy is worthless if the patient does not eat! The following points should be considered:

- Review the patient's food likes and dislikes and the cultural and religious beliefs that influence his or her eating habits. Relay the findings to the dietary department as needed. Allow the patient's family to bring favorite foods from home, if permitted, under nursing supervision.
- Encourage the patient to make dietary choices when possible to increase the diet's palatability.
- If the patient wears dentures, be sure they are in place before serving the meal. Patients with ill-fitting dentures or few teeth may require a soft diet to provide adequate nourishment (discuss findings with dietitian and physician to identify a suitable diet form).
- Provide comfort measures as needed before meals (e.g., the patient with a distended bladder may need to be catheterized; the patient in pain may require an analgesic).
- Place the tray within easy reach of the patient.
- Assist the patient in preparing the tray if necessary (e.g., open milk cartons, pour coffee, take utensils out of cellophane, cut up food). Remember that a weak or partially paralyzed patient, or one with an IV device in the hand, cannot easily perform these activities.
- Elevate the head of the bed to 80° or 90°, if allowed, to facilitate swallowing.
- Give the patient uninterrupted time to eat. The not-too-eager appetite can be easily discouraged by the poor planning of nursing activities.

- Feed patients in an unhurried manner, allowing patients sufficient time to chew and swallow comfortably. Offer liquids and solids alternately in manageable amounts.
- Teach patients with dysphagia (swallowing difficulties) the importance of neck flexion while tilting the body forward as a method to minimize aspiration of food and liquids into the trachea. This maneuver provides a passage to the esophagus while leaving the trachea protected by the back of the tongue (Larsen, 1973).
- Provide aids such as straws, special cups, or plates.

Helping *neurologically impaired patients* to eat is often problematic because they have defective swallowing reflexes. As indicated in the case study at the beginning of this chapter, there is a tendency to avoid feeding such individuals because of the fear of choking; this practice can lead to serious problems if another route of feeding is not initiated. Before initiating another route of feeding, it is helpful to try to help improve the ability to swallow. In practice, it has been observed that patients with dysphagia can swallow solids more easily than thin liquids. For this reason, patients who have suffered strokes and have swallowing difficulties are usually started on frozen popsicles rather than water. It has been noted that many patients will automatically throw their heads back to facilitate swallowing. Yet, this action provides a direct pathway to the trachea and should be avoided. As indicated earlier, dysphagic patients should be taught the importance of neck flexion while tilting the body forward, thereby providing a bypass to the esophagus, leaving the trachea protected by the back of the tongue (Larsen, 1973). Others also recommend ventral flexion of the neck, with the torso elevated 80° to 90° (Zimmerman and Oder, 1981).

ADMINISTERING ENTERAL TUBE FEEDING

The procedure for administering nasogastric enteral feedings is described in the next section. Presented here are some principles to promote patient safety during enteral feedings.

Confirming Proper Tube Position Prior to Feeding

It is imperative to confirm proper tube position on initial placement before introducing any substance (formula or medications) through the tube; the obvious danger is that the tube may have been inadvertently positioned in the lung instead of the gastrointestinal tract. It is also important to check tube placement before intermittent feedings and at regular intervals during continuous feedings to be sure that the tube has not moved from its intended position. Events such as pulling of the tube during movement or intentional tugging by patients, as well as coughing, retching, and vomiting, may cause tube dislodgement.

The most effective way to confirm correct placement of small-bore feeding tubes is an abdominal x-ray film. Unfortunately, no presently available bedside test is as accurate as radiography. Review agency policy to find if x-ray films to determine proper placement are used.

Two bedside methods are most helpful: aspirating gastric secretions and air insufflation.

Aspiration. Withdrawing fluid from the feeding tube and observing its appearance and pH is quite helpful. Gastric aspirates are likely to be greenish or off-white or tan and to have a low pH (<6, and probably ≤ 4). In contrast, intestinal aspirates are likely to be golden yellow and to have a pH more than 6. The pH can easily be checked using paper test strips. Aspirates from feeding tubes inadvertently positioned in the lung often bear characteristics of the fluid from that region—they include mucus if from the tracheobronchial tree and serous fluid or blood if from the pleural space (Metheny et al, 1990a). The fluids aspirated may be difficult to identify as to source because the fluids may be similar in appearance.

Insufflation and Auscultation. The auscultatory method (consisting of listening over the epigastric region with a stethoscope while injecting air through the feeding tube) is often used. Because this method is misleading, it should not be used as the sole method for confirming tube placement, because sounds can usually be heard even when the tube is in the lung or pleural space. However, this method can help indicate when a tube is in the esophagus because patients are likely to belch when air is insufflated (Metheny et al, 1989). Also, faint to absent sounds may indicate that the tube is coiled in the back of the throat or is kinked.

Maintaining Correct Tube Position

After it is determined that the tube is correctly placed, it is anchored firmly with tape and its exit site from the nose is marked with permanent ink. This position should be monitored every 4 hours, because confused patients sometimes pull at their tubes or the tubes are accidentally dislodged during movement and performance of nursing procedures. The tube may be taped with flesh-colored (instead of white) tape to make it less obvious.

If the mark indicates that the tube's position has changed, the tube will need to be repositioned or replaced. Recall that the internal end of the tube can become dislodged upwardly during violent coughing or retching even though the external portion remains taped in place. A nasogastric tube that is inadvertently displaced into the esophagus, of course, predisposes to aspiration. Similarly, an intestinal tube that is inadvertently moved upward into the stomach also increases the risk for aspiration.

Detecting Pulmonary Aspiration

This complication is seldom obvious. In fact, it is difficult to detect, causing clinicians to rely on observations made on tracheobronchial secretions. If tube-feeding formula is present in tracheobronchial secretions, it is evidence of aspiration of gastric contents into the lung. However, tube-feeding formula is usually a creamy white or tan color, much like the color of respiratory mucus, making it difficult to determine if formula is present. Therefore, some nurses aseptically add a small quantity of blue food coloring to the tube-feeding formula to make it easier to detect if it is aspirated. However, there is some indication that this method is a poor indicator of aspiration (Potts et al, 1993), and there are some reports of problems associated with this practice (e.g., contamination of the formula, discoloration of the patient's skin and body fluids, possible allergic reactions, and interference with interpreting guaiac tests performed on stool specimens).

A less problematic method for detecting pulmonary aspiration is the testing of tracheobronchial secretions for glucose content with glucose oxidase reagent strips. Theoretically, tracheobronchial secretions contain less than 5 mg/dl of glucose; therefore, the presence of glucose greater than this amount could indicate the aspiration of glucose-rich tube-feeding formula (Winterbauer et al, 1981). Generally, tracheobronchial glucose secretion levels greater than 20 mg/dl are thought to be significant. However, this method may also not be specific for aspiration because there may be reasons other than aspiration for glucose to be present in tracheobronchial secretions (Kinsey et al, 1994). Both the food coloring and glucose detection methods require direct access to the tracheobronchial secretions through an artificial airway (e.g., a tracheostomy or an endotracheal tube). Because not all tube-fed patients have this access, these methods are not helpful in all tube-fed patients.

All tube-fed patients should be monitored for signs of respiratory problems, such as dyspnea, tachypnea (respiratory rate >20 breaths per minute), tachycardia (heart rate >100 beats per minute), fever (>38°C), elevated white blood count, and purulent sputum. Although these signs are not specific for aspiration pneumonia, they are frequently associated with it. Chest x-ray films and sputum cultures are often used to determine the origin of pulmonary problems in tube-fed patients displaying respiratory symptoms.

If aspiration of formula is witnessed, the feeding should be turned off and suction used to remove the formula from the patient's mouth and upper respiratory tract. Suctioning also stimulates coughing and helps clear the respiratory tract. The physician should be notified immediately because further treatment will be necessary.

Minimizing Pulmonary Aspiration

Even more important than detection of pulmonary aspiration is its prevention. Fortunately, there are a number of things that can be done by nurses to minimize this complication.

Elevating the Head of the Bed. At least two research studies have demonstrated the great value associated with keeping the head of the bed elevated to at least 30° during feedings (Ibanez et al, 1992; Torres et al, 1992). By gravity, this position reduces refluxing of formula into the mouth where it could be inhaled into the respiratory tract of unconscious patients or those with impaired gag reflex and swallowing ability.

Monitoring Gastric Residual Volumes. It is important to monitor for high gastric residuals during continuous feedings and before each intermittent feeding. This is because patients are at greater risk for pulmonary aspiration if they have distended stomachs. Although there is no general agreement as to what is an excessive residual volume, one clinical study cites 200 ml for a patient with a nasogastric tube and 100 ml for an adult patient with a gastrostomy (McClave et al, 1992). To measure gastric residual volumes, it is necessary to use a large syringe (e.g., 60-ml syringe). Clinicians differ over whether to return the aspirate to the stomach or discard it. Probably the best action is to return the aspirate (with its electrolytes, fluid, nutrients, and perhaps even medications) through the tube back to the patient unless the volume is quite large.

Other methods to monitor for decreased gastric emptying include measuring the abdominal girth with a millimeter tape and asking the patient if nausea and discomfort are present. In addition, assessing for hypoactive bowel sounds helps to indicate when the gastrointestinal tract is functioning normally.

Choosing the Optimum Feeding Site. Most clinicians believe that it is prudent to place a feeding tube in the intestine instead of the stomach in patients at high risk for aspiration; however, there is not complete agreement on this in practice settings. Those who favor intestinal feedings hypothesize that the pyloric sphincter offers added protection against reflux of fluid into the respiratory tract. As previously stated, high-risk patients are those who are unconscious and/or have impaired swallowing and gag reflexes. Refluxing of formula is less likely when the tube feeding is introduced into the distal duodenum/proximal jejunum (Gustke et al, 1970). For ambulatory patients who are alert and who have normal gastrointestinal function, the gastric site is preferable because it allows intermittent bolus feedings, which facilitates patient mobility.

Preventing Tube Clogging

Small-bore feeding tubes will not clog if they are properly handled. Among the most important maneuvers to prevent tube clogging is regular flushing with water. For example, a reasonable protocol might call for flushing the tube with 10 to 30 ml of water every 4 hours during continuous tube feedings and after each intermittent feeding. Some authors recommend cranberry juice as an irrigant, although there is no scientific evidence of its effectiveness. No irrigant has been shown to be superior to water; yet water has been shown to be superior to cranberry juice in maintaining tube patency. Therefore, water is the preferred irrigant because it is readily available.

Proper administration of medications through small-bore feeding tubes is crucial to prevent tube clogging. When possible, medications should be administered in liquid form. If pills must be crushed for administration through feeding tubes, it is important to finely pulverize the pill and dissolve it in an appropriate solvent. Of course, enteric-coated tablets should not be crushed because their coatings are insoluble and will clog the feeding tube; also, enteric-coated medications are designed to dissolve slowly in the gastrointestinal tract. When more than one medication must be administered, it is important to give each one separately, followed by the injection of 5 ml of water through the tube. This avoids chemical and physical interactions between the medications that could further increase the possibility of tube clogging. It is helpful to have a standard hospital protocol for medication administration through small-bore tubes; such a protocol should be jointly developed by pharmacists, nurses, and physicians.

It is better to use enteral feeding pumps when available to help maintain a steady flow of formula through feeding tubes. Gravity flow rates are notoriously difficult to maintain; when the rate inadvertently slows, the incidence of tube clogging is greater. For this reason, it is necessary to check gravity flow rates frequently and to readjust the rate as indicated to maintain the desired flow rate.

Prevention of tube clogging is preferable to dealing with a tube after it has clogged. However, small-bore tubes do occasionally clog and a variety of procedures may be tried. The first thing to try is irrigation with warm water. If irrigation with warm water does not unclog the tube, probably the best substance to instill into the tube is pancreatic enzyme that has been activated to an alkaline pH with sodium bicarbonate (Marcuard et al, 1989); however, a specific protocol is needed for use of these substances. At times, specialized mechanical devices are available to insert through the feeding tube to help remove the clogged substance.

PREVENTING CONTAMINATION OF FORMULA AND EQUIPMENT

Good handwashing is by far the most important way to prevent contaminating formulas and administration setups. Also, the equipment should be handled as little as possible. If prefilled ready-to-use delivery sets are available and appropriate for the patient's needs, they should be used because they minimize the risk of contamination that accompanies handling of formula during mixing and transfer to the administration set (Vaughn et al, 1988). Today most formulas are administered undiluted, which reduces the contamination risk compared with earlier practice in which all formulas were diluted with water before administration.

Most enteral formulas can be hung at room temperature for 8 to 12 hours without fear of contamination if properly handled (Kohn and Keithley, 1989). Exceptions include formulas with perishable ingredients (such as hospital-blended formulas), which should hang no longer than 4 hours, and prefilled ready-to-use delivery sets, which can probably hang safely for 24 hours.

Reusable delivery sets should be changed at least every 24 hours or more frequently if known to be contaminated (Schroeder et al, 1983). The delivery set should be rinsed thoroughly with water before adding formula to avoid contaminating the new formula and infusing traces of a previous (possibly contaminated) formula.

Reducing the Risk of Diarrhea

Many causes of diarrhea (such as antibiotic use) are beyond the province of nursing to prevent. However, some nursing interventions can help minimize certain causes of diarrhea. For example, dilution of hyperosmotic medications (e.g., suspensions and elixirs) before administering them by bolus through feeding tubes can be helpful (Niemec et al, 1983). Also, avoiding contamination of formula and the apparatus is helpful in preventing diarrhea related to infectious agents.

Each tube-feeding formula should be evaluated as a possible cause of diarrhea. For example, lactose intolerance is a cause of diarrhea in selected patients. Even though very few formulas contain lactose, this factor should be considered. Also, the fat content of formulas should be considered as a possible contributor to diarrhea. As discussed earlier, diarrhea is more common when high-fat formulas are used. Although controversial, there is some evidence that fiber-enriched formulas may help normalize stool consistency of tube-fed patients with diarrhea.

Monitoring for Metabolic Complications

To detect metabolic disorders in tube-fed patients, it is necessary to monitor the patient's intake and output, body weight, urine and possibly capillary glucose levels, blood urea nitrogen, and serum electrolytes at regular intervals. These observations are usually made daily in the first 1 or 2 weeks of tube feedings and then less frequently afterward as the patient's condition stabilizes.

Glucose. Observation for elevated urinary or blood glucose levels is necessary to detect intolerance to the glucose in the feeding formula. Elevated glucose levels signal that the intake of glucose has exceeded the body's ability to produce insulin. If allowed to continue unchecked, the patient is likely to develop severe polyuria (excessive amounts of urine) and fluid volume deficit, which may progress to a serious condition known as hyperosmolar nonketotic hyperosmolar coma.

Nitrogen. A markedly elevated blood urea nitrogen value signals fluid volume deficit due to protein overloading with inadequate water intake.

Electrolytes. Many types of fluid and electrolyte imbalances can occur with tube feedings; such imbalances may reflect the patient's underlying disease condition. Regular monitoring of laboratory values is indicated to detect developing metabolic problems. For example, potassium, phosphorus, and magnesium deficiencies are likely if a high-calorie feeding is initiated suddenly in a previously malnourished patient. Modification of the formula's electrolyte content may be indicated for individual patients. For example, potassium and phosphates may need to be reduced in patients with advanced renal disease but who are not yet on dialysis; sodium may be reduced in patients with heart disease. Observations for sodium imbalance (both hyponatremia and hypernatremia) are indicated and need to be correlated with fluid intake.

BOX 22-1
CALCULATING IV FLOW RATES

Use the following formula to determine the desired flow rate:

$$\text{Drip/minute} = \frac{\text{Total volume to be infused} \times \text{Drop factor}}{\text{Infusion time in minutes}}$$

Example: Infuse 1000 ml of fluid over 8 hours, using a set furnishing 15 drop/ml

1000 ml = Total volume
15 drops/ml = Drop factor
480 minutes = Total time in minutes (8 × 60)

$$\text{Drops/minute} = \frac{1000 \times 15}{480} = 31$$

The desired flow rate is approximately 31 drops/min.

ADMINISTERING PARENTERAL FLUIDS

Over 85 percent of all hospitalized patients receive IV fluid therapy, mostly by means of vascular access devices. IV fluid administration can lead to both local and systemic complications. Whereas local complications are more frequent, systemic complications are more serious. Examples of local complications are dislodgement of an IV needle, resulting in infusion of the solution into subcutaneous tissue, and phlebitis (irritation of the venous wall) by either mechanical or chemical means.

Monitoring for Infiltration

Infiltration of fluid into tissues surrounding the venipuncture site is the most common complication of IV fluid delivery. It can occur when the device punctures the venous wall owing to patient movement or vein fragility, allowing fluid to infiltrate into the surrounding tissue. It is important to check for infiltration at least every 2 hours when giving fluids in a peripheral vein. The most common symptoms include swelling, blanching, and coolness at the site and a decreased fluid flow rate if the fluid is administered by gravity. The latter occurs when the fluid meets greater resistance from the tissue than previously encountered when the needle was correctly positioned in the vein. Flow rate will remain at the designated rate when a pressure infusion pump is used; this is unfortunate because more severe tissue injury will result as the fluid continues to flow at its usual rate into the site.

Managing Phlebitis

The specific nursing interventions for phlebitis vary with the cause and degree of phlebitis. Among the possible interventions are discontinuing the IV device at the involved site, elevating the involved extremity, applying warm moist packs for 20 minutes four times daily, and culturing the IV device and drainage to determine the type of infective organism (Perucca and Micek, 1993). It is important to remember that infusion-related phlebitis is a common but often preventable complication associated with IV therapy.

In review, *phlebitis* is defined as the inflammation of a vein; it is characterized by tenderness, pain, erythema, edema, streak formation, and sometimes a palpable cord and purulence at the site (Bennet and Brachman, 1992). Stages of phlebitis can range from 0 to 5+, with 0 representing no pain, redness, or edema at the IV site and 5+ representing the most severe form (with purulent drainage plus signs of criteria for 4+ phlebitis). Criteria for 4+ phlebitis include painful IV site with redness, edema, induration, and a palpable cord more than 3 inches above the IV site (Perucca and Micek, 1993).

Monitoring for Metabolic Complications

The metabolic complications that can accompany IV fluid and nutrient delivery are numerous and complex. The most important interventions in this area include:

- Reviewing the types of fluids the patient is receiving and consider what electrolytes and nutrients are contained in them
- Monitoring laboratory values for significant abnormalities
- Performing the assessments for fluid/electrolyte and nutrition status described earlier in this chapter
- Discussing any significant findings with the primary nurse caring for the patient

Great care must be exercised when administering IV fluid therapy because it is possible to seriously alter plasma electrolyte concentrations with the infusion of parenteral fluids. For example, the excessive administration of D_5W can cause a below-normal plasma sodium level, and the excessive administration of 0.9 percent sodium chloride can cause fluid volume excess. Virtually any fluid and electrolyte disturbance can occur with TPN. The most likely is fluid volume deficit after administration of highly concentrated TPN solution. Because of the high dextrose concentration in the formula, too-rapid administration can lead to hyperglycemia, which, in turn, causes excessive urinary output. Fluid volume deficit can thus follow, accompanied by a multitude of electrolyte abnormalities, such as deficits of the primary cellular electrolytes (potassium, magnesium, and phosphorus). It is common practice to closely monitor plasma electrolytes during TPN administration to allow early detection of abnormalities.

Central Vein Cannulation Complications

The administration of parenteral nutrients and fluids through central veins has gained broad acceptance in multiple settings; because of this, the nurse is increasingly involved in educating patients and in monitoring for the clinical and mechanical complications associated with these infusions (Richardson and Bruso, 1993). Among the possible complications of inserting a catheter into one of the large central veins are air embolism, pneumothorax (presence of air in the pleural space between the lung and chest wall), hemothorax

RESEARCH HIGHLIGHT

PREDICTORS OF DIETARY INTAKE IN AN ELDERLY POPULATION IN THE COMMUNITY

Elderly people, particularly those suffering from chronic diseases, are vulnerable to caloric and nutritional deficits. Deficiencies are found more frequently among institutionalized elderly than in healthy noninstitutionalized elderly. Improving the nutritional status of the elderly appears to have an effect on reducing morbidity of this population group. Recent studies have associated the level of dependency in activities of daily living with the quality of nutritional intake. The few studies undertaken of noninstitutionalized elderly suggest that poor health is associated with low dietary intake, which leads to undernutrition that is difficult to reverse. Predictors of dietary intake in healthy elderly include living alone or in social isolation, limited financial resources, declining physical or mental health, and functional limitations. Payette and associates (1995) conducted a study to identify predictors of the energy and protein intake in a group of high-risk older adults. The goals of the study were to estimate the energy and macronutrient intake of a group of community-living older adults with loss of autonomy and to relate energy and protein intake to socioeconomic indicators, food-related behaviors, and health status.

THE STUDY

Elderly people living in publicly financed home care services in Sherbrooke, Quebec, Canada, were included in the study population. The 145 subjects were between the ages of 60 and 94 and enrolled in three home care programs. Interviews were conducted to measure sociodemographic, health status, and food-related behaviors. Dietary intake information was collected over three nonconsecutive 24-hour periods. Data included dietary habits, social networks, food beliefs, recent stressful life events, health status, medication use, lifestyle habits, height, weight, and weight changes. A home interview and follow-up telephone calls were used to collect the information. A theoretical model was formulated to analyze the data.

THE RESULTS

The overall age of the population group was 78.8. Over half of the participants (51 percent) reported feeling lonely, even though they had frequent contact with relatives, friends, or neighbors. Half of the subjects stated that their health status was fair or poor. The reported number of illnesses was high. Many participants indicated that they experienced a high number of stressful incidents. Eighty-six percent of the men and 91 percent of the women wore dentures. One third of the group reported difficulty with shopping, and 69 percent of the men and 26 percent of the women never prepared their own meals. Ninety percent of the participants consumed three meals a day. A large number reported poor appetites. Very few used vitamin or mineral supplements. A large number of the subjects indicated that they had poor vision. Forty percent of the men and 32 percent of the women were at high risk of health problems because of low body weight.

Nutrient intake of a large number of the subjects was not adequate; more than 50 percent did not meet the recommended level of daily intake of protein, and intake of saturated fat was slightly elevated. The study *did not* find that social or friendship networks or financial resources were predictors of dietary intake. Also, dentition was not a predictor. Occurrence of stressful events *did* affect dietary intake, as did chronic and acute disease episodes. Dependency in activities of daily living was identified as a risk factor and therefore a predictor of dietary intake. Decline in vision was also a determinant. The results of the study indicate that the diet of the participants in regard to nutrients was balanced but total intake was low.

IMPLICATIONS FOR NURSING PRACTICE

The importance of obtaining an accurate nutritional assessment, especially of the elderly, cannot be overstated. The study defines the risk factors or predictors that affect dietary intake and lead to malnutrition. Attention should be given to the following while planning for the care of an elderly patient:

- Presence of a chronic disease
- Ability to conduct activities of daily living
- Poor appetite
- High level of stressful events
- Poor vision.

The nutritional assessment is an important nursing activity and should be completed regardless of the setting where the patient is located. This study was conducted in a home care setting; however, the results are of equal significance in long-term care facilities and in hospitals. Inadequate nutrient intake leads to deterioration of the patient's physical and mental status, reduces the quality of life, or may be life threatening.

(presence of blood in the pleural cavity), air embolus, and arterial puncture (Richardson and Bruso, 1993). Nursing responsibilities include observing for these complications and relaying the information quickly to the physician so that a chest tube can be inserted if indicated.

Air Emboli. Although an infrequent occurrence, air emboli can enter the central circulation through the catheter or administration set. It can occur after the insertion or removal of central venous catheters (Sing et al, 1995). Although it is more likely to occur with a central venous line, it can also happen with a peripheral line. If large enough, emboli can cause serious illness or death. Air may enter the vascular system during the time of catheter insertion, during periods when the catheter is separated from the infusion (at tubing changes), and on catheter removal. Clinically it has been noted that this complication is most likely to occur during

PATIENT TEACHING
TEACHING PATIENTS HOW TO AVOID SWALLOWING PROBLEMS

The greatest risk to oral ingestion is the potential to aspirate food or liquids into the trachea, particularly in patients who have dysphagia (difficulty swallowing). For patients with dysphagia it may be necessary to modify the diet to accommodate the swallowing difficulties. The likes and dislikes of the patient in relation to food types should also be considered. The patient's ability to comprehend and cooperate in his or her own dietary intake must also be assessed.

SPECIFIC TOPICS TO TEACH THE PATIENT

- Explain the process to be used and what is expected of the patient.
- Select foods that have a consistency that is soft but able to be picked up with an eating utensil (fork or spoon). Special utensils such as straws, cups with lids, or plates with suction cups may be helpful. Avoid foods such as peanut butter that adhere to the oral tissues.
- If patient is bed fast, adjust the patient to a high Fowler position or at home prop the patient with pillows.
- Instruct the patient to point the chin toward the midline with head forward (flexion). If appropriate, have patient insert dentures.
- Place the food within easy reach of the patient.
- Tell the patient to smell the food before eating, take time to hold the food in the mouth, and think about the swallowing process. Instruct the patient to try to stimulate and to collect saliva to moisten the food and assist in swallowing.
- Instruct the patient to take adequate time to eat. Rushing may cause choking.
- Teach the patient to remain upright for a period of time after eating. Gravity aids the patient to swallow more easily.
- Teach family members the same information provided to the patient.
- Provide mouth care after the meal.

CLINICAL DECISION MAKING

Mrs. Mary Smith, as described in the case study, was confined to a nursing home. While in the nursing home she suffered a stroke and became debilitated. She had difficulty swallowing, suffered from dehydration, and was malnourished. She was also mentally confused. Because of increasing deterioration, Mrs. Smith was moved to an acute care hospital where she was treated for her problems. What are the factors that need to be considered in planning for Mrs. Smith's care?

FACTORS TO CONSIDER

- Frail elderly individual
- Institutionalized nursing home living arrangement
- Difficulty swallowing
- Dehydration due to limited fluid intake
- Removal from nursing home to a new unfamiliar environment
- Intravenous therapy
- Malnutrition
- Presence of a nasogastric tube and tube feedings
- Status of family and social support system
- Effects of physical therapy on frail patient
- Status of patient mobility and determination of physical condition to perform activities of daily living

GOAL

Assist Mrs. Smith to return to her highest level of competence, both physically and mentally, through planned nursing interventions.

INTERVENTIONS

The nursing care of Mrs. Smith is planned and coordinated with the physician, dietitian, physical therapist, pharmacist, and members of the nursing staff. The nurse assumes responsibility for coordination.

Some specific nursing interventions to consider to assist Mrs. Smith:

- Discuss the plans for Mrs. Smith's care with her (and family members if available).
- Consider Mrs. Smith's confused mental status and continue to reinforce the elements of the care plan.
- Establish routines to maintain patency of the gastric tubes, tube-feeding schedules, and IV therapy.
- Together with the physical therapist, assist in carrying out the rehabilitation program to help Mrs. Smith regain her ability to swallow.
- Determine the status of Mrs. Smith's mobility and evaluate how she is able to perform activities of daily living and develop greater independence. Aid her to develop the skills she is lacking.
- Ascertain the involvement of Mrs. Smith's support system; and if family members or significant others are available and interested, assist them in understanding and participating in Mrs. Smith's care.
- Provide mental stimulation to help Mrs. Smith in maintaining mental competence. At periodic intervals, assess Mrs. Smith's mental state to detect presence or absence of confusion.
- Before the return of Mrs. Smith to the nursing home, confer with nursing home staff to provide for continuity of care after discharge from the acute care facility. Specifically, plan for a long-term dietary and fluid program.

tubing changes or when connections of the administration apparatus are not air tight.

To protect against air embolism, it is important to prime all IV tubing carefully and to tape all IV connections securely; also, the entire IV system should be inspected at least once per shift for possible disconnections (Bohony, 1993). Air embolism is a very serious complication that must be guarded against during situations in which air might enter the catheter. Symptoms can include chest pain, dyspnea, hypoxia, tachycardia, and hypotension. Nursing interventions to prevent air embolism may include:

- Having the patient lie flat when the system is being opened (as during tubing change)
- Having the patient perform the Valsalva maneuver when the system is being opened (as during tubing change)
- Being sure all connectors in the system are air tight
- Placing the patient in the supine position for catheter removal

Pneumothorax. *Pneumothorax* (accumulation of air or gas in the pleural cavity of the lung) occurs in approximately 5 percent of patients whose central catheters are inserted by the direct subclavian approach; symptoms may include pain on respiration, dyspnea, and diminished breath sounds over the involved side (Richardson and Bruso, 1993). Clinical indicators of hemothorax are essentially the same as those for pneumothorax except the initial signs are usually dyspnea and tachycardia instead of pain (Richardson and Bruso, 1993).

Procedures

Nursing actions related to nutrition and fluid administration include the following procedures:

- Measuring intake and output (Procedure 22–1)
- Assisting a patient with oral feeding (Procedure 22–2)
- Inserting a nasogastric tube (Procedure 22–3)
- Administering an enteral tube feeding (Procedure 22–4)
- Changing IV tubing and adding an IV container (Procedure 22–5)
- Regulating IV flow rate on gravity infusions (Procedure 22–6)

PROCEDURE 22-1

Measuring Intake and Output

Objectives

Measure quantities and types of fluids taken in by the patient.
Measure quantities and types of fluids eliminated by the patient.
Provide a written summary of fluid intake and output for use in fluid balance assessment.

Terminology

gastric suction drainage—drainage withdrawn from the stomach by means of a large-diameter tube placed in the stomach and attached to suction.
liquids—all substances that are in a fluid state at room temperature.
oliguria—urine output less than 500 ml in 24 hours in the typical adult or less than 30 ml/hr for several consecutive hours in the adult patient.
oral fluids—fluids ingested by mouth.
parenteral fluids—fluids received by the intravenous or subcutaneous route.
surgical tube drainage—drainage from a tube placed during surgery to drain fluids from the surgical site.
wound drainage—fluid from a break in the skin or from a body cavity usually collected in a dressing or container.

Critical Elements

Before measuring intake and output, it is important to determine what routes are used for fluid intake in each patient and what routes exist for elimination of body fluids.

Intake and output should be accurately measured in order to facilitate evaluation of the patient's fluid status.

Weighing the patient daily, along with accurately measured intake and output, will assist in facilitating subsequent planning of fluid intake and maintenance of fluid balance.

Equipment

Calibrated container—small or large
Calibrated urine container
Intake and output record
Sign: "Intake and Output"

Special Considerations

Fluid intake and output must be evaluated in relation to other important observations regarding fluid balance, including vital signs, skin turgor, and daily weights.

continued on next page

PROCEDURE 22-1 (cont'd)

A reference of relevant menu items and their liquid equivalents should be posted or incorporated into the intake and output record.

Assessment of fluid intake and output is essential because disease processes and drug therapies may disturb fluid balance in a variety of ways.

Some patients are able to cooperate in the maintenance of fluid intake and output measurement whereas others may need constant assessment to maintain accuracy.

Record intake from ice chips as approximately half of the volume of the ice chips because water expands when it is frozen.

If the patient is incontinent of urine or liquid feces, attempt to estimate the volume of fluid rather than documenting "incontinent." Also describe the amount of perspiration lost in clothing and bed linen as well as the amount of drainage on wound dressings because estimates of fluid loss are helpful in planning fluid replacement.

To evaluate fluid balance status, it is frequently necessary to assess intake and output for several consecutive days to determine a pattern in fluid gains and losses.

Action	*Rationale*
1. Assemble all equipment.	1. Promotes successful task completion.
2. Prepare an "Intake and Output Record" with the patient's identification data (Fig 22–15).	2. Provides a written form for accurate record keeping.
3. Identify the patient.	3. Provides patient safety.
4. Place the "Intake and Output Record" in a prominent location in the patient's room.	4. Provides a visual reminder for the nurse.
5. Explain the procedure for measuring intake and output to the patient.	5. Promotes patient compliance and accuracy of measurement.
6. Provide graduated collection devices in the patient's room for intake and output.	6. Provides nurse with accurate measurement devices.
7. Measure all fluids gained or lost in the appropriate graduated container.	7. Prevents inaccurate measurement of small amounts of fluids.

Documentation

Document all fluid volume gained and lost on the Intake and Output Record.

Documentation may be hourly or at the end of each shift depending on the condition of the patient. In addition to actual fluid volumes, it is important to record types of fluids because some require different fluid replacement than others.

Elements of Patient Teaching

Instruct the patient and family regarding the importance of accurate measurement of all fluids. Demonstrate measuring techniques and which graduated containers to use.

Instruct the patient or family to either record the fluid information or to notify the nurse so an entry can be made on the intake and output record.

continued on next page

PROCEDURE 22-1 (cont'd)

Intake and Output Documentation Form

BED | DATE

	INTAKE			OUTPUT					
	TIME	PO/NG	AMOUNT	TIME	URINE	STOOL	EMESIS/GASTRIC	OTHER	OTHER
N									
I									
G									
H									
T									
	NIGHT TOTAL ▶			NIGHT TOTAL					
D									
A									
Y									
	DAY TOTAL ▶			DAY TOTAL					
E									
V									
E									
N									
I									
N									
G									
	EVENING TOTAL ▶			EVENING TOTAL					

Figure 22–15. Sample intake and output record form.

PROCEDURE 22-2

Assisting with Oral Feeding

Objectives

Provide an environment conducive to eating.

Provide suitable nutrients that are acceptable to the patient.

Assist the patient in overcoming disabilities that make eating difficult.

Terminology

dysphagia—difficulty swallowing.

tracheal aspiration—accidental introduction of food or fluids into the trachea during swallowing.

Critical Elements

Determine the amount of assistance that the patient will need at meal time. Factors to consider include level of consciousness and physical impediments to self-feeding.

Whenever possible, patients should eat in an upright position. If the patient cannot sit, a lateral position is preferred over a supine position.

Patients who have difficulty handling objects or have poor vision should never be given hot foods or liquids to prevent potential burn incidents.

The greatest risk to oral intake for the patient with dysphagia is the potential for tracheal aspiration of food and fluids. The extent of the problem should be assessed before initiating feeding.

Equipment

Diet tray, as ordered

Special feeding equipment if necessary (Fig. 22–16)

Suction (if dysphagia is a problem)

Oral hygiene equipment

Towel and washcloth

Special Considerations

For special dietary problems, the dietitian should be consulted for nutritional counseling.

Assess the patient's food preferences including cultural and religious factors. Allow food choices when possible.

Patients should be encouraged to feed themselves whenever possible. The patient's family should be encouraged to participate in assisting patients who are dependent or confused.

Treatments such as deep breathing and coughing should be avoided just before or after meals when possible.

Foods should be served at the proper temperature so arrangements should be made to feed patients requiring assistance when the food arrives.

If the patient wears dentures, be sure they are in place before serving the meal.

Provide comfort measures as needed before meals, such as assisting with urination or defecation or providing pain medication.

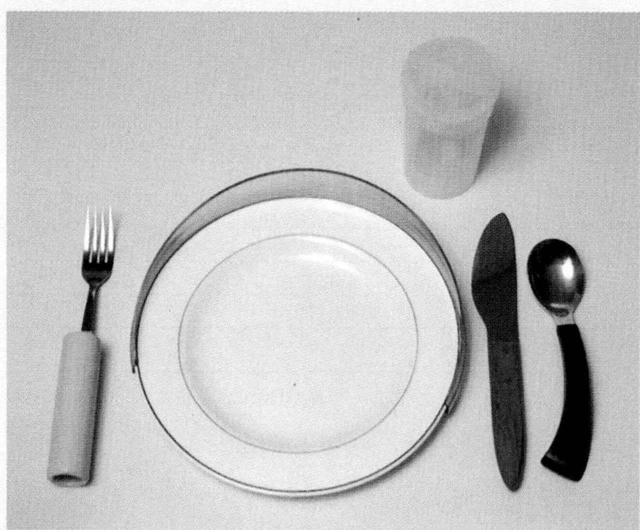

Figure 22–16. Eating aids for patients with disabilities.

continued on next page

PROCEDURE 22-2 (cont'd)

Action	*Rationale*
1. Prepare the environment and the patient for meal time by providing an uncluttered eating area and assisting with oral hygiene and handwashing.	1. Promotes appetite and nutritional intake.
2. Assist the patient to an upright position or into a chair.	2. The sitting position facilitates swallowing.
3. Verify that the tray is the correct diet for the patient.	3. Promotes patient safety.
4. Place the tray within easy reach of the patient.	4. Promotes patient compliance with eating.
5. Remove food protectors and prepare the food as necessary, including cutting food, opening containers, and pouring liquids.	5. Provides easy access to food and liquids.
6. Protect the patient's chest and lap with a napkin or towel.	6. Provides protection for clothing and improves self-esteem.
7. Assist the patient with feeding, allowing for rest periods as necessary. Allow patient to choose the order and type of foods.	7. Promotes a pleasant eating experience with minimal discomfort to the patient.
8. Remove the tray and note portions of food eaten and fluid intake.	8. Provides documentation of intake for caregivers.
9. Assist the patient with oral care and repositioning after the meal.	9. Promotes patient comfort.

Documentation

Record dietary intake including amount of food and fluids and an assessment of the patient's ability to eat. Describe on the nursing care plan measures required to promote eating.

Elements of Patient Teaching

Instruct patient and family regarding special eating devices if needed. If dysphagia is a problem, teach the patient the importance of neck flexion while tilting the body forward as a method of minimizing aspiration of food and fluid.

PROCEDURE 22-3

Inserting and Removing a Nasogastric/Nasoenteric Tube

Objective

Provides a route for administering nutrients, fluid and/or medication. Provides a means for applying suction to remove air and/or fluid from the gastrointestinal tract.

Terminology

nasoenteric (duodenal/jejunal) tube—a tube that is passed through the nose, the pharynx, down the esophagus, through the stomach into the first few inches of the small intestines.

nasogastric tube—a tube that is passed through the nose, the pharynx, down the esophagus to the stomach.

Critical Elements

Never force a nasogastric or nasoenteric tube during the placement process. Slight pressure may be necessary when passing the tube through the back of the nose to the nasopharynx but never force the tube. If unable to pass the tube through one naris, then remove the tube and use the other naris.

The type of tube used should be chosen based on the physician order, purpose for the tube, and size of the patient. As a rule, the larger bore (>14 French) nasogastric tubes are used for suction purposes.

continued on next page

PROCEDURE 22-3 (cont'd)

Suction tubes may have a second small tube built into the tube that functions as a vent. This helps prevent the tip of the tube from adhering to the side of the gastrointestinal tract and possibly causing damage during the suctioning process. Tubes that do not have this feature are usually used only with intermittent suction.

Smaller-bore tubes are usually used for the administration of nutrients, fluid, and medication. Certain of these smaller tubes come with a weighted tip and a stylette in place that assist in the placement of the tube. Mercury-weighted tubes for intestinal insertion are placed by the physician. Tubes with weighted tips are used for nasoenteric/duodenal use. The weighted tip helps the tube pass through the pyloric valve into the small intestines. The tubes usually have the stylette wires left in the tube until placement is verified by radiologic examination. Once this is done, the stylette wire is removed before using the tube. The stylette wire should not be reintroduced into the tube while the tube is in place (unless done by a physician under fluoroscopic examination). An attempt to reintroduce the stylette with the tube in place may result in the stylette wire puncturing the side of the tube, resulting in injury to the patient. Small-bore tubes are also used for patients who are at higher risk of aspiration.

No nasogastric or nasoenteric tube should be used until placement is verified. *Always check your facility's policy for tube use and tube placement before beginning the procedure.* Tube placement may be verified by:

1. Aspiration of gastric secretions. This may not be effective because the tip of the tube may be against the wall of the stomach, therefore preventing aspiration of contents.
2. Injecting air into the tube while listening over the stomach with a stethoscope. A "whooshing" sound will be heard. This may not be effective because the whooshing sound may also be heard if the tube is in the lower half of the esophagus or in the duodenal area of the small intestines.
3. Checking the pH of fluid aspirated from the tube. The gastric pH is usually between 2 and 3 (but may be as high as 6). This may be altered by pH-altering medications. Intestinal fluid is usually 7.5 to 8, whereas pleural fluid is approximately 7.4. Because both pleural fluid and intestinal fluid are close in pH this is not a good test for a nasoenteric tube.
4. Checking for choking or coughing. This may be a good test with the large-bore tubes. These symptoms are usually present if the tube is in the trachea. However, this may not be a symptom if a small-bore tube is in the trachea or if the patient has decreased or no tracheal irritation reflex.
5. Having the patient speak or hum. This may not be possible if the tube is in the trachea but is not always a reliable indicator if a small-bore tube is used.

Equipment

- Nasogastric or nasoenteric tube
- Gloves
- Water-soluble lubricant
- Glass of water and straw
- Tissue
- Safety pin
- Tube plug (if indicated)
- Stethoscope
- Towel
- Emesis basin
- 30- to 50-ml syringe or irrigation set
- pH paper
- Tongue blade
- Flashlight
- Tape
- Plastic bag (for removal)

Special Considerations

This procedure may be unpleasant for the patient due to the gag reflex. There may also be psychosocial issues raised by the fact that the patient cannot eat during the time the tube is in place.

Frequent oral care is necessary during this time. It is also necessary to clean around the tube at the naris to prevent the buildup of secretions. The tape fastening should be checked at this time.

Before inserting the tube, the care provider should test the air flow of both nares by having the patient blow out of each side of the nose while the other side is held closed. The side having the greatest air flow should be used for insertion. It is also helpful to inspect the nares with a flashlight to check for any obvious structural abnormalities in the nasal passages that may impede passage of the tube.

Rubber tubes may be stiffened to aid in insertion by placing in an emesis basin of ice for a few minutes. Plastic tubes may be softened by placing in warm water for a few minutes before insertion.

All tubes should be measured before placement (Figs. 22–17 and 22–18). This is done by holding the tip of the tube at the tip of the nose, reaching back with the tube to the tip of the ear lobe, and continuing down to the xiphoid process. For duodenal tubes add approximately 9 inches or 23 cm to this measurement.

continued on next page

PROCEDURE 22-3 (cont'd)

The location of the tip of the tube should always be noted in the patient record. This location will influence the type of feeding and/or medications that can or will be administered. If the patient is unable to sit up for this procedure, place the patient in a right side-lying position with a slight elevation of the head.

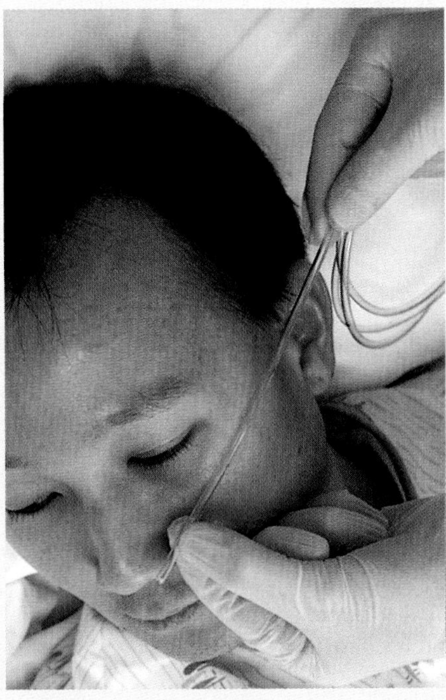

Figure 22–17. Measuring nasogastric tube from ear to nose.

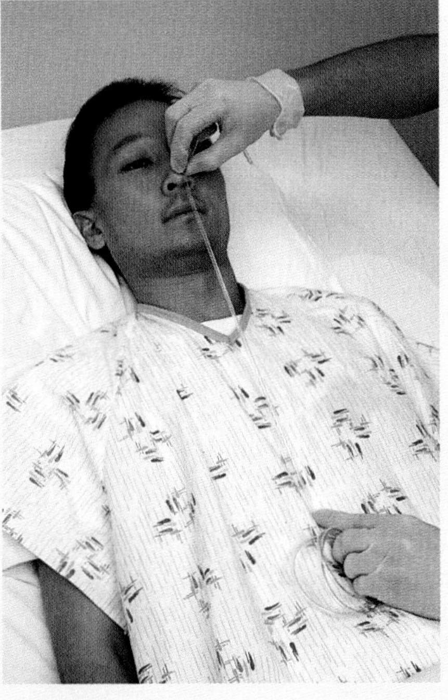

Figure 22–18. Measuring nasogastric tube from nose to sternum.

Action	*Rationale*
Tube Insertion:	
1. Verify order.	1. Ensures correct procedure.
2. Assemble supplies	2. Promotes good task organization.
3. Identify patient.	3. Provides patient safety.
4. Explain procedure to patient.	4. Promotes patient compliance.
5. Assist patient to Fowler's position and put towel across patient's upper chest.	5. Reduces risk of aspiration, positions patient for optimal swallowing effort, and allows gravity to assist with insertion procedure.
6. Cut 3-inch length of tape and secure within easy reach.	6. Prepares for point when tube must be secured, therefore avoiding displacement.
7. Measure tube length and note that point on length of tube with tape or by identification of tube markings.	7. Provides guideline for amount of tube to be inserted.
8. Don gloves.	8. Protects care provider from contact with blood or body fluids and prevents transmission of microorganisms from one patient to another.

continued on next page

PROCEDURE 22-3 (cont'd)

9. Lubricate tube with water-soluble lubricant or dip tip of prelubricated tube in water (according to manufacturer's directions). *Do not* use petroleum-based lubricant products.	9. Enables smoother passage of tube and use of water-soluble lubricant is safer if tube accidentally is placed in trachea.
10. Note natural curvature of tube and insert tube through appropriate naris with curve downward.	10. Facilitates passage of tube in conjunction with nasopharyngeal anatomy.
11. Have patient tilt head forward and take sips of water as tube is passed through back of pharynx.	11. Facilitates glottis closure while tube is passed over this area.
12. If persistent gagging occurs, check back of mouth with flashlight. Also note if patient has difficulty breathing or severe coughing.	12. Provides means to note if tube is being curled in back of pharynx or slips into trachea so it may be removed and insertion process restarted.
13. Wrap around tube and secure to nose after advancement of tube to proper point is achieved. Additional tape can be placed several inches from nose and tube may be pinned to patient's gown.	13. Ensures that tube stays in proper position and prevents accidental removal.
14. After tube placement is verified: Plug tube or hook up to suction or feeding as indicated.	14. Promotes safety by verifying location of tube before use.
15. Return or discard equipment in appropriate place.	15. Ensures clean, organized work area.
Tube Removal:	
1. Verify order.	1. Ensures correct procedure is done.
2. Identify patient.	2. Provides patient safety.
3. Assemble equipment.	3. Promotes task organization.
4. Don gloves.	4. Protects care provider from contact with blood or body fluids and prevents transmission of microorganisms from one patient to another.
5. Disconnect tube from suction or feeding, remove safety pin, and remove tape from patient's nose.	5. Prepares tube for removal.
6. Instill 30 to 50 ml of air into tube (optional).	6. Removes all liquids from tube to lessen potential for tracheal aspiration during removal process.
7. Have patient take deep breath and hold it; then pull tube quickly and smoothly from nose.	7. Closes glottis to protect trachea.
8. Place tube into plastic bag after checking whether tube is intact.	8. Prevents contamination from microorganisms on tube and ensures whole tube has been removed.
9. Give patient tissue to wipe nose, offer oral care, and return to position of comfort.	9. Promotes patient hygiene and comfort.
10. Return or discard equipment in appropriate receptacle.	10. Ensures clean, organized work area.

Documentation

Record in the patient record the time of the procedure, type of tube used, and placement location. Note how tube placement was verified as well as a description and amount of any fluid aspirated. Note on the patient's Intake and Output Record amount of fluid removed. Record the assessment of the patient's abdomen at the time of placement and the patient's response to the procedure.

Elements of Patient Teaching

Instruct the patient and family members regarding the purpose of this procedure. Inform them of eating/drinking restrictions during the time the tube is in place. The need for frequent oral care should also be stressed. If the patient or family members will be administering nutrients/fluid or medication through the tube they will need careful instruction along with a time to perform a return-demonstration so the care provider can evaluate their ability to perform the procedure safely.

PROCEDURE 22-4

Administering an Enteral Feeding

Objective

Provide intermittent or continuous fluid and nutrition into the stomach or small intestines.

Terminology

closed feeding system—feeding container with formula added by the manufacturer.

continuous feeding—feeding administered at a slow and steady rate over a 24-hour period.

intermittent or bolus feeding—feeding given at intermittent times over a relatively short period of time.

open feeding system—feeding container and tubing that is opened for the purpose of adding tube-feeding formula.

residual volume—amount of fluid remaining in the stomach after the time when most of the feeding should have emptied into the small intestines.

Critical Elements

Before starting this procedure, refer to your facility's policy regarding the length of time formulas may be stored and how many hours of formula may be hung at one time.

Patients with enteral feeding should have abdominal assessments, including the presence of abdominal distention, quality of bowel sounds, and complaints of discomfort, completed at least every 8 hours or as the patient's condition requires.

The physician will prescribe the nutritional formula to be used, the rate and frequency of the feedings, any laboratory tests, and amount of water to be administered to the patient. The formula used will be based on the nutrients necessary to maintain the appropriate body weight and fluid and electrolyte balance. Commercial formulas or blended products made by your facility may be used.

The care provider should always assess the contents of the formula for any food allergies that the patient may have. The expiration date of the product should also be noted. Most formulas (both commercial and blended) must be discarded after 24 hours.

Formulas are usually administered at room temperature unless otherwise ordered. If needed, a bag of ice may be hung surrounding the feeding container to keep the formula cool. It is also advisable to hang only a few hours (usually 4 hours) of formula at a time.

Feeding pumps are often used for continuous feeding or for those that must instill at a slow rate. Some of these pumps have an automatic water flush as one of the features. The nurse should calculate how much free water will be delivered in this manner and verify with the physician if this feature is to be used. When using a feeding container, be sure to flush the tubing before attaching it to the nasogastric or nasoenteric tube so no air is forced into the patient with the feedings.

Equipment

- Feeding solution
- 30- to 50-ml syringe
- Emesis basin
- Feeding bag/container (if indicated)
- Prefilled bottle (if indicated)
- Towel
- Water
- Feeding pump (if indicated)

Special Considerations

Placement location (intestinal or gastric) of the tube should always be noted because since this may influence what medications and what formulas are used.

Patients receiving enteral feeding are at risk for aspiration and should be placed with the head of the bed elevated at least 30° during and for 45 to 60 minutes after intermittent feedings and at all times for patients with continuous feedings. If this position is contraindicated by the patient's condition, place the patient in the right side-lying position with the head slightly elevated.

Intermittent feedings should not be administered too quickly and should be given over 15 to 30 minutes (depending on the amount). If administered too quickly, the patient may experience flatus, cramping pains, or reflux vomiting.

Before intermittent feedings and at regular intervals during continuous feedings, the care provider should assess for residual volume in the stomach. Refer to your facility's policy on how much residual volume constitutes a need to hold the feeding or reduce the rate and whether the residual amount removed should be reinstilled. These decisions will also be influenced by physician order.

All equipment used should be cleaned after each use and changed every 24 hours. Food coloring is sometimes added to the feeding to ascertain whether aspiration of gastric contents is occurring. If tracheal suctioning shows the presence of the food coloring, aspiration should be considered and should be reported to the physician immediately.

continued on next page

PROCEDURE 22-4 (cont'd)

Action	*Rationale*
1. Verify order.	1. Ensures correct procedure is done.
2. Assemble equipment.	2. Promotes task organization.
3. Identify patient.	3. Provides patient safety.
4. Explain procedure.	4. Promotes patient compliance.
5. Place patient in Fowler's position (or if contraindicated may use right side-lying position with head slightly elevated).	5. Reduces risk of aspiration.
6. Place a towel under area where end of tube will be opened.	6. Protects patient and linens from accidental spill/drips.
7. Assess tube placement (refer to Procedure 22–3: Inserting and Removing a Nasogastric/Nasoenteric Tube)	7. Ensures tube in proper placement before instilling feeding.
8. Assess for residual volume by aspirating gastric contents.	8. Enables evaluation of how gastric contents are emptying.

Bolus Feeding:

1. Remove plug from end of tube and attach syringe or feeding bag (Figs. 22–19 and 22–20), crimping tubing just below tip.	1. Prepares equipment for feeding procedure while keeping air from entering system.
2. Add feeding to syringe or container if not using closed feeding system.	2. Places formula in container for administration.

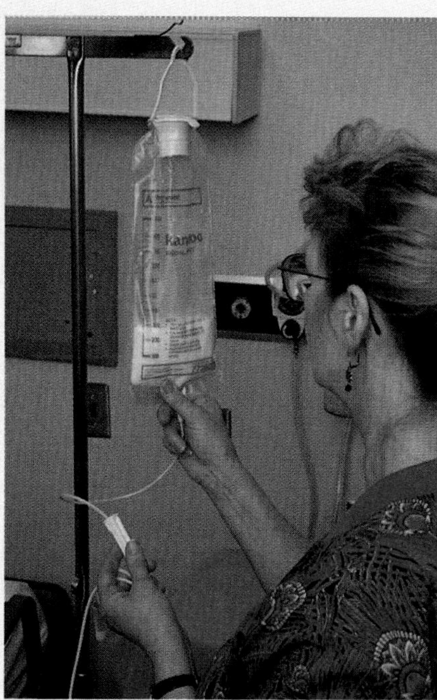

Figure 22–19. Attaching feeding bag tubing to nasogastric tube.

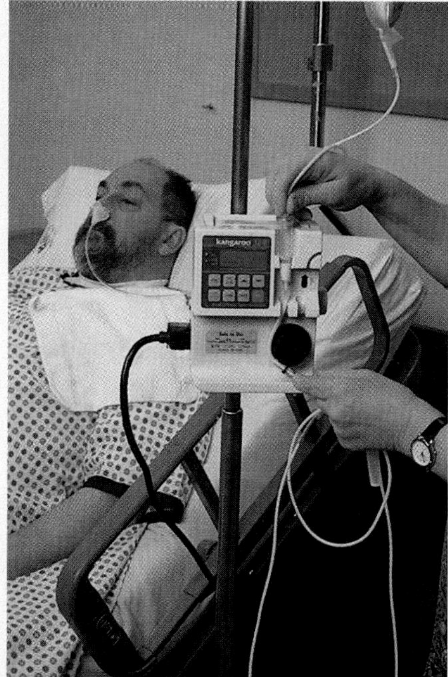

Figure 22–20. Attaching gavage tubing to infusion pump.

continued on next page

PROCEDURE 22-4 (cont'd)

3. Elevate syringe or container 12 to 18 inches above patient and allow fluid to start to flow, refilling syringe or container as necessary. Rate may be adjusted by crimping tube below syringe or by roller clamp on container tubing.	3. Provides height where fluid will flow at slow steady rate.
4. After feeding is completed, flush line with 30 to 50 ml of water.	4. Prevents buildup of formula in tube, which may cause tube to occlude.
5. Return patient to position of comfort.	5. Promotes patient comfort.
6. Clean and *return* or *discard* equipment to appropriate place.	6. Promotes clean, organized work area.

Continuous Feedings:

1. Hang container and attach to nasogastric or nasoenteric tube.	1. Prepares container for feeding administration.
2. If infusion pump (Fig. 22–21) is in use, attach container to pump and program pump according to manufacturer's instructions and physician order.	2. Provides means to administer slow, steady feeding.
3. Add formula to container and regulate flow with roller clamp or pump rate.	3. Provides formula for feeding at proper rate.
4. Monitor patient and assess tolerance of feeding by assessment and checking residual volume (refer to your facility's policy).	4. Evaluates patient's tolerance of enteral feeding.
5. Refill container as indicated and change container every 24 hours.	5. Provides for continuous administration of feeding.

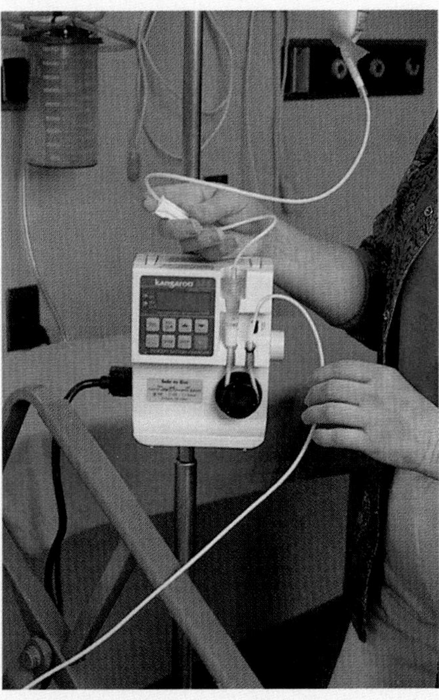

Figure 22–21. Infusion pump.

continued on next page

PROCEDURE 22-4 (cont'd)

Documentation

Record in the patient record the time of feeding, amount given, type of formula, residual volume (if any), and patient tolerance. The assessment of the patient's abdomen should also be recorded. All intake should also be noted on the patient's Intake and Output Record.

Elements of Patient Teaching

Instruct the patient or family members regarding the purpose for administering nutrition by the enteral method. Also instruct the patient to report any nausea, vomiting, abdominal distention, cramping, or diarrhea immediately. If the patient or family members will be administering the feedings, they should be instructed and provided with a time for a return-demonstration so the care provider can evaluate whether they can safely perform the procedure.

PROCEDURE 22-5

Changing IV Tubing and Adding an IV Container

Objective

Provide a means to change IV tubing or add a container while maintaining sterile technique and line function.

Terminology

air embolism—air allowed entry into the circulatory system that travels and may cause cardiovascular complications and/or death.

catheter embolism—portion of IV catheter inadvertently damaged, broken off, and allowed to enter the circulatory system.

central vein—a large vein in the trunk of the body such as the subclavian vein

infiltration—escape of fluid intended for IV delivery into the surrounding tissues, which usually occurs from dislodgement of needle or catheter from the vein.

infusion container port—access site on container that allows connection of IV tubing.

infusion set—plastic drip chamber, tubing, and a spike connector, made to attach to the IV container, as well as an elongated adaptor to attach to the venipuncture device (needle or plastic catheter).

peripheral vein—a vein in the hand or arm that is readily visible and can be entered with a short needle or catheter.

phlebitis—inflammation of a vein that is manifested by redness and swelling at the site of venipuncture or along the path of the vein.

Critical Elements

Before initiating a tubing or container change, refer to your facility's policy of frequency of tubing change and how long any one IV container may be allowed to hang. Most facilities will not allow a container to hang longer than 24 hours, making replacement necessary whether it is empty or not.

It is extremely important to maintain sterility throughout the tubing and IV container change procedure. It is also important to prevent air from entering the circulatory system during this procedure because an air embolism may result. This is more of a risk with a central line than with a peripheral line.

The care provider should also assess any allergy to latex as well as clarifying whether the tubing being used has any latex components. This is very important because a latex allergy reaction can be very severe and may result in death.

The drop factor should also be noted so that the correct drops per minute can be calculated. If the tubing has needless ports, the care provider should choose equipment accordingly.

Each time the tubing is changed, the IV site should be assessed. If signs of phlebitis are noted in a peripheral vein, the site should be changed. In addition, central vein sites should be assessed for any signs of site infection and, if present, should be reported to the physician.

If the infusion is a gravity infusion, the IV container should be marked with tape or commercial IV container

continued on next page

PROCEDURE 22-5 (cont'd)

measuring tape to provide a reference point of accuracy of IV infusion rate. All IV intake should be recorded on the appropriate portion of the patient record.

If the IV container is soft vinyl/plastic, the tubing does not need to be vented to allow the contents to infuse. However, if the container is hard plastic or glass, the tubing must be vented to allow the contents to infuse. Many tubings have the option of being vented by opening a vent cap.

Equipment

IV infusion set
IV infusion container
Tape
Bandages
Sterile 2 × 2-inch gauze pads
Gloves

Special Considerations

Because this procedure may expose the care provider to blood/body fluids, all necessary universal blood and body fluid (UBBF) precautions should be used. All used equipment from this procedure should be disposed of using UBBF precautions.

When changing the tubing on a central vein site (Fig. 22–22), it is preferable to have the patient lie flat, as well as using any slide clamp closures on the central line itself, to minimize the risk of air embolism.

Whenever caring for a patient receiving IV fluids, frequent assessments should be made of potential fluid imbalance such as presence of edema, abnormal lung sounds, or inadequate or excessive urine output.

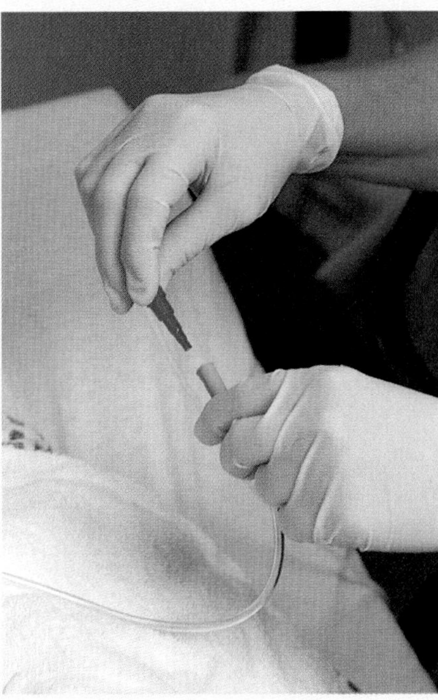

Figure 22–22. Changing IV tubing on vein cannula.

Action	*Rationale*
1. Verify order (if hanging new container).	1. Ensures correct procedure is done.
2. Assemble equipment.	2. Promotes task organization.
3. Identify patient.	3. Provides patient safety.
4. Explain procedure.	4. Promotes patient compliance.
5. Position patient to expose site.	5. Allows access to site for procedure.

continued on next page

PROCEDURE 22-5 (cont'd)

Changing Tubing and Container:

1. Attach tubing to container.

   1. Provides means to change both tubing and container at one time.

2. Fill drip chamber on tubing with appropriate amount (usually about half full); flush tubing and close roller clamp. Hang container on IV pole.

   2. Protects patient from air embolism by purging air from line.

3. Cut lengths of tape necessary to secure line when done and have within easy reach.

   3. Facilitates securing tubing at end of procedure.

4. Don gloves.

   4. Protects care provider from contact with blood and body fluids.

5. Close roller clamp on tubing currently in use.

   5. Prevents free flow of fluid when tubing is disconnected.

6. Loosen tape around tubing, taking care not to loosen actual needle/catheter at site and slip a 2 × 2-inch gauze pad under point where tubing connects to needle/catheter.

   6. Prepares tubing for removal.

7. Holding new tubing in your nondominant hand, remove protective covering over end of tubing, taking care to maintain sterility of tubing end. Place tubing between fingers of nondominant hand.

   7. Prepares tubing for attachment to needle/catheter.

8. Using dominant hand, remove old tubing from needle/catheter while stabilizing needle/catheter to prevent dislodgement from vein.

   8. Removes old tubing and prepares for attachment of new tubing.

9. Quickly take new tubing and attach to needle/catheter, then open roller clamp.

   9. Attaches new tubing to needle/catheter and allows any blood that may have collected in needle/catheter during this time to be flushed out before it can clot.

10. Secure new tubing with tape.

    10. Ensures stability of intravenous site (Fig. 22–23).

11. Dispose or return supplies to appropriate place.

    11. Promotes clean, organized work area.

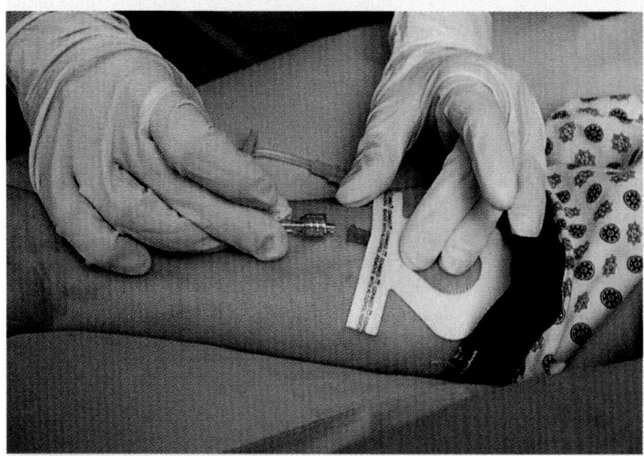

Figure 22–23. Peripheral line with dressing in place.

continued on next page

PROCEDURE 22-5 (cont'd)

Changing Container Only:

1. Close roller clamp on tubing.	1. Prevents free flow of fluid or air entering line during changing process.
2. Hang new container on IV pole.	2. Places container within reach in preparation for change procedure.
3. Remove port covering on container taking care to maintain sterility of port.	3. Readies port for spiking with tubing spike.
4. Remove tubing spike from old container and spike it into new container.	4. Removes old container from tubing and connects new tubing.
5. Open roller clamp and adjust rate.	5. Reestablishes correct flow rate for IV fluid.
6. Dispose of old container in appropriate receptacle.	6. Provides clean, organized work area.

Documentation

Record in the patient record the time of the procedure and the patient response. Note the assessment of the IV site as well as any pertinent assessment regarding the patient's fluid balance state. Note the IV intake on the patient Intake and Output Record.

Elements of Patient Teaching

Instruct the patient and family members regarding the purpose of the procedure and to immediately report any pain or swelling at the IV site or any other problems with IV infusion.

PROCEDURE 22-6

Regulating IV Flow Rate on Gravity Infusion

Objective

Infuse IV fluids at the prescribed, appropriate rate.

Terminology

gravity flow—allowing IV fluid to flow under the force of gravity into the circulatory system via IV tubing.

gravity rate controller—a device made for the purpose of adding to the infusion set, usually close to the IV needle/catheter, that provides adjusted control over the rate of the fluid.

infusion pump—a mechanical device (see Fig. 22–21) that applies positive pressure to the IV tubing to deliver fluid into the patient's circulatory system.

macrodrip—an IV infusion set that consists of tubing and drip chamber that provides a drop size of 10 to 15 drops/ml.

microdrip—an IV infusion set that consists of tubing and a drip chamber that provides a drop size of approximately 60 drops/ml.

roller/slide clamp—a device on IV infusion set used to control the flow of fluid through the tubing by compressing the tubing as it is rolled/slid back and forth (Figs. 22–24 and 22–25).

Critical Elements

The rate of flow of the IV fluid is prescribed by the physician. The care provider must know the drop factor of the tubing being used and should calculate the drops per minute before starting the procedure. Before choosing either macrodrip or microdrip IV tubing, the care provider should evaluate the type of fluid including its contents, prescribed rate, and patient condition. Microdrip tubing is often used for pediatric patients as well as medications where small amounts of fluid and rigid control are indicated.

The care provider should also evaluate whether the fluid should be delivered by gravity or by an infusion pump. In some instances, infusion pump use is often dictated by institutional policy; therefore, the facility's policy should be consulted before proceeding. In some in-

continued on next page

PROCEDURE 22-6 (cont'd)

stances, an infusion pump is clearly indicated because of the IV needs of the patient (such as a very slow rate, a positional IV line, or a hemodynamically compromised patient). Whenever using an infusion pump, the care provider should review the manufacturer's directions before use.

Gravity rate controllers, although less accurate than an infusion pump, may be added to an IV infusion line as a cost-containment measure for noncritical situations. Consult your facility's policy before using this device. Taping and marking the side of the IV container will help the care provider establish whether the infusion is going at the correct rate. Plain tape with handwritten markings or commercially made stick-on tapes may be used. All gravity intravenous fluid infusions should be assessed frequently by the care provider to make sure they are running at the prescribed rate. If the fluid should infuse too quickly or too slowly there is danger of fluid and electrolyte imbalance.

The care provider should also be aware of the contents of the IV fluid in relation to any allergies the patient may have. The care provider should assess for any patient allergy to latex as well as clarifying whether the tubing being used has any latex components. This is very important because a latex allergy reaction can be very severe and may result in death.

All IV fluid should be recorded on the patient's Intake and Output Record.

Equipment

- IV infusion set
- Infusion pump (if indicated)
- Gravity rate controller (if indicated)
- Paper/pencil (if drop calculations are needed)

Special Considerations

Whenever working with a patient receiving IV fluids frequent assessments should be made of potential fluid imbalance such as presence of edema, abnormal lung sounds, or inadequate or excessive urine output.

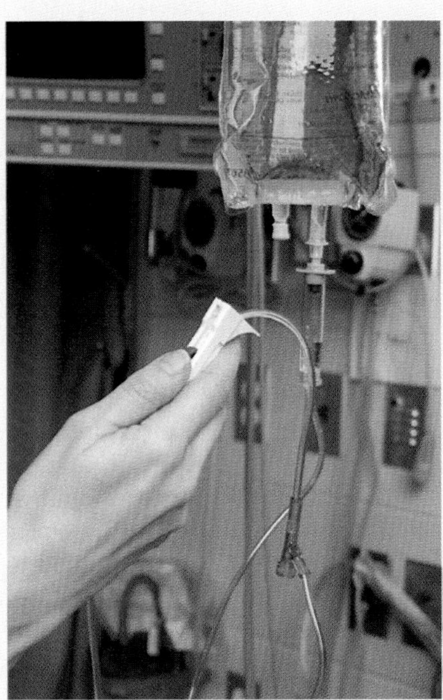

Figure 22–24. Adjusting roller clamp.

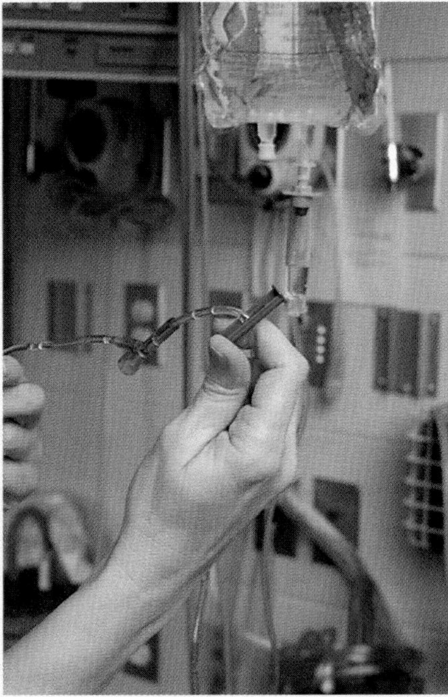

Figure 22–25. Adjusting slide clamp.

continued on next page

PROCEDURE 22-6 (cont'd)

Action	*Rationale*
1. Verify order.	1. Ensures correct procedure is done.
2. Calculate IV drop rate.	2. Provides correct drop rate is available for regulation of fluid flow.
3. Identify patient.	3. Provides patient safety.
4. Explain procedure.	4. Promotes patient compliance.
5. Adjust roller clamp while counting drops per minute until correct count is reached *or* set infusion rate on an infusion pump or gravity rate controller.	5. Ensures fluid infuses at prescribed rate.
6. Assess rate of flow at least every hour.	6. Ensure fluid continues to infuse at prescribed rate.

Documentation

Record on the patient record the time the IV fluid is initiated, the type of IV fluid, the volume of fluid, and the rate of flow of the IV fluid. Record the amount of fluid infused on the patient's Intake and Output Record. The assessment of the patient's fluid status as well as any pertinent assessment observations of the IV site should also be recorded. The IV rate and fluid are also noted on the patient's medication administration record in most health care settings.

Elements of Patient Teaching

Instruct the patient and family members regarding the purpose of the procedure and to report immediately any pain or swelling at the IV site or any other problems with the IV infusion.

CHAPTER HIGHLIGHTS

- Adequate fluid and nutrients, either by mouth, feeding tube, or through the IV route, need to be provided to every patient.
- Determining indicators of inadequate nutrition, fluid and electrolyte imbalance, and monitoring fluid and nutrition intake are essential aspects to be included in nursing care.
- Providing adequate nutrition to patients is a team effort including physicians, dietitians, nutritionists, and health educators.
- Proper nutrition is required for normal growth, reproduction, and maintenance of life processes, normal organ development and function, and resisting and recovering from infections, disease, and body injuries.
- There is a steady growth in the body of knowledge relating to functioning of the gastrointestinal system, nutrition, and diet therapy.
- Metabolism comprises all the physical and chemical processes of cellular nutrition. Metabolism is a chemical engine.
- Foods provide three basic classes of essential nutrition: carbohydrates, proteins, and fats. Digestion reduces the nutrients to sugars, amino acids, fatty acids, and glycerol.
- Water is essential for all metabolic activities. Patients must be provided with adequate fluid intake to maintain body processes.
- Recommendations for prudent diets have been made by several national health organizations.
- Nursing care of all patients, regardless of the setting, requires attention to adequate dietary and fluid intake. Nutritional needs include attention to the patient's age, individual food habits, cultural and religious influences, and socioeconomic status.

REFERENCES

Adams, F. (1988). How much do elders drink? *Geriatric Nursing, 8,* 218–220.

Akerlund, B., Norberg, A. (1985). An ethical analysis of double blind conflicts as experienced by care workers feeding severely demented patients. *International Journal of Nursing Studies, 22*(3), 207–216.

Alpers, D., Stenson, W., Bier, D. (1995). *Manual of Nutritional Therapeutics,* 3rd ed. Boston: Little, Brown & Co.

American Dietetic Association. *Cost Effectiveness of Nutritional Support.* Report to Congress, 1986.

Anderson, K., Norris, D., Godfrey, B., et al. (1984). Bacterial contamination of tube-feeding formulas. *Journal of Parenteral and Enteral Nutrition, 8,* 673–678.

Ashton, J., Gibson, V., Summer, S. (1990). Effect of heparin versus saline solution on intermittent infusion device irrigation. *Heart Lung, 19,* 608–612.

Bennet, J., Brachman, P. (eds.). (1992). *Hospital Infections.* Boston: Little, Brown, & Co., pp. 850–852, 855–858.

Bivens, B., Rapp, R., Powers, P., et al. (1980). Electronic flow control and roller clamp control in intravenous therapy. *Archives of Surgery, 115,* 70–72.

Blackburn, G., Maini, B., Bistrian, B., et al. (1976). Cyclic hyperalimentation—an optimal technique for preservation of visceral protein mass. *Acta Chirurgica Scandinavica* Supplementum, *466,* 50–1.

Bohony, J. (1993). Nine common IV complications and what to do about them. *American Journal of Nursing, 93*(10), 45–49.

Bowman, M., Eisenberg, P., Katz, B., Metheny, N. (1989). Sodium imbalances in tube-fed patients. *Critical Care Nurse, 9*(1), 22–28.

Breach, C., Saldanha, L. (1988). Tube feedings—a survey of compliance to procedures and complications. *Nutrition in Clinical Practice, 3,* 230–234.

Brinson, R., Kolts, B. (1987). Hypoalbuminemia as an indicator of diarrheal incidence in critically ill patients. *Critical Care Medicine, 15,* 506–509.

Capron, A. (1991). The implications of the Cruzan decision for clinical nutrition teams. *Nutrition in Clinical Practice, 6*(3), 89–94.

Chernoff, R. (1990). Physiologic aging and nutritional status. *Nutrition in Clinical Practice, 5*(1), 8–13.

Chernoff, R., Lipshitz, D. (1990). Enteral feeding and the geriatric patient. In J. Rombeau and M. Caldwell (eds.): *Clinical Nutrition: Enteral and Tube Feeding,* 2nd ed. Philadelphia: W.B. Saunders.

Ciocon, J., Silverstone F., Graver, L., Foley, C. (1988). Tube feedings in elderly patients: Indications, benefits, and complications. *Archives of Internal Medicine, 148,* 429–433.

Coben, R., Weintraub, A., Marino, A., Cohen, S. (1994). Gastroesophageal reflux during gastrostomy feeding. *Gastroenterology, 106,* 13–18.

Consensus Report on the Ethics of Foregoing Life-Sustaining Treatments in the Critically Ill. (1990). Task force on ethics of the Society of Critical Care Medicine. *Critical Care Medicine,* 18, 1435–1439.

Coward, D. (1988). Hypercalcemia knowledge assessment in patients at-risk of developing cancer-induced hypercalcemia. *Oncology Nursing Forum, 15*(4), 471–476.

Detsky, A., Smalley, P., Change, J. (1994). Is this patient malnourished? *Journal of the American Medical Association, 27* (1), 54–58.

Don, B., Sebastian, A., Cheitlin, M., et al. (1990). Pseudohyperkalemia caused by fist clenching during phlebotomy. *New England Journal of Medicine, 322,* 1290–1292.

Dougherty, D., Bankhead, R., Kushner, R., et al. Nutrition care given new importance in JCAHO standards. *Nutrition in Clinical Practice, 10*(1), 26–31.

Dresser, R. (1985). When patients resist feeding: Medical, ethical and legal considerations. *Journal of American Geriatric Society, 33*(1), 790–794.

Eisenberg, P., Spies, M., Metheny, N. (1987). Characteristics of patients who remove their feeding tubes. *Clinical Nurse Specialist, 1*(3), 94–98.

Flynn, K., Norton, L., Fisher, R. (1987). Enteral tube feeding: indications, practices and outcomes. *Image, 19,* 16.

Foreman, M. (1989). Confusion in the hospitalized elderly: Incidence, onset, and associated factors. *Research in Nursing & Health, 12,* 21–29.

Gaspar, P. (1988). What determines how much elders drink? *Geriatric Nursing, 8:*221–224.

Gershan, J., Freeman, C., Ross, M., et al. (1990). Fluid volume deficit: Validating the indicators. *Heart Lung, 19,* 152–156.

Gottschlich, M., Warden, G., Michel, M., et al. (1988). Diarrhea in tube-fed patients: Incidence, etiology, nutritional impact, and prevention. *Journal of Parenteral & Enteral Nutrition, 12*(4), 338–345.

Gross, C., Lindquist, R., Woolley, A. (1992). Clinical indicators of dehydration severity in elderly patients. *Journal of Emergency Medicine, 10,* 267–274.

Guenter, P., Settle, R., Permutter, S., et al. (1991). Tube-feeding related diarrhea in acutely ill patients. *Journal of Parenteral & Enteral Nutrition,* 15(3), 277–280.

Gustke, R., Varma, R., Soergel, K. (1970). Gastric reflux during perfusion of the proximal small bowel. *Gastroenterology, 59,* 890–895.

Guyton, A. (1991). *Textbook of Medical Physiology,* 8th ed. Philadelphia: W.B. Saunders.

Haddad, A., Keefer, K., Stein, J. (1993). Teamwork in home infusion therapy: The relationship between nursing and pharmacy. *Home Healthcare Nurse, 11*(1), 40–46.

Hanson, R. (1979). Predictive criteria for length of nasogastric tube insertion for tube feeding. *Journal of Parenteral and Enteral Nutrition, 3*(3), 160–163.

Hassett, J., Sunby, C., Flint, L. (1988). No elimination of aspiration pneumonia in neurologically disabled patients with feeding gastrostomy. *Surgery, Gynecology & Obstetrics, 167,* 383–388, 1988.

Herron, D.G. (!991). Strategies for promoting a healthy dietary intake. *Nursing Clinics of North America, 26,* 875–884.

Heitkemper, M., Martin, D., Hansen, B., et al. (1981). Rate and volume of intermittent enteral feeding. *Journal of Parenteral & Enteral Nutrition, 5*(1), 125–129.

Hur, T. (1994). Survival skills: A patient teaching model for home intravenous therapy. *Ostomy/Wound Management, 40*(3), 58–67.

Ibanez, J., Penafiel, A., Raurich, J., et al. (1992). Gastroesophageal reflux in intubated patients receiving enteral nutrition: Effect of supine and semirecumbent positions. *Journal of Parenteral and Enteral Nutrition, 16,* 419–422.

Inadomi, D., Kopple, J. (1994). Fluid and electrolyte disorders in total parenteral nutrition. In Narins, R. (ed.): *Clinical Disorders of Fluid and Electrolyte Metabolism,* 5th ed. p. 1438. New York, McGraw-Hill, p 1438.

Kagawa-Busby, K., Heitkemper, M., Hansen, B., et al. (1980). Effect of diet temperature on tolerance of enteral feedings. *Nursing Research, 29*(5), 276–280.

Kaplan, D., Murphy, U., Linsheer, W. (1985). Percutaneous endoscopic jejunostomy: Long-term follow-up of 23 patients. *Gastrointestinal Endoscopy, 35,* 403–406.

Kinsey, G., Murray, M., Swensen, S. (1994). Glucose content of tracheal aspirates: Implications for the detection of tube feeding aspiration. *Critical Care Medicine, 22,* 1557–1562.

Kohn, C., Keithley, J. (1989). Enteral nutrition: Potential complications and patient monitoring. *Nursing Clinics of North America, 24,* 339–353.

Krzywda, E., et al. (1993). Glucose response to abrupt initiation and discontinuance of total parenteral nutrition. *Journal of Parenteral and Enteral Nutrition, 17*, 64–67.

Larsen, G. (1973). Conservative management for incomplete dysphagic paralytics. *Archives of Physical Medicine and Rehabilitation, 54,* 180–185.

Lickley, H. (1978). Metabolic responses to enteral and parenteral nutrition. *American Journal of Surgery,* 135, 172.

Mahon, S. (1987). Symptoms as clues to calcium levels. *American Journal of Nursing, 87,* 354–355.

Malcolm, R., Robson, J., Vanderveen, T., O'Neil, P. (1980). Psychosocial aspects of total parenteral nutrition. *Psychosomatics, 21*(2), 115–125.

Marcuard, S., Stegall, K. (1990). Unclogging feeding tubes with pancreatic enzyme. *Journal of Parenteral and Enteral Nutrition, 14*(2), 198–200.

Marcuard, S., Stegall, K., Trogdon, S. (1989). Clearing obstructed feeding tubes. *Journal of Parenteral and Enteral Nutrition, 13*(1), 81–83.

Masoorli, S. (1996). Nursing issues. *Intravenous Nursing Newsline, 17*(1), 5.

McCann, R., et al. (1994). Comfort care for terminally ill patients: The appropriate use of nutrition and hydration. *Journal of the American Medical Association, 272,* 1263–1266.

McClave, S., Snider, H., Lowen, C., et al. (1992). Use of residual volume as a marker for enteral feeding intolerance: Prospective blinded comparison with physical examination and radiographic findings. *Journal of Parenteral and Enteral Nutrition, 15,* 99–105.

Metheny, N., Dettenmeier, P., Hampton, K., et al. (1990a). Detection of inadvertent respiratory placement of small-bore feeding tubes: A report of 10 cases. *Heart Lung, 19,* 631–638.

Metheny, N., Eisenberg, P., McSweeney, M. (1988). Effect of feeding tube properties and three irrigants on clogging rates. *Nursing Research, 37*(3), 165–269.

Metheny, N., Eisenberg, P., Spies, M. (1986a). Aspiration pneumonia in patients fed through nasoenteral tubes. *Heart Lung,* 15(3), 256–261.

Metheny, N., McSweeney, M., Wiersema, L., Wehrle, M. (1990b). Predicting feeding tube placement by the auscultatory method. *Nursing Research,* 39(5), 262–267.

Metheny, N., Merritt, S., Myers, J. (1991). Testing of alteration in potassium balance: Hypo- and hyperkalemia as nursing diagnoses. *Classification of Nursing Diagnoses: Proceedings of the Ninth Conference of the North American Nursing Diagnoses Association.* Philadelphia: J.B. Lippincott, pp 294–295.

Metheny, N., Reed, L., Berglund, B., Wehrle, M. (1994). Characteristics of aspirates from feeding tubes as a method for predicting tube location. *Nursing Research, 43*(5), 282–287.

Metheny, N., Reed, L., Wiersema, L., et al. (1993a). Effectiveness of pH measurements in predicting feeding tube placement: An update. *Nursing Research, 42*(6), 324–331.

Metheny, N., Reed, L., Worseck, M., Clark, J. (1993b). Aspiration of fluid from small-bore feeding tubes. *American Journal of Nursing, 93*(5), 86–88.

Metheny, N., Spies, M., Eisenberg, P. (1986b). Frequency of nasoenteral tube displacement and associated risk factors. *Research in Nursing and Health, 9*(3), 241–247.

Metheny, N., Williams, P., Wiersema, L., et al. (1989). Effectiveness of pH measurements in predicting feeding tube placement. *Nursing Research, 38*(5), 280–285.

Mickschi, D., Davidson, L., Flournoy, D., Parker, D. (1990). Contamination of enteral feedings and diarrhea in patients in intensive care units. *Heart Lung, 19,* 362–370.

Mumma, C. (1986). Withholding nutrition: A nursing perspective. *Nursing Administration Quarterly, 10*(3), 31–38.

Niemec, P., Vanderveen, T., Morrison, J. (1983). Gastrointestinal disorders caused by medications and electrolyte solution osmolality during enteral nutrition. *Journal of Parenteral and Enteral Nutrition, 7,* 387–389.

Nightingale, F. (1859). *Notes on Nursing: What it is and What it is Not.* London: Harrison & Sons.

Ordway, C. (1974). Air embolus via central venous pressure catheter without positive pressure. *Annals of Surgery, 179,* 479.

Padilla, G., Grant, M., Wong, H., et al. (1979). Subjective distresses of nasogastric tube feedings. *Journal of Parenteral and Enteral Nutrition, 3*(2), 53–57.

Payette, H., Gray-Donald, K., Cyr, R., Boutier, V. (1995). Predictors of dietary intake in a functionally dependent elderly population in the community. *American Journal of Public Health, 85*(5), 677–683.

Perez, S., Brandt, K. (1989). Enteral feeding contamination: Comparison of diluents and feeding bag usage. *Journal of Parenteral and Enteral Nutrition, 13*(3), 306–308.

Perucca, R., Micek, J. (1993). Treatment of infusion-related phlebitis. *Journal of Intravenous Nursing, 16*(5), 282–286.

Pestana, C. (1989). *Fluids and Electrolytes in the Surgical Patient,* 4th ed. Baltimore: Williams & Wilkins.

Petrosino, B., Christian, B., Becker, H. (1989). Implications of selected problems with nasoenteral tubes. *Critical Care Nursing Quarterly,* 12(3), 1–18.

Pflaum, S. (1979). Investigation of intake-output as a means of assessing body fluid balance. *Heart Lung, 8*(3), 495–498.

Phillips, P., Phil, M., Rolls, B., et al. (1984). Reduced thirst after water deprivation. *New England Journal of Medicine, 311,* 753–759.

Pierson, M., Funk, M. (1989). Technology versus clinical evaluation for fluid management decisions in coronary artery bypass (CABG) patients. *Image, 21,* 192–195.

Powell, K., Marcuard, S., Farrior, E., Gallagher, M. (1993). Aspirating gastric residuals causes occlusion of small-bore feeding tubes. *Journal of Parenteral and Enteral Nutrition, 17*(3), 243–246.

Potts, R., Zaroukian, M., Guerrero, P. (1993). Comparison of blue dye visualization and glucose oxidase test strip methods for detecting pulmonary aspiration of enteral feedings in intubated adults. *Chest, 103,* 117–121.

Rains, B. (1981). The non-hospitalized tube-fed patient. *Oncology Nursing Forum, 8,* 8–13.

Richardson, D., Bruso, P. (1993). Vascular access devices: Management of common complications. *Journal of Intravenous Nursing, 16*(1), 44–49.

Robinson, S., Demuth, P. (1985). Diagnostic studies for the aged: What are the dangers? *Journal of Gerontological Nursing, 11*(6), 6.

Rosofsky, W., Bell, S., Blackburn, G. (1990). The challenges of feeding the elderly. *Nutrition in Clinical Practice, 5*(1), 6–7.

Sanville, M. (1994). Initiating parenteral nutrition therapy in the home. *Journal of Intravenous Nursing, 17*(3), 119–126.

Savage, S., Wilkinson, M. (1994). Patient weights: From physician complaints to improved nursing practice through quality improvement. *Gastroenterology Nursing, 16*(6), 264–268.

Scanlan, M., Frisch, S. (1992). Nasoduodenal feeding tubes: Prevention of occlusion. *Journal of Neuroscience Nursing, 24*(5), 256–259.

Schlegal-Pratt, K., Heizer, W. (1990). The accuracy of scales used to weigh patients. *Nutrition in Clinical Practice, 6*(6), 254.

Schroeder, P., Fisher, D., Volz, M., Paloucek, J. (1983). Microbial contamination of enteral feeding solutions in a community hospital. *Journal of Parenteral and Enteral Nutrition, 7,* 364–368.

Shock, N., Gruelich, R., Andres, R. (1984). Normal human aging: The Baltimore longitudinal study of aging. Washington, DC: US Department of Health and Human Services, NIH publication No. 84-2450.

Silberman, H. (1989). *Parenteral and Enteral Nutrition,* 2nd ed. Norwalk, CT: Appleton & Lang.

Sing, R., Steffe, T., Branas, C. (1995). Fatal air embolism after removal of a central venous catheter. *Journal of the American Osteopathic Association, 95,* 204–205.

Smith, C., Marien, L., Brogdon, C., et al. (1990). Diarrhea associated with tube feeding in mechanically ventilated critically ill patients. *Nursing Research, 39*(3), 148–152.

Standards of Practice. (1995). Standards for nutritional support in hospitalized patients. *Nutrition in Clinical Practice, 10*(6), 20–218.

Stebor, A. (1989). Posturination time and specific gravity in infants' diapers. *Nursing Research, 38*(4), 244.

Taylor, N., Huthinson, E., Milliken, W., Larson, E. (1989). Comparison of normal versus heparinized saline for flushing infusion devices. *Journal of Nursing Quality Assurance, 3*(4), 49–55.

Taylor, S. (1992). Lost in the system. *Journal of Intravenous Nursing* Supplement, *15*(March/April)., 522–527.

Thompson, D., Jowell, N., Folwell, A., Sutton, T. (1989). A trial of povidone-iodine antiseptic solution for the prevention of cannula-related thrombophlebitis. *Journal of Intravenous Nursing, 12*(2), 99–102.

Torres, A., Serra-Batlles, K., Piera, C. (1992). Pulmonary aspiration of gastric contents in patients receiving mechanical ventilation: The effect of body position. *Annals of Internal Medicine, 16,* 419–422.

Twomey, P. (1990). Cost-effectiveness of enteral nutrition. In J. Rombeau and M. Caldwell (eds.): *Clinical Nutrition: Enteral and Tube Feeding,* 2nd ed. Philadelphia: W.B. Saunders.

Vaughn, L., Manore, M., Winston, D. (1988). Bacterial safety of a closed-administration system for enteral nutrition solutions. *Journal of American Dietetic Association, 88,* 35–37.

Viall, C., Crocker, K., Hennessy, K., Orr, M. (1995). High tech home care: Surviving and prospering in a changing environment. *Nutrition in Clinical Practice,* 19(1), 32–36.

Wagman, L., Newsome, H., Miller, K., Thomas, R. (1986). The effect of acute discontinuation of total parenteral nutrition. *Annals of Surgery, 204,* 524.

Walike, B., Walike, J. (1977). Relative lactose intolerance: A clinical study of tube-fed patients. *Journal of the American Medical Association, 238,* 948–951.

Watson, K., O'Kell, R., Joyce, J. (1983). Data regarding blood drawing sites in patients receiving intravenous fluids. *American Journal of Clinical Pathology, 79,* 119.

Weinsier, R., Bacon, J., Butterworth, C. (1982). Central venous alimentation: A prospective study of the frequency of metabolic abnormalities among medical and surgical patients. *Journal of Parenteral and Enteral Nutrition, 6,* 421.

Weinsier, R., Heimburger, D., Butterworth, C. (1989). *Handbook of Clinical Nutrition.* St. Louis: C.V. Mosby.

Williams, E., Kelman, G., Jacox, M. (1994). A regional survey of intravenous therapy practices. *Journal of Intravenous Nursing, 17*(4), 195–199.

Wilson, M., Haynes-Johnson, V. (1987). Cranberry juice or water? A comparison of feeding tube irrigants. *Nutritional Support Services, 7*(7), 23–24.

Winterbauer, R., Durning, R., Barron, E. (1981). Aspirated nasogastric feeding solutions detected by glucose strips. *Annals of Internal Medicine, 95,* 67–68.

Worthington-Roberts, B. (1985). Eating disorders in women. *Focus on Critical Care, 12*(4), 32–41.

Yeakel, A. (1969). Lethal air embolism from plastic blood storage containers. *Journal of the American Medical Association, 204,* 267.

Yucha, C., Hastings-Tolsma, M., Szeverenyi, N. (1993). Differences among intravenous extravasations using four common solutions. *Journal of Intravenous Nursing, 16*(5), 277–281.

Zerwekh, J. (1997). Do dying patients routinely really need IV fluids? *American Journal of Nursing, 97*(3), 26–30.

Zimmaro, D., Rollandelli, R., Kopuda, M., et al. (1987). Isotonic tube feeding formula induces liquid stool in normal subjects: Reversal by pectin. *Journal of Parenteral and Enteral Nutrition 13*(2), 117–123.

Zimmerman, J., Oder, L. (1981). Swallowing dysfunction in acutely ill patients. *Physical Therapy, 61,* 1755–1764.

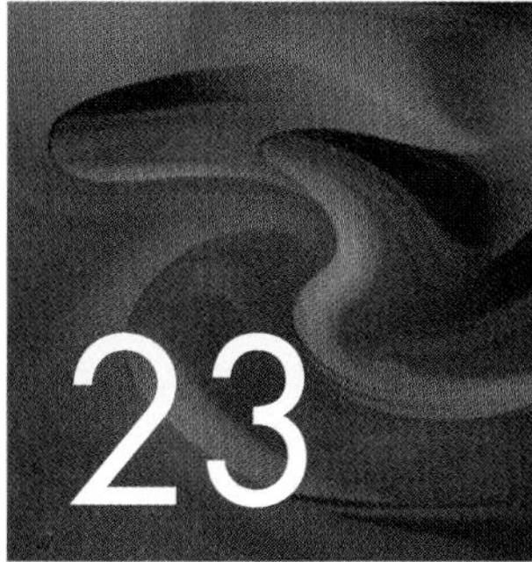

Intestinal Elimination 23

Margaret A. Martin and Diane Krasner

Nancy Waller is a 36-year-old elementary school teacher. She has been married for 9 years and is the mother of two children. Nancy has had distressing gastrointestinal (GI) symptoms for the past 4 years. She has intermittent episodes of both diarrhea and constipation. She occasionally feels bloated and experiences excessive belching. She has attempted to discuss this with her family physician, who attributes her complaints to a stressful, busy life. Nancy acknowledges that she is very busy, sometimes eating on the run. She worries about proper nutrition for her family, but realizes she is often unable to give the same attention to her own nutrition needs. Lately Nancy's symptoms have become worse. The diarrhea occurs several times a week, and is sometimes accompanied by severe cramping and mucus in her stool. Nancy read an article in a magazine about lactose intolerance and believed that was the basis of her problems.

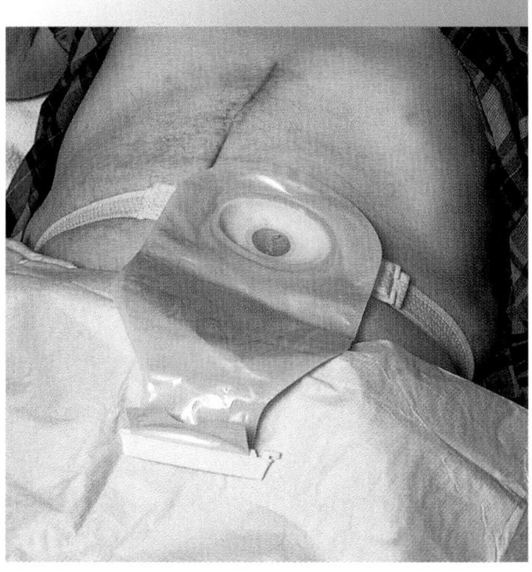

She eliminated all dairy products from her diet. At first, this seemed to help. But after a few days, her symptoms resumed. Nancy returned to her physician. After a complete physical and numerous GI studies, including a barium enema and a sigmoidoscopy, her doctor informed her that she has irritable bowel syndrome. Nancy was told that this chronic condition would require both dietary and lifestyle changes in order to manage the symptoms and improve her quality of life.

OBJECTIVES

After studying this chapter, students will be able to:

- **describe the normal eliminative functions of the intestinal system.**
- **explain the effects of intrinsic and extrinsic factors on intestinal elimination and what interventions can minimize these effects.**
- **describe the eliminative alterations caused by certain pathologic conditions and the nurse's role in assessing and facilitating management of these situations.**
- **relate advances in medical and nursing research that lead to improving conditions for persons with alterations in elimination.**
- **describe and perform specific nursing procedures related to normal and abnormal elimination.**

SCOPE OF NURSING PRACTICE

Elimination of the waste products of digestion from the body is essential to health. Adequate elimination involves proper functioning of the small and large bowel. Normal defecation has two aspects: the pattern or frequency of defecation and the normal color, odor, and consistency of the stool. Important measures that influence defecation include diet, fluid intake, regularity of meals, exercise, privacy, and a regular time for defecation.

Common problems of defecation include constipation, fecal impaction, diarrhea, flatulence, and anal incontinence. Certain pathologic conditions can alter patterns of intestinal elimination. These include carcinoma of the bowel, the inflammatory bowel diseases (Crohn's disease and ulcerative colitis), and irritable bowel syndrome. Nursing interventions are aimed at maintaining the person's usual pattern of bowel functioning and assisting the patient with management of any alteration in function.

Intestinal elimination is essential for supporting normal living. Elimination refers to the process of excreting the body's wastes and the byproducts of metabolism. Alterations in the eliminative process are common and range from simple, one-time bouts of diarrhea to more serious scenarios as described in Nancy's case. Nurses are often involved in helping people alleviate GI symptoms. In all settings—acute care, long-term care, and home care—the nurse is usually the first health care professional that a person confides in and is, therefore, the first to perform an assessment of eliminative disruptions. The nurse may be the first person to identify a silent symptom, such as a stool specimen that is suspicious for blood.

The need for normal elimination or regular bowel movements is a matter of great cultural concern for people in North American culture. Advertising concerned with laxatives and descriptions of fatigue due to bowel irregularity bombard people daily. In addition, eliminative problems are often embarrassing for people to talk about, thus complicating their confusion regarding what is normal or abnormal. Nurses who are equipped with a thorough understanding of the normal eliminative system and its common alterations as well as nursing practice and research related to intestinal elimination can optimize the care of all patients.

KNOWLEDGE BASE

Basic Science

Essential to the maintenance of life and health is the elimination of the waste products of digestion from the body. These waste products, called feces or stool, consist of bile pigments, mucus, unabsorbed minerals, undigested fats, cellulose, meat protein toxins, shredded epithelial cells, potassium, chloride, sodium, bicarbonate, and water. Fecal composition is three-fourths water and one-fourth solid matter (Hampton and Bryant, 1992). The usual brown color of feces is due to the presence of bile pigments and the action of bacteria. The passage of feces out of the body is known as defecation or, more commonly, "having a bowel movement."

GASTROINTESTINAL SYSTEM

The *gastrointestinal system,* which performs digestion, absorption of nutrients, and storage and elimination of wastes, is divided into two parts: the alimentary canal and the accessory organs. (See Chapter 22, Nutrition and Fluids, for more details on GI system structure and function.) The alimentary canal is the tube extending from the mouth to the anus: mouth, esophagus, stomach, small intestines, large intestines, rectum, and anus. *Accessory organs* are those outside the alimentary canal that contribute to digestion: liver, gallbladder, and pancreas (Hampton and Bryant, 1992). The intestines, as the terminal portion of the alimentary canal, are responsible for the storage and elimination of fecal wastes. Two distinct portions, the *small intestines* and the *large intestines,* make up this portion of the GI system (Fig. 23–1).

Approximately 22 feet long, the small intestine extends from the pylorus of the stomach to the cecum of the large intestines. It consists of three distinct parts: the duodenum (10–12 inches long), the jejunum (8–9 feet long), and the ileum (12 feet long). The diameter of the small intestine averages 1 inch. The average adult has abut 7600 cm of absorptive surface in the small intestine. It is the major organ for digestion and absorption of nutrients (Guyton, 1991).

The large intestine, or colon, is 5 to 6 feet long. Its function is to absorb water and to store and eliminate stool. It extends from the ileocecal valve at the distal end of the small intestine to the anus. The adult colon varies in width from 1 to 2½ inches. It consists of seven distinct parts: cecum, ascending colon, transverse colon, descending colon, sigmoid colon, rectum, and anus.

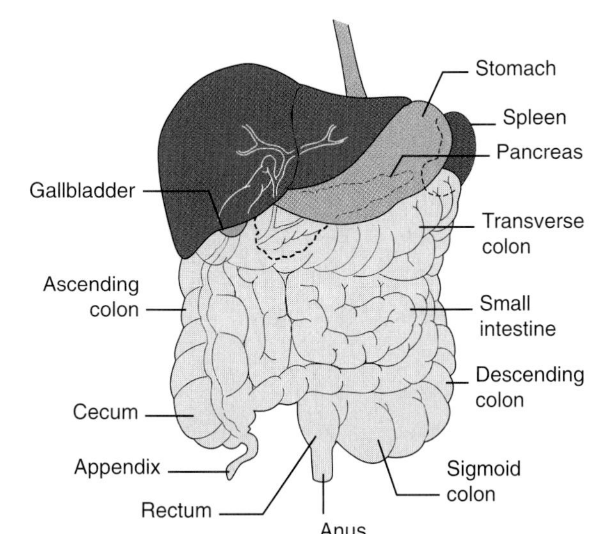

Figure 23–1. Anatomy of the lower GI system.

The muscular fibers of the colon are circular and longitudinal and can contract in both width and length. The longitudinal muscle segments are shorter than the circular ones, forming the typical pouches or *haustra* of the large intestines. The longitudinal and circular muscles work together, creating a synchronous activity that propels fecal material through the colon. This movement is called *peristalsis.*

In addition to its absorptive and transporting functions, the colon also provides protective properties. Cells in the inner lining of the colon secrete mucus that protects the intestinal wall from irritation and bacterial invasion. This mucus also binds and lubricates the fecal material, thereby facilitating defecation.

The process of movement through the GI system begins as ingested food and fluids are mixed in the stomach with gastric secretions and converted to a semifluid material called *chyme.* Together the small and large intestines transport this food mass, chyme, from the pyloric *sphincter* at the distal end of the stomach to exit the body through the anus. Approximately 1500 ml of chyme is transferred into the intestines every 24 hours. Because of the absorptive properties of the two intestines, only about 80 to 200 ml eventually leaves the body as waste (Guyton, 1991).

The rectum is the distal continuation of the colon. It is 12 to 15 cm long and is larger in diameter than the colon. The most distal end of the rectum, the anus, is where stool exits the body (Fig. 23–2). The anorectal sphincter, which includes an internal and external component, enables a person to voluntarily retain the stool until defecation is appropriate. This is accomplished by contraction of the sphincter and is called continence (Doughty, 1996).

DIGESTION

Numerous digestive enzymes secreted throughout the GI tract are required for digestion. Mechanical digestion of nutrients begins in the mouth with the process of chewing, which breaks the food into smaller particles and increases the surface available for enzymatic activity. Enzymatic digestion of carbohydrates is initiated in the mouth by the action of salivary amylase. Only a small percentage of carbohydrates are digested in the mouth, because most are covered with cellulose, which blocks enzymatic contact with the surface of the carbohydrate. In the stomach, the breakdown of starches is interrupted because the stomach's acidic environment inactivates the salivary amylase.

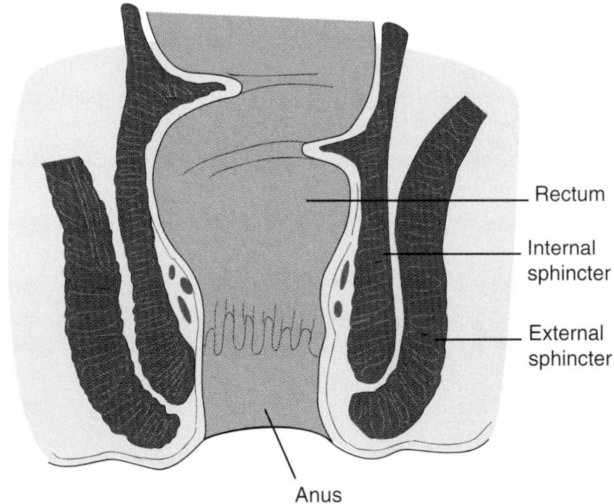

Figure 23–2. The rectum and anus.

The acidic environment of the stomach initiates protein digestion, however. The *hydrochloric acid (HCl)* of the stomach converts *pepsinogen* to *pepsin,* an enzyme that breaks down protein. Minute quantities of *gastric lipase* for beginning digestion of fats and milk protein are also secreted by the stomach. As the chyme formed in the stomach moves into the intestinal tract, enzymes control the rate and continue the digestive process. The duodenum accepts only the amount of chyme that can be accommodated by liver-produced bile released into the duodenum. Thus, a diet high in fat, requiring a lot of bile to digest it, moves slowly. The enzyme *enterogastrone* is responsible for this slowing (Broadwell and Jackson, 1982). Highly acidic chyme emptied into the duodenum automatically stops further progression of food from the stomach until pancreatic enzymes have neutralized it. The presence of the acidic chyme in the duodenum causes the release of secretin, which stimulates the pancreas to secrete a fluid with *bicarbonate.* This fluid drains through the pancreatic duct into the duodenum to neutralize the chyme. The presence of fats in the duodenum stimulates the delivery of bile from the liver, which also neutralizes the acidic chyme. Bile emulsifies the fats, making them more susceptible to enzymatic breakdown.

The small intestine contains several enzymes that continue the digestive process: *amylase* for carbohydrate digestion; *lipase* for fat digestion; *lactose* for milk sugars, and *trypsin, chymotrypsin,* and *carboxypeptidase* for the breakdown of proteins (Hampton and Bryant, 1992). In addition, a hormonal mechanism helps determine the types of enzymes secreted. *Enterocrinin,* a mixture of hormones, stimulates the intestinal glands to secrete appropriate enzymes for digesting the foods in the small intestine (Broadwell and Jackson, 1982).

Normal secretion of gastric enzymes is necessary for the digestion of food and natural elimination of wastes. Some studies show that with aging, the quantity of digestive enzymes produced decreases, which may lead to an increase in the rate of intestinal complications in the elderly (Cox et al., 1989).

NORMAL ELIMINATION

Normal elimination depends on various factors:

- The coordinated delivery of stool to the rectum from the colon
- Expulsive forces that propel the stool from the distal GI tract
- Sensory awareness of rectal distention and contents

- Voluntary sphincter control
- Access to toilet facilities (Doughty, 1991a, 1996)

DEFECATION

Normal defecation begins with mass movements in the left colon, which propel stool toward the rectum. When stool reaches the rectum, the sudden distention causes relaxation of the internal sphincter and activates stretch receptors within the wall of the rectum. These events alert the person to impending defecation. Normal sensory awareness includes the ability to discriminate between gas, liquid, and solid rectal contents. If defecation is not convenient, the person contracts the external sphincter, which interrupts the peristaltic force from the colon and allows the rectum to relax around the stool.

Voluntary defecation is initiated by the relaxation of the external sphincter and contraction of abdominal muscles. This causes a drop in anal canal pressure and an increase in rectal pressure that forces the stool out. This force is lost when defecation is delayed; thus, optimal elimination occurs by prompt response to the sensory signals of impending defecation (Doughty, 1996).

Most people defecate on a regular basis, often following meals. Approximately 30 minutes after eating, in response to food entering the stomach, the colon is stimulated to proceed with evacuation. This is known as the *gastrocolic reflex* (Guyton, 1991). Stool frequency varies from one to three movements a day to once every 3 days for adults. Infants may have one to six movements a day. Normal adult stools are soft, formed, and brown. Infant stools are yellow, soft, and pasty. The color and consistency of stools can vary depending on diet and physical condition. For example, illness and decreased fluid intake can cause constipated, hard stools; whereas some illnesses (e.g., flu or GI virus) can cause loose, watery stools. Some foods such as red beets change the color of stool, whereas foods such as onions and fish cause a strong, foul odor.

FACTORS AFFECTING ELIMINATION

The process of elimination can be significantly altered by both intrinsic and extrinsic factors. *Intrinsic* factors are those processes operating within a person, such as diet, age, medications, neurologic status, exercise, regular time for meals and elimination, and psychological factors. *Extrinsic* factors are external factors that affect the person; these include diagnostic testing, anesthesia, and surgery.

Intrinsic Factors

Diet and Fluid Intake. Diet and fluid intake have a major effect on bowel elimination. Sufficient bulk, obtained from high-fiber foods such as whole grains, fruits, and vegetables, is necessary to provide fecal bulk that increases the rate of transit time through the intestine. This contributes to regularity of bowel movements. Low-fiber foods, such as most processed foods, slow the rate of transit, allowing more fluid to be reabsorbed through the intestinal wall. This results in *constipation.* Chronic constipation of dry, hard stools leads to muscle atrophy and, therefore, a continuation and worsening of the difficult elimination.

The volume of fluid a person takes in determines the moisture and mobility of the feces. Adults should drink six to eight glasses (1500 to 2000 ml) a day, unless contraindicated for some other medical reason. If fluid intake is low or output of fluid in the form of urine or vomitus is high, the stools become hard and difficult to pass. Once again, movement is slowed, increasing fluid reabsorption and increasing drying of the stools.

Spicy foods, spoiled or contaminated foods, or irregularly eaten foods can irritate the mucosal lining of the intestine and produce bowel symptoms. Most often such irritants cause *diarrhea, flatus,* or both. Gas-producing foods include cabbage, onions, beans, carbonated and alcoholic beverages, and chewing gum. Milk or milk products present a problem for people with *lactose intolerance.* These people are unable to produce the digestive enzyme *lactase* that is needed to digest *lactose,* a simple sugar found in milk. Symptoms such as diarrhea, distention, and cramping can be avoided by adding lactase to the diet, limiting milk products, or both. Some foods such as bananas and rice tend to bind the stool.

Age. Age can affect both the character and control of fecal elimination. The very young are unable to control their elimination until the neuromuscular system is developed. This usually occurs between age 2 and 3 years. The changes that occur with aging also affect bowel elimination. As people age, muscle tone is decreased, resulting in lack of tone of the smooth muscles of the colon. This can result in slower peristalsis. The decreased tone of the abdominal muscles decreases the pressure that can be exerted during defecation. These changes can lead to chronic constipation and painful, difficult elimination for the elderly person. In addition, digestive enzyme production decreases, leading to slowed digestion. The loss of teeth, resulting in difficult chewing and poorly chewed food, also contributes to slow digestion and stool transit. Some elderly people also have a problem of decreased control over the anal sphincter muscles, which can result in an urgency to defecate or the involuntary passages of stool—incontinence (Doughty, 1996).

Medications. Certain medications can affect the consistency and pattern of elimination. Some drugs can alter the normal process of intestinal elimination. Some cause diarrhea, others cause constipation. Table 23–1 lists medications that commonly alter patterns of intestinal elimination.

Some medications are specifically intended to directly affect elimination. *Laxatives* are medications used to stimulate bowel activity. *Stool softeners* soften the feces and facilitate elimination. Medications used to treat diarrhea slow down colon function.

Neurologic Status. Neurologic status or changes in a person's sensory or motor function can affect intestinal elimination. For example, decreased muscle tone reduces colonic

TABLE 23-1 Medications That Commonly Alter Intestinal Elimination

Medication Class	Example	Common Side Effect(s)
Antacids	Maalox Mylanta	Constipation
Antibiotics	Ampicillin Ceftin	Diarrhea
Anticholinergics and adrenergics	Atropine	Constipation
Antidepressants	Prozac	Constipation
Antidiarrheals	Donnatal Lomotil	Constipation with overuse
Anti-Parkinsonian drugs	Cogentin	Constipation
Anti-psychotic drugs	Haldol	Constipation
Barium sulfate	Oral barium for x-ray visualization	Constipation
Bismuth salts	Pepto-Bismol	Constipation
Cathartics and laxatives	Milk of Magnesia	Diarrhea or dependence with overuse
Calcium carbonate	Os-Cal	Constipation
Iron	Ferrous sulfate	Constipation; dark green or black discoloration of stool
Narcotic analgesics	Morphine Codeine	Constipation
Sedatives	Seconal	Constipation
Stool softeners	Colace	Diarrhea with overuse
Tranquilizers	Valium	Constipation

peristalsis. In addition, decreased innervation of the abdominal muscles decreases the pressure that can be exerted to assist with defecation. If a person's sensory functions are impaired, such as in spinal cord–injured or stroke patients, the sensory stimulation for defecation may be absent. Dementias and other changes in levels of consciousness may mean that a person is not able to adequately respond to the signal to defecate.

Exercise. Exercise serves to maintain muscle tone. The abdominal and pelvic muscles and the diaphragm are important for defecation. Activity stimulates peristalsis and facilitates the movement of chyme through the colon. Inactivity decreases muscle tone and depresses colonic mobility.

Regular Mealtimes. Regular mealtimes affect the pattern and functioning of the GI tract. Regular mealtimes enhance normal defecation by providing the body with a regularly timed, physiologic response to the intake of food. The intake of food stimulates the peristaltic activity in the colon. This process, the gastrocolic reflex, thus aids in establishing a pattern for elimination.

Regularity. Establishing a regular time for elimination ensures the response to the physiologic urge to defecate, which occurs once the stool has entered the rectum. Delaying elimination once the urge is felt leads to difficult defecation resulting from the absence of the propulsive force created by the intestinal movements that initially move the stool into the rectum.

Psychological Factors. Psychological factors such as stress and anxiety affect the pattern of elimination as well as the consistency of stool. Stress and anxiety can increase peristaltic activity in the colon, which causes diarrhea. Depression, which tends to cause a decrease in all activity, can affect eating patterns and leads to constipation.

Extrinsic Factors

Diagnostic Tests. Diagnostic testing and radiologic procedures can affect defecation by interrupting a person's eating pattern. Most testing requires that a person withhold food and fluids for a specified time before the procedure. This leaves the intestinal system without bulk or food to digest and without fluid. The physiologic responses to eating are absent, although the GI system continues to secrete some enzymes and maintain some mobility.

Patients may also receive laxatives or enemas or be given contrast materials to drink. All of these can alter normal elimination patterns. After the administration of certain contrast materials, such as barium sulfate, patients are given laxatives to facilitate the movement of barium out of the intestine. It may take several days after diagnostic testing and the resumption of a regular diet before bowel functioning returns to normal.

Anesthesia and Surgery. Anesthesia and surgery can interrupt the normal pattern of elimination. General anesthesia slows peristalsis in the colon by blocking the neurologic transmission of stimulation to the muscles in the colon. Surgery and handling of the intestine can also decrease peristalsis, resulting in a phenomenon called *paralytic ileus* (Handerhan, 1991). Signs and symptoms include loss of intestinal motility (the ability to move spontaneously), failure to pass stool or flatus, distention of the abdomen due to retention of flatus and stool, abdominal tenderness, and absent bowel sounds on abdominal auscultation. When the bowel is functioning normally, a variety of sounds can be heard when a stethoscope is placed on the abdomen. These sounds, which are gurgling in nature, are called *bowel sounds* and are an indication of movement within the intestinal tract. (See Chapter

15, Patient Assessment, for information on auscultating bowel sounds.)

Laboratory work performed on a person with *paralytic ileus* reveals electrolyte imbalances. The condition usually lasts 24 to 48 hours after surgery and usually resolves spontaneously. Other causes of ileus include certain medications (e.g., anesthetics and narcotics), abdominal infections, trauma, and neurologic impairment. If ileus does not resolve spontaneously, treatment may include fluid and electrolyte replacement, *total parenteral nutrition* (replacement of nutrients intravenously), and the placement of a nasogastric tube to facilitate the removal of excess fluid from the GI tract. (See Chapter 22, Nutrition and Fluids, for more information on total parenteral nutrition.) If not properly managed, ileus can result in bowel edema, bowel rupture, death of bowel tissue (necrosis), or a combination of these. Pain medications, immobility, and limited diet also contribute to slowed intestinal patterns following surgery.

ABNORMAL ELIMINATION

ALTERED STOOL APPEARANCE

Disruptions in the intestinal tract and alterations in bowel elimination are characterized by a wide range of signs and symptoms. Appearance of the stool can be an indication of alterations within the bowel. Changes in the color of the stool have many origins. For example, black, tar-like stools, known as melena, can be caused by darkened blood pigments and are suggestive of bleeding in the upper GI system (mouth, esophagus, stomach). Stools become tan or clay-colored if there is a deficiency or absence of bile, as in biliary obstruction. Red stools or the visible presence of bright-red blood indicate bleeding in the lower GI system (intestine, rectum) or hemorrhoids. Certain foods can also change the color of stool temporarily, most notably beets (red or green) red Jell-O, strawberries, licorice, and red food coloring.

Consistency of stools changes with diet and disease processes. Foamy stools may be due to increased fats in the stool or to infection. Fatty stools are often associated with cystic fibrosis, gallbladder disease, pancreatic disorders, sprue, and excessive dietary intake of fat. Malodorous stools can be caused by infection, drugs (such as antibiotics), or ingestion of certain foods. Mucous stools are often observed with the inflammatory bowel diseases, such as Crohn's disease and ulcerative colitis.

Changes in the shape of the stool, such as pencil-like stools, may be due to changes in the lumen of the bowel. This may indicate bowel stricture or a growth or tumor.

ABDOMINAL DISTENTION AND PAIN

Symptoms of abdominal distention and abdominal or anorectal pain are indications of an abnormality within the intestinal tract. The stretching of the abdominal wall can be indicative of constipation, fecal impaction, food intolerance, flatulence, or intestinal obstruction. Abdominal pain varies from mild to severe and ranges from dull, to aching, to sharp. Cramping is a spasmodic pain due to muscular contractions, as in irritable bowel syndrome. Colicky pain, a severe spasmodic cramping, is typical in obstruction. Anorectal pain is most commonly caused by hemorrhoids.

CONSTIPATION

Constipation refers to the passage of small, dry, hard stools or the passage of no stool for a period of time. It occurs when the movement of forces through the large intestine is slow, thus allowing time for additional reabsorption of fluid from the large intestine. Associated with constipation is the difficult evacuation of stools and increased effort and straining of the voluntary muscles of defecation. Constipation is determined in relation to the person's regular elimination patterns. Some people defecate only a few times a week and are not constipated when they miss a day or two. Other people normally defecate more than once a day and can be constipated when they have no bowel movement for 1 day.

Certain patterns of daily living can predispose a person to constipation. These include irregular eating and bowel habits, low-fiber diets or diets high in processed foods, inadequate fluid intake, lack of exercise, regular use of medications with constipating side effects (e.g., morphine, codeine, iron supplements), and overuse of laxatives, which tends to inhibit the natural defecation reflexes. Elderly persons with poor muscle tone and sphincter tone may have chronic constipation. Table 23–2 lists common causes of constipation.

Several disease conditions of the bowel can also produce constipation. Among these are bowel obstruction, paralysis (which inhibits the person's ability to bear down to evacuate stool), and pelvic inflammatory conditions that create paralysis or atony of the bowel.

Constipation can be accompanied by nausea, vomiting, loss of appetite (anorexia), flatulence, foul breath, abdominal distention, colicky pain, headaches, irritability, anxiety, and weakness. Prolonged constipation is known as *obstipation*. *Terminal reservoir syndrome* refers to the condition, common in immobilized or paralyzed persons, in which the lower colon is never completely emptied.

Preventing constipation depends on regular dietary habits with adequate fluid intake and fiber, which is found in whole grains, bran, cereals and breads, fruits, and vegetables. Regular exercise improves the condition by stimulating intestinal peristalsis. If conservative methods fail, alternative actions can be instituted. These actions include the use of laxatives or enemas. Laxatives can stimulate the intestinal movement, provide bulk to encourage more rapid movement, or both. Stool softeners can be added to soften the stools for more ease of evacuation. Enemas promote elimination by increasing the pressure within the bowel, thereby stimulating an increase in peristalsis in the body's effort to empty the colon, which is overfilled. All of these methods demand caution in use. All of them, if used frequently, can inhibit the natural urge to defecate. In addition, chronic laxative use can result in serious fluid and electrolyte depletion.

RESEARCH HIGHLIGHT

CONSTIPATION IN LONG-TERM CARE

Harari. (1994). Assessment of constipation in long-term care residents. Journal of the American Geriatric Society, *42, p 947.*

The prevalence of self-reported constipation among older adults is estimated to be 23 to 53 percent. Harari studied residents in a long-term care facility and compared self-reports of constipation with nursing assessments. The researcher also analyzed prescribing and use patterns of common therapies.

The study included 694 elderly residents. The residents' clinical and functional status, bowel-related symptoms, and medications were determined from medical and nursing records. Two thirds of the study subjects and their respective nurses were interviewed separately. Symptom-specific constipation was defined as no more than two bowel movements per week, straining on more than one fourth of bowel movements, or both. Fifty percent (367) of the residents used a stool softener, laxative, or enema at least once daily. Of the laxative users, 55% took more than 60 doses per month. Forty-seven percent of the 456 residents interviewed reported having constipation. Only 62% of the 213 residents who reported constipation actually met the study's definition of constipation. The residents who reported constipation took almost twice the medications (laxatives, softeners) as did those who did not report constipation. Correlation between residents and nurses' reports regarding constipation was slight to fair.

The author concluded that nearly half of nursing home residents may have constipation even though daily use of laxatives, stool softeners, and enemas is common. Current management of constipation may be clinically ineffective or become ineffective over time. The discrepancy between resident and nursing evaluation of constipation demonstrates the need for a more systematic approach to the evaluation and management of constipation in the long-term care setting.

FECAL IMPACTION

Fecal impaction is defined as a mass or collection of hardened feces in the rectum due to prolonged retention and accumulation of fecal material. In severe cases, the feces accumulate and extend well into the sigmoid colon and beyond, causing massive obstruction. Fecal impaction is recognized by the passage of liquid fecal seepage and no normal stools. The liquid portion of the feces seeps out around the impacted mass. Impaction can be felt by digital examination. The patient with a fecal impaction has a frequent urge to defecate, but is unable to do so, and the effort is accompanied by rectal pain. If the condition is not resolved, the person becomes weak, the abdomen becomes distended, and nausea and vomiting may occur.

Fecal impaction usually can be traced to poor defecation habits. Contributing factors may include inadequate fluid intake, insufficient bulk intake, lack of activity, and inability to bear down at defecation. Although in some people impactions tend to occur regardless of measures to prevent them, they are mostly preventable (Wrenn, 1989).

TABLE 23–2 Common Causes of Constipation and Diarrhea

Constipation	Diarrhea
Anorexia nervosa	Allergy to foods (e.g., dairy products)
Bowel stricture or obstruction	Antibiotics (e.g., ampicillin, tetracycline)
Cancer	Anxiety
Chronic laxative abuse	Cancer
Dehydration	Celiac disease (malabsorption)
Dementia	Contaminated water
Depression	Fecal impaction with paradoxical diarrhea
Diabetes	Food intolerances (e.g., rich foods, coffee, alcohol, strong seasonings)
Dietary deficiencies of fiber, bulk	Gastroenteritis
Fecal impaction	Inflammatory bowel disease
Hemorrhoids	Irritable bowel syndrome
Hypothyroidism	Lactose intolerance
Ileus	Laxative abuse
Immobility	Malabsorption syndrome
Irritable bowel syndrome	Medications (see Table 23–1)
Medications (see Table 23–1)	Radiation therapy
Muscle weakness	Stress
Neglecting the urge to defecate	Tube feedings
Neurologic disorders	
Paralysis	
Pelvic inflammatory disorders	
Stress	

Impactions can be relieved by a series of low-volume phosphate enemas given once or twice a day for 7 to 10 days or until clear (Jensen, 1990). Impactions can also be relieved manually by a process known as *disimpaction,* or digital removal of stool. Because disimpaction can cause mucosal trauma, pain, or cardiac arrhythmias, this procedure should be undertaken only by a trained health care professional such as a nurse. Patients should be cautioned never to perform this themselves or to allow family members to disimpact. After disimpaction, follow-up treatment with suppositories or enemas is common practice. Efforts to prevent future impactions, such as changes in diet and mobility, should be instituted.

DIARRHEA

The rapid movement of fecal material through the intestines, diarrhea is characterized by liquid, frequent stools, poor intestinal absorption, mucous stools, and generalized weakness. Often patients experience an urgency to defecate and they may even suffer urge *incontinence* (involuntary passage of stool). Stools may be blood-tinged, and crampy pain may accompany the diarrhea. The loss of electrolytes, especially potassium, is a common side effect that can lead to electrolyte imbalance. The patient may also experience nausea and vomiting. Table 23–2 lists some of the common causes of diarrhea. Proper diagnosis is imperative if prompt, appropriate treatment is to be initiated (Smith et al., 1990).

To prevent dehydration, fluid and electrolyte imbalances, and acid-base imbalances during bouts of diarrhea, attention must be given to fluid and electrolyte replacement, either parenterally or orally. Patients experiencing chronic diarrhea must be watched for anemia and malnutrition. At home, fluid replacement may be accomplished with homemade preparations of salt, bicarbonate of soda, and high-potassium fruit juices, or with commercial preparations such as Gatorade (Candy, 1987). Solid foods should be withheld for at least 24 to 48 hours after diarrhea subsides.

Certain symptoms of diarrhea, such as pain, abdominal cramping, and distention, can be controlled with medications. Certain antidiarrheal drugs inhibit bowel motility, reducing peristalsis, pain, and cramping. Other medications coat and protect the intestinal mucosa or absorb flatus and bacterial toxins. Strict attention to perineal skin care is needed to prevent skin irritation and breakdown. The perineal area should be cleansed gently after each episode of diarrhea and a moisture barrier ointment applied to protect the skin.

FISTULA

A fistula is an abnormal connection or tract between two internal organs or between an internal organ and the surface of the body. Examples of fecal fistulas include enterocutaneous fistulas, draining from the small intestines to the skin; enterovaginal fistulas, draining from the small intestines to the vagina; and enterovesical fistulas, draining from the small intestines into the bladder. Fistulas are often the result of chronic bowel diseases or are a postoperative complication.

Fistulas commonly drain stool, pus, blood, or a combination thereof, causing skin irritation and breakdown. Although some fistulas may close spontaneously with careful conservative management, many require surgery and some never resolve.

FLATUS

Flatus is intestinal air or gas. The formation of excessive amounts of air or gas in the intestines is called *flatulence.* Common causes include the production of gas by bacteria; the formation of carbon dioxide when bicarbonate interacts with hydrochloric or fatty acid; the diffusion of gases from the blood into the GI tract; swallowing of air; constipation; and gas-forming foods and medications. Patients often experience postoperative distention following abdominal surgery due to anesthesia, narcotics, and immobility.

Anti-gas medications, such as simethicone and hydroxide antacids, can be taken after meals. Gas-forming foods, such as beans, cabbage, onions, and carbonated beverages, should be eliminated from the diet, and drinking with a straw should be avoided. The person with flatulence should remain erect following meals to facilitate the belching of gas from the stomach. Ambulation to increase peristalsis and move gas through the GI tract should be encouraged. If these measures are not successful, a rectal tube may be inserted for approximately 20 minutes to relieve distention by flatulence.

FECAL INCONTINENCE

Fecal incontinence is the loss of voluntary control over defecation (Madoff et al., 1992). An estimated 1 in 200 community-living adults suffer from fecal incontinence. In extended care facilities, the rate may be as high as 50% (Jensen, 1990). Whenever the complex coordination between the neuromuscular control mechanisms is thrown off balance, fecal incontinence can occur. Common causes include a malfunctioning or incompetent anal sphincter, damage to the pelvic nerves as a result of anal or rectal surgery or childbirth, weakening of the muscles of the pelvic floor, and neurologic disorders, such as paralysis or multiple sclerosis. Confused or demented persons may no longer be aware of the urge to defecate and may experience fecal incontinence (Tobein, 1986). Persons experiencing limitations in their mobility may have functional or environmentally induced incontinence due to their inability to maintain a tightly closed sphincter until they are able to reach a commode (Henry, 1981).

Careful assessment of the pattern of incontinence and a physical examination of the abdomen, rectum, and anal sphincter should be undertaken prior to any nursing intervention for incontinence. After a complete history and physical examination, further testing may be needed to determine which component of continence is affected: sensory, motor, or rectal capacity and compliance (Doughty, 1991a).

Certain pathologies can result in disruptions in intestinal elimination. The most common include bowel carcinoma, diverticulosis/diverticulitis, hemorrhoids, the inflammatory bowel diseases, ulcerative colitis and Crohn's disease, and irritable bowel syndrome. All of these disorders are characterized by alterations in bowel elimination, and they are often accompanied by bleeding, pain, anorexia, weight loss, and anemia.

BOWEL CANCER

The incidence of bowel carcinoma in the United States is second only to lung cancer, with more than 157,000 new cases each year. Every year approximately 56,000 people die in the United States from colon and rectal cancer. Yet, with early detection and prevention strategies, colorectal carcinoma is one of the most curable forms of cancer (Executive Health, 1995). The etiology of colorectal cancer is not yet understood but may include a combination of factors including genetic predisposition, autoimmune changes, and environmental factors. The most common symptoms of bowel cancer are any change in bowel habits or blood in the stool. These may be accompanied by cramping pain, distention, a palpable mass, pencil-shaped stools, or obstruction.

Barium enema and endoscopy with biopsy are used to confirm the diagnosis. Fifty percent of all colon carcinomas occur in the rectum and sigmoid colon (Daher, 1995). The American Cancer Society recommends the following preventive measures against bowel carcinoma:

- Digital rectal examination every year after age 40
- Stool blood test every year after age 50
- Proctosigmoidoscopy every 3 to 5 years after age 50, based on physician advice

People with a family history of colorectal cancer, inflammatory bowel disease, or polyps are at increased risk and may need these tests more frequently.

Treatment for bowel cancer includes surgical excision of the lesion, chemotherapy, and radiation. New surgical procedures often spare the rectum and avoid the need for colostomy surgery, which diverts the bowel to an opening on the abdomen for stool to exit the body Fig. 23–3. Figure 23–4 illustrates two procedures that provide mechanisms for containing the waste within the body. The *ileoanal reservoir* connects the small intestine to the anus, allowing for passage of waste from the body through the anus. The *Kock continent ileostomy* creates an internal pouch that is emptied by insertion of a catheter through an opening *(stoma)* in the abdominal wall. Although these procedures, and other similar surgeries, are a result of 50 years of development, they continue to carry a high complication rate and require careful consideration as treatment.

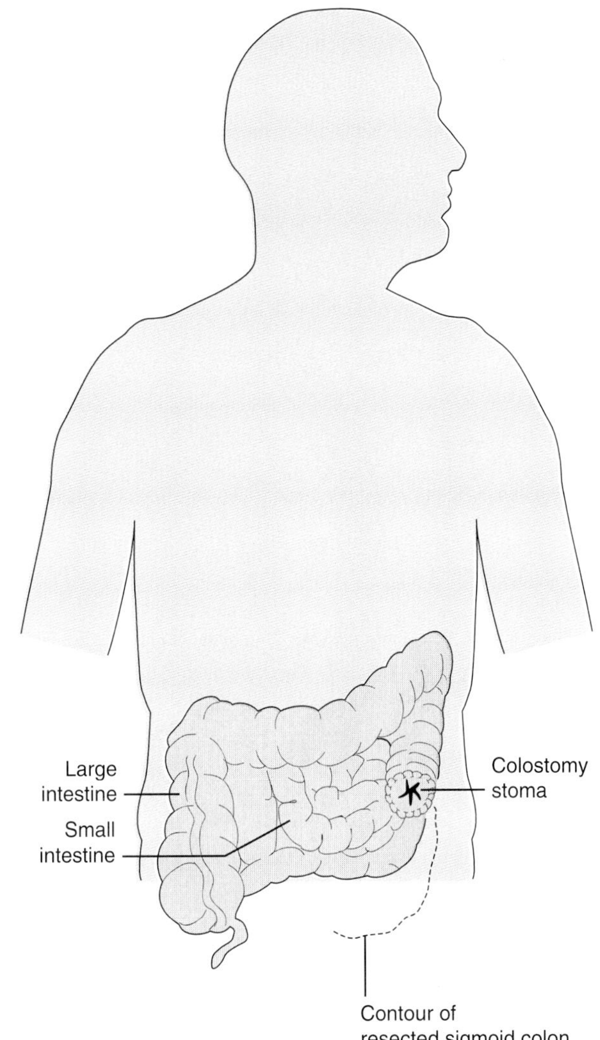

Figure 23–3. Colostomy.

DIVERTICULITIS

Diverticula are mucosal sacs that protrude outward through the bowel wall. They are usually numerous and occur most often in the sigmoid colon. When diverticula are present but not inflamed, the condition is known as diverticulosis. This condition is usually asymptomatic. Diverticulitis occurs when the sacs become inflamed, usually because of fecal material lodged within the sac. Symptoms include pain, nausea, vomiting, bleeding, fever, abdominal distention, and alternating constipation and diarrhea. This condition is usually associated with high-fat, low-fiber diets and diets high in processed foods. These diets tend to decrease the transit time of stool through the large intestines, allowing for the fecal matter to adhere to the outward protruding sacs (Coellen, 1989).

Diverticular disease is confirmed by barium enema. Mild disease can be treated with dietary modifications. Severe disease may require surgical intervention to remove the inflamed bowel tissue, possibly resulting in a temporary colostomy.

HEMORRHOIDS

Dilated veins that lie beneath the anal canal lining and the perianal skin, hemorrhoids result from repeated pressure or straining. Hemorrhoidal disease affects 50% of the population over 50 and is one of the most common afflictions of Western

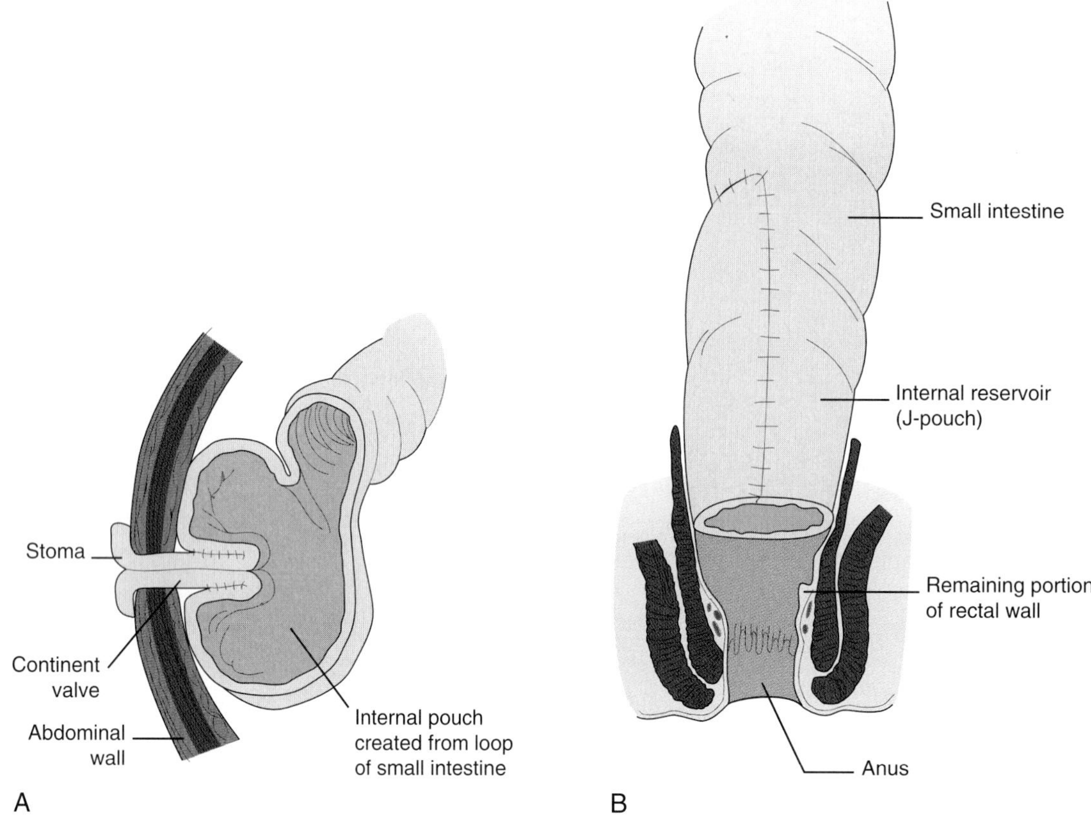

Figure 23-4. Continence-preserving surgery. **A**, Kock continent ileostomy; **B**, ileoanal resevoir.

civilization (Gyetvan et al, 1995). Common causes include habitual straining at stool, chronic constipation, and pregnancy. Signs and symptoms include bleeding from the distended veins, internal or external bulging of vessels, pain, and infection. Diagnosis is confirmed by rectal examination and proctoscopy.

Lifestyle changes can significantly improve the management of hemorrhoids. Proper cleansing following defecation, sitz baths, a nonconstipating diet high in bulk fiber, and regular exercise can all improve this condition. Topical preparations to reduce itching, swelling, and pain are also helpful. Nursing care involves teaching perineal hygiene and symptom control.

Rectal temperatures should be taken cautiously, so as not to irritate or traumatize distended rectal veins or mucosa. If conservative management of hemorrhoids fails, surgical removal by ligation or excision—hemorrhoidectomy—may be necessary. Other treatments include dilation of the anus, cryotherapy, and injection therapy.

INFLAMMATORY BOWEL DISEASE

Inflammatory bowel disease (IBD) refers to inflammatory conditions of the intestines, most notably Crohn's disease and ulcerative colitis. Although these conditions have many symptoms in common, they are significantly different and should be differentiated whenever possible. *Crohn's disease* is a chronic, relapsing disorder characterized by pain, diarrhea, fever, and weight loss. Usually the ileum is involved, but any segment of the alimentary tract may be affected. In Crohn's disease, all layers of the bowel wall (transmural) are involved. Other characteristic symptoms include nodules on the bowel that look like cobblestones, bowel obstruction or stenosis, fistulas, abscesses, and ulcerations. Systemic symptoms often accompany Crohn's disease, including arthritis, inflammatory disorders, liver or renal disorders, and skin problems. A familial tendency toward Crohn's disease is observed, and it has been suggested that the cause may be autoimmune or genetic. The estimated prevalence is 10 to 50 cases per 100,000 population (Sartor, 1995).

Diagnosis is confirmed by barium enema and endoscopy with biopsy. Medically, Crohn's disease is managed with medications. Nutritional support is indicated to provide nutrients that cannot be absorbed by the diseased bowel. This may be in the form of special feedings or intravenous nutritional supplements. If this management fails, surgical resection of the diseased portion of the intestine or an ostomy may be necessary (Bayless, 1989; Brandt and Steiner-Grossman, 1989; Steiner-Grossman et al., 1992).

Ulcerative colitis is a chronic bowel disease characterized by ulceration and inflammation of the colon and rectum. In colitis only the mucosal and submucosal layers of the bowel are involved. Symptoms range from mild to severe and include increased bowel motility, frequent diarrheal stools, fever, pain, hemorrhages of the mucosa and submucosa resulting in bloody stools, cramping, crypt abscesses, thrombi, perforation, and peritonitis. Systemic symptoms often accompany ulcerative colitis, including arthritis, biliary tract disease, uveitis, and skin problems. A familial tendency toward ulcerative colitis is observed, and it has been suggested that the cause may be autoimmune or genetic. The estimated prevalence is 40 to 100 cases per 100,000 population (Sartor, 1995).

Diagnosis is confirmed by barium enema and endoscopy with biopsy. Medical management includes control of symptoms by diet and medication.

IRRITABLE BOWEL SYNDROME

Irritable bowel syndrome (IBS) is a disorder of GI function characterized by persistent abdominal pain and alterations in bowel habits. The bowel alterations consist of chronic or episodic constipation, diarrhea, or both (Caudell, 1993). IBS accounts for approximately one half of all visits to gastroenterologists in the United States and Great Britain (Heitkemper, Sharver, and Mitchell, 1988). It is estimated to occur in 18% of the U.S. population (Caudell, 1993).

The case study at the beginning of this chapter illustrates some of the typical characteristics and symptoms of IBS. The symptoms usually present in the third and fourth decades of life, and there is a 2 : 1 greater incidence in females (Bonis and Norton, 1996). The etiology is unknown, but studies indicate that it is a syndrome that involves the entire GI tract and results from a combination of physiologic, psychological, and behavior factors. The major physiologic factors involve alterations in motility along the entire length of the GI tract and a hypersensitivity to stimuli such as stool or flatus. Psychological factors include depression and anxiety, whereas behavioral factors include irregular dietary and activity habits (Caudell, 1994).

Management of IBS remains controversial. Studies reveal conflicting results regarding dietary significance. For example, many believe that IBS is caused by a diet high in refined carbohydrates and low in dietary fiber; however, there is evidence that IBS occurred before the advent of highly refined carbohydrates (Caudell, 1994). Nurses who provide care for patients with IBS must help them to develop methods to manage their symptoms. These include stress reduction, nutritional counseling, and instituting regular patterns of meals and elimination. Stress management, including relaxation exercises, can help patients cope when exposed to a stressful situation. Nutritional counseling advises the person to avoid dairy products, gas-forming foods, highly spiced foods, coffee, and alcohol. These foods can act as irritants to the sensitive digestive tract. Additionally, fiber increases may be beneficial to those persons with frequent constipation.

Relevant Research

The amount of research related to intestinal elimination has increased in the 1990s. Much of this research has been initiated in an attempt to identify causes and cures for devastating intestinal disorders such as colon cancer and IBD (Bueno, 1993; Daher, 1995; Finne, 1991; Hillemieri, 1995; Kodner, 1993; Pierre, 1996). As the normal functioning of the GI system is more clearly understood, the management and remedy for alterations in that function become more feasible.

NURSING RESEARCH

Traditionally, nurses have taken a holistic approach to patients, concerned with the experience of the illness in a person's life and not just the illness itself. This approach is reflected in nursing research. Nursing research related to intestinal elimination spans from management of alterations to psychological and quality-of-life investigations. Considerations for patient teaching, in many instances, can be found in nursing research.

Nursing research has identified the importance of nutritional consultation in the management of alterations in intestinal elimination (Ellett et al., 1993). It has identified interventions, such as tube feedings, for alterations related to environmental factors (Smith et al., 1990). Nursing research has identified strategies to manage intestinal alterations due to disease processes such as cancer. These strategies include identifying all factors that place the patient at risk for bowel dysfunction (e.g., radiation therapy, chemotherapy, antibiotic administration, bowel resection surgery) and then treating the resulting dysfunction, such as diarrhea or constipation, with a variety of methods such as dietary manipulation, medications, and suppositories or enemas (Doughty, 1991b).

Several nursing research studies have yielded significant findings related to assessment and diagnostic tests. An early study that reviewed patients' emotional responses to undergoing barium radiography (Barnett, 1978) indicated that patients who were informed prior to receiving a barium enema reported significantly lower levels of anxiety than those patients who were not informed. With the barium swallow procedure, in contrast, there was no significant difference in response between informed patients and uninformed patients. It was suggested more recently that a patient's predisposition to acquiring information and the varying levels of desire for control need to be considered when preparing him or her for a barium enema. In another study, Pieper (1992) evaluated the physiologic effects of upper GI and barium tests. The study results indicated that physiologic symptoms were reduced through patient teaching and attending to the patient's total needs.

Nursing research studies have consistently demonstrated that informed, educated patients cope better than patients who are not informed (Blaylock, 1991; Mihalopoulos, 1996). In addition, nursing research clearly identifies the important role of the nurse in promoting adequate patient adaptation to alterations in lifestyle resulting from disruptions in elimination patterns.

The role of the nurse in reducing patient concerns and stress through education and support has been verified in a

PATIENT TEACHING
DIET AND COLON CANCER

Evidence indicates that people may reduce colon cancer risk by observing these nutritional guidelines:

- Maintain a desirable weight; persons who are 40% or more overweight increase their risk of colon cancer.
- Eat a varied diet, including plenty of vegetables and fresh fruit.
- Eat more high-fiber foods, such as whole-grain cereals, breads, and pasta.
- Daily consumption of a small dose of aspirin seems to decrease the risk of colon cancer; calcium and vitamin D may have the same effect.
- Cut down on total fat intake.
- Limit consumption of alcohol and salt-cured, smoked, and nitrite-cured food (Daher, 1995).

number of studies of persons with specific pathology: the concerns of the GI cancer patient (Coe and Kluka, 1990; Oberst and Scott, 1988; Ramer, 1992), patient stress related to IBD (Joachim, 1983; Milne et al., 1986), psychological factors associated with IBS (Caudell, 1993), and coping strategies for the ostomy patient (Gloeckner, 1994; Martinsson and Josefsson, 1991; Mihalopoulos et al., 1996; Reaume and Gooding, 1991; Ramer, 1992; Wade, 1990).

The importance of promoting independence and facilitating self-care has been identified by nursing research as one of the optimal strategies for the ongoing care of most people with alterations in intestinal elimination (Blaylock 1991; Ewing, 1989; Trainor, 1982). Nursing research supports the theory that promotion of independence and ability to maintain usual lifestyle contributes to a person's overall quality of life. The successful management of alterations in intestinal elimination can significantly affect this ability.

RESEARCH FROM OTHER FIELDS

Medical research has had a major impact on knowledge of disease process and ultimately treatment and management. Studies have revealed information regarding the normal function and motility of the GI system (Bassotti et al., 1995; Bueno, 1993; Proano et al., 1990). In addition to understanding the neurohormonal aspects of control of intestinal transit (Bueno and Fioramonti, 1994), studies have identified conditions that may alter this function, including environmental or lifestyle factors such as nicotine, which can damage GI mucosa (Endoh and Leung, 1994), and diet, particularly dietary fiber, which keeps waste material moving smoothly, allowing absorption without slowing transit (Hillemeier, 1995).

The study of IBD and IBS has made some significant progress (Toosan et al., 1995). Studies of IBD suggest genetic susceptibility and inflammatory mediator profiles (Sartor, 1995). Although the actual cause and precise immunoregulatory defects are not known, research offers the promise of being able to identify genetically susceptible hosts and, one hopes, triggering events that will enable early treatment and delay of devastating complications (Sartor, 1995).

Despite extensive research, the pathophysiology underlying IBS remains a mystery (Green, 1995). Several areas of investigation suggest that there are measurable differences between persons with IBS and those without the disorder (Green, 1995; Sartor, 1995). These areas are alteration in bowel motility (Garard and Farthing, 1994), GI hypersensitivity to pain (Mayer and Gebhart, 1994), and stress and the connection with neurohormones and the brain (Baber et al., 1989; Farthing, 1995; Svensson, 1987).

The research related to colon cancer has yielded means to identify the disease at an early phase. When detected and treated early, the average 5-year survival rate is 90 percent (Daher, 1995). Although early detection is important, research related to prevention of colon cancer indicates that there is much a person can do to decrease the risk of developing this disease (Daher, 1995; Endoh and Leung, 1994). In the 1990s, research has shown that diet and other environmental factors play a predominant role in the development of colon and rectal cancer (Daher, 1995; Finne, 1991) (see Patient Teaching). In addition, surgical techniques have im-

PATIENT TEACHING
PROMOTING HEALTHY INTESTINAL ELIMINATION

For promotion of overall healthy intestinal elimination, encourage patients to follow these guidelines:

- Minimize highly processed foods, such as frozen dinners and fast foods.
- Maintain a regular schedule for meals. Sit down and eat meals in a relaxed and unhurried atmosphere.
- Drink 6–8 glasses of noncaffeinated fluids each day.
- Establish a pattern of daily moderate exercise such as a brisk 10-minute walk.
- Remain within easy assessibility to a bathroom for 1 hour after meals to facilitate response to the normal physiologic urge to defecate after eating. Try not to suppress this normal urge.
- Avoid overusing laxatives.

proved and treatment, including radiation, chemotherapy, and biotherapy, holds promise of increasing survival for cancer patients (Finne, 1991; Kodner, 1993; Rieger, 1994).

Relevant Theory

Theoretical concepts important to intestinal elimination are those concerned with promoting normal patterns of elimination. The concept of dietary importance continues to be demonstrated in research studies, but certain pathologic conditions are yielding conflicting results related to diet—for example, the controversy over processed foods and irritable bowel (Caudell, 1994). The theoretical concepts of promoting regularity of bowel movements through regular, healthy eating and elimination practices and providing private, accessible toilet facilities guide management and intervention strategies related to alterations in intestinal elimination. The theoretical concept of regularity as a daily bowel movement, although inaccurate, is accepted by most people in the United States. This concept, driven and promoted by media advertising, causes undo concern and stress and may even cause physical and functional impairment as a person strives to achieve this accepted "regularity."

Another, as yet unproven, theoretical concept that can be damaging is the belief that IBS is strictly a psychological disorder. Although studies demonstrate psychological aspects associated with the condition, it does not constitute the entire etiology (Sartor, 1995). Belief that this condition is purely psychological not only adds stress to the patient but may also delay interventions such as diet changes that may help.

FACTORS AFFECTING CLINICAL DECISIONS

Various factors can affect clinical decisions regarding elimination. Some of these factors alter expectations, whereas others include assumptions or particular ritual regarding the eliminative process.

Age

Age affects the character and control of fecal elimination and, consequently, the expectation for bowel function. Infants are unable to control their elimination until the neuromuscular system is developed, which normally occurs at age 2 to 3 years. The development of the neuromuscular system and the child's growing ability to correlate actions with response make bowel training possible. This correlation of action and response occurs in stages:

- Awareness of discomfort created by incontinent bowel movement
- Identification that the elimination function is the reason for the discomfort
- Awareness of the body sensation that indicates a need for defecation
- Desire to avoid the discomfort caused by involuntary defecation

Bowel training, commonly called *toilet training,* is successful as it follows these stages. The methods used to accomplish this training vary, but they must incorporate the involvement of a significant person in the child's life. Communication between the child and this person is paramount, along with the child's desire to please this person. Daytime bowel control is usually attained by age 30 months.

Although loss of bowel control is common in the elderly, it is not a normal consequence of aging. Decreased muscle tone and decreased control over the anal sphincter muscles can result in an urgency to defecate, but incontinence is not a necessary result. This symptom should be diagnosed and appropriately treated (Doughty, 1992).

Gender

Pregnancy often results in alterations in bowel elimination due to increased intra-abdominal pressure and hormone changes and may result in urgency, constipation, hemorrhoids, or a combination thereof (Baron et al., 1993). Many women experience diarrhea during their menstrual cycles. Women with endometriosis may experience cyclic bouts of diarrhea, constipation, or both (Heitkemper et al., 1988). Women are twice as likely as men to suffer from IBS (Caudell, 1994).

Individual and Family Values

EDUCATIONAL BACKGROUND AND SOCIOECONOMIC STATUS

A person's educational background and socioeconomic status can have an effect on clinical decisions regarding elimination. To ensure the patient's understanding of health teaching, the nurse must know and present information at a level relative to the patient's comprehension. For many people, an adequate understanding of GI functioning can be based on simplified anatomy and physiology. Simple diagrams depicting the movement of food through the alimentary tract can be used for instruction with most people.

CULTURE AND ETHNICITY

Culture and ethnic backgrounds affect many of the intrinsic and extrinsic factors and determine many practices of daily living that can influence intestinal elimination. For example, the choice of diet is often culturally determined and deeply ingrained. Different cultures approach the act of fecal elimination differently. In some societies, defecation is performed sitting; in other cultures it is performed squatting. Toilet facilities reflect these cultural differences. Middle Eastern people squat over floor-level openings and expect to find water to cleanse with

CLINICAL DECISION MAKING

Nancy Waller, the patient in the case study at the beginning of this chapter, is concerned about her diagnosis of irritable bowel syndrome. She is concerned that her family and friends will think "it's all in her head." She is also concerned about her ability to manage her condition. She feels that she has little time to devote to altering her diet and states she has no ability to alter her lifestyle. She must work and this has a direct affect on her stress, time, energy, and eating habits. In addition, her family is used to meals based on red meat and very little fiber. Unable to prepare two separate meals, she wonders how she will manage.

The clinical decisions for this patient involved teaching lifestyle adaptations without causing her additional stress and anxiety. This includes basic education regarding irritable bowel syndrome and the fact that management is individual and may take time to determine. Dietary changes will need to be made, and with the help of a dietician and some literature, changes can be made that can be modified so that the preparation of one meal will be acceptable to her family and therapeutic for her.

Instruction in stress-reduction techniques is indicated in this situation. When considering the management of this patient's condition, all aspects must be accounted for: physical, psychological (stress), financial (the need to work), and lifestyle, which includes her relationship with family and friends.

after defecation, instead of toilet paper. In most cultures, privacy during defecation is practiced and valued. Additionally, most cultures have a strong taboo about the discussion of fecal elimination. Denial of problems and failure to seek help are common consequences of these cultural attitudes.

Regularity, defined by some as a daily bowel movement, is valued and promoted in Western culture. Advertisements suggest that the way to achieve regularity is by the use of over-the-counter products. This has led to the overuse and abuse of these products by many people.

Throughout the world, different cultures have developed unique approaches to handling elimination problems. Many of these methods incorporate herbs, whole grains, and other products such as sprouts, seaweeds, fruits, vegetables, and soured milk products (yogurt, kefir, buttermilk, and whey).

Special enemas have been used throughout history to facilitate elimination. Folk healers continue to recommend the use of honey, molasses, chamomile, or fenugreek in enema preparations. The use of garlic for intestinal disorders dates back to the ancient Egyptians and Babylonians. Today garlic is used in many parts of the world for treating constipation. Allicin in garlic stimulates peristalsis. Garlic is also known to be antibacterial.

Setting in Which Care Is Delivered

In all care settings, careful attention to the needs for privacy is a major factor in assisting persons with intestinal disruptions. In the hospital and long-term care setting, privacy can be difficult to achieve. When planning for a patient's discharge from the hospital, the setting to which he or she is returning must be carefully assessed in light of the patient's elimination needs.

In the home, the accessibility of the bathroom is an important issue. If the patient is unable to climb stairs and the bathroom is on the second floor, other accommodations such as a portable (bedside) commode must be made. With the use of a bedside commode, facilitating privacy becomes more difficult. Social services, discharge planning, and home health care agencies may be required to determine and provide essentials for care at home.

Ethical Considerations

Ethical, esthetic, and epidemiologic problems are serious concerns mostly in developing countries. Some areas of the world have inadequate elimination facilities that can result in waste material contaminating drinking water. This can lead to the spread of serious diseases such as cholera.

Epidemiologic concerns can exist in modern society as well. Disease can be spread by poor hygiene practice. This can occur in situations where facilities are inadequate or people are cared for by personnel with inadequate hygiene practices.

Ethical and esthetic concerns relate to the access to clean, private elimination facilities. Though this is mostly a concern in developing countries, once again, the lack of clean private facilities can exist anywhere. These ethical, esthetic, and epidemiologic issues must be considered in clinical decisions. The nurse must attempt to address these issues and implement measures to provide access to elimination facilities, adequate hygiene, and privacy.

Financial Considerations

Financial considerations are important when the patient needs to purchase medications or supplies in order to manage intestinal alterations. This concern is most common for persons with ostomies. The total cost for ostomy supplies averages around $1000 per year.

FUTURE DEVELOPMENTS

With improved diagnostic testing and better-informed consumers of health care, many disorders of the GI tract are being detected earlier. The result has been fewer surgeries and better outcomes for many people (Daher, 1995; Executive Health,

1995; Kodner, 1993). Because of a strong push by health care professionals and community service organizations, information and materials about preventive health practices are being widely distributed. One hopes that increased screening for colon cancer will result in reduced rates of the disease.

New surgical techniques, such as plastic surgery for fecal incontinence and the development of an artificial sphincter, hold great promise for restoring continence (Madoff et al., 1992). In addition, continued improvement of surgical techniques to maintain continence in persons without colons or rectums is improving the quality of life for many patients (Weiss and Wexner, 1995).

Medical research continues to investigate the causes of colon cancer and other GI diseases. New discoveries related to the genetic link for colon cancer and IBD can significantly affect the treatment of these disorders. Although the etiology of IBS has yet to be determined, continued study in this area is leading toward an understanding of the pathology. This could result in better, more reliable management of this distressing condition (Bonis and Norton, 1996).

New technical developments, such as polymer-filled, super-absorbent products, make containment more effective. Ergonomically designed bedside commodes have recently appeared in the marketplace. An inflatable bedpan, which can easily be positioned under the patient in the deflated mode, then inflated with the patient in position, allows one caregiver to assist the patient with ease.

NURSING CARE ACTIONS

Principles and Practices

Principles, both research-based and non–research-based (tradition, culture), are the basis for all nursing actions. In relation to intestinal elimination, the principles based on the structure and function of the GI system and the cultural considerations surrounding the eliminative process guide nursing interventions.

ASSESSMENT

An assessment of the patient's usual elimination pattern reveals whether or not the person is experiencing an alteration in his or her pattern. This is based on the principle of normal individual patterns of elimination. Recent changes in bowel functioning may be significant.

The use or abuse of laxatives should be determined. This can cause severe problems with elimination. Understanding the normal functioning of the intestines and the effect of laxatives determines the nurse's ability to educate the patient regarding the use of these substances.

An abdominal assessment can provide clues to any intestinal abnormality. Abdominal assessment includes visual inspection of the abdomen to observe for distention or visible peristalsis. This is performed with the patient lying flat. Auscultation with a stethoscope should be performed daily to evaluate the quantity and quality of bowel sounds. (See Chapter 15, Patient Assessment, for details on how to auscultate for bowel sounds.) Auscultation is performed in all four quadrants of the abdomen. The absence of bowel sounds may indicate an ileus. Extremely high-pitched sounds may indicate an obstruction.

Rectal examination, usually performed by a physician, nurse practitioner, or clinical nurse specialist, involves inserting a lubricated, gloved finger beyond the anal sphincter. Sphincter tone can be evaluated, low rectal masses palpated, and stool specimens obtained. Patients are usually positioned in a side-lying position. Deep breathing and relaxation can ease the discomfort of the exam. See Chapter 15, Patient Assessment, for more details on performing a rectal examination.

FACILITATION OF NORMAL ELIMINATION

Providing for a patient's elimination needs encompasses both scientific and cultural principles. To facilitate the normal eliminative process and to meet the primary needs, a number of nursing actions must be employed. Bedpans are receptacles used to collect waste when a person is unable to get out of bed and go to the bathroom. A portable or bedside commode can be used for patients who can get out of bed but cannot reach the toilet. Raised toilet seats can be obtained for patients who can reach the toilet but who have difficulty lowering themselves down onto the seat. Plastic bedpans can be kept from sticking to the skin and causing friction trauma by lightly sprinkling them with cornstarch prior to positioning them under the patient. Toilet paper, disposable wet wipes, or washclothes and towels should be provided for clean-up after defecation.

ENSURING PRIVACY

Attention to privacy and comfortable positioning are of the utmost importance. The call light should be placed within easy reach of the patient whenever the nurse leaves the room to provide privacy.

CLEANSING

When removing a bedpan or emptying the container of a bedside commode, universal precautions should always be followed. Because of the possibility of exposure to body fluids, nonsterile gloves must be worn. Receptacles are rinsed with water, detergents are used as necessary, and then receptacles are dried and stored within reach of the patient. Hand washing for the patient and the nurse is the last step in the process.

The skin should be cleansed as soon after defecation as possible. Warm water and soap are adequate, although the newer pH-balanced cleansers are preferable, especially with frequent incontinence that predisposes a patient's skin to irritation (Krasner, 1990). To protect the skin, moisturizing lotions and moisture barrier ointments such as A & D ointment or zinc oxide may be used. For some patients with severe, liquid fecal incontinence, fecal collectors can be applied to collect and contain the stool. These collectors are plastic pouches with pectin-based wafers that adhere to the perianal skin. Other containment methods involve the use of absorbent briefs or diapers. New products on the market more closely resemble undergarments and thus maintain the patient's dignity.

INSTITUTING A BOWEL PROGRAM

To regulate defecation in patients who cannot eliminate regularly because of neurologic or other deficits, bowel programs or bowel retraining can be implemented. This involves assessing the person's defecation pattern for several days to 1 week. After this, the first action is to assist the patient onto the commode prior to the time defecation is expected. Additional actions are then employed to encourage defecation to occur at this time: providing a drink of hot coffee or tea to stimulate peristalsis, administering oral stool softeners daily, or administering a suppository 30 minutes prior to expected defecation time. Bowel retraining requires patience; these actions may continue for several weeks before defecation is regulated.

Procedures

ADMINISTERING A CLEANSING ENEMA

For many diagnostic tests of the intestines, including endoscopic and radiologic examinations, visualization depends on an empty intestine. Traditionally, a series of enemas or solutions instilled into the lower bowel, laxatives, or cathartics are given to thoroughly cleanse the bowel. Procedure 23–1 describes how to administer a cleansing enema.

OBTAINING A STOOL SPECIMEN

Stool specimens are sometimes evaluated in the laboratory for bacterial content, fat, foreign bodies, or blood. A single specimen or all of the fecal matter excreted within a 24-hour period may be required. Specimens should be collected in a plastic container, with a lid, and must be uncontaminated by urine. Procedure 23–2 details the steps involved in collecting a stool specimen and testing it for the presence of occult (hidden) blood.

PROVIDING OSTOMY CARE

Surgical diversion or bypasses of the large or small intestine are frequently required in the presence of bowel pathology. A *colostomy* is created when an end of the colon is exteriorized on the abdominal surface. The exteriorized end is referred to as a *stoma.* An *ileostomy* is created when an end of the small intestine (the ileum) is exteriorized on the abdominal surface. Temporary ostomies are common after traumatic injury, whereas permanent ostomies are frequently performed for cancer, ulcerative colitis, or congenital defects.

Stool patterns of ostomies differ according to location. The more large bowel that the person retains, the more formed the stool will be. The output from an ileostomy is liquid and continuous because the person has no large bowel for fluid absorption.

Persons with ostomies wear plastic pouches to contain the waste. Today most pouches are disposable and adhere to the skin with an adhesive gelatin wafer. Care must be taken to keep the *peristomal skin,* skin around the stoma, clean and protected. Most people accomplish this with the use of soap and water at the time of pouch change. Some people with very low colostomies who have retained most of their large intestines can regulate their bowel movements with diet and irrigation or an enema through the stoma, and will not wear a pouch.

A balanced diet with adequate fluid intake (8–10 8-oz. glasses a day) is important for all persons with intestinal ostomies. For persons with colostomies, a diet with fiber foods, both soluble and insoluble, helps maintain normal bowel activity. Food tolerances and sensitivities must be assessed. Fiber-rich foods must be added gradually to the diet, and the patient must avoid excessive amounts at any one meal—which may cause increased flatulence (gas) or a high volume output of stool (Price, 1995).

Persons with ileostomies must be more cautious with their diets. Adequate fluid intake and foods high in electrolytes are recommended. Never delete salt from their diet. One of the main functions of the colon is to absorb fluid and electrolytes. It takes time for the small bowel to adapt to the loss of the

BOX 23-1
COMMUNITY RESOURCES FOR PERSONS WITH OSTOMIES

American Cancer Society (ACS)
1599 Clifton Road NE
Atlanta, GA 30329
1-800-ACS-2345

Crohn's & Colitis Foundation of America, Inc. (CCFA)
444 Park Avenue South
New York, NY 10016-7374
1-800-343-3637
212-685-3440 for NY

United Ostomy Association, Inc. (UOA)
36 Executive Park
Suite 120
Irvine, CA 92714-6744
800-826-0826

Wound, Ostomy, and Continence Nurses Society, An Association of ET Nurses (WOCN, formerly IAET)
2755 Bristol Street
Suite 110
Costa Mesa, CA 92626
714-476-0268

colon and to take over some of the large intestine's functions. For this reason, electrolyte balance through food and fluid consumption is critical.

Persons with illeostomies should limit fats and insoluble-fiber foods. Their diet may contain some soluble fibers, starting with small amounts. Some persons with ileostomies are prone to food blockage in the stoma. This occurs when insoluble fiber or coarse food travels quickly through the GI system and is not digested upon excretion from the body. To prevent this, the person should chew all foods well, drink plenty of fluids, and avoid foods that may cause a problem, such as raw vegetables, popcorn, and nuts (Price, 1995).

Infants and children with ostomies and their parents have special learning needs and concerns. Referral to specialized support groups is often helpful.

Nurses are very involved with assisting the ostomy patient to adjust to this alteration in eliminative functioning. Along with providing care for the ostomy appliance and site, counseling, education, and referrals to support groups are important aspects of the nursing role. Box 23–1 lists support organizations for patients with ostomies. Procedure 23–3 details the steps involved in changing an ostomy pouch; Procedure 23–4 explains how to irrigate a colostomy.

PROCEDURE 23-1

Administering an Enema

Objective

Administer prescribed solution into the colon for the purpose of removing feces, stimulating peristalsis, or administering medication.

Terminology

- **Enema:** the introduction of a solution into the rectum and sigmoid colon to remove feces, flatus, or both.
- **Hypertonic:** having an osmotic pressure greater than that of the solution with which it is compared.
- **Osmotic pressure:** amount of pressure necessary to stop flow of water across a membrane.

Critical Elements

Enemas are administered by physician's order.

Many enemas come commercially prepared. Always read the manufacturer's recommendations prior to use. Some commercially prepared disposable enemas are hypertonic solutions (having a greater osmotic pressure than that of body fluids). Their action is to distend the colon and rectum and to irritate the mucous membranes, thus stimulating peristalsis. The amount of solution is only about 120 ml. Because it is hypertonic, it draws fluid into the bowel from the circulation, thus increasing the fluid volume in the colon and rectum.

Liquid castile soap should be used (no more than 5 ml/1000 ml water) for a soap-suds enema.

Tap water and normal saline solutions are commonly used for enemas for adults but should not be used for infants because of the danger of electrolyte imbalance. Repeated tap water or saline enemas in adults can result in water absorption in the colon with the possibility of fluid overload and electrolyte imbalance. For the saline, tap water, and cleansing enemas, the volume administered is 500–1000 ml.

Some enemas are given for the purpose of administering medication such as sodium polystyrene (Kayexalate), neomycin, or steroid preparations.

Other retention enemas are given for the purpose of softening stool (oil) or promote the expelling of flatus (milk and molasses).

When enemas are prepared, the temperature of the solution should be 105–110° Fahrenheit (40.5°–43° Celsius). The solution should be prepared just prior to administering so that the temperature remains warm.

All air should be purged from the tubing prior to administration so that no air is administered into the colon. For nonretention enemas, the patient should be encouraged to hold the solution at least 10 minutes. Retention enemas (those meant to soften stool or for medication administration) should be held 20–30 minutes.

If any obstruction is encountered upon insertion of the tube, it should be withdrawn and reported.

For most enemas, the container of solution should be no higher than 12 inches above the level of the bed. The higher the container, the greater the force with which the solution flows into the patient. If the solution infuses too rapidly it can cause abdominal cramping. The solution should take about 15 minutes per 1000 ml of fluid.

continued on next page

PROCEDURE 23-1 (cont'd)

Contaminated disposable and reusable equipment should be cleansed or discarded properly according to the infection control policy of the facility.

Equipment (Fig. 23–5)

- Gloves
- Enema bag with solution prepared as ordered or commercially prepared enema product
- Lubricant
- Bed protector underpad
- Bedpan or commode (if necessary)
- Bath thermometer

Special Considerations

Patients should be positioned for safety and comfort. Privacy should be provided during this procedure unless it is dangerous to leave the patient alone. The call light should always be left within the patient's reach.

The patient's ability to safely and independently go to the bathroom should be assessed. If ambulating independently is not safe, a bedpan or bedside commode may be required. It may also be necessary for the nurse to accompany the patient to the bathroom.

It should be remembered that repeated enemas can be very tiring to the patient. Therefore if "enemas until clear" are ordered, do not give more than three enemas. If the return is not clear at that time, notify the physician for further instructions. Repeated enemas may also irritate hemorrhoids and possibly cause vagal stimulation with resultant cardiac problems.

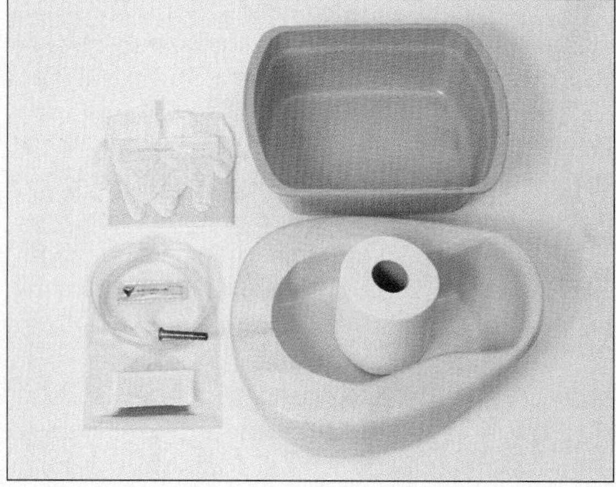

Figure 23–5. Equipment for an enema.

Action	*Rationale*
1. Verify order.	1. Ensures that correct procedure is performed
2. Assemble and prepare equipment.	2. Promotes task organization.
3. Identify patient.	3. Promotes patient safety.
4. Explain procedure to patient, including deep breathing to be used in case of abdominal cramping.	4. Promotes patient compliance.
5. Close door/curtain.	5. Provides privacy.
6. Don gloves.	6. Protects patient care provider from contact with body fluids.
7. Assist patient to a left lateral position.	7. Provides best anatomic position for flow of fluid into descending colon.
8. Place bed protector under patient's buttocks.	8. Provides protection from soiling bed linens.
9. Lubricate first 4–6 inches of tube with water-soluble lubricant, then insert tube smoothly and slowly into rectum after informing patient (Fig. 23–6).	9. Facilitates insertion of tube through anal sphincter.

continued on next page

PROCEDURE 23-1 (cont'd)

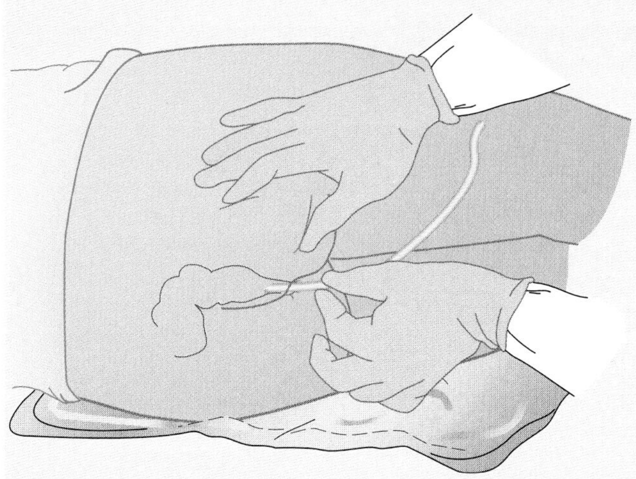

Figure 23–6. Inserting a rectal tube.

10. Instill solution: • When using an enema bag, by opening clamp on tubing and holding bag about 12 inches above bed. • When using a commercially prepared product, by squeezing or otherwise emptying product by manufacturer's recommendations.	10. Instills solution into colon.
11. After solution has been administered, clamp tubing (if using an enema bag) and remove from anal opening.	11. Prevents backflow of solution into empty container.
12. Advise patient on length of time to hold enema and leave call light within reach of patient.	12. Promotes patient safety.
13. Assist patient to bathroom, commode, or bedpan as necessary. If using toilet, instruct not to flush. Assist back to bed when finished.	13. Promotes patient safety.
14. Assess enema results.	14. Ensures accurate evaluation of effectiveness of procedure.
15. Assist patient to position of comfort.	15. Promotes patient comfort.
16. Return or discard equipment as necessary.	16. Promotes clean, organized work space.

Documentation

Record in the patient record the type and amount of enema administered. Note the patient's response to the procedure, including any assessment of the results.

Elements of Patient Teaching

Instruct patient and family as to the purpose of the enema(s). Instruct the patient to call when ready to evacuate the enema and to not flush the toilet until the care provider has assessed the results. Also inform the patient that he or she may have additional results from the enema for the next few hours.

PROCEDURE 23-2

Collecting a Stool Sample and Measuring Occult Blood

Objective

Identify presence or absence of occult blood in the stool.

Terminology

- **Occult blood:** blood that is not grossly visible in the specimen.

Critical Elements

This test is usually performed in response to physician order; however, in some facilities it may be initiated because of nursing judgment. Review the policy of your facility.

Gastrointestinal bleeding may be intermittent. Because of this it is recommended that hemoccult testing be performed on three consecutive stool specimens. Contamination of the specimen by menstrual blood or blood from hemorrhoids may give a false-positive result on this test. Stool specimens should be prevented from being contaminated with urine because this too can lead to an inaccurate reading.

Equipment

- Hemoccult test kit
- Gloves
- Specimen container
- Tongue blade

Special Considerations

Always review the expiration date on both the paper and the solution in your test kit. Never use expired products. Read manufacturer's instructions prior to using product.

If the patient is unable to defecate, the specimen may be obtained by digital examination. Presence of any blue coloring on the card while reading indicates a positive result.

Action	*Rationale*
1. Verify order.	1. Ensures proper procedure.
2. Assemble equipment.	2. Organizes work and facilitates task.
3. Identify patient.	3. Promotes patient safety.
4. Explain procedure.	4. Promotes patient compliance.
5. Collect specimen in specimen container.	5. Provides specimen in an uncontaminated holder.
6. Don clean gloves.	6. Protects care provider from contact with potential contamination.
Collecting a Specimen in a Container	
7. Smear specimen on appropriate spots on card using a tongue blade.	7. Provides specimen for testing.
Collecting a Specimen Using a Digital Examination	
8. Insert gloved finger into rectal area and smear stool from examination glove on appropriate spots on card (Fig. 23–7).	8. Provides specimen for testing using digital examination method.

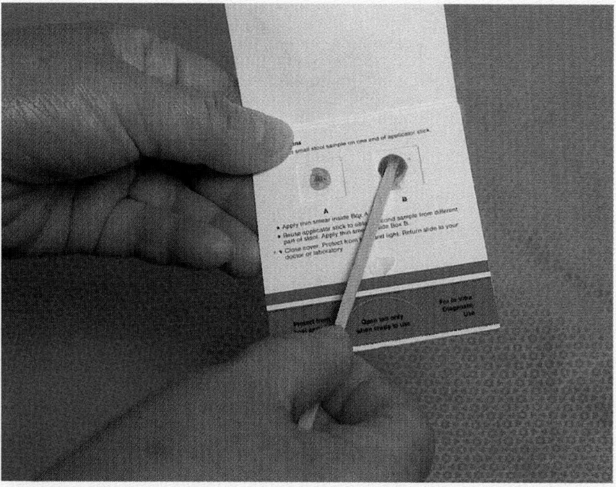

Figure 23–7. Applying smear of stool on Hemoccult slide.

continued on next page

PROCEDURE 23-2 (cont'd)

9. Remove exam glove, discard, and reapply new examination glove.	9. Prevents transmission of organisms to other clean areas.
10. Close card, turn card over, and open back developing window.	10. Provides access to section of card used for applying developing solution.
11. Apply developing solution per manufacturer's instructions, wait 30 seconds, and read.	11. Completes the developing process.
12. Discard equipment in appropriate container.	12. Promotes an organized and clean work area.
13. Wash hands.	13. Prevents transmission of organisms.

Documentation

Report test results to the appropriate person. Record test results and reporting of test results in the patient record. Record a complete description of the stool specimen, including amount, color, and consistency.

Elements of Patient Teaching

Explain to patient and family the purpose of the test as well as the instructions for collecting the specimen.

PROCEDURE 23-3

Pouching a Colostomy or Ileostomy

Objective

Provide a means to contain stool while protecting the peristomal area from skin breakdown.

Terminology

- **Peristomal area:** the skin immediately surrounding the stoma.
- **Colostomy:** an opening in the colon that provides a temporary diversion of stool or a permanent means to evacuate the bowel.
- **Ileostomy:** a permanent opening in the ileum portion of the bowel that provides for evacuation of the bowel after removal of the colon.
- **Stoma:** an artificial opening made in an internal organ, bringing it to the surface.
- **Mucocutaneous line:** the incisional line where the stoma is attached to skin.
- **Wafer:** portion of pouch that adheres to skin.

Critical Elements

The proper fitting of the ostomy pouch around the stoma is critical. Use the correct size of appliance. The stomal opening should be cut not more than ⅛ inch larger than the stoma to fit properly.

Change the appliance regularly to avoid leakage and skin irritation. Any excrement that comes in contact with skin will cause itching and burning if not removed quickly, causing skin irritation.

An appliance may be left in place as long as a proper seal is maintained around the stoma. The stoma should be assessed each time the wafer is changed or the bag is emptied. A new stoma shrinks dramatically in size during the first 6 months.

Assess the stoma every 4 hours during the first postoperative day and daily for 1 week postoperatively. Immediately report any color change in stoma. Dark purple, black, or pale color may indicate impaired circulation to the area.

Keep a record of daily output.

A variety of ostomy appliances are available that patients may want to try before deciding on the type that meets their long-term needs. Watch for sensitivities and allergies to adhesive or pouch material. They can develop days, weeks, or years after use of a product. Initially, while the size of the stoma is changing, the patient will want to use a cut-to-fit appliance. Eventually, a premeasured ostomy appliance may be more appropriate for use.

continued on next page

PROCEDURE 23-3 (cont'd)

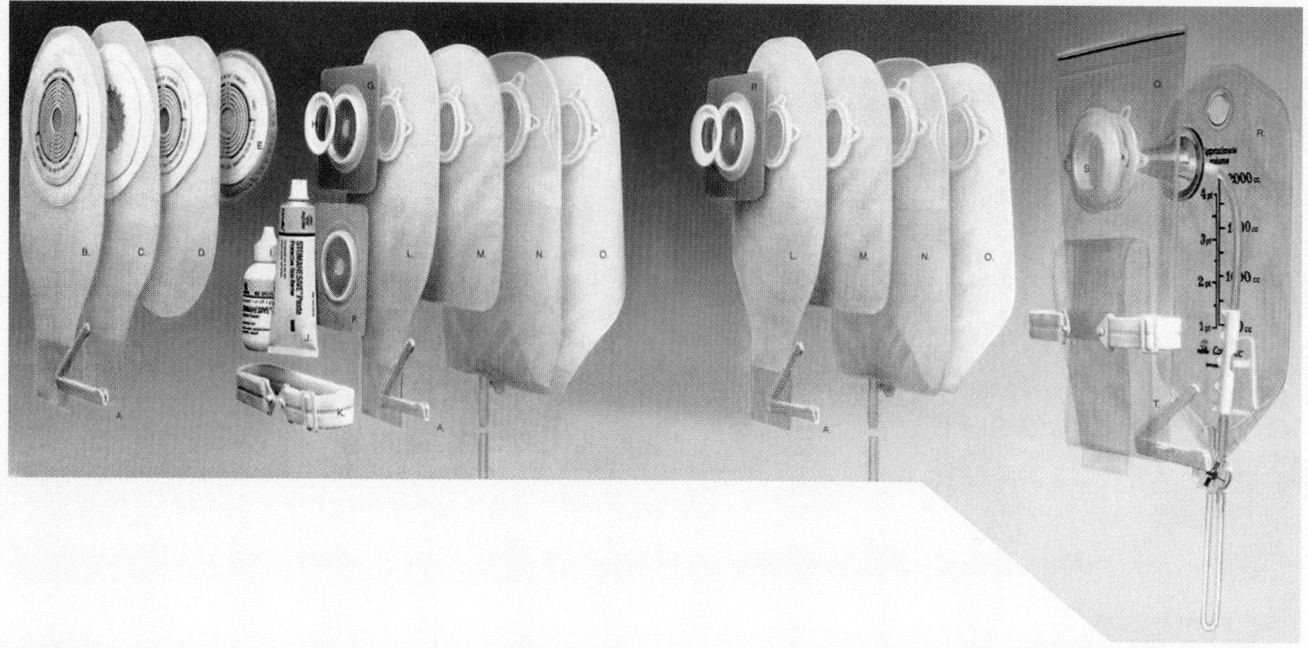

Figure 23–8. Equipment for ostomy pouching. These are examples of the various types of colostomy equipment that patients may use. *A*, Active Life/Sur-Fit Tail Closure; *B*, Active Life One-Piece Drainable Custom Pouch; *C*, Active Life One-Piece Drainable Pouch with precut openings; *D*, Active Life One-Piece Closed-End Pouch; *E*, Active Life One-Piece Stoma Cap; *F*, Sur-Fit Flexible; *G*, Stomahesive Wafer with Sur-Fit Flange; *H*, Sur-Fit Disposable Convexinsert; *I*, Stomahesive Protective Powder; *J*, Stomahesive Paste; *K*, Adjustable Belt; *L*, Sur-Fit Drainable Pouch; *M*, Sur-Fit Closed-End Pouch; *N*, Sur-Fit Urostomy Pouch; *O*, Sur-Fit Urostomy Pouch with Accuseal Tap; *P*, Durahesive Wafer with Flange; *Q*, Sur-Fit Irrigation Sleeve; *R*, Visi-Flow Irrigation System; *S*, Sur-Fit Adapter Faceplate; *T*, Sur-Fit Irrigation Sleeve Tail Closure. (Courtesy of Convatec, Princeton, NJ.)

Equipment (Fig. 23–8)

- Stoma measuring guide
- Ostomy appliance (with clip if necessary)
- Skin barrier paste
- Washcloth and soap
- Gloves
- Skin cleanser (optional)
- Skin preparation wipes (optional)
- Scissors
- Hy-tape (optional)

Special Considerations

The ostomy appliance should be changed immediately if the patient complains of itching or burning or if leaking is noted. The pouch should be emptied when one-third to one-half full. Allowing the pouch to become too full may cause the seal to loosen.

Never use cream or ointment (other than the ostomy skin preparation products) on the peristomal area.

The appliance may be changed most easily when the bowel is quiet, such as in the early morning or 2 to 4 hours after a meal. If the patient is on bedrest, the pouch should be angled over to the patient's side so as to facilitate drainage.

Ostomy patients should be monitored for possible nutritional problems, fluid and electrolyte imbalance, skin breakdown at the peristomal area, and weight change.

The patient should be allowed to express his or her feelings regarding the change in body image. The patient care provider should have a positive, accepting attitude that may help the patient with acceptance of this change.

Action	*Rationale*
1. Gather supplies.	1. Organizes work.
2. Identify patient.	2. Promotes patient safety.
3. Explain procedure.	3. Promotes patient compliance.

continued on next page

PROCEDURE 23-3 (cont'd)

4. Position patient as flat as possible with protective bed pad under the patient.

4. Provides flat access to peristomal area and protects bed.

5. Don gloves.

5. Provides protection for patient care provider from contact with patient body fluids.

6. Remove pouch by grasping inner upper corner of appliance with dominant hand, gently peeling back appliance while pressing downward on skin with nondominant hand (you may want to use a moistened 4 × 4 when pressing down on skin in order to assist in loosening the appliance) (Fig. 23–9). *Note:* save the clamp if appliance has this type of closure.

6. Provides means to remove pouch while guarding against spills and protecting skin.

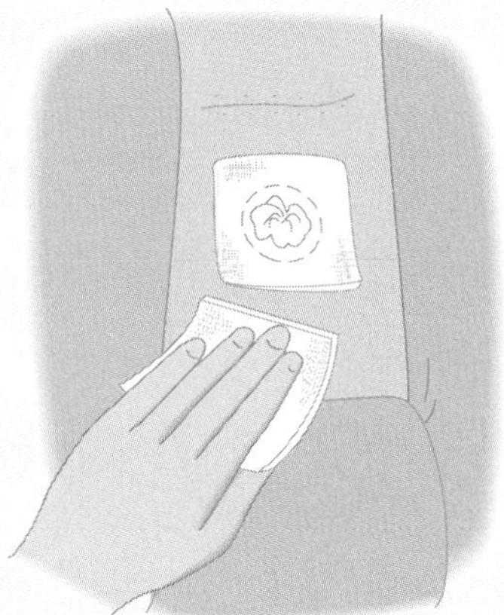

Figure 23–9. Gently remove the old pouch, and clean the peristomal area with moist gauze.

7. Assess skin, stoma, and mucocutaneous line.

7. Provides opportunity to identify potential skin or stomal problems or incisional separation.

8. Cleanse the peristomal area with soap and water or skin cleanser (optional). Rinse and dry thoroughly. Apply skin preparation (optional).

8. Protects skin from irritation by any possible contamination from bowel contents.

9. Measure stoma with stoma measuring guide (Fig. 23–10). If skin barrier wafer is not the correct size, cut to size by using stoma measuring guide to trace pattern on back of wafer barrier. Then cut wafer to ⅛ inch larger than stoma.

9. Ensures good fit of appliance to stoma, therefore protecting peristomal area from potential irritation from stool.

10. Apply skin barrier paste to the back of wafer. Then apply wafer, adhesive side to skin, gently pressing to secure edges. (If wafer and pouch are separate pieces, snap pouch to wafer at this time.) (Fig. 23–11) (Fig. 23–12)

10. Provides for a secure seal between wafer and skin.

11. If pouch is open at end, apply clamp to tail of pouch, folding pouch over clip.

11. Secures closure to end of pouch until it is necessary to open and drain.

12. Return patient to position of comfort.

12. Promotes patient comfort.

13. Return or dispose of supplies in appropriate area.

13. Provides clean and organized work space.

14. Remove and dispose of gloves in appropriate container, then wash hands.

14. Prevents transmission of microorganisms from one patient to another.

continued on next page

PROCEDURE 23-3 (cont'd)

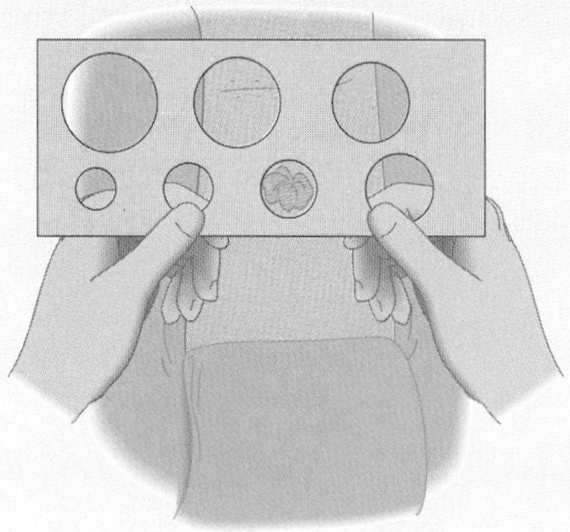

Figure 23–10. Measure the stoma with a stoma template.

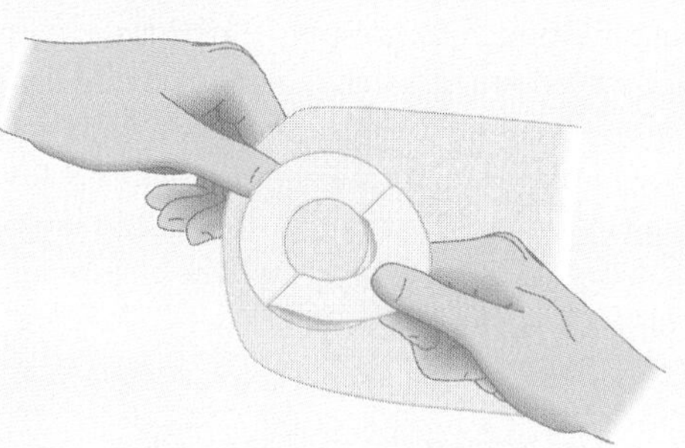

Figure 23–11. Remove backing from the adhesive surface of the disposable ostomy pouch.

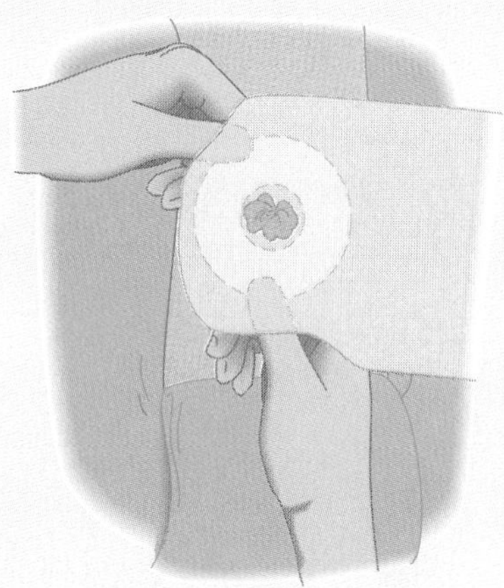

Figure 23–12. Center the pouch opening over the stoma and seal, making sure the seal is tight.

Documentation

Record change of appliance in patient record. Record the assessment of the patient's stoma, peristomal skin condition, mucocutaneous line, and amount, color, and consistency of stool. Also record patient's response to procedure, including any patient family teaching done.

Elements of Patient Teaching

Instruct patient/family in the correct steps for changing an ostomy appliance. Assist patient/family as necessary until such time as they can perform this function independently.

PROCEDURE 23-4

Irrigating a Colostomy

Objective

Stimulate peristalsis while aiding in the evacuation of the colon.

Terminology

- **Stoma:** artificial opening made in an internal organ, bringing it to the surface.
- **Colostomy irrigation:** an enema given through an ostomy into the colon.

Critical Elements

The colostomy irrigation should be performed in the bathroom if at all possible. It may, however, be performed with the patient in bed using the bedpan to collect drainage. It is preferable to perform this procedure at the same time each day. It is a clean (not sterile) procedure. For a new ostomy patient, irrigation is often performed 7–10 days after the surgery.

Irrigation of a sigmoid or descending colostomy can assist in establishing a regular evacuation pattern. Because stool in the ascending and transverse colostomies is much more liquid, it is less likely that a consistent evacuation pattern can be established. A variety of irrigation products are available so that patient choice of equipment may be individualized.

Equipment

- Irrigation appliance
- Cone/tube irrigation set
- Gloves
- Washcloth
- Soap
- Towel
- Water-soluble lubricant
- Bedpan (if procedure is performed in bed)
- Closure clip

Special Considerations

Firm stool or anxiety may make insertion of the irrigation catheter tip or cone difficult. Never force the insertion because this may cause damage to the bowel wall.

The evacuation process may take 45–60 minutes to complete. Gently massaging the abdomen or drinking warm fluids may stimulate peristalsis. If evacuation does not proceed, assess the stoma for the presence of hard stool. Use 500 ml for the first irrigation with gradual increases up to 1000 ml (unless otherwise ordered by the physician).

Action	*Rationale*
1. Verify order.	1. Ensures that proper procedure is performed.
2. Identify patient.	2. Promotes patient safety.
3. Explain procedure.	3. Promotes patient compliance.
4. Gather and prepare equipment.	4. Provides organized work area.
5. Position patient: • Sitting on toilet or chair next to toilet. • Lying supine in bed with bedpan next to patient.	5. Ensures proper positioning to complete procedure.
6. Fill irrigation bag with warm tap water and flush tubing.	6. Use of warm water helps stimulate peristalsis.
7. Don gloves.	7. Protects care provider from contact with body fluids.
8. Remove ostomy appliance.	8. Provides access to stoma.
9. Assess stoma.	9. Ensures the stoma shows sign of good circulation.
10. Gently insert lubricated gloved finger into stoma. (*Note:* Never force finger into stoma.)	10. Dilates stoma in preparation for irrigation procedure.
11. Apply irrigation sleeve putting end of sleeve into toilet (if patient is seated in bathroom) or in bedpan (if patient is in bed).	11. Prepares ostomy for irrigation.
12. Lubricate cone/catheter tip and insert into stoma. • ½ to 1 inch for cone • 4–6 inches for catheter tip (*Note:* Never force cone/catheter into stoma)	12. Provides means to deliver irrigation fluid.

continued on next page

PROCEDURE 23-4 (cont'd)

13. Holding bag 12–18 inches above stoma, allow fluid to slowly enter stoma. This should take 5–10 minutes.	13. Assists in preventing cramping that may occur if fluid is administered too quickly.
14. Remove catheter tubing/cone and clamp bottom of sleeve. Encourage patient to ambulate if possible.	14. Promotes peristalsis through movement.
15. Open clamp and drain contents after evacuation is completed.	15. Allows for drainage of bag before removal.
16. Remove sleeve, rinse it out, and hang it up to dry. Wash skin around stoma with soap and water.	16. Prevents skin breakdown by removing fecal material from skin around stoma.
17. Apply ostomy appliance.	17. Provides means to capture any fecal material from stoma.
18. Return patient to position of comfort.	18. Promotes patient comfort.
19. Return or dispose of supplies in appropriate area.	19. Provides clean and organized work space.
20. Remove and dispose of gloves in appropriate container, then wash hands.	20. Prevents transmission of microorganisms from one patient to another.

Documentation

Record procedure in patient record. Note assessment of stoma and amount of fluid used as well as amount, color, and consistency of stool. Also record the patient's response to procedure.

Elements of Patient Teaching

Explain procedure to patient and family. Allow patient/family to assist with procedure. Continue to supervise patient/family in procedure until they are independent.

CHAPTER HIGHLIGHTS

- Elimination of waste products of the digestive system from the body is essential to maintain health.
- Elimination refers to the process of excreting the body's waste and the byproducts of metabolism.
- The digestive system includes the alimentary canal (mouth, esophagus, stomach, small intestines, large intestines, rectum, and anus) and accessory organs (liver, gallbladder, and pancreas).
- A major function of the intestines is to complete the digestive process through absorption of water, nutrients, and electrolytes.
- Defecation is influenced by intrinsic and extrinsic factors. Intrinsic factors include diet, fluid intake, regularity of meals, exercise, privacy, and a regular time for defecation. Extrinsic factors include diagnostic testing, anesthesia, medications, and surgery.
- Disruptions in the intestinal tract and alterations in bowel elimination may be characterized by many different symptoms, including changes in appearance of the stool, abdominal distention and pain, constipation, diarrhea, flatus, and fecal incontinence or impaction.
- Pathological conditions of the intestinal system include carcinoma, ulcerative colitis, diverticulitis, and hemorrhoids.
- Nursing research has identified strategies to manage intestinal alterations due to disease processes.
- Nursing interventions are aimed at maintaining the person's usual pattern of bowel functioning and assisting the patient with management of any alteration in function.

REFERENCES

Baber, N.S., Dourish, C.T., Hill, D.R. (1989). The role of CCK, caerulein, and CCK antagonists in nociception. *Pain, 39,* 307–328.

Barnett, J.W. (1978). Patients' emotional response to barium x-ray. *Journal of Advanced Nursing, 3,* 37–46.

Baron, T.H., Ramirez, B., Richter, J.E. (1993). Gastrointestinal motility disorders during pregnancy. *Annals of Internal Medicine, 118* (5), 366–375.

Bassotti, G., Germani, A., Morelli, A. (1995). Human colonic motility. *International Journal of Colorectal Disease, 10* (3), 173–180.

Bayless, T.M. (1989). *Current Management of Inflammatory Bowel Disease*. Toronto: B.C. Decker.

Blaylock, B. (1991). Enhancing self-care of the elderly client: Practical tips for ostomy care. *Journal of Enterostomal Therapy Nursing, 18* (4), 118–121.

Bonis, P., Norton, R. (1996). The challenge of irritable bowel syndrome. *American Family Physician, 53* (3), 1229–1239.

Brandt, L.J., Steiner-Grossman, P. (1989). *Treating IBD: A Patient's Guide to the Medical and Surgical Management of Inflammatory Bowel Disease*. New York: Raven Press.

Broadwell, D.C., Jackson, B.S. (1982). *Principles of Ostomy Care*. St. Louis: C.V. Mosby.

Bueno, L. (1993). Involvement of brain CCK in the adoption of gut motility to digestive status and stress. *Journal of Physiology (France), 87* (5), 301–306.

Bueno, L., Fioramonti, J. (1994). Neurohormonal control of intestinal transit. *Reproductive Nutrition (France), 34* (6), 513–525.

Candy, C.E. (1987). Recent advances in the care of children with acute diarrhea: Giving responsibility to the nurse and parents. *Journal of Advanced Nursing, 12*, 95–99.

Caudell, K. (1993). Psychophysiological factors associated with irritable bowel syndrome. *Gastroenterology Nursing, 17* (2), 61–67.

Coe, M., Kluka, S. (1990). Comparisons of concerns of clients and spouses regarding ostomy surgery for treatment of cancer. *Journal of Enterostomal Therapy, 17* (3), 106–111.

Coellen, D. (1989). Understanding diverticular disease. *Journal of Enterostomal Therapy, 16* (4), 176–181.

Cox, H.C., Hinz, M.D., Lubno, M.A., et al. (1989). *Clinical Applications of Nursing Diagnosis*. Baltimore: Williams & Wilkins.

Daher, M. (1995). Worldwide cancer of the colon. *Ostomy Quarterly, 32* (4), 72–75.

Doughty, D.B. (1991a). *Urinary and Fecal Incontinence*. St. Louis: Mosby Year Book.

Doughty, D. B. (1991b). Maintaining normal bowel function in the patient with cancer. *Journal of ET Nursing, 18* (3), 90–94.

Doughty, D. (1992). A step-by-step approach to bowel training. *Progressions, 4* (2), 12–23.

Doughty, D. (1996). A physiologic approach to bowel training. *Journal of Wound, Ostomy and Continence Nursing, 23* (1), 46–56.

Endoh, K., Leung, F.W. (1994). Effects of smoking and nicotine on the gastric mucosa: A review of clinical and experimental evidence. *Gastroenterology, 107* (3), 864–878.

Ellett, M.L., Fitzgerald, J.F., Winchester, M. (1993). Dietary management of chronic diarrhea in children. *Gastroenterology Nursing*, February 170–177.

Ewing, G. (1989). The nursing preparation of stoma patients for self-care. *Journal of Advanced Nursing, 14*, 411–420.

Executive Health (1995). Social stigma of colon and rectal problems thwarts life saving cancer treatment. *Executive Health's Good Health Report, 32* (1), 1–2.

Farthing, M.J. (1995). Irritable bowel, irritable body, or irritable brain. *British Medical Journal, 310* (6973), 171–176.

Finne, C.O. (1991). Advances in colorectal cancer. *Journal of ET Nursing, 18* (3), 82–87.

Garard, D.A., Farthing, M.J. (1994). Intestinal motor function in irritable bowel syndrome. *Digestive Diseases, 12*, 72–84.

Gloeckner, M.R. (1994). Perceptions of sexual attractiveness following ostomy surgery. *Research in Nursing and Health, 7*, 87–92.

Green, D. (1995). Gut issue: The search for a bowel-distress cure. *The Financial Post, 8* (26), 86.

Guyton, A.C. (1991). *Textbook of Medical Physiology*. Philadelphia: W.B. Saunders.

Gyetvan, M.C., Schilling, O., McCann, J., Tscheschlog, B., Burlen, C. (1995). *Professional Guide To Diseases*. Springhouse, PA: Springhouse Corporation.

Hampton, B.G., Bryant, R.A. (1992). *Ostomies and Continent Diversions*. St. Louis: Mosby Year Book.

Handerhan, B. (1991). Protecting your patient from ileus. *Nursing 91*, April, 92–95.

Harari, D. (1994). Constipation: assessment and management in an institutionalized elderly population. *Journal of the American Geriatrics Society, 42*(a). 947–952.

Heitkemper, M.M., Sharver, J.F., Mitchell, E.S. (1988). Gastrointestinal symptoms and bowel patterns across the menstrual cycle in dysmenorrhea. *Nursing Research, 37* (2), 108–113.

Henry, M.M. (1981). Incontinence of feces. *British Journal of Hospital Medicine, 28* (3), 232, 234–235.

Hillemeier, C. (1995). An overview of the effects of dietary fiber on gastrointestinal transit. *Pediatrics, 96, 997–999.*

Jensen, L.L. (1990). Fecal Incontinence. In Jeter, K.F., Faller, N., Norton, C. (eds.): *Nursing for Continence*. Philadelphia: W.B. Saunders, pp 223–240.

Joachim, G. (1983). The effects of two stress management techniques on feeling of well-being in patients with inflammatory bowel disease. *Nursing Papers, 15* (4), 5–19.

Kodner, I.J. (1993). Twenty-five years in colon and rectal surgery: Changes and progressions. *Journal of ET Nursing, 20* (3), 98–100.

Krasner, D. (1990). Incontinence in varied settings. In Jeter, K.F., Faller, N., Norton, C. *Nursing for Continence*. Philadelphia, W.B. Saunders.

Madoff, R.D., Williams J.G., Caushaj, P.F. (1992). Fecal incontinence. *The New England Journal of Medicine, 326* (15), 1002–1007.

Martinsson, E.S., Josefsson, M., Ed, A. (1991). Working capacity and quality of life after undergoing ileostomy. *Journal of Advanced Nursing, 16*, 1035–1041.

Mayer, E.A., Gebhart, G.E. (1994). Basic and clinical aspects of visceral hyperalgesia. *Gastroenterology, 107*, 271–293.

Mihalopoulos, N.G., Trunnell, E., Ball, K., Moncur, C. (1996). The psychological impact of ostomy surgery on persons 50 years of age and older. *Journal of Wound, Ostomy and Continence Nursing, 21* (4), 149–155.

Milne, B., Joachim, G., Niedhardt, J. (1986). A stress management program for inflammatory bowel disease patients. *Journal of Advanced Nursing, 11, 561–567.*

Oberst, M.T., Scott, D.W. (1988). Post discharge stress in surgically treated cancer patients and their spouses. *Research in Nursing and Health, 11*, 223–233.

Pieper, B. (1992). A study of persons undergoing outpatient gastrointestinal radiography. *Journal of ET Nursing, 19* (2), 54–58.

Pierre, R. (1996). Ileal pouch/anal anastomosis for Crohn's disease. *The Lancet, 347* (9005), 854.

Price, A.L. (1995). Ostomy surgery general guidelines for nutritional health. *Ostomy Quarterly, 32* (4), 24–27.

Proano, M., Camilleri, M., Phillips, S., et al. (1990). Transit of solids through the human colon. *American Journal of Physiology, 258* (6), 856–862.

Ramer, L. (1992). Self-image changes with time in the cancer patient with a colostomy after operation. *Journal of ET Nursing, 19* (6), 195–203.

Reaume, A., Gooding, B.A. (1991). Social support, coping strategies, and long-term adaptation to ostomy among self-help group members. *Journal of Enterostomal Therapy, 18* (1), 11–15.

Rieger, P. (1994). Biotherapy for colon cancer: Promise or progress? *Journal of Wound, Ostomy and Continence Nursing, 21* (3), 111–119.

Sartor, R.B. (1995). Current concepts of the etiology and pathogenesis of ulcerative colitis and Crohn's disease. In Peppercorn, M.A. (ed.): *Gastroenterology Clinics of North America: Inflammatory Bowel Disease, 24* (3), 475–507.

Smith, C.E., Marlen, L., Brogdon, C., et al. (1990). Diarrhea associated with tube feeding in mechanically ventilated critically ill patients. *Nursing Research, 39* (3), 148–152.

Steiner-Grossman, P., Banks, P.A., Present, D.H. (1992). *The New People Not Patients: A Source Book for Living with Inflammatory Bowel Disease.* New York: Crohns & Colitis Foundation of America.

Svensson, J.H. (1987). Peripheral, autonomic regulation of locus coeruleus noradrenergic neurons in brain: Putative implications for psychiatry and psychopharmacology. *Psychopharmacology, 92,* 1–7.

Tobein, G.W., Brocklehurst, J.C. (1986). Fecal incontinence in residential homes for the elderly: Prevalence, aetiology and management. *Age and Ageing, 15,* 41–46.

Toosan, J., DeWayne D., Varilek C., Gary, B. (1995). Inflammatory diseases of the colon: Narrowing a wide field of symptoms and possible causes. *Postgraduate Medicine, 98* (5), 46–58.

Trainor, M.A. (1982). Acceptance of ostomy and the visitor role in a self-help group for ostomy patients. *Nursing Research, 31* (2), 102–106.

Wade, B.E. (1990). Colostomy patients: Psychological adjustment at 10 weeks and 1 year after surgery in districts which employed stoma-care nurses and districts which did not. *Journal of Advanced Nursing, 15,* 1297–1304.

Weiss, E.G., Wexner, S.D. (1995). Surgical treatment for ulcerative colitis. In Peppercorn, M.A. (ed.): *Gastroenterology Clinics of North America: Inflammatory Bowel Disease, 24* (3).

Wrenn, K. (1989). Fecal impaction. *The New England Journal of Medicine, 321* (10), 658–661.

Urinary Elimination 24

Loretta Filitske and Diane Krasner

Mrs. Harris is a 74-year-old widow who lives alone. She is a mother of four children and grandmother of 13. After a stroke 2 years ago, Mrs. Harris regained 90 percent of her function through intensive rehabilitation. She was able to return home to independent living.

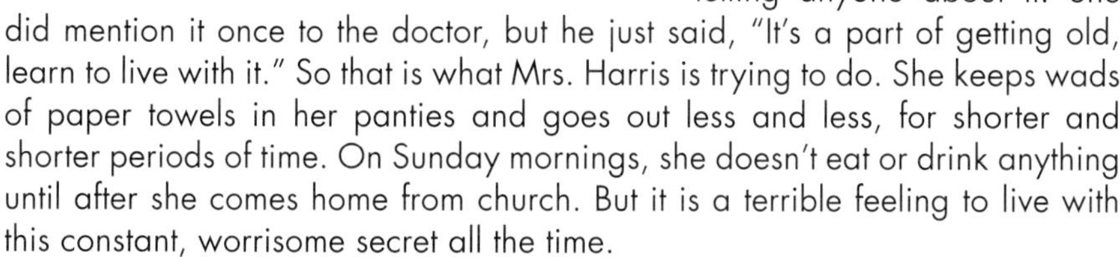

One problem that did not resolve after the stroke was her bladder trouble. Mrs. Harris can never seem to get to the toilet on time without having an accident. It always takes her too long to get there, too long to get her clothes undone, and too long to get into position.

Mrs. Harris is so self-conscious about this problem that she won't even think of telling anyone about it. She did mention it once to the doctor, but he just said, "It's a part of getting old, learn to live with it." So that is what Mrs. Harris is trying to do. She keeps wads of paper towels in her panties and goes out less and less, for shorter and shorter periods of time. On Sunday mornings, she doesn't eat or drink anything until after she comes home from church. But it is a terrible feeling to live with this constant, worrisome secret all the time.

Mrs. Harris heard a public service announcement on the radio about a self-help group for people with incontinence. When she got up the courage to call the 800-number, she found a supportive and informative volunteer counselor on the other end of the line. Upon recommendation of the counselor, she saw a urogynecologist and went through urodynamic testing (the holding or storage of urine in the bladder, the facility with which it empties, and the rate of movement of urine out of the bladder during micturition). Her diagnosis of mixed, urge-functional incontinence was confirmed.

OBJECTIVES

After studying this chapter, students will be able to:

- **assess a patient's elimination patterns and identify deviations from normal and risk factors associated with incontinence.**
- **collaborate with the patient and family, as appropriate, to identify goals and appropriate nursing interventions to help the patient reach these goals.**
- **implement appropriate nursing procedures related to urinary elimination.**
- **identify and discuss the various types of urinary diversions.**
- **implement counseling and supportive interventions to prevent or delay incontinence in high-risk persons.**

SCOPE OF NURSING PRACTICE

Nurses have a major role in preventing and managing urinary elimination problems. This includes conditions of urinary incontinence (UI), urinary retention, urinary tract infections (UTIs), and urinary diseases requiring medical intervention, surgical intervention, or both. UI is the most prevalent of all these conditions.

Approximately 13 million Americans, the majority of them female, suffer from incontinence (Agency for Health Care Policy and Research [AHCPR], 1996). Incontinence can cause UTIs, falls, pressure ulcers, social isolation, guilt, shame, and loss of self-esteem. Appropriate management of incontinence can significantly reduce health care costs, prevent nursing home admissions, and improve the quality of life.

Nurses are in a unique position to prevent or delay the development of incontinence and manage the problem if it occurs. Through a caring nurse-patient relationship, persons with incontinence or at high risk for the problem can be identified. These persons and their family can be educated regarding techniques for prevention and management of the problem. The nurse can also serve as care manager, coordinating cost-effective, quality care in a multidisciplinary setting.

KNOWLEDGE BASE

Basic Science

Urinary elimination is the process by which the body excretes liquid wastes, byproducts of metabolism, and materials in excess of bodily needs. The kidneys filter the blood, eliminating waste, excess acids or bases, and any other unwanted substances they detect. Urine is transported into the bladder via the two ureters, where it is stored until eliminated through the urethra by a process known as urination, voiding, or micturition.

A normal urinary elimination system is efficient and effective. Alterations in urination can produce problems ranging from disturbances in lifestyles, as described in the case study about Mrs. Harris, to life-threatening situations, such as urinary retention (inability to empty the bladder).

ANATOMY AND PHYSIOLOGY

The urinary tract comprises the kidneys, ureters, bladder, and urethra (Fig. 24–1). The kidneys are responsible for the production of urine. The other structures transport, store, and excrete urine. Normally the urinary tract is sterile and the urine is free of microorganisms.

Regulation of the organs of the urinary tract is under control of the central nervous system. Reflex and voluntary control involves the brain and the autonomic nervous system (sensory and motor; parasympathetic and sympathetic) (Guyton and Hall, 1997).

KIDNEYS

The two kidneys lie on the posterior abdominal cavity to the right and left of the lumbar spine and are level with the T12 and the L1 to L3 vertebrae. The kidney is composed of an outer cortex, a central medulla, and the internal calices and pelvis. Each kidney is composed of approximately 1 million neurons, each capable of forming urine. The renal pelvis begins at the hilum and, as it proceeds downward, narrows and becomes the ureter (Fig. 24–2). The walls of the calices, pelvis, and ureters contain contractile elements that move the urine toward the bladder.

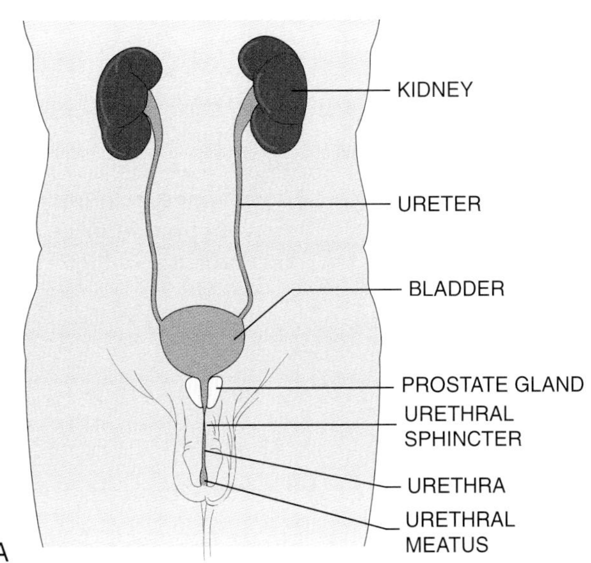

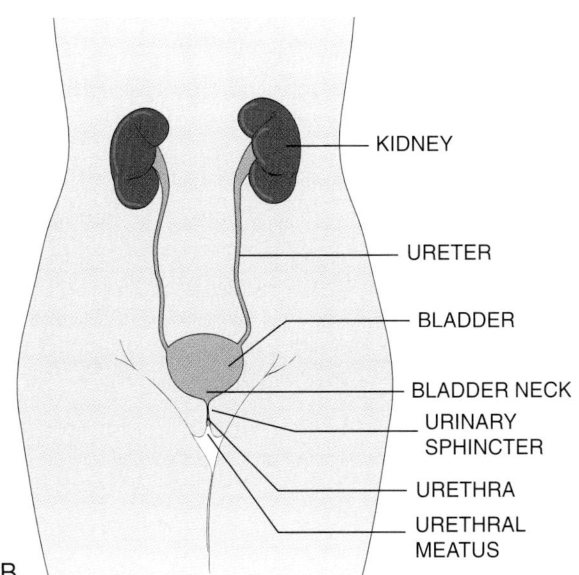

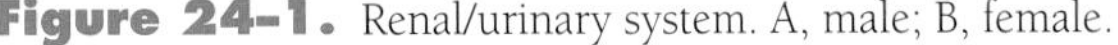

Figure 24–1. Renal/urinary system. A, male; B, female.

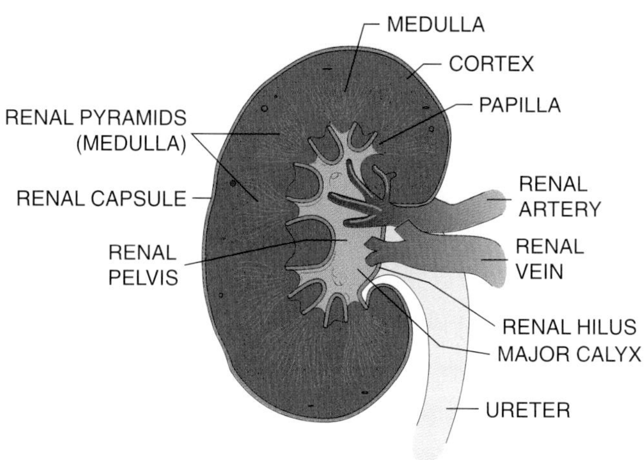

Figure 24–2. The kidney.

Two important functions of the kidney are relevant to this chapter:

- Through filtration, rid the body of waste material ingested or produced by metabolism
- Control the volume and composition of body fluids to balance intake and output

The kidneys also serve these other important functions, however:

- Regulation of acid-base balance
- Regulation of arterial pressure
- Secretion of hormones
- Synthesis of glucose (Guyton and Hall, 1997)

URETERS

From the pelvis of the kidney, urine is transported through the ureters by gravity and peristalsis into the bladder. Each ureter is 25 to 30 cm (10–12 inches) long and 1.7 cm (0.5 inches) wide at the widest point. It is composed of flexible smooth muscle and an inner mucous membrane. The ureters enter the posterior corners of the floor of the bladder obliquely. This angle as well as a fold of mucous membrane (the trigone) in the bladder wall close off the entrance of the ureters. This reduces the risk of urine flowing back towards the kidney, a phenomenon called *urinary reflux* or *backflow*.

URINARY BLADDER

The ureters enter into a hollow muscular organ known as the bladder. The bladder stores urine until it is emptied by micturition. The bladder is located behind the symphysis pubis, in front of the uterus and vagina in women and in front of the rectum in men. When distended or filled like a balloon with urine, the bladder can stretch up as high as the level of the umbilicus. The average bladder capacity is 250 to 400 ml (8–13 oz).

The bladder has two parts: the body and the bladder neck. The body has four layers: serosa, muscular, submucosa, and mucosa. The muscular layer composed of longitudinal and circular muscles is known as the detrusor. When the bladder fills with between 150 and 250 ml (5–8 oz) of urine, a person feels the desire to void because stretch receptors in the detrusor respond when the tension reaches a certain threshold value.

At the base of the bladder is a circular layer of smooth muscle tissue that forms the internal urinary sphincter. This sphincter is controlled involuntarily.

URETHRA

The urethra is the tube that transports urine from the floor of the bladder to exit the body. In the adult male the urethra also transports semen. The male urethra is approximately 20 cm (8 inches) long and has two parts: anterior and posterior. The female urethra is 3 to 5 cm (1.5 inches).

Located within the urethra is a layer of skeletal muscle that forms the external urinary sphincter. This sphincter is under voluntary control of the cortex, midbrain, and medulla. The exit of the urethra from the body is the urinary meatus (opening or passage). The pelvic floor muscles that support the bladder and urethra are known as the pelvic sling. These muscles assist with continence by tightening under voluntary control.

MICTURITION

Normal micturition (urination or voiding) has two components: storage of urine and emptying of the bladder. Both components are under control of the central nervous system.

When the adult bladder fills with 150 to 250 ml of urine, the normal person perceives the desire to urinate. This occurs because as the bladder fills with urine, pressure within the bladder (intravesical pressure) rises and stretch receptors in the detrusor are activated. This signals the spinal micturition center, located at spinal cord levels S2, S3, and S4, which sends signals up to the midbrain and pons via the parasympathetic nervous system (Fig. 24–3).

If the time and place are appropriate for voiding, voluntary control permits micturition to occur. The internal urinary sphincter relaxes, the detrusor muscle contracts, the muscles of the abdominal wall also contract to assist, the diaphragm is lowered, the external urinary sphincter relaxes, and micturition occurs. If the time and place are not right, voluntary control takes over. The sphincters remain contracted, the muscles of the pelvic floor tightened, and micturition does not occur. The micturition reflex may remain in an uninhibited state for up to an hour or more. Then another micturition reflex occurs.

Characteristics of Normal Urine

Color and Clarity. Urine is normally clear and light yellow but may range from pale yellow to dark brown. High fluid intake may dilute the urine, causing the pale color. Dark urine

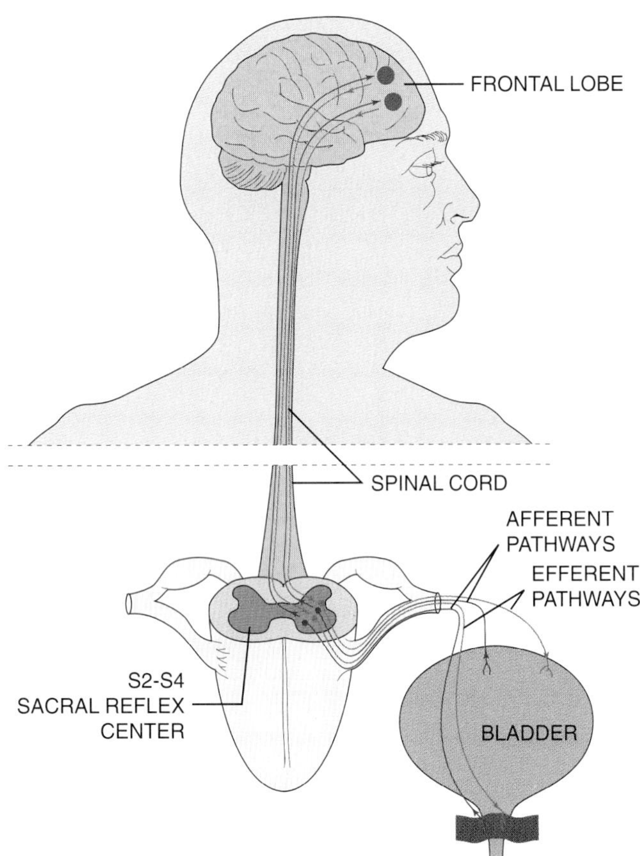

Figure 24-3. Structures involved in micturition.

is concentrated, usually indicating low fluid intake. Urine color can be altered by food intake, medication, or blood in the urine (Table 24–1).

Urine should be clear without sediment. Sediment may indicate kidney or bladder dysfunction. Urine left standing may become cloudy.

Volume. The average daily urinary output for a normal healthy adult is 1000 to 1500 ml. Fluid output varies depending on body size, general health status, fluid intake, and fluid loss. Catheterized patients excrete approximately 30 ml/hour.

Odor. Urine has a slight aroma; if concentrated it may have a stronger odor. Food and medication can affect its odor.

Chemistry. Urine pH ranges from 4.8 to 7.5; its specific gravity (the weight of a substance compared with the weight of an equal volume of water) ranges from 1.005 to 1.025. Specific gravity below 1.005 yields *dilute* urine; specific gravity greater than 1.025 yields *concentrated* urine. Normal urine should be free of protein, glucose, and red or white blood cells.

Characteristics of Abnormal Urine

Disruptions of the urinary tract and alterations in urinary elimination are characterized by a wide range of symptoms. Familiarity with the most common symptoms can sharpen nursing assessment skills.

BOX 24-1
COMMON ALTERATIONS IN URINE

Albuminuria: albumin in the urine
Bacteriuria: bacteria in the urine
Glucosuria: glucose in the urine
Hematuria: blood in the urine
Pyuria: pus (white blood cells) in the urine

Color and Clarity. Changes in urine color or transparency may be due to foods, drugs, disease processes, and abnormal hydration states (see Table 24–1). Box 24–1 lists terms commonly used to describe alterations in the urine.

Odor. Certain foods, such as asparagus and garlic, and certain medications, such as vitamins, can change the odor of the urine. If the urine is left standing, urea in the urine decomposes, releasing ammonia. This causes urine to have a typical ammonia odor. In a person with diabetes mellitus, the urine may have a "sweet" odor due to the presence of acetone. Foul-smelling urine may be a sign of a UTI.

Frequency and Volume. Some conditions can alter the total amount of urine produced. For example, in acute nephritis totals may only reach 200 to 500 ml or less in 24 hours. Medications such as diuretics are given to cause diuresis when a person is in fluid overload. Box 24–2 lists common terms used to describe alterations in urinary elimination.

FACTORS AFFECTING URINARY TRACT FUNCTION

The process of elimination can be altered by both intrinsic and extrinsic factors. *Intrinsic factors,* or processes operating within the individual, include fluid intake, age, medications, neurologic status, psychological factors, and immobility. *Extrinsic factors* (factors in the environment) include diagnostic testing, trauma, anesthesia, surgery, and environmental barriers.

BOX 24-2
ALTERATIONS IN URINARY ELIMINATION

Anuria: total urine output less than 100 ml/24 hours
Oliguria: scanty urine output
Polyuria: urine output exceeding 2000 ml/24 hours
Nocturia: awakening at night to urinate
Dysuria: painful urination
Pneumaturia: excretion of urine containing air or gas
Enuresis: urination while sleeping
Tenesmus: painful straining in an attempt to urinate
Urgency: sudden, strong desire to urinate
Hesitancy: delay in starting voluntary urination
Diuresis: increased urinary output
Incontinence: involuntary loss of urine flow from the bladder
Retention: inability to empty the bladder
Overflow incontinence: the bladder fills but the signal to empty is absent or inadequate and some urine leaks out

TABLE 24–1 Foods and Medications That Alter Urinary Color

Color	Medication or Diet	Other Causes
Colorless or pale yellow	Diuretics Alcohol	Dilute urine due to diabetes insipidus, diabetes mellitus, overhydration, chronic renal disease, nervousness
Bright yellow	Riboflavin (multiple vitamins)	None
Dark amber to orange	Phenazopyridine HCl (Pyridium, Azo Gantanol, Azo Gantrisin) Nitrofurantoin (Macrodantin) Sulfasalazine (Azulfidine) Docusate calcium; phenolphthalein (Doxidan) (in alkaline urine) Thiamin (multiple vitamins) Excessive carotene (e.g. carrots)	Concentrated urine due to dehydration or increased metabolic state Urobilinogen Bilirubin
Pink to red	Phenothiazines Phenolphthalein (laxatives) (in alkaline urine) Phenytoin (Dilantin) Rifampin Phenolsulfonphthalein (PSP) dye (in alkaline urine) Cascara (in alkaline urine) Senna (X-Prep, Senokot) Beets Blackberries Rhubarb (in alkaline urine)	Hemoglobin Porphyrin Red blood cells Myoglobin Menstrual contamination
Brown	Cascara (in acid urine) Metronidazole (Flagyl) (if left standing)	Extremely concentrated urine due to dehydration or increased metabolic state Urobilinogen Porphyrin Bilirubin Red blood cells
Blue or green	Triamterene (Dyrenium) Amitriptyline (Elavil) Phenylsalicylate Methylene blue Indigo carmine Vitamin B complex	Bilirubin-biliverdin *Pseudomonas* infection
Dark brown to black	Nitrofurantoin (Macrodantin) Iron preparations (if left standing) Levodopa (if left standing) Methocarbamol (if left standing) Phenacetin Quinine Cascara (in acid urine) Senna (X-Prep, Senokot) Methyldopa (Aldomet)	Melanin Porphyrin Red blood cells (old blood) Hemogentisic acid in alkaptonuria

From Karlowicz, K.A. (ed.) (1995). *Urologic Nursing: Principles and Practice.* Philadelphia: W.B. Saunders, p. 41.

INTRINSIC FACTORS

Fluid Intake

Output depends on intake. Persons in fluid homeostasis, however, have less output than input. In the summer, profuse sweating can reduce urinary output. In the winter, people tend to urinate more frequently; they also tend to perspire less. In cases of diseases in which urine output is excessive, fluid intake also increases, e.g., diabetes.

Medications

Many medications alter urinary elimination. Whenever there is a change in a person's urinary elimination patterns, the medication regimen, including both prescription and nonprescription drugs, should be investigated. Table 24–2 lists common medications and their effects on urinary elimination.

Neurologic Status

Changes in the neurologic innervation to the urinary tract can cause retention (inability to empty bladder), incontinence (involuntary loss of urine from the bladder), and overflow incontinence (the bladder fills but the signal to empty is absent and some urine leaks out). Neurologic conditions that affect a person's mobility can also cause functional incontinence. Dementias and other mental changes may block the response to cues to void.

TABLE 24-2 Medications That Commonly Alter Urinary Elimination

Class of Medication	Common Side Effect(s)
Alcohol	Diuresis, incontinence
Anticholinergics (atropine sulfate, scopolamine, belladonna, hyoscyamine)	Retention, overflow incontinence
Antidepressants (amitriptyline, imipramine)	Incontinence
Calcium channel blockers (verapamil, diltiazem hydrochloride)	Diuresis
Cold capsules (Contac, Dristan)	Retention, overflow incontinence
Decongestants (Tylenol cold medication, phenylephrine hydrochloride)	Retention, overflow incontinence
Diuretics (furosemide, bemitradine)	Diuresis, incontinence
Sedative hypnotics (zolpidem tartrate)	Incontinence
Antispasmodics (dicyclomine, Donnatol)	Incontinence

Adapted from Agency for Health Care Policy and Research (1992). *Urinary Continence in Adults: Clinical Practice Guideline.* (AHC PR Publication No. 92-0038.) Washington, D.C., U.S. Government Printing Office.

Psychological Factors

Patients who are depressed or who have given up hope may no longer be concerned with trying to maintain continence. Lonely persons who are institutionalized have used incontinence as an attention-obtaining device, i.e., the resident gets attention by setting up a situation in which the staff must change the resident's clothing, bedding, or continence products repeatedly.

Immobility

Prolonged immobility can have dire consequences on urinary elimination. The prone position decreases drainage from the kidneys to the ureters, and urine can pool in the bladder. This can lead to urinary stasis, UTI, incontinence, retention, and renal or urinary calculi (stone) formation (Krasner, 1992).

Immobility causes calcium to move out of the bones into the bloodstream. This is known as *immobilization hypercalcemia.* Increased calcium excretion begins within 2 days of bed rest, reaches a maximum level by 5 weeks, and stays elevated as long as the person is immobilized. This phenomenon can result in *disuse osteoporosis* and can also predispose the immobilized person to stone formation (Issekutz et al., 1965; Steinburg, 1980).

EXTRINSIC FACTORS

Diagnostic Testing

Diagnostic tests such as some ultrasound studies that involve the consumption or infusion of large quantities of fluids can cause transient diuresis or acute incontinence. Medications (e.g., diuretics) or dyes (e.g., methylene blue) injected for testing may alter urinary elimination patterns, the color of the urine, or both.

Anesthesia and Surgery

Urinary elimination is both a reflex and a voluntary activity, so any situations that interfere with reflex or voluntary actions of the nerves or muscles affect normal micturition. Medications used during anesthesia, lengthy surgical time, large fluid volumes, and long-acting spinal anesthetics can contribute to postoperative urinary retention (Wren and Wren, 1996).

Environmental Barriers

Unclearly marked bathrooms, poor lighting, siderails, restraints, lack of privacy, buttons, zippers, and layers of clothing are just a few environmental barriers that can slow a person's progress toward the toilet and possibly cause incontinence and retention (Garcia et al., 1988; Sherman and Umlauf, 1994).

URINARY SYSTEM DYSFUNCTIONS

INCONTINENCE

Urinary incontinence is an involuntary loss of urine that is sufficient to be a problem (AHCPR, 1992; Newman et al., 1991). UI is a symptom, not a disease. It can be due to problems with the anatomy and or physiology of the urinary system. Some additional factors influencing urinary elimination are mobility, medications, mental status, constipation, diabetes, stroke, hormonal changes, and muscle weakness (Kennedy et al., 1995). The following is a brief discussion of the various types of incontinence and some possible measures for control of the problem.

Acute, transient, or *reversible incontinence* is usually of short duration. Possible causes include infection, medications, and constipation.

Chronic incontinence is a persistent, long-term problem that usually involves a change in the person's internal functioning. In the case study, Mrs. Harris has been experiencing chronic, mixed incontinence (age and stress incontinence) since her stroke. Other common causes of chronic incontinence include structural problems (such as spina bifida and spinal cord injury) and neurologic diseases (such as multiple sclerosis and Parkinson's).

Chronic UI is subdivided into specific categories. It is not uncommon for people to suffer from more than one of these types at the same time, resulting in *mixed incontinence.* Eighty-five percent of incontinent people have stress, urge, or mixed incontinence.

Stress incontinence is the involuntary loss of urine that occurs with increased intra-abdominal pressure. People complain of dribbling or losing urine when coughing, sneezing, laughing, bending, lifting, exercising, or changing position. The amount of urine lost is usually small. Other symptoms may include urinary frequency and urgency.

Stress incontinence occurs most often in women (Turner and Plymat, 1988) from two causes. Childbirth places a strain on the pelvic floor muscles and can weaken or damage them, resulting in chronic stress incontinence. Second, postmenopausal women may experience a thinning of the pelvic floor muscles and of the urethral tissue due to a drop in estrogen levels, which results in stress incontinence. Stress incontinence may occur in men after prostate or urethral surgery.

Other causes of stress incontinence include trauma, congenital urinary sphincter weakness, decreased sphincter tone in the proximal urethra, and certain medications, e.g., alpha-antagonists.

Medications can sometimes improve stress incontinence. (Bourcier and Juras, 1995). Alpha-adrenergic agonists (e.g., ephedrine and pseudoephedrine) produce smooth muscle contraction at the bladder outlet. Estrogens in postmenopausal women may improve urgency and frequency. If medication therapy fails or if the person prefers, surgical interventions may be considered. Such interventions include the following:

- Bladder suspension (raising the bladder neck and decreasing mobility of the urethra)
- Sling procedure (surgical attachment of a piece of tissue to elevate the urethra and decrease mobility)
- Artificial sphincter implantation (a device consisting of a cuff and pump with the cuff around the urethra and the pump in the testicle)
- Uretheral bulking procedure (injection of material around the urethra)

With *urge incontinence,* the person senses an abrupt need and strong desire to void (urgency). Causes of urge incontinence include neurologic problems (such as dementias, multiple sclerosis, Parkinson's, spinal cord lesions, and stroke), bladder cancer, bladder tumors, calculi, and diabetes mellitus.

Drugs such as anticholinergics (e.g., propantheline), antispasmodics (oxybutynin), and imipramine are especially beneficial for urge incontinence. Estrogens may be useful for postmenopausal urge incontinence in women. Surgery may be indicated in cases of cancer, tumors, or calculi.

Reflex incontinence is an involuntary loss of urine with no sense of urgency. Causes include bladder stones, fecal impaction, chemotherapy, radiation therapy, prostatic hyperplasia, neoplasms, and neurologic disorders.

Overflow incontinence is the voluntary loss of urine associated with bladder overdistention. The bladder never empties completely and can become distended. Excess urine overflows the bladder. People with overflow incontinence lose small to moderate amounts of urine frequently throughout the day and night. After passing small amounts of urine, they may still feel as if the bladder is full.

Causes of overflow incontinence include prostatic hyperplasia, bladder outlet obstruction, neurologic disorders, medications, and fecal impaction.

Interventions include clean intermittent catheterization (CIC), i.e., a scheduled insertion of a catheter to drain the bladder; changing medications (avoidance of large amounts of narcotics, anticholinergics, and hypnotics); improving intestinal elimination (constipation can prevent the bladder from emptying); prostate surgery (surgery to relieve bladder outlet obstruction); or surgery to relieve other obstructions (stones or trauma).

Total incontinence is the continuous, uncontrolled loss of urine. The person experiences no sense of bladder filling or awareness of the need to void. The bladder drains urine constantly. Causes include birth defects (spina bifida or bladder extrophy), structural damage following surgery, spinal cord injury, and fistulas. Interventions include CIC, containment devices, or surgery (artificial urinary sphincter, urostomy, or fistula repair).

Functional incontinence occurs when a person who is normally continent is unable or unwilling to get to the toilet. These people have normal urinary tract physiology; some other reason is causing their incontinence.

Environmental barriers are often the cause of functional incontinence. Difficulties in moving or transferring, inaccessible call buttons, inaccessible toilets, beds that are too high, siderails, restraints, poor lighting, or restrictive clothing are examples of common environmental conditions that can cause or exacerbate an incontinence problem (Krasner, 1990). Other causes of functional incontinence include musculoskeletal disorders, impaired dexterity, arthritic disorders, sedation, medications, fear of falls, and psychological disorders (anxiety, depression).

In the case study, Mrs. Harris exhibited symptoms of mixed, urge-functional incontinence after her stroke. She could not reach the toilet fast enough once she perceived the need to void (urge incontinence). In addition, when she did reach the toilet, she could not get her clothes undone or seat herself fast enough (functional incontinence). Interventions for Mrs. Harris, if they are to be successful, must address both of the causes of her incontinence.

URINARY RETENTION

Urinary retention is the inability to empty the bladder completely when voiding or the inability to void after 10 to 12 hours. This may be an acute or chronic condition. The flow of urine may be blocked anywhere between the kidneys and the meatus (Gibbs, 1995; Karlowicz, 1995). Urinary retention can often be detected by palpation in the suprapubic abdominal area.

Common mechanical causes include a stone (calculus), a stricture, or in men an enlarged prostate. Swelling at the meatus after childbirth can cause a mechanical obstruction. Functional retention can be caused by neurologic disorders, psychological problems, medications, or environmental barriers.

Symptoms of urinary retention include pain, bladder/abdominal distention, feeling of fullness, frequency, and overflow incontinence. An "overflow" may happen if the bladder becomes distended and can no longer hold the urine. Diagnosis to determine the exact cause is critical because, if left untreated, retention can cause serious problems.

URINARY TRACT INFECTION

UTIs are caused by numerous microorganisms and may be acute or chronic. UTIs are one of the most frequent *nosocomial,* or hospital-acquired, infections. Infection can ascend from the bladder to the kidneys, causing pyelonephritis or sepsis. *Urinary stasis,* or the pooling of urine in the bladder, promotes bacterial growth and is a common cause of UTIs. Stretching of the bladder with overdistension decreases the bladder's resistance to infection. The bacteria *Escherichia coli* commonly reaches the urinary tract from the gastrointestinal tract, causing infection. Other causes of UTI include catheterization and immunosuppressive medications.

Signs and symptoms of UTI may include the following:

- Frequency
- Urgency
- Voiding in small amounts
- Odor, cloudiness, or sediment in the urine
- Lower back, flank, or suprapubic pain
- Fever, shaking, or chills
- UI
- Pyuria (>100,000 colonies/ml of urine)
- Increased bladder spasticity in patients with spinal cord injury
- Hematuria
- Increased urine pH

When these symptoms appear, a culture and sensitivity of the urine is obtained. Based on the results, appropriate antibiotic therapy is prescribed. Urinary analgesic medications can be used to control irritative symptoms, such as burning, itching, frequency, or urgency. Recurrent UTIs can cause fibrotic changes in the bladder wall, resulting in decreased bladder capacity.

DIAGNOSTIC TESTS

The goals of diagnostic testing include identifying potentially reversible situations that can cause urinary elimination problems and identifying conditions that require further evaluation or treatment. Initially, a complete history and physical is performed. (See Chapter 15, Patient Assessment, for details.) This includes a medication profile because prescription and nonprescription medications may be the cause of urinary problems. The physical examination should include the rectum, genitalia, and abdomen to rule out bladder or prostate enlargement, fecal impaction, or structural abnormalities.

URINE SPECIMENS

Urinary diagnostic testing includes many different types of urinary specimens.

- *Urinalysis* is the baseline test used in most physical assessment examinations. The test is performed to determine the presence of bacteria (bacteriuria), blood (hematuria), or pus in the urine (pyuria).
- *Culture and sensitivity* (C&S) determines organisms present in the urine and their sensitivity to a variety of medications used to treat the condition (antibiotics and antimicrobials).
- Urinary *cytology* is performed when patients with hematuria have a negative urine culture. A sterile specimen is needed for the culture and sensitivity and cytology test.
- A *24-hour urine specimen* is collected to determine the type of substances being excreted over a designated time period.
- *Specific gravity* testing determines the weight or concentration of the urine.
- *Reagent strips* are used to measure the amount of substances such as glucose, protein, or ketones in the urine.

Nursing responsibilities in collection of urine specimens is further discussed under Nursing Care Actions.

Serum blood specimens are collected to determine the presence of kidney disease. Abnormal amounts of blood urea nitrogen (BUN) and serum creatinine may indicate the presence of kidney dysfunction. The results of these tests do not necessarily indicate kidney disorders because the BUN and creatinine levels may be affected by low fluid intake, high protein intake, and infectious processes.

ENDOSCOPY AND RADIOLOGY

Visualization of the inside of the bladder using a *cystoscope* (telescope-like instrument) is called a cystoscopy. It may be performed in a physician's office or in the hospital.

Imaging techniques may be used to evaluate urinary tract abnormalities. Contrast media may or may not be used. *Kidney-ureter-bladder (KUB)* radiography is used to determine the position, size, and structure of the urinary tract organs. Calculi, foreign bodies, and other gross abnormalities can sometimes be detected.

Intravenous pyelography (IVP), also known as *excretory urography,* is a radiologic examination that allows visualization of the structural details of the urinary tract after administration of the contrast medium. Abnormalities of the kidney, ureters, and bladder can be diagnosed. Abnormal-appearing KUB radiographs or IVPs may be followed up with computed tomography (CT), magnetic resonance imaging (MRI), ultrasound studies, or other scans of the urinary tract.

URODYNAMIC TESTS

Several distinct diagnostic studies are often collectively called *urodynamic tests.* The goal of all of these screening tests is to evaluate the anatomical and functional status of a patient's usual voiding process. Diagnosis of voiding disorders, such as retention, ureteral reflux, and incontinence can be made. Urodynamic tests include the following:

- Cystometrography (CMG): measurement of bladder pressures

- Electrophysiologic sphincter testing (EMG): studies of urethral nerve function during bladder filling and emptying
- Filling studies: a procedure in which the bladder is filled with water and the person is then asked to urinate
- Urethral pressure profilometry (UPP): measurement of resting and dynamic urethral pressures
- Urine flow studies (uroflowmetry): tests to detect reduced or abnormal urine flow
- Video urodynamic evaluation: combination of urodynamic studies and fluoroscopy
- Voiding cystourethrography: radiographs of bladder and urethra performed during voiding

TREATMENT MODALITIES

Once the type of incontinence has been identified, goals and interventions can be determined. There are three categories of interventions: medication, surgery, and behavioral techniques. Behavioral techniques are discussed under Nursing Care Actions.

MEDICATIONS

Certain types of urinary problems lend themselves better to pharmacologic treatment than do others. For example, the treatment of choice for acute incontinence due to a UTI is antibiotic therapy. Chronic incontinence due to weakening of the urinary sphincter in a postmenopausal woman can often be successfully treated with oral or topical estrogen. Urge incontinence and bladder spasms have been effectively managed with medications that relax the bladder, decrease bladder spasms, or tighten the sphincter and pelvic floor muscles.

Medications commonly used for incontinence management include the following:

- Anticholinergics, which inhibit detrusor (the external longitudinal layer of the muscular coat of the bladder) contraction and may increase bladder capacity—for urge incontinence
- Antispasmodics, which relax the bladder smooth muscle—for urge incontinence
- Imipramine (a tricyclic antidepressant), which has anticholinergic and muscle relaxant effects—for urge incontinence
- Alpha-adrenergic agonists, which cause smooth muscle contraction at the bladder outlet—for stress incontinence
- Estrogens—for postmenopausal women to improve urgency and frequency in stress incontinence (AHCPR, 1992)

Some of these medications have undesirable side effects, including dry mouth, dry eyes, exacerbation of eye problems such as glaucoma, urinary retention, constipation, and confusion. The use of these medicines should be carefully monitored by a physician, especially in the elderly.

SURGICAL PROCEDURES

Surgical repair of blockages or structural problems is often necessary. Mechanical blockages due to calculi, prostatic hypertrophy, or tumor can be relieved by removal or excision of the material causing the blockage. Structural repairs involve tightening ligaments or supportive structures. Weakened pelvic muscles can be reinforced or replaced (urethral sling procedures). This is especially effective in cases of pure stress incontinence. Bladder augmentation involves enlarging the bladder to increase its capacity by adding segments of bowel. For patients who have sphincter dysfunction after surgery (such as a radical prostatectomy) or due to sphincter denervation, an artificial sphincter can be implanted (Fig. 24–4). Although the success rate for this procedure is very high (70 to 80 percent), the complication rate is also high (over 20 percent) and reoperation is frequently required (AHCPR,

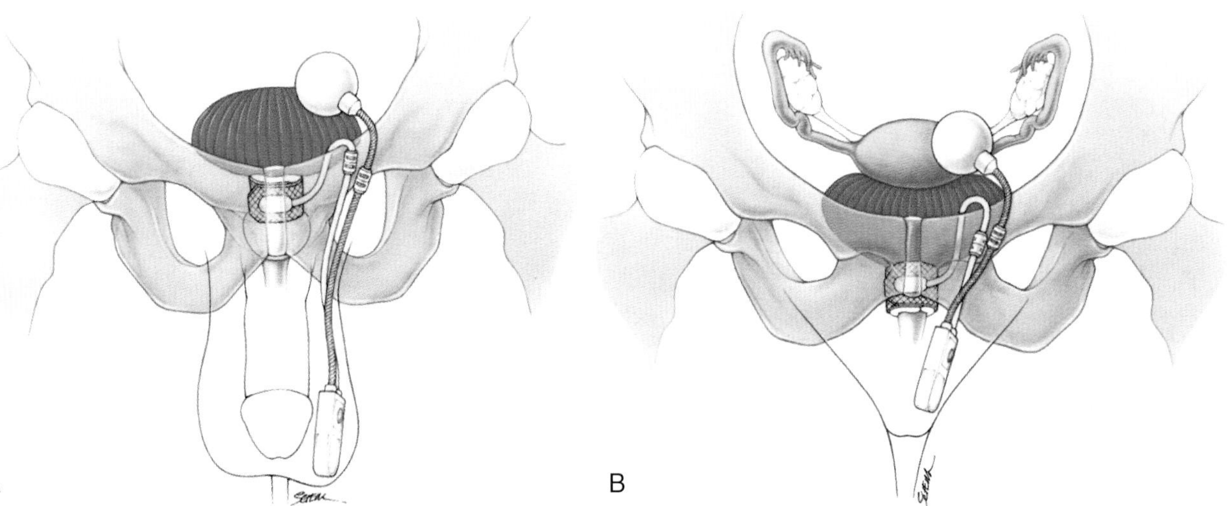

Figure 24–4. Artificial urinary sphincter. A, male; B, female. (Courtesy of American Medical Systems, Inc.)

1992). In cases of advanced bladder cancer, in which cystectomy is necessary, and in cases of severe intractable incontinence, ostomy surgery may be performed.

Surgical diversion of the ureters, known as *urostomy,* with or without removal of the bladder, is sometimes needed in the presence of urinary tract pathologies. Invasive carcinoma of the bladder is the most common reason for urostomy surgery. Congenital abnormalities, severe injuries, interstitial cystitis, obstruction, and intractable incontinence are other reasons for performing urostomy surgery. Most urostomies are permanent. When a temporary urostomy is reversed, this is known as an *undiversion.* Common forms of urostomy surgery include ureterostomy, ileal conduit, Kock pouch, and continent vesicostomy (Fig. 24–5).

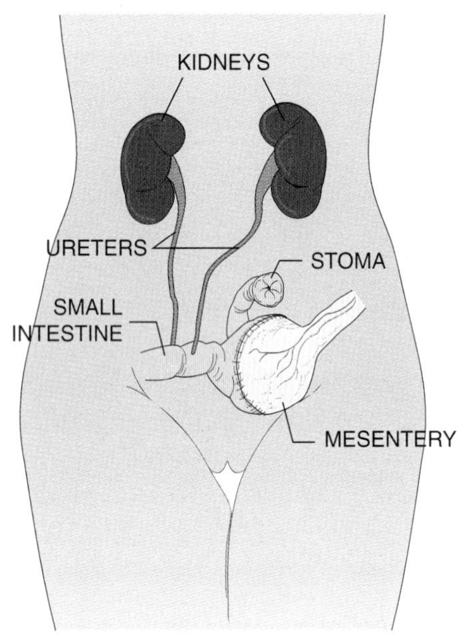

A. The Kock ileostomy pouch is adapted for use as a urinary diversion and is emptied via a catheter

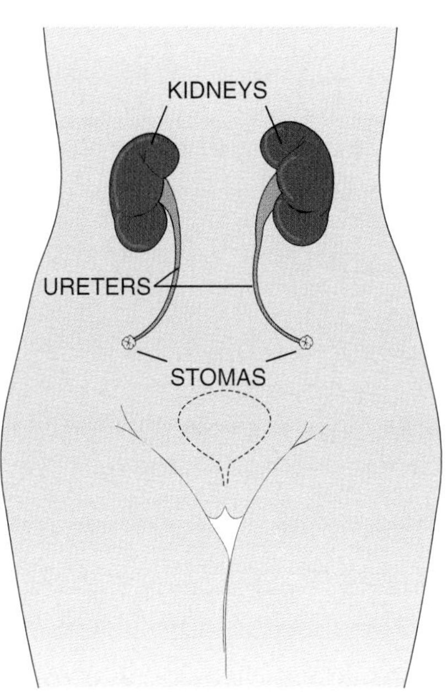

B. Ureterostomy brings the distal end of the ureter (or in a bilateral procedure, the ureters) out through the abdominal wall, creating one or two stomas, from which urine flows directly into a drainage appliance

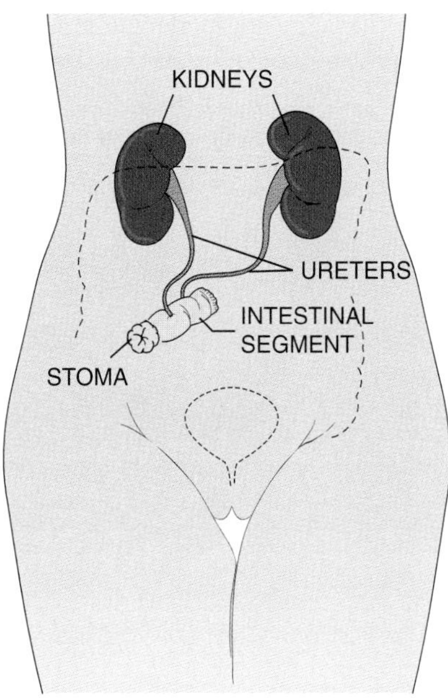

C. Ileal conduit uses a segment of the intestine (usually, the terminal ileum) as a conduit through which urine is emptied through a stoma in the abdominal wall

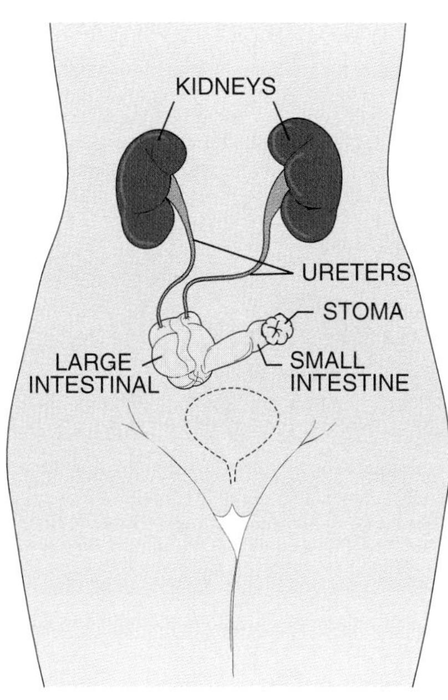

D. The Indiana pouch uses the ileocecal segment of the bowel as an internal pouch and is emptied via a catheter

Figure 24–5. A to D, Urinary diversions.

A *ureterostomy* is created when the ends of the ureters are brought out onto each side of the abdominal wall. The bladder may or may not be removed. Urine flows out continuously from the small exit holes on either side of the body and is collected in urostomy pouches or bags that can be changed by the patient or their caregiver. Urine reflux can become a problem. After surgery, the ureters are prone to stricture that can cause obstruction. Furthermore, because there is a direct route of entry for microorganisms that can ascend to the kidney, pyelonephritis is a common and serious chronic complication.

Intestinal (ileal)/conduit surgery was developed to address the problems with ureterostomy just described. The ileal conduit is performed when a portion of the ileum is removed and the ends of the intestines are reattached. A pouch is created from the portion of the ileum that was removed. One end of the intestine is closed (sutured) and the other end is brought through the abdominal wall. A stoma is created on the end that is extended through the abdominal wall (Fig. 24–6). The ureters are planted into the pouch. The bladder may be removed depending on the patient's diagnosis.

Following conduit surgery, *stents* or plastic tubes are frequently threaded from the stoma, up each ureter, into the renal pelvis of the kidney (Fig. 24–7). The stents stabilize the anastomoses and ensure patency of the system during the postoperative period when swelling is likely. The stents are usually left in place for 7 to 14 days after surgery.

An intestinal conduit stoma should be bright red, moist, and protruding. Urine flow from the stoma is almost constant. Initially, the urine drainage is blood-tinged. Strands of mucus are normally found in the urine of the urostomy patient because the goblet cells of the mucosa of the intestinal conduit continue to produce mucus.

During the last several decades, just as surgeons have improved continent procedures for ileostomy, the *Kock pouch* has also been perfected. A replacement bladder or reservoir is created with sections of small intestine. A small, one-way nipple valve is created and brought onto the abdominal surface. Every 3 to 4 hours, the person inserts a catheter into the pouch (reservoir) and drains the urine out.

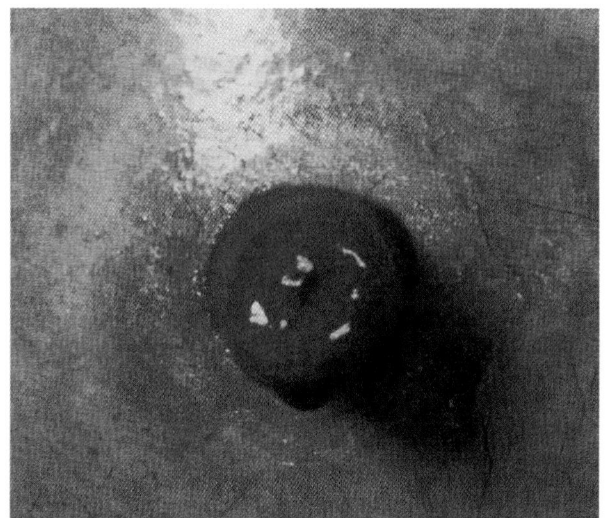

Figure 24–6. End stoma. (Courtesy of Convatec.)

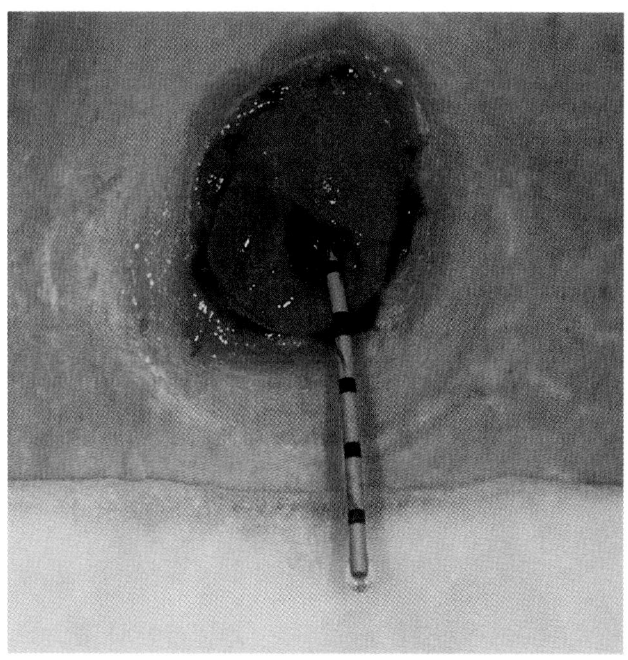

Figure 24–7. Ileal conduit stoma with stent.

In the *continent vesicostomy,* the neck of the bladder is sutured shut. The anterior wall of the bladder is brought forward and sutured to the abdominal wall. An incision is made through the abdominal wall into the bladder, and the bladder wall is formed into a stoma. There is constant drainage of urine from the bladder, requiring a urinary collection device to be worn. This surgical procedure is similar to the Kock pouch in that a nipple value can be created from the bladder wall. In this case, the patient requires catheterization.

Other urinary diversions that are performed include the following:

- Nephrostomy: transcutaneous catheter into the renal pelvis
- Cystostomy: transcutaneous catheter into the bladder
- Ureterosigmoidostomy: ureters draining into the sigmoid colon

Relevant Research

Until recently, little was known about the assessment and management of UI. In the early 1980s, research on UI began appearing in the health care literature. Because of the significance of the problem and the lack of research, the National Institute on Aging (NIA) made UI a priority. From 1984 to 1989 the NIA and DHHS Division of Nursing (now the National Institute on Nursing Research) sponsored a multisite clinical trial on the behavioral management of UI. In 1988, the National Institutes of Health (NIH) held a consensus conference on UI that led to publication of a summary of current knowledge (Wyman, 1992).

AGENCY FOR HEALTH CARE POLICY AND RESEARCH

In 1992, the Agency for Health Care Policy and Research (AHCPR) published a clinical practice guide for UI in adults. A second guideline was published in 1996. Guidelines are developed by a panel of experts along with consultants and peer-reviewers. Guidelines are research-based and tested before being published. Each guideline is published in three versions: a patient's guide, a quick reference guide for clinicians, and the full clinical practice guideline. Copies of guidelines can be obtained from the AHCPR Publications Clearinghouse (see Box 24–4).

A new classification for continence, based on an Australian model, has been developed:

- *Independent:* able to maintain continence without assistance
- *Dependent:* the physically and mentally impaired kept dry through help of others
- *Social:* dependent on absorbent products, collection devices, or both

In an effort to help professional and nonprofessional caregivers, the AHCPR has released the following documents:

- Helping People with Incontinence
- Establishing, Implementing, and Continuing an Effective Continence Program in a Long Term Care Facility (Newman, 1996)

RESEARCH ON INTERMITTENT CATHETERIZATION AND BEHAVIORAL TECHNIQUES

Here, research in the areas of intermittent catheterization and behavioral techniques is reviewed to illustrate the impact of such research on nursing practice.

INTERMITTENT CATHETERIZATION

No-touch (sterile) intermittent catheterization was originally advocated by Sir Ludwig Guttman for managing spinal cord patients during and after World War II (Guttman, 1973). Research on CIC began in the early 1970s. Since then, a series of studies has demonstrated that clean (nonsterile) intermittent catheterization is an effective management technique for selected patients experiencing UI (Barnes, 1986; Champion, 1976; Gray et al., 1995; Lapides et al., 1976; Plunkett and Braren, 1979).

The effect of these studies has been to reverse the practice of sterile intermittent catheterization, which once limited the practicability and availability of the technique for patient care. CIC has proven to be safe and cost-effective. Today, it is taught by nurses and other health care professionals and used extensively by outpatients, including the very young and the very old. Limitations in the use of intermittent catheterization may be due to patient morbidity and cognitive and mobility deficits. Some complications that occur with intermittent catheterization are urethral strictures, urethral inflammations, false passage, hydronephrosis, and epididymitis (Webb et al., 1990).

A research article advances the theory that by microwaving the catheters used for intermittent catheterization, aseptic technique could be accomplished without using a new catheter each time (Silber et al., 1989). The question of whether such aseptic intermittent catheterization would reduce bacteriuria and UTI rates has yet to be investigated. Microwaved catheters should always be allowed to cool thoroughly to avoid a burn. Another issue that needs to be addressed relates to the modifications in the CIC technique that should be made when it is carried out in an institutional setting. In current practice, most experts recommend that a sterile, no-touch procedure be used and that new, sterile catheters be used for each catheterization. Research on this matter is needed.

Finally, it was recognized early on by Lapides and associates (1976) and others that the success of CIC is based on the patient's acceptance of its benefits and ease in learning the procedure. The role of the nurse in building patient trust and acceptance is vital. Nursing research concerning the teaching techniques and supportive interventions that prove most successful in accomplishing these goals would provide a research base for nursing practice (see Research Highlight).

BEHAVIORAL TECHNIQUES

The four major behavioral techniques used for incontinence management (bladder training, habit training, prompted voiding, and pelvic muscle exercises) have been researched extensively over the last several decades (see Burgio and Burgio, 1986; Petrilli et al., 1988; and Wheeler et al., 1992 for reviews of this research). One clear observation that emerges from the research literature is that in addition to the type of incontinence, a number of other variables (such as cognition, mobility, and patient desire for continence) affect the success of the behavioral techniques. Feedback or praise to the patient for success with the intervention is extremely important. A successful outcome is affected by a long-term, positive relationship between the patient and the health care practitioner who supervises the intervention.

Another observation is that although some of these techniques may significantly reduce the frequency, volume, and overall number of incontinent episodes, incontinence is often not totally eliminated; yet the techniques are considered "successful." The implication of this observation for nursing management is that measures to control incontinent episodes will still be needed.

It is difficult to predict which specific behavioral techniques will work best for a particular patient or type of incontinence. So, a certain amount of trial and error is required. Research on bladder training (retraining or drill) shows that proper bladder training can restore normal bladder functioning in selected patients. Physiologic lengthening of the

RESEARCH HIGHLIGHT

Patterned Urge Response Toileting for Urinary Incontinence: A Clinical Trial By Joyce Colling, Betty Jo Hadley, Joan Eisch, Emily Campbell, and Joseph G. Ouslander (1992). In S.G. Funk, E.M. Tornquist, M.T. Champagne, and R.A. Wiese (eds.): Key Aspects of Elder Care. *New York: Springer, pp. 169–186.*

These researchers tested the effects of a noninvasive behavioral treatment called patterned urge response toileting (PURT) on urge/functional urinary incontinence among nursing home residents. The study differs from other "scheduled toileting program" research, which use fixed toileting schedules (e.g., every 3 hours) in that individualized toileting prescriptions were developed and implemented.

SUBJECTS

From four nursing homes in different parts of the United States, 113 residents met the criteria for inclusion in the study and agreed to participate. Of those 113 subjects, 88 completed the entire 9-month study. In each nursing home, one or two units were selected to implement the experimental intervention, and one or two units far away from the experimental units served as controls. An ambulatory electronic monitoring device was used to obtain the exact timing of voiding occurrences for three consecutive 24-hour days for each experimental subject.

NURSING INTERVENTION

Staff on the experimental units followed these instructions for toileting residents in the PURT program:

- At times shown on the toileting sheet, approach each resident. State: "Mr./Mrs., it is time to go to the bathroom/use the commode."
- Assist resident to toilet even if found wet.
- Provide privacy for resident, allow 15 minutes for toileting.
- If resident voided correctly, state: "Good, Mr./Mrs., you were able to use the toilet." Or make some other positive comment.
- Engage briefly in social conversation while making resident feel comfortable.
- If resident did not void correctly, remove from toilet after 15 minutes. Do not comment negatively or positively or engage in social conversation. Make resident comfortable and leave resident's room.

Staff on the experimental units attended staff development classes, enabling them to implement the procedures correctly and consistently.

DATA ANALYSIS

Data were collected on urinary incontinence and volume, incidence of complications, psychosocial well-being of the residents, behavioral capabilities of the residents, and costs for incontinence care. The data analysis showed that there was some degree of improvement in 83% of the residents involved in the PURT program. In 33% of those residents, continence improved by more than 20%. There was also a statistically significant improvement in behavioral capabilities for elimination. These residents became more independent and less dependent in initiating toileting activities. The data also supported the cost-effectiveness of PURT.

IMPLICATIONS FOR NURSING PRACTICE

Combining information about the person's specific urinary pattern with a structured toileting routine can lead to improvement in urinary elimination.

voiding times can be obtained and dryness achieved with persistence and patience. It is clear from the literature that a highly motivated, cognitively alert patient or caregiver is needed if this method is to be successful.

Unlike bladder training, habit training and prompted voiding do not restore normal bladder functioning. These interventions strictly help to avoid incontinent episodes. Once the interventions are stopped, the incontinence returns. Yet, when consistently implemented, these techniques have been demonstrated to have promising, although variable, rates of success, even with cognitively impaired patients (Colling et al., 1992; Jirovec, 1991; McCormick et al., 1992; Ouslander et al., 1988; Schnelle et al., 1989; Warkentin, 1992). What emerges from the research literature is the need for sufficient, highly motivated staff and an adequate nurse/patient ratio for implementation of these types of programs (Burgio et al., 1988).

Pelvic muscle or Kegel exercises have been shown in numerous studies to have a significant effect on reducing rates on incontinence, particularly in selected, screened patient populations. For example, in one study of patients with stress incontinence, continence rates were improved by 60 to 90 percent (Pannill, 1989). The addition of medications or biofeedback has also been shown to improve the efficacy of this technique (Ouslander and Bruskewitz, 1989).

AREAS FOR FUTURE RESEARCH

Wyman (1992), after assessing the current bases for UI practice, identified the following priorities for nursing research:

- Basic research on the mechanisms underlying the etiology, exacerbation, and response to treatment of specific forms of UI
- Epidemiologic studies, with emphasis on the identification of risk factors for development of UI, its occurrence in specific populations (particularly men, nonwhites, persons under the age of 65, acutely hospitalized patients, and homebound adults), and the

natural history of the various clinical and physiologic subtypes
- Longitudinal studies on the prevention of incontinence in high-risk populations
- Development and refinement of instruments to measure physiologic and psychosocial variables (including quality of life) associated with incontinence status and development of noninvasive techniques to assess lower urinary tract function, particularly for cognitively impaired adults
- Studies on the psychosocial impact of UI on affected persons and caregivers, including examination of factors involved in help-seeking behavior
- Development and testing of new strategies using innovative techniques for the treatment of UI, particularly in nursing home patients, frail or homebound adults, and patients whose incontinence is intractable to traditional forms of therapy
- Development and testing of nursing care delivery systems in acute and long-term care settings that foster staff participation in and compliance with incontinence management programs
- Randomized clinical trials on interventions, including longitudinal follow-up evaluation, algorithms for the systematic assessment and management of incontinent patients, and specific behavioral or pharmacologic interventions, either alone or in combination
- Identification of factors that predict treatment success in order to target specific treatments to particular client characteristics and investigation into adherence to interventions and strategies that promote optimal compliance
- Comparative clinical trials of products and equipment involved in the management of refractory incontinence
- Studies of the natural history of bacteriuria in the use of condoms and intermittent catheters
- Investigations into indwelling catheter–related problems such as leakage around catheters and bladder retraining after catheterization
- Economic studies that examine the costs and benefits associated with incontinence treatment, with attention to the level of improvement experienced by incontinent persons
- Development of strategies to disseminate research innovations into clinical practice, with emphasis on nurses' involvement in the assessment and management of UI

FACTORS AFFECTING CLINICAL DECISIONS

Age, gender, individual and family values, care setting, and financial resources are thought to influence clinical decisions regarding urinary elimination. To date, however, research has provided little insight into the effects of age, gender, or ethnicity differences on the perceived impact of UI (Wyman, 1992). By carefully assessing each patient's particular urinary pattern and responses, the nurse can help to develop an effective plan of care.

Age

Incontinence may be temporary or permanent and affect any age group. With the normal aging process, there is a loss of muscle tone, motor and sensory loss, and an actual decrease in the number of nephrons in the kidney. Age-related changes can include bladder capacity, prostatic enlargement, atrophic urethritis, or vaginitis. The frequency of uninhabited bladder contractions increases and residual urine decreases (Meyer, 1989).

Other age-related changes that affect clinical decisions include visual acuity, manual dexterity, mobility, and cognitive changes. For example, physically impaired patients with intact cognition may benefit from behavioral techniques but require that caregivers help them to the toilet (AHCPR, 1996). Half of all adult women experience a loss of bladder control at sometime in their lives (National Institute on Aging, 1991).

Many of the structures that support the bladder weaken with aging. If women have had multiple pregnancies, they may have had structural damage, which can lead to anatomic changes (cystocele, urethrocele, prolapsed uterus) that can cause alterations in urinary elimination.

Gender

Women have a decreased bladder capacity and may develop stress incontinence during pregnancy due to the anatomic changes that occur. Frequent emptying of the bladder can aid in avoiding overdistension and stress incontinence. Many experts suggest that pregnant women be taught pelvic muscle exercises. It is also common for pregnant women to experience UTIs. Urinary frequency, burning on urination, dysuria, and cloudy, foul-smelling urine should be reported to the appropriate health care practitioner. During childbirth, damage to pelvic structures can occur that results in chronic incontinence problems.

Postmenopausal women may experience stress incontinence or transient UI due to atrophic urethritis or vaginitis. Treatment with oral or topical estrogen can be helpful.

In older men, prostatic hyperplasia can cause urinary retention and overflow incontinence. Medications, such as over-the-counter cold preparations (alpha-agonists and anticholinergic agents), may exacerbate the condition, compounding the urinary retention.

Individual and Family Values

Bladder control is not a topic of daily conversation with men and women. Some persons think of incontinence as a social or hygiene problem. Because of people's myths and misconceptions about incontinence and health care professionals' general lack of knowledge, disinterest, and discomfort with the subject, incontinence is often under reported, underdiagnosed, and untreated (AHCPR, 1992; Goldstein et al., 1992).

Greater than 50 percent of nursing home residents experience more than one episode of incontinence a day. Incontinence can result in social isolation, loss of self-esteem, depression, skin irritation, and pressure ulcers (Mitteness, 1987).

Incontinence is a common problem. Unfortunately, most persons are too embarrassed to discuss their problem with others. Today's elderly population were raised in a society with strict codes of decency and morality. Bodily functions were not discussed. These persons may blame themselves for their loss of control—saying, for example, "I'm just old, I move too slow."

They may become apathetic and develop feelings of guilt, anger, embarrassment, or passive acceptance. Social isolation may occur. Marital problems, altered sexual relationships, elderly abuse, and child abuse may occur. Family members who are direct caregivers may feel trapped or they may ignore the situation (mutual pretense). Social isolation may occur because of odor or soiled clothing, furniture, and rugs.

It is important that dialogue and educational opportunities be provided. Informational brochures about elimination problems should be made available in all health care settings. When discussing incontinence with patients it is important to use language and questions they can understand. The patient's guide from the AHCPR is available for free from the AHCPR Clearinghouse.

Setting in Which Care Is Delivered

Not every incontinent person is hospitalized. UI affects 15 to 30 percent of noninstitutionalized persons over 60 and at least half of nursing home residents (AHCPR, 1992). Care settings can include the home, acute care hospital, extended care or rehabilitation facility, nursing home, assisted living home, or personal care home.

Privacy, mobility, clothing, accessible toilets, nonslip floors, good lighting, and availability of assistive devices can aid in developing continence. Privacy can be maintained by closing doors or curtains when toileting patients. Assistive devices may include walkers, grab bars, good lighting, and accessible toilets. Physical and occupational therapy may be needed to improve dexterity and mobility.

Staff and family attitude toward incontinence can be addressed through education and sensitivity training. Soiled clothing should be changed in private. Management of incontinence can improve the quality of life and allow many patients to become productive members of society.

Financial Considerations

Incontinence is expensive. One must pay careful attention to what the patient can afford in continence care. In 1988, the National Institutes of Health estimated the cost for incontinence to be $10.3 billion a year in the United States. On a comparative basis, in 1996, $16 billion or more was spent on caring for adults with UI and an additional $1 billion was spent on disposable absorbent products (Canavan, 1996).

Disposable absorbents have an annual cost of $1600 to $2100. The average price of condom catheters with leg bags is $900 to $1200 annually (Convatec). Penile compression devices are $10 to $45 per device.

In addition to incontinence product cost, one also needs to consider the cost of laundry and dry cleaning, replacement of damaged clothing, and cleaning and replacement of soiled furniture and carpeting. A recent estimate of the direct costs of caring for persons of all ages with incontinence is more than $15 billion annually (AHCPR, 1996).

FUTURE DEVELOPMENTS

There is still much to learn about urinary disorders and their management. New surgical procedures are continually being developed. Procedures that strengthen the urethra by injecting collagen materials around it have already been shown to be effective for stress incontinence (AHCPR, 1996; Fournier and Corcos, 1996). Improved techniques for urostomy surgeries will have higher success rates and be performed more frequently. A new female continence device has been developed and is available for use (AHCPR, 1996).

Other areas for future research include intervention research on protocols for skin care and prevention of skin breakdown for incontinent patients, preoperative and postoperative management techniques for patients with continent ostomies, and management and coping strategies for patients and caregivers of patients with alterations in urinary elimination.

One hopes that the future will also bring improved opportunities for all people with urinary elimination problems to obtain a careful and thorough assessment and diagnosis of the problem. With heightened awareness of the extent and complexity of urinary elimination problems, more referrals by health care professionals and by people themselves will be made. The critical roles of the AHCPR, the National Institute on Aging, the National Institutes of Health, professional health care organizations, and self-help groups in promoting an understanding of these problems cannot be underestimated. It is only through heightened awareness that these problems can be addressed and people's lives improved.

NURSING CARE ACTIONS

The AHCPR guidelines define a strong role for nursing in the prevention, detection, diagnosis, and management of incontinence. Nurses have an equally important role in other aspects of urinary elimination, such as retention and UTIs.

Principles and Practices

Basic science knowledge, nursing science, multidisciplinary research, and insights of expert clinicians support the following principles to remember when caring for patients with abnormalities in urinary elimination:

- Assessment of individual patterns of elimination is essential because of the wide range of patterns that are considered normal.
- Assessment and identification of the causes of alterations in elimination can reflect a wide range of problems and must precede interventions and treatments.
- Elimination patterns should be assessed routinely and documented, noting any specific relevant detail.
- Individual practices related to elimination should be assessed and, if appropriate, opportunities provided for them whenever possible.
- Nursing diagnoses (or other classification techniques) reflecting the holistic nature of problems in elimination should be written for each patient.
- Nursing interventions may be short-term or long-term, beginning during diagnostic testing and continuing with routine follow-up or preoperative and postoperative interventions or with chronic care.
- Education of the patient and family to optimize independence and effective eliminative functioning should be a nursing goal.
- Sensitivity to the psychosocial needs of patients with alterations in elimination is vital to their adaptation and coping.

PREVENTION

UI differs from many other health problems in that it triggers major changes in a person's life, from social isolation to admission to a long-term care facility. Families that are willing to care for a continent family member at home find they cannot do so if the person becomes incontinent. A person's self-esteem and sense of independence are altered when the bladder no longer can be controlled. Prevention of incontinence is a significant component of nursing care.

RISK FACTORS

Table 24–3 provides criteria for continence and risk for incontinence factors identified through an extensive literature review (Pearson and Larson, 1992). The table also lists health-promoting behaviors associated with each risk factor.

NURSING ACTIVITIES

Prevention involves assessment of risk factors followed by education. A condensed form of a continence history is shown in Box 24–3. The educational process must be designed to build on the individual's motivation and empower the person to be an agent of his or her own care. (See Chapter 36, Health Promotion and Self-Care, for more information.) Patients must see the connection between what they do and the outcomes they desire, e.g., doing pelvic floor muscle exercises and experiencing greater control over starting and stopping urination.

Self-care instructions for interventions related to risk factors are provided in the Patient Teaching boxes. Teaching of pelvic floor muscle exercises is treated with a Patient Teaching box and text later in this chapter.

ASSESSMENT

The general nursing history should always include an assessment of a person's elimination patterns. Because many patients are reluctant to discuss urinary tract problems, assessment should begin with open-ended questions. Examples of such questions include the following:

- "Do you have trouble with your bladder?"
- "Do you have trouble holding your urine?"

TABLE 24–3 Criteria for Continence, Risk Factors, and Treatments

Criteria for Continence	Risk for Incontinence	Interventions
Liquid intake of ½ oz/lb body weight/day	Liquid intake less than ½ oz/lb body weight/day	Increase fluid intake
Ability to wait 10 min or longer to void after urge strikes	Inability to wait 10 min to void after urge strikes	Regular toileting schedule
Recognition of bladder fullness	No sense of bladder fullness	Pelvic floor muscle exercise regimen
Recognition of when urination begins	No sense of when urination begins	Pelvic floor muscle exercise regimen
Urination 5–8 times a day	Frequency of daytime urination <5 or >8	Regular toileting schedule
Nocturia = or less than 1 time per night	Nocturia more often than 1 time per night	Regular toileting schedule
No dribbling	Dribbling	Pelvic floor muscle exercise regimen
Ability to start and stop urine flow	Inability to stop and start urine flow	Pelvic floor muscle exercise regimen
No burning on urination	Burning on urination	Increase fluid intake; provide proper perineal care; obtain urinalysis
No bowel constipation	Bowel constipation	Increase fluid and fiber intake; establish a postmeal defecation schedule
Moist vagina	Dry vagina	Vitamins B and E

From Pearson, B.D., Carson, J.M. (1992). Urine control by elders. In S. Funk, E.M. Tornquist, M.T. Champagne, R.A. White (eds.): *Key Aspects of Elder Care.* New York: Springer, pp. 154–168.

BOX 24-3
CONTINENCE HISTORY (CONDENSED FORM)

Date:	**Name:**	**Birthdate:**
	Address:	**Telephone:**

Medical Diagnosis(es):
Medications: Prescription and nonprescription
Ability to follow directions:
Environmental: Properly fitted requisite devices (e.g., walking, chair, toilet), suitable clothing (for finger dexterity), adequate lighting
Mobility: Ambulatory, walking aid, chair, bed

REMEDIAL RISK FACTORS

1. Average 24 hour fluid intake: _______ ounces
2. Once you are aware you need to urinate, how long can you wait?
3. Can you tell when your bladder is full?
4. Can you tell when your urine begins to come?
5. How often do you urinate during the day?
6. How often do you urinate during the night?
7. Do you ever dribble urine when you cough, sneeze, or change position?
8. Can you stop your urine and start it again once you have begun to urinate?
9. Do you ever have burning when you pass urine?
10. Do you have a problem with a decrease in the frequency of your bowel movements accompanied by difficulty in emptying your bowels? How often?
11. (Females only). Are you experiencing a "dry" vagina, poor lubrication of the vagina?

Diagnostic: Do you ever lose your urine at times or places you do not want to? How often? (e.g., once a month? once per day?)

OTHER

1. Do you do anything that makes it easier for you to control your urine? Your bowels?
2. Is there anything that makes it harder for you to control your urine? Your bowels?

- "Do you ever lose urine when you don't want to?"
- "Do you ever wear a pad or other protective device to collect your urine?" (AHCPR, 1992, p. 13)

Time, frequency, amount, and characteristics of the urine should be determined. Recent changes in urinary functioning, such as a change in comfort or control, may be significant and should be noted. Medications, including prescriptions and over-the-counter drugs, should be assessed. The nurse should determine whether the patient has undergone any previous genitourinary surgery or any other surgery that would affect urinary elimination (Tucker et al., 1988).

If urinary tract problems are noted, a thorough history, physical examination, and urinalysis are required for diagnosis. Additional data that might be helpful in the assessment phase include the following:

- A "voiding record or diary" in which the frequency, timing, and amount of urination and other factors associated with urinary problems are noted (Fig. 24–8).
- Evaluation of environmental and social factors, such as access to toilets, living arrangements, social contacts, and caregiver involvement.
- Observation of voiding to determine hesitancy and control.

The nursing assessment and diagnoses should be carefully documented in the patient's medical record. Failure to do so has legal and fiscal implications related to quality-of-care issues (Palmer et al., 1992).

Remember that a holistic approach must be used during assessment. The patient's cognitive and physical status must be considered as well as his or her environmental context. A urinary tract problem may be a symptom of another disease process.

COLLECTING URINE SPECIMENS

Different types of urine specimens are required for different urine tests. Nursing responsibilities include the collection of specimens. Procedure 24–1 details the steps involved in collecting urine specimens.

ROUTINE URINALYSIS

For a routine urinalysis, a clean, randomly collected specimen is required. The specimen can be collected in a clean specimen pan or container from a clean urinal or from a patient's indwelling catheter. External collection devices, such as condom catheters or female external collection devices, can be used to collect routine specimens when patients are incontinent or cognitively impaired. The specimen should not be contaminated with stool. Some institutions use a *midstream urine collection technique,* also know as a *clean-catch technique,* to obtain a routine urine specimen. This involves cleansing the external meatus area with an antimicrobial solution and voiding a small amount into the toilet before starting to collect the specimen in a container.

For a *catheterized* specimen, a rubber, nylon, or clear plastic *catheter* or tube is inserted into the external meatus and then into the bladder via sterile technique. Urine is drained into a sterile container and transported to the laboratory for analysis. If the patient has an indwelling urinary catheter, the sterile specimen may be obtained from an access port in the drainage bag tubing. It is vital that sterile technique be followed for this procedure and that the closed system remain intact to avoid the risk of introducing organisms that can cause a UTI. *Culture and sensitivity* (C&S) and *urine cytology* tests also require a sterile specimen.

TWENTY-FOUR-HOUR URINE COLLECTIONS

Twenty-four-hour urine collections are required for certain laboratory tests. All the urine excreted over a 24-hour period

PATIENT TEACHING
INCREASING LIQUID INTAKE

1. Drink a minimum of ½ ounce of liquid for each pound of body weight each day (24 hours). Your requirement is ________ ounces.
2. Drink a glass of water, a cup of some juice or other liquid of your choice about every 2 hours.
3. If you are not drinking this much, increase the amount you drink gradually. Drink an additional ½ cup, about 4 ounces a day, then in 4 days increase another 4 ounces for 4 days and so on until you reach your required amount.
4. One easy method to keep track of the amount you are drinking each day is to place two containers of the amount of liquid you require in your refrigerator in the morning. These should be empty at bedtime. Another method is to mark down on a pad of paper each time you drink something.

You should gradually increase to the amount you require and continue to drink that amount.

This is a typical day and amount of liquid taken:

Rising	7 ounces or more of water (1 glass)
Breakfast	7 ounces or more of coffee (1 cup)
	4 ounces water (½ glass)
	4 ounces juice
	4 ounces milk
10:00 A.M.	7 ounces water or juice or other beverage
Noon meal	7 ounces water
	7 ounces beverage
	4 ounces milk
	3½ ounces soup
3:00 P.M.	7 ounces beverage
Evening meal	7 ounces beverage
	4 ounces water
Bed Time	3½ ounces water

In addition, you may take on your own any of these items:

extra juice = 4 ounces	martini = 3½ ounces
can of beverage = 12 ounces (1½ cups)	ice cream = 3½ ounces
Jell-O = 3½ ounces	wine = 3½ ounces
broth = 3½ ounces	sherbet = 3½ ounces
beer = 7 ounces	and others

From Pearson, B.D., Larson, J.M. (1992). Urine control by elders. In S. Funk, E.M. Tornquist, M.T. Champagne, R.A. White (eds.): *Key Aspects of Elder Care*. New York: Springer, pp. 154–168.

PATIENT TEACHING
REGULAR TOILETING: INSTRUCTIONS FOR PERSONS EMPTYING THEIR BLADDERS LESS THAN FIVE TIMES A DAY

Emptying your bladder regularly, 5 to 8 times a day, increases your control of urine and decreases the likelihood you will urinate involuntarily. To do so, you must have drunk adequate amounts of liquids (½ ounce of liquid per pound of body weight).

1. Empty your bladder immediately on arising from bed.
2. Empty your bladder before each meal.
3. Empty your bladder immediately before retiring to bed.
4. Empty your bladder one time each night, if necessary.

Each time you do so, celebrate the fact that you have control of your urine. Drink ½ cup of water each time you go to the bathroom at night.

5. Urinate at least every 2–3 hours during the day.

Example		
	6:00 A.M.	1:00 P.M.
	7:00 A.M.	4:00 P.M.
	9:00 A.M.	7:00 P.M.
	11:00 A.M.	9:00 P.M. (bedtime)

From Pearson, B.D., Larson, J.M. (1992). Urine control by elders. In S. Funk, E.M. Tornquist, M.T. Champagne, R.A. White (eds.): *Key Aspects of Elder Care*. New York: Springer, pp. 154–168.

is collected in a container. The test begins by having the patient empty his or her bladder. The time is noted and urine collection begins, continuing for 24 hours. The urine should be kept on ice during the entire period. Sometimes the laboratory supplies preservatives to be added to the specimen. If renal function needs to be evaluated or other complicating factors exist, serum (blood) studies may be performed in addition to urine tests.

The nurse needs to obtain the specimen appropriately. Sterile techniques must be used for sterile specimens. Timed specimens (24-hour or 19-hour specimens) need to be collected accurately and in appropriate containers. The nurse must always inform and instruct the patient and family to ensure compliance.

RECORDING INTAKE AND OUTPUT

Intake and output records, or *I&Os*, show the amount and frequency of urine voided over a 24-hour period. When possible, output is measured for each void by collecting it in a

PATIENT TEACHING
REGULAR TOILETING: INSTRUCTIONS FOR PERSONS EMPTYING THEIR BLADDERS MORE THAN EIGHT TIMES A DAY

Emptying your bladder more than 8 times a day increases your chances of losing control of urine. To urinate only 8 times a day, you must have drunk adequate amounts of liquids (½ ounce per pound of body weight).

1. Empty your bladder immediately on arising from bed.
2. Empty your bladder after each meal.
3. Follow the instructions for pelvic floor muscle exercises. Do these a total of 60 times a day.
4. Instead of rushing to the toilet in response to need to empty your bladder, pause, sit or stand quietly, relax your abdominal muscles, tighten your pelvic floor muscles; then walk at a normal pace to the toilet.
5. During the day, try to extend the length of time between emptying your bladder. You will probably find you can increase the length of time gradually.
6. Your goal is to empty your bladder ONLY every 2 to 3 hours during the day.

Do not be discouraged; changes take time. It may take you several months to achieve a frequency of only every 2 to 3 hours.

From Pearson, B.D., Larson, J.M. (1992). Urine control by elders. In S. Funk, E.M. Tornquist, M.T. Champagne, R.A. White (eds.): *Key Aspects of Elder Care.* New York: Springer, pp. 154–168.

PATIENT TEACHING
PREVENTING CONSTIPATION

1. Drink a minimum of ½ an ounce of liquid per pound of body weight each day (24 hours).
2. Once a day eat 3 or 4 dried prunes, or drink 4 ounces of prune juice.
3. Eat a serving of bran cereal each day, or eat 2 slices of bran bread (you may toast it if you prefer).
4. Set a regular time each day to have a bowel movement.
5. Do some type of physical exercise for at least 20 minutes. Walk if you can; if not, try tightening and relaxing your abdominal muscles 25 times after you go to bed.

From Pearson, B.D., Larson, J.M. (1992). Urine control by elders. In S. Funk, E.M. Tornquist, M.T. Champagne, R.A. White (eds.): *Key Aspects of Elder Care.* New York: Springer, pp. 154–168.

PATIENT TEACHING
GUIDELINES FOR PURCHASING AND TAKING VITAMIN B COMPLEX AND VITAMIN E

NOT RECOMMENDED IF YOU HAVE ENDOMETRIOSIS OR ARE TAKING ESTROGEN.

1. Read the label of vitamin B complex available at your usual drugstore, or show these guidelines to your pharmacist.
2. Purchase vitamin B complex whose label lists B_1, B_2, and so forth, or thiamine, riboflavin, niacin, and so forth, as no more than 100% of daily requirements. Vitamins are effective regardless of whether they are labeled natural or not. Take one each day after breakfast. Note that you may find your urine bright yellow the next time you pass urine. This is okay; it is not harmful.
3. Purchase vitamin E that is labeled 400 IU or 400 units. Take one tablet each day after breakfast. If you have diabetes, request aqua vitamin E from your pharmacist. (It is made by Armour and available from Nature Made or Valu-Rite.)
4. If you forget to take your vitamins after breakfast, they may be taken after lunch. DO NOT take 2 of each if you have missed a day.

DO NOT expect immediate results. Some women need several months before these vitamins are helpful.

From Pearson, B.D., Larson, J.M. (1992). Urine control by elders. In S. Funk, E.M. Tornquist, M.T. Champagne, R.A. White (eds.): *Key Aspects of Elder Care.* New York: Springer, pp. 154–168.

urinal, bedpan, or specimen pan and measuring it in a graduated container.

If a patient has an indwelling catheter, one usually measures I&Os every 4 or 8 hours by emptying the accumulated urine from the gravity urinary drainage bag. Patients may be asked to keep a voiding diary or record during an incontinence workup (see Fig. 24–8). The patient is instructed to record leakage episodes and their severity/symptoms on a chart or tablet.

NAME: ______________________________

DATE: ______________________________

INSTRUCTIONS: Place a check in the appropriate column next to the time you urinated in the toilet or when an incontinence episode occurred. Note the reason for the incontinence and describe your liquid intake (for example, coffee, water) and estimate the amount (for example, one cup).

Time interval	Urinated in toilet	Had a small incontinence episode	Had a large incontinence episode	Reason for incontinence episode	Type/amount of liquid intake
6–8 a.m.					
8–10 a.m.					
10–noon					
Noon–2 p.m.					
2–4 p.m.					
4–6 p.m.					
6–8 p.m.					
8–10 p.m.					
10–midnight					
Overnight					

No. of pads used today: __________ No. of episodes: ______________________

Comments: ______________________________

AHCPR Quick Reference Guide for Clinicians Number 2, 1996 Update

Figure 24-8. Sample bladder record.

CARE OF PATIENTS UNABLE TO USE NORMAL URINATION FACILITIES

In general, it is common practice for people who are ambulatory to use sanitary depositories for urinary elimination. Most civilized cultures provide some type of toilet for this purpose. Toilets are automatic water flushing devices, chemical chambers, or "outhouses" or latrines where body waste is deposited into an excavated pit.

Toilets vary from an opening or slit in the floor, requiring the person to use a squatting position to urinate or defecate, to an elevated bowl that allows elimination in a sitting position. Some elevated water flushing toilet facilities may provide for a bidet, a flushing device that cleanses the perineum. Urinals for males may or may not have water-flushing capabilities.

When persons are incapacitated they may be unable to use the usual toilet facilities, necessitating their adapting to other waste-collection methods. Patients with illnesses requiring home, hospital, or long-term care will need special assistance in eliminating body wastes.

Under all circumstances it is important to respect the patient and provide privacy. Patient rooms should be equipped with curtains or screens that ensure that they are accorded respect. Hand washing facilities also need to be provided to all patients after they eliminate body wastes.

Nurses must be aware of the possibility of cross-infections when handling body wastes. Universal precautions need to be exercised, and gloves should be worn under most circumstances. Equipment should be individualized and never shared between patients unless properly sterilized. Most institutions use disposable personal hygiene equipment. (See Chapter 26, Personal Hygiene, for more information.)

AMBULATORY PATIENTS

When patients have bathroom privileges, care must be taken to assess their ability to get in and out of bed and ambulate to and from the bathroom. Weakened, sedated, or disoriented patients should not be allowed to go to the bathroom without assistance. Many patient falls occur when patients are on their way to the bathroom (Garcia et al., 1988). Patients with urinary urgency may have an accident on the way to or in the toilet, slip, fall, and break a hip or do other serious damage. Bathroom doors should not be locked, and all bathrooms should have an alarm system within easy reach of the patient.

IMMOBILE PATIENTS

Because most men urinate in the standing position and most women do so in the sitting or squatting position, people often experience difficulties urinating when confined to bed. For bedridden patients, devices other than toilets are used to collect body wastes.

Urinals

Urinals are collection devices used when normal urinating facilities are not available to the patient. There are male and female urinals. Obviously the urinals are designed differently. Urinals may be plastic, metal, or glass (Fig. 24–9).

Female urinals are useful for immobilized women, for example, following hip or pelvic surgery or for women at complete bedrest or who are unable to void into a bedpan.

Male urinals may be used by ambulatory or immobilized male patients. If the male patient's condition allows, the nurse may assist the patient in sitting up and dangling the legs over the side of the bed or stand at the bedside.

When permitted by the patient's condition, those confined to bed may be assisted in voiding by elevating the head of the bed (Fowler's position). Nurses may need to hold the urinal in place if the patient is unable to do so.

The nurse should assess the characteristics of urine when emptying a urinal. Urinals need to be handled carefully after use to avoid soiling the patient's bed and emptied immediately after use. Patients should be provided with the opportunity to wash their hands after using the urinal.

Bedside Commode

In the event the patient is unable to ambulate to the bathroom or no toilet facilities are available, a portable toilet or bedside commode can be provided. The commode is a chair, with a toilet-like seat, equipped with a receptacle for the deposit of body waste.

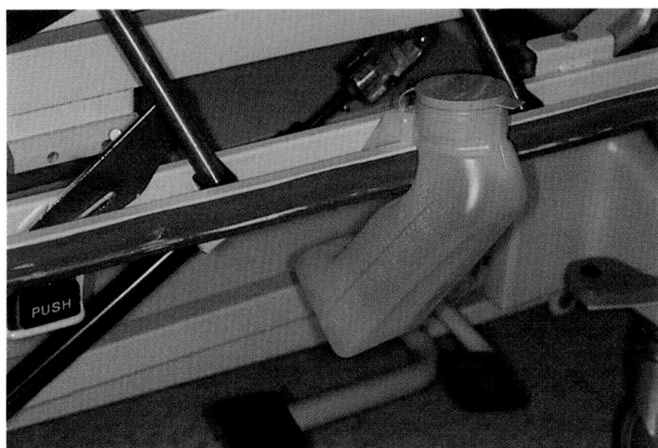

Figure 24–9. Urinal hung on bed frame.

The patient must be able to transfer safely from the bed to the commode. Furthermore, the patient should be carefully observed to determine if there is sufficient energy to be able to use the commode and provided with help when deemed necessary.

Bedpan

Bedpans tend to be more frequently used by female patients; however, males also use them for defecation purposes. Bedpans are of two types: a rounded elevated receptacle with a toilet-seat–like top or a fracture bedpan with a lower, flattened back and a toilet-like seat. A fracture pan is used for patients who are unable to elevate the buttocks, for example, persons with hip surgery or pelvic injuries. Bedpans are made from plastic or metal.

Patients that need to use a bedpan usually require nursing assistance. If the patient's condition allows, the head of the bed should be elevated and the patient instructed to flex the knees. The bedpan is placed under the hips of the patient in the most comfortable position possible. Care should be taken to prevent spillage when the bedpan is removed.

Urination in bed can be difficult. Techniques to assist the patient in urinating include pouring warm water over the perineum (assuming intake and output measuring are not required), discussing falling water, and placing the patient's hands in warm water. These techniques need to be validated through research.

CARE OF PATIENTS WITH URINARY DYSFUNCTION

Urinary disruptions can result from many different causes, such as infections, obstructions, neurologic injuries, surgery, and pregnancy. Under these circumstances, UI or retention can require catheterization of the patient or the patient may be catheterized for diagnostic reasons, i.e., collecting a sterile urine specimen. *Internal* catheterization is the process of inserting a plastic or rubber tube through the urinary meatus and urethra into the urinary bladder. An *external* catheter can be applied to the vulva or penis.

INTERNAL CATHETERIZATION

A *single-lumen catheter* is used for internal catheterization to remove urine from the bladder for the purposes of collecting a sterile urine specimen or to temporarily relieve acute urinary retention. The procedure may be performed via a sterile technique or may be a CIC in which the equipment is clean but not sterile.

CIC is a technique for managing acute or chronic urinary retention (*Renal and Urologic Disorders*, 1984). The patient or caregiver inserts a catheter through the urethra into the bladder to empty out the stored urine. The procedure is performed on a routine scheduled basis, usually every 3 to 6 hours. For most patients, catheterizing every 3 to 6 hours is sufficient. Research has demonstrated that nonsterile, clean CIC technique is a safe and effective management method

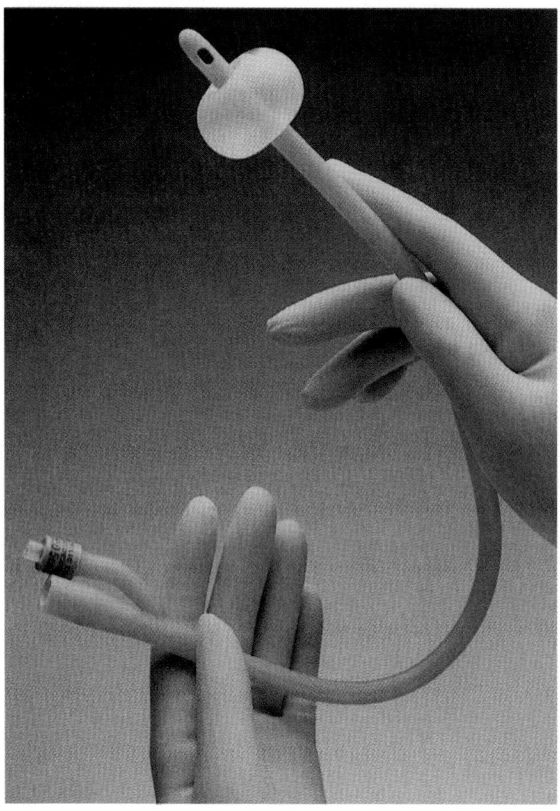

Figure 24–10. Two-way Foley catheter with balloon inflated. (Courtesy of Bard.)

(AHCPR, 1992). Infrequent complications include urethritis, UTI, stricture, epididymitis, and bladder stones. The patient may be taught the proper method to insert the catheter and relieve bladder retention.

A *double-lumen catheter* is used when an indwelling catheter is required (Fig. 24–10). Indwelling or Foley catheters are inserted and left in position. A balloon at the end of the catheter is inflated to keep the catheter in position in the bladder. Urine drains by gravity into a collection unit. The system is a closed, sterile system. Indwelling catheters can be used for monitoring output for bladder drainage or for controlling incontinence. Although long-term use of indwelling catheters (more than 2–4 weeks) is sometimes necessary to control chronic problems, the practice is discouraged because of the high rate of bacteriuria, UTI, and other complications associated with this practice (AHCPR, 1996; Clifford, 1982; Hart, 1985). Procedure 24–2 outlines the method for inserting an indwelling urinary catheter.

The catheter is attached to tubing and a bedside gravity drainage or collection bag. The bag is attached to the frame of the bed. Maintaining these systems as closed systems to minimize the introduction of organisms reduces infection rates (Roe et al., 1988). The tubing should always be kept lower than the bladder to facilitate gravity drainage. To minimize tension and drag on the external meatus, a leg strap or tape should be used to stabilize the tubing leading to the collection unit. This also prevents the tubing from becoming kinked or twisted.

In the past, catheter care was performed routinely on all patients with indwelling catheters. This procedure involved the use of topical antimicrobials at the insertion site. Today, perineal hygiene is generally considered sufficient to maintain an indwelling catheter (see Procedure 24–3). Gross build-up of mucus or other secretions may need extra attention such as intermittent irrigations (see Procedure 24–4).

To decrease the risk of introducing bacteria into the urinary tract, all equipment used during the indwelling catheterization procedure should be sterile. Strict aseptic technique is followed. The retention catheter, drainage bag, and tubing should be changed often to prevent blockages in the system. The presence of sediment in the drainage bag is an indication of the need to change the equipment. The drainage bag needs to be emptied as necessary but at least every 8 hours. Hand washing by all health care personnel who come in contact with the catheter and the urinary drainage is critical to help prevent UTI (Larson, 1989; Roe, 1990; Roe et al., 1988).

A *triple-lumen catheter* is used when there is need for an indwelling catheter, a lumen for drainage, and a lumen to irrigate or instill medication into the bladder. This type of catheter is primarily used following bladder or prostatic surgery (Procedure 24–5).

Indwelling catheters are removed by deflating the balloon in one of the lumens. It is important to carefully remove the catheter so that injury to the urethra is avoided.

EXTERNAL CATHETERIZATION

Male Collection Device

A condom (or Texas) catheter is used on male patients as a urine collection device. The condom is placed on the penis, attached to drainage tubing, and connected to a bedside or leg drainage bag (Procedure 24–6). The devices are made from latex or polyvinyl silicone and are either self-adhesive or have an adhesive band that fits around the penis. External catheters must be carefully sized or they will not stay in place. Improper sizing can lead to skin damage or penile damage if the catheter is too tight around the shaft, impeding circulation. Most manufacturers of external devices provide measuring guides with the product. The catheter should be changed every 24 hours. The skin underneath the catheter can be protected from the catheter adhesive or maceration with a skin sealant. Research suggests that there is an increased incidence of UTI associated with the use of external catheters (AHCPR, 1992; Ouslander, et al., 1987).

Female Collection Devices

Several external collection devices for women have been developed in recent years (Pieper, et al., 1989). Female anatomy makes this option much more difficult for women than for men. One currently available device for immobilized females is a modified ostomy pouch with a wafer barrier that is shaped to fit the labia majora. The labia must be carefully prepared, with the pubic hair trimmed back prior to application of the pouch. The device can be attached to a leg bag or to a gravity drainage bag. A second type of device for mobile women is made of a small silicon cup with tubing that fits between the labia and covers the urinary meatus. The device is held in place by stretch panties, and the tubing attaches to the leg bag. For selected mobile and dexterous female patients, the device can maximize control, convenience, and well-being.

CARE OF INCONTINENT PATIENTS

As previously discussed, there are many different types of incontinence. Care of the incontinent patient involves assisting patients to prevent or reduce the incidents in which incontinence occurs and caring for the skin and providing the incontinent patient with containment devices (see Clinical Decision Making box).

BEHAVIORAL TECHNIQUES TO PREVENT OR MINIMIZE URINARY INCONTINENCE

Behavioral techniques are noninvasive treatments used for the management of UI (Burgio and Burgio, 1986). Through this process, patients become more aware of their anatomy and can improve their control over the detrusor muscle and the pelvic floor muscles. This can improve incontinence control. Application of behavioral techniques is preceded by a thorough assessment of symptoms with appropriate diagnostic testing. Specific interventions are carried out. Positive feedback or reinforcers complete the process, which is based on the principles of operant learning.

Four major behavioral techniques are used for incontinence management:

- Bladder training (retraining)
- Habit training (timed voiding)
- Prompted voiding
- Pelvic muscle exercises

Other techniques that may be used alone or in combination with the behavioral techniques include the following:

- Biofeedback
- Vaginal cones
- Electrical stimulation

Behavioral techniques can also be combined with other treatment modalities, such as medications or surgery. In general, behavioral techniques have no side effects and can be used to treat most types of incontinence, except overflow incontinence. Behavioral techniques are the safest of all interventions.

Some techniques work better than others for particular individuals (McCormick and Burgio, 1984). Success rates vary. The success rate depends on the person's motivation, his or her cognitive ability, and the experience and skill of the health care practitioner teaching the technique. It may take weeks or months for patients to achieve results, and they must continue the techniques in order to maintain the benefits. As the AHCPR Guideline states:

> As a general rule, the least invasive and least dangerous procedure that is appropriate for the patient should be the first choice. For many forms of UI, behavioral and/or pharmacologic

CLINICAL DECISION MAKING
CARE OF THE INCONTINENT PATIENT

SITUATION

Mrs. Harris, an elderly widow who lives alone, has been diagnosed with mixed urge-functional incontinence. She is embarrassed about her problem and has refused to leave her house except to see the doctor. Yet, Mrs. Harris has said repeatedly that she wants to be independent in her activities of daily living and to interact with her friends socially. The nurse has been asked to develop a plan of care to help Mrs. Harris accomplish these goals.

FACTORS THAT INFLUENCE CARE

The nurse knows that age, mobility, dexterity, expectations, and social support systems are factors that will influence the plan of care for Mrs. Harris. Specific data needed from Mrs. Harris include:

- Documentation of episodes of wetness
- Environmental barriers
- Toileting habits/schedule
- Medication history
- Dietary habits

INTERVENTIONS

The nurse met with Mrs. Harris and reviewed the information. As she did so, she listened carefully to Mrs. Harris's definition of her problem and goals. The nurse understood why it was important to Mrs. Harris to be able to interact socially with her friends. Together they created a plan that included the following:

- A regular, frequent toileting schedule
- Assessment of her prescribed medication regimen
- Review of information regarding absorbent products to protect clothing
- Clothing adaptations
- Tentative schedule for brief trips to the grocery store, church, and lunch with friends

SELF-ASSESSMENT

The nurse found that she had associated Mrs. Harris with her own mother because they are similar in age and appearance. The nurse concluded that this association had not affected the plan of care.

REFLECTION

The nurse realized that for the immediate time period she would have to provide support to Mrs. Harris by calling her and asking questions regarding the effectiveness of the plan of care. The embarrassment experienced by Mrs. Harris is likely to keep her from contacting the nurse or anyone else for the necessary support.

interventions may help, but more research is required to determine the optimum treatment combinations in specific patient groups (AHCPR, 1992, p. 27).

Research suggests that behavioral techniques may significantly improve the incontinence of patients with dementia or mobility impairment (Heller et al., 1989).

Bladder Training or Retraining

Bladder training and retraining is a technique that teaches patients to void regularly and frequently. Positive reinforcement is provided. Usually, patients begin voiding every hour during the daytime, then gradually increase the interval to every 3 hours over a period of several weeks. Delay tactics, distractions, and relaxation techniques are used to increase the time interval between voiding. Bladder training helps both stress and urge incontinence. From 10 to 57 percent of patients treated this way report benefit from the treatment (Fantl et al., 1991).

Habit Training or Timed Voiding

Habit training or timed voiding is when toileting is scheduled at regular intervals (Criner, 1994). The voiding times are matched to the person's natural voiding schedule. A number of research studies demonstrate significant improvement in incontinence when this technique is used.

Prompted Voiding

Promoted voiding is a technique wherein the caregiver reminds the patient to void and then praises the patient for success. This method is useful for dependent and cognitively impaired patients. Frequent checks for dryness and prompting are made (usually every 1–2 hours). The use of prompted voiding in extended-care facilities has been shown in numerous trials to significantly reduce incontinent episodes.

Pelvic Muscle Exercises

Pelvic muscle exercises, also known as *Kegel exercises* (Brink et al., 1989; Kegel, 1949, 1951; Sampselle and DeLancey, 1992), strengthen the muscles of the pelvic floor and the periurethral muscles. These exercises help with both stress and urge incontinence. The prescribed exercise program is based on a pelvic-floor muscle evaluation and the severity of urinary incontinence. The exercise program is typically done two or three times a day for an indefinite period (see Patient Teaching: Pelvic Floor Muscle Exercises). Periodic reevaluation of the exercise program is needed, and benefits may not be noticed for 3 to 4 months. Reports of benefits range from 30 to 90 percent. Nurse specialists and physicians can teach these exercises to patients with or without *biofeed-*

PATIENT TEACHING
PELVIC FLOOR MUSCLE EXERCISES

RECOGNIZING THE CORRECT MUSCLES

Before you begin exercising the muscles supporting the abdominal contents from below (called the floor of the pelvis or pelvic floor), you must be certain that you are exercising the correct muscles. The following instructions labeled A, B, and C will teach you to recognize the correct muscles. You will want to lie on your back while you learn to identify the correct muscles.

A. Lubricate one finger (water works well) and place it in your vagina or your rectum. Now tighten your abdominal muscles and notice how this changes what you are feeling. THIS IS NOT WHAT YOU WILL FEEL WHEN TIGHTENING THE CORRECT MUSCLES.

B. Now with your abdominal muscles relaxed and while you are blowing air through your mouth, pull in around your lubricated finger as if you were trying to stop a bowel movement. THESE ARE THE MUSCLES YOU DO WANT TO TIGHTEN. Do not tighten your leg muscles.

C. Next time you need to urinate, sit on the toilet with your knees spread apart. Start to urinate, then stop; then start, then stop; then finish. When your muscles are strengthened, this can be done easily.

PELVIC FLOOR MUSCLE EXERCISES

Do these exercises THREE TIMES A DAY, one set while sitting, standing, and lying down. You may do these anytime—any place that is convenient for you.

A. Tighten your pelvic floor muscles; hold for 1 second; relax for 1 second; repeat about 10 times. Next, tighten your pelvic floor muscles; hold for about 10 seconds; relax for about 10 seconds; and repeat about 10 times. (You should tighten these muscles about 60 times a day.)

B. While practicing and using this exercise, make certain that you are keeping your abdominal muscles relaxed. If you also tighten the abdominal muscles, you will put pressure on the urinary bladder and it may empty. It is easier to keep the abdominal muscles relaxed if you breathe out while tightening the pelvic floor muscles. As you tighten your pelvic floor muscles, think about moving these muscles up an elevator, one floor at a time.

C. You should tighten these muscles:

1. immediately upon getting the urge to urinate, and before moving any other muscles in your body, walking, or changing your position;
2. before you start to get up from a chair;
3. before you move to get out of bed;
4. before and during lifting heavy objects.

DO NOT expect immediate results. Some women and men have done the exercises as directed for 2 to 6 months before they could laugh, cough, sneeze, or lift without leaking urine.

From Pearson, B.D., Larson, J.M. (1992). Urine control by elders. In S. Funk, E.M. Tornquist, M.T. Champagne, R.A. White (eds.): *Key Aspects of Elder Care*. New York: Springer, pp. 154–168.

back. The biofeedback equipment gives patients visual and audio feedback to help them to identify and use their muscles most effectively. A booklet with audiotape describing the exercises is available from HIP (see Box 24–4).

Biofeedback

Biofeedback uses sophisticated visual and auditory equipment to teach patients to gain improved control over their continence control mechanisms. Patients learn to identify their detrusor, abdominal muscles, and sphincter. They can improve their continence control. Biofeedback may be combined with pelvic muscle exercises, medications, or both. Reports of benefits range from 20 to 30 percent (Tries, 1990).

Vaginal Cones

Weighted vaginal cones are used as an adjunct to pelvic muscle exercises for women. A set of cones of identical shape and size, but increasing weight, are given to the woman. She inserts the cones intravaginally to increase the strength of the contraction needed when performing pelvic muscle exercises. This increases pelvic muscle strengthening.

Electrical Stimulation

This technique has several different applications. For example, electrical stimulation can be used to stimulate pelvic muscles, to induce bladder contractions, or to reduce detrusor overactivity. The treatment may cause pain or discomfort, and more research is needed to ascertain which parameters for electrical stimulation are most effective when combined with other management techniques.

SKIN CARE AND CONTAINMENT DEVICES

Skin Care

The skin should be cleansed as soon after urination as possible. Urine that is left on the skin decomposes, releasing ammonia. Ammonia is a skin irritant and cause dermatitis (McMullen, 1991), skin maceration (softening), and skin erosion.

As mentioned previously, warm water and soap are traditional cleansers, which while adequate for cleansing may cause irritation with repeated use or vigorous scrubbing. The newer pH-balanced perineal washes are preferable, especially with frequent incontinence. The abrasive effects of washcloths and the drying effects of soaps are avoided when perineal washes are used. Moisturizing lotions and moisture barrier ointments are recommended by most experts to protect the skin from maceration and breakdown. The nurse should follow universal precautions when performing skin care. More nursing research is needed to validate whether current nursing practices can be modified to minimize incontinence-related skin problems (Lyder et al., 1992).

Containment Devices

Total incontinence requires CIC and containment devices. Functional incontinence may be due to environmental barriers. A careful nursing assessment can call attention to these problems, and modifications can be identified and implemented. Other interventions for functional incontinence include prompt toileting and the use of adaptive equipment to assist with voiding transfers and dressing. If behavioral techniques are not sufficient to cure or manage the problem, medications or surgery are other options for people with alterations in urinary elimination.

A variety of devices are available to contain urine: self-adhesive external catheters, external collection devices for women, superabsorbent pads and garments, just to name a few. The most effective, least invasive, and least expensive device should be chosen.

A variety of absorbent products are available for managing incontinence. The most effective products whisk moisture away from the skin and prevent maceration. There are disposable and reusable products. Patients should be encouraged to buy products designed specifically for incontinence control and not sanitary napkins, which are less effective and more costly in the long run (Gartley, 1985).

CARE OF PATIENTS WITH URINARY RETENTION

Urinary retention has a variety of causes. Nursing care actions include monitoring the surgical patient, using methods to stimulate urination, measuring intake and output of body fluids to determine the presence of urinary retention, and preventing infections of the urinary system.

PRESURGICAL CARE

Anesthesia, hypnotics, and narcotics all depress neuromuscular function and can cause decreased urine production, delayed bladder emptying, and urinary retention. For these reasons, as well as to allow the outpatient to be carefully monitored, patients undergoing general anesthesia and surgery may require catheterization to accurately monitor output.

PROMOTING URINATION

Nursing measures that assist in promoting urination due to retention include the following:

- Offering fluids, especially warm drinks
- Warming the bedpan or urinal
- Running water from the tap within earshot of the patient
- Pouring warm water over the perineum
- Placing the patient's hands in warm water
- Performing intermittent catheterization (may require a physician order)

PREVENTING URINARY INFECTIONS

Urinary infections are a common cause of urinary retention. Preventing infections reduces the incidence of urinary retention. Nursing activities to reduce infections include the following:

- Using proper hand washing technique before and after voiding or caregiving (Larson, 1989)

- Using proper perineal hygiene, wiping from front to back
- Drinking adequate amounts of fluids to keep the urine dilute
- Voiding regularly so that the bladder does not become overdistended
- Avoiding bladder irritants, such as caffeine and alcohol
- Acidifying the urine by taking vitamin C supplements
- Wearing cotton underwear
- Avoiding perfumed soaps, fragrances, hygiene sprays, and toilet paper

CARE OF UROSTOMY PATIENTS

Urostomies are surgical diversions of the ureters. As previously discussed, there are different types of urostomies and the care of the patient depends on the type of urostomy performed; however, there are general procedures used for most cases. Procedure 24–7 details the steps involved in providing urostomy care.

POUCHING

Pouching for skin protection is particularly important for urostomy patients because the flow of urine is almost continuous. Prevention of peristomal skin maceration or erosion is critical. After the area around the stoma is cleaned, a gelatin wafer is applied. Pouches should always have skin wafers or rings attached to them. Many pouches have antireflux valves that reduce the backflow of urine onto the skin when the patient lies down. Pouches must fit with a tight seal so that no skin is exposed. Pouches should be emptied when they are approximately half full so that they do not pull off. Frequent drainage prevents urinary stasis in the pouch that can lead to bacteria buildup in the pouch.

Urostomy pouches have spigots or spouts at the bottom for emptying the urine. At night, people generally attach the pouch to a bedside gravity drainage system so they do not have to be awakened during the night. The urinary tube should be kink-free to prevent urine from backing up in the tubing. A catheter strap should be attached to the patient's leg to further eliminate kinking. To prevent a vacuum from forming, a small amount of urine should be left in the drainage bag. A dilute vinegar solution, a bleach solution, or a commercial cleaner can be used to clean the drainage bag used during the night.

The length of time between changing pouches varies with the patient but usually is 2 to 5 days. If the patient has a poor response to the pouch, if leakage is a problem, or if other complications develop, the patient should be examined by an experienced health care professional.

UROSTOMY DIETS

Certain foods are known to increase the odor of the urine, such as asparagus, garlic, and seafood. For patients with urostomies, it is critical that they maintain an adequate fluid intake of 1800 to 2400 ml per day unless contraindicated for some other medical reason (Hampton and Bryant, 1992). This amount of fluid intake helps to prevent the development of urinary calculi, UTIs, encrustations, and crystals. Normal dilute urine does not have a strong odor. A strong odor may be the first sign of a UTI (Smith and Babaian, 1989; Williamson, 1986). Concentrated urine suggests that the person's fluid intake is inadequate. The urine should be slightly acidic. If it is highly acidic or too basic, the person's diet may have to be regulated to prevent the formation of urinary stones or crystals. Vitamin C is often added prophylactically to the diet to acidify the urine.

PSYCHOSOCIAL CARE

Successful adjustment to urostomy surgery requires participation of the patient from the preoperative period through postoperative recovery (Smith and Babaian, 1989). The changes in self-image and lifestyle that may be required demand understanding, careful counseling and technically precise patient education. Early postoperative experiences, whether positive or negative, can have a lasting effect on a person's adjustment to ostomy surgery and on the mastery of tasks involved in self-care.

Both men and women experience changes in sexuality following urostomy surgery. Counseling, education, and referrals to support groups are important aspects of the nurse's role. People may also be referred to the organizations listed in Box 24–4.

BOX 24–4
COMMUNITY RESOURCES FOR PERSONS WITH ALTERATIONS IN URINARY ELIMINATION

AHCPR Clearinghouse
Agency for Health Care Policy and Research
Center for Research Dissemination and Liaison
P.O. Box 8547
Silver Spring, MD 20908
800-358-9295, 301-227-8364

Alliance for Aging Research
2021 K Street NW
Suite 305
Washington, DC 20006

HIP, Inc.
Help for Incontinent People, Inc.
P.O. Box 8306
Spartanburg, SC 29305
800-BLADDER, 803-579-7900

National Institute on Aging
9000 Rockville Pike
Bethesda, MD 20892
301-496-1752

The Simon Foundation for Continence
P.O. Box 815
Wilmette, IL 60091
800-23-SIMON, 708-864-3913

REFERRALS TO SELF-HELP GROUPS

There are two national self-help groups in the United States that supply information about incontinence and urinary management: Help for Incontinent People, Inc. (HIP) and the Simon Foundation. Both HIP and the Simon Foundation have newsletters, videos, and local support groups in many cities across the United States. Many of the support groups are led by nurses who have a special interest in incontinence. The message from the self-help groups for people is twofold: you are not alone, and there is hope and help (see Box 24–4).

When Mrs. Harris mustered up the courage to call the 800-number of the self-help group, she found a supportive and informative volunteer counselor on the other end of the line. Upon recommendation of the counselor, she saw a urogynecologist and went through urodynamic testing. Her diagnosis of mixed, urge-functional incontinence was confirmed.

The doctor started Mrs. Harris on a medication that decreased her uninhibited bladder contractions and increased her bladder capacity. A clinical nurse specialist taught her ways to modify her clothing with Velcro and obtained a toilet seat elevator for her. In addition, Mrs. Harris ordered protective liners for her panties to catch accidents. Now, 2 months later, she hardly has any problems, only an occasional dribble every now and then . . . for which she is extremely grateful.

Procedures

PROCEDURE 24-1

Collecting Urine Specimens (Sterile and Clean-Catch)

Objective

Obtain an uncontaminated urine specimen.

Terminology

- **Clean-catch specimen:** a midstream urine specimen collected after cleansing of urinary meatus.
- **Sterile specimen:** a urine specimen obtained by sterile catheterization of the bladder.
- **Urinary meatus:** the opening of the urethra at the perineum through which urine is eliminated from the bladder.

Critical Elements

This procedure requires a physician's order. Refer to the order for any specific details related to the procedure.

Prior to obtaining any urine specimen, the care provider should assess the patient's bladder. After the specimen is obtained, the urine should also be assessed for color, clarity, and odor.

Prior to either collection procedure, the perineum should be washed with soap and water.

Any procedure involving exposure of the genitourinary area is potentially embarrassing to the patient. The care provider should provide privacy and maintain patient dignity as much as possible throughout the procedure.

Clean-catch Specimen

The purpose of this procedure is to obtain a specimen that is free of the contamination found around the urinary meatus.

The care provider must evaluate the patient's ability to perform this procedure. The patient must be able to understand the instructions as well as have the manual dexterity to do the cleansing, use the equipment, and understand sterile precautions. If the patient cannot meet these requirements, the care provider needs to provide assistance.

If using a commercially prepared kit, the care provider should read the manufacturer's instructions prior to beginning. Some of the kits have instructions with illustrations that may be given to the patient.

Sterile Specimen

The purpose of this type of procedure is to obtain a sterile specimen directly from the bladder with a catheter. The physician may order the size of the catheter and amount of urine to be obtained (specimen only or drain the bladder).

This is always a sterile procedure. Whenever bladder catheterization is performed, there is a risk of introducing microorganisms into the urinary system. Because of this risk, it is important to complete the cleansing steps and to maintain sterile technique at all times.

Commercially prepared kits may be used for this procedure. In some kits the catheter is actually connected to the specimen container. The care provider should read the manufacturer's instructions prior to the procedure.

continued on next page

PROCEDURE 24-1 (cont'd)

Equipment

Clean-catch Specimen

(These items may be part of a commercially prepared kit. Some equipment is shown in Fig. 24–11.)

- Sterile gloves
- Cotton balls*
- Antiseptic solution*
- Water-soluble lubricant
- Specimen container
- Towel/washcloth

Sterile Specimen

(These items may be part of a commercially prepared kit.) (Fig. 24–12)

- Sterile gloves
- Cotton balls*
- Antiseptic solution*
- Water-soluble lubricant
- Specimen container
- Catheter
- Towel/washcloth

*Antiseptic wipes may be included instead of cotton balls/antiseptic solution.

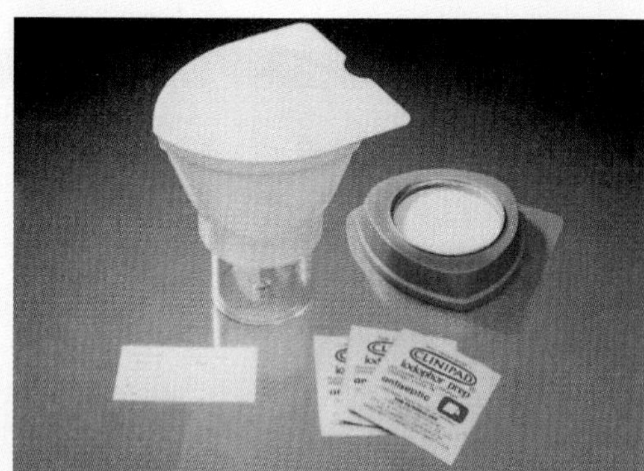

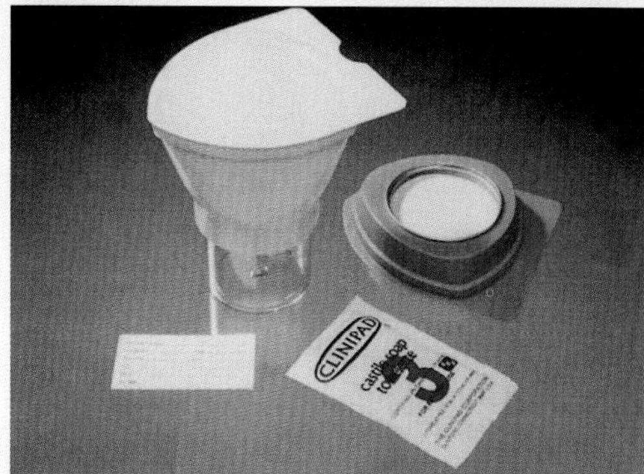

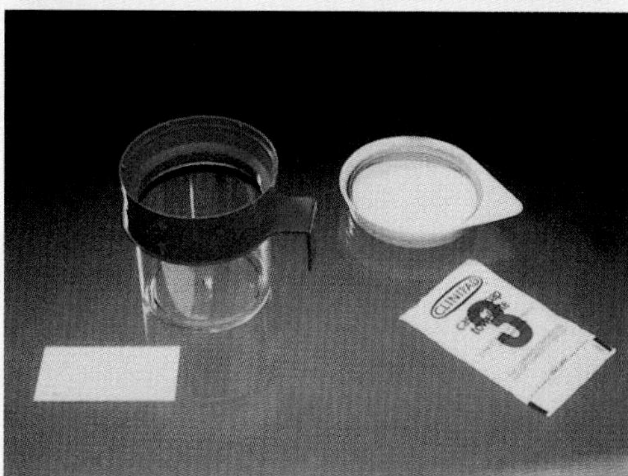

Figure 24–11. Equipment for midstream sample collection. (Courtesy of Bard.)

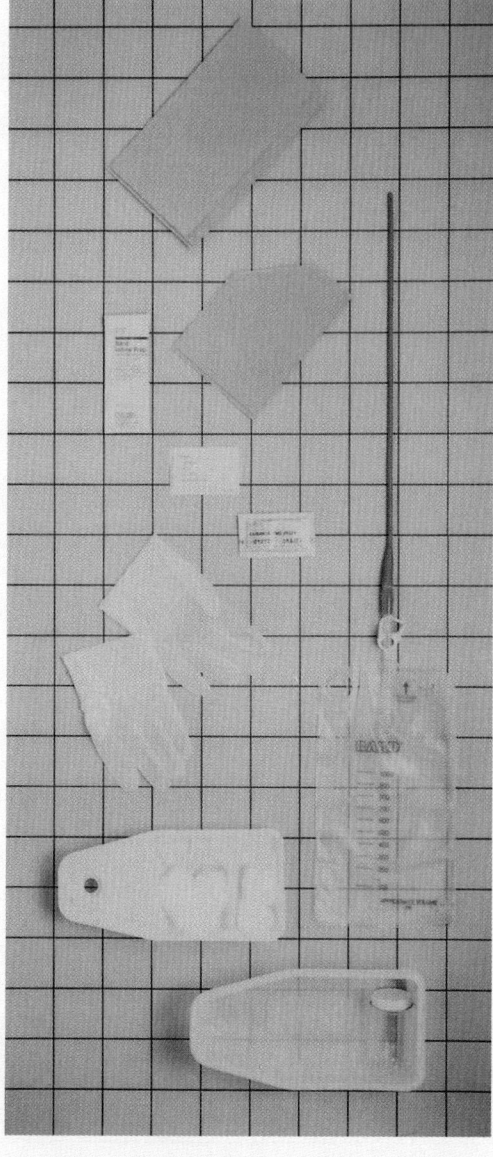

Figure 24–12. Urethral catheterization tray with drainage bag. (Courtesy of Bard.)

continued on next page

PROCEDURE 24-1 (cont'd)

Special Considerations

Depending on the patient's fluid balance status, it may be necessary to encourage the patient to take increased fluids in order to obtain the specimen.

When obtaining any specimen, care must be taken to ensure that the specimen is labeled properly and is accompanied by the specimen slip that reflects the test ordered by the physician. Specimens must be delivered to the laboratory promptly because allowing them to wait prior to testing may alter the results.

Sterile Specimen

When obtaining a sterile catheter specimen, the care provider should know whether the specimen should be the only urine obtained or if the bladder should be emptied. If draining the entire bladder remember that removing volumes greater than 750 ml at one time may lead to hypovolemic shock. Refer to your facility's policy on this issue or obtain physician orders clarifying this point prior to the procedure.

Action	***Rationale***
1. Verify order.	1. Ensures that proper procedure is performed.
2. Assemble equipment.	2. Promotes task organization.
3. Identify patient.	3. Provides patient safety.
4. Explain procedure.	4. Promotes patient compliance.

Clean-catch Specimen

1. Assist patient to bathroom/commode; close door/curtain.	1. Provides patient with privacy and maintains dignity.
2. Provide patient with all supplies within easy reach.	2. Allows patient easy access to supplies during procedure.
3. Don gloves.	3. Protects care provider from contact with blood or body fluids.
4. Perineal preparation.	4. Cleanse area, working from area of least contamination to greatest contamination while keeping labia from contacting meatus and recontaminating area.

Female Patient

Hold labia apart with nondominant hand (Fig. 24–13) (and continue to hold apart during entire procedure). Wipe with cotton balls soaked with antiseptic solution or antiseptic wipes. Using dominant hand, wipe first from front to back over area of meatus and then on each side.

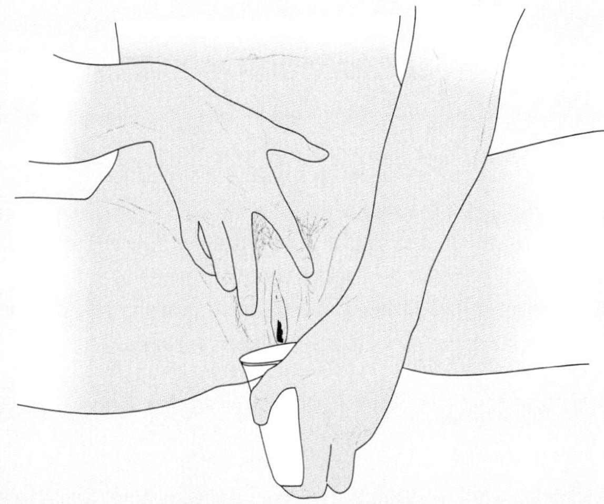

Figure 24–13. Technique for midstream sample collection: female.

continued on next page

PROCEDURE 24-1 (cont'd)

Male Patient

Hold penis firmly in nondominant hand (Fig. 24–14). Using cotton balls soaked with antiseptic solution or antiseptic wipes, wipe in circular motion around meatus and then around head of penis.

Cleanses area working from area of least contamination to greatest contamination.

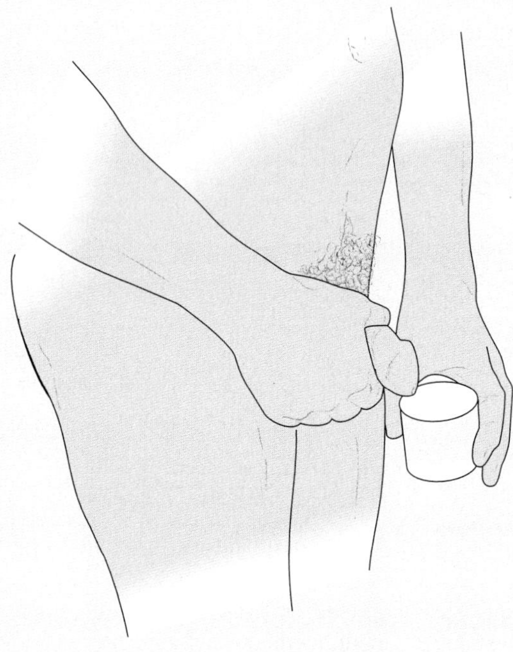

Figure 24–14. Technique for midstream sample collection: male.

5. Have patient start voiding, then place specimen cup under urine stream to catch specimen after first urine is eliminated.

5. Allows any remaining contamination to be washed off with initial urine stream, providing a specimen as free from contamination as possible.

6. Cover specimen container with sterile lid while allowing patient to finish voiding.

6. Protects specimen from contamination.

7. Dry perineal area and return patient to bed/chair.

7. Provides for patient comfort.

8. Discard or return supplies to appropriate area.

8. Provides clean, organized work area.

9. Send properly labeled specimen to laboratory promptly. Include all necessary laboratory slips for test ordered.

9. Ensures that proper test is performed and reported to proper patient record.

Sterile Specimen

Female Patient

1. Place patient on back with knees bent and legs apart; fold top linens back and cover abdomen and chest with bath blanket or sheet.

1. Positions patient so perineum can be accessed for procedure.

continued on next page

PROCEDURE 24-1 (cont'd)

2. Place catheterization tray between patient's legs. (*Note:* it may be necessary to use an overbed table placed over foot of bed if patient is in danger of touching tray during procedure.)

2. Allows easy access to supplies for care provider.

3. Remove sterile under drape, being sure to touch only corners in order to maintain sterility, and place under patient's hips.

3. Creates sterile field for procedure.

4. Don sterile gloves.

4. Protects patient from contamination by microorganisms during procedure and protects care provider from contact with blood or body fluids.

5. Set up supplies (Fig. 24–15):
   - Remove protective covering from catheter (if indicated).
   - Open antiseptic solution and pour onto cotton balls or open antiseptic wipes.
   - Open lubricant and squeeze onto area of tray that may be easily accessed.
   - Remove lid from specimen container.

5. Prepares supplies for use.

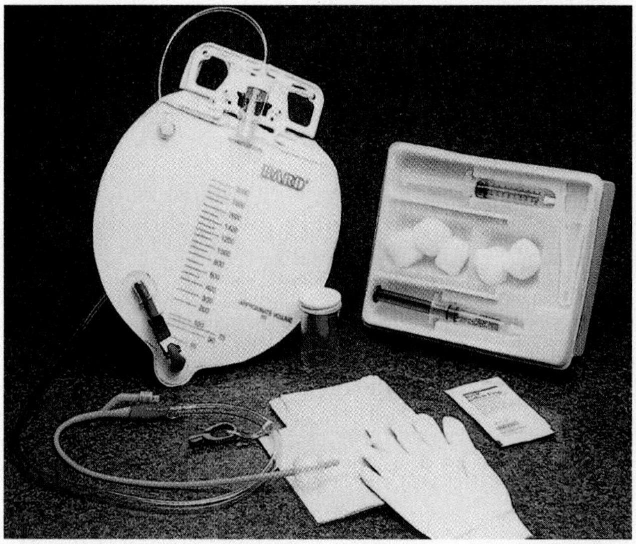

Figure 24–15. Equipment for indwelling catheterization. (Courtesy of Bard.)

6. Place fenestrated drape over perineal area with meatus exposed.

6. Creates sterile field for procedure.

7. Separate labia with nondominant hand. Continue to hold labia apart during entire procedure.

7. Allows visualization of urinary meatus.

8. Using a dominant hand, take cotton balls soaked with antiseptic solution or antiseptic wipes and wipe down over meatus from anterior to posterior, then discard cotton ball after each wipe. Then wipe each side of meatus using same process (Fig. 24–16).

8. Cleanses area to decrease possibility of microorganisms being introduced into urinary system during procedure.

continued on next page

PROCEDURE 24-1 (cont'd)

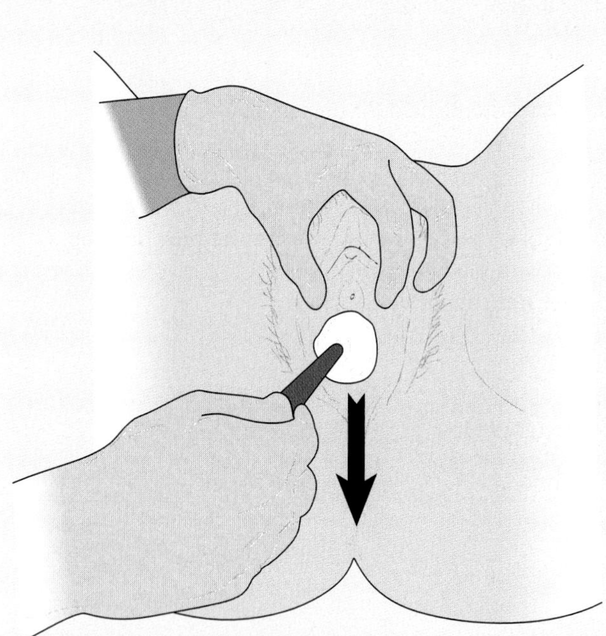

Figure 24–16. Cleansing labial folds and urinary meatus.

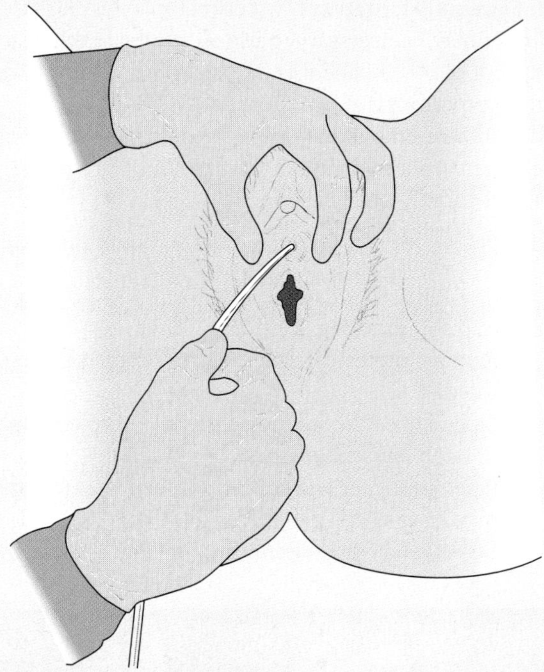

Figure 24–17. Inserting catheter: female.

9. Holding catheter in dominant hand lubricate tip of catheter for approximately 2–3 inches.

9. Facilitates introduction of catheter into urethra.

10. Gently insert catheter into meatus until urine begins to flow (Fig. 24–17).

10. Ensures catheter is in bladder.

11. If no urine is obtained:
    - Leave catheter in place.
    - Obtain second catheter.
    - Reglove.
    - Prepare perineum as indicated above.
    - Insert catheter using procedure above.

11. Allows first catheter to indicate improper position (usually catheter has been inserted into vagina) while attempting insertion of catheter into urinary meatus.

12. When urine begins flowing, obtain specimen in sterile container. Place lid on container after urine obtained.

12. Protects specimen from contamination.

13. Remove catheter while pinching tubing.

13. Prevents urine from catheter being left in urethra during removal process.

14. Return patient to position of comfort and cover with top linens.

14. Provides patient comfort and warmth.

15. Discard or return equipment to appropriate place.

15. Provides clean, organized work area.

16. Send properly labeled specimen to laboratory promptly. Include all necessary laboratory slips for test ordered.

16. Ensures that proper test is performed and reported to proper patient record.

Male Patients

1. Place patient on back with knees slightly flexed.

1. Positions patient for procedure.

2. Open set and place sterile drape over patient's thighs.

2. Creates a sterile field for procedure.

continued on next page

PROCEDURE 24-1 (cont'd)

3. Don sterile gloves.

3. Protects patient from contamination from microorganisms during procedure and protects care provider from contact with blood or body fluids.

4. Set up supplies:
   - Remove protective covering from catheter (if indicated).
   - Open antiseptic solution and pour onto cotton balls or open antiseptic wipes.
   - Open lubricant and squeeze onto area of tray that may be easily accessed.
   - Remove lid from specimen container.

4. Prepares supplies for use.

5. Place fenestrated drape so patient's penis is in opening.

5. Creates sterile field for procedure.

6. Grasp penis firmly in nondominant hand, holding at 90° angle to body.

6. Allows access to urinary meatus and straightens urethra in preparation for catheter insertion, while firm grasp helps decrease chance of erection.

7. Take cotton ball soaked with antiseptic solution and cleanse with a circular motion around the meatus, then dispose of the cotton ball. Repeat with a new cotton ball, going from the area around the meatus down the penis (Fig. 24–18).

7. Cleanses area to decrease possibility of microorganisms being introduced into urinary system during procedure.

8. Holding catheter in dominant hand lubricate first 3–4 inches of catheter.

8. Facilitates introduction of catheter into urethra.

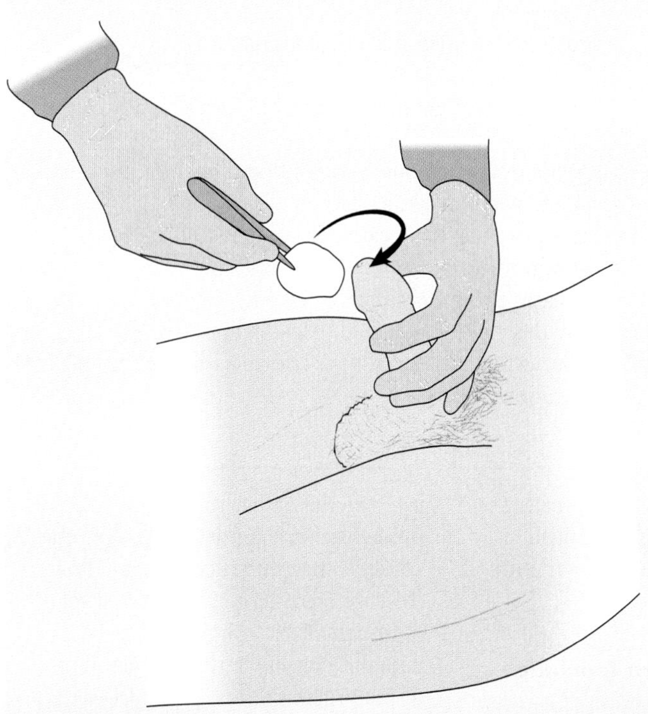

Figure 24–18. Cleansing penis.

continued on next page

PROCEDURE 24-1 (cont'd)

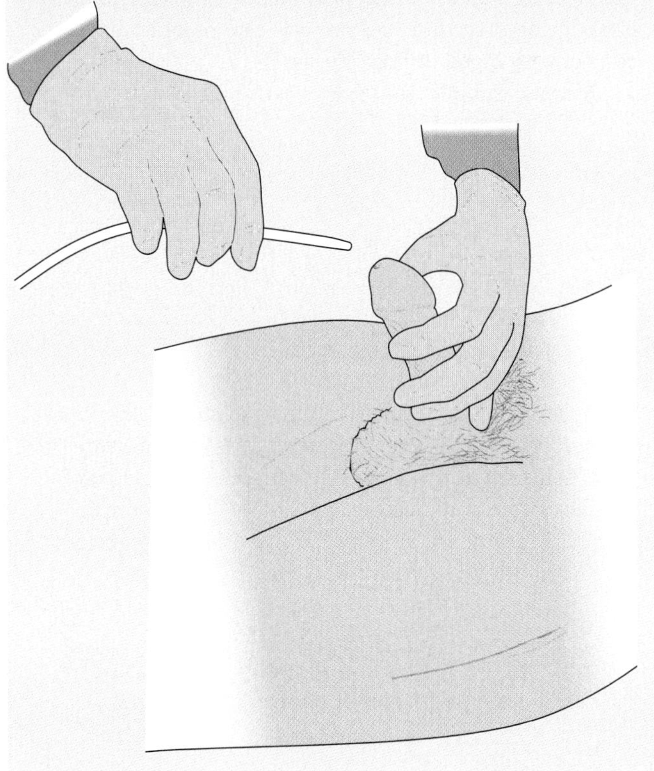

Figure 24–19. Inserting catheter: male.

Action	Rationale
9. Gently insert catheter until urine is obtained (Fig. 24–19). Collect specimen and cover container with lid.	9. Protects specimen from contamination.
10. If unable to insert catheter, gently pull upward on penis.	10. Facilitates straightening of urethra for easier insertion.
11. If still unable to insert catheter, remove catheter and notify physician.	11. Avoids excess trauma to urethra and enables physician to evaluate need for coudé catheter.
12. Remove catheter while pinching tubing.	12. Prevents urine from catheter being left in urethra during removal process.
13. Return patient to position of comfort.	13. Provides patient comfort.
14. Discard or return equipment to appropriate place.	14. Provides clean, organized work area.
15. Send properly labeled specimen to laboratory promptly. Include all necessary laboratory slips for test ordered.	15. Ensures that proper test is performed and reported to proper patient record.

Documentation

Record in the patient record that the procedure is done, time completed, amount of urine obtained, and patient response to the procedure. Note whether the bladder has been emptied when taking catheter specimens. Also note the assessment of the bladder (if pertinent) and the assessment of the urine. All output should be recorded on the patient's intake and output record.

Elements of Patient Teaching

Instruct the patient/family regarding the purpose of the procedure. Assess the patient's ability to perform the procedure independently. Having the patient repeat instructions can allow the care provider to assess the level of understanding. Instruct the patient/family regarding all elements of the procedure, including the need for sterile technique.

PROCEDURE 24-2

Inserting and Removing an Indwelling Urinary Catheter

Objective

Provide a mechanism to drain urine continuously from the bladder and/or manage urinary incontinence. Measure accurate intake and output.

Terminology

- **Urinary meatus:** the opening of the urethra at the perineum through which urine is eliminated from the bladder.
- **Coudé catheter:** a urinary catheter that has a curved tip and is stiffer than an ordinary catheter; often used for catheterization of males with prostatic hypertrophy.
- **Three-way catheter:** a urinary catheter that has three lumens: one for urine drainage, one for filling the balloon tip, and one for continuous/intermittent irrigation.
- **Foley catheter:** an indwelling urinary catheter used for continuous bladder drainage.

Critical Elements

This procedure requires a physician's order. The order also indicates whether irrigation will be continuous so that a three-way catheter can be obtained if indicated. The choice of catheter size depends on patient anatomy and physical condition (i.e., patients undergoing urinary surgery who may have bloody urine and clots may need a larger-lumen catheter). The order may also indicate the size of the balloon on the catheter. Most catheters have a 5- to 10-ml balloon, but some have a 30-ml balloon. The larger balloon is often used after prostatic surgery in order to help provide hemostasis to the prostatic fossa. Noting the balloon size on the catheter also is important in order to select the appropriate size of syringe for balloon deflation during the catheter removal process.

Urinary catheter insertion is always a sterile procedure because there is always a risk of introducing microorganisms into the urinary system during the procedure. During the time that the indwelling catheter is in place, there is also a danger of infection; therefore, the following precautions should be taken: (*Note:* if the patient/family will be caring for the catheter or if the patient is ambulatory while carrying the urine drainage bag, instructions should be given regarding the following issues.)

1. The catheter should be cleansed daily to remove any secretions that may collect around the catheter at the urinary meatus.
2. The urine drainage system should not be opened because this may allow the introduction of microorganisms into the system (the exception to this is opening the drainage bag for the purpose of emptying).
3. The drainage bag should be kept below the level of the bladder at all times to prevent backflow of urine into the bladder from the bag or tubing.

Assess the patient for any latex allergy prior to choosing a catheter. Many Foley catheters are made of latex. If an allergy to this substance exists, the care provider must obtain a plastic/vinyl catheter. Latex allergy reactions can be severe and even lead to death.

When the patient has an indwelling Foley catheter, the care provider should always assess the urinary meatus for any signs of infection such as unusual drainage, redness, or swelling. In addition the bladder should be palpated and the urine should be assessed at this time. Note any signs or symptoms of urinary infection or retention such as fever, foul-smelling urine, cloudy urine, hematuria, suprapubic or flank pain, or distended bladder.

Changing an indwelling catheter may require a physician's order. Refer to your facility's policy for guidance.

When emptying the urinary drainage bag, the care provider should make sure to accurately total and record the output. An assessment of the bladder and urine drainage should also be noted.

Never force the catheter into the meatus during the insertion procedure. It may be necessary to use gentle pressure to ease the catheter into the male urethra if there is prostatic hypertrophy. If gentle pressure is not sufficient, stop the procedure and notify the physician. A coudé catheter may be indicated.

Equipment

- Bath blanket/sheet
- Waste receptacle (the plastic wrapper from the catheterization tray is often used for this purpose)

These Supplies Are Usually Part of a Commercial Urinary Catheterization Set (see Fig. 24–15)

- Sterile gloves
- Under drape
- Fenestrated drape
- Cotton balls
- Antiseptic solution
- Water-soluble lubricant
- Foley catheter
- Drainage bag and tubing
- Specimen container
- Syringe filled with sterile water

For the Removal of a Catheter

- Gloves
- 10- to 20-ml syringe
- Bed protector underpad/towel

continued on next page

PROCEDURE 24-2 (cont'd)

Special Considerations

The care provider should assess the balloon on the catheter prior to inserting it in the patient. This is done while setting up the contents of the catheterization set.

Procedures dealing with the genitourinary area may be embarrassing to the patient. Care should be taken to provide privacy and comfort to the patient throughout the procedure. In order to increase patient comfort, an order for use of lidocaine jelly (for use as a lubricant) may be obtained from the physician.

Prior to starting the procedure, the care provider should assess the patient's ability to maintain the necessary position. If it is thought that the patient will be unable to do this, pillows may be used to assist the patient or a second person may be needed in order to maintain the proper position. This is important because patient movement during the procedure may lead to contamination, which may in turn cause the inadvertent introduction of microorganisms into the urinary system.

It may be necessary to use clean gloves to inspect the female perineal area in order to locate the urinary meatus prior to the beginning of the procedure. This may be indicated if there has been prior perineal surgery or trauma that may cause difficulty in visualizing the meatus.

Some facilities recommend taking a urine specimen at the time of catheter removal (refer to your facility's policy).

Action	*Rationale*
1. Verify order.	1. Ensures proper procedure is performed.
2. Assemble supplies.	2. Promotes task organization.
3. Identify patient.	3. Provides for patient safety.
4. Explain procedure.	4. Promotes patient compliance.
5. Close door/curtain.	5. Provides patient privacy and maintains dignity.

Catheter Insertion

For Female Patient

1. Place patient on back with knees bent and legs apart; fold top linens back and cover abdomen and chest with bath blanket or sheet.	1. Positions patient so perineum can be accessed for procedure.
2. Place catheterization tray between patient's legs. (*Note:* it may be necessary to use an overbed table placed over foot of bed if patient is in danger of touching tray during procedure.)	2. Allows easy access to supplies for care provider.
3. Set up supplies in tray: • Remove protective covering from catheter (if indicated). • Open antiseptic solution and pour over cotton balls. • Open lubricant and squeeze onto area of tray that may be easily accessed. • Test balloon of catheter by filling then deflating with sterile water and syringe.	3. Prepares supplies for use.
4. Remove sterile under drape being sure to touch only corners, in order to maintain sterility, and place under patient's hips.	4. Creates sterile field for procedure.
5. Don sterile gloves.	5. Protects patient from contamination by microorganisms during procedure and protects care provider from contact with blood or body fluids.
6. Place fenestrated drape over perineal area with meatus exposed.	6. Creates sterile field for procedure.

continued on next page

PROCEDURE 24-2 (cont'd)

7. Separate labia with nondominant hand. Continue to hold labia apart during entire procedure.	7. Allows visualization of urinary meatus.
8. Using dominant hand, take forceps from tray, pick up cotton ball soaked with antiseptic solution, wipe down over meatus from anterior to posterior, then discard cotton ball. Repeat, wiping with new cotton ball for each wipe, going down on each side of meatus (see Fig. 24–16).	8. Cleanses area to decrease possibility of microorganisms being introduced into urinary system during procedure.
9. Holding catheter in dominant hand, lubricate tip of catheter for approximately 2–3 inches.	9. Facilitates introduction of catheter into urethra.
10. Gently insert catheter into meatus until urine begins to flow.	10. Ensures that catheter is in bladder.
11. If no urine is obtained: • Leave catheter in place. • Obtain second catheter. • Reglove. • Prepare perineum as indicated above. • Insert catheter using procedure above.	11. Allows first catheter to indicate improper position (usually catheter has been inserted into vagina) while one is attempting insertion of catheter into urinary meatus.
12. When urine is visualized, fill balloon and gently pull on catheter. (*Note:* if patient complains of pain while balloon is filled, deflate balloon and insert catheter further and try filling again.)	12. Provides means to maintain catheter in bladder; pulling gently will test this.
13. Tape catheter to patient's thigh (Fig. 24–20).	13. Protects urinary meatus from trauma due to pulling on catheter tubing.

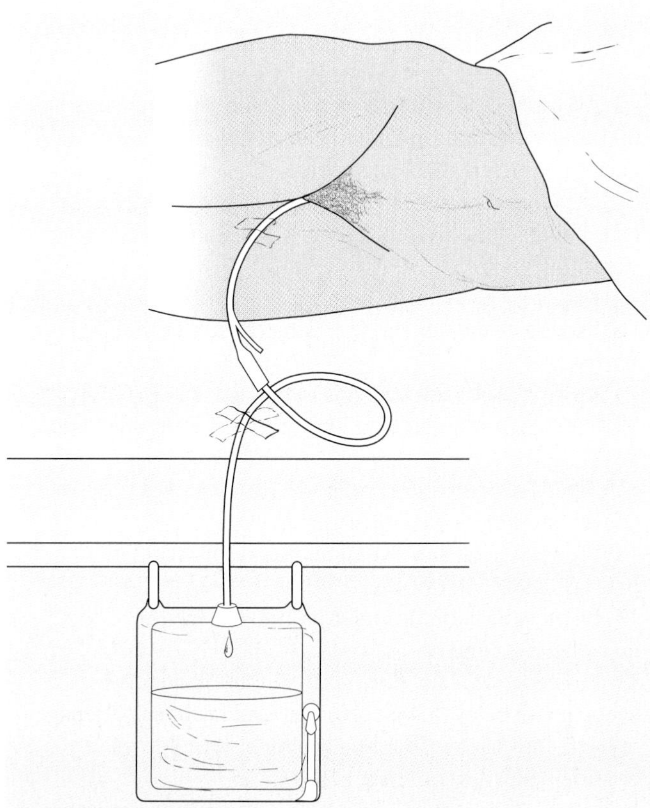

Figure 24–20. Securing catheter to female patient's thigh.

continued on next page

PROCEDURE 24-2 (cont'd)

Action	Rationale
14. Hang bag at bedside below level of bladder, placing tubing on bed (see Fig. 24–22).	14. Protects from back flow of urine into bladder by keeping bag below level of bladder and facilitates drainage of urine into bag by avoiding tubing hanging down at bedside below level of bag.
15. Pull up top linens and return patient to position of comfort.	15. Provides for patient comfort.
16. Discard or return supplies to appropriate place.	16. Provides clean, organized work area.
For Male Patient	
1. Place patient on back with knees slightly flexed.	1. Positions patient for procedure.
2. Open set and remove sterile under drape placing it over patient's thighs.	2. Creates a sterile field for procedure.
3. Set up supplies in tray: • Remove protective covering from catheter (if indicated). • Open antiseptic solution and pour onto cotton balls. • Open lubricant and squeeze onto area of tray that may be easily accessed. • Test balloon of catheter by filling and then deflating with sterile water and syringe.	3. Prepares supplies for procedure.
4. Don sterile gloves.	4. Protects patient from contamination from microorganisms during procedure and protects care provider from contact with blood and body fluids.
5. Place fenestrated drape so patient's penis is in opening.	5. Creates sterile field for procedure.
6. Grasp penis firmly in nondominant hand, holding at 90° angle to body.	6. Allows access to urinary meatus and straightens urethra in preparation for catheter insertion, while firm grasp helps decrease chance of erection.
7. Take cotton ball soaked with antiseptic solution and cleanse with circular motion around meatus, then dispose of cotton ball. Repeat with new cotton ball, going from area around meatus down penis (see Fig. 24–18).	7. Cleanses area to decrease possibility of microorganisms being introduced into urinary system during procedure.
8. Holding catheter in dominant hand, lubricate first 3–4 inches of catheter.	8. Facilitates introduction of catheter into urethra.
9. Gently insert catheter until urine is obtained.	9. Ensures that catheter tip is in bladder.
10. If unable to insert catheter, gently pull upward on penis.	10. Facilitates straightening of urethra for easier insertion.
11. If still unable to insert catheter, remove catheter and notify physician.	11. Avoids excess trauma to urethra and enables physician to evaluate need for coudé catheter.
12. When urine is visualized, fill balloon and gently pull on catheter.	12. Provides means to maintain catheter in bladder; pulling gently will test this.
13. Tape catheter to patient's thigh or leg (Fig. 24–21).	13. Protects urinary meatus from trauma due to pulling on catheter tubing.
14. Hang bag at bedside below level of bladder, placing tubing on bed (Fig. 24–22).	14. Protects from backflow of urine into bladder by keeping bag below level of bladder and facilitates drainage of urine into bag by avoiding tubing hanging down at bedside below level of bag.

continued on next page

PROCEDURE 24-2 (cont'd)

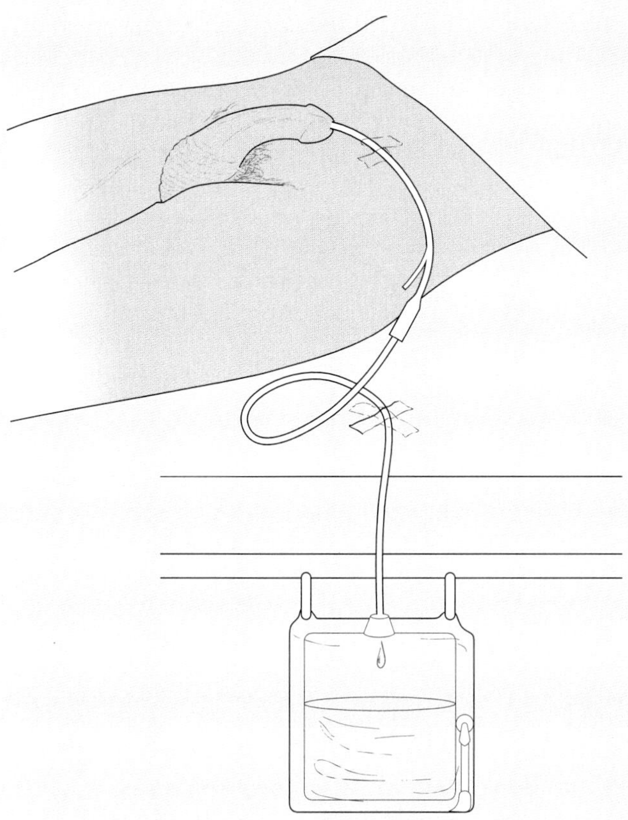

Figure 24–21. Securing catheter to male patient's abdomen.

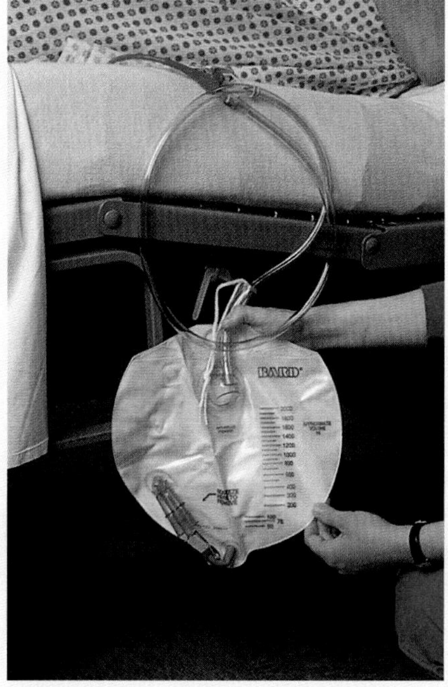

Figure 24–22. Securing drainage setup.

15. Pull up top linens and return patient to position of comfort. — 15. Provides for patient comfort.

16. Discard or return supplies to appropriate place. — 16. Provides clean, organized work area.

Catheter Removal

1. Inspect catheter for markings. — 1. Determines size of catheter balloon so that appropriate size of syringe may be used.

2. Place patient in supine position; female patients should have knees bent and legs separated. Fold top linens back and place bed protector pad under patient's hips for female or towel just under penis for males. — 2. Positions patient for procedure.

3. Don gloves. — 3. Protects care provider from contact with blood and body fluids.

4. Attach syringe to Leur lock valve on catheter and withdraw all solution from balloon. — 4. Collapses balloon on tip of catheter in preparation for removal.

5. While pinching catheter, gently remove from urethra. — 5. Avoids possibility of urine in catheter being deposited in urethra during removal procedure.

6. Pull up top linens and return patient to position of comfort. — 6. Provides for patient comfort.

7. Discard or return equipment to appropriate place. — 7. Provides clean, organized work area.

continued on next page

PROCEDURE 24-2 (cont'd)

Documentation

Record in the patient record the time the procedure was done along with the patient's response. Note assessment of the bladder as well as assessment of urine, including color, clarity, and presence of any unusual substance such as blood. All urine output should also be noted on the patient's intake and output record. Note in the patient record if a specimen was sent to the laboratory.

Elements of Patient Teaching

Instruct patient/family on purpose of the procedure. If patient will be ambulating with catheter in place, instruct on the importance of keeping drainage bag lower than the bladder. Also instruct on need for catheter care. If patient/family will be performing this procedure, allow time in the instruction process to have a return demonstration in order to ascertain patient/family competence. Encourage increased fluid intake unless otherwise contraindicated.

At the time of catheter removal, assure the patient that it is not unusual to feel the urge to void immediately after the catheter is removed. In addition, instruct the ambulatory patient to save the first voiding (or all voidings if on intake and output measurement) and provide a means to collect this urine, such as an in-toilet measuring container. Also inform the patient that the first voiding may be uncomfortable.

PROCEDURE 24-3

Providing Indwelling Catheter Care

Objective

Minimize catheter-associated urinary tract infection through the cleansing of the catheter at the urinary meatus.

Terminology

- **Urinary meatus:** the opening of the urethra at the perineum through which urine is eliminated from the bladder.
- **Foley catheter:** an indwelling urinary catheter used for continuous bladder drainage.

Critical Elements

Catheter care should be a part of patient hygiene each day. As such, it is usually performed at the same time as bathing. Policies regarding the frequency and use of special cleansing solutions (i.e., povidone-iodine solution) vary from facility to facility. Refer to your facility's policy prior to proceeding.

Infection from the presence of a Foley catheter is one of the greatest problems with an indwelling catheter. Because of this, the following precautions should be taken. (*Note:* if the patient/family will be caring for the catheter or will be ambulating while carrying the urine drainage bag, they too should be instructed regarding these issues.)

1. The catheter should be cleansed to remove any secretions that may collect around the catheter at the urinary meatus.
2. The urinary drainage system should not be opened because this may allow the introduction of microorganisms into the system (the exception to this is opening the drainage bag for the purpose of emptying).
3. The urinary drainage bag should be kept below the level of the bladder at all times to prevent backflow of urine into the bladder from the bag or tubing.

The urinary meatus should be observed for any signs of infection, such as unusual drainage, redness, or swelling. In addition, the bladder and the urine should be assessed at this time. Note any signs or symptoms of urinary infection in the patient, such as fever, foul-smelling urine, cloudy urine, hematuria, or suprapubic or flank pain.

Equipment

- Wash cloth
- Towel
- Soap
- Gloves
- Sheet/bath blanket (if indicated)

Special Considerations

Procedures dealing with the genitourinary area may be embarrassing to the patient. Care should be taken to provide privacy and comfort to the patient throughout the procedure.

continued on next page

PROCEDURE 24-3 (cont'd)

Action	*Rationale*
1. Assemble equipment.	1. Promotes task organization.
2. Identify patient.	2. Provides for patient safety.
3. Explain procedure.	3. Promotes patient compliance.
4. Close door/curtain.	4. Provides patient privacy and maintains dignity.
5. Fold back top linen (if not already done such as during bath) and cover top of patient with sheet or bath blanket.	5. Exposes area for procedure while still providing warmth to patient.
For Female Patient	
1. Hold labia apart and wash with warm, soapy wash cloth around urinary meatus and down catheter. Dry thoroughly after washing.	1. Cleanses site of catheter insertion to help inhibit microorganisms from traveling up catheter to bladder.
2. Wash and dry rest of perineal area. (*Note:* all washing strokes should use a separate, clean portion of wash cloth and go from anterior area to posterior.)	2. Provides cleansing with uncontaminated cloth to each area as well as from area of least contamination to area of greatest contamination.
3. Return patient to position of comfort and cover with top covers.	3. Provides comfort and warmth.
4. Discard or return equipment to appropriate place.	4. Provides clean, organized work area.
For Male Patient	
1. Grasp penis firmly and wash with a warm soapy wash cloth around urinary meatus and down catheter. Dry thoroughly after washing.	1. Cleanses site of catheter insertion to help inhibit microorganisms from traveling up catheter to bladder.
2. Cleanse and dry rest of penis, going from tip to base.	2. Provides cleansing from area of least contamination to area of greatest contamination.
3. Return patient to position of comfort and cover with top covers.	3. Provides comfort and warmth.
4. Discard or return equipment to appropriate place.	4. Provides clean, organized work area.

Documentation

Record the procedure in the patient record. Note the assessment of the bladder, urine (color, clarity, presence of any unusual substance such as blood), and perineal area. Note patient's response to the treatment.

Elements of Patient Teaching

Instruct patient/family regarding the purpose of catheter care. If patient/family will be performing this task, allow time for a return demonstration so the care provider can assess competency. If the patient will be ambulating with the catheter in place, instruct on importance of keeping drainage bag lower than the bladder. Encourage increased fluid intake unless otherwise contraindicated.

PROCEDURE 24-4

Irrigating an Indwelling Urinary Catheter

Objective

Provide intermittent irrigation of urinary catheter to maintain patency.

Terminology

- **Foley catheter:** an indwelling urinary catheter used for continuous bladder drainage (see Fig. 24–10).

Critical Elements

This procedure usually requires a physician's order. Refer to your facility's policy prior to proceeding. The order often states the frequency of irrigation, solution to be used, and amount to be used.

This is a sterile procedure. Sterile technique is important in order to keep from introducing microorganisms into the urinary tract system. Infection from the presence of a Foley catheter is one of the greatest problems with an indwelling catheter. Because of this, the following precautions should be taken. (*Note:* if the patient is ambulatory or if the family will be caring for the catheter, they too should be instructed regarding these issues.)

1. The catheter should be cleansed daily to remove any secretions that may collect around the catheter at the urinary meatus.
2. The urinary drainage system should be opened only when necessary because interrupting the system may allow the introduction of microorganisms into the system (the exception to this is opening the drainage bag for the purpose of emptying).
3. The urinary drainage bag should be kept below the level of the bladder at all times to prevent backflow of urine into the bladder from the bag or tubing.

When caring for a Foley catheter, always observe the urinary meatus for any signs of infection, such as unusual drainage, redness, or swelling. In addition, the bladder and the urine should be assessed at this time. Note any signs or symptoms of urinary infection in the patient, such as fever, foul-smelling urine, cloudy urine, hematuria, or suprapubic or flank pain.

Intermittent irrigation is often used after urologic surgery. Always note the color of the urine prior to and after the irrigation. If blood is in the urine, the amount of bleeding should decrease over time. If this does not occur, report this to the physician. The care provider should also note and report significant changes in laboratory values that may indicate the extent of blood loss.

If you are unable to irrigate the Foley catheter, do not try to force the irrigation solution. Stop the procedure and notify the physician. If the patient complains of pain during procedure, stop and call the physician.

Equipment

- Bath blanket
- Sterile gloves
- Alcohol wipes (or solution recommended by facility policy)
- Sterile tubing cap
- Irrigation solution (per order or policy)
- Sterile basin*
- 30- to 60-ml sterile syringe*
- Sterile drape*
- Graduated solution container*

*May be part of an irrigation set.

Special Considerations

Irrigation solution should not be included as part of the urinary output. If the irrigation solution introduced into the Foley catheter does not return at the time of irrigation, be sure to note this in the patient record as well as deleting it from the urinary output totals.

Procedures dealing with the genitourinary area may be embarrassing to the patient. Care should be taken to provide privacy and comfort to the patient throughout the procedure.

Action	*Rationale*
1. Verify order.	1. Ensures that correct procedure is performed.
2. Assemble equipment.	2. Promotes task organization.
3. Identify patient.	3. Provides patient safety.
4. Explain procedure.	4. Promotes patient cooperation.
5. Place patient in supine position.	5. Provides position of comfort for procedure.
6. Fold top linen back to expose catheter and urinary drainage tube connection and place bath blanket over patient's chest and abdomen.	6. Provides for patient privacy and warmth while allowing access to connection site.

continued on next page

PROCEDURE 24-4 (cont'd)

7. Cleanse connection site with alcohol wipe and place sterile drape under tubing connection site.

7. Reduces chance of microorganisms entering when system is opened.

8. Open irrigation set and fill solution container with irrigation solution.

8. Prepares equipment for use.

9. Don sterile gloves.

9. Reduces transmission of microorganisms.

10. Place sterile basin next to patient's thigh.

10. Provides container for irrigation drainage.

11. Disconnect drainage tubing from Foley catheter and cover tubing end with sterile cap and allow urinary catheter to drain into sterile basin.

11. Maintains sterility of tubing.

12. Draw up 30 ml (or amount ordered by physician) into sterile syringe, attach syringe to catheter, and gently instill solution into catheter (Fig. 24–23).

12. Provides irrigation of catheter while gentle action decreases chance of bladder spasms.

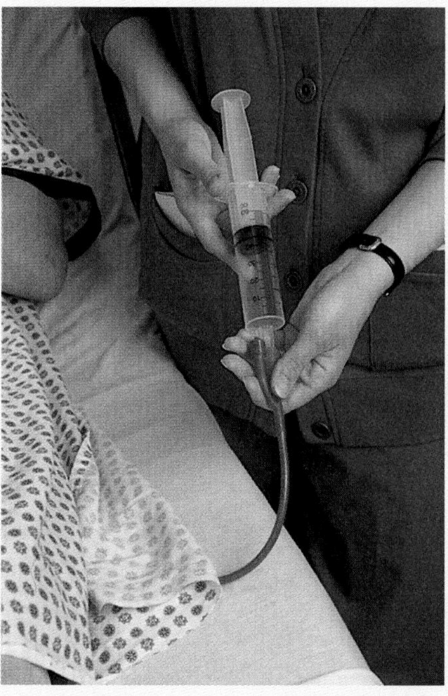

Figure 24–23. Instilling irrigating solution into catheter port.

13. Disconnect syringe from catheter and allow solution to drain into basin. Repeat irrigation solution instillation as necessary.

13. Provides means to drain irrigation solution from catheter by gravity method.

14. If solution does not drain, try to gently withdraw solution with syringe. If solution still does not return, stop procedure and call physician.

14. Provides means to remove clots or debris that may block catheter.

15. Remove sterile protective cap from drainage tubing and cleanse end of tubing with alcohol wipe (or solution recommended per facility policy) and reconnect to catheter.

15. Reduces risk of contamination to system by microorganisms.

continued on next page

PROCEDURE 24-4 (cont'd)

16. Measure amount of solution in basin and subtract amount of irrigation used.	16. Provides means to accurately assess urine output.
17. Cover patient with top linen and return to position of comfort.	17. Provides warmth and comfort for patient.
18. Discard or return equipment to appropriate place.	18. Provides for clean, organized work area.

Documentation

Record in patient record the time procedure was done, the type and amount of solution used, the color of urine before and after, the amount and character (clots, debris) of return, the ease or difficulty of irrigation, and how the patient tolerated the procedure. Note any other assessments of the urine and bladder. Always note accurate urinary output on the patient record as well as intake/output record, including the difference in irrigation solution instilled and returned.

Elements of Patient Teaching

Explain to the patient/family the reason for the procedure. Also instruct the patient/family in the importance of maintaining sterility in the drainage system and how to keep the drainage bag below the level of the bladder. The patient should be encouraged to drink fluids, if this is not contraindicated. If this procedure is being taught the patient or family, they should be provided with an opportunity to do a return demonstration so the care provider can accurately assess their competence.

PROCEDURE 24-5

Performing Continuous Urinary Catheter/Bladder Irrigation

Objective

Provide continuous catheter/bladder irrigation without interruption of the closed urinary drainage system (Fig. 24–24).

Terminology

- **Three-way catheter:** an indwelling urinary catheter with one lumen used for continuous bladder drainage, one lumen used for irrigation, and one lumen used to inflate balloon tip.

Critical Elements

This procedure requires a physician's order. Refer to your facility's policy prior to proceeding. The order states the frequency of irrigation, solution to be used, and amount to be used. Continuous irrigation is often ordered to be delivered at a rate to keep the catheter open and the urine free from clots. Frequent assessment of the patient's bladder and urine color are necessary in order to maintain the proper rate of solution delivery.

Continuous irrigation is often used after urologic surgery. Always note the color of the urine prior to and after irrigation. If blood is in the urine, the amount of bleeding should decrease over time. If this does not occur, report this to the physician. The care provider should also note and report significant changes in laboratory values that may indicate the extent of blood loss.

This is a sterile procedure. Sterile technique is important in order to keep from introducing microorganisms into the urinary tract system. Infection from the presence of a catheter is one of the greatest problems with an indwelling catheter. Because of this, the following precautions should be taken. (*Note:* if the patient will ambulate while carrying the drainage bag or if the patient/family will be caring for the catheter, they too should be instructed regarding these issues.)

continued on next page

PROCEDURE 24-5 (cont'd)

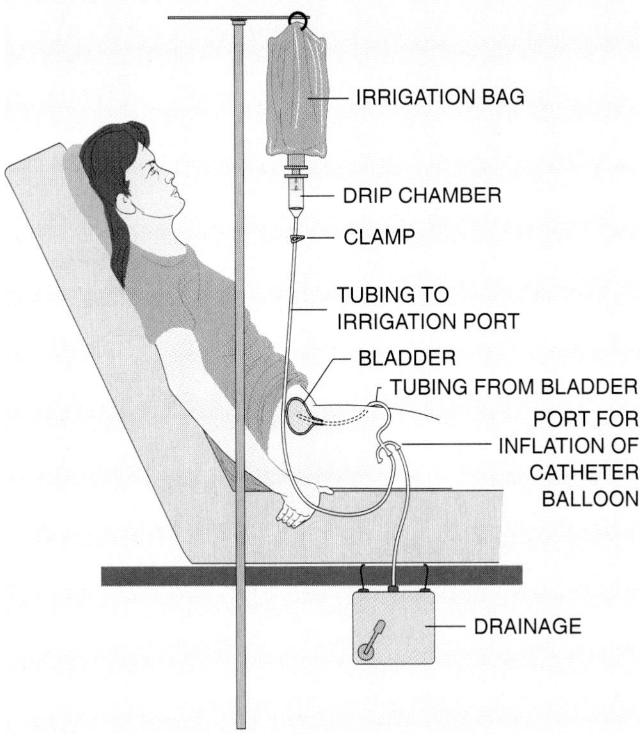

Figure 24–24. Patient with closed irrigation setup.

1. The catheter should be cleansed daily to remove any secretions that may collect around the catheter at the urinary meatus.
2. The urine drainage system should be opened only when necessary because interrupting the system may allow the introduction of microorganisms into the system (the exception to this is opening the drainage bag for the purpose of emptying).
3. The urinary drainage bag should be kept below the level of the bladder at all times to prevent backflow of urine into the bladder from the bag or tubing.

When caring for the catheter, always observe the urinary meatus for any signs of infection, such as unusual drainage, redness, or swelling. In addition, the bladder and the urine should be assessed at this time. Note any signs or symptoms of urinary infection in the patient, such as fever, foul-smelling urine, cloudy urine, hematuria, or suprapubic or flank pain.

Equipment

- Three-way catheter (see Fig. 24–25)
- Irrigation solution
- Tubing for connection from irrigation port to irrigation solution
- Bath blanket

Special Considerations

Frequently note the amount of drainage in the collection bag and the amount of solution in the irrigation bag. Also assess the bladder. If it appears that the irrigation solution is being retained in the bladder and not draining through the catheter, stop the irrigation solution and notify the physician.

Irrigation solution should not be included as part of the urinary output. If the irrigation solution introduced into the Foley catheter does not return at the time of irrigation, be sure to note this in the patient record as well as delete it from the urinary output totals.

Procedures dealing with the genitourinary area may be embarrassing to the patient. Care should be taken to provide privacy and comfort to the patient throughout the procedure.

continued on next page

PROCEDURE 24-5 (cont'd)

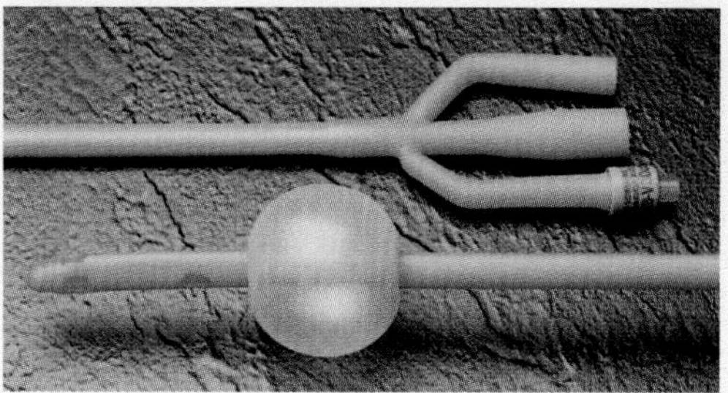

Figure 24–25. Three-way Foley catheter. Three-way catheters are used when continuous bladder irrigations are required. (Courtesy of Bard.)

Action	*Rationale*
1. Verify order.	1. Ensures that correct procedure is performed.
2. Assemble equipment.	2. Promotes task organization.
3. Identify patient.	3. Promotes patient safety.
4. Explain procedure to patient.	4. Promotes patient compliance.
5. Place patient in supine position.	5. Provides position of comfort for procedure.
6. Fold top linen back to expose irrigation tubing port and cover chest and abdomen with bath blanket.	6. Protects patient privacy and provides warmth.
7. Remove port cover from irrigation solution and spike cover from tubing. Spike tubing into irrigation bag port, flush tubing, then close roller or slide clamp.	7. Prepares irrigation solution for delivery.
8. Remove port cover from irrigation port on three-way catheter and protective cap from end of tubing. Attach tubing to irrigation port on three-way catheter.	8. Establishes connection of irrigation solution to three-way catheter.
9. Open slide or roller clamp on tubing until irrigation solution is running at prescribed rate.	9. Allows irrigation solution to enter catheter and bladder.
10. Assess patient bladder, level of irrigation solution, and drainage bag amounts frequently. If solution is not draining, stop irrigation solution and notify physician.	10. Protects patient from bladder distention related to solution retention.
11. Cover patient with top linens and return to position of comfort.	11. Provides for patient warmth and comfort.
12. Discard or return equipment to appropriate place.	12. Provides for clean, organized work space.

Documentation

Record in patient record the time procedure was done, the type and amount of solution used, the color of urine before and after irrigation, the amount and character (clots, debris) of return, the ease or difficulty of irrigation, and how the patient tolerated the procedure. Note any other assessments of the urine and bladder. Always note accurate urinary output on the patient record as well as the intake/output record.

Elements of Patient Teaching

Explain to the patient/family the reason for the procedure. Also instruct the patient/family in the importance of maintaining sterility in the drainage system and how to keep the drainage bag below the level of the bladder. If not contraindicated, the patient should be encouraged to drink fluids. If this procedure is being taught to the patient or family, they should be provided with an opportunity to do a return demonstration so the care provider can accurately assess their competence.

PROCEDURE 24-6

Applying and Removing a Condom Catheter

Objective

Provide external urinary catheter drainage without invasion of the urinary tract.

Terminology

- **Condom catheter:** a sheath covering the penis, connected to a drainage tube and collection bag, that provides external urinary catheter drainage.
- **Paraphimosis:** retraction and swelling of the foreskin.

Critical Elements

Application of a condom catheter may require a physician's order. Consult your facility's policy prior to proceeding.

This type of urinary drainage can protect the patient's skin integrity and allow for accurate intake. It also reduces the risk of infection because there is no invasion of the urinary tract.

In order to reduce the chance of infection, both the care provider and the patient/family should adhere to the following precautions:

1. The condom catheter should be removed daily followed by skin care/perineal care. Assess for signs of skin irritation at this time.
2. The urine drainage bag should not be raised above the level of the bladder.

Observe the meatus for any signs of infection, such as unusual drainage, redness, or swelling. In addition, the bladder and the urine should be assessed at this time. Note any signs or symptoms of urinary infection, such as fever, foul-smelling urine, cloudy urine, hematuria, or suprapubic or flank pain.

Assess the patient for latex allergy prior to choosing a catheter. Many condom catheters are made of latex. If an allergy to this substance exists, the care provider must obtain a nonlatex product or use another method of urinary drainage collection.

Always read the manufacturer's instructions prior to use of the product. Prior to choosing a condom catheter, the care provider should assess the sizes of product available and the size needed for the patient. Some products provide a sizing guide that may be used.

When emptying the urinary drainage bag, the care provider should make sure to accurately total and record the output.

Equipment

- Condom catheter
- Drainage tubing and bag
- Gloves
- Scissors/razor (if indicated)
- Bath blanket
- Towel/washcloth

Special Considerations

Prior to applying a condom catheter, the care provider should assess the skin around and on the penis. With the uncircumcised male, the foreskin should be left in place in order to prevent paraphimosis. There should be at least 1 inch of space between the end of the penis and the tip of the condom.

Condom catheters that have adhesive at the end of the condom may stick to the patient's hair during the removal process. For this reason, it may be necessary to clip or shave the hair at the end of the penis prior to application of the condom catheter.

If the condom catheter is secured with an elastic strap, the care provider should assess the penis 20 to 30 minutes after the application process in order to ensure that circulation has not been compromised by the application of the strap. Any swelling or change in color may indicate that the strap is too tight and that it must be removed and reapplied.

Procedures dealing with the genitourinary area may be embarrassing to the patient. Care should be taken to provide privacy and comfort to the patient throughout the procedure.

Action	*Rationale*
Application of Condom Catheter	
1. Verify order (if indicated).	1. Ensures that correct procedure is performed.
2. Assemble equipment.	2. Promotes task organization.
3. Identify patient.	3. Protects patient safety.
4. Explain procedure.	4. Promotes patient compliance.
5. Close door/curtain and position patient in supine position.	5. Maintains patient dignity and privacy.
6. Fold back top covers exposing perineal area. Cover patient's trunk with bath blanket.	6. Minimizes patient exposure during procedure.

continued on next page

PROCEDURE 24-6 (cont'd)

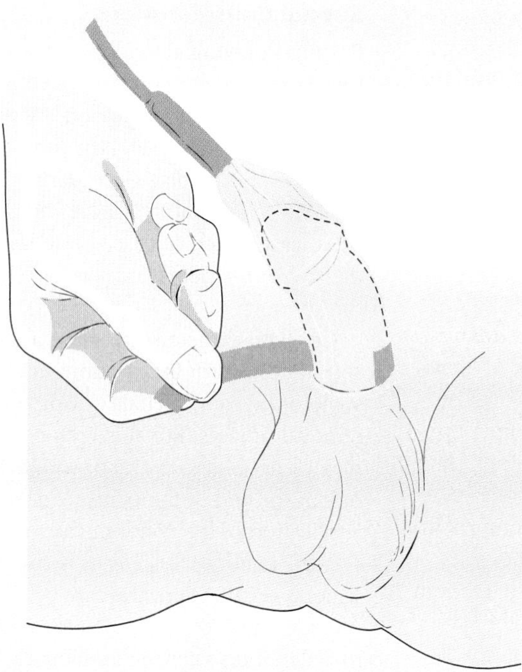

Figure 24–26. Applying a condom catheter.

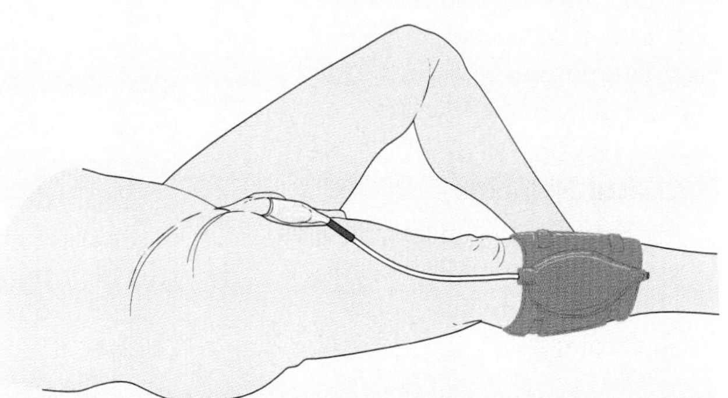

Figure 24–27. Securing leg bag.

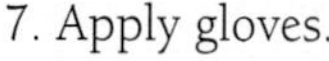

7. Apply gloves.	7. Protects care provider from contact with blood or body fluid.
8. Provide perineal care if indicated.	8. Promotes skin integrity.
9. Hold penis firmly but gently in your nondominant hand and roll condom over penis with dominant hand, being sure to leave 1 inch of space between end of penis and tip of condom (Fig. 24–26).	9. Provides for proper application of condom catheter.
10. Connect drainage tubing to end of condom catheter and to the leg drainage bag (Fig. 24–27) or collection bag at side of bed.	10. Provides means to collect urine.
11. Return patient to position of comfort and replace top linens.	11. Provides for patient comfort.
12. Discard or return equipment to appropriate place.	12. Provides clean organized work area.

Removal of Condom Catheter

1. Close door/curtain.	1. Maintains patient privacy and dignity.
2. Fold top linen to expose perineal area and cover trunk of body with bath blanket.	2. Provides patient warmth.
3. Loosen adhesive area of condom or remove elastic strap.	3. Prepares condom for removal.
4. Gently roll condom forward from base of penis until it is completely removed.	4. Removes condom from penis.
5. Provide skin/perineal care and assess skin integrity.	5. Promotes skin integrity.

continued on next page

PROCEDURE 24-6 (cont'd)

6. Return patient to position of comfort and cover with top linens.	6. Promotes patient comfort and privacy.
7. Accurately total and record output in drainage bag.	7. Provides accurate data collection.
8. Discard or return equipment to appropriate place.	8. Provides clean, organized work area.

Documentation

Record in the patient record the application or removal of the condom catheter. Note the skin assessment, urine assessment, and any signs or symptoms of infection. Record the patient's response to the procedure.

Elements of Patient Teaching

Instruct the patient/family in the daily removal process and skin care necessary with a condom catheter. Instruct them on the importance of keeping the drainage bag lower than the level of the bladder.

They should also be instructed on how to recognize the signs and symptoms of a urinary tract infection and the importance of reporting these symptoms promptly. If the patient/family will be performing the application/removal independently, they should be given an opportunity to do a return demonstration so the care provider can assess competency in performing the procedure.

PROCEDURE 24-7

Providing Urostomy Pouch Care

Objective

Provide maintenance care to a urostomy pouch.

Terminology

- **Urostomy:** a form of urinary diversion in which the bladder or the ureters empty through a stoma that is formed on the abdominal wall.
- **Stoma:** an artificial opening made in an internal organ, bringing it to the surface.

Critical Elements

The correct-size appliance should always be used because the proper fitting of the ostomy pouch around the stoma is critical. The stomal opening should be cut not more than ⅛ inch larger than the stoma to fit properly.

Change the appliance regularly to avoid leakage and skin irritation. Any urine that comes in contact with skin will cause itching and burning if not removed quickly, causing skin irritation. Assess for sensitivities and allergies to adhesive or pouch materials that can develop days, weeks, or years after use of a product.

An appliance may be left in place as long as a proper seal is maintained around the stoma. The stoma should be assessed each time the wafer is changed or the bag is emptied. A new stoma shrinks dramatically during the first 6 months.

Assess the stoma every 4 hours during the first postoperative day and daily for 1 week. Report immediately any pale, dark-purple, or black color changes in the stoma that could indicate impaired circulation to the area.

Keep a record of daily output.

A variety of ostomy appliances are available that the patient may want to try before deciding on the type that meets a long-term need. Initially, while the size of the stoma is changing, the patient will want to use a cut-to-fit appliance. Eventually, a premeasured ostomy appliance may be more appropriate for use.

continued on next page

PROCEDURE 24-7 (cont'd)

Equipment

- Towel
- Washcloth
- Scissors (if indicated)
- Precut wafer and pouch
- 4×4 gauze or small tampon (deodorant-free or unscented)
- Tape (optional)
- Skin prep wipe (optional)
- Skin barrier paste (optional)
- Gloves

Special Considerations

When working with the urostomy patient, the care provider should note the color, odor, and clarity of the urine as well as any signs or symptoms of urinary tract infection.

The ostomy appliance should be changed immediately if the patient complains of itching or burning or if leaking is noted. The pouch should be emptied when one-third to one-half full. Allowing the pouch to become too full may cause the seal to loosen. The pouch may be easier to change upon arising in the morning when urine output is decreased.

Never use cream or ointment (other than the ostomy skin preparation products) on the peristomal area.

The patient should be allowed to express his or her feelings regarding the change in body image. The patient care provider should have a positive, accepting attitude that may help the patient with acceptance of this change.

Action	*Rationale*
1. Assemble equipment.	1. Promotes task organization.
2. Identify patient.	2. Provides for patient safety.
3. Explain procedure.	3. Promotes compliance.
4. Close door/curtain and fold top linen to expose ostomy appliance.	4. Provides privacy and allows access to ostomy site.
5. Don gloves.	5. Protects care provider from contact with blood or body fluids.
6. Gently remove old pouch/wafer by pushing down on skin while lifting edge of seal upward. Moisten with warm water if pouch difficult to remove.	6. Maintains skin integrity during removal process.
7. Apply rolled 4×4-inch gauze or tampon to stoma.	7. Contains any urine drainage so skin may be cleansed and dried.
8. Wash skin surrounding stoma with warm water (if using soap, be sure to rinse well).	8. Maintains skin integrity because urine on skin may be corrosive.
9. Using sizing guide, measure stoma and cut wafer to fit allowing no more than ⅛ inch between stoma and wafer. If using presized product, assess that sizing is still appropriate.	9. Provides wafer that fits appropriately in order to protect skin from urine drainage.
10. Wipe skin around stoma with skin prep pad *(optional)*.	10. Prepares skin for application of wafer.
11. Remove backing from wafer and apply to skin (skin barrier paste may be applied around wafer opening if indicated).	11. Applies wafer to skin around stoma.
12. If using two-piece ostomy product, snap bag portion of appliance to wafer at this time.	12. Provides urine collection receptacle.
13. Make sure urine drainage spout is closed.	13. Ensures that urine will stay in bag and not leak.
14. Pull top linens back in place and return patient to position of comfort.	14. Provides for warmth and comfort.
15. Discard or return supplies to appropriate place.	15. Maintains clean, organized work area.

continued on next page

PROCEDURE 24-7 (cont'd)

Documentation

Record in the patient record the time the procedure was completed and the patient response. Note the type and size of appliance used, as well as assessment of the urine, stoma, and skin. Accurately record the urine drainage in the patient's chart and intake/output record.

Elements of Patient Teaching

Instruct the patient/family in the steps necessary to perform the procedure. Stress the importance of assessing the stoma, skin, and urine routinely and reporting any unusual changes. Provide an opportunity for the patient/family to perform a return demonstration of the procedure so that the care provider can accurately assess the patient/family's competence in completing the procedure.

CHAPTER HIGHLIGHTS

- Alterations in urinary elimination can be attributed to multiple causes: physical, environmental, psychological, or a combination of these factors. A comprehensive approach to symptom management is needed.
- Careful attention should be given to the assessment of urinary elimination and identification of abnormalities and appropriate interventions.
- Normal intestinal and urinary elimination is an indicator of general biopsychosocial wellness.
- Assessment of individual patterns of elimination is essential because of the wide range of patterns that are considered normal.
- Assessment and identification of the causes of alterations in elimination can reflect a wide range of problems and must precede interventions and treatments.
- Alterations in elimination can result in changes not only in the elimination system but also in many other body functions, such as fluid and electrolyte balance, nutritional status, and skin integrity.
- Elimination patterns should be assessed routinely and documented, noting any specific relevant detail.
- Individual practices related to elimination should be assessed and, if appropriate, opportunities provided for them whenever possible.
- Nursing diagnoses reflecting the holistic nature of problems in elimination should be written for each patient.
- Nursing interventions may be short- or long-term, beginning during diagnostic testing and continuing with routine follow-up or preoperative and postoperative interventions or with chronic care.
- Education of the patient and family to optimize independence and effective eliminative functioning should be a nursing goal.
- Sensitivity to the psychosocial needs of patients with alterations in elimination is vital to their adaptation and coping.

REFERENCES

Agency for Health Care Policy and Research (1992). *Urinary Incontinence in Adults: Clinical Practice Guideline.* (AHCPR Publication No. 92-0038.) Washington, D.C.: U.S. Government Printing Office.

Agency for Health Care Policy and Research (1996). *Urinary Incontinence in Adults: Acute and Chronic Management.* (AHCPR Publication No. 96-0682). Washington, D.C.: U.S. Government Printing Office.

American Nurses Association, Divison on Medical-Surgical Nursing Practice & American Urological Association Allied (1977). *Standards of Urologic Nursing Practice.* Kansas City: American Nurses Association.

Barnes, S.H. (1986). The development of a comprehensive instructional package for teaching intermittent self-catheterization. *The Journal of Enterostomal Therapy, 13,* 238–241.

Bourcier, A.P., Juras, J.C. (1995). Nonsurgical therapy for stress incontinence. *Urologic Clinics of North America, 22* (3), 613–627.

Brink, C.A., Sampselle, C.M., Wells, T.J., et al (1989). A digital test for pelvic muscle strength in older women with urinary incontinence. *Nursing Research, 38* (4), 196–199.

Burgio, K.L., Burgio, L.D. (1986). Behavior therapies for urinary incontinence in the elderly. *Clinics of Geriatric Medicine, 2,* 809–827.

Burgio, L.D., Jones, L.T., Engel, B.T. (1988). Studying incontinence in an urban nursing home. *Journal of Gerontological Nursing, 14* (4), 40–45.

Canavan, K. (1996). ANA endorses guidelines for smoking cessation, urinary incontinence. *American Nurse, 28*(5), 8.

Champion, V.L. (1976). Clean technique for intermittent self-catheterization. *Nursing Research, 25* (1), 13–18.

Clifford, C.M. (1982). Urinary tract infection: A brief selective review. *International Journal of Nursing Studies, 19* (4), 213–222.

Colling, J., Hadley, B.J., Eisch, J., et al (1992). Patterned urge response toileting for urinary incontinence: A clinical trial. In

S. Funk, E.M. Tornquist, M.T. Champagne, R.A. White (eds.): *Key Aspects of Elder Care.* New York: Springer, pp. 169–186.

Colling, J.C., Ouslander, J.G., Hadley, B.J., et al (1992). The effects of patterned urge-response toileting (PURT) on urinary incontinence among nursing home residents. *Journal of the American Geriatrics Society, 40,* 135–141.

Criner, J.A. (1994). A nursing management protocol for incontinence. *Rehabilitation Nursing, 19* (3), 141–144.

Fantl, J.A., Wyman, J.F., McClish, D.K., et al (1991). Efficacy of bladder training in older women with urinary incontinence. *Journal of the American Medical Association, 265* (5), 609–613.

Fournier, C., Corcos, J. (1996). Collagen injections in difficult cases of stress urinary incontinence: Study results. *Urologic Nursing, 16* (4), 135–139.

Garcia, R., Cruz, M., Reed, M., et al (1988). Relationship between falls and patient attempts to satisfy elimination needs. *Nursing Management, 19* (7), 80V–80X.

Gartley, C.B. (1985). *Managing Incontinence.* Ottawa, IL: Jameson Books.

Gibbs, T.D. (1995). Health assessment of the adult urology patient. In K.A. Karlowicz (ed.): *Urologic Nursing: Principles and Practice.* Philadelphia: W.B. Saunders, pp. 33–85.

Goldstein, M., Hawthorne, M.E., Engeberg, S., et al (1992). Urinary incontinence: Why people do not seek help. *Journal of Gerontological Nursing, 18* (4), 15–20.

Gray, M., Rayome, R. Anson, C. (1995). Incontinence and clean intermittent catheterization following spinal cord injury. *Clinical Nursing Research, 4* (1), 6–21.

Guyton, A.C., Hall, J. (1997). *Physiology and Mechanism of Disease,* 6th ed. Philadelphia: W.B. Saunders.

Guttman, Sir L. (1973). *Spinal Cord Injury: Comprehensive Management and Research.* Oxford, England: Blackwell Scientific Publications, pp 345–356.

Hampton, B.G., Bryant, R.A. (1992). *Ostomies and Continent Diversions: Nursing Management.* St. Louis: Mosby Year-Book.

Hart, J.A. (1985). The urethral catheter: A review of its implication in urinary-tract infection. *International Journal of Nursing Studies, 22* (1), 57–70.

Heller, B.R., Whitehead, W.E., Johnson, L.D. (1989). Incontinence. *Journal of Gerontological Nursing, 15* (5), 16–23.

International Association for Enterostomal Therapy. (1987). *Standards of Care: Urinary Incontinence.* Irvine, CA: International Association for Enterostomal Therapy.

Issekutz, B., et al (1965). Effect of prolonged bed rest on urinary calcium output. *Journal of Applied Physiology, 21* (3), 1013–1020.

Jirovec, M.M. (1991). Effect of individualized prompted toileting on incontinence in nursing home residents. *Applied Nursing Research 4* (4); 188–191.

Karlowicz, K.A. (ed.) (1995). *Urologic Nursing: Principles and Practice.* Philadelphia: W.B. Saunders.

Kegel, A.H. (1949). Physiologic treatment of poor tone and function of genital muscles and of urinary stress incontinence. *Western Journal of Surgery, 57,* 527.

Kegel, A.H. (1951). Physiologic therapy for urinary stress incontinence. *Journal of the American Medical Association, 146,* 915–917.

Kennedy, K.L., Steidle, C.P. Letizia, T.M. (1995). Urinary incontinence: The basis. *Ostomy-Wound Management, 41* (7), 16–30.

Krasner, D. (1990). Incontinence in varied settings. In Jeter, K.F., Faller, N., Norton, C. (eds.): *Nursing for Continence.* Philadelphia: W.B. Saunders.

Krasner, D. (1992). *Urinary system: Effects of immobility.* Charleston, SC: Support Systems International.

Lapides, J., Diokno, A.C., Gould, F.R., Lowe, B.S. (1976). Further observations on self-catheterization. *The Journal of Urology, 116,* 169–171.

Larson, E.L. (1989). Handwashing: It's essential—even when you use gloves. *American Journal of Nursing, 89* (7), 934–939.

Lyder, C., Clemes-Lowrance, C., Davis, A., et al (1992). Structured skin care regimen to prevent perineal dermatitis in the elderly. *Journal of ET Nursing, 19,* 12–16.

McCormick, K.A., Burgio, K.L. (1984). Incontinence: An update on nursing care measures. *Journal of Gerontological Nursing, 10* (10), 16–23.

McCormick, K.A., Burgio, L.D., Engel, B.T., et al (1992). Urinary incontinence: An augmented prompted void approach for the demented. *Journal of Gerontological Nursing, 18* (3), 3–10.

McMullen, D. (1991). *Candida albicans* and incontinence. *Dermatology Nursing, 3* (1), 21–24.

Meyer, B.R. (1989). Renal function in aging. *Journal American Geriatric Society, 37,* 791–800. (From *The Yearbook of Urology,* 1990, pp. 36–37.)

Mitteness, L.S. (1987). The management of urinary incontinence by community-living elderly. *The Gerontologist, 27* (2), 185–193.

National Institute on Aging/Alliance for Aging Research (1991). *Clinical Bulletin: Treating Patients with Urinary Incontinence.* Bethesda, MD, Department of Health and Human Services, National Institutes of Health.

Newman, D.K. (1996). Aging and the problem of urinary incontinence: AHCPR's 1996 clinical practice guideline. *Urologic Nursing, 16,* (4), 123–126.

Newman, D.K., Lynch, K., Smith, D.A., Cell, P. (1991). Restoring urinary continence. *American Journal of Nursing, 91* (1), 28–36.

Ouslander, J.G., Blaustein, J., Conner, A., Pitt, A. (1988). Habit training and oxybutynin for incontinence in nursing home patients: A placebo-controlled trial. *Journal of the American Geriatrics Society, 36,* 40–46.

Ouslander, J.G., Bruskenitz, R. (1989). Disorders of micturition in the aging patient. *Advances in Internal Medicine, 34,* 165–190.

Ouslander, J.G., Greengold, B., Chen, S. (1987). External catheter use and urinary tract infections among incontinent male nursing home patients. *Journal of American Geriatrics Society, 35* (12), 1063–1070.

Palmer, M.H., McCormick, K.A., Langford, A., et al (1992). Continence outcomes: Documentation on medical records in the nursing home environment. *Journal of Nursing Care and Quality, 6* (3), 36–43.

Pannill, F.C. (1989). Practical management of urinary incontinence. *Medical Clinics of North America, 73,* 1423–1439.

Pearson, B.D., Larson, J.M. (1992). Urine control by elders: Noninvasive strategies. In S. Funk, E. M. Tornquist, M.T. Champagne, R.A. White (eds.): *Key Aspects of Elder Care.* New York: Springer, pp. 154–168.

Petrilli, C.O., Traughber, B., Schnelle, J.F. (1988). Behavioral management in the inpatient geriatric population. *Nursing Clinics of North America, 23* (1), 265–277.

Pieper, B., Cleland, V., Johnson, D.E., O'Reilly, J.L. (1989). Inventing urine incontinence devices for women. *Image, 21* (4), 205–209.

Plunkett, J.M., Braren V. (1979). Clean intermittent catheterization in children. *The Journal of Urology, 121*, 469–471.

Renal and Urologic Disorders. (1984). Nurse's Clinical Library. Nursing 84 Books. Springhouse, PA: Springhouse Corporation.

Roe, B.H. (1990). Study of the effects of education on the management of urine drainage systems by patients and carers. *Journal of Advanced Nursing, 15*, 517–524.

Roe, B.H., Reid, F.J., Brocklehurst, J.C. (1988). Comparison of four urine drainage systems. *Journal of Advanced Nursing, 13*, 374–382.

Sampselle, C.M., DeLancey, J.O.L. (1992). The urine stream interruption test and pelvic muscle function. *Nursing Research, 41* (2), 73–77.

Schnelle, J.F., Traughber, B., Sowell, V.A., et al (1989). Prompted voiding treatment of urinary incontinence in nursing home patients: A behavior management approach for nursing home staff. *Journal of the American Geriatrics Society, 37*, 1051–1057.

Sherman, S., Umlauf, M.G. (1994). Urinary incontinence in community dwelling elders. *Urologic Nursing, 13* (4), 120–127.

Silber, E.C., Cicmanec, J.F., Burke, B.M., Bracken, R.B. (1989). Microwave sterilization: A method for home sterilization of urinary catheters. *The Journal of Urology, 141*, 88–89.

Smith, D.B., Babaian, R.J. (1989). Patient adjustment to an ileal conduit after radical cystectomy. *Journal of Enterostomal Therapy, 16* (6), 244–246.

Steinberg, F.U. (1980). *The Immobilized Patient: Functional Pathology and Management.* New York: Plenum Medical Book Company.

Tries, J. (1990). Kegel exercises enhanced by biofeedback. *Journal of Enterostomal Therapy, 17* (2), 67–76.

Tucker, S.M., Canobbio, M.M., Paquette, E.V., Wells, M.F. (1988). *Patient Care Standards: Nursing Process, Diagnosis, and Outcomes.* St Louis: Mosby.

Turner, S.L., Plymat, K.R. (1988). As women age: Perspectives on urinary incontinence. *Rehabilitation Nursing, 13* (3), 132–135.

Warkentin, R. (1992). Implementation of a urinary continence program. *Journal of Gerontological Nursing, 18* (1), 31–36.

Webb, R.J., Lawson, A.L., Neal, D.E. (1990). Clean intermittent self-catheterization in 172 adults. *British Journal of Urology, 65* (1), 20–23.

Wheeler, J.S., Walter, J.S., Niecestro, R.M., Scalzo, A.J. (1992). Behavioral therapy for urinary incontinence. *Journal of ET Nursing, 19* (2), 59–65.

Williamson, J.A. (1986). Pharmacologic considerations in treating urinary tract infections in patients with urinary diversions. *Ostomy/Wound Management*, Winter, 37–42.

Wren, K.R., Wren, T.L. (1996). Postsurgical urinary retention. *Urological Nursing, 16* (2), 45–47.

Wyman, J.F. (1992). Managing incontinence: The current bases for practice. In S. Funk, E.M. Tornquist, M.T. Champagne, R.A. White (eds.): *Key Aspects of Elder Care.* New York: Springer, pp. 135–153.

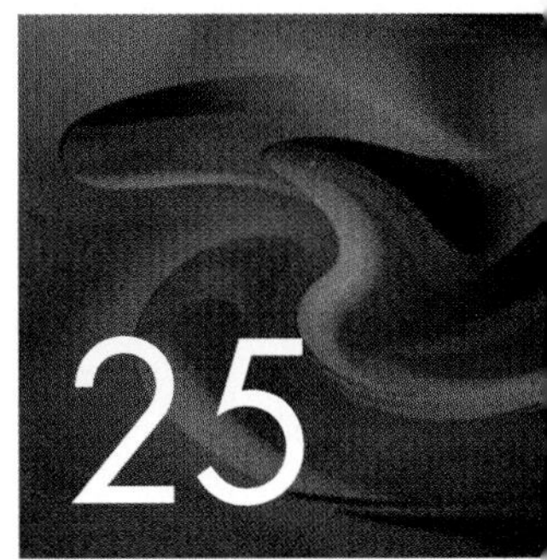

Rest and Sleep 25

Kathryn A. Lee

Mrs. Cameron, a 79-year-old widow, was admitted to a semiprivate room on the orthopedic unit with pain in her left hip lasting several months caused by degenerative joint disease. She will have hip replacement surgery tomorrow. She has never been hospitalized before, but spent a great deal of time in hospitals caring for her husband before his death. Considering individual differences that influence normal sleep patterns, the nurse determined that this patient might have difficulty getting to sleep and staying asleep for several reasons. First, she is experiencing a change in her usual sleep environment. Second, her anxiety about being hospitalized and having surgery is likely to interfere with sleep. Third, her hip pain is likely to interrupt her sleep. The nurse administers the prescribed sleeping pill to Mrs. Cameron at her normal bedtime after a relaxing back massage.

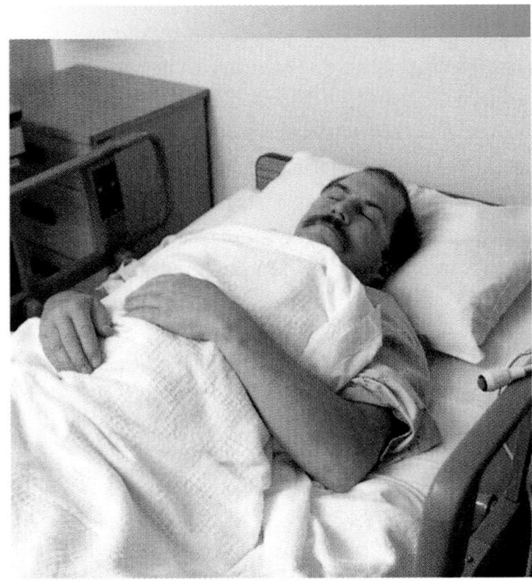

On the morning of surgery, Mrs. Cameron stated that she slept well, but awakened twice because of her roommate's light snoring. When planning for the next evening of care, the nurse will use strategies known to be effective in reducing sleep disturbances. The nurse might consider moving Mrs. Cameron or her roommate, pulling the curtain between the beds to reduce the sound transmitted, or providing Mrs. Cameron with earplugs. The nurse will also attend to Mrs. Cameron's postoperative pain to preclude that from disturbing her sleep. Mrs. Cameron's anxiety will also be monitored. With these strategies, Mrs. Cameron will be less likely to experience disturbed sleep, will feel more rested, and will have more energy during her recovery from surgery.

OBJECTIVES

After studying the content of this chapter, students will be able to:

- **contrast a patient's sleep pattern with the normal sleep cycle**
- **assess a patient and determine factors that could produce sleep disturbance**
- **distinguish disorders of initiating and maintaining sleep from disorders of excessive daytime sleepiness and parasomnias (movements or behaviors during sleep that may not be normal but seldom cause arousal such as sleepwalking or talking)**
- **identify and implement appropriate nursing interventions for people with problems initiating or maintaining sleep**
- **identify and implement appropriate nursing interventions for people with disorders of excessive daytime sleepiness**

SCOPE OF NURSING CARE

Changes in sleep are inevitable whenever illness occurs or the sleeping environment is altered. The total amount of sleep may be reduced or the quality of the sleep diminished because of interruptions in sleep. Sleep can be interrupted because of external environmental factors, such as noise or unfamiliar surroundings. Sleep can also be interrupted because of internal factors, such as pain or breathing problems.

Falling asleep can be especially difficult for the elderly and for any hospitalized patient. Residents in nursing homes frequently complain of sleep disturbances resulting from a physical condition or changes in the environment. Patients receiving home care may describe excessive sleepiness during the day resulting from chronic sleep-related health problems.

Regardless of the setting in which the person is receiving care and the actual or potential sleep disturbance, good nursing assessment, management, and evaluation will promote the quality and quantity of a patient's sleep. With adequate rest and restorative sleep, patients will have more energy for coping with their health problem or preventing adverse health outcomes.

KNOWLEDGE BASE

Rest and sleep are two of our most basic human needs. To feel rested, we spend about one quarter to one third of our lives sleeping. Scientists are busy studying animals and humans to understand why we sleep. So far, they have only been able to describe cycles of sleep for healthy and ill populations and what happens when someone is deprived of sleep for short or long periods of time. This research provides data that relate directly to nursing research and patient care. For example, nurses can apply this knowledge to patient care activities and examine how the scheduling of activities, treatments, and medications might interfere with sleep and how patients are affected by interrupted sleep. This knowledge is then used by the nurse to provide safe, professional patient care.

Basic Science

NORMAL SLEEP

Sleep is defined as a period of diminished responsiveness to external stimuli that regularly alternates with periods of wakefulness. It is a behavior that is usually taken for granted unless there is an inadequate amount of sleep or the individual does not feel rested on awakening.

The stages of sleep are most clearly recognized by recording the brain's electrical activity with electroencephalography (EEG), eye movements with electrooculography (EOG), and muscle activity with electromyography (EMG). Sleep is described as "active" or "quiet" and as "light" or "deep" on the basis of these EEG, EOG, and EMG findings. As shown in Figure 25–1, very distinct EEG patterns are used to distinguish one stage of sleep from another. When eyes are simply closed, alpha waves (8–12 cycles/second) appear on the EEG tracing. By definition, sleep begins at the point at which alpha waves give way to theta waves (3–7 cycles/second). Sleep spindles (12–14 cycles/second) and K complexes are characteristic of Stage 2, the predominant component of sleep. Slow EEG waves (0.5–2 cycles/second) with high amplitude (greater than 75 μV) are characteristic of deep sleep (Stages 3 and 4). Fewer delta waves in a designated time frame indicate Stage 3 deep sleep, and a predominant number of delta waves in the designated time frame indicate Stage 4 deep sleep.

ACTIVE (RAPID EYE MOVEMENT) SLEEP

Active sleep is more commonly known as rapid eye movement (REM) sleep, or dream sleep. The EEG waveforms are very similar to an awake state (see Fig. 25–1). During this stage of sleep, a careful observer will notice activity that includes bursts of eye movements and some twitching of small facial muscles. During REM sleep, large muscle groups are actually paralyzed, and the sleeper is unable to move or act out dreams.

A person awakened during a REM period is likely to report dreaming. Although newborns spend about 50% of their sleep time in REM, actual dreams begin to occur at the age when cognitive function (thinking) becomes apparent (Cartwright, 1994). REM periods still occur in persons who are sensory impaired. Those who are congenitally blind or blind before the fifth year of life report primarily auditory dreams, whereas deaf persons report using sign language in their dreams (Pivik, 1994).

Until recently, it was thought that all dreams occurred during REM sleep. It is now known that some dreaming, of a more realistic, repetitive nature, occurs in other stages of sleep (Cavallero et al, 1992). Recalling dreams is not of major importance, because the function of REM sleep is still fulfilled regardless of recall.

QUIET (NON RAPID EYE MOVEMENT) SLEEP

The quiet phase of sleep is often called non rapid eye movement (NREM) sleep, but has also been called synchronized sleep. As one progresses through the four NREM stages, sleep becomes progressively deeper (Fig. 25–2). During Stage 1, usually less than 5% of a person's total sleep time, a person has eye movements, but they are slow and have a rolling pattern. Subjects awakened from this stage report drowsiness but do not feel as though they were asleep. Therefore, Stage 1 is classified as a very light state of sleep and is defined as a subjective state of drowsiness.

Stage 2 sleep is where most (50–55%) of our sleep occurs. Although it is more difficult to arouse someone from Stage 2 than Stage 1 sleep, Stage 2 is still classified as light sleep. Stages 3 and 4 are the deepest stages and represent about 20% of total sleep time in a young, healthy person. Because of their waveforms on the EEG, Stages 3 and 4 are collectively called slow-wave or delta wave sleep. Awakening someone from Stage 4, in which delta waves are more dense than in Stage 3 sleep, is the most difficult.

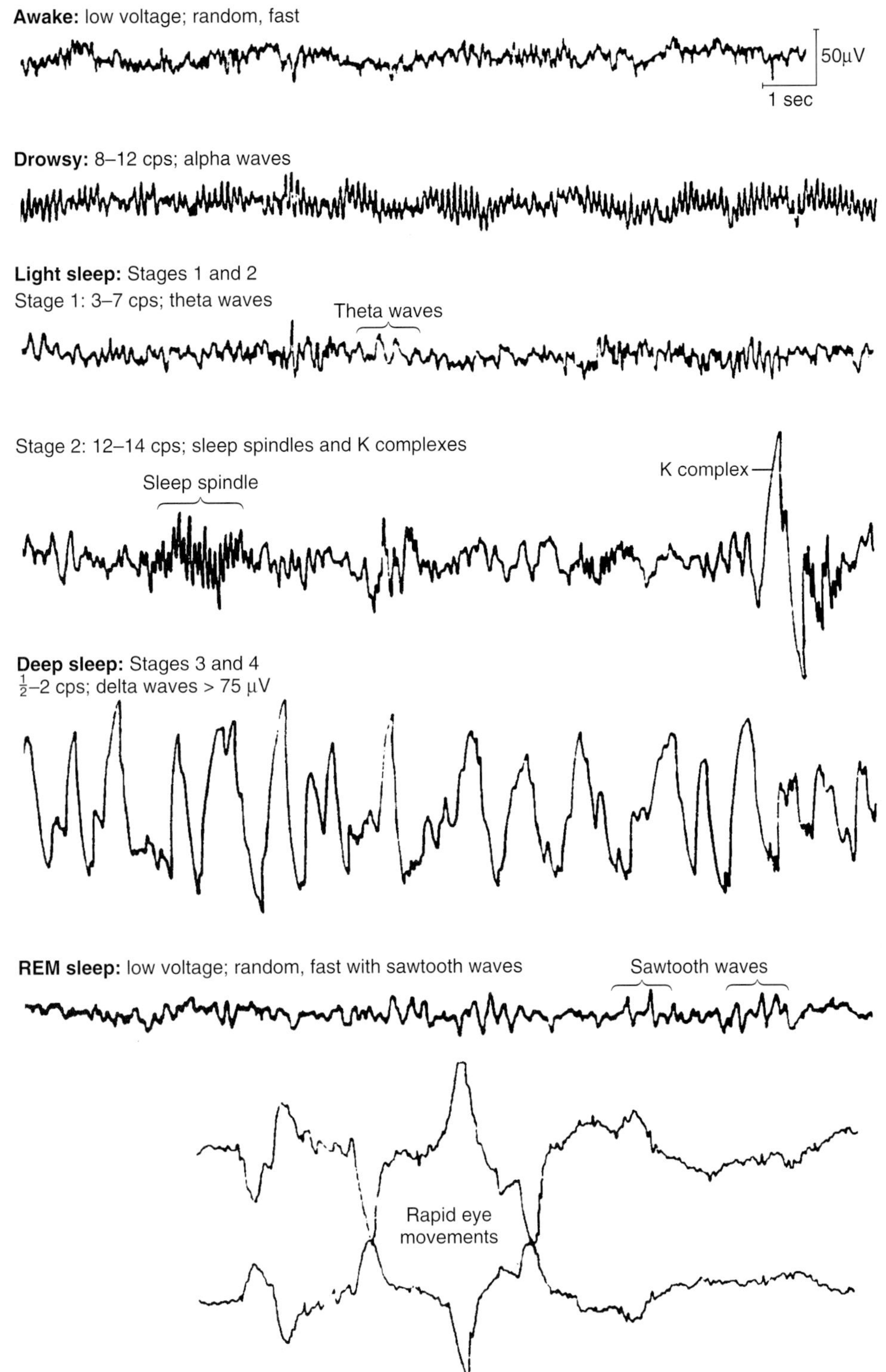

Figure 25–1. Human sleep stages (cps = cycles per second; REM = rapid eye movement)

CYCLES OF SLEEP

One sleep cycle includes both quiet and active sleep stages and repeats itself four or five times during a typical 7 or 8 hours of sleep. The length of a sleep cycle and the number of cycles vary with the individual and time of night. An uninterrupted cycle ranges from 60 minutes during the early part of the night to 120 minutes toward the end of a night's sleep.

NREM sleep dominates the early half of the night. As sleep progresses, delta wave sleep may be absent, whereas REM periods become longer and occur closer together. There is a stepwise progression from wakefulness through NREM to

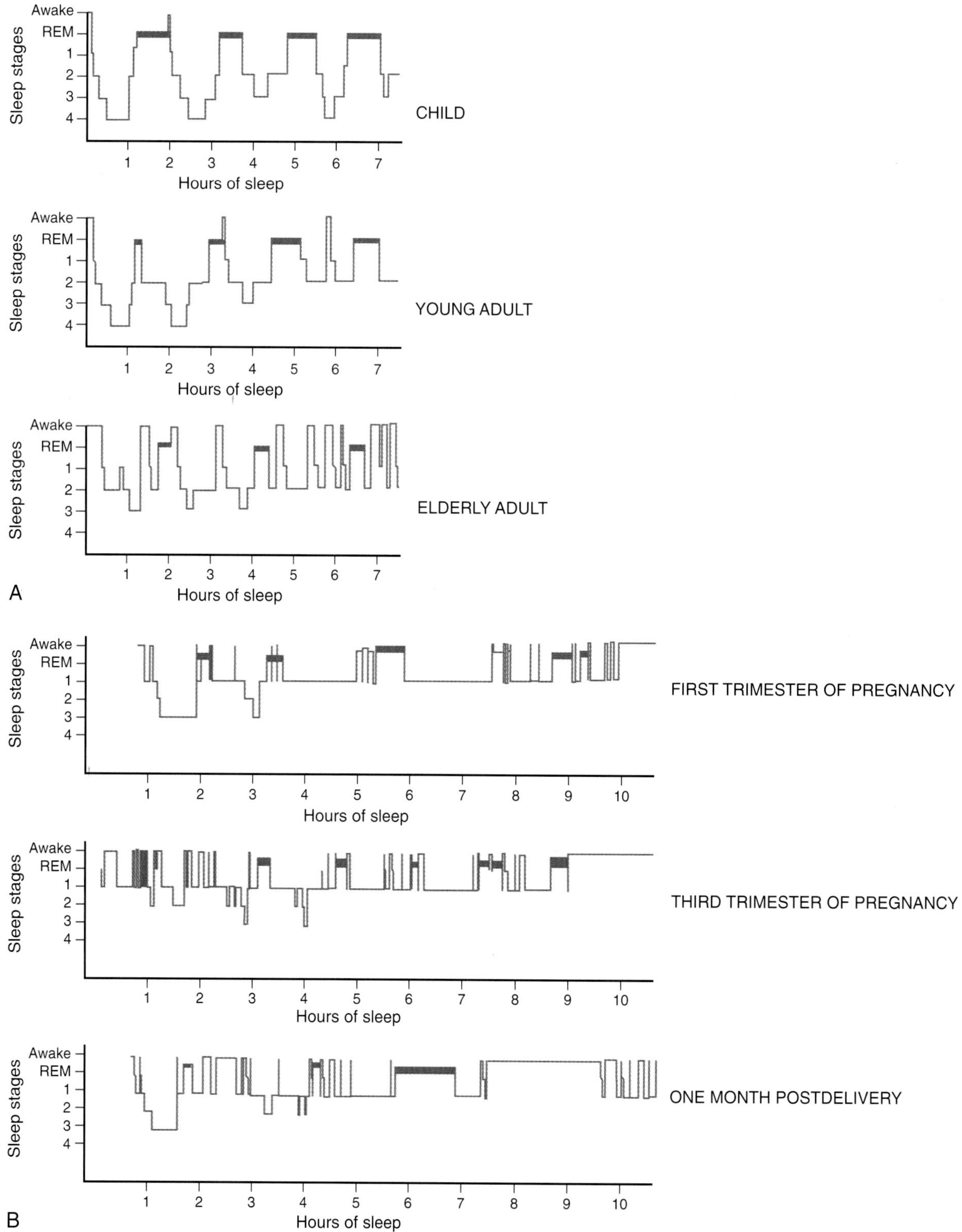

Figure 25–2. Diagrammatic representation of a typical night's sleep by age group *(A)* and during pregnancy *(B)*. (REM = rapid eye movement)

Stage 4 and then back up to Stage 2 and into REM. This cyclic pattern will continue through the night until the sleeper is awakened. When a sleeper is awakened, perhaps by the sound of an alarm clock, the sleep cycle does not resume from where it is interrupted (descending Stage 2, in this example) but begins again at Stage 1. Figure 25–2 shows the effect of certain physiologic changes (e.g., pregnancy and aging) on sleep patterns.

RESEARCH HIGHLIGHT
DIFFERENCES IN SLEEP EFFICIENCY AMONG PREGNANT WOMEN

PURPOSE

The purpose of this study was to describe the differences in sleep efficiency between 12 primigravidae and 19 multigravidae during the third trimester and during the first month postpartum.

HYPOTHESIS

Multigravidae will experience significantly lower sleep efficiency than primigravidae.

METHODS

This was a secondary analysis of data from a convenience sample of pregnant women participating in a longitudinal study of sleep and fatigue before conception until the third postpartum month. Subjects ranged in age from 22 to 40 years. They had EEG monitored for 2 consecutive nights in their home. Sleep efficiency was defined as the total percentage of REM and NREM sleep occurring during the time spent in bed trying to sleep (minus the percentage of awake time). Sleep efficiency can range from 0% (no NREM or REM sleep at all) to 100% (no awake time during the night of sleep).

RESULTS

There was no significant difference in sleep efficiency between primigravidae (90%) and multigravidae (87%) during the third trimester. At 1 month postpartum, the primigravidae experienced significantly lower sleep efficiency (77%) compared with the multigravidae (84%). The primiparae experienced significantly poorer sleep during their postpartum period compared to their own third-trimester sleep, $F(1, 27) = 25.2$, $P < .001$, and to the multigravidae during the postpartum period, $F(1,.58) = 8.7$, $P < .0047$.

DISCUSSION

These results suggest that maternal role acquisition results in more disrupted sleep than maternal role expansion. Nurses need to provide anticipatory guidance to primigravidae to help them smooth the transition from pregnancy to new motherhood.

CRITIQUE

Generalizing these findings to all pregnant women is limited by the small convenience sample of women planning a pregnancy who volunteered to participate in a sleep study before conception. Generally, those who volunteer for a sleep study are fairly good sleepers and do not mind the idea of having wires glued to their heads while they sleep. Studying subjects for 2 consecutive nights allows for the first night to be an adaptation to the monitoring equipment, but the environmental noises in the home interfere with sleep. Although subjects' sleep could have been better if a soundproof sleep laboratory setting was used, monitoring sleep in the home environment provides data in a natural and familiar setting.

Waters, M.A., Lee, K.A. (1996). Differences between primigravidae and multigravidae mothers in sleep disturbances, fatigue, and functional status. *Journal of Nurse-Midwifery, 41(5)*, 364–367.

These sleep cycles also occur during daytime naps. However, naps taken in the morning hours resemble the type of sleep seen in the last half of the night's sleep pattern and include more REM sleep stages. Those naps taken in the afternoon or early evening resemble the first part of the night's sleep and include more NREM sleep stages (Carskadon and Dement, 1994).

PHYSIOLOGIC CHANGES DURING SLEEP

Physiologic changes during sleep differ by sleep stage. Changes during NREM and REM sleep primarily involve autonomic nervous system effects on the cardiovascular and skeletomuscular systems, but many other systems are indirectly affected. Table 25–1 outlines many of the physiologic changes that have been observed during sleep (Dickerson et al, 1993; Parmeggiani, 1994; Orr, 1994).

The cardiopulmonary changes noted during REM sleep are explained by bursts of sympathetic nervous system activity. This may be responsible for the increased incidence of arrhythmia (irregular heartbeat), angina (chest pain), nocturnal asthma and cerebrovascular accidents (stroke) documented during REM sleep (Dickerson et al, 1993). However, an increased incidence of these conditions has also been noted during NREM sleep, perhaps because of a sustained hypotension (low blood pressure).

Body movements occur unconsciously during NREM sleep but are totally absent during REM sleep. The absence of muscle tone during REM sleep is thought to be a protective mechanism to prevent individuals from actually acting out their dreams. Gastric motility and smooth muscle contractions appear to occur in 100-minute cycles but are not related to stage of sleep (Orr et al, 1984). Gastric secretions are unaffected by sleep stages in normal individuals. However, patients with gastric ulcers have increased gastric secretions and report epigastric pain primarily during REM sleep (Orr, 1994).

Changes in hormone levels and brain biochemistry occur before sleep onset. Sleep onset is heavily influenced by melatonin secretion. Melatonin secretion from the pineal gland is suppressed by daylight and only secreted during the dark. When melatonin secretion is high, serotonin secretion is low. Both of these hormones are involved in initiating and maintaining sleep. NREM sleep involves serotonin pathways, which are prevalent in the area of the brain known as the reticular formation activating system, and it is this area of the brain that is responsible for an individual's arousal threshold or level of consciousness (Jones, 1994). (See Fig. 25–3.)

TABLE 25-1 Physiologic Changes During Phases of Sleep

Variable	NREM (Primarily Stages 3 and 4)	REM
Circulatory		
Heart rate	Diminished 5–10%	Increased and more variable
Blood pressure	Reduced 20%	Increased and higher than when awake
Central venous pressure	Reduced slightly	Increased and higher than when awake
Cerebral blood flow	Diminished	Increased
Vessel diameter	Peripheral vasodilation	Peripheral vasoconstriction
Genitourinary system	No change	Penile erection, increased vaginal blood flow
Respiratory		
Respiratory rate	Decreased	Increased and higher than when awake
Apneic episodes (normals)	Occasional at sleep onset lasting less than 10 seconds	Frequent minor episodes with bursts of REMs lasting 15–30 seconds
Motor		
Skeletal muscle tone	Diminished	Completely relaxed
Activity	Bursts of large body movements just before entering REM	Integrated fine motor activity; twitching and jerky movements
Extraocular movements	Absent	Present
Genitourinary systems	Intermittent bladder contractions	No change
Deep tendon reflexes	No change	Absent knee jerk
Hormonal-biochemical		
Growth hormone secretion	Present	Absent
Prolactin secretion	Absent	Present
Antidiuretic hormone secretion	No change	Decreased urine output
Adrenocorticotropic hormone and glucocorticoid secretion	Lowest	Highest
Serotonin concentration	High	No change
Catecholamine concentration	No change	High
Gastric secretions		
Normals	No change	No change
Patients with duodenal ulcers	No change	Increased secretion

NREM, non-rapid eye movement; REM, rapid eye movement.

Growth hormone is secreted primarily during delta wave sleep; the largest release from the pituitary occurs about 1 hour after sleep onset. In fact, reversing the sleep cycle and allowing individuals to sleep during the daytime still results in growth hormone secretion peaks during delta wave sleep (Born et al, 1988). The nocturnal secretion of growth hormone is absent in the elderly and in persons with some pituitary or hypothalamic disorders such as short stature, thyroid disorders, and obesity. Compared with growth hormone, secretion of prolactin (stimulates mammary glands) follows a similar wake-sleep pattern, but cortisone (steroid hormone) secretion is highest during the early morning hours just before awakening and appears to be more dependent on time of day rather than wake-sleep cycles (Weitzman et al, 1983).

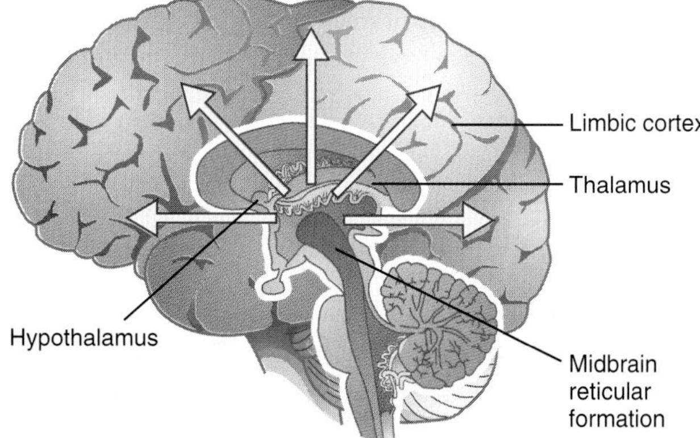

Figure 25-3. The reticular activating system in the brain.

In animals, an increase in skin and bone marrow cell division has been shown to occur during inactivity, rest, and sleep (Fisher, 1968; Scheving, 1959). This helps to explain why adequate rest promotes wound healing and restores and maintains health. A dramatic example is described in *All Things Bright and Beautiful* by James Herriot (1973). Unknown to a farmer, Dr. Herriot gave a very large dose of barbiturates to a sheep who was badly infected and suffering. To his bewilderment when he returned a week later, the animal was doing just fine after sleeping continuously for 48 hours.

Because metabolism is slowed during sleep, body temperature naturally decreases during NREM sleep. However, even for people on bed rest or awake for 24 hours, body temperature fluctuates in a circadian (24-hour-day) pattern. It can vary between 0.5°C and 1.5°C, with a peak during the afternoon

TABLE 25-2 Sleep Stage Characteristics

Stage	Description
1 (NREM)	Lightest sleep stage Presence of theta waves on EEG Transitional state between wakefulness and deeper sleep Lasts only a few minutes in normal persons Person very easily awakened by sensory stimulation such as touch or noise Slow, rolling eye movements Sensation of drowsiness and relaxation Vital signs (pulse, blood pressure, and respirations) gradually decrease Body temperature and metabolism declining Constitutes about 5% of normal sleep time Increases in those with chronic illness and in the elderly
2 (NREM)	Light-sleep stage Presence of sleep spindles and K complexes on EEG Person not as easily awakened Vital signs (pulse, blood pressure, and respirations) decreased Body temperature and metabolism continue to decline Constitutes about 50–55% of normal sleep time
3 (NREM)	Deep-sleep stage Presence of some delta waves on EEG Person difficult to arouse Vital signs (pulse, blood pressure, and respirations) decreased Body temperature and metabolism low Constitutes about 10–15% of normal sleep time in young adults Reduced or absent in chronic illness and in the elderly
4 (NREM)	Deepest-sleep stage Delta waves predominant on EEG Person very difficult to arouse Vital signs (pulse, blood pressure, and heart rate) lowest Body temperature very low Probably responsible for feeling rested on awakening Constitutes about 5–10% of normal sleep time in young adults Reduced or absent in chronic illness and in the elderly
REM	Fast, low-amplitude random EEG waves, similar to the awake state Normally first occurs about 90 minutes after falling asleep Occurs earlier than 90 minutes in the elderly and major depression Occurs at onset of sleep in persons with narcolepsy REM periods normally get longer and closer together as the night progresses Rapidly darting eye movements visible Visible twitching of small facial muscles Skeletal muscle paralysis Periods of oxygen desaturation in persons with diminished respiratory muscle function (i.e., chronic obstructive pulmonary disease) Vivid dreaming reported if awakened from this stage Vital signs increase and widely fluctuate Hypothalamus unable to regulate body temperature (cannot thermoregulate) Probably responsible for mental alertness and memory recall Constitutes about 20–25% of normal sleep time in the adult Constitutes more than 50% of normal sleep in the newborn and infant

NREM, non-rapid eye movement; REM, rapid eye movement; EEG, electroencephalogram

and a trough during the early morning hours. Increased body temperature before sleep, such as with a warm bath or afternoon exercise, results in more NREM sleep (Kupfer et al, 1985). During REM sleep, however, thermoregulation (self-regulation of body temperature) is absent so shivering and heating cannot occur (Glotzbach and Heller, 1994). The newborn infant, who spends half of its sleep time in REM sleep, is particularly vulnerable to environmental temperature changes.

Table 25–2 summarizes physiologic changes that occur during each sleep stage.

FUNCTION OF SLEEP

Although the exact purpose of sleep is unknown, most sleep researchers agree that NREM sleep is an anabolic state needed for synthesizing new proteins (Borbely, 1994; Horne,

1988). In an anabolic state, energy is produced when simple substances are converted into more complex matter. Examples are normal growth and development and tissue replacement. Support for this theory comes from the knowledge that more NREM occurs after exercise (a time of increased catabolism or chemical release of energy) and that the peak secretion of growth hormone occurs during NREM (Born et al, 1988; Edinger et al, 1993). This theory is also supported in studies with children and the elderly. Children, with high requirements for anabolism, sleep more than adults, whereas the elderly spend very little time in deep sleep (see Fig. 25–2). The body's priority need for deep sleep is demonstrated when Stages 3 and 4 delta waves take precedence over REM sleep during recovery from sleep deprivation. There is a much higher percentage of delta wave sleep compared with REM sleep during the first night of sleep after sleep deprivation (Horne, 1988).

The function of REM sleep remains unclear. One researcher hypothesized that REM sleep was necessary to maintain vision in both eyes (Berger, 1970). Others suggested that REM sleep allows the brain to process all of the day's experiences and consolidate information into memory. Support for this theory is based on the following phenomena:

- More REM sleep occurs after days of stress or intense learning.
- REM sleep diminishes throughout the lifespan.
- REM sleep is reduced in persons who are mentally impaired.

REM sleep may provide the opportunity for the nervous system to use all the proteins synthesized during NREM and restructure synapses so that learning takes place. Other researchers (Crick and Mitchison, 1983) hypothesized that REM sleep is actually the way the brain "unlearns" or dumps information to prevent overloading memory storage centers. Current research data indicate a lack of certain cell activity during periods of REM sleep. Inactivity of these cells prevents receptor sites from becoming sensitized (Siegel, 1994).

REM sleep is also necessary for hypothalamic functioning (Zepelin, 1994). In studies of individuals deprived of REM sleep, complaints include increased appetite, anxiety, irritability, hyperactivity, difficulty concentrating, and difficulty coping with new environmental stressors. Rats deprived of REM sleep also have an increased appetite but begin to lose body fat, experience stomach ulcers, and are less able to retain body heat (Everson et al, 1986). These symptoms are all related to the function of the hypothalamus.

DISTURBANCES IN SLEEP PATTERNS

Sleep pattern disturbances can occur in individuals who are hospitalized, living in institutional settings, or living at home. These disturbances can be classified as disorders of initiating and maintaining sleep (DIMS), disorders of excessive somnolence (daytime sleepiness) (DOES), and dysfunctions associated with abnormal behaviors during sleep (parasomnias). DIMS and DOES have particular relevance for nursing practice. DIMS are particularly common in the elderly and in hospitalized patients. DOES are the result of chronic sleep-related health problems that manifest themselves as excessive sleepiness during the daytime.

DISORDERS OF INITIATING AND MAINTAINING SLEEP

The ability to initiate and maintain sleep can be disturbed in many ways and for many different reasons. Rapid crossing of time zones, working night shifts, daylight savings time, nocturia (excessive urination at night), a snoring bed partner, depression, a strange environment, and drug dependency or sudden withdrawal can adversely affect sleep. We know that a particular amount of uninterrupted sleep is necessary for normal functioning of the human body because of various physical and psychological changes that occur when a person is deprived of sleep. Some differential nursing diagnoses related to initiating and maintaining sleep may include insomnia, sleep deprivation, and altered sleep-wake cycles.

Insomnia. Difficulty falling asleep (longer than 20 minutes), frequent awakenings, awakening too early, or any combination of these conditions is referred to as insomnia. Insomnia, affecting one of every three adults, is the most prevalent of the sleep disorders (Kales and Kales, 1984). It is particularly detrimental because the sleeper cannot rely on a good night's sleep to get through the next day's activities. Persons at risk for insomnia include those experiencing discomfort or pain associated with medical conditions, those under stress, those who are anxious or depressed, and those ingesting drugs such as caffeine or reserpine (an antihypertensive medication for high blood pressure and nerve disorders) that stimulate the central nervous system.

Sleep Deprivation. After approximately 4 days of total sleep deprivation, healthy people begin to display psychological symptoms such as increased fatigue, difficulty concentrating, confusion, disorientation and misperception, feelings of persecution, general irritability, personality changes, and hallucinations. Physical signs include tremors, diminished reaction time, and decreased attention span. These signs and symptoms are more rapidly induced by strenuous physical activity during the period of sleep deprivation. Box 25–1 summarizes the known physiologic and psychological effects of sleep deprivation.

Because these symptoms are not found in all people who are sleep deprived, it is believed that certain individuals may be more susceptible than others and that these symptoms may not be an inevitable result of total deprivation. On recovery nights after total deprivation, there is less light sleep (Stage 2), whereas deep sleep (Stages 3 and 4) increases twofold and REM sleep also increases (Carskadon and Dement, 1994). Even if individuals are deprived only of REM sleep, it is only recovered after any missing Stage 4 sleep is replaced. After 8 hours of sleep, the sleeper's cyclic pattern usually returns to normal.

BOX 25-1
SIGNS AND SYMPTOMS OF SLEEP DEPRIVATION

PHYSIOLOGIC

- Hand tremors
- Decreased reflexes
- Slowed response time
- Impaired word memory
- Decreased reasoning, judgment, and association
- Cardiac dysrhythmias
- Decreased auditory and visual alertness

PSYCHOSOCIAL

- Disorientation
- Irritability
- Decreased motivation
- Fatigue
- Sleepiness
- Hyperactivity
- Agitation

It is easy to see how normal sleep patterns would be disrupted by admission to the hospital or nursing home. During hospitalization, the environment is new and the stressors are many. The patient must cope with restricted positioning, pain and discomfort, anxiety over finances or family welfare, fear of dying, and poorly coordinated nurse-patient activities. Problems with nutritional status (nothing by mouth after midnight), elimination status (urinary frequency or diarrhea), respiratory status (orthopnea, or difficulty breathing when lying down), mobility, integumentary (skin, hair, glands) status (turning every 2 hours to prevent bedsores), and comfort status (unable to sleep in usual prone position because of abdominal surgery) are a few of the many risk factors related to initiating and maintaining sleep.

Any institution's environment can be a source of sensory overload from bright lights and strange noises, new experiences, and unknown outcomes. The environment can also be a source of sensory deprivation, particularly when Universal Precautions to guard against infection are in place for patients. When deprived of sensory stimuli, Wood (1962) found an increase in REM sleep and a delay in the onset of the first REM period. The increase in REM, together with frequent awakenings, can result in patients reporting increased dreams and restlessness in the hospital setting compared with sleeping at home.

Because REM sleep occurs at the end of an average 90-minute sleep cycle, and because the majority of REM occurs during the latter half of the night (see Fig. 25–2), REM deprivation probably occurs clinically when patients are allowed to sleep only for short periods (less than 1 hour), when they only sleep a total of 3 to 4 hours in a 24-hour period, or when they are awakened too early in the morning. REM sleep deprivation also occurs with REM-suppressant medications (see Drug Therapy).

Observers in intensive care units (ICUs) have described a syndrome known as postcardiotomy, or intensive care, delirium. Although first recognized with postcardiotomy patients, the cause has not been definitely established. This syndrome is likely to occur after any patient has been in an ICU for approximately 3 to 5 days. Defining characteristics, similar to those discussed in total deprivation, include illusions, hallucinations, and even psychosis or paranoia. It has been associated with sleep deprivation, sensory deprivation, age, severity of preoperative illness, duration of surgery, and time spent on the heart-lung bypass machine (Easton and MacKenzie, 1988).

Some of the first sleep studies conducted by nurse researchers involved patients in ICUs (Hilton, 1976; McFadden and Giblin, 1979; Walker, 1972; Woods, 1972). Nursing studies have documented that a patient's sleep while in an acute care unit is frequently interrupted by medical and nursing procedures as well as the noise of staff and equipment (Richards and Bairnsfather, 1988; Webster and Thompson, 1986; Woods and Falk, 1974). Researchers have found that a patient in an ICU may spend as much as 40 to 50% of their sleep time awake and as little as 3 to 4% of their sleep time in REM sleep (Deamer et al, 1972; Richards and Bairnsfeather, 1988). Intensive care (postcardiotomy) delirium, like other types of sleep deprivation, commonly disappears after a full night's sleep, regardless of the cause.

A thorough assessment of a patient's normal sleep patterns and sleeping environment should be made on admission to the hospital. Because each individual's sleep pattern is unique, an initial nursing assessment is necessary to help patients cope with sleep pattern disturbances resulting from health problems.

Altered Wake-Sleep Cycles. Altered wake-sleep cycles result in sleep deprivation, even when the same number of hours are spent in bed. For shift workers who work at night and sleep during the day, wake-sleep cycles tend to become altered during their work week and revert back to normal on days off. Consequently, employees who work at night or rotate shifts have been found to be chronically deprived of sleep, as noted in a classic nursing research study of nurses who rotated shifts (Felton, 1975). Night workers have more Stage 4 sleep than the normal young adult, a decreased amount of time from onset of sleep to the first REM period, less REM sleep, and fewer body movements (Akerstedt, 1985).

Rapid jet travel westward or eastward across time zones, between San Francisco and London, for example, is also an example of altered wake-sleep patterns that commonly manifest as "jet lag" (Fig. 25–4). Disturbances in sleep patterns are similar to REM deprivation: more Stage 4 sleep, less REM sleep, and more early morning awakenings during the first 5 days after arriving in the new time zone (Moline et al, 1992).

With some older persons, a condition of nocturnal delusions, disorientation, and agitation has been observed. It is often called sundown syndrome because it occurs in people who are alert and oriented during the day but manifest confusion and disorientation during the evening and night, particularly when placed in a strange environment. Although it is

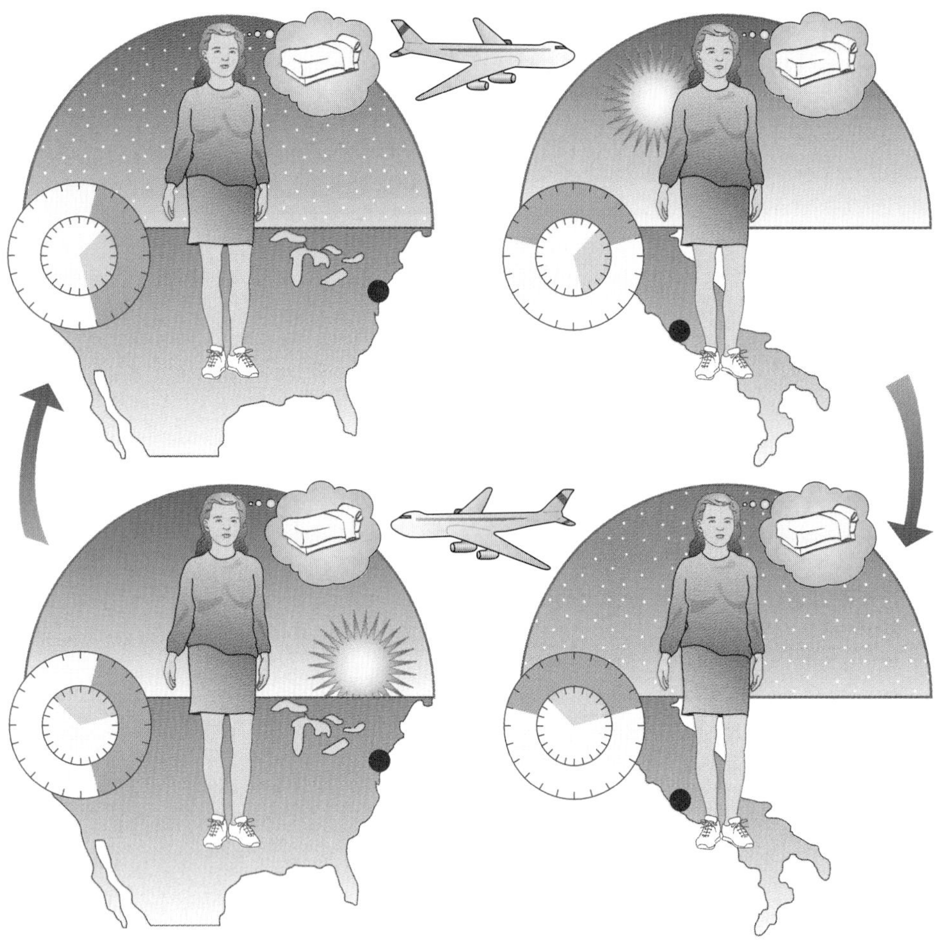

Figure 25-4. This illustration depicts a typical disruption in a person's circadian rhythms caused by travel from one time zone to another. The person who leaves New York City and flies to Rome will experience a period of adjustment as sleep-wake patterns align with the body's circadian rhythms, commonly known as "jet lag." On return to New York City, the person must readjust the now-altered sleep-wake patterns to local time.

very common in persons with dementia (Cohen-Mansfield et al, 1990) who become more confused and disoriented at night, it can be a result of undetected changes in circulatory, respiratory, nutritional, or fluid and electrolyte status in an otherwise alert person. It can also be a direct result of medications and the side effects unique to the elderly population.

Persons with certain types of *depression* exhibit increased amounts of REM sleep; the first REM period occurs earlier than normal after falling asleep at night. These patients respond to REM deprivation. REM sleep can be suppressed with tricyclic antidepressants, or the nurse can limit the patient to just the first half of the night's sleep until tricyclic antidepressants achieve their therapeutic effect (Kupfer et al, 1991). The therapeutic effect of REM deprivation is often a dramatic improvement in mood state, but the effect is only temporary, and the depressed person must be deprived of REM sleep every few days if drug therapy is not used.

A genetically inherited sleep disorder known as *narcolepsy* is also a clinical example of altered wake-sleep cycles. In this case, the appearance of REM sleep is altered. Narcolepsy is diagnosed only from a formal sleep study that documents REM sleep beginning within 15 minutes after sleep onset. The main symptom of narcolepsy is abrupt and unexpected sleep onset during the day, with a REM sleep episode intruding on wakefulness. Unlike other disorders of daytime sleepiness caused by frequent nocturnal arousals, this disorder is related to a change in the pattern of REM sleep. This disorder begins in early adulthood, and both sexes are equally at risk. Their sleep attacks occur with sudden stimulation (loud noise or bright lights) or sudden emotions (laughing or anger). The narcoleptic event may consist only of cataplexy or the loss of muscle tone that normally occurs during REM sleep, and the person may still be consciously aware of the environment (Guilleminault, 1994).

DISORDERS OF EXCESSIVE SOMNOLENCE

Excessive daytime sleepiness most always indicates chronic sleep deprivation or interrupted nocturnal sleep. Many physiologic processes (breathing, gastric secretions, muscle tone) can malfunction during sleep, disrupt sleep stages, and cause disorders of excessive sleepiness (DOES). The disruptions consist of brief, but frequent, arousals from NREM or REM sleep. Because of their brief duration, there may be no recall of these arousals. In fact, it is usually the bed partner or family member who provides the data for diagnosis of the problem.

Disorders of excessive sleepiness are devastating to quality of life because they affect a person's ability to maintain a job; they also have an impact on the person's family. DOES can be life threatening because people who suffer from them are at extreme risk of falling asleep while in hazardous work situations or while driving an automobile. The main causes of these disorders are obstructive sleep apnea, periodic movements in sleep, and gastroesophageal reflux (gastric acids in the esophagus).

Obstructive Sleep Apnea Syndrome. One of the most common causes of disturbed sleep at night, obstructive sleep apnea syndrome (OSAS) primarily affects older men (usually after age 40) who have a history of loud snoring and excessive daytime sleepiness. Affected persons have a tendency to become extremely overweight because the chronic sleep deprivation leaves little energy for daytime activities or exercising. Even if they are not overweight, they often have hypertension because of the nocturnal increases in pulmonary arterial pressure with repetitive snoring and hypoxemia (lack of oxygen in arterial blood) (Stoohs et al, 1993). A summary of clinical signs and symptoms of OSAS appears in Table 25–3.

Snoring is an essential indicator of sleep apnea and occurs because the narrowed opening of the airway causes the soft palate to vibrate loudly during inspiration (Fig. 25–5). During sleep, this narrowing episodically obstructs the airway. If these obstructive apneic events occur for longer than 10 seconds and more than five times per hour, the patient is usually diagnosed by a formal sleep diagnostic test as having OSAS. With each obstructive event, the low oxygen saturation levels arouse the central nervous system and stimulates breathing to resume. Not only are these individuals in danger of falling asleep during daytime activities, they are also at risk for respiratory failure during sleep if they have taken any CNS depressant medication, including anesthetics or alcohol. A variety of therapies are offered: nasal administration of continuous positive airway pressure (CPAP), a weight reduction program, dental appliances, corrective surgery to the throat and palate, maxillofacial (upper jaw and face) surgery, or tracheostomy (Kryger, 1994). However, long-term effectiveness from these procedures is not well known.

TABLE 25-3 Common Clinical Features of Sleep Apnea

Examination of the Awake Patient	Examination of Sleeping Patient
Frequently obese	Loud, intermittent snoring, "resuscitative" snort
Short, fat neck	Repetitive apneas, hypopneas terminated by arousal
Upper airway abnormalities: large uvula, low-hanging soft palate, large tonsils, adenoids	Sleep continuity interrupted
Micognathia-retrognathia	Usually 30+ apneas per hour
Upper airway tumors, cysts	Usually over 50% of sleep time apneic
High blood pressure	Increased motor activity during sleep
Polycythemia (increased concentration of red blood cells)	Nocturnal cardiac dysrhythmias
	Decreased "deep" (Stages 3, 4) sleep
	Decreased rapid eye movement sleep

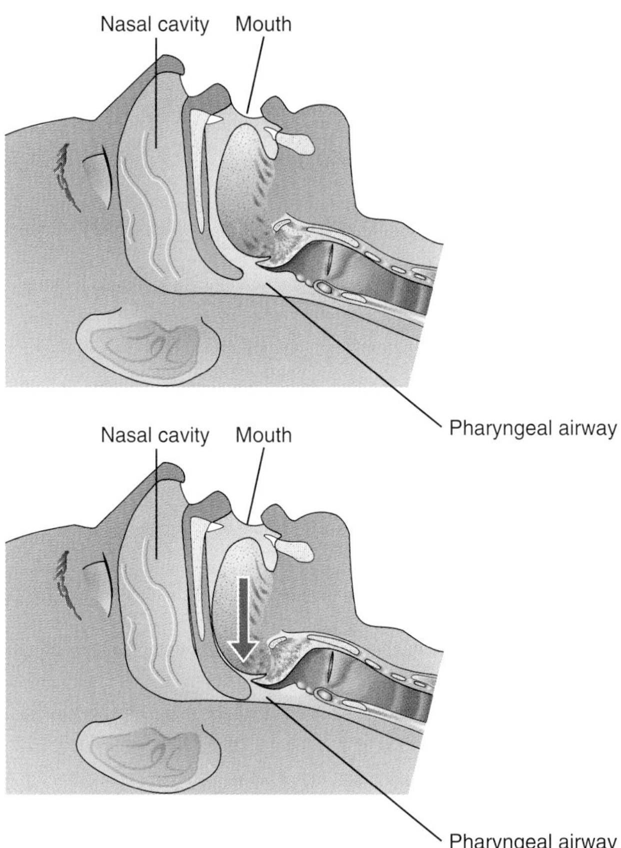

Figure 25-5. How obstructive sleep apnea occurs. The predisposed person has a small pharyngeal airway. During sleep, the pharyngeal muscles relax, causing the airway to close and producing an apneic episode.

Myoclonus. Periodic leg movements during the night (nocturnal myoclonus) can also result in frequent and brief arousals from sleep and excessive daytime sleepiness. Periodic leg jerks are most often seen as a sleep disorder in the elderly population (Ancoli-Israel et al, 1985; Bixler et al, 1982). Bursts of leg muscle activity are evident when EMG is recorded from the anterior tibialis (outside muscle of the lower leg) (Fig. 25–6). These periodic leg movements cannot be reduced by medications, but arousals from the myoclonus

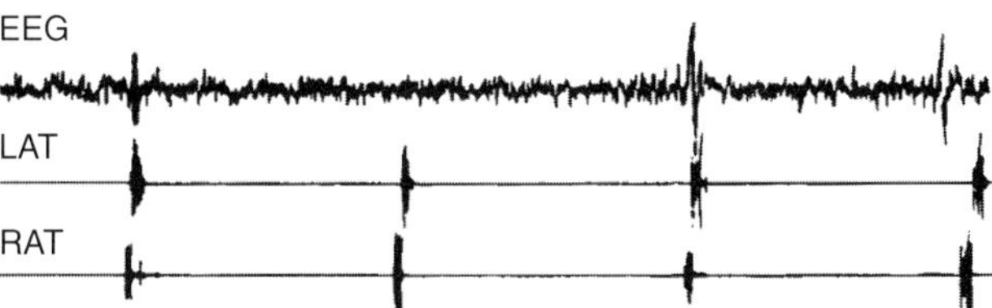

Figure 25-6. Polysomnogram readings showing periodic movements of sleep. The electroencephalographic reading reflects patterns of brain activity during sleep. The left anterior tibialis (LAT) and right anterior tibialis (RAT) readings show periodic bursts of electrical activity recorded by electrodes on the patient's left and right legs, reflecting muscle movements during sleep.

have been reduced with short-acting benzodiazepines (sleeping medication). Although medications that increase dopamine (L-dopa or bromocriptine) may prove useful in treating this disorder, tolerance may develop, and side effects of nausea or leg movements during the day may render this therapy unfeasible (Becker et al, 1993).

Gastroesophageal Reflux. Nocturnal gastroesophageal reflux, a condition in which a person complains of heartburn or a tightness in the chest on awakening, can result from the low pressure at the esophageal sphincter while sleeping in a reclined posture. Without treatment, sleep is unknowingly fragmented by frequent arousals from nocturnal gastric acid secretion and reflux, laryngopharyngitis (inflammation of the throat and larynx) is common, and aspiration is a constant danger (Orr, 1994).

PARASOMNIAS

In addition to the two categories of sleep pattern disturbances just discussed, there are several other sleep-related disorders categorized as parasomnias. Parasomnias are movements or behaviors during sleep that may not be normal but seldom cause arousals. Parasomnias include enuresis (bed wetting), somnambulism (sleep walking), sleep terrors, and bruxism (teeth grinding) and occur primarily during the early portion of the night, when NREM sleep predominates. Parasomnias are frequently seen in children, but tend to disappear at puberty. Adults who exhibit parasomnias should be evaluated for evidence of nocturnal epilepsy (Rauch and Stern, 1986), abnormal stress and anxiety, or psychiatric disturbances (Kales and Kales, 1984).

FACTORS AFFECTING CLINICAL DECISIONS

Age

The total amount of sleep per night decreases from birth to adulthood (Fig. 25–7). REM sleep comprises as much as 50% of an infant's sleep (Haslam, 1984) but diminishes to between 20% and 25% in the young adult and to about 15% in the older adult. REM sleep often begins as soon as a newborn falls asleep, whereas it typically begins about 90 minutes after an adult falls asleep. The amount of REM sleep remains approximately the same for young adults and the elderly during the first half of the night. During the second half of the night, young adults increase their REM sleep 300%, whereas the older adult's REM increases only 50% (Bliwise, 1994; Kramer, 1994).

The average length of each sleep cycle increases from about 50 minutes in newborns to about 90 minutes in adults. In adults there is no significant change in the hours of sleep, but older adults have much less deep sleep (delta waves) and more Stage 2 light sleep (Bliwise, 1994). This helps to explain why elderly clients awaken more easily and more frequently

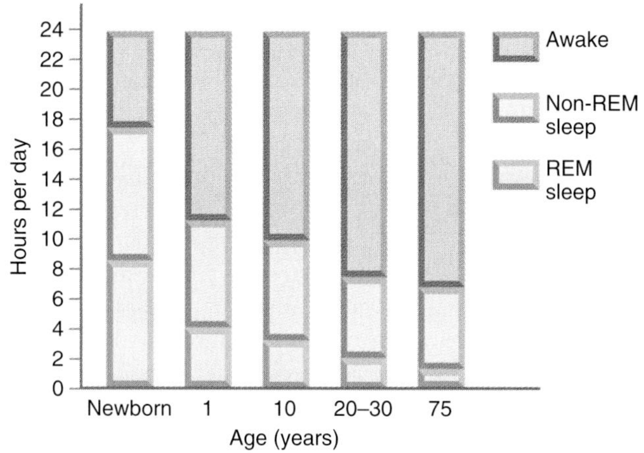

Figure 25–7. Typical changes in sleep patterns with aging.

than young adults (Pacini and Fitzpatrick, 1982). Although changes in sleep are expected with increasing age, Hayter (1983) found wide variations in self-reported bedtime hour, time to get to sleep, number of awakenings, the time of awakening, total sleep time, and napping behavior in the elderly. The results of her study demonstrate the need for gathering accurate baseline information about the elderly patient's sleep pattern before initiating a nursing intervention. Sleep patterns according to age are summarized in Table 25–4.

Nutritional Status

Another factor that influences sleep patterns is one's state of nutrition (Schneider-Helmert, 1986). The need for NREM sleep increases when overeating and gaining weight or dieting and losing weight. During periods of increased catabolism (chemical release of energy) such as starvation or hyperthyroidism (overactive thyroid) or when tissue is damaged, there is an increased need for Stage 3 and 4 deep sleep. In cases of untreated hypothyroidism (slowed metabolism), delta wave sleep may be decreased or totally absent (Evans, 1983).

Foods high in protein induce sleep more rapidly without distorting the normal sleep cycle. Protein food sources contain L-tryptophan, an amino acid important for initiating sleep. Adults normally consume 1 to 2 g of L-tryptophan in their daily diets. In addition to meat, poultry, and fish, a variety of nuts have large amounts of this amino acid. Ingestion of 1 g (there are approximately 10 mg in 1 g of protein) has been shown to reduce sleep-onset time by 50%. Clinical studies indicate that L-tryptophan's effect on sleep is limited to only 1 or 2 nights (Sallanon et al, 1983) and higher doses can cause liver dysfunction.

Melatonin supplements, available in various doses from health food stores, are proving helpful to some individuals with insomnia-related sleep problems. However, the effective dosage remains unknown, and the melatonin is often packaged in a mixture of other nutrients, such as vitamin B6 or amino acids.

TABLE 25-4 Sleep Patterns According to Age Group

Age Group	Normal Sleep Pattern
Newborn	About 14–18 hours of sleep a day 50% REM sleep Most of the remaining time in Stage 3 and 4 NREM sleep Sleep cycles of 45–60 minutes duration
Infant	About 12–14 hours of sleep a day 20–30% REM sleep Increased sleep at night (8–10 hours), with a scheduled pattern of naps At 12 months, one or two naps a day
Toddler	About 10–12 hours of sleep a day 25% REM sleep Generally sleeps during the night Decrease in midmorning naps Normal sleep-wake cycle usually established at age 2 or 3 years
Preschooler	About 11 hours of sleep at night 25% REM sleep Second nap usually eliminated by age 3 Daytime naps discontinued around age 5, except in cultures in which an afternoon nap or siesta is customary
School-age child	About 10 hours of sleep at night 25% REM sleep 20% Stage 3 and 4 sleep Sleep time remains relatively constant
Adolescent	About 10 hours of sleep at night 25% REM sleep 20% Stage 3 and 4 sleep
Young adult	About 7–9 hours sleep at night 20 to 25% REM sleep 20% Stage 3 and 4 sleep 50% Stage 2 sleep
Middle-aged adult	About 7 hours of sleep at night About 20–25% REM sleep 5% Stage 1 sleep
Elderly adult	About 6 hours of sleep at night 20% REM sleep 10–15% Stage 1 sleep Stage 4 sleep markedly decreased, sometimes absent First REM period occurs earlier May awaken more often during the night

REM, rapid eye movement; NREM, non-rapid eye movement

Exercise Pattern

Activity level may also affect sleep patterns, probably by increasing body temperature. Subjects placed on bed rest for 5 weeks had increased Stage 3 and 4 sleep, decreased light sleep (Stages 1 and 2), and no alteration in REM sleep (Ryback et al, 1971). In comparison with normal boys, boys immobilized with muscular dystrophy also have more Stage 3 and 4 sleep (Redding et al, 1985). Exercising near bedtime can be detrimental to adequate rest because it stimulates metabolism. Daytime exercise may increase delta wave sleep, increase total sleep time, and decrease REM sleep in some healthy individuals, but may have no effect on sleep in trained athletes (Kupfer et al, 1985; Edinger et al, 1993).

Stress Level

A person's current level of stress can temporarily alter sleep patterns. It appears that people working at heavy labor (physical stress) may get more consolidated delta sleep, with less light sleep Stages 1 and 2. The result is a reduction in total sleep time and feeling more rested compared with those who work at heavy thinking (psychological stress). During times of psychological stress, more time is sent in light sleep Stages 1 and 2 and in trying to initiate sleep. Anxiety can result in a delayed onset of sleep and less REM sleep (Monroe et al, 1992). As the anxiety diminishes or the individual adapts to the new situation, these alterations disappear. Other stress-related factors, such as waking up to get to work early versus sleeping in later on weekends, can also influence sleep patterns by altering the body's normal circadian clock.

Drug Therapy

Medications can have profound and long-lasting effects on sleep patterns. Sedative-hypnotics deactivate the reticular activating system (area in Figure 25–3 responsible for arousal), allowing more rapid onset of sleep with fewer awakenings. However, suppression of REM sleep can occur with drugs such as hypnotics, narcotics, L-dopa (to treat Parkinson's disease), alcohol, antidepressants, stimulants, and marijuana. Individuals may report better sleep the first few nights, but tolerance increases, and these REM-suppressant drugs tend to lose their effect after about 2 weeks. If these drugs are abruptly withdrawn after long-term use, REM rebound (a marked increase in REM sleep) occurs. This rebound may last several days and can even be passed on to the unborn fetus. In addition, patients with REM rebound often complain of nightmares, restlessness, anxiety, depression, and disrupted sleep (Hartmann, 1994; Nicholson et al, 1994). The effects on sleep of commonly prescribed drugs are summarized in Table 25–5.

Fortunately, prescriptions for barbiturates have been declining. Short-acting benzodiazepines (sleeping medications), such as triazolam, are the most widely prescribed group of drugs on the market today for complaints of disturbed sleep. These drugs may increase total sleep time, but they suppress Stage 4 and REM sleep, have a wide variation in rate of onset and elimination times, cause a rebound effect of increased daytime anxiety, and have a high tendency toward addiction and short-term memory loss (Ashton, 1984). Therefore, only short-term, intermittent usage is recommended (Gaillard, 1994; Syvalahti, 1985; Lader, 1986). The pharmacology of commonly used sleeping medications is summarized in Table 25–6.

TABLE 25-5 Commonly Used Drugs That Affect Sleep

Drug	Action
Alcohol	Speeds onset of sleep Causes frequent arousals resulting in fragmented REM and NREM sleep Suppresses REM sleep
Antidepressants and stimulants	Suppress REM sleep
Beta-blockers	Cause nightmares Cause insomnia Fragment sleep
Caffeine	Delays falling asleep Fragments sleep by increasing awakenings during night
Diuretics	Cause voiding during the night if taken in the evening
Narcotics	Suppress REM sleep If discontinued abruptly, can increase risk of cardiac dysrhythmias because of "rebound REM" periods Cause increased awakenings and daytime drowsiness
Sedative-hypnotics	Provide only temporary (1 week) help to fall asleep Cause "hangover" during day: drowsiness, confusion, decreased energy May exacerbate sleep apnea in older adults
Diazepam (Valium)	Decreases Stages 2, 4, and REM sleep Decreases awakenings

REM, rapid eye movement; NREM, non-rapid eye movement

Stimulants, such as caffeine, will delay sleep onset and decrease total sleep time (Stavric, 1992). Sleepers who drank the equivalent of four cups of coffee about 30 minutes before bedtime had disruptions in REM sleep. Drinking two cups of coffee (300 mg of caffeine) can result in 2 hours less total sleep time, delayed sleep onset, and twice as much wakefulness during the sleep period (Kales and Kales, 1984). It is important to assess caffeine intake from all sources (e.g., medications, teas, colas, chocolate) in all patients complaining of sleep disturbance.

Sociocultural Considerations

Sociocultural factors can greatly affect sleep. Personal habits termed "bedtime rituals" are culturally derived and consist of certain routine behaviors that are believed (either spiritually, socially, or culturally) to improve the quality of sleep. People use many rituals to help them fall asleep and sleep well. Patients may have a bedtime ritual that nurses need to consider when assisting them to prepare for sleep at bedtime. Drinking warm milk, taking a warm bath, quiet reading in bed, praying, starting out in a certain supine position, or even counting sheep are just some of the more common bedtime rituals.

A major sociocultural consideration for sleep behavior is that of "cosleeping" or sleeping in a family bed. Variations range from sleeping with a newborn in the parents' bed to sleeping in close proximity but in separate beds. Ethnographers Barry and Paxson (1971) studied cosleeping behaviors in various cultures and found that mother and infant share the same bed in 76 cultures and sleep in the same room in 42 cultures. In most cultures, a child is raised with a value of closeness and sleeps with the mother well into toddlerhood (Morelli et al, 1992).

Very little is known about cosleeping in Western culture. In the United States, Anglo parents are socialized to value independence, and beginning at birth it becomes desirable for newborns to sleep alone in a separate bedroom (Morelli et al, 1992).

Setting in Which Care Is Delivered

A tired infant or young child can usually sleep anywhere, anytime, and in any position, whereas an exhausted adult is more sensitive to the sleep environment and cannot fall asleep unless the environment is precisely arranged. Adult sleep is disturbed whenever the environment is altered by changes in light, noise, bed surface characteristics, or room temperature. All of these changes occur when a person is admitted to the hospital or transferred to a new setting. Prescribing a sleeping medication (see Table 25–6) may be appropriate for a patient with a sleep disturbance occurring during temporary changes in the environment.

A new sleep environment's effect is clearly shown when research subjects are admitted into a sleep laboratory and studied for a few nights. The first night is almost never used in

TABLE 25-6 Commonly Prescribed Drugs to Aid Sleep

Generic Name	Trade Name	Onset of Action	Dosage	Indications
Alprazolam	Xanax	15–45 min	0.25–0.5 mg tid	Anxiety
Flurazepam	Dalmane Apo-Flurazepam	15–45 min	15–30 mg at bedtime	Insomnia
Temazepam	Restoril	25–27 min	15–30 mg at bedtime	Insomnia
Triazolam	Halcion	15–30 min	0.25–0.5 mg at bedtime	Insomnia
Zolpidem	Ambien	10–15 min	5–10 mg	Insomnia

reports of research findings because of the delayed sleep onset and frequent awakenings that occur. Only subsequent nights more accurately reflect typical sleep patterns in the home environment.

Certain noises in the environment will create sleep disturbances. There is wide variation in the sensitivity of individuals to noise. The elderly are more sensitive to nighttime noises, perhaps because they spend more time in light sleep stages. The significance of the noise is another important factor. A new mother, for example, will hear a whimper from her infant but may not hear the alarm clock.

For human beings functioning in a daytime world, light is a major cue that one should be awake and alert, whereas darkness is a cue that one should be tired or sleeping. Those who work at night and sleep during the day have disturbed sleep patterns because of the light that enters through windows in the sleep setting. Those who experience total daylight or total darkness in geographic areas above the Arctic Circle also have disturbed sleep patterns that sometimes result in seasonal affective disorder, or winter depression.

Environmental temperature has an important influence on sleep. During REM sleep, the environmental temperature has a direct effect on a person's internal temperature because thermoregulation is absent, so shivering or sweating cannot occur in response to cold and heat. When the environment is too cold or too hot (i.e., not thermoneutral [optimum with minimal requirement of energy and oxygen] at 29°C), REM sleep is decreased (Glotzbach and Heller, 1994).

FUTURE DEVELOPMENTS

In an era of health care reform, managed care, and cost containment, more major illnesses are now treated on an outpatient basis, with minimal time spent in acute care hospitals. As a result, health problems are primarily managed in the home by family members rather than by professional nurses employed in health care settings. Family members may take on this new caregiving role in addition to a regular paying job. The results of caring for family members during the night while maintaining full-time employment will be evident in decreased work performance and social interactions with work colleagues, friends, and family members. Without respite care for family members, these caregivers will also begin to suffer from inadequate and disturbed sleep.

NURSING CARE ACTIONS

Each situation or health problem dictates which of the patient's usual routines for initiating and maintaining sleep will remain useful and which will need modification and nursing management. Relevant nursing care principles and practices, including assessment and interventions to promote adequate sleep, allow the nurse to teach patients and their caregivers about healthy sleep patterns and discuss alternative actions to improve the quality of their sleep.

Research supports three principles of nursing care that apply to all patient care encounters.

1. Adequate rest and sleep are essential to maintain health and recover from illness.
2. Sleep disturbances can result from various factors such as discomfort, pain, stress, anxiety, depression, and the environment (lighting, noise, unfamiliar surroundings).
3. Until the patient and family are able to manage factors associated with sleep disturbances, the nurse must implement interventions appropriate to the patient and the situation.

Any nursing intervention must be based on an assessment of the patient and the situation. Components of a good sleep history are presented in Box 25–2. From a careful sleep history, the nurse should be able to evaluate and categorize the patient's sleep problem as DIMS or DOES. From this distinction, an appropriate plan of nursing care can be developed and implemented. Nursing actions for specific sleep disturbances are presented next.

Disorders of Initiating and Maintaining Sleep

Insomnia. Factors that place a person at risk for insomnia are usually related to either sensory overload or sensory deprivation. A careful assessment of the daily routine may be helpful when a client expresses difficulty in going to sleep or remaining asleep or shows a dependence on drugs. In the initial assessment, the exact nature of the problem (whether it is due to sensory overload or deprivation), its origin, duration, and characteristics should be determined. The nurse should also ask about the patient's usual daily activities. Examples of questions to ask the patient who complains of insomnia and other DIMS can be found in Box 25–3.

When insomnia is due to sensory deprivation, measures can be taken to increase external stimuli. Possible actions include the following:

- A sedentary or relatively inactive lifestyle can be modified to include more exercise and activity during daytime hours.

BOX 25-2
COMPONENTS OF A SLEEP HISTORY

- Patient's typical normal sleep pattern
- Description of the patient's current sleep problem
- Description of any physical illness that the patient may be experiencing
- Review of the patient's current life events for stressors
- Patient's emotional and mental status
- Patient's usual bedtime rituals

BOX 25-3
QUESTIONS TO ASK WHEN ASSESSING FOR DISORDERS OF EXCESSIVE DAYTIME SLEEPINESS

SLEEP APNEA

1. Has anyone recently told you that you snore loudly?
2. Has anyone ever told you that you stop breathing when you sleep?
3. Do you wake up suddenly coughing or choking?
4. Do you have difficulty staying awake during the day?
5. If so, under what circumstances?
   - Sitting in front of the television?
   - While reading a book?
   - While eating a meal?
   - While working at your desk?
   - While in the middle of a physical activity?
   - While driving?

MYOCLONUS

1. Has anyone ever told you that your legs jerk while you are sleeping?

ESOPHAGEAL REFLUX

1. Do you wake up suddenly coughing or choking?
2. Do you frequently awaken suddenly with an acid taste in your mouth?

- A sleep program that consists of a regular bedtime hour, only going to bed when sleepy, and not staying in bed if not sleepy, can be implemented (Zarcone, 1994).
- Increasing stimulation (exercise, noise from television or radio) right before bedtime has proven helpful. It is hypothesized that increasing stimuli may actually produce a rebound effect that makes the person sleepy.
- When measures such as the above do not relieve the insomnia, psychological counseling should be recommended (Hauri, 1994). Psychological disturbance has been identified in as many as 85% of those reporting insomnia (Kales and Kales, 1984).

When insomnia is due to sensory overload, measures should be taken to limit external stimuli, for example:

- Evening hours should be occupied with relaxing, uncomplicated, and nonstressful activities to prevent excitation.
- Bedtime rituals that the patient used at home should be followed as closely as possible.
- A good book, a warm bath, and a hot drink are helpful to many people (Horne and Reid, 1985).
- Providing an environment that is quiet and tidy, has subdued lighting, and suitable ventilation will help initiate and maintain sleep.
- A comfortable bed, freedom from pain, and knowing how to summon help if necessary will help some patients fall asleep more easily.
- Keeping bed rails up will help a patient who is afraid of falling out of a narrow hospital bed feel more secure and sleep more easily.
- Stress and anxiety can be reduced by allowing the patient time to ask questions and discuss fears.
- Sleep medications should be taken after nursing care is completed and the patient is ready for sleep.
- Aspirin has been shown to be as effective in initiating sleep as barbiturates and other potent sedative-hypnotics without affecting the normal sleep cycle (Hauri and Silbergard, 1979).

Evaluation of interventions is essential. It is important to note the patient's subjective feelings on awakening. Whether or not sleep is evaluated as "good" depends on the perception of how long it takes to fall asleep, the number of remembered awakenings during the night, and the patient's total sleep time (Kales and Kales, 1984, pp. 104–105). Individuals are unable to remember brief arousals from sleep and are unlikely to remember awakenings that last less than 3 minutes.

Physiologic and behavioral changes that occur during sleep can be helpful in evaluating whether or not sleep was successfully initiated and maintained. Lack of purposeful movement and speech, closed eyelids, heavy, slow breathing, and decreased response to external stimuli should be observed during sleep. Any one of these changes alone will not indicate that the patient is sleeping; however, if all are observed, it will be reasonable to conclude that sleep is in progress and nursing interventions were successful. Using these data to validate sleep may be questionable if the patient is dependent on a respirator and cannot speak, if the patient has a heart pacemaker and heart rate does not change during sleep, or if the

BOX 25-4
METHODS TO REDUCE ENVIRONMENTAL DISTRACTIONS

- Close the door of the patient's room.
- Pull curtains around the patient's bed.
- Unplug the telephone or reduce volume of nearby telephone and paging equipment.
- Provide soft music.
- Reduce or eliminate lighting; provide a night-light.
- Match the patient with a compatible roommate.
- Wear rubber-soled shoes.
- Turn off bedside equipment that is not in use (e.g., oxygen, suction equipment).
- Avoid abrupt loud noise such as flushing a toilet or moving a bed.
- Keep unnecessary conversations at low levels, particularly at night.
- Conduct discussions or nursing reports in a private, separate area away from patient rooms.
- Turn off the television or radio unless the patient prefers soft music.

CLINICAL DECISION MAKING
PLANNING FOR ADEQUATE REST IN A POSTOPERATIVE SITUATION

Mrs. Cameron, a 79-year-old widow, was admitted yesterday to a semiprivate room on the orthopedic unit. She suffers from degenerative joint disease and had surgery today on her left hip. Last night, Mrs. Cameron slept reasonably well but awakened twice because of her roommate's light snoring. What factors does the nurse consider in planning care that will help Mrs. Cameron obtain adequate rest after her surgery?

FACTORS

The following factors influence sleep:

- Age
- Nutrition
- Exercise
- Stress level
- Drug therapy
- Sociocultural considerations
- Setting-environment

GOALS

1. Create a setting that is most conducive to initiating and maintaining sleep.
2. Help Mrs. Cameron cope with stress and postoperative pain so she can sleep better.
3. Plan nutrition and exercise or activities that will help Mrs. Cameron obtain adequate rest.
4. Mrs. Cameron's sleep is interrupted only once during the night for voiding and vital signs.
5. Mrs. Cameron obtains enough rest to remain alert and oriented during the day.

INTERVENTIONS

The nurse knows it will be more difficult for Mrs. Cameron to initiate and maintain sleep in a hospital setting, especially with postoperative pain. To plan her care effectively, the nurse needs a thorough patient history. This includes age, nutritional status, activity, routine medications (actions and adverse effects), exercise regimen, usual retiring and awakening times, and bedtime rituals before the onset of her health problem. The nurse also needs to understand what value sleep has for Mrs. Cameron, how she perceives an altered sleep pattern, what coping mechanisms she uses, and what stressors are present in the hospital environment relative to her usual environment. Comparing preillness data with an assessment of the current situation will help the nurse determine the potential for disruption of Mrs. Cameron's rest and sleep patterns. Because Mrs. Cameron awoke last night as a result of her roommate's light snoring, the nurse should pay special attention to her environment and do everything possible to reduce noise.

The nurse is able to arrange for Mrs. Cameron to have a new roommate. In addition, the nurse schedules treatments, activities, and medications to allow Mrs. Cameron a quiet period for relaxation before bedtime and to avoid awakenings during the night. The nurse helps Mrs. Cameron stay comfortable by administering pain medications prescribed by the physician and helps reduce her anxiety with a massage and with a radio playing soft music.

SELF-ASSESSMENT

Nurses must be aware of their experiences, values, and attitudes toward sleep while planning care and interacting with a patient. For example, a nurse who has no difficulty falling asleep in a noisy environment may have a hard time understanding why a patient does. Nurses must be empathetic to patients who have sleep requirements different from their own.

REFLECTION

The nurse should evaluate Mrs. Cameron's sleep patterns each day and decide whether changes should be made to the nursing care plan.

patient has a motor or sensory impairment and cannot respond to external stimulation.

In the case presentation of Mrs. Cameron, an assessment of the effectiveness of nursing management related to disorders of initiating and maintaining sleep could include the following:

- Verbalized slept well: at least 6 on a scale of 1 to 10 (with 10 being exceptionally well)
- States that she fell asleep within 15 minutes after lights turned out
- Lack of purposeful movement and eyes closed when checked at 0200, 0430, and 0600 hours

Sleep Deprivation. Although sleep deprivation can occur in any setting, it is a particular problem in the hospital and nursing home setting. In the institutional setting, a very common and irritating environmental disturbance is conversation and laughter from staff members in the halls and nursing station. This is especially true for elderly clients who have less deep sleep and awaken more easily because of lower auditory thresholds (sensitivity to noise) during their lighter sleep (Hayter, 1983). If the patient is in a multiple-bed room, attention should be given to the compatibility of the roommates. Box 25–4 lists some ways to reduce noise and other factors that may disturb the patient's sleep. The chapter feature Clinical Decision Making: Planning for Adequate Sleep in a Postoperative Situation also addresses how the nurse can help in this regard.

The primary nursing action to minimize sleep deprivation is to plan and organize care to maintain sleep patterns. Treatments, activities, and medications should be scheduled to allow a quiet period for relaxation before bedtime and to avoid awakenings during the night. Visiting hour policy may need to be reexamined. If manifestations of REM sleep are observed, the patient should be allowed to complete that stage before awakening if possible to ensure a complete sleep cycle. If arousal is unavoidable, it should be planned so that several things are done in less than 3 minutes. Taking vital signs, giving the nighttime dose of antibiotic, and the as-needed sleeping pill at the same time are indicators of good nursing management.

The rationale for routines that require waking a patient should be examined to determine whether or not these routines are logical and whether they should be retained or revised. Why are patients in some settings routinely awakened for vital signs at 5 A.M.? Instead, the nurse can make necessary assessments when the patient awakens spontaneously.

A nurse can learn to observe the condition of a sleeping patient without disturbing him or her. For example, the nurse can note increasing restlessness, which may indicate pain or shock, count respirations and note their quality, and, with some patients, obtain pulse rate. The nurse can also obtain some of this information from electronic monitors without touching the patients, but alarms on the equipment should be directed away from the patient's head. The nurse can use this information to decide whether the person should be disturbed for further assessment or allowed an uninterrupted sleep period.

Although patients in pain experience even more discomfort with body movement, these body movements occur without awareness during NREM sleep, and the frequency is not altered by sleeping on a firm mattress or waterbed (Rosekind, 1976). However, patients with chronic pain may benefit from sleeping on surfaces such as sheepskins and waterbeds, which distribute their body weight more evenly and relieve pressure.

In addition to pain, patients in the hospital setting often experience changes in medication regimens. Knowledge of the effects of medications on sleep patterns will enable the nurse to counsel clients about these effects. To minimize REM-rebound effects, REM-suppressant drugs should not be discontinued suddenly, but rather tapered off slowly at the rate of one therapeutic dose every 5 to 6 days. Slow discontinuation is especially important for patients with angina (chest pain), hypertension, peptic ulcer disease, or cerebrovascular disease (stroke) who may suffer from increased severity of their condition during a REM-rebound period. During the process of withdrawal, clients should be informed that severe changes (e.g., nightmares, anxiety, depression) may occur and that these changes are not long-lasting psychological problems but are directly related to the physiologic effects of drug withdrawal. If total withdrawal of the REM-suppressing drug is not possible, gradual replacement with a medication that does not suppress REM sleep should be considered.

When determining whether or not a nursing plan of care is effective, results should be evaluated in relation to certain predetermined expected outcomes. In the example of Mrs. Cameron, expected outcome might include sleep disrupted only at 0400 hours for voiding and vital signs.

Altered Wake-Sleep Cycles. Nursing management of sundown syndrome (senile nocturnal agitation) is aimed at minimizing the dangers inherent in nocturnal disorientation. Unnecessary medications should be slowly discontinued under medical supervision, routine activities minimally altered, and frequent simple explanations for procedures provided. The patient should have a constant, familiar environment with limited extraneous personnel and minimal transfers to other rooms. Measures to minimize sensory deprivation and nocturnal isolation (a clock, radio, night-light, colorful calendar, photographs, paintings, and familiar visitors) should be part of the patient's plan of care. To promote deeper sleep, the elderly patient should be kept active during the day with self-care and group activities. If the nocturnal agitation is prolonged, it may be necessary for the physician to prescribe antipsychotic (haloperidol) therapy (Kales and Kales, 1984).

Narcolepsy is medically treated with central nervous system stimulants to promote alertness and with REM suppressants (tricyclic antidepressants) for the associated cataplexy (sudden muscle weakness). However, nurses can educate persons with narcolepsy about the importance of scheduled naps (Rogers and Aldrich, 1993) to reduce inappropriate sleep events. Nurses can also explain the increased risk for accidents if the person falls asleep while operating hazardous equipment or driving. Working night shift is especially hazardous for the person with narcolepsy because of the added effects of chronic sleep deprivation and reverse wake-sleep cycles. Narcoleptic patients can also benefit from weekend "drug holidays" to delay their tolerance to the prescribed medications.

BOX 25-5
COMFORT MEASURES TO PROMOTE SLEEP

- Encourage the patient to wear comfortable, loose-fitting night wear.
- Keep bed linen clean and dry.
- Provide a comfortable mattress.
- Remove any irritants against the patient's skin, such as moist or wrinkled sheets or drainage tubing.
- Position and support body parts as needed to protect pressure points and aid muscle relaxation.
- Offer a massage just before bedtime.
- Provide a cap and socks for older patients and others prone to cold, and provide additional blankets for warmth.
- Provide or assist the patient with necessary personal hygiene measures.
- Encourage the patient to void before going to sleep.
- Administer analgesics or sedatives about 30 minutes before bedtime, or apply warm or cool applications or supportive dressings or splints to painful areas.
- Schedule administration of other medications, especially diuretics, to prevent nocturnal awakenings.
- For patients with breathing problems, administer prescribed medications such as bronchodilators before bedtime and position the patient appropriately (e.g., semi-Fowler's position) to facilitate breathing.
- Listen to the patient's concerns and deal with problems as they arise.

PATIENT TEACHING
HELPING PATIENTS SLEEP BETTER

You can help patients sleep better by teaching them about nutrition, exercise, and other daily living habits that help to promote sleep.

NUTRITION

Encourage patients to eat foods high in protein such as meat, poultry, fish, and nuts. These foods induce sleep more rapidly without distorting the normal sleep cycle.

All these protein sources contain L-tryptophan, an amino acid important for initiating sleep. Eating 1 g of protein has been shown to reduce sleep-onset time by 50%.

It should be noted that clinical studies show that L-tryptophan's effect on sleep is limited to only 1 or 2 nights (Sallanon et al, 1983), and higher doses can cause liver dysfunction.

Melatonin supplements, available in various doses from health food stores, are proving helpful to some individuals with insomnia-related sleep problems. Melatonin can be purchased by itself, but it is often packaged in a mixture of other nutrients, such as vitamin B6 or amino acids. The effective dosage remains unknown.

Patients should avoid stimulants, such as caffeine, because they will delay sleep onset and decrease total sleep time. Caffeine is found in chocolate, tea, cola, some analgesics, and even in decaffeinated coffee. Its stimulatory effects are known to last between 6 to 8 hours in healthy adults; it is not known how long it affects children and elderly people.

EXERCISE

Activity level may also affect a person's sleep pattern, probably by increasing body temperature. Extreme fatigue (e.g., from too many hospital visitors) or exercising near bedtime can make it more difficult for the patient to obtain adequate rest because both stimulate the patient's metabolism.

A quiet period in the evening before bed with relaxing activities such as reading or taking a warm bath can help the patient unwind and fall asleep more easily.

Sometimes patients may have so little activity that they are understimulated and find it equally difficult to fall asleep. In that case, they should be encouraged to exercise or become involved in activities during the day. Watching television or listening to the radio near bedtime may also help.

Nursing measures to promote uninterrupted sleep and improve the quality of sleep are summarized in Box 25–5. The chapter feature Patient Teaching: Helping Patients Sleep Better provides information that the nurse can pass on to patients and their families.

Disorders of Excessive Sleepiness

DOES are an indication of inadequate total sleep. If sleep deprivation is due to frequent but brief arousals, the patient may not be able to provide accurate data about sleep pattern disturbances. In these cases, the family or sleeping partner should be consulted. If no data source is available, the person's age, gender, family history, and symptoms experienced immediately on awakening will provide clues to potential disorders of excessive sleepiness. Box 25–6 lists some questions to ask the patient about DOES. Because many disorders can appear as excessive daytime sleepiness, a careful history is very important. Narcolepsy may appear as excessive sleep during the daytime, but sleepiness is not experienced before the sudden onset of REM sleep. Sleep apnea patients appear sleepy and often struggle to stay awake in a variety of circumstances.

In the case of sleep apnea, when surgical intervention is necessary to restore normal sleep patterns, the nurse's role in patient management becomes that of routine postoperative care. If medical interventions, such as nasal CPAP or a weight-loss program, are initiated before surgical intervention, nurses become primary managers of patient care by teaching patients how to carry out the medical therapy effec-

BOX 25-6
QUESTIONS TO ASK WHEN ASSESSING DISORDERS OF INITIATING AND MAINTAINING SLEEP

- Have you noticed any change in your sleep patterns lately?
- Describe your typical sleep period. When do you go to bed and get up on work (school) days?
- On days off (weekends)?
- How long does it usually take you to fall asleep?
- Do you take anything to help you fall asleep?
- How often do you have trouble sleeping?
- How often do you take naps?
- How often do you travel by airplane?
- Does your work involve night shifts or rotating schedules?
- How many caffeinated beverages (e.g., cola, coffee, chocolate, tea) do you drink on a typical day? Do you drink caffeine to help stay awake?
- How much alcohol do you drink on a typical day? Do you drink alcohol to help you fall asleep?
- What medications are you taking routinely? Have you recently stopped taking a medication?
- How often do you find yourself waking up during your sleep period? What do you think wakes you up? What do you do when you wake up in the middle of the night?
- How often do you wake up too early and cannot get back to sleep? Why do you think you are waking up so early?
- Are you able to carry out your normal daytime activities without feeling exhausted or taking a nap?

tively. Repeated nightly use of nasal CPAP causes most patients to complain of dry and irritated nares (nostrils) as well as nasal congestion. These complaints are minimized with presleep use of normal saline mist into the nares and an ultrasonic nebulizer (device that makes a fine spray) at the bedside. Nurses cannot overly emphasize the precautions that must be taken in preventing persons with excessive sleepiness from falling asleep in hazardous situations. Scheduled naps throughout the day are often more effective measures than stimulants like caffeine because of the rebound sleepiness that occurs when caffeine is eliminated from the body. A major role for nurses is support for family members who have dealt with a chronically sleepy person who suddenly becomes energetic after treatment.

Potential sleep disorders related to excessive daytime sleepiness are evaluated in terms of daytime functioning and quality of life. The overriding goal of nursing management in these cases is early identification of the disorder and referral to appropriate medical specialists for diagnosis and intervention.

CHAPTER HIGHLIGHTS

- Adequate sleep and rest are essential to maintain health and recover from illness.
- Sleep is defined as a period of diminished responsiveness to external stimuli that regularly alternates with periods of wakefulness.
- Basic science research has provided an understanding of the stages of normal sleep.
- Sleep pattern disturbance can be classified as disorders of maintaining sleep (DIMS), disorders of daytime sleepiness (DOES), and dysfunctions associated with abnormal behaviors during sleep (parasomnias).
- Age, nutritional status, exercise patterns, stress level, drug therapy, sociocultural factors, and the setting in which care is delivered influence an individual's sleep pattern.
- A wide range of potential nursing actions directed toward either the patient or the environment has been identified through research and practice.
- The evaluation of nursing actions includes both subjective and objective data.
- Educating the patient and family to minimize sleep deprivation is more important than ever as more and more families deliver care in the home.

REFERENCES

Akerstedt, T. (1985). Shifted sleep hours. *Annals of Clinical Research, 17,* 273–279.

Ancoli-Israel, S., Kripke, D.F., Mason, W., Kaplan, O.J. (1985). Sleep apnea and periodic movements in an aging sample. *Journal of Gerontology, 40,* 419–425.

Ashton, H. (1984). Benzodiazepine withdrawal: an unfinished story. *British Medical Journal, 288,* 1135–1140.

Barry, H., Paxton, L. (1971). Infancy and early childhood: cross-cultural codes. *Ethnology, 10,* 466–508.

Becker, P.M., Jamieson, A.O., Brown, W.D. (1993). Dopaminergic agents in restless legs syndrome and periodic limb movements of sleep: response and complications of extended treatment in 49 cases. *Sleep, 16,* 713–716.

Berger, R.J. (1970). REM sleep and mechanisms of oculomotor control. *International Psychiatric Clinics, 7,* 277–294.

Bixler, E.O., Kales, A., Vela-Bueno, A., et al. (1982). Nocturnal myoclonus and nocturnal activity in a normal population. *Research Communications in Chemical Pathology and Pharmacology, 36,* 129–140.

Bliwise, D.L. (1994). Normal aging. In M.H. Kryger, T. Roth, and W.C. Dement (eds.): *Principles and Practice of Sleep Medicine.* Philadelphia: W.B. Saunders, pp. 26–39.

Borbely, A.A. (1994). Sleep homeostasis and models of sleep regulation. In M.H. Kryger, T. Roth, and W.C. Dement (eds.). *Principles and Practice of Sleep Medicine.* Philadelphia: W.B. Saunders, pp. 309–320.

Born, J., Muth, S., Fehm, H.L. (1988). The significance of sleep onset and slow wave sleep for nocturnal release of growth hormone (GH) and cortisol. *Psychoneuroendocrinology, 13,* 233–243.

Cartwright, R.D. (1994). Dreams and their meaning. In M.H. Kryger, T. Roth, and W.C. Dement (eds.): *Principles and Practice of Sleep Medicine.* Philadelphia: W.B. Saunders, pp. 400–406.

Carskadon, M.A., Dement, W.C. (1994). Normal human sleep: an overview. In M.H. Kryger, T. Roth, and W.C. Dement (eds.): *Principles and Practice of Sleep Medicine.* Philadelphia: W.B. Saunders, pp. 16–25.

Cavallero, C., Cicogna, P., Natale, V., et al. (1992). Slow wave sleep dreaming. *Sleep, 15,* 562–566.

Cohen-Mansfield, J., Marx, M.S., Rosenthal, A.S. (1990). Dementia and agitation in nursing home residents: how are they related? *Psychology of Aging, 5,* 3–8.

Crick, F., Mitchison, G. (1983). The function of dream sleep. *Nature, 304,* 111–114.

Deamer, R.M., Scharf, M., Kales, A. (1972). Sleep patterns in the coronary care unit. *U.S. Navy Medicine, 59,* 19–23.

Dickerson, L.W., Huang, A.H., Thurnher, M.M., et al. (1993). Relationship between coronary hemodynamic changes and the phasic events of rapid eye movement sleep. *Sleep, 16,* 550–557.

Easton, C., MacKenzie, F. (1988). Sensory-perceptual alterations: delirium in the intensive care unit. *Heart & Lung, 17,* 229–235.

Edinger, J.D., Morey, M.C., Sullivan, R.J., et al. (1993). Aerobic fitness, acute exercise and sleep in older men. *Sleep, 16,* 351–359.

Evans, F.J. (1983). Sleep, eating, and weight disorders. In R.K. Goodstein (ed.): *Eating and Weight Disorders.* New York: Springer, pp. 147–156.

Everson, C., Bergmann, B., Fang, V.S., et al. (1986). Physiological and biochemical effect of total sleep deprivation in the rat. *Sleep Research, 15,* 216.

Felton, G. (1975). Body rhythm effects on rotating work shifts. *Journal of Nursing Administration, 5,* 16–19.

Fisher, L.B. (1968). The diurnal mitotic rhythm in the human epidermis. *British Journal of Dermatology, 80,* 75–80.

Gaillard, J.M. (1994). Benzodiazepines and GABA-ergic transmission. In M.H. Kryger, T. Roth, and W.C. Dement (eds.): *Principles and Practice of Sleep Medicine.* Philadelphia: W.B. Saunders, pp. 349–354.

Glotzbach, S.F., Heller, C. (1994). Temperature regulation. In M.H. Kryger, T. Roth, and W.C. Dement (eds.): *Principles and Practice of Sleep Medicine.* Philadelphia: W.B. Saunders, pp. 260–275.

Guilleminault, C. (1994). Narcolepsy syndrome. In M.H. Kryger, T. Roth, and W.C. Dement (eds.): *Principles and Practice of Sleep Medicine.* Philadelphia: W.B. Saunders, pp. 549–561.

Hartmann, E. (1994). Nightmares and other dreams. In M.H. Kryger, T. Roth, and W.C. Dement (eds.): *Principles and Practice of Sleep Medicine.* Philadelphia: W.B. Saunders, pp. 407–410.

Haslam, D. (1984). *Sleepless Children: A Handbook for Parents.* New York: Pocket Books.

Hauri, P. (1994). Primary insomnia. In M.H. Kryger, T. Roth, and W.C. Dement (eds.): *Principles and Practice of Sleep Medicine.* Philadelphia: W.B. Saunders, pp. 494–499.

Hauri, P., Silbergard, P.M. (1979). The effects of aspirin on the sleep of insomniacs. *Sleep Research, 7,* 100.

Hayter, J. (1983). Sleep behaviors of older persons. *Nursing Research, 32,* 242–246.

Herriot, J. (1973). *All Things Bright and Beautiful.* New York: St. Martin's Press.

Hilton, B.A. (1976). Quantity and quality of patient's sleep and sleep disturbing factors in a respiratory intensive care unit. *Journal of Advanced Nursing, 1,* 453–468.

Horne, J. (1988). *Why We Sleep: The Functions of Sleep in Humans and Other Mammals.* New York: Oxford University Press.

Horne, J.A., Reid, A.J. (1985). Night-time sleep EEG changes following body heating in a warm bath. *Electroencephalography and Clinical Neurophysiology, 60,* 154–157.

Jones, B.E. (1994). Basic mechanisms of sleep-wake state. In M.H. Kryger, T. Roth, and W.C. Dement (eds.): *Principles and Practice of Sleep Medicine.* Philadelphia: W.B. Saunders, pp. 145–162.

Kales, A., Kales, J.D. (1984). *Evaluation and Treatment of Insomnia.* New York: Oxford University Press, p. 149.

Kramer, M. (1994). The scientific study of dreaming. In M.H. Kryger, T. Roth, and W.C. Dement (eds.): *Principles and Practice of Sleep Medicine.* Philadelphia: W.B. Saunders, pp. 394–399.

Kryger, M.H. (1994). Management of obstructive sleep apnea: overview. In M.H. Kryger, T. Roth, and W.C. Dement (eds.): *Principles and Practice of Sleep Medicine.* Philadelphia: W.B. Saunders, pp. 736–747.

Kupfer, D.J., Ehlers, C.L., Frank, E. (1991). EEG sleep profiles and recurrent depression. *Biological Psychiatry, 30,* 641–655.

Kupfer, D.J., Sewitch, D.E., Epstein, L.H., et al. (1985). Exercise and subsequent sleep in male runners: failure to support the slow wave sleep-mood-exercise hypothesis. *Neuropsychobiology, 14,* 5–12.

Lader, M. (1986). A practical guide to prescribing hypnotic benzodiazepines. *British Medical Journal, 293,* 1048–1049.

McFadden, E., Giblin, E. (1979). Sleep deprivation in patients having open heart surgery. *Nursing Research, 20,* 249–254.

Moline, M.L., Pollak, C.P., Monk, T.H., et al. (1992). Age-related differences in recovery from simulated jet lag. *Sleep, 15,* 28–40.

Monroe, S.M., Thase, M.E., Simons, A.D. (1992). Social factors and the psychobiology of depression: Relations between life stress and rapid eye movement sleep latency. *J Abnormal Psychology* 101(3): 528–537.

Morelli, G.A., Rogoff, B., Oppenhein, D., Goldsmith, D. (1992). Cultural variation in infants' sleeping arrangements: questions of independence. *Developmental Psychology, 28,* 604–613.

Nicholson, A.N., Bradley, C.M., Pascoe, P.A. (1994). Medications: effect on sleep and wakefulness. In M.H. Kryger, T. Roth, and W.C. Dement (eds.): *Principles and Practice of Sleep Medicine.* Philadelphia: W.B. Saunders, pp. 364–372.

Orr, W.C. (1994). Gastrointestinal disorders. In M.H. Kryger, T. Roth, and W.C. Dement (eds.): *Principles and Practice of Sleep Medicine.* Philadelphia: W.B. Saunders, pp. 252–259.

Orr, W.C., Johnson, L.F., Robinson, M.G. (1984). The effect of sleep on swallowing, esophageal peristalsis, and acid clearance. *Gastroenterology, 96,* 814–819.

Pacini, C.M., Fitzpatrick, J.J. (1982). Sleep patterns of hospitalized and nonhospitalized aged individuals. *Journal of Gerontological Nursing, 8,* 327–332.

Parmeggiani, P.L. (1994). The autonomic nervous system in sleep. In M.H. Kryger, T. Roth, and W.C. Dement (eds.): *Principles and Practice of Sleep Medicine.* Philadelphia: W.B. Saunders, pp. 193–204.

Pivik, R.T. (1994). The psychophysiology of dreams. In M.H. Kryger, T. Roth, and W.C. Dement (eds.): *Principles and Practice of Sleep Medicine.* Philadelphia: W.B. Saunders, pp. 384–393.

Rauch, P.K., Stern, T.A. (1986). Life-threatening injuries resulting from sleepwalking and night terrors. *Psychosomatics, 27,* 62–64.

Redding, G.J., Okamoto, G.A., Guthrie, R.D., et al. (1985). Sleep patterns in nonambulatory boys with Duchenne muscular dystrophy. *Archives of Physical Medicine and Rehabilitation, 66,* 818–821.

Richards, K.C., Bairnsfather, L. (1988). A description of night sleep patterns in the critical care unit. *Heart & Lung, 17,* 35–42.

Rogers, A.E., Aldrich, M.S. (1993). The effect of regularly scheduled naps on sleep attacks and excessive daytime sleepiness associated with narcolepsy. *Nursing Research, 42,* 111–117.

Rosekind, M. (1976). Effects of waterbed surface on sleep: a pilot study, *Sleep Research, 5,* 132.

Ryback, R.S., Lewis, O.F., Lessard, C.S. (1971). Psychobiologic effects of prolonged bed rest (weightlessness) in young healthy volunteers. *Aerospace Medicine, 42,* 529–535.

Sallanon, M., Janin, M., Buda, C., Jourvet, M. (1983). Serotonergic mechanisms and sleep rebound. *Brain Research, 268,* 95–104.

Schneider-Helmert, D. (1986). Nutrition and sleeping behavior. *Bibliotheca Nutritio et Dieta, 38,* 87–93.

Scheving, L.E. (1959). Mitotic activity in the human epidermis. *Anatomical Record, 135,* 7–20.

Siegel, J.M. (1994). Brainstem mechanisms generating REM sleep. In M.H. Kryger, T. Roth, and W.C. Dement (eds.): *Principles and Practice of Sleep Medicine.* Philadelphia: W.B. Saunders, pp. 125–144.

Stavric, B. (1992). An update on research with coffee/caffeine (1989–1990). *Food Chemical Toxicology, 30,* 533–555.

Stoohs, R.A., Guilleminault, C.A., Dement, W.C. (1993). Sleep apnea and hypertension in commercial truck drivers. *Sleep, 16,* S11–S14.

Syvalahti, E.K.G. (1985). Drug treatment of insomnia: indications and complications. *Annals of Clinical Research, 17,* 265–272.

Walker, B. (1972). The postsurgery heart patient: amount of uninterrupted time for sleep and rest during first, second, and third postoperative days in a teaching hospital. *Nursing Research, 21,* 164–169.

Webster, R.A., Thompson, D.R. (1986). Sleep in hospital. *Journal of Advanced Nursing, 11,* 447–457.

Weitzman, E.D., Zimmerman, J.C., Czeisler, C.A., et al. (1983). Cortisol secretion is inhibited during sleep in normal man. *Journal of Clinical Endocrinology and Metabolism, 56,* 352–358.

Wood, P.B. (1962). *Dreaming and Social Isolation* (doctoral dissertation). Chapel Hill: University of North Carolina.

Woods, N.F. (1972). Patterns of sleep in post-cardiotomy patients. *Nursing Research, 21,* 347–352.

Woods, N.F., Falk, S.A. (1974). Noise stimuli in the acute care area. *Nursing Research, 23,* 144–150.

Zarcone, V.P. (1994). Sleep hygiene. In M.H. Kryger, T. Roth, and W.C. Dement (eds.): *Principles and Practice of Sleep Medicine.* Philadelphia: W.B. Saunders, pp. 452–546.

Zepelin, H. (1994). Mammalian sleep. In M.H. Kryger, T. Roth, and W.C. Dement (eds.): *Principles and Practice of Sleep Medicine.* Philadelphia: W.B. Saunders, pp. 69–80.

ADDITIONAL READINGS

Cole, R.M. (1986). *Wide awake at 3:00* A.M. New York: W.H. Freeman.

Dement, W.C. (1974). *Some Must Watch While Some Must Sleep.* San Francisco: W.H. Freeman.

Ferber, R. (1985). Sleep, sleepiness, and sleep disruptions in infants and young children. *Annals of Clinical Research, 17,* 227–234.

Hindmarch, I., Ott, H., Roth, T. (1984). *Sleep, Benzodiazepines and Performance.* New York: Springer-Verlag.

Kleitman, N. (1963). *Sleep and Wakefulness.* Chicago: University of Chicago Press.

Kryger, M.H., Roth, T., Dement, W.C. (eds.). (1994). *Principles and Practice of Sleep Medicine.* Philadelphia: W.B. Saunders.

Monk, T.H. (ed.). (1991). *Sleep, Sleepiness and Performance.* New York: Wiley.

Waterhouse, J.M., Minors, D.S., Waterhouse, M.E. (1990). *Your Body Clock: How to Live with It, Not Against It.* New York: Oxford University Press.

Williams, R.L., Karacan, I. (eds.). (1978). *Sleep Disorders: Diagnosis and Treatment.* New York: Wiley.

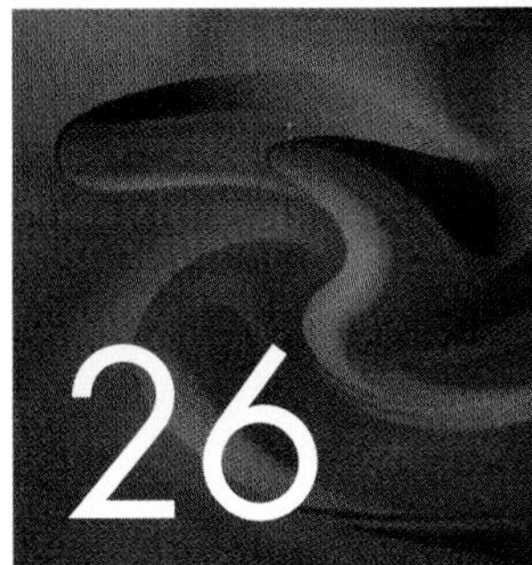

Personal Hygiene 26

Anita Catlin

Gladys Carpenter, a 61-year-old homemaker, is admitted with a diagnosis of recurrent urinary tract infection. Her history reveals diabetes mellitus with retinopathy (damage to her vision due to diabetes), hypertension (elevated blood pressure), and rheumatoid arthritis (joint inflammation). She has a seventh-grade education and was married at age 16 to her current husband; they have four children, now all married. Mrs. Carpenter's health and vision problems have kept her from performing many household chores and some activities of daily living that relate to her own health and hygiene needs. Her husband, a retired truck driver, does much of the household work and most of the cooking. The Carpenters live on his modest retirement income in a small trailer.

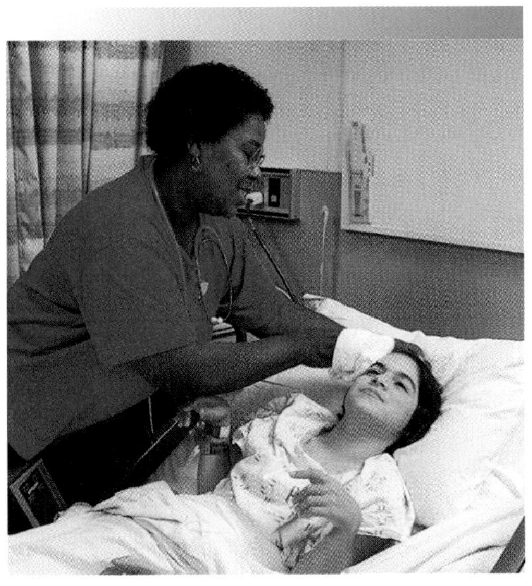

Physical assessment of Mrs. Carpenter reveals a somewhat disheveled appearance. She has noticeable body odor, unclean clothes and undergarments, and signs of skin irritation. She is 157 cm tall (5 feet 2 inches) and weighs 86.5 kg (190 lb). She presents with poor dental hygiene, and her fingernails and toenails are thickened, overgrown, and cracked. Her hair is rather oily, thinning, gray, and pulled back with a rubber band. She is alert to person, place, and time and cooperates with the staff during admission procedures.

OBJECTIVES

After studying this chapter, the student will be able to:

- **provide personal hygiene to any patient, within the health care continuum**
- **maintain appropriate infection control during provision of hygiene**
- **compare and contrast hygiene measures on the basis of patient needs, ability, and diagnosis**
- **relate the research on patient energy expenditure during hygiene care**
- **provide a bed bath, towel bath, and shower in shower chair**
- **anticipate and provide appropriate safety measures when the patient is in a shower or tub bath**
- **provide at least two examples of topics in hygiene care that need a better research base**

SCOPE OF NURSING PRACTICE

Personal hygiene care comprises measures to ensure patient cleanliness and comfort and prevent infection. Promoting personal hygiene in patients has always been considered an important nursing activity. Some patients are unable to provide hygiene for themselves and must rely on nurses for assistance with hygiene care. Reasons that a person might not be able to provide his or her own hygiene include limits on activity tolerance, pain, musculoskeletal impairment, neuromuscular impairment, mobility impairment, and the inability to access a water source (McKeighen et al, 1990).

In its most basic form, personal hygiene care consists of cleansing the patient's skin, hair, nails, eyes, ears, nose, mouth, teeth, and perineum. Other aspects of care often incorporated in personal hygiene care include

- Performing physical assessment
- Stimulating circulation
- Exercising stiff joints by performing range of motion exercises
- Promoting relaxation
- Enhancing self-esteem

The Nursing Interventions Classification group at the University of Iowa has accepted bathing, hair care, nail care, and oral hygiene as crucial nursing activities for all persons under a nurse's care (Titler et al, 1991).

In providing personal hygiene care, the nurse first assesses the patient's hygiene needs and plans for appropriate care. The nurse then gathers the necessary supplies and equipment and provides this care. Finally, the nurse evaluates the impact of the hygienic measures on the patient and adjusts the plan of care accordingly. While providing personal hygiene care, the nurse can also assess a patient's physical condition and establish a trusting relationship with the patient and the patient's family through observation and purposeful conversation.

This chapter focuses on the assessment, planning, provision, and evaluation of personal hygiene care to patients in a nurse's care. The chapter describes how the nurse makes decisions when providing personal hygiene care to patients. It shows how decision making must be both flexible and interactive, depending on time of day, level of patient assistance needed, the patient's type of illness, and the method of bathing and other hygienic measures needed. Relevant nursing research studies involving hygiene are presented to help guide nursing practice. Hygiene care is discussed in context, specific to patient age, physical condition, and cultural background. It is also discussed in terms of various care settings—the hospital, the home, and long-term care settings. Relevant safety, ethical, and financial considerations are explored as well.

This chapter is crucial to mastering nursing in today's increasingly restrictive managed-care environment. Providing personal hygiene care often occupies a very large portion of patient care hours, and all of these hours are accounted for when planning adequate staffing to provide care. As more and more nursing care is being delegated to others, those nursing care actions allowing close patient interaction, assessment, and provision of comfort need to be cherished and retained.

KNOWLEDGE BASE

Historical Perspective

The role of hygiene in medicine has been recognized throughout history. From Greek mythology comes the tale of Asclepius, the god of healing and the first physician. Asclepius and his wife, Epigone, "the soothing one," had five daughters associated in myth with five different aspects of health. They were "Hygeia, "goddess of health"; Panacea, "restorer of health"; Aegle, "light of the sun"; Medtrina, "preserver of health"; and Laso, "recovery from illness." Hygeia was worshiped and represented in works of art as a virgin holding a snake in her hand. The famous Hippocratic oath, which tells us to "do no harm," was originated by Greek physicians who swore by Apollo, Asclepius, Hygeia, Panacea, and all the Greek gods (Ostwalt, 1969)

A more modern discussion of hygiene care begins with Florence Nightingale, the founder of scientific nursing. Her writings show that she nursed, watched, thought, and wrote about the importance of cleanliness and the patient's environment. In her book, *Notes on Nursing,* published in 1860, are chapters of advice on how to bathe, feed, comfort, clean, and observe a patient and organize his or her room. Today, 100 years later, hygienic care is largely practiced as it was in Nightingale's time. However, according to nurse theorists, we now call this same work "assistance in self-care deficit" and "performing physical assessment."

Nightingale worked in the same era as Dr. Ignaz Semmelweis, an important contributor to hygienic care and theory. Semmelweiss discovered and wrote about the need to wash hands between patient care activities—in his case, between performing autopsies and delivering babies (see Chapter 17). Because of his work, women no longer were at risk of death immediately after childbirth from systemic infection. Joseph Lister, another nineteenth century surgeon, is credited with formulating the germ theory of antisepsis. Because of him, patient care areas and operating rooms are routinely cleaned and disinfected. Nightingale's discussion of cleanliness, Semmelweis's handwashing, and Lister's management of the hospital environment form basic tenets of hygienic practice today.

Basic Science: Anatomy and Physiology–Based Hygiene Care

Knowledge of anatomy and physiology allows the nurse to inspect body parts and assess for hygiene needs. The following sections present descriptions of specific hygiene needs for various body areas.

SKIN

Nursing assessment of the patient's hygiene needs is most evident while assessing the patient's skin. The skin, its glands, and its appendages—the hair and nails—together form the integument. The body's largest organ system, the integument functions to provide or regulate protection, sensation, temperature control, fluid balance, vitamin synthesis, and esthetics (see Chapter 28).

Complete assessment of skin integrity can be made during the bathing of patients. Any break in the epidermis may necessitate alternative hygiene measures and specific wound care. Maintaining cleanliness of the skin provides a more natural environment to facilitate the skin's protective processes. Thicker areas of the epidermis, such as the sole of the foot, are usually more exposed to environmental surfaces and may require soaking as well as extra cleansing. More delicate, thinner areas may require extra care during cleansing to prevent skin tears and maintain skin integrity. This is especially true for the very young and the very old, as well as those patients whose skin integrity may be compromised as a result of a disease process, drug therapy, or immobility.

Temperature control is a vital function of the skin, and perspiration is a means of heat dissipation. Hygiene measures are necessary to ensure that the patient's sweat glands are free of debris and obstruction and that the patient's comfort and esthetic needs are met. The nurse should avoid excessive powdering of the patient's axillary area to prevent caking of the sweat glands.

Patient sensitivity to touch, pressure, and temperature or complications resulting from a skin reaction with itching or pain present a challenge to the nurse in providing appropriate hygiene measures. Patients who cannot provide symptomatic or subjective responses reflecting pain or pressure are to be guarded. These patients are in danger of serious injury from water temperature or improper positioning.

Vitamin synthesis, another of skin's vital functions, requires exposure to sunlight. The nurse should check the patient's chart for medications that may cause sun sensitivity, a side effect of several prescription drugs. Patients must be protected against overexposure to sunlight, as this can cause burns and has been linked to skin cancer. Time spent during bathing can be used for patient teaching regarding skin sensitivity and the use of sunscreen lotions.

Continual shedding of the outer epidermal cells occurs when a person bathes regularly using moderate friction along with nonirritating soaps or cleansers. Hormonal changes can bring about changes in the texture of the skin, especially the epidermal layers. The nurse can acquire information related to hormonal changes by means of assessing the patient and obtaining a thorough nursing database, including hormonal prescriptions the patient may be taking.

Concern is directed toward assessment of the evenness of color distribution on the patient's skin. Variations signal potential pathology. One example would be a condition referred to as vitiligo, which is a condition in which melanocytes are destroyed in small or large circumscribed areas, resulting in patches of depigmentation with a hyperpigmented border. Although this condition is not uncommon and is generally of no significance in respect to the general health of the patient, it can be extremely disfiguring and problematic in dark-skinned persons. This condition tends to progress slowly (Fitzpatrick et al, 1987).

Signs and symptoms of inflammation of the skin are fairly easily recognized. Erythema over intact skin that blanches when pressure is applied and reappears when pressure is released is the first stage indicating potential skin impairment. The patient may complain of pain or tenderness at the site. Hygiene measures may need to be modified if such signs and symptoms exist, as any further signs of pressure could result in a break in the epidermis.

Skin integrity is frequently assessed in relation to the skin's strength and toughness, as well as the skin's resiliency and turgor. A loss of this quality necessitates a need for alternative and more gentle hygiene measures. The measurement of skin turgor, which is done by gently pinching together the skin over the clavicle or dorsal surface of the forehand, can give information on the presence or absence of good hydration. When a patient loses excessive fluid, the subcutaneous tissues dehydrate and lose elasticity. A dehydrated patient's skin will adhere together as opposed to hydrated skin, which "bounces" quickly back into place.

Observation and palpation of the skin can determine skin temperature, the presence or absence of diaphoresis, and configuration and color of skin nevi and lesions. Symmetry in underlying body structure can also be observed. Because the skin provides insulation and absorbs mechanical shock, the nurse should consider the need to provide a warmer environment during hygiene care of a patient who has less subcutaneous insulation.

The skin also provides a reserve for calories, and special care must be provided for those who are emaciated; they have a potential for skin impairment and poor tissue regeneration. Such patients have little reserve in terms of nutrients in the subcutaneous tissue layers.

Occasionally when inspecting the skin, the nurse may find areas circled in ink on the patient's forearm or back. These inked areas should not be washed off: They are used by the nurse to indicate sites of tuberculin or allergy screening tests. The nurse may also find transdermal patches on the patient's skin. The nurse must likewise take care not to remove these patches during bathing.

HAIR

Hair follicles are located in the skin's dermal layers and extend out into the epidermis. In each follicle are hair roots, composed of many tiny blood vessels that provide nourishment for hair. Hair grows at an approximate rate of 1 mm every 3 days; an adult sheds between 10 and 100 hairs daily. Hair color is determined by the amount of melanin contained in the hair cells. Hair color and texture are related to genetic components. Changes in health and illness affect the rate of hair growth and loss. Some medications, particularly medications for cancer that kill rapidly dividing cells, cause hair loss. This type of hair loss due to a disease process or medication is called *alopecia.*

Shampoo and grooming of hair are determined by patient condition, preference, and nursing assessment. Dry shampoo sprays, such as the starch compound made by Clairol (presently called Psssst!), are available for those patients whose condition does not allow their head to get wet. It is important to gently release all tangles from matted hair.

The nurse inspects for pediculosis (head lice) or fungal infections of the scalp, such as *Trichophyton violaceum* (ringworm). The nurse washes, rinses, conditions, and combs the hair. Braids and ponytails should be used cautiously, as there have been reported cases of "traction alopecia" and hair breakage from hair gathered together too tightly (Spector, 1991).

NAILS

The finger- and toenails are hard, keratinized layers of epidermis. The cells form a clear, solid covering over the terminal portions of the fingers and toes for the purpose of protection. Functionally, fingernails also assist in grasping and manipulating small objects. Fingernails grow about 1 mm per week, and toenails grow slightly slower than that. Nurses are concerned with keeping the free edges of the nails clean of dirt, which can harbor microorganisms. Nurses may trim fingernails as needed, but toenails are trimmed only after assessing that a patient has good circulation and does not have peripheral vascular disease or diabetes.

ORAL CAVITY

Oral care is another area requiring nursing intervention. Patients often require special care when disease processes affect the oral cavity. The oral cavity essentially consists of the lips, teeth, tongue, taste buds, cheeks, roof and floor of the mouth, and salivary glands. The oral mucosa should be observed for moistness, color, and any abnormal signs of inflammation, ulcerations, abrasions, or lesions.

Dental caries and periodontal disease are frequent problems, leading to tooth loss. Dental plaque, which consists essentially of bacteria embedded in a dense matrix, adheres to the teeth, eventually destroying the enamel and resulting in cavitation if left untreated, or uncleaned. Periodontal disease leads to the destruction of the supporting structures (periodontium) of the teeth. Tooth loss results from atrophy of the periodontium.

The tongue is normally pink and moist, with minimal coating. There should be no unpleasant odor from the mouth. There should be a moderate amount of clear saliva, and the lips should be soft and smooth.

EYES

The eyes are spheric organs situated within bony sockets (orbits) that protect most of each eye, except for the anterior portion. This anterior portion has a cornea (clear window), which allows light to enter for visionary interpretation through the posterior (inner) structures and the brain. Each eye has muscles around its circumference that extend to the back of each orbit. These muscles help support the eyes and allows for eye movement to facilitate vision from various directions.

In addition to the protective structure of the bony sockets, the eyes receive protection from the eyelids and eyelashes, which close or cover the eyes purposefully or reflexively. The lacrimal glands, including their ducts, produce tears to lubricate and wash the eyes' outer surface. The conjunctiva is a delicate mucous membrane that lines the eyelids and covers the exposed surface of each eye. The color of the conjunctiva is inspected, as a pale conjunctiva may indicate anemia. The color of the sclera is also assessed. Sclera having a red or pink shiny appearance may indicate bacterial infection, and sclera with yellow appearance (jaundice) may indicate hepatic dysfunction.

Eyelashes of ill patients may be matted with secretions. Gentle cleansing with warm water will be needed.

EARS

The ears are also important sensory organs, used for hearing and maintaining a sense of balance and equilibrium. The ear is divided into three parts: external ear, middle ear, and inner ear. Hygiene care of the ears includes cleansing measures of the external ear. The external ear consists of the pinna or auricle (external projection of each ear), the external auditory canal, and the tympanic membrane (eardrum).

Careful assessment of the external ear is necessary to determine specific hygiene measures needed. The external auditory canal, which is approximately 2.5 to 3.75 cm long, may have an accumulation of cerumen (ear wax), foreign matter, pus, or secretions. The internal canal opens approximately halfway into the canal (approximately 1.25 to 1.89 cm), and the nurse may provide gentle cleansing up to this point. Hair sometimes grows from the external auditory canal, and is trimmed when it appears unsightly.

NOSE

The nose has two nostrils (nares), which are separated by the nasal septum. Beyond the nares are nasal cavities located between the roof of the mouth and the frontal, ethmoid, and sphenoid bones. The lateral walls of each nasal cavity have three projections or turbinate bones (superior, middle, and inferior), which provide an increased mucous membrane surface area with which air comes in contact as part of an air-conditioning process. These turbinates are sometimes referred to as *conchae* because of their shell shape.

The nasal cavities have a vascular membrane, as circulating blood helps deliver moisture and heat to further help condition the air we breathe. The blood supply to the nose is derived from the internal and external carotid vessels. Because the nasal passages have a rich blood supply and the internal sinus structure lies in very close proximity to the cranium, infected acne and lesions around the nose are treated vigorously to prevent the spread of systemic infection.

The external structure of the nose is made up of cartilage, whereas the walls of the nasal cavities are made up of bone with a mucous membrane covering. The external nose folds to the sides of the nares are frequent sites for skin cancers, and all lesions here should be inspected. The nasal passages, or vestibules, are lined with skin and contain nasal hairs or vibrissae. Occasionally the nurse must trim excessive nasal hair if it is interfering with the provision of hygiene. The respiratory mucosa secrete mucus, which traps bacteria and pollutants, and ciliary movements normally carry this mucus to the back nasopharyngeal area, where it is expectorated or swallowed.

As a filtration organ, the nose entraps minute dust particles and other contaminants such as smoke, pollen, and bacteria. The nose is a direct pathway for airborne contaminants, and if the patient's overall condition is compromised, opportunistic infections can find their way into the patient's body via the nose. Hygiene measures can help prevent such infections from invading the patient's bodily systems.

PERINEUM

Hygiene care of the perineal area is required for patients who cannot cleanse this area themselves. The female perineum contains the external genital organs within the vulva, including the labia majora, labia minora, clitoris, vaginal opening, sebaceous glands, urethra, Skene's glands, and Bartholin's glands. The anus is posterior to the vulva (see Chapter 33).

The vaginal vault and the perineum have their own lubrication. The menstrual flow passes out from the uterus through the vaginal canal. The sebaceous glands in this area secrete sebum to help lubricate the skin. Apocrine sweat glands communicate with the hair follicles in the perineal area. The Bartholin's glands, located on each side of the vaginal opening, secrete mucus, particularly during sexual arousal, to lubricate the inner labia for intercourse. The Skene's glands are located posteriorly to the external urethral meatus and secrete mucus for the purpose of keeping the urethral opening lubricated. Both the Bartholin's and Skene's glands are subject to infection and obstruction. The nurse must take precautionary measures while cleansing the perineal area to always clean from front to back, going from the cleaner urethra to the rectal area, which is considered contaminated. This precaution prevents the possibility of transference of bacteria present in the rectal area to the patient's urethral and/or vaginal area. The gonococcus germ may infect the male or female urethra, the vagina, or the rectum; this is another reason to be very cautious to prevent cross-contamination between any of these four areas.

The male genitourinary organs include the penis, prostate, urethra, testes, and scrotum (see Chapter 33). The rectum is posterior to the scrotum. The glands of Littre, located along the urethra, secrete mucus as a lubricant. The bulbourethral glands, located just below the prostate gland, produce an alkaline secretion that also provides lubricating fluid during sexual arousal. Male patients may be circumcised or uncircumcised, depending on their age, culture, and country of origin. The uncircumcised penis needs special hygiene care, as described in the Procedures section.

Hygiene measures for both male and female patients involving the perineal areas require sensitivity to the patient's right to privacy and avoidance of embarrassment.

Relevant Research

Personal hygiene care as we now know it has evolved from the nineteenth-century work of Nightingale, Lister, and Semmelweiss. Much of the hygiene care provided to patients has been taught to nursing students exactly as their instructors learned it in their schools of nursing, possibly decades ago. Only in the last 20 years or so have nurse researchers attempted to systematically analyze hygiene care—not just practice it according to institutional and traditional requirements.

Nursing research and research from other fields related to personal hygiene care has focused on the following areas:

- Minimizing adverse physiologic responses of the patient to hygiene care
- Maximizing patient comfort
- Ensuring safety during hygiene care
- Providing hygiene care to patients with special needs
- Ensuring safe and effective personal hygiene products and supplies
- Maximizing the cost-effectiveness of hygiene care
- Promoting a positive nurse-patient relationship during hygiene care

MINIMIZING ADVERSE PHYSIOLOGIC RESPONSES TO HYGIENE CARE

FATIGUE STUDIES

Piper (1986) advises nurses to assess the patient's level of physical functioning, patterns of activity and exercise, and rest and sleep requirements before planning hygiene care. How fatigue affects hygiene has been assessed by many nurses (Cohen and Hardin, 1989; Crosby, 1989; Jamar, 1989; Piper et al, 1989; Potempa, 1989; Srivastava, 1989). For example, although it may appear that the patient who stays in bed most of the day is well rested, he or she may be exhausted by the day's activities. The patient may have spent considerable energy worrying, being transported for x-rays and other examination procedures, exercising in physical therapy, or physically recovering from illness or trauma. Thus, the patient may be very fatigued when the nurse tries to provide or assist with personal hygiene care. It is sometimes difficult to balance the nurse's desire to provide care or promote independence with the patient's feelings of fatigue and illness. The nurse can try to "cluster" care, so that activities can be grouped together to then allow for long periods of rest.

Researchers have examined the actual amounts of energy that patients expend when performing and receiving personal hygiene care (Thaney, 1981). The amount of oxygen required by the body (measured in terms of venous oxygen saturation, or VO_2) during various activities was expressed by Thaney in terms of metabolic equivalents (METs). A patient receiving a bed bath typically expends 0.5 to 1.5 METs; a patient giving himself or herself a partial bath with nursing assistance expends 1.5 to 2.0 METs; and a patient bathing himself or herself while sitting on the side of the bed, 3.0 METs. The nurse assesses the patient's fatigue level and provide the type of hygienic care that will cause the least amount of stress.

CARDIOVASCULAR RESPONSE TO BATHING

Various research studies have investigated the effects of bathing and other personal hygiene care measures on the patient's body. A patient's use of upper body strength during bathing (particularly, in lifting himself or herself in and out of the bathtub) can produce a rise in both systolic and diastolic blood pressure and an increase in myocardial workload. To minimize these effects, the bathtub should be equipped with grip bars, and the nurse should always help the patient in and out of the tub. Vasodilation caused by immersion in a hot-water bath or shower can also influence cardiovascular response.

In two studies comparing basin baths, tub baths, and showers, one study found no significant difference in patients' cardiovascular response to the three different bathing methods (Winslow et al, 1985; Winslow and Smith, 1991). The patients did express a preference for showering over basin baths. Some patients in all the groups experienced tachycardia (abnormally rapid heartbeat) and/or dysrhythmias while bathing. Winslow recommends that bath or shower temperature be kept at 95 to 98°F to help prevent tachycardia changes from occurring. Winslow also found that blood pressure changed the least after basin baths, as compared with after tub or shower baths but that the differences were not statistically significant.

Turning and moving patients in bed can cause cardiovascular effects. One study found that turning critically ill adults caused adverse changes in oxygen saturation and heart rate (Winslow et al, 1990a). Another study measured the differences in cardiac activity occurring when making the patient's bed with the patient in it (occupied bed) versus transferring the patient into a chair to make the bed (unoccupied bed) (Harrell et al, 1990). It was found that patients tolerated unoccupied bed making better than the rolling from side to side of occupied bed making. When the physical effects from using bedpans versus toileting were measured, no significant difference in oxygen consumption or cardiovascular response was found (Winslow et al, 1990b). The inference that these studies make is that getting a patient out of bed for hygiene measures may be easier on the patient than providing hygiene in bed. Also, if there are no significant differences in the cardiovascular responses to being up in the shower as opposed to being given a complete bed bath and patients prefer to take showers, nurses should make the effort to shower rather than bathe patients, as the shower is much more cost effective in terms of nurse's time. However, it is essential that ill patients never be left in the shower alone.

Some critically ill patients tolerate personal hygiene care very poorly (White et al, 1990). Using a pulse oximeter to measure mixed VO_2, researchers estimated how much oxygen was consumed—a reliable stress indicator—for each nursing intervention. A bed bath caused a 23 percent increase in the oxygen consumed, a position change caused a 31 percent increase, and a back rub required a 6 percent increase, with associated tachycardia (Tyler et al, 1990). These studies suggest that very ill patients need close observation to determine their tolerance of routine nursing actions and that a pulse oximetry monitor be used to provide information about how well a critically ill patient tolerates basic care.

MAXIMIZING PATIENT COMFORT DURING HYGIENE CARE

Studies exploring patient comfort during hygiene care found that patients who are nauseated, fatigued, or in pain are poor participants in their own care. The nurse should take measures to relieve a patient's nausea or pain, which may include providing analgesics or antiemetics, before providing or assisting with hygiene care (Funk, 1989; Piper et al, 1989).

ENSURING SAFETY WHILE PROVIDING HYGIENE CARE

PREVENTING FALLS

Researchers have studied ways to prevent injuries to patients and nurses during hygiene care. One study of patient safety and nurse comfort while transferring patients from bed to shower chair evaluated five different transfer techniques (Garg et al, 1991). The method that proved safest for both patient and nurse was the two-person walking belt, using a gentle rocking motion to transfer the patient from bed to belt and a mechanical transfer aid called the Ambulift. Another study evaluated various mechanical patient transfer lifts. It found that a new lifting device using ceiling tracks and a portable power pack best allowed one-person transfers. The ceiling track model was perceived to cost less and required the least effort (Holliday et al, 1994).

Two new types of gait belts are increasingly utilized in health care facilities to provide back support to the nurse when transferring patients in the provision of hygiene care (Heeschen, 1989). One is a canvas strip placed around the patient, which the nurse grasps for extra support while transferring the patient to a shower chair. Such transfer techniques are described in Chapter 20. The second belt is worn by the nurse to protect his or her back when transferring the patient into a shower chair or to the toilet. This nylon webbed belt goes around the nurse's back and has shoulder straps to provide support during lifting.

PREVENTING TRANSFER OF MICROORGANISMS

When the nurse is bathing the patient and changing the bed, the risk is run of coming into contact with microorganisms and fungi. Universal precautions, as discussed in Chapter 17, are always followed. One study documented the spread of tinea corporis (ringworm) to hospital personnel in close contact with either an infected patient or his or her bed linen (Arnow et al, 1991). To prevent such organism transfer, the nurse does not gather linen and soiled clothing against the body or uniform, and hand washing is scrupulously observed. If the nurse is bathing a patient with methicillin-resistant staphylococcus, it has been suggested that washing his or her hands afterwards with mild iodine soap can prevent the spread of this organism (Shovein and Young, 1992).

It is important to use supplies such as combs, wash basins, soap bars, drinking cups, and electric razors on one patient only. Skewes (1996) warns of the spread of gram-negative organisms from patient to patient through reuse of unsterilized metal or plastic bath basins. Personal supplies should not be shared with other patients. If, however, equipment must be reused among patients due to lack of supplies, time, and other constraints, the equipment must be sanitized between the patients with an antiseptic, bacteriolytic cleanser. The antiseptic solution **must** be used in the proper dilution for the proper period to be effective. Alternatively, plastic items can be put through a gas sterilizer and metal items autoclaved.

PROVIDING HYGIENE CARE TO PATIENTS WITH SPECIAL NEEDS

Certain categories of patients require hygiene care that is specialized for their needs. Although all patients need the generalized bathing, hair care, and oral hygiene, it may be neccessary to adapt procedures to the special needs of the following patients.

PATIENTS WITH CARDIOVASCULAR DISORDERS

The effect of hygiene on patients with myocardial infarctions has been studied. Braun and Holm (1989) recommend careful assessment of patients with recent heart damage before and after bathing. They suggest that all activity be stopped, or at least decreased in intensity, in the event of any of the following parameters:

- Cardiac discomfort or breathlessness
- Dizziness, confusion, faintness
- Marked pallor
- Cold sweats
- Ataxia
- Severe fatigue
- Heart rate greater than 110 beats per minute
- Decrease or no change in heart rate with physical activity
- Fall in systolic blood pressure of 10 mm Hg or more during effort
- Increase in systolic blood pressure of 40 mm Hg or more, for any reason
- Changes in the cardiogram pattern seen on the cardiac monitor

Another study evaluating the effects of bathing on patients with cardiac disease (Robichaud-Ekstrand, 1991) found no real difference in whether the first bath after myocardial infarction was done with the patient sitting up at the sink or sitting in the shower. However, as in other studies, this study did find significant physical responses to bathing, such as changes in blood pressure and heart rate. Every cardiac patient should have individualized assessment when hygiene care is being planned.

PATIENTS WITH HEAD OR SPINAL INJURIES

Patients with increased intracranial pressure (ICP) or spinal cord injury require hygiene care that does not exacerbate their injuries. One study explored the effect of personal hygiene care on patients with increased intracranial pressure and found that turning the patient to change the linen was associated with a rise in ICP (Rising, 1993). This study suggests that nurses caring for patients with head injuries should limit the number of times the patient is turned during hygiene care. Bathing patients with increased ICP, by conventional bed bath or by towel bath (Barsevick and Llwellyn, 1982) was not found to raise ICP and in some cases actually lowered it. Rising (1993) suggests that a warm, relaxing bath has the effect of vasodilating and relaxing the patient, which can lower ICP.

Patients with spinal cord injuries have special needs and considerations that the nurse needs to consider during personal hygiene care (Barker and Higgins, 1989). Some of these include

- Logrolling. These patients need to be "log-rolled" when they are turned during bathing or bedmaking. To logroll a patient, several nurses place their hand beneath the patient and turn the patient as one straight unit (see Chapter 20).
- Condom catheter. Male patients with spinal cord injuries are usually fitted with a condom catheter, worn external to the penis (see Chapter 24). One study found that less-than-adequate cleansing under condom catheters in spinal cord injured males was a potential cause of urinary sepsis (Taylor and Waites, 1993). The nurse should remove the condom catheter and clean the genital area daily, as the warm and wet area under the condom could provide a host to pathogens. Similar concerns regarding long-term indwelling catheters for such patients are discussed in Chapter 24.
- Decubitus ulcers. Pressure sores are common in spinal-cord–injured patients because of pressure, friction, and shearing. The nurse should examine such patients' skin carefully, especially around the coccyx,

hips, ankles, and elbows. Prevention through intermittent turning, cushioning, and other intermittent pressure relief is the best course of treatment (see Chapter 28).

PATIENTS WITH ENTERAL FEEDING TUBES

A research study was done regarding hygiene of patients with implanted feeding tubes. The suggestion was made that patients have less skin breakdown and hygiene needs with the use of an antireflux valve, which keeps stomach or intestinal contents from leaking out (Tucker et al, 1991). With less seepage, patients needed fewer linen changes and hygienic interventions.

PATIENTS RECEIVING RADIATION THERAPY

Patients receiving radiation therapy to treat cancer have special hygiene needs (Petton, 1985) and require special considerations. For instance, the radiation oncologist marks the skin with a dark ink to identify the target area. The nurse must not wash this mark off, or he or she risks altering the entire course of treatment. The patient may also have skin reactions in the areas under treatment. Hair may fall out, for instance, and irritation may range from bright red erythema to blistering and scabbing. The nurse should avoid using bath salts, oils, perfumes, hot water bottles, or heating pads on any radiated areas. Radiated areas should be treated with extreme gentleness and bathed with plain cool water.

PATIENTS WITH DIABETES

The condition of the patient's skin may be affected by the amount of circulating blood sugar in the body. Skin care and hygiene measures are especially important for patients with diabetes, because elevated blood sugar levels can make the patient prone to yeast and other skin infections such as furuncles, or boils. Assessing the skin would be a high nursing priority for a patient like Mrs. Carpenter (see the case study).

Patients with diabetes also need special attention to foot care. The nurse should teach proper foot care at every encounter with a diabetic patient; this should be part of Mrs. Carpenter's care. Further, a diabetic patient with poor vision should have an assigned foot "inspector" to check his or her feet for ulcerations or other abnormalities (Christensen et al, 1991).

OTHER PATIENTS WITH SPECIAL NEEDS

It is important that special care be given to patients receiving hemodialysis. The use of extra hand washing and gloves prior to bathing the patient's vascular access site lessens the possibility of sepsis and infection (Kaplowitz et al, 1988).

Patients with acquired immunodeficiency syndrome may be in an extremely weakened condition. Their high risk for falls requires these patients to have special assistance with bathing, transfers to tub or shower, and toileting (Odell et al, 1991). Patients with HIV or AIDS will also require special attention to mouth care as they may have painful oral lesions from thrush infections.

ENSURING SAFE AND EFFECTIVE PERSONAL HYGIENE PRODUCTS AND SUPPLIES

The safety and effectiveness of bathing, showering, and preoperative cleansing products have been extensively researched. One study reviewed the historical use of soap and found skin infection and illness to increase when soap was scarce (Brumberg, 1989). A more detailed study of shower soaps compared chlorhexidine gluconate (Hibiclens), povidone-iodine (Betadine), and standard lotion soap (Kaiser et al, 1988). Chlorhexidine gluconate worked significantly better to lower bacterial counts preoperatively, and lotion soaps were associated with increased bacterial colony counts after showering.

Other studies have investigated the effect of bed linens on hygiene care. Patients with sensitive skin may develop a contact dermatitis rash when in contact with hospital bed linens. One study found 30 cases of reported allergy to the various dyes and permanent press resins found in hospital sheets (Brown, 1990). This and soap residue left on sheets may be the cause of many unexplained skin reactions in the hospital. Most hospitals have the ability to order hypoallergenic sheets or sheets washed without soap from their service laundries. A Swedish study evaluated the absorption difference between linen sheets and cotton/polyester sheets (Larsson and Berg, 1991). The far more costly linen sheets were found to absorb perspiration slightly better in diaphoretic patients, but not enough to be statistically significant. The study recommended using cotton-blend sheets, 15 times less costly than linen—an important suggestion in today's cost-conscious managed care environment.

MAXIMIZING COST-EFFECTIVENESS OF HYGIENE CARE

Studies have been looking at the cost-effectiveness of giving a towel bath, in which a large, wet towel is draped across the patient and used for the bath, versus the traditional basin-at-the-bedside bed bath. Wright (1990) compared patient preference, time requirements, and cost analysis for each of these two methods and found that towel baths were preferred by both patients and nurses and were more cost-effective, too. Skewes (1996) also described the lowered cost-benefit of a prepackaged disposable towel for giving towel baths.

Another study of hygienic cost-effectiveness compared using traditional bed padding with towels versus disposable diapers for incontinent patients (Grant, 1982). The author compared patients' skin condition, time factors, cost factors, safety, and esthetics and was unable to prove that using disposable diapers was better in any of the five examined areas.

The type of hygiene provided patients is a major factor in determining the amount of nursing care allotted. Using time studies and other work-measurement tools, institutions have developed models to measure nursing care requirements of patients (Cleland, 1990), grouping patients into nursing requirement prototypes such as self-care, assisted care, moderate care, and critical care.

One important study has determined the amount of time it takes a nurse to perform each action of providing hygiene (Deines, 1985). According to Deines' estimates, caring for the patient with total care needs requires 58 minutes of nursing time a day: bath and occupied bed, 18 minutes; physical observation during bath, 10 minutes; back care, 3 minutes; mouth care, 3 minutes; shampoo, 8 minutes; nail care, 3 minutes; perianal care, 3 minutes; combing hair, 2 minutes; getting a patient up into a chair, 4 minutes; performing range of motion exercises, 6 minutes; putting up side rails, 1 minute; positioning essential surrounding items such as the call bell, 1 minute; and housekeeping the patient's unit, 2 minutes. Deines showed that development of a nurse staffing system must take into consideration time allotted for the amount of hygiene care needed per patient.

PROMOTING A POSITIVE NURSE-PATIENT RELATIONSHIP DURING HYGIENE CARE

Nurses enter into a special type of helping relationship when providing hygiene care or personal grooming for a patient. Henderson and Nite (1978) attempt to explicate this relationship in their often-quoted definition of nursing:

> Nursing is primarily helping people (sick or well) in the performance of those activities contributing to health or its recovery (or to a peaceful death) that they could perform unaided if they had the necessary strength, will, or knowledge. It is likewise the unique contribution of nursing to help people to be independent of such assistance as soon as possible.

Harder (1992) found patients to be truly appreciative of this help that Henderson and Nite describe. The following excerpt from Harder's study of hospital nursing care in Denmark depicts these feelings:

> It was after breakfast. I did not eat as much as I wanted to. I felt surprised because I couldn't mobilize my will, I leaned back, as if I had used my body for hours. Suddenly she was there again, a nurse that had spent a lot of time with me the day before. She was smiling, full of energy. She went straight to the point, leaned onto the table and offered to help me have a shower in the bathroom. It seemed like climbing a mountain, but she was so convincing that I agreed. She explained the whole procedure, how she would cover the wound with plastic, etc. It began to sound like heaven. I had confidence in her, she seemed to have been doing this for a hundred years. And it was heaven, Never had I thought that I would appreciate water running down my body as I did that morning. I was sitting on a chair, and the nurse was next to me. I relaxed. She had a special way of offering her help in concrete ways like washing my back and feet, which I literally could not reach that morning. "I suggest to you . . . " and "what you could do is turn your body," yes she was assisting me, never taking over. I was in command, I felt. I mattered. Even though the only thing I could manage was steering the shower handle.

Harder's work indicates to us the essential connection that comes about between nurses and patients in a caring setting. This is verified by the research of Wolf (1993) in her historic review of the bath as a ritual of closeness between nurse and patient.

USING TOUCH THERAPEUTICALLY

Many experienced nurses are now developing this essential connection between patient and nurse through the therapeutic use of touch. This practice is based on the theory that human contact releases stress and may promote healing. Such touch may range from a nurse's normal physical contact with a patient to a back rub after bathing. The essential component is always the nurse's sincere desire to help the patient (see Chapter 32).

Not surprisingly, one study found that elderly subjects had less anxiety and were calmer for days after a back rub (Simington and Laing, 1993). Another far more specific study found that a therapeutic back rub was able to measurably increase patients' immunoglobulin A response time, compared with a control group that received no back rub (Groer et al, 1994). Immunoglobulin A is the principal antibody protein in mucus, saliva, and tears, protecting mucosal surfaces from bacterial and viral invasion. This could mean that a nurse may actually help increase a patient's physiologic immune response through the therapeutic use of touch.

PROMOTING PATIENT COMFORT WITH THE INTIMATE NATURE OF HYGIENE CARE

How the patient feels about his or her body, the changes it has undergone due to medical conditions or treatments, and how it currently looks and feels are vital to providing hygiene care. Six factors have been described (Bower, 1980) that can influence a patient's response to a change in appearance due to medical causes:

- Functional significance of the body part
- Importance of physical appearance
- Visibility of the part involved
- Feasibility and availability of rehabilitation
- Speed at which the change occurred
- Patient's previous coping patterns

Changes in appearance may cause the patient great distress. While providing hygiene care, the nurse needs to be acutely aware and supportive of the patient's feelings. Body image changes commonly described are those of loss of limb (amputation), loss of breast (mastectomy), or change in facial structure (such as from laryngectomy, burns, or radical neck dissection). A problem less often described is when an elderly person begins to be incontinent of urine (Brink, 1980). In all cases, the nurse can set the tone for positive self-perception in the patient. Studies have shown that a patient's feelings about changes in appearance are directly related to the nurse's initial response.

PROMOTING NURSE COMFORT WITH THE INTIMATE NATURE OF HYGIENE CARE

Providing personal hygiene care for others can at times cause the nurse unease. The nurse is expected to undress, examine, wash, and groom the patient, who is usually a stranger. These most intimate actions are often among the first duties that nursing students are asked to perform. A study of nursing students found that actions such as bathing, touching, and caring for patients who are incontinent caused them discomfort and fear (Bradby, 1990). Nurses are performing the most intimate procedures for patients and yet are expected to do so in a professional, nonsexual manner (Savage, 1989). Instructors and experienced nurses can nurture and support students entering into the new role of personal care providers and teach them what to expect and how to deal with these new responsibilities.

On occasion, during a bathing activity, a patient may behave in a way that proves embarrassing or uncomfortable to the nurse, such as touching the nurse or touching himself or herself in a sexual way. Displaying sexual behavior toward nurses is not uncommon in hospitalized or institutionalized patients (Poorman and Smith, 1988). Patients who act or talk seductively are probably not really asking to engage in sexual activity as much as they are looking for reassurance. These patients may be trying to verify that even with their new body image or changes in health state, they are still acceptable to others as a sexual being. The nurse should reaffirm caring for the patient while rejecting a specific behavior (Poorman and Smith, 1988).

In some cases, what a nurse interprets as a patient's inappropriate sexual behavior may in fact be a simple physiologic response with no underlying sexual intent. For instance, in a male patient an erection during a bed bath may simply be a healthy nervous system response to mechanical stimulation. The same could apply to nipple stimulation in a female patient during bed bathing with a washcloth. The nurse should be careful to differentiate such normal physiologic responses from inappropriate behavior. If such a response occurs, the nurse can matter-of-factly continue with hygiene care or take a short break and resume care when the response has subsided.

Very little has been written about nurses' sexual feelings and attraction to patients. Feelings of sexual attraction and fantasy are part of the human experience and can occur just as easily in nurses as in patients (Poorman and Smith, 1988). It is not abnormal for a nurse to feel a sexual attraction to a patient; however, the nurse must always strive to maintain an ethical and appropriate relationship with all patients in her or his care. A request for an assignment change in an uncomfortable situation would be honored.

Relevant Theory

One non-nurse theorist whose work has helped shape how patient care is delivered is Abraham Maslow (1954). Maslow's Hierarchy of Needs, an ordering or classification of basic human needs in ascending order of importance (air, water, food, health, belonging, self-actualization), can help guide nurses in recognizing and prioritizing patients' needs. Cleanliness, comfort, and safety are basic to feeling good about oneself. Thus, the patient's bath must be warm, safe, and comforting. The patient must feel that the nurse will keep him or her safe from falls, slips in the tub room, unnecessary exposure, or improper technique. When these basic needs are met, the patient is free to go on to achieve Maslow's higher-level goals, such as meeting needs for self-esteem and self-actualization. Here, too, the nurse can help by showing the patient respect as a vital, worthwhile human being who can contribute to society, regardless of the degree of injury, illness, or condition.

Swanson (1991, 1993) has developed a middle-range theory of caring in the nursing role. This model depicts five components of the nurse's role: *knowing, being with, doing for, enabling,* and *maintaining belief.* Applied to the provision of personal hygiene for another, the nurse knows what the patient's limitations are, can be with the patient on an emotional level, do for by assisting with bathing and grooming, enable the patient to look fresh and feel renewed, and maintain belief that the patient may be able to regain some degree of self-care in the future.

Self-care has been explored as a theoretical model in nursing. Nurse theorists have developed this model in which patients are helped to independently direct their own care (Orem, 1985; Steiger and Lipson, 1985). Steiger and Lipson's text presents a new model of nurse-patient interaction in which the nurse is far more a teacher and facilitator than caregiver, allowing the patient to "achieve, maintain, and promote maximum health." An example of a patient's desire for self-care was found in one research study of critically ill patients (Ziemann and Dracup, 1990). These researchers found that even the most ill patients wished to have control over their hygiene care, even if they could just choose the timing of the care when unable to provide it themselves.

Nurse theorist Imogene King's goal attainment model (1981), which allows for mutual interaction between the nurse and the patient, provides another theoretical model for the delivery of hygiene care. According to this theory, the patient is not a passive participant but actively contributes to the direction and input of the plan of care. King states that nurses who are able to accurately perceive what is happening to patients and family members, who are able to make that "essential connection," are most successful in providing meaningful care.

FACTORS AFFECTING CLINICAL DECISIONS

Age

CHILDREN, ADOLESCENTS, AND YOUNG ADULTS

The hygiene needs of the very young and the elderly who may be unable to care for themselves are, in many cases, obvious: complete hygiene care. Less obvious may be the need for assistive hygiene in adolescents, young adults, and adults. The nurse should carefully assess patients of all ages to determine their specific hygiene needs because these patients' physical limitations are not always evident. The young adult may need as much nursing support and assistance as an older patient.

One special need of adolescents and young children is the need to respect their extreme modesty in front of strangers. Care must be taken to provide privacy when providing personal care, such as keeping body parts covered, allowing the wearing of cotton underwear into the operating room, keeping doors and curtains closed, and allowing as much self-care as possible.

Safety is another imperative in providing hygiene for adolescents and children. One nurse researcher described a case of a 15-year-old girl who slipped in the shower and received penetrating injuries from broken glass in the shower door (Kelly, 1986). It is also extremely important that children are never left in or near bathwater unattended.

In the care of young children, nurses must help prevent the development of dental caries in their teeth. A study of the incidence of dental caries in children in various populations found that as many as 50 percent of children had decayed teeth (Griffen and Goepferd, 1991). Diet, fluoridation, oral hygiene measures, and frequent professional dental care are the keys to preventing decay. Another important preventive measure is avoiding prolonged exposure of teeth to carbohydrates, such as occurs when a baby bottle is left in an infant's mouth for an extended time ("baby bottle caries").

Providing oral hygiene during the first years of life may only require that the nurse use a clean washcloth to wipe plaque from baby teeth. In a toddler, a nurse should encourage him or her to use a soft child's toothbrush as soon as the toddler is capable of handling one. Toothpaste is initially unnecessary because the taste and foaming action may be objectionable to children, and fluoridated toothpastes may contribute to excess fluoride intake. While it has been conclusively proven that the application and ingestion of fluoride **will** prevent caries, some children have developed dental staining—enamel fluorosis—from excessive ingestion of fluoride. Nurses should teach parents the benefits of fluoride, making certain that the proper dosage has been prescribed by the pediatrician or dentist, and that this medication is not used when a city has already added fluoride to the drinking water. When teaching young children self-care measures, the nurse can demonstrate first on a doll or teddy bear. This may decrease fear and engage young children's participation in hygienic care.

OLDER ADULTS

Many researchers have studied hygiene care in the elderly. A recent study of elderly residents reported that many physical barriers existed that stood in the way of their providing their own hygiene care, and that their sense of usefulness would increase if they could be more active in their own bathing and grooming (Lindgren and Linton, 1991). Another study of 175 elderly patients in England receiving home care found that many families were unable to bathe their elderly family members more than once every 2 weeks due to problems such as Alzheimer's disease (Penn et al, 1989). Many factors contribute to this hygienic deficit, notably the confusion, poor balance, and striking out at caregivers often characterizing Alzheimer's patients. Having a skilled home-care nurse available to bathe these patients was found by the families to meet one of their greatest needs.

As patients age into their 80s and 90s, they may also develop incontinence. These patients have special hygiene needs (Demmerle and Bartol, 1980). For instance, the risk of skin breakdown is very great. Every time that the patient is changed, it is important to wash the perineal area well with soap and water and dry thoroughly. A lubricating lotion in the water will help prevent skin dryness. It is likewise very important to maintain skin integrity and prevent infection by turning the patient every 2 hours and changing wet bedding or clothing frequently.

Other studies have found that a majority of elderly patients have dry skin (Frantz and Kinney, 1986). The researchers were unable to determine the causes for skin dryness but did find that skin dryness increased with age. They also discovered that accepted nursing practices such as bathing elderly patients less frequently and putting emollients in the bath water did not prove to have any statistical influence on skin dryness. Fluid hydration, nutrition, and body temperature were far more important in maintaining healthy skin.

A study that assessed dry skin in elderly patients found that using superfatted soaps (Dove brand, in this case), patting rather than rubbing skin dry, and applying mineral oil to the body after bathing significantly resolved skin dryness (Hardy, 1990). The author found that when these treatments were discontinued, dry skin returned. Thorough rinsing of soap from all parts of the body has also been found to be important. A study of hospitalized elderly women reported perineal discomfort due to residual soap remaining in the labia area after baths. The researchers suggest that using soap with a low acid content and ensuring that all soap is completely rinsed from the female labia will prevent such discomfort (Lindell and Olsson, 1990).

For nurses providing home care, elderly patients living on their own may have special hygiene needs. Limited vision or mobility may preclude the ability to safely meet hygiene needs. The section on home care offers suggestions for necessary assistance.

Gender

Bath blankets, closed curtains, and cover gowns or robes can help ensure privacy, modesty, and dignity for male and female patients alike during the provision of personal care.

The nurse should be prepared for menses in hospitalized women patients of child-bearing age. In particular, this means ensuring ready access to a supply of sanitary napkins. Hospitals do not allow the use of tampons as a precautionary measure against toxic shock syndrome. A patient who is sedated or given pain medication or anesthesia may forget or be unable to remove the tampon in a timely manner, which can cause this serious systemic infection (Creehan, 1995).

Individual and Family Values

EDUCATIONAL BACKGROUND

The patient's developmental level, education, and literacy levels are important in determining the level of teaching a nurse provides (Doak et al, 1985). Teaching the patient and his or her significant others is vital in ensuring continuity of hygiene care measures. For very young patients, it may be necessary to teach hygiene measures to the patient's parents or primary guardian. For patients with developmental disabilities, it may be possible to establish a behavior modification program, with rewards for assisting with personal grooming. Patients with visual, hearing, or motor function incapacities may require social workers and occupational and rehabilitation specialists. The nurse can assess the level of need and then provide the necessary referral.

To establish a formal teaching plan for patient hygiene, the nurse

- Assesses the patient's strengths and weaknesses
- Plans objectives with inclusion of patient input
- Implements and evaluates the plan
- Follows up by documenting the results of patient teaching in the patient's chart
- Determines what follow-up care is necessary at discharge to continue these care measures at home

Consider Mrs. Carpenter (see the case study). Her diabetic condition, aggravated by visual and motor function difficulty, might require several teaching sessions conducted with sensitivity and vocabulary appropriate to her seventh-grade level of education. If at all possible, Mr. Carpenter should be included in these sessions.

SOCIOECONOMIC STATUS

Hygiene habits differ from person to person and culture to culture. In the United States, many people bathe daily by washing at the sink, showering, or bathing. Most American homes have access to warm, running water and soap. This is not the case for all persons in a nurse's care.

Disenfranchised patients, such as those who misuse alcohol or drugs or are homeless or mentally ill, may have hygiene needs far greater than the norm. Alcohol abuse may lead to or stem from poverty; these patients may have a high level of self-neglect manifested by poor hygiene, lice, dental caries, bruises and unhealed lesions, and malnutrition. The alcoholic patient may present with liver enlargement, abdominal tenderness, and ankle edema, which could affect the method of bathing. Clotting difficulties may be present due to alcoholic liver dysfunction. The nurse needs to take special precautions in bathing and shaving a patient with clotting problems. Additionally, the patient suffering from delirium tremens may not be able to participate in personal hygiene care without sedation.

A patient who is abusing drugs may exhibit similar signs of self-neglect. There may be infected skin lesions at points of needle entry, requiring cleansing, débriding, and bandaging. The nurse uses universal precautions for all patients but is especially cognizant that intravenous drug users are at high risk of carrying hepatitis and human immunodeficiency virus. A patient abusing oral or inhaled substances may have similar health problems, including lack of the judgment needed to allow showering alone safely.

Homeless patients may present significant hygienic needs (Memmott and Young, 1993; Vredevoe et al, 1992). A study of mothers and children in a homeless shelter found hygiene requirements to be one of their most expressed needs (Memmot and Young, 1993), and another study found homeless persons to place great emphasis on the need for a place to shower and wash their clothes (Vredevoe et al, 1992). Deficits of those who live on the streets may include dental caries, extremely poor personal hygiene, wounds, trauma, lice, scabies, leg ulcers, and gangrenous toes from prolonged exposure to cold (Fernsebner, 1980). These groups of patients, without financial means, may have neither the funds available for toothbrushes, soap, and combs nor a place to use them. Establishing the means for a homeless patient to provide hygienic self-care may be one of the most significant hygiene measures a community nurse can provide such patients. The nurse working in an inpatient facility will hopefully have access to the proper supplies and be able to provide the ultimate in good hygiene care to such patients. These patients may not have the opportunity to receive another bath for a long time.

Patients with chronic mental illness may also have significant self-care deficits. The nurse may have to provide hair cleaning, dental assessment, nail trimming, pediculosis assessment, foot care, and skin care for this group of patients. One nurse researcher described teaching and assisting hygienic self-care to institutionalized chronic mentally ill and schizophrenic patients (Wong et al, 1988).

CULTURE AND ETHNICITY

Whenever feasible, the nurse includes family members in planning and providing a patient's personal hygiene care. The family unit today may represent a wide variety of both legal and presumptive relationships. The term *significant other* is derived from psychology and describes the person of primary importance in a patient's life. A patient's significant other is considered his or her family, whether or not blood relationship or marriage exists, and may include heterosexual boyfriends and girlfriends, gay and lesbian partners, roommates, and teenage friends of emancipated minors. The astute nurse simply asks both the patient and his or her guests who is available to help with care, respecting and including all persons who lovingly wish to participate in a patient's care.

Providing hygienic care of children may present special challenges when multiple family sets are involved. These may include the child's natural parents and their respective spouses or significant others, stepparents, and several sets of grandparents. In some cultures, the nurse should consult the father for all decision making; in other families, the grandmother. When in doubt, the nurse simply asks.

Family tradition is as great a part of hygiene care as any other aspect of culture. Many cultures require that multiple family members remain with the patient at all times (Leininger, 1991). It might be only in the Western culture that a patient is "surrendered" to the hospital and treated in isolation. In some cultures, such as traditional Filipino, it might be considered a disgrace for the family to depend on the nurse to provide a bath. In others, such as traditional Hispanic, a husband might be very uncomfortable if his wife were to be bathed in his absence. Many cultures are sensitive to male nurses caring for female patients or to anyone undressing a female patient without her husband's presence and consent.

Research has validated the value of using the patient's ethnic support system to blend traditional healing with modern medical care (Marchione and Stearns, 1991). Asian patients, for example, may insist on wearing special amulets or bracelets of yarn at all times (Spector, 1991). The Hmong of Southeast Asia believe that the soul of a person resides in the head (Rairdan and Higgs, 1992); thus, the nurse should ask permission before washing or assessing a patient's hair and head.

Many cultures, such as Native American, Japanese, African, and Scandinavian, have used bathing for cleansing and healing purposes (Vogel, 1970). The popular use of hot tubs and saunas stems from these groups' practices. Native American use boiled herbs and vapors in the bath as a restorative. Japanese bathe outside the tub, rinsing their bodies before entering a hot communal tub for physical and mental relaxation (Silberman, 1962).

America is a land of multiple ethnic strands and points of origin, with different individuals and cultures, many practicing unique hygiene. Some hygiene practices may be symbolic, ritualistic, or religious. These practices may not necessarily be grounded in any scientific principle or theory but may be handed down throughout the generations. Cultural sensitivity and assessment of the patient's family and home situation is vital. Assessment determines how much the patient and family can and want to care for the patient, how much is culturally appropriate, and how much assistance and education the nurse needs to provide (Kelly et al, 1991). A willingness to recognize cultural differences and incorporate these differences into hygienic care and patient teaching is a hallmark of a thoughtful and sensitive nurse.

SPIRITUALITY AND RELIGIOUS PRACTICES

Cleansing and ceremonial hygiene have long been incorporated into spiritual beliefs. For example, Christian baptism, the use of fonts of holy water and its sprinkling, and the shaking of branches made of white paper (called Haraiaguishi) over followers of the Shinto religion all represent a symbolic act of cleansing the body and soul of evil, allowing rebirth, or reawakening to a more spiritually pure state. Dipping in ritual bathwater at critical times, such as before the Sabbath or when converting to Judaism, is a traditional custom of Orthodox Jews (Kolatch, 1981).

A patient receiving traditional Catholic or Episcopal communion should be bathed or showered prior to these special blessings. Such ceremonial acts represent important and meaningful rites of passage to both patient and family. The nurse who can respectfully and sincerely assist patients with these beliefs and ceremonies in a hospital or clinical setting contributes greatly to the patient's physical and mental comfort.

Setting in Which Care Is Delivered

INPATIENT SETTINGS

Hospital environments can be new, strange, and frightening for any patient, whatever his or her age, culture, or ethnicity. When entering a patient's room in any acute or long-term setting to provide hygiene care, the nurse assesses the patient's environment for excessive noise or human traffic, uncomfortable temperature or humidity, lack of safety, and or poor esthetics. All these factors can interfere with the therapeutic environment, and the nurse should minimize them to the largest extent possible.

The patient's room may be too cold during bathing, for example, or too many people—clinical or extended family—may be entering and leaving the room during the bath, disregarding the patient's needs for privacy and modesty. Cold temperatures and lack of privacy may also characterize a shower room in a long-term care facility. Nurses should ensure that the patient care setting is optimal for delivering hygiene care with privacy, dignity, and at a temperature appropriate for that patient.

The nurse adjusts room temperature and humidity in conjunction with the hospital's engineering department, ensuring adequate ventilation. The nurse minimizes noise, a potent stressor, by keeping doors partially closed and keeping telephones and televisions at the lowest practical setting. Although visitors are no longer limited in most patient care areas, the nurse should consider the patient's fatigue and ask visitors to shorten visits as necessary.

The nurse also orients the patient to safety features in the room, such as call lights, emergency lights, side rails, grip bars, electric bed positioning, overhead frames, and trapeze bars. The nurse further ensures patient safety by having personal electrical appliances such as shaving razors or hair dryers tested by the engineering department prior to use, to make certain no potentially hazardous electrical malfunctions will occur.

The patient's room should be neat and sanitary before beginning the bath. Preparation includes

- Removing all uneaten food and used food dishes
- Rinsing all used instruments in cold water and sending them to the decontamination area

- Double-bagging dressings and garbage for disposal and removing them from the room
- Regularly emptying all linen hampers
- Controlling odor by using canned or spray deodorizer and promptly removing body waste products
- Changing water in flowers daily to prevent decomposing odors

Patients may wish to personalize their rooms with pictures and other belongings, which the nurse should encourage, labeling them to prevent loss. Every patient care setting should also include a wall clock and calendar. Promptly answered call lights, adequate lighting, and rapid elimination of any spills on the floors further ensure patient safety during bathing.

LONG-TERM CARE SETTINGS

The nurse is often the supervisor of hygiene care providers rather than the primary caregiver in a long-term care facility. The nurse directs and monitors the physical care provided by ancillary staff. However, the nurse is legally responsible for knowing and communicating the patient's condition to all relevant personnel and following up on any identified problems.

Shower chairs are the main bathing vehicle in long-term facilities (Fig. 26–1). The nurse assesses that qualified care providers have properly transferred and positioned the patient in the chair, properly covered him or her, and properly transported him or her down the hallways. A more complete discussion of shower chair baths is included in Procedure 26–1.

HOME CARE SETTINGS

Home care nursing offers challenges and services far beyond those of simply providing hygiene in a hospital setting. The nurse going out to a home to assist in personal care is doing far more than cleaning a patient; the nurse constantly assesses the total picture of the patient's life and ensures that the home is safe from harm. Examples of safety and lifestyle monitoring questions the nurse asks include

- Are there dangerous substances or medications lying about?
- Are there small rugs or pieces of furniture over which a person with impaired vision could trip?
- In what physical and mental condition is the patient?
- Is there food in the house? What kind?
- Is the house clean, or does it represent a hazard to the patient's health?
- Does the community provide "Meals on Wheels" for the homebound? Can the patient receive meals if he or she is housebound?
- What is the condition of the patient's skin?
- Do the caregivers know how to and practice turning a bedridden patient frequently and provide high-protein foods to prevent decubitus ulcers?
- Would a different type of patient bed be more appropriate?

Taking baths in the home is often comforting for the patient, who is in familiar surroundings, using familiar equipment. To increase patient safety at home, nurses may recommend portable shower chairs (see Fig. 26–1), installation of

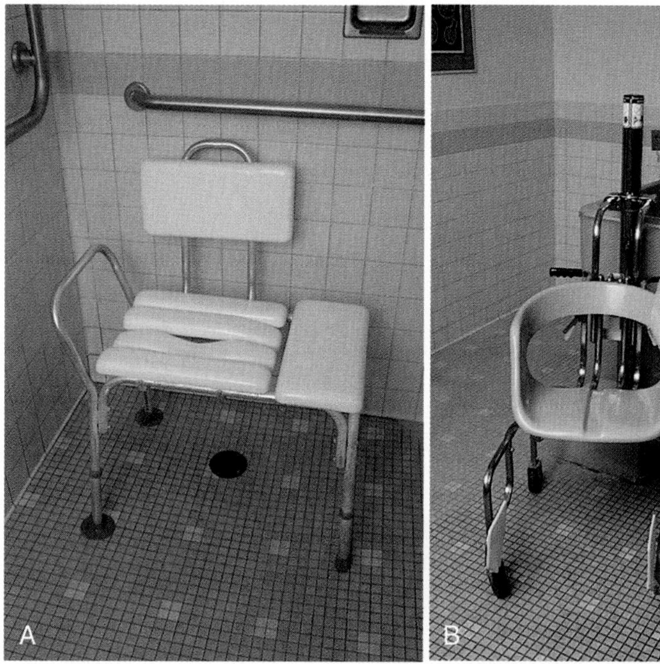

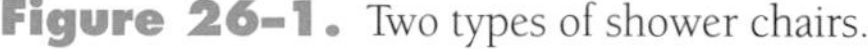
Figure 26–1. Two types of shower chairs.

hand grip bars in the tub and shower, and removal of the bathroom rug to prevent falls. Home care nurses provide physical assessment during provision of personal hygiene care because they are often the only link between the patient and potentially life-saving medical intervention.

Legal and Ethical Considerations

ACCOUNTABILITY

Who should actually be responsible for the patient's personal care? This is a chief ethical dilemma related to hygiene care. Some nurse advocates feel that only licensed nurses should provide hands-on patient care. Others advocate that ancillary personnel, such as unit assistants or nurse's aids, should provide hygiene care to free the nurse for more complex duties.

In many cases, the setting influences this decision. Nurses always perform hygiene intervention in a critical care unit, for example, but rarely in a long-term care facility. Each facility has policies to determine whose job it is to provide patient hygiene. When the nurse is not providing hygiene care, however, he or she remains responsible for the effectiveness of other staff members' work and is held accountable for any breach or deficit in hygiene. Nurse educators can teach students to appreciate that the time spent in bathing the patient allows for complete assessment of the patient's physical and emotional status.

CONFIDENTIALITY

Any time the nurse enters into such an intimate encounter as physical assessment and bathing, he or she may discover or be told details highly personal in nature. All communications are maintained within the bounds of nurse-patient confidentiality (see Chapter 8). If, however, when disrobing the patient or during the bath, the nurse believes that he or she is viewing signs of possible physical abuse on the patient's body, he or she must collect more data to rule out or verify these suspicions and then discuss this with an instructor or supervisor. The nurse is required by law in the United States to report signs of physical abuse. The nurse should also let the patient or, if a minor, the patient's guardian know that this information is going to be shared with appropriate authorities. One researcher maintains the absolute necessity for health care providers to address and never ignore possible domestic violence, because this intervention may save a life (Warshaw, 1993).

PATIENT'S RIGHTS

Another ethical dilemma arises when the patient refuses to participate in hygiene. Since Nightingale, nurses have traditionally viewed bathing as an integral part of the patient's recovery; indeed, a substantial portion of nursing time is devoted to hygiene. The nurse needs superb assessment skills when the patient refuses to bathe or be bathed.

The nurse needs to assess the reasons for such refusal. Are cultural considerations involved? Is the patient too fatigued to participate? Is the patient anxious about his or her condition? Is the patient waiting for visitors and afraid of missing them while bathing? Does the patient normally bathe or shower daily? At what time does the patient normally shower—morning, evening? Is this an issue of control, in which a patient whose life is rapidly changing due to illness or injury wants **something** he or she can say "no" to?

Mrs. Carpenter of the case study may resist some care measures and embrace others. She may, for instance, be unwilling to wash her hair but will cheerfully clean her fingernails. The nurse works in small steps, accomplishing bit by bit, and accommodating to each patient within the limits possible.

A 91-year-old man living in a California veteran's institution refused daily bathing, offering a group of nursing students their first ethical dilemma (Simpson, L.S., personal communication, 1992). What guidelines may the nurse use? Patients who undergo little physical exertion and who are continent can probably bathe or be bathed much less often. Patients whose clothes are soiled with fecal matter or urine, on the other hand, will suffer serious skin consequences if they are not cleaned up. Odors offensive to other patients in a shared room may necessitate more forcefulness than in the case of a patient at home who does not wish to bathe.

American law provides the patient the right to refuse treatment (see Chapter 8). The student nurse or new nurse may find it difficult to sort through the reasons for refusal and determine an approach to take in response. One researcher suggests that bathing by towel represents a kinder, less-invasive approach than going to a cold shower room, which may seem like an assault to a confused patient (Rader, 1994). Here, too, the nursing instructor can provide guidance. Courtesy, respect, and ingenuity are the essential nursing qualities to meet this challenge.

LEGAL EXPECTATIONS THAT PERSONAL HYGIENE CARE WILL BE DELIVERED

Keeping residents in nursing homes clean is not an ethical or theoretical concern but a legal requirement in most states. Thus, it is the nurse's duty to try to secure patient compliance and active participation to the greatest degree possible, using the qualities discussed previously. One study of 853 personal care complaints made to the Texas Department of Health, which monitors long-term care facilities in that state, found that the largest percentage of complaints (27 percent) concerned bathing and personal hygiene deficits (Wagnild, 1986). These deficits can have severe legal repercussions for the facility and the nurse, including (but not limited to) termination of employment, suspension of license, and fines.

Financial Considerations

Today's nurses operate in a dramatically different fiscal environment than their predecessors. Nurses must strive to

CLINICAL DECISION MAKING
PROVIDING HYGIENIC CARE

Each step of providing hygiene should be done with privacy and courtesy. When providing hygiene and doing a physical assessment of Mrs. Carpenter, teaching can be supplied along the way. Mrs. Carpenter's hygiene care will be complex, based on the nurse's understanding of her current and past medical history. Mrs. Carpenter has a history of diabetes mellitus with retinopathy and healing problems. And because Mrs. Carpenter cannot see well, there will be areas of her body with which she will need assistance cleaning.

The nurse must carefully assess her extremities, especially the feet, because patients with diabetes often have poor circulation. Further, the nurse is alert for and reports any redness or heat (signs of infection) or darkened tissue (lack of circulation). If Mrs. Carpenter is able to see well enough, she should be taught to inspect and dry her feet well after bathing. If she is not able, the teaching should be directed to her husband. The nurse is aware that any special nail care can be performed only by a podiatrist.

Mrs. Carpenter also has a recurrent urinary tract infection. The nurse must teach her special precautionary care in providing her own perineal care. She must be taught to cleanse herself from front to back to avoid contamination of her urinary tract. The nurse uses simple words and directions and asks for return demonstrations. Mrs. Carpenter's groin area should be inspected for redness, which could be a sign of mycosis (*Candida* infection), prevalent in diabetic women.

Mrs. Carpenter is also in need of oral and hair care. Because of her limited mobility from arthritis, she may not be able to raise her arms easily to shampoo, comb, and groom her hair. Her matted hair must be washed and then carefully combed. Mrs. Carpenter can probably provide her own oral care when supplied with the proper equipment. Because the nurse also knows that Mrs. Carpenter is overweight, the nurse should inspect under her breasts and in abdominal folds for irritation where, with sufficient irritation, mycosis may occur.

deliver cost-effective care and compare costs through research as the health care system adapts to managed care. Today, nursing actions must be competitive in terms of quality and efficiency (Harrington, 1995). As described in the research section, use of the towel bath for bedbound patients and the shower for those with more mobility has proven to be more cost effective in terms of nurses' time and are preferred by patients as well.

Financial considerations are also reflected in the use and cost of hygiene products. Many facilities supply necessary items; some do not. When essential care products are not available, the nurse faces a dilemma. Does the nurse borrow these items from another patient, buy patient supplies with his or her own money, ask the patient to supply money, or provide less care to those unable to afford more? There is no simple solution. Nurses today must become patient advocates and active participants in finding necessary funding for their institutions to provide adequate patient care. Providing health care may increasingly be the domain of cost-conscious businesses, but the nurse's primary loyalty must be to ensure patient recovery.

FUTURE DEVELOPMENTS

In the future, hygienic care will demand better products and equipment to provide cleansing. More nurses will be aware of hygiene research, and practices will change: Fewer bed baths and more towel baths or showers will be given, for example, and fewer occupied beds will be made. Newer hospital beds and lift systems will be used to provide easier transport and transfer from bed to tub or shower. New hygiene care products will allow the nurse to work more productively; for example, Skewes' (1996) towel and soap bag requires no rinsing. Patient care areas will all have tubs with built-in hydrotherapy to aid patient circulation.

New technologies developed by nurse researchers will also dramatically shape the personal care of tomorrow. An electric sensory device can now assess and alert a paralyzed individual that his or her bladder is full, and a practical female urinal may soon become a reality (Pieper et al, 1989).

The future will also find nurses assuming greater responsibility for prescribing appropriate hygiene measures and collaborating with physicians when questions arise. Nurses will continue to be responsible for providing cost-effective care and must become more sophisticated in demonstrating this care in terms of dollars and cents to hospital administrators, regulatory agencies, and the public. More families will participate in the patient's care, and home care will be provided and supervised by home care or public health nurses. In long-term care facilities, nurse practitioners will assume responsibility for much of the care.

NURSING CARE ACTIONS

Principles and Practices

Nursing research tests what is known, introduces what is new, explores what is unknown or poorly understood, and adds guidelines for practice and rationales for action. In hygiene care, some of what nurses traditionally do is validated by research. But much of what nurses do, such as providing bed baths, has been shown to be potentially harmful. In all instances, nursing research must guide practice. Nurses providing personal hygiene care in hospitals, long-term care facilities, home care settings, and outpatient settings must read, inquire, practice, and follow current research.

Nursing students should ask of each practice they are taught, "Has this been studied?" "Has it been tested?" "What does the literature say?" and "How much does it cost?" Nursing practice will be based on scientific data collected by those closest to the delivery of care—nurses.

ASSESSING PATIENTS' HYGIENE NEEDS AND PLANNING APPROPRIATE CARE

The studies cited in the Research section demonstrate that careful physical assessment is necessary before providing hygiene care and that potentially stressful, even fatal, physiologic changes can occur during bathing, especially during turning. They clearly contraindicate some elements of traditional practice—proving, for example, that a bed bath may be more stressful than a shower for a severely ill patient. These study findings are equally important to providing more cost-effective care; for instance, showers and making an unoccupied bed are far more cost effective than their alternatives and thus should be done whenever possible.

The nurse needs to assess the patient's level of physical functioning, patterns of activity and exercise, and rest and sleep requirements before planning hygiene care (Piper, 1986). The nurse also needs to determine how much assistance with hygiene care each patient needs. Physician's orders may specify limits on the patient's activity or position; these orders should be checked and a complete report obtained from the previous shift. Alert, confused, unconscious, immobilized, or critically ill patients may have dramatically different needs. Whenever possible, the patient and his or her significant others can guide the nurse in determining the amount of care needed.

ALERT PATIENTS

Alert and oriented patients with stable mobility may need only to be provided with towels and clean clothes and directed to the shower. An alert patient who has recently delivered a baby, has undergone surgery, or has limited mobility needs more assistance, and should be provided with a chair to sit on in the shower and closer supervision. Such patients may need assistance in cleansing themselves at the bathroom sink or in bed as well.

CONFUSED PATIENTS

Confused patients need nursing supervision while bathing to ensure their safety. The nurse stays with such patients in the shower at all times and uses the shower chair and seat belt to prevent falls. The bed rails of a confused patient's bed are locked in place during bed bathing, and very close attention is paid to water temperature to prevent burns. Several nurse researchers have suggested that the towel bath method is a soothing measure for the confused patient (Rader, 1994; Wright, 1990).

UNCONSCIOUS PATIENTS

Unconscious, comatose, or completely immobilized patients require bed bathing. These patients further require extensive range of motion exercises as an integral part of bathing (see Chapter 21). Special gurneys equipped with drains have also been used to shower patients who are in long-term persistent vegetative states. Such patients must be moved slowly and gently. These patients might become hypotensive if moved too quickly. Even if the nurse sees no signs of comprehension, he or she always explains to the patient what is being done. Care is taken to place the body in anatomic alignment.

CRITICALLY ILL PATIENTS

Patients in intensive care units are bathed only as their condition allows. The Research section discussed several studies of the potential oxygen deficits that may result from turning and bathing a patient. Judicious use of the pulse oximeter and the list provided by Braun and Holm (1989) assist in keeping the patient from overexertion during the critical periods.

PROVIDING HYGIENE CARE AT DIFFERENT TIMES OF DAY

At different times of the day, different types of hygiene care are needed. Most commonly, hospitalized patients and those living in long-term care facilities are given the following types of care:

EARLY MORNING CARE

Early morning care is provided by the night shift or very early morning nurses. Patients are assisted with toileting, using a bed pan, urinal, or commode. Hands are washed (Fig. 26–2). The nurse may assist with oral care. The patient is rolled up in bed for breakfast.

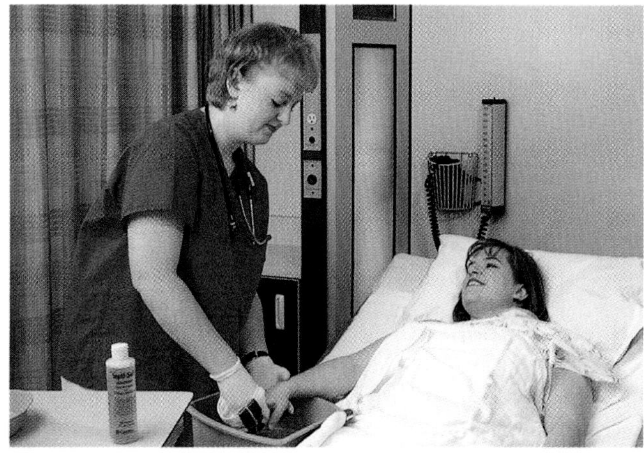

Figure 26–2. Washing the hand.

MORNING CARE

After breakfast, the nurse assists with bathing in one of the many ways to be described. The bed bath, partial bath, shower in a shower chair, shower standing in the shower, bath in a whirlpool tub, bath in a bathtub, or towel bath are all options discussed in this chapter. Oral care, hair care, nail care, leg washing (Fig. 26–3) and foot care are included. Range of motion exercises are done. Male patients are shaved. The patient is given a back massage (Fig 26–4) and clean clothes, pajamas, or a gown is provided. Patients receiving intravenous therapy should be provided with special gowns with sleeves that snap or velcro open, as intravenous lines should never be opened or disconnected to change gowns. The patient's area is straightened, soiled dressings and linen are removed from the room, tables are left clean, and call lights are left in place. If the patient is able to sit up in a chair, a transfer is done, and the patient sits in a chair while the unoccupied bed is being made. If the patient is on bed rest, turn, cough, and deep breathing exercises are done, and an occupied bed is made. The bed linen is changed as needed and per facility policy.

MID-DAY CARE

Hands are washed before and after meals. Patients are offered toileting during the day, and hands are washed afterward. The nurse uses universal precautions to dispose of any body fluids. Sheets are tightened and cleaned of crumbs during the day. Patients in bed are turned frequently. Patients up in wheelchairs have their positions shifted once an hour.

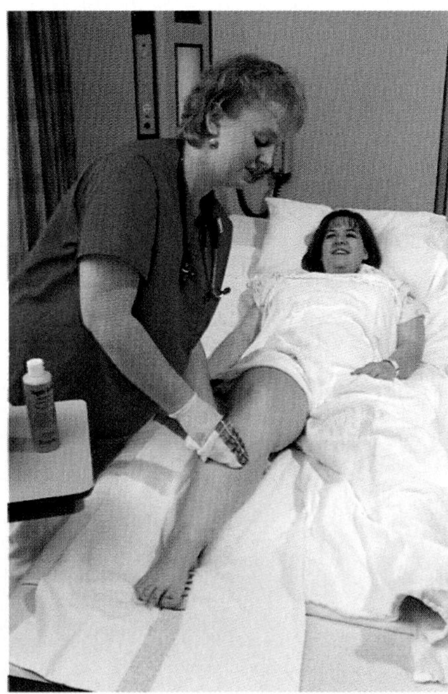

Figure 26–3. Washing the leg.

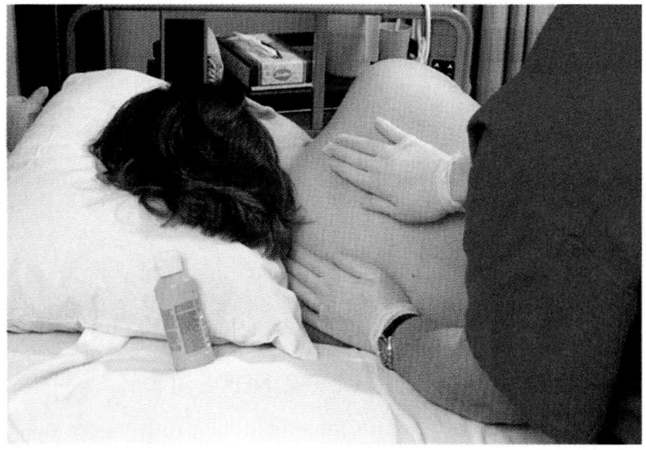

Figure 26–4. Giving a back rub after bathing.

HOUR OF SLEEP CARE

Before bedtime, the patient is assisted to the bathroom or commode or offered a urinal or bedpan. Clean bedclothes are offered. Sheets are cleaned or tightened. Hands and face are washed. Oral hygiene is provided. The nurse gives a backrub to assist relaxation (see Fig. 26–4). Pain medication or a sedating sleeping pill may be offered.

Procedures

BATHING

The nurse may choose from different methods of bathing the patient. These include the shower, shower chair, whirlpool tub, tub bath, tepid bath, colloidal bath, sitz bath, bed bath, and towel bath. Each has drawbacks and advantages; each bathing method should be tailored to each individual patient's needs. Procedure 26–1 outlines the steps involved in bathing a patient in bed and assisting a patient with showering.

SHOWER

Some patients may walk into and stand up in the shower. However, it is preferred that the patient sit on a shower chair. Hot water can cause vasodilation and potentiate syncope (loss of consciousness, or fainting).

The nurse ensures that the call light is readily available and does not leave the patient alone during showering for any period. The nurse may make the bed outside the shower or check on another patient in the room but must be stationed nearby to continually supervise any patient in the shower. This is especially true of patients with anemia, whose low hemoglobin (oxygen-carrying capacity of blood), combined with vasodilation, may cause syncope; patients with convulsive disorders, who may experience seizure; and young children or the elderly, who may be more sensitive to hot water on their skin and for whom the nurse must carefully regulate water temperature. The physician may also wish to order an antiseptic cleanser for the patient going to surgery to decrease surface bacteria.

The nurse then dries the patient or assists in drying and makes certain that adequate warmth is provided after the shower. The patient should be dressed warmly when leaving the shower room to prevent chills. The nurse ensures that there is a bath mat in the bathing room to prevent slips and sees to it that the patient wears shoes or nonskid slippers to prevent falls and possible contamination from hospital floors. The patient may be extremely fatigued after a shower and need to return to bed; the nurse escorts him or her back to bed.

SHOWER CHAIR

Shower chairs on wheels are available for patients with poor balance or mobility in most facilities (see Fig. 26–1A and B). To use one, the nurse transfers the patient from the bed into the chair, using good body mechanics or a mechanical lift (see Chapter 21). The patient should be adequately clothed, and the wheels of the chair should be locked for safety when not in motion. The patient should also wear a safety belt to prevent falls.

While transporting the patient to the shower, the nurse should take care to raise the patient's feet off the floor to prevent lacerations or abrasions on the patient's heels. All of the other precautions for showers discussed previously are applicable here. If possible, a bedpan should be placed under the shower chair during transport to the shower room in case of incontinence. Patients using continuous oxygen via cannula can be transported in their own portable-oxygen-tank-equipped wheelchairs and transferred into the shower chair when directly under the water.

WHIRLPOOL TUB

Whirlpool tubs are used for bathing immobilized patients and are available in many facilities. The nurse may take the patient to the physical therapy department for a Hubbard tank or whirlpool bath for therapy if indicated. The whirlpool tub must be carefully cleaned between patients with an antiseptic solution. Extreme caution must be taken to prevent burns in a whirlpool tub. Elderly patients have very fragile and sensitive skin and can suffer severe burns very easily. All tubs should have working thermometers. Water should be kept at 85 to 90°F, and cool water is added if this feels too warm. The patient must be removed immediately if his or her skin appears reddened. The water temperature should never be higher than 105°F for any patient.

BATHTUB

Hospitals may also have a regular bathtub available. When bathing a patient in a bathtub, the nurse ensures that the patient is agile enough to get in and out of the tub safely, using hand grips, and assists as necessary. The nurse never leaves a patient in a tub alone, observing and supervising all patients but particularly children and those who have recently undergone rectal surgery, in whom heat and vasodilation can cause syncope or bleeding. The tub must be cleaned thoroughly between patients, using an antiseptic solution.

TEPID BATH

A tepid bath is a hydrotherapeutic measure used to lower body temperature. The nurse uses lukewarm water (85 to 92°F) to continuously sponge the patient to increase body heat evaporation and conduction.

One researcher reviewing therapeutic measures to lower fever found that adding ice or isopropyl alcohol, 70 percent, to bathwater quickly lowered fever but was perceived as uncomfortable. Morgan (1990) found that a simple tepid bath, combined with acetaminophen given orally was most effective in reducing fever. The method recommended for sponge baths is to continuously stroke the patient with a washcloth, employing a rubbing motion over the trunk and extremities using some friction, and keeping a thin film of tepid water over the trunk and extremities at all times. If a tepid bath does not bring a patient's fever down within 30 minutes, the physician must be notified to institute further cooling measures (Morgan, 1990).

COLLOIDAL BATH

A colloidal bath is one in which a soothing agent such as gelatin, starch, or oatmeal is added to bathwater to relieve skin irritation and itching. The nurse obtains and follows package directions for use from the pharmacy. The nurse always dries the patient with irritated skin by patting, not rubbing.

SITZ BATH

A sitz bath is another form of hydrotherapy designed to cleanse and provide comfort to the perineal area after childbirth or for rectal, vaginal, or bladder surgery or discomforts. The nurse places the patient in a tub, filling it with warm water and a prescribed dose of medication to just above the patient's hips. Sitz baths must be supervised at all times, as vasodilation could cause syncope. The perineal area is submerged and allowed to soak for 20 minutes; the patient is then extracted from the tub, rinsed, and patted dry.

Occasionally, patients are instructed to attempt to empty their bladder or bowel while submerged in a bath. This is a common therapy when extremely painful genital herpes lesions have entered the urethra and for the first defecation after extensive rectal surgery. Always diligently clean the tub after such procedures using gloves and bactericidal solution.

The nurse may also offer women abbreviated sitz baths with a spray bottle. The nurse mixes warm water with an antiseptic, and continuously sprays the solution over the perineal area for cleansing and comfort.

BED BATH

Nurses have traditionally given immobilized patients bed baths using a basin of water placed on the bedside table. Research studies discussed previously, however, have shown bed baths to be more fatiguing than previously thought and sometimes even compromising to the patient's health. Thus, the nurse should towel bathe or shower the patient in a shower chair whenever feasible.

For a patient with heart or respiratory problems, who may not be able to lay flat for the bath, the orthopnea position is preferred. The orthopnea position is an upright one with pillow support or the arms laid across the bedside table to assist chest expansion and reduce respiratory effort. When performing a bed bath on these patients, the strokes of the washcloth should always go in the direction of venous return to the heart. This prevents edema or further circulatory problems.

Before beginning the bath, the nurse should explain to the patient what he or she is about to do and gain his or her input and cooperation. The patient is encouraged to do as much for himself or herself as possible and should not be rushed. The nurse must ensure proper body mechanics when bathing, moving, and lifting patients (see Chapter 20). The nurse asks for help and uses hydraulic lifts when attempting to move patients larger and heavier than himself or herself to avoid back injury.

The nurse uses universal precautions by wearing gloves during the bath if the patient has any open wound or draining body fluids. Gloves are always worn when providing oral or perineal care, too, or if the nurse has any open lesions on his or her hands or skin.

During the bed bath, the side rails remain up any time the nurse is not directly at the patient's bedside and are put back up any time when leaving the bedside for linen, supplies, or any other reason. If a patient is wearing restraints that are loosened to provide hygienic care, they must be replaced safely and comfortably when the bath is completed.

The nurse respects the patient's privacy and modesty by closing curtains and using bath blankets to cover patients who are undressed and closing the door during the bath.

TOWEL BATH

To bathe a bedbound patient by towel, the nurse obtains a large (7-foot) warm towel that has been presoaked in a 110°F solution of water and cleansing and softening agents. The towel is placed over the entire body, and the nurse gently rubs the patient's body. No rinsing is needed. This procedure has proven to be an effective and desirable method of hygiene among patients and nurses and far safer than bed baths. One company is now manufacturing disposable towel baths (Skewes, 1996).

HAIR CARE

The nurse should wash and comb the patient's hair daily or as needed. There may be occasions, however, when a patient is not allowed to get his or her head wet, such as after cranial or spinal surgery or after a head injury. In these instances, the nurse should use dry shampoo sprays with starch components. Dry shampoo is sprayed on the hair, allowed to absorb the oil, then gently combed out.

The nurse washes, rinses, conditions, and combs the patient's hair. It is important to gently release all the tangles from matted hair. For example, Mrs. Carpenter in the case study requires such care. Patients with alopecia must have their hair washed very gently with baby shampoo to prevent further loss. The nurse should provide emotional support during the procedure, as hair loss commonly has a damaging effect on a patient's body image. Braiding and making ponytails should likewise be performed with care—there have been reported cases of "traction alopecia," hair breakage caused by hair gathered or pulled too tightly (Spector, 1991).

While washing or combing the patient's hair, the nurse should also inspect for pediculosis. Pediculosis is an infestation of lice, which attach themselves to mammals and live by piercing the mammals' skin and removing blood for nutrition. They can be found in the hair on the head, beard, eyebrows, and lashes. Baby eggs, called nits, attach themselves to the hair shaft. Lice are capable of spreading bloodborne pathogens, such as typhus. The lice may be in the pubic hair (*Phthirus pubis,* crab louse) or on the body (*Pediculus humanus corporis,* body louse). Both nits and lice can be destroyed by applications of 1 percent gamma benzene hexachloride, then by removing the nits with a fine-tooth comb. Clothes of the patient must also be specially laundered to stop the further spread of lice residing in the clothing. Fungal infections such as *Trichophyton violaceum* (ringworm) may also appear in the hair. The physician should be contacted for recommendations to kill this organism.

CULTURAL INFLUENCES

Culture influences hair care and hair removal a great deal. Black patients usually have very thick hair, for which a wide-toothed comb or pik is used. If hair is braided into "corn rows" and/or has beads braided throughout, the hair is shampooed without removing or unbraiding these. Patients may wish to have oil applied to their hair or scalp.

A condition called pseudofolliculitis may be seen in black patients as a result of being shaved too closely with an electric or straight razor (Spector, 1991). The sharp point of the hair may enter the skin and cause a type of foreign body reaction, resulting in papules, pustules, and keloids or enlarged scar tissue.

The nurse may find patients with different beliefs about hair removal. There may be Muslim patients and Orthodox Jewish women who shave hair for religious reasons. It is interesting that many American women shave axillary hair and leave pubic hair, and many European women do just the opposite. Muslim patients may shave the hair of an infant soon after birth and also after a pilgrimage to Mecca. A strict Sikh will keep body and scalp hair uncut, and this may present a problem if a preoperative shave is ordered (McAvoy and Donaldson, 1990). The Hmong culture might find it unacceptable for a nurse to touch the head without permission (Rairdan and Higgs, 1992). Traction alopecia, as described previously, may occur in Libyan women, who often hold their hair tightly bound in place with a scarf (Spector, 1991).

SHAVING

Shaving a male patient is an important part of daily grooming. Electric razors must be approved by the facility engineering department prior to use to ascertain that there is no sparking, which could cause combustion. Disposable razors and shaving cream are the equipment most often used for shaving; however, there are patients for whom a razor with a sharp cutting edge would be contraindicated. These include

- Patients with blood dyscrasias, such as platelet disorders involving clotting, hemophilia, or liver failure
- Patients receiving anticoagulant drugs
- Patients with mood disorders, on suicide precautions, or who exhibit violent behavior
- Patients whose risk of spreading bloodborne pathogens is very great, such as patients with the hepatitis B virus or human immunodeficiency virus.

The patient should be assessed for manual dexterity and the ability to shave himself or herself prior to being given a safety razor to use on his or her own.

Female patients may wish to shave their axillary area or legs during hospitalization. All the same precautions apply.

NAIL CARE

Care of the patient's nails is an essential hygiene measure, as various forms of infectious agents can be transmitted by scratching and touching with the fingers and nails. Care would include soaking, scrubbing, and gently cleaning with an orange stick. Any dirt, stool, or blood must be removed from under the nails. Clipping or cutting a patient's fingernails must be done with caution. Mrs. Carpenter in the case study is a good example on someone in need of nail care.

One fashion trend for women is to have long, painted nails that may be natural or artificial. Acrylic or wrapped fingernails are painted or polished, making assessment and cleaning difficult. The nurse must inspect these nails for fungal or bacterial infection. Artificial nails have been associated with onycholysis, a condition in which the nail plate separates from the nailbed and an air pocket forms beneath the nail plate, allowing contaminants to enter this pocket and infection to develop.

The nurse must clean under the fingernails to remove microorganisms when preparing patients for surgery. The nurse also may visually inspect fingernail beds to assess oxygenation levels; a bluish or darkened color indicates a lack of oxygen. Polish should be removed from at least one finger on each of the patient's hands using acetone; some surgeons may wish to have all polish or artificial nails removed. Using a pulse oximeter to measure oxygen saturation rate requires that very long nails be shortened. The oximeter does not work unless the clamp is properly positioned, and long nails interfere with clamp placement. Also, an oximeter cannot read through blue, black, brown, or green nail polish. The nurse should be aware that many nail polishes have blue tints, which will likewise affect oximeter readings (Nellcor, Inc., 1986). Light-colored polish and short acrylic or wrapped nails do not appear to influence oximetry readings.

FOOT CARE

Care of the toenails involves cleansing with a brush, emery board, soap, and water; lubrication; and then trimming. Thick, hard nails require soaking to soften them for trimming. Nurses should not attempt to correct an ingrown toenail or cut the nails of anyone with peripheral vascular disease or diabetes. The nurse should consult a podiatrist for this and any other invasive foot care procedure.

Patients with diabetes need to pay extra attention to foot care (Christensen et al, 1991). Patients with poor vision need an assigned "inspector." The nurse must inspect the feet, discuss the feet, and teach foot care in every encounter with diabetic patients.

ORAL CARE

Many patients need assistance with oral hygiene (see Figs. 26–7, 26–8, and 26–9). Care measures include brushing and flossing the teeth or cleaning dentures (see Procedure 26–2). While providing oral care, the nurse inspects the oral mucosa for moistness, changes in color, and any sign of inflammation, ulcerations, abrasions, or lesions. Gloves should be worn. Caution should be used when placing fingers inside the mouth of a confused patient, as he or she might bite down and injure the nurse.

If the patient is unconscious or has lost his or her gag reflex, he or she should be positioned on the side with the head slightly lowered during oral care. The gag reflex can be checked by placing a tongue depressor in the back of the patient's throat, against the pharynx. If this does not cause gagging, the patient is at high risk for aspirating any contents used for cleaning the oral cavity.

The nurse provides specialized mouth care for any patient whose condition may cause mouth ulcers or infections. This may include patients receiving chemotherapy, undergoing bone marrow transplant, or suffering from acquired immunodeficiency syndrome. Patients living with a nasogastric, gastrostomy, or jejunostomy tube are also prone to developing parotitis (inflammation of the parotid salivary glands) and mouth ulcers. For these patients, the nurse must provide the gentlest oral care, augmented as needed with physician ordered lidocaine gel. When a patient is severely immunosuppressed (lacks the ability to ward off infection), the nurse should use only mouthwash, rather than brushing or flossing, which could cause bacteria to enter the bloodstream and further weaken the patient (Ezzone et al, 1993).

Specific measures are available to comfort a thirsty patient with orders for nothing to be given by mouth (Woodtli, 1990). These measures include performing oral hygiene more often; providing sugarless hard candy, gum, or ice chips; lubricating the lips; and rinsing the mouth frequently. The nurse may also provide various juices or other liquids for the patient to sip or make ice chips that are diet-appropriate to specific medical problems.

If the patient wears dentures, these are removed and cleaned as a part of oral hygiene. The sink is padded when cleansing the dentures to prevent breakage if dropped. When not worn, teeth are stored in cool water in a covered and labeled container.

EYE CARE

Eyes require special hygienic care. When the patient is unable to care for his or her eyes, the nurse can be of great assistance. Patients who are comatose without eye movement or a blink reflex, for instance, are in danger of developing corneal abrasions. The nurse can prevent this by eye lubrication or patching the affected eye.

In addition to cleaning the outer lid surfaces of each comatose patient's eye, the nurse may find it necessary to provide artificial teardrops. This ensures adequate eye lubrication to prevent the damaging effects of drying.

When eye care is given, each eye is considered a separate entity. Potential infection can easily spread from one eye to the other. The nurse cleans eyes from the corners closest to the nose outward (inner to outer canthus), and a separate side of the washcloth must always be used for each eye.

Eye irrigation may be necessary to remove foreign matter, such as hazardous irritants, which may have come in contact with the eyes. Irrigation, too, is always done from inner canthus to outer, with the patient's head turned so that the solution flows away from the face and is not allowed to contaminate the other eye.

The nurse can also help the patient clean his or her contact lenses or glasses. Lenses and glasses should always be kept in a labeled container on the patient's bedside table when not in use. Patients with prosthetic eyes require special care.

EAR CARE

The ears are sensory organs used not only for hearing but also for maintaining balance and equilibrium. Hygiene of the patient's ears usually refers to cleaning only the external ear and the first portion of the external auditory canal gently, with a washcloth. The canal may have accumulated significant amounts of cerumen (ear wax), foreign matter, pus, or other secretions.

Beyond the external canal, the epithelial lining over bony structure is very thin and sensitive, so a physician's or specialist's guidance is usually necessary to clean this inner half of the ear canal. Prescription eardrops and ear irrigations may also be required to remove any obstructive or infectious matter.

Young children or adults may have tympanostomy tubes inserted into their ear drums to treat recurring ear infections. These tubes open an area normally sealed to outside air and water. The nurse should ensure that patients with such ventilation tubes wear ear plugs when bathing or showering to prevent any water from entering the internal ear structures, complicating an existing or provoking a new ear infection.

NOSE CARE

Cleaning the patient's nose with soap, water, and a washcloth is part of the hygienic process. Patients may blow their nose gently into tissue to clear nostrils. The nurse should keep in mind that many small blood vessels are located in the underlying tissues of the nares and hygienic measures not performed with gentle care can provoke nosebleeds, which can be serious in patients with hemophilia and other blood dyscrasias.

Specialized care becomes necessary when the patient is intubated via the nose and secretions form at the external nares. Excessive secretions should be gently wiped away with a tissue. Patients receiving continuous oxygen via nasal cannula, nasogastric intubation, or continuous humidification by mask often require more frequent cleaning of the nostrils and outer surface of the nose. If tape has been used over the nose to hold tubes in place, gummy residue often remains on the patient's nose. Special pads have been developed that can be used to loosen and remove tape.

The nurse should familiarize himself or herself with substances such as tincture of benzoin, which protect the skin underneath the tape and help the tape to stick better. When benzoin is used on the nose, care must be taken to prevent any from entering the patient's eye.

PERINEAL CARE

The nurse should allow a patient to cleanse his or her own perineal area for privacy and dignity reasons but provide perineal hygiene for patients who cannot do it for themselves. To do this, the nurse

- Visually assesses that the patient has been cleansed adequately
- Inspects to ascertain that no pressure areas or rashes have formed

When cleaning the perineum, always clean and teach the patient to clean from front to back to prevent contamination by rectal area germs to the urinary tract. Procedure 26–3 discusses the steps involved in perineal care.

The nurse must exercise great caution if a patient is known to have any sexually transmitted disease. The gonorrhea bacillus, for example, or virus from an open herpes lesion may cross-contaminate or spread the infection from one part of a patient's body to another. If the patient is infected in one area, such as the urethra, for instance, the nurse may inadvertently spread these contaminants to the vagina or rectum.

PATIENT TEACHING
PREVENTING CROSS-CONTAMINATION IN PERINEAL CARE

The nurse teaches patients to always clean from front to back of the perineal area, from the upper urethral area to the lower rectal area. This allows the urethral area, considered to be contaminant free, to be cleaned prior to moving on to washing the rectal area, considered to be contaminated. This precaution helps prevent transfer of bacteria present in the rectal area to the patients's urethral or vaginal area. Microorganisms such as *Escherichia coli,* normally present around the rectum and in stool, can cause urinary tract infections if brought up to the urethra. Female patients can be taught to use this method for wiping themselves with toilet tissue after toileting.

A separate washcloth should be used for each area and disposed of after each use, along with all bed linen and any other objects that may have come into contact with the infected area, in special body fluid precaution bags marked "Infectious Waste."

Male patients may be circumcised or uncircumcised, depending on their age, culture, and country of origin. If a patient is not circumcised, the nurse washes or has the patient wash under the glans penis by rolling it gently up, cleansing underneath, and rolling it back after hygiene care is given. This hygienic care measure is a prime example of a case in which being attuned to the patient's desire for privacy and avoidance of embarrassment and providing it to the greatest degree possible are important.

GIVING A BACK RUB

Back rubs are used to induce relaxation and sedation. The back rub also helps identify and prevent any pressure area forming over bony prominences on the back, in the sacral or scapular areas. The patient should be well covered to protect privacy. Hands and lotion should be warmed before starting. The lotion bottle can be placed in the bath basin of warm water prior to use. Back rubs are generally given with the patient lying in the prone position (see Fig. 26–4). If the patient is unable to lie flat, lateral positioning can also be used (see Chapter 20).

BEDMAKING

Linen on the patient's bed is normally changed after hygiene care is given. If the patient can be gotten out of bed, it is easier to make an unoccupied bed (see Procedure 26–4, Fig. 26–13). For the nurse's safety, the bed is placed at a proper working height. If the patient cannot be out of bed, the linen is changed by moving the patient from side to side (see Procedure 26–5, Figs. 26–14, 26–15, and 26–16). Remember the research results of the energy needed for side-to-side turning: The patient must be allowed to rest during the bath and bed changing process.

PROCEDURE 26-1

Bathing

Objective

Provide cleansing of the patient's skin while stimulating circulation and allowing skin assessment.

Terminology

- Bed bath—bathing of the patient completed entirely by the care provider, without patient assistance
- Partial bath—bathing done in part by the patient, with the assistance of the care provider for that which the patient is unable to do
- Shower bath—bathing by use of a shower facility

Critical Elements

The type of bath should be determined by the patient condition. The care provider should encourage as much independence as possible while still maintaining safety. Be sure to raise the bed to the care provider's level so proper body mechanics may be used.

Limitation on patient mobility should be considered (i.e., traction, casts, paralysis, orthopnea) when assisting with bathing.

Bathing provides the opportunity for skin assessment and is an optimal time for linen change.

Prior to using any skin products be sure to check for patient allergies. Skin cleansing products that do not have to be rinsed from the skin are available. These are preferable for giving a bath out of a basin.

Gloving is essential for perineal care and may be necessary if the care provider may be exposed to any

continued on next page

PROCEDURE 26-1 (cont'd)

blood or body fluids on either the patient or the linens.

The use of a shower bath may require a physician order. Refer to your facility's policy for clarification.

Equipment

- Bath basin
- Soap
- Towels and washcloth
- Hospital gown or own nightwear
- Bath blanket
- Toilet articles (optional)
- Skin care products (as necessary)
- Gloves

Special Considerations

Bathing can be a relaxing time for the patient. It can also be a time when the care provider can interact with the patient and therefore assess a variety of things such as orientation, emotional state, or other needs. When possible, the patient's own personal care items (i.e., toothbrush, toothpaste, deodorant, skin cream) should be used.

When giving the bath, the care provider should proceed from face and neck down the body. The perineal area should be last. Water temperature should be 105 to 110°F. Care should be taken to ensure that the patient does not become chilled. A bath blanket should be used to cover the patient.

Towels should be positioned under the part being washed to protect the bed linens and may be used to cover the body part being washed. The washcloth should be folded around the hand, forming a mitt, so the ends of the cloth are not loose and flapping as the care provider washes the patient. Firm strokes are recommended to stimulate circulation.

Action	*Rationale*
1. Assemble equipment.	1. Promotes task organization.
2. Identify patient.	2. Ensures patient safety.
3. Explain procedure.	3. Promotes patient compliance.
4. Close door and/or curtain.	4. Maintains privacy.

For Bed Bath/Partial Bath

1. Remove top linens and cover patient with bath blanket.	1. Provides warmth and maintains privacy and dignity.
2. Remove patient gown or patient's own nightclothing.	2. Prepares patient for bathing.
3. Don gloves at this time (if indicated).	3. Protects care provider from contact with blood or body fluids.
4. Begin bathing patient or assisting patient to bathe, starting with face, placing towel under body part being bathed.	4. Protects linen from bath water.
5. Dry skin on each part bathed prior to proceeding.	5. Prevents chilling from exposure of damp skin to air.
6. Turn patient to side for back care.	6. Positions patient so back care may be done.
7. Don gloves.	7. Protects care provider from contact with blood or body fluids.
8. Wash and dry well around hips and then around rectal area, remembering to wash from just behind scrotum or vagina back to area of hips.	8. Provides cleansing from area of least contamination to most contamination.
9. Position patient on back in position of comfort.	9. Provides patient comfort.

Perineal Care

1. Position patient on back a. Female—with knees flexed and well apart (Fig. 26–5). b. Male—with knees apart (Fig. 26–6)	1. Provides optimal position for perineal care.
2. Don gloves.	2. Protects care provider from contact with blood or body fluids.

continued on next page

PROCEDURE 26-1 (cont'd)

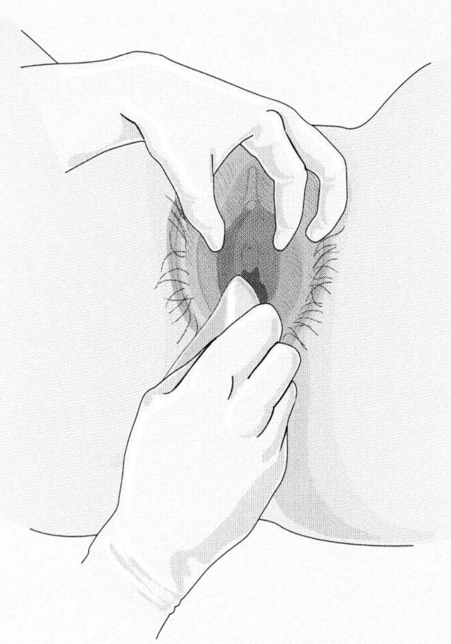

Figure 26–5. Providing perineal care: Female.

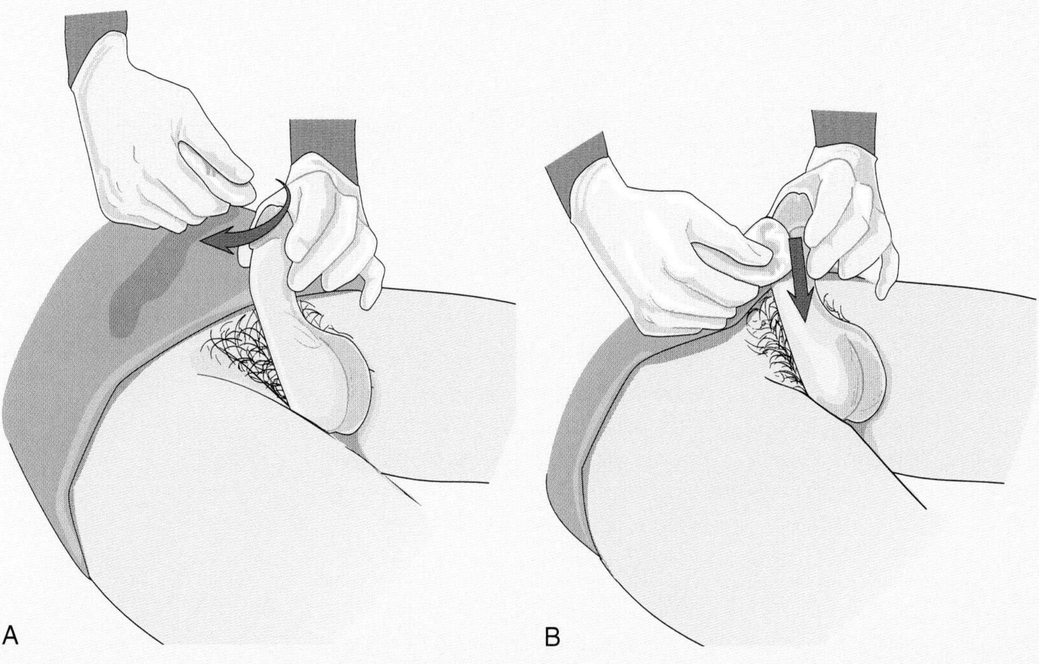

Figure 26–6. Providing perineal care: Male.

continued on next page

PROCEDURE 26-1 (cont'd)

Steps	Rationale
3. Using clean washcloth, wash perineal area from front to back.	3. Provides cleansing from area of least contamination to most contamination.
4. Female patients—spread labia (both majora and minora). Use a separate area of washcloth for each stroke (not reusing same portion of cloth more than once). Note: for women experiencing menses, you may want to use cotton balls or gauze. Rinse well and then dry. Patient may be rinsed by pouring water over area while patient is on a clean bedpan (see Fig. 26–5).	4. Prevents cross-contamination between areas being cleaned.
5. Male patients—wash and dry with firm strokes.	5. Reduces chance of erection with firm strokes.
6. If an uncircumcised male patient, gently retract foreskin and wash underneath it; replace foreskin over glans after cleansing.	6. Removes secretions, which may collect under foreskin and facilitate bacterial growth.
7. Return or dispose of items as necessary.	7. Provides a clean and organized work area.
Shower	
1. Assist patient to shower; robe and/or slippers may be indicated if shower is not in patient's room. Place bathmat on floor to prevent patient from slipping	1. Promotes safety and comfort.
2. Wrap any cast, dressing, or intermittent intravenous device with plastic wrap and secure with tape.	2. Protects cast, dressing, or intermittent intravenous device.
3. Assist patient into shower; may use chair or stool for seating while patient is in shower.	3. Promotes patient safety.
4. Instruct patient on use of call light.	4. Promotes patient safety.
5. Place soap, washcloth, and/or other personal care items within patient reach.	5. Facilitates independence of patient in performing shower.
6. Assess patient frequently during bathing process.	6. Promotes patient safety.
7. Assist patient from shower and with drying and dressing as necessary.	7. Promotes patient safety.
8. Assist patient back to bed or chair.	8. Provides patient comfort.
9. Dispose or return equipment to appropriate place.	9. Provides clean and organized work area.

Documentation

Record procedure in patient record along with patient's response. Note skin assessment and any specific skin care given.

Elements of Patient Teachings

Instruct patient regarding necessary safety precautions for procedure. Also instruct regarding any personal hygiene techniques including patient participation.

PROCEDURE 26-2

Providing Oral Hygiene

Objective

Removal of food particles/plaque while preventing sores or infection of oral tissues.

Terminology

- Dentures—artificial teeth that are able to be removed from the mouth
- Plaque—a soft film found on the enamel of the teeth, containing bacteria, epithelial cell remnants, saliva, and leukocytes

Critical Elements

When giving oral care, it is important to inspect the mouth carefully. Note the presence of any sores, bleeding, dental caries, or food particles present. If dentures are worn, the care provider should assess any problems with the fit of the dentures.

Toothbrushing should be preceded by flossing. Oral care using a soft, moistened toothbrush should be offered prior to breakfast and after every meal.

Patients with oxygen running or those who are taking nothing by mouth have a greater need for oral care because their oral mucosa becomes dry easily. Patients receiving chemotherapy, undergoing bone marrow transplant, or suffering from acquired immunodeficiency syndrome may need specialized mouth care (often with special physician-prescribed mouthwash preparations).

Equipment

- Toothbrush
- Toothpaste
- Small towel
- Cup of water
- Dental floss
- Emesis basin
- Gloves
- Denture cleanser (if applicable)
- Denture cup (if applicable)
- Piece of gauze (if applicable)
- Mouthwash (optional)

Special Considerations

Gloves should be worn for this procedure. Prior to placing fingers in the patient's mouth, care should also be taken with those patients who are confused, as they may bite.

Patients who are unable to move the toothbrush in an adequate manner may use an electric toothbrush. If the patient is unable to sit up, assist the patient in rolling to the side or turning the head to expectorate in the emesis basin. A swab may be used to provide oral care for an unconscious patient. (Fig. 26–7.)

When performing denture care over a sink, line the sink with a soft, clean towel. If the dentures should be dropped, there is less chance of breakage with this precaution. If storing dentures in a denture cup, be sure to label the cup with the patient's full name and identification number.

Always follow manufacturer's recommendations for use of commercial preparations of toothpaste, denture cleansers or soaking agents, or denture adhesives.

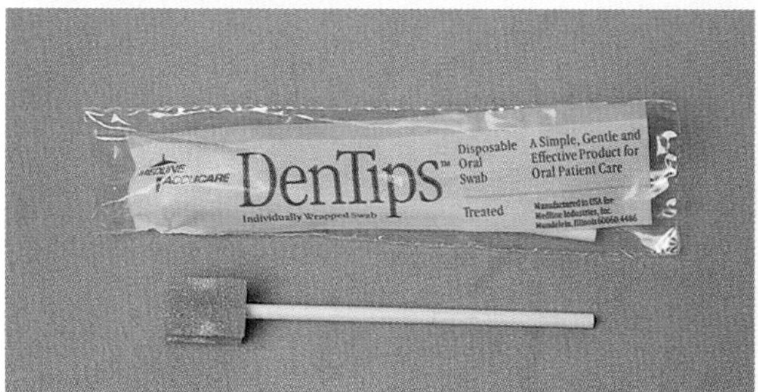

Figure 26–7. Swab for providing oral hygiene to an unconscious patient.

Action	*Rationale*
1. Assemble equipment.	1. Promotes task organization.
2. Identify patient.	2. Provides patient safety.
3. Explain procedure.	3. Promotes patient compliance.
4. Close door and/or curtain.	4. Provides privacy.

continued on next page

PROCEDURE 26-2 (cont'd)

For Patients Who Are Independent with Oral Care

1. Assist patient to a semi-Fowler's or high Fowler's position.	1. Places patient in optimal position for oral care.
2. Place supplies on overbed table in front of patient.	2. Allows supplies to be within patient's sight and reach.
3. Don gloves.	3. Protects care provider from contact with blood or body fluids.
4. Place small towel on patient's chest.	4. Protects patient gown from drips or spills.
5. Assist patient only as necessary with brushing and flossing.	5. Promotes patient independence.
6. Provide mouthwash or water for patient to rinse mouth and expectorate in emesis basin.	6. Removes remaining toothpaste and loosened food particles from mouth while freshening mouth and providing moisture.
7. Rinse patient's toothbrush under running water after use.	7. Removes toothpaste and other contamination from brush.
8. Clean area and return equipment after use.	8. Provides clean, organized work space.

For Patient Needing Assistance with Oral Care (Fig. 26–8)

1. Assist patient to semi-Fowler's or Fowler's position.	1. Places patient in optimal position for oral care.
2. Assist patient in turning head to side if unable to be in semi-Fowler's or high Fowler's position.	2. Positions patient so that fluids may run out of mouth into emesis basin without being swallowed or causing choking.

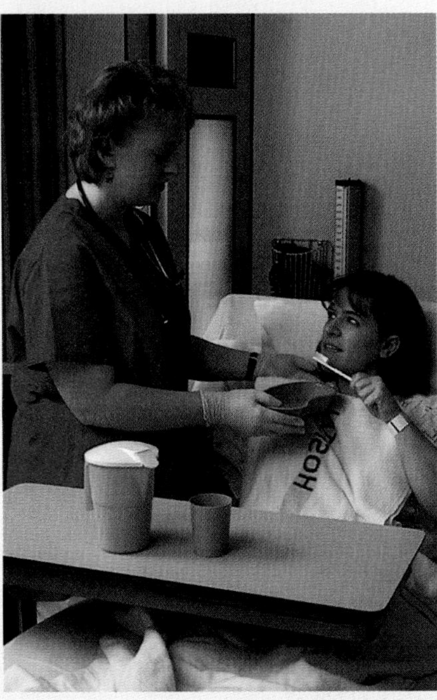

Figure 26–8. Assisting conscious patient with toothbrushing in bed.

continued on next page

PROCEDURE 26-2 (cont'd)

3. Assist patient in flossing by wrapping one end of floss around middle fingers of both hands and pulling tight.

3. Prepares floss for procedure.

4. Slip floss between teeth and use thumb and forefinger to move floss up and down. Use a new section of floss each time it is placed between teeth.

4. Removes food particles from between teeth.

5. Apply toothpaste to toothbrush and moisten with water. Brush teeth with toothbrush at a 45° angle (Fig. 26–9), moving in small, circular motions from gum to bottom of tooth. Repeat on both inner and outer surfaces of teeth. Use a back-and-forth motion on chewing surface of molars.

5. Cleanses enamel of teeth and gums and provides stimulation of gums.

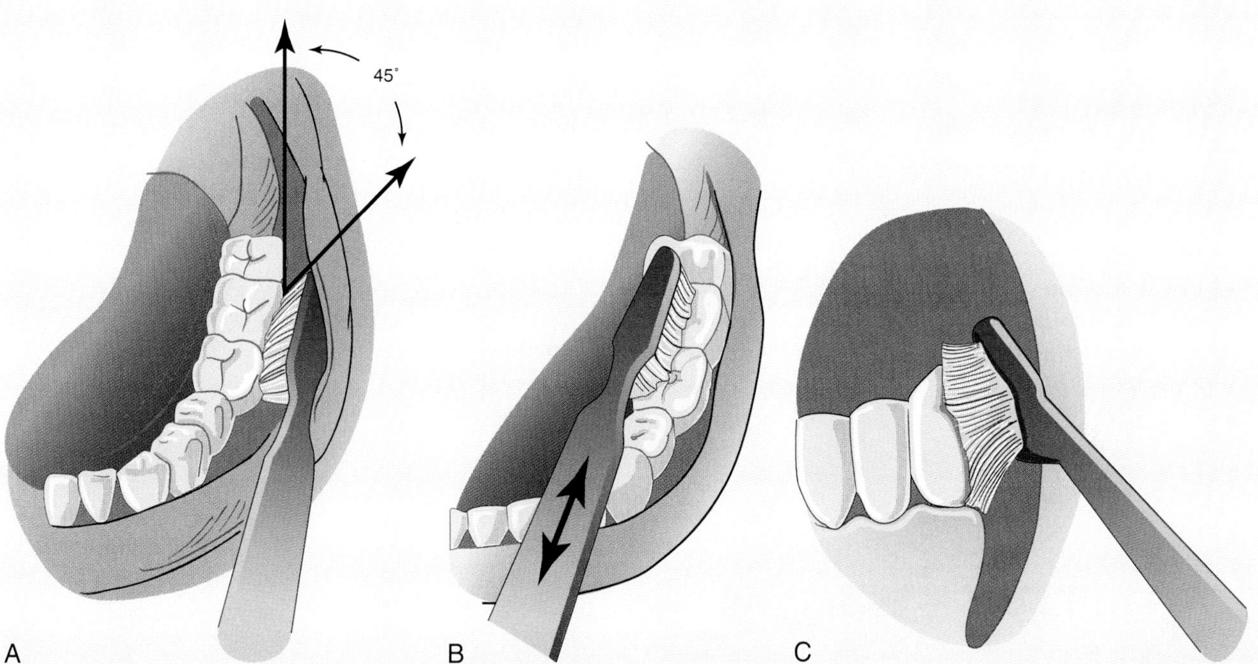

Figure 26–9. Proper brushing technique.

6. Assist patient to rinse mouth with mouthwash or tepid water and expectorate into emesis basin held at edge of chin. If patient is lying flat, then emesis basin may need to be held under corner of mouth.

6. Removes remaining toothpaste and loosened food particles from mouth while freshening mouth and providing moisture.

To Provide Denture Care

1. Grasp upper denture with clean gauze if patient is unable to remove own dentures. Move dentures slightly up and down to loosen, and remove from patient's mouth. Repeat for lower dentures.

1. Allows movement to break suction between dentures and patient's gums.

continued on next page

PROCEDURE 26-2 (cont'd)

2. Place fingers on both sides of partial dentures and gently remove from mouth if patient has a partial denture in place.	2. Protects partial dentures from twisting and breaking, which may occur if only one side is grasped.
3. Take dentures to sink lined with small towel. Brush with toothbrush and toothpaste and rinse with tepid water.	3. Cleanses dentures while protecting from damage.
4. Allow patient to rinse mouth with mouthwash or water.	4. Removes remaining toothpaste and loosened food particles from mouth while freshening mouth and providing moisture.
5. Gently slip dentures in place, taking care to prevent injury to patient's lips when returning dentures to patient's mouth.	5. Returns dentures to cleansed, moistened mouth.
6. Place dentures in denture cup with cool water if leaving dentures out of patient's mouth. Some patients may wish to have their dentures soaked in a commercial preparation of their choice.	6. Allows commercial preparation to remove stains and keeps dentures moist.
7. Cleanse toothbrush under running water and return equipment to appropriate place.	7. Promotes clean, organized work space.

Documentation

Record procedure in patient record. Note patient's response to procedure, as well as his or her ability to assist with procedure. Also note assessment of oral cavity and report any abnormal findings.

Elements of Patient Teaching

Instruct patient or family regarding the appropriate method and times to perform oral care. Also instruct them to report immediately any bleeding, sores, problems with chewing, tooth pain, or other unusual symptoms.

PROCEDURE 26-3

Assisting with a Bedpan

Objective

Provide means for bedfast patient to evacuate bowel and/or bladder.

Terminology

- Fracture pan—a special bedpan with a low profile and a wedgelike rim that requires less pelvic movement for placement than a regular bedpan; used for patients with fractures, body casts, spinal injuries, or restricted movement
- Defecation—elimination of wastes and undigested food, as feces from the rectum
- Urinal—a receptacle for urine
- Void—to evacuate urine from the bladder

Critical Elements

If the patient only has the need to void, then a urinal may be placed or offered instead of a bedpan.

Patients should be positioned for both safety and comfort. If the patient is left unattended during use of the bedpan or urinal, be sure to have siderails up and the bed in the low position.

Privacy must be maintained, both for patient dignity and to facilitate the elimination process. Have the call light within reach at all times. If the patient's condition warrants, the nurse may need to stay with the patient during this process.

Contaminated disposable and reusable equipment should be cleansed or discarded properly ac-

continued on next page

PROCEDURE 26-3 (cont'd)

cording to the infection control policy of the facility. Reusable equipment should be stored out of sight.

Careful cleansing of the skin is necessary after using the bedpan. This is also a good time for skin assessment. Special products are available for perineal skin.

Equipment

- Bedpan or urinal
- Gloves
- Underpad
- Toilet tissue
- Washcloth and towel
- Specimen container (optional)
- Room deodorizer (optional)

Special Considerations

Assessing the needs of each individual patient is important so that the patient may complete the evacuation of bowel or bladder with privacy and dignity.

It is important to assess the patient's ability to move, remembering any movement restrictions due to his or her condition. It is also important to note any change in bowel or bladder patterns, as well as abnormal findings in the stool or urine.

Action	*Rationale*
Placing Bedpan	
1. Assemble equipment (Fig. 26–10)	1. Promotes task organization.
2. Provide for patient privacy by closing door and/or drawing curtain.	2. Maintains patient privacy and dignity.

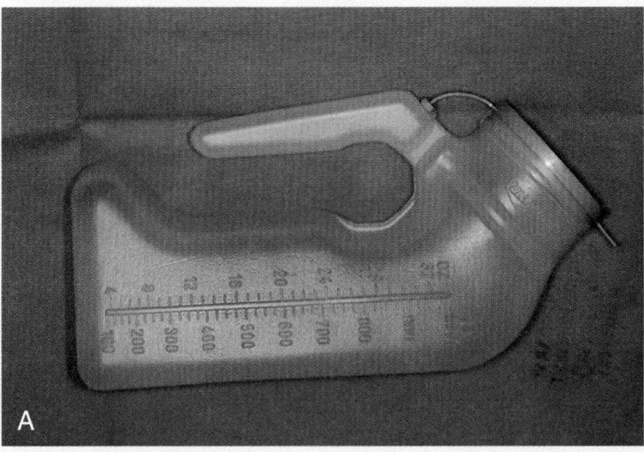

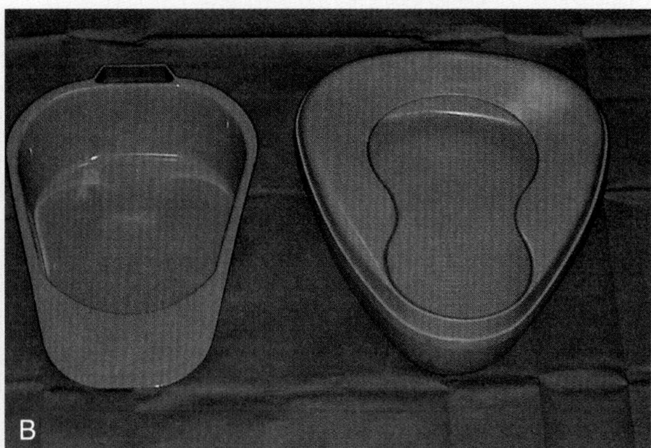

Figure 26–10. Urinal (A) and bedpan (B).

Action	*Rationale*
3. Explain procedure to patient.	3. Promotes patient compliance.
4. Wash hands and don gloves.	4. Protects care provider from potential contamination with body fluids.
5. Place a bed protector under patient's buttocks and elevate bed about 30° (if permitted by patient's condition).	5. Protects bed linen from accidental spillage from bedpan or urinal.
6. Sprinkle cornstarch or powder on rim of bedpan.	6. Reduces risk of shearing forces on skin while placing and removing bedpan.

continued on next page

PROCEDURE 26-3 (cont'd)

7. Position patient on bedpan (Fig. 26–11).
If patient can lift pelvic area:
Slip bedpan under patient while patient lifts pelvic area off bed.
If patient cannot lift pelvic area:
While bed is flat, roll patient to one side, place bedpan against buttock, and roll patient back onto bedpan adjusting bedpan as necessary (Fig. 26–12)

7. Provides means to place bedpan in position while recognizing patient mobility and limitations.

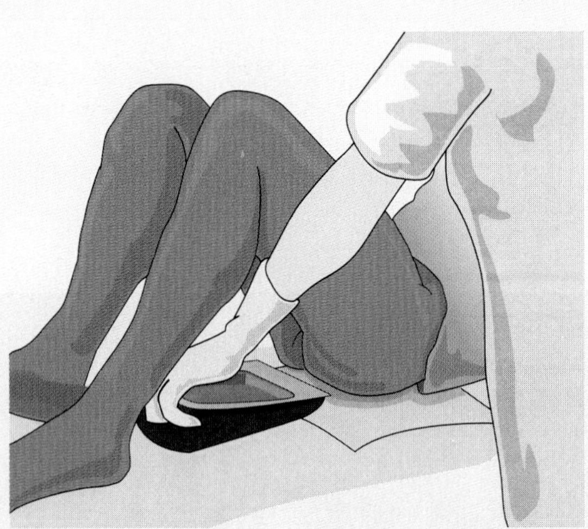

Figure 26–11. Placing bedpan under patient's buttocks.

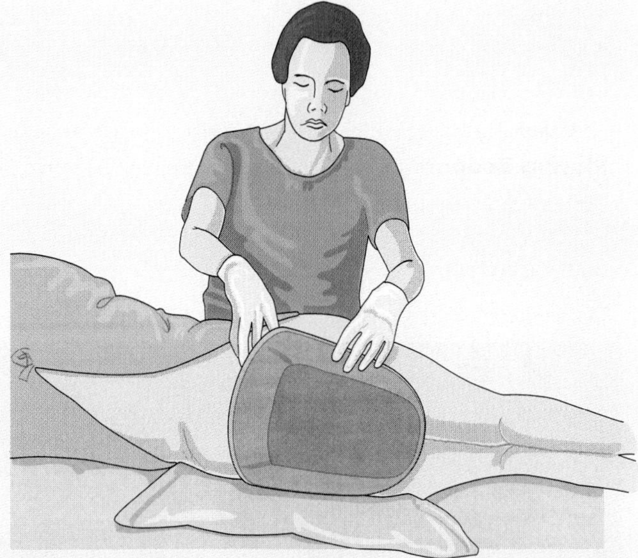

Figure 26–12. Placing bedpan with patient in side-lying position.

8. When pan is positioned, raise head of bed (if permitted by patient's condition) so that patient is in a sitting position. **Note:** If head of bed cannot be elevated, then a small pillow or towel roll at small of back may provide patient comfort.

8. Provides position as close as possible to anatomic position assumed when using a toilet.

9. Cover patient, provide toilet tissue, and make sure call light is within reach.

9. Provides for patient privacy.

10. Remove and dispose of gloves in proper receptacle and wash hands.

10. Prevents transmission of microorganisms from one patient to another.

Removing Bedpan

1. Don gloves.

1. Protects care provider from potential contamination with body fluids.

2. Lower head of bed.

2. Provides better position for removal of bedpan.

continued on next page

PROCEDURE 26-3 (cont'd)

3. While holding bedpan with one hand, do the following. *If patient can move pelvic area:* Have patient lift pelvic area off pan, then slip pan from under patient. *If patient cannot move pelvic area:* Roll patient to one side, holding pan flat. Remove pan once patient is far enough to side.	3. Secures position of pan and prevents spilling,
4. Cleanse perineum with toilet paper or a washcloth moistened with warm water and cleanser if patient is unable to perform task.	4. Prevents possible skin breakdown related to leaving feces on perineal area.
5. Inspect perineal skin area.	5. Identifies any actual or potential areas of skin breakdown.
6. Give patient a washcloth or towel for his or her hands.	6. Prevents spread of microorganisms.
7. Assess color, odor, and consistency (measure if liquid) of feces and urine.	7. Identifies any change in stool or urine appearance.
8. Empty, cleanse, and store bedpan in appropriate manner.	8. Prevents potential contamination of others with patient's excrement.
9. Remove and dispose of gloves and wash hands.	9. Prevents transmission of microorganisms.

Documentation

Record in the patient record assessment the color, odor, consistency, and amount of feces or urine. Note the skin assessment as well as the response to the procedure. Record the appropriate information on the patient's intake and output record.

Elements of Patient Teaching

Instruct the patient and family in the proper procedure for the placement of the bedpan, as well as the appropriate universal precautions. Also instruct them to inform staff of any change in bowel and bladder habits.

PROCEDURE 26-4

Making an Unoccupied Bed

Objective

Provide a clean, comfortable bed for patient use.

Terminology

- Waterproof pad—a paper or linen pad that may be placed under the patient, which in turn protects the bed from body fluids

Critical Elements

The unoccupied bed is made when the patient is able to be out of the bed for any reason. Linen change is usually done after bathing the patient and as necessary.

Soiled linens should be deposited directly into a soiled linen container to protect the care provider's clothing and the floor from potential contamination.

The level of the bed should be adjusted so the care provider avoids back strain and can utilize proper body mechanics. Always leave the bed in the low position for patient safety.

Equipment

- Bottom sheet
- Top sheet
- Drawsheet (if indicated)
- Waterproof pad (if indicated)
- Pillowcase
- Blanket (if indicated)
- Soiled linen receptacle

continued on next page

PROCEDURE 26-4 (cont'd)

Special Considerations

To conserve time and energy, the unoccupied bed is first made on one side (applying all linens) and then completed on the second side.

Always don gloves to remove sheet, which may have been contaminated with blood or body fluids. Should the patient be on an airflow mattress or airflow overlay product, consult manufacturer's recommendations regarding use of bottom sheet and type of waterproof pad.

Action	*Rationale*
1. Assemble equipment.	1. Provides organized work area.
2. Identify patient.	2. Promotes patient safety.
3. Explain procedure.	3. Promotes patient compliance.
4. Assist patient out of bed if necessary.	4. Promotes patient safety.
5. Lower side rails, return bed to flat position, and raise bed to working level.	5. Provides comfortable access to bed.
6. Don gloves if linens are soiled with blood or body fluids.	6. Protects care provider.
7. Loosen linen around bed, remove, and deposit in soiled linen receptacle. (**Note:** fold and save any linens that will be reapplied, such as blankets.)	7. Prepares bed for application of clean linen.
8. Wash hands.	8. Reduces risk of transfer of microorganisms.
9. Apply bottom sheet to first side of bed, fold second half of sheet to middle of the bed. **If indicated:** Apply and tuck in drawsheet or underpad over middle section of bed, folding remaining half of drawsheet or pad to the center of the bed.	9. Promotes conservation of energy to work from one side of the bed at a time.
10. Apply top sheet (seam side up), making sheet even with top of mattress. Place any blankets or additional top linen in the same manner. Tuck top linens under bottom of mattress. Miter corner of top covers at bottom corner of mattress.	10. Secures top covers at bottom of mattress.
11. Move to second side of bed. Pull second half of bottom sheet over remainder of mattress and tuck in. **If indicated:** Pull second half of drawsheet or pad over remainder of mattress. Pull drawsheet tight and tuck in. Center pad on bottom sheets.	11. Completes application of bottom linens.
12. Pull second half of top linens over, tuck in under bottom of mattress, miter the bottom corner of top linens (Fig. 26–13).	12. Secures top linens at bottom of mattress.
13. Fanfold top linen to bottom of the bed.	13. Prepares linens for patient to get back into bed.
14. Apply pillowcase to pillow by grasping closed end of pillowcase, inverting pillowcase over this same hand, grasping end of pillow with this hand, and slipping pillowcase on pillow.	14. Provides means to apply pillowcase without having pillow or linens contacting care provider's clothing.

Postanesthesia Bed

1. Apply bottom linen as in making an unoccupied bed.	1. Provides means to apply bottom linen.
2. Apply top linen to bed, but do not tuck in place. Fanfold linen to side of bed.	2. Provides clear access to move postanesthesia patient into bed without interference from top linen.

continued on next page

PROCEDURE 26-4 (cont'd)

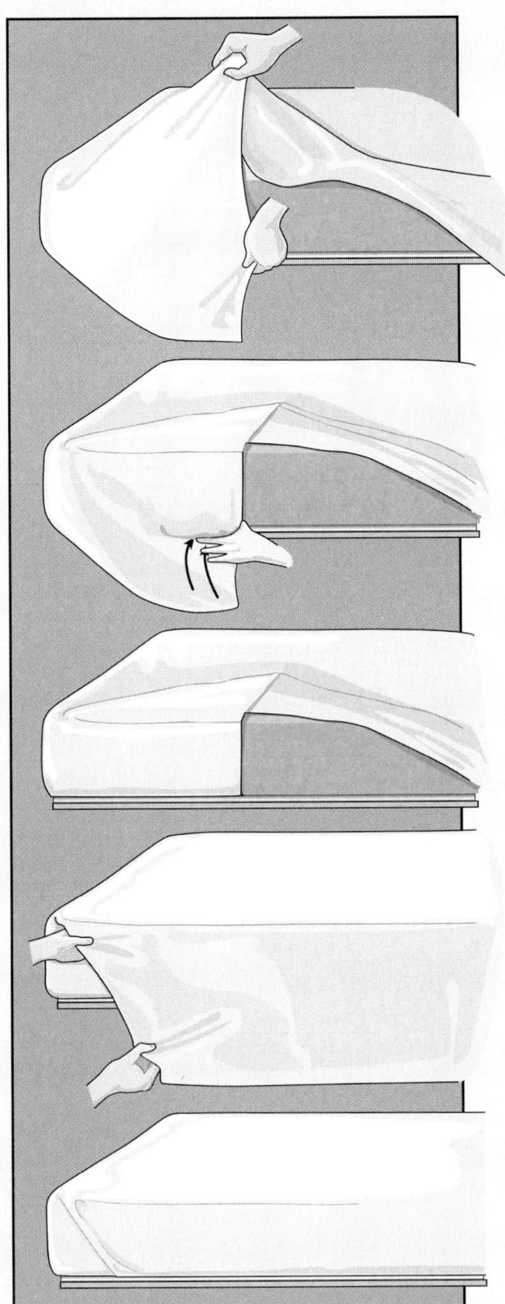

Figure 26–13. Mitering corners of bottom sheet.

Documentation

Record patient response, if any, to procedure. Also record any skin assessment done.

Elements of Patient Teaching

Explain procedure to patient and/or family. Be sure to explain activity or position restrictions necessary when assisting patient from the bed.

PROCEDURE 26-5

Making an Occupied Bed

Objective

Provide a clean, comfortable bed for the patient.

Terminology

- Waterproof pad—a paper or linen pad that may be placed under the patient, which in turn protects the bed from body fluids.

Critical Elements

When a patient is on bedrest, the care provider must make an occupied bed. Linen change is usually done after bathing the patient and as necessary. Soiled linens should be deposited directly into a soiled linen container to protect the care provider's clothing and the floor from potential contamination.

The level of the bed should be adjusted so the care provider avoids back strain and can utilize proper body mechanics. Always leave the bed in the low position for patient safety. Keep the patient covered during this procedure to provide both warmth and patient privacy.

Equipment

- Bottom sheet
- Top sheet
- Draw sheet (if indicated)
- Waterproof pad (if indicated)
- Pillowcase(s)
- Dirty linen receptacle
- Blanket (if indicated)

Special Considerations

Making the occupied bed provides an opportunity to do a head-to-toe skin assessment. An evaluation of the patient's condition must be done prior to turning.

A second person may be needed to assist the patient to turn and stay on his or her side during linen change. If the patient's condition prohibits turning (i.e., traction) the bed may be made from head to toe. For the patient in traction, it is important not to disrupt traction weights. Should the patient be on an airflow mattress or airflow overlay product, consult manufacturer's recommendations regarding use of bottom sheet and type of waterproof pad.

Action	*Rationale*
1. Identify patient.	1. Ensures correct patient.
2. Gather equipment.	2. Provides organized work environment.
3. Explain procedure to patient.	3. Promotes patient compliance.
4. Wash hands. Don gloves if linens are contaminated with blood or body fluids.	4. Reduces risk of organism transmission.
5. Lower side rails on side next to care provider, making sure that opposite side rails are in the up position	5. Provides means to access the mattress for linen change procedure.
6. Loosen top linen at bottom of bed.	6. Allows linens to be moved to side for linen change procedure.
7. Assist patient to roll to side away from care provider.	7. Removes patient from half of the bed so linens may be removed.
8. Loosen all bottom linen on side of bed next to care provider and roll soiled linen as close to patient as possible, with soiled side inward.	8. Removes soiled linen from half the bed while preparing area for application of clean linen.
9. Apply bottom sheet on cleared side of bed (Fig. 26–14). Drawsheet or waterproof pad should be applied if applicable. Roll other half of clean linens with top side inward up against roll of soiled linens.	9. Provides means to apply clean linens to half the bed.
10. Assist patient to roll over linens in middle of bed until lying on side on the clean linens (Fig. 26–15).	10. Provides means to access remainder of bed to complete linen change.
11. Raise side rail.	11. Provides patient safety and support.
12. Lower side rail on opposite side of bed and remove all soiled linens, placing in soiled linen receptacle.	12. Clears bed of all soiled linen.
13. Unroll clean linen (Fig. 26–16) and secure to bed as necessary.	13. Completes application of clean bottom linen.

continued on next page

PROCEDURE 26-5 (cont'd)

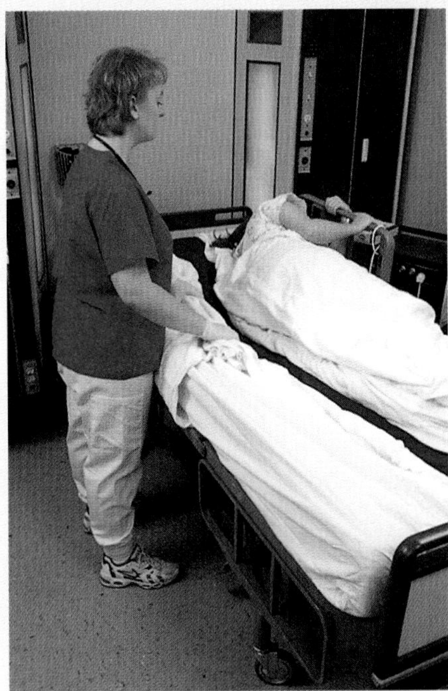

Figure 26–14. Applying bottom sheet on cleared side of bed.

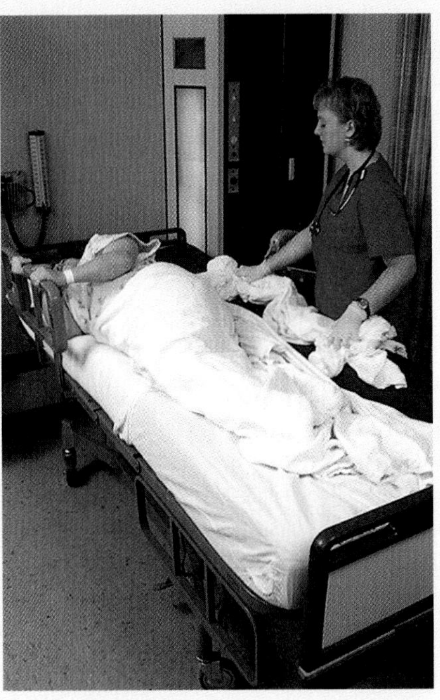

Figure 26–15. Fanfolding soiled top linens close to patient.

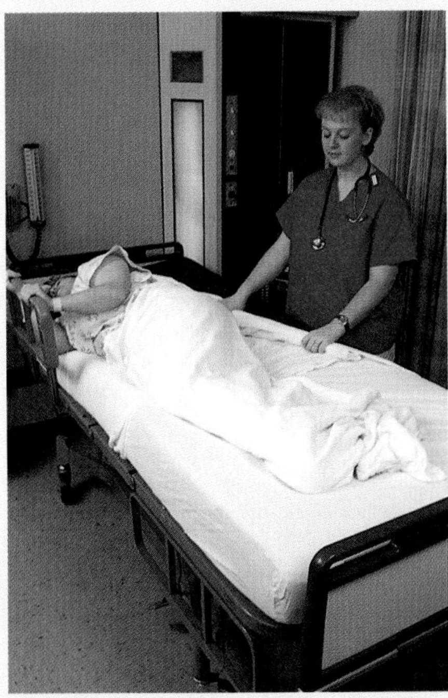

Figure 26–16. Aligning clean bottom sheet on half of bed.

continued on next page

PROCEDURE 26-5 (cont'd)

14. Assist patient to supine position, then remove top linen and apply clean linen as soiled linen is being removed. Remember to keep patient covered through this process.	14. Completes removal of top linen while providing patient privacy.
15. Adjust top linen to provide space for feet.	15. Provides space for patient to move feet freely and keep pressure off patient's toes.
16. Gently remove pillow and apply pillowcase to pillow by grasping closed end of pillow case, inverting pillowcase over this same hand, grasping end of pillow with this hand, and slipping pillowcase on.	16. Provides means to apply pillowcase without having pillow or linens contacting care provider's clothing.
17. Assist patient to position of comfort.	17. Promotes patient comfort.

Documentation

Record patient response, if any, to procedure. Also record skin assessment.

Elements of Patient Teaching

Explain procedure to patient and/or family. Be sure to explain activity or position restrictions.

CHAPTER HIGHLIGHTS

- Personal hygienic care includes measures to ensure patient cleanliness and comfort and prevent infections.
- Basic nursing includes assisting or providing personal hygienic care to patients. Hygienic care consists of cleansing the patient's skin, hair, nails, eyes, ears, nose, mouth, teeth, and perineum.
- Hygienic care has been documented throughout the history of mankind. Greek mythology includes descriptions of the god of healing and the first physician.
- Florence Nightingale, the founder of modern nursing, wrote of the importance of cleanliness and a clean environment in her *Notes on Nursing* published in 1860.
- Knowledge of the anatomy and physiology of skin, glands, and its appendages provides the basis for the nurse to assess the hygienic needs of the patient.
- Research studies have been conducted on cardiovascular response, fatigue, and the energy expended during personal hygienic care. Studies have also included improving patient safety by preventing patient falls and reducing the spread of microorganisms. Other studies involve care of spinal cord injury patients, patients undergoing radiation, and those suffering from diabetes.
- Nurses enter into a special relationship with a patient while providing personal hygiene. The nurse is expected to undress, examine, wash, and groom the patient, who is usually a stranger.
- Various nursing theories include proposals involving hygienic care.
- Hygienic care involves all age levels and both genders. The patient's health care and hygienic habits may be affected by his or her educational, cultural and ethnic background; religious and spiritual practices; and socioeconomic status.
- Personal hygiene is essential for all patients regardless of where they may reside.
- Nurses are legally responsible for safeguarding the patient. Nurses must be advocates for and ensure that the patient is provided essential basic hygienic nursing care.

REFERENCES

Arnow, P.M., Houchins, S.G., Pugliese, G. (1991). An outbreak of tinea corporis in hospital personnel caused by a patient with *Trichophyton tonsurans* infection. *Pediatric Infectious Disease Journal, 10* (5), 355–359.

Barker, E., Higgins, R. (1989). Managing a suspected spinal cord injury. *Nursing 89, 19* (4), 52–59.

Barsevick, A. and Llewellyn, J. (1982) A comparison of the anxiety reducing potential of two techniques of bathing. *Nursing Research* 31(1), 22–27.

Bower, F. (ed.). (1980). *Distortions in Body Image in Illness and Disability.* New York: Wiley Nursing Concept Modules, John Wiley and Sons.

Bradby, M.B. (1990). Status passage into nursing: Undertaking nursing care. *Journal of Advanced Nursing, 15* (12), 1363–1369.

Braun, L.T., Holm, K. (1989). Prevention of ischemic myocardium through activity management. *Journal of Cardiovascular Nursing, 3* (4), 39–48.

Brink, C. (1980). Assessing the problem (incontinence). *Geriatric Nursing, 1,* 242.

Brown, R. (1990). Allergy to dyes in permanent press bed linen. *Contact Dermatitis, 22* (5), 303–304.

Brumberg, E. (1989). Five ways to clean your face. *Health, 21* (8), 84–85, 92.

Christensen, M.H., Funnell, M.M., Ehrlich, M.R., et al. (1991). How to care for the diabetic foot. *American Journal of Nursing, 91* (3), 50–56.

Cleland, V. (1990). *The Economics of Nursing.* Norwalk, CT: Appleton and Lange.

Cohen, F.L., Hardin, S.B. (1989). Fatigue in patients with catastrophic illness. In S. Funk (ed.): *Key Aspects of Comfort: Management of Pain, Fatigue and Nausea.* New York: Springer Publishing Company, pp. 208–216.

Creehan, P. (1995). Toxic shock syndrome: An opportunity for nursing intervention. *Journal of Obstetric, Gynecologic, and Neonatal Nursing, 24* (6), 557–561.

Crosby, L.J. (1989). Fatigue, pain, depression and sleep disturbance in rheumatoid arthritis patients. In S. Funk (ed.): *Key Aspects of Comfort: Management of Pain, Fatigue and Nausea.* New York: Springer Publishing Company, pp. 299–302.

Deines, E. (1985). Coping with PPS and DRGs: The levels-of-care approach. *Nursing Management, 16* (10), 43–52.

Demmerle, B., Bartol, M.A. (1980). Nursing care for the incontinent person. *Geriatric Nursing, 1,* 246–250.

Doak, C.C., Doak, L.G., Rout, J.H. (1985). *Teaching Patients with Low Literacy Skills.* Philadelphia: J.B. Lippincott.

Ezzone, S., Jolly, D., Replogle, K., et al (1993). Survey of oral hygiene regimens among bone marrow transplant centers. *Oncology Nursing Forum, 20* (9), 1375–1381.

Fernsebner, B. (1980). Transcultural aspects. *Perioperative Nursing.* St. Louis: Mosby, pp. 465–475.

Fitzpatrick, T.B., Eisen, A.Z., Wolff, L., et al (1987). *Dermatology in General Medicine.* New York: McGraw-Hill.

Frantz, R.A., Kinney, C.K. (1986). Variables associated with skin dryness in the elderly. *Nursing Research, 35* (2), 98–100.

Funk, S. (ed.) (1989). *Key Aspects of Comfort: Management of Pain, Fatigue and Nausea.* New York: Springer Publishing Company.

Garg, A., Owen, B., Beller, D., Banaag, J. (1991). A biomechanical and ergonomic of patient transferring tasks: Wheelchair to shower chair and shower chair to wheelchair. *Ergonomics, 34* (4):407–419.

Grant, R. (1982). Washable pads versus diapers: Cost study procedure of incontinent care. *Geriatric Nursing, 3,* 248–251.

Griffen, A.L., Goepferd, S.J. (1991). Preventive oral health care for the infant, child and adolescent. *Pediatric Clinics of North America, 38* (5), 1209–1225.

Groer, M., Mozingo, J., Droppleman, P., et al (1994). Measures of salivary secretory Immunoglobulin A and state anxiety after a nursing back rub. *Applied Nursing Research, 7* (1), 2–6.

Harder, I. (1992). *The World of the Hospital Nurse: Nurse Patient Interactions—Body Nursing and Health Promotion* [doctoral dissertation]. Aarhus, Denmark: University of Aarhus.

Hardy, M.A. (1990). A pilot study on the diagnosis and treatment of impaired skin integrity: Dry skin in older persons. *Nursing Diagnosis, 1* (2), 57–63.

Harrell, J.S., Futrell, A., Adams, L.A., Forst, S. (1990). Cardiac output and other cardiovascular responses to two methods of bedmaking. *Key Aspects of Recovery.* New York: Springer Publishing Company, pp. 260–274.

Harrington, R.C. (1995). Health care reform: Impact of managed care on perinatal and neonatal care delivery. *Journal of Perinatal and Neonatal Nursing, 8* (4), 47–58.

Heeschen, S.J. (1989). Getting a handle on patient mobility. *Geriatric Nursing, 10* (3), 146–147.

Henderson, V., Nite, G. (1978). *Principles and Practice of Nursing.* New York: Macmillan Publishing.

Holliday, P.J., Fernie, G.R., Plowman, S. (1994). Impact of new lifting technology in long term care. *AAOHN, 42* (120), 582–589.

Jamar, S.C. (1989). Fatigue in women receiving chemotherapy for ovarian cancer. In S. Funk (ed.) *Key Aspects of Comfort: Management of Pain, Fatigue and Nausea.* New York: Springer Publishing Company, pp. 224–228.

Joyner, M. (1988). Hair care in the black patient. *Journal of Pediatric Health Care, 2,* 281–287.

Kaiser, A.B., Kernodle, D.S., Barg, N.L., Petracek, M.R. (1988). Influence of preoperative showers on staphylococcal skin colonization: A comparative trial of antiseptic skin cleansers. *Annals of Thoracic Surgery, 45* (1), 35–38.

Kaplowitz, L.G., Comstock, J.A., Landwehr, D.M., et al (1988). A prospective study of infections in hemodialysis patients: Patient hygiene and other risk factors for infection. *Infection Control and Hospital Epidemiology, 9* (12), 534–541.

Kelly, R., Zyzanski, S.J., Alemagno, S.A. (1991). Predictors of motivation and behavior change following health promotion. *Social Science Medicine, 32* (3), 311–320.

Kelly, S.B. (1986). Penetrating injury of rectum caused by fall in shower. *Archives of Emergency Medicine, 3,* 115–118.

King, I.M. (1981). *A Theory for Nursing: Systems, Concepts, Process.* New York: John Wiley & Sons.

Kolatch, A.J. (1981). *The Jewish Book of Why.* Middle Village, NY: Jonathan David Publishers, Inc.

Larson, E. (1989). Innovations in health care: Antisepsis as a case study. *American Journal of Public Health, 79,* 92–99.

Larsson, G., Berg, V. (1991). Linen in the hospital bed: Effects on patients' well-being. *Journal of Advanced Nursing, 16* (8), 1004–1008.

Leininger, M. (1991). Transcultural nursing: The study and practice field. *Imprint, 38* (2), 55, 57, 59–63, 66.

Lindell, M.E., Olsson, H.M. (1990). Personal hygiene in external genitalia of healthy and hospitalized elderly women. *Health Care for Women International, 11,* 151–158.

Lindgren, C.L., Linton, A.D. (1991). Problems of nursing home residents: Nurse and resident perceptions. *Applied Nursing Research, 4* (3), 113–121.

Marchione, J., Stearns, S.J. (1991). Ethnic power perspectives for nursing. *Nursing and Health Care, 11* (6), 296–301.

Maslow, A. (1954). *Motivation and Personality.* New York: Harper and Row.

McAvoy, B.R., Donaldson, L.J. (1990). *Health Care for Asians.* New York: Oxford Press.

McKeighen, R.J., Mehmert, P.A., Dichel, C.A. (1990). *Nursing Diagnosis, 1* (4), 155–161.

Memmott, R.J., Young, L.A. (1993). An encounter with homeless mothers and children: Gaining an awareness. *Issues in Mental Health Nursing, 14* (4), 357–365.

Morgan, S.P. (1990). A comparison of three methods of managing fever in the neurologic patient. *Journal of Neuroscience Nursing, 22* (1), 19–24.

Nellcor Incorporated Users Manual for Nellcor N-10 Portable Pulse Oximeter (1986). Hayward, California: Nellcor.

Nightingale, F. (1860; 1969). *Notes on Nursing: What It Is and What It Is Not.* Toronto, Ontario, Canada: Dover Publications.

Odell, M.W., Crawford, A., Bohi, E.S., Bonner, F.J. (1991). Disability in persons hospitalized with AIDS. *American Journal of Physical Medicine and Rehabilitation, 70* (2), 91–95.

Orem, D.E. (1985). *Nursing: Concepts of Practice.* New York: McGraw-Hill.

Ostwalt, S.G. (1969). *Concise Encyclopedia of Greek and Roman Mythology.* Chicago: Follett Larousse Publishers.

Penn, N.D., Belfield, P.W., Marcie-Taylor, B.H., Mulley, G.P. (1989). Old and unwashed: Bathing problems in the over 70's. *British Medical Journal, 298,* 1158–1159.

Petton, S. (1985). Your role in radiation therapy. *RN, 48* (2), 32–37.

Pieper, B., Cleland, V., Johnson, D.E., O'Reilly, J.L. (1989). Inventing urine incontinence devices for women. *IMAGE, 21* (4), 205–209.

Piper, B.F. (1986). Fatigue. In L. Carrieri and P. West (eds.): *Pathophysiological Phenomena in Nursing.* Philadelphia: W.B. Saunders Company, pp. 219–234.

Piper, B.F. (1989). Fatigue: Current bases for practice. In S. Funk (ed.): *Key Aspects of Comfort: Management of Pain, Fatigue and Nausea.* New York: Springer Publishing Company, pp. 187–198.

Piper, B.F., Lindsey, A.M., Dodd, M.J., et al (1989). The development of an instrument to measure the subjective dimension of pain. In S. Funk (ed.): *Key Aspects of Comfort: Management of Pain, Fatigue and Nausea.* New York: Springer Publishing Company, pp. 199–207.

Poorman, S.G., Smith, J.G. (1988). Changes in sexuality related to institutionalization. In *Human Sexuality and the Nursing Process.* East Norwalk, CT: Appleton and Lange, pp. 123–142.

Potempa, K. (1989). Chronic fatigue: Directions for research and practice. In S. Funk (ed.): *Key Aspects of Comfort: Management of Pain, Fatigue and Nausea.* New York: Springer Publishing Company, pp. 229–233.

Pritchard, V., Hathaway, C. (1988). Patient handwashing practice. *Nursing Times, 84* (36), 68–72.

Rairdan, B., Higgs, Z. (1992). When your patient is a Hmong refugee. *American Journal of Nursing, 92* (3), 52–55.

Rader, J. (1994). To bathe or not to bathe: That is the question. *Journal of Gerontological Nursing, 20* (9), 53–54.

Rising, C.J. (1993). The relationship of selected nursing activities to ICP. *Journal of Neuroscience Nursing, 25* (5), 302–308.

Robichaud-Ekstrand, S. (1991). Shower versus sink bath: Evaluation of heart rate, blood pressure, and subjective response of the patient with myocardial infarction. *Heart Lung, 20,* 375–382.

Savage, J. (1989). Sexuality, an uninvited guest. *Nursing Times, 85* (5), 25–28.

Shovein, J., Young, M.S. (1992). MSRA, Pandora's box for hospitals. *American Journal of Nursing, 92* (2), 48–52.

Silberman, B.S. (1962). *Japanese Character and Culture.* Tucson: University of Arizona Press.

Simington, J.A., Laing, G.P. (1993). Effects of therapeutic touch on anxiety in the institutionalized elderly. *Clinical Nursing Research, 2* (4), 438–450.

Skewes, S.M. (1996). Skin care rituals that do more harm than good. *American Journal of Nursing, 96* (10), 33–35.

Spector, R.E. (1991). *Cultural Diversity in Health and Illness.* Norwalk, CT: Appleton-Lange.

Srivastava, R.H. (1989). Fatigue in end-stage renal disease patients. In S. Funk (ed.): *Key Aspects of Comfort: Management of Pain, Fatigue and Nausea.* New York: Springer Publishing Company, pp. 217–223.

Steiger, N.J., Lipson, J.G. (1985). *Self-Care Nursing: Theory and Practice.* Bowie, MD, Brady Communications.

Swanson, K.M. (1991). Empirical development of a middle range theory of nursing. *Nursing Research, 40* (30), 161–166.

Swanson, K.M. (1993). Nursing as informed caring for the well being of others. *Image, 25* (4), 352–357.

Taylor, T.A., Waites, K.B. (1993). A quantitative study of genital skin flora in male spinal cord injured outpatients. *American Journal of Physical Medicine and Rehabilitation, 72* (3), 117–121.

Thaney, K.M. (1981). *Prevention of Immobility. Proceedings of the Third National Conference on Cancer, American Cancer Society, New York.* In *Pathophysiological Phenomena in Nursing,* Philadelphia: W.B. Saunders Company, p. 229.

Titler, M.G., Pettit, D., Bulechek, G.M., et al (1991). Classifications for nursing interventions for care of the integument. *Nursing Diagnosis, 2* (2), 45–56.

Tucker, K., Kaiser, S., Ahrens, T. (1991). Clinical effectiveness of a GI anti-reflux valve. *Heart Lung, 20* (3), 304.

Tyler, D.O., Winslow, E.H., Clark, A.P., White, K.M. (1990). Effects of a 1-minute back rub on mixed venous oxygen saturation and heart rate in critically ill patients. *Heart-Lung, 19* (5, part 2), 562–565.

Vogel, V.J. (1970). *American Indian Medicine.* Noran, OK: University of Oklahoma Press.

Vredevoe, D.L., Brecht, M.L., Shuler, P., Woo, M. (1992). Risk factors for disease in homeless population. *Public Health Nursing, 9* (4), 263–269.

Wagnild, G. (1986). Personal care complaints: A descriptive study. *Journal of Long Term Care Administration, Fall,* 27–29.

Warshaw, C. (1993). Domestic violence: Challenges to medical practice. *Journal of Women's Health, 2* (1), 73–80.

White, K.M., Winslow, E.H., Clark, A.P., Tyler, D.O. (1990). The physiological basis for continuous mixed venous oxygen saturation monitoring. *Heart-Lung, 19* (5, part 2), 548–551.

Willington, F.L., Yarnell, J., Sweetman, P.M. (1981). Cleansing incontinent patients: An evaluation of the use of non-ionic detergents compared to soap. *Journal of Advanced Nursing,* March; 6(2), 107–109.

Winslow, E.H., Clark, A.P., White, K.M., Tyler, D.O. (1990a). Effects of a lateral turn on mixed venous oxygen saturation and heart rate in critically ill adults. *Heart Lung, 19,* 557–561.

Winslow, E.H., Lane, L.D., Gaffney, F.A. (1985). O_2 Uptake and cardiovascular response in control adults and acute myocardial infarction patients during bathing. *Nursing Research, 34* (3), 164–169.

Winslow, E.H., Lane, L.D., Gaffney, F.A. (1990b). Oxygen consumption and cardiovascular response in patients and normal adults during in-bed and out-of-bed toileting. In S.G. Funk: *Key Aspects of Recovery.* New York: Springer Publishing Company, pp. 248–259.

Winslow, E.H., Smith, J. (1991). Effects of basin baths, tub baths, and showers on cardiovascular responses in 51 healthy men and women. *Cardiovascular Nursing, 27* (5), 25–30.

Wolf, Z.R. (1993). The bath: A nursing ritual. *Journal of Holistic Nursing, 11* (2), 135–148.

Wong, S.E., Flanagan, S.G., Kuehnel, T.G., et al (1988). Training chronic mental patients to independently practice personal grooming skills. *Hospital and Community Psychiatry, 39* (8), 874–879.

Woodtli, A.O. (1990). Thirst: A critical care nursing challenge. *Dimensions of Critical Care Nursing, 9* (1), 6–15, 22.

Wright, L. (1990). Bathing by towel. *Nursing Times, 86* (41), 36–39.

Ziemann, K.M., Dracup, K. (1990). Patient-nurse contracts in critical care: A controlled trial. *Progress in Cardiovascular Nursing, 5* (3), 98–103.

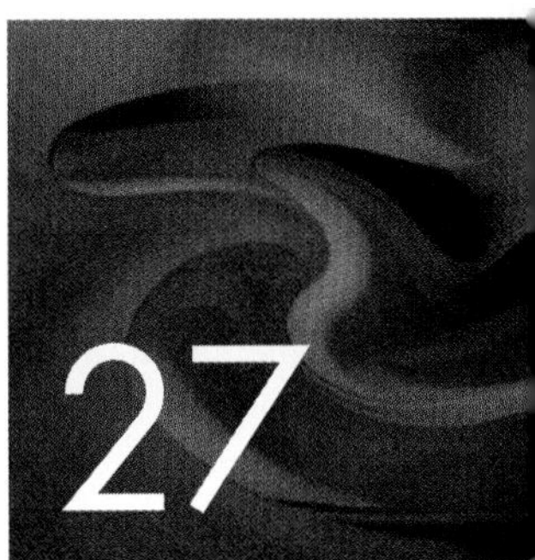

Pain and Comfort 27

Marilee I. Donovan

Paul, an 18-year-old white male, has sustained a fractured left leg and possible head injury in a motor vehicle accident. Yesterday, he underwent surgery on his leg, during which pins were inserted to stabilize the fracture. Today, he reports pain of varying intensity in four sites: left leg, left ankle, left knee, and right knee. His mental status appears stable; his parents report no apparent alterations. Paul's medical history reveals mild juvenile rheumatoid arthritis (JRA) treated with nonsteroidal anti-inflammatory drugs (NSAIDs) and narcotic and alcohol abuse. He is currently enrolled in a drug rehabilitation program and is taking methadone.

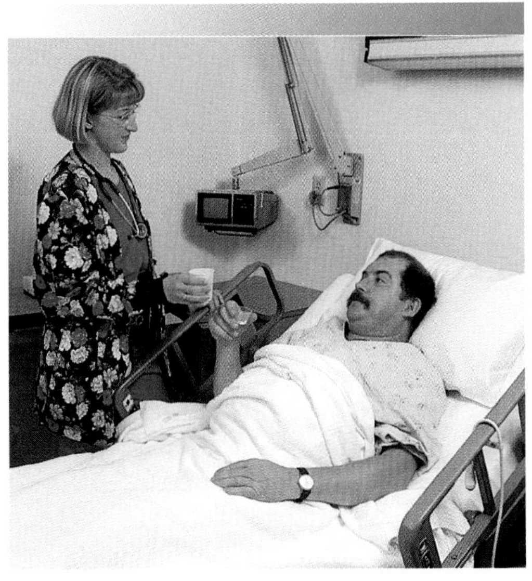

Paul needs to receive adequate pain relief so that he can participate in recovery from his injuries. Paul and his parents need teaching about the nature of his pain and methods of relieving it. All interventions must address Paul's multiple problems: long-term chronic pain from JRA, recovering from alcohol and narcotic abuse. Paul's plan of care will need to be revised daily as his recovery progresses and then again when he leaves the hospital for the home setting.

PRACTICE OBJECTIVES

After studying this chapter, the student will be able to:

- **identify the anatomy and physiology relevant to the individual pain experience**
- **explain to a patient how pain is transmitted and altered on its path from the peripheral nervous system to the brain**
- **conduct a basic assessment of a patient in pain to select individualized interventions**
- **select a combination of pharmacologic and nonpharmacologic pain relief methods likely to be effective for a given patient**
- **identify the sites of action of pharmacologic and nonpharmacologic pain relief methods**
- **teach a patient how to use nonanalgesic pain relievers properly**
- **evaluate the outcomes of pain relief therapy**

SCOPE OF NURSING PRACTICE

Pain is a diverse, subjective experience. That is, two patients with pain caused by the same injuries may experience it entirely differently. Conversely, two patients experiencing pain in different areas of the body may describe it similarly. For example, the pain of two women with a 20-year history of migraine headaches may be less alike than the pain of a patient with herpes zoster (shingles) of the head and neck and that of a patient with foot pain of unknown origin.

Pain is also a widespread phenomenon, indeed a cornerstone of human existence. In a telephone survey, conducted for a pharmaceutical company, of the frequency, severity, and costs of pain, more than half of the 1254 subjects reported headache, backache, or joint pain within the past year. Abdominal pain, menstrual pain, and dental pain were also common (Vincenti, 1989). Other studies have consistently demonstrated the pervasiveness and undertreatment of postsurgical, trauma-related, and cancer pain (American Pain Society [APS], 1995). Research has found that pain

- Is a physiologic stressor resulting in deleterious cardiovascular effects
- Interferes with activities of daily living (ADLs)
- Impairs mood and cognition
- Sensitizes the nervous system to future pain, thus setting the foundation for the development of chronic pain
- Is the primary reason that chronically ill patients seek assisted suicide (Foley, 1991)

Comfort is difficult to define. It is more than the absence of pain, and individuals have their own definitions of comfort. Comfort is, most fundamentally, the opposite of suffering and includes the absence of pain, nausea, fatigue, itching, depression, anxiety, insomnia, and dyspnea (difficulty breathing). These aggravants are multidimensional and interrelated; although it is the nurse's responsibility to isolate and treat these phenomena, they are considered secondary within the context of this chapter. This chapter explores the concept of pain as the most fundamental concept related to comfort.

Comfort measures must be part of any plan of care and are often the only treatments given to terminal patients in the final days of life. What are comfort measures? They can be defined as those activities, approaches, or therapies that yield an acceptable level of comfort to the individual patient. These activities may include positioning, counseling activity, distraction, anxiety reduction, dietary modifications or removal of dietary restrictions, medication, cessation of treatment causing discomfort, or simply being in the presence of another human being. All these comfort techniques must be individualized to the patient's needs. All comfort measures also include these related principles:

- Subjective experience. The patient is the ultimate authority on personal comfort.
- Assessment and evaluation. These are essential to individualizing a plan of care.
- Combinations of interventions. Research and practice clearly demonstrate that combinations of comfort measures provide better outcomes than single interventions used in sequence.
- Frequent reevaluation and continuous modification of the nurse's plan of care.

Pain is often inadequately treated. For instance, more than 23 million surgical operations are performed annually in the United States (Peebles and Schneiderman, 1991), yet in a study of patient satisfaction in university hospitals in which 9000 patients were asked about their pain experience, 86 percent reported feeling pain while hospitalized, and 22 to 39 percent reported experiencing severe pain (University Hospital Consortium, 1992).

Further, the Agency for Health Care Policy and Research (AHCPR) Consensus Panel on Cancer Pain concluded that cancer pain is common and inadequately treated despite the availability of therapies to easily control more than 90% of cancer patients' pain (AHCPR, 1994). The World Health Organization (WHO) estimates that a minimum of 3.5 million people suffer from cancer-related pain each day (WHO, 1985).

Fear of pain and lack of pain relief are commonly expressed by patients. By virtue of knowledge, skill, and patient contact, the nurse is uniquely situated to help patients avoid sources of pain, minimize painful stimuli, address their realistic and unrealistic fears, and treat the pain to achieve maximal comfort.

KNOWLEDGE BASE

Basic Science

PAIN DEFINED

Pain can be defined from various perspectives. The broadest and most widely accepted definition of pain is the one developed by the International Association for the Study of Pain: "an unpleasant sensory and emotional experience associated with actual or potential tissue damage or described in terms of such damage" (Merskey, 1986). The Consensus Development Conference on The Integrated Approach to Management of Pain, sponsored by the National Institutes of Health (1987) suggested three major categories of pain based on its underlying cause:

- Pain after acute injury (*acute* pain)
- Pain associated with cancer or other progressive disorders (*chronic malignant* pain)
- Pain associated with progressive or healing tissue injury (*chronic nonmalignant* pain)

There are other commonly considered characteristics of the pain:

- Its degree of severity (intensity)
- Whether it is aching, burning, stabbing in nature (quality)

- Whether it is felt in other areas around or distant from the original pain (referred pain)

Any of these types of pain (acute, chronic malignant, and chronic nonmalignant) has these characteristics, and they can be very useful in selecting the appropriate treatment. Previously, it was thought that the intensity and quality related to the category of pain; for instance, chronic nonmalignant pain was moderate in intensity and burning or that chronic malignant pain was severe and stabbing. Research findings now confirm that these characteristics are unique to an individual's experience of pain. All levels of severity, all qualities of pain, and the phenomenon of referred pain can occur with any of the categories of pain.

ANATOMY AND PHYSIOLOGY

Because pain can occur in any body region or any body part, the important anatomy is that of the peripheral and central nervous system:

- The peripheral nerve cells *(nociceptors)* experience the injury and alert the rest of the nervous system.
- Nerves are composed of many nerve fibers, like bundles of wire carrying electricity into your house. The fibers that carry pain and the fibers that carry messages that block pain may be together in the same nerve.
- Nerves carry the message of injury-pain *(neurotransmission)* to the spinal cord. These nerves are composed of myelin covered A-delta fibers and unmyelinated C fibers.
- Nerves carry messages to block the pain (A-beta fibers).
- The cells in the dorsal horn of the spinal cord *(SG cells for spinal gate)* integrate a variety of incoming neurotransmissions.
- The cells in the dorsal horn of the spinal cord send the neurotransmission to the brain *(T cells).*
- The ascending nerve pathways in the spinal cord carry this neurotransmission to the midbrain, thalamus, and cortex.
- The peripheral motor and sympathetic nerves carry the messages from the spinal cord to the area of injury.
- The muscles, blood vessels, and noninjured cells in the area of injury respond to the local and central nervous system (CNS) response.
- The midbrain and thalamus add to the response begun in the spinal cord by initiating emotional reactions and modifying the neurotransmission sent to the cortex.
- The cortex recognizes, assigns meaning, and initiates a variety of responses to the message that has been perceived as pain.
- The descending nerve pathways in the spinal cord carry the neurotransmission from the cortex, midbrain, and thalamus to the spinal cord and area of injury.

PAIN TRANSMISSION AND SENSATION

When a body part is injured by pressure, cutting, intense heat or cold, chemicals, or lack of oxygen, the injured cells release a variety of substances that are normally intracellular. When these intracellular substances are released into the extracellular space around the nociceptors, these neurons are depolarized (excited), and the nerve impulse begins to move along the nerve fiber (neurotransmission). More than 40 substances have been identified as playing a role in this process of exciting nociceptors; these substances are called *neurotransmitters.* Among the most common of these substances are prostaglandins, substance P, epinephrine, and potassium. In addition to depolarizing the nociceptors, these neurotransmitters also

- Dilate blood vessels in the injured area
- Increase *edema* (fluid accumulation in the injured area)
- Increase *hypersensitivity* (excessive or heightened sensitivity to pain or even touch in the area surrounding the original injury) (Coderre et al, 1993; Mao et al, 1995; Paice, 1988).

This neurotransmission is then carried over A-delta or C fibers to the dorsal horn of the spinal cord. The nerve fibers then release more neurotransmitters, which carry the pain message to *T cells,* neurons in the spinal cord. If the chemical message is strong enough, these T cells then provoke the following series of events:

- The pain message is transmitted up to the midbrain, thalamus, and cortex
- A message is sent to the nervous system's periphery to protect the injured area by increasing muscle tone by muscle spasm and increasing hypersensitivity
- *Inflammation,* or vascular dilation of injured tissue, results, bringing cells and chemicals to start the process of healing.

The body also has the capacity to send messages over the A-beta fibers to minimize or block the pain in the spinal cord. In general, these blocking or modulating processes occur by raising the threshold of the next nerve cell so that it takes more input to depolarize or excite the next nerve cell. For example, if it takes 10 units of input to depolarize the neurons in the spinal cord and the pain impulse is 12 units, then they will be depolarized and send on the pain transmission. However, if the threshold for excitation of the second neurons can be raised to 13 units, no pain transmission will occur, even though the periphery is still sending in a message of 12 units. We now know that some of this occurs without conscious control but that it can also be stimulated by instinctive responses such as rubbing, or application of ice. This process is called *neuromodulation.* In addition to the input from the periphery, there are also modulating processes that occur among the cells in the spinal cord and processes that are initiated by the midbrain and cortex, which reduce the transmission of pain from one cell in the spinal cord to the next. Without these normal processes of neuromodulation, an individual is hypersensitive to pain. It has been proposed that many chronic pain problems are the result of impaired neuromodulation or a combination of impaired neuromodulation and hypersensitization.

Even if the patient receives a general anesthetic, pain impulses carried from the periphery to the spinal cord stimulate the sensitization process directed by the spinal cord. However, if the patient receives a general anesthetic *and* a local anesthetic, this sensitization is minimized, and patients report less postoperative pain (Woolf, 1991).

If neurotransmission exceeds neuromodulation in the dorsal horn of the spinal cord and the pain message is transmitted to the midbrain and cortex, additional interactions occur that result in

1. Recognition of the sensation as pain: "Ouch, that hurts!"
2. Identification of the site of pain: "I stubbed my *right great toe.*"
3. Emotional reaction to pain. The emotional reaction to pain is largely governed by
   - An individual's family culture: do these family members cry easily? Withdraw when upset? Express anger when frightened? Show little emotion at any time?
   - The individual's personality: Is he or she anxious or fearful? Quiet? Outgoing?
   - The context of the injury: "Who left that box in the middle of the hall?" "How long before I will be able to go back to work?" "Is it cancer?" "Will the pain ever get better?"
   - Activation of the stress response (Cousins, 1989).
   - Initially vasodilatation, edema, white blood cells in the area, and increased heart rate, respirations, and blood pressure; these eventually decrease.
   - After several days or weeks of a stress like pain, the body's response is often vasoconstriction, muscle tension, rare vital sign changes, or gastrointestinal distress.
   - Suppression of the immune response (Liebeskind, 1991a; Page, 1996)
   - Pain decreases the activity of some of the white blood cells responsible for eliminating cancer cells from the body; in animal studies, pain increases the development of cancer and the risk and rate of metastases.
   - Increased messages to the dorsal horn of the spinal cord; these can either increase neuromodulation or neurotransmission.
   - An example of how the cortex can increase neuromodulation: a person practices deep breathing and relaxation. This reduces muscle tension, producing less nociceptive input; it increases oxygenation, which reduces the amount of injury from hypoxia; it increases blood flow, which removes neurotransmitters from the peripheral area of injury and from around the neurons in the dorsal horn of the spinal cord. It also is thought to raise the threshold for activation of the T cells in the dorsal horn of the spinal cord. When the threshold for activation is raised, more neurotransmission is needed to excite this next neuron.
   - An example of how the cortex can increase neurotransmission: depressed patients often have insufficient serotonin produced in their brain. Without sufficient serotonin, the neurons in the spinal cord are depolarized at a lower than normal level. Pain is felt from sensations that would not normally be interpreted as pain, and painful sensations are felt more intensely.

For readers who desire to explore the pathophysiology of pain in more detail, the articles by Coderre (1993) and Mao (1995) and their colleagues are the clearest we have found.

PSYCHOSOCIAL ASPECTS OF PAIN

Contemporary research indicates that emotions, psychological factors, and individual characteristics may increase or decrease the pain experience (Gamsa, 1994). John Liebeskind, former president of the American Pain Society, warned that it is as foolish to consider pain a psychological problem as it is to ignore the psychological aspects of pain (Liebeskind, 1991b).

Increasingly, research shows that psychological states are affected by some of the same neurotransmitters involved in the physiologic transmission and modulation of pain. For instance, many forms of depression are associated with decreased serotonin levels. (Serotonin is a key neurotransmitter involved in the transmission and modulation of pain.) It is thus not surprising that antidepressants, which alter serotonin levels, alter pain perception as well. In some patients, depression can increase perceptions of pain and decrease perceptions of general quality of life.

Anxiety is the most common emotion associated with acute pain, and depression the most common emotion associated with chronic pain. However, research has indicated that the patient's emotional reaction to pain is far more variable than this. Caregivers tend to overestimate their patients' anxiety and underestimate the extent of their depression. The nurse should systematically assess mood in all patients with pain.

When pain is not as easily relieved as the physician or nurse anticipates, the patient is often labeled "anxious" and an antianxiety medication is ordered. Such medication will often sedate the patient sufficiently to reduce the expression of pain but seldom relieve the pain itself. It is more likely that the pain is causing the patient to be anxious than that the anxiety is producing unrelieved pain; for many patients, not knowing the cause of the pain is in itself anxiety provoking. If the cause of the pain can be identified and discussed, the anxiety may be relieved.

Pain for which no known cause can be found or pain associated with a progressive illness is usually more stressful than pain that has a clear, treatable cause. Nurses and physicians should generally defer treatment of anxiety with medication until an aggressive approach is made to control the pain. Research has shown that the anxiety will often disappear when the pain is controlled (McCaffery and Beebe, 1989).

Relevant Theory

There are a variety of theories regarding the physiology of pain, the process of assigning meaning to pain, and the various therapies. No single theory of pain or pain therapy completely explains all that is observed about pain production, transmission, perception, reaction, and relief. The gate control theory of pain and Loesser's model of pain are the most useful for understanding and planning interventions to reduce pain and increase comfort.

GATE CONTROL THEORY

The gate control theory of pain, originally proposed by Melzack and Wall in 1965, is the most comprehensive explanation of the phenomenon of pain proposed so far (Fig. 27–1). They identified two types of nerve fibers entering the cord from the periphery: the A-delta and C fibers (also called small nerve fibers) carrying pain transmission and the A-beta fibers (also called large nerve fibers) carrying sensations that were capable of blocking pain. Before the chemicals responsible for neurotransmission and neuromodulation had been identified, Melzack and Wall proposed that there was a "gating" mechanism in the dorsal horn of the spinal cord. In this area of the cord, input from the brain and midbrain is combined with input from the peripheral neurotransmitters and the peripheral neuromodulators. The balanced neurotransmitters and neuromodulation determine whether the pain transmission ascends to the brain or is blocked by the "gate" in the cord. This theory was the first to begin to explain how cortical processes like fear, memory, and a variety of psychosocial variables could affect pain transmission. It also was the first to begin to explain how such diverse therapies as breathing techniques, massage, opiates, and ice can produce pain relief.

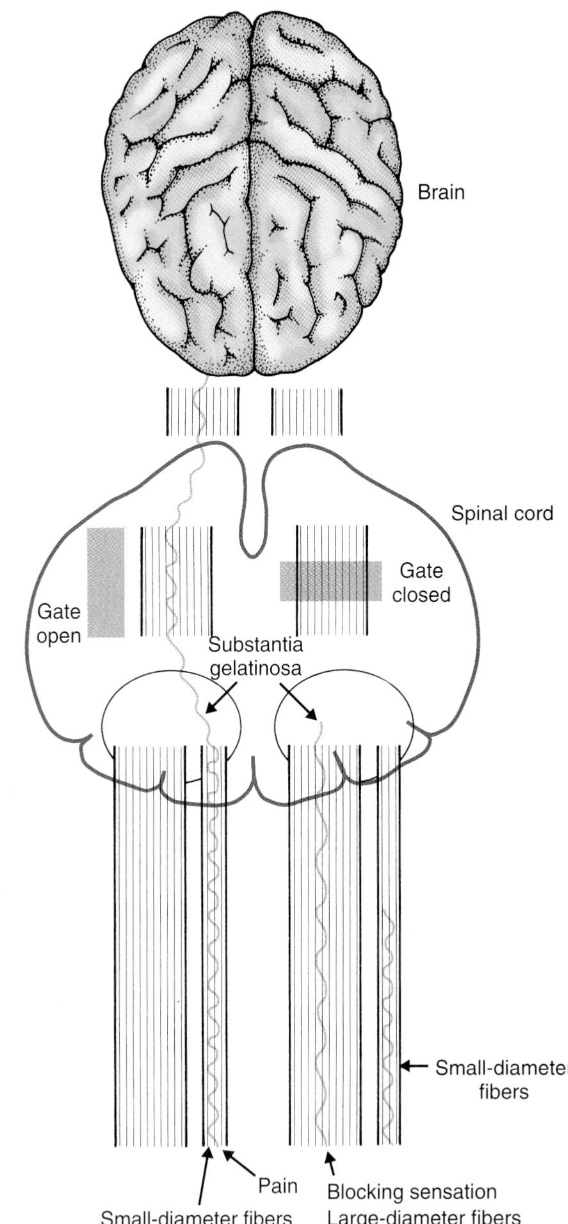

Figure 27–1. The gate control theory of pain. From Ignatavicius, D., Workman, M.J., Mishler, M. (1999). *Medical-Surgical Nursing: Care Across the Continuum,* 3rd ed. Philadelphia: W.B. Saunders. Used with permission.

LOESSER MODEL OF PAIN

A multilayered model of pain was developed by John Loesser, director of the Pain Clinic at the University of Washington, in 1986. Loesser's model includes four factors: nociception, suffering, pain experience, and pain behaviors. *Nociception* refers primarily to the processes of neurotransmission and neuromodulation described above. *Suffering* is a cortical activity and involves such diverse functions as memory, emotion, meaning of the pain to the individual, depression, and fear. The following examples illustrate how suffering can vary a great deal based on the meaning of the pain and emotional responses and how the overall pain experience is unique to the individual:

- Perineal pain: A 35-year-old woman who has a long, exhausting labor, resulting in the delivery of a healthy baby, whom she and her spouse have tried to have for 10 years, may suffer very little from her perineal pain. A 35-year-old woman whose vaginal hysterectomy showed a rapidly growing cancer that had spread beyond the uterus is likely to be suffering a great deal from her perineal pain.
- A broken leg: A 25-year-old construction worker who dislikes his job may experience no suffering from his

broken leg. A 25-year-old pilot who cannot take her long-awaited flight test for the newest jet airplane may suffer increased pain, frustration, anger, and anxiety about her future.

Nociception, suffering, and the pain experience are internal processes and can be known to the nurse only through the patient's pain behaviors. Pain behaviors include both verbal reports and nonverbal expressions of pain.

DONOVAN'S ADAPTATION OF LOESSER'S MODEL

Another theory of pain proposes that to understand pain and pain relief, the nurse must add up the pain the patient expresses to family, friends, and health care providers (Donovan, 1990) (Fig. 27–2). These system responses shape how much pain the patient will tolerate and report and the actions performed in response to this report (Strauss, 1974). For instance, most subcultures in the United States expect men to be strong, so men are more likely to deny or minimize their pain. A family who believes that pain is punishment from God may be hesitant to treat pain, because it would be interfering with the will of God. A nurse who believes that a patient is a drug seeker may consistently undermedicate that patient.

Relevant Research

NURSING RESEARCH

INADEQUATE KNOWLEDGE AND ATTITUDES OF CAREGIVERS

Many researchers have documented a significant lack of knowledge about pain assessment and management among nurses, other caregivers, and nursing faculty (Donovan, 1992; Edwards, 1990; Marks and Sachar, 1973; Von Roenn et al, 1993; Vortherms et al, 1992; Watt-Watson, 1987). In fact, a study of the knowledge and attitudes of nursing faculty revealed that up to 57 percent of faculty members have inadequate or erroneous knowledge in several key areas despite excellent knowledge in related areas (Ferrell, et al, 1992):

- 57 percent did not know the duration of action of common opiates. **Fact:** this misinformation could result in too-frequent dosing with long-acting opiates or too-infrequent dosing with short-acting opiates.

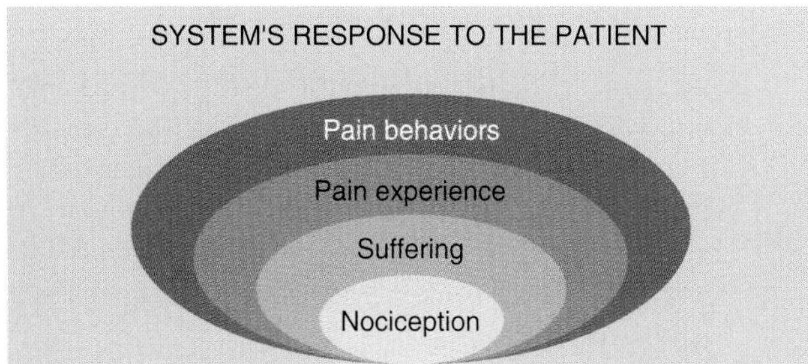

Figure 27–2. Donovan's adaptation of Loesser's pain model.

- 45 percent expected that chronic pain would be localized. **Fact:** research indicates that chronic pain is constantly changing, and the most painful site often varies from day to day.
- 35 percent did not know that the risk of respiratory depression is minor in patients taking large doses of opiates for a long time. **Fact:** tolerance to the respiratory side effects of opiates develops early; the true risk of respiratory depression is with the first few doses at a new dosage.
- 25 percent did not have complete pain relief as a goal. **Fact:** nurses may not always achieve complete pain relief, but if they do not even try, it most definitely will not be achieved.
- 31 percent thought that patient clock watching was a sign of addiction. **Fact:** clock watching is usually a sign of medication being given less frequently than the duration of action of the ordered analgesic.

EFFECTS OF PAIN ON INFANTS

Research has indicated that infants not only experience pain but that the experience is actively harmful. Stress responses and immune suppression occur even in a premature neonate. One experimental study demonstrated that infants who received a higher concentration of analgesics as part of surgical care had fewer complications and a lower mortality rate than those who received less analgesic (Anand and Hickey, 1987).

The most common sources of childhood pain are lacerations, infections, insect bites, burns, sprains, sore throats, stomach aches, headaches, and earaches (Ross and Ross, 1988). In a health care setting, the most common causes of pain are blood draws, insertion of intravenous catheters, injections, and postoperative pain (Wong and Baker, 1988).

ASSESSMENT OF PAIN

Several studies have demonstrated that patients, physicians, and nurses do not agree as to the intensity of a patient's pain (Donovan et al, 1989; Grossman et al, 1991). Some have shown that nurses and physicians underestimate the amount of pain experienced by patients (Grossman et al, 1991; McGuire and Yarbro, 1987). A study of 270 patients with cancer indicated that these patients often did not report their pain because they wanted to be good patients and that they were reluctant to use analgesics (Ward et al, 1993).

RESEARCH FROM OTHER FIELDS

UNDERTREATMENT OF PAIN

Undertreatment of patients with pain is a well-documented phenomenon (APS, 1995; Donovan et al, 1987; Marks and Sachar, 1973). Investigators have proposed several reasons for this continuing dilemma:

- Inadequate knowledge and attitudes of caregivers (physicians, nurses, patients, and families)

- Fear of addiction to narcotics
- Fear of developing tolerance to the medication, reducing its effectiveness
- Fear of respiratory depression
- Failure to assess patients at risk of pain
- Failure to evaluate the outcomes of therapy

SCIENTIFIC EVIDENCE FOR TREATMENTS

In the past 5 years, there have been federally sponsored multidisciplinary guideline panels and a consensus conference related to pain and pain therapies. Guidelines are systematically developed statements to guide practice; they are based on a thorough review of the empirical evidence available.

The AHCPR Guideline on Management of Cancer Pain (1994) reported research findings in support of encouraging the patient to be active, thus preventing prolonged immobilization, and to participate in self-care, behavioral and cognitive therapies, relaxation and imagery, and patient education. The guideline panel also reported expert opinion but limited research in support of the application of heat or cold, massage, exercise and positioning, transcutaneous electrical nerve stimulation (TENS), and acupuncture. They also stressed that, in general, these therapies are in addition to pharmacologic, surgical, or radiotherapeutic treatments, and are not substitutes for them.

An extensive literature survey by the AHCPR Guideline on Acute Low Back Problems in Adults indicated scientific data supporting patient education, spinal manipulation within the first 4 weeks of pain if there are no symptoms of neurologic deficit, and return to normal activities as quickly as possible. In addition, they report expert opinion but limited research in support of NSAIDs like acetaminophen or ibuprofen, heat or cold as self-care therapy, shoe insoles, low-stress aerobic exercise, and gradual conditioning of back muscles.

In 1996, the National Institutes of Health held a technology assessment conference on integration of behavioral and relaxation approaches in the treatment of chronic pain and insomnia. They reported strong evidence for the effectiveness of the following therapies: relaxation, hypnosis, cognitive-behavioral therapies, and biofeedback. They concluded that there is no evidence to suggest that one of these therapies is superior to another, that in a given individual "one approach may indeed be more appropriate than another."

FEAR OF ADDICTION, TOLERANCE, AND RESPIRATORY DEPRESSION

Fear of addiction is common among patients, family members, nurses, and physicians. The majority of physicians, nurses, and patients surveyed in many studies believe that a patient who takes narcotics regularly will become addicted (Marks and Sachar, 1973; McCaffery et al, 1990; Ward et al, 1993; Watt-Watson, 1987). The available scientific evidence strongly disputes this belief, however. In a study published in the *New England Journal of Medicine,* only 4 of 11,882 patients treated with narcotics for postoperative pain became addicted (Porter and Jick, 1980). Another survey reported that in a major headache treatment center, only 3 of 2369 patients were abusing narcotics. Each year, additional studies are published indicating that drug abuse and drug addiction in the patient with pain are extremely rare (Portenoy, 1990).

In a patient like Paul, discussed earlier, the nurse may hesitate to administer an ordered long-acting opiate for fear of a "high" or euphoric state. This is yet another myth: opiates of long duration, like methadone, do not create euphoric states and so are less likely to reactivate a recovering addict's craving.

Fear of respiratory depression has become a fear as common and as unrealistic as the fear of addiction. The belief that morphine produces life-threatening respiratory depression is reinforced in most textbooks and pharmacology lectures (Ferrell et al, 1992). Certainly, all opiates are capable of producing respiratory depression. However, adjusting the dose of pain medication for an individual to achieve optimal pain relief with minimal side effects minimizes the risk of respiratory depression.

FAILURE TO ASSESS

Research has consistently indicated that caregivers do not know the extent of pain being experienced by their patients, and so overestimate the degree of relief patients achieve with ordered medications (APS, 1995; Donovan et al, 1989; Rankin and Snider, 1984; Teske and Cleeland, 1983; Von Roenn et al, 1993). Acting on erroneous assumptions is especially prevalent in the care of children and the elderly (Beyer et al., 1992; Ferrell and Ferrell, 1989).

The implication is clear: patients and caregivers do not have adequate means of communication as a result of caregiver reluctance to explore patient pain thoroughly or patient failure to express it. In any case, the nurse should not assume that a patient's pain is adequately relieved and should develop methods to assess, evaluate, and document pain.

FACTORS AFFECTING CLINICAL DECISIONS

Age

INFANTS AND CHILDREN

Pain in children was virtually ignored before the mid-1970s. The conviction was widespread among researchers, practitioners, and laypersons alike that the younger the child, the less was his or her ability to sense pain neurologically, interpret noxious stimulus as pain, and experience pain as adults do. Studies during this time documented the lack of pain medications being administered to postoperative children compared with a similar adult group (Beyer et al, 1992).

Interest in childhood pain has risen sharply since the 1980s. One researcher demonstrated that not only do newborn infants experience pain, but that adequate pain relief in newborns actually reduced the death rate after heart surgery (Anand and Hickey, 1987). Today, nurses, physicians, and psychologists are investigating the effects of pain, assessment of pain, and effects of many different therapies on pediatric patients. Figure 27–3 shows the Oucher pediatric pain assessment tool.

Infants and children warrant special consideration in pain assessment and management. Some health care providers actually believe that because their neurons are not yet fully myelinated (equipped with the protective sheath around nerve axons), young children cannot experience pain. One survey showed that only 59 percent of surgeons believe that 2-year-olds experienced pain like an adult (Schecter and Allen, 1986). However, even in adults, nociceptive impulses are carried by unmyelinated C fibers. The lack of myelination, therefore, does not indicate lack of pain transmission. These and other such myths may harm younger patients (Table 27–1).

Research has shown that neurotransmitters appear as early as 8 to 10 weeks of gestation; nerve tracts develop between 22 and 30 weeks; and the cortex is completely developed by 20 weeks. Descending *modulating tracts,* bundles of nerve fibers, may not develop until after birth. Infants may, therefore, be *more* sensitive to pain because their neurotransmitting systems are intact, but they lack adult neuromodulating systems. Alhough infants may respond more slowly and differently than adults, they do respond to pain (Johnston and Stevens, 1992). The long-term effects of infant pain are just beginning to be explored.

Other studies clearly indicate that pain in young patients is significantly undertreated (Beyer et al, 1992). Children, with reduced access to pain behaviors and less experience vocalizing pain, are even more likely than adults to be overwhelmed by unrelieved pain; and anger, frustration, helplessness, and fatigue can compound the problem. The nurse must be sensitive and responsive to a juvenile's expression of pain and minimize invasive procedures as much as institutional policy allows.

ELDERLY ADULTS

Elderly patients also need special consideration. It is a misconception that the elderly should expect to have pain; research on the effects of age on pain perception and behaviors is contradictory, however.

A frequently cited case describes a 101-year-old patient who stated that his left leg hurt. His physician suggested that left leg pain was to be expected at age 101. The man then asked the physician to explain why his right leg, which was also 101 years old, did not hurt a bit! One researcher exploring the problem of pain among residents of nursing homes found pain interfered with most ADLs, such as:

- Enjoyable activities (54 percent)
- Ambulation (52 percent)
- Sleep (45 percent)
- Appetite (14 percent)
- Dressing and grooming (8 percent) (Ferrell et al, 1990).

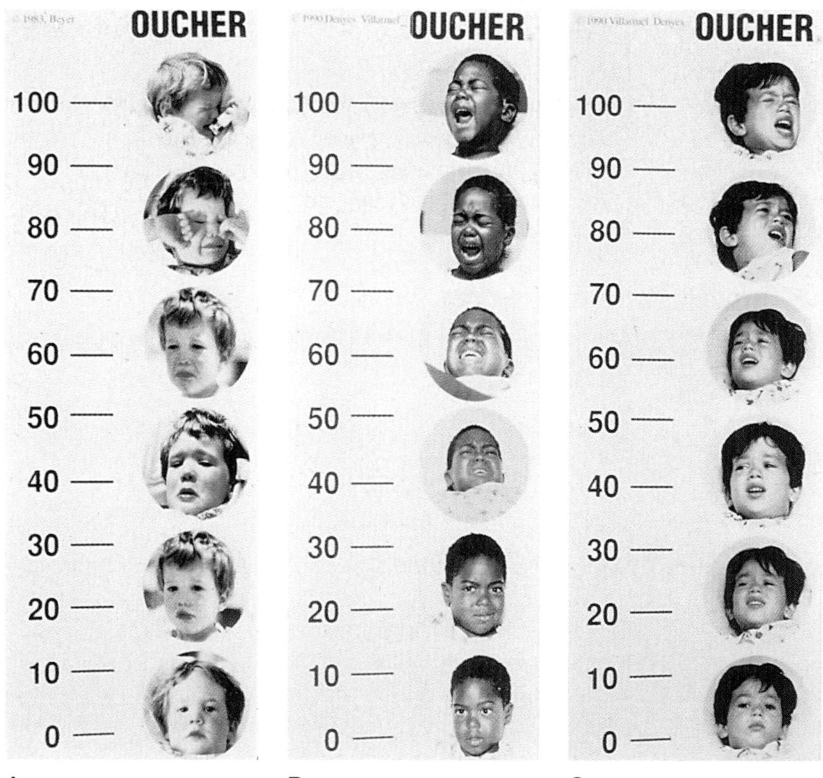

Figure 27–3. The Oucher pediatric pain assessment tool: *(A)* white version; *(B)* African American version; *(C)* Hispanic version. A, developed and copyrighted by Judith E. Beyer, Ph.D., R.N., 1983; B, developed and copyrighted by Mary J. Denyes, Ph.D., R.N., and Antonia M. Villarruel, Ph.D., R.N., 1990; C, developed and copyrighted by Antonia M. Villarruel, Ph.D., R.N., and Mary J. Denyes, Ph.D., R.N. Used with permission.

TABLE 27-1 Myths of Pain in Children

Myth	Fact
Children do not feel pain.	Children do feel pain, perhaps more intensely than adults.
Narcotics depress respiration and cause more problems in children than in adults.	Side effects of opiates, such as depressed respiration, are variable in both children and adults.
Children metabolize opiates differently than adults.	Metabolism of all medications is highly variable in all ages, not just in children. Ongoing assessment of effects and side effects is essential.

Furthermore, elderly patients are likely to have multiple medical problems compounding pain and its perception. The nurse must perform a thorough assessment of the elderly patient to rule out other underlying and less obvious medical problems that may be the source of the pain or affect pain therapy. These may include

- Changes in sensation, such as hypersensitivity or abnormal sensations
- Impaired motor function or range of motion
- Inflammation of soft tissue of joints
- Reduced circulation evidenced by lack of peripheral pulses, cool skin, and dusky color
- Memory deficits and cognitive impairments
- Depression
- Reduced liver function
- Reduced renal function

The nurse should be aware that many of these problems interact, may contribute to cognitive deficits, and may intensify the duration and side effects of a variety of medications.

Over- and undermedication of the elderly are both common problems. The *therapeutic window*—the range between unacceptable side effects on one end and lack of relief on the other—becomes narrower with increasing age. The response of the frail elderly patient to medication is especially variable and varies more from person to person. In general, all drug interactions are more problematic in this group, and multiple diagnosed and undiagnosed health issues are also more common, compounding the problem. For instance, analgesics reported to cause confusion in younger patients (e.g., pentazocine or meperidine) may cause extreme confusion in elderly patients. In addition, the constipating side effects of opiates and the gastric irritation associated with most NSAIDs are also more common in elderly patients.

Nonpharmacologic interventions can be effective in elderly patients as long as appropriate modifications are made for each individual. TENS may be difficult to manage for a patient with cognitive impairment or arthritis, for instance. Heat, cold, massage, and physical therapy are appropriate for the older patient if used gently and cautiously. Biofeedback, hypnosis, and distraction techniques depend on cognitive ability rather than age or physical capabilities.

The nurse must also be aware that elderly patients have long-established beliefs and patterns of behavior that may be extremely difficult to change. The principle of matching the intervention to the needs, beliefs, and patterns of the patient becomes particularly relevant to elders. This individuation of intervention increases the individual's sense of control and increases acceptance of the course of treatment as well as acceptance of the caregivers. Religious services, favorite television shows, and conversations with significant others may well be patterns of distraction far more helpful than any intervention devised by caregivers. Future research is warranted in all these facets of pain treatment in the elderly.

Gender

The first observations were that women reported painful conditions more often than men. Originally, this was thought to be the result of the differences in the way boys and girls are raised. However, more recently, it was discovered that women are more sensitive to neurotransmission of painful impulses than men. The exact mechanisms for this difference in neurosensitivity are unknown. Currently, research at the University of California at San Francisco has uncovered that women and men respond differently to analgesics. For instance, drug A may be very effective in women and not very effective in men, whereas drug B will be very effective in men but not so in women. Because these differences occur despite the phase of the menstrual cycle, they do not appear to be hormonally controlled. The reasons for these differences are unclear (Gear et al, 1996).

Culture and Ethnicity

The meaning of and reaction to pain varies from family to family, culture to culture, and in the same patient over time. The nurse should anticipate expressive behavior in cultures or settings in which screaming and moaning are expected and reinforced (e.g., some labor rooms or in Italian, Jewish, African-American, and other expressive cultures). In many Asian cultures, on the other hand, such open expression is essentially nonexistent.

A patient's behavior may not correlate with his or her verbal responses to questions about pain either. Some patients may deny the existence of pain and instead use words that express pain peripherally, such as burning, discomfort, and soreness. Such patients may be afraid to display too much or too little pain, depending on their cultural or family-instilled responses and the response of health care professionals.

When the client cannot speak English, the nurse faces greater difficulty in interviewing and completing an effective assessment. It is also more difficult to understand the individual's cultural attitude toward pain if communication is impeded. To obtain an accurate assessment of the pain, the nurse may wish to use an unbiased interpreter rather than relying exclusively on family members in communication.

To complicate the issue further, cross-cultural studies performed in the clinical setting are limited. The works of Zbrowski (1969) are classic studies of cross-cultural pain responses in hospitalized groups of more established American ethnic groups: Anglo-Saxon patients many generations after immigration and Italian, Irish, and Jewish patients. Zbrowski reached the following conclusions: Anglo-Saxon and Irish patients showed little emotion confronted with pain and tended to withdraw from other people when experiencing pain. Italian and Jewish patients, in contrast, freely expressed pain by crying, moaning, complaining, and being more demanding. These latter patients preferred family or health care workers around them when experiencing pain.

It is clear that culturally accepted pain behaviors vary widely. Nurses observe great differences between members of the same culture and between members of different cultural groups. The reactions of any individual are a result of an elusive and often unexpressed meld of culture, age, beliefs, and experiences of the subculture of a given environment. Paul's addiction therapy subculture, for instance, may have adopted a stoic reflex to pain and not concede the true degree of pain experienced to nurses, families, or anyone but each other.

Important patient beliefs related to pain and illness that the nurse should explore to establish pain beliefs addressed in Box 27–1 and include

- What a patient believes is necessary to maintain health
- How the patient believes that he or she is expected to act when sick
- Which symptoms must be treated and which may be ignored
- Who helps the patient when he or she falls ill
- Expected outcomes or treatment
- What folk remedies and curing techniques the patient habitually uses
- The patient's degree of trust, spoken or implicit, in both the health care provider and the system

Setting in Which Care Is Delivered

Pain can occur in any health care setting. Research indicates that more than 50 percent of patients in acute care hospitals experience pain greater than 6 on a scale ranging from 0 to 10 at some time during their hospital stay. It has been suggested that 5 percent of the population experiences significant ongoing pain. Whether the nurse works in intensive care, obstetrics, pediatrics, an extended-care facility, an outpatient setting, or in home care, pain relief will be a constant challenge. Even the

BOX 27–1
HISTORIC PERSPECTIVES OF PAIN

From the biblical reference in which the Lord said to Eve, "I will greatly multiply your pain in childbearing; in pain you shall bring forth children" (Genesis 3:16), through the much-publicized "Say no to drugs" campaign of the 1980s, societal beliefs and fears have influenced what patients are willing to do about and what caregivers are willing to provide (e.g., no drugs). In sixteenth-century Europe, pain was widely viewed as punishment for sins, possession of the devil, or the will of God. It is likely that many early settlers of the United States were proponents of this belief system. One researcher suggested the enduring legacy of this belief: Even today, some patients, families, and caregivers act as if pain is a sign of moral weakness and that suffering pain has some redeeming value (Kilwein, 1983). The practice of withholding analgesics from patients with a history of substance abuse is often predicated on the belief that "he did it to himself; so he'll just have to suffer."

Philosophical and scientific views of pain have equally reflected societal views and current research and likewise persist today. As early as the fourth century B.C., Aristotle taught that pain was not a sensation but an emotion. Debate continues among pain specialists regarding the extent to which particular types of pain are related primarily to the mind or to the body.

In 1664, French philosopher and mathematician René Descartes described pain as a bell ringing a warning. To treat pain was to interfere with this warning. Today, this belief lingers, even among highly trained personnel. Emergency room and critical care unit staff report that some practitioners continue to withhold analgesics from patients with injuries such as fractures, acute abdominal, or even chest pain because it might mask the symptoms and interfere with diagnosis.

In 1822, the identification of the role of the spinal cord in carrying pain messages gave birth to a more overtly biologic view of pain. In the late twentieth century, the identification and reversal of acute illness processes have been replaced by the need to understand and manage chronic illnesses and their long-term effects. Many of these illnesses are accompanied by pain, yet the pathophysiology, treatment, and relief of pain have only recently been adequately treated in nursing and medical texts.

Pain treatment as a specialty is barely 25 years old. Pain clinics emerged in the early 1960s but developed slowly in the 1970s, and the International Association for the Study of Pain (IASP) was founded in 1974. National IASP chapters and regional groups began to develop in the late 1970s. The first hospice in the United States was founded in 1974. Hospices began as lodging for travelers, the sick, or the underprivileged in the Middle Ages run by religious orders, but are today facilities providing a caring environment for the terminally ill. The American Pain Society was formed in 1978, and the World Health Organization made a formal commitment to worldwide cancer pain relief in 1985.

high-technology interventions for pain relief (pumps to deliver opiates or antispasmodics into the epidural space around the spinal cord, portable patient-controlled analgesia (PCA) pumps to allow the patient to provide intravenous analgesics as needed) are now appearing in the home care setting. Special programs for treatment of chronic pain have moved beyond the tertiary referral centers and are now appearing in primary care group offices. The nursing interventions described in this chapter are appropriate for any setting. They are generally based on scientific evidence of what is effective and on the principles for effective use. Modifications are needed for each individual whether in an acute care setting, outpatient, or at home. The needs of the individual are responsible for more modifications than the setting in which care is delivered.

Regulatory Considerations

The wording of laws throughout the country and the procedures for implementing those laws are effective barriers to the effective treatment of pain. Although the Federal Controlled Substance Act of 1970 does not include a patient with chronic pain in its definition of addict, some state definitions are written so even a terminally ill cancer patient taking narcotics is classified as an addict (Joranson, 1995). The nurse should check with her or his state regulatory board for appropriate definitions and classifications. Because it is illegal to prescribe narcotics for an addict, these laws or regulatory board interpretations can place the physician, nurse, and patient in a very difficult position. Patients with advanced cancer as well as chronic nonmalignant pain may well be denied essential opiate analgesics.

A 1992 survey by Joranson and associates indicated that state boards of medical examiners rely on outdated knowledge related to pain management and the appropriate use of opiates. In addition, fear of being sued for pain management resulting in significant side effects, fear of being censured, and fear of having one's practice restricted for helping patients achieve relief with opiates are also effective deterrents to the aggressive treatment of pain.

Yet undermedication may also bear legal consequences. In 1990, a nursing home was sued for having failed to provide a patient adequate pain medication. A nurse at the facility had concluded that the patient was addicted to morphine and proceeded to reduce the analgesic dose without consulting the physician. The patient's family demanded $15 million for unnecessary pain and suffering; an unspecified settlement was reached (Cushing, 1992). The nurse hesitating to fully medicate Paul, the recovering addict in the case study, should bear this in mind. If such legal actions become more common, the nurse can anticipate a policy shift toward more aggressive treatment of pain. Many normative policies and procedures are likely to stay in place, however. For instance, any medication must always benefit the patient; because Paul has a suspected head injury, meperidine is contraindicated as a result of the risk of seizures.

The AHCPR, established by the U.S. Congress to improve the quality, appropriateness, and effectiveness of health care services, is charged with developing and disseminating clinical practice guidelines. These guidelines are designed to assist practitioners in the prevention, diagnosis, and treatment of specific clinical conditions. In 1990, a panel on acute pain management convened to review the literature and solicit testimony of expert practitioners and patients alike. The panel's review led to the publication of the clinical practice guideline *Acute Pain Management: Operative or Medical Procedures and Trauma* in 1992. Two additional AHCPR pain guidelines have been released: a clinical practice guideline for cancer pain in 1994 and a guideline for low back problems in 1995.

In general, these guidelines support the following strategies:

- A collaborative, interdisciplinary approach, which includes the patient as part of the team
- An individualized pain control plan focused on prevention, developed jointly by patient and caregivers
- A systematic assessment of patient pain, with frequent reassessment of pain, pain relief, and highly visible documentation
- More knowledgeable use of both pharmacologic and nonpharmacologic methods of pain relief
- A formal, institution-wide approach to pain assessment and treatment.

These guidelines are now being implemented and tested at hospitals throughout the country. Professional nursing associations have taken a strong, positive stand on pain relief in the past few years as well. In February 1992, the American Nurses' Association published a position statement on pain, clearly defining the nurse's role in the titration (determination of appropriate amount of analgesic to produce pain relief). The following statement, related to pain in the terminally ill patient, is representative of their stance:

> Nurses shouldn't hesitate to use full and effective doses of pain medication for the proper management of pain in the dying patient. The increasing titration of medication to achieve symptom control, even at the expense of life, thus hastening death secondarily, is ethically justified. (American Nurses' Association, 1992)

Before the development of this statement, many nurses were hesitant and fearful that they could be held culpable for any act of pain relief that could be viewed as hastening death.

In 1990, the Oncology Nursing Society (ONS) published a position papers (1990a–c) on cancer pain, extensively reviewing the subject and cataloging the knowledge needed to implement the ONS' position:

> Individuals with cancer pain have a right to obtain optimal pain relief. Nurses caring for them have an ethical obligation to ensure exploration of everything possible within the scope of nursing practice to provide this relief. (Oncology Nursing Society, 1990)

STATE CANCER PAIN INITIATIVES

In 1984, Wisconsin developed what has become known as the State Cancer Pain Initiatives. These initiatives are a voluntary joint venture of the state's public regulatory agencies, legislators, patients and families, health care professionals, care agencies, and institutions of higher education to improve management of cancer pain. The impetus for these initiatives was based on the finding that poor cancer pain relief was related to lack of knowledge and the prevalence of unrealistic fears among health care professional and patients, not to any lack of effective analgesics.

These state initiatives focus on three primary goals:

- Public and professional education
- A network of professional resources
- Regulatory changes

State Cancer Pain Initiatives are rapidly becoming a powerful force to balance society's need to control access to and use of opiates and pain patients' need for access to opiates for treatment of pain and promotion of comfort (Joranson and Dahl, 1989). More than half of the states now have State Cancer Pain Initiatives.

Ethical Considerations

Pain is dehumanizing and can destroy a person's sense of autonomy and self-esteem. Adequate pain control is, therefore, the ethical responsibility of all health care professionals. However, pain control therapies may impair patients' alertness and ability to control their life, produce side effects such as constipation, and cost up to thousands of dollars monthly.

A balance must, therefore, be struck. One researcher (who is also a priest) proposed that pain control is a dramatic example of the ethical tension between the twin goals of prolonging life and alleviating suffering (Lisson, 1987).

An ethical dilemma occurs when a proposed nursing action seems to meet some ethical principles but violates others. What can a nurse use as ethical guideposts? The four major principles used for making ethical decisions are *nonmaleficence, beneficence, justice,* and *autonomy.* Nonmaleficence states that a nursing action should never do harm. Beneficence requires the nurse to act to benefit the individual. Justice, in a nursing context, addresses the distribution of beneficial actions fairly among all patients. Autonomy requires that individuals be given the opportunity to participate in all decisions and actions that affect them.

In addition to providing pain relief itself (beneficence), the nurse faces the additional responsibility of producing minimal side effects and aggressively treating any side effects that may appear (nonmaleficence).

One investigator discovered that a lack of accurate knowledge about pain treatment and inadequate communication among caregivers contributed to both a critical problem-solving deficit and a poor resolution of ethical dilemmas (Bosek, 1992) (Box 27–2).

BOX 27-2
FOLLOWING ETHICAL PRINCIPLES IN PAIN MANAGEMENT

To ensure adherence to ethical pain management principles, Bosek (1992) encouraged nurses to

- Improve their knowledge of pain management approaches
- Improve their communication with other nurses, physicians, patients, and families
- Develop questioning and problem-solving skills critical to managing patients in pain (and, indeed, the entire nursing process)

Inaccurate knowledge and fears have led many caregivers to withhold opiate analgesics in the belief that withholding them supports nonmaleficence and beneficence. Research, however, clearly indicates that unrelieved pain does not benefit the patient and, in fact, causes immense short- and long-term harm (Cousins, 1989; Dubner and Hargreaves, 1989), directly causing maleficence and nonbeneficence.

Many health care practices have been developed to delay a patient from obtaining pain relief. For instance, analgesics are often ordered every 4 to 6 hours, when the actual medication duration of action is 2.5 to 3 hours. In addition, well-meaning caregivers often give the lowest dose in an ordered range to prevent addiction or tolerance rather than determining the most effective dose for the individual patient.

These practices, based on lack of knowledge, violate the principles of beneficence. They do active harm by contributing to hypersensitization and causing physical and mental distress. These practices also fail to acknowledge autonomy, the patient's right to decide what constitutes adequate pain relief. Use of a placebo, a much less common practice today than in the past, also challenges autonomy (in denying the patient's right to necessary information) as well as the related ethical principles of *veracity* (telling the truth) and *fidelity* (keeping one's promises).

Ethical dilemmas may at times be unresolvable. For instance, being totally honest with a patient (veracity) may produce psychological harm (violation of beneficence), and giving the patient all the information that is needed to make an informed decision may be impossible when that patient is sedated. However, such unresolvable ethical dilemmas are more likely if the patient, family physician, or nurse harbors inaccurate information about pain management or unrealistic fears related to opiate use or if they are not effectively communicating with one another. See Chapter 9, Ethics in Nursing Practice for additional information regarding ethical issues.

No patient should ever suffer needlessly because of false assumptions, poor information, lack of commitment to ensuring pain control, and caregivers' inability to address conflicting priorities. Many state boards of medicine and of nursing are working with the APS to draft guidelines that balance the needs of suffering patients with the boards' concerns about diversion, drug abuse, and addiction.

Financial Considerations

Research related to the financial aspects of pain management is very rare. Whedon and Ferrell (1991) indicated that the high-technology interventions currently used for pain relief (home PCA, epidural analgesia, and implantable delivery systems) can cost up to $4000 per month. Increasingly, all health care providers must consider the costs and benefits of each alternative therapy.

Insurers have evinced a clear bias toward high-cost, high-technology alternatives, so there has been little incentive to conduct these studies in the past. It has been common for an insurance company, for instance, to refuse to pay for oral analgesics taken by the patient at home while unquestioningly paying for home nursing to maintain a PCA pump delivering the same or similar analgesics intravenously (Box 27–3).

As cost becomes a primary driver of technology, however, it behooves nurses to understand better the costs and benefits of alternative therapies. They can then quickly change to a less costly low-tech option if it is equally beneficial, or they can lobby against discontinuing a high-tech therapy if its benefits are clearly superior. For instance, a nurse who clearly understands and can demonstrate that administering analgesics around the clock, on schedule, is as effective as PCA can help ensure high-quality care if PCA use is curtailed for any reason, including cost. Alternatively, a clinical nurse who understands that unrelieved pain increases hypersensitivity and provokes more pain can more persuasively argue for ensuring 7-day pharmacy coverage, so that patients do not run out of needed analgesics on weekends or holidays.

FUTURE DEVELOPMENTS

Research in the past decade has changed the way nurses and health care organizations view pain and treatment alternatives. Some of these findings include the identification of neurotransmitters that sensitize the nervous system, leading to chronic pain. Research is now focusing on developing ways to block these neurotransmitters.

No single psychological factor is consistently related to pain or to the outcomes of pain treatment based on 20 years of studies. Instead, personal characteristics—needs, expectations, style—may be essential in individualizing truly effective treatment programs.

Pain medication's Holy Grail has been the development of an analgesic with none of the addictive or other side effects of opiate analgesics, yet is as effective in relieving pain. In the nineteenth century, morphine was initially heralded as the answer to the problems associated with heroin use; then by 1928 it was condemned in some publications. In the latter half of this century, pentazocine (Talwin), propoxyphene (Darvon), butorphanol (Stadol), and nalbuphine (Nubain) were reported to be potent analgesics equal to morphine but with no side effects. They have all been shown to have equally distressing and limiting side effects, such as dependence and the development of symptoms mimicking psychosis (e.g., paranoia, dementia, and hallucinations). Research continues to try to develop analgesics that control severe pain over long periods of time with few undesirable side effects. Because we now know that cells, nerves, and processes involved in pain transmission are not specific to pain alone, it is unlikely that medications that block pain will be able to do so without effects on the other processes served by these nerves, cells, or chemical substances.

New, alternative methods of delivering analgesics may see broader applications in the future. *Epidural* (in the dura, the outer membrane covering the spinal cord) and *intrathecal* delivery of analgesics, especially those in which the drug is delivered by an implanted device, have been shown to be valuable in the 5 to 10 percent of patients for whom extremely high doses of oral or parenteral narcotics are no longer effective (i.e., those who develop tolerance). PCAs, intradermal or subcutaneous continuous infusions of opiates or lidocaine, transdermal patches (fentanyl), and sublingual administration are all accepted routes to pain relief, regardless of coexisting problems, such as an inability to swallow or maintain a stable blood level of analgesic by other methods. These high-technology methods of opiate delivery avoid the peaks and troughs of as-required (prn) dosing, and reinforce the benefits of a stable blood level maintained through around-the-clock dosing.

BOX 27–3
COMPARING COSTS OF METHADONE AND MORPHINE HOME TREATMENT

Methadone and morphine are two therapies with comparable analgesic effects. Both can be administered po (*per os*, by mouth). How do they compare when one is administered po and the other by the far more labor- and technology-intensive patient-controlled analgesia (PCA) pump at home?

- Methadone, 30 mg tid (three times a day) po. Typical cost/month = $50/mo (average wholesale cost + 30%)
- Morphine, 90 mg, PCA pump. Cost/month should reach $4000/mo (per Ferrell and Rhiner, 1994)

NURSING CARE ACTIONS

Principles and Practices

ASSESSING PAIN

Pain is a complex, multidimensional psychophysiologic process fully known only to the person experiencing it. Any assessment must, therefore, be multidimensional, subjective, and regularly repeated over the period in which pain is likely to occur. Nurses perform clinical pain assessment for two specific reasons:

- To aid in the selection of pain relief measures, including the elimination of painful stimuli whenever possible

- To provide the basis for evaluating the efficacy of any measures used

Many methods of measuring pain have been developed. However, research has consistently demonstrated that a systematic assessment of pain is rarely performed (Donovan et al, 1987). Such an assessment becomes all the more urgent considering that patients, nurses, and physicians often disagree about the severity of the pain that the patient is experiencing (Donovan et al, 1989; Grossman et al, 1991).

Any sentiment that such formal assessment of pain is not necessary (e.g., that an experienced nurse can assess pain based on experience alone) has been disproven. In one study, more than one third of patients surveyed reported multiple sites of pain (Donovan et al, 1987). Other studies have indicated that the amount of medication taken by the patient is generally about one quarter of what could have been taken, based on written orders (Donovan et al, 1987; Marks and Sachar, 1973). Institutional quality improvement plans designed to identify and correct these patterns are currently being implemented across the country (APS, 1995).

Clinical judgment is crucial to any assessment, but particularly so to pain assessment; novice practitioners often need guidance and supervision. A two-level clinical assessment provides a systematic method applicable to a variety of settings (Donovan, 1992): a basic pain assessment and a more in-depth, comprehensive pain assessment. Special consideration is given to patients requiring more detailed assessment, such as pediatric patients. The novice can use this two-tiered method to assess all patients at risk of experiencing pain.

This method of assessment also guides the nurse in designing and implementing a plan to alleviate most uncomplicated acute pain, and meets the standards established by the AHCPR (1992, 1994) and the APS (1995). If the pain does not respond to initial efforts, then comprehensive pain assessment may be needed.

Frequent reassessment to determine patterns of pain and effects of interventions on pain relief is essential, whether the patient is an infant, child, or adult, and regardless of the method of assessment used. Further, any method used to record pain and pain relief data must be visible to the patient, the family, and all caregivers (APS, 1995; Max, 1990). Bedside and wall charts in the patient's room have both been found useful to this effect and help transform the subjective experience of pain into a concrete phenomenon that all concerned parties can monitor together.

BASIC PAIN ASSESSMENT

To perform basic pain assessment, the nurse follows the acronym PAIN (Table 27–2). The patient must be alert, responsive, and cooperative, and the nurse needs two assessment tools: a human body outline and an age-appropriate pain scale.

Various scales have been developed to quantify pain intensity (Fig. 27–4). Any of these three standard scales are adequate for clinical assessment. For patients with impaired mental status, the nurse may use the simple categorical scale or one of the pediatric scales (such as the one shown in Fig. 27–3), to assess pain intensity. Each AHCPR guideline, available from the AHCPR and covering a variety of clinical settings and conditions, contains examples of valid assessment tools that the AHCPR recommends for clinical use.

The scales in Figure 27–4 include measurements of pain relief. Most standard pain assessments do not have such scales, however. If the nurse's facility lacks pain relief scales, an easy-to-use relief scale can be developed using the same format as the pain intensity scale.

The nurse should keep in mind that a patient may fail to report the presence and extent of pain accurately. A major reason for this is the fear that physicians, nurses, and family will conclude that the pain is psychological in origin. Patients are thus often hesitant to report pain relief from nonpharmacologic interventions such as distraction, massage, and heat and cold therapies, even though these techniques are proven and effective. The nurse must formulate specific questions to elicit this information such as, "What other things do you do that help you feel more comfortable?"

Some institutions are beginning to assess patient satisfaction with care and outcomes of pain therapy. Many are using 0–10 scales similar to those for pain intensity and relief. Researchers have reported that most patients report satisfaction even when reporting high pain intensity scores (APS, 1995). Ware suggested that it is important to assess separately satisfaction with the caregiving process and also satisfaction with the outcomes of care (Ware and Hays, 1988).

How to explain this paradox? Research has suggested that satisfaction scores measure the caring attitudes of the staff

TABLE 27-2 Basic (Level 1) Pain Assessment

Aspects of Pain Management	Assessment Questions
P = place/location of pain	Where is the pain? Point with one finger to indicate the site(s) of pain on a figure of human body.
A = amount/intensity of pain	How much pain do you have right now? What is the worst pain you've experienced in the past 24 hours? Use the facility's pain scale.
I = interactions (factors that increase the pain)	What makes the pain worse? List any contributing factors, no matter how trivial: position, movement, weather, temperature, feelings, procedures, time of day, and any other events that affect the pain.
N = normalizers (factors that reduce the pain to normal levels)	What have you used in the past to relieve your pain? When did and how often did you use them? How much relief did you obtain with that factor? Are you satisfied with the relief you are obtaining? (Again, use the appropriate scale.)

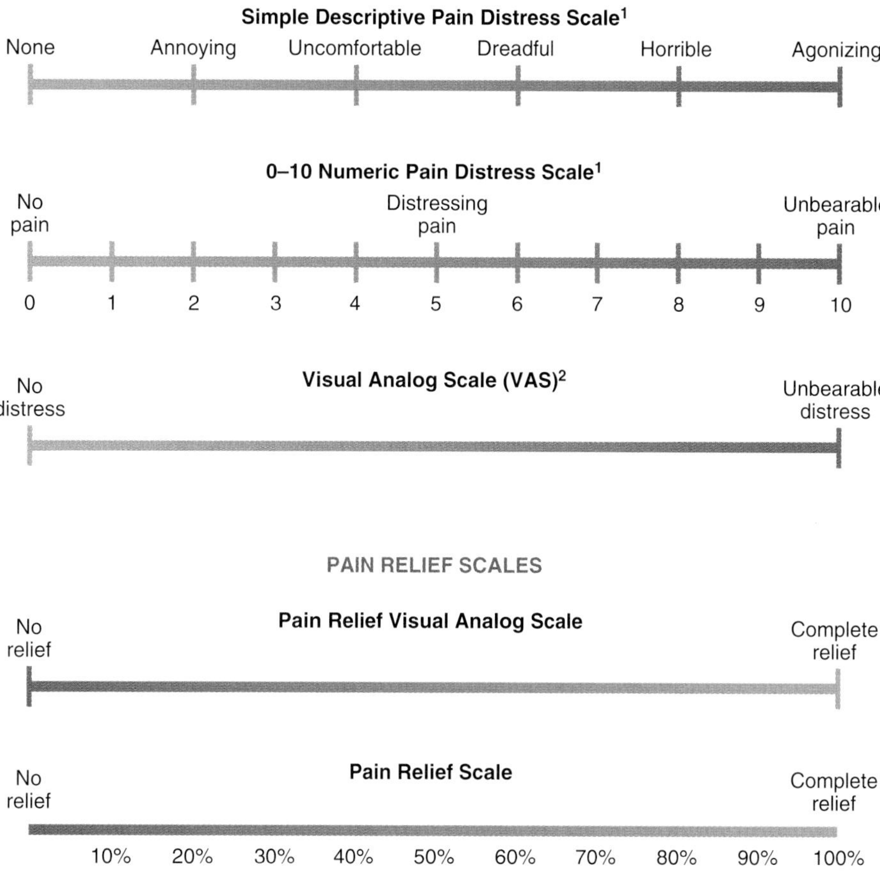

Figure 27-4. Pain rating scales.

rather than satisfaction with pain therapy or relief. The nurse should thoroughly explore both satisfaction with care and satisfaction with pain relief with the patient and family (Ward and Gordon, 1996), and never assume that pain is controlled.

COMPREHENSIVE PAIN ASSESSMENT

If pain relief, as defined by the patient, is not adequate, a more extensive assessment is indicated. As with the basic assessment, this more focused assessment is warranted to identify and eliminate factors intensifying the pain and to design a more effective plan of care to modify the pain experience.

Nurses use this comprehensive assessment to elicit the following information:

- The patient's expectation of pain and of pain relief (how much, when)
- Acceptable levels of pain and pain relief
- The meaning of pain (pain can mean increased risk of death, need to change life, a transitory annoyance, an excuse to skip class, the treatment may need to account for the meaning)
- How the patient and family have dealt with pain in the past and the patient's health coping mechanisms
- Indicators of depression or anxiety (see Chapter 31, Stress and Anxiety, for more information)
- Observation of interactions with family and others: do these interactions relieve or aggravate the pain?
- Nonverbal expressions of pain
- Trends in vital signs
- Extent to which pain interferes with ADLs, such as the ability to work, sleep, relate to others, and enjoy life

The Wisconsin Brief Pain Inventory (Daut et al, 1983) is an excellent tool for systematically assessing these functions.

Patients with unrelieved chronic pain require even more extensive assessment. This assessment should consider

- Financial impact of medical care, hospitalization, treatments, medications, and loss of income on the patient and family
- Patient and family travel expenses and barriers to obtaining treatment
- Cognitive, psychological, and behavioral evaluations

- Family dynamics, particularly regarding pain behaviors
- Complete physical examination

More invasive procedures are often prescribed in response to such exams, to diagnose or rule out a more treatable illness, often to satisfy the patient or family.

PAIN ASSESSMENT IN CHILDREN

Special approaches and strategies are needed to assess and evaluate pain and pain relief in infants and children (Box 27–4). Children in pain are often restless, agitated, and not easily distracted; refuse to eat or play; or have an extremely short attention span. This makes assessment of the pain experience that much more problematic and resistant to accurate quantification by an objective observer.

A number of studies, however, have documented the use of physiologic measures as reliable infant pain indicators: heart rate, vagal tone, transcutaneous oxygenation, and palmar sweating (Gedaly-Duff, 1989; Johnston and Stevens, 1992). The nurse should be aware that these physiologic measures display a great deal of variation from infant to infant and allow for individuation.

Facial expression, crying, and body movements have also been identified as indicators of pain. There have even been attempts to differentiate the cry of pain from the cry of hunger and fussiness. Research has identified the cry of pain as high-pitched, harsh or without sound, or intense (Johnston and Stevens, 1992). A variety of body movements have been identified in response to painful stimuli as well; changes in facial expression provide the most consistent measure of pain. In one study, the typical responses of infants to heel lances were rapid facial grimaces consisting of lowered brows, eyes squeezed shut, deepening of the nasolabial furrow, and open lips (Grunua et al, 1990).

The nurse should be alert to far more subtle signs too. Changes in a given infant's behavior are often far more meaningful than any single observation. When a child's behaviors are not obvious pain avoidance behaviors (e.g., grimacing, shut eyes) but are unusual for that child, the nurse should consider whether a "well" child would exhibit these behaviors. If not, could these behaviors be signs of discomfort or pain? As is true in adults, children's behavioral reactions and the degree of physical pain are not always correlated (Hester et al, 1992b).

The physiologic changes associated with pain are even more variable in the child than in the infant. Current behavioral assessments have limited applicability to the clinical situation since their reliability, validity, and use over time have not yet been well established (Hester et al, 1992a).

A variety of research-based assessment instruments have been developed specifically for young children (see Fig. 27–3). *Pain maps* or figures on which the child can mark his or her pain sites, giving it concrete form by *drawing* the pain (e.g., as a black cloud, a monster, or a jumble of dark-colored scribbles) are also helpful in determining the site, or multiple sites, of pain (Hester et al, 1992b).

Although the pain assessment scales are easily administered and well accepted by adult patients, there are little data on scales' acceptance in children of different ages. One team conducted a study comparing the validity, reliability, and preference of pain intensity assessment scales in different-aged children (Wong and Baker, 1988). Their results indicated that children age 3 to 8 *prefer* one of the faces scales over other scales. However, these researchers also reported that no one scale demonstrated superiority in validity and reliability.

Verbal communication about pain may be further hampered in children because of a child's limited vocabulary. Adults may fluently and lucidly describe their pain, but a child's vocabulary may be limited to a single word, such as "hurt" or "owie." Older children and adolescents, however, are capable of completing questionnaires or answering direct questions about their pain. Nurses should ask their superiors for such questionnaires or seek out reliable sources for them. The assessment described for adults, for instance, is generally effective in assessing pain in these patients.

BOX 27–4
NINE STRATEGIES TO IMPROVE CHILDREN'S PAIN

Many nurses feel helpless when presented with a juvenile patient in pain. Indeed, it may be one of the most stressful aspects of a nursing assignment. Here are nine concrete methods to make a juvenile patient's pain more bearable:

1. Make pain relief a distinct, separate goal.
2. Differentiate between apprehension and pain, and treat each separately.
3. Assess pain systematically and regularly.
4. Use noninvasive pain management techniques whenever feasible (avoid injections).
5. Use analgesics appropriately (titrate to effect and administer regularly, not as needed).
6. Use nonpharmacologic techniques liberally and appropriately (hypnosis, distraction, music, humor).
7. Do not be afraid to try new pain management techniques.
8. Avoid myths and misinformation making decisions about a child's pain. Base decisions on facts.
9. Keep trying to control the pain. Do not give up.

Data from the works of Beyer, J., et al (1992) and McCaffery and Beebe (1989).

MANAGING PAIN

The overall goal of pain management is helping the patient control pain and learn effective strategies to control future pain. Hence, thorough patient teaching is essential in pain management, as in few other areas that the nurse will encounter. To this end, it is imperative that the nurse actively

RESEARCH HIGHLIGHT
EFFECTIVE PAIN MANAGEMENT

The complexity associated with effective pain management is illustrated by the recent findings of Ward and Gordon (1996). Similar findings have also been reported from other settings. The study was conducted to increase understanding of why patients are satisfied with pain management despite continuing to experience pain. Data were gathered from patients after 2 years of a series of programs to improve pain management had been implemented in this medical center. The data were gathered by patient survey (n = 360), telephone interview (n = 869), and chart review (n = 112). The current data were compared with data from 2 years previously (before the pain management improvement program).

FINDINGS

- There were no significant differences in patient satisfaction from before the "improvements" 2 years prior to now after the improvements. However, both groups of patients were overwhelmingly positive about their pain management.
- There were no differences in worst pain reported by the "before" group and the "now" group. However, the intensity of pain was an average of 7 (on a 0–10 scale).

CONCLUSIONS

Most orders continue to be written prn (as needed). This creates a pattern of peaks of pain followed by relief. Because the patients continued to experience the expected pattern, they were very satisfied even though the amount of pain they experienced was considerably less than what would be physiologically beneficial and in most cases less than what was reasonably possible.

IMPLICATIONS FOR PRACTICE

Patient education must include

- Why pain relief is necessary to reduce the effects of stress on the body and to prevent, if possible, the development of hypersensitivity
- The value of scheduled analgesics to prevent pain rather than prn to respond to pain
- An assessment of the patient-family beliefs regarding these concepts, which may be seem very strange to them
- A plan for what to do if the current pain management plan does not effectively relieve the pain (e.g., call health care provider, use nonpharmacologic therapies)
- A method for the patient to easily report pain in the future (but more important is to be aware that one can never assume that lack of reporting pain means lack of pain)

Research conducted and reported by Ward, S., Gordon, D. (1996). Patient satisfaction and pain severity as outcomes in pain management: a longitudinal view in one setting's experience. *Journal of Pain Symptom Management, 11*(4), 242–251.

involve both patient and family members in the selection and implementation of all pain interventions. However, no intervention, no matter how successful in theory or actual clinical practice, will truly reduce pain without the full cooperation of the patient and the patient's support system of family, friends, and significant others (if an adult).

Patient education materials are available from a variety of sources: marketing, public affairs, or outpatient services programs of the nurse's facility; pharmaceutical companies; the U.S. Department of Health and Human Services; the AHCPR; the American Cancer Society; Arthritis Foundation; hospice organizations; and State Cancer Pain Initiatives.

Clinical experience in a variety of diagnoses, problems, and settings suggests that multiple interventions used at different sites of action are far more effective than single interventions and have fewer side effects. Multiple pharmacologic and nonpharmacologic interventions in the treatment of pain are not only gaining wider acceptance but are supported by the gate control theory of pain. Simply, the more sites that are stimulated, the less likely the pain is to traverse the "gate." The theory suggests four sites at which clinicians may intervene to reduce the pain experience:

- Peripheral site of the painful stimulus
- Spinal gate
- Thalamus and midbrain
- The cortex

REMOVING PAINFUL STIMULI

Initial interventions involve identifying and removing all possible pain-producing factors. Common pain-producing factors include

- Position (caused by patient's staying in one position for hours during surgery, inability to move independently, sitting, fear of moving, or fatigue)
- Certain ADLs (e.g., getting out of bed, tying one's shoes, riding in a car)
- Certain procedures (venipuncture, dressing change)

Changes in position, splinting and support of the painful body part with a soft cervical collar, brace, or use of a cane, and frequent gentle stretching are often overlooked interventions. The nurse should be aware that transferring a patient to a chair or ambulation are activities that may significantly increase pain for some patients.

In all cases, the nurse's own informed clinical judgment is essential in determining benefit or harm from the activity in view of the pain generated. The nurse should consider alternatives. The pain-producing activity may not be the only method of ensuring the desired outcomes; turning and the use of incentive spirometry (measured deep breathing with the nurse providing visual and vocal stimuli), for example, may be less painful and equally effective as moving the patient to a chair to ensure adequate lung expansion in a patient with bone metastases for whom movement is painful. Caregivers must, therefore, carefully select effective methods of controlling the patient's pain during any activity.

BLOCKING CHEMICAL PAIN TRANSMITTERS

Several methods, both pharmacologic and nonpharmacologic, effectively block the chemical transmission of painful impulses. The most commonly used and successful strategies include application of cold, heat, and massage to the area of injury; administration of local anesthetics to the injured area; and administration of nonopiate analgesics, an underused group of oral medications that have systemic effects.

Cold, Heat, and Massage. Local application of cold interferes with the production of the chemicals needed to transmit pain from one nerve cell to the next. One specific effect is related to the effects of cold on inflammation. Cold reduces the ability of cells to produce the chemicals responsible for initiating and maintaining the inflammatory response. The lack of inflammation results in less stimulation of the peripheral nerve endings and less transmission of pain. If muscle spasm is a component of the pain experience, local application of heat produces local muscle relaxation, vasodilatation, and removal of pain transmitters from the area of pain with resultant pain relief. These techniques can be applied as often as 15 minutes every 2 hours. McCaffery and Beebe (1989) described many different techniques for the use of cold, heat and massage.

Massage techniques, such as shiatsu, Swedish, and deep-muscle massage, as well as therapeutic touch, seem to produce increased relaxation and a sense of well-being. This, in turn, increases local circulation and removes locally produced transmitters of pain. (See Chapter 32, Touch, for more information on these therapies.)

Local Anesthetics. Research has indicated the value of local anesthetics, with or without general anesthetic, for surgical procedures. Local anesthetics, such as bupivacaine or lidocaine, prevent local nerve cells from communicating with neurons in the spinal cord, also preventing hypersensitization of the nervous system (Woolf, 1991), thus both blocking existing pain and reducing the potential for future pain. The local application of ice or a local anesthetic cream or spray before injections or other painful procedures is a simple way to use these principles in daily practice. They can also help reduce the hypersensitivity associated with some chronic pain syndromes.

Nonopiate Analgesics. Analgesics are the mainstay of acute pain management in the institutional environment and in the lives of millions of Americans. Aspirin, acetaminophen, and NSAIDs operate at the peripheral site of the injury. That is, these drugs interfere with the production of neurotransmitters at the site of injury or trauma, effectively blocking pain. NSAIDs are especially effective when inflammation is a significant factor, such as in osteoarthritis, bony metastases, dysmenorrhea, and headaches. (Acetaminophen, however, has no anti-inflammatory effects.) Most NSAIDs need to be taken every 4 to 6 hours (piroxicam, whose primary indications are osteoarthritis and rheumatoid arthritis, taken in one dose daily is the exception) and are effective for mild to moderate pain (see Fig. 27–7).

Studies have demonstrated that administering acetaminophen 30 minutes before dental procedures reduces postprocedural pain. Other research indicates that treatment with NSAIDs, because of their anti-inflammatory effect, are superior to treatment with acetaminophen or even the opiate oxycodone (Dubner and Hargreaves, 1989).

Nonopiate analgesics are underused, however, despite their proven effectiveness. Several interlocking reasons are responsible:

- Patient resistance. NSAIDs are not prescription drugs, so patients may not believe they are as effective.
- Underdosing. The dose patients routinely take or are administered is well below the therapeutic dose. For instance, 1000 mg of aspirin is the therapeutic dose for an adult, but the patient habitually takes only 325 to 650 mg.
- As-needed dosing. NSAIDs are often taken as needed when scheduled dosing is both more appropriate and effective.
- Risk of Reye's syndrome. Development of this deadly respiratory-CNS syndrome in children with viral infections has been definitely linked to aspirin use since the early 1960s. Aspirin, if used at all, must always be administered cautiously in children.
- Gastrointestinal side effects. These side effects, including bleeding gastric ulcers, are common.

Table 27–3 presents an overview of common NSAIDs. Box 27–5 discusses general guidelines for analgesic use.

CLOSING THE SPINAL GATE

Shutting the gate to a major source of pain transmission, the spinal cord, is one of the four generally accepted methods

BOX 27–5
GENERAL GUIDELINES FOR ANALGESIC USE

- First and foremost, listen to the patient.
- Individualize therapy based on a systematic assessment.
- Follow the concepts of the World Health Organization's three-step analgesic ladder.
- Know the duration of effect, pharmacology, and equianalgesic doses of any drugs given.
- Administer analgesics regularly, not as needed.
- Combine nonpharmacologic and pharmacologic interventions.
- Titrate dose up or down to maximize pain relief with minimal side effects.
- Be persistent. Nonpharmacologic interventions, in particular, may demand significant patient learning curves.
- Treat side effects aggressively.
- Taper slowly if analgesic is no longer needed.

CLINICAL DECISION MAKING
WHAT IS THE BEST PLAN OF CARE FOR PAUL'S PAIN?

SITUATION

Paul, an 18-year-old high school senior and recovering addict, suffered multiple fractures of his left leg and a possible head injury in a motor vehicle accident yesterday. He had surgery last night to insert pins and stabilize his leg. He has a history of juvenile rheumatoid arthritis treated effectively with ibuprofen, 600 mg four times daily, and application of heat. He seems slightly depressed as well. The nurse performs a systematic assessment to understand the pain experience from Paul's perspective and implement a plan to control Paul's pain. The nurse concludes that Paul has two types of acute pain in addition to his chronic pain: ankle and leg pain. His knee pain is the result of his arthritis. His left ankle pain is caused by pressure from the end of the cast and varies with position, and his left leg pain is related to his acute injury and surgery. The nurse also assesses Paul's fear of readdiction, if opiates are prescribed, and notes his parents' fears.

Goals: Based on what Paul and his parents relate about his chronic and acute pain and his potential head injury, the nurse concludes that the plan of care will need to address these goals:

1. Provide relief of the three different pains.
2. Teach Paul a variety of techniques he can use to control his own pain.
3. Establish clear communication concerning pain and pain relief.
4. Develop alternative methods of relieving stress.
5. Decrease fears related to addiction (his and his parents).
6. Relieve depression.
7. Recognize any mental changes.
8. Continue his addiction recovery.

PATIENT FACTORS

The nurse knows the following factors are likely to affect Paul's perception of and reaction to pain and the effectiveness of any interventions:

- Age and developmental state
- Expectations, beliefs, values, and fears of the various groups of which Paul is a part (his family, his schoolmates and peers, his arthritis treatment program) regarding (1) illness and recognition of pain; (2) what constitutes acceptable therapy. Paul reports a fear of redeveloping addiction. Paul's parents are present and express ambivalence; they want Paul to be free of pain but do not want to risk his developing a new drug problem.
- Gender. Paul's peer group believes that it is important to be strong and never complain.
- Guilt. Was the motor vehicle accident his fault? Was anyone else hurt?
- Spirituality. Paul describes the solace of a walk in the woods when under stress and the peace it brings.
- Effects of chronic pain. Because Paul's arthritic pain has existed for years, it is possible that these nerves are hypersensitive; Paul could experience more intense pain than would a person who had not experienced chronic pain in the same site.
- Effects of acute pain. The acute episode of a trauma and leg fracture will generally produce symptoms of stress. Because Paul also lives with chronic pain, the nurse acknowledges the difficulty of predicting how his body will respond to his additional pain, which symptoms will develop, and how long they will last.
- Baseline mental capacity; mental changes related to head injury
- Depression related to interference with his normal activity because of unrelieved pain

INTERVENTIONS

Paul will be discharged the following day, so the nurse moves swiftly to establish a care plan and ensure that these interventions are suitable for the home environment as well as for the hospital. They include

- An orthopedic consultation to remove the source of the ankle pain; avoiding positions provoking pain until his cast is adjusted; teaching Paul how to recognize early signs of cast irritation or of the cast being too tight
- A combination of analgesics, which includes his usual ibuprofen regimen and a mild narcotic analgesic taken orally every 4 hours for 3 days, then every 6 hours for 2 days, and then every 8 hours for 2 days.
- Education of Paul and his parents regarding regular, around-the-clock medication with analgesics and how analgesics encourage recovery and minimize the development of chronic pain
- Frank discussion with Paul and his parents of the minimal risk of addiction from taking narcotic pain medications; structure a schedule of narcotic analgesics to make it easier for them to see that the narcotic regimen is short in duration, and allow them to follow a specific set of written directions for using narcotic analgesics.
- Application of ice or heat to the right knee to relieve pain (15–20 minutes every 2 hours)
- Listening to music or humor with a personal cassette player (parents or friends are encouraged to bring in cassette player and favorite tapes). Knowing his love of nature, the nurse encourages listening to forest sounds or watching videos of wooded scenes to replace walks in the woods. These relaxation and distraction techniques also ease Paul's slight depression and increase his sense of control.
- Assessment of mental status and changes per institutional head trauma protocol, and teaching his family the signs of a change in mental status: inability to arouse him from sleep, memory deficits, and any weakness or changes in sensation other than those related to the fractured leg and cast

continued on next page

CLINICAL DECISION MAKING
WHAT IS THE BEST PLAN OF CARE FOR PAUL'S PAIN? (cont'd)

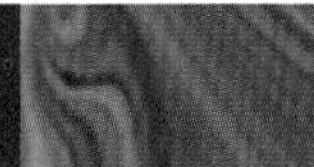

- Evaluation of the effectiveness of this pain therapy, three times daily in the hospital and daily after discharge. This evaluation must include pain level, pain relief, satisfaction with pain relief, and any problems or side effects that arise. The nurse gives Paul and his family written instructions regarding who to call if any of these questions or problems arise.
- Involving Paul's family in all aspects of care and patient teaching; may reduce their feelings of guilt and fears of readdiction and increase their commitment to continued use of all techniques after discharge

SELF-ASSESSMENT

The nurse must guard against making assumptions about adolescents who are involved in motor vehicle accidents, addiction, chronic and acute pain, how pain should be expressed, and what is appropriate therapy. Every patient must be assessed individually, especially when an individual has strong beliefs and when he or she has multiple pathologic processes interacting, like Paul. The nurse with significant negative experience or beliefs about narcotics needs to guard against letting patients reticent to express pain continue to experience high levels of unrelieved pain. The nurse who believes that narcotics should be freely used to relieve pain must guard against not recognizing and appreciating those fearful of addiction as a result. The nursing challenge is providing effective pain relief within the framework acceptable to a given patient.

REFLECTION

An assumption becomes evident after Paul's discharge: that the discharge instructions to Paul and his family would provide satisfactory pain relief without unacceptable side effects at home. No provision was made to evaluate the effects of the plan of care at home after Paul's discharge. On reflection, the nurse schedules a follow-up phone call the next day to see if there are any questions, to evaluate the effectiveness of the plan, and to be certain that Paul has an appointment to see the orthopedic surgeon in 7–10 days. If Paul or his family have encountered any difficulties, scheduling a home health visit may be necessary. The nurse also suggests that Paul contact his addiction counselor.

of minimizing the pain experience. Three methods of closing the spinal gate are commonly used: one squarely in the tradition of orthodox, institutionalized, Western medicine (epidural and spinal anesthetics); another still considered largely investigational after nearly two decades of use (TENS) and a third, often-dismissed Asian technique backed by centuries of use (acupuncture and acupressure).

Epidural and Spinal Anesthetics. Physicians and surgeons may inject epidural and spinal analgesics into the epidural space around the spinal cord (less often, the intrathecal space) during surgery, labor, or postoperatively. These analgesics temporarily block the transmission of painful impulses up the spinal tract from the dorsal horn to the cortex (AHCPR, 1995; Dubner and Hargreaves, 1989). Spinal anesthetics (most often bupivacaine) delivered into the epidural space block sensory nerves; at higher concentrations, spinal anesthetics block autonomic and motor nerves as well. The combination of spinal anesthetic and spinal opiate also in-

TABLE 27-3 Overview of Common Nonsteroidal Anti-inflammatory Drugs

Variable	Aspirin	Acetaminophen	Ibuprofen	Toradol
Adult dose	650–975 mg every 4 hours	650–975 mg every 4 hours	400 mg every 4–6 hours	25–75 mg every 6–8 hours
Pediatric dose	10–15 mg/kg every 4 hours	10–15 mg/kg every 4 hours	10 mg/kg every 6–8 hours	Not approved
Maximum dose	4000 mg/24 hours	4000 mg/day		5 days maximum
Antipyretic	Yes	Yes		
Anti-inflammatory	Yes	Yes	Yes	Yes
GI toxicity	Yes		Yes	Yes
Impairment of platelet aggregation	For 1 or more weeks	—	Yes, but reversible	Wound bleeding
Allergic reactions	Yes	Yes	Yes	Yes
Tinnitus	Yes		Yes	Yes
Renal toxicity	Yes	Yes	Yes	Yes
Liver toxicity		Potentially severe	Yes	Yes
Anemia		Yes	Yes	

GI, gastrointestinal; IM, intramuscular.

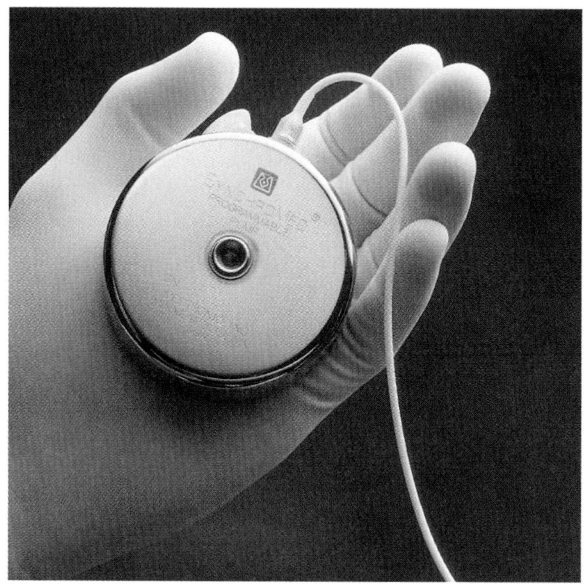

Figure 27-5. The SynchroMed implantable pump, which delivers a preset dosage of intraspinal analgesic. (Courtesy of Medtronic, Inc., Minneapolis, MN.)

creases the incidence of side effects, such as respiratory depression (Naber et al, 1994).

Spinal drugs (Fig. 27–5) are delivered through a catheter inserted into the epidural space. There is less danger of infection, meningitis, or encephalitis with this method than the intrathecal administration. For continuous long-term use when standard methods of analgesia have proven ineffective, permanently implanted catheters attached to an internal or external pump delivery system may be used to deliver a predetermined rate of analgesic.

With these methods, medications are concentrated in the spinal cord, and the number and severity of side effects are limited. The nurse must check labeling to ensure that the drug is preservative free, however; even small amounts of preservative can damage the spinal cord. In addition, appropriate personnel should inject medications as high in the spinal cord as is commensurate with safety. Research now indicates that drugs administered low in the spinal cord spread upward in the intrathecal space and can result in nausea, vomiting, urinary retention, pruritus, somnolence, respiratory depression, hypotension, and cardiotoxic effects. Further, the greater the volume of fluid containing the opioid or anesthetic and the higher the rate of injection, the greater is the risk of supraspinal spread of the opiate. Spinal opiates and spinal anesthetics are contraindicated when the patient has a systemic infection, is receiving anticoagulant therapy, or has a local injury to the spinal cord because of increased risk of complications, such as septicemia from an infected catheter or hemorrhage resulting from inadequate clothing (Naber et al, 1994).

TENS. This is an electrical device that stimulates large nerve fibers in the skin via cutaneous electrodes. (Fig. 27–6)

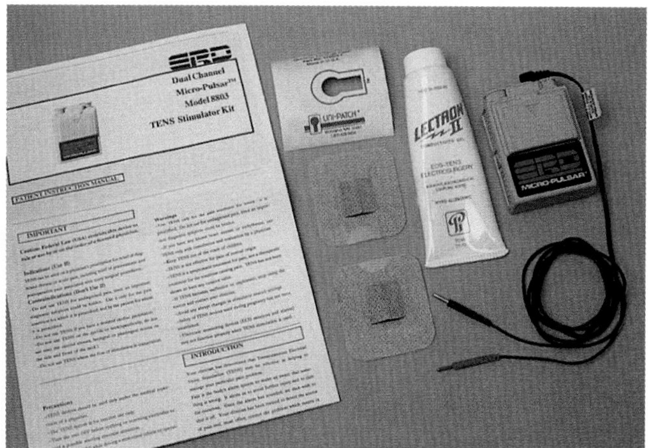

Figure 27-6. TENS unit.

The patient adjusts the type and intensity of stimulation delivered via a small (approximately 3 in^2) controller. The stimulated large nerve fibers in the skin then release neuromodulators in the dorsal horn of the spinal cord, blocking pain transmission at the spinal gate. Some research indicates that TENS activates deep fibers, leading to the release of endorphins, a specific neuromodulator similar to morphine that blocks the transmission of pain at the site of pain in the spinal cord and in the cortex.

TENS has broad applications: during labor; postoperatively for incisional pain; treatment or prevention of ileus (intestinal obstruction resulting from muscular paralysis, obstruction, surgery, and other causes); during painful procedures; and treatment of recurrent, acute pain such as dysmenorrhea (pain associated with menstruation), headaches, and reduction of twitching and spasms associated with some chronic pain syndrome. TENS is contraindicated for pregnant patients or certain cardiac patients in pain, however (Edgar and Smith-Hanrahan, 1992), because the electrical stimulation it produces has never been shown to be safe for the developing fetus and because there is concern that it might interfere with the pace signal. No research has ever been performed to support or refute these concerns.

Persistent, methodical patient teaching is essential in TENS therapy. Patients often become frustrated and give up on TENS without an adequate trial. Finding the right placement of electrodes and settings for electrical stimulation is currently a process of trial and error with each patient. Nurses who regularly care for patients using TENS units need to develop skill in helping patients persevere in trying different combinations (McCaffery and Beebe, 1989).

Acupuncture and Acupressure. Acupuncture (needles inserted into prespecified points along the meridian lines throughout the body (Fig. 27–7), acupressure (application of pressure rather than needles at acupuncture points), and vibration (use of any of a variety of vibrators from hand-held to chairs and cushions) may act by stimulating large fibers leading to the dorsal horn of the spinal cord, thus blocking

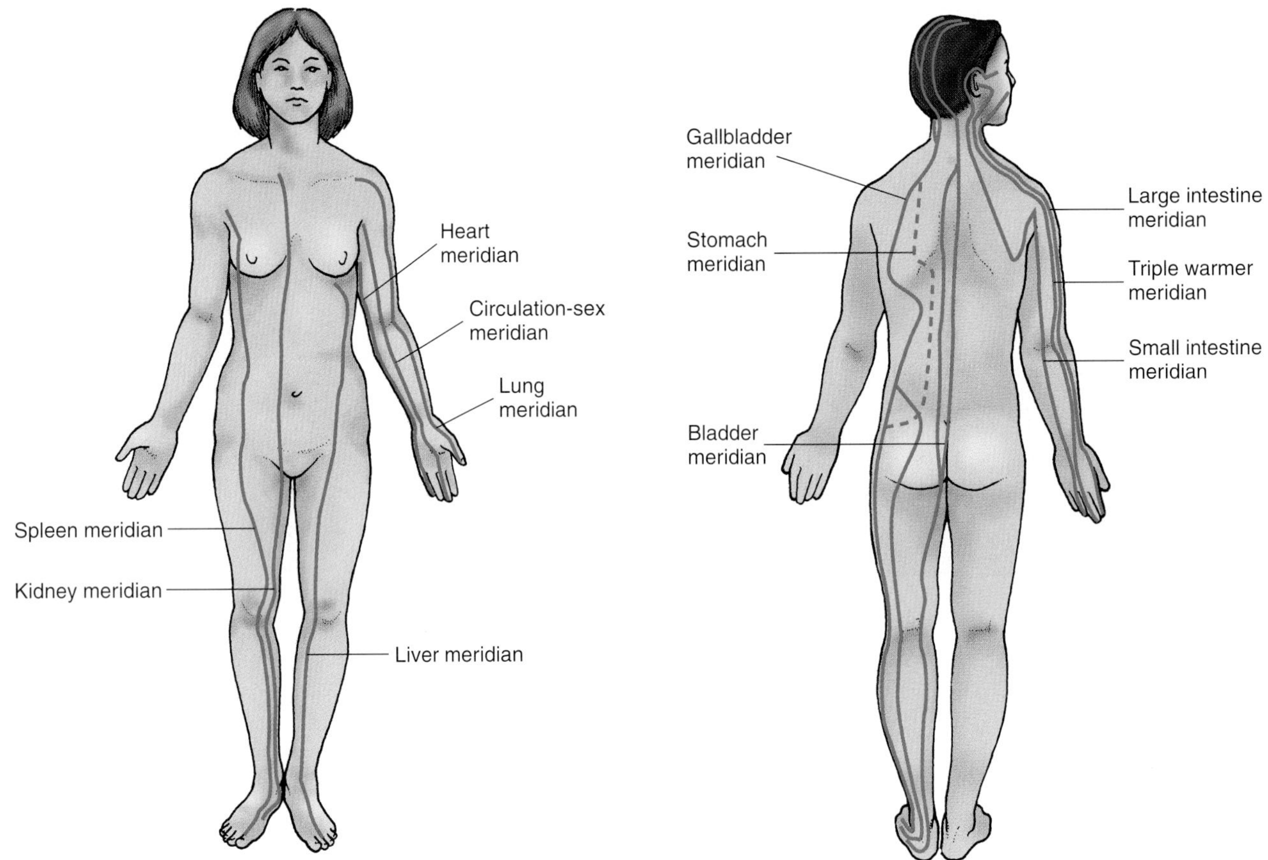

Figure 27–7. Acupuncture meridians. (From Ignatavicius, D., Workman, M.J., Mishler, M. (1999). *Medical-Surgical Nursing: Care Across the Continuum*, 3rd ed. Philadelphia: W.B. Saunders. Used with permission.)

the spinal gate (AHCPR, 1992; McCaffery and Beebe, 1989; Wright, 1987). In many states, acupuncturists are licensed health care providers and treat a variety of illnesses, including pain. Acupressure is often taught to patients and family members to use as needed to combat pain. Theracare is a device invented to help patients to use acupressure or trigger point massage by themselves whenever they need to. Nurses can readily acquire these techniques through community education programs, and then use these skills to reduce pain impulses in infants as well as children and adults.

ALTERING THE PAIN EXPERIENCE

Therapies that alter patients' emotional response to or meaning of the pain experience can also dramatically affect their perception of or aversion to intensity of pain. These therapies include analgesics and adjuvant (or auxiliary) drugs (Box 27–6). They also include nonpharmacologic methods such as distraction, relaxation techniques (imagery, rhythmic breathing, hypnosis, and biofeedback), and cognitive techniques (sensory education, cognitive rehearsal, and modeling). Significant numbers of patients have reported use of and benefit from nonpharmacologic treatment of pain:

- 44 to 68 percent report relief with application of heat
- 49 to 67 percent report relief with massage
- 35 to 89 percent report relief with distraction
- 18 to 25 percent report relief with exercise (Donovan et al, 1987).

Analgesics. Weak opiates (codeine, oxycodone, hydrocodone) and strong opiates (fentanyl, hydromorphone, levorphanol, meperidine, methadone, morphine, and oxymorphone) are called *opiate agonists.* Opiate agonist-antagonists include buprenorphine, butorphanol, nalbuphine, and pentazocine. Both agonists and agonist-antagonist analgesics act by attaching to one or several opiate receptors on neurons in the CNS, preventing the transmission of pain impulses to the next neuron (see Fig. 27–7). Table 27–4 provides a brief overview of these analgesics' key characteristics. Table 27–5 summarizes key interventions to alleviate common opiate side effects.

Nurses should be cautious administering opiate agonist-antagonists. These medications may precipitate acute withdrawal symptoms if, like Paul, a patient has been using (or abusing) an agonist narcotic. Agonist-antagonist opiates are, therefore, best used before any agonist opiate. Although agonist-antagonist narcotics produce less respiratory depression than agonists, as a class they frequently produce psychomimetic side effects such as delusions, hallucinations, and psychotic ideation.

TABLE 27-4 Opiates Used for Severe Pain (Step 3 WHO Ladder) (see Fig. 27-7)

Generic Name	IM Dose = 10-mg Morphine IM	PO Dose = 10-mg Morphine IM	Half-Life	Administration/Mechanism of Action Considerations
Agonist				
Fentanyl (Duragesic)	1.1 mg	NA		Transdermal patch delivering fentanyl at the rate of 25–50 μg/hour is equal to 30 mg sustained-release morphine; 12 hours delay in onset of peak relief after patch is applied; 12 hours for skin accumulation to be used up after removal of patch; fever increases rate of drug absorption from the skin.
Hydromorphone (Dilaudid)	1.5 mg	7.5 mg	2.5–3 hours	Less nausea and vomiting; 1 mg po = 60 mg codeine + 600 mg aspirin; 3 mg is usual rectal dose. Available in high-potency formulation for injection (10 mg/ml).
Levorphanol (Levo-Dromoran)	2 mg	4 mg	12–16 hours	Good oral potency. Because of long half-life, it accumulates over 2–3 days; first sign of accumulation is increased sedation; observe patient closely for 24–96 hours. Less constipation; more sedation.
Meperidine (Demerol)	75–100 mg	300 mg	2–3 hours	A toxic metabolite that accumulates with repeated dosing, especially in renal impairment; may result in seizures. Irritating to tissues. Do not give to patients taking MAOIs
Methadone	10 mg	20 mg	24–36 hours	Because of long half-life, methadone accumulates over several days; peak risk is 3–5 days. First sign of accumulation is increasing sedation. Less nausea and vomiting or constipation than with morphine. Inexpensive.
Morphine	10 mg	30–60 mg	3 hours	Sustained-release preparation releases drug over 8–12 hours. Rectal suppositories available in 5, 10, 20, 30 mg. Use cautiously in patients with impaired respiratory status, bronchial asthma, increased intracranial pressure, or liver failure.
Oxymorphone (Numorphan)	1 mg	NA	2–3 hours	Not recommended in children. Rectal suppositories available. Less constipation and sedation and more nausea, vomiting, and euphoria than with morphine.
Mixed Agonist-Antagonists				
Butorphanol (Stadol)	2 mg	NA	2.5–3.5 hours	Likely to precipitate withdrawal in patients currently taking opiates; hallucinations and other psychomimetic symptoms. Contraindicated in patients with cardiac disease. Less euphoria than with pentazocine.
Nalbuphine (Nubain)	10 mg	NA	5 hours	Likely to precipitate withdrawal in patients currently taking an opiate. Incidence of psychomimetic symptoms lower than with pentazocine. Sedating at higher doses.
Pentazocine (Talwin)	60 mg	180 mg	2–3 hours	Likely to precipitate withdrawal in patients taking an opiate. Psychomimetic effects, including hallucinations, in 25% of population; contraindicated in patients with cardiac diseases.

WHO, World Health Organization; IM, intramuscular; NA, not applicable; po, orally; MAOIs, monoamine oxidase inhibitors
Data from American Pain Society (1992) and Agency for Health Care Policy and Research (1994).

TABLE 27-5 Treatment of Common Opiates' Side Effects

Common Side Effect	Cause	Treatment to Minimize Side Effect
Sedation	Opiates bind to receptors in brain stem	Is most pronounced when patient is sleep deprived as a result of pain; decreases over time and with sufficient rest. Dextroamphetamine (2.5–10 mg) or methylphenidate (5–10 mg) each A.M. can be helpful if necessary (American Pain Society, 1992).
Respiratory depression	Opiates bind to receptors in respiratory center in brain stem	As carbon dioxide increases, the breath stimulus is triggered; giving oxygen prevents this reflex, potentiating this side effect. Coach patient to breathe. Tolerance to this side effect develops after several doses. May need to reduce dose by 10%. Greatest risk is with the first dose in a patient who has not recently received any opiate medication. Naloxone is the antagonist. (Mix 0.4 mg naloxone in 10 ml normal saline, and give intravenously slowly to improve respirations and not precipitate the immediate return of pain. Because half-life of naloxone is only 30 minutes, naloxone may need to be given every 20–30 minutes for 3–4 hours in an acute overdose.)
Nausea and vomiting	Opiates stimulate the chemoreceptor trigger zone to varying degrees	Increases with movement, decreases with bed rest; also likely to decrease over time. It responds to treatment with prochlorperazine or metoclopramide. Response to standard antiemetics is variable (Foley and Inturrisi, 1987).
Constipation	Opiates bind to receptors in the wall of the intestines	Little tolerance develops to this most common side effect. All patients taking opiates should be on a high-fluid, high-fiber diet, be exercising daily, and be on a bowel regimen, which includes a daily stool softener and laxative (such as senna) (Paice,1988; Portenoy, 1990).
Biliary colic	Opiates increase smooth muscle tone	Meperidine and fentanyl (Sublimaze) are most likely to produce this side effect. It is also more likely to occur in patients with a history of gallbladder disease (Jaffe and Meutin, 1985).
Urinary retention	Opiates increase smooth muscle tone	Most likely to occur in patients with known risk factors (especially prostatic hypertrophy). Monitor output carefully. Catheterization may be needed.
Pruritus	Opiates can cause the release of histamine	Diphenhydramine 25–50 mg is effective in treating this side effect (Bayless, et al, 1987).

BOX 27-6
OTHER MEDICATIONS THAT REDUCE PAIN

- **Phenothiazines.** Promethazine (Phenergan) actually is an antianalgesic. Phenothiazines in general do not potentiate the analgesic properties of analgesics, but do potentiate their sedative and respiratory depressant side effects, preventing the patient from reporting lack of pain relief. Only hydroxyzine (Vistaril) has analgesic action.
- **Benzodiazepines.** These drugs relax muscle spasms and relieve pain if a muscle spasm is a precipitating or contributing cause of pain. Limiting their use to 7 to 10 days is strongly recommended because their efficacy declines with time, and physiologic dependence can occur.
- **Tricyclic antidepressants.** These drugs increase certain neuromodulators and make the spinal neurons less sensitive to neurotransmission. They also help relieve depression often associated with chronic pain.
- **Corticosteroids.** These drugs reduce inflammation. They may be useful alone, with a nonsteroidal anti-inflammatory drug, or with an opiate for bone pain or pain related to inflammation.
- **Anticonvulsants.** These drugs increase neuromodulation by raising the threshold for excitation of the spinal neurons. They are most effective in relieving pain caused by damaged nerves (neuropathies).

Principles for Analgesic Use. The WHO suggested a three-step ladder approach to the treatment of cancer pain (Fig. 27–8). WHO recommends that adjuvant drugs such as tricyclic antidepressants, NSAIDs, anticonvulsants, and corticosteroids be used at each step, if needed, to enhance the effects of the primary analgesic (WHO, 1985).

A pain management plan sheet is shown in Figure 27–9.

Heated debate about the appropriateness of using opiates for chronic nonmalignant pain has raged for years (Portenoy, 1994). Psychological counseling and physical retraining of patients with chronic pain have shown improved functioning, and patients taking opiates are less successful than those not taking opiates. Other studies suggest that patients in these programs still suffer from residual pain and would benefit from the addition of opiates to the pain management program. Research clearly demonstrates that patients who have severe pain at the beginning of a pain management program are less likely to be successful than those with mild to moderate pain.

Apparently, the intensity of the pain is a more important factor than whether the pain is being treated with opiates. One investigator also questioned whether current treatments of chronic pain (based on pain center models of pain management) are as cost effective as the judicious use of opiate and other pain medications (Portenoy, 1990). Whatever treatments or therapies the nurse may be asked to participate in, implement, or assess, the nurse should always consider the patient's needs paramount and advocate opiates, as necessary.

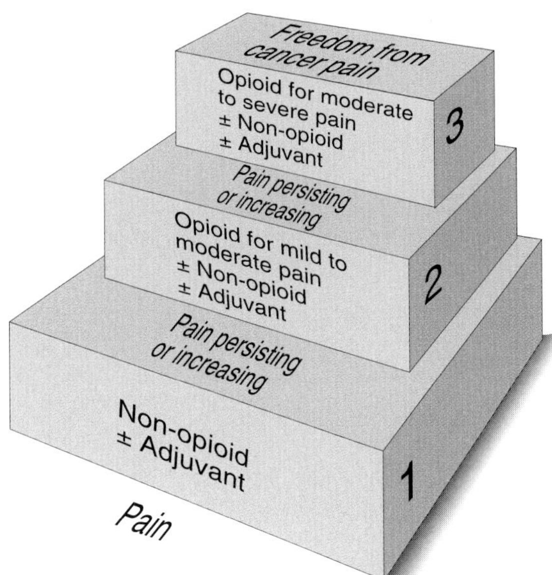

Figure 27–8. The World Health Organization (WHO) three-step ladder approach to treating cancer pain. Reproduced by permission of WHO, from *Cancer Pain Relief,* 2nd ed. Geneva: World Health Organization, 1996.

However, rigorous clinical trials are still needed to determine the effects, side effects, benefits, and costs of opiate use for chronic pain. The health care reform movement, with its focus on cost containment, may be the stimulus required to move forward with these clinical trials.

Common Misperceptions About Analgesic Use. Health care providers' failure to appreciate the risks and benefits of NSAIDs often interferes with their appropriate use. Misunderstanding of the meaning and risks of tolerance, respiratory depression, and addiction interfere with the effective use of opiate analgesics. Here are some common misconceptions of NSAIDs and opiates, with their corresponding facts:

- NSAIDs are not very effective analgesics. **Fact:** given in the correct dose, NSAIDs can be highly effective for mild to moderate pain; they are, in fact, often more effective than opiates for inflammatory pain.
- NSAIDs are safer than opiates. **Fact:** NSAIDs have significant side effects, among them life-threatening gastric bleeding and liver failure; and the risk of these side effects increases with the total daily dose and the duration of time the medication is used.
- Tolerance develops quickly to the analgesic effects of an opiate. **Fact:** tolerance—the need for an increased dose of a substance to obtain the same effect—develops to the euphoric, sedative, and respiratory depression side effects of opiates very quickly after a stable dose is reached (very slowly, if at all, to constipation). Observations or long-term elderly hospice patients, cancer patients with pain not in hospices, and small numbers of chronic pain patients receiving opiates over several years have shown that development of tolerance to the analgesic effects of opiates is relatively rare. Most patients, if treated aggressively and effectively for pain relief, stabilize at an analgesic dose that relieves their pain. Between 5% and 10% of patients require increased doses; research into this phenomenon continues. Undertreatment of pain resulting in *hyperalgesia,* excessive sensitivity to pain, is today thought to be a critical factor in the development of tolerance (Mao et al, 1995).
- Patients taking high doses of opiates are likely to experience respiratory depression, which is not easily reversible. **Fact:** Patients are at greatest risk for respiratory depression between, generally, the first and eighth doses. However, narcotic-induced respiratory depression, unlike the side effects of most drugs, is easily reversible. Coaching the patient to breathe is an immediate and highly effective intervention to counteract respiratory depression. The nurse must follow this emergency intervention immediately by administering naloxone, an opiate antagonist. Naloxone should be given slowly to reverse respiratory depression, yet avoid nullifying the desired analgesic actions (Foley and Inturrisi, 1987). Again, there is no substitute for knowledge. Familiarity with the duration of action of each opioid alerts the nurse to when respiratory depression and other noxious side effects are likely to occur.
- Many patients in pain become addicted to opiates. **Fact:** Even highly trained caregivers often confuse addiction, physical dependence, and regular use of an opiate. *Physical dependence* means that if a drug is abruptly stopped, the individual taking it will experience symptoms related to its cessation. More than a few doses of analgesia will almost always result in some form of physical dependence. We know this to be true of opiates, insulin, prednisone, caffeine, nicotine, alcohol, and most drugs that affect the nervous system. Just as the discontinuation of insulin or prednisone requires a tapering-off process, so do opiates or many drugs whose primary site of action is the CNS. *Addiction,* however, may include no drug dependence whatsoever; rather, it is characterized by drug use for its euphoric effects despite any physical or psychological harm that may occur as a result. This may include self-neglect as dire as malnutrition, related to a failure to eat; arrest, resulting from robbery to obtain drugs; and cessation or severe disruption of social, civic, or economic activities such as personal relationships or jobs. Many patients whom caregivers or society label as drug seeking are actually seeking pain relief.

Patient-Controlled Analgesia. PCA describes any number of patient-controlled (not institutionally) intravenous and, more recently, epidural methods of delivering narcotics. PCA's goal is simple: to relieve pain by maintaining a stable level of analgesic in the blood or epidural space by giving the patient control of the delivery of analgesic.

In all PCA pumps, the patient pushes a control device, which delivers a predetermined dose of analgesic. Each injected dose and lockout interval (the time interval that must elapse between injections) is preset to prevent accidental overdosing. Like all pain interventions, however, caregivers must adjust PCA for each individual; research indicates that the dose required for relief is not related to age, sex, weight, or type of surgery. Although PCA has demonstrated superiority to prn analgesia in many settings, reports indicate that scheduled administration of analgesics is as effective as PCA.

The common factor in both PCA and scheduled analgesic administration is the maintenance of a stable blood level. Even though the patient is self-administering the medication with PCA, the nurse's pain assessment, evaluation of efficacy, and prevention of and management of side effects are the same whether the patient receives the analgesic by mouth, parenterally, or PCA (Hauer et al, 1995). In the home setting, a variety of medications (morphine, baclofen, lidocaine) may be given by PCA or continuous infusion pump to control pain. The pump used in the home setting is often pocket sized to encourage maintaining normal activity. Patient education is vital in the home setting where the patient (or family member) is the caregiver as well as the care receiver. It is especially important in the home setting that the patient and a responsible other person understand

- Why the intravenous infusion is used and the medications and doses involved
- How the system delivering the medication works and how to problem solve and treat the common problems that can occur with the pump or the intravenous catheter
- Skillful care of the intravenous catheter, the pump, and the medication (including cleaning, checking for problems, changing bags of medication, changing settings on the pump)
- The signs of inadequate or excessive administration of medication
- How to quickly obtain advice or assistance from the home nursing service.

See Procedure 27–1 for information on assisting a patient with PCA.

Distraction Techniques. Distraction helps reduce pain by several of the neuromodulating mechanisms described in the gate control theory of pain

- Promotes relaxation, reduces muscle spasm, and increases oxygenation, thereby reducing the amount of neurotransmission coming to the spinal cord from the periphery
- Increases production and release of neuromodulating chemicals from the brain, which are responsible for the *emotional* reaction to pain; these chemicals also can assist in "closing" the gate in the spinal cord and blocking pain
- Lessens anxiety, which leads to reduced muscle spasm, and alters the chemical environment in the brain so that there is more neuromodulation and less neurotransmission
- Alters the patient's perception of pain by redirecting the mind's focus and sending messages to the gate in the spinal cord that the situation is under control, thereby decreasing the sensitivity of the spinal cord neurons to incoming neurotransmission.

A common caregiver misconception is that effective pain relief from distraction means the patient's pain is psychological. This is definitely false. As can be seen, distraction is an effective means of increasing neuromodulation and blocking neurotransmission regardless of the site or reason for the pain. Distraction strategies, however, cannot be based on light or less attention-demanding activities such as watching television or reading a book. Puzzles and other games, storytelling, conversation, humorous movies, and music have all been reported to be effective sources of distraction (AHCPR, 1992).

Once again, though, the nurse must carefully individualize any distraction techniques. For instance, the wrong music is an annoyance rather than a distraction or method of relaxing. Paul, the young patient in the case study, for instance, may react with hostility, bewilderment, or boredom to music the nurse considers soothing and distracting, such as classical or light jazz. A patient like this may respond for the better to loud, raucous—and to older ears, atonal—alternative rock. A personal cassette player may be most appropriate in this situation. Letting Paul choose his own music gives him more control and respects his adolescent need for autonomy. Similarly, a comedy tape humorous to one patient may be offensive to another.

Cognitive Therapies. Cognitive approaches for treatment of acute pain include sensory education, cognitive rehearsal, and modeling. An extensive literature review (of more than 10,000 articles) performed by the AHCPR panel developing guidelines on acute pain indicates that such strategies as imagining the painful event (cognitive rehearsal) provides the patient greater control over the pain. The nurse can help the patient imagine a painful event such as starting an intravenous catheter, then practice deep breathing while continuing to image the painful event and feeling as though the event is being mastered. Alternatively, the nurse may help the patient relax and imagine being someplace else doing something pleasant while experiencing a painful procedure. Patients can use tape-recorded imagery exercises at home or even in the hospital or clinic when a nurse or family cannot be present to coach them through the imagery exercise. Patients who use imagery report less distress associated with painful procedures. Similarly, patients who see another patient experience a painful event with composure and with few demonstrated pain behaviors (modeling) may consequently report less pain and distress when they undergo the procedure themselves. Nurses can encourage patients who are about to undergo a procedure to talk with someone who has successfully undergone the same procedure recently. Many self-help books and lay magazines include a variety of cognitive-behavioral techniques; the nurse is wise to know at least some

PATIENT TEACHING
DEEP BREATHING TO REDUCE PAIN AND STRESS

Pain and stress produce tension, often serious muscle spasm. Even the stressors of daily life may send pulse, respiration, and other vital indicators soaring.

1. Goal: deep breathing can help minimize everyday tension-producing situations and relieve muscle spasm. In a patient like Paul, this technique may also allay his fears and ease his depression. The nurse would teach Paul along the following lines:
2. Teaching: Place one hand on your chest, and one hand on your stomach. Notice which hand moves when you breathe. The goal is to take a deep breath which moves the hand on your stomach, and barely moves the hand on your chest. Inhale through your nose and relax your stomach muscles. Let the air fill your lungs and move the hand resting on your stomach. Exhale through your mouth while relaxing. Be patient. If you are used to breathing only with your chest, this can take some time to master. Practice three slow deep breaths each hour, and you will eventually be able to do this almost automatically.

   Learn to deep breathe for daily stress. When confronted with a stressful situation, practice deep breathing for three to four breaths. This will require regular practice. Develop a routine for regular use (e.g., every time you are waiting for an elevator, practice two deep breaths; set your clock to chime at each hour and practice two deep breaths each time; use deep breathing for 1 to 2 minutes to prepare for sleep at bedtime).

   Guard against side effects. The major side effect is hyperventilation. This may happen if you are breathing very deeply but too rapidly. If you become light-headed, experience tingling sensations of your fingers or around your mouth, stop deep breathing, sit down, and breath normally. Within a few breaths you should feel fine again. Hyperventilation happens occasionally when you are first learning deep breathing for relaxation; expect it. It's normal. You are concentrating on your breathing and may tend to breathe a bit too rapidly. When you really start to relax with this technique, your breathing becomes slow and deep. and hyperventilation seldom occurs.

   Let us practice three deep breaths together.
3. Follow-Up: The nurse returns to see whether Paul is deep breathing and assesses his technique. If inadequate or if he is hyperventilating, the nurse reteaches. The nurse is never insistent or impatient and recognizes that deep breathing may not be appropriate for some patients.

of these common strategies. Community education programs often offer 4- to 16-hour courses on such topics as anger management, meditation, stress management, and yoga.

Relaxation Techniques. Relaxation is a form of distraction and of cognitive therapy that promotes specific muscle relaxation, reduced sympathetic activation, and increased oxygenation. Although relaxation is a form of distraction and distraction often promotes relaxation, they are usually addressed as separate techniques. For instance, when certain types of music are used for distraction, little relaxation may occur; when music is selected to enhance a relaxation technique, a much greater state of relaxation can occur. Relaxation techniques commonly include rhythmic or deep breathing, guided imagery, and biofeedback.

The most basic relaxation technique is deep abdominal breathing (see Patient Teaching: Deep Breathing to Reduce Pain and Stress). As easy as it sounds, it takes most people several practice sessions to be able to breathe deeply using the abdomen rather than the chest. Initially, the patient should do this only four to five times because they commonly hyperventilate when they are first learning this. They can gradually increase to several minutes two to three times daily. Nurses can use this technique to coach patients through brief painful procedures.

Guided imagery is the process of using a pleasant image to enhance relaxation (see Patient Teaching: Relaxation with Guided Imagery). Various "relaxation" tapes are available in bookstores, libraries, and even bed and bath shops. These are effective for some people, but the most effective imagery tape is one made by or for the individual patient. This tape can progress at a pace that is comfortable for the individual and can focus on this individual's very unique image.

Relaxation techniques are ideal for the home setting because they require little special equipment and can be independently done by most patients. Imagery may also produce cognitive changes that alter the patient's perception of pain. Some studies suggest that the pain relief associated with imagery is caused by the release of endorphins (internal opiates), which block pain transmission (AHCPR, 1992; Blanchard and Ahles, 1990; Edgar and Smith-Hanrahan, 1992; McCaffery and Beebe, 1989).

Exercise. Research supports that exercise has several essential roles in pain management; it is essential to prevent the complications of disuse, increase oxygenation of tissues, prevent shortening and spasms of muscles, and increase endurance. It is also a form of distraction and for some people a form of relaxation. The adage "no pain, no gain!" has no place in the use of these techniques. Exercise should begin with gentle stretching done frequently without causing pain. (See Patient Teaching: Basic Exercises to Reduce or Prevent Neck Pain.) Because any body part can experience pain, an overview of exercises that can be helpful for pain is beyond the limits of this chapter. Regardless of the site of pain, the principles for use of exercise to reduce pain are

- Start with a few gentle stretches that do not cause pain and increase slowly.

PATIENT TEACHING
RELAXATION WITH GUIDED IMAGERY

Guided imagery is a relaxation technique whereby the patient imagines him- or herself in a completely stress-free environment—floating on a raft in the ocean, watching a tropical sunset, or, in Paul's case, walking through the forest—with every detail elaborated and each part of the body relaxed in turn. This technique

Reduces muscle tension and spasms
Reduces psychological tension, stress, and anxiety
Reduces pain
Increases the patient's ability to increase his own comfort.

Patient Readiness

For a patient like Paul, the nurse first explores his interest in learning relaxation with guided imagery. If interested, the nurse then explains that relaxation sends messages to the muscles to reduce muscle spasm and reduces anxiety (Paul cannot be concentrating on relaxation and also be anxious or tense at the same time). At the very least, it provides a brief "time out." Relaxation also reduces some of the chemicals that transmit pain (neurotransmitters), thereby reducing some of the pain, and increases some of the chemicals that block pain (neuromodulators).

If Paul is amenable, the nurse helps him into a comfortable position with all body parts supported well; to prevent falling asleep, a sitting position is usually better than a lying position. Because many patients experience vasodilatation with relaxation, the nurse covers Paul with an extra-light blanket.

Next, the nurse individualizes the technique for the patient; if, unlike Paul, the patient has a history of respiratory problems, teaching does not focus much on breathing. The nurse asks Paul to fully describe a forest, eliciting input for all senses: sight, hearing, smell, touch, taste, emotional reaction, presence of others, the overall experience. Some patients give a great deal of detail; others have only a general impression. The nurse modifies the approach based on the patient's success in mentally recreating a peaceful scene; if it works well, the nurse models her approach after it. If it worked poorly, the nurse improvises.

The basic script (presented next) is usually acceptable. The nurse remembers that any image, direction, or pacing is more effective if it matches the patient's own images, and watches the patient's nonverbal cues during the experience (e.g., shifting about may indicate problems with relaxation and a need to slow down or speed up the pace, and visible signs of muscle relaxation warrant a comment on how well the patient is doing). If a significant other is to be coaching the patient in future relaxation experiences, the nurse ensures that that person has a copy of the script and is sitting where he or she can see and hear what is occurring.

Following a Script

The nurse may use this basic script, improvising according to the patient's reaction:

Get into as comfortable a position as you can get . . . head and arms and back and legs supported comfortably. Move around a bit to get as comfortable as you can be. Close your eyes and focus on a particular spot [such as Paul's forest].

Take a deep breath, let it out slowly and relax. Relax. Take another deep breath, and as you exhale, relax more. You may already begin to notice that your body is beginning to calm itself. There are muscles all over your body that hold tension and contribute to pain. You are relaxing these muscles and becoming more comfortable. Identifying this tension is the first step in getting rid of it.

Focus on different body parts. Identify any tension, what it feels like, and then relax those muscles. Begin with your hands. Think about your right hand. Make a fist . . . tight as you can. Notice what it feels like. The next time you exhale, relax your right hand. Now make a fist with both hands. Notice how the tension feels. Exhale. Relax. Notice how it feels. There may be feelings of warmth or coolness, heaviness or lightness, or other changes in sensation. These are signals that you are starting to relax.

Now think about your forearms. Notice any tension there. As you exhale, relax. Allow both arms and hands to relax. Allow those special feelings of relaxation that you identified in your hands to move up your arms. Even when you think you are relaxed, your muscles can relax even more. Try it. And still more.

Now focus on your forehead, face, neck, and shoulders. This is an area where many people keep a lot of tension. Imagine the tension being wiped away by a warm towel. Let your scalp relax and your face and neck and shoulders, too. Squeeze your eyes tightly together and then relax, open your mouth really wide, stick out your tongue, and then relax. Let the relaxation and comfort that started in your hands when you released your fists flow down over your head and face one muscle at a time. Each time you exhale, relax.

Focus on your neck, shoulders, and upper back. Imagine the tension as knots in big ropes. You can untie those knots. Take a moment now to imagine one of those knots just effortlessly untying itself. Feel the relaxation moving from muscle to muscle, one muscle at a time. Not all of the tension will disappear at once; as you get more skillful at relaxation, you will discover that you can become more relaxed more easily. Just allow your neck and shoulders and back to become more relaxed each time you exhale. Relax.

Notice any tension in your chest or abdomen. As you exhale, relax. Each time you inhale, feel that relaxation that started in your hands flowing from muscle to muscle. And each time you exhale, blow more and more tension out of your body and relax. Think about the muscles of your lower back and pelvis. Exhale and relax. Focus on your hips, buttocks, and upper legs. Exhale and relax. Now your legs, knees, ankles, feet, and toes. Relax and blow away more tension. And still more.

Now refocus on each group of muscles briefly, and let go of even more tension. Relax each time you exhale.

PATIENT TEACHING
RELAXATION WITH GUIDED IMAGERY (cont'd)

Arms relax . . . head and face relax . . . neck and back relax . . . chest and abdomen relax . . . back relax . . . legs and feet relax.

While you are relaxing your muscles, revel in your special place. Begin by imagining that special place. Experience it as vividly as you can: smell, sight, temperature, everything. [Describe the image the patient described to you during preparation; do not add or delete anything.] Notice how calm and relaxed you feel. Each time you exhale, you are becoming more and more comfortable, more and more relaxed.

Continue to stay in that special place, becoming as relaxed as possible, even drift off to sleep if you wish. Or become more alert, and return to your life. It is your choice. To become more alert and aware now, begin counting backward from 4 to 1. Allow just a bit more muscle tone to return with each number. Become just a little more alert as 4 becomes 3. Begin to move your arms and legs a bit as you count from 3 to 2. Feel completely alert and comfortable as you count from 2 to 1. Now you're fully alert, capable of dealing with anything.

As you need to become less tense and more comfortable throughout the day, take a deep breath, hold it for the count of 3 and then slowly exhale while relaxing. Take a deep breath, hold it for the count of three, and exhale slowly, thinking R-E-L-A-X.

Follow-Up

Review with the patient what the process of relaxation feels like, where the pacing was too fast or too slow, what seemed to work well, any problems, the degree of relaxation, and pain relief experienced. Then incorporate this input into the script for the next coached relaxation with this patient. Review with the patient the signs observed when the patient was beginning to relax an area, and answers the patient's or coach's questions.

If the patient wants an audiotape of the relaxation with guided imagery, arrange to make the tape during the second session, incorporating the improvements suggested previously. If the patient is using imagery to achieve rest and even sleep, close the door and put up a "do not disturb" sign.

- Do a limited number of exercises hourly rather than many repetitions only once or twice daily.
- Stop if pain increases.

AMERICAN PAIN SOCIETY RECOMMENDATIONS

In its 1995 guidelines, the APS suggested that health care institutions must redirect their protocols if pain relief is to improve in the future.

Make Pain Visible. The APS believes that pain should be considered the fifth vital sign, as visible in the patient record as is pulse, respiration, blood pressure, and temperature. (Figure 27–9 illustrates three ways the nurse can do this.) Some institutions post a large plastic graph or table on the wall of the patient's room. Every 4 hours, caregivers chart both pain intensity and pain relief scores there and in the patient record.

Develop Methods to Facilitate Changing Caregivers' Pain Management Behaviors. Lack of knowledge about pain, analgesics, and the correct doses is common among

PATIENT TEACHING
BASIC EXERCISES TO REDUCE OR PREVENT NECK PAIN

Neck pain and tension-induced headaches are among the most common causes of pain. Simple exercises can help:

- Reduce spasm in the neck muscles and the associated pain
- Improve the strength of the neck muscles, making spasm less likely
- Increase flexibility by stretching the muscles

Provide the following instructions to the patient:

While seated with shoulders directly above hips and head and neck squarely above the line of shoulders, look straight ahead and tuck chin in (most people will get two to three double chins if they do this correctly). Hold this position for the count of 5 and then relax. The goal is to feel tension and then relax. Do not do this so strongly that it causes any increase in pain. Repeat one to three times each hour. Increase by one repetition each day if the previous day's exercise did not increase pain.

Develop a routine of doing this exercise 5 to 12 times daily.

If pain increases, decrease repetitions by 1 per hour.

If pain persists despite decreasing repetitions, see your primary health care provider.

A

TIME												
F C												C F
103.1 39.5												39.5 103.1
102.2 39.0												39.0 102.2
101.3 38.5												38.5 101.3
100.4 38.0												38.0 100.4
99.5 37.5												37.5 99.5
98.6 37.0												37.0 98.6
97.7 36.5												36.5 97.7
96.8 36.0												36.0 96.8
95.9 35.5 95.0 35.0												35.5 95.9 35.0 95.0
PULSE RADIAL												**PAIN LEVEL**
PULSE APICAL												
RESP.												0-NONE
B/P												10-SEVERE
PAIN												

B

Pain Management Flow Sheet

	Date	March 3, 1997			
	Time	0800	1200	1600	2000
	R	16	14	16	16
	O_2 Sat	—	—	—	—
	Pain Score (0-10)	2	2	4	2
	Arousal Score	Alert	Dozing	Restless	Dozing
	Side Effects	Nausea	Ø	Ø	Ø
PCA	Drug Morphine				
PCA	Basal Rate 1 mg/hr	———	———	———	——>
PCA	Patient injections 1 mg				
PCA	Lockout 10 min				
PCA	Attempts/Injections				
PCA	Total Dose 7 mg/hr	20 mg/4h	20 mg/4h	10 mg/4h	27 mg/4h

Figure 27–9. Three methods of documenting pain and pain relief: *A,* As the fifth vital sign on the graphic sheet; *B,* on a pain management flow sheet.

Continued

nurses, physicians, and pharmacists, as we have documented. Education of all individuals intimately involved in providing comfort is obviously essential. Methods of providing easy access to necessary, behavior-changing information in day-to-day practice should include

1. An easy-to-use chart to convert from one analgesic to another without compromising the amount given the patient
2. An easy and consistent way of assessing and documenting pain intensity and relief
3. Ready access to the latest information, packaged with the medication cart in an easy-to-review, easy-to-understand format: clinical updates from the pharmacy on current, common questions or problems on a specific drug, for instance.

Implement Procedures to Ensure That Patients Have a Key Role in the Assessment, Treatment, and Evaluation of Their Pain Relief. Regular assessment by the patient of pain and relief is the first essential step in this process. APS also recommended a process in which a sample of patients are interviewed about their pain, pain relief, length of time they waited for pain relief, expectations related to pain and pain relief, how pain has affected ability to function, and satisfac-

C **Brief Pain Inventory (Short Form)**

Date: ______/______/______

Time: ________________

Name: ____________________ ____________________ __________

Last First Middle Initial

1) Throughout our lives, most of us have had pain from time to time (such as minor headaches, sprains, and toothaches). Have you had pain other than these everyday kinds of pain today? 1. Yes 2. No

2) On the diagram, shade in the areas where you feel pain. Put an X on the area that hurts the most.

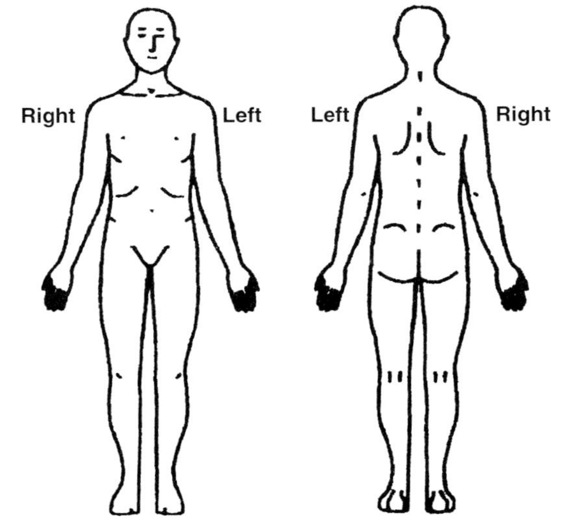

3) Please rate your pain by circling the one number that best describes your pain at its **worst** in the past 24 hours.

0 1 2 3 4 5 6 7 8 9 10
No pain ... Pain as bad as you can imagine

4) Please rate your pain by circling the one number that best describes your pain at its **least** in the past 24 hours.

0 1 2 3 4 5 6 7 8 9 10
No pain ... Pain as bad as you can imagine

5) Please rate your pain by circling the one number that best describes your pain on the **average.**

0 1 2 3 4 5 6 7 8 9 10
No pain ... Pain as bad as you can imagine

6) Please rate your pain by circling the one number that tells how much pain you have **right now.**

0 1 2 3 4 5 6 7 8 9 10
No pain ... Pain as bad as you can imagine

7) What treatments or medications are you receiving for your pain? ____________________

____

8) In the past 24 hours, how much **relief** have pain treatments or medications provided? Please circle the one percentage that most shows how much relief you have received.

0% 10% 20% 30% 40% 50% 60% 70% 80% 90% 100%
No relief ... Complete relief

9) Circle the one number that describes how, during the past 24 hours, pain has **interfered** with your:

A. General activity

0 1 2 3 4 5 6 7 8 9 10
Does not interfere ... Completely interferes

B. Mood

0 1 2 3 4 5 6 7 8 9 10
Does not interfere ... Completely interferes

C. Walking ability

0 1 2 3 4 5 6 7 8 9 10
Does not interfere ... Completely interferes

D. Normal work (includes both work outside the home and housework)

0 1 2 3 4 5 6 7 8 9 10
Does not interfere ... Completely interferes

E. Relations with other people

0 1 2 3 4 5 6 7 8 9 10
Does not interfere ... Completely interferes

F. Sleep

0 1 2 3 4 5 6 7 8 9 10
Does not interfere ... Completely interferes

G. Enjoyment of life

0 1 2 3 4 5 6 7 8 9 10
Does not interfere ... Completely interferes

Source: Pain Research Group, Department of Neurology, University of Wisconsin-Madison

Figure 27–9. *Continued* *C,* on a pain inventory form that the patient completes. (C, from the Pain Research Group, Department of Neurology, University of Wisconsin-Madison.)

tion with caregivers and with pain relief. The APS recommended that this information be gathered quarterly and used to improve the processes of delivering care.

Increase Clinical Accountability. This process begins when the information gathered in Step 3 is fed back to inpatient, home care, hospice, clinic, same-day surgical, and other care delivery units in a timely manner. These practitioners then have the information their facility needs to hold them accountable for improving their quality of care. It also requires, however, an administrative commitment to hold the practitioners responsible for determining what changes need to be effected and then implementing them. Although it is true that improvement is difficult without feedback, it is equally true that actually doing so is impossible without the commitment to improve.

Proceed with Demonstration Projects to Accomplish the Warranted Changes. Practitioners who wait for the perfect documentation method or protocol may not only be waiting in vain. They do so at the patient's expense, when taking one simple tentative step forward would improve the patient's pain. For example, many nurses improvised a way of making pain visible on the patient record, by writing "pain" or "pain relief" into any blank space they can find, while the Forms Committees debated this temporary expedient's validity. The information these nurses obtained about the intensity of pain and lack of pain relief with their "write-in" campaign was often exactly the information necessary to get permanent changes implemented.

Participate Jointly with Federal and State Regulatory Agencies to Change Policies or Practices That Interfere with Adequate Pain Relief. Recently, the Joint Commission on the Accreditation of Health Care Organizations, the body responsible for the accreditation of hospitals, home care programs, and ambulatory care centers, changed its focus from *checking* on quality assurance to *facilitating* quality improvement. That is, instead of checking how often something is done *poorly,* the commission recommends quality improvement approaches that analyze the processes by which care is given to continuously improve them and achieve or exceed patient comfort. The AHCPR guidelines and the APS standards also support this approach. If this broad institutional approach is followed, the future will indeed be better for patients experiencing pain because

- Pain will be assessed *with,* not independent of, the patient.
- Interventions appropriate for the individual patient will be selected, implemented, and evaluated.
- If pain relief is inadequate or side effects are unacceptable, the treatment plan will be swiftly modified to continuously improve patient relief and satisfaction.

PROCEDURE 27-1

Providing Patient-Controlled Analgesia

Objective

Provide pain relief with the least amount of narcotic analgesic necessary while providing the patient with the opportunity to manage delivery of medication.

Terminology

- **Patient-controlled analgesia (PCA) pump:** a mechanical device used to administer preprogrammed doses of narcotic analgesic medication intravenously (it may sometimes be used for subcutaneous and epidural administration also) (Fig. 27–10)
- **Intravenous heparin-saline lock:** intermittent infusion needle or catheter that provides direct access to venous system and may be used intermittently; is filled with saline-heparin between uses
- **Primary catheter:** intravenous tubing that provides direct access to the venous system while delivering continuous fluid therapy
- **Loading dose:** initial dose of narcotic analgesic given to help reach a therapeutic blood level of medication
- **Patient-initiated dose:** incremental doses of narcotic analgesic administered by the patient via the pump for the purpose of pain relief
- **Continuous dose:** amount of medication delivered consistently by the pump as programmed by the care provider or pharmacist
- **Lockout:** time interval between patient-initiated doses

Critical Elements

The parameters of medication administration allowed by the PCA pump are determined by a physician order. These parameters are programmed into the pump by the pharmacist or the licensed care provider. Refer to your facility's policy on the use of PCA pumps to determine which care providers may program or supervise the use of this device and the medication delivered by this device.

Before using a PCA pump, assess the patient to determine the suitability of using the pump as a pain

continued on next page

PROCEDURE 27-1 (cont'd)

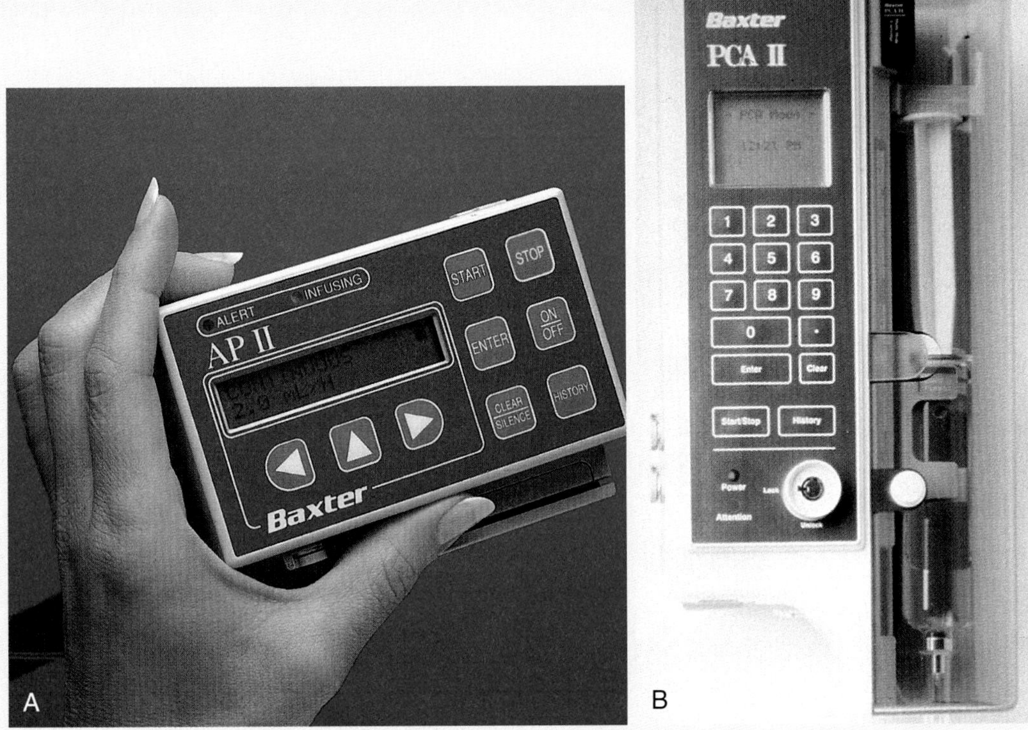

Figure 27–10. Two patient-controlled analgesic infusion pumps. (Courtesy Baxter Healthcare Corporation, Round Lake, IL.)

control device. This assessment should include respiratory status, mental status, and manual dexterity. For those patients who will receive the medication by intravenous route, it should also include whether there is an appropriate intravenous access.

Another aspect of assessment is instruction and discussion of expected outcomes. This will include

- Acceptable pain relief
- Understanding of cause of pain and reasons for treatment
- Ability to report pain on scale of 0 to 10
- Effective patient use and satisfaction with PCA

Also teach use of the pain intensity or pain relief scale, and ascertain the patient's understanding of it. Be certain the patient knows what it feels like to push the control button, and has the coordination and strength to do so. Arrange for special interpretive services if needed for a patient with inadequate English skills. If the patient cannot read, develop a creative communication plan to assess pain and pain relief.

Assess for patient allergies before administering any new medication.

For reasons of cost containment and documented decreased incidence of medication errors, the pharmacy in many facilities now dispenses medications by the unit dose method and mixes the majority of subcutaneous and intravenous solution medication cartridges with the patient-controlled dispensing unit. However, the nurse actually giving the medication is still responsible for all aspects of medication administration. When giving any medication, observe the five rights of medication administration:

- Right medication
- Right dosage
- Right time
- Right route
- Right patient

Before administering any medication, make sure you know

- Desired therapeutic effect
- Reason for administering the drug
- Usual dosage and route
- Any potential for drug/food interactions
- Potential adverse side effects

Triple-check labels

continued on next page

PROCEDURE 27-1 (cont'd)

- When removing medication cartridge from shelf, refrigerator, or drawer
- While attaching the medication cartridge to the pump.
- When checking the medication before activation of the medication administration pump

Medication expiration dates should always be checked and outdated medication discarded or returned to the pharmacy.

Most manufacturers of intravenous products now make ports for needleless access. Ports may be covered with a sterile port cap or may need to be cleansed with an alcohol pad before use. Refer to the manufacturer's recommended method of use before using equipment.

Equipment

- PCA pump
- Medication cartridge with extension tubing
- Alcohol wipe (if indicated)
- Medication flow sheet

Preparation of equipment is determined by each different pump manufacturer. A set of troubleshooting instructions should be attached to each pump and training videos available from the manufacturer. Even nurses who use pumps regularly may need to review training tapes periodically for special features of the pump that that individual nurse seldom uses.

Special Considerations

Before initiating PCA therapy, assess the intravenous catheter for patency and inspect the site for signs of phlebitis and infiltration. When the pump is delivering only patient-initiated dose medication, it is necessary to have a running maintenance intravenous solution because patient-initiated dosing delivered into an intravenous saline or heparin lock may not be sufficient to keep the catheter patent and may cause discomfort at the infusion site. For this reason, the PCA pump should be attached to a primary intravenous catheter port. Before attaching the pump, the care provider should always review the compatibility of the medication with the solution in the intravenous catheter.

Assess the patient closely for any signs of adverse reactions because the intravenous route of medication administration provides quick action or reaction to medication. Note any manufacturer's recommendations for intravenous administration of PCA medications.

Action	*Rationale*
1. Verify order.	1. Ensures proper medication is given
2. Assemble supplies.	2. Promotes task organization
3. Identify patient.	3. Promotes patient safety
4. Explain procedure.	4. Promotes patient compliance
5. Determine patency of intravenous catheter.	5. Ensures patent intravenous access is available
6. Attach medication cartridge to pump, and verify drug administration parameters.	6. Prepares PCA for use
7. Connect PCA tubing to intravenous tubing, making sure that all tubing attached to the PCA cartridge is flushed.	7. Provides means to deliver medication into venous system
8. Open slide clamps on tubing.	8. Provides an open flow for medication
9. Deliver loading dose (if ordered) per manufacturer's direction.	9. Provides initial dose of medication
10. Instruct patient on use of pump for delivery of patient-initiated doses.	10. Enables patient to use pump for pain medication administration
11. Monitor patient closely for response to medication.	11. Promotes patient safety and determines level of pain relief
12. Discard or return supplies to appropriate place.	12. Maintains clean, organized work area

continued on next page

PROCEDURE 27-1 (cont'd)

Evaluation/Documentation

Assess vital signs, pain relief, and level of sedation every hour for 12 hours; every 2 hours for the next 12 hours; then, if the patient is using PCA correctly, every 4 hours. Evaluate the patient's pain on a pain intensity scale, ensure that PCA is connected and operational, and that intravenous tubing is not kinked. If the patient is dozing and not using PCA, consider alternatives (e.g., obtain an order to increase the basal rate, obtain an order for a different route until patient is awake). Also evaluate the patient's alertness level and difficulty arousing, if any. If the patient cannot be aroused, stop PCA, check respiratory rate, obtain oxygen saturation, and notify appropriate personnel immediately. If patient cannot be aroused and respiratory rate is 6 or less, stop PCA, administer oxygen via mask at 6 L/min, administer naloxone per protocol, and notify appropriate medical personnel immediately.

Record procedure in patient record, including time of PCA pump activation and medication used.

Record pump parameters on the PCA medication flow sheet or medication administration record, or both. Note assessment of patient's pain and effect of medication.

Elements of Patient Teaching

Instruct the patient and family on the purpose and use of the PCA pump. Caution the family that, before assisting the patient with a bolus dose, the pain status along with the level of orientation must be assessed to avoid overdosing the patient. Also instruct the patient and family to inform the care provider regarding the effect of the medication, any unusual symptoms, or problems associated with the intravenous site.

Instruct the patient on basal rate and rate of intravenous analgesic being administered, whether the patient is using the control button to administer additional injections or not. Then teach about lockout, the period after the patient administers an injection during which subsequent attempts do not deliver any additional analgesic. This is preordered by the physician and preset by the nurse to eliminate the hazard of unintentional overdosing by an anxious patient who pushes the control device multiple times successfully.

Also teach the patient how to

- Confirm that the pump is connected and operating
- Confirm that the intravenous tubing is not kinked
- Review the manufacturer's instructions
- Obtain replacement pump
- Calculate the proper dose
- Recognize side effects, such as excess sedation and respiratory depression, itching, and nausea, and contact a physician or trained nurse immediately
- If good pain relief has been achieved with the current analgesic, the first patient teaching efforts should focus on controlling the side effects; if poor pain relief has been achieved, the first efforts include treating the side effects and obtaining orders for an alternative analgesic.

CHAPTER HIGHLIGHTS

- This chapter provided a current description of pain transmission based on the latest research findings.
- Myriad factors lead to the undertreatment of pain.
- This chapter provided a review of the history of the development of pain management.
- Some analgesics that are not effective for men are effective for women.
- Ethical dilemmas are posed by pain and pain therapy.
- Basic pain assessment techniques exist for adults and children.
- Nursing actions use multiple interventions applied at different sites simultaneously to increase effectiveness and reduce overlapping side effects.
- Myths and actual facts regarding pain and pain management are delineated.

REFERENCES

Agency for Health Care Policy and Research (1992). *Acute Pain Management: Operative or Medical Procedures and Trauma. Clinical Practice Guideline* (AHCPR #92-0032). Rockville, MD: Author.

Agency for Health Care Policy and Research (1994). *Management of Cancer Pain. Clinical Practice Guideline* (AHCPR #94-0592). Rockville, MD: Author.

Agency for Health Care Policy and Research (1995). *Acute Low Back Problems in Adults. Clinical Practice Guideline* (AHCPR #95-0642). Rockville, MD: Author.

American Nurses Association (1992). *Statement on use of opiates.* Washington, D.C.: American Nurses Association.

American Pain Society (1992). *Principles of Analgesic Use in the Treatment of Acute Pain and Cancer Pain.* Skokie, IL: American Pain Society.

American Pain Society, Quality of Care Committee. (1995). Quality improvement guidelines for the treatment of acute pain and cancer pain. *Journal of the American Medical Association, 274*(23), 1874–1880.

Anand, K.J.S., Hickey, P.R. (1987). Pain and its effects in the human neonate and fetus. *New England Journal of Medicine, 317,* 1321–1347.

Barbour, L.A., McGuire, D.B., Kirchoff, K.T. (1986). Nonanalgesic methods of pain control used by cancer outpatients. *Oncology Nursing Forum, 13,* 56–60.

Bayless, J.M., Stanley, T.H., Hare, B.D. (1987). Pain in the ICU: Using analgesics effectively. *Journal of Critical Illness, 2*(1): 19–27.

Bedder, M.D., Soifer, B.E., Mulhall, J.J.V. (1991). A comparison of patient-controlled analgesia and bolus PRN intravenous morphine in the intensive care environment. *Clinical Journal of Pain, 7*(3), 205–208.

Beyer, J.E., DeGood, D.E., Ashley, L.C., Russell, G.A. (1983). Patterns of postoperative analgesic use with adults and children following cardiac surgery. *Pain, 17,* 71–81.

Beyer, J. et al. (1992). Clinical judgment in managing the crisis of children's pain. In J.H. Watt-Watson and M.I. Donovan (eds.): *Pain Management: Nursing Perspective.* St. Louis: C.V. Mosby, pp. 295–347.

Blanchard, E.B., Ahles, T.A. (1990). Biofeedback therapy. In J.J. Bonica (ed.): *The Management of Pain, Vol. I.* Philadelphia: Lea & Febiger, pp. 1722–1732.

Bond, M.R., Charlton, J.E., Woolf, C.J. (eds.). (1991). *Proceedings of the VIth World Congress on Pain.* New York: Elsevier.

Bosek, M.D. (1992). Ethical decision-making. In J. Watt-Watson and M.I. Donovan (eds.): *Pain Management: Nursing Perspective.* St. Louis: C.V. Mosby, pp. 93–123.

Broome, M.E., et al. (1989). Pain interventions with children: a meta-analysis of research. *Nursing Research, 38,* 154–158.

Burckhardt, C.S. (1990). Chronic pain. *Nursing Clinics of North America,* 25(4), 863–870.

Callister, L. (1992). *Pain Management. Understanding BME's Newest Guidelines.* BHE Report. Portland, OR: Board of Medical Examiners.

Coderre, T.J., Katz, J., Vaccarino, A.L., Melzack, R. (1993). Contribution of central neuroplasticity to pathological pain: review of clinical and experimental evidence. *Pain, 52,* 259–285.

Cousins, M. (1989). Acute and postoperative pain. In P.D. Wall and R. Melzack (eds.): *Textbook of Pain.* New York: Churchill Livingstone, pp. 284–305.

Crooke, J., Rideout, E., Browne, G. (1984). The prevalence of pain complaints in a general population. *Pain, 18,* 299–316.

Cushing, M. (1992). Pain management on trial. *American Journal of Nursing, 92,* 21–23.

Dahl, J. (1993). State cancer initiatives. *Journal of Pain and Symptom Management, 8*: 372–375.

Daut, R.L., Cleeland, C.S., Flanery, R.C. (1983). Development of the Wisconsin Brief Pain Questionnaire to Assess Pain in Cancer and Other Diseases. *Pain, 17,* 197–210.

Derogatis, L.R., Abelfoff, M.D., McBeth, C.D. (1976). Cancer patients and their physicians in the perception of psychological symptoms. *Psychosomatics, 17,* 197–201.

Donovan, M.I. (1990). Acute pain relief. *Nursing Clinics of North America, 25*(4), 851–861.

Donovan, M. (1992). A practical approach to pain assessment. In J. Watt-Watson and M.I. Donovan (eds.): *Pain Management: Nursing Perspective.* St. Louis: C.V. Mosby, pp. 59–78.

Donovan, M., Dillon, P., McGuire, L. (1987). Incidence and characteristics of pain in a sample of medical-surgical inpatients. *Pain, 30,* 69–78.

Donovan, M.I., Slack, J., Wright, S., Faut, M. (1989). Factors Associated with the Inadequate Management of Acute Pain (abstract). Presented at the Eighth Annual Scientific Meeting of the American Pain Society, Phoenix, AZ, October 26–29.

Dubner, R., Hargreaves, K.M. (1989). The neurobiology of pain and its modulation. *Clinical Journal of Pain, 5,* 51–56.

Edgar, L., Smith-Hanrahan, C.M. (1992). Non-pharmacological pain management. In J. Watt-Watson and M. Donovan (eds.): *Pain Management—Nursing Perspective.* St. Louis: Mosby–Year Book, pp. 162–199.

Edwards, W.T. (1990). Optimizing opioid treatment of postoperative pain. *Journal of Pain and Symptom Management, 5*(1), S24–S36.

Elliott, T.E., Elliott, B.A. (1992). Physician attitudes and beliefs about use of morphine for cancer pain. *Journal of Pain and Symptom Management, 7*(3), 141–148.

Evans, F.J. (1989). Hypnosis and the management of clinical pain. *Pain Management, 2*(5), 247–255.

Faries, J.E., et al. (1991). Systematic pain records and their impact on pain control: a pilot study. *Cancer Nursing, 14*(6), 306–313.

Ferrell, B.A., Ferrell, B.R. (1989). Assessment of chronic pain in the elderly. *Geriatric Medicine Today, 8,* 123–134.

Ferrell, B.A., Ferrell, B.R., Osterwell, D. (1990). Pain in the nursing home. *Journal of the American Geriatric Society, 38,* 9–14.

Ferrell, B.R., Donovan, M.I., McGuire, D. (1992). Knowledge and beliefs regarding pain in a sample of nursing faculty. *Journal of Professional Nursing, 9*(2), 79–88.

Ferrell, B.R., Ferrell, B.A., Ahn, C., Trn, K. (1994). Pain management for elderly patients with cancer at home. *Cancer, 74*(7), 2139–2146.

Ferrell, B.R., McCaffery, M. (1991). Clinical decision making and pain. *Cancer Nursing, 14*(6), 289–297.

Ferrell, B.R., McCaffery, M., Rhiner, M. (1992). Pain and addiction: an urgent need for change in nursing education. *Journal of Pain and Symptom Management, 7*(2), 117–124.

Ferrell, B.R., Rhiner, M. (1991). High-tech Comfort: ethical issues in cancer pain management for the 1990s. *Journal of Clinical Ethics, 2*(2), 108–117.

Ferrell, B.R., Rhiner, M. (1994). Use of technology in the management of cancer pain. *Journal of Pharmaceutical Care in Pain and Symptom Control, 2*(1), 15–35.

Foley, K.M. (1989). Controversies in cancer pain. *Cancer, 63*(11), 2257–2265.

Foley, K.M. (1991). The relationship of pain and symptom management to patient requests for physician-assisted suicide. *Journal of Pain and Symptom Management, 6*(5), 289–297.

Foley, K.M., Inturrisi, C.E. (1987). Analgesic drug therapy in cancer pain: principles and practice. *Medical Clinics of North America, 71,* 207–232.

Foley, K.M., Payne, R.M. (1989). *Current Therapy of Pain.* Philadelphia: B.C. Decker.

Funk, S.G., et al. (1989). *Key Aspects of Comfort.* New York: Springer.

Gamsa, A. (1994). The role of psychological factors in chronic pain: II. A critical appraisal. *Pain, 57,* 17–29.

Gear, R.W., et al. (1996). Gender differences in analgesic response to the kappa opioid, pentazocine. *Neuroscience Letter, 205*(3), 207–209.

Gedaly-Duff, V. (1989). Palmar sweat index (PSI) use with children in pain research. *Journal of Pediatric Nursing, 4,* 3–8.

Gobel, B.H., Donovan, M.I. (1987). Depression and anxiety. *Seminars in Oncology Nursing, 3*(4), 267–276.

Grass, J.A. (1992). Sufentanil: clinical use as postoperative analgesic—epidural/intrathecal route. *Journal of Pain and Symptom Management, 7*(5), 271–286.

Grossman, S.A., Sheidler, V.R. (1989). *The Johns Hopkins Oncology Center's Narcotic Conversion Program* (computer program). Philadelphia: Lea & Febiger.

Grossman, S.A., Sheidler, V.R., Mylenski, J., Piantadosi, S. (1991). Correlation of patient and caregiver ratings of cancer pain. *Journal of Pain and Symptom Management, 6*(2): 53–57.

Grunua, R.V.E., Johnson, C.C., Craig, K.D. (1990). Facial and cry responses to invasive and non-invasive procedures in neonates. *Pain, 42,* 295–305.

Hamilton, J., Edgar, L. (1992). A survey examining nurses' knowledge of pain control. *Journal of Pain and Symptom Management, 7*(1), 18–26.

Hauer, M., Cram, E., Titler, M., et al. (1995). Intravenous patient-controlled analgesia in critically ill postoperative/trauma patients: research-based practice recommendations. *Dimensions of Critical Care Nursing, 14*(3), 144–153.

Henderson, V. (1964). The nature of nursing. *American Journal of Nursing, 64*(8), 62–68.

Hester, N.O., (1992a). Excerpts from Guidelines for The Management of Pain in Infants, Children and Adolescents Undergoing Operative and Medical Procedures. MCN, 17, 146–162.

Hester, N.O., Foster, R.L., Beyer, J.E. (1992b). Clinical judgment in assessing children's pain. In J.H. Watt-Watson and M.I. Donovan (eds.): *Pain Management: Nursing Perspective.* St. Louis: C.V. Mosby, pp. 236–294.

Hyman, R.B. et al. (1989). The effects of relaxation training on clinical symptoms: a meta analysis. *Nursing Research, 38*(4), 216–220.

Jaffe, J.H., Meutin, W.R. (1985). Opioid analgesics and antagonists. In A.G. Gilman, et al (eds.): *Goodman and Gilman's: The Pharmaceutical Basis of Therapeutics,* 7th ed. New York: Macmillan Co., pp. 491–531.

Johnston, C., Stevens, B. (1992). Pain in infants. In J.H. Watt-Watson and M.I. Donovan (eds.): *Pain Management: Nursing Perspective.* St. Louis: C.V. Mosby, pp. 230–235.

Joranson, D.E. (1995). Intractable pain treatment laws & regulation. *APS Bulletin, 5*(2), 1-3+.

Joranson, D.E., Cleeland, C.S., Weissman, D.E. (1992). Opioids for chronic cancer and non cancer pain: a survey of State Medical Boards (abstract). Presented at the Eleventh Annual Scientific Meeting of the American Pain Society, San Diego.

Joranson, D.G., Dahl, J. (1989). Achieving balance in drug policy: The Wisconsin model. In C.S Hill, W.S. Fields (eds.): *Advances in Pain Research and Therapy,* Vol. 11. New York: Raven Press, pp. 197–204.

Kachoyeanos, M.K., Friedhoff, M. (1993). Cognitive and behavioral strategies to reduce children's pain. *MCN, 18,* 14–19.

Kilwein, J. (1983). Valium and values. *American Pharmacy, NS23*(12), 5–7.

Lander, J., Fowler-Kerry, S., Oberle, S. (1992). Children's venipuncture pain: influence of technical factors. *Journal of Pain and Symptom Management, 7*(6), 343–349.

Latimer, E.J. (1991). Ethical decision-making in the care of the dying and its application to clinical practice. *Journal of Pain and Symptom Management, 6*(5), 329–336.

Lehmann, K.A., Zech, S. (1992). Transdermal fentanyl: clinical pharmacology. *Journal of Pain and Symptom Management, 7*(3S), S8–S16.

Liebeskind, J.C. (1991a). Pain can kill. *Pain, 44,* 3–4.

Liebeskind, J.C. (1991b). President's message. *APS Bulletin, 1*(2), 2–3.

Lindley, C.M., Dalton, J., Fields, S.M. (1990). Narcotic analgesics—clinical pharmacology and therapeutics. *Cancer Nursing, 13*(1), 28–38.

Lisson, E.L. (1987). Ethical issues related to pain control. *Nursing Clinics of North America, 22*(3), 649–659.

Loesser, J. (1986). *Pain and Its Management. An Overview—NIH Consensus Development Conference. In the Integrated Approach to Management of Pain.* Presented at the NIH meeting, Bethesda, MD, May 19–21.

Mansson, M.E., Fredrikson, B., Rosberg, B. (1992). Comparison of preparation and narcotic-sedative premedication in children undergoing surgery. *Pediatric Nursing, 18*(4), 337–342.

Mao, J., Price, D.D., Mayer D.J. (1995). Mechanisms of hyperalgesia and morphine tolerance: a current view of their possible interactions. *Pain,* 62(3):259–274.

Marks, R., Sachar, M. (1973). Undertreatment of medical inpatients with narcotic analgesics. *Annals of Internal Medicine, 78,* 173–181.

Max, M. (1990). Improving outcomes of analgesic treatment: is education enough? *Annals of Internal Medicine, 113*(11), 885–889.

McAlary, P. (1988). Relieving pain with heat or cold. *Nursing '88, 18,* 64K–64N.

McCaffery, M., Beebe, A. (1989). *Pain: Clinical Manual for Nursing Practice.* St. Louis: C.V. Mosby.

McCaffery, M., et al. (1990). Nurses' knowledge of opioid analgesics and psychological dependence. *Cancer Nursing, 13,* 21–27.

McCauley, V., et al. (1993). Patient-related barriers to management of cancer pain. *Pain, 74,* 2139–2145.

McGuire, D.B. (1992). Comprehensive and multidimensional assessment and measurement of pain. *Journal of Pain and Symptom Management, 7*(5), 312–319.

McGuire, D.B., Yarbro, C.H. (eds). (1987). *Cancer Pain Management.* Orlando, FL: Grune & Stratton.

Melzack, R. (1975). The McGill Pain Questionnaire: major properties and scoring methods. *Pain, 1,* 297–299.

Melzack, R. (1990). The tragedy of needless pain. *Scientific American, 262*(2), 27–33.

Melzack, R., Wall, P.D. (1965). Pain mechanisms: a new theory. *Science, 150,* 971–979.

Merskey, H. (1986). International Association for the Study of Pain—pain terms: a current list with definitions and notes on usage. *Pain, 3*(Suppl), S1–S225.

Miaskowski, C., et al. (1992). Interdisciplinary guidelines for the management of acute pain: implications for quality improvement. *Journal of Nursing Care Quality, 7*(1), 1–6.

Naber, L., Jones, G., Halm, M. (1994). Epidural analgesia for effective pain control. *Critical Care Nurse, 14,* 69–83.

National Institutes of Health (1987). The integrated approach to the management of pain—a Consensus Development Conference statement. *Journal of Pain and Symptom Management, 2,* 35–44.

National Institutes of Health Technology Assessment Panel (1996). Integration of behavioral and relaxation approaches to treatment of chronic pain and insomnia. *Journal of American Medical Association, 76*(4), 313–318.

Oncology Nursing Society (1990). Position paper on cancer pain. Parts I, II, and III. *Oncology Nursing Forum, 17,* 595–614, 751–760, and 943–955.

Page, G.G. (1996). The medical necessity of adequate pain management. *Pain Forum,* 5: 227–233.

Paice, J. (1988). The phenomenon of analgesic tolerance in cancer pain management. *Oncology Nursing Forum, 15,* 455–460.

Paris, J.J., Reardon, F.E. (1986). Dilemmas in intensive care medicine: an ethical and legal analysis. *Journal of Intensive Care Medicine, 1,* 75–90.

Peebles, R.J., Schneiderman, D.S. (1991). *Socio-economic Economic Factbook for Surgery. 1991–92.* Chicago: American College of Surgeons.

Pert, C., Snyder, S. (1973). Opiate receptor: demonstration in nervous tissue. *Science, 179,* 1001–1014.

Portenoy, R.K. (1990). Chronic opioid therapy in nonmalignant pain. *Journal of Pain and Symptom Management, 5*(1, Suppl), S46–S62.

Portenoy, R. (1994). Opioid therapy for chronic nonmalignant pain: current status. In H.L. Fields and J.C. Liebeskind (eds.): *Progress in Pain Research and Management. Vol. I. Pharmacological Approaches to the Treatment of Chronic Pain: New Concepts and Critical Issues.* Seattle: IASP, pp. 247–287.

Porter, J., Jick, H. (1980). Addiction rare in patients treated with narcotics. *New England Journal of Medicine, 302,* 123.

Rankin, M., Snider, B. (1984). Nurses' perceptions of cancer patients' pain. *Cancer Nursing, 1,* 149–155.

Ross, D., Ross, S. (1988). *Childhood Pain: Current Issues, Research and Management.* Baltimore: Urban & Schwarzenberg.

Rowat, K.M. (1992). Living with chronic pain: a family perspective. In J.H. Watt-Watson and M.I. Donovan (eds.): *Pain Management: Nursing Perspective.* St. Louis: C.V. Mosby, pp. 79–92.

Schecter, N., Allen, D. (1986). Physicians' attitudes toward pain in children. *Developmental Behaviors in Pediatrics, 7,* 350–354.

Shapiro, C. (1989). Pain in the neonate: assessment and intervention. *Neonatal Net,* 8(1), 6–21.

Smith, C.M., et al. (1986). The effects of transcutaneous electrical nerve stimulation on post-cesarean pain. *Pain, 27,* 181–193.

Stambaugh, J.E. (1989). The use of nonsteroidal anti-inflammatory drugs in chronic bone pain. *Orthopaedic Review, 18*(Suppl), 54–60.

Strauss, A., Fagerhaugh, S., Glaser, B. (1974). Pain: an organizational-work-interactive perspective. *Nursing Outlook, 22,* 560–566.

Teske, R., Cleeland, C.S. (1983). Relationship between nurse's observations and self-report of pain. *Pain, 16:* 289–296.

Thomas, I.L., et al. (1988). An evaluation of transcutaneous electrical nerve stimulation for pain relief in labour. *Australian Journal of Obstetrics and Gynaecology, 28,* 182–189.

University Hospital Consortium (1992). *Patient Satisfaction in UHC Hospitals Reported—Pilot Study Completed.* Chicago: University Hospital Consortium News.

Valenta, S.M. (1991). Using hypnosis with children for pain management. *Oncology Nursing Forum, 18*(4), 699–704.

Vincenti, P.I. (1989). The Nuprin report: a summary. *Pain, 37,* 295–299.

VonKorff, M., et al. (1987). An epidemiological comparison of pain complaints. *Pain, 32,* 173–183.

Von Roenn, J., Cleeland, C.S., Gonin, R., et al. (1993). Physician attitudes and practice in cancer pain management. *Annals of Internal Medicine, 199,* 121–126.

Vortherms, R., Ryan, P., Ward, S. (1992). Knowledge of, attitudes toward, and barriers to pharmacologic management of cancer pain in a statewide random sample of nurses. *Research in Nursing and Health, 15,* 459–466.

Wall, P.D. The prevention of postoperative pain. *Pain, 33,* 289–290.

Ward, S.E., et al. (1993). Patient-related barriers to management of cancer pain. *Pain, 52,* 319–324.

Ward, S.E., Gordon, D.B. (1996). Patient satisfaction and pain severity as outcomes in pain management: a longitudinal view in one setting's experience. *Journal of Pain and Symptom Management, 11*(4), 242–251.

Ware, V.E., Hays, R.D. (1988). Methods for measuring patient satisfaction with specific medical encounters. *Medical Care, 26:* 393–402.

Watt-Watson, J. (1987). Nurses' knowledge of pain issues: a survey. *Journal of Pain & Symptom Management, 2,* 207–211.

Watt-Watson, J.H., Donovan, M.I. (1992). *Pain Management: Nursing Perspective.* St. Louis: C.V. Mosby.

Whedon, M., Ferrell, B.R. (1991). Professional and ethical considerations in the use of high-tech pain management. *Oncology Nursing Forum, 18,* 1135–1143.

Wild, L. (1992). Transition from pain to comfort: managing the hemodynamic risks. *Critical Care Nursing Quarterly, 15*(1), 46–56.

Wilkie, D.J., Keefe, F.J. (1991). Coping strategies of patients with lung cancer-related pain. *Clinical Journal of Pain, 7,* 292–299.

Wong, D., Baker, C. (1988). Pain in children: comparison of assessment scales. *Pediatric Nursing, 14,* 9–17.

Woolf, C.J. (1991). Central mechanisms of acute pain. In M.R. Bond, J.E. Charlton, and C.J. Woolf (eds.): *Proceedings of the VIth World Congress on Pain.* New York: Elsevier, pp. 25–34.

World Health Organization (WHO) (1985). *Cancer Pain Relief.* Geneva, Switzerland: Author.

Wright, S. (1987). The use of therapeutic touch in the management of pain. *Nursing Clinics of North America, 22*(3), 705–714.

Zbrowski, M. (1969). *People in Pain.* San Francisco: Jossey-Bass.

Skin Integrity 28

Carolyn E. Carlson, Rosemarie B. King, and Irene B. Alyn

Clara Larson, a 72-year-old retired school teacher, has been admitted to the rehabilitation unit following acute care for a right hemisphere cerebrovascular accident (stroke), resulting in left hemiplegia. She is a childless widow and lives with her sister, who visits her frequently in the hospital.

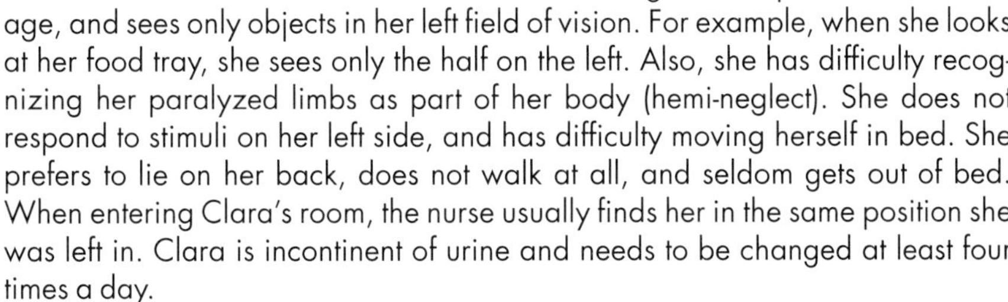

Clara has lost 15 pounds since her stroke and is not eating well. A typical day's intake includes a piece of buttered toast with jelly, four ounces of orange juice, four ounces of yogurt, half a meat patty, a green salad, and half a potato. She has difficulty swallowing and refuses supplements.

Clara also has disruption in her visual field, common with right hemisphere brain damage, and sees only objects in her left field of vision. For example, when she looks at her food tray, she sees only the half on the left. Also, she has difficulty recognizing her paralyzed limbs as part of her body (hemi-neglect). She does not respond to stimuli on her left side, and has difficulty moving herself in bed. She prefers to lie on her back, does not walk at all, and seldom gets out of bed. When entering Clara's room, the nurse usually finds her in the same position she was left in. Clara is incontinent of urine and needs to be changed at least four times a day.

After an admission assessment, the nursing staff recognize that Clara is at risk for developing pressure ulcers, and plan a specific program to protect Clara's skin. The nurses involve Clara in the planning. Their assessments, planning, and teaching are based on their knowledge of the etiology, prevention, and treatment of pressure ulcers and needs, preferences, and characteristics of Clara. Nurses explain to Clara that she needs to change position to relieve pressure over bony prominences at least every hour. They work out a schedule in such a way that she will be sitting in a chair for meals and will be facing the TV for her favorite programs.

OBJECTIVES

After studying this chapter, the student will be able to:

- **perform a skin assessment**
- **perform a risk assessment for pressure ulcers**
- **assess and document characteristics of wounds**
- **describe a plan of care to decrease risk of infection for existing wounds**
- **describe a plan of care to decrease risk of pressure ulcers**
- **describe individual differences to take into account in planning care for a person with actual or potential disruption of skin integrity**

SCOPE OF NURSING PRACTICE

Interruption in skin integrity is a frequent occurrence in many areas of nursing practice. Lacerations, surgical incision, pressure ulcers, and burns may be part of patient assessment and care in the emergency department, intensive care unit, medical-surgical unit, rehabilitation unit, home, outpatient clinics, or any other care setting. Treatment of pressure ulcers entails much time, cost, and patient discomfort.

Skin integrity is important to maintain and restore health, and nurses play a vital role in assessing and intervening to prevent skin integrity disruptions and promote wound healing when disruptions have occurred. Nurses prepared with knowledge, skills, and motivation needed for skin integrity assessment and intervention can contribute a great deal to the health and quality of life of the individuals committed to their care. Knowledge of persons at risk for burns, pressure ulcers, or other wounds has implications for public education, types and frequency of assessments to be done in health care settings as well as resources needed for prevention and treatment. Prevention of wounds prevents discomfort as well as loss of time at work, school, and other important activities.

KNOWLEDGE BASE

Basic Science

ANATOMY AND PHYSIOLOGY

Approximate the total mass of skin by looking at a pile of your jeans, heavy long-sleeved shirt, socks, and shoes. Estimate the square feet that the clothing covers. How much do these items weigh, five to eight pounds? Look at yourself. Note that you have nails, hair, and pores in your skin. Why? Pinch yourself hard, lightly brush your fingertips over your arm, and put your hand into warm or cold water. Your skin contains several types of receptors to detect somatic sensations.

The skin and its accessory structures of hair, nails, and glands comprise the integumentary system, the largest structure in the body. The skin weighs 6 to 8 pounds and covers a 20-square-foot area in the average adult (Davis, 1986; Fitzpatrick et al, 1993). The skin in most regions of the body is 1 to 5 mm (1/4 inch or less) thick. The skin on the palms of the hands, soles of the feet, eyelids, and back vary in skin thickness, turgor, and the type and quantity of appendages: nails, hair, glands. The type of receptor (pain, touch, or temperature) also differs in various areas of the skin.

The skin is a highly visible organ. Astute observation and palpation yield much data about the general physical and emotional condition of an individual. The facial skin, for example, reflects embarrassment, fear, anxiety, and anger. Skin turgor is used to assess hydration and nail beds. Other skin areas are used to assess capillary filling time.

Each skin surface is designed to meet specific body needs. That is, various areas of skin have distinct but interrelated functions.

SKIN STRUCTURE

The skin consists of three layers: epidermis, dermis, and an inner layer of subcutaneous tissue connecting the dermis with the muscle layer (Fig. 28–1). Each layer's efficiency increases with development (child to adult), then decreases with aging.

Epidermis. The epidermis is the outermost layer of the skin and consists of five layers. The innermost layer, stratum germinativum, is a single layer of specialized cells called basal cells (keratinocytes) that constantly replace the cell population. The older cells move outward toward the stratum corneum. These cells flatten and alter until they form dead, scalelike keratin flakes that continually slough off the surface of the skin. The epidermal barrier thus prevents dehydration from loss of body fluids and bars entrance of foreign environmental hazards. The acid pH of the skin provides a chemical barrier by retarding the growth of certain fungi and bacteria. Tissues that do not regenerate are replaced by scar tissue.

The dermal appendages, glands, and hair follicles invaginate the originating epidermis and dermis. If a large area of the epidermis is damaged, the epithelial cells lining the dermal appendages regenerate the epidermal layer (Table 28–1).

Dermis. The dermis is connected to the epidermis by a convoluted layer of cells composed primarily of collagen and elastin fibers that allow the skin to stretch and contract with body movement. Interspersed in the dermis is a rich supply of blood vessels, nerve fibers, lymph vessels, hair follicles, sebaceous glands, and sweat glands. The skin is thickest on the soles of the feet and palms of the hands, and thinnest over the eyelids.

The dermis serves the epidermis as an undergirding structure and as a source of nutrition. Changes in the dermis are more difficult to observe by inspection. This fact is especially important in assessing pressure ulcers, in which tissue damage to the dermis may occur prior to any observable change in the epidermis.

Cells in the dermis include fibroblasts, mast cells, and macrophages. Fibroblasts secrete connective tissue (collagen and elastin), mast cells release histamine, and macrophages participate in the immune response through phagocytic action (Davis, 1986).

The *dermal appendages* are variably distributed in the body and include the nails, hair follicles, sebaceous glands, and eccrine and apocrine sweat glands. The nails and hair consist of keratin and serve as protective plates over the distal ends of fingers and toes. Nails grow at a rate of approximately ¼ inch or less per week. All humans have hair at birth, but the amount and texture varies. Newborn scalp hair is replaced by thicker, darker hair as the child grows. At puberty, hair growth in the axillary and pubic areas (and chest and facial areas in men) is stimulated by androgenic hormones. Many men and some women lose scalp hair with aging. Hair growth

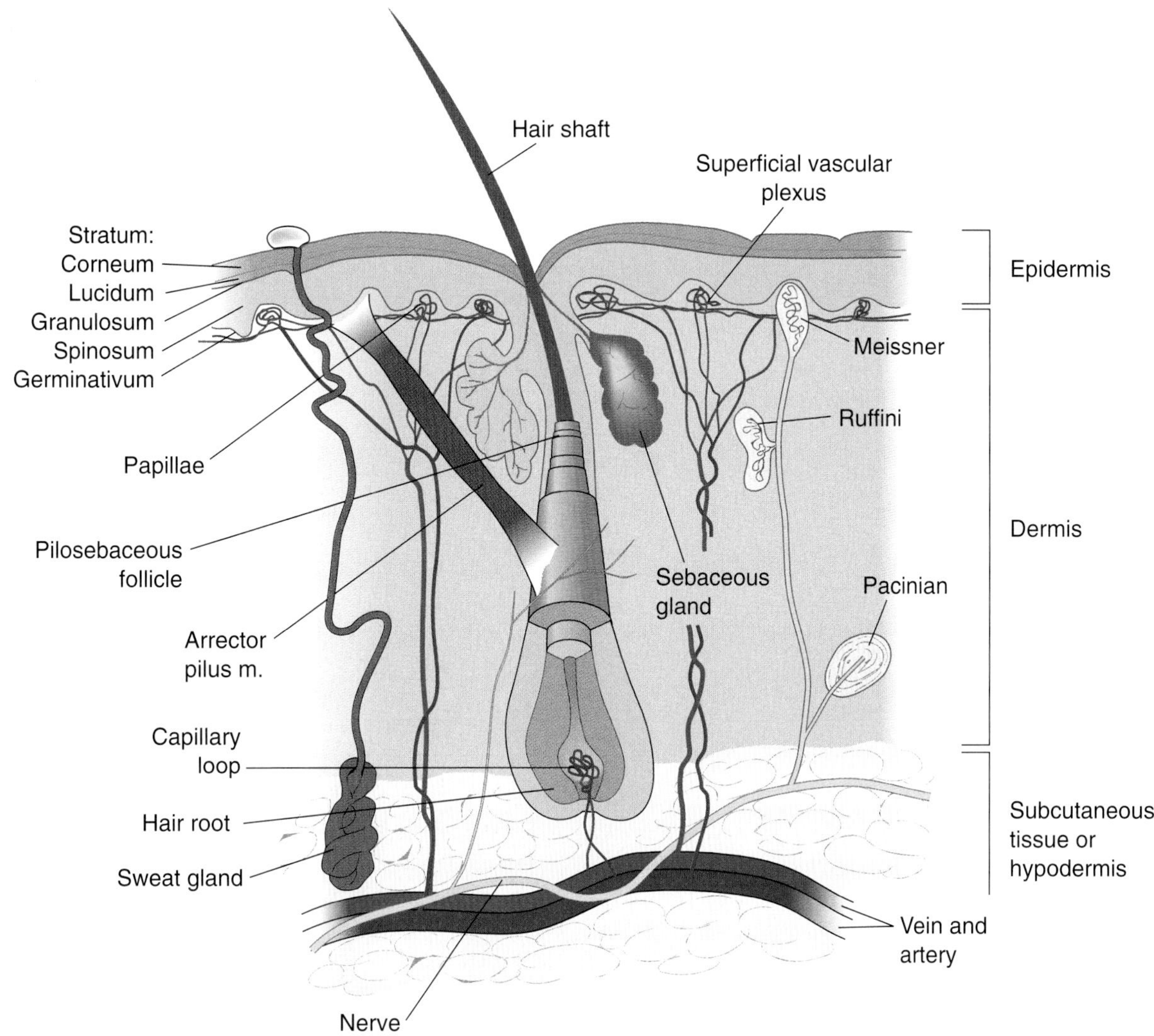

Figure 28–1. Cross-section of normal skin.

is not constant and varies over different body surfaces. Hair follicles have an arrector pilus muscle (see Fig. 28–1) that straightens the follicle when contracted, causing the hair to "stand up."

Hair follicles, sebaceous glands, and *apocrine sweat glands* comprise an integrated unit (see Fig. 28–1). The sebaceous glands open onto the skin surface through the hair to follicle channels. The function of the sebaceous glands is to produce a fatty secretion called sebum that reduces water content loss and keeps the skin supple. An increase in androgen increases sebum production. Sebaceous glands are located in greatest numbers on the scalp, face, and genitals, and are less numerous on the trunk and extremities. They are not located on the soles or palms.

The *apocrine sweat glands* are located mainly in the axillary and genital areas and are inactive until puberty. Bacteria acting on sweat from these glands cause body odor.

Eccrine sweat glands function primarily as a heat-regulating mechanism and, to a much lesser extent, contribute to electrolyte balance. A newborn has the same number of eccrine sweat glands as an adult, so, due to the infant's smaller body surface area, the density of gland concentration is high. However, while the eccrine sweat glands function in the newborn, they do not reach maximal performance until puberty (Wong, 1995).

Sweat glands are innervated by sympathetic cholinergic nerve fibers and can be stimulated by both acetylcholine and norepinephrine/epinephrine.

Sweat is secreted in a bulb of the gland and its ion concentration resembles plasma except it contains no proteins. The unacclimated (to a hot environment) person, exposed to hot weather, can produce about 700 ml of sweat per hour, which often results in losses of 15 to 30 grams of sodium chloride per day. The acclimated person can produce about 2000 ml of sweat per hour, with a loss of 3 to 5 grams of sodium chloride per day. The body's adaptability to environmental extremes is remarkable. At room temperature, the normal person loses 100 ml of water in sweat per day, increasing to 1400 ml per

TABLE 28-1 Characteristics and Cells of Skin Layers

Layer of the Skin	Characteristics	Key Cells Contained in the Layer
Epidermis 0.3 to 1.5 mm thick	The epidermis is the outermost layer of the skin and consists of five layers (see Fig. 28–1). The innermost layer of the epidermis contains keratinocytes, which produce keratin. The keratinocytes migrate toward the skin surface. They become flattened and keratinized. This keratinization prevents water loss and dehydration of the deeper skin layers. The stratum corneum, or outermost layer of the epidermis, constantly sloughs off from the surface of the body. This layer protects against dehydration of the dermis and subcutaneous tissue. The epidermal renewal cycle takes about 30 days. A chemical barrier is provided by the acidic pH of the epidermal surface.	Keratinocytes—produce keratin, a main component of skin, hair, and nails. Melanocytes—secrete melanin, which gives color and shields against ultraviolet light. Melanin protects against skin cancer. Langerhans' cells—macrophages that initiate an immune response and serve as a defense against antigens Merkel's cells—touch receptors.
Dermis 1 to 4 mm thick	The dermis constitutes the bulk of the skin and has invagination by epidermal structures: Hair follicles and glands (see Fig. 28–1). Interwoven in the layer of fibrous, elastic connective tissue (i.e., collagen) are blood vessels, lymphatics, nerve fibers, sebaceous glands, sweat glands, and hair follicles.	Fibroblasts—secrete connective tissue. Mast cells—release histamine causing vasodilation. Macrophages—phagocytic cells that participate in the immune response.
Subcutaneous Tissue	The subcutaneous tissue connects the dermis to the muscle layer underneath. This layer is composed of connective tissue, larger blood vessels, lymph vessels, and nerve trunks. The subcutaneous tissue serves as a depot for fat storage (which determines the body contour). The fat provides a cushion and an insulation layer.	Fat cells.

day in hot weather, and as much as 5000 ml per day with prolonged heavy exercise. The insensible water loss from skin in all these situations remains constant at 350 ml per day (Guyton, 1995).

Subcutaneous Tissue. The subcutaneous tissue connects the dermis to the muscle layers underneath and tissue is composed of loose connective tissue, fat cells, lymph vessels, nerve fibers, and larger blood vessels. The blood vessels supply oxygen nutrients to the skin and aid in temperature regulation. The fat cells serve as a depot for fat storage, which determines body contour. Fat provides a cushion and an excellent insulation layer for the body because fat conducts heat only one third as rapidly as other body tissues (Guyton and Hall, 1995). Fat also serves as a calorie/energy depot during starvation or illness.

SKIN FUNCTION

Thinking about the anatomy of the skin helps ascertain the purpose of each specific structure. Included in the major functions of the skin are protection, regulation of body temperature, maintenance of fluid and electrolyte balance, synthesis of vitamin D, and expression of feelings.

Protection. The skin serves as a protection against mechanical, chemical, thermal, and radiant trauma. The layer of tightly packed keratinocyte cells forms a mechanical barrier between the underlying tissue and the environment. The relatively dry, oily, and slightly acidic skin limits the growth of bacteria. Bacteria that invade the hair follicles are removed by sebum. Fat-soluble substances can penetrate the oily skin. Aged skin contains fewer hair follicles, is less oily, and thus is less permeable to fat-soluble substances.

The skin contains pain, temperature, and several types of touch receptors (*sensory*). The impulses from these receptors elicit their sensation by conducting impulses through several types of nerve fibers (free nerve endings, A and C fibers).

Regulation of Body Temperature. The skin, subcutaneous tissues, and fat provide heat insulation for the body, vasoconstriction, and shivering, and are an effective means of maintaining normal internal core body temperature. The body employs three mechanisms to reduce body heat when the temperature is too high: vasodilatation, sweating (see previous sections), and decrease in heat production. Full vasodilatation of skin blood vessels can increase the rate of heat transfer to the surface of the skin as much as eightfold, because blood flow into the venous plexus in the subcutaneous tissue can increase to as great as 30 percent of cardiac output (Guyton and Hall, 1995). This high rate of blood flow in vasodilated vessels very efficiently conducts heat from the core of the body to the skin surface.

Fluid and Electrolyte Balance Maintenance. Few substances are able to penetrate the skin easily. The skin seals the body from the environment. The effectiveness of the skin barrier is demonstrated by the profuse fluid loss that follows damage to the epidermis by injury, burns, and dermatitis (e.g., poison ivy). Water and electrolytes normally are lost through the pores only.

Vitamin D Synthesis. Synthesis of vitamin D takes place in the skin by irradiation from ultraviolet rays from the sun. Vitamin D is essential to absorb calcium and phosphorus.

Expression of Feelings. Facial skin reflects embarrassment (blushing), anger (redness), fear (blanching), and anxiety (sweating). The skin is entwined with a person's body image because it is so immediately visible to others.

DISRUPTIONS IN SKIN INTEGRITY AND WOUND HEALING

A *wound* is a disruption in the continuity and regulatory processes of the skin and/or underlying tissues. The type and extent of the wound and the resources of the victim determine the process of healing and management.

Healing a wound is a complex sequence of tissue repair. The process includes several phases: coagulation, inflammation; fibroplasia or granulation tissue production; and matrix contraction and maturation. All of these are measurable components of wound healing. Intrinsic factors (e.g., age, nutritional status, oxygenation, chronic diseases, and infection) and extrinsic factors (e.g., moist or dry environment, wound-cleansing solutions, antimicrobials, type of dressing) influence the rate of healing and the amount of scarring. Wound healing may or may not restore cellular functioning in all tissues damaged. The type of injury and the location of the wound influence the subsequent repair.

WOUND CLASSIFICATION

Wounds are classified as **open or closed, superficial or deep,** by **mechanism of injury, degree of contamination,** and/or as **those with or without tissue loss.** A wound is classified as *open* if the skin has been disrupted and *closed* if the skin surface remains intact. Wounds that are *superficial* disrupt epidermal tissue only, whereas *deep* wounds damage the dermis, subcutaneous tissue, and underlying structures (organ, muscle, bone). *Mechanisms of injury* include surgical incisions (open wound) and contusion wounds made by a blunt force that does not break the skin (closed wound). A *clean* wound made by surgical incision is theoretically aseptic, or not contaminated. *Contaminated* wounds are exposed to bacteria in a variety of ways (usually by a break in aseptic technique). Preexisting infections or perforated viscera contribute to *infected* wounds that retain bacteria and necrotic tissues. An example of a wound without tissue loss is a surgical incision. Wounds with tissue loss include full-thickness burns, severe pressure ulcers, and lacerations.

BURNS

Burns are classified by depth and surface involved. The depth of the burn is traditionally divided into the major categories of **superficial** (first-degree) **burns, partial-thickness** (second-degree) **burns,** and **full-thickness** (third-degree) **burns.** The terms relate to the amount or layers of the skin destroyed or disrupted. The color, surface moisture, blister formation and size, and type of tissue exposed are evident through observation of the burned areas. Touching the wounds (with sterile gloves) reveals the presence or absence of capillary filling, indicating whether circulation is intact. Absence of sensation and blanching and refilling indicate a full-thickness burn. Hair is easily pulled out of a full-thickness burn. All categories of burns may appear red but only the full-thickness burn is red, white, black, or brown. The red color indicates tissue erythema and viability. Small blisters appear on superficial-thickness burns, and large blisters on deep partial-thickness burns. Blisters are not present on full-thickness burns.

PRESSURE ULCERS

"*Pressure ulcers,* also called decubitus ulcers, bedsores, and pressure sores, are localized areas of tissue necrosis that tend to develop when soft tissue is compressed between a bony prominence and an external surface for a prolonged period of time" (National Pressure Ulcer Advisory Panel [NPUAP], 1989). The terms pressure ulcer or pressure sore call attention to the essential risk factor in the development of this type of wound: pressure.

Pressure ulcers are generally classified using a staging system recommended by the National Pressure Ulcer Advisory Panel (NPUAP, 1989). There are four stages; however, the numbers do not necessarily imply any progression.

- Stage I: Nonblanchable erythema of intact skin, the heralding lesion of skin ulceration. In individuals with darker skin, discoloration of the skin, warmth, edema, induration, or hardness may also be indicators (Fig. 28–2). Nonblanchable erythema in a light-skinned person is a reddened area that does not turn white when pressure is applied to it. It signifies damage to blood vessels.
- Stage II: Partial-thickness skin loss involving the epidermis, dermis, or both. The ulcer is superficial and presents clinically as an abrasion, blister, or shallow crater.
- Stage III: Full-thickness skin loss involving damage to or necrosis of subcutaneous tissue that may extend down to but not through underlying fascia. The ulcer presents clinically as a deep crater with or without undermining of adjacent tissue.
- Stage IV: Full-thickness skin loss with extensive destruction, tissue necrosis, or damage to muscle, bone, or supporting structures (e.g., tendon, joint capsule). Undermining and sinus tracts also may be associated with stage IV pressure ulcers (see Fig. 28–2).

Note that erythema in a burn wound indicates tissue viability. In a stage I pressure ulcer nonblanchable erythema (does not turn white or lighter when pressed on) is indicative of disruption in blood flow.

WOUND HEALING

Process. All wounds are not the same. Wound healing is a continuous process and measuring wound repair lacks objec-

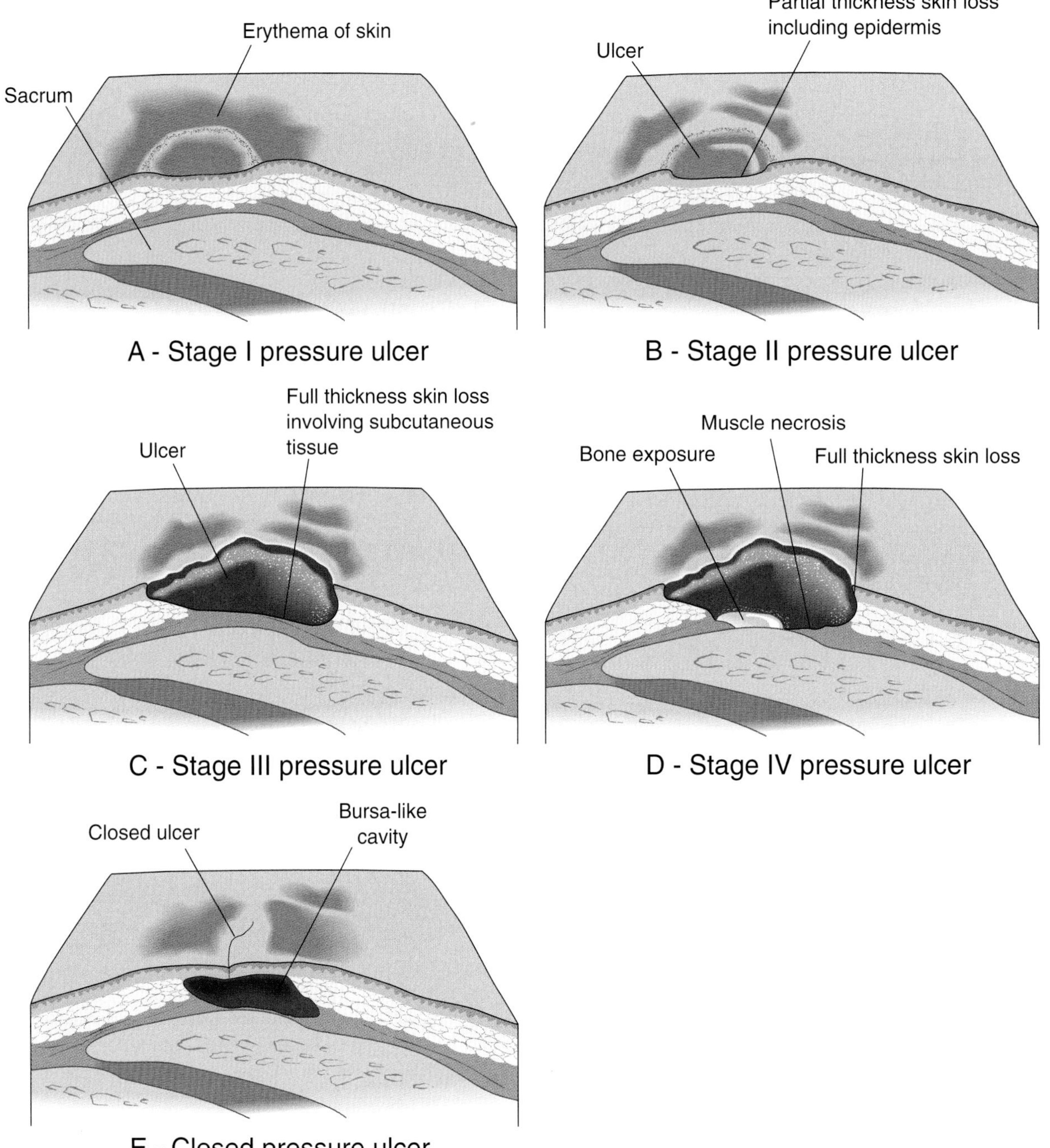

Figure 28–2. Stages of pressure ulcers.

tivity. Recall from reading previous sections of this chapter that the type of injury (e.g., surgical injury versus pressure ulcer), kind of tissues damaged, blood supply, and location of the wound all have major impact on wound healing.

Methods. The goal of wound healing is restoration of normal structure and function with minimal scarring in as brief a time as possible. Wounds heal by two methods: regeneration and repair (McCance and Heuther, 1996). The method of healing varies with the type of body cell damaged, the amount of tissue lost, and the blood supply to the area. Healing varies primarily because body cells differ in their ability to regenerate (by mitosis). Central nervous system neurons and myocardial cells do not regenerate. Most other body cells have, in varying degrees, the capacity for mitosis.

Wounds that heal by *regeneration* (also called healing by *primary intention*) are superficial wounds without tissue loss, to cells that regenerate. Only epithelial tissue is damaged and no large blood vessels are interrupted. For example, in a surgical incision, all wound layers are approximated by suturing and heal with little scarring. Granulation tissue is not visible because rapid replacement by cells similar to those destroyed occurs. Epithelial cells migrate from the wound edges toward the center, and stop when contact is made with epithelial cells migrating from other sides.

Wounds in tissue unable to regenerate *repair* by substituting fibrous connective tissue for damaged or necrotic cells. This scar tissue is dissimilar to the original tissue, and serves as a patch to replace tissue lost to injury. These wounds are left open and not sutured. Granulation tissue grows inward and upward from surrounding healthy connecting tissue to eventually approximate the wound edges. In stage III or IV pressure ulcers, lacerations, and full-thickness burns, damage occurs to cells in deeper skin layers that cannot regenerate. Therefore, these wounds repair or heal by *secondary intention.* The process takes longer and results in more scar tissue than in wounds that heal by regeneration.

Suturing of a contaminated wound (e.g., puncture wound) may be delayed to allow removal of infection prior to closure. Healing by this method is called repair by *tertiary intention.*

Phases. Although the phases of wound healing are described differently by nurses and basic science writers, each describes a sequential process that begins with inflammation. The generally accepted phases of wound healing are:

- coagulation and inflammation
- fibroplasia
- matrix contraction and maturation (Hunt, 1990; Kerstein, 1997)

Cell types involved in wound healing are reviewed in Table 28–2; time and functions of each phase of wound healing are reviewed in Table 28–3.

Coagulation and inflammation are vascular and cellular responses that prepare tissues for subsequent repair. Immediately after cellular injury, blood vessels constrict and then vasodilate, bringing more blood to the area and causing heat, redness, swelling, and pain characteristic of inflammatory response. The increased blood flow in the injury elevates the hydrostatic pressure to a pressure greater than the colloid oncotic pressure (regulated by the concentration of plasma proteins) in the capillaries. This pressure imbalance pushes exudate out of the vasculature into the tissues. Fibrinogen, platelets, and leukocytes in the exudate (lymphocytes, neutrophils, monocytes, and granulocytes) enter the wound.

TABLE 28–2 Cells and Their Function in Wound Healing

Cells/Agents	Category	Function in Wound Healing
1. Coagulation and Inflammation		
Fibrinogen	Plasma protein	Synthesized by the liver. Contained in plasma. Precursor of fibrin.
Fibrin	Protein blood-clotting factor	Formed from the interaction of fibrinogen and thrombin.
Platelets	Fragments of precursor WBCs	Assist in blood clot formation. Platelet degranulation releases cytokines.
Neutrophils	Granulocytic leukocyte (WBC) accounts for 50–70% of WBCs	Phagocytic. Early control of infection in wound site.
Monocytes	Agranulocytic leukocytes (WBCs)	Phagocytic cells that are few in number but ingest more particles and live longer in an inflammation than neutrophils.
Macrophages	Transformed monocytes Phagocytic cells	Macrophages have a key role in modulating wound healing. Major phagocytes in wounds that engulf foreign substances and cellular debris. Release growth factors (angiogenesis factor and fibroblast-stimulating factor) that accelerate various aspects of wound healing. Excess exogenous stimulation of macrophage activators may be destructive to a wound site.
Lymphocytes	Agranulocytic leukocytes (WBCs)	Phagocytic cells. Synthesize immunoglobulinemia: B cells (humoral immunity) and T cells (cellular immunity). Contribute to wound healing, primarily in chronic inflammation.
Cytokines	Chemoattractants	Cause motion in cells. Recruit macrophages to the wound site. Stimulate macrophages to release "growth factors." Cytokines have chemotactic, proliferative, and mitogenic functions (Cromack et al, 1990).
Epithelial cells	Cells	Cells of the epidermis and lining of respiratory, digestive, and genitourinary systems.
2. Fibroplasia (Granulation and Tissue Synthesis)		
Fibroblasts	Immature connective tissue cells	Major source of matrix proteins: collagen, elastin, granulation tissue consists of fibroblasts, macrophages, ground substance, blood vessels in the collagen matrix.
3. Matrix Contraction and Maturation		
Collagen	Protein	Collagen is synthesized and degraded throughout wound healing. Collagen forms the scaffolding or matrix for wound repair and contributes to the strength of the wound.

WBCs = white blood cells.

TABLE 28-3 Phases of Wound Healing

Phases of Wound Healing	Time	Function
1. Coagulation and inflammation	Immediately and lasts for 1–5 days.	Platelets and fibrin aid in clot formation to wall or seal the wound. Plasma exudate that fills the wound and contains proteins (complement) and leukocytes that remove foreign substances and debris. Fibrin clot provides a framework for wound repair and epithelial cell migration.
2. Fibroplasia (granulation and tissue synthesis) • Matrix deposition • Angiogenesis • Epithelialization	Begins on day 2 after injury and continues 5 to 28 days.	Fibroblasts secrete collagen, which forms the matrix for the new tissue and eventually scar tissue. Capillaries form and grow along the fibrin matrix. The new blood flow across the wound brings oxygen and nutrients necessary for healing. Blood flow in the capillaries gives the wound a pink color. Epithelial cells formed at the wound edges migrate "leap frog" fashion over each other across the top of the wound. When cells from each edge come in contact, this growth stops and the wound has a barrier to the external environment.
3. Matrix contraction and maturation	Begins 6–12 days after injury. Lasts 21 days to months to years.	Collagen continues to be deposited by the fibroblasts and degraded and the scar is remodeled and retracted. The synthesis and lysis of collagen must be balanced. The color of the scar changes to silver white. The tissue regains 80% of its original tensile strength (Rote, 1990).

Fibrinogen/fibrin mesh created by coagulation traps platelets and creates a tight seal for the wound. The fibrin seal forms a barrier against bacterial invasion, helps approximate the wound edges, and provides a framework for collagen and epithelial cells to fill the wound after the clot is dissolved. Inflammation is an essential phase in wound healing. Without it, healing cannot occur. Because inflammation can occur only in vascularized, perfused tissue, an inflammatory response occurs only at the wound edges of a pressure ulcer or other perforative injury. In other words, the blood supply must not be restricted by mechanical pressure in the soft tissue between a bony prominence and external surface (mattress, chair, etc.).

Fibroplasia and matrix deposition (granulation or proliferation) make up the second phase of healing and last 5 to 28 days. The fibroblasts secrete matrix proteins (collagen), which form the framework of the new tissue. Fibroblasts migrate along the fibrin strands toward the wound edge, apparently pulled there by chemoattractants. The platelets in the inflammatory exudate release cytokines (e.g., growth factors and interferons) that act as chemoattractants for endothelial cells and fibroblasts, essential for wound repair.

Clot debridement by macrophages and neutrophils may be followed either by simple resolution with regeneration of destroyed cells or by repair with granulation tissue, which grows inward from the surrounding connective tissue (McCance and Heuther, 1996). Collagen is continually synthesized and degraded in the wound-healing process.

Inflammatory response is crucial to fibroplasia. Good nutrition and oxygenation are important for fibroblast replication and collagen deposition in wounds (Hunt, 1990).

Wound healing depends on blood perfusion. *Angiogenesis* is the proliferation of a new microcirculation (blood vessel network) to replace that which was destroyed through injury. As collagen is being synthesized by fibroblasts, capillaries form and stretch across the supporting fibrin matrix. Macrophages make a channel by secreting lytic enzymes and lead each advancing capillary. Macrophages also release an angiogenic factor and chemoattractants to endothelial cells. The combination of capillary development and proliferating fibroblasts assumes a granular appearance and is called granulation tissue. Irradiation destroys or impairs capillary development.

Researchers are attempting to induce angiogenesis (Knighton et al, 1990). The ability to manipulate collagen deposition, and therefore angiogenesis, would be of great benefit to injured patients.

The growth of epithelial cells over raw, repairing tissue is called *epithelialization.* A thin layer of epithelial cells is advanced over the surface of the wound by "flowing." That is, one cell anchors and the next cell advances over it and anchors (from the peripheral edges of the wound). The force or motion that attracts the cells is not known. Growth factors may accelerate wound epithelialization. The source of mitotic activity is the epithelial cells of the hair follicles in partial-thickness wounds or from deeper tissue in more severe injury such as pressure ulcers and full-thickness burns. Epithelialization of the wound begins 1 to 2 days after injury. The rate of epithelialization depends on vascularization and oxygen supply (Hunt, 1990). Because epithelial cells move best in a moist environment, moist dressings enhance healing (Kerstein, 1997; Maklebust and Sieggreen, 1991; Rote, 1990). Epithelial cells can move under a scab because these cells secrete lytic enzymes that create a space for advancing and anchoring of the cells (Hunt, 1990). Contact with epithelial cells flowing and anchoring from the opposite side of the wound causes migration and proliferation to cease. Acceleration of epithelialization is desirable clinically. Why proliferation ceases and how suppression of angiogenesis and fibroplasia occur are not understood, but are currently being researched (Eisinger et al, 1988).

Matrix contraction and maturation occur in the last phase of the construction phase of wound healing. This phase begins

TABLE 28–4 Wound Healing Process

Phase	1. Coagulation and Inflammation	2. Fibroplasia	3. Matrix Contraction and Maturation
Time	Injury to day 5	Day 2 after injury to 28 days	Day 6–12 after injury to 2 years
Cells/Protein	**Platelets** and clot formation **Fibrin** and clot formation **Lymphocytes** produce immunoglobulins **Neutrophils** phagocytize debris (pus cells) **Epithelial cells** comprise the layers of the skin and dermal appendages **Monocytes** are precursors of macrophages		
	Macrophages are phagocytes that secrete "growth" factors crucial to wound healing ⟶	⟶ Macrophages ⟶	⟶ Macrophages
	Complement consists of proteins contained in the plasma that lyse bacterial cell walls or coat antigens with antibodies.		
		Fibroblasts ⟶ Stimulate production of connective tissues collagen elastin glycoproteins	⟶ Fibroblasts

approximately 6 to 12 days after injury and continues for months to years until the wound matures. During contraction, collagen continues to be deposited and organized, and regeneration and lysis of collagen are balanced. The interaction of the new collagen and fibroblasts draws the periphery toward the center of the wound. Recent research shows that myofibroblasts may not be required for contraction and maturation of wounds (Ehrlich, 1988).

As the scar is remodeled, capillaries are compressed and disappear. During this process, the color of the scar changes from red to white-silver and the size decreases. Normal wound healing results in tissue that regains 80 percent of its original tensile strength (Rote, 1990). The phases of wound healing, time, and the functions of the cells involved in the healing process are shown in Table 28–4.

Relevant Research

The knowledge base for nursing patients with wounds or patients who are at risk of preventable wounds such as pressure ulcers comes from research and expert opinion from several fields such as nursing, medicine, anatomy and physiology, engineering, and biomechanics.

INCIDENCE (PRESSURE ULCERS)

Incidence is especially important in pressure ulcers because these frequently occur in persons being treated for other conditions. Reports of incidence of pressure ulcers in hospitalized patients have ranged from 2.7 percent (Gerson, 1975) to 29.5 percent (Clarke and Kadhorn, 1988). Certain subgroups of patients have been found to be more at risk: 40 percent of patients with spinal cord injury (Young and Burns, 1982); 66 percent of elderly patients with femoral fractures; and 33 percent of critical care patients (Bergstrom et al, 1987b) developed pressure ulcers. Although there are problems in measuring incidence, the numbers support the need to learn to prevent and treat this type of wound.

PREVENTION OF NONSURGICAL WOUNDS

Injuries from any source incur multidimensional consequences. Prevention can save much pain, disability, and economic stress. Understanding the etiology of wounds, risk factors, and factors that improve or interfere with healing can result in improvement in prevention and treatment.

Burns. Burn prevention is routinely advocated through health education. However, burn prevention programs have not resulted in large decreases in burn injuries (Linares and Linares, 1990), a reminder that knowing and doing are different phenomena.

The Health Belief Model, modified by Becker and colleagues (1974), specifies that burn prevention programs must increase the individual's perceived susceptibility to burn injury and heighten his or her sensitivity to the immense concomitant psychological and physiologic complications of burns. A comprehensive burn prevention program includes control of the environment (smoke detectors, sprinklers, fire alarms, low temperature for water heaters, inflammability of fabric, doors in public buildings swinging outward, product safety) and modification of products through legislation and consumer pressure (Linares and Linares, 1990). To accomplish these goals, causes and methods to modify risk factors must be integrated.

It is well documented that young children (especially 6 months to 2 years) and the elderly are burned more frequently than middle-aged adults. Boys and men are more likely than girls and women to be burned. The majority of burn injuries occur in the home, especially in the kitchen. Burns to children trigger intense emotions: compassion for the agony the child is enduring, and anger at the persons who "allowed" the burn. Even in homes where children are loved and properly supervised, burns occur accidentally. In dysfunctional families, children may be burned deliberately as a form of punishment. Most children's burns are from scalds or contact with hot objects.

Young children are curious, do not perceive their susceptibility to a burn, and do not have the ability to react quickly to avert harm. Children are fascinated with fire. At times setting a fire is used to communicate distress or rebellion.

Falling asleep while smoking cigarettes causes a number of fires and burns in adults. The elderly often sustain burns because of decreased reaction time; reduction in mobility, visual acuity, and accurate perception of the extent of the danger of thermal injury; and poor living conditions.

Public health nurses are in the unique position to assist in the reduction of burns in the home and in the development of burn prevention programs for communities. In the home, nurses can assess for safety and injury risk for all occupants. Some communities have health education programs that involve all members of the health care team.

Pressure Ulcers. To prevent and treat pressure ulcers, nurses must understand how they occur, how they can be prevented, and how healing can be promoted. Understanding of factors that contribute to individual vulnerability to ulcers and environmental conditions that influence pressure ulcer development enables the nurse to take action to prevent ulcer development. Pressure at the site of contact between a surface and soft tissue over a bony prominence is the key factor in development of pressure ulcers (Husain, 1953). Personal (intrinsic) and environmental (extrinsic) factors can increase or decrease risk of developing ulcers; therefore, the nurse can influence pressure ulcer development and healing by identifying pressure risk and taking action to decrease risk (where alterations can be made). Prevention of pressure ulcers is a major goal for nursing.

Research in the basic sciences has focused primarily on learning the cause of pressure ulcers (etiology), in particular the role of pressure. Less emphasis has been directed toward the study of external factors, such as shear, friction, and humidity.

The current knowledge base includes findings from research done many years ago. Despite the prevalence of the problem of pressure ulcers, there is a dearth of research. Guidelines for prevention and treatment of pressure ulcers were proposed by the Panel for Prediction and Prevention of Pressure Ulcers in Adults, and were based on evidence which required "one or more of the following: (1) results of one controlled trial; (2) results of at least two case series/descriptive studies on pressure ulcers in humans; or (3) expert opinion" (Bergstrom et al., 1994; Panel for Prediction and Prevention of Pressure Ulcers in Adults, 1992).

Etiology. A pressure ulcer begins and progresses as the results of ischemia of skin and underlying soft tissue. Pressure greater than capillary pressure exerted on the capillary wall creates tissue ischemia by occluding capillary blood flow, as shown in Figure 28–3. Arteriolar capillary pressure necessary for adequate tissue perfusion is generally accepted to be 30 to 32 mmHg (Landis, 1930), although there is evidence that pressure approximating diastolic pressure is necessary to occlude capillary circulation (Holstein et al, 1979).

Soft tissues over bony prominences are particularly vulnerable to pressure because tissue is compressed between the bone and the external contact surface (e.g., chair or mattress). The most common areas vulnerable to pressure are shown in Figure 28–4.

On release of pressure, vasodilation occurs and the reactive hyperemic response can be observed on the skin. The response includes increased localized temperature and flushing (redness or other change in color depending on skin color) due to compensatory dilatation of blood vessels and increased capillary blood flow. The flushing is difficult to detect in darkly pigmented skin. This reactive hyperemic response is a physiologic response to compensate for the occlusion of blood flow.

Duration and Intensity of Pressure. During the first half of the twentieth century, Lewis and Grant (1925) reported that ischemia persists one half to three quarters as long as the pressure. This study was based on responses in healthy adults who experienced occlusion of blood flow for brief periods. More information is needed on the expected duration of

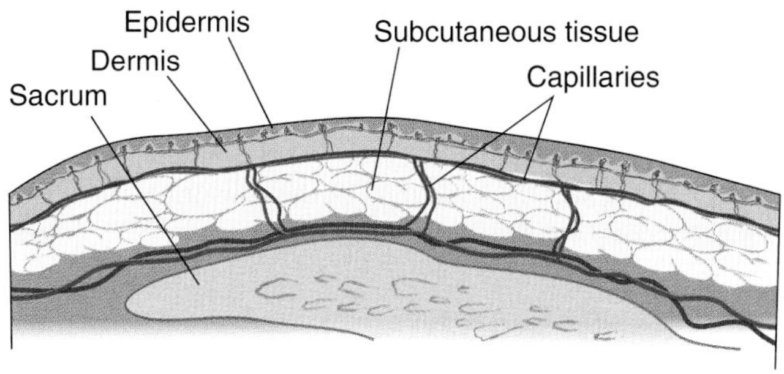

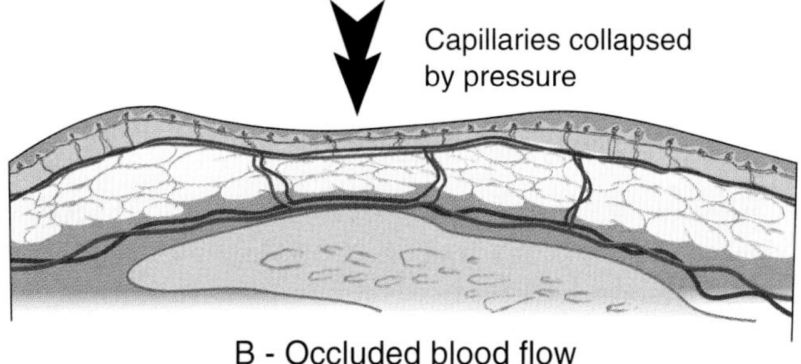

Figure 28–3. Normal capillary blood flow *(A)* and occlusion of capillary blood flow due to pressure from a bony prominence *(B)*.

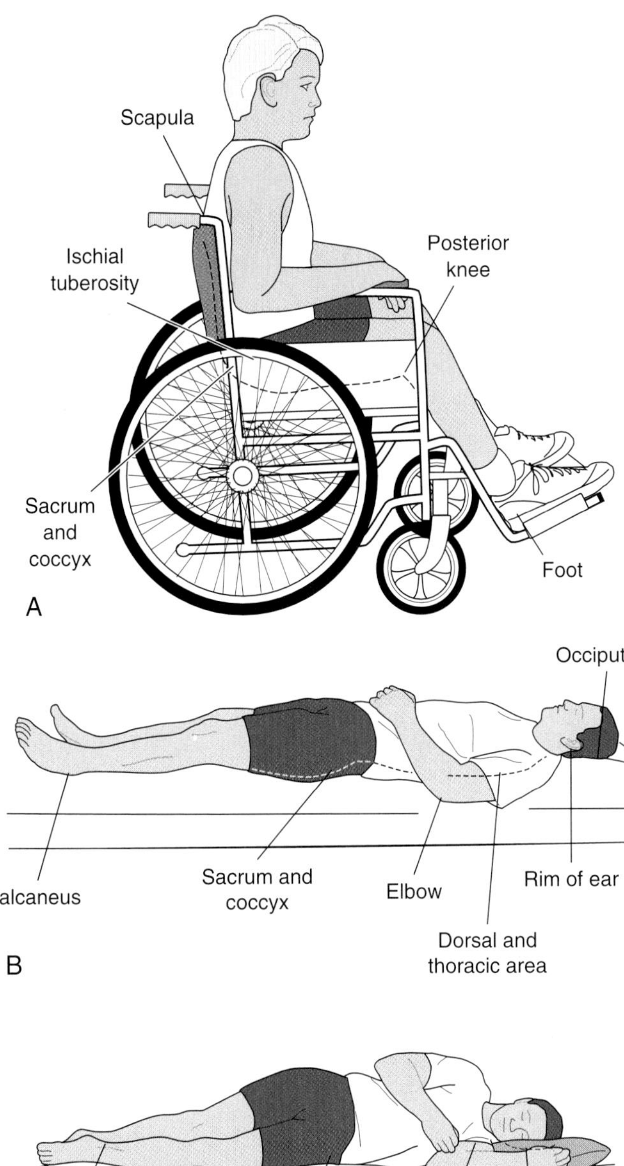

Figure 28–4. Pressure points in sitting *(A)*, prone *(B)*, and side-lying *(C)*, positions.

visual reactive hyperemia when prolonged periods (1 or 2 hours) of partial and total occlusion occur. Failure to relieve pressure at intervals sufficient to provide for tissue nutrients results in cell death and pressure ulcers (Groth, 1942; Kosiak, 1959).

Investigations have been performed on animals and humans to determine the effects of pressure duration and intensity on soft tissues. Pathologic changes in soft tissue of animals have been reported in response to pressures of 60 to 70 mmHg exerted less than 1 hour (Husain, 1953; Kosiak, 1959). Pressures in excess of these values have been reported for tissues over bony surfaces such as the trochanter, heel, and ischium (Lindan et al, 1965). Research on animals showed an inverse relationship between pressure duration and intensity and soft tissue damage (Kosiak, 1959). In other words, high pressures caused damage in shorter time periods than did low pressures. On the other hand, low pressures were tolerated for longer durations before causing cell damage.

Risk Factors. Clinical research has focused on identifying risk factors associated with pressure ulcers in hospitalized patients and patients in nursing homes, the evaluation of tools used to predict patients at risk of developing pressure ulcers, and programs for prevention of pressure ulcers. The following factors have most consistently been found to be associated with risk of pressure ulcers:

- activity or mobility deficit
- moisture/incontinence
- nutritional deficit (Panel for Prediction and Prevention of Pressure Ulcers in Adults, 1992)

Mobility is the ability to change and control body position; *activity* relates to the degree of physical activity. Both influence the duration and intensity of pressure over body surfaces. Any condition that reduces mobility/activity and thereby prolongs pressure over bony prominences such as being chair-bound, confined to bed with restricted ability to turn, weakness, paralysis, or immobilization by restraints, casts, or braces has the potential to increase or prolong pressure on soft tissues. Research findings consistently demonstrate that immobility is associated with the development of pressure ulcers. Two early studies support an inverse relationship between spontaneous movement of elderly persons in bed and development of pressure ulcers (Exton-Smith and Sherwin, 1961) and a lower incidence of pressure ulcers in patients who were turned frequently (Norton et al, 1962). Results of more recent studies have supported the association between pressure ulcer development and immobility in patients in chronic care hospitals (Berlowitz and Wilking, 1989), in orthopedic patients (Goldstone and Goldstone, 1982), in patients in long-term medical units (Ek et al, 1985), and in recurrence of pressure ulcers in patients with spinal cord injuries (Niazi et al, 1997).

Clara, in the case study at the beginning of the chapter, has mobility limitations. She does not change positions often, prefers lying on her back, and is paralyzed on her left side. Clara is at risk for excessive pressure over several bony prominences unless preventive nursing care plans are developed and implemented.

Numerous studies have compared properties of *support surfaces* such as mattress toppers, mattresses, and beds of various types, and sitting-surface cushions as they relate to the prevention of pressure ulcers. Those that compared the standard hospital mattress to a water mattress, foam, or air mattress consistently reported higher incidence of pressure ulcers with the standard mattress (Carlson and King, 1990; King and French, 1990; Panel on Prediction and Prevention of Pressure Ulcers, 1992). Studies comparing various types of nonstandard mattresses or overlays have demonstrated that pressure-reducing devices can decrease incidence of pressure ulcers, but no type has been determined to be superior (Conine et al, 1990).

In a study by DeLateur and colleagues (1976), each of seven wheelchair cushions studied resulted in reactive hyperemia and thus some degree of tissue ischemia after 30 minutes of sitting. Ring cushions should not be used, as they have been found to be more likely to promote pressure ulcers than to prevent them (Crewe, 1987).

More detail on characteristics of surfaces and their effectiveness in preventing or promoting healing of pressure ulcers is available in the technical reports of the Agency for Health Care Policy and Research panels on prediction and prevention and treatment of pressure ulcer guidelines (Bergstrom et al, 1994; Panel for Prediction and Prevention of Pressure Ulcers in Adults, 1992). A summary of characteristics of mattress and bed types designed to reduce pressure is shown in Table 28–5.

Sensory perception has been defined in different ways including neurologic impairment of sensation and altered level of consciousness. In the Braden scale (an assessment scale for prediction of the probability of development of a pressure ulcer), sensory perception refers to the ability to respond meaningfully to pressure-related discomfort. Impaired sensation, level of consciousness, or mental status may contribute to pressure ulcers because of altered awareness of the need to change positions or altered ability to move. Consider the number of times that you change position when you are sitting in class. Generally, these position shifts occur in response to stimuli out of conscious awareness. Little research has been done on the relationship between sensory perception and the development of pressure ulcers. Berlowitz and Wilking (1989) found altered level of consciousness to be significantly associated with pressure ulcers; however, method of measurement of level of consciousness was not provided.

Clara also shows evidence of a sensory perception problem. She has a limited visual field and does not recognize part of her body as her own. Absence of sensory signals indicating the need to change position may also influence nutrition if Clara is unable to see the food on her tray. The nursing care plan for Clara needs to address ways to compensate for these perceptual problems.

The role of *friction* and *shear* in the development of pressure ulcers has been investigated. *Friction* is the rubbing of two surfaces against each other, such as skin being pulled across a bedsheet, which may result in skin abrasion. Dinsdale (1974) found that the combination of friction and pressure resulted in significantly greater susceptibility to skin ulceration in animals than pressure alone. *Shear* is a stress resulting from applied forces that cause two contiguous parts of the body to slide parallel to each other. *Thrombosis* and *ischemia* result from this stretching and angulation of blood vessels (Guyton and Hall, 1995; McCance and Heuther, 1996). Take a piece of transparent tape and place it lengthwise on the end of your finger. Pull horizontally and notice the blanching of the skin. This represents shear. The most common example of shear occurs in the sacral area when the head of the bed is raised less than 90 degrees but greater than 30 degrees and the trunk slides down and the skin over the sacrum stays in the same position (Fig. 28–5).

Skin surface *moisture* from perspiration or incontinence of urine or feces, or moisture from other sources may influence integrity of skin by making it more vulnerable to friction or chemicals. Studies have shown a relationship between incontinence and pressure ulcers (Allman et al, 1986; Goldstone and Goldstone, 1982; Lowthian, 1976; Manley, 1978); however, others have failed to demonstrate any association (e.g., Ek et al, 1985; Gosnell, 1973; Williams, 1972). In many reports, authors do not report whether their findings relate to fecal, urinary, or both types of incontinence. Clara is incontinent of urine, which adds to her risk of pressure ulcer development.

Nutrition is significant to the health of all living tissue and is measured using various blood indices, calorie or protein intake, weight, etc. Low serum albumin, a measure of nutritional status, has been associated with pressure ulcers in adult inpatients (Allman et al, 1986) and patients in nursing homes (Pinchofsky-Devin and Kaminski, 1986) but not in adult surgical patients (Kemp et al, 1990; Stotts, 1987). Higher caloric intake and higher protein intake have been associated with healing of pressure ulcers in malnourished patients in nursing homes. Vitamin and mineral deficiencies have been identified in a great number of nursing home

TABLE 28–5 Selected Characteristics of Support Devices

	Support Device					
Performance Characteristics	*Air-Fluidized*	*Low-Air-Loss*	*Alternating Air*	*Static Flotation (air or water)*	*Foam*	*Standard Mattress*
Increased support area	Yes	Yes	Yes	Yes	Yes	No
Low moisture retention	Yes	Yes	No	No	No	No
Reduced heat accumulation	Yes	Yes	No	No	No	No
Shear reduction	Yes	?	Yes	Yes	No	No
Pressure reduction	Yes	Yes	Yes	Yes	Yes	No
Dynamic	Yes	Yes	Yes	No	No	No
Cost per day	High	High	Moderate	Low	Low	Low

Bergstrom, N., Bennett, M.A., Carlson, E. C., et al (December 1994). *Treatment of Pressure Ulcers.* Clinical Practice Guideline, No. 15, Rockville, MD: U.S. Department of Health and Human Services. Public Health Service, Agency for Health Care Policy and Research. AHCPR Publication No. 95-0652, p. 38.

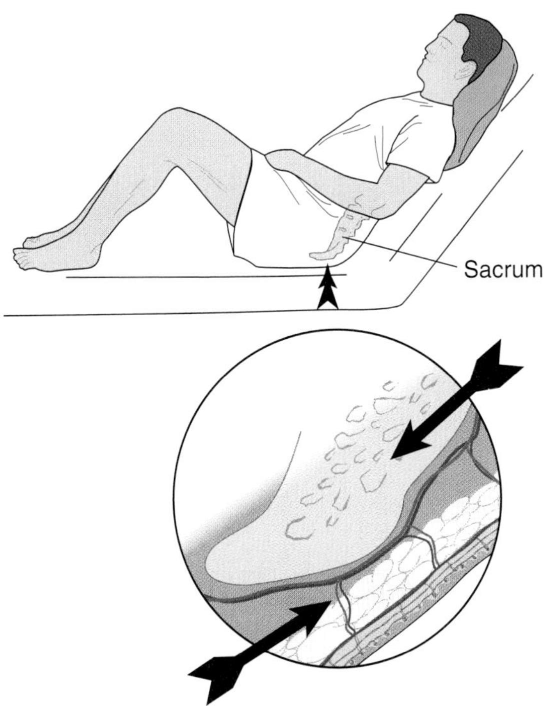

Figure 28–5. Shearing forces in sacral area. Blood vessels are being closed off because of forces of tissues going in opposite directions.

residents (Bergstrom and Braden, 1992); see Research Highlight. Clara in the case study is at risk; her caloric and protein intake are inade-quate. Normal serum albumin ranges between 3.5 and 5.0. According to Kaminski and colleagues (1989) and Flanigan (1994), serum albumin less than 3.5 g/dl is low and signals the need for further complete nutritional evaluation. A level below 2.5 g/dl is associated with protein depletion.

Risk Prediction. Assessment of risk of developing pressure ulcers can be done using valid, reliable tools such as the Braden (Fig. 28–6) or Norton scales (Bergstrom and Braden, 1992; Norton et al, 1962; Panel on Prediction and Prevention of Pressure Ulcers in Adults, 1992). Accuracy of these tools has received much attention in nursing research since accurate identification of those at risk will enable nurses to use staff and material resources more efficiently. When using a tool to measure risk, it is important to measure risk consistently and accurately (reliability) and to measure the concepts it is designed to measure (validity). Also, when a person evaluates how well the tool identifies persons at risk of developing pressure ulcers, it is important to know how often it overpredicts or underpredicts risk. If a tool overpredicts, costs of care will increase due to increased caregiving time, equipment, etc. If a tool underpredicts those at risk, the patient may not get necessary interventions and resources, such as staff and pressure reduction devices.

Although a number of risk prediction scales are available, only two, the Norton and the Braden scales, have been examined extensively. The Norton scale includes an assessment of local moisture or continence, perception of pressure, activity, mobility, and physical condition or nutrition. The Braden scale adds assessment of friction and shear. The reliability and validity of the Braden scale have been tested in several clinical settings, such as rehabilitation units of skilled nursing facilities, institutionalized elderly, medical-surgical units of teach-

RESEARCH HIGHLIGHT
RISK FACTORS FOR PRESSURE ULCERS

Bergstrom and Braden (1992) conducted a study to determine if nutritional status, dietary intake, and other variables are risk factors for the development of pressure ulcers in elderly persons such as Clara in the case study. They studied 200 residents who were over 65 years old, had a Braden scale score ≤17, expected to stay in the nursing home for more than 10 days, and were currently free of pressure ulcers.

The outcome measure (variable) of primary interest was presence or absence of pressure ulcers and their stage. The other variables were skin assessment; Braden scale score; blood pressure; body temperature; anthropometrics (body weight, knee height, stature, wrist and mid-arm muscle circumference, tricep skinfold thickness); complete blood count (CBC), serum albumin, protein, iron, zinc, copper, and vitamin C levels; and iron-binding capacity. These variables were studied weekly for 4 weeks and biweekly for 8 weeks.

Findings. 70 residents (35 percent) developed stage I pressure ulcers and 77 (38.5 percent) developed stage II or worse. Age was positively associated with pressure ulcers. Those with ulcers had lower systolic and diastolic pressure ($p < .001$), and a higher body temperature ($p < .001$) than those without pressure ulcers. Residents with pressure ulcers had lower dietary intake of nutrients than those without. The best predictors of pressure ulcers were: Braden scale score; diastolic blood pressure; body temperature; protein intake; and age.

Implications for Nursing Practice. Risk assessments should be done when residents are admitted to nursing homes, then weekly for at least a month. Variables included in assessment of risk factors include age, condition of the skin, activity, mobility, nutrition (especially protein intake), sensory perception, moisture, friction, shear, diastolic blood pressure, and body temperature. The Braden scale is one prediction tool that can be used to assess several of the variables that place an elderly person at risk for development of pressure ulcers.

Bergstrom, N., Braden, B. (1992). A prospective study of pressure sore risk among institutionalized elderly. *Journal of the American Geriatric Society, 40,* 747–758.

Client's name ______________________ Evaluator's name ______________________

					Date of assessment	
Sensory perception Ability to respond meaningfully to pressure-related discomfort	**1. Completely limited** Unresponsive to painful stimuli (does not moan, flinch, or grasp) because of diminished level of consciousness or sedation OR limited ability to feel pain over most of body surface	**2. Very limited** Responds only to painful stimuli; cannot communicate discomfort except by moaning or restlessness OR has a sensory impairment that limits the ability to feel pain or discomfort over half of the body	**3. Slightly limited** Responds to verbal commands but cannot always communicate discomfort or need to be turned OR has some sensory impairment that limits ability to feel pain or discomfort in one or two extremities	**4. No impairment** Responds to verbal commands; has no sensory deficit that would limit ability to feel or voice pain or discomfort		
Moisture Degree to which skin is exposed to moisture	**1. Completely moist** Skin is kept moist almost constantly by perspiration, urine; dampness is detected every time the client is moved or turned	**2. Moist** Skin is often but not always moist; linen must be changed at least once a shift	**3. Occasionally moist** Skin is occasionally moist, requiring an extra linen change approximately once a day	**4. Rarely moist** Skin is usually dry; linen requires changing only at routine intervals		
Activity Degree of physical activity	**1. Bedfast** Confined to bed	**2. Chairfast** Ability to walk severely limited or nonexistent; cannot bear own weight and must be assisted into chair or wheelchair	**3. Walks occasionally** Walks occasionally during the day but for very short distances, with or without assistance; spends the majority of each shift in bed or chair	**4. Walks frequently** Walks outside the room at least twice a day and inside the room at least once every 2 hours during waking hours		
Mobility Ability to change or control body position	**1. Completely immobile** Does not make even slight changes in body or extremity position without assistance	**2. Very limited** Makes occasional slight changes in body or extremity position but unable to make frequent or significant changes independently	**3. Slightly limited** Makes frequent though slight changes in body or extremity position independently	**4. No limitations** Makes major and frequent changes in position without assistance		
Nutrition Usual food intake pattern	**1. Very poor** Never eats a complete meal; rarely eats more than a third of any food offered; eats two servings or less of protein (meat or dairy products) per day; takes fluids poorly; does not take a liquid dietary supplement OR is NPO or maintained on clear liquids or IV for more than 5 days	**2. Probably inadequate** Rarely eats a complete meal and generally eats only about half of any food offered; protein intake includes only three servings of meat or dairy products per day; occasionally will take a dietary supplement OR receives less than optimal amount of liquid diet or tube feeding	**3. Adequate** Eats over half of most meals; eats a total of four servings of protein (meat, dairy products) each day; occasionally will refuse a meal, but will usually take a supplement if offered OR is receiving tube feeding or total parenteral nutrition, which probably meets most nutritional needs	**4. Excellent** Eats most of every meal; never refuses a meal; usually eats a total of four or more servings of meat and dairy products; occasionally eats between meals; does not require supplementation		
Friction and shear	**1. Problem** Requires moderate to maximum assistance in moving; complete lifting without sliding against sheets is impossible; frequently slides down in bed or chair, requiring frequent repositioning with maximum assistance; spasticity, contractures, or agitation leads to almost constant friction	**2. Potential problem** Moves feebly or requires minimum assistance during a move; skin probably slides to some extent against sheets, chair, restraints, or other devices; maintains relatively good position in chair or bed most of the time but occasionally slides down	**3. No apparent problem** Moves in bed and in chair independently and has sufficient muscle strength to lift up completely during move; maintains good position in bed or chair at all times			
				Total score		

Scoring system: 15–16 = mild risk, 12–14 = moderate risk, <11 = severe risk. (Modified from Barbara Braden and Nancy Bergstrom. Copyright 1988.)

Figure 28–6. The Braden scale. (Courtesy of Barbara Braden and Nancy Bergstrom. Copyright 1988.)

ing hospital (Bergstrom et al, 1987a, 1987b; Bergstrom and Braden, in press). The scale has six subscales: sensory perception, activity, mobility, moisture, friction, and nutrition. Five of the six subscales are evaluated on a scale from 1 (least favorable) to 4 (most favorable). Friction and shear subscale are rated from 1 to 3. Scores range from 6 to 23. The lower the score, the greater the risk. A score below 16 has been used in several studies as the cut-off for predicting risk (Bergstrom et al, 1987a); however, the effective cut-off point for prediction may vary with different patient populations.

Other factors, such as older age, arteriolar pressure, edema, elevated body temperature, smoking, soft tissue atrophy, dry skin, and psychological and social variables have been studied as potential risk factors less consistently (Bergstrom and Braden, 1992). The nurse must be aware of factors that theoretically may influence nutrients reaching cells through increasing duration or intensity of pressure or reducing tissue tolerance of pressure. For instance, low blood pressure results in less resistance of blood vessels to pressure; elevated body temperature or local skin temperature increases metabolic needs.

WOUND HEALING (TREATMENT)

Clinicians are concerned with promoting healing and preventing the occurrence of conditions that will promote infection or failure of wound healing. Whether the wound be a surgical incision, pressure ulcer, burn, or other type of wound it is important to consider intrinsic and extrinsic factors that may influence healing. Research related to risk factors described previously is relevant to healing also. For example, stage of pressure ulcer has been shown to be correlated with deficits in nutrition, especially low protein intake or low serum albumin (Bergstrom and Braden, 1992; Berlowitz and Wilking, 1989; Breslow et al, 1991). Breslow and colleagues (1993) reported that pressure ulcer healing may be improved in malnourished nursing home patients given high-protein diets with increased calories. Many patients in nursing homes have been shown to have vitamin and mineral deficiencies (Bergstrom and Braden, 1992). When such deficiencies exist, supplementation of vitamin C and zinc may facilitate healing (Taylor et al, 1974). When deficiencies of water-soluble vitamins are identified, it has been documented that amounts considerably higher than recommended daily allowances (RDAs) may be needed to remove the deficiencies (Cruz Santiago et al, 1981; Williams et al, 1988).

Support surfaces have been found to influence pressure ulcer healing as well as promote prevention. Results of studies comparing static support surfaces (Conine et al, 1990; Ferrell et al, 1993; Warner, 1992) have shown healing to improve when such surfaces are used. However, there is no evidence that any one of the static surfaces is more effective than the other. If the support surface is foam, it should be at least three or four inches thick (Kemp and Krouskop, 1994).

INFECTION CONTROL, WOUND CLEANSING, AND DEBRIDEMENT

Prevention of Infection. All wounds except perhaps surgical wounds are contaminated with bacteria that cause an infection if they invade surrounding viable tissue. When the bacterial concentration is greater than 100,000 organisms/gram of tissue, a local wound infection exists (Baxter and Mertz, 1990). The density of bacteria in a grossly necrotic or stage I wound is in the millions, and it is reduced to the hundreds for healing stage II wounds (Sapico et al, 1986). Bacteria most commonly found in grossly necrotic draining wounds were gram-positive aerobes (e.g., *Enterococcus, Staphylococcus aureus*), gram-negative aerobes (e.g., *Escherichia coli, Pseudomonas aeruginosa*), gram-positive anaerobes *Peptostreptococcus,* and gram-negative anaerobes (e.g., *Bacteroides fragilis*). Infection from gram-negative rods is often associated with sepsis, which has a high mortality rate.

Wounds need to be cleansed adequately, with nurses' hands washed properly and clean/sterile technique maintained to decrease the extent of a wound infection. Enhancement of the patient's nutrition and circulation to the tissues decreases the risk of infection and aids wound healing.

Wound infection is characterized by an increase in erythema, edema, change in color of exudate and/or presence of pus, and an uncharacteristic odor; fever; elevated white blood count; and pain. Patients with circulatory/respiratory problems or immunocompromised patients may not manifest all these signs; pain may be the only symptom. High bacterial counts in wounds delay healing (Harding, 1990).

Wound Cleansers. Studies have demonstrated that wound cleansers need to be diluted to not destroy cells (Burkey et al, 1993; Foresman et al, 1993). Normal saline is the preferred agent.

Wound irrigation pressures have been studied to determine the pressure that will enhance cleansing of the wound without causing trauma to cells (see Fig. 28–10) (Brown et al, 1978; Longmire et al, 1987). The range of safety is from 4 to 15 pounds per square inch (psi).

Wound Debridement. Removal of necrotic tissue and infection control must be accomplished before optimal wound healing can occur. Debridement can reduce bacterial counts within a wound. Antiseptics, antimicrobials, and/or antibiotics are used to treat infected wounds.

Until recently, debridement was accomplished mechanically with scalpel and forceps, and/or with saline-soaked gauze allowed to dry before removal. Both methods of debridement caused pain and damaged healthy tissue. Surgical debridement may also cause bacteremia (Corum, 1993; Glenchar et al, 1981). Chemical debridement using proteolytic enzymes (e.g., collagenase, fibrinolysin, trypsin, and papain) is slower than mechanical debridement, and also can damage healthy tissue. Hydrocolloid dressings, e.g., DuoDerm, decrease bacterial counts in wounds resulting in better healing than wet-to-dry dressings and increase the rate of angiogenesis (Bolton et al, 1990).

TABLE 28-6 Intrinsic Factors that Influence Wound Healing

Factor	Effect on Healing	Nursing Assessment/Action
Oxygenation of the wound	Inflammatory response is essential to wound healing and inflammation can occur only in perfused tissue. Lack of oxygenation at the wound site impairs healing. Adequate blood flow to the wound is required to supply nutrients, oxygen, WBCs (white blood cells), and to remove debris from the wound. Oxygen is required for fibroblast replication and collagen deposition in wounds.	Assess for: • capillary refill, nonblanchable erythema • redness, swelling, and warmth of wound • low hemoglobin (low hemoglobin interferes with O_2 delivery) Prevent pressure to the wound site. Prevent mechanical disruption of the wound. Provide fluids to maintain blood volume. Elevate the injured area, if possible. Keep the environment warm to prevent vasoconstriction. Protect wounds from irradiation, which destroys or impairs capillary development. Ambulate QID or to patient's tolerance.
Nutritional status	Preinjury and postinjury nutritional status influence wound healing.	Calculate the correct amount of calories needed. Use formula for estimating basal energy requirements. Adjust for activity, growth, stress, and other factors. Calculate the correct amount of protein for the body size and age to build new tissue. Low serum albumin is a late sign of protein deficiency. Adult Requirements: (Food and Nutrition Board, 1998) • Normal = 0.8 to 1.0 g/kg/day • Moderate stress (infection, fracture, surgery) = 1.0 to 2.0 g/kg/day • Severe stress (burns, multiple fractures) = 2.0 to 2.5 g/kg/day
Deficiencies of proteins	Deficiency of protein results in less amino acids for tissue repair.	Give any assistance required to provide a high-protein, high-calorie diet.
Deficiency of calories	Insufficient caloric intake results in breakdown of protein to meet energy needs. Less protein is then available for tissue repair.	Discuss needs for nutritional supplements or total parenteral nutrition when nutritional intake is inadequate.
Deficiencies—Vitamin C, A	Deficiency of vitamins C and A results in decreased fibroplasia and collagen synthesis and capillary development.	Provide vitamin supplements as indicated.
Low plasma zinc concentration	Epithelization is impaired in persons with low plasma zinc concentration.	Administer zinc supplements as prescribed.
Obesity	Adipose tissue has poor blood perfusion. Adipose tissue does not hold sutures well.	Turn, ambulate frequently to prevent pressure that contributes to the formation of pressure ulcers and delays wound healing. Assess for dehiscence of suture wounds.
Corticosteroid release or exogenous administration	Corticosteroids impair the inflammatory response which is required for wound healing. Corticosteroids impair phagocytosis by decreasing the WBC numbers.	Assess carefully for wound infection because corticosteroids mask usual signs of infection. Administer vitamin A as prescribed because vitamin A counteracts the anti-inflammatory effect of steroids, and so it may be given to patients who have wounds and who require steroids for treatment of other disease processes (Sporn & Roberts, 1990). Minimize stress because stress causes endogenous release of corticosteroids.
Age	Children normally have good blood perfusion and hydration, rapid epidermal growth, and skin elasticity. Elderly individuals frequently experience reduced blood perfusion and tissue cell proliferation, and so have a marked reduction in wound healing.	Encourage and assist in eating the proper diet for wound healing and drinking fluids to maintain blood volume. Protect the skin/wound from contamination and infection.

TABLE 28–6 Intrinsic Factors that Influence Wound Healing *Continued*

Factor	Effect on Healing	Nursing Assessment/Action
Disease processes		
Diabetes	Persons with diabetes often have impaired circulation and thus decreased collagen synthesis in injury. Hyperglycemia impedes phagocytosis.	Assist the patient to maintain normal blood glucose concentrations.
Anemia	Reduced RBCs (red blood cells) result in less oxygen supply to the tissues.	Encourage eating iron-rich foods. Correct anemia by administering hematins and blood transfusions as prescribed.
Infection	Infection impairs wound healing by increasing wound destruction. Infection increases the inflammatory response. Healing cannot progress until all necrotic tissue is removed from a wound.	Assess for the presence, amount, type of exudate. Assess for systemic signs of infection, e.g., fever, elevated WBC count. Keep wound clean, dry and/or moist as prescribed. Administer antibiotics selectively (as per physician order). Follow physician prescription for wound debridement.
Pain	Releases catecholamines that cause vasoconstriction. Results in release of corticosteroids.	Assess the nature, cause of pain. Immobilize the injured area. Administer pain medication (per order). Apply cold compresses when appropriate to reduce swelling.
Impaired circulation	Impaired circulation delays nutrient delivery to the wound and removal of debris from the wound.	Determine underlying cause of impaired circulation. Administer cardiac drugs as prescribed. Turn immobile patients every 2 hours or more frequently.

Topical Antiseptics and Antibiotics. Both systemic antibiotics and topical antiseptics are used to control colonization of microorganisms. Systemic antibiotics may predispose patients to diarrhea and development of resistant bacteria, so should be avoided or used cautiously. Several topical antibiotics are available to treat wounds and pressure ulcers (e.g., Bactroban, Silvadene, and Flagyl). Generally, clinicians do not recommend them because they are expensive and have not been proven to be superior to commonly used disinfectant solutions such as povidone-iodine or saline irrigation (Patterson and Bennett, 1995). Use of topical antiseptics has been reported to destroy or inhibit the growth of fibroblasts and thus impede wound healing. However, prospective studies are inconclusive. Povidone-iodine solution was found to lower bacterial counts in wounds without delaying wound healing (Goldenheim, 1993). Patterson and Bennett (1995) also found povidone-iodine solution effective in treating wounds with odoriferous and purulent drainage, but recommended that clinicians avoid hydrogen peroxide, detergent-containing Betadine surgical scrub, and alcohol-based products. Antiseptics should only be used in initial wound cleansing and should be discontinued when the wound is clean and granulating.

Directions in Wound Treatment. Wounds present three major problems: hemorrhage, tissue disruption, and infection. Hemorrhage and disruption of normal tissue are obvious problems to even the casual observer. Minor hemorrhage was controlled with cautery, and wounds were sutured as early as 2000 B.C. (Caldwell, 1990). However, infection is insidious and invisible and remains somewhat a mystery even today. Early empiric methods of managing wound infections included lint, honey, oil, wine, and metallic salts. Today, the mechanisms of normal wound repair can be studied in the absence of infection. Current research includes study of inflammatory cells in the repair process, action of growth factors in wound healing, importance of direct versus indirect angiogenesis in the healing wound, influence of the extracellular matrix in stimulating wound healing, and management of larger surface wounds.

Research has resulted in the application of topical growth factors obtained from the patient's own platelets (Baxter and Mertz, 1990; Brown et al, 1989), and cultured epithelial allographs in clinical management of surgical incisions, burns, or pressure ulcers. In the future, understanding of normal tissue inflammation, regeneration, and repair may lead to understanding and manipulation of tumor formation.

Summary of Factors that Influence Wound Healing. The healing of a wound demonstrates the innate drive of the body toward healing and/or health. Numerous intrinsic and extrinsic factors may influence the rate and completeness of the wound healing.

Intrinsic factors, the processes operating within the person that influence wound healing, include nutritional status, circulation or oxygenation, stress, corticosteroids, age, presence of disease and/or infection, and the type and location of the wound (Table 28–6). Intrinsic factors are controlled primarily by the patient. The nurse can play a key role in facilitating individual actions that promote healing such as assessing the individual on these intrinsic factors, analyzing data to determine action that needs to be taken, teaching importance of each, and taking action that will encourage wound healing.

TABLE 28-7 Extrinsic Factors that Influence Wound Healing

Factor	Effect on Healing	Nursing Assessment/Action
Cleansing agents, debridement, and infection control	Reducing the amount of bacteria in the wound reduces the amount of infection and enhances wound healing.	Flush the wound with saline solution using a piston syringe (35 ml) and an angiocatheter (19 gauge) (Corum, 1993; Lehmann & Konstautindes, 1989). The irrigation pressure produced (8 pounds per square inch [psi]) is sufficient to remove bacteria without forcing bacteria deeper into the tissue. Use other wound cleansing agents cautiously. Apply proteolytic enzymes as prescribed. Place the patient in whirlpool as ordered. Administer antiseptics, antimicrobials, or antibiotics as prescribed.
Protective dressings and ointments	Effects include: • providing a barrier to bacteria • reducing pain • protecting healthy tissue • keeping the wound moist, which promotes granulation	Apply an occlusive dressing, petroleum gauze dressing, or semipermeable dressing film as prescribed. Apply protective ointments as prescribed.
Pressure relief	Capillary filling pressure > 32 mmHg impedes the flow of oxygen and nutrients to tissues and removal of debris from the wound.	Avoid pressure over wounds and bony prominences. Reposition the patient every 2 hours or more often. Place an immobile patient on a low-air-loss bed or air-fluidized bed. Do not elevate the head of the bed for a patient who does not have the strength to consistently maintain an upright position.

Nutritional requirements, for example, increase with wounds, infection, elevated temperature, growth, and activity. Requirements need to be calculated and explained to the person (see Table 28–6).

Extrinsic factors, the environment of the wound, influence the rate and completeness of wound healing. These include the agents used to cleanse the wound, the amount of debridement, the type of dressing placed on the wound, pressure from surface in contact with skin, and other characteristics of the external environment (Table 28–7). Of course, the extrinsic factors are managed primarily by nurses and physicians.

Included in Tables 28–6 and 28–7 are the intrinsic and extrinsic factors that influence wound healing and their specific impact on healing. Also included are the nursing assessments and actions designed to influence the rate and completeness of wound healing.

Relevant Theory

Bergstrom and Braden have collaborated to develop a conceptual schema to facilitate the understanding of how intrinsic and extrinsic variables influence the prevention or the development of a pressure ulcer (Braden and Bergstrom, 1987) (Fig. 28–7). This model is not the only conceptual schema, framework, or theory related to skin integrity; however, it is based on considerable research in an area where research-based nursing care can make a tremendous difference in outcomes for patients. The two major variables in this schema are *pressure* and *tolerance.* Nurses can decrease pressure by in-

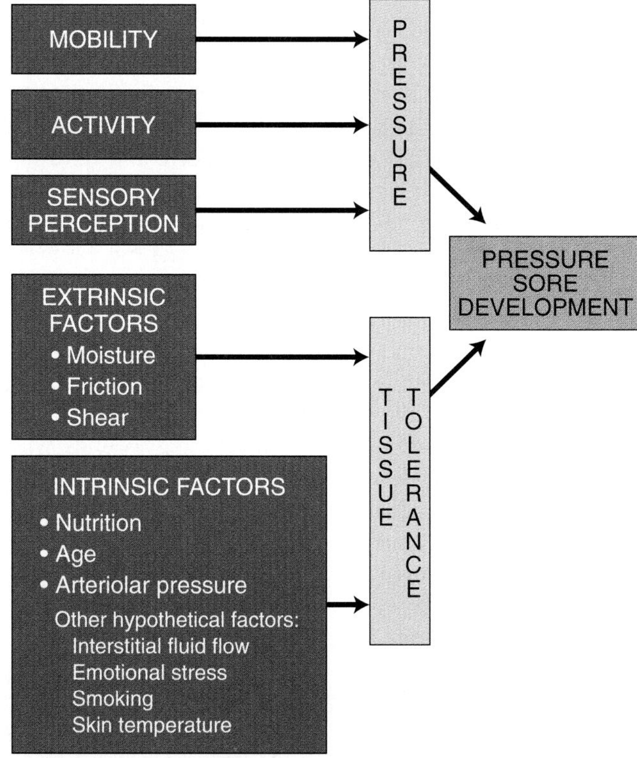

Figure 28-7. Conceptual model of the etiology of pressure ulcers.

creasing patients' mobility and activity or addressing problems with sensory perception. Tissue tolerance to pressure can be enhanced by avoiding or removing moisture, preventing friction and shear, improving nutrition, decreasing emotional stress, etc. The schema provides a framework for practice and research that can promote further development of the knowledge base for nursing practice.

The schema is the conceptual model for the Braden risk prediction scale and subsequent research to validate the scale (see Fig. 28–6). Use of the scale for predicting patients at risk of developing pressure ulcers is described later in the chapter.

As Henderson has suggested (George, 1995) nurses assist the sick or well individual to carry out actions that will contribute to maintaining intact skin or healing of wounds when they exist. It is assumed that these activities would be performed by the patient if he or she had the strength and knowledge required. If the patient understood the importance of preventing pressure and the factors contributing to wound healing and had the ability to perform needed actions, he or she would do them.

The Braden and Bergstrom schema identifies major factors contributing to pressure ulcers. Some of these factors overlap with Henderson's 14 components of basic nursing care (George, 1995). Four needs based on components that are particularly relevant are: eat and drink adequately; move and maintain posture; keep body clean and well groomed; and avoid dangers in the environment.

As described in the Clinical Decision Making box, the nurse assesses the patient on needs suggested by Henderson as well as variables included in Braden and Bergstrom's conceptual schema. Based on the assessment, decisions are made regarding help that the patient may need to maintain skin integrity or to promote wound healing. A plan is developed, implemented, and continually evaluated and adjusted as needed. The plan includes assisting with actions that the patient is unable to carry out on his or her own. It also includes teaching the patient and family/caregivers what needs to be done and why and encouraging participation in implementing the plan.

Systematic incorporation of relevant research and nursing theory in individual patient care results in relevant planning and action.

FACTORS AFFECTING CLINICAL DECISIONS

Individual patient differences are well documented and include intrinsic factors such as nutritional status, sensation, moisture (sweating, urinary and fecal incontinence, mobility), and extrinsic factors such as bed or chair surface. The reader is challenged to think of illnesses and circumstances that involve these and other factors. For example, consider what conditions disrupt nutritional status. Stroke, anorexia nervosa, quadriplegia, and advanced stages of malignancy are only a few of many; however, the nature of the problem will influence the type of solution that is appropriate. Nutritional status may be compromised by any condition that affects the ability to acquire or prepare food; ingest food; or digest, absorb, and transport nutrients. Think about other factors such as mobility and conditions that may reduce the person's desire or ability to move. Such thinking is vital to effective nursing.

Other factors that have the potential for influencing risk and/or response to treatment are discussed briefly below. For the most part, these individual differences need to be attended to in any caregiving situation.

Age and Gender

Burns happen more frequently to the very young and the elderly, and more often to males than females. There also is evidence showing an association between older age and incidence of pressure ulcers, although findings have been inconsistent. Perhaps these populations are at risk for burns and other injuries because the young tend to be unaware of many dangers or are high risk takers and the elderly have diminished reflexes and perceptual abilities.

CLINICAL DECISION MAKING
REDUCING THE RISK OF PRESSURE ULCERS

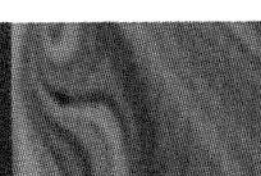

Figure 28–6 shows the process of assessing risk factors for Clara based on the minimal information we have from the case study, making a decision about risk for developing pressure ulcers, planning interventions to reduce risk, and expected outcomes of interventions to reduce risk. The conceptual schema developed by Braden and Bergstrom is included in the figure.

Decision making includes the patient, family, other health care team members, and the consideration of multiple characteristics of the patient. For example, when making plans for improving nutrition, the nurse needs to take into account swallowing difficulties, patient likes and dislikes, perceptual deficits, need for socialization, and difficulty in changing positions. A skillful nurse who carefully assesses patients, identifies risks, and thinks through actions to take to reduce risks can greatly reduce the incidence of pressure ulcers.

Individual and Family Values

Individual and family values in all clinical decisions must be considered. The patient and family members are team members who should be incorporated in planning, decision making, and performance of procedures whenever feasible. As hospital stays continue to decrease in length, many preventive and treatment practices involving wounds will take place in the home by the person with the actual or potential wound or a family member.

Family and friends can provide help with tasks as well as contribute to the patient's psychological welfare. Prevention and treatment of pressure ulcers and treatment of burns often require a long-term care commitment. Successful outcomes are enhanced when the nurse assesses the patient's family/friend resources and involves them in learning and participating in patient care early.

Educational background and learning style may influence the type of patient and family teaching that will be effective. Demonstrations along with written instructions of, for example, a turning schedule or dressing change, are generally helpful. It is important not to make assumptions about level of understanding, learning style, preferences, and resources, based on formal education. Look and listen and learn.

Socioeconomic status and insurance coverage may influence such decisions as method of relieving pressure to prevent or heal pressure ulcers. There is wide variation in cost of mattress toppers, mattresses, and special types of beds. The clinician needs to consider economic issues when making decisions about choices of other supplies and caregiving methods. For example, an individual who has the economic means to hire someone to care for him or her may not desire to learn how to carry out particular caregiving tasks.

Culture and *ethnicity* both refer to interrelated patterns of beliefs, attitudes, and practices of a large or small group. Ethnicity generally refers to characteristics such as race or religion. Gross and subtle differences exist between individuals with variation in cultural and/or ethnic background. It is always important to be observant of clues to individual perceptions about the body, illness, methods of treatment, authority, etc. For example, educational efforts may be more effective if they are directed to the person in a family who is viewed as the authority according to a cultural pattern. The reader is cautioned not to generalize from global descriptions of ethnic and cultural groups. There are many individual differences within cultures.

Spirituality and *religious practices* are often overlooked in planning care. Spirituality is central to an individual's view of him/herself and the meaning of life, the existence of and nature of God, goals in life, and virtually all aspects of life. It is what drives the individual. Often, spirituality is defined simply in terms of religious preference or rituals of a specific religion; however, one's spirituality cannot be confined to rituals. An individual's beliefs influence that person's practices, behaviors, attitudes, values, and choices. One's spirituality influences perception of vulnerability to injury, risk-taking behaviors, and the meaning given to gunshot wounds, burns, or other wounds.

Understanding of a person's spirituality helps the caregiver to plan care that respects the patient's beliefs and to refer persons to a chaplain or someone else of common belief for counsel.

Setting in Which Care Is Delivered

Wound prevention and wound care are given in multiple settings including the home. The diligent nurse is consistent in taking into consideration variations in resources, burdens, and demands in the specific settings. When planning for discharge from a health care agency, for example, the nurse needs to be aware of resources available in the home and in the local environment. Awareness of obstacles is also important. For example, is the environment clean or are there sources of potentially infectious bacteria?

Interagency referrals when the setting for care changes need to include written information about the individual and the wound care required so no disruption in care occurs.

Ethical Considerations

Plans of care need to carefully consider the goals and anticipated outcomes of care, patient desires, and patient comfort. Prevention of pressure ulcers and treatment of ulcers, surgical wounds, burns, and other wounds can result in extreme patient discomfort (frequent turning, removal of dressings, debridement, nutritional interventions, etc.). If the anticipated outcome or goal is peaceful death, aggressive, uncomfortable preventive activities may be inappropriate. On the other hand, if the goal is to maintain current function or to improve it, aggressive, painful treatments may be desirable.

Petro (1990) has identified four ethical issues encountered in pressure ulcer prevention and treatment:

- costs, risks, and burdens of treating risk factors
- choices on use of limited resources (such as expensive support surfaces)
- decision to treat pressure ulcers conservatively or surgically
- factors and values influencing clinical decisions

Financial Considerations

Costs of treatment are important to health care agencies, third-party payers, patients, and families. Costs include equipment, time, energy, and any other disruptions in goal attainment important to individuals, families, or agencies. Preventive skin care and treatment of wounds can be very costly.

As with other aspects of nursing, the nurse makes decisions about the use of products consistent with patient and family goals and means. The goal for the nurse is to find the most economical plan of prevention and treatment that fits within the individual and family lifestyles. For example, when limited financial support is available, a family may choose to change a patient's position manually using a standard support surface such as a mattress, rather than purchase special beds that alternate or reduce pressure.

In addition to financial cost considerations in developing a care plan, time and energy costs need to be taken into account. A patient may be able to carry out all care requirements without special equipment; however, the time required makes it impossible to work, go to school, or pursue other goals. The nurse is in an excellent position to help patients and family members make decisions about caregiving that will best meet their needs.

FUTURE DEVELOPMENTS

Although much research has been done to understand mechanisms of skin breakdown and healing, a great deal remains to be done to improve our understanding and our practices. Infection remains somewhat of a mystery. It is insidious and invisible. Further knowledge is needed on the inflammatory cells, the repair process, and the effects of growth factors on wound healing. The relationship of specific nutritional factors and skin breakdown and healing need further study. Early studies indicated zinc (Abbott et al, 1968) and ascorbic acid (Hunter and Rajan, 1972; Taylor et al, 1974) may promote healing of pressure ulcers. Current knowledge is not sufficient to develop specific recommendations for practice.

Few of the possible risk factors associated with pressure ulcer development and wound healing have been investigated sufficiently to be labeled a risk factor. Research findings on age, temperature, blood pressure, muscle wasting, etc., have been inconsistent. Further research needs to be done to identify variables that influence pressure ulcer development and wound healing in general.

Validation of current nursing practice methods is also needed. Although visual reactive hyperemia (VRH) is the common observation used to measure tissue tolerance to pressure, its reliability has yet to be determined. Even if VRH is reliable, methods need to be developed to measure this reactive response in persons with dark skin.

Clinicians believe that psychosocial variables are important in the development and treatment of pressure ulcers, especially in the population with spinal cord injury. Social support, stress, coping methods, and other variables logically influence the help available, the help required, and perhaps motivation. More needs to be learned about these relationships and how nurses can address them in practice.

Patient and family education are vital to patient understanding and follow-through. Research needs to determine the most effective ways of assessing patient and family readiness to learn, and to present essential knowledge and skills to patients, family, and staff. Major wounds require understanding of healing principles and commitment to follow them.

Clinicians are in the position to carry out preventive actions, treat wounds, and observe patient responses. These observations are critical to future research questions that will result in improved clinical practice.

NURSING CARE ACTIONS

Principles and Practices

PREDICTION AND PREVENTION

Nursing care designed to prevent or treat wounds is planned and implemented using knowledge of research, personal experience, sensitivity to individual differences, limitations related to other clinical conditions, and other factors. This section discusses the key principles and practices based on research outlined previously.

It is important to know the parameters of roles of health care workers in different states and health care facilities. Some of the nursing care described below, such as encouraging patients to change position to relieve pressure, or eat nourishing food, can be carried out independently by nurses without a physician's order. On the other hand, dressing changes and application of any solution, ointment, or other substance to a wound generally require a physician's order. Also, all of the goals of patient care need to be considered when planning skin care. For example, Clara in the case study has paralyzed limbs, perceptual problems, and is incontinent. Clara will need help in changing positions, her paralyzed limbs will need to be supported, and her skin will have to be kept dry.

Nurses have a major responsibility to predict risk of pressure ulcers and prevent them. Once a wound has occurred, responsibilities for prevention of other wounds continues, with added responsibilities.

The Clinical Practice Guideline for Prediction and Prevention of Pressure Ulcers in Adults (Panel for Prediction and Prevention of Pressure Ulcers in Adults, 1992) includes four basic goals:

- Identify at-risk individuals needing prevention and the specific factors placing them at risk.
- Maintain and improve tissue tolerance to pressure to prevent injury.
- Protect against adverse effects of external mechanical forces: pressure, friction, and shear.
- Reduce the incidence of pressure ulcers through educational programs.

The panel recommended several guidelines for prediction and prevention based on research and expert opinion. Many of the guidelines are incorporated in the sections that follow. The Braden scale (see Fig. 28–6) is helpful in understanding nursing practice actions. The purpose of recommended actions is to reduce pressure on soft tissues, or increase tissue tolerance using knowledge derived from research and experience.

RESEARCH-BASED PRINCIPLES AND PRACTICES

Persons with impaired ability to change position (e.g., chair-bound or bed-bound) should be assessed for other risk factors such as immobility, incontinence, adequacy of nutrition, level of consciousness, and sensation. Such an assessment using a validated instrument should be done on admission to the health care facility and should be repeated periodically. The Braden scale is an example of such an instrument that has been tested for reliability and validity. It is important to follow its specific instructions. Using Clara from the case study as an example, the nurse evaluates Clara on each of six risk factors. Four descriptions are given for all but one factor (friction and shear). First, **sensory perception** is evaluated (the ability to respond meaningfully to pressure-related discomfort). The nurse believes that description 2 (very limited) best fits Clara's response; therefore, she places a score of 2 in the column to the right of the scale. **Moisture** is the second variable to evaluate (the degree to which skin is exposed to moisture). Clara is incontinent and needs to be changed at least two times per shift. She is thus rated 2, very moist. Since Clara is confined to bed, she is scored 1, bedfast, on **activity** (degree of physical activity). **Mobility** is the ability to change and control body position. Clara is rated 2, very limited. (From the description, she is not totally immobile; however, mobility is very limited.) **Nutrition** is defined as usual food intake pattern. From the information provided on Clara, her intake pattern is scored 1, very poor. **Friction and shear** has three possible classifications. The nurse gives Clara a score of 2, a potential problem. Adding up the score gives Clara a total risk score of 10. This is considered high risk. Any person with a score under 16 is considered at risk. It is important that the form be dated so that comparisons can be made at a later time.

The panel recommended that massage over bony prominences be avoided because there is research evidence of damage from such practice. Further, exposure to moisture from incontinence, perspiration, or drainage from a wound should be minimized. When the moisture cannot be prevented, products that absorb and draw moisture away from the skin are recommended. Topical agents that serve as barriers to moisture can also be useful. Further information on managing urinary incontinence is available from the Agency for Health Care Policy Research (Urinary Incontinence Guideline Panel, 1992).

The panel also recommended that any person assessed to be at risk for developing a pressure ulcer should be repositioned at least every 2 hours if such a practice does not interfere with overall patient goals. Further, it was recommended that a written schedule be used for systematically turning and repositioning. Such a schedule will facilitate communication among staff caring for the person. Small body rotations instead of full turns shift the site of pressure and can be accomplished with decreased effort. Positioning the superior leg posterior to the inferior leg has been reported to significantly decrease pressures compared with traditional positioning techniques (Garber et al, 1982).

Similarly, it is recommended that uninterrupted sitting be avoided for a person at risk of developing pressure ulcers. The panel recommended that the person be repositioned at least every hour or put back to bed, depending on overall patient goals. If the person in a chair or wheelchair is able, it is recommended that weight be shifted every 15 minutes. Foam, gel, air, or combination pressure-reducing cushions are recommended for persons who are chair-bound. Donut-type devices are to be avoided because they cause edema.

NON–RESEARCH-BASED PRINCIPLES AND PRACTICES

The panel recommended that all individuals found to be at risk of developing pressure ulcers have a systematic skin inspection at least daily with particular attention given to bony prominences (see Fig. 28–4). The intergluteal cleft, other skinfolds, and penis (when using an external or an indwelling catheter) need to be assessed. Assessment also includes general characteristics of the skin such as cleanliness, elasticity, skin hydration, edema, and identification of abnormalities including blisters, hyperemia, induration, scars, rashes, excess moisture, burns, and other open areas (Table 28–8). Results of inspection should be documented on the patient's record and should include time of inspection, grade, and characteristics of any wound. It is also important to assess objects in the environment that may contribute to pressure, such as wrinkled sheets, clothing, tape (external catheter), shoes, casts, and braces.

The panel further recommended that skin be cleansed at the time of soiling and at routine intervals. Hot water should be avoided and a mild cleansing agent used to reduce irritation and dryness of the skin. Force and friction applied to the skin should be minimized in cleansing.

Nurses should also minimize the possibility of skin injury due to friction or shear forces when transferring or turning patients. Patients should be lifted rather than dragged across sheets or other surfaces. (Use sheets or other lifting devices as needed.) Lubricants such as corn starch and creams and protective films such as transparent film dressings and skin sealants, protective dressings, and protective paddings can be used to protect against friction. Maintaining the head of the bed at the lowest degree of elevation possible consistent with the patient's medical condition or other restrictions and limiting the time that the head of the bed is elevated are recommended to prevent or minimize shearing forces (Panel for Prediction and Prevention of Pressure Ulcers in Adults, 1992).

For persons in bed, the panel recommended that positioning devices such as pillows or foam wedges be used to keep bony prominences such as knees or ankles from direct contact with one another. Whether the patient is in bed or in a wheelchair, position extremities to avoid increased pressure. The heels are prone to intense pressures even when pressure reduction mattresses are used. Position heels free of the mattress by bridging (Fig. 28–8). Also, special boots are available to reduce pressures over heels and ankles. Positioning techniques can

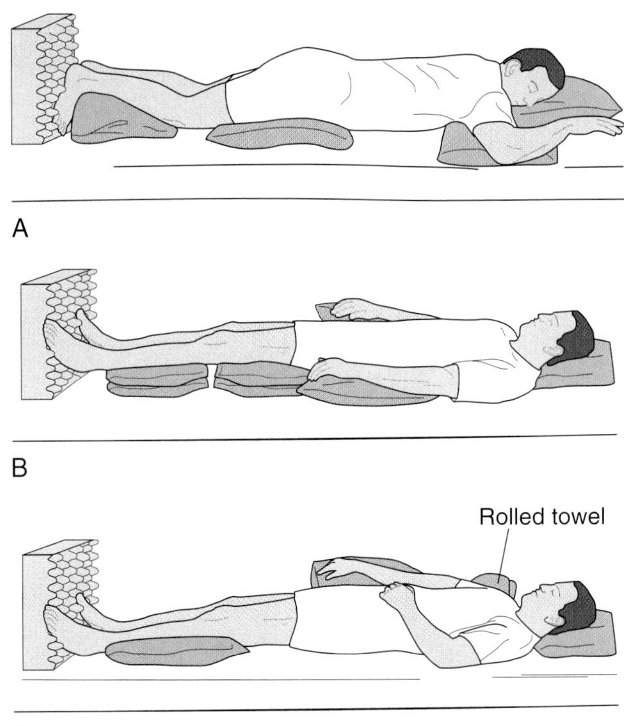

Figure 28–8. *A–C,* Bridging with pillows to prevent or reduce pressure over bony prominences.

alter intensity and location of pressure; however, little research has been done on pressure reduction effectiveness of various positions. Again, a written plan is recommended. It is also recommended that when a person is in a side-lying position, positioning directly on the trochanter should be avoided.

Frequent position monitoring is necessary for patients who remove positioning supports and repeatedly resume one position. Assess comfort by questioning and observing the patient. If the patient is sitting, arrange for pressure relief through "push-ups" (Fig. 28–9), or lifting by the caregiver. An individual should not be repositioned on a hyperemic or erythemic area. Such an area should be protected from pressure.

The health care team must carefully monitor the nutritional state of patients. The nurse shares responsibility with the physician and dietitian in determining nutritional needs through laboratory data, food intake, weight, and observation. Too often, nutrition is overlooked, which can have devastating consequences. Eating while in bed or in a bedroom is generally not part of a person's pattern of living. It is a challenge to the team to create an environment conducive to eating and to recognize when assistance with eating is necessary. Food and fluid intake need to be assessed and documented consistently for those at risk of pressure ulcers.

Many beds, mattress toppers, wheelchair cushions, and other materials are available to reduce pressure. They vary in performance characteristics and cost. The nurse should document risk of pressure ulcer development and report the need for support devices to the physician.

PATIENT EDUCATION

Patient and family education about maintenance of skin integrity and treatment of skin conditions is an important ingredient in promoting independence, completeness, and wholeness. Prevention of pressure ulcers requires a team effort among health caregivers and the patient. The nurse has a limited span of contact with a given patient and family. If the nurse gives expert care without teaching why and how it is being done, continuity of care may be lost when the patient goes home, to another unit, or to another agency. Knowledge and skill in prevention of pressure ulcers does not guarantee compliance; however, it gives the patient and family the po-

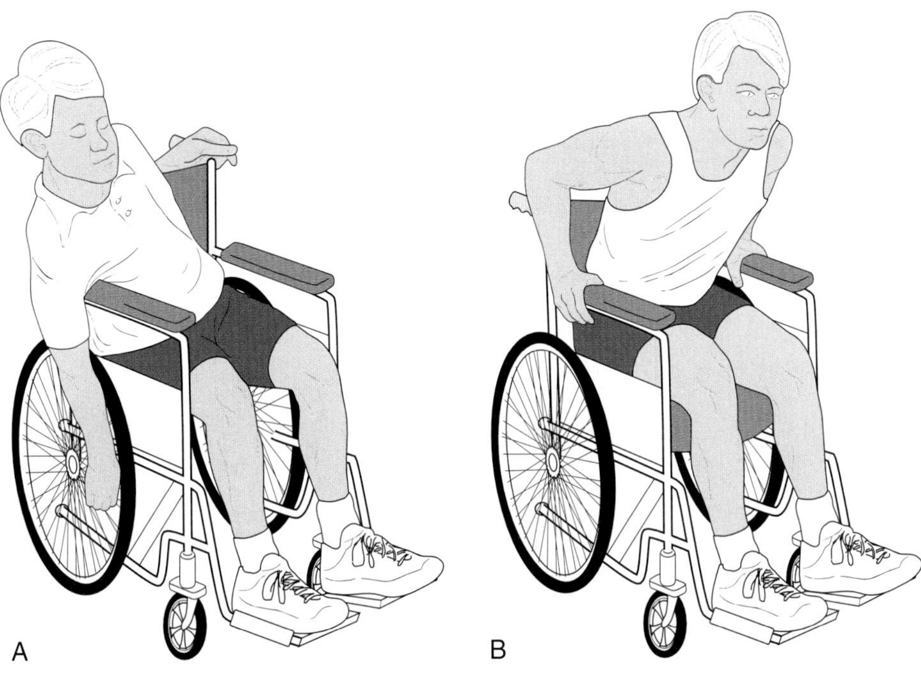

Figure 28–9. *A & B,* Wheelchair pressure relief.

TABLE 28-8 Skin Assessment

Characteristic	Action		
General Characteristics		*Objects in Contact with Skin*	
Cleanliness	Assess	Bed linens	Observe for and remove wrinkles, crumbs, or other objects causing pressure on skin
Elasticity	Assess		
Edema	Assess		
Abnormalities		Clothing	Observe for tightness, wrinkles; make necessary adjustments
Blisters	Assess, describe size, location, color	Tape	Observe for tightness (i.e., tape of catheter, tape that can cause tourniquet effect) and signs of irritation; report
Redness	Assess, describe location, time required for resolution, blanchable or nonblanchable		
Induration	Palpate and note hardness of tissue	Surface (mattress, cushion)	Note type of mattress, cushion being used
Scars	Assess, describe characteristics and location	Shoes	Assess fit of shoes and report those that fit improperly
Rashes	Assess, describe characteristics and location	Casts/orthoses/prostheses	Assess skin around casts and under orthoses and prostheses; note signs of impaired circulation
Excess moisture	Note source, time, location		
Burns	Note location and characteristic		
Open areas	Assess and describe using institutional staging system	Braces	Assess skin at any points where brace is in contact with skin; report any irregularities in skin
Drainage	Describe location, amount, color, odor	External catheter	Observe skin for redness and edema

tential to do so or to teach others the care that is required. The importance of patient and family teaching of basic information and skills required for managing risk factors and preventing pressure ulcers cannot be overemphasized. Any plan for education needs to include an evaluation method to determine if learning has occurred.

WOUND CARE

The nurse should follow prevention principles to prevent other pressure ulcers and promote wound healing and consider the effects of pressure on any wound over bony prominences, since circulation may be compromised. A pressure ulcer is shown in Figure 28–10.

The general goal in wound treatment is to allow the body to heal by removing or attenuating influences that interfere with normal wound healing, prevent further damage to the wound and surrounding viable tissue, remove the cause of the wound, prevent complications, and relieve pain. Box 28–1 summarizes key principles and practices related to wound healing and wound care.

During the past two decades research on wound healing has changed clinicians' understanding and drastically altered healing interventions. Specific changes in treatment of wounds are detailed in Table 28–9.

PATIENT TEACHING
PRESSURE ULCER PREVENTION AND TREATMENT

Successful wound prevention or wound care programs require education and involvement of the patient and all current and future caregivers early in the treatment program. Hospital care of persons with pressure ulcers is given primarily by an interdisciplinary team. However, nurses and physicians need to take every opportunity to describe to patients and families or friends what they are doing while giving patient care. Teach the patient and caregivers why the patient is eating a particular food, being repositioned, having the wound cleansed/debrided, and having specific dressings applied.

Seventy-eight percent of wounds healed in patients cared for at home by nurses specially trained in wound care, but only 36.3 percent of wounds healed in patients not cared for by specially trained nurses (Arnold & Weir, 1994). If education improves the outcomes of care, it is highly probable that education of the patient's caregivers postdischarge can have the same result. Further, continuity of care and cost-effectiveness can result from educating *all* caregivers to diligently follow the treatment protocol or critical path for wound care. Successful quality assurance programs to reduce pressure ulcer incidence and/or wound infection incidence must rely on a multidisciplinary, collaborative approach for the early reporting of new skin lesions, data collection and analysis, reallocation of resources, and more effective prevention and treatment strategies.

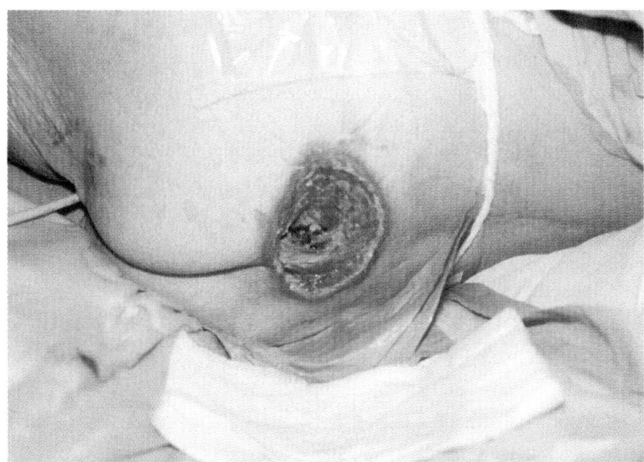

Figure 28–10. A pressure ulcer. (From Black, J., Matassarin-Jacobs, E. [1997]. Medical-Surgical Nursing: Clinical Management for Continuity of Care, 5th ed. Philadelphia: W.B. Saunders.)

INTRINSIC FACTORS IN WOUND HEALING

Research related to the *intrinsic* factors that influence wound healing has been discussed previously in this chapter. These intrinsic factors include oxygenation of the wound, nutritional status, corticosteroid release, age, and disease processes (diabetes, anemia, circulatory problems, infection, and pain). See Table 28–6 for a summary of these factors and the nursing assessment and/or actions to facilitate optimal wound healing.

EXTRINSIC FACTORS IN WOUND HEALING

Extrinsic factors related to wound healing are designed to protect healthy tissue and promote granulation (see Table 28–7). Treatment of wounds is based on wound assessment and underlying intrinsic and extrinsic factors. The goals are to

BOX 28–1
WOUND CARE: PRINCIPLES AND PRACTICES

- No debridement, cleansing agent, dressing, mattress, or any other product can eliminate the need for caregivers' vigilance in applying principles designed to maintain skin integrity.
- Caregivers must schedule systematic interventions to maintain/regain skin integrity.
- Moist skin is more likely than dry skin to sustain friction injury and to colonize bacteria. However, once a nonsurgical wound has occurred, it heals best in a moist environment.
- Necrotic tissue must be removed and infection controlled before optimal wound healing will occur.
- No wound should be irrigated with any solution caustic to tissue or with pressure greater than 15 pounds per square inch (psi).
- Pressure is the main cause of pressure ulcers. Nurses need to assess both the intensity of the pressure on the skin and the amount of time the pressure is maintained.
- Many wound care products are on the market. Many of these have not been researched adequately to determine their therapeutic value. In some cases, studies report conflicting data. Nurses must maintain an open attitude and keenly observe patients using any of these products.
- Nutrients and oxygen are transported to the wound via the circulatory system and are essential for collagen formation.
- Nurses must evaluate all patients with limitations of movement for risk of pressure ulcers using a valid and reliable method.
- Nurses must take action to eliminate or reduce risk factors when possible.

TABLE 28–9 Changes in Wound Treatment

Outdated	Current Treatment
Dressings	
Maintain dry environment in the wound to promote eschar formation. Eschar prevents wound contraction. Example: Allow wound to dry. Healed in 25–30 days.	Promote a moist wound environment that prevents eschar formation and enhances migration of epithelial cells across the wound. Example: Cover nonsurgical wound with an occlusive dressing. Heals in 12–15 days.
Debridement	
Mechanical debridement with wet-to-dry gauze or scalpel and forceps.	Chemical debridement with occlusive dressing to promote autolysis (body releases enzymes to lyse eschar). Commonly used occlusive dressings include polyurethane hydrocolloids.
Topical Therapy	
Topical application of corticosteroids, zinc.	Topical application of epidermal growth factors.
Wound Cleansing	
Cleanse wound with hydrogen peroxide.	Cleanse wound with normal saline.
Relieve Pressure	
Turn q 12 hr or when possible.	Turn more frequently than q 2 hr. Keep pressure off wound.

relieve pressure, remove necrotic tissue, control local infection, promote granulation, protect healthy tissue, and assess the impact of intrinsic factors on wound healing.

Pressure Relief. Examples of pressure-relieving devices are mattresses (foam overlay, alternating pressure, low-air-loss mattresses), special beds (low-air beds, air-fluidized beds), and heel protectors (standard cushioning, special devices), seat cushions (standard cushioning, special padding). See the section on prevention for a more detailed discussion.

The patient must also be turned as indicated by his or her skin and wound condition. The air-fluidized bed equalizes pressure (less than 10 mmHg) over all surfaces in contact with the bed; its actual effectiveness remains unclear.

Removal of Necrotic Tissue and Infection Control. Necrotic tissue must be debrided and infection controlled prior to progression of wound healing. Chemical debridement is accomplished with enzymatic products (Elase, Santyl, Granulex). A whirlpool bath provides debridement of loose necrotic tissue.

Wounds with purulent drainage are treated with topical antimicrobials, topical antiseptics, and systemic antibiotics. These are used sparingly and with caution because many topical antiseptics are destructive to fibroblasts and impede wound healing.

Protection of Healthy Tissue and Granulation Promotion. Occlusive dressings aim to primarily provide a moist environment for optimal healing and protect healthy tissue surrounding the wound. Examples of commonly used dressings include polyurethane films (e.g., Tegaderm), hydrocolloids (DuoDerm), and hydrogels (Vigilon). Avoid use of these occlusive dressings on grossly infected wounds. Occlusive dressings are used to protect the wound and/or provide autolytic debridement, to provide some pain relief, and provide moist healing environment. Dressings are removed if leakage occurs or after a specified time interval. Teach patients that the yellow gel forming under the hydrocolloid dressing is normal exudate and not pus.

Petroleum gauze dressings and transparent semipermeable dressing films (e.g., Op-Site, Tegaderm) are used for superficial wounds because they protect and do not damage surrounding viable tissue or developing epithelium when removed. These dressings also allow wound visibility and contain any serous exudate in the wound, thus aiding healing and maintaining a dry environment for viable surrounding tissue.

Hydrocolloid dressings are especially useful in decreasing bacterial counts and increasing angiogenesis. Selection of the type of dressing agent, dressings, antiseptics, and/or antimicrobials is often based on physician/institutional preference and/or economic considerations. These solutions also vary with the stage of wound healing (Table 28–10).

Procedures

The steps involved in caring for pressure ulcers are outlined in Procedure 28–1.

TABLE 28-10 Mechanisms of Action of Different Types of Dressing*,†

Dressing	Mechanism of Action	Stage I	Stage II	Stage III	Stage IV
Dry gauze	Wicks drainage away from wound surface	O	O	X	X
Moist-to-dry gauze	Maintains a moist wound environment while wicking drainage from surface	O	O	XO	XO
Polyurethane film	Traps serous exudate and provides a moist wound environment	X	X	O	O
Hydrocolloid	Reacts with wound fluid to create a soft gel that encourages granulation and epithelialization	O	X	XO	O
Polyurethane foam	Absorbs exudate and maintains a moist wound environment	O	X	XO	O
Absorptive dressings	Absorbs exudate and debris while maintaining a moist environment	O	O	X	XO
Hydrogel	Maintains a moist environment	O	X	X	O

*Selection of the appropriate dressing is based on wound assessment.

†Examples of types of dressings:

Gauze

Polyurethane film: Tegaderm, Op-Site, Bioclusive, Polyskin

Hydrocolloid: DuoDerm, Intact, J&J Ulcer Dressing, Restore, Intrasite

Polyurethane foam: Lyofoam, Epilock, Synthaderm

Absorptive dressings: Bard Absorption Dressing, Debrisan, Hydragran, Hollister Wound Exudate Absorber, Kaltostat, Sorbsan

Hydrogel: Vigilon, Geliperm

X = may use; O = not recommended; XO = requires clinical judgment; depends on amount and type of wound drainage.

From Maklebust, J., Sieggreen, M. (1991). *Pressure Ulcers: Guidelines for Prevention and Nursing Management.* West Dundee, IL: S-N Publication.

PROCEDURE 28-1

Pressure Ulcer Care

Objective

Promote wound healing, prevent infection, and protect adjacent skin surfaces.

Terminology

epithelialization—skin regrowth that occurs over the wound as part of the healing process

eschar—a dry crust or scab that forms after excoriation of the skin

granulation—soft pink tissue with many capillaries that forms during the wound healing process

tunneling—the undermining of surrounding tissue creating pockets of tissue destruction not readily visible when first looking into the wound

Critical Elements

Care of a pressure ulcer may require a physician's order. Refer to your facility's policy prior to the procedure.

Each patient should be assessed for pressure ulcer risk factors and steps should be taken to reduce or eliminate these risk factors whenever necessary. These risk factors include decreased sensory perception, excessive moisture, decreased physical activity and/or mobility, poor nutrition, decreased circulation, and potential for friction and/or shear.

The wound and surrounding tissue should be assessed each time the dressing is changed. If the patient has an occlusive dressing, adjacent tissues should be assessed at least every 8 hours. When assessing the wound, the care provider should note the size and depth of the wound as well as the presence of necrotic tissue, exudate, granulation tissue, and wound epithelialization. The wound should also be assessed for tunneling. Surrounding tissue should be assessed for edema, induration, and color.

Pressure ulcers are staged in four groups and include:

Stage 1—the skin is intact, red, and does not blanch

Stage 2—there is superficial skin loss of the epidermis and/or dermis; it may look like a blister, abrasion, or very shallow crater

Stage 3—there is full-thickness skin loss, damage and possible necrosis of the subcutaneous tissue; it appears as a deep crater without undermining of any of the adjacent tissues

Stage 4—there is full-thickness skin loss with extensive tissue destruction including necrosis or damage to muscle, bone, or supporting structures; tunneling or undermining of adjacent tissue is often present at this stage

During dressing changes the care provider should maintain strict aseptic technique. Universal blood and body fluids precautions should be used when working with the patient if drainage or body secretions are present. Selected wound cultures may indicate the need for isolation procedures.

Normal saline is used to cleanse/irrigate deep and draining wounds unless otherwise ordered by the physician. Irrigation is often essential for cleansing of undermined areas. When using solutions, document the date and time the solution is opened. Refer to your facility's policy for length of use of opened solutions.

When applying dressings, fine mesh gauze is most often used in the presence of granulation tissue during a dressing change. Wide mesh gauze is usually used for mechanical debridement. If the wound adheres to the wound bed and you are not using a wet-to-dry dressing, the dressing may be moistened with saline to decrease the possibility of trauma when removed.

The dressing should be selected based on the depth of the ulcer, amount of drainage, presence of infection or presence of necrotic tissue or eschar. The type of dressing may often be prescribed by the physician. Your facility may have policies regarding the use of specific dressings for different types/stages of pressure ulcers. Refer to your facility's policies prior to proceeding.

Prior to using any premanufactured product, read the manufacturer's instructions. Assess the patient for possible allergies to any of the products being used. When taping the dressing, try to alternate the taping pattern to avoid irritation to the skin. If the area has decreased tactile sensation, tape should be avoided and an alternate method of securing the dressing in place should be considered.

Equipment

Gloves
Sterile gloves
Dressing materials (as indicated)
Sterile normal saline
Irrigation syringe*
Irrigation solution container*
Waterproof underpad*
Sterile cotton tip applicator (if indicated)
Measuring tape or other measuring device
Tape (if indicated)
Protective paste (if indicated)

---

*These items may be part of an irrigation set.

continued on next page

PROCEDURE 28-1 (cont'd)

Special Considerations

The need for pain medication should be assessed prior to any procedure for pressure ulcer care.

Pressure areas often occur over areas of bony prominence. Frequent position changes are an important preventive measure. Positioning to avoid pressure to areas of known skin breakdown is also important.

Special beds are often used for patients with potential or actual skin breakdown. A physician's order may be required for the use of these beds. Refer to your facility's policy prior to using.

When treating necrotic wounds, topical agents that assist with tissue debridement and granulation are often used. Antiseptics that reduce bacterial growth are often used with infected wounds. Wounds that need cleansing are often treated with oxidizing agents and are especially effective with anaerobic bacteria. If using enzyme agents, care should be taken to avoid getting these agents on surrounding skin since they may cause tissue damage. Other treatments that may be used for wound care include the whirlpool baths and hand-held wound irrigation devices.

Hands must be washed before and after every patient contact.

Action	*Rationale*
1. Verify order.	1. Ensures proper procedure is done.
2. Assemble equipment.	2. Promotes task organization.
3. Identify patient.	3. Promotes patient safety.
4. Explain procedure.	4. Promotes patient compliance.
5. Close door/curtain.	5. Provides privacy and maintains dignity.
6. Position patient so pressure ulcer area is exposed, remembering to keep patient covered as much as possible.	6. Maintains dignity and warmth.
7. Wash hands. Open supplies, pour solutions, and set up sterile field as indicated.	7. Organizes work area so aseptic technique may be maintained.
8. Don gloves.	8. Protects care provider from contact with blood and/or body fluids.
9. Remove soiled dressing and dispose in appropriate container.	9. Exposes pressure ulcer for assessment and treatment.
10. Measure wound size and assess for tunneling (if indicated).	10. Provides information used to determine progress of wound healing.
11. Wash skin around wound with soap and water. Rinse and dry well.	11. Reduces microorganisms on surrounding skin.
12. Remove and dispose of gloves and wash hands. Don sterile gloves.	12. Prepares care provider for use of aseptic technique.
13. Using irrigation syringe, draw up solution and thoroughly irrigate wound. NOTE: If tunneling is present be sure to irrigate into this area.	13. Removes loose debris from wound.
14. Apply any prescribed agents to wound.	14. Provides appropriate agent for wound healing.
15. Cover wound with appropriate dressing material. Tape in place or secure with other non-tape devices.	15. Provides protection for wound during healing process.
16. Return patient to position of comfort, not on wound area, and replace top linens.	16. Provides for patient comfort and privacy.
17. Return or dispose of equipment in appropriate place. Wash hands.	17. Provides a clean, organized work area.

continued on next page

PROCEDURE 28-1 (cont'd)

Documentation

Record in the patient record the location, size, and appearance of the pressure ulcer. Record the assessment of any tunneling, exudate, granulation or epithelialization, and the condition of the surrounding skin. Record the patient's response to the treatment. Note the positioning used to keep patient off the pressure ulcer area and the type of special bed used if indicated.

Elements of Patient Teaching

Explain the purpose of the procedure to the patient/family. Reinforce the importance of prevention measures that should be used to prevent further skin breakdown. Encourage the use of positions that will prevent further pressure on the ulcer area. If the family will be doing the procedure for the patient, allow time for a return demonstration so competency may be assessed.

CHAPTER HIGHLIGHTS

- No debridement, cleansing agent, dressing, mattress, or any other product can eliminate the need for caregivers' vigilance in applying principles designed to maintain skin integrity.
- Caregivers must schedule systematic interventions to maintain or regain skin integrity.
- Moist skin is more likely than dry skin to sustain friction injury and to colonize bacteria. However, once a nonsurgical wound has occurred, it heals best in a moist environment.
- Necrotic tissue must be removed and infection controlled before optimal wound healing will occur.
- No wound should be irrigated with any solution caustic to tissue or with pressure greater than 15 psi.
- Pressure is the main cause of pressure ulcers. Nurses need to assess both the intensity of the pressure on the skin and the amount of time the pressure is maintained.
- Many wound care products are on the market. Many of these have not been researched adequately to determine their therapeutic value. In some cases, studies report conflicting data. Nurses must maintain an open attitude and keenly observe patients using any of these products.
- Nutrients and oxygen are transported to the wound via the circulatory system and are essential for collagen formation.

REFERENCES

Abbott, D.F., Exton-Smith, A.N., Millard, P.H., Temperley, J.M. (1968). Zinc sulphate and bedsores. *British Medical Journal, 2* (607), 763.

Allman, R.M., Laprade, C.A., Noel, L.B., et al (1986). Pressure sores among hospitalized patients. *Annals of Internal Medicine, 105* (3), 337–342.

Arnold, N., Weir, D. (1994). Retrospective analysis of healing in wounds cared for by ET nurses versus staff nurses in a home setting. *Journal of Wound, Ostomy, & Continence Nursing, 21* (4), 156–160.

Bankert, K., Daughtridge, S., Meehan, M., Colburn, L. (1996). The application of collaborative benchmarking to the prevention and treatment of pressure ulcers. *Advances in Wound Care, 9* (2), 21– 29.

Baxter, C., Mertz, P.M. (1990). Local factors that affect wound healing. In W.H. Eaglstein (ed.): *New Directions in Wound Healing*. Princeton: ER Squibb and Sons, pp. 25–37.

Becker, M.H., Drachman, R.H., Kirscht, J.P. (1974). A new approach to explaining sick role behaviors in low income populations. *American Journal of Public Health, 64,* 205–216.

Bennett, M.A. (1995). Report and the task force on implications for darkly pigmented intact skin in the prediction and prevention of pressure ulcers. *Advances in Wound Care,* 8 (6), 34–35.

Bergstrom, N., Bennett, M.A., Carlson, C.E., et al (1994). Treatment of Pressure Ulcers. Clinical Practice Guideline, No. 15. Rockville, MD: U.S. Department of Health and Human Services. Public Health Service, Agency for Health Care Policy and Research. AHCPR Publication No. 95–0652.

Bergstrom, N., Braden, B.(1992). A prospective study of pressure sore risk among institutionalized elderly. *Journal of Geriatric Society.*

Bergstrom, N., Braden, B.J., Laguzza, A., Holman, V. (1987a). The Braden Scale for predicting pressure sore risk. *Nursing Research, 35,* 205–210.

Bergstrom, N., Demuth, P.J., Braden, B.J. (1987b). A clinical trial of the Braden Scale for predicting pressure sore risk. *Nursing Clinics of North America, 22,* 417–428.

Berlowitz, D.R., Wilking, S.V.B. (1989). Risk factors for pressure sores: A comparison of cross-sectional and cohort-derived data. *Journal of the American Geriatric Society, 37* (11), 1043–1050.

Bolton, L., Pirone, L., Chen, J., et al (1990). Dressings effect on wound healing. *Wounds: Compendium of Clinical Research Practice, 2,* 126–134.

Braden, B., Bergstrom, N. (1987). A conceptual schema for the study of the etiology of pressure sores. *Rehabilitation Nursing, 12,* 8–12.

Breslow, R.A., Hallfrisch, J., Goldberg, A.P. (1991). Malnutrition in tubefed nursing home patients with pressure sores. *Journal of Parenteral Enteral Nutrition, 15,* 663–668.

Breslow, R.A., Hallfrisch, J., Guy, D.G., et al (1993). The importance of dietary protein in healing pressure ulcers. *Journal of American Geriatric Society, 41* (4), 357–362.

Brown, G.L., Nanney, L.B., Griffen, J., et al (1989). Enhancement of wound healing by topical treatment with epidermal growth factor. *New England Journal of Medicine, 321,* 76–79.

Brown, L.L., Shelton, H.T., Bornside, G.H., Cohn, I., Jr. (1978). Evaluation of wound irrigation by pulsatile jet and conventional methods. *Annals of Surgery, 187* (2), 170–173.

Burkey, J.L., Weinberg, C., Brenden, R.A. (1993). Differential methodologies for the evaluation of skin and wound cleansers. *Wounds, 5* (6), 284–291.

Caldwell, M.D. (1990). Topical wound therapy—an historical perspective. *The Journal of Trauma, 30* (12) Supplement, 116–122.

Carlson, C.E., Griggs, W.P., King, R.R. (1990). *Rehabilitation nursing procedures manual.* Rockville, MD: Aspen.

Carlson, C.E., King, R.B. (1990). Prevention of pressure sores. In J.J. Fitzpatrick, R.L. Taunton, J. Benoliel (eds.): *Annual Review of Nursing Research,* Vol. 8. New York: Springer.

Clarke, M., Kadhorn, H.M. (1988). The nursing prevention of pressure sores in hospital and community patients. *Journal of Advanced Nursing, 13* (3), 365–373.

Conine, T.A., Daechsel, D., Choi, A.K., Lau, M.S. (1990). Costs and acceptability of two special overlays for the prevention of pressure sores. *Rehabilitation Nursing, 15* (3), 133–137.

Corum, G.M. (1993). Characteristics and prevention of wound infection. *Journal of ET Nursing, 20* (1), 21–25.

Crewe, R.A. (1987). Problems of rubber ring nursing cushions and a clinical survey of alternative cushions for ill patients. *Care Sci Pract, 5* (2), 9–11.

Cromack, O.T., Porras-Reyes, B., Mustoe, T.A. (1990). Current concepts in wound healing: Growth factor and macrophage interaction. *The Journal of Trauma, 30* (12) Supplement, 129–133.

Cruz Santiago, G., Kaminski, M.V., Jr., Palencia Salainas, C. (1981). Adequacy of vitamin C supplementation in total parenteral nutrition [abstract]. *Journal of Parenteral and Enteral Nutrition, 5* (6).

Davis, J.T. (1986). Integumentary system. In U. Bloom, D.S. Fawcett (Eds.): *A Textbook of Histology,* 11th ed. Philadelphia, W.B. Saunders.

DeLateur, B., Berni, R., Hongladarom, T., Giaconi, R. (1976). Wheelchair cushions designed to prevent pressure sores: An evaluation. *Archives of Physical Medicine and Rehabilitation, 57,* 129–135.

Dinsdale, S.M. (1974). Decubitus ulcers, role of pressure and friction in causation. *Archives of Physical Medicine and Rehabilitation, 55,* 147–152.

Ehrlich, H.P. (1988). Wound closure: Evidence of cooperation in fibroblasts and collagen matrix. *Eye,* 2, 149–157.

Eisinger, M., Sadan, S., Soehnehen, R., Silver, I.A. (1988). Wound healing by epidermal-derived factors: Experimental and preliminary clinical studies. *Progress in Clinical Biological Research, 266,* 291–302.

Ek, A.C., Gustavsson, G., Lewis, D.H. (1985). The local skin in blood flow in areas at risk for pressure sores treated with massage. *Scandinavian Journal for Rehabilitation Medicine, 17,* 81–86.

Exton-Smith, A.N., Sherwin, R.W. (1961). The prevention of pressure sores: The significance of spontaneous bodily movements. *Lancet 2,* 1124–1126.

Ferrell, B.A., Osterweil, D., Christenson, P. (1993). A randomized trial of low-air-loss beds for treatment of pressure ulcers. *JAMA, 269* (4), 494–497.

Fitzpatrick, T.B., Eisen, A.Z., Wolff, K. (eds.) (1993). *Dermatology in General Medicine,* 4th ed. Philadelphia, W.B. Saunders.

Flanigan, K.H. (1997). Nutritional aspects of wound healing. *Advances in Wound Care, 10* (3), 48–52.

Food and Nutrition Board, National Research Council, National Academy of Science. (1998). *Recommened Dietary Allowances,* 10th ed. Washington, D.C.

Foresman, P.A., Payne, D.S., Becker, D., et al (1993). A relative toxicity index for wound cleansers. *Wounds, 5* (5), 226–231.

Garber, S.L., Campion, L.T., Krouskop, T.A. (1982). Trochanteric pressure in spinal cord injury. *Archives of Physical Medicine and Rehabilitation,* 63, 549–552.

George, J.B. (1995). *Nursing Theories,* 4th ed. Norwalk, CT: 1995.

Gerson, L.W. (1975). The incidence of pressure sores in active treatment hospitals. *International Journal of Nursing Studies, 12* (4), 201–204.

Glenchar, J., Patel, B.S., Pathmarajah, C. (1981). Transient bacteremia associated with debridement of decubitus ulcers. *Military Medicine, 146,* 432–433.

Goldenheim, P.D. (1993). An appraisal of povidone-iodine and wound healing. *Postgraduate Medical Journal, 69* (Suppl 3), S97–105.

Goldstone, L.A., Goldstone, J. (1982). The Norton score: An early warning of pressure sores? *Journal of Advanced Nursing, 7,* 419– 426.

Gosnell, D.J. (1973). An assessment tool to identify pressure sores. *Nursing Research, 22,* 55–59.

Groth, K.E. (1942). Experimental studies on decubitus. *Nordic Medicine, 15,* 2423–2428.

Guyton, A., Hall, J.E. (1995). *Textbook of Medical Physiology,* 9th ed. Philadelphia, W.B. Saunders.

Harding, K.G. (1990). Wound care: Putting theory into clinical practice. In Krasner, D. (ed.): *Chronic wound care.* King of Prussia, PA: Health Management Publications, pp. 19–30.

Henderson, V. (1964). The nature of nursing. *American Journal of Nursing, 64* (8), 62–68.

Holstein, P., Nielsen, P.E., Barras, J. (1979). Blood flow cessation at external pressure in the skin of normal human limbs. *Microvascular Research, 17,* 71–79.

Hunt, T.K. (1990). Basic principles of wound healing. *The Journal of Trauma, 30* (12) Supplement, 122–128.

Hunter, T., Rajan, K.T. (1972). The role of ascorbic acid in the pathogenesis and treatment of pressure sores. *Paraplegia, 8*(4), 211–216.

Husain, T. (1953). An experimental study of some pressure effects on tissues with reference to the bedsore problem. *Journal of Pathology and Bacteriology, 66,* 347–358.

Kaminski, M.V., Jr., Pinchofsky-Devin, G., Williams, S.D. (1989). Nutritional management of decubitus ulcers in the elderly. *Decubitus, 2* (4), 20–30.

Kemp, M.G., Keithly, J.K., Smith, D.W., Morreale, B. (1990). Factors that contribute to pressure sores in surgical patients. *Research in Nursing and Health, 13,* 293–301.

Kemp, M.G., Krouskop, T.A. (1994). Pressure Ulcers: Reducing the incidence and severity by managing pressure. *Journal of Gerontolic Nursing,* 20(9), 27–34.

Kerstein, M.D. (1997). The scientific basis of healing. *Advances in Wound Care, 10*(3), 30–36.

King, R.B., French, E. (1990). Procedures to maintain and restore tissue integrity. In Carlson, C.E., Griggs, W.P., King, R.B. (eds.): *Rehabilitation Nursing Procedures Manual.* Rockville, MD: Aspen, pp. 195–197.

King, R., Boyink, M., Keenan, M. (eds.) (1977). *Rehabilitation Guide.* Chicago: Rehabilitation Institute of Chicago.

Knighton, D.R., Phillips, G.D., Fiegel, V.D. (1990). Wound healing angiogenesis: Indirect stimulation by basic fibroblast growth factor. *The Journal of Trauma, 30* (12) Supplement, 134–144.

Kosiak, M. (1959). Etiology and pathology of ischemic ulcers. *Archives of Physical Medicine and Rehabilitation, 40,* 62–68.

Landis, E.M. (1930). Micro-injection studies of capillary blood pressure in human skin. *Heart, 15,* 209–228.

Laufman, H. (1989). Current use of skin and wound cleanser and antiseptics. *American Journal of Surgery, 157* (3), 359–365.

Lawrence, J.C. (1997). Wound Irrigation: An update on irrigating fluids and their effect on wounds. *Journal of Wound Care, 6* (1), 23–26.

Lehmann, S.L., Konstautindes, N.N. (1989). Wound healing and management. *Critical Care Nursing Currents, 1* (3), 9–12.

Lewis, T., Grant, R.T. (1925). Observations upon reactive hyperemia in man. *Heart, 12,* 73–120.

Lilienfeld, D.E., et al (1988). Obesity and diabetes as risk factors in postoperative wound infections after cardiac surgery. *American Journal of Infection Control, 16* (1), 3–6.

Linares, A.Z., Linares, H.A. (1990). Burn prevention: The need for a comprehensive approach. *Burns, 16* (4), 281–285.

Lindan, O., Greenway, R., Piazza, J. (1965). Pressure distribution on the surface of the human body. *Association of Physical Medicine and Rehabilitation, 46,* 378–385.

Longmire, A.W., Broom, L.A., Burch, J. (1987). Wound infection following high-pressure syringe and needle irrigation [Letter]. *American Journal of Emergency Medicine, 5* (2), 1779–1781.

Lowthian, P. (1979). Pressure sore prevalence: A survey of sores in orthopedic patients. *Nursing Times, 75,* 358–360.

Lowthian, P.T. (1976). Underpads in the prevention of decubiti. In R.M. Kenedi and J.T. Scales (eds.): *Bedsore Biomechanics.* London: MacMillan, 142–145.

Maklebust, J., Sieggreen, M. (1991). *Pressure Ulcers: Guidelines for Prevention and Nursing Management.* West Dundee, IL: S-N Publication.

Manley, M.T. (1978). Incidence, contributory factors, and costs of pressure sores. *South American Medical Journal, 53,* 217–222.

McCance, K.L., Heuther, S.E. (1996). *Pathophysiology. The Biologic Basis for Disease in Adults and Children,* 3rd ed. St. Louis: Mosby.

Merbitz, C.M., King, R.B., Bleiberg, J., Grip, J.C. (1985). Wheelchair push-ups: Measuring pressure relief frequency. *Archives of Physical Medicine and Rehabilitation, 66,* 433–438.

Moore, F.A., Moore, E.E., Jones, T.N., et al (1989). TEN versus TPN following major abdominal trauma—Reduced septic morbidity. *The Journal of Trauma, 29,* 916–923.

National Pressure Ulcer Advisory Panel (1989). Pressure ulcers prevalence, cost and risk assessment: Consensus development conference statement. *Decubitus, 2* (2), 24–28.

Niazi, Z.B.M., Salzberg, A., Byrne, D.W., Viehbeck, M. (1997). Recurrence of initial pressure ulcer in persons with spinal cord injuries. *Advances in Wound Care, 10* (3), 38–42.

North, A. (1990). The effect of sleep on wound healing. *Ostomy/Wound Management, 27,* 57–58.

Norton, D., McLaren, R., Exton-Smith, A.N. (1962). *Pressure sores. An investigation of geriatric nursing problems in hospital.* London: The National Corporation for the Care of Old People.

Panel for Prediction and Prevention of Pressure Ulcers in Adults (1992). *Pressure Ulcers in Adults: Prediction and Prevention.* Clinical Practice Guideline. AHCPR Publication No. 92–0047. Rockville, MD: Agency for Health Care Policy and Research, Public Health Service, U.S. Department of Health and Human Services.

Patterson, J.A., Bennett, R.G. (1995). Prevention and Treatment of Pressure Sores. *Journal of the American Geriatric Society,* 43 (8), 919–927.

Petro, J.A. (1990). Ethical dilemmas of pressure ulcers. *Decubitus, 3* (2), 28–31.

Pinchofsky-Devin, G., Kaminski, M.V., Jr. (1986). Correlation of pressure sores and nutritional status. *Journal of American Geriatric Society, 34*(6), 435–440.

Polaski, A.L., Tatro, S.E. (1996). *Luckmann's Core Principles and Practice of Medical-Surgical Nursing.* Philadelphia: W.B. Saunders.

Roberts, B.V., Goldstone, L.A. (1979). A survey of pressure sores in the over sixties on two orthopaedic wards. *International Journal of Nursing Studies, 16*(4), 355–364.

Rodeheaver, G. (1988). Controversies in topical wound management. *Ostomy/Wound Management, 20* (Fall), 58–68.

Rodeheaver, G., Bellamy, W., Kody, M., et al (1982). Bactericidal activity and toxicity of iodine-containing solutions in wounds. *Archives of Surgery, 7* (11), 115.

Rodeheaver, G.T., Pettry, D., Thacker, J.G., et al (1975). Wound cleansing by high pressure irrigation. *Surgery Gynecololgy and Obstetrics, 141* (3), 357–362.

Rote, N.S. (1990). Inflammation. In K.L. McCance and S.E. Heuther (eds.): *Pathophysiology. The Biologic Basis for Disease in Adults and Children.* St. Louis: Mosby Year Book, 217–248.

Sapico, F.L., Ginunas, V.J., Thornhill-Joynes, M., et al (1986). Quantitative microbiology of pressure sores in different stages of healing. *Diagnostic Microbiology and Infectious Disease, 5,* 31–38.

Schneider, D., Hebert, L. (1987). Subcutaneous gas from hydrogen peroxide administration under pressure. *American Journal of Diseases of Children, 141,* 10–11.

Sporn, M.B., Roberts, A.B. (1990). The Transforming Growth Factor-Betas: Past, Present, and Future. *Annals of New York Academy of Science,* p. 593.

Sporn, M.B., Roberts, A.B. (1993). A major advance in the use of growth factors to enhance wound healing. *Journal of Clinical Investigation, 92,* 2565–2566.

Stotts, N.A. (1987). Age-specific characteristics of patients who develop pressure ulcers in the tertiary-care setting. *Nursing Clinics of North America, 22,* 391–398.

Taylor, T.V., Rimmer, S., Day, B., et al (1974). Ascorbic acid supplementation in the treatment of pressure sores. *Lancet, 2* (7880), 544–546.

Thomas, C. (1988). Nursing alert: Wound healing halted with the use of povidone iodine. *Ostomy/Wound Management, 18,* 30–33.

Thompson, J.M., McFarland, G.K., Hirsch, J.E., et al (1989). *Mosby's Manual of Clinical Nursing,* 2nd ed. St. Louis: Mosby Year Book.

Urinary Incontinence Guideline Panel (1992). *Urinary Incontinence in Adults: Clinical Practice Guideline.* AHCPR Publication No. 92–0038. Rockville, MD: Agency for Health Care Policy and Research, Public Health Service, U.S. Department of Health and Human Services.

Warner, D.J. (1992). A clinical comparison of two pressure-reducing surfaces in the management of pressure ulcers. *Decubitus, 5*(3), 52–55, 58–60, 62–64.

Whitney, J.D. (1989). Physiologic effect of tissue oxygenation in wound healing. *Heart and Lung, 18* (5), 466–467.

Whitney, J.D., Fellows, B., Larson, E. (1984). Do mattresses make a difference? *Journal of Gerontological Nursing, 10* (9), 20–25.

Williams, A. (1972). A study of factors contributing to skin breakdown. *Nursing Research 21,* 238–243.

Williams, C., Lines, C., McKay, E. (1988). Iron and zinc status in multiple sclerosis patients with pressure sores. *European Journal of Clinical Nutrition, 42* (4), 321–328.

Wong, D.L. (1995). *Whaley and Wong's Nursing Care of Infants and Children,* 5th ed. St. Louis: Mosby.

Yarkony, G., Matthews-Kirk, P., Carlson, C.E., et al. (1991). Classification of pressure ulcers. *Archives of Dermatology, 126,* 1218–1219.

Young, J.S., Burns, P.E. (1982). Pressure sores and the spinal cord injured. In J.S. Young, P.E. Burns, A.M. Bowen, and R. McCutchen (eds.). *Statistics: Experience of the Regional Spinal Cord Injury System.* Phoenix: National Spinal Cord Injury Data Research Center, pp. 95–105.

Social Support 29

Virginia P. Tilden and Christine A. Nelson

Becky, an African American high school student, has just been diagnosed with diabetes. In her high school, the school nurse leads a diabetes support group, which Becky has decided to join. The school nurse plays an important role in helping Becky adjust to her new diagnosis, learn to cope with a long-term condition, modify existing relationships, and form new relationships to provide the social support she needs. In assessing and developing a plan of care for Becky, the nurse draws on a knowledge of the physiologic and psychosocial aspects of diabetes, of growth and development during adolescence, and social support as a way to reduce stress and promote coping.

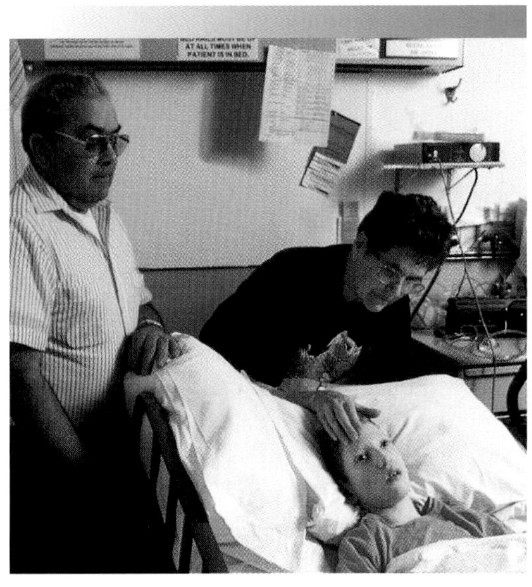

For Becky, the nurse considers factors that may affect care such as Becky's age and developmental stage, how long she has lived in the community, her ethnic and cultural background, and her family. The nurse knows that Becky is at risk for social isolation because of the stigma of having a chronic condition. The nurse works to help Becky adjust to the necessary changes in diet, exercise, and stress management, while keeping in mind Becky's relationships with family and friends that will affect her adjustment.

In the diabetes support group, the nurse and the other group members help Becky learn about diabetes and how to live with it. The nurse also encourages group members to help Becky with rides to school functions and loans of good books about living with diabetes. Being in the support group will help meet Becky's needs for ventilation, normalization, problem solving, peer support, and socialization. By applying the principles of social support, the nurse helps Becky gather the support she needs, minimize conflict in the network, avoid people who burden rather than benefit her, and reciprocate support to others.

OBJECTIVES

After studying this chapter, the student will be able to:

- **identify factors related to social support that can affect a patient's care**
- **assess a patient's access to social support**
- **use a convoy map to help a patient evaluate social support assets and deficits**
- **teach a patient about the relationship between social support, coping, and stress reduction**
- **implement the concept of social support cost-effectively in patient care**

SCOPE OF NURSING PRACTICE

Knowledge of social networks and social support plays a central role in contemporary nursing practice for several reasons. First, current trends in health care delivery mean that social networks must shoulder much of the responsibility for the care of patients, who now have briefer hospital stays, longer lives, and more chronic conditions than ever. Second, health care delivery has become more oriented to health maintenance and promotion. Public health programs encourage people to be socially involved to help protect their health. Social involvement means staying active with family, friends, and the community, as well as participating in self-help and mutual aid groups, when appropriate.

Third, the consumer movement has brought family and friends into health care because patients now refuse to be separated from their loved ones during health or illness events. Families are now commonly present during births, deaths, and other health events. Therefore, the nurse must include the patient's social network when providing care. For example, the school nurse in the introductory case study can encourage Becky to invite her parents to a group session so that they can meet the group and understand Becky's involvement with it. This is vital because Becky's success in adjusting to diabetes depends in part on her family's involvement.

Fourth, ample research shows that social support reduces stress, promotes coping, and is associated with decreased morbidity and mortality. Therefore, nurses now routinely assess the social network and its stability, resilience, and support-providing capacity. Finally, social support is beneficial for nurses who experience stress related to their practice, especially in intensive care, psychiatric, and trauma settings.

This chapter discusses social support, including its definitions, research base, and clinical applications. It is based on the idea that nursing care includes attention to the patients' psychosocial needs and network of relationships.

Nurses take a holistic approach to caring for their patients. This means that they view patients as having physical, psychological, spiritual, emotional, and social aspects. Nurses know that all of these aspects are interrelated: If a patient has a problem with one aspect, the others can be affected.

Nursing has three basic areas of focus:

- helping individuals with daily activities, such as eating, sleeping, and communicating
- helping patients and families with health problems, such as abnormal respiration or elimination
- helping patients with illnesses that require long-term care (Henderson, 1979)

In each area, the nurse must draw on knowledge of social support to promote the patient's adaptation and recovery.

THE KNOWLEDGE BASE

The social sciences have contributed much to our understanding of human beings as social animals with needs for social support. Recent research by nurses and others has explored the effects of social support on health.

Basic Science

SOCIAL RELATIONSHIPS

Humans are social animals. As *Homo sapiens* evolved, the social nature of the species formed the cornerstone of its mental and emotional life. Through interconnectedness came protection and comfort in hostile environments. As human cultures developed, social relationships took on ever greater importance. Today, all of the world's cultures stress the importance of interdependence, reciprocity, mutuality, and caretaking of loved ones as well as strangers in need. To understand social relationships, the nurse must be aware of basic psychosocial concepts related to the individual, family, and community. See Chapter 6 for more information on these basic concepts.

THE NATURE OF SOCIAL SUPPORT

There has been confusion about the nature of social support and its ability to reduce stress and protect health. In part, this confusion stems from the effort to turn such a common human experience into a scientific variable. It also is due to inconsistency among health scientists in defining and measuring social support and related concepts, such as social network and social interactions.

Our present understanding of social support evolved primarily from the writings of several theorists, which are summarized in Table 29–1. For the purposes of this chapter, social support means interpersonal transactions among members of a social network in which the reciprocal, informal, and usually spontaneous exchange of beneficial supplies occurs. Social support supplies consist of:

- emotional support, which includes feelings of empathy, caring, love, liking, trust
- appraisal support, which includes feedback or information that allows a person to compare self to others and therefore leads to self-correction, which leads to enhanced self-confidence and self-esteem
- informational support, which includes information or advice that a person can use in coping with and solving problems
- instrumental support, which includes tangible aid (services, money, time, food, shelter, or other direct help)

These four types of social support can be categorized as *affective* (emotional, appraisal, informational) or *tangible* (instrumental). In the introductory case study, the group offers

TABLE 29-1 Descriptions of Social Support*

Theorist	Conception of Social Support
James House (1981)	Social support consists of: • emotional support (trust, concern, love, listening) • appraisal support (feedback that builds self-confidence and self-esteem) • informational support (advice, suggestions, and directions) • instrumental support (labor, money, time, services, tangible aid)
Robert Kahn (1979)	Social support consists of: • affect (feeling liked or loved) • affirmation (feeling acknowledged and respected) • aid (direct services, supplies, or tangible help)
Sidney Cobb (1976)	Social support is information that one is: • cared for • loved, esteemed, and valued • part of a caring network
Gerald Caplan (1974)	Social support aids in coping with stress by helping to: • mobilize psychological resources • master emotional burdens • share tasks • provide guidance and tools
Robert Weiss (1974)	Social support aids in coping with situational crises and has six commodities: • attachment • social integration • opportunity to nurture another person • reassurance of worth • sense of reliable alliance • guidance in times of need

*Various theorists have conceived of social support in different ways. House's description of social support is the most widely accepted.

Becky tangible support by providing rides to school. It also offers affective support by sharing information and giving Becky an opportunity to express her feelings.

A few points require additional explanation. When people are asked to identify supportive others, they most often name informational sources of support, such as a spouse or partner, friends, neighbors, relatives, and work or school colleagues. They are less likely to name formal sources of support, such as physicians, nurses, clergy members, and counselors, though they may speak highly of these professional helpers (Gottlieb, 1978; House, 1981). So, social support usually refers to "noncontractual" relationships. In such relationships, exchanges are spontaneous, rather than purchased (such as when one visits a physician) or formally prescribed by social custom (such as when one visits a minister).

Further, when people are asked to describe supportive relationships, they expect reciprocity, a mutual give-and-take of support (Tilden et al, 1990a). Social support rarely is provided selflessly; even a parent caring for an infant usually anticipates a future give-and-take relationship with that child (House, 1981). Both giving and receiving usually involve implicit expectations of reciprocity. Costs of time, energy, or goods are kept in mind for later exchanges. Reciprocity appears to be an essential ingredient of supportive relationships. However, not all support provided by others is viewed as helpful and supportive by the receiver. Such unsupportive "support" includes discouraging ventilation, encouraging false optimism, minimizing a person's problem, glossing over a person's concern, falling back on platitudes, making unhelpful comparisons, and refusing reciprocity. Therefore, support provided is not synonymous with support perceived. A person's opinion about the supportiveness of others' behaviors is critical to the health benefits of that support. Each person's network can have nonsupportive relationships as well as supportive relationships that are stressful at times. People who are ill often have particular difficulty with nonsupportive relationships; for instance, well-meaning friends who say "don't worry" or "get well soon" to a patient with cancer (Wortman and Conway, 1985).

Thus, social support usually refers to the emotional and tangible help that a person gives and receives from informal relationships in everyday interactions—in person and by long-distance, such as via telephone and correspondence. To be effective, these interactions must convey a message of worth or affirmation to both parties in the exchange, and they must provide aid in coping with life's problems. To illustrate these concepts, consider the introductory case study. The school nurse should teach Becky the importance of receiving—and giving—the emotional support of listening and ventilating, the affirmational support of enhancing self-esteem, the informational support of exchanging advice, and the tangible support of sharing rides, gifts, food, and other things. By encouraging Becky to reciprocate with the group, the nurse promotes the mastery of an essential social skill and helps Becky achieve her health goals.

DIMENSIONS OF SOCIAL SUPPORT

Social support has two main dimensions: structural and functional.

STRUCTURAL DIMENSION

The structural dimension of social relationships is called the *social network*. This term refers to all those people known by the focus person or patient, usually consisting of close family, relatives, friends, acquaintances, neighbors, and work, school, or other activity-related associates.

Social network can be envisioned as a convoy of helping relationships that travel and evolve with a person across the lifespan (Kahn and Antonucci, 1980). As shown in Figure 29–1, the convoy can be represented by concentric circles around the focal person. Close supporters occupy inner circles of the convoy, and distant relationships occupy outer

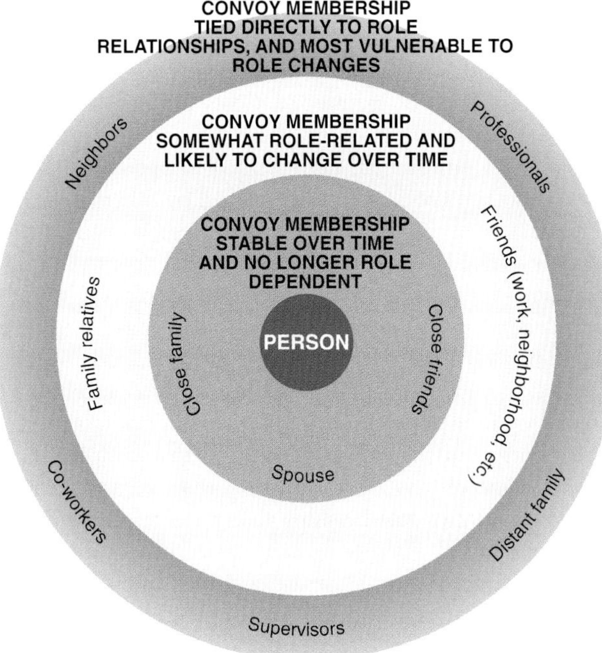

Figure 29–1. Social network as a convoy. This figure illustrates a convoy, with the focal person (P) at the center, close supporters in the inner circles, and distant relationships in the outer circle. (Redrawn from Kahn, R.L., Antonucci, T.C. [1980]. Convoys over the life course: Attachment, roles, and social support. In P.B. Baltes and O.G. Brim, Jr. (eds.): *Life-Span Development and Behavior,* New York: Academic Press.)

circles. Life events, transitions, and developmental stages affect the convoy, and circle memberships change with the phases of the life cycle. Figure 29–2 represents convoy changes at two different ages in a hypothetical person's life.

Most people relate to 6 to 10 people intimately, see an additional 30 or more persons regularly, and have access to about 100 distant acquaintances who could be called on for specific needs or in an emergency (Erickson, 1984).

Of course, not everyone known by a person, and technically within their social network, provides support. In fact, as Figure 29–3 illustrates, the social network is much larger than that part of the network that actually provides support. Also, support provided is not always seen as supportive by the receiver. People in a network—even those who usually are considered supportive—sometimes act in ways that cause stress even though they may mean well; this is called *conflicted support.* Finally, people outside of a social network, such as health professionals, often provide support temporarily. Their support is called *surrogate support.* Also, support occasionally is provided by strangers, such as a fellow airline passenger who offers information, advice, affirmation, or a listening ear during a flight (Norbeck, 1988a). These concepts can be useful in clinical practices. For example, in the introductory case study, the nurse talks with Becky about her social network, and together they identify people who provide, or can provide, the support Becky needs. They also identify conflicted supporters and discuss strategies for handling these people, such as avoiding them or modifying interactions with them.

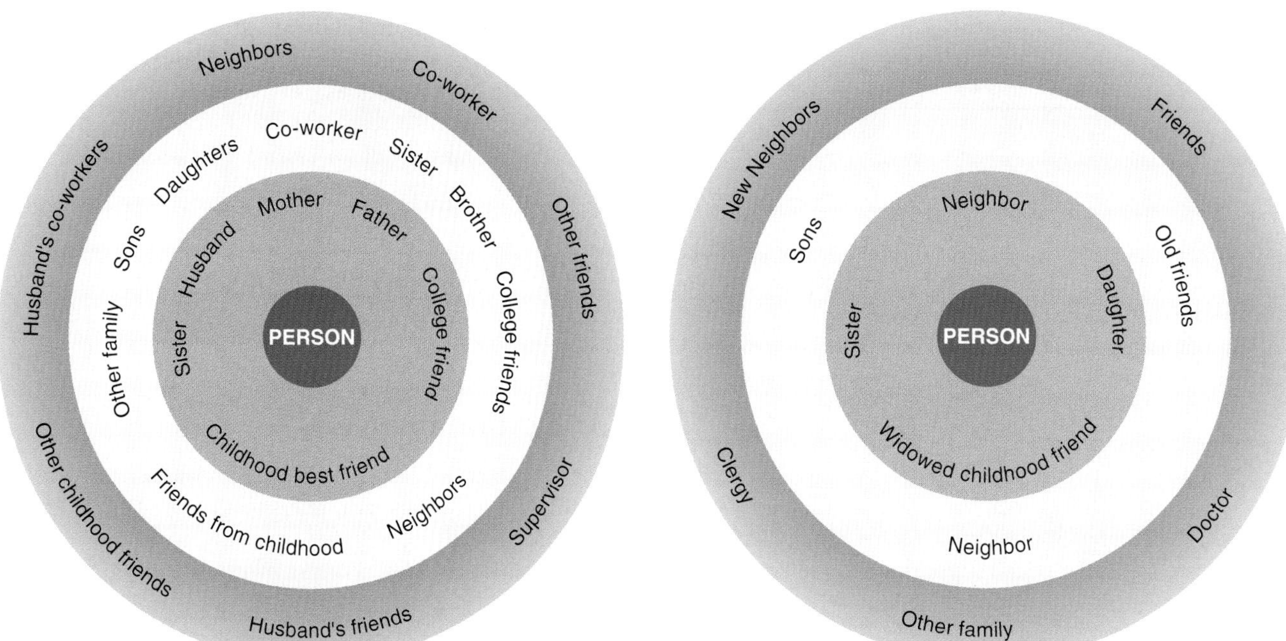

Figure 29–2. Possible changes in convoy composition. The sample convoys shown here compare the social network of a woman at two distinct times in her life. (Redrawn from Kahn, R.L., Antonucci, T.C. [1980]. Convoys over the life course: Attachment, roles, and social support. In P.B. Baltes and O.G. Brim, Jr. (eds.): *Life-Span Development and Behavior.* New York: Academic Press.)

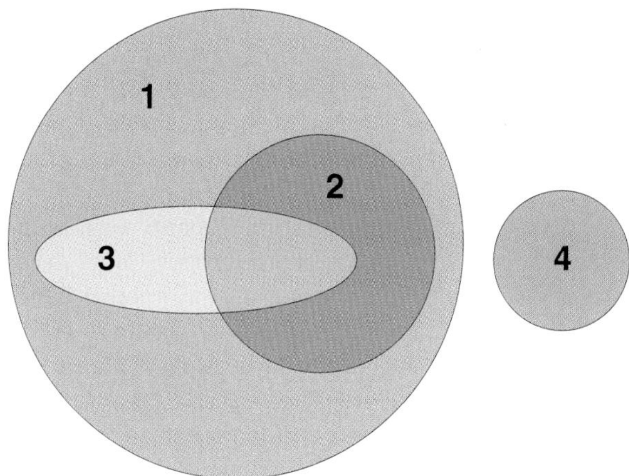

Figure 29–3. Components of the social network. A person's social network (area 1) is larger than his or her social support network (area 2). Some network members may provide conflicted support (area 3). People outside the network, such as a health care professional or sympathetic stranger, may provide surrogate or stranger support (area 4). (Redrawn from Norbeck, J.S., Barnes, L.E. [1988]. Social support. In H.S. Wilson and C.R. Kneisl (eds.): *Psychiatric Nursing,* 3rd ed. Menlo Park, CA: Addison-Wesley.)

Social networks can be described in structural terms, including:

- size (total number of people in the network)
- source (the type of support person, such as friend, relative, or coworker)
- density (the extent to which network members know or are interconnected with each other)
- clusters (portions of the network with high density, such as family or church groups)
- durability (duration of relationships)
- multiplexity (number of kinds of support one person provides, such as a friend who provides emotional *and* tangible support versus another friend who only provides emotional support)
- directionality (direction of support, whether given, received, or both)
- frequency of contact (Hall and Wellman, 1985).

A social network's density can dramatically affect social support. Network density can range from low to high, as shown in Figure 29–4. People whose networks are large in number but low in across-cluster density enjoy better health and well-being. Among young widows and older women returning to college, those with less dense networks reported significantly better support and better mental health (Hirsch, 1980). Their multiplex friendships correlated with their perceived support and mental health. Among women undergoing separation and divorce, those with the best psychosocial adjustment had slightly larger networks, less overlap of support sources with their husbands' networks, and less dense networks than women who showed poor adjustment (Wilcox, 1981). These findings suggest that highly dense, close-knit networks with few sources of support can jeopardize mental health by reinforcing maladaptive patterns. Among substance-abusing families, violent families, and single-mother families whose children are placed in foster care, highly dense, close-knit networks were common (Van Meter et al, 1987). In dense networks, people may be so much alike that they provide a narrow range or role models, information, and advice. In some situations, such as an interracial marriage, a strong family network may not promote adjustment to the marriage. In fact, the reverse may be true. When a cluster in the network is self-destructive, as in a substance-abusing or violent cluster, such negative behaviors tend to be reinforced by cluster members. This allows less opportunity for changing the behavior or investing in sources of support not connected to the cluster.

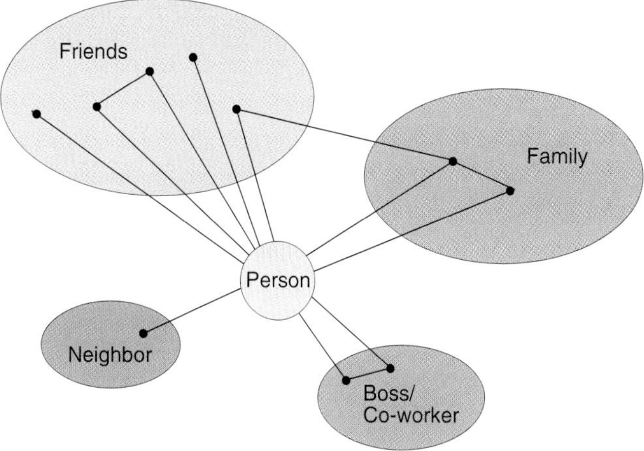

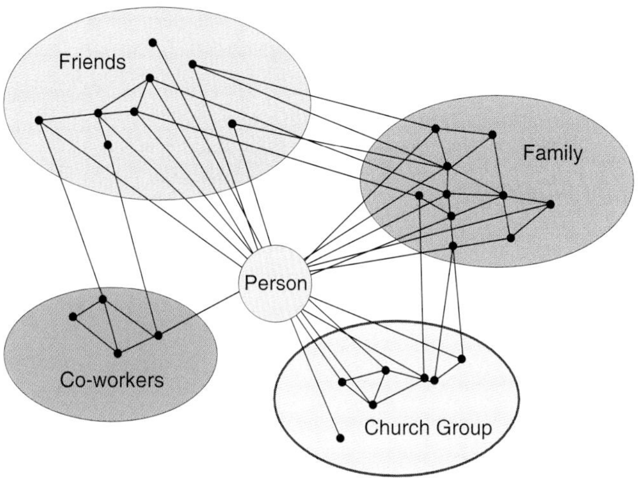

Figure 29–4. Social network density. The social network on the left shows four small clusters of support sources and is characterized by low density between clusters. In contrast, the network on the right shows four large clusters of support and is characterized by high density within and across clusters.

In the introductory case study, the nurse can use these structural concepts by encouraging Becky to have many sources of support, not just her family and diabetic support group. The nurse should urge Becky to explore interests via school clubs and community activities, which can lead to new sources of support. The more diverse Becky's support, the more likely she is to benefit from it and to develop effective coping skills.

FUNCTIONAL DIMENSION

The functional dimension of social support reflects the person's perception or experiences of social support. Usually, nurses try to understand social support from the perspective of the focal person or patient. One reason that perceived (subjective) is more important than actual (objective) support is that social support can be helpful just by being perceived as available if needed. Social support functions if a person perceives it as:

- available. The person thinks that he or she is reliably connected to others who will provide support if and when needed.
- enacted. The person experiences actual support from another person.
- satisfying. The person is pleased or satisfied with the support that is available or enacted.
- fitting. The person perceives a close match between the support enacted or available and the support that he or she feels is needed (Barrera, 1986).

Relevant Research

The issues of research into social support can be captured in a single question: Who gives what to whom regarding which problems and with what effects (House, 1981; Pearlin, 1985). In terms of the patient in the introductory case study, this question could be restated as: Among Becky's everyday relationships, who will be helpful to her? How will they be helpful? How will their help be used by Becky as she adjusts to her health condition? Research findings and theories can help answer this questions.

RESEARCH FROM NON-NURSING FIELDS

Although "caring," "friendship," and "support" are concepts as old as human relationships, the concept of social support is relatively new. It first emerged in the health sciences in the early 1970s, when numerous human and animal studies on the health effects of social interactions and social isolation found that individuals in a caring social network were physically and psychologically healthier (Caplan, 1974; Cassel, 1976; Cobb, 1976).

Also in the early 1970s, psychotherapists discovered that emotionally disturbed patients improved more rapidly and remained stable longer when the whole family was included in therapy. Family therapists who studied the influence of social milieu on mental illness also concluded that patients should be treated within the context of the family system. During the same period, treatment of hospitalized psychiatric patients changed. Mental health professionals learned that the ward environment, or group culture, had a powerful impact on patients and could be manipulated for therapeutic effects (Jones, 1953, 1968). These changes in treatment for psychiatric patients resulted from the growing awareness that social groups—including families and fellow patients—contribute significantly to an individual's mental and physical health and well-being.

For most of the 1980s, research about social support focused descriptively on its characteristics. More recently, non-nursing investigators have focused on whether interventions based on social support can make a difference in patient outcomes. For example, one study evaluated the extent to which peer support via telephone could boost morale and reduce depression in low-income, community-based elderly women (Heller et al, 1991). Such intervention studies are difficult to do, because effects due to social support must be distinguished from those due to other factors, such as initiating medication therapy or making a major change in housing or health status. In general, intervention studies have not shown major effects of social support on health outcomes (Stewart, 1989b).

NURSING RESEARCH

The early, tentative hypotheses that social support helps people maintain health and protects them from the effects of stress led to a great deal of research by professionals from various health and behavioral sciences, including nursing. Today, virtually every illness and health event has been studied in relation to social support. Most studies have shown that the more social support a person reports, the better his or her state of health and well-being. For example, nurse researchers have documented that social support relates to improved outcomes of pregnancy (Norbeck and Tilden, 1983), teenage mothering (Mercer et al, 1984a, 1984b), breastfeeding (Hewat and Ellis, 1984), self-care practices in elderly patients (Hubbard et al, 1984), rape trauma (Burgess and Holmstrom, 1978), hospitalization (Ahmadi, 1985), hysterectomy (Webb and Wilson-Barnett, 1983), mastectomy (Woods and Earp, 1978), cancer (Lindsey et al, 1985; Mishel and Braden, 1987), and head injury (Hermansen-Williams, 1990) (see Research Highlight).

Armed with such research findings, the nurse in the introductory case study should be able to improve Becky's chances for successful adaptation to her condition by promoting her use of the existing social network and by adding new support resources.

Most of the tools for measuring social support were designed for research, not clinical, purposes. Some 21 measuring tools have been developed by nurses alone (Stewart, 1989a). Three of the most important research measures are the Norbeck Social Support Questionnaire (NSSQ), the Personal Resource Questionnaire (PRQ), and the Interpersonal Relationship Inventory (IPRI).

The NSSQ measures several dimensions of social network and social support, including size, duration, and loss of rela-

RESEARCH HIGHLIGHT
HEAD INJURY SUPPORT GROUPS PROVE BENEFICIAL

In one study, 77 members of head injury support groups were surveyed concerning the impact and benefits of their support group membership. According to the respondents, the support groups helped them obtain information about available resources, allowed them to share experiences with others in a similar situation, and helped enhance their ability to cope (Hermansen-Williams, 1990).

tionships; frequency of contact of network members; and perceived affect, affirmation, and aid (Norbeck et al, 1981, 1983). It is based on the concept of the social network as a convoy of relationships that travel with an individual throughout the lifespan, providing affect, affirmation, and aid to the focal person. Nine questions evaluate each of these dimensions for each person in the network. The measure is a paper-and-pencil questionnaire, is self-administered, and takes about 20 minutes to complete.

The PRQ measures both available support resources and perceived social support (Brandt and Weinert, 1981; Weinert, 1987). It is a self-administered pencil-and-paper questionnaire in two parts. The first part presents 10 life situations in which a person might need assistance (such as being ill) and asks who from a list of support sources (such as a parent, spouse, or neighbor) would be available to help. The second part is a global measure of perceived social support based on Weiss's (1974) definition of support as six commodities or provisions. The respondent marks 25 statements about social support on a 7-point scale from "strongly agree" to "strongly disagree." The measure is self-administered and takes about 20 minutes to complete.

Unlike other tools, the IPRI measures not only network structure and perceived social support, but also reciprocity and interpersonal conflict. (Tilden et al, 1990a, 1990b). It is based conceptually on social exchange theory. This theory says that interpersonal relationships within social networks depend on reciprocal exchanges of emotional and tangible supplies. The IPRI is a self-administered questionnaire that consists of several social network items (size of the network, type of support relationships, size of household, and proximity of relatives) and three separate scales to measure support, reciprocity, and conflict. Each of the three scales consists of 13 statements that the respondent rates from 1 to 5 as "agree-disagree" or "never-frequently." For example, to the statement "There is someone I can turn to for helpful advice about a problem," the respondent would mark one of the following options: "strongly disagree," "disagree," "neutral," "agree," or "strongly agree." The instrument takes about 15 minutes to complete.

Relevant Theory

Many social scientists have proposed theories to explain the supportive functions of interpersonal relationships. Four theories have gained the widest acceptance: social exchange theory, social comparison theory, self-esteem theory, and personal control theory.

SOCIAL EXCHANGE THEORY

Social exchange theory says that human relationships are based on the same exchange of goods, services, rewards, and costs as economic transactions. However, instead of money and goods being exchanged, human relationships include exchanges of esteem, affection, love, status, information, advice, and nurturance in addition to tangible goods and services. As in economic transactions, reciprocity (give and take) is expected, and rewards should be proportional to investments and costs.

In the introductory case study, for example, the school nurse knows to encourage Becky to *provide* support to group members as soon as she is able. This reciprocity is essential to successful support transactions.

Social exchange theory effectively explains friendships. However, it does not explain intimate couple relationships, such as parent-child and spousal relationships very well. It may be helpful to distinguish between *exchange* relationships (those with neighbors, friends, or work asso-ciates) and *communal* relationships (those between intimate couples). In communal relationships, interpersonal behavior is governed more by a desire to respond to the other's need and less by the demands of fair exchange.

SOCIAL COMPARISON THEORY

Social comparison theory describes two types of support: affirmational and informational support. This theory says that people obtain *affirmational support* when they compare their perceptions, experiences, performances, and opinions to those of others in an effort to validate them. It also states that people obtain *informational support* when they receive cognitive information that allows them to correct misperceptions and learn new behaviors. Affirmational and informational support affect the experience of stress and thus reduce its negative effects.

In the introductory case study, for example, the school nurse expects Becky and the other group members to exchange opinions and provide feedback, which should help combat isolation, correct misinformation, improve self-esteem, and help normalize experiences. The nurse's role is to facilitate and encourage this exchange of affirmational and informational support.

SELF-ESTEEM THEORY

Similar to social comparison theory, self-esteem theory holds that *self-esteem* is a basic human social drive, and that maintenance of it occurs within interpersonal relationships. By comparing oneself to others who are worse off, a person can obtain a sense of self-enhancement. Likewise, messages of esteem and competence from supportive others during times of stress can bolster one's sense of ability to cope.

For example, as Becky becomes confident that others in the support group believe in her, she will be more likely to believe in herself.

PERSONAL CONTROL THEORY

Personal control theory holds that psychological well-being depends on one's perception of control and sense of mastery (self-efficacy) over events. To have this sense of mastery, a person needs to believe that he or she has sufficient "safety nets" for support should disaster strike. This feeling of having sufficient safety nets comes from perceiving that one is part of a social network of reliable and trustworthy relationships that could be called on if needed. A sense of mastery is the opposite of the powerlessness and helplessness that a person may feel when facing a crisis without a supportive network.

As illustrated in the case study, Becky's membership in the diabetes support group can help her develop a sense of mastery by giving her a network of peers who understand her condition. She can turn to the group members whenever she feels misunderstood by nondiabetic students, relatives, and others.

THEORIES ABOUT THE EFFECTS OF SOCIAL SUPPORT

Several theories have tried to explain exactly how social support acts to prevent stress, alleviate its negative effects, and promote health. The stress-diathesis model says that stress negatively affects health by suppressing the endocrine and immune systems in vulnerable individuals (Ader, 1980). Social support protects against this through the action of the neurohormones (Pilisuk and Parks, 1986).

There are three main hypotheses regarding the mechanisms by which social support protects and promotes health: the preventive function, the buffering function, and the health-promotion function (Fig. 29–5). The hypothesized mechanisms of action reflected in Figure 29–5 are simplified for clarity. In reality, social support acts on stress and health, but stress and health can also affect the social network and the support it provides. For example, a social network that mobilizes to help a person whose home is destroyed in a fire will be affected by the situation as much as it affects the situation. Perhaps the person will need to move in with relatives until he or she can find another home, thus dramatically changing the relatives' lives. The relatives may feel the strain of an additional mouth to feed; may be crowded with another person in the home; may feel resentful about their loss of privacy; or may leave the home because the changes are too unwelcome. Thus, stress can create changes in social support just as social support can affect stress.

The simplified Figure 29–5 also assumes that stress is a discrete event that affects everyone equally. Actually, individuals react to stress uniquely, based on their personal characteristics

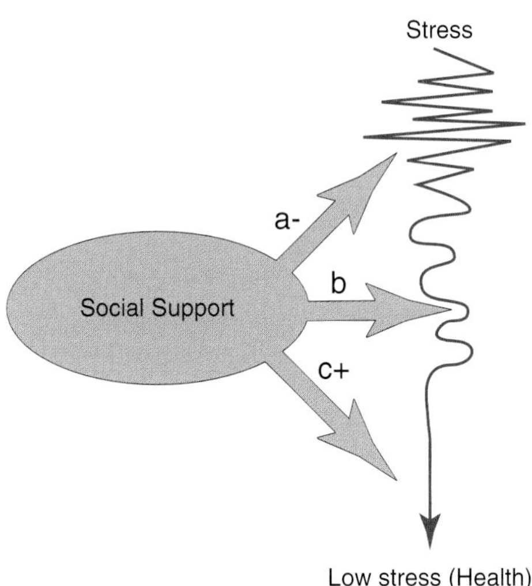

Figure 29–5. Simplified action of social support on stress and health. The model shown here illustrates three ways in which social support promotes health. First, arrow a− indicates that social support may have a direct effect on stress. When social support is ample, a person will experience fewer stressors. The minus sign indicates this inverse relationship; when one is high, the other is low. Thus, social support may act directly to prevent stressful events from happening. For example, a person with good support is unlikely to be homeless or without resources. This is called the preventive function, because social support helps prevent stressful events.

Second, social support may buffer stress that occurs, as indicated by arrow b. Although stressful events occur, their debilitating effects on health are lessened. For example, a person whose home burns in a fire is buffered from many resulting stresses by a supportive social network that mobilizes to help the person by providing shelter and other tangible support, expressing care, helping with insurance forms, and mobilizing emergency services. This intermediate action of social support between stress and health is called the buffering function.

Third, social support may have a direct effect on health that is unrelated to stress, as indicated by arrow c+. Through this mechanism of action, people with ample support enjoy better health because the support network encourages them to adhere to health-related regimens, such as proper management of diabetes or hypertension, and to practice healthy behaviors, such as eating well, using seat belts, obtaining immunizations, and performing breast self-examinations.

Perhaps people with ample support have more incentive to stay healthy longer in life, and therefore they engage in more, and more effective, self-care activities. In this hypothesis, support and health have a positive relationship; when one is high, the other is also high, as indicated by the plus sign.

and subjective appraisal of the stressor, which determine the degree of threat perceived (Lazarus and Folkman, 1984). Thus, stress does not affect people equally. Rather, stressful events precipitate a unique appraisal by a person about his or her ability to respond to the stress effectively. When the person perceives that the situation exceeds personal coping resources, then lowered self-esteem, perceptions of low self-efficacy, and perceived lack of control over events are likely to follow. These demoralized states can actually depress the immune system, leading to physiologic changes and, eventually, health changes. In other works, negative health effects are likely to occur. For example, for the person whose home burns in a fire, the answers to the following questions determine the effect of stress on health:

- How does this person view the stressor of the fire and the loss of the home?
- What is the meaning of the fire and loss to that person?
- To what extent does this person experience lowered self-esteem, lowered self-efficacy, and loss of control in the face of the fire and loss of the home?

Therefore, a more sophisticated model is needed to describe the actions of social support, as in Figure 29–6.

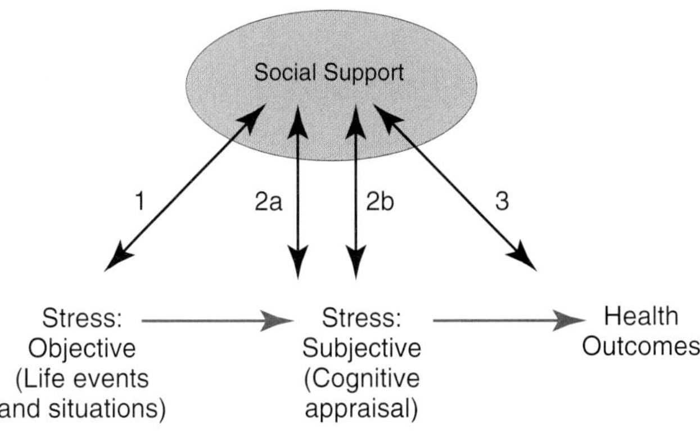

Figure 29–6. Detailed action of social support on stress and health. The model shown here illustrates the interaction between social support, stress, and health, and the intermediate role of cognitive appraisal. The bi-directional arrows (1, 2a, 2b, and 3) indicate that the effects of variables go both ways. Stress no longer has a single, direct relationship with health. Instead, it goes through an intermediate step called cognitive appraisal. Social support affects the link between objective stress and subjective (perceived) stress, as shown by arrow 2a. Support also affects the link between subjective stress and health outcomes, as shown by arrow 2b. Social support still may affect stress and health directly, as shown by arrows 1 and 3. However, stress and health can now affect social support. A stressful event, such as a fire that strips a family of its home, affects the social network initially by causing network members to increase their offers of social support. But if this stress becomes long-term (for example, if the family becomes permanently homeless), it may cause social network exhaustion and a progressive *decrease* in social support. Finally, health can affect social support. A healthy, mobile, and emotionally stable person can evoke more support and maintain a wider network than a person who is restricted by health problems.

FACTORS AFFECTING CLINICAL DECISIONS

Characteristics of each individual determine in large part the amount and kinds of social support needed, the network's structure and function, and the effects of social support on the person's health and well-being.

Age and Developmental Stage

A patient's age and developmental stage affect his or her roles, relationships, needs, and behaviors. They also determine the membership of his or her social network. For example, the social relationships and support interactions of an adolescent differ greatly from those of an elderly person. Because age-related changes in the social network often coexist with age-related health changes, the nurse should be aware of the complex interactions between health, age, developmental stage, and social relationships.

Age seems to have little effect on the need for social support. Among adults of all ages, no differences were found in support and reciprocity (Tilden et al, 1990b). Also, network size and frequency of contact, especially with close kin, remain fairly stable across the lifespan. However, differences may exist in social network composition and other factors.

INFANTS AND CHILDREN

Social networks of infants and children are defined almost entirely by the family and neighborhood, broadening out to encompass school ties as a child ages. In fact, social support of infants and young children is often described in terms of their parents' social support. For example increased mother-infant attachment is associated with greater social support from family and friends (Cranley, 1984). Women with ample social support experience significantly fewer complications of pregnancy and delivery, and deliver healthier infants than women with inadequate support (Norbeck and Tilden, 1983). Among pregnant adolescents, informational support and the father's presence during labor and delivery enhance the new mother's ability to attach to her infant (Mercer et al, 1984a, 1984b).

ADOLESCENTS

During adolescence, the social network exerts more influence on behaviors and values than at any other stage of the life cycle. Same-aged peer groups have tremendous influence over adolescents, who gradually separate from the family by rebelling against the family's values and requirements. When parents divorce, their adolescent children are at risk for conflicted relationships with parents and siblings and for depletion of their peer network (Gottlieb, 1985).

As a school nurse, the nurse in the introductory case study is an expert in adolescent development. The nurse knows the special needs of adolescents for approval from peers, separation from family, and recognition from teachers and other adults. Therefore, the nurse assesses Becky and plans nursing interventions with her and the other support group members from the standpoint of adolescent development.

ADULTS

For young adults, parents are the main source of tangible aid, and friends are the main source of informational and emotional support. Other relatives play a secondary role.

As young adults, many people become parents, which can alter their social network. For example, from early pregnancy through 6 months postpartum, new parents change their networks to include people who are also parents (Cronenwett, 1985a, 1985b). Those who adapted best to parenthood had emotional and instrumental support from a large network with low density, but a relatively high percentage of kin. Gender differences in network and support variables were noted postpartum. After the birth of the baby, husbands listed more network members that overlapped with their wives, and more husbands than wives were satisfied with the amount of support available to them. Wives substituted coworker contacts for contacts with friends so that the total frequency of contacts with network members was unchanged. Most wives perceived an increased need for support at 5 months postpartum.

Among low-income, single mothers with preschool children, those who had no one close to confide in displayed more parenting problems. Also, their children displayed more behavioral problems when the mothers did not have a close family member (Norbeck and Sheiner, 1982).

For middle-aged adults, the spouse or partner is the primary provider of tangible aid and emotional support. Friends, colleagues, and neighbors provide most of the informational support. However, conflict is likely to occur. Adults age 30 to 39 reported significantly greater conflict than older adults (age 64 and older). This may be true because the early middle years are characterized by establishing families and work roles and, therefore, may be more vulnerable to discord and stress in the social network (Tilden et al, 1990b).

ELDERLY

For the elderly, adult children and the spouse or partner (if living) provide most of the tangible aid. Informational and emotional support comes from various sources, including children, friends, formal organizations such as a church or synagogue, and special support groups such as widowhood and Alzheimer's disease support groups. However, social relationships may vary.

As with younger people, older adults have social support needs. If these needs are not met, poor health and institutionalization can occur. For example, widowers who lived alone and believed that family and friends were not supportive had a higher rate of poor health outcomes than other widowers (O'Brien, 1985). Most elderly people receive supportive care from family members and use few community resources (Lindsey and Hughes, 1981). Lack of such social support is the variable that most accurately predicts institutionalization (Brock and O'Sullivan, 1985).

Among institutionalized older adults, friendships in the institution can serve as a buffer against staff changes and other stressful events. Sometimes emotional ties to family members make it difficult for elderly persons to accept institutional activities and relationships. Social support helps enhance self-esteem in daily interactions (Powers, 1985).

ROLES

Different ages and development stages carry differing role expectations. As individuals move through the life cycle, they assume various age-related roles, such as student, worker, parent, and caregiver. They learn behavior appropriate for the role from others who are in the role. The social network facilitates this process by giving the individual feedback about how he or she is performing that role. Such supportive role modeling provides affirmational and informational support.

Age-related and stage-related roles, such as parent, worker, and caregiver, influence the amount and kind of social support given and received. For example, the demands placed on young mothers by household members can reduce their opportunities to meet their own needs for companionship and counseling (Fischer, 1982).

People who work may have job-related stress as well as job-related social support. Among female critical care nurses, married nurses reported significantly more support from their spouses, family, and relatives than unmarried nurses. Unmarried nurses received more support from friends than their married counterparts. Support from the workplace was most important for married nurses in reducing job stress. Married nurses more than unmarried nurses said that small support groups at work were valuable in dealing with problems and coping with stress (Norbeck, 1985a). Of particular interest from this study was the finding that the global scores of social support were less able to statistically predict psychological distress than knowing the specific types and sources of social support reported by the nurses. This finding suggests that global measures of social support might be less useful in research than situation-specific measures.

Lack of social support was found to be a key contributing factor (along with intense job stress and other stressful life changes) to burnout among nurses (Cronin-Stubbs and Brophy, 1985; Cronin-Stubbs and Rooks, 1985).

People's roles in their social networks often influence the social support they are expected to give and receive. For example, a caregiver for a frail elderly parent or a chronically ill family member may give a lot of unreciprocated support to the care receiver over time. Such a caregiver also may suffer reduced socialization, increased isolation, and financial strain, all of which increase the caregiver's risk for social support deficiencies. A person who depends on a network member for care may feel pressure to not upset the relationship for fear of losing that support.

Gender

Men and women tend to have differing social networks and social support exchanges and to be affected differently by social support. Women report larger networks and greater perceived need for social support, as well as more burden, overinvolvement, and network conflict. Men typically describe a network that includes only a spouse and perhaps adult children, despite the fact that they may have kin, neighbors, and work-related associates (Tilden and Galyen, 1987).

Among men and women enrolled in health education classes, women's mental health was more positively affected by social support and reciprocity and more adversely affected by conflict in the social network. Also, women reported significantly more social support, reciprocity, and network conflict than men (Tilden et al, 1990b). They talked about network members in more detail and included hurtful people in their network, such as an abusing spouse or villainous mother-in-law. Men, on the other hand, tended to describe their networks briefly and did not include past network members who had wronged them (Tilden et al, 1990a).

Women's networks tend to be more diverse and lower in density than men's, and their network members usually furnish multiple types of support. However, women often pay a price for having larger networks, such as increased demands for caregiving services. The more their services are demanded, the less satisfied women may feel with their social network (Antonucci, 1989). In rural and urban social networks, women more often play the role of counselor; men more typically provide practical or financial aid (Fischer, 1982). A feeling of having no one to confide in is more common in older unmarried men than in older unmarried women.

Unlike age, which has a highly variable effect on social networks and social support, the effect of gender on social support (and vice versa) tends to be consistent. Women tend to want and accept more support, have larger and less dense social networks, and are more burdened by network demands. They also receive greater benefits to their mental health from network support and sustain greater damage to their mental health by conflict in the network.

Family Status

For most people, the family is the single most enduring source of social support throughout their lives. Family ties of affiliation, mutual obligation, nurturance, and intimacy are strong in all cultures. However, cultural norms shape the specific support behaviors. Families clearly demonstrate the extent of interdependence and reciprocity that characterizes us as human. Caregiving and care receiving permeate all family relationships—with children, parents, and grandparents assuming the roles of caregiver and care receiver at different times.

CHILDREN

In families, support begins with the earliest parent-infant interactions (Boyce, 1985). The infant is born with sophisticated abilities for social interaction, including visual acuity that allows focusing, following, and exhibiting visual preferences, such as selectively attending to the human face. The infant's motor and auditory systems also are organized for responsive interactions even in the first few days of life. These abilities quickly develop into the infant's smiling recognition, clinging protests on separation, and enthusiastic greeting. This capacity for social interaction allows the attachment and reciprocity that is vital to the formation of the parent-infant bond. This bond forms the foundation for all subsequent social relationships (Boyce, 1985).

Children are strongly affected by patterns of the parents. Parents who provide a strong foundation of support raise children who, as adults, can do the same. Children who were raised by adequate parents and had positive relationships with them are later perceived as being trustworthy and skilled in dealing with social problems; conversely, children who were raised by abusive parents tend to perpetuate that pattern as adults (Crittenden, 1985; Sarason et al, 1986).

COUPLES

The long-held notion that married people have greater social support than single, divorced, and widowed people has been shown to be false. In fact, unhappily married persons are worse off than unmarried people, because an unhappy marriage tends to restrict access to other sources of social support and because unmarried people often have large networks of supportive friends.

However, even adequate marriages do not necessarily provide high levels of support. For example, only about one third of married women would go to their husbands first for support if they had a serious problem, such as depression, nervousness, or anxiety (Brown and Gary, 1985). Only one third of women named their husbands as one of the three people closest to them (Rubin, 1984). More men than women considered their spouses to be their best friend. Among older married couples, men are more likely than women to name their spouses as people in whom they confide; women are more likely to perceive less emotional support in marriage than men (Depner and Ingersoll-Dayton, 1985). Further, only 39 percent of men and 28 percent of women confide in their partners (Lee, 1988).

Men and women differ in the type of support they desire from their partner. Husbands tend to be pleased by wives' instrumental support, such as meal preparation; wives tend to be pleased by husbands' displays of affection, such as saying "I love you" (Wills et al, 1974).

Even though married people do not necessarily derive large amounts of support from their spouses, most married people have healthier lifestyles than single, divorced, or widowed people. Married people are more likely to quit smoking and eat balanced meals, probably because spouses pressure them to do so (Ross et al, 1991).

DIVORCE AND WORK

Divorce disrupts social networks through the loss or change of friends, kin, and socializing patterns (Ambert, 1988). Family members play a key role in adjustment to divorce, especially among women (Gerstel, 1988). Separated and divorced people are more likely to seek professional help, such as counseling, than are married, single, or widowed people. In fact, 54 percent of separated and divorced women and 46 percent of men sought help from health care professionals, compared with 28 percent of married women and 18 percent of men (Veroff et al, 1981).

When divorce occurs in the later years, social isolation may result. Divorced elderly people may have limited social interactions and feel discrimination and alienation because of the divorce (Kitson et al, 1980). Further, the divorce of adult children may drastically change the kinship network of elderly parents. Older people may suddenly need to provide more support for their divorced children, and grandparent and in-law relationships may be damaged (Johnson, 1988).

Family relationships and social support can also be affected by work. Before the twentieth century, families tended to work together on family farms. Today, family members usually work in separate settings, often at great distances from home. Isolation and high work stress (or the stress of unemployment and economic uncertainty) can erode a family's sense of shared mission and common goals. Often high work stress overwhelms family relationships and reduces the family members' ability to provide social support for each other.

ELDERLY

Families are the major source of support to elderly persons. Also, large numbers of families in the United States care for a family member with serious health problems in the home. Although the ill family member may be any age, often the person is elderly and can no longer live independently. Usually, the primary caregiver is an adult daughter. This situation, commonly called "women in the middle" and "sandwich generation," characterizes millions of American women who are raising their own children while also caring for an elderly parent. Although this situation has the potential to be overwhelming, family caregivers who feel prepared to cope and who feel a sense of predictability and control usually do well with its demands (Archbold et al, 1990).

Educational Background and Socioeconomic Status

Differences in education and socioeconomic factors result in unequal access to social support (Fischer, 1982; Antonucci, 1989). Higher education is associated with greater diversity of sources of support, access to helpful information, and opportunity to connect with needed resources. People with more education depend less on kin and more on friends to broaden opportunities for jobs and companionship. People who have little education and low socioeconomic status have fewer overall resources and may be at risk for social support deficits. Their networks are likely to contain a high percent of kin and to be denser and less adaptive, due to the economic and emotional stresses of their lower socioeconomic status.

Problems such as alcoholism, drug dependency, and family violence can be associated with the socioeconomics of unemployment, underemployment, and economic deprivation. These problems obviously affect relationships in the social network.

Culture and Ethnicity

The characteristics of social networks and the social norms that govern the exchange of support vary widely across cultures. Primarily, they are determined by such cultural factors as religiosity, level of industrialization, kinship patterns, and the roles of men and women (see Research Highlight).

Because most of our knowledge about social support is based on studies of white, middle-class Westerners, it cannot be generalized to other cultural, ethnic, and socioeconomic groups. Instead, the nurse should *assume* differences and should gain an understanding of the norms that influence each patient's support systems. Information important for assessment includes how a patient's culture views individual autonomy versus group responsibility, when and why an individual is labeled dysfunctional, and what is seen as helpful behavior (Pearson, 1990).

The introductory case study illustrates this process. The school nurse makes no assumptions about cultural or ethnic characteristics of Becky or her family because acculturation or blending of cultures is common in the United States. Instead, the nurse listens carefully to Becky's views, ideas, and descriptions of her family. From this data, the nurse can assess Becky's social support and social network in a way that is culturally sensitive and individually tailored.

Spirituality

In the United States, when people are asked to name network members who provide the most support, they commonly include a spiritual being, such as God or Jesus. This is especially true of African American people, who consistently display higher levels of religiousness than whites (Taylor, 1988). Organized religion and personal spirituality provide a great deal of support for many people. A spiritual figure may even be included in their inner support network. The nurse's role to accept and encourage whatever personal spirituality the patient indicates is important.

Chronic Illness

Persons with chronic illness, whether at home, in the hospital, or in a nursing home, have special needs and problems related

RESEARCH HIGHLIGHT
SOCIAL SUPPORT VARIES ACROSS CULTURES

Several studies have provided insights into cultural factors relevant to social support. For example, the social networks of Taiwanese cancer patients consist overwhelmingly of family and extended relatives. They include few friends, unlike the support networks of Westerners, which usually consist equally of family and friends. Traditional Asian society emphasizes reciprocity, and perceives family members as the predominant—almost sole—sources of support during a major illness (Lindsey et al, 1985).

In the Japanese culture, the term for social support is *amae,* which also means interdependence. Very traditional and rigidly prescribed roles between generations are related to *amae.* For example, young people honor their elders, and grandparents expect to be cared for by their adult children (Minami, 1989).

Ethnicity can shape families' responses to stressful events. For example, compared with Anglo families, Latino families tend to depend more on extended families and less on the husband-wife relationship for aid in coping with childhood cancer. They also depend less on counselors, other parents of children with cancer, and the health care team (Friedman, 1985).

The social networks of African American and Hispanic families typically differ somewhat from those of Anglo families. In African American and Hispanic networks, the extended family is pervasive. Kin are more prevalent than nonkin, and relationships are characterized by high rates of visiting and exchange (Taylor et al, 1991; Vega, 1991). Like Anglos, African American and Hispanic adults with supportive family and friends have heightened self-esteem, greater self-efficacy, and reduced psychological distress.

to their social networks (Tilden and Weinert, 1987). Due to pain, fatigue, disfigurement, and other problems, illness usually increases the need for social support (Wortman and Conway, 1985). This may be compounded by difficulty in obtaining support that really helps. Three quarters of patients with cancer reported feeling that people treated them differently after learning that they had cancer (Peters-Golden, 1982). People with chronic disability conditions often report feeling misunderstood, avoided, and feared by others. Others may act overly optimistic and cheerful, may avoid open discussion, or may appear strained. Hemodialysis patients reported that the quality of their interactions decreased over time as their feelings of alienation and estrangement increased. Unsupportive responses by support network members may occur because of the particular disease. For example, cancer may engender repulsion over physical changes; acquired immunodeficiency syndrome (AIDS) commonly engenders fear of contagion and homophobia (Wortman and Conway, 1985). Therefore, physically ill people may find that their social network members not only fail to buffer them from the stress of the illness, but also become an additional source of stress (Wortman and Conway, 1985).

Serious illness of a network member can affect the social network. Typically, network members rally during the immediate crisis, providing various forms of support to the ill individual or immediate family. However, when health problems are chronic, network members may become worn out and may not be able to provide long-term support. Caregiving to a chronically ill or frail elderly person usually falls to immediate family members, putting them at risk for social isolation and emotional and physical burnout. Among wives of myocardial infarction patients, 50 percent reported not receiving adequate information for home care, and 17 percent reported receiving no support from family members or health care professionals (Hentinen, 1983).

An additional problem is the inability of the ill person to return support. For chronically ill and elderly persons receiving care in the home, the inability to reciprocate—not the need for assistance—undermines their morale (Stoller, 1985). The inability to reciprocate also is a major factor in deterring homeless people from seeking help (Antonucci, 1989).

Ethical Considerations

Although some cross-cultural research exists on social behaviors, social support as a health concept is based on studies of Western, Caucasian, middle-class people. This fact raises an ethical concern because indiscriminate application of this knowledge to all people could result in culturally insensitive care and could harm patients through ignorance. To avoid this ethical problem, the nurse should learn about each patient's culture before drawing conclusions about the need for and use of social support, and before performing interventions.

Although assessing a patient's culture may sound easy, it often challenges the nurse to think beyond personal convictions and values. A patient's culture includes ethnic identity, religion, and lifestyle preferences, such as sexual orientation. These aspects of culture help determine how an individual's network provides and receives social support. Nurses often interact with the social network, especially with the family who gathers by the patient's bedside during health crisis. Therefore, nurses have an ethical obligation to withhold judgment about who should be in the family or social network and how network members should provide support. For example, the family of the person with AIDS may consist of the lover and numerous close friends whom the patient considers to be as close as kin. The nurse's ethical duty is to accept the patient's views and decisions about his or her social network, and to affirm the patient's right to self-determination and full personhood as he or she defines it.

For example, the nurse in the introductory case study should note how each group member describes her or his family. The nurse should listen closely to learn who is considered inside the family and what types of support they do or do not provide. Also, the nurse should remember that affective or "feeling" relationships may be more important then formal relationships. For example, the boyfriend of a student's mother may be a more important part of the student's world than the student's biologic father.

Financial Considerations

Because informal social support is given and received without formal contracts and payment, social support is often praised as a cost-free way to promote health and prevent disease. It is particularly appealing to the government, which is seeking more cost-effective ways to help people due to the huge national debt and financially strained health and human service systems. Consequently, families and extended social networks increasingly are expected to provide care for ill, disabled, or frail elderly family members. At the same time, support for such caregivers, such as financial aid, respite programs, and educational programs, is dwindling. This can lead to exhaustion and burnout for many caregivers if their emotional and tangible resources become overwhelmed by the demands of caregiving.

So although social support *is* a cost-effective approach to preventing health problems, it is not an automatic solution to providing care for ill people. Because the costs of capitalizing on social networks tend to be low compared with the costs of other health care strategies, it becomes easy to exploit or abuse social networks.

FUTURE DEVELOPMENTS

In the future, nurses and other health care professionals should be able to apply their knowledge of social support in new and creative ways to help people enhance their health. Social support interventions have already been designed for:

- individual patients
- categories of patients, such as women with breast cancer and people with AIDS
- large communities, such as Friends Can Be Good Medicine (Taylor et al, 1984).

More such social support interventions are likely to be developed in the future. Communities of the future may become "helping networks," where neighbors join forces to stop crime, protect children and the elderly, employ culture-specific health services for the community, and serve as mutual-aid communities where people feel connected, supported, and valued (Froland et al, 1981).

Support Programs

Large-scale community support programs have already been developed. In California, a state health program called "Friends Can Be Good Medicine" gave citizens information about how social support can promote health and prevent disease (Taylor et al, 1984). In this program, messages on radio, television, flyers, billboards, shopping bag ads, and town hall meetings encouraged people to keep a network of friends who made them feel supported. The program was very successful in disseminating the message; most of the public had heard the message, and some had taken action to implement it. In Canada, two community-based support programs successfully increased self-esteem and decreased life stress and suicide thoughts among people who had previously admitted thinking about suicide (De Man and Labreche-Gauthier, 1991).

Alternate Sources of Support

Although social support traditionally has been supplied by humans, it may be supplied by nonhumans—specifically computers, other electronic devices, and animals—in the future. To date, these innovations have been limited to specific populations.

COMPUTERS

In psychotherapy, computers have been used as therapists with patients who are inhibited by the presence of a human therapist. By interacting with a specially programmed computer, such patients obtain the same increased sense of well-being and decreased anxiety as with a human therapist. However, they have more anonymity than they would with a human therapist (Colby et al, 1989; Slack et al, 1990). For depressed patients, therapist-administered cognitive behavioral therapy and computer-administered cognitive behavioral therapy equally reduced depression, compared with patients who received no therapy (Selmi et al, 1990). For patients with sexual dysfunction who are particularly embarrassed or worried about confidentiality, a rule-based expert computer can assess and treat sexual dysfunction. It has met with high rates of patient acceptance and therapeutic response (Binik et al, 1988).

People who want to stay healthy longer in life may benefit from health-promotion computer software that can be accessed at work or at home. For example, the Stanford Health Net is an interactive computer program that provides self-care and disease prevention strategies to residents of Stanford, California. Health Net users used the program for several reasons: curiosity and a desire for general health education, help in evaluating current symptoms, and anonymity of information (Robinson, 1989). Teaching the importance of maintaining a healthy social network could be a component of such programs in the future.

OTHER ELECTRONIC DEVICES

Telephones also can be used to promote social support for special populations. In one rural community, an education and support program linked patients with AIDS by telephone conference calling to group members in their homes (Rounds et al, 1991). The program consisted of six telephone group sessions designed to increase information and social support, reduce isolation, and enhance individual coping with living with AIDS. In the future, visual display terminals on telephones will allow people to give and receive nonverbal messages. This should increase the telephone's usefulness as a vehicle for social support.

ANIMALS

Many of the beneficial effects of social support on health can be produced through animal-human bonding. To date, human–pet dog interactions have been shown to lower blood pressure and improve psychological well-being (Vormbrock and Grossberg, 1988). In the future, patients may receive a prescription to obtain a pet as routinely as they receive prescriptions for medications or special diets (Wilkes et al, 1989). Pet therapy may be especially cost-effective for people with limited mobility and those who suffer from age-related social isolation, such as the elderly. However, the benefits of human-pet bonding are likely to extend to all age groups. For example, having a pet has been shown to affect development in children. Children with pets in the home scored higher on social competency and empathy than children who did not (Poresky and Hendrix, 1990).

The presence of an animal affects not only its owner but also others in the environment. Children in wheelchairs received more social acknowledgments (such as friendly glances, smiles, and conversations) from strangers when a service dog was present than children in wheelchairs with no dog (Mader et al, 1989). This may be true because service dogs help normalize social interactions for children with disabilities.

Elderly people with pets who experience high stress made fewer calls to physicians than elderly people experiencing high stress without pets (Siegel, 1990). Dog owners, in particular, had a lower need to call a physician during stressful periods. They also reported spending more time with their pets and felt that their pets were more important to them. More than other pets, dogs provided their owners with companionship and an object of attachment.

Among nursing home residents, smiling and alertness were increased by three types of visiting programs: people alone, people with pets, and pets alone (Hendy, 1987). Six weeks after a resident dog was introduced onto the unit, staff members and nursing home residents showed a significant increase in interactive behaviors. At 22 weeks, behaviors for residents reverted to baseline levels, but remained high for staff members (Winkler et al, 1989).

Pets or animal-assisted therapy has consistently been shown to be effective in nursing homes. It should be implemented only after a careful nursing and activity assessment of the unit (Gammonley and Yates, 1991).

NURSING CARE ACTIONS

Principles and Practices

The following principles summarize nursing care related to social support:

- Social support depends on the patient's ability to attract and receive support, reciprocate support, and otherwise maintain a functioning social network. To assess these factors, the nurse must gather information about the patient's characteristics, capacities, abilities, needs, and history of using social support.
- Social support also depends on characteristics of the social network, such as size, density, proximity, and duration of relationships. The nurse must assess these factors and note the extent to which the social network can meet the patient's present needs.
- Social support problems may reside with the patient (patient barriers), the system (system barriers), or both. The nurse must analyze assessment data to determine the source(s) of the problem and plan effective care.
- To increase social support and promote improved functioning, the nurse should intervene with the patient, system, or both as needed. Interventions may include assisting with communication and networking, locating new sources of support such as a self-help group, facilitating connections and increased knowledge among network members, modifying the network's views of the patient's health problem, consulting with an agency or school system to promote better relations with the patient, and educating the community about the ability of supportive networks to promote health.
- The nurse should use outcome criteria to determine if an intervention has been successful. The overall outcome criterion for determining an intervention's effectiveness is that the patient perceives the network as more supportive and can better maintain its supportive component.

To illustrate these principles at work, consider the introductory case study. In it, the nurse assesses Becky's individual characteristics and interpersonal skills by observing her interactions in the diabetes support group. Also, the nurse listens carefully to Becky's descriptions of relationships with her high school peers and others (Fig. 29–7). From these two sources of data (observations of Becky and Becky's own descriptions), the nurse forms an assessment of Becky's ability to obtain, main-

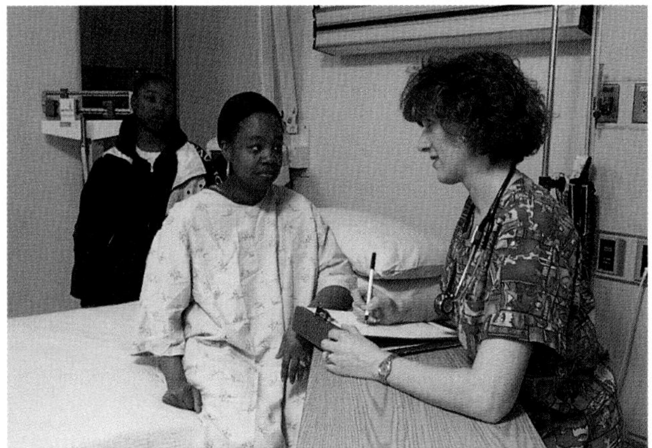

Figure 29–7. Careful assessment of a patient's social support network includes an interview, with family or other network members present if possible.

tain, and reciprocate support. Based on Becky's sadness and withdrawal from relationships since the onset of diabetes, the nurse determines that *social isolation* is an appropriate diagnosis. The nurse also decides that social support barriers exist in Becky—and her high school peers. Becky's barriers are feelings of being different, sick, and "weird," which cause her to withdraw from friends. The barriers of high school peers (the system around Becky) are peer pressure to be "normal" and discomfort with illness and differences among people. The nurse can intervene by facilitating processes in the support group that should decrease Becky's social isolation and by increasing the understanding of diabetes among the high school students. Later, the nurse will evaluate the effectiveness of these interventions by making note of Becky's emotional state, behavior, and knowledge base as expressed through her self-care behaviors.

ASSESSING A PATIENT'S SOCIAL SUPPORT

Nurses assess an individual's social network and the support it provides by gathering information about the person's individual differences, capacities, abilities, and needs (Fig. 29–8). The nurse considers whether the network is providing emotional, affirmational, informational, and tangible support to enhance the patient's physical and psychological well-being. If not, the nurse identifies any deficiencies or dysfunctions in the network or in the patient's ability to access support from, and maintain relationships in, the network.

Various tools can be used to conduct a complete social support assessment; see Box 29–1 for examples of questions to consider when interviewing a patient. To organize assessment data, the nurse may use a diagram to map the support network, as shown in Figure 29–9.

ANALYSIS

Based on the assessment data, the nurse determines whether the source of the problem is with the patient (patient barrier) or the system around the patient (system barrier). A

BOX 29–1
ASSESSING A PATIENT'S SOCIAL SUPPORT

The nurse can use these questions as a guide to assessing a patient's social support:

- Who are the patient's primary sources of support? Who are the most distant, yet still available, sources? Does the size of the support network seem adequate given the patient's situation?
- What are the network properties of the patient's sources of support? (Consider frequency of contact, density, duration of relationships, multiplexity, and recent losses.)
- What specific behaviors of support sources are supportive or nonsupportive to the patient?
- Is the patient satisfied with the perceived amount of available and enacted support?
- What other formal or informal sources of support are available but not being used by the patient? Why not?
- Are there any patient barriers or system barriers to the delivery or acceptance of social support?
- Is the patient at high risk for problems related to social support? For example, has the patient recently moved or been widowed, or is the patient elderly or mentally ill?
- Do the patient's health problems affect the availability of social support? Do they affect the social network's ability to provide support to the patient?
- What is the patient's history of using the social network during times of stress?

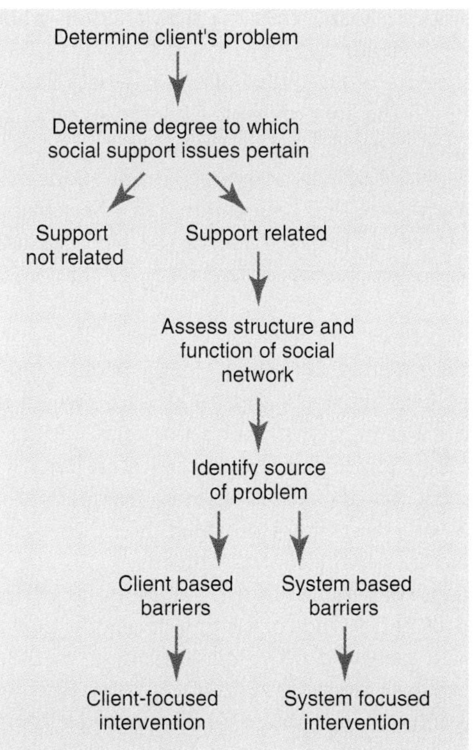

Figure 29–8. Social support assessment and intervention. (Redrawn from Pearson, R.E. [1990]. *Counseling and Social Support.* Newbury Park, CA: Sage p. 22.)

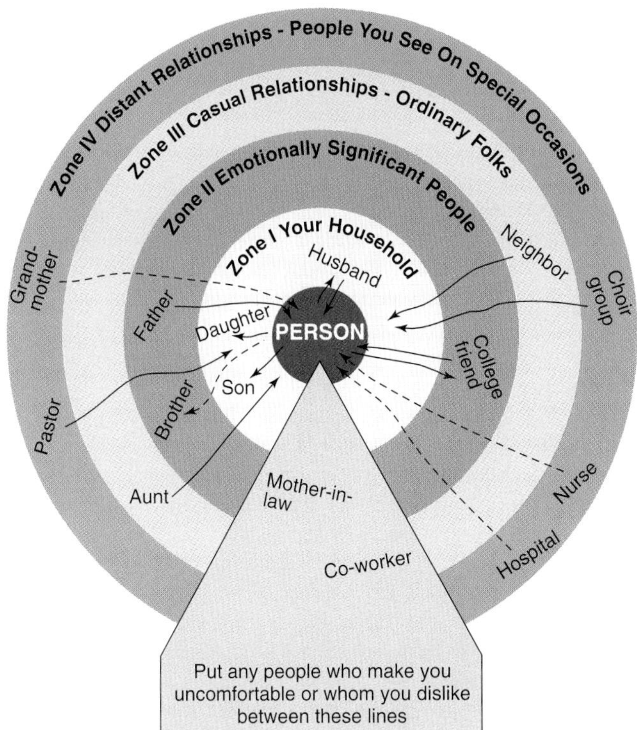

Figure 29-9. Convoy mapping. To map a patient's social network, or convoy, have the patient fill out the map below. (If the patient is ill or disabled, complete the map for him or her.) Keep in mind that a convoy map is designed to show, at a glance, the people in the patient's network as well as their frequency of contact, closeness of relationship, type of support provided, and other aspects, such as conflicted support. To demonstrate the level of support, use solid lines (representing continuous support) and dotted lines (representing intermittent support) to connect the support persons to the patient, as shown in the completed sample convoy map here. (Redrawn from Pilisuk, M., Parks, S.H. [1986]. *The Healing Web.* Hanover, NH: University Press of New England.)

patient barrier is any cause of a social support deficit caused by an individual's difficulty in developing or using supportive relationships. A *system barrier* is any cause of a social support deficit caused by a problem in the system outside of the individual, such as the support system, hospital system, school system, or family system. The nurse also determines areas of strength within the support network.

If appropriate, a nursing diagnosis can be used to guide plans for the patient's care. Two nursing diagnoses relate directly to social support: social isolation and impaired social interaction. Both have been added by the North American Nursing Diagnosis Association (NANDA) since 1980, reflecting the recent increased consideration of social support in nursing practice.

Social isolation refers to a negative state of aloneness or to dysfunctional or diminished participation in social relationships. Its defining characteristics include a social network deficit or withdrawal from social relationships, inappropriate and extreme aloneness, expressions of loneliness or rejection, and feelings of sadness or withdrawal. Many factors may contribute to social isolation: an altered physical appearance or mental status, altered health, developmental delays, and inadequate personal resources, such as those caused by financial depletion.

Impaired social interaction refers to ineffective or dysfunctional social interaction. Its defining characteristics include discomfort in social situations, dysfunctional communication patterns, or unsuccessful social behaviors. Common contributing factors include lack of knowledge of skill related to appropriate social behaviors, self-concept disturbances, and major emotional disorders.

These two diagnoses are related, and future NANDA conferences may rephrase them to increase their distinction or may consider adding a new diagnosis: *Social support deficit* (Yenny, 1990). A person with a support deficit perceives a lack of the support needed to reduce the effects of a problem. Although *Social support deficit* is not yet an official nursing diagnosis, it is currently widely used by nurses in clinical practice.

INTERVENTIONS TO ENHANCE SOCIAL SUPPORT

Based on analysis of the patient's needs, the nurse performs interventions that address the individual patient or the patient's network.

INDIVIDUAL INTERVENTIONS

As discussed earlier, nursing research on specific interventions to enhance or support social support has been limited (see Research Highlight). The following interventions have been used in research, but their effectiveness has not been determined. They are offered here as suggestions:

- conducting educational programs about social support (Gray-Toft and Anderson, 1983)
- providing surrogate support; that is, providing those activities missing from the individual's support network (Barnard et al, 1984)
- providing educational programs focusing on esteem-building, positive feedback, and affirmation (Doyle and Straub, 1985)
- using trained volunteers who offer concrete information and personal support (Vachon et al, 1980)

NETWORK INTERVENTIONS

Network intervention programs attempt to improve the functioning of the network around a person. These include:

- family systems therapy, which includes the nuclear family and significant others
- neighborhood organization, which includes the residents of a geographic area as in Neighborhood Watch programs
- system consultation, which includes members of an organization and addresses interpersonal problems that impede work productivity and satisfaction
- supportive consultation with natural helpers or volunteer linking, which includes patients or families with

RESEARCH HIGHLIGHT
INTERVENTIONS TO ENHANCE SOCIAL SUPPORT HAVE MIXED, BUT PROMISING, RESULTS

Nurse researchers have studied various types of individual interventions to enhance social support. Here are some examples.

A group of spouses of patients with cardiac disorders were taught about social support. These spouses showed better psychological well-being—and their cardiac patient spouses demonstrated better compliance with their medical regimens—than people in the control group (Gray-Toft and Anderson, 1983).

A program of surrogate support was provided for 60 new mothers who were deemed to be at risk for social support deficits because their partners were uninvolved, they had a low income, and they had few reliable family members or friends. A nurse provided surrogate support to replace that support missing from the usual support network. Each patient received a partially individualized program of support based on a structured protocol. However, only 27 of the 60 new mothers found the support useful. Some felt that they did not need the extra support; six mothers who were highly stressed reported that they could not use the support during the brief time it was offered. Researchers concluded that high-risk mothers had special needs that varied greatly, and that interventions needed to be more completely individualized (Barnard et al, 1984).

In another study, trained volunteers who were widows were offered as sources of support to women who had just experienced the loss of their spouse. These volunteers provided practical advice about community connections, supportive telephone calls, and personal contact. A control group of new widows did not have contact with the volunteers. At 6, 12, and 24 months, the new widows were evaluated for adjustment to widowhood. Those in the experimental group adjusted significantly better than those in the control group, demonstrating the effectiveness of the intervention (Vachon et al, 1980).

An educational program was provided for adults at high risk for health problems due to a combination of extensive life changes and low social support. This program included self-esteem building, feedback, and affirmation. Although the subjects did not report a perceived increase in social support, the rate of illness for the experimental group was lower than that for the control group (Doyle and Straub, 1985).

Thus, growing evidence demonstrates that interventions to enhance social support can improve health and well-being—especially when the patient's individual needs are addressed.

common concerns, such as an illness or health condition, and provides education and mutual support
- community empowerment, which includes community leaders in local task forces and forums for meeting community needs (Chapman and Pancoast, 1985; Froland et al, 1981; Pilisuk and Parks, 1986)

Nurse practitioners and other nurses in advanced practice use social support principles to treat patients with special problems, such as alcoholism or mental illness. When network therapy is appropriate, nurse therapists bring together in small groups patients' family members, coworkers, friends, professional helpers, and concerned neighbors to help the patient with problem solving. Other advanced practice nurses act as consultants for agencies, such as nursing homes or group homes, that care for specific patient populations. Consultations may facilitate the staff's understanding of social networks and social support or help the staff identify ways to enhance peer support among the patients.

EVALUATION

The nurse uses outcome criteria to evaluate the success of social support interventions. Successful social support interventions should:

- improve the patient's mental and physical health
- increase the patient's functioning
- decrease loneliness
- increase problem-solving skills
- increase communication and reciprocity among network members
- increase recognition of behaviors that are supportive and of those that are unhelpful
- increase the patient's ability to maximize supportive and minimize nonsupportive behaviors of network members
- improve the match between the patient's need for support and the social network's capacity to provide support (Stewart, 1989b)

PROCEDURES

In hospital and nursing home settings, the nurse plays an important role in monitoring a patient's social support with respect to visitors (Fig. 29–10). The nurse cannot assume that visitors are either a positive or a negative factor for the patient. Procedure 29–1 outlines nursing responsibilities for visitation.

PROCEDURE 29-1

Visitation

Objectives

- Decrease the patient's isolation and enhance sense of reliable alliance and connection within a support network
- Increase patient's motivation to maintain or regain maximum health potential
- Foster patient's coping responses, such as problem solving and use of humor
- Assess structure of network by noting composition and characteristics of visitors
- Assess function of the network by noting impact of visitors on patient
- Educate visitors about patient's condition and needs
- Motivate visitors to maximize supportive and minimize nonsupportive communications and behaviors

Terminology Specific to Skill

Type of visitor as source of support: immediate family, extended family, neighbor, friend, work or school associate, peer counselor (e.g., self-help group member), professional helper (e.g., clergy, case worker).

Type of support provided during visit: emotional, affirmational, informational, instrumental.

Critical Elements/Risk Factors

Common nonsupportive communications of visitors: discouraging ventilation, overencouraging optimism, minimizing the patient's problem, glossing over points the patient is worried about, making unhelpful comparisons (e.g., "others are worse off"), using platitudes (e.g., "tomorrow is a new day"), telling the patient that they know how he or she feels.

Reciprocity imbalance between patient and visitors: patient may experience lowered self esteem if he or she perceives self as unable to reciprocate support.

Preparation of Equipment

Not applicable.

Special Considerations

Assess needs of the individual patient

- Readiness for visitors
- Purpose of visit
- Timing and length of visit
- Type of visitor

Visiting (or lack of visitors) provides opportunity for the nurse to observe the patient in social interaction and to use these observations to determine whether a nursing diagnosis is appropriate.

Nursing Interventions

Actions	*Rationale*
1. Talk with patient about visitors prior to visit	1. To assess patient's readiness for visit and any concerns about visit or visitors
2. Talk with visitors prior to visit (Fig. 29–10)	2. To educate visitors about patient's condition and needs; to assess structure and function of the social network
3. Talk with visitors after visit	3. To elicit visitors' perception of patient's progress
4. Talk with patient about visitors after visit	4. To assess impact of the visit on the patient

Evaluation/Documentation/Reporting

Chart and Report on:

- Structure and function of visiting social network
- Impact of visit on patient
- Information about the patient learned from visitors

Compare the effect of visit with outcome criteria related to objectives for patient:

- Decreased isolation/loneliness
- Increased motivation to maximize health
- Enhanced coping
- Enhanced knowledge of resources

Compare the effect of visit with outcome criteria related to objectives for visitors:

- Increased knowledge about patient's condition, situation, and needs
- Increased understanding of supportive and nonsupportive communications and behaviors

Elements to be Included in Patient Teaching

With patient, write in members of social network on diagrams (see Fig. 29–9) to illustrate current social network. With patient, recognize supportive and nonsupportive communication patterns and behaviors of network members. With patient, identify any deficits in support, and problem-solve ways to ameliorate, such as referral to community center, self-help group, volunteer linking.

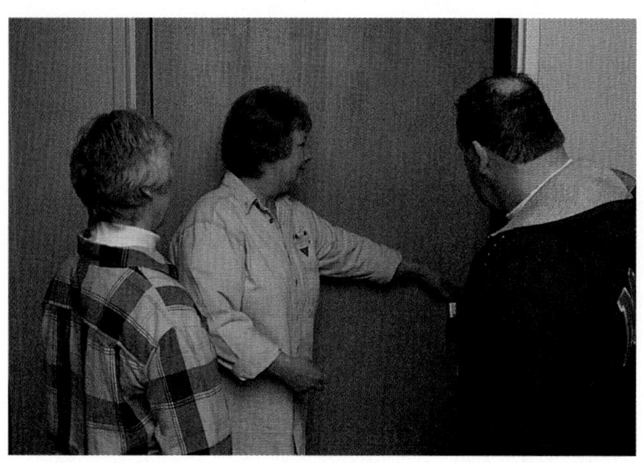

Figure 29-10. The nurse monitors visits from the patient's family members, friends, and others.

CHAPTER HIGHLIGHTS

- Knowledge of social networks and social support plays a central role in contemporary nursing practice. Research has shown that social support reduces stress, promotes coping, and is associated with decreased morbidity and mortality.
- Social support is defined as the interpersonal transactions among members of a social network in which reciprocal information and spontaneous exchange of beneficial supplies occur.
- Social support consists of emotional support, appraisal support, informational support, and instrumental support.
- Age, developmental status, spirituality, culture and ethnicity, family status, and gender influence the effects of social support
- Assessment of an individual's social network and support includes the person's unique characteristics, capacities, abilities, and needs.
- Nursing actions include both individual interventions and network interventions.

REFERENCES

Ader, R. (ed.) (1980). *Psychoneuroimmunology.* New York: Academic Press.

Ahmadi, K.S. (1985). The experience of being hospitalized: Stress, social support and satisfaction. *International Journal of Nursing Studies, 22,* 137–148.

Ambert, A. (1988). Relationships with former in-laws after divorce: A research note. *Journal of Marriage and the Family, 50,* 679–686.

Antonucci, T. (1989). Social support and social relations. In R. Bristock and L. Georg (eds.): *The Handbook of Aging and the Social Sciences.* Orlando: Academic Press.

Archbold, P.G., Stewart, B.J., Harvath, T., Greenlick, M.R. (1990). Mutuality and preparedness as predictors of caregiver role strain. *Research in Nursing and Health, 13,* 375–384.

Barnard, K., Snyder, C., Spietz, A. (1984). Supportive measures for high-risk infants and families. In K. Barnard, P. Brandt, B. Raff, and P. Carroll (eds.): *Social Support and Families of Vulnerable Infants.* New York: March of Dimes Birth Defects Foundation, pp. 291–315.

Barrera, M. (1986). Distinctions between social support concepts, measures, and models. *American Journal of Community Psychology, 14* (4), 413–445.

Binik, Y.M., Servan-Schreiber, S., Freiwald, S., Hall, K.S. (1988). Intelligent computer-based assessment and psychotherapy: An expert system for sexual dysfunction. *Journal of Nervous and Mental Disease, 176* (7), 387–400.

Boyce, W.T. (1985). Social support, family relations, and children. In S. Cohen and S.L. Syme (eds.): *Social Support and Health.* Orlando: Academic Press, pp. 151–173.

Brandt, P.A., Weinert, C. (1981). The PRQ-A social support measure. *Nursing Research, 30,* 277–280.

Brock, A., O'Sullivan, P. (1985). A study to determine what variables predict institutionalization of elderly people. *Journal of Advanced Nursing, 10,* 533–537.

Brown, D.R., Gary, L.E. (1985). Social support network differentials among married and nonmarried females. *Psychology of Women Quarterly, 9,* 229–241.

Burgess, A.W., Holmstrom, L.L. (1978). Recovery from rape and prior life stress. *Research in Nursing and Health, 1,* 165–174.

Caplan, G. (1974). *Support Systems and Community Mental Health.* New York: Behavioral Publications.

Cassell, J. (1976). The contribution of the social environment to host resistance. *American Journal of Epidemiology, 104,* 107–123.

Chapman, N., Pancoast, D. (1985). Working with the informal helping networks of the elderly: The experience of three programs. *Journal of Social Issues, 41,* 47–63.

Chiriboga, D.A., Jenkins, G., Bailey, J. (1983). Stress and coping among hospice nurses: Test of an analytic model. *Nursing Research, 32,* 294–299.

Cobb, S. (1976). Social support as a moderator of life stress. *Psychosomatic Medicine, 38,* 300–314.

Colby, K.M., Gould, R.L., Aronson, G. (1989). Some pros and cons of computer-assisted psychotherapy. *Journal of Nervous and Mental Disease, 177* (2), 105–108.

Cranley, M. (1984). Social support as a factor in the development of parents' attachment to their unborn. In K. Barnard, P. Brandt, B. Raff, and P. Carroll (eds.): *Social Support and Families of Vulnerable Infants.* New York: March of Dimes Birth Defects Foundation, pp. 99–109.

Crittenden, P.M. (1985). Social networks, quality of child rearing, and child development. *Child Development, 54,* 1299–1313.

Cronenwett, L. (1984). Social networks and social support of primigravida mothers and fathers. In K. Barnard, P. Brandt, B. Raff, and P. Carroll (eds.): *Social Support and Families of Vulnerable Infants.* New York: March of Dimes Birth Defects Foundation, pp. 167–186.

Cronenwett, L. (1985a). Network structure, social support, and psychological outcomes of pregnancy. *Nursing Research, 34* (2), 93–99.

Cronenwett, L. (1985b). Parental network structure and perceived support after birth of first child. *Nursing Research, 34* (6), 347–352.

Cronin-Stubbs, D., Brophy, E. (1985). Burnout: Can social support save the psychiatric nurse? *Journal of Psychosocial Nursing, 23* (7), 9–13.

Cronin-Stubbs, D., Rooks, C.A. (1985). The stress, social support and burnout of critical care nurses: The results of research. *Heart and Lung, 14,* 31–39.

deLaszlo, V.S. (1959). *The Basic Writings of C.G. Jung.* New York: Random House.

De Man, A., Labreche-Gauthier, L. (1991). Suicide ideation and community supports: An evaluation of two programs. *Journal of Clinical Psychology, 47* (1), 57–60.

Depner, C.E., and Ingersoll-Dayton, B. (1985). Conjugal social support: Patterns in later life. *Journal of Gerontology, 40,* 761–766.

Dimond, J. (1979). Social support and adaptation to chronic illness: The case of maintenance dialysis. *Research in Nursing and Health, 2,* 101–108.

Doyle, E., Straub, V. (1985). An intervention to improve social supports in a high risk population. In R. O'Brien (ed.): *Social Support and Health: New Directions for Theory Development and Research* (Proceedings). New York: University of Rochester, pp. 221–224.

Ellison, E. (1983). Social networks and the mental health caregiving system: Implications for psychiatric nursing practice. *Journal of Psychiatric Nursing and Mental Health Services, 21* (2), 18–24.

Erickson, G. (1984). A framework and themes for social network intervention. *Family Process, 23,* 187–198.

Fischer, C. (1982). *To Dwell Among Friends. Personal Networks in Town and City.* Chicago: University of Chicago Press.

Friedman, M. (1985). The impact of stress and social support on family conflict among Anglo and Latino families with childhood cancer. In R. O'Brien (ed.): *Social Support and Health: New Directions for Theory and Research* (Proceedings). New York: University of Rochester, pp. 180–184.

Froland, C., Pancoast, D.L., Chapman, N.J., Kimboko, P.J. (1981). *Helping Networks and Human Services.* Beverly Hills, CA: Sage.

Gammonley, J., Yates, J. (1991). Pet projects: Animal assisted therapy in nursing homes. *Journal of Gerontological Nursing, 17* (1), 12–15.

Gerstel, N. (1988). Divorce and kin ties: The importance of gender. *Journal of Marriage and the Family, 50,* 209–219.

Gottlieb, B. (1985). Marshalling and augmenting social support of medical patients and their families. In R. O'Brien (ed.): *Social Support and Health: New Directions for Theory and Research* (Proceedings). New York: University of Rochester, pp. 107–148.

Gottlieb, B.H. (1978). The development and application of a classification scheme of informal helping behaviors. *Canadian Journal of Behavioral Science, 10,* 105–115.

Gray-Toft, P., Anderson, J. (1983). A hospital support program: Design and evaluation. *International Journal of Nursing Studies, 20,* 137–147.

Hall, A., Wellman, B. (1985). Social networks and social support. In S. Cohen and S.L. Syme (eds.): *Social Support and Health.* Orlando: Academic Press, pp. 23–41.

Heitzmann, C.A., Kaplan R.M. (1988). Assessment of methods for measuring social support. *Health Psychology, 7* (1), 75–109.

Heller, K., Thompson, M., Trueba, P., Hogg, J., Vlachos-Weber, I. (1991). Peer support telephone dyads for elderly women: Was this the wrong intervention? *American Journal of Community Psychology, 19*(1), 53–74.

Henderson, V. (1964). The nature of nursing. *American Journal of Nursing, 64* (8), 62–68.

Henderson, V. (1979). In a technologic age. *Nursing Times, 75* (48), 2056–2058.

Henderson, V. (1985). The essence of nursing in high technology. *Nursing Administration Quarterly, 9* (4), 1–9.

Hendy, H.M. (1987). Effects of pet and/or people visits on nursing home residents. *International Journal of Aging and Human Development, 25* (4), 279–291.

Hentinen, M. (1983). Need for instruction and support of the wives of patients with myocardial infarction. *Journal of Advanced Nursing, 8,* 519–524.

Hermansen-Williams, M. (1990). The self-help movement in head injury. *Rehabilitation Nursing, 15*(6), 311–315.

Hewat, R.J., Ellis, D.J. (1984). Breastfeeding as a maternal-child team effort: Women's perceptions. *Health Care for Women International, 5,* 437–452.

Hirsch, B.J. (1980). Natural support systems and coping with major life changes. *American Journal of Community Psychology, 8,* 159–172.

House, J.S. (1981). *Work Stress and Social Support.* Reading, MA: Addison-Wesley.

Hubbard, P., Muhlenkamp, P.A., Brown, N. (1984). The relationship between social support and self-care practices. *Nursing Research, 33,* 266–270.

Jackson, B. (1985). Role of social resource variables on life satisfaction in black climacteric hysterectomized women. *Nursing Papers, 17,* 4–22.

Johnson, C.L. (1988). Postdivorce reorganization of relationships between divorcing children and their parents. *Journal of Marriage and the Family, 50,* 221–231.

Jones, M. (1953). *The Therapeutic Community: A New Treatment Method in Psychiatry.* New York: Basic Books.

Jones, M. (1968). *Beyond the Therapeutic Community: Social Learning and Social Psychiatry.* New Haven: Yale University Press.

Kahn, R.L. (1979). Aging and social support. In M.W. Riley (ed.): *Aging from Birth to Death: Interdisciplinary Perspectives.* Boulder, CO: Westview Press, pp. 77–99.

Kahn, R.L., Antonucci, T.C. (1980). Convoys over the life course: Attachment, roles and social support. In P.B. Baltes and O.G. Brim Jr. (eds.): *Life-Span Development and Behavior,* Vol. 3. New York: Academic Press, pp. 253–286.

Kahn, R.L., Antonucci, T.C. (1984). Social supports of the elderly: Family, friends, professionals. Final report to the National Institute on Aging, Grant No. AG1632-01.

Kitson, G., Lopata, H., Holmes, W., Meyering, S. (1980). Divorcees and widows: Similarities and differences. *American Journal of Orthopsychiatry, 50,* 291–301.

Klinger, M. (1984). Compliance and the post-MI patient. *The Canadian Nurse, 81* (7), 32–38.

Lasching, S. (1984). The relationship of social support to health in elderly people. *Western Journal of Nursing Research, 6,* 341–350.

Lazarus, R., Folkman, S. (1984). *Stress, Appraisal, and Coping.* New York: Springer.

Lee, G.R. (1988). Marital intimacy among older persons: The spouse as confidant. *Journal of Family Issues, 9,* 273–284.

Lindsey, A., Dodd, M.J., Chen, S. (1985). Social support networks of Taiwanese cancer patients. *International Journal of Nursing Students, 22* (2), 149–164.

Lindsey, A., Hughes, E. (1981). Social support and alternatives to institutionalization for the at-risk elderly. *Journal of the American Geriatrics Society, 29,* 308–315.

MacFarland, G., Wasli, E. (1986). *Nursing Diagnoses and Process in Psychiatric Mental Health Nursing.* Philadelphia: J.B. Lippincott.

McLane, A.M. (ed.). (1987). Classification of nursing diagnosis: Proceedings of the 7th conference. St. Louis: C.V. Mosby.

Mader, B., Hart, L.A., Bergin, B. (1989). Social acknowledgements for children with disabilities: Effects of service dogs. *Child Development, 60* (6), 1529–1534.

Mercer, R.T., Hackley, K.C., Bostrom, A. (1983). Relationship of psychosocial and perinatal variables to perception of childbirth. *Nursing Research, 32,* 202–207.

Mercer, R.T., Hackley, K.C., Bostrom, A. (1984a). Social support of teenage mothers. *Birth Defects: Original Article Series, 20,* 245–290.

Mercer, R.T., Hackley, K.C., Bostrom, A. (1984b). Social support of teenage mothers. In K. Barnard, P. Brandt, B. Raff, and P. Carroll (eds.): *Social Support and Families of Vulnerable Infants.* New York: March of Dimes Birth Defects Foundation, pp. 245–272.

Minami, H. (1989). Cross cultural view of social support. Keynote address: Second International Nursing Research Conference on Social Support (pp. 1–10) (Proceedings). San Francisco, CA: University of California San Francisco School of Nursing.

Mishel, M.H., Braden, C.J. (1987). Uncertainty: A mediator between support and adjustment. *Western Journal of Nursing Research, 9, 43–57.*

Murphy, S. (1987). Self-efficacy and social support: Mediation of stress and mental health following a natural disaster. *Western Journal of Nursing Research, 9,* 58–86.

Nikolaisen, S., Williams, R. (1980). Parents' view of support following the loss of their infant to sudden infant death syndrome. *Western Journal of Nursing Research, 2,* 593–601.

Norbeck, J. (1982). The use of social support in clinical practice. *Journal of Psychosocial Nursing and Mental Health Services, 20* (12), 22–29.

Norbeck, J., Sheiner, M. (1982). Sources of social support related to single parent functioning. *Research in Nursing and Health, 5,* 3–12.

Norbeck, J. (1985a). Types and sources of social support for managing job stress in critical care nursing. *Nursing Research, 34* (4), 225–230.

Norbeck, J. (1985b). *Perceived Job Stress, Job Satisfaction and Psychological Symptoms in Critical Care Nursing.* (Report No. 0160-6891/55-030253-07.) Dallas: American Association of Critical Care Nurses National Teaching Institute.

Norbeck, J., Barnes, L. (1988). Social support. In H. Wilson and C. Kneisl (eds.): *Psychiatric Nursing,* 3rd ed. Menlo Park, CA: Addison-Wesley, pp. 148–167.

Norbeck, J.S. (1988a). Social support. *Annual Review of Nursing Research, 6,* 85–109. New York: Springer.

Norbeck, J.S. (1988b). Challenges in social support research. The Eighth Helen Nahm Research Lecture. University of California School of Nursing, San Francisco.

Norbeck, J.S., Lindsey, A.M., Carrieri, V.L. (1981). The development of an instrument to measure social support. *Nursing Research, 30,* 264–269.

Norbeck, J.S., Lindsey, A.M., Carrieri, V.L. (1983). Further development of the Norbeck social support questionnaire: Normative data and validity testing. *Nursing Research, 32,* 4–9.

Norbeck, J.S., Tilden, V.P. (1988). International nursing research in social support: Theoretical and methodological issues. *Journal of Advanced Nursing, 13,* 173–178.

Norbeck, J.S., Tilden, V.P. (1983). Life stress, social support and emotional disequilibrium in complications of pregnancy: A prospective multivariate study. *Journal of Health and Social Behavior, 24,* 30–46.

Northouse, L. (1981). Mastectomy patients and the fear of cancer recurrence. *Cancer Nursing, 4,* 213–220.

Nuckolls, K.B., Cassel, J., Kaplan, B.H. (1972). Psychosocial assets, life crisis and the prognosis of pregnancy. *American Journal of Epidemiology, 95,* 431–441.

O'Brian, M.E. (1980). Hemodialysis regimen compliance and social environment: A panel analysis. *Nursing Research, 29,* 250–255.

O'Brien, R. (1985). Social support and health maintenance during early bereavement. In R. O'Brien (ed.): *Social support and health: New directions for theory development and research* (Proceedings). New York: University of Rochester, pp. 203–207.

Pagel, M., Erdly, W., Becker, J. (1987). Social networks: We get by with (and in spite of) a little help from our friends. *Journal of Personality and Social Psychology, 12, 37–52.*

Pearlin, L.I. (1985). Social structure and processes of social support. In S. Cohen and S.L. Syme (eds.): *Social Support and Health.* Orlando: Academic Press, pp. 43–60.

Pearson, R. (1990). *Counseling and Social Support.* Newbury Park, CA: Sage.

Peters-Golden, H. (1982). Breast cancer: Varied perceptions of social support in the illness experience. *Social Science and Medicine, 16,* 483–491.

Pilisuk, M., Parks, S.H. (1986). *The Healing Web: Social Networks and Human Survival.* Hanover, NH: University Press of New England.

Poresky, R.H., Hendrix, C. (1990). Differential effects of pet presence and pet-bonding on young children. *Psychological Reports, 67* (1), 51–54.

Powers, B. (1985). Social networks, social support, and elderly institutionalized people. In R. O'Brien (ed.): *Social Support and Health: New Directions for Theory Development and Research* (Proceedings). New York: University of Rochester, pp. 190–193.

Robinson, T.N. (1989). Community health behavior change through computer network health promotion: Preliminary findings from Stanford Health-Net. *Computer Methods and Programs in Biomedicine, 30* (2–3), 137–144.

Rook, K. (1984). The negative side of social interactions: Impact on psychological well-being. *Journal of Personality and Social Psychology, 46* (5), 1097–1108.

Ross, C.E., Mirowsky, J., Goldsteen, K. (1991). The impact of the family on health: The decade in review. In A. Booth (ed.): *Contemporary Families: Looking Forward, Looking Back.* Minneapolis, MN: National Council of Family Relations, pp. 341–360.

Rounds, K.A., Galinsky, M.J., Stevens, L.S. (1991). Linking people with AIDS in rural communities: The telephone group. *Social Work, 36* (1), 13–18.

Rubin, L. (1984). *Intimate Strangers: Men and Women Together.* New York: Harper and Row.

Sarason, I., Sarason, B., Shearin, E. (1986). Social support as an individual difference variable: Its stability, origins, and relational aspects. *Journal of Personality and Social Psychology, 50,* 845–855.

Schulz, R., Rau, M.T. (1985). Social support through the life course. In S. Cohen and S.L. Syme (eds.): *Social support and health.* Orlando: Academic Press, pp. 129–149.

Selmi, P.M., Klein, M.H., Greist, et al (1990). Computer-administered cognitive-behavioral therapy for depression. *American Journal of Psychiatry, 147* (1), 51–56.

Siegel, J.M. (1990). Stressful life events and use of physician services among the elderly: The moderating role of pet ownership. *Journal of Personality and Social Psychology, 58* (6), 1081–1086.

Slack, W.V., Porter, D., Balkin, P., et al (1990). Computer-assisted soliloquy as an approach to psychotherapy. *MD Computing, 7* (1), 37–42.

Stewart, M.J. (1989a). Social support instruments created by nurse investigators. *Nursing Research, 38* (5), 268–275.

Stewart, M. (1989b). Social support intervention studies: A review and prospective of nursing contributions. *International Journal of Nursing Studies, 26* (2), 93–114.

Stewart, M. (1989c). Target populations of nursing research on social support. *International Journal of Nursing Studies, 26* (2), 115–129.

Stewart, M. (1990). From provider to partner: A conceptual framework for nursing education based on primary health care premises. *Advances in Nursing Sciences, 12* (2), 9–27.

Stoller, E.P. (1985). Exchange patterns in the informal support networks of the elderly: The impact of reciprocity on morale. *Journal of Marriage and the Family, 47,* 335–342.

Storm, H. (1972). *Seven Arrows.* New York: Ballantine.

Taylor, R.J. (1988). Structural determinants of religious participation among Black Americans. *Review of Religious Research, 30,* 114–125.

Taylor, R.J., Chatters, L.M., Tucker, M.B., Lewis, E. (1991). Development in research on Black families: A decade review. In A. Booth (ed.): *Contemporary Families: Looking Forward, Looking Back.* Minneapolis: National Council on Family Relations, pp. 275–296.

Taylor, R.L., Lam, D.J., Roppel, C.E., Barter, J.T. (1984). Friends can be good medicine: An excursion into mental health promotion. *Community Mental Health Journal, 20* (4), 294–303.

Tilden, V.P. (1985a). Cross cultural perspectives of nursing research in social support. *Closing Address for the 1st International Nursing Conference on Social Support,* Tel Aviv, Israel.

Tilden, V.P. (1985b). Issues in conceptualization and measurement of social support in the construction of nursing theory. *Research in Nursing and Health, 8,* 199–206.

Tilden, V.P., Galyen, R.D. (1987). Cost and conflict: The darker side of social support. *Western Journal of Nursing Research, 9* (1), 9–16.

Tilden, V.P., Nelson, C.A., May, B.A. (1990a). Use of qualitative methods to enhance content validity. *Nursing Research, 39* (3), 172–175.

Tilden, V.P., Nelson, C.A., May, B.A. (1990b). The IPR Inventory: Development and psychometric characteristics. *Nursing Research, 39* (6), 337–343.

Tilden, V.P., Weinert, C. (1987). Social support and the chronically ill. *Nursing Clinics of North America, 22* (3), 613–619.

Turner, S. (1979). Disability among schizophrenics in a rural community: Services and social support. *Research in Nursing and Health, 2,* 151–161.

Vachon, M., Lyall, W., Rogers, J., et al (1980). A controlled study of self-help intervention for widows. *American Journal of Psychiatry, 137,* 1380–1384.

Van Meter, M.S., Haynes, O.M., Kropp, J.P. (1987). The negative social work network: When friends are foes. *Child Welfare League of America, 66* (1), 69–75.

Vega, W.A. (1991). Hispanic families in the 1980s: A decade of research. In A. Booth (ed.): *Contemporary Families: Looking Forward, Looking Back.* Minneapolis: National Council on Family Relations, pp. 270–306.

Veroff, J., Kulka, R.A., Douvan, E. (1981). *Mental Health in America: Patterns of Help-Seeking from 1957 to 1976.* New York: Basic Books.

Vormbrock, J.K., Grossberg, J.M. (1988). Cardiovascular effects of human-pet dog interactions. *Journal of Behavioral Medicine, 11* (5), 509–517.

Webb, C., Wilson-Barnett, J. (1983). Hysterectomy: A study in coping with recovery. *Journal of Advanced Nursing, 8,* 311–319.

Weinert, C. (1987). A social support measure: PRQ85. *Nursing Research, 36,* 273–277.

Weiss, R. (1974). The provision of social support. In Z. Rubin (ed.). *Doing unto Others.* Englewood Cliffs, NJ: Prentice-Hall.

Wilcox, B.L. (1981). Social support in adjusting to marital disruption: A network analysis. In B.H. Gottlieb (ed.): *Social Networks and Social Support.* Beverly Hills, CA: Sage, pp. 98–115.

Wilkes, C.N., Shalko, T.K., Trahan, M. (1989). Pet Rx: Implication for good health. *Health Education, 20* (2), 6–9.

Wills, T.A. (1985). Supportive functions of interpersonal relationships. In S. Cohen, and S.L. Syme (eds.): *Social Support and Health.* Orlando: Academic Press, pp. 61–82.

Wills, T.A., Weiss, R.L., Patterson, G.R. (1974). A behavioral analysis of the determinants of marital satisfaction. *Journal of Consulting and Clinical Psychology, 42,* 802–811.

Winkler, A., Fairnie, H., Gericevich, F., Long, M. (1989). The impact of a resident dog on an institution for the elderly: Effects on perceptions and social interactions. *Gerontologist, 29* (2), 216–223.

Woods, N., Earp, J. (1978). Women with cured breast cancer. *Nursing Research, 27,* 279–285.

Worthouse, L. (1988). Social support in patients' and husbands' adjustment to breast cancer. *Nursing Research, 37,* 91–97.

Wortman, C.B., Conway, T.L. (1985). The role of social support in adaptation and recovery from physical illness. In S. Cohen and S.L. Syme (eds.): *Social Support and Health.* Orlando: Academic Press, pp. 281–302.

Wortman, C.B., Lehman, D.R. (1985). Reactions to victims of life crises: Support attempts that fail. In I. Sarason and B. Sarason (eds.): *Social Support: Theory, Research, and Applications.* Dordrecht, Netherlands: Martinus Nijhoff, pp. 463–489.

Yenny, S. (1990). Development and validation of a new nursing diagnosis: Social support deficit. Unpublished master's thesis, Creighton University, Omaha, NE.

Zachariah, R. (1985). Intergenerational attachment and psychological well-being during pregnancy. In R. O'Brien (ed.): *Social Support and Health: New Directions for Theory and Research* (Proceedings). New York: University of Rochester, pp. 168–174.

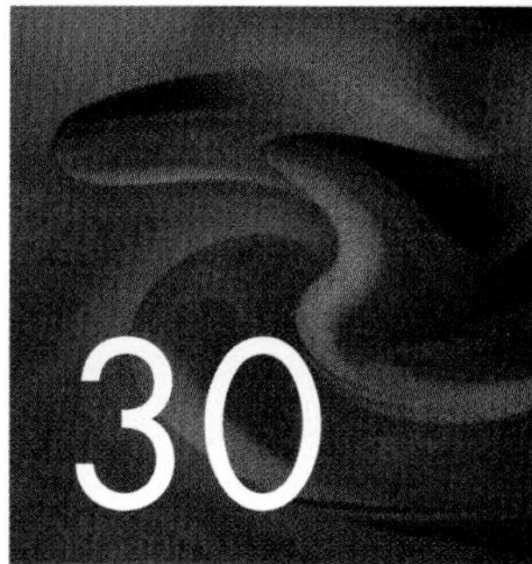

Environment and Health

Margaret Ovitt

With contributions by Margaret Topf, PhD, RN, Associate Professor; School of Nursing, University of Colorado Health Sciences Center

Mr. T., age 65, was admitted to a hospital intensive care unit with an acute asthmatic attack. After the acute asthmatic crisis had been resolved, he was transferred to the general medical unit. His room is across from the nurses' station, and the lights from the station are on all the time. The window in his room is small and looks out onto another hospital wing. He cannot see out of it anyway, because the curtains are always pulled between his bed and his roommate's. The temperature of the room is about 72°F. Mr. T.'s blanket is not always tucked in and is removed or moved aside whenever care is administered. Mr. T. hears numerous sounds close by and in the background, many of which he cannot identify. These include staff talking, the telephone ringing, IV alarms, paging system in the hallway, a baby crying, equipment being dropped, the ice machine, a computer printer, cellular phones, and so forth. Although his condition has improved, Mr. T. is still occasionally short of breath. This, in combination with unidentified sounds, increases his level of anxiety. He has trouble getting a good night's sleep, and as his stay progresses, he becomes increasingly confused and has trouble remembering things. He forgets where he is and what time of day it is, although he knows who he is and recognizes staff. He improves rapidly when the nurses begin taking him outside in the afternoons.

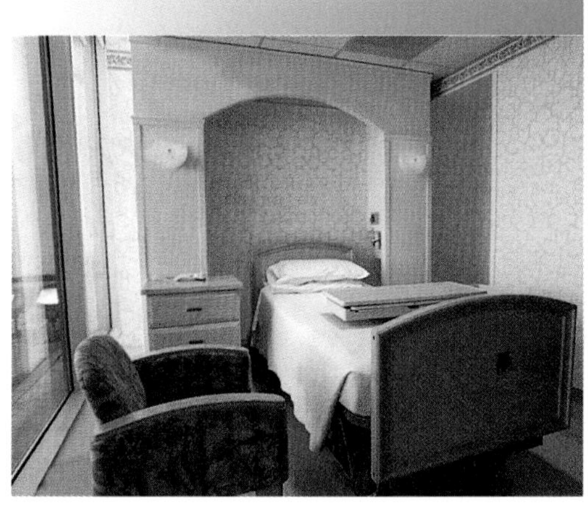

OBJECTIVES

After studying this chapter, the student will be able to:

- **assess the impact of various environmental pollutants on health of patients**
- **evaluate both the workplace environment of adults and the play environments of children for potential hazards**
- **intervene when the physical environment has real or potential negative health effects on patients**
- **educate patients about the need for following preventive health measures to lessen or nullify the harmful effects of the environment**
- **perform a nursing procedure for at least one potential ambient stressor for patients**

SCOPE OF NURSING PRACTICE

Historically, the physical environment as it affected patient care was of great importance in nursing practice. Nightingale discussed at length the impact of fresh air, control of noise, cleanliness, natural light and views, warmth, and an orderly environment on the health of the patient.

Williams (1988) noted that as infection control, heating, and construction methods of hospitals have improved, and as the maintenance and housekeeping tasks have been delegated to non-nursing personnel, nursing practice became less directly involved with environmental concerns. Now the problems facing the nurse with respect to patient care and the physical environment include the global environment and its impact on the health of individuals and populations, as well as the impact of the built environment on health.

The physical environment contains both natural and manmade elements (Williams, 1988), and this chapter discusses impacts of the manmade as it applies to hospital unit design and of the natural such as air, water, and environmental quality issues.

Community-based nurses, such as nurses working in home care and public health settings, are fortunate in that they can observe the patient in his or her home. If the patient has a history of upper respiratory illnesses, then the nurse knows to inquire about pollution. Is there a factory nearby? Does someone in the household smoke? Are there smog alerts and does the patient take appropriate precautions? Is there a history of asthma? What is the patient's occupation?

Nurses who work in industry are constantly monitoring the effects of the environment (such factors as noise and air pollution and exposure to chemicals) on workers' health, as well as assessing the overall safety of the workplace. In urban hospitals, nurses who work in emergency departments (EDs) and outpatient services notice an increase in patients with a history of chronic pulmonary disease and asthma presenting with acute respiratory conditions during smog alerts or just during periods of warm weather. Assessment of the patient's condition is very important, as it is not unusual for a patient with asthma to underestimate how quickly this crisis can progress.

Contaminants are not restricted to the outside air. Neurotoxic symptoms from eating contaminated fish or being exposed to formaldehydes and other vapors associated with the building industry can also be seen in the office or ED patients.

Finally, if the patient is hospitalized, the hospital's physical environment affects the patient in yet another way. A patient must adjust to unfamiliar technology and terminology of the modern medical environment. Routines of daily life are scrambled, and there are no familiar sites or sights to help one find one's way. Diurnal rhythms are upset. And the patient does not feel well. The nurse has the opportunity to help the patient on many levels when the principles as laid out in this chapter are put into practice.

KNOWLEDGE BASE

Basic Science of Environmental Health

Hazards associated with environmental health affect all aspects of life and nursing practice. Thousands of new chemical compounds have been introduced into the environment since the early 1950s. It is estimated that 72,000 chemicals are now used in commerce (including food additives, drugs, cosmetics, and pesticides). Many of the chemicals have had limited testing for their effect on humans. The Surgeon General's Report on Health Promotion and Disease Prevention in 1979 indicated that there were virtually no major chronic diseases that were not affected by environmental factors. The link between environmental hazards and adverse health effects has been established. Environmental hazards can be found in health care settings, homes, work places, and in the community. There are several pathways: air, water, soil, and food. Routes of exposure include inhalation such as dust or fumes, soil, and water; ingestion such as pesticides, or microorganisms; and radiation (such as sun and manmade toxic materials) (Institute of Medicine, 1995).

Several systems for classifying environmental hazards have been proposed. Table 30–1 illustrates a system of classifying hazards recommended by the Institute of Medicine (1995). Also see Chapter 18 for additional information relating to environmental hazards. The major environmental hazards associated with nursing practice include air pollution, water pollution, noise pollution, and other factors such as light and temperature control.

AIR POLLUTION

The respiratory system contains the structures that extract oxygen from the air and expel the waste product carbon dioxide from the body. Poor environmental air quality can have a significant effect on this basic physiologic function. Normally, the lungs expand to fill with air and, during expiration, contract to expel waste products. In persons with abnormal airway resistance such as asthma or increased lung size as in emphysema, the normal air exchange functions are compromised. Chemical irritants can cause the constriction of the smooth muscles of the airways, thus narrowing the airway openings in order to prevent such compounds reaching normal lungs. But in an asthmatic, for example, who already has increased difficulty in inhalation due to abnormally narrowed airways, the chemicals in smog can cause airways to shut down completely. Also, certain lifestyle choices such as smoking tobacco can compromise respiratory system function to such a degree that air pollution that would normally be just an irritation can trigger an acute respiratory episode requiring treatment and possibly hospitalization. Of all the bodily systems, the respiratory system is the most seriously affected by air pollution.

Air pollutants can be either gases or particulates (small separate particles), and particulates can be solid or liquid (Philp,

TABLE 30-1 Examples of Environmental Health Hazards

Area	Problems
Living problems	Environmental tobacco smoke
	Noise exposure
	Urban crowding
	Residential lead-based paint
Work hazards	Toxic substances
	Machine-operating hazards
	Repetitive motion injuries
	Carcinogenic work exposures
Atmospheric quality	Greenhouse gases and global warming
	Depletion of the ozone layer
	Aerial spraying of herbicides and pesticides
	Acid rain
Water quality	Contamination by human waste
	Oil and chemical spills in waterways
	Pesticide/herbicide contamination of groundwater and runoff to local waterways
	Aquifer contamination by industrial pollutants
	Toxic contamination of fish and seafood
Housing	Rodent and insect infestations
	Particulates from woodburning stoves
	Houses and buildings with poor ventilation systems—sick building syndrome
	Off-gases from carpets and plastics used in home construction
Food quality	Bacterial contaminants
	Pesticide residues on fruits and vegetables
	Disruption of food chain by pollutants
	Chemical food additives
	Hormone supplements and antibiotic residues in animal food products
Waste control	Use of nonbiodegradable products
	Contamination of air, soil, and waters due to poorly designed solid waste dumps and inadequate sewage systems
	Transport and storage of hazardous waste
	Illegal dumping of industrial waste
	Abandoned hazardous waste sites (including Superfund sites)
Radiation	Nuclear facility emissions
	Radioactive nuclear waste
	Radon gas seepage in homes and schools
	Nuclear testing
	Excessive exposure to x-rays
	Ultraviolet radiation (UVB) due to global depletion of stratospheric ozone
Violence	Proliferation of handguns
	Pervasive images of violence in the media
	Violent acts against women and children
	Excessive incidents of violence in work places, schools, and community settings

Data from Institute of Medicine, 1995.

1995). Pollution can result from human activities and from natural sources. Historically, air pollutants such as dust, soot, smoke (including tobacco smoke), caustic soda (sodium hydroxide, NaOH), and acids (sulfuric acid, H_2SO_4; hydrochloric acid, HCl) have been recognized as having deleterious effects on human health (Dubos, 1977). Certain occupations, such as coal and bauxite mining, are also known to cause health problems from inhalation of particulate matter. During the past 20 years, organic compounds such as carbon dioxide (CO_2), which is emitted when gasoline or coal is burned, methane (formed by decomposing landfills and vented to the air), chlorofluorocarbons (CFCs), polycyclic aromatic hydrocarbons (PAHs), polychlorinated biphenyls (PCBs), and dioxins have become the main concerns of those who monitor air quality.

When air pollutants accumulate to form smog (a term derived from the words "smoke" and "fog"), health consequences can be serious, sometimes even fatal. Smog is a term that describes a mixture of gaseous and particulate pollutants and is visible as a sort of brownish-yellow haze mainly over cities. Smog is held close to the ground during a thermal inversion (the trapping of cold air under a layer of warm air). Normally, updrafts of the warm air at the ground rise toward the cooler air above, keeping pollutants from concentrating at ground level. During an inversion, a cold layer of air is trapped by a warm layer that has formed at a high altitude. Pollutants are concentrated at the ground, where they cause various kinds of problems.

Most people are aware of the irritation of the eyes and mucous membranes that occurs during a "smog alert," when air pollutants reach hazardous levels. People at greatest risk during smog alerts are the very young and the elderly, as well as those with cardiopulmonary disease and heavy smokers. Acute effects include irritations as mentioned above as well as respiratory irritation. Chronic effects can result in or aggravate chronic bronchitis, bronchial asthma, and pulmonary emphysema.

Tests have consistently revealed that exposure to air pollutants invariably causes disturbances in respiratory rates and increased pulmonary flow resistance. Such exposure slows down or stops the beating motion of the cilia in the respiratory passages, just like what happens in the bronchi of smokers. So for people with an existing pulmonary pathology, air pollution is a serious matter, and the advice to stay indoors during a smog alert is crucial. Even with precautions, however, people can develop an acute respiratory crisis and need to be hospitalized for treatment.

Ozone (O_3) is a major part of photochemical smog and a potent respiratory irritant (Bates, 1994). Ozone occurs naturally in the stratosphere to provide a protective layer high above the earth, but at the ground level, it is highly unstable and poisonous and the prime ingredient of smog. Levels as low as 1 part per million (ppm) are lethal in 6 hours for laboratory animals made to exercise for a few minutes each hour. Human volunteers exposed to 3 to 6 ppm by weight also exhibit symptoms. These include headache, chest pain and a marked decrease in vital capacity after 1 hour (Dubos, 1982).

Two recent studies have noted an increase in asthma attacks in the elderly and children during high ozone days (Rosenberg, 1997). The children in the first study, campers at an asthma camp in Connecticut, were found to suffer symptoms 40 percent more frequently when the ozone level exceeded 160 parts per billion (ppb). Children are most at risk to ozone exposure because their respiratory systems are still developing and they breathe more air per pound of body weight than adults. Ground-level ozone is a summertime problem, and that is precisely the time when children are active outside (U.S. Environmental Protection Agency [EPA] Health and Environmental Effects of Ground-Level Ozone [Online]. July 17, 1997).

A second study that looked at hospital emergency room visits of persons age 64 and older found a 21 percent increase in visits when the ozone levels were high. Based on these and several studies over recent years, the EPA has recommended a new standard for ozone levels of 80 ppb averaged over an 8-hour period that went into effect September, 1997. The major source of the nitrogen oxide that forms the ozone of photochemical smog comes from automobiles, power plants, and other sources of combustion. Volatile organic compounds (VOCs) that react with sunlight to form ozone are emitted from a variety of sources, including chemical factories, motor vehicles, refineries, factories, and other industrial sources (U.S. EPA Fact Sheet).

Along with asthma, other upper respiratory diseases aggravated by air pollution include bronchitis, emphysema, and chronic obstructive pulmonary disease (COPD). COPD is usually defined by clinical criteria such as airway obstruction, dyspnea (shortness of breath) on exertion, and, less frequently, a chronic productive cough with repeated bronchopulmonary infections.

In the upper atmosphere, the protective ozone layer is thinning, owing to the actions of pollutants such as nitric oxide (NO). Ozone thinning is of concern because it contributes to climactic change by allowing short-wave ultraviolet (UV) radiation to penetrate the atmosphere and reach the earth's surface. UV radiation is associated with an increase in skin cancer, especially in places near the equator where the ozone layer is thinnest. Light-skinned people are at greatest risk, and the recommendation of the use of sunscreens of a factor of 20 or more is standard health teaching for those living in the southern part of the United States (Philp, 1995).

Particulate matter (PM) is the term used for the mix of solid particles and liquid droplets found in the air. Coarse particles (>2.5 micrometers) come from such sources as windblown dust and grinding operations. Fine particles (<2.5 micrometers) mostly come from fuel combustion, power plants, and diesel buses and trucks. These are so small that several thousand of them could fit on the period at the end of this sentence. They are a health concern because they can easily reach deep into the lungs. Some of the observed health effects from a multitude of studies of particles—especially the fine particles—include respiratory problems, aggravated asthma, chronic bronchitis, and absences from work and/or school (U.S. EPA Fact Sheet on Health and Environmental Effects of Particulate Matter, July 17, 1997).

Another way that these fine particles pollute is that they remain suspended in the air for a long time, contributing to the haze that has reduced visibility in many parts of the United States. These particles also contribute to acid rain, which will be discussed later in this chapter.

NOISE POLLUTION

The health of our hearing is often taken for granted. Yet increasing noise levels in the modern world are affecting the quality of life for many (see Patient Teaching box). The frequencies of sound that we hear are measured in decibels (dB) and are usually designed as the "A" scale. So 30 dBA and 90 dBA are measurements of sound levels. To grasp what these measurements mean, 30 dBA is the typical level found in a house at night from a refrigerator, furnace fan, crickets outside, and so forth. At the other extreme, 90 dBA is a level that could cause permanent hearing damage if exposed to it for more than 30 minutes at a time. A jackhammer is an example of this level of noise. A rock concert can easily maintain such a high level that people complain of their ears ringing for days afterward. A busy office of people talking, telephones ringing, and printers, copiers, and faxes all operating can generate a noise level of 70 dBA.

Figure 30–1 illustrates typical sound pressure levels for common sounds in the environment. Sound waves travel into the ear canal where they vibrate, causing reverberation against

PATIENT TEACHING
PRECAUTIONS TO PROTECT HEARING

Hearing protection is probably one of the least stressed and practiced health preventive measures that patients receive teaching about. Yet, it is easy to do and is applicable across populations and ages and genders.

Occupations such as dentistry, construction work, musician (classical or contemporary), and working around airports or traffic (think of bicycle couriers) are all at risk for contributing to a patient's hearing loss.

The nurse can determine while interviewing the patient what type of occupation the patient has, the environment that the patient lives in, and the social activities the patient enjoys. This information is usually sufficient to begin to introduce the concept of hearing protection. An excellent resource of the nurse is an audiologist who will have information to show and explain to the patient. Teaching will be more successful when the environment is a quiet and nonstressful one, such as a quiet alcove away from the main activity of the clinic or ward.

There are earmolds that are specific for almost every situation and are comfortable and practically invisible. So finding out if the patient has objections to wearing ear protection and what they might be is often a help in gathering the kind of information you will want to stress. An array of sample products that the patient can examine and try on might be very helpful. Information about the long-term effects of his or her specific situation on their hearing would also be needed.

Scheduling an appointment for a hearing evaluation might be advisable, especially for some whose occupations put them at high risk. Often a person's loss may be so gradual that it is not even noticed, and a testing is able to demonstrate that to the patient.

the tympanic membrane. The tympanic membrane will move according to the force and velocity of the waves that hit it. The membrane then transmits energy through the middle ear to the fluid-filled inner ear where the receptors (hair cells) are located. The hair cells transform the sound energy (pressure waves) into action, or the sound we hear. The hair cells are very sensitive to high-intensity noises such as amplified rock music, jet plane engines, and revved-up motorcycles. In cases of long exposure to loud sounds, hair cells and their supporting cells completely degenerate. Much lesser noise levels also cause damage if exposure is chronic (Vander et al, 1980).

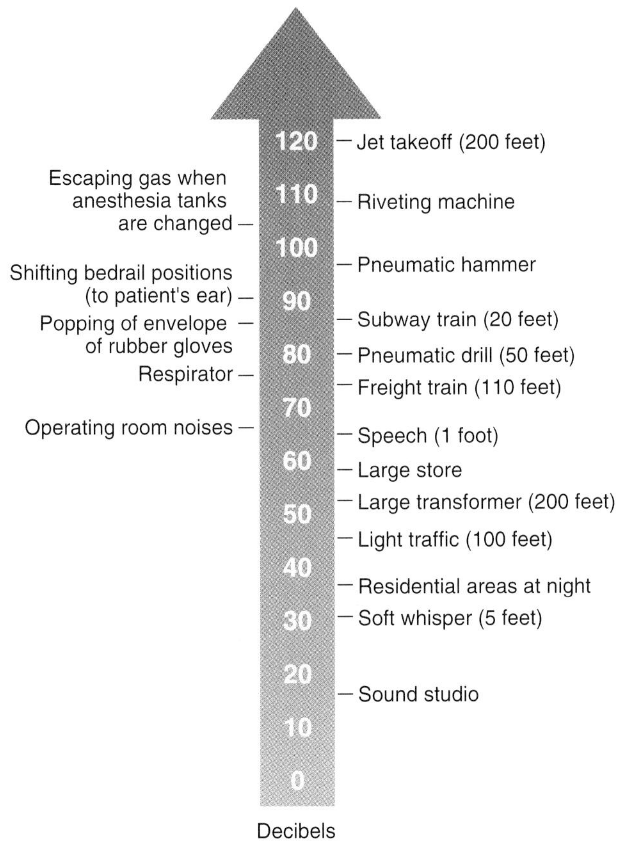

120 — Jet takeoff (200 feet)
Escaping gas when anesthesia tanks are changed — 110 — Riveting machine
100 — Pneumatic hammer
Shifting bedrail positions (to patient's ear) — 90
Popping of envelope of rubber gloves — Subway train (20 feet)
80 — Pneumatic drill (50 feet)
Respirator — Freight train (110 feet)
70
Operating room noises — Speech (1 foot)
60 — Large store
50 — Large transformer (200 feet)
— Light traffic (100 feet)
40 — Residential areas at night
30 — Soft whisper (5 feet)
20 — Sound studio
10
0
Decibels

Figure 30-1. Typical sound pressure levels of common sounds in the environment.

WATER POLLUTION

The neurologic system—the brain, spinal cord, peripheral and autonomic nerves—not only regulates life-sustaining functions such as body temperature, heartbeat, and respiration, but also is the very essence of cognition and affect. It relies on input from various sensory mechanisms to help it regulate bodily functions and actions. Numerous pollutants are toxic to the nervous system—particularly the heavy metals, including mercury, cadmium, arsenic, and lead. Heavy metal toxicity can cause mental retardation, nerve dysfunction, and other serious neurologic disorders.

Major water pollutants can be classified as follows:

- oxygen-depleting (those that contribute to eutrophication)
- synthetic organic chemicals (detergents, paints, plastics, petroleum products, solvents)
- inorganic chemicals (salts, heavy metals, acids)
- radioactive wastes from nuclear plants (Philp, 1995)

Water quality also has been shown to deteriorate from the effects of acid rain. The rainwater leaches toxic metals from the soil as it percolates down to the groundwater. Acid rain can also contribute to the creation of methylmercury from mercury. A study by the Health and Welfare of Canada has shown that acid rain can cause lead to be leached from the solder in plumbing found in existing houses and cottages

(Philp, 1995). One of the health problems of acid surface water with a pH of 5 or less is that aluminum can be leached from the soil and not only will be toxic to fish but also can cause osteomalacia and symptoms of dementia in humans. Microcytic-hypochromic (i.e., small pale cells) anemia (deficiency of red blood corpuscles) can occur, as has been observed in hemodialysis patients due to the leaching of aluminum from the dialyzer into the patient's bloodstream and from aluminum hydroxide contained in over-the-counter antacids. Aluminum also appears in treated drinking water from the use of alum to precipitate suspended organic matter in the third stage of water treatment (Philp, 1995).

Additionally, the various chemicals and waste products of industries, agricultural institutions, and domestic uses all contribute to water pollution on varying levels and at varying degrees of toxicity. These pollutants may be solids, liquids, gases, or sludges and can be flammable, corrosive, radioactive, and biologically toxic.

TOXIC METALS

Mercury. Ingestion of heavy metals occurs via the respiratory and digestive systems. The metal mercury occurs naturally in the environment in several forms. Metallic mercury is used in thermometers and barometers and other consumer products. Inorganic mercury is the main form in the air, and it occurs naturally from the degassing of the Earth's crust and oceans. Degassing is an ongoing process in which naturally occurring soil gases (which consist of air, water vapor, and natural and synthetic contaminants that are found in the spaces between soil particles and cracks in bedrock) and ocean gases are released during chemical reactions caused by weather and atmospheric changes. Additionally, 2000 to 3000 tons are released into the atmosphere each year by human activities, primarily from the burning of coal and waste (Foulke, 1994).

Air usually contains 2.4 parts of mercury per trillion parts of air (ppt), but levels near some industrial areas can rise to nearly 1800 ppt. It will stay in the environment for a long time, and can change between organic and inorganic forms (Agency for Toxic Substances and Disease Registry [ATSDR], 1990b).

There are small amounts of mercury in the water; bacteria can transform it into the organic form called methylmercury, a more toxic form. Fish absorb methylmercury as they feed and also as the water passes over their gills. Large predator fish ingest mercury from their prey, where it binds tightly to the protein in muscle and tissue. Levels in the water are usually less than 25 ppt. However, levels in water samples taken from contaminated Superfund sites are about 200 ppt on average (ATSDR, 1990b).

Mercury can enter the body by breathing in the vapor, or eating contaminated fish or other foods. It can also be ingested by drinking contaminated water. Mercury in all forms can enter the body directly through the skin. It leaves mainly by urine and feces, but once ingested, stays in the body for months. It is almost completely absorbed from the intestine into the blood, is distributed throughout the body, and passes into the brain to reach nerve cells. Long-term exposure to either organic or inorganic mercury can permanently damage the brain, kidneys, and developing fetus. Organic mercury exposure comes from eating contaminated fish or grain and causes greater harm to the brain and developing fetus. For this reason, mercury poses special concerns for the developing fetus and young children (Minnesota Dept. of Health [MNDH], 1997).

Early symptoms of mercury exposure are fine tremors in the fingers, eyelids, and lips (ATSDR, 1990b). With increased exposure, the tremors in the hands and arms may interfere with such activities of handwriting. Difficulty in walking and talking and constriction of the visual fields are some of the symptoms of more exposure (Foulke, 1994). Some of the behavioral effects observed are depression, irritability, insomnia, and exaggerated responses to stimuli (Centers for Disease Control, Mortality Morbidity Weekly Report [CDC:MMWR], 1996).

Several government agencies have developed recommendations on mercury exposures. These are called minimal risk levels (MRL). An MRL is an estimate of the daily human exposure to a chemical that is likely to be without appreciable risk of deleterious (noncarcinogenic) effects during a specified period of exposure (ATSDR, 1990b). The EPA has limited the level of inorganic mercury in lakes and rivers to 144 parts per trillion (ppt). The food and drug administration (FDA) limits levels of mercury to 2 ppb in a liter of water and 1 part per million (ppm) in fish. The Occupational Safety and Health Administration (OSHA) has set a limit of 1.2 ppb of organic mercury in workroom air (0.01 mg/m^3) and exposures over an 8-hour shift to protect workers. However, at this time, no studies have shown at what level exposure affects a fetus. Studies are in progress and the results should be known in the near future, since it is known that even low levels of mercury exposure in pregnant women can have effects on the cognitive function of children. The FDA has advised that pregnant women, nursing mothers, and women of childbearing age limit their intake of fish to no more than once a month. The Minnesota Department of Public Health recommends that pregnant women and women who are planning to become pregnant not eat shark or swordfish, and also should not eat more than 7 ounces of tuna a week (MNDH, 1997).

In the poisoning episodes in Japan in the 1960s and 1970s, mercury levels in fish were considerably higher. In the Minimata case (see Box 30–1), over 900 people died, mostly from nervous system damage from eating fish daily from waters that were severely polluted with methylmercury. In a similar incident in Nigata, Japan, where 120 persons were poisoned, it was shown that the symptoms can progress over years after exposure has ended. Mercury levels in fish in both areas ranged from 9 ppm to 24 ppm; in Minimata, some fish had levels as high as 40 ppm (Foulke, 1994).

A recent report aired on National Public Radio stated that the EPA has warned consumers not to eat fish from more than

BOX 30-1
MINIMATA DISEASE

Minimata, Japan, is a small fishing village located on Minimata Bay. In the 1950s, Japan was entering a phase of rapid economic growth. A manufacturer of industrial chlorides, Chisso, was the largest producer of vinyl chlorides in the country and was located on Minimata Bay. Its production needed large quantities of mercury as a catalyst, and this mercury was dumped into the bay as waste after it was used.

A doctor at the Minimata plant's hospital, Dr. Hosokawa, noticed a series of patients who were ill with what seemed to be a combination of epilepsy and paralysis. He suspected that factory effluent might be the cause of these mysterious symptoms, and in July 1959, he began conducting experiments with the discharge from the factory. He sprinkled the effluent on food fed to cats, and the cats were stricken with the same convulsions and motor disorders that he had observed in his patients.

When he reported his results to Chisso executives, he was told to stop the experiments and the rest of the cats were destroyed. He repeatedly tried to get the company to publish the results of his tests but was turned down. In 1962, he resigned from Chisso. In 1970, dying from terminal cancer, he revealed what had happened in 1959.

Chisso not only suppressed all word of the experiments but continued pumping 500 tons of effluent an hour into Minimata Bay. This bay was the source of fish and other seafood that the local people relied on for their livelihood. The set of symptoms that people developed came to be known as Minimata disease, and was the result of mercury poisoning.

By the mid-1990s, more than 900 people had died, and 5000 others were suffering the chronic effects of mercury poisoning.

1700 lakes and rivers because the fish were contaminated with high levels of chemicals, including PCBs, mercury, and DDT. The warning was even more specific for pregnant women and children under 15 about not eating more than one meal per month of bass, yellow perch, or northern pike from any of Michigan's reservoirs, lakes, or Great Lakes. Also specifically targeted were lake trout and Chinook salmon from Lake Ontario (NPR, July 1996).

PCBs. PCBs are a group of 209 synthetic chemicals that were widely used as coolants in electrical transformers, capacitors, and other electrical equipment. Because they can withstand temperatures up to 800°C, they were used in brake fluid, hydraulic fluid, and other industrial products. The accumulating evidence of the environmental threat to humans and wildlife from PCBs led to their production being banned in 1976 (MNDH, Fish and Your Health, June 1993).

Because they are such stable compounds, they degrade very slowly and are often detected where they have been improperly disposed of and are seeping into groundwater and soil. Nationwide, PCBs have been found in at least 286 Superfund sites listed by the EPA. They are not soluble in water, but are present in the sediment or some of the suspended organic matter in the water. They are ingested by aquatic organisms resulting in increasing levels of PCBs in the successive steps of a lake or river food chain (MNDH, June 1993). High levels of PCBs (5–20 ppm) have been detected in Lake Ontario fish, and all of the Great Lakes fish are considered contaminated. Although various types of toxicity have been reported in phytoplankton, mammals, and birds, the data are not clear for human toxicity (Philp, 1995).

Lead. In spite of the fact that lead was removed from household paint and gasoline 20 years ago, millions of tons of lead remain in the environment. It is a common element in the earth's crust. Even though it is regulated in household paint, it is not limited in industrial paint. According to the Centers for Disease Control (CDC), lead poisoning is one of the most common pediatric health problems and is the most preventable (House Report, 1992).

Young children under six are the most frequent victims. The playground equipment in many schoolyards is painted with industrial paint. As it flakes off and becomes ground to dust in the soil, children can ingest it as they play. Children can get high blood levels by ingesting a paint chip the size of the top of a pencil eraser (Living on Earth [LOE], May 30, 1997). It is still present in the layers of paint in old houses. Activities such as scraping off the paint in preparation for repainting can leave lead deposits on the ground around the building, thereby creating a hazard for young children playing in the area. Also, lead deposits remain in the soil from decades of exhaust from leaded motor fuel. Paint is the main source of lead poisoning in children, but water can also contain lead. It can leach out of old municipal water tanks and can come from the solder in copper plumbing installed until the late 1980s. Older homes can even have lead pipes.

Even though it is now illegal to use lead in the glaze for pottery and crockery, it is present in high levels in some of the imported crockery from Latin America and Asia. According to Neil Gandel of Consumer Action (LOE, June 1997), government agencies just cannot keep up with the illegal merchandise.

Exposure to lead at work is another way people get lead poisoning. In 1996, twenty-five states reported almost 27,000 adults had dangerously high blood lead levels. Industries such as battery manufacturing, foundries, house painting, gun firing ranges and radiator repair shops all have conditions that can potentially expose workers to high lead concentrations. The industry affecting the highest number of people is painting. Until 1950, paint contained as much as 50 percent lead by weight. That paint is still on millions of buildings across the United States. In a city such as San Francisco, 95 percent of the houses have lead paint. Painters disturb the paint when they scrape, wash, sand, or burn off the old layers. Unless the painters use safe painting practices, the painters can expose not only themselves but also the occupants of the building and the neighbors to lead dust. Safe practices include wearing respirators and washing hands before eating or drinking.

High-power washers are not used, and the painters all wear protective clothing (LOE, June 13, 1997).

Lead has been known for a long time to have toxic effects. There are no obvious symptoms of low-level lead poisoning, but lead can adversely affect every system in a child's body. Low levels can shorten physical stature, impair kidney development, and alter red blood cell metabolism and vitamin D synthesis. The most significant effects, though, are found in the development of the nervous system. Low levels can reduce intelligence and impair perception, hearing, and speech as well as cause behavior problems such as hyperactivity (House Report, 1992). Tiny microscopic doses in children not only lower intelligence, but cause a sixfold increase in learning disabilities in later life. Children with moderate blood levels are seven times more likely to drop out of school. When the bones of a group of 12-year-old boys were x-rayed for lead exposure, it was found that the boys who had high bone lead levels, indicating past exposure, had more attention disorders, more aggressive behavior, and were more likely to be delinquent (LOE, June 6, 1997).

Scientists at Dartmouth College say the presence of lead and another heavy metal, manganese, is directly correlated to rates of violent crime (such as homicide, aggravated assault, sexual assault, and so on). Their team looked at countries that had no environmental pollution from either lead or manganese and found a crime rate of 278 per 100,000 per year. In countries with both kinds of pollution present, the crime rate was 578 per 100,000. One of the members of the research team also noted that the effect of alcohol on a brain already impaired by heavy metal exposure is much greater than in the unexposed brain. They found that in countries with high rates of alcoholism and release of both toxins, the crime rate is three times the national average (LOE, June 6, 1997).

In adults, high blood lead levels can damage kidneys and the brain, as well as increase blood pressure in middle-aged men. High levels can also damage sperm and other parts of a man's reproductive system. It has also been shown that lead can damage an unborn child (ATSDR, Public Health Statement: Lead 1990a).

With the introduction of the 1970 Lead Paint Poisoning Prevention Program, the CDC regarded a blood level of 60 micrograms per deciliter (μg/dl) as the threshold for childhood lead poisoning. Since then, the threshold has been lowered four times. In the CDC's "Strategic Plan for the Elimination of Childhood Lead Poisoning," the agency said that there is compelling evidence that adverse health effects can occur in young children with blood levels as low as 10 μg/dl, and there should be community prevention activities triggered when these levels are found. Additionally, all children with levels of 15 μg/dl need medical evaluation and individual case management, including nutritional and educational interventions. Medical evaluation and environmental investigation and remediation should be done for all children with blood lead levels greater or equal to 20 μg/dl (House Report, 1992).

Relevant Research

Ambient Stressors. It is interesting to note that Florence Nightingale (1859) wrote in her *Notes on Nursing* about the health-promoting aspects of the physical environment, including fresh air, cleanliness, light, and variety. She also emphasized the importance of a quiet environment, writing some 15 paragraphs on the *kind* of noise that is disturbing to a patient. Her keen observations have been borne out by subsequent researchers, both in nursing and other fields.

What Nightingale was observing and writing about was what could be described today as environmental stress. Nightingale (1859, p. 5) noted:

> All disease, at some period or other of its course, is more or less a reparative process . . . In watching disease, . . . the thing which strikes the experienced observer most forcibly is this, that the symptoms or the sufferings generally considered to be inevitable and incident to the disease are very often not symptoms of the disease at all, but of . . . the want of fresh air, or of light, or of warmth, or of quiet, or of cleanliness, or of punctuality and care in the administration of diet, of each or of all of these.

Environmental stressors are usually thought of as arising from the physical environment. Noise, light, temperature extremes and poor air quality are classified as *ambient stressors.* Ambient stressors are defined as chronic, negatively valued environmental conditions that are uncontrollable by occupants (Campbell, 1983).

Noise. Excessive and constant noises have been identified as sources of stress (see Chapter 31). The abundance of equipment such as monitors and computers has led to concern by health care givers over the effects of high sound levels on patient care, especially in areas such as intensive care units where this type of equipment is concentrated.

According to Nightingale (1859, p. 25), it is rarely the loudness of the noise that appears to affect the sick, but rather the intermittent noise, or sudden and sharp noise that "affects far more than continuous noise." In the hospital, this might be an equipment alarm, a pager, a telephone, equipment moving past the room, a sudden laugh, and so forth—all this against a background of continuous conversation and movement. Nightingale also noted that a patient "cannot bear the talking, still less the whispering, especially if it be of a familiar voice, outside his door" (1859, p. 25).

Hospital noise is one of the more heavily researched environmental stressors, perhaps because of the recognized importance of rest and sleep in patient recuperation. Noise is usually defined as any sound that is subjectively or physically arousing to people (Anastasi, 1964). Some of the studies of noise include measurement of patient's subjective and physiologic stress, patient's sleep and health, as well as measurement of sound levels in various hospital areas.

The EPA recommends a 24-hour average sound level of 45 dBA to prevent annoyance and interference with activities in the hospital. This is slightly higher than the typical level in a house at night (35 dBA). Studies of hospital levels reveal that operating room sounds (e.g., suctioning of patient trachea, continuous suction bottle, and surgeon's conversation) range from 55 to 86 dBA (Shapiro and Berland, 1972). Equipment sounds (e.g., ice machine, suction machine, telephone, respirator alarm in the recovery room) range from about 49 dBA to 80 dBA, with more than one half above 65 dBA (Falk and Woods, 1973). Sound levels in adult coronary care units (CCUs) from IV and cardiac monitor alarms, ice machines, personnel beepers, ventilator beepers, the moving of x-ray equipment, and other sources range from 58 to 78 dBA (Baker, 1984; Hilton, 1985).

With all the noisy pieces of equipment around, it is definitely appropriate to ask how all this affects patients (and health care workers). It is well known that sleep is a restorative process that returns the body to a former state of vigor and/or well-being (Horne, 1988; Nightingale, 1859). Sleep problems have been identified due both to noise, and to another environmental stressor—continuous artificial light.

A study of 15 CCU patients found that the patients took longer to fall asleep, slept less during the night, had more changes in sleep stages, and spent more time in the early stage of sleep (stage 1) than age- and gender-matched normal subjects who slept in a laboratory (Culpepper-Richards and Bairnsfather, 1988). Ten normal female volunteers who were exposed to an audiotape of CCU sounds while attempting to sleep in a laboratory exhibited increased cardiac rates and poorer sleep, as measured by a questionnaire of sleep, compared with two nights when the volunteers slept without the tape (Snyder-Halpern, 1985). Because these studies did not have large numbers of subjects and did not use a random method of assignment to groups, it is hard to draw firm conclusions on sleep disturbance due to noise.

More recently, data were collected in an overnight laboratory study (Topf, 1992b). Thirty-five female volunteers who slept in a quiet condition slept better than 70 subjects divided into two groups exposed to audiotapes of hospital noise from a CCU. In another study done in a hospital with postoperative patients, it was reported that patients who scored the highest on reported stress also had more machines running by their bedsides. It is interesting to note that the most disturbing noise to the patients was other people's conversations (Topf, 1985a).

Another way that noise takes a toll is in the arena of performance. Noise seems to reduce the efficiency of short-term memory and forces people to either make an extra effort to perform the task or accept a lower level of performance (Hockey, 1984). Thus, if the nurse is trying to explain a procedure or test to a patient against a background of noise, the chance of misunderstanding is greater than it would be if the explanation were done in a quiet environment.

Light. According to Nightingale (1859, p. 34), "little as we know about the way in which we are affected by form, colour, and light, we do know this: They have an actual physical effect." Light is essential in the hospital if patients are to read, visitors find their way, and nurses observe their patients and perform their tasks. Windows, light levels, type and placement of illuminating devices, glare from reflective surfaces, and even the timing and quality of darkness are all important in the quality of the hospital environment and the health of the patients. Glare can be a stressor for elderly patients (Williams, 1989). Bright, direct glare, such as that produced by television and/or monitor screens located next to patient beds, can actually be painful.

It is important to note that not all light is understood by our minds and bodies as being equal. When a trend toward building windowless hospitals, office buildings, and schools developed in the 1960s and 1970s, several researchers focused on the effects of such a design, especially in hospitals. Some early studies looked particularly at windowless intensive care units (ICUs), which were considered by some to be habitable because the patients are unconscious and unaware of their surroundings (Fig. 30–2).

Patients in an artificially lit unit are not aware of the time of day or night and are also subjected to a sensory deprivation from the lack of daylight stimulus. One of the first research studies done on the effects of lack of light on ICU patients compared data from the charts of patients treated in two hospitals' ICUs, one with windows and the other windowless

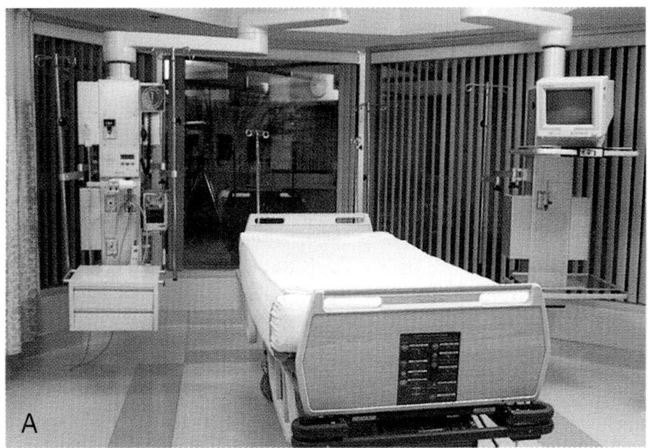

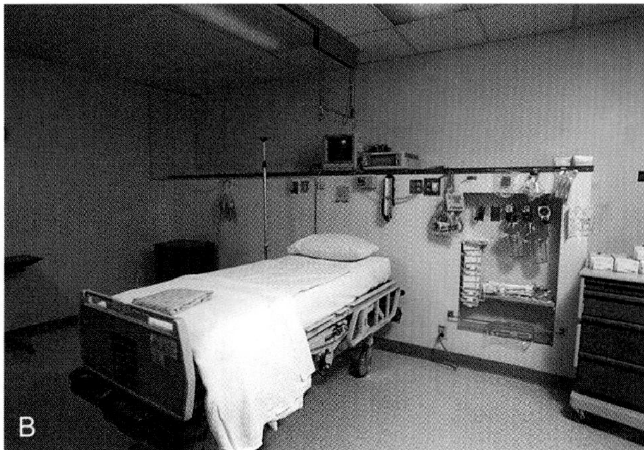

Figure 30–2. Two contrasting intensive care units (ICUs): one with windows *(A)* and the other without *(B)*.

(Wilson, 1972). Both hospitals were served by the same medical staff and offered similar services, and the age of the patients and the postoperative temperatures of the units were practically identical. The incidence of postoperative delirium in the patients who stayed 72 hours in the units without windows was more than double (40 percent) that of patients with similar lengths of stay in the unit with windows (18 percent).

Another pioneer study surveyed patients who had stayed in either a windowed or windowless ICU for at least 48 hours (Keep, 1977). Hallucinations and delusions were reported by more than twice the number from the windowless unit (48.3 percent) than the windowed unit (23.6 percent). Disorientation and loss of memory were also more frequent in the windowless unit. The researcher concluded that windows are able to convey necessary information about times of day as well as provide an important link with normality.

Among the findings of a study of windows in six rehabilitation units in Chicago were that some spaces are considered virtually windowless, even when minimum architectural and code standards for windows are met in technical terms (Verderber, 1986). Windows that occupy less than 15 percent of the wall area and were long and narrow (vertically or horizontally) or that had a monotonous view such as a brick wall or building or just sky or automobile parking were assessed by subjects as windowless. Also, sills that were high above the floor (over 80 inches) and closed curtains had the effect of visually disconnecting the interior and exterior environments.

The researcher noted that an absence of meaningful contact with the outside world is an unwarranted barrier in an era of barrier-free design (Fig. 30–3). For the hospitalized person, a window is "a constant reminder of the society to which one belongs and hopes to return to as soon as possible" (Verderber, 1986, p. 464).

The preceding research noted that it was important to subjects not only to have windows, but also to have something to look at outside the window—a view, in other words. The research reinforces another one of the insights by Florence Nightingale (1859, p. 34), who said, "Among the kindred effects of light I may mention, from experience, as quite perceptible in promoting recovery, the being able to see out of a window, instead of looking against a dead wall; the bright colors of flowers. . . ."

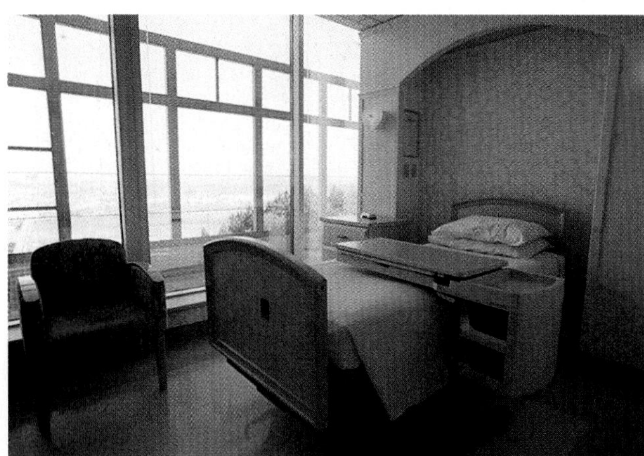

Figure 30–3. A pleasantly decorated, well-lit, and well-windowed patient room.

Some studies of more recent times uphold the validity of Nightingale's experiences. A 1984 study reported that a view of nature for patients following gallbladder surgery may have influenced their recovery (Ulrich, 1984). The lengths of stay and use of potent analgesics (painkillers) following gallbladder surgery were compared in patients who stayed at the same hospital and who were matched in age, sex, weight, and smoking history. One group stayed in rooms that had views of a brick wall; the other, in rooms with views of a small grove of trees. The group with the tree view had a significantly shorter postoperative stay, had fewer negative comments written about them in the nurses' notes, and took fewer potent analgesics than the group without the view.

A study focusing on ICU nurses reported on the effect of a view of nature on the stress levels and performance of ICU nurses at two Midwestern hospitals (Ovitt, 1996). One hospital had a windowless lounge for their ICU staff; the other had a lounge with large windows overlooking trees, buildings, and parking. After the nurses had completed a task and assessed their mood and arousal levels at work in the morning, they repeated the same task and assessment in their lounges after their noon break. The nurses who took their break in the windowed lounge were significantly less stressed and made fewer errors on their tasks than the nurses whose lounge had no windows. This is especially interesting because the nurses who worked in the unit with the windowed lounge reported being much busier and more stressed than the other group.

Temperature. The inability to have their personal preference for temperature met during their hospital stay can be stressful for patients. Some hospitals do not have air conditioning. Other hospitals have automatic heat and cooling temperatures set to change with the seasons rather than with individual patient needs. Some patient rooms can be situated with west sunlight exposure but without temperature control to handle this. Patients are thus often forced to accommodate to personally incompatible temperature regulation regardless of their acute physical needs, such as chills or fever, for warmer or cooler environments (Shumaker and Reizenstein, 1982).

Phillips and Skov (1988) reviewed articles about and identified a number of nursing temperature interventions for postoperative cardiac patients. The risk for hypothermia is great for these patients due to cold operating rooms and multiple unwarmed procedures. Postoperative care includes using warming lights, warm blankets, and increasing room temperature.

Research on hospital temperature is scarce. Only one nursing study was found on temperature regulation among adult patients. This study investigated the use of reflective blankets (lightweight metallic blankets developed in the space program) to prevent hypothermia. Eighteen postoperative patients were randomly assigned to an experimental or control group (Crayne and Miner, 1988). All subjects received routine postoperative attention to temperature, getting a warm cotton blanket, a head turban, and so on. Subjects in the experimental group also got a reflective blanket on top of the warm one. The reflective blanket was withheld from the control group. Each patient's temperature was recorded postoperatively every 15 minutes until it reached 96°F. The patients in the two groups did not differ significantly in thermal stress over the 15-minute data collection points. The investigators noted that the nonsignificant results may have been due to the small sample size.

Even though the results for the aforementioned study were not significant in terms of measurement of thermal stress, another study on body temperature yielded some interesting results. Body temperatures of surgical patients typically drop about 4° below normal due to the coolness of the operating rooms and general anesthesia. A study of 200 surgical patients concluded that keeping a patient's body temperature near normal reduces infections, speeds healing, and shortens hospital stays (Coile, 1996).

Air Quality. According to Nightingale (1859, p. 8), "the very first canon of nursing . . . is this: To keep the air [the patient] breathes as pure as the external air without chilling him." Although the external air is sometimes not as pure now as it once was, the indoor air has suffered as well. Today, indoor air quality (IAQ) research has identified many pollutants that can adversely affect health. A syndrome known as "sick building syndrome" does not have a universally accepted definition, but is generally accepted as referring to such poor indoor air quality that various symptoms are noted.

One of the major reasons for poor indoor air quality has been the change in building and technologic advances in the last half of the twentieth century. New building and engineering technologies developed in the 1960s that allowed a building's heating and cooling to be entirely managed by automatic thermostats and fans. Windows that were permanently sealed were installed or, in some cases, no windows were installed at all. Heating, ventilation, and air-conditioning (HVAC) systems can have profound impacts on the quality (or lack thereof) of the indoor environment. Other factors in the air quality indoors are the same as those outdoors—pollutants. Cigarette smoke, chemicals such as formaldehyde, volatile organic compounds (VOCs), ozone, carbon monoxide, and microorganisms can impact indoor air (OSHA Technical Manual, 1995).

One study evaluated indoor air quality and levels of common bacteria for a 5-month period at a university library (Au Yeung et al, 1991). The library staff were interviewed to elicit their subjective feelings about the indoor environment and also the prevalence of low-level symptoms. The sensory reactions were ones that the World Health Organization (WHO) has classified:

- sensory irritation in eyes, nose, and throat
- skin irritation
- neurotoxic symptoms
- unspecified hyperreactions
- odor and taste complaints

The researchers found that the indoor conditions were within acceptable limits as laid down by the WHO and the American Society of Heating, Refrigerating and Air Conditioning Engineers (ASHRAE) Standard (62-1989) except for four sections of the library, in which high formaldehyde levels were detected. In these areas, plywood, fabrics, and carpets were identified as potential sources of the excessive formaldehyde levels. Symptoms reported in those areas included headache (a neurotoxic finding), lethargy, and nasal dryness and stuffiness (even though the ambient humidity ranged from 60 to 80 percent during the testing period). The most symptoms per person were recorded in the section where the CO_2 level was highest. It was also noted that prevalence of symptoms increased if the working environment was completely sealed to the outside.

In the fall of 1994, nurses left their jobs at Brigham and Women's Hospital in Boston over the issue of indoor air quality. More than 300 of the hospital's 1800 nurses reported ailments that they blamed on the poor indoor environment. Symptoms included rashes, asthma, bronchitis, sinusitis, chest pain, headaches, and nausea (R.N.'s Battle, 1995).

A hospital in England was forced to close just 3 weeks after it opened because staff became incapacitated by reactions to the formaldehyde-based glue used to fasten the carpet. Babies, children, the elderly, and people with debilitating illnesses are "predisposed to aggravation by indoor air contaminants" (Weber, 1995, p. 45).

Hospital odors are another aspect of indoor air quality and might provide a clue as to the adequacy of the ventilation system. A number of hospitals have begun experimenting with natural fragrancing not only to improve the air but also to enhance healing. A consultant noted that "when essential oils (as distinct from synthetic perfumes) are diffused into the air, they affect both the body and mind. On the one hand, they are antibacterial and antifungal; some are even antiviral. On the other hand, they are antidepressant, sedative and uplifting" (Weber, 1995, p. 45).

The National Aeronautics and Space Administration (NASA) is deeply interested in artificially heated and cooled environments and has hired researchers from various scientific backgrounds to examine air cleanliness. NASA discovered it needed to deal with air quality because the Skylab prototype emitted more than 100 chemicals. William Wolverton, a former senior scientist at NASA, experimented with the air-cleansing properties of plants by sealing them in chambers that had been filled with formaldehyde, benzene, xylene, and ammonia (Raver, 1994). He discovered that plants indeed have remarkable air-purifying characteristics. Among some of his findings are that microorganisms in both the plant leaves and root zone break down chemicals. Not only do the plants remove chemicals, but in more of his recent research he has demonstrated that certain plants also emit a substance that removes spores, molds, and fungi from the air. Even the soil microorganisms were actively removing harmful molds and spores from the atmosphere. A room full of tropical plants not only humidifies the air, but also makes it cleaner and healthier.

Relevant Theory

Nightingale (1859) was the first nurse to publish the health-promoting aspects of the physical environment. Other early nurse theorists from 1900 to 1950 emphasized keeping the environment safe and clean for patients. From 1950 to the 1970s, many nurse theorists (Patterson and Zderod, 1976; Weidenbach, 1964) devoted their attention to the nurse-patient relationship with little focus on the physical environment. Most nurse theorists writing in the 1970s and 1980s viewed the environment primarily as a potential negative influence on patient recovery that needed to be controlled or adapted to (Johnson, 1980; King, 1971; Neuman, 1974; Orem, 1971; Roy, 1976). In 1983, Rose and Killian wrote about the dynamic relationship between the patient and the environment and how risk for negative outcomes was due to patient vulnerability, such as constitutional and/or acquired factors.

A more global and unified view of the patient and physical environment was advanced by Rogers (1970) and nurse theorists building on her contentions, such as Parse (1981) and Newman (1987). An underlying principle of Rogers' theory is that the individual and the environment are continuously exchanging matter and energy with each other. Although she did not define exactly what was meant by the physical environment, many of her students studied the effects of factors such as light and sound on health (Williams, 1988). Thus, the physical environment can be either supportive in the sense of it being a delightful place to be in, or distressing (Kaufman, 1969). A polluted and noisy environment is an example of physical environment that has the potential to be distressing, whereas access to natural light, fresh air, and views of nature creates examples of supportive environments. More recent authors (Davidson and Ray, 1991) have emphasized that the person-environment relationship is a complex phenomenon that may require complex methods to study it.

The interrelatedness of the natural and built environments with human behavior interests researchers in a variety of fields (Williams, 1988). Two researchers have pioneered studies in the effect that nature might have on persons in the built environment. They are Roger Ulrich of Texas A&M and the team of Rachel and Stephen Kaplan at the University of Michigan. These researchers' approaches have differed; the Kaplans have developed a theory based on a cognitive pathway, whereas Ulrich and his researchers have studied the stress reduction effect of nature via the affective pathway.

Briefly, the Kaplans note that we use our cognitive pathways to make sense out of our everyday world; how to find our way around cities and buildings (wayfinding), listening to lectures or directions, learning how to do various skills and so on. When our cognition tires and we want to rest, the most effective way we can relax and return to work refreshed, according to the Kaplans, is to include nature in our break time. It can be as simple as a view of nature from a window at work to a vacation at the beach or in the mountains, but the key here is that somehow nature is included (Kaplan, 1983).

Ulrich's research focuses on the calming effects of nature via the affective path. In his model, stress reduction results from viewing nature. For example, if an individual is under stress from whatever source—a final exam coming up, a move to another city or job—that person's stress will be reduced if nature is included in some daily activity (Ulrich et al, 1991).

FACTORS AFFECTING CLINICAL DECISIONS

An important consideration in the planning of nursing care is that although patients may be alike in many ways, they are also characterized by specific individual differences. This is true with respect to patients' reactions to ambient stressors and the way the patient responds to nursing actions to reduce stress. Individual differences of particular importance include age and developmental stage; the meaning of specific environmental stressors; mental status; and the specific needs of patients in settings other than the hospital. Additional factors that may affect nursing care include gender, culture and ethnicity, religious beliefs, and educational background.

Age

Elderly populations have decreasing cardiac, renal, pulmonary, and immune system processes. As a result, elderly individuals have lowered defense mechanisms and changes in the functioning of the immune system. Skin changes increase the likelihood of increased absorption of chemicals. As a result of the changes, the elderly may be more susceptible to and experience adverse health outcomes (Institute of Medicine, 1995).

Children are also highly susceptible to environmental health hazards. Because children have higher metabolism rates, absorption of toxins is greater. Children are also closer to the floor where dust, dirt, and toxic metals such as lead are present (Institute of Medicine, 1995).

Generally speaking, the young and the elderly are less able to handle environmental insults such as toxic chemicals than are older children and adults of young and middle age. Illnesses resulting from exposure to toxic chemicals in the environment are especially critical for the young. Cells in a state of growth as exists in childhood are more susceptible to damage (Sherman, 1994).

Infants and the elderly can also be expected to experience greater light-induced stress than other age groups in the hospital. Williams (1988) noted that glare can actually be painful for elderly patients. Sources of glare are the television and monitor screens and the way sunlight reflects off a highly polished hospital floor.

Some of the hearing changes that occur with age are the loss of the range of sounds in the higher frequencies, and also the finding that the noise most annoying to people is in the lower frequencies (Au Yeung et al., 1991). In light of this, the room assignment for an elderly person might be in a quieter part of the unit, and the assignment for a teenager could be in a noisier spot.

Elderly and infants are also more susceptible to changes in temperature (Williams, 1988). Most elderly are likely to prefer more warmth in winter and be less able to endure the summer heat. They are less likely to be aware of dangerous changes in temperature levels and, at the same time, less able to tolerate such changes (Carpman et al, 1986).

All age levels are susceptible to the results of radiation from the sun. Actinic keratosis, a precancerous skin condition, results from excessive exposure to the sun, particularly in light-skinned individuals.

Gender

Perhaps the most obvious difference in impact of the physical environment with regard to gender is in reproductive health. In the acute care setting, hospitals and birthing centers are responding to the demands of patients for alternative birthing practices that do not fragment the family as a traditional setting does. Such features include rooming-in, labor and delivery room design that looks more homelike with indirect lighting, soft colors, and much of the equipment hidden behind partitions and doors. Although studies have not found any differences in stress of mothers delivering in either setting, women do report a higher satisfaction with and a greater sense of participation in the birth experience in the alternative setting than in the conventional labor and delivery room setting (Williams, 1988).

Although the research is beginning to release results of studies of the effects of environmental chemicals on hormones of men, as of this writing, the evidence is suggestive only that decreased sperm counts are related to environmental pollution.

What is much more certain is that some pollutants definitely affect fetal development and health. As discussed earlier in this chapter, heavy metals such as mercury and lead and inert compounds such as PCBs pose dangers to healthy and normal fetal development.

Individual and Family Values

Educational Background. Part of the analysis of census data includes educational level attained and annual earnings. A college education is usually required for most jobs that have long-term earnings potential. In 1996, the unemployment rate for adults who did not complete high school was 8.7 percent compared with 4.7 percent with a high school diploma and 2.2 percent for college graduates (U.S. Dept. of Education, 1997).

The types of jobs that are most likely to expose workers to chemical hazards are those usually, but not always, involving manual labor. These jobs are usually taken by those with less than high school preparation. Foundry and steel workers, oil drillers, gas station workers, miners, workers with solvents, dry cleaning workers, carpenters, plumbers, farmers, and so on are some of the occupations that have had known risks associated with them (Sherman, 1994). One exception is in the health care industry, where the anesthetists and persons handling drugs and chemotherapeutic agents take precautions with those agents.

Another factor is that information on environmental hazards is not necessarily stressed in high school or in college. Many workers who are exposed to hazardous chemicals do not have an opportunity to learn about them and are unaware of the risks that are present.

Socioeconomic Status. Persons and families who earn less typically live in neighborhoods that are at higher risk for environmental risk. Old houses with lead-based paint, as was discussed earlier, are in the older neighborhoods, and roads and highways have had years of leaded gasoline vapors deposited in the soils.

Poor nutritional status also is a factor in lead poisoning in children. Lack of proper nutrition is more prevalent in poorer families. A key factor in the absorption of lead seems to be deficiencies in calcium and zinc. If the body has enough calcium and zinc, the body does not absorb the lead (LOE, Part 2).

The ability to provide a comfortable physical environment is often driven by financial reality. Accounts of a patient with a respiratory illness who will not turn on the air conditioning during periods of ozone alerts or an elderly person who cannot afford to heat during frigid weather and freezes to death are reported every year. Financial considerations definitely play a part in a family's ability or lack thereof to buy winter coats, gloves, and hats for children. In colder parts of the country, exposure to the cold leading to frostbite and hypothermia occurs every winter.

Another aspect of the physical environment that affects health is crowding. People living in crowded conditions have higher stress levels, which can contribute to illness and also retard healing. Research (Zimring, 1982) has shown that people who do not have their own well-defined private space tend to be more withdrawn and less social than those who have such a space available. Anecdotal reports suggest that children who live in crowded homes suffer fewer ill effects if there is a private place they can go to or if they can play outside. The nurse can help the patient find some degree of privacy to help minimize psychological distress in a crowded living arrangement.

Culture and Ethnicity. It is not uncommon for a patient's culture and/or ethnic background to dictate certain behaviors that place their health at risk. In spite of all that is known about the relationship between skin cancer and sun exposure, the cultural norm that a tan is much healthier than white untanned skin is still the prevalent one, at least among young adults. Even though tanning ages the skin faster and causes an increased incidence in skin cancers and melanoma, to some tanned skin is preferred. People living in areas of the country such as in southern climates are more vulnerable to sun damage owing to being closer to the equator and receiving the sun rays in a more direct and intense manner.

Look at the instance of a father and his son who go fishing at the local pier because that is how the father related to his father and he wants to pass on the tradition. The nurse is aware that any fish caught from those waters is likely to be contaminated and that consuming it would be potentially dangerous to the child's health, yet does not want to put a stop to this activity. Making the family aware of the kind of contaminants and the guidelines for how often, if at all, they can safely eat the fish will prevent future illness. If the family is not dependent on the fish to supplement their meals, the safest action would be to catch and release. People from northern countries, Southern Asia, and Native Americans who traditionally eat larger amounts of fish than the general population are at greater risk for long-term health effects because they are particularly susceptible to contaminants in fish.

Spirituality and Religious Practices. Persons who use metallic mercury in ethnic folk medicine and for religious practices are placing themselves at risk. Mercury is sold under the name *azogue* in stores that specialize in religious items used in Esperitismo (a spiritual belief system from Puerto Rico), Santeria (a Cuban-based religion), and voodoo. The use of azogue in religious practices is recommended in some Hispanic communities by a spiritual leader. The azogue is prepared by the spiritual leader and either placed in a sealed pouch to be worn, or sprinkled in the home or automobile. Some of the stores that sell it suggest mixing the azogue in bath water or perfume and placing it in devotional candles (ATSDR, June 27, 1997).

Setting in Which Care Is Delivered

Although most nursing care is delivered in the acute and long-term care setting, this is rapidly changing. Community-based care is one of the fastest growing settings for nursing practice, especially the advanced practice nurse. More and more nursing care will be administered in the community—homes and clinics—as the paradigm shifts away from institutional-based care to community-based care. Some of the settings include not only the familiar ones of industry and public health but also a rural clinic, an urban home health agency, and a multi-specialty clinic that draws clients from all over. Nurses are now taking management positions in managed health care organizations, home health agencies, and group practice areas. The emphasis is shifting from the management of the acute condition to that of preventive care.

Financial Considerations

At this time, millions of children and adults are not covered by any health care insurance. This means more emergency department visits for acute crises such as acute asthmatic attacks or respiratory problems because the preventive or palliative care was not affordable.

As more children grow up in poverty, nutritional requirements that are so important to young growing minds and bodies are often not met. Research indicates that the relationship between lack of basic nutrients and learning disorders and delinquency has a solution. Experts have estimated it would take $30 billion to clean up the household lead hazard and that it would soon pay for itself in a smarter and safer society (LOE, part 4).

People who subsist on fish out of economic necessity are at greater risk, as already mentioned. Again, the importance of not exposing the developing fetus to contaminated fish cannot be overemphasized.

FUTURE DEVELOPMENTS

Costs are a major factor in planning future health care facilities. Energy-efficient buildings are going to be more common in the future in an effort to reduce operating costs. One design change is that of incorporating natural light deep into spaces with 10-foot ceilings. Not only does this help save on artificial lighting but also, by incorporating natural light, productivity is improved and patients' comments on surveys are more positive (Coile, 1996).

A survey of patients in two hospitals in Wales (Singleton, 1992) that were designed with courtyard gardens and an abundance of natural light yielded some insightful remarks from the patients and the nurses. Patients were unequivocally positive about the hospitals' design. For example, one noted ". . . this is the first time I've had such contentment in any hospital . . . brought about by all this—the plants taking away that terrible coldness and fear . . . " and "It's life . . . all those plants . . . and birds . . . If they want patients to get better more quickly and to release beds for other people, that's what they must do . . . people want to be in a position that when they are starting to . . . [heal] they get better much more quickly by being able to go away from the sickness into life, and . . . life is . . . the water garden courtyard" (Singleton, 1992, p. 87). Patients' visitors were also very positive. They commented that the hospital and its garden setting was an asset to the community. They were happy their relatives were being looked after in such a "friendly, lovely place."

The above comments are quite different from the typical stereotypical hospital as perceived by the public. The *Æsclepius* newsletter (Coile, 1996) cited the following description

> Most hospitals are dismally inhospitable. A weakened patient and traumatized family are greeted by harsh lights and cold stainless steel, labyrinths of white corridors, thumping equipment, and acrid mysterious smells. The sick rarely have access to information, privacy or a quiet place for quiet talk and grieving. The resulting sense of anxiety and helplessness is the worst imaginable place to promote healing.

Developing a caring attitude and projecting that attitude to the public through a hospital's or nursing home's design has become important to the health care industry, which is, after all, a service industry. "Humanistic design must be more than just an afterthought. It must move health facility design from its 'hospital green' image to a sense of caring for the whole person" (Carpman et al, 1986, p. 16).

Futurist and former hospital administrator Leland Kaiser states, "if a hospital is to be a healing place as well as a curing place, healthcare architects must design for the spiritual, mental and emotional dimensions of patients as well as for their bodies. Good design is in itself an experiential therapeutic intervention" (Weber, 1995, p. 43). The same statement can also apply to nursing homes.

PRINCIPLES AND PRACTICES

Historically, the nurse has monitored the patient's physical environment to promote the optimal healing environment. Nightingale was an environmentalist before the term was ever coined. Her two published works, *Notes on Nursing* and *Notes on Hospitals,* both contain guidelines for ensuring the optimal physical environments for health and healing. In the book on hospitals, she gives detailed instructions on unit design so that patients are in clean, safe, and attractive surroundings. Her ward design soon became known as the Nightingale ward.

According to Williams (1988), early nursing leaders in the United States addressed hospital construction and environment and the nurses' responsibility for participating in the planning of hospitals. But as building practices changed and more non-nursing personnel took over many maintenance tasks, environmental concerns became less important in hospital nursing.

Today, the physical environment is once again becoming a prominent factor in many areas of health and illness. As buildings became more and more designed for the housing of the rapid increase in the technological side of patient care—or so it seemed—the attention to the comfort of the patient became subservient to efficiencies in lighting, temperature control, and so forth. The consequences of 24-hour lighting, monitors, ventilators, beepers, and other noises, and such concerns as indoor air quality have once again brought the environment to the forefront.

The pollution of the outdoor physical environment resulting in physical health impacts is another area that has grown in importance over recent decades. As nursing moves from the acute care setting into more community-based positions, the impact of the environmental pollution and its effects on families and the workforce becomes paramount. For certain populations such as the poor and the elderly, a nurse may be the sole health care provider located in the neighborhood. Nursing needs to reclaim the heritage left by Nightingale and once again include effects of the environment in nursing care of patients.

Nurses in every practice setting can help bridge the gap between the scientific understanding and public understanding of environmental health risks. The role of the nurse in improving environmental health is an important one and nurses should be competent in this arena. Nursing has historically been concerned about this issue as evidenced by the American Nurses' Association's inclusion of environmental issues in its publication *Scope of Nursing Practice* (see Chapter 1).

Focus has also been placed on nursing and the environment by the national Institute of Medicine (IOM). The IOM appointed a Committee on Enhancing Environmental Health Content in Nursing Practice in 1993. A study was conducted by the committee that resulted in the following themes:

- The environment is a primary determinant of health, and environmental health hazards affect all aspects of life and all areas of nursing practice.
- Nurses are well positioned for addressing environmental health concerns of individuals and communities. Nurses are the largest group of health professionals; they have great variety in their settings and locations of practice; environmental health is a good fit with the values of the nursing profession regarding disease prevention and social justice; and nurses are trusted by the public.
- There is a need to enhance the emphasis and awareness of environmental threats to the health of populations served by all areas of nursing practice. This will require changes in practice, education, and research (IOM, 1995, p. vi).

The Committee also determined that there was a need to develop environmental health competencies for nurses and adapted the competencies of the International Council of Nurses (IOM, 1995). Box 30–2 lists the general environmental health competencies for nurses.

Institutional Settings

By now, it is hoped, this overview of the relationship between the physical environment and health has served as an introduction to the complexity of our existence in both the natural and built environments. The research data presented in this chapter are supportive of some of the earliest nursing principles as laid down by Nightingale (1859) in her farsighted and insightful notes. Nightingale identified noise, light, pure fresh air, temperature, and diet as essential components of healing. These very basic nursing care principles are increasingly supported by research, by nurses and others, that supports their importance in nursing practice. Attention to the physical environment is just as important now as it was historically.

AMBIENT STRESSORS REVISITED

Recall that ambient stressors are chronic, negatively valued environmental conditions that are perceived as uncontrollable by affected persons (Campbell, 1983). A concept central to dealing with stressors is **coping strategies.** A common coping strategy is **personal control**—an individual's ability to exer-

BOX 30-2
GENERAL ENVIRONMENTAL HEALTH COMPETENCIES FOR NURSES

BASIC KNOWLEDGE AND CONCEPTS

All nurses should understand the scientific principles and underpinnings of the relationship between individuals or populations, and the environment (including the work environment). This understanding includes the basic mechanisms and pathways of exposure to environmental health hazards, basic prevention and control strategies, the interdisciplinary nature of effective interventions, and the role of research.

ASSESSMENT AND REFERRAL

All nurses should be able to successfully complete an environmental health history, recognize potential environmental hazards and sentinel illnesses, and make appropriate referrals for conditions with probable environmental etiologies. An essential component of this is the ability to access and provide information to patients and communities, and to locate referral sources.

ADVOCACY, ETHICS, AND RISK COMMUNICATION

All nurses should be able to demonstrate knowledge of the role of advocacy (case and class), ethics, and risk communication in patient care and community intervention with respect to the potential adverse effects of the environment on health.

LEGISLATION AND REGULATION

All nurses should understand the policy framework and major pieces of legislation and regulations related to environmental health.

Data from Institute of Medicine, 1995, p. 62.

cise some control over stressors (Lazarus and Folkman, 1984). Personal control involves the expectations that one can influence (decrease or increase) a stressor and/or the stress linked with a stressor. Examples of personal control behaviors include informing oneself about a stressor, learning cognitive methods of managing a stressor, devising alternative ways to manage a stressor (decisional control), and taking steps to directly reduce a stressor (behavioral control) (Averill, 1973; Thompson, 1981). Throughout the literature, nurses (Davidson and Ray, 1991; Dracup, 1988; Topf, 1984) have emphasized the importance of personal control over ambient stressors for patient well-being.

Instruction in control involves teaching patients ways to enhance behavioral and other types of control over stressors (Krantz, 1980)—in this case, ambient stressors. An example of instruction in information control includes nurses informing patients about ambient stressors, such as identifying sounds for patients and explaining why the lights are on at night. Teaching patients relaxation/meditation techniques is a form of instruction in cognitive control to decrease stress. Instruction in decisional control involves providing patients with choices (e.g., think about something else) to deal with ambient stressors. Finally, instruction in behavioral control might involve teaching patients behavioral responses; for example, requesting a sleep medication and asking visitors at the bedside to lower their voices, to deal with the ambient stressor of excessive noise (Topf, 1993).

Authors have discussed how control over a stressor may result in stress reduction. One contention is that exercising control over a stressor is positively reinforcing and thus reduces the stress that is linked with ambient stressors. Even if the intensity of the stressor does not change, when a patient senses that he or she can do something about this source of irritation, he or she feels better (Janis and Rodin, 1979). Consequently, some (Sherrod et al, 1977) claim that the more control one has over ambient stressors, the better.

Some studies evaluating the effects of instructing patients in personal control over ambient stressors have been limited to patient control over hospital noise (Griffin et al, 1988; Topf, 1985b, 1992a, 1992b). The tested interventions have included instructions in the use of earplugs (behavioral control), turning on a sound conditioner to block out noise (behavioral control), and progressive muscle relaxation (cognitive control). These attempts proved unsuccessful in helping patients deal with stressors effectively.

Studies such as these provide some insight into how to best instruct patients in ways to exert personal control over ambient stressors in the hospital setting. The intensity of some stressors may outweigh a patient's attempts to cope with them, however. Furthermore, some authors have argued that instruction in control can fail when exercising control requires too much effort (Thompson et al, 1988). It is easy to understand that such simple tasks as asking for a sleep medication or turning over in bed to ask that annoying noise be quieted might be a burden for an acutely ill patient. According to the "environmental docility hypothesis," as personal competence decreases, the probability that behavior will be influenced by environmental constraints (ambient stressors) or facilitators increases (Lawton, 1974; Williams, 1989). It seems reasonable to assume that all institutionalized patients, including adults, the elderly, children, and infants, would have less than personal competence. There is a crucial need for nursing awareness and action to reduce environmental constraints and enhance patient coping (Topf, 1993).

Reduction has shown that noise is a stressor, and that hospitals are noisy. All nursing care plans need to include noise control measures. The actions might range from the nursing staff learning to talk more quietly to the goal of placing machines that alarm away from the head of the patient's bed. Orienting the patient to hospital or equipment sounds will also help in recognition of the various noises and thereby help in reducing stress.

CLINICAL DECISION MAKING

THE SITUATION

Mr. T., the patient discussed in the case study, was exhibiting signs of disorientation. He is 65 years old. Mr. T. was admitted with an acute attack of asthma. He is confined to a room that is in a noisy, lighted area. He has no opportunity to relate to an outdoor environment because the window in his room is small and looks out at another building. He has trouble sleeping. He is increasingly becoming disoriented as to time, place, and recognizing people.

FACTORS POSSIBLY INFLUENCING THE PROBLEM

Mr. T.'s age and physical condition
Excessive noise from staff, paging system, and equipment usage
Excessive lights
Cool temperature in the room
Medication side effects
Oxygen depletion due to asthmatic condition.
Lack of physical orientation to the outdoors
Sensory deprivation
Insomnia

GOALS

The causes of Mr. T.'s disorientation need to be discovered and proper treatment initiated. The first question to ask is what is known about the causes of disorientation that might be applicable in this situation. A next step is to identify factors contributing to the problem.

Each factor should be carefully examined to ascertain how it applies to Mr. T. For example, check each side effect of the patient's medications as well as interactions between medications. Determine if the dosage is proper for Mr. T.'s age. Review the factors identified and determine how and what they contribute to the patient's disorientation.

By checking the patient's medications, history, oxygen saturation, environmental factors, and nursing notes for sleep patterns, the nurse can accumulate a body of data. The results of the data collection indicate that a lack of sleep has possibly caused a temporary situational disorientation.

NURSING INTERVENTIONS

Appropriate nursing actions need to be taken. These might include passing on the information to the night nurses, moving the patient to another room away from the nurses' station and the light in the hallway, pulling his door closed at night, and opening the curtain between the beds so he can see out during the day. He might need to just be able to get out of his room to a sitting area by a window or outside the unit. The nursing staff needs to provide added stimulation by interacting more often with Mr. T. and alerting his family to visit him more frequently.

EVALUATE THE RESULTS OF THE INTERVENTIONS

Once the patient starts sleeping better, his disorientation should disappear. The patient's disorientation to time and place should be frequently assessed. If symptoms are not alleviated, the process used to decide the appropriate nursing intervention should be reinstituted with other solutions proposed.

Lighting is another part of the physical environment that is sometimes difficult to change. Most patient rooms have indirect lighting fixtures that can be used instead of the overhead fluorescent ones. However, patients who have to travel on carts to other areas might end up looking at the ceiling lights for extended periods of time. The nurse should ask the patient if the light is distracting and provide the patient with eye covers to protect his or her eyes. It is necessary to remember that elderly people have an increased adaption time from light to dark, so patients who use the eye protectors need to be instructed to take them off ahead of time before getting off the cart so they can see clearly.

THE THERAPEUTIC ENVIRONMENT

The concept of the role the physical environment might have in facilitating therapeutic goals has given rise to the idea of the therapeutic environment. An example might be in using the physical environment in dealing with the stress of hospitalization in acute or long-term care facilities. By introducing such items of ordinary and familiar reassurance as plants and natural light, the nurse is helping the patient deal with one of the potential sources of stress. A hospital is visually stressful, with unfamiliar and rather forbidding-looking equipment and interior spaces, so the inclusion of familiar and nonthreatening parts of everyday life is reassuring. There is a growing body of research showing that using natural lighting and incorporating aspects of nature into the care and discharge planning of patients are important to patients' healing. The inclusion of a nurturing and loving environment as expressed by spaces that are wonderful to be in should be a top priority for someone who is not well. The sounds, smells, tastes, and sights of the modern health care institutions are foreign to most people and are not conducive to tapping into healing mechanisms.

Mr. T., who was described in the case presentation, is a candidate for nursing interventions to moderate the effects of a nonsupportive physical environment. The nurse can assess the physical environment with regard to noise, light, and access to natural light. Mr. T. might not be able to explain how well he sleeps at night, and so the communication between nurses about his sleeping behavior is very important. The nurse also needs to control noise. Background noise is especially distracting for an older person, who might have some

RESEARCH HIGHLIGHT
ATTENTIONAL FATIGUE AND RESTORATION IN PATIENTS WITH CANCER

Cimprich noted that "for individuals who have cancer, it is vitally important for them to deal effectively with diagnostic and treatment events, therapeutic self-care and interpersonal relationships. . . . Nursing approaches that may help conserve or restore (directed) attention would have significant therapeutic value" (p. 26).

The restorative intervention Cimprich designed was threefold, involving:

- increasing the subjects' understanding of nature and the purpose of the restorative experience
- assisting the subjects to identify and select preferred restorative activities, such as gardening, bird-watching, walking in a park
- contracting with subjects to engage in restorative activities three times a week.

The subjects were 32 women with early-stage breast cancer. All subjects were tested for attentional capacity and randomly assigned to receive the experimental restorative intervention or to receive no intervention. Intervention was initiated before hospital discharge. Repeated measures were used to allow following changes over time.

Some of the important findings of this study were as follows:

- A significant proportion of the women exhibited severe impairment on the attentional measures at the first testing, about three days post-surgery. These attentional deficits were still present at the start of adjuvant therapy, two to three weeks following surgery.
- Lower scores on attentional tests early in treatment suggest that attentional effort is prolonged and intense in the pretreatment phase of the illness.
- An unexpected finding was that mastectomy and breast conservative surgery groups did not differ significantly in attentional capacity, even though it is popularly thought that conservative surgery has distinct psychological advantages over mastectomy.
- The restorative intervention appeared to have a beneficial effect over time. This group showed greater gains and less decline in attentional scores, and older subjects especially benefited from the intervention. Conversely, older subjects in the nonintervention group showed the greatest losses in attentional capacity over time, suggesting that these subjects had greater difficulty dealing with the demands of long-term radiation therapy.
- An unexpected finding was the reporting of taking on new projects by the intervention group during the study period. None were reported by the other group.
- All subjects in the intervention group who were employed outside the home had returned to work full-time during the study period. Of the 11 women who were employed in the other group, two had not returned to work and two reverted from full-time to part-time employment.

Data from Cimprich, B. (1990). Attentional fatigue and restoration in individuals with cancer. Dissertation Abstracts International, 51, (04), 1740B (University Microfilms No. Dex 9023531).

hearing loss in the higher frequency range. Observations about daylight can be made easily, and being aware of the position of the curtain and the covers is as important an observation as are ones on the physical condition of the patient. Supportive actions include ensuring the patient has access to daylight, preferably with a view of nature, for part of his day. If the patient does not have a view from the window in his room, nursing actions might be moving him out of his room to a place where there is a view, providing plants, and hanging artwork depicting natural scenes in his room where the patient can easily see them.

RESTORATIVE ACTIONS

Cimprich (1990), in her research on restorative interventions, noted that Nightingale (1859) observed the need for providing patients with activities that would offer some relief from "painful ideas" as well as bodily pain. In calling out the "varieties of relief" Nightingale says: "A little needlework, a little writing, a little cleaning would be the greatest relief the sick could have if they could do it" (p. 36). Other "varieties of relief" that Nightingale observed to be effective included "a real laugh," plants, flowers, pets (and if the patient can care for them, "so much the better"), and "engravings of choice that might be hung in view and changed when desired" (p. 27).

Cimprich (1990, p. 95) also notes (see Research Highlight) that the findings in her study on decreased attentional functioning underscore the need for nurses to "create a supportive health care environment . . . that would eliminate barriers to make it possible for people to help themselves." Cimprich notes that nurses control many of the aspects of the patient's immediate environment, such as "irritating distractions (noise, people traffic), unpredictable schedules of care, multiple caregivers, impersonal or monotonous surroundings, clumsy arrangements of furniture, bedside clutter and lack of privacy, to name a few" (p. 96).

As noted earlier, data show that supportive, healing environments are beneficial to patient and staff functioning. The design expression of these data are beginning to show up in health care facilities. It is not hard to design indirect lighting, put windows in walls, have indoor and outdoor spaces for all who use the facility to enjoy, and reduce noise. It does take health care professionals committed to the very best for their patients and the community.

Cimprich (1990) noted that in teaching patients about cancer, nurses rely typically on specific content while ignoring the nonsupportive environment that constrains learning. Most patient education protocols are designed around specific content, and there are relatively few, if any, that specify the physical environment as part of attaining the desired outcome. Knowing that views of nature or some sort of vegetation are nonthreatening and supportive, perhaps a period of meditation or quiet time in a garden or at a window would be a prerequisite for beginning the teaching. Inclusion of nature-related therapies after discharge would ensure that the patient is given the opportunity to decrease stress levels and promote healing.

Another interesting practice that flies in the face of research is that of not allowing plants in certain areas of the hospital, especially critical care units. The principle is one of the contamination of the unit by microorganisms in the soil—the "jumping bacteria" theory. Research done by and for NASA has shown convincingly that plants and soil microbes actually cleanse the air; the irony is that formaldehyde-based adhesives such as those used for putting down carpet and tile are far more contaminating than plants and soil and yet are routinely permitted.

Community Setting

Nurses in community clinics might be asked to do risk management, pollution assessment, and even some epidemiology. Other actions include participating in lead abatement programs or other community programs in health promotion and education.

Nursing actions definitely include patient education about the risks involved in lead ingestion in children as well as exposure at the work place. Blood lead levels of children under the age of 6 should be routinely tested. Teaching mothers that children need to wash their hands before eating, or taking some sort of wipes to the playground to wipe off the child's hands, will go a long way to preventing any swallowing of the dust that might be contaminated. Nutrition education is also important. The child's body will substitute lead in the place of calcium or iron if those are inadequate in the diet. In old buildings with chipping paint, it is important to sample the paint and then take preventive actions. If there is an active lead abatement program in the community, a crew can be sent in to repaint the areas. Other actions include covering the chipping areas with shelf paper or tape, and also wiping down areas with a wet sponge or rag and then disposing of it (LOE, Part 4).

The practice areas of the public health nurse and home health nurse might overlap when it comes to teaching about keeping healthy in the home. Part of a home assessment for potential toxic risks could be a standard for the employing agency. For example, the patients might not realize that there is metallic mercury in the home, even though it is present in thermostats, fluorescent light bulbs, glass thermometers, and some blood pressure machines. If there is a mercury spill, the patient needs to know how to safely contain the mercury as in a spill from a broken thermometer. Never vacuum it up; remove children from the area, provide plenty of clean air, and roll the mercury onto a sheet of paper or suck it up with an eye dropper. This should all be put into an airtight container. Allow a minimum of 1 hour for ventilation (ATSDR, June 27, 1997).

Knowledge and understanding of the impact of the physical environment on both work place safety and individual health practices of the workforce will be important for these areas of practice. Activities such as monitoring the noise levels and understanding the chemicals that are used in the work place are essential in the occupational setting. Asking workers to keep a journal of the chemicals they work with on a day-to-day basis is one way of keeping track of valuable information for a medical history. See Chapter 18 for additional information.

Additionally, the nurse needs to be observant and understand the physical environment of the community where the clients live. For example, if there are a large number of inland lakes around, the potential for eating contaminated fish from one of these lakes could be a serious threat to pregnant women and children. Each state sets standards for protection of health, and the nurse will draw on these as a guide and basis for teaching clients.

Are there industrial plants that might be contaminating the air or are there old waste sites that could be potential hazards for groundwater or as children's play areas? The ATSDR estimates that about one in four American children lives within 4 miles of a hazardous waste site. Children often have greater exposures and greater potential for health problems and less ability to avoid the hazards (ATSDR, Child Health Programs Home Page, 1998–1999). The nurse needs to be informed about the local environment.

By monitoring air quality alerts and patients with impaired respiratory function, nurses teach of the need for a safe environment during periods of poor air quality alerts. If the home does not have air conditioning, then the nurse needs to assist in locating a shelter for the patient and instruct the patient about the need to go there at these times. Children with asthma who want to be outside during periods of smog alerts also need to be instructed in the importance of either staying indoors or going to community-provided shelter.

Effects of environmental hazards on the community as a whole often cause controversy resulting in citizens organizing to protect the health and welfare of all living in the area. An example of such community involvement occurred at the Love Canal, New York, in the 1960s. Residential property in the area was contaminated with dangerous toxic waste products. People living in the neighborhood banded together and sought professional help from health and scientific experts. As a result of these activities, a major social movement evolved that has led to a national environmental focus. Other such movements involving water pollution, pesticide pollution, and oil spills were subsequently undertaken (Institute of Medicine, 1995).

CHAPTER HIGHLIGHTS

- The need for consideration of the environment as an essential part of nursing and health care was addressed by Florence Nightingale in her many writings.
- The physical environment includes both natural and man-made components.
- The Surgeon General's report on Health Promotion and Disease Prevention indicated that almost all chronic diseases are affected by environmental factors.
- Environmental hazards can be found in health care settings, homes, work places, and the community.
- Hazards include air pollution, noise pollution, water pollution, and toxic metals.
- Ambient stressors in the environment include noise, light, temperature extremes, and poor air quality.
- Environment is considered a major element in nursing theories.
- Environmental hazards affect individuals of all ages and both genders in specific ways. There are certain occupations and living conditions in which exposure to environmental hazards are very high.
- Cultural traditions may include practices that are environmentally hazardous.
- Structural and architectural designs affect the environment of persons who occupy the buildings.
- Nursing care includes environmental concerns such as noise suppression, light, temperature control, noncontaminated food, and fresh air with control of air-borne contaminants.

REFERENCES

Agency for Toxic Substances and Disease Registry, Office of Children's Health (1998). *Child Health Programs: 1998–1999.* [Homepage of Agency for Toxic Substances and Disease Registry—Child Health] [Online]. Available: NHP://atsdr.gov:8080/child/[1998: August 9].

Agency for Toxic Substances and Disease Registry (ed.) (1990a, December—last update). *Public Health Statement: Lead.* [Homepage of Agency for Toxic Substances and Disease Registry] [Online]. Available: http://www.atsdr.atsdr.cdc.gov:8080/atsdrhomehtml/[1997, July 23].

Agency for Toxic Substances and Disease Registry (ed.) (1990b, December—last update). *Public Health Statement: Mercury.* [Homepage of Agency for Toxic Substances and Disease Registry] [Online]. Available: http://www.atsdr.atsdr.cdc.gov:8080/atsdrhomehtml/[1997, July 23].

Agency for Toxic Substances and Disease Registry Office of Policy and External Affairs (ed.). (June 27, 1997). *National Alert: A Warning About Continuing Patterns of Metallic Mercury Exposure.* [Homepage of Agency for Toxic Substances and Disease Registry] [Online]. Available: http://www.atsdr.atsdr.cdc.gov.8080/atsdrhome.html/[1997, August 19].

Anastasi, A. (1964). *Fields of Applied Psychology.* New York: McGraw-Hill.

Au Yeung, Y., Chow, W., Lam, Y. (1991). Sick building syndrome—A case study. *Building and Environment, 26,* 319–327.

Averill, J. (1973). Personal control over aversive stimuli and its relationship to stress. *Psychological Bulletin, 80,* 286–303.

Baker, C. (1984). Sensory overload and noise in the ICU: Sources of environmental stress. *Critical Care Quarterly, 6,* 66–80.

Bates, D. (1994). *Environmental health risks and public policy decision making in free societies.* Seattle: University of Washington Press.

Baum, A., Singer, J., Baum, C. (1981). Stress and the environment. *Journal of Social Issues, 40,* 150–155.

Berry, W. (1995, September–October). Health is membership. *The Utne Reader,* pp. 60–63.

Campbell, J. (1983). Ambient stressors. *Environment and Behaviour, 15,* 355–380.

Carpman, J.R., Grant, M.A., Simmons, D. (1986). *Design That Cares: Planning Health Facilities for Patients and Visitors.* Chicago: American Hospital Publishing, Inc.

Center for Disease Control (May 24, 1996). *Mortality, morbidity weekly report.* 45, pp. 422–424. U.S. Government Printing Office (1996–733–175/47005 Region IV).

Cimprich, B. (1990). Attentional fatigue and restoration in individuals with cancer. *Dissertation Abstracts International, 51,* (04), 1740B (University Microfilms No. Dex 9023531).

Coile, Jr., R. (1996). Essay: Healthcare design 1996–2000. *Æsclepius, 5,* 5–7.

Crayne, H., Miner, D. (1988). Thermoresuscitation for postoperative hypothermia. *Association of Operating Room Nurses, 47,* 222–227.

Culpepper-Richards, K., Bairnsfather, L. (1988). A description of night sleep patterns in the critical care unit. *Heart & Lung, 17,* 35–42.

Curtin, L. (1990, July). Touch-tempered technology [editorial]. *Nursing Management, 21,* 7–8.

Davidson, A., Ray, M. (1991). Studying the human-environment phenomenon using the science of complexity. *Advances in Nursing Science, 14,* 72–85.

Dracup, K. (1988). Are critical care units hazardous to health? *Applied Nursing Research, 1,* 14–21.

Dubos, R. (1977). *Man Adapting.* New Haven: Yale University Press.

Evans, G. (1982). *Environmental Stress.* New York: Cambridge University Press.

Falk, S., Woods, N. (1973). Hospital noise levels and potential health effects. *The New England Journal of Medicine, 289,* 774–781.

Foulke, J. (1994). Mercury in fish: Cause for concern? *FDA Consumer,* 5–8.

Griffin, J., Myers, S., Kopelke, C., Walker, D. (1988). The effects of progressive muscular relaxation on subjectively reported disturbance due to hospital noise. *Behavioral Medicine, 14,* 37–42.

Hilton, B. (1985). Noise in acute patient care areas. *Research in Nursing & Health, 8,* 283–291.

Hockey, R. (1984). Varieties of attentional state: The effects of environment. In R. Parasuraman and D. R. Davies (eds.): *Varieties of Attention.* Orlando: Academic Press, pp. 29–62.

Hoffman, M. (1993). Chemical pollution of the environment: Past, present and future. In J. Lake, G. Bock (organizers), and K. Ackrill (eds.): *Environmental Change and Human Health:*

A Ciba Foundation Symposium 175. Chichester: John Wiley & Sons Ltd, pp. 23–41.

Horne, J. (1988). *Why we sleep*. Oxford: Oxford University Press.

House Report #102-852 (1992). *Lead Exposure Reduction Act*. Washington, D.C.: U.S. Government Printing Office.

Institute of Medicine (1995). *Nursing, Health and the Environment—Strengthening the Relationship to Improve the Public's Health*. Washington, D.C.: National Academy Press.

Janis, L., Rodin, J. (1979). Attribution, control, and decision-making: Social psychology and health care. In G. Stone, F. Cohen, and N. Adler (eds.): *Health Psychology*. San Francisco: Jossey-Bass, pp. 487–521.

Johnson, D. (1980). The Johnson behavioral system model for nursing. In J. Riehl and C. Roy (eds.): *Conceptual Models for Nursing Practice*, 2nd ed. New York: Appleton-Century-Crofts, pp. 207–216.

Kaiser, L. (1996). *Health Care in the 21st Century*. (Available from Estes Park Institute, P.O. Box 400, Englewood, CO 80151.)

Kaplan, S. (1983). A model of person-environment compatibility. *Environment and Behavior, 15*, 311–332.

Kaplan, S. (1992). The restorative environment: Nature and human experience. In D. Relf (ed.): *The Role of Horticulture in Human Well-Being and Social Development: A National Symposium*. Portland, OR: Thirber Press, pp. 134–142.

Kaufman, M. (1969). A time, stress, perception model for theory development. In C. Norris (ed.): *Proceedings First Nursing Theory Conference*. Kansas City, MO: University of Kansas, pp. 23–32.

Keep, P. (1977). Stimulus deprivation in windowless rooms. *Anaesthesia, 32*, 598–600.

King, I (1971). *Toward a theory for nursing*. New York: John Wiley.

Kleinjans, J., van Maanen, J., van Schooten, F. (1993). Human respiratory disease: Environmental carcinogens and lung cancer risk. In J. Lake, G. Bock (organizers), and K. Ackrill (eds.): *Environmental Change and Human Health: A Ciba Foundation Symposium 175*. Chichester: John Wiley & Sons Ltd, pp. 171–181.

Krantz, D. (1980). Cognitive processes and recovery from heart attack: A review and theoretical analysis. *Journal of Human Stress, 6*, 27–38.

Lawton, M. (1974). The human being and the institutional building. In J. Lang, C. Burnette, W. Moleski, and D. Vachon (eds.): *Designing for Human Behavior: Architecture and the Behavioral Sciences*. Stroudsburg, PA: Dowden, Hutchinson & Ross, pp. 60–71.

Lazarus, R., Folkman, S. (1984). *Stress Appraisal and Coping*. New York: Springer.

Living on Earth Transcript (May 30, 1997). *Lead Poisoning: The Silent Epidemic, Part One, Protecting Kids From Lead*. [Homepage of Living on Earth] [Online]. Available: http://loe.npr.org/[1997, July 3].

Living on Earth Transcript (June 6, 1997). *Lead Poisoning: The Silent Epidemic, Part Two, Crime and Heavy Metal*. [Homepage of Living on Earth] [Online]. Available: http://loe.npr.org/[1997, July 3].

Living on Earth Transcript (June 13, 1997). *Lead Poisoning: The Silent Epidemic, Part Three, Lead in the Workplace*. [Homepage of Living on Earth] [Online]. Available: http://loe.npr.org/[1997, July 3].

Living on Earth Transcript (June 30, 1997). *Lead Poisoning: The Silent Epidemic, Part Four, Hidden Lead*. [Homepage of Living on Earth] [Online]. Available: http://loe.npr.org/ [1997, July 3].

Minnesota Department of Health (1997). *An Expectant Mother's Guide to Eating Minnesota Fish*. St. Paul, MN: Author.

Minnesota Department of Health (1993). *Fish and Your Health: Environmental Exposure to PCBs in Fish*. St. Paul, MN: Author.

Minnesota Department of Health (March 1997). *Fish Facts: Mercury in the Environment* (IC #141-0627). St. Paul, MN: Author.

Minnesota Department of Health (April 1996). *To Your Health: Eating Lake Fish in Minnesota* (IC #141-0370). St. Paul, MN: Author.

Mishima, A. (1992). *Bitter Sea: The Human Cost of Minamata Disease*. (Trans. by R. Gage and S. Murata). Tokyo: Kosei Publishing Co. (Original work published 1977. *Nake, Shiranui, no Umi: Minimata mi Sasageta Chinkon no Tatakai*.)

National Public Radio (1996, July). *Why Pregnant Women Shouldn't Eat Fish* (NPRAT 2245-5). Washington, D.C.

Neuman, B. (1974). The Betty Neuman health-care systems model: A total person approach to patient problems. In J. Tiehl and C. Roy (eds.): *Conceptual Models for Nursing Practice*. New York: Appleton-Century-Crofts, pp. 99–114.

Newman, M. (1987). *Health as Expanding Consciousness*. St. Louis: C.V. Mosby.

Nightingale, F. (1859). *Notes on Nursing*. New York: Dover Publications.

Occupational safety and health administration (Sept. 22, 1995). *OSHA technical manual*. Section II: Chapter 2, indoor air quality investigation (OSHA instruction Ted.1.15).

Orem, D. (1971). *Nursing Concepts for Practice*. New York: McGraw-Hill.

Ornish, D. (1984). *Stress, Diet and Your Heart*. New York: Penguin.

Ovitt, M. (1996). *The Effect of a View of Nature on Performance and Stress Reduction of ICU Nurses*. Unpublished master's thesis, University of Illinois, Urbana-Champaign.

Parse, R. (1981). *Man-Living Health: A Theory of Nursing*. New York: Wiley.

Patterson, J., Zderod, L. (1976). *Humanistic Nursing*. New York: Wiley.

Phillips, R., Skov, P. (1988). Rewarming and cardiac surgery: A review. *Heart & Lung, 17*, 511–519.

Philp, R. (1995). *Environmental Hazards and Human Health*. Boca Raton: Lewis Publishers.

Raver, A. (1994). Need an air freshener? Try plants. *The New York Times*, February 13, p. 19.

R.N.'s battle poor indoor air quality. (1995, winter). *Æsclepius*, 4, p. 1.

Rogers, M. (1970). *An Introduction to the Theoretical Basis for Nursing*. Philadelphia: F.A. Davis.

Rose, M., Killian, M. (1983). Risk and vulnerability: A case for differentiation. *Advances in Nursing Science, 5*, 60–73.

Rosenberg, N. (1997, March 10). Asthma attacks in kids, seniors linked to high ozone. *Milwaukee Journal Sentinel*, p. 2G.

Roy, C. (1976). *Introduction to Nursing: An Adaptation Model*. Englewood Cliffs, NJ: Prentice-Hall.

Shapiro, R., Berland, T. (1972). Noise in the operating room. *The New England Journal of Medicine, 287*, 1236–1238.

Sherman, J. (1994). *Chemical Exposure and Disease.* Princeton Scientific Publishing Co., Inc.

Sherrod, D., Hage, J., Halpern, P., Moore, B. (1977). Effects of personal causation and perceived control of responses to an aversive environment: The more control the better. *Journal of Experimental Social Psychology, 13,* 14–27.

Shumaker, S., Reizenstein, J. (1982). Environmental factors affecting inpatient stress. In G. Evans (ed.): *Environmental Stress.* New York: Cambridge University Press, pp. 179–223.

Singleton, D. (1992). Case study on therapeutic benefits: The therapeutic value of landscape design [Appendix 11]. In *Health Building Note 45: External Works for Health Buildings,* Department of Health, author. London: HMSO, pp. 80–88.

Snyder-Halpern, R. (1985). The effect of critical care unit noise on patient sleep cycles. *Critical Care Quarterly, 7* (4), 41–51.

Thompson, S. (1981). Will it hurt less if I can control it? A complex answer to a simple question. *Psychological Bulletin, 90,* 89–91.

Thompson, S., Cheek, P., Graham, M. (1988). The other side of perceived control: Disadvantages and negative effects. In S. Spacapan, S. Oskamp (eds.): *The Social Psychology of Health.* Beverly Hills: Sage, pp. 69–93.

Topf, M. (1984). A framework for research on aversive physical aspects of the environment. *Research in Nursing & Health, 7,* 35–42.

Topf, M. (1985a). Personal and environmental predictors of disturbance due to hospital noise. *Journal of Applied Psychology, 70,* 22–28.

Topf, M. (1985b). Noise-induced stress in hospital patients: Coping and nonauditory health outcomes. *The Journal of Human Stress, 11,* 125–134.

Topf, M. (1992a). Stress effects of personal control over hospital noise. *Behavioral Medicine, 18,* 84–94.

Topf, M. (1992b). Effects of personal control over hospital noise on sleep. *Research in Nursing and Health, 15,* 19–28.

Topf, M. (1993). Theoretical considerations for research on environmental stress and health. Manuscript submitted for publication.

Ulrich, R. (1979). Visual landscapes and psychological well-being. *Landscape Research, 4,* 17–23.

Ulrich, R. (1984). View through a window may influence recovery from surgery. *Science, 224,* 420–421.

Ulrich, R., Simons, R., Losito, B., et al (1991). Stress recovery during exposure to natural and urban environments. *Journal of Environmental Psychology, 11,* 1–23.

United States Department of Education, National Center for Education Statistics (1997) (NCES 98–105) Washington, D.C.

United States Environmental Protection Agency (July 17, 1997—last update). *Health and Environmental Effects of Ground-Level Ozone.* [Homepage of Office of Air & Radiation] [Online]. Available: http://www.epa.gov/oar/[1997, August 5].

United States Environmental Protection Agency (July 17, 1997—last update). *Health and Environmental Effects of Particulate Matter.* [Homepage of Office of Air & Radiation] [Online]. Available: http://www.epa.gov/oar/[1997, August 5].

Vander, A., Sherman, J., Luciano, D. (1980). *Human Physiology: The Mechanisms of Human Function,* 3rd ed. New York: McGraw-Hill Book Co.

Verderber, S. (1986). Dimensions of person-window transactions in the hospital environment. *Environment and Behavior, 18,* 450–466.

Weber, D. (1995). Environments that heal. *The Healthcare Forum, 38,* 39–49.

Weidenbach, E. (1964). *Clinical Nursing: A Helping Art.* New York: Springer Publishing.

Williams, M. (1988). The physical environment and patient care. *Annual Review of Nursing Research, 6,* 61–84.

Williams, M. (1989). Physical environment of the intensive care unit and elderly patients. *Critical Care Nursing Quarterly, 12,* 52–60.

Wilson, L. (1972). Intensive care delirium. *Archives of Internal Medicine, 130,* 225–226.

Zimring, C. (1982). The built environment as a source of psychological stress: impacts of building and cities on satisfaction and behavior. In G.E. Evans (eD.): *Environmental stress.* Cambridge: Cambridge University Press.

Stress and Anxiety 31

Joan Stehle Werner

Viola Stenson, age 62, has been admitted to the hospital for joint replacement surgery of the left knee. She was widowed 2 years ago when her husband of 40 years died of a heart attack. She retired from her position as a dietary worker at the local high school 6 months ago. Her two grown daughters live several states away and visit once or twice a year with their families.

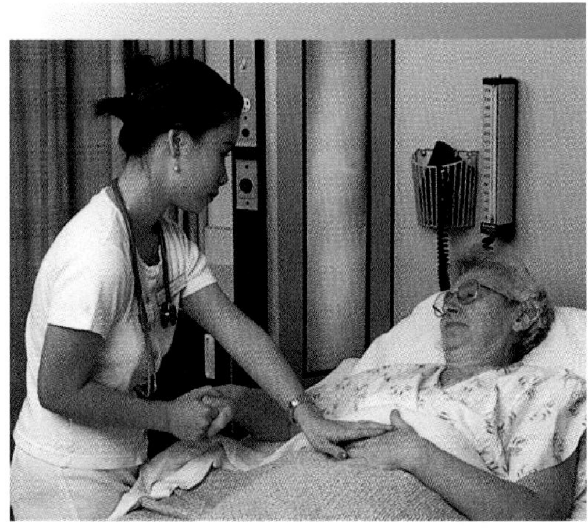

Mrs. Stenson's medical diagnoses include degenerative joint disease of the left knee and right elbow, status post–aortic valve replacement, and a history of chronic vertigo. Because of these diagnoses, Mrs. Stenson usually walks with a cane. She has been transported to the surgical unit by wheelchair, accompanied by the neighbor who brought her to the hospital.

During the admission interview with the nurse, Mrs. Stenson holds a handkerchief, which she moves quickly from one hand to the other. Tremors of her hands and facial muscles are obvious, and her face appears pale. As she speaks, her speech rate increases and her voice pitch heightens. She repeatedly sighs during the interview, and also asks the nurse to repeat her questions several times.

As the nurse asks about her worries, Mrs. Stenson expresses numerous financial concerns. She relates that she had just purchased a $2000 furnace and a new car battery, and that she needs a new kitchen floor. She says that she does not want to dip into her life savings any further, because she is saving the money for her grandchildren's education. She states that her insurance will cover only a portion of her hospital bill and that all of these expenses are very worrisome, since she receives only Social Security and a small pension. In addition, she says that making major decisions has been very difficult since her husband died, and that she worries a great deal about them.

OBJECTIVES

After studying this chapter, the student will be able to:

- **discuss current definitions and causative factors associated with stress and anxiety**
- **describe symptoms and behaviors that nurses are likely to observe in a person experiencing stress or anxiety**
- **state aspects of the stress process that nurses should recognize in a stressed individual**
- **describe health- and illness-related events in which stress and anxiety are likely to occur**
- **demonstrate beginning competence in clinical judgment and interpretation of stress and anxiety by identifying appropriate nursing diagnoses, remaining questions, and areas for ongoing assessment**
- **identify nursing interventions that are usually effective in reducing stress and anxiety**
- **state the desired outcomes regarding health that are related to stress and anxiety**

Sincere appreciation to Kathleen Shadick, R.N., M.S.N., Valerie Hutton, Kathleen Kiltenen, and Karen Krenz for assistance with library work for this chapter and to Mary Jo Fehr for her diligence and efficiency in secretarial support.

As the nurse continues to build rapport with this patient and ask about her obvious discomfort and her reasons for admission, Mrs. Stenson haltingly expresses fear of dying during surgery. She explains that she had undergone heart surgery five years ago and now has an "animal valve." She asserts that the prospect of "being put to sleep" causes her great distress and that she has delayed surgery on her knee for 4 years because she is afraid her "heart will stop" while she is asleep during surgery. Mrs. Stenson also confides that her best friend died 6 years ago during surgery and that this event has been on her mind since her own surgery was scheduled 2 weeks ago. She reports no one with whom to discuss her fears.

During the interview, the nurse notes other signs of stress and anxiety in the patient. Mrs. Stenson reports having trouble concentrating and difficulty catching her breath. She also states that she has been feeling very tired lately, yet is unable to sleep well at night. She says that her mouth is very dry and that she has a tension headache. Her facial expression is fearful, and her eyes continually dart about. Her anxiety about the scheduled surgery, along with her fears of "going broke" and "going to the poor house," dominate the remainder of her conversation with the nurse. (Later, the nurse learns that Mrs. Stenson in fact has substantial savings that will easily cover her financial needs for the rest of her life.)

SCOPE OF NURSING PRACTICE

Stress and anxiety are important concerns for nurses who adhere to Virginia Henderson's view of nursing: "to assist the individual, sick or well, in the performance of those activities contributing to health or its recovery (or to a peaceful death)" (Henderson and Nite, 1978, p. 95). Because the prevention or reduction of stress and anxiety can contribute to health or its recovery, it is of paramount concern to both nurses and patients.

Stress and anxiety are natural or instinctive responses to events in which individuals feel threatened or insecure. The awareness of the threat may be perceived consciously or unconsciously. Because health is so highly valued, any threat to health and well-being (or any medically related event, such as a diagnostic test) can precipitate stress and anxiety. Since they care for people with various health- and illness-related concerns, nurses must be prepared to deal with stress and anxiety in any patient at any time. In fact, nurses diagnose anxiety more frequently than any other condition except pain (Levin et al, 1989).

Numerous professionals and scientists from a wide range of disciplines study and treat stress and anxiety. Nurses, because they deal intimately with individuals in all walks of life, are in key positions to identify, label, and treat stress and anxiety. Contrary to many common notions, stress is not always imposed upon people from the environment. There are many aspects of stress that arise within a person. Therefore, much of the time, stress can be reduced or even prevented, thereby assisting in restoring or preserving health.

Likewise, anxiety is very real. When severe, it is not something people can ignore or "just snap out of." Think of how fast your heart beats when you are about to give a speech or take a risk. In many cases, as anxiety rises, people become unable to control this rise in tension. Although anxiety is a normal reaction meant to alert human beings to actual danger, it can become problematic if it outlasts the danger or is of greater intensity than necessary for the situation. Intense anxiety and stress have even been associated with sudden death (Dolnick, 1989; Mollica et al, 1987).

Because of the widespread experience of stress and anxiety in a myriad of situations, nurses must be knowledgeable about them. Nurses should be alert for signs of agitation, restlessness, sympathetic nervous system effects, and changes in perception. They need to focus on helping people to engage in adaptive coping behaviors. They also need to learn nursing actions that can reduce the great discomfort in stress and anxiety, such as offering realistic assurance, providing a quiet atmosphere, helping the patient clarify thinking, or using music or relaxation techniques. Finally, they need to learn to appraise and allay their own stress and anxiety in order to give effective nursing care.

KNOWLEDGE BASE

Basic Science

STRESS

A number of theories contribute to our current understanding of stress. The work of three early scientists, Cannon, Selye, and Wolff, is particularly significant for nurses.

In the early twentieth century, physiologist Walter Cannon referred to the steady state of the body's internal environment as *homeostasis.* He defined homeostasis as "the coordinated physiologic processes which maintain most of the steady states in the organism" (Cannon, 1932, p. 333). Cannon's research led to an understanding of how the sympathetic nervous system stimulates a "fight or flight" response (the body's reaction to either resist an invader or escape). This ancient response, which serves to help people and animals handle threats, still forms the basis for much of our knowledge about physiologic anxiety and stress today. Researchers presumed that homeostasis was desirable and the response of fighting or fleeing—a departure from steady state—led directly to physiologic stress. Emotional factors were also believed to be important contributors to stress (Cannon, 1935).

Another major concept of stress emphasized the body's responses to various noxious (harmful) stimuli, such as infection, trauma, surgery, or strong emotion (Selye, 1956, 1974).

One significant aspect of Selye's theory is the general adaptation syndrome (GAS), which involved three stages: an alarm reaction, a stage of resistance, and a stage of exhaustion (Fig. 31–1). Selye believed that disease and possibly even death could result from prolonged stress.

Still another theory defined stress as an internal state and as a dynamic (changing) process (Wolff, 1953). Wolff, a physician, linked stress in life with disease. He spoke of the person as adapting to demands with the purpose of restoring balance. These ideas are the basis for many current viewpoints of stress and its results, such as the negative outcome of disease, or the potential benefit of growth through reducing stress.

ANXIETY

Anxiety is often studied in conjunction with stress because it is a frequent and common reaction to stress. If left unchecked, anxiety can reach levels where a person becomes disorganized and debilitated. It is important for nurses to study anxiety to prevent patients from enduring the turmoil and disorganization that can occur. For example, psychiatric patients who experience panic levels of anxiety can become suicidal or homicidal. In these cases, it is imperative for the anxiety to be reduced to prevent these extreme cases of disorganization.

Anxiety is generally defined as a reaction to an unreal, imagined, or as yet unidentified source (Taylor and Arnow, 1988). Recent efforts have been made to distinguish between anxiety in response to some unknown source, and anxiety in response to something real. Two chief types of anxiety have been proposed. The first type, *endogenous anxiety,* arises from within the person. The other type, *exogenous anxiety,* is triggered by stressors in the environment (Emery and Tracy, 1987).

Anxiety also has been described as both a state and a trait. *State anxiety* is a feeling of anxiety in a specific, current situation; *trait anxiety* is an overall, nonspecific feeling of anxiety (Spielberger, 1971, 1979).

Historically, three major historical perspectives regarding anxiety include the psychodynamic, learning, and biologic perspectives. The psychodynamic view of anxiety originated with Freud. He believed that anxiety occurred within the "psyche" (mind) of the person and that it was dynamic, and thus psychodynamic in nature (Freud, 1926, 1936, 1953). He also theorized that anxiety occurs unconsciously in a person and signals an underlying traumatic situation, such as loss or separation. He proposed that anxiety produces symptoms that, if left unchecked, result in defense mechanisms (unhealthy modes of cognitive coping) such as repression (keeping disturbing thoughts or feelings out of awareness) or rationalization (construction of a more acceptable thought), which become unhealthy.

Learning theories explain anxiety as a conditioned or learned response to various situations. Building on Pavlov's ideas of classical conditioning, some scientists proposed that human anxiety, fear, and phobia result from a conditioned fear response. According to this theory, fear motivates an individual to reduce the fear through certain behaviors, such as keeping things in precise and impeccable order or refusal to leave the house in extreme cases. The subsequent reduction in fear following the behavior feeds back to the person's psyche, telling him or her that because the behavior reduced the anxiety, there must be something to fear. This reduction in fear then reinforces the behavior, maintaining the presence of anxiety (Dollard and Miller, 1950).

Biologic or neurophysiologic views of anxiety describe what occurs within the body during the anxiety response. This knowledge has its origin in the works of Darwin (1872),

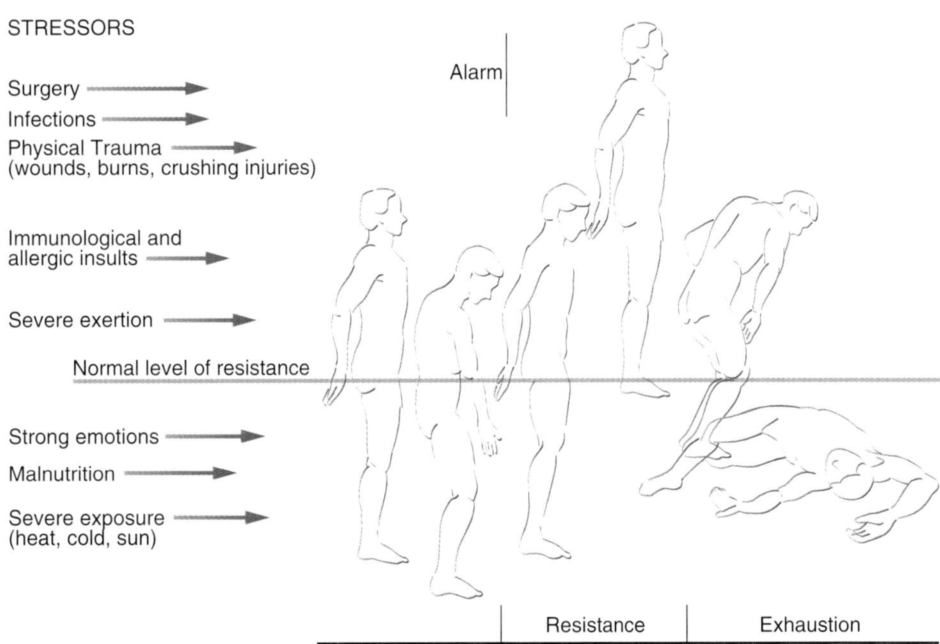

Figure 31–1. Selye's general adaptation syndrome. (From Byrne, M.L., & Thompson, L. [1978]. *Key Concepts for the Study and Practice of Nursing.* St. Louis: Mosby.)

who believed anxiety to be an instinct. Darwin's concept of anxiety contributed to Cannon's theory of fear producing the "fight or flight" response.

PHYSIOLOGIC PROCESSES IN STRESS AND ANXIETY

Stress and anxiety are interrelated processes that result from very complicated physiologic mechanisms. The major body systems involved in stress and anxiety are the endocrine, nervous, and immune systems. These systems communicate with each other through neuropeptides (chemical transmitters of the nervous system that excite or inhibit neurons), hormones (chemical messengers produced in glands), and cytokines (products from immune system cells). These communications, in turn, direct changes and activities in the cells of each system. Figure 31–2 illustrates the body systems involved in the stress process.

The stress process begins with the occurrence of a stressor from either outside the body (such as extreme cold or lack of basic nutrition), or inside the body (intense emotion, such as fear or anger). The presence of such a stressor is processed through the hypothalamus in the brain and is communicated to the rest of the body by hormones from the pituitary and adrenal glands and by the sympathetic nervous system.

Increased hypothalamic activity stimulates the release of hormones from the anterior pituitary gland, the adrenal cortex, and the adrenal medulla. These hormones weaken the immune response so that the body can coexist with the stressor. They also increase the blood's ability to clot in case of injury. They convert blood glucose and protein into sources of available energy to meet the demands of the stressor.

At the same time, increases occur in heart rate, blood pressure, blood flow to the muscles, and perspiration, enhancing the body's functioning and stability. Increased blood supply to vital organs causes the skin to become cool and pale and slows gastrointestinal tract activity. Several feedback mechanisms also operate during this process. These responses to stress galvanize bodily functions that are essential to life, while subduing nonessential functions. Box 31–1 summarizes the major physiologic changes that occur in response to stress. Figure 31–3 illustrates the principal neuroendocrine pathways involved in human stress. This figure relates the stress process to Selye's GAS.

Meanwhile, the parasympathetic nervous system also activates responses, causing the characteristic fearful facial expression, altered voice, increased heart rate, and bronchodilation (dilating of bronchioles in the lungs). In extreme cases, parasympathetic activity can lead to lower bowel evacuation. If anxiety is severe or pathologic, or reaches the panic level,

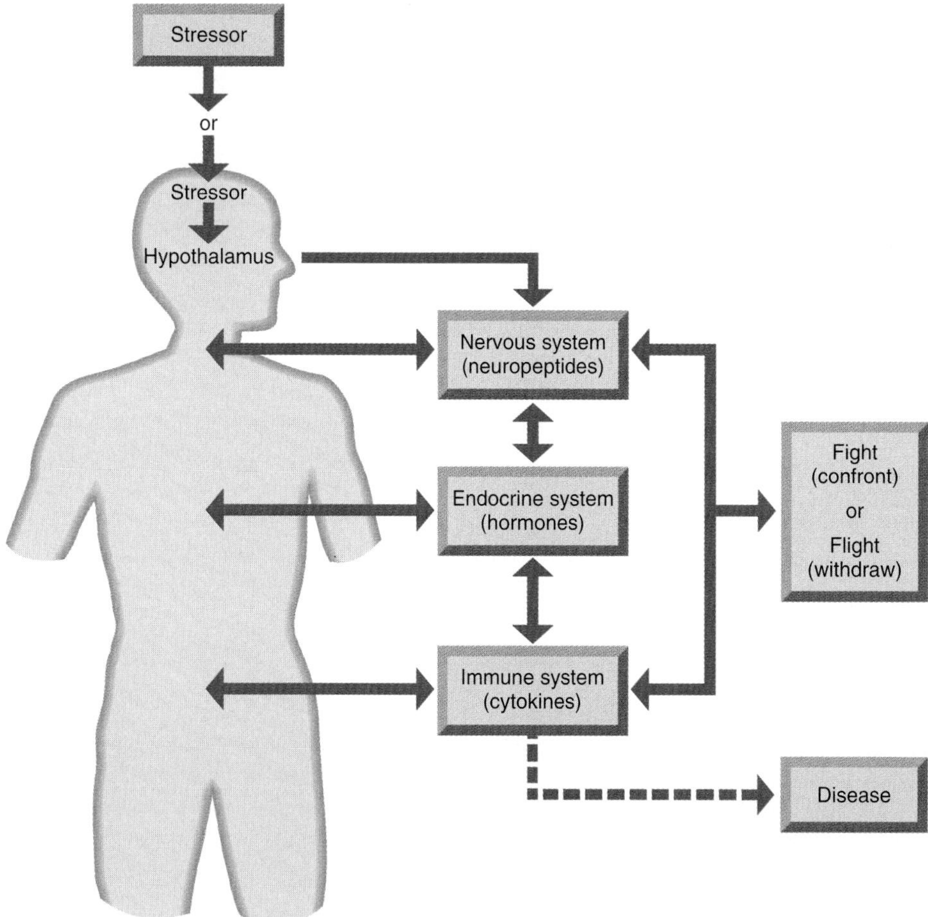

Figure 31–2. Major body systems involved in the stress response.

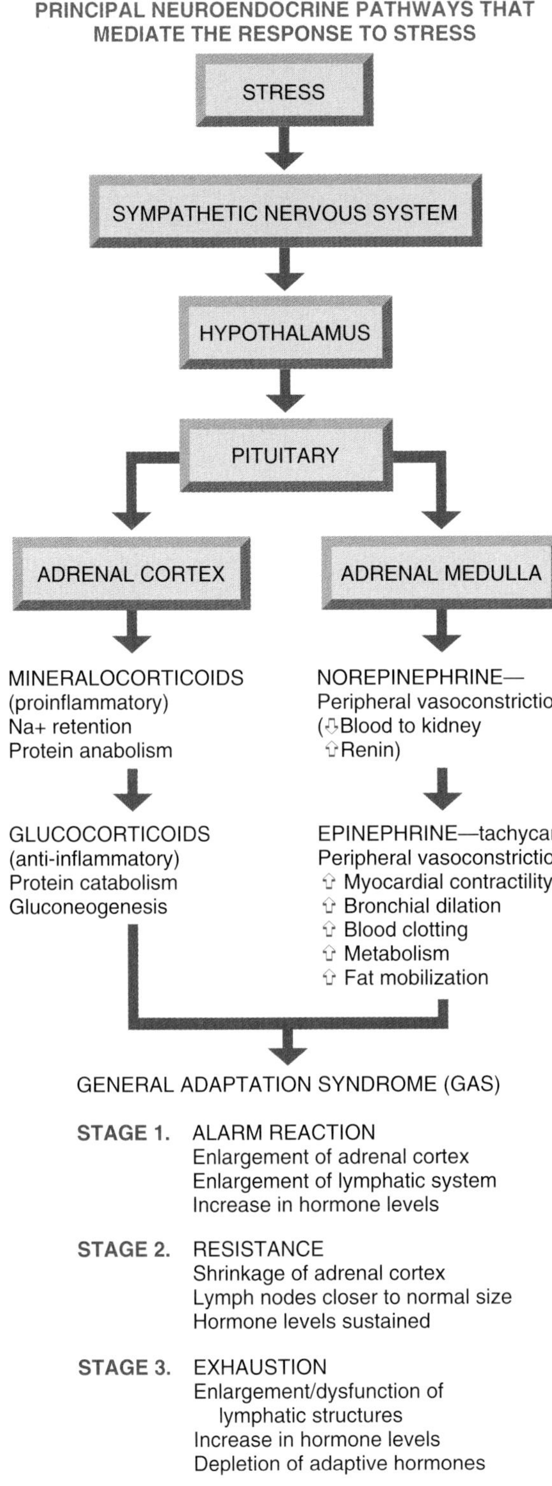

Figure 31–3. Principal neuroendocrine pathways that mediate the response to stress. (From Smith, M.J., & Selye, H. [1979]. Effects of stress, reducing the negative. *American Journal of Nursing, 79*[10], 1953–1964.)

BOX 31–1
SUMMARY OF MAJOR BODY CHANGES DURING STRESS

Increases in (Essential Functions):
Clotting ability of the blood
Energy from glucose and protein
Heart rate
Blood pressure
Blood to muscles and vital organs
Perspiration
Bronchodilation

Decreases in (Nonessential Functions):
Immune response
Blood to skin
Gastrointestinal activity

several somatic (bodily) symptoms are usually present. These symptoms include muscular pain, twitching, tremors, sometimes spasms; blurred vision, flushing or sweating; heart palpitations, chest pain, feeling faint; choking or sighing; difficulty swallowing, nausea or vomiting; need to urinate; dry mouth, giggling, or tension headache. Some people tend to freeze, some tend to faint, and some withdraw (Beck, 1985; Doswell, 1989; Taylor and Arnow, 1988).

In addition, studies have indicated that the body's stress response and associated distress can alter immune system function (Cohen and Williamson, 1991; Kiecolt-Glaser and Glaser, 1991). Therefore, consequences of stress can cause or contribute to disease. Scientists in the field of psychoneuroimmunology (psyche = mind, emotions; neuro = nervous system; immunology = immune function) are currently studying these relationships.

PSYCHOLOGICAL PROCESSES IN STRESS AND ANXIETY

Understanding stress and anxiety from a psychological viewpoint requires a framework for organizing this knowledge. One such framework, developed on the basis of hundreds of research studies, was proposed by the Institute of Medicine in its report on *Research on Stress and Human Health* (Elliott and Eisdorfer, 1982); they call it a "Framework for Interactions between the Individual and the Environment" (Fig. 31–4). This framework conceptualizes stress and anxiety as a "person-environment" interaction in which the experience of stress and anxiety is explained by four major concepts:

- stressors
- reactions
- consequences
- mediators

STRESSORS

The first concept in the Institute of Medicine's framework is *stressors*, or "potential activators" (Elliott and Eisdorfer, p. 19). Stressors are stimuli or initiators of the stress process that

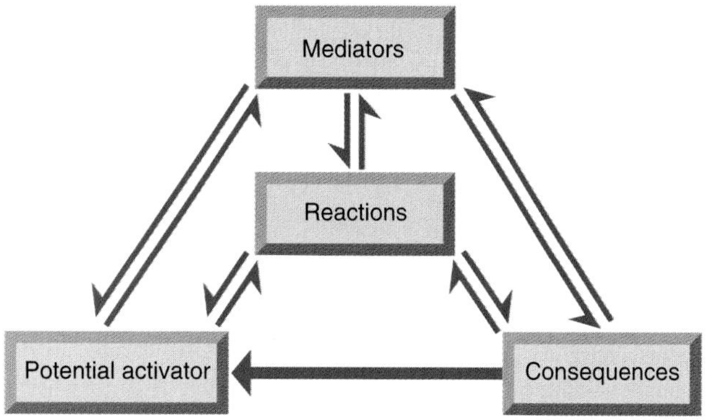

Figure 31–4. Framework for organizing current knowledge about stress and anxiety. (From Elliot, G., & Eisdorfer, C. [Eds.] [1982]. *Stress and Human Health.* New York: Springer.)

sometimes result in anxiety. A stressor is defined as an "internal or external event condition, situation, or cue that has the potential to bring about or actually activates" reactions, which may be physical or psychological (Werner, 1993, p. 15). For Mrs. Stenson of the chapter opening case study, major stressors include the prospect of impending surgery, her history of heart problems, her grief over the loss of her husband and best friend, and several recent expenditures. Additional stressors are her fear of dying during surgery and her degenerative joint disease and related mobility problems.

REACTIONS

Reactions are the responses of an individual to a stressor. They may include psychological reactions such as fear or anger, and bodily responses such as sympathetic nervous system activity. Reactions vary from individual to individual. Some may be severe or persistent enough to produce harmful consequences. Many of the observations made by the nurse in the interview with Mrs. Stenson, such as sighing, fidgeting, tremors, and increased speech rate and pitch, illustrate anxious reactions. Other notable responses were her reports of intense worry and fear about dying, trouble concentrating, and sensation of breathlessness.

CONSEQUENCES

Consequences are negative outcomes that generally occur over time, following intense or prolonged reactions to stress. Consequences may be biologic, such as rheumatoid arthritis (Anderson et al, 1985), or psychological, such as depression or unremitting anxiety. For Mrs. Stenson, it is important to reduce her stress and anxiety so that negative consequences do not develop. It is also possible that Mrs. Stenson is experiencing depression due to bereavement following the deaths of her husband and friend. Indications of depression are her reports of fatigue and trouble sleeping. Further assessment would be needed to explore the possibility of clinical depression.

MEDIATORS

Mediators are traits, resources, and situations that act as "filters" or cushions for stress, thereby changing or lessening the effect of stressors on reactions and consequences (Elliott and Eisdorfer, 1982). Mediators can be biologic, such as factors passed down through the genes from generation to generation, or psychological, such as the thinking process of denial. An individual's environment or setting can also be a mediator, as can the availability of supportive people. Other potential mediators include personality traits, prior coping abilities, age, gender, and religious beliefs and spirituality (Fig. 31–5).

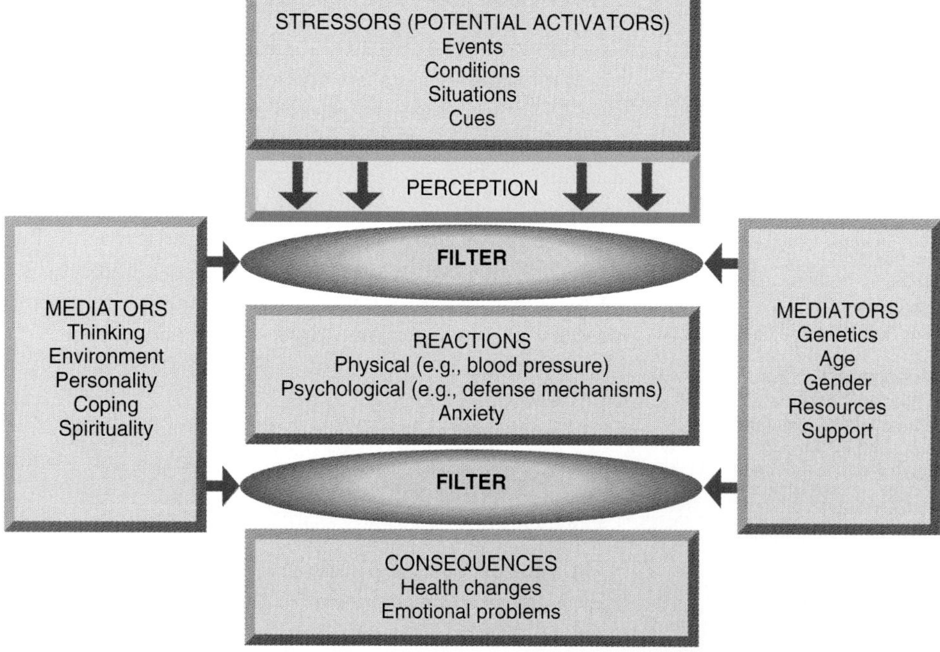

Figure 31–5. Framework for assessing stress and anxiety. This framework illustrates the four major concepts of the stress process: stressors, reactions, consequences, and mediators. It also shows the role of the mediators as filters (or cushions), crucial elements in the stress process.

Mediators help explain why some people experience stressors without having any apparent negative responses, while others react strongly and experience numerous reactions and consequences. For Mrs. Stenson, protective mediators include her prior experience coping with surgery before and her adequate financial resources. A mediator that might worsen her stress and anxiety, however, is her lack of accessible, supportive persons in her life (since her husband and best friend are deceased and her daughters are geographically distant). The possibility of the neighbor being a source of support is an issue that the nurse will assess further.

Relevant Research

RESEARCH FROM OTHER FIELDS

Thanks to numerous research studies, our understanding of stress and anxiety has increased greatly since the 1950s. In part, the increased research interest in these phenomena may be due to concerns about the rapid, often dislocating, pace of change in today's world. In addition, the general increase in wealth and improved living conditions of developed societies has freed people to concern themselves with their well-being rather than only with basic survival.

STRESSORS

Much recent research on the stress process has been concerned with stressors. A stressor is often referred to as the stimulus to a stressful reaction. Although early researchers such as Selye identified noxious agents as stressors, more recent research has delved more deeply into the ways in which life events or changes and demands made on an individual by the environment contribute to development of the vulnerability for illness (Holmes and Rahe, 1967; Holmes and Masuda, 1974).

More recent research has shown that many external and internal factors can trigger stress reactions. Internal factors can be pain or illness itself (Hertzman, 1990; Prugh and Thompson, 1990). External factors might be work pressures or exposure to excessive noise. Stressors range from *catastrophic events,* such as natural disasters or death of a loved one, to more minor events and circumstances such as food additives and intense cold. Figure 31–6 illustrates examples of biophysical, chemical, psychosocial, and cultural stressors.

Another type of stressor is called "daily hassles" (Lazarus and Folkman, 1984, p. 13). Hassles are minor irritating events that occur frequently, such as having to stop at red lights, minor family conflicts, and being ignored by a coworker. Hassles influence health because they are cumulative—they build up over time.

The major assumption of much of the research on major life events and minor daily hassles is that an accumulation of stressful life events will ultimately lead to a decline in physical health or mental health or both. The associations between major life events and ill health have not been exceedingly strong, but they are consistently present. Daily hassles have

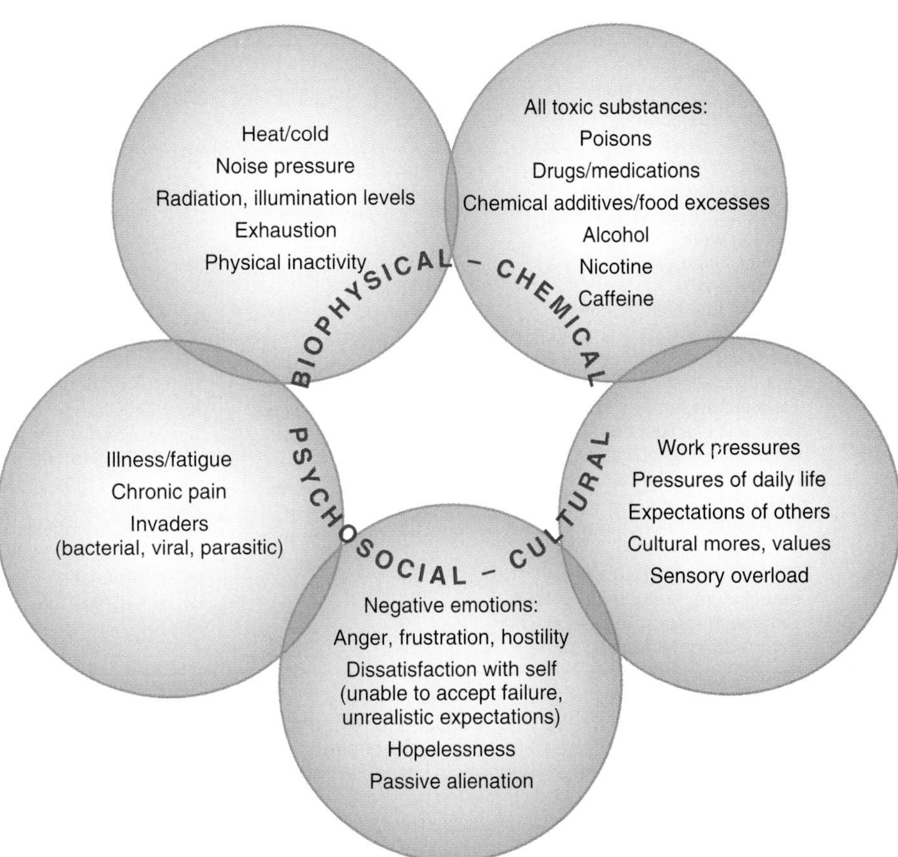

Figure 31–6. Various types of stressors. (From Sutterly, D.C. [1979]. Stress and health: A survey of self-regulation modalities. *Topics in Clinical Nursing, 1,* 6.)

been shown to have greater impact on health decline than major life stressors (DeLongis et al, 1988; Landreville and Vezina, 1992).

Many instruments have been developed to investigate stressful life events. The grandfather of these tools is the Social Readjustment Rating Scale (SRRS) developed by Holmes and Rahe (1967). This scale presents a list of possible stressful life events, rated according to their likely impact on the individual. These events range from those with major impact, such as the death of a spouse, to those with relatively minor impact, such as taking a vacation. Responders add up their life event ratings to get a total score. Presumably, the higher the score, the greater the chance that a negative health consequence will occur during the coming months (Fig. 31–7).

The same types of external stressors that are linked to stress are often related to anxiety. These include (1) developmental factors, such as childhood separation; (2) traumatic life events, such as loss of a loved one, assault, rape, accident, natural disaster, or the prospect of one's own death; and (3) medical crisis events, such as hospitalization, surgery, diagnosis, or pain. In addition, once a traumatic event has passed, repetitious memories of trauma can occur with or without external stimuli. In this way, memories of the event may actually become a stimulus to further anxiety (Horowitz, 1993). In some cases the person is anxious but a stimulus cannot be identified.

REACTIONS AND CONSEQUENCES

Reactions and consequences refer to the pattern of anxiety responses in a person who has encountered troubling or demanding stressors. Physiologic measures such as blood pressure, pulse, galvanic skin response, and urinalysis have been used to indicate reactions. Research on reactions has enjoyed a resurgence of interest in the past few years, due in part to a growing concern about individual differences in stress responses. For example, when two people are exposed to the same stressor, why does one person become ill while the other remains healthy? A second reason for this renewed research focus is a revitalized interest in psychosomatics, the study of physiologic disorders whose causes are linked to emotional factors.

Psychological reactions to stressors can result in long-term pathologic consequences. The fourth edition of the Diagnostic and Statistical Manual of Mental Disorders (DSM-IV) (American Psychiatric Association, 1994) classifies the major types of anxiety disorders as follows:

- anxiety disorders due to medical conditions
- generalized anxiety disorders
- panic disorders
- phobias (intense fear of specific things)
- obsessive-compulsive disorder

Rank	Life Event	Life Change Units	Your Score	Rank	Life Event	Life Change Units	Your Score
1	Death of spouse	100	_____	24	Trouble with in-laws	29	_____
2	Divorce	73	_____	25	Outstanding personal achievement	28	_____
3	Marital separation	65	_____	26	Wife begins or stops work	26	_____
4	Jail term	63	_____	27	Begin or end school	26	_____
5	Death of close family member	63	_____	28	Change in living conditions	25	_____
6	Personal injury or illness	53	_____	29	Revision of personal habits	24	_____
7	Marriage	50	_____	30	Trouble with boss	23	_____
8	Fired at work	47	_____	31	Change in work hours or conditions	20	_____
9	Marital reconciliation	45	_____	32	Change in residence	20	_____
10	Retirement	45	_____	33	Change in school	20	_____
11	Change in health of family member	44	_____	34	Change in recreation	19	_____
12	Pregnancy	40	_____	35	Change in church activities	19	_____
13	Sex difficulties	39	_____	36	Change in social activities	18	_____
14	Gain of new family member	39	_____	37	Mortgage or loan less than $10,000	17	_____
15	Business readjustment	39	_____	38	Change in sleeping habits	16	_____
16	Change in financial state	38	_____	39	Change in number of family get-togethers	15	_____
17	Death of close friend	37	_____	40	Change in eating habits	15	_____
18	Change to different line of work	36	_____	41	Vacation	13	_____
19	Change in number of arguments with spouse	35	_____	42	Christmas	12	_____
20	Mortgage over $10,000	31	_____	43	Minor violations of the law	11	_____
21	Foreclosure of mortgage or loan	30	_____			TOTAL	_____
22	Change in responsibilities at work	29	_____				
23	Son or daughter leaving home	29	_____				

Scoring

Add up your score. If your total for the year is under 150, you probably won't have any adverse reaction. A score 150–199 indicates a "mild" problem, with a 37 percent chance you'll feel the impact of stress with physical symptoms. From 200–299, you qualify as having a "moderate" problem with a 51 percent chance of experiencing a change in your health. A score of over 300 could really threaten your well-being.

Figure 31–7. Social readjustment rating scale (SRRS). (Adapted from Holmes, T.H., & Rahe, R.H. [1967]. The social readjustment rating scale. *Journal of Psychosomatic Research, 11*[2], 213.)

- posttraumatic stress disorder
- acute stress disorder

These major, severe consequences of anxiety are generally assessed and treated by mental health professionals such as psychiatric clinical nurse specialists, psychiatrists, psychologists, and social workers. However, all nurses need to be aware of these disorders, which can affect any patient. If the nurse suspects that a patient has an anxiety disorder, he or she should refer the patient to a mental health professional.

When anxiety is severe, some individuals use psychological cognitive (thinking) processes that help them block out the stressor or distressing responses. These processes are known as *defense mechanisms*. Most people use defense mechanisms in their day-to-day life to reduce anxiety. These mechanisms can become pathologic, however, when reality is greatly distorted, or when they are used for a lengthy period, thereby preventing helpful learning and coping efforts. They occur unconsciously, and probably represent the most adaptive response the person can muster in a particular situation at that particular time. The most common defense mechanisms are denial, selective inattention, and isolation. Table 31–1 defines and discusses the most common defense mechanisms, and provides examples of these mechanisms that nurses may encounter in practice.

Nurses in general practice are more likely to encounter *normal* anxiety than clinical anxiety in day-to-day practice. It has yet to be determined when anxiety passes the threshold from normal to clinical, or what specific grouping of symptoms represents normal or clinical anxiety. Presumably, the more numerous and severe the symptoms, the more severe the anxiety. In the case of Viola Stenson, her excessive worry about impending death related to surgery and unrealistic concerns over financial ruin may alert the nurse to the possibility of an anxiety disorder. In this case the nurse will refer the patient to a professional skilled in detecting anxiety disorders.

Subjective Symptoms. Whether they are experiencing mild or severe anxiety, most people are able to describe their responses in some way. Terms that patients use frequently to describe their subjective symptoms of anxiety include anxious, apprehensive, helpless, nervous, fearful, lacking in confidence, out of control, tense, unable to relax, unreal, and threatened (Carpenito, 1993; Taylor and Arnow, 1988).

Cognitive Symptoms. Individuals experiencing anxiety also report various thoughts in relation to their distress. Expressions such as "I'm going to die of a heart attack," "I can't cope," and "I'll make a fool of myself" are common in anxious persons (Taylor and Arnow, 1988). Other common thought patterns include lack of concentration, lack of awareness, forgetting, repetitive thoughts, frequent thoughts about the past, and increased attentiveness or alertness (Carpenito, 1993; Sarason, 1985). Persons with severe anxiety disorders experience several of these symptoms, whereas those with normal anxiety exhibit a few.

Behavioral Symptoms. People experiencing severe anxiety are likely to exhibit certain behaviors, including impatience or anger, crying, blaming, hypervigilance and startle reaction, criticism of self or others, withdrawing or avoiding, perspiring, trembling, and wearing a fearful facial expression (Carpenito, 1993; Marks, 1987; Taylor and Arnow, 1988). In normal anxiety, some of these symptoms may be present in milder forms, or none may occur.

MEDIATORS

The study of mediators in the stress and anxiety process has two major foci: (1) the person-environment transaction in producing stress, and (2) the role of coping as a mediator to reactions and consequences.

Person-Environment Transaction. The cornerstone of person-environment stress research and theory is the *psychological impact* of stressors on a person. In this transactional view of stress, the person and his or her environment are studied in a mutual relationship, emphasizing the role of perception (Lazarus and Folkman, 1984). Perceptions of the stressor and its "demand" on the person are viewed as *subjective* (filtered through perception) rather than objective (directly observable). People continuously assess stressors through the *primary appraisal* process. The stimulus is perceived as stressful if it has importance for the person as harm/loss, threat, or challenge (Table 31–2). Harm/loss occurs if the stimulus has already produced damage to the person. Threat is the belief that harm or loss has not yet taken place but will occur. Challenge refers to a situation perceived to represent potential for growth (Lazarus and Folkman, 1984).

Another important part of the mediator process is called secondary appraisal. Secondary appraisal involves assessing what a person can do to handle the stressor—his or her coping strategies. In this stage of the process, an individual "takes into account which coping options are available, the likelihood that a given coping option will accomplish what it is supposed to, and the likelihood that one can apply a particular strategy or set of strategies effectively" (Lazarus and Folkman, 1984, p. 35).

Coping. The other major mediator is *coping*, a person's attempt to control, manage, or live with a stressful situation. Coping strategies can be either problem-focused or emotion-focused. *Problem-focused* coping involves effort to solve the problem or meet the demand directly. *Emotion-focused* coping occurs when nothing can be done directly, or when the person perceives that nothing can be done and turns to cognitive processes such as distancing, wishful thinking, or self-blame (Folkman and Lazarus, 1980, 1985; Lazarus and Folkman, 1984).

Based on their investigations of coping, Lazarus and colleagues developed an instrument for assessing coping strategies. The Ways of Coping Checklist consists of items categorized into eight subscales. These subscales represent various problem-focused and emotion-focused strategies that people characteristically use to cope with stress (Table 31–3). This tool has been shown to be valid and reliable and is used the world over in research on stress and coping.

TABLE 31-1 Defense Mechanisms and Nursing Care Examples

Defense Mechanism	Description	Examples in Nursing Care
Rationalization	Assigning logical reasons or plausible excuses for what we have done impulsively or for motives that we do not wish to acknowledge; serves to maintain self-respect and prevents feelings of guilt.	A person is extremely rude and demanding; he thinks to himself that it is all right for him to behave this way because he is sick; he thus excuses his behavior.
Projection	Attributing to others exaggerated amounts of undesirable qualities that we have but do not wish to recognize in ourselves.	The rude, demanding individual may not recognize his behavior; instead he thinks the nurse is behaving in this way, thus projecting his feelings onto her; actually her behavior is misinterpreted by him, since she has not been rude or demanding.
Repression	Involuntarily forgetting about unacceptable ideas, impulses, or events; serves to protect us from being constantly aware of anxiety-producing situations.	A person had a sudden strong urge to defecate and was incontinent before the nurse could help her onto the bedpan; the patient was extremely embarrassed by the situation; a month later she had totally forgotten about the incident and did not remember it again.
Suppression	Consciously putting unacceptable ideas, impulses, or events out of mind; the material can readily be recalled.	An individual has been told by her physician that she needs to undergo surgery; this thought is upsetting to her; she leaves the physician's office and says to herself, "I won't think about it now; I'll do some shopping instead."
Regression	Returning to an earlier level of emotional adjustment; an unconscious process.	A person is usually quite self-sufficient when he is feeling well; however, with his illness he becomes somewhat more dependent than his physical condition necessitates; thus, he returns to an earlier level of dependency.
Identification	Unconsciously adopting the personality characteristics of another individual whom the subject admires—the opposite of projection; not consciously trying to be like someone else.	Two individuals with multiple sclerosis share a room in the hospital for several weeks; one admires the other very much and over a period of time her attitude toward her illness becomes similar to that of the friend she admires. A nurse's professional, kind attitude with people is unconsciously adopted by other members of the staff who admire her.
Compensation	A conscious or unconscious attempt to overcome real or imagined inferiorities.	A person paralyzed from the waist down works hard to develop the muscles in his trunk and arms to compensate for his inability to use his legs.
Denial	Unconsciously refusing to acknowledge to oneself a known fact that is uncomfortable to accept; not consciously lying to oneself.	An individual is proved to have cancer and is told the diagnosis by her physician; the patient does not consciously admit to herself that she has cancer; she denies the diagnosis.
Reaction formation	A forbidden motive or behavior is denied, and the individual develops behavior displaying the opposite motive.	A person is fearful of surgery but instead of appearing fearful he acts unconcerned and nonchalant about it; he jokes about surgery and says, "There's nothing to it. I don't know why some guys are such babies about going."
Sublimation	The "socialization of energy" by diverting unacceptable impulses into socially accepted behavior.	An individual is angry because he was hit by a car, was injured, and is hospitalized for several weeks; he is missing work and his wife is home taking care of their three young children by herself; he directs his "angry energy" into pounding designs into leather and selling the purses, wallets, etc.; he sends home the small amount of money he makes and thus has a sense of contributing to his home and family.
Displacement	Emotion or behavior is redirected from the original object or person to a more acceptable substitute object.	A person hopes to go home but is told by her physician that she probably cannot be discharged for some time; the person is angry at what the doctor says but doesn't want to appear angry at the doctor; the rest of the day she is short-tempered with the nurses; she thus displaces her anger from the physician to the nurses.
Selective inattention	Excluding from awareness those situations that provoke anxiety.	A woman denies the presence of a breast lump.
Isolation or depersonalization	Removing feeling from what one perceives as stressful.	Laughing and joking about an upcoming breast biopsy.

TABLE 31-2 Stressful Primary Appraisals

Appraisal	Definition	Example
Harm/Loss	Person-environment transaction in which damage has occurred in an area or situation important to the person.	Loss of self-esteem due to a job layoff.
Threat	Person-environment transaction in which harm/loss (damage) is likely to occur, or is anticipated.	Anticipated loss of good academic standing in college after failing three final exams.
Challenge	Person-environment transaction appraised as providing oportunity for growth or gain.	Being told by a health care provider that one is obese and needs to lose weight.

Data from Burns and Egan, 1994; Lazarus and Folkman, 1984.

Coping behaviors are considered successful if, when reappraised, the stressor or threat is absent or more manageable. Common indicators of effective coping are perceived helpfulness, reduction of anxiety and emotional distress, and reduction or elimination of the problem.

The external resources of social support and financial means are also very important in coping (Artinian, 1993). Other factors that influence coping include personal characteristics such as age, gender, and internal resources, notably the personality dimensions of hardiness, sense of coherence, and self-efficacy. *Hardiness* is a personality factor made up of three components (the Three C's): high commitment, control, and challenge (Ouellette, 1993). Commitment refers to an attitude of involvement and a belief that goals and values are very important. Control is defined as the belief by a person that he or she can influence events and their outcomes. Challenge is the perception that change presents an opportunity for growth (Kobasa, 1979). *Sense of coherence* is an overall life perspective in which the world is viewed as comprehensible, manageable, and meaningful (Antonovsky, 1987). *Self-efficacy* is an appraisal of self as able to actively confront and handle challenging situations (Bandura, 1989).

Finally, *self-regulation,* a process rather than a strategy or a resource, focuses on how clarifying thinking about stressful situations aids in coping. This theory proposes that clear and objective information about events helps the person form a mental structure (cognitive schema) that closely represents actual experience. This clear mental picture helps reduce the difference between what is expected (such as when a person experiences threat), and what is actual. It thus helps people to better predict occurrences and interpret experiences realistically (Leventhal and Johnson, 1983). Armed with clear information and accurate mental images, people are then able to go against any natural tendency they may have to respond in a characteristic way that may be unhealthy. They may still experience the impulse to behave in a certain way, but learn to override it (Heatherton and Renn, 1995). Since education and practice can assist in providing clear information and therefore in self-regulation, it is an important area to consider when caring for patients.

TABLE 31-3 Ways of Coping Subscales and Typical Items—Revised Version

Subscale	Item
1. Confrontive Coping	I stood my ground and fought for what I wanted.
2. Distancing	I went on as if nothing happened.
3. Self-Control	I tried to keep my feelings to myself.
4. Seeking Social Support	I talked to someone who could do something concrete about the problem.
5. Accepting Responsibility	I criticized or lectured myself.
6. Escape-Avoidance	I wished the situation would go away or somehow be over with.
7. Planful Problem-Solving	I knew what had to be done, so I doubled my efforts to make things work.
8. Positive Reappraisal	I found new faith.

From Lazarus, R. (1991). Stress, coping, and illness. In H. Friedman (ed.): *Personality and Disease.* New York: Wiley.

NURSING RESEARCH

Nursing's interest in stress and anxiety began in the 1950s and has grown steadily. Stress and anxiety are major topics of nursing research because they are so widely experienced by the general population and by patients facing harm, hospitalization, disease, and medical procedures. Anxiety and stress are often viewed by nurses as patterns of human responses to health or illness (American Nurses' Association, 1995). Nurses also study these phenomena because stress and anxiety contribute to illness and disease, and can be modified to promote health. Nurse researchers have examined all aspects of the stress process, including stressors, mediators, reactions, and consequences.

STRESSORS

Diagnosis-Related Stressors. The experience of awaiting or receiving a medical diagnoses can be a powerful stressor for individuals and their families, especially in the case of life-threatening conditions (Halm, 1990; Nyamathi et al, 1992). For example, breast biopsy is very stressful and often represents a crisis to women undergoing this procedure. During this critical period, general reasoning ability is substantially lower than normal, and anxiety and perception of threat are high (Hilton, 1989).

Shock is the most common response to the stressor of receiving a diagnosis of cancer. Two thirds of persons receiving this diagnosis describe the experience in such terms as terror, horror, surprise, sense of unreality, anger, hopelessness, and doom. Following the initial shock, many cancer patients report fear, sorrow, hopelessness, depression, and bitterness. A few actually describe relief at confirming their own suspicions (Krause, 1993). For many, the perceived recurrence of cancer through recognition of one's own symptoms, or the actual return of cancer that has been in remission, is more upsetting than the initial diagnosis (Mahon et al, 1990).

Disease-Related Stressors. One major area of nursing research is the association between stress and disease outcomes. In many cases, disease contributes to stress; in other cases stress appears to exacerbate illness and disease. Conditions such as rheumatoid arthritis, cardiac diseases, cancer, diabetes, and chronic obstructive pulmonary disease (COPD) have been shown to be associated with stress.

Emotional stress, along with the number and severity of daily hassles, has been related to rheumatoid arthritis activity. In one study, patients with rheumatoid disease were most concerned about health-related issues such as lack of energy, difficulty relaxing, and declining physical health (Crosby, 1988). An implication of this study is that nursing interventions aimed at reducing stressors may also help reduce disease-related symptoms.

Anxiety, panic, and worry have been shown to occur in conjunction with the shortness of breath occurring in such disorders as bronchitis, emphysema, and asthma. Women with COPD report stress arising from shortness of breath, fatigue, and loneliness, which in turn contribute to increased depression and restricted activities. Dyspnea (difficulty breathing) in COPD is also related to significant anxiety. Lower life satisfaction is another outcome. For example, wives of men with COPD report higher perceived stress, less life satisfaction, and lower perception of health than wives of men without COPD (Gift and Cahill, 1990; Sexton and Munro, 1988).

Considerable nursing research has investigated the stress associated with *acute myocardial infarction* (MI). Medical research suggests that stressful life events preceding an MI are perceived by people experiencing an MI as being more negative and uncontrollable than those same events experienced by persons who do not have an MI (Gupta and Verma, 1989). As a stressful life event itself, acute MI is frequently associated with significant personal stress. The increased catecholamine secretion commonly triggered by stress may in turn cause complications to an already damaged cardiovascular system. The stress of having suffered an MI is particularly hazardous to cardiac patients because of the potential for significant sympathetic nervous system arousal and the resulting potential for lethal arrhythmias (irregular heart beat), exacerbated pain, worsened heart failure, and disrupted sleep and rest.

Although perceptions of stress are individual, several consistent stressors have been identified within the experience of acute MI. Particularly stress producing are the pain and distress during the MI itself, the diagnosis, and the sick role assumed by patients, which typically involves decreased personal and family responsibilities, decreased independence, and increased dependence on others for assistance. Anxiety, anger and depression are also common (Buchanan et al, 1993). Lack of information about the hospital environment and the prognosis, anticipation of pain as a result of treatment, and unfamiliar medical language also contribute to stress. Moreover, many MI patients have a chance to ruminate on their negative feelings due to their isolation in the critical care unit.

Several studies have also examined the stress experienced by spouses of patients who had recent MIs. Highly stressful are the possibility of the partner's death, seeing him or her ill, and losses associated with the disorder (Caplin and Sexton, 1988). In some cases, spouses report significantly higher subjective stress than patients (Mardsen and Dracup, 1991).

One month following hospitalization, persons having experienced an MI still report stress. Stressors at this point focus most on the harm that has occurred to them and the losses they have sustained. Especially stressful are "physical health, inability to partake in gratifying behaviors, job responsibilities, and guilt about not exhibiting expected behaviors" (Miller et al, 1990, p. 308).

Cancer as a chronic illness is extremely stressful. In addition to high emotional distress following diagnosis, beginning radiotherapy or chemotherapy, or having surgery are stress producing treatment aspects. As the disease continues, the particular stressors change.

In one study, 60 percent of gynecological cancer survivors had concerns or worries about recurrence of cancer following surgery. For most, the fear did not diminish with time, and for 13 percent this worry increased with time. In general, the more recent the surgery, the higher the fear of recurrence (Corney et al, 1992). After a cancer recurrence, patients experience shock, uncertainty, grief, a sense of injustice with resulting anger, and fear of death (Chekryn, 1984). All aspects of the ongoing cancer experience have been found to be distressing for both patients and significant others (Oberst et al, 1989).

Pain can be caused or exacerbated by multiple factors, including anxiety. For example, chest pain frequently results from anxiety, and headache pain has also been shown to increase when a person is anxious. For postoperative patients, the higher the anxiety, the greater the pain (Oberle et al, 1990). At the same time, the ongoing or intermittent pain associated with chronic illness can be a continuing stressor. In this way anxiety is precipitated by pain.

Stressors related to severe illness and disease include physical, psychological, and social components. Pain, weakness, and other symptoms tend to worsen stress, whereas stress in turn may exacerbate physical problems. Consequences of disease may also include changes in the body, stigma, lack of control, threat of future physical limitations, work and financial problems, and changes in family roles and relationships.

The greater the potential for lifestyle changes, the greater the stress likely to be experienced by patients. Often, the patient is unable to adequately appraise the situation and choose appropriate coping methods. The nurse can and should assist patients in adjusting to their changing situation, since chronic stress can hinder recovery from illness.

Threatening Medical Events. Nurse researchers have also examined the stress of threatening medical events. Some of the more stressful diagnostic procedures include barium enema, endoscopic examination, colposcopy, pelvic examination, femoral arteriography, intravenous pyelography (x-ray of the ureter and kidney), nasogastric intubation and feeding, and ongoing hemodialysis (Clark and Gregor, 1988; Barsevick and Johnson, 1990; Hjelm-Karlson, 1989). In addition to the diagnostic procedures themselves, the period following such procedures before an actual diagnosis is made or negated is highly stressful, as uncertainty is extremely high during this period.

Nursing research is also beginning to address the stress associated with ongoing therapy. In patients undergoing hemodialysis, the stressors of fatigue, food and fluid restrictions, boredom, and physical activity limitations are ongoing. Additional stressors include decrease in social life and uncertainty about the future. Physiologic aspects are more stressful than the psychological aspects (Bihl et al, 1988; Gurklis and Menke, 1988, 1995; Lok, 1996). As time on hemodialysis increases, patients are more apt to use problem-oriented coping, such as seeking out social support from others, than emotion-oriented coping strategies, such as withdrawal. It also appears that high anxiety is related to a high incidence of complications for hemodialysis patients.

Hospitalization. Hospitalization itself has been found to trigger stress and anxiety in patients. In a long-term study of stressors in hospitalized patients, Volicer and colleagues identified numerous important stressful hospital factors, including unfamiliar surroundings, loss of independence, separation, and isolation (Ballard, 1981; Volicer, 1974, 1977; Volicer and Bohannon, 1975; Volicer and Burns, 1977; Volicer and Volicer, 1977). Based on these findings, they developed the Hospital Stress Rating Scale (HSRS) (Volicer and Bohannon, 1975) displayed in Table 31–4. Using this scale, various hospital events are assessed to determine how stressful they are for a particular patient. Whether or not the nurse uses the HSRS, knowledge of the major stressors listed can be useful in the nurse's overall assessment of hospitalized patients. Usually, illness-related stressors are significantly more stressful than hospital factors (Miller et al, 1990; Werner, 1993).

Hospitalization in a *critical care unit* (CCU) poses unique stressors. Critical care patients are generally barraged with many confusing stimuli: medical jargon, continuous beeping, alarms, and unfamiliar people. This disorienting experience is often exacerbated by the patients' immobility, dependence on machines, and limited visitation by significant others. Meaningful explanation of their condition and prognosis is frequently withheld for fear of increasing anxiety. Pain, thirst, isolation, insomnia, and presence of oral or nasal tubes add to CCU stress, as do the generally reduced capacity to control situations and missing one's spouse (Omalley and Menke, 1988; Soehren, 1995). Thus, when caring for critical care patients, the nurse should assess for stressors unique to this specialized setting.

Within the area of critical care, some nurses are studying a phenomenon called *anxiety transmission*. Anxiety transmission is defined as "anxiety which arises by intuitive communication from one person to another" (Laughlin, 1967, p. 12) or, stated more simply, anxiety arising in an individual through communication with others. Some research indicates that family visits tend to increase anxiety in patients with cardiac disease (Frederickson, 1989). This is problematic for the critical care nurse because other research has shown that the presence of family is extremely important for patients and that visiting is a top priority for family members (Leske, 1986). Evidence suggests that when the nurse gives information and support to family members prior to visitation, patient anxiety is less likely to increase during or following the visit.

Nursing research has also investigated the parental stress associated with *pediatric intensive care* hospitalization (Carter and Miles, 1982; Carter et al, 1985; Graves and Ware, 1990; Miles et al, 1992). Findings indicate that more stress is associated with the parent's role and relationship to the child and with the child's behavior, emotions, and appearance than with the intensive care unit (ICU) environment itself. Adequate preparation for ICU hospitalization is related to lower stress, whereas unexpected emergency hospitalization produces more stress. Although it is as yet unclear whether mothers or fathers experience more overall stress (Perehudoff, 1990), mothers do report greater stress related to the parenting role, whereas fathers in one study rated the overall ICU experience more stressful than did mothers (Heuer, 1993). The degree of anxiety is similar in mothers and fathers (Miles et al, 1992), and both are stressed by separation from their child (Heuer, 1993). Parents of children who are intubated have been found to be more distressed by painful procedures than parents of nonintubated children (Haines et al, 1995). Further research is needed to identify the most stressful experiences for the hospitalized children themselves. The overall experience and procedures of the pediatric intensive care unit are overwhelming to the vast majority of people. Nurses need to provide education and support to the parents from the moment of admission. If the admission is planned, parents should receive information prior to admission. Teaching parents should proceed from general to specific, and from least to most threatening (Philichi, 1988).

Noise is another significant stressor for hospitalized patients, especially in critical care (Baker, 1992; Snyder-Halpern, 1985; Topf, 1985, 1992). In an early study of surgical ICU patients, noise ranked among the top five environmental sources perceived to induce anxiety (Ballard, 1981). Sources of noise include equipment, alarms and buzzers, staff, other patients, visitors, and background noise, including radios and televisions (Gast and Baker, 1989). However, the mere presence of noise does not necessarily

TABLE 31-4 Hospital Stress Rating Scale

Factor	Stress Scale Events	Assigned Rank
Unfamiliarity of surroundings	Having strangers sleep in the same room with you	01
	Having to sleep in a strange bed	03
	Having strange machines around	05
	Being awakened in the night by the nurse	06
	Being aware of unusual smells around you	11
	Being in a room that is too cold or too hot	16
	Having to eat cold or tasteless food	21
	Being cared for by an unfamiliar doctor	23
Loss of independence	Having to eat at different times than you usually do	02
	Having to wear a hospital gown	04
	Having to be assisted with bathing	07
	Not being able to get newspapers, radio, or TV when you want them	08
	Having a roommate who has too many visitors	09
	Having to stay in bed or the same room all day	10
	Having to be assisted with a bedpan	13
	Not having your call light answered	35
	Being fed through tubes	39
	Thinking you may lose your sight	49
Separation from spouse	Worrying about your spouse being away from you	20
	Missing your spouse	38
Financial problems	Thinking about losing income because of your illness	27
	Not having enough insurance to pay for your hospitalization	36
Isolation from other people	Having a roommate who is seriously ill or cannot talk with you	12
	Having a roommate who is unfriendly	14
	Not having friends visit you	15
	Not being able to call family or friends on the phone	22
	Having the staff be in too much of a hurry	26
	Thinking you might lose your hearing	45
Lack of information	Thinking you might have pain because of surgery or test procedures	19
	Not knowing when to expect things will be done to you	25
	Having nurses or doctors talk too fast or use words you can't understand	29
	Not having your questions answered by the staff	37
	Not knowing the results or reasons for your treatments	41
	Not knowing for sure what illnesses you have	43
	Not being told what your diagnosis is	44
Threat of severe illness	Thinking your appearance might be changed after your hospitalization	17
	Being put in the hospital because of an accident	24
	Knowing you have to have an operation	32
	Having a sudden hospitalization you weren't planning to have	34
	Knowing you have a serious illness	46
	Thinking you might lose a kidney or some other organ	47
	Thinking you might have cancer	48
Separation from family	Being in the hospital during holidays or special family occasions	18
	Not having family visit you	31
	Being hospitalized far away from home	33
Problems with medications	Having medications cause you discomfort	28
	Feeling you are getting dependent on medications	30
	Not getting relief from pain medications	40
	Not getting pain medication when you need it	42

From Volicer, B.J., Bohannon, W. (1975). A Hospital Stress Rating Scale. *Nursing Research, 24,* 356.

result in anxiety. An investigation of 150 postoperative patients found that a person's sensitivity to noise in general was a predictor of the degree of disturbance a patient would experience in response to noise (Topf, 1985). Because unit sounds are associated with poorer sleep (Topf, 1992), nurses should attempt to remove or lessen unnecessary noise, especially during nighttime hours.

Surgery. Nursing research has shown that patients undergoing surgery typically experience greater anxiety than medical patients. The most common preoperative stressors for anxiety are pain and discomfort, not knowing what to expect, not being told the whole truth about diagnosis, damage to body image, separation from family, worries about how the family will cope, financial worries, and the possibility of death. Other concerns relate to the disruption of life plans, loss of control associated with anesthesia, dependency, and fear due to previous surgical experiences (Biley, 1989). Ramsay (1972) found the anesthesia induction technique (when the patient is put to sleep) to be particularly threatening. Some patients are also afraid of waking up in the middle of the operation and of feeling pain. One study found that women anticipating gynecologic surgery experienced greater anxiety than preoperative patients awaiting either orthopedic or general surgery (Nyamathi and Kashiwabara, 1988). Postoperatively, the higher the anxiety, the more intense the pain (Oberly et al, 1990).

Cardiac surgeries, such as coronary artery bypass surgery, valve replacement, pericardiectomy (removal of a portion of the membrane covering the heart), and cardiac transplant, are especially stressful for both patients and their family members or significant others (Knapp-Spooner and Yarcheski, 1992; Moore, 1994). Because of the serious, sometimes even life-threatening nature of such surgeries, they are associated with numerous stressors. For example, patients undergoing coronary artery bypass were found to experience four major illness-related stressors (having cardiac surgery, prospect of resuming lifestyle, pain and discomfort, and fear of dying) and one major hospitalization-related stressor (being absent from home and/or business) (Carr and Powers, 1986; Yarcheski and Knapp-Spooner, 1994). Perhaps not surprisingly, even waiting to undergo cardiac surgery is very stressful (Bresser et al, 1993). Because illness-related stressors are most stressful to patients, nurses should focus on the management of these as a priority, before giving attention to reduction of hospital-related stressors (Yarcheski and Knapp-Spooner, 1994).

Developmental Events. Anxiety related to pregnancy, birth, and parenting outcomes has been the focus of considerable nursing research. In a series of studies, high-risk women hospitalized during pregnancy and their mates reported greater anxiety than those in low-risk situations. In addition, having a premature baby is typically experienced as a crisis, with accompanying high anxiety levels (Gennaro, 1988; Gennaro et al, 1993; Mercer, 1986; Mercer and Ferketich, 1988). Several nurse investigators also have found that psychological states such as anxiety can have negative effects on adaptation to labor and delivery and on the progress of labor. Prenatal anxiety has also been linked to poorer interactions between mothers and their infants (Lederman et al, 1981; Norbeck and Anderson, 1989; Tilden, 1984). Because stress and anxiety are related to several negative parent and child outcomes, nursing interventions need to focus on reducing parental stress during all stages of pregnancy, labor, delivery, and parenting.

Many reactions and consequences of stress have been studied by nurse researchers. Some of the consequences most studies include:

- psychological distress, also called psychosocial adjustment or outcome (Alfonso et al, 1994; Bohachick et al, 1992; Hilbert, 1994; Leonard et al, 1993)
- symptom distress or symptoms (Grady et al, 1992; Redeker, 1993)
- depression (Dimond et al, 1994)
- quality of life (Zacharias et al, 1994)
- pain perception (Broome et al, 1994)
- physiologic response such as neuroendocrine and immunologic activity (Caudell and Gallucci, 1995), and heart rate variability (Buchanan et al, 1993)
- coping (Bossert, 1994; Cayse, 1994) and health (Gennaro et al, 1993; Taylor and Walkey, 1994/95).

For example, Leonard and coworkers (1993) studied the *psychological distress* of parents resulting from taking care of "medically fragile" children at home. They report that 59 percent of mothers and 67 percent of fathers reported distress at the level of needing psychiatric intervention. This distress was mainly associated with increased family responsibilities.

Hilbert (1993), studying MI patients and their spouses, found that both experienced significantly higher *emotional distress* when compared with people not having a stressful medical event. Those who were satisfied with family functioning reported better affect. Hilbert's results indicate that assessing family functioning and distress of both spouses is important when an MI occurs.

Regarding depression, Dimond and coworkers (1994) found that for a small sample of adults over age 55 who had lost a spouse, depression was intensified in those who reported life change events more frequently. In general, for the majority of outcomes, as stress increases or is more frequent, the outcome measure becomes more negative.

Numerous studies by nurse researchers have focused on anxiety as a reaction in the overall stress process (Buchanan et al, 1993; Nugent et al, 1993; Redeker, 1993). For example, in patients experiencing acute MI, Crowe and colleagues identified that in the hospital immediately after the MI, 10 percent of the 785 patients in the sample had state anxiety scores higher than psychiatric patients' average scores. Anxiety levels remained high over a year of follow-up. Nine percent had moderate to severe depression. This study found no relationship between anxiety and depression, and there were no differences in anxiety or depression based on sex (Crowe et al, 1996).

In another example, Nugent and colleagues (1993) found that the experience of having to undergo a colposcopy (the examination of vaginal and cervical tissue by means of an instrument) following an abnormal Pap smear evoked anxiety. Younger women with additional life stressors were more anxious than older women with less life stress.

REACTIONS AND CONSEQUENCES

In recent years nurses have also begun to explore the linkages between anxiety and certain outcomes. For example, the relationship between anxiety and cognitive thinking abilities has been examined in patients undergoing same-day surgery. In one study, 25 percent of patients had high anxiety scores preoperatively; of those highly anxious patients, 75 percent had low scores in critical thinking. The investigators concluded that as anxiety levels rise, cognitive abilities diminish (Nyamathi and Kashiwabara, 1988). This may have important implications for the content and timing of preoperative patient teaching. Other studies suggest that high anxiety and low self-esteem are associated with decreased compliance with medical treatment regimens, and that anxiety and anger impede coping.

MEDIATORS

In addition to an awareness of stressful events themselves, nurses need to be aware of mediators to help their patients manage stress more effectively. Three major mediators of stress have been topics of substantial nursing research: uncertainty, social support, and coping.

Uncertainty. Defined as the "inability to determine the meaning of events, and occurs in a situation where the decision-maker is unable to assign definite values to objects and events and/or is unable to accurately predict outcomes" (Mishel and Braden, 1988, p. 98), uncertainty is an important influence on the degree of stress experienced by hospitalized and ill patients (Mishel, 1984). Uncertainty is a contributing factor in the perception of novel events as stressful, such as the experience of discharge for a patient recovering from myocardial infarction (Christman et al, 1988). In addition, uncertainty can impede coping efforts. Major contributors to uncertainty, and consequently to stress, include the ambiguity of the illness, the complexity of the treatment, lack of information, and the unpredictability of the diagnosis and/or prognosis (Mishel, 1981). Also contributing to uncertainty are unfamiliar medical jargon, diagnostic studies, monitoring equipment, unfamiliar symptoms, hospital routines, and questionable ability to return to a normal lifestyle (Mishel, 1981, 1984).

More recently, Mishel (1988, 1990) has extended her theory from the events of acute illness and deteriorating medical conditions to chronic illness. In some cases, it appears that uncertainty is harmful, whereas in others it is beneficial and a natural cognitive factor in coping. For example, for hospitalized adults with an acute medical situation such as a myocardial infarction, "Uncertainty hampers the formation of a cognitive structure, which in turn limits the person's ability to adequately appraise a situation" (Mishel, 1981, p. 259). When situations cannot clearly be appraised, the person experiences more stress because the person is unsure of how to cope, than if events are clearly appraised (Mishel, 1981). However, in situations where there is a high proportion of dangerous or negative results, such as the potential outcome of death with cancer, the role of uncertainty may be different. Here uncertainty is more welcome, since uncertainty offers hope, versus the certainty of one's own demise (Mishel, 1990).

Social Support. Social support generally refers to the helpful assistance and emotional comfort received from important people in one's life. The availability of social support has been shown to directly reduce adverse psychological and physical outcomes of the stress process (Artinian, 1993). In some cases, the perception of having support available, rather than the actual use of such support, is more important for patient coping (McNett, 1987).

Patients with many different disease states, medical conditions, and life situations have been studied in relation to social support (Artinian, 1993). Social support has been found to be a particularly important mediator in the stress process for persons with multiple sclerosis (Wineman, 1990), disabled persons bound to wheelchairs (McNett, 1987), burn victims (Brown et al, 1988), and women with chronic illness (Lambert et al, 1989; Primono et al, 1990). Numerous studies with pregnant women indicate that social support reduces stress associated with pregnancy and childbirth (Norbeck and Anderson, 1989; Reece, 1993).

In addition to support from family network members, social support from the nurse has also been shown to be important to patients (Gardner and Wheeler, 1987). Moreover, spouses of ill patients also have been shown to benefit from social support (Stanley and Frantz, 1988). The reader should refer to Chapter 29 for more detail.

Coping. The third major mediator investigated in nursing research is coping. The nursing research on coping and adaptation has increased dramatically in the last few years. In general, people have been found to use a combination of problem-focused and emotional-focused coping strategies (Jalowiec, 1993). Through such strategies, individuals attempt to gain mastery over their illness. Mastery is defined as "a human response to difficult or stressful circumstances in which a person gains competence, control, and dominion over the experience" (Younger, 1993, p. 68). Younger has developed a theory (Younger, 1991) and a tool to measure this outcome of coping. The theory and tool focus on four defining aspects of mastery: achieving a sense of control, finding the answer to a question, recovering self-esteem, and finding alternative sources of satisfaction to replace anything that has been lost. In other words, Younger (1991, 1993) sees elements of mastery as certainty, change, acceptance, and growth. Younger's view is that these are outcomes nurses can help facilitate during client coping.

Immediately following a diagnosis, many patients use emotion-oriented coping strategies, such as optimism, acceptance, and wishful thinking, to manage stressors (Krause, 1993). In addition, the defense mechanism of denial may be beneficial in initial coping with some illnesses (Lazarus, 1983). As the situation progresses, patients may try to increase their control over conditions through problem-oriented coping (Jalowiec, 1993).

One promising method for assessing patient coping is the Jalowiec Coping Scale (JCS). This scale was originally developed to determine how people cope with various stressors and was designed for use in assessing both general and specific coping behaviors (Jalowiec et al, 1984). Jalowiec's original tool has been revised and now consists of eight major coping methods:

- confrontive, acting to solve the problem
- evasive, avoiding the situation
- optimistic, being positive
- fatalistic, feeling pessimistic or hopeless
- emotive, expressing emotions
- palliative, increasing one's general feeling of well-being
- supportant, relying on support systems
- self-reliant, relying on the self for support

Table 31–5 includes an example item from each of the eight major subscales.

The JCS has been used to examine coping in long-term (over 5 years) cancer survivors. These mostly female, married, white, middle-aged and elderly survivors reported using optimistic, supportive, and confrontive strategies more than other types of coping (Halstead and Fernsler, 1994). This and other ongoing research will give nurses valuable knowledge about effective coping strategies for patients and survivors.

TABLE 31–5 Eight Subscales and Sample Items from the Jalowiec Coping Scale

Subscale	Sample Item
Confrontive (facing up to the problem)	(I) tried to change the situation
Evasive (avoiding the situation)	(I) waited to see what would happen
Optimistic (having a positive outlook)	(I) tried to think positively
Fatalistic (pessimistic, hopeless)	(I) prepared for the worst that could happen
Emotive (ventilating feelings)	(I) got mad and let off steam
Palliative (reducing or controlling distress by trying to make self feel better)	(I) ate or smoked more than usual
Supportant (relying on support systems)	(I) depended on others to help out
Self-reliant (relying on self, not others)	(I) preferred to work things out myself

From Jalowiec, A. (1987) *Changes in the Revised Version of the Jalowiec Coping Scale.* Unpublished manuscript. Loyola University of Chicago.

ANXIETY AS A NURSING DIAGNOSIS

Anxiety was first cited as a nursing diagnosis by the North American Nursing Diagnosis Association (NANDA) in 1973 (Gebbie and Lavin, 1975). In the ensuing years, research on Anxiety as a nursing diagnosis has included studies with patients and with expert nurses to validate the diagnosis. The current nursing diagnosis of Anxiety is defined as "a vague uneasy feeling whose source is often nonspecific or unknown to the individual" (NANDA, 1994, p. 87). It is differentiated from the diagnosis of Fear, which is defined as "a feeling of dread related to an identifiable source which the person validates" (NANDA, 1994, p. 87).

The sole critical defining characteristic of Anxiety listed by NANDA is the objective indicator of sympathetic (nervous system) stimulation. Other recent research, however, has identified other defining characteristics of anxiety. Whitley (1992) identified four critical attributes: (1) a vague feeling of dread; (2) an unknown cause; (3) psychological and behavioral subjective responses that contribute energy; and (4) physiologic, psychological/behavioral, and cognitive objective indicators. Another study had expert nurses rate anxiety characteristics on frequency (occurrence of the characteristic when the diagnosis occurs), importance (of the characteristic to the diagnosis), and competency (of the nurse to identify the characteristic) (Kinney and Guzzetta, 1989). They determined five critical characteristics. These are listed in Table 31–6 under Quartile 1; other characteristics not as crucial to the diagnosis are listed under Quartiles 2 and 3.

NURSING ACTIONS TO REDUCE STRESS AND ANXIETY

Some nurses have investigated interventions to reduce stress. Probably the most notable program of nursing research in this area focuses on the reduction or prevention of distress during or after a troubling or painful procedure by preparing the patient for what he or she is likely to experience (Johnson, 1973). In this intervention, called *preparatory sensory information,* the nurse describes what the patient will feel, hear, see, taste, and smell during the upcoming procedure (Fig. 31–8). Ongoing research has shown that the intervention of preparatory sensory information is effective in reducing stress in patients undergoing surgery and such procedures as barium enema, pelvic examination, and cast removal.

For example, in one study that examined four different nursing actions for patients with prostate cancer undergoing radiation therapy, preparatory sensory informational interventions most successfully enhanced coping outcomes "because they decrease the discrepancy between expectations and actual experience, and they increase patients' understanding of their experience" (Robinson, 1990, p. 939). Others have found that a combination of teaching about procedures and providing preparatory sensory information is effective in reducing stress.

Other nursing interventions aimed at reducing stress under investigation can be grouped into four categories: relaxation

TABLE 31-6 Defining Characteristics of Anxiety: Results of Magnitude Estimation Scaling

Quartile 1	Quartile 2	Quartile 3
1. Mildly to severely expressed anxiety	1. Tachycardia	1. Elevated voice pitch
2. Verbal complaints of anxiety	2. Involuntary motor activity	2. Lack of eye contact
3. Mild to severe motor activity	3. Increased respiration	3. Increased elimination
4. Mild to severe nail or lip biting, or drumming of fingers, shaking leg, pulling hair (i.e., any nervous habit)	4. Muscle tension	4. Darting eyes
5. Mildly to severely apprehensive	5. Diaphoresis	5. Sighing
	6. Reactive to surroundings	6. Nausea/vomiting
	7. Increased heart rate	
	8. Increased blood pressure	
	9. Accelerated speech	
	10. Mild to severely verbose	
	11. Strained facial appearance	
	12. Loud speech	

From Kinney, M., Guzzetta, C.E. (1989). Identifying critical defining characteristics of nursing diagnoses using magnitude estimation scaling. *Research in Nursing and Health, 12,* 378.

techniques; educational and information provision; time, environment/person (use of empathy, spending time with patients, and use of touch); and social strategies (such as support groups) (Snyder, 1993). Because study samples and methods have varied greatly, it is yet unclear which interventions work best for which situations. However, it does appear that relaxation techniques are effective in a variety of situations (Snyder, 1993).

Relaxation Techniques. For reducing stress and anxiety, *biofeedback techniques* are relatively new technologies. Katkin and Goldband (1980, cited in Snyder, 1985, p. 537) define biofeedback as the uses of "instrumentation to provide a person with immediate and continuous signals concerning bodily functions of which that person is not normally conscious." Therefore, biofeedback is the use of instruments to increase personal awareness of bodily functions that are often not in awareness. These instruments or machines immediately signal the person about his or her internal conditions.

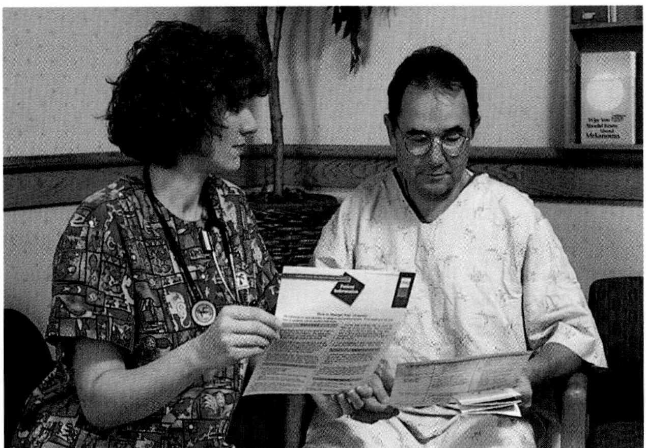

Figure 31-8. The nurse provides preparatory sensory information to the patient before a scheduled procedure.

Feedback to patients has been provided by a number of measures, including electrocardiography (ECG), electromyography (EMG), blood pressure measurements, electroencephalography (EEG), and galvanic skill response (GSR). While attached to the particular instrument, persons attempt to reduce or increase internal processes that signify a more relaxed state. The nurse should ensure that the patient using biofeedback is knowledgeable about the particular device used and about the hazards of using electrical equipment, and has received proper training in biofeedback.

Another advance in reduction of stress or anxiety is *relaxation training.* This technique has evolved into several procedures, including:

- autogenic training: suggestions of feeling "heavy" and "warm" given to the patient
- simple relaxation: use of comforting voice and environment along with deep breathing and calming images
- progressive muscle relaxation: instructions for tensing and releasing muscles progressively throughout the body (McCloskey and Bulechek, 1992)

For example, in a study involving patients with COPD, those who participated in taped relaxation training experienced significantly lower anxiety and dyspnea than those who received no taped relaxation training (Gift et al, 1992). This and other research supports that relaxation training is effective in reducing stress and anxiety for both hospitalized patients and outpatients.

Other promising relaxation-promoting techniques for reducing stress and anxiety include meditation and guided imagery, music therapy, and back massage (McCloskey and Bulechek, 1992; Meek, 1993) (see Research Highlight). Meditation involves the continual focusing of conscious attention toward a single reference point, which alters awareness and in turn tends to reduce autonomic nervous system activity.

RESEARCH HIGHLIGHT
SLOW-STROKE BACK MASSAGE TO PROMOTE RELAXATION

A study examined the effects of slow-stroke back massage on relaxation in a group of 30 adult patients in a home care hospice program. In this study, slow-stroke back massage was performed as follows. The patient was helped to a comfortable position. The clinician warmed her hands, applied massage oil, and massaged the patient's back, using slow, rhythmic hand strokes from head to sacrum. Each massage session lasted 3 minutes, and massage was given on 2 consecutive days. Physiologic parameters—heart rate, blood pressure, and skin temperature—were recorded before and after each massage session.

RESULTS

In all subjects, physiologic measurements indicated increased relaxation after each massage session. Heart rate and blood pressure decreased, and skin temperature increased. The researchers concluded that slow-stroke back massage "is a cost-effective treatment which adds to the comfort of hospice clients" (Meek, 1993, p. 17).

IMPLICATIONS FOR PRACTICE

With the many technological advances in nursing, many nurses have forgotten the comfort and relaxation that can be achieved with the common back rub. Following the bath, or before sleep at night are ideal times for giving a back rub. As with any optional procedure, the nurse should ask the patient if he or she desires a back rub. Patients who are unfamiliar with the back rub can be given information on the positive results that most patients experience.

Meek, S.S. (1993). Effects of slow-stroke back massage on relaxation in hospice clients. *Image: Journal of Nursing Scholarship, 25,* 17–21.

Guided imagery is a mental process of conjuring up positive images and fantasies to reduce stress or anxiety. Guided imagery may be effective in helping bolster immune function, enhancing coping with cancer, and reducing pain.

Music therapy is the "systematic application of music to produce relaxation and desired changes in emotions, behavior, and physiology" (Dossey et al, 1995, p. 670). Music has been found to be effective, for example, in reducing anxiety for ambulatory surgery patients (Augustin and Hains, 1996), and in improving mood in patients receiving coronary artery bypass surgery (Barnason et al, 1995).

Back massage is a form of touch intervention. Nurses have used the back rub for decades as part of routine care of patients. Back massage aids in circulatory stimulation and also in producing relaxation. It may also aid in reducing pain (McCloskey and Bulechek, 1996). There are several types of back massages. One of these, the slow-stroke back massage, has been described as a particularly effective technique in relaxation (Snyder, 1992).

In 1991, the U.S. government established the Office of Alternative Medicine (OAM) within the National Institutes of Health (NIH) to explore unconventional medical practices. This office's goal is "to facilitate the fair, scientific evaluation of alternative therapies that could improve many people's health and well being" (Workshop on Alternative Medicine, 1992, p. xi). Relaxation to reduce stress and anxiety is one area currently being explored by the OAM.

Relevant Theory

One measure of the importance of a phenomenon for a discipline is its degree of inclusion in the discipline's theories. Theory development in nursing has included important work on both stress and anxiety.

STRESS

Nursing theoreticians have developed a number of models to explain stress and its management. One prominent framework is a *systems model* that depicts an individual, a family, or a community as an open system in need of protection and fortification from noxious stressors (Neuman, 1989). The nurse's responsibility in intervention is to facilitate stability of the system through primary prevention (averting stressors), secondary prevention (identifying responses to stress), and tertiary prevention (intervening to reduce negative outcomes). The nurse works with the patient to identify stressors and assists with coping.

Another framework that incorporates stress as a central concern is the *modeling and role modeling* theory (Erickson and Swain, 1982; Erickson et al, 1983). This framework adapts Selye's view of stress as physiologic response. This theory directs the nurse to carry out an interpersonal process with the client, based on the client's perception of the world and his or her immediate situation. Modeling is a process whereby nurses strive to understand the world, including stressors, from the client's viewpoint. Role-modeling represents efforts of the nurse to intervene with the goal of assisting clients to reach their human potential (promoting the client's own control over his or her life), while enhancing their health (Erickson et al, 1983).

Three other nursing theorists have included stress in their models, although stress is not the central concern. Adaptation is the major focus of the theoretical model developed by Callista Roy (1984, 1988). In her view, adaptation is a person-environment interaction in which health is achieved through effective adaptation to internal and external influencing stimuli or stressors that produce a *stress response*.

Dorothy Johnson describes nursing as care provided to persons, healthy or ill, who experience either internal or external stressors (Johnson, 1959, 1980). A stressed person experiences disequilibrium. To Johnson, *stressors* are positive or negative stimuli that have the capability of disrupting system equilibrium. Stability or equilibrium of the human system is the goal of nursing. The nursing process is used to promote facilitation of behavioral and biologic system integrity, through reducing stimuli (stressors) or supporting the adaptation of the client to stressors.

In Benner and Wrubel's (1989) theoretical framework, nursing is viewed as the care and study of a person's life experiences of health, illness, and disease, and his or her relationships with others. Stress is viewed as a disruption in the meaning of life that occurs in illness, whereas coping is how the person deals with this disrupted meaning. Their view of stress is that it is disruption in which "harm, loss, or challenge is experienced, and sorrow, interpretation, or new skill acquisition is required" (Benner and Wrubel, 1989, p. 59).

The nurse assists the person through helping to interpret the event or illness or through teaching and facilitating the acquisition of new skills. Nursing theorists King (1981) and Orem (1991) also focus on coping as essential in meeting health goals and needs.

ANXIETY

One of the earliest nursing theories focused on patient anxiety and the interpersonal process of nursing. Nurse theorist Hildegard Peplau (1952, 1968) viewed all behavior as directed toward decreasing anxiety stemming from unmet needs. Peplau theorized that people experience levels of anxiety depending on their perception of the degree of threat and their individual bodily responses. A person experiencing *mild anxiety* has enhanced ability to perceive stimuli and to learn. In *moderate anxiety,* the ability to perceive narrows, and the focus is on specifics of a situation. A person with *severe anxiety* experiences increased discomfort, both physically and emotionally, and the ability to perceive constricts further. In the *panic* phase, perception often becomes distorted, is very restricted, and the person is unable to think logically. He or she may seem immobilized. The ability to learn is minimal, and immediate assistance from others is imperative to lessen anxiety (Peplau, 1963).

Because severe or panic anxiety prevents an individual from acting rationally to cope with the situation, the nurse steps in to provide a safe calm environment. The nurse may need to take direct action on behalf of the patient if the patient cannot act on his or her own behalf.

Nursing theorists have also modified theories from other disciplines in order to understand anxiety and stress. Some nurses have modified theories about crises from psychology and psychiatry for application to nursing care. Crisis theory defines crisis as an event or situation that causes great disequilibrium and disorganization (Caplan, 1964). Nurse theorists who have modified crisis theory for nursing include Hall and Weaver (1974), who describe nursing care for both situational (event) and maturational (developmental) crises, and Narayuan and Joslin (1980), who propose a holistic nursing model of crisis. Aguilera and Messick (1984) center on crisis intervention as a problem-solving process across nursing practice.

In each of these viewpoints, a crisis follows an actual stressful event that is perceived by the person or family to have a very important meaning. The coping mechanisms used are inadequate for the situation. This causes anxiety to rise. If left unchecked, high anxiety can bring about a state of disequilibrium. The nurse or other health professional engaged in crisis intervention assists the person or family to clarify what the precipitating event is and what it means. Then the nurse assists with coping by helping the person (family) to obtain and use needed resources and to plan appropriate action (Aguilera and Messick, 1984).

FACTORS AFFECTING CLINICAL DECISIONS

Age and Developmental Level

Many individual differences in stress and anxiety are rooted in developmental level and age. Different life events and circumstances tend to occur at various developmental levels, and stressors may be perceived and managed differently according to an individual's age and developmental level.

CHILDREN AND ADOLESCENTS

Research on normal life stressors for children is sparse (Ryan-Wenger, 1989). However, Sorenson (1994) identified differences in daily stressors and coping behaviors between a group of rural children and a group of suburban children, aged 4 to 11. Suburban children were found to be stressed more by external stressors such as school, chores, and activities. Rural children reported more internal stressors such as disappointment, emotional discomfort (fear), and physical symptoms. The boys from both groups also differed in common coping responses, with suburban boys reporting more submission and rural boys coping through activities and problem solving.

In another study of the meaning of stressful life experiences for normal children, 14 children aged 9 to 11 expressed stress related to loss, feelings of threat to self, and feelings of being hassled as their major types of stressful situations (Jacobson, 1994).

Research also indicates that various medical-related events experienced by children are associated to stress. Children in ICUs rank physical stressors as most distressing, followed by environmental, social, and psychological factors (Tichy et al, 1988). In another study, Hockenberry-Eaton and coworkers (1994) studied acute and chronic stressors of 48 children undergoing treatment for cancer during two clinic visits. They also studied protective factors (perceptions that reduce the stress) and responses (physiologic and psychological). Findings indicated increased physiologic responses (abnormally elevated epinephrine levels) in response to the prolonged stressors of perceptions related to having cancer and having to undergo treatment. Anxiety as a psychological response, however, was not high during either visit. Family environment, self-esteem, and social support were important protective factors. More research is needed, however, on how children's perceptions of stressors differ from those of adults, and on the rapid changes that occur during childhood.

Approximately one third of adolescents express a high number of stressful events. These generally relate to interpersonal relationships, with girls expressing greater concern regarding this stressor than boys (Stark et al, 1989). Boys, however, do report relationship stressors related to parents and siblings (Groer et al, 1992). Barron and Yoest (1994) report that middle and late adolescent boys are stressed by parents, but also by girlfriend relationships. Higher levels of emotional distress in their sample were found in male adolescents with greater use of coping in the forms of worrying, crying, expecting the worst, getting angry and "taking tensions out on someone or something" (p. 17). The greater the life changes for adolescents, the more likely they are to experience what Beard (1980) calls nervous tension, which they commonly express in such behaviors as depression, anger, and eating disorders. In one study of children and adolescents with diabetes, adolescents were found to cope less effectively and be more depressed and anxious than preadolescents. They also were less well adjusted and less in control of their blood sugar (Grey et al, 1991). Findings such as these can assist nurses in identifying adolescents who are at risk for anxiety and emotional distress.

ADULTS

In adulthood, new stressors arise. For young women in the general population, personal time issues are often extremely stressful. Personal time issues are situations in which women feel they do not have enough time to fulfill all the roles expected of them such as mother, wife, employee, community member, etc. For women at midlife (age 35 to 65), health issues are more likely to become stressors. In middle-aged women, the perception that life has, or has not, gone as it should has been found to be an influencing factor in whether or not stressful experiences contribute to midlife illness (Dixon et al, 1989). Those whose life had not gone as they expected reported more illnesses.

Young adult men have been found to perceive significantly more control over life events than early middle- and late middle-aged men (Mulvy and Dohrenwend, 1983). Usually, the greater the perception of control, the less stress experienced. Significantly, for both sexes, death anxiety has been found to be more prevalent in middle age than in the elderly (Shamoian, 1991).

Most medical-related stress and coping research has been conducted with adults. In general, older adults have been found to report more stress. One notable exception to this generalization was found in a study of the association between anxiety and age in 399 individuals with chronic heart disease (Nickel et al, 1990). When these subjects were studied 8 to 9 years after hospitalization for an acute coronary episode, one third reported considerable anxiety and one fourth reported taking anti-anxiety medications. The strongest predictor of anxiety was "heart-associated disability." Subjects age 65 or older were less likely than younger persons to report anxiety. Similarly, in a study of preoperative anxiety, younger adult patients indicated significantly more situational anxiety than did older adult patients (Wells et al, 1986). One explanation for this finding may be that the older patients had more experience with surgical procedures than the younger patients. Another explanation is that older people have learned to cope with many varied stressors, and therefore cope better generally than younger individuals. These findings emphasize the need to fully assess stressors, anxiety, and coping in all age groups because it is still unclear which situations will be likely to cause increased anxiety and coping needs. Nurses should be prepared to identify stressors and reduce anxiety with any age group.

Adults of childbearing age face some unique stressors. For example, families with young children have been shown to experience moderate levels of family stress stemming from personal and lifestyle factors. In these families, everyday stressors (daily ongoing hassles) are more strongly associated with child behavior problems than major stressful life events (Tobey and Schraeder, 1990). Illness and medical diagnoses have been shown to be very stressful to families dealing with these hardships (Anderson, 1994; Turk and Kerns, 1985).

ELDERLY ADULTS

For the elderly, stress often arises in response to an accumulation of functional losses, such as failing eyesight and decreased mobility. In addition, traumatic events increasingly attend this stage of life. Two major types of stressful life events are those involving *loss* of health, relationships, economic resources, and *conflict,* events involving issues of power, either interpersonally or intrapersonally. Examples of interpersonal conflict refer to stress from "a domineering spouse, domineering children, or from a domineering sibling" (Manfredi and Pickett, p. 105). Intrapersonal conflicts include concerns within one's self such as worries about children. The most stressful major life event for elderly persons is commonly the loss of a child or spouse. However, daily hassles have been found to be as stressful in the elderly as they are in other age groups (Manfredi and Pickett, 1987; Stokes and Gordon, 1988). In addition, elderly individuals returning from the hospital to home care are considerably stressed by early discharge, heavy home care demands, poorly adapted home settings, and inadequate resources such as the need for caregivers, finances, and equipment (Wagnild and Grupp, 1991). Physiologically, stress takes a greater toll on the immune system for the elderly than for younger people (Schleifer et al, 1989).

Gender

Probably the most clear-cut individual difference factor affecting anxiety and stress is gender. Although men and women in the general population experience no significant differences in the number of stressful life events, research has repeatedly indicated that women report higher levels of emotional stress than men (Staats and Staats, 1983; Thoits, 1982). Most of the potent life stressors for women are in the family arena, such as worries about child safety, and responsibility for work, home, and family welfare. Women also respond to stress with more illness, work loss, medicine use, and medical or mental health consultations than men. Men are more likely to use alcohol and to develop hypertension in response to stress. Overall, discrepancies in gender-related stress research may be due to women's tendency to perceive stressful events as more threatening than men tend to do, as well as women's greater willingness to acknowledge and seek help for stress-related problems (Dimond et al, 1987).

Other research has explored gender and stress in relation to medical conditions and treatments. In the case of anxiety induced by myocardial infarction, for example, women have been shown to experience greater distress than men. The same is true for persons with chronic heart disease, with younger women experiencing significantly more anxiety than younger males (Nickel et al, 1990). Toth (1993), however, found no difference in either stress or stressors at the time of hospital discharge for men and women after acute myocardial infarction. Regarding surgical anxiety, research again indicates that female patients report significantly more anxiety than male patients (Domar et al, 1989; Simpson and Fellett, 1987). However, it should be noted that many studies compare women undergoing gynecologic surgery with men undergoing abdominal surgery. It is possible that the type of surgery affects anxiety ratings, rather than gender alone.

Individual and Family Values

ROLE

Meaningful differences in the experience of medically related stress and anxiety occur according to an individual's role. Research has shown differences between those in the role of patient or spouse, between those in the parental role of mother or father, and between patients and nurses. Box 31–2 explores some of these differences.

MARITAL STATUS

Repeatedly, unmarried persons report more stress than do married persons, and married persons tend to cope better (Bennett, 1993). In the general population, single men report significantly more stressful life events than married men. Regarding both men and women, there is a positive association between the number of roles a person holds (such as spouse, parent, employee, etc.) and psychological well-being (Barnett, 1993; Crosby, 1984). The break-up of a marriage is more stressful for men than for women (Wallerstein and Kelley, 1980). Because of these findings, the nurse will need to pay special attention to the stress and anxiety of single adults whether male or female. Likewise, nurses need to be particularly mindful of stress and anxiety in divorced male patients.

SUPPORT OF OTHERS

Another factor closely related to marital status is the presence of supportive others. For example, in pregnant women with high life stress, those with highest anxiety had less support from partners and others (Norbeck and Anderson, 1989). Many other nursing research studies have shown that partner support reduces stress, buffers the effect of stressors, or assists in coping (Bennett, 1993). It is as yet unclear whether conflict in a relationship adds to stress, or remains supportive despite the conflict (Barrera and Baca, 1990).

EDUCATIONAL BACKGROUND AND SOCIOECONOMIC STATUS

Generally, those with more education, greater income and affluence, and more prestigious occupations experience less stress than those with less education, lower socioeconomic status, and blue collar work (Murata, 1994; Thoits, 1982). Similarly, those with lower socioeconomic status and less prestigious jobs exhibit more anxiety (Nickel et al, 1990). Regarding education, patients with less education report significantly more situational anxiety that patients with higher educational levels (Arellano et al, 1989). At present, the research has not identified why these trends occur.

CULTURE AND ETHNICITY

While stress and anxiety are present in all cultures, one's cultural, racial, or ethnic background appears to influence how they are experienced. Researchers have begun to explore some relationships between culture, stress, and anxiety but because of the limited scope of the research, the results have as yet limited value for nursing practice.

It does appear, however, that single-parent, low-income, black families living in inner-city environments are particularly stressed by family relationships and lack of social support (Murata, 1994). Neighbors and colleagues have identified that black families are generally more stressed than white middle class citizens, and that these stressors often relate to family conflict and financial problems. Low-income blacks experience these stressors more intensely than those with more ample finances (Neighbors et al, 1983).

Other more specific studies are beginning to address aspects of stress and anxiety for various groups. Smyth and Yarandi (1992) found that southern black women who were assessed as having Type A (impatient, aggressive, competitive) personalities exhibited less effective coping and higher stress responses than those with Type B (more easygoing) personalities. These Type A women had higher blood pressures (one

BOX 31-2
STRESS: THE IMPORTANCE OF ROLE

Studies on the impact of marital status have shown that spouses of cancer patients undergoing surgery experienced significantly higher anxiety before discharge and at 3 months post-discharge than did the patients themselves (Oberst and Scott, 1988). Likewise, spouses of coronary artery bypass surgery patients perceived significantly higher stress than the patients 3 to 8 days following surgery (Gillis, 1984). For women with breast cancer and their husbands, the most stressful time was the diagnostic phase before surgery. After surgery, both women and their husbands were most stressed by survival concerns (Northouse, 1989).

Regarding the role of the parent, there are mixed results when investigating the stress associated with having a child in a pediatric intensive care unit (ICU). In some studies, mothers have found the experience as significantly more stressful than have fathers (Miles et al, 1992; Perehudof, 1990). In another study, "fathers rated their overall intensive care experience as more stressful than the mothers" (Heuer, 1993). Parents often differ in the specific factors perceived to cause stress. Mothers report greater problems from the changes in their parental role and in the child's behavior and emotions than do fathers (Carter et al, 1985; Miles et al, 1992). In Heuer's study fathers rated suctioning of their child as significantly more stressful to them than did mothers—perhaps because they were present in the ICU less frequently than the mothers and therefore had not become as familiar with the procedure. In the same study, having tubes in their children was the most stressful procedure investigated (for both parents). Interestingly, environmental ICU aspects were not highly stressful to either parent (Carter et al, 1985; Miles et al, 1992).

In another study, mothers of pediatric patients perceived uncertainty as being more stressful than did fathers, whereas both mothers and nurses reported feeling more stress associated with the child's discomfort than did fathers (Graves and Ware, 1990). In coping with stress associated with having a child with spina bifida, mothers were more likely to respond with crying, diversionary activities, ignoring their stress, and removing themselves from sources of stress than were fathers (Van Cleve, 1989). It is as yet unclear whether these differences relate to danger to the child, or to parental role. Leonard, Brust, and Nelson (1993) found that 59 percent of mothers and 67 percent of fathers identified significant distress while caring for a medically fragile child at home.

The differing roles of patient and nurse also affect perceptions of stress. Generally, nurses and patients differ in their estimation of the severity of various stressors for patients, with nurses usually rating stressors as more distressing than patients. This difference has been found in research with coronary bypass surgery patients and their nurses (Carr and Powers, 1986; Yarcheski and Knapp-Spooner, 1994), with ICU patients and nurses (Cochrane, 1989), with pediatric patients and nurses (Hayes and Knox, 1984), and with elderly hospitalized patients and nurses, with the greatest discrepancy occurring in the area of hospital environment and routine (Davies and Peters, 1983). However, some researchers have found that nurses' perceptions of patient stress do correlate positively with those of the patients themselves (Caplin and Sexton, 1988; Tichy et al, 1988). While research outcomes in this area are not entirely consistent, they do emphasize the need to assess stress from the patient's perspective instead of relying on the nurse's own assumptions about the patient's experience.

physiologic measure of stress) than other groups. Blood pressure is, therefore, a very important measure of stress for nurses to obtain, especially in people who seem irritable and impatient.

Interestingly, several recent nursing research studies have focused on the stress of Indochinese (Southeast Asian) refugees living in the United States (Erickson et al, 1994; Frye and D'Avanzo, 1994; Kemp, 1985; Muecke and Sassi, 1992; Thompson, 1991). Between 1975 and 1990, over 959,000 Indochinese (Cambodian, Vietnamese, Thai, and Laotian) refugees resettled in the United States following the Vietnam War. These refugees report many troubling memories of war trauma, torture, and escape (Mollica et al, 1987), in addition to the deaths of family and friends. Results of the stress experienced by these cultural groups are reported to be suicide, somatization (physical symptoms as primary stress responses), and even sudden unexpected death (Mollica et al, 1987). Other stressors here in the United States include financial problems and family conflicts. These are often accompanied by difficulty in coping (D'Avanzo et al, 1994).

Different ethnic/cultural groups also may have distinctive ways of describing and expressing stress and anxiety. For instance, "nerves" is an expression used by rural Appalachian populations to describe a group of symptoms that characterize anxiety (Van Schaik, 1989). Cambodian refugees describe a stress response of "koucharang," or "thinking too much" (Frye, 1991). Koucharang refers to intense mental concentration on stressors resulting in depression or depressive behaviors such as isolation. Hispanic and Asian cultural groups in America often express their stress exhibiting somatic (physical) characteristics of stress and anxiety (Koss, 1990). These culturally specific responses to stress suggest that with all ethnic and cultural groups, it is important for the nurse to be sensitive to the culture at hand. Listening and keen observational skills are necessary. Additional education on particular cultures and their specific values and practices should be obtained if the nurse practices in a setting with clients from various cultures. At times, the nurse may have to arrange for a translator in order to carry out clinical decision making with culturally diverse patients. Finally, it is important for the nurse to remember that knowledge of cultural trends is only an aid to clinical decision making. Each individual should still be individually assessed for his or her unique pattern of stressors, and responses to stress.

SPIRITUALITY AND RELIGIOUS PRACTICES

Religious practices assist individuals in understanding and forming their reactions to stressful events. Religious beliefs, for many, aid in coping (Ochberg, 1992). In the United States, 50 percent of people studied indicate that religious beliefs and practices are important in coping with stress (Pargament et al, 1990). These religious practices may include, among others, seeking the help of clergy, prayer, confession, or focusing on life after death.

A possible influencing factor for stress and anxiety now being examined by nurse researchers is spirituality (Dossey and Guzzetta, 1994). Spirituality has been defined as "the human capacity to transcend self . . . reflected in three basic spiritual needs": self-acceptance, relationships with others and with God, and "the need for hope" (Highfield, 1992, p. 2). In a study of spirituality in cancer patients and nurses, nurses tended to underestimate the spiritual health of their patients, which was relatively high. Highfield hypothesized that this finding was due to cancer patients' using spiritual resources to cope with disease, utilizing spiritual resources because of advancing age, and utilizing these resources because of the terminal nature of their disease (Highfield, 1992).

For achievement of spiritual health and its use in coping, patients often turn to clergy, significant others, friends, nurses, and other health care providers. Nurses can assist these patients by establishing honest and open communication with patients, by addressing and accepting the spiritual needs of the patient, and by identifying patients who may be in danger of spiritual distress. Patients who are in spiritual distress often question their own beliefs regarding life, death, or suffering; describe despair; express no reason for continuing to live; and show detachment from self, others, or their deity (Carpenito, 1995). This and other related topics are now beginning to be addressed in more depth by nurse researchers.

Setting in Which Care Is Delivered

Many settings in which stress, anxiety, and coping have been studied for patients relate to the hospital, intensive care units, surgery, clinics, and other health care settings. Aspects of stress in these settings have already been addressed in previous sections of this chapter. For patients experiencing stress and anxiety in any of these settings, the stressors are most often related to the illness, disease, need for surgery, losses that have been or will be incurred, and changes in roles, rather than in environmental aspects of the particular setting (Werner, 1993).

Other settings of care, such as home care and area of residence as it relates to stress and anxiety, are just beginning to be studied. For example, in regard to home care, a survey of 178 Medicare-certified home care agencies identified four major stressor categories for patients. These included early hospital discharge, acuteness of the illness with accompanying demands in the home, unsafe environments, and inadequate resources (Wagnild and Grupp, 1992).

Preliminary support for residential setting as a differentiating characteristic has been reported by Preston and Crawford (1990). In a large sample of community-dwelling elderly, those living in small urban communities reported more stress in the areas of finances and health than did those in rural areas. Area of residence has not been well studied in nursing, but appears to be important in life-related stress.

Ethical Considerations

Ethics has become a topic of increasing concern for all health professions. Overarching ethical principles regarding any nursing action, including intervention in stress and anxiety, are difficult to develop, because our knowledge of health and illness underscores the individuality of each patient. What is ethically sound for one patient may prove to be unethical for another. Therefore, the nurse's judgment must be relied on to determine the ethics involved in each individual case (Donahue, 1990).

Two general principles should guide the nurse-patient relationship when the patient is experiencing stress or anxiety. The first is to refrain from adding to the patient's stress if at all possible. This principle is based on the concept of nonmaleficence, which is refraining from adding risk (Beauchamp and Childress, 1979), and requires the nurse to carefully assess an individual patient's stress level. Some patients, for example, may benefit from thorough instruction on what to expect (Freel, 1990), whereas for others, the instruction itself may increase stress. Similarly, the decision to subject patients to lengthy and/or complex assessment procedures requires careful judgment. For some patients who are obviously anxious it may be more important to induce a calm, restful environment than to use technologically advanced assessment techniques that may lead to greater fatigue and anxiety.

The second principle guiding ethical care of the stressed patient is respect for the privacy and integrity of the individual. Denial is a case in point. For some patients, denial may be the initial response to an anxiety-producing situation. Although the nurse may want to reduce denial to encourage realistic, conscious coping, it may be more ethical to allow the patient to continue using denial, unless it becomes clearly problematic. For example, a patient with acute MI who wants to exercise despite activity restrictions is an example of denial that may be detrimental, whereas denial resulting in lower pulse and blood pressure during the acute episode of MI may actually promote initial physiologic stabilization.

In these situations it is clear that careful nursing judgment geared to each individual situation must be used. The nurse should reflect upon the best course of action for each patient. In all cases, a genuine and informed concern for the patient's overall welfare is the most reliable ethical guideline.

Financial Considerations

Many studies of stress and anxiety include finances, often within the topic of socioeconomic status, as a variable of interest. Finances or economic status is often considered a resource or a mediator in the stress process. If finances are lacking, this lack may become an important stressor itself. The majority of studies indicate that those with higher levels of financial resources are not as stressed as those with less resources (Catalano and Dooley, 1977; Murata, 1994; Thoits, 1982).

It is therefore important for the nurse to assess the level of financial resources available to the patient or family. In some cases, the perception of this stressor changes over time. For example, even in families who report having adequate finances, a lengthy hospital stay coupled with lack of insurance or only partial coverage, may be a stressor that was unexpected by the patient or family. In some cases, it is the perception of these resources that can be stressful, rather than the actual economic situation.

FUTURE DEVELOPMENTS

Several areas of nursing research in the fields of stress and anxiety are promising, but need more investigation. One such area is the impact of mediators (influencing factors) on the stress response. While numerous investigations have been conducted into the effects of social support on stress, more research is needed to clearly determine whether and what type of support prevents stress from occurring, modifies the intensity of stress or anxiety experienced, or helps a person or family handle stress once it occurs. More information is also needed on the types of support that may *not* be helpful, or may even be harmful.

Family stress also warrants further study. While it has become increasingly clear that families of patients tend to experience considerable stress and anxiety (Anderson, 1994; McCubbin, 1989; Figley and McCubbin, 1983), future research will help pinpoint the specific factors that cause and exacerbate distress. Research is also needed regarding interventions to reduce family stress. Initial research has been conducted on methods of reducing stress in parents of children in pediatric intensive care (Curley, 1988; Melnyk, 1994) and on support groups for families of critically ill patients, which have been shown to be beneficial in reducing stress (Halm, 1990).

Stress related to outpatient surgery is just beginning to be studied. For example, in a small study of patients undergoing outpatient extracorporeal piezolithotripsy (noninvasive removal of kidney stones), 42 percent experienced significant agitation, which may have been related to the fact that the patients were conscious and experienced more pain than was expected (Brown, 1990a). In a follow-up study, anxiety measured by palmar sweat was lower postoperatively in patients who had outpatient surgery with anesthesia, whereas it remained the same for patients operated on while they were conscious (Brown, 1990b). More research into same-day surgery will help to clarify the factors that cause and mediate anxiety.

The effectiveness of *nursing interventions* to relieve anxiety and stress is being explored by nursing researchers and by scientists in other fields. Promising research is under way on the topics of pet or animal-assisted therapy (Baun et al, 1991; Kongable et al, 1989), and therapeutic touch (Quinn and Strelkauskas, 1993; Simington and Lang, 1993). Newer therapies, such as aromatherapy, are only now beginning to be studied.

NURSING CARE ACTIONS

Assessing Stress and Anxiety

Stress and anxiety influence health and illness. It is therefore essential that the nurse assess the patient's and family's stress and anxiety and intervene effectively. The desired outcome of care is a person and family with stress and anxiety levels that facilitate health.

When assessing a patient's stress and anxiety, the nurse must consider:

- stressors impinging on the patient
- the patient's perception of the stressors and the degree of harm/loss threat, or challenge imposed
- the patient's perceptions of mediators and resources
- the patient's coping skills

STRESSORS

In general, we know that many health- and illness-related conditions precipitate stress and therefore affect the nurse's clinical decisions. Stressors related to disease states, symptoms, illness, hospitalization, and surgery, as well as specific medical treatments, have been shown to affect patients and should be assessed. The stressors previously described can be the basis for interview questions designed to address which stressors are most troublesome for a particular patient.

For example, for the patient facing coronary bypass surgery, the nurse may ask about cardiac disease and its effects on the patient, such as perceived losses (of roles, etc.). The nurse can also inquire as to what aspects of hospitalization are most distressing. To provide more structure, major factors included in Volicer's (1977) instrument can be addressed. These include unfamiliar surroundings, issues of dependence, separation from spouse or family, finances, isolation, need for information, effects of the illness, and medication problems.

Pain can also be a stressor. To assess pain and its relationship to anxiety, a number of issues can be addressed with the patient to determine the role of pain. Questions for the patient include:

- Describe the location, quality and severity of the pain you experience.
- Describe the tension (anxiety) you are experiencing.

- Do you notice any relationship between increasing tension and pain?
- How often do you have pain?
- How often are you tense?
- What helps to reduce your pain?

PATIENT'S PERCEPTION OF STRESSORS

Since no two individuals will perceive a stressor in exactly the same manner, it is very important to assess the meaning identified stressors have for patients. For example, the prospect of surgery is a stressor for most surgical patients. Therefore, the nurse will want to address surgery as a stressor, but will also want to inquire as to what surgery means to the individual. For some patients it may indicate a change in body image; for others the prospect of losing control over one's body and consciousness may be most troubling. For some, the fear of death during surgery may be paramount (such as in the case example of Mrs. Stenson at the beginning of this chapter). And for still others, surgery may be perceived of as a relief for long-standing pain, troubling only in the sense that the patient will have to miss a certain amount of work, or experience a few days of pain. There are no instruments which are capable of assessing all of the various perceptions regarding potential stressors. Therefore the best method of assessing meaning is through an interview with the patient.

MEDIATORS AND RESOURCES

Various mediators have been shown to moderate perceptions of stress, and the nurse should also engage in an assessment of these resources. Topics include personal characteristics such as optimistic or pessimistic outlook, and proneness to anxiety. Social support is also a topic for assessment. Does the patient have support of others? Are these persons readily available to the patient? Does the patient perceive that these others are available if needed? Is the support others give perceived as beneficial? Are the financial resources of the patient adequate? Spiritual support is another important resource for some individuals and can be inquired about in a nonjudgmental way.

Another topic to explore is whether or not the patient has prior experience with particular stressors such as hospitalization. Does this prior experience help? The nurse may also ask what the patient perceives to be the resources needed in a particular situation. For example, the question "What would be of help to you in this situation?" may elicit ideas for resources that the nurse might either provide for, or attempt to assist with. Another question the nurse can ask is "Do you have close relatives or friends who can help you through this situation?"

ANXIETY RESPONSE

Attempts to recognize and measure anxiety must address the multiple ways in which anxiety can be displayed. Anxiety and fear are experienced in similar ways physically. Anxiety is viewed as a response to an unknown or unconscious threat, although considerable research on anxiety includes identifiable threats. Although anxiety commonly occurs in patients with certain medical diagnoses, in those awaiting a diagnosis after having diagnostic tests, and in those hospitalized and/or undergoing surgical procedures, the extent of anxiety necessary for pathology is yet unclear. A single assessment method may not fully capture the phenomenon.

There is physiologic information available to the nurse that may assist in assessing anxiety. Vital signs can point to anxiety, if the pulse and blood pressure are elevated. The nurse can hold the patient's hand to see if perspiration is present, or if there is a tremor. McCleane and Watters (1990) examined the relationship between the changes in anxiety experienced by surgical patients and any subsequent alterations in the concentrations of serum potassium. They demonstrated small decreases in serum potassium in a study of 200 preoperative patients who had an increase in anxiety and concluded that the potassium changes were caused by alterations in the amount of adrenaline secreted by the patient. Serum potassium is one index included in typical preoperative blood studies and this information should be available on the patient's chart.

In addition, it is important to note that the defense mechanism of denial can dramatically affect assessment of observable anxiety. MI patients classified as "deniers" acknowledge less anxiety on admission to a CCU than is typical of normal, nonstressed individuals whereas those classified as "nondeniers" usually report a much higher level of anxiety. Therefore, using the patient's laboratory values as indicators of potential anxiety is warranted.

In appraising anxiety the nurse will also want to engage in evaluation of subjective symptoms, cognitive symptoms, behavioral symptoms, and the defining characteristics of the nursing diagnosis of anxiety. Particular attention should be paid to the characteristics of verbal expressions of anxiety, motor activity, nervous habits, and expressions of apprehension.

COPING SKILLS

Assessment of an individual's coping skills is a crucial step in the determination of that individual's response to stress. No two patients will cope in the same manner to a given stressor. Attempting to predict an individual's response to stress and planning care based on that prediction would lead to inaccurate and nonspecific nursing intervention. Assessment of an individual's coping behaviors can proceed by asking the patient how he or she typically handles stress. Use of the Ways of Coping Scale or Jalowiec Coping Scale may be valuable. If the tools are not available, the nurse can inquire about each of the coping styles contained in the tools. It is also wise to ask about use of problem-focused and emotion-focused coping because patients who report more problem-focused strategies have generally better adjustment (Keckeisen and Nyamathi, 1990).

Analyzing Stress and Anxiety

After assessment, the nurse will draw conclusions regarding the patient's stress and anxiety, and possible health changes or emotional problems. Some of these conclusions may be stated as questions for further consideration. For example, the nurse may note that the patient denies any concerns regarding surgery. Yet the nurse noted that the patient looked tense during the discussion. Therefore the nurse is not certain whether or not the patient is concerned about the surgery. The nurse considers this an issue to be pursued with ongoing assessment.

Some of the conclusions will be stated as direct quotes from the patient. For example, the patient stated, "I am very worried about the costs of my hospital stay. I just don't know what my insurance covers. There have been so many changes in health insurance lately."

Some of the conclusions will be stated as nursing diagnoses. Nursing diagnoses related to stress include:

- Anxiety
- Fear
- Fatigue
- Hopelessness
- Ineffective Coping
- High Risk for Injury
- Sleep Pattern Disturbance

See Figure 31–5 for major areas to be assessed.

Reducing Stress and Anxiety

Outcome-oriented interventions aimed at reducing a patient's stress and anxiety include:

- eliminating stressors or reducing their occurrence
- assisting the patient in perceiving the stressors differently
- providing for or assisting the patient in obtaining necessary resources or support
- decreasing or modifying the patient's anxiety response
- enhancing the patient's ability to cope

Eliminating or reducing the incidence of stressors is one way in which nurses can assist patients. For example if heat or cold is a stressor, the nurse can institute measures to eliminate the stressor. If the presence of a certain roommate is a stressor, the nurse can be instrumental in a room change. Of course there are some stressors that cannot be eliminated. The fact of having to be hospitalized or having a disease obviously cannot be immediately changed. However, eliminating stressors that can be changed frees more energy to deal with other stressors.

Because pain is one stressor many patients experience, nurses should institute measures to reduce this stressor. Frequent, adequate pain medication should be given. Proper positioning and body alignment can also reduce pain. Thirst as a stressor can also be reduced by moistening the mucosa, or by offering oral fluids to those who may have them.

For certain stressors, the nurse may be of assistance in *modifying the person's perception*. Cognitive appraisal of some stressors can be changed to make them less threatening. For example, to a patient who perceives time away from his or her job as threatening, it may be suggested that this absence may provide a needed period of rest and recuperation that will assist the person in doing a better job once he or she returns to work. Certain stressors can be explained as presenting a challenge or an opportunity for growth. Giving procedural and preparatory sensory information eliminates uncertainty about the effects of threatening procedures.

Assisting in providing additional resources is another type of nursing intervention for patients experiencing stress. Some measures to improve resources may be to attempt to increase social support for the patient. Examples are communicating needs to family members, increasing visiting times for patients in the ICU, and arranging for attendance of a priest, rabbi, shaman, minister, or mullah for spiritual resources, or a social worker for financial concerns.

One common resource that can be provided is information. For many patients stress is worsened by a lack of information in a certain area. It is first necessary to ascertain how much knowledge the person has, and to assess the patient's readiness to learn. Then patient teaching or provision of information can proceed.

Decreasing the anxiety response will likely be a priority for many patients, particularly if the anxiety is at moderate or severe levels (Guzzetta, 1989). Reducing panic levels of anxiety is an absolute necessity that often calls for medical interventions such as medications that bring about relaxation. Anxiety disorders require referral to mental health professionals.

Other interventions for the hospitalized patient include familiarizing the patient with surroundings and routines of the unit or clinic. This type of structuring will often increase the patient's security. The nurse should also provide the type of support the patient desires. This may involve sitting with the patient, touching the patient, or listening to the patient, based on the patient's wishes.

Music has been shown to be an anxiety- and stress-reducing intervention for most patients studied, particularly in acute care settings (see Patient Teaching box). Lueders-Bolwerk (1990) showed that the state anxiety in MI patients who heard three sessions of relaxing music was reduced significantly in 2 days. However, state anxiety was also significantly less in the control group presumably because of physiologic improvement, sedatives, and other unidentified factors. Anxiety is lessened by the therapeutic use of music for cancer patients, ICU surgical patients (Kaempf and Amodei, 1989; Steelman, 1990; Updike, 1990), and patients with heart attacks (White, 1992). Conflicting results have been reported in coronary care (Zimmerman et al, 1988), yet generally, the research supports music as relaxing to patients. Patients do better if given a type of music they enjoy. Music they do not enjoy could itself be a stressor.

PATIENT TEACHING

PATIENT TEACHING WITH THE PATIENT EXPERIENCING ANXIETY REGARDING IMPENDING SURGERY

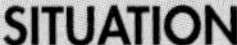

SITUATION

Surgery has been shown to produce anxiety in most patients. In fact, anxiety is described as the most frequent nursing diagnosis identified preoperatively by nurses. For Mrs. Stenson, additional stressors are present, and the nurse's assessment indicates that she experiences anxiety frequently. Therefore the nurse institutes patient teaching in the area of music for reduction of anxiety. Patient teaching on using music for relaxation, and on the benefits of music, will help now as Mrs. Stenson faces surgery, and for the future so that she can benefit from music in other situations.

PATIENT READINESS

Part of the nurse's assessment focuses on Mrs. Stenson's readiness for learning the anxiety-reducing strategy. In this situation, the nurse assesses that Mrs. Stenson enjoys music very much, but has never thought of it as an adjunct to trying to relax. As the nurse introduces the idea of listening to quiet calming music, Mrs. Stenson states she has never thought about it but would like to try it. Because Mrs. Stenson's anxiety is so uncomfortable to her, she appears ready to learn new ways of handling it.

TEACHING

After the patient's initial anxiety is reduced to a manageable level, the nurse begins to teach her verbally about the therapeutic effects of music, stating principles in simple, direct, short statements. The major points taught include:

- Music has been shown to be effective in reducing tension.
- Calm music works better than fast, exciting music.
- Music can be effective, whether or not headphones are used.

The nurse then provides Mrs. Stenson with a small audiocassette player and a tape of a slow, calming musical piece, matching her preference for classical, new age, or instrumental music. This musical piece has a regular rhythm, predictable dynamics, and consonance in its harmony (Steelman, 1990). The nurse also provides a set of headphones, which Mrs. Stenson can try for comfort. If these headphones are not comfortable, she is not required to use them.

EVALUATION

Following 10 minutes of listening to music, the nurse reassesses Mrs. Stenson and her anxiety. The outcomes the nurse attends to include a reduction in facial tension, less fidgeting, reduction in darting eye movements, better facial color, decreased blood pressure, and increased ability to talk calmly with the nurse. In addition, it is very important that the nurse ask Mrs. Stenson how she is feeling, what her tension level is, and if she feels more relaxed.

FOLLOW-UP

Following surgery, the nurse institutes a plan to reinforce the teaching already done with Mrs. Stenson. The nurse also explores the use of music with Mrs. Stenson to increase relaxation and thereby reduce pain postoperatively. The nurse reteaches as necessary, and continues to evaluate Mrs. Stenson's response to music in each new situation. When discharge planning takes place, the use of music for relaxation is included in the plan, so that its value can carry on after Mrs. Stenson leaves the hospital.

Other research has shown that *supportive educative counseling* for MI patients and their partners significantly reduces anxiety. In one study, coronary care nurses provided the counseling, which had five aspects: (1) reducing uncertainty by explaining the illness and ramifications; (2) discussing sensations and complications; (3) providing continuous psychological support through an ongoing trusting relationship; (4) involving the couple in decisions about care; and (5) listening attentively to concerns. Anxiety was significantly reduced in 4 days (Thompson, 1989). This study illustrates the importance of nurse support in reducing anxiety.

Moreover, in a large review of 102 intervention studies with surgical patients, Devine and Cook (1986) found that psychoeducational interventions were successful in assisting recovery, lowering pain, and increasing both well-being and satisfaction with care. These interventions included psychological support or educational interventions such as providing information (see Clinical Decision Making box). It is also noteworthy that provision of unnecessary or inappropriate information may increase patient anxiety. In a study of medical surgical patients and nurses, Olson (1995) obtained a strong relationship between the empathy of the nurses, and reduced distress (anxiety, depression, and anger) of the patients.

The final type of intervention for reducing stress is to *enhance patient coping*. This may involve assisting direct actions of the patient to remove or lessen stressors or increase resources (problem-focused coping), or to facilitate affective methods such as expressing emotions (emotion-focused coping). Teaching coping strategies such as relaxation or use of guided imagery also helps the patient cope, in addition to reducing anxiety.

ASSESSING AND INTERVENING IN ANXIETY IN PATIENTS WITH HEART DISEASE

The importance of assessing and intervening in anxiety upon admission to the hospital, especially in MI patients, cannot be overstated. For example, in coronary care patients,

CLINICAL DECISION MAKING

ESTABLISHING PRIORITIES WITH A PATIENT EXPERIENCING BOTH ANXIETY AND STRESS

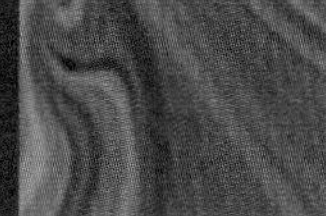

SITUATION

Viola Stenson, a 62-year-old white retired widowed female patient, has just been admitted to the hospital for planned knee surgery. Upon admission, the nurse assesses several characteristics of anxiety, including restlessness, hand tremors, facial twitches, pale skin color, darting glances, rapid speech, sighing, and high voice pitch. The nurse also assess several stressful life events and ongoing stressors. These include:

- death of husband 2 years ago
- retirement 6 months ago
- death of best friend during surgery 6 years ago
- both daughters living at great distance
- immobility due to joint disease
- having had heart surgery
- financial concerns
- fear of dying during surgery

NURSE'S LONG-TERM MEMORY

The nurse knows that it is important before surgery to prepare the patient for what will occur after surgery, and to teach her what to do. Important areas to be covered include:

- mobility after surgery
- pain and pain relief
- avoiding dislocation through proper movement
- avoiding medical complications such as thrombosis

The nurse also knows that people experiencing high levels of anxiety are not able to listen and remember well. In addition, their perception narrows, and they tend to focus on a limited number of items. The nurse also reflects on knowledge that major life stressors cannot be solved in a short period of time, but often take an increase of resources such as social support, a change in meaning, or a gradual resolution over time.

GOALS

In this situation, the nurse does not have Mrs. Stenson establish her own goals, because high anxiety inhibits this process. Instead, the nurse decides the first and foremost goal is reduction of Mrs. Stenson's anxiety. After anxiety has been reduced, the nurse can reassess Mrs. Stenson to determine if mutual goal setting can occur, and to institute teaching and preparation for what will occur after surgery. The nurse's short-term goal, therefore, is:

- to reduce anxiety

The nurse knows that anxiety reduction is a must to prevent physiologic complications and to increase Mrs. Stenson's ability to set further goals with the nurse.

As the nurse institutes interventions to reduce anxiety, she or he reflects on other potential areas for mutual goal setting once the anxiety has been reduced. These include:

- Reduce the stress stemming from fear of dying.
- Prepare for surgery.
- Teach about pain reduction, mobility, and recuperation.
- Increase coping resources including social support.
- Assist Mrs. Stenson through the grieving process.

INTERVENTIONS

The nurse takes immediate steps to reduce Mrs. Stenson's anxiety. These include:

1. Provide a calm, reassuring presence.
2. Provide a safe quiet environment.
3. Develop rapport with Mrs. Stenson.
4. Collaborate with a physician to provide anxiety-reducing medication.
5. Offer reassurance and support.
6. Continue to develop trust throughout the interaction.
7. Avoid additional stressors; for example, avoid use of medical jargon that cannot be easily understood.
8. Use short simple sentences.
9. Encourage ventilation of feelings if patient is ready.
10. Use music for relaxation.

SELF-ASSESSMENT

The nurse maintains an attitude of self-assessment during care with Mrs. Stenson. This includes assessing his or her own anxiety level. If the nurse's anxiety is high, this often increases the patient's anxiety. In this case it is appropriate to request the assistance of another nurse. The nurse also examines his or her own feelings about surgery and death in order to be of utmost assistance to each individual client.

REFLECTION

The nurse regularly thinks through decisions made and evaluates goals for their relevance. During this reflection process, areas for further assessment often surface. Once Mrs. Stenson's anxiety has been reduced, the nurse makes a judgment as to whether or not Mrs. Stenson can assist in identifying further goals. The nurse at this point may reassess Mrs. Stenson's fear of dying, her need for social support, her readiness for surgery, and her knowledge of what to expect following surgery. Perhaps in this case, Mrs. Stenson's fear of death during surgery needs attention. Helping Mrs. Stenson to modify her perception may be an additional goal. The nurse can assist by explaining the nature of the surgery and that qualified experienced personnel including nurses, physicians, and anesthesiologists will be present. The nurse also focuses on the resulting increased ability to move without pain as a desirable outcome of the surgery. In this way, the nurse may help Mrs. Stenson to modify her perception of the stressor. Once these priorities are addressed, the nurse and patient can move on to further reflection and planning.

psychological stress (as well as physical exertion) has been shown to aggravate changing heart abnormalities (Medich et al, 1991). There is a well-established relationship between psychological stress and decreased survival following an MI (Malan, 1992). Nurses are in a position to reduce stress upon admission and therefore to intervene in the process by which stress activates the sympathetic nervous system. This is particularly important for patients with cardiac disease, since the cardiopulmonary system is already overtaxed.

CLOSE COMMUNICATION AMONG MEMBERS OF THE HEALTH CARE TEAM ABOUT THE PATIENT'S CARE

It is also essential that assessment information, conclusions, and plan of care be communicated at shift report or to other involved health care personnel. Progress made in reducing stress and anxiety must be communicated from shift to shift. It should be given as high a priority as any other condition. Without communication, assessment and other planning efforts may be duplicated, a process that can increase stress and anxiety.

REASSESSMENT OF STRESS AND ANXIETY AT CRITICAL POINTS IN THE PATIENT'S RECOVERY PROCESS

As discharge approaches it is also essential that a reassessment and discharge planning take place. In addition to medical condition, self-care, follow-up, and other teaching, stress and anxiety should be reassessed and planned for because the prospect of returning home can initiate new stressors, especially in today's era of short hospital stays and increasing responsibilities of home care (Wagnild and Grupp, 1992). Where to get help is an important topic for patient teaching as discharge draws near. Unusual or unexpected reactions or conditions once the patient is at home can dramatically increase the patient's overall stress and anxiety. The nurse should provide specific sources of help and telephone numbers through which patients can receive immediate attention for unexpected symptoms. If the patient is referred to an outside agency, home care, or public health nurse, information about stress and anxiety should be communicated in the referral. Planning and intervention should be guided by the acceptability of the client (Bulechek and McCloskey, 1989).

EVALUATING OUTCOMES FOCUSED ON INCREASED ABILITY TO COPE WITH STRESSORS, REDUCTION OF ANXIETY, AND ENHANCED HEALTH

Finally, the nurse will need to appraise his or her interventions in terms of their effectiveness in increasing the patient's ability to cope with stressors. Additional questions the nurse may ask are: Has the perception of stressors changed? Have appropriate resources been obtained or put to use? Has positive support been given? Has anxiety been reduced to a more manageable level? All of these questions will help the nurse to evaluate whether or not the health of the patient has been enhanced.

CHAPTER HIGHLIGHTS

- Cannon's concept of homeostasis, Selye's General Adaptation Syndrome, and Wolff's representation of restoring balance through adaptation are foundational to today's knowledge of stress.
- Three major historical perspectives on anxiety include psychodynamic, learning, and biologic aspects.
- The major body systems involved in stress and anxiety are the endocrine, nervous, and immune systems, which communicate via neuropeptides.
- The Institute of Medicine's "Framework for Interactions Between the Individual and the Environment" contains four major concepts: stressors, reactions, consequences, and mediators.
- Stressors can be anything that activates the stress response, including internal and external stimuli.
- When anxiety is severe, some individuals use the cognitive processes, defense mechanisms to reduce anxiety.
- Primary and secondary appraisal, and problem-focused and emotion-focused coping are psychological processes identified as operational when people experience stress.
- Major stressors identified in nursing research are concerned with diagnosis of a medical condition, disease, threatening medical events, hospitalization, surgery, and developmental transitions.
- Reactions and consequences to stress studied in nursing include psychological distress, symptoms, depression, quality of life, pain, physiologic responses, and coping, as well as anxiety.
- Mediators include uncertainty, social support, and coping.
- Nursing interventions to reduce stress and anxiety fall into the categories of relaxation; education and information; time, environment-person; and social strategies.
- Nursing theories that address stress and/or anxiety include those of Neuman (1989), Erickson, Tomlin, and Swain (1983), Roy (1988), Johnson (1980), and Benner and Wrubel (1989).
- Nurse theorist Hildegard Peplau describes four levels of anxiety: mild, moderate, severe, and panic.
- The following factors influence nurse clinical decision making regarding stress and anxiety: age/developmental level, gender, individual and family values (marital status, support, and role), education, socioeconomic status, culture/ethnicity, spirituality or religious beliefs and practices, setting, ethics, and finances.
- Nurses assess stressors, perception, anxiety, and coping.
- Nurses intervene to eliminate or reduce stressor occurrence, change perceptions, increase support, decrease anxiety, and enhance coping.
- Evaluation of outcomes focuses on reduced stress and anxiety and enhanced health.

REFERENCES

Affonso, D.D., Maybery, L.S., Paul, S. (1994). Cognitive adaptation to stressful events during pregnancy and postpartum: Development and testing of the CASE instrument. *Nursing Research, 43,* 338–343.

Aguilera, D.C., Messick, J.M. (1984). *Crisis Intervention: Theory and Methodology,* 4th ed. St. Louis: C.V. Mosby.

American Nurses' Association (1995). *Nursing: A Social Policy Statement.* Washington, D.C.: Author.

American Psychiatric Association (1994). *Diagnostic and Statistical Manual of Mental Disorders,* 4th ed. Washington D.C.: Author.

Anderson, K.H. (1994). Family sense of coherence: As collective and consensus in relation to family quality of life after illness diagnosis. In H. McCubbin, E. Thompson, A. Thompson, and J. Fromer (eds.): *Sense of Coherence and Resiliency.* Madison, WI: The University of Wisconsin System, pp. 169–187.

Anderson, K.O., Bradley, L., Young, L., et al (1985). Rheumatoid arthritis: Review of psychological factors related to etiology, effects, and treatment. *Psychological Bulletin, 98,* 358–387.

Antonovsky, A. (1987). *Unraveling the Mystery of Health.* San Francisco: Jossey-Bass.

Arellano, R., Cruise, C., Chung, F. (1989). Timing of the anesthetist's preoperative outpatient interview. *Anesthiologist Analogue, 68* (5), 645–648.

Artinian, N.T. (1993). Resources: Factors that mediate the stress-outcome relationship. In J. Barnfather and B.L. Lyon (eds.): *Stress and Coping: State of the Science and Implications for Nursing Theory, Research and Practice.* Indianapolis: Center Nursing Press, Sigma Theta Tau International, pp. 95–111.

Augustin, P., Hains, A. (1996). Effects of music on ambulatory surgery patients' preoperative anxiety. *AORN Journal, 63,* 753–756.

Baker, C.F. (1986). *The Effects of Noise on Heart Rate and Annoyance in Postoperative Patients in Intensive Care.* Doctoral dissertation, The University of Texas at Austin, Austin, Texas.

Ballard, K.S. (1981). Identification of environmental stressors for patients in a surgical intensive care unit. *Issues in Mental Health Nursing, 3* (3), 89–108.

Bandura, A. (1989). Self-regulation of motivation and action through internal standards and goal system. In L. A. Pervin (ed.): *Goal Concepts in Personality and Social Psychology.* Hillsdale, NJ: Erlbaum.

Barnason, S., Zimmerman, L., Nieveen, J. (1995). The effects of music interventions on anxiety in the patient after coronary artery bypass grafting. *Heart & Lung, 24,* 124–132.

Barnett, R.C. (1993). Multiple roles, gender, and psychological distress. In L. Goldberer and S. Breznitz (eds.): *Handbook of Stress: Theoretical and Clinical Aspects.* NY: The Free Press, pp. 427–445.

Barnett, R.C., Marshall, N.L., Singer, J.D. (1992). Job experiences over time, multiple roles, and women's mental health: A longitudinal study. *Journal of Personality and Social Psychology, 64,* 634–644.

Barnfather, J., Lyon, B., Artinian, N., et al (1991). *Synthesis Conference Working Bibliography.* Unpublished Manuscript, Midwest Nursing Research Society Stress and Coping Research Section.

Barrera, M., Baca, L. (1990). Recipient reactions to social support. *Journal of Social and Personal Relationships, 1,* 541–551.

Barsevick, A.M., Johnson, J.E. (1990). Preference for information and involvement, information seeking and emotional responses of women undergoing colposcopy. *Research in Nursing and Health, 13,* 1–7.

Beard, M. (1980, November). Interpersonal trust, life events and coping in an ethnic adolescent population. *Journal of Psychiatric Nursing and Mental Health Services,* 12–20.

Beauchamp, T.L., Childress, J. (1979). *Principles of Biomedical* Ethics. New York: Oxford University Press.

Beck, A.T. (1985). Theoretical perspectives on clinical anxiety. In A.H. Tuma and J.D. Maser (eds.): *Anxiety and the Anxiety Disorders.* Hillsdale, NJ: Erlbaum.

Benner, P., Wrubel, J. (1989). *The Primacy of Caring: Stress and Coping in Health and Illness.* Menlo Park: Addison-Wesley.

Bennett, S.J. (1993). Relationships among selected antecedent variables and coping effectiveness in postmyocardial infarction patients. *Research in Nursing and Health, 16,* 131–139.

Bihl, M.A., Ferrans, C.E., Powers, M.J. (1988). Comparing stressors and quality of life of dialysis patients. *American Nephrology Nurses' Association Journal, 15* (l), 27–36.

Biley, F.C. (1989). Nurses' perception of stress in preoperative surgical patients. *Journal of Advanced Nursing, 14,* 575–581.

Bohachick, P., Anton, B., Wooldridge, P., et al (1992). Psychosocial outcome six months after heart transplant surgery: A preliminary report. *Research in Nursing and Health, 15,* 165–173.

Bowlby, J. (1973). *Attachment and loss: Vol. II. Separation, anxiety, and anger.* New York: Basic Books.

Bresser, P.J., Sexton, D., Foell, D. (1993). Patient's responses to postponement of coronary artery bypass graft surgery. *Image: Journal of Nursing Scholarship, 25,* 5–10.

Broome, M.E., Bates, T., Lillis, P., McGahee, T. (1994). Children's medical fears, coping behavior patterns and pain perceptions during a lumbar puncture. *European Journal of Cancer Care, 3,* 31–38.

Brown, B., Roberts, J., Browne, G., et al (1988). Gender differences in variables associated with psychosocial adjustment to a burn injury. *Research in Nursing & Health, 11,* 23–30.

Brown, S.M. (1990a). Perioperative anxiety in patients undergoing extracorporeal piezolithotripsy. *Journal of Advanced Nursing, 15,* 1078–1082.

Brown, S.M. (1990b). Quantitative measurement of anxiety in patients undergoing surgery for renal calculus disease. *Journal of Advanced Nursing, 15,* 962–970.

Browne, G., Byrne, C., Roberts, J., et al (1988). The Meaning of Illness Questionnaire: Reliability and validity. *Nursing Research, 37,* 368–373.

Buchanan, L.M., Cowan, M., Burr, R., et al (1993). Measurement of recovery from myocardial infarction using heart rate variability and psychological outcomes. *Nursing Research, 42,* 74–78.

Bulechek, G.M., McCloskey, J.C. (1989). Nursing interventions: Treatments for potential nursing diagnoses. In R.M. Carroll-Johnson, *Classification of Nursing Diagnoses: Proceedings of the Eighth Conference*. Philadelphia: Lippincott.

Burns, K.R., Egan, E. (1994). Description of a stressful encounter: Appraisal, threat, and challenge. *Journal of Nursing Education, 33* (l), 21–28.

Cannon, W.B. (1932). The *Wisdom of the Body.* New York: Norton.

Cannon, W.B. (1935). Stresses and strains of homeostasis. *American Journal of the Medical Sciences, 189,* 1–14.

Caplan, G. (1964). *Principles of Preventive Psychiatry.* New York: Basic Books.

Caplin, M.S., Sexton, D.L. (1988). Stresses experienced by spouses of patients in a coronary care unit with myocardial infarction. *Focus on Critical Care, 15* (5), 31–40.

Carpenito, L.J. (1995). *Nursing Diagnosis: Application to Clinical Practice,* 6th ed. Philadelphia: Lippincott.

Carpenito, L.J. (1993). *Nursing Diagnosis: Application to Clinical Practice.* Philadelphia: Lippincott.

Carr, J.A., Powers, M.J. (1986). Stressors associated with coronary bypass surgery. *Nursing Research, 35,* 243–246.

Carroll-Johnson, R.M. (ed.) (1989): *Classification of Nursing Diagnoses: Proceedings of the Eighth Conference.* Philadelphia: Lippincott.

Carter, M.C., Miles, M.S. (1982). Parental stressor scale: Pediatric intensive care units. *Nursing Research, 31,* 121.

Carter, M.C., Miles, M.S., Buford, T.H., Hassanein, R.S. (1985). Parental environmental stress in pediatric intensive care units. *Dimensions of Critical Care Nursing, 4* (3), 180–188.

Catalans, R., Dooley, D. (1977). Economic predictors of depressed mood and stressful life events in a metropolitan community. *Journal of Health and Social Behavior, 18,* 292–307.

Caudell, K.A. Gallucci, B. (1995). Neuroendocrine and immunological responses of women to stress. *Western Journal of Nursing Review, 17,* 672–692.

Chekryn, J. (1984). Cancer recurrence: Personal meaning, communication, and marital adjustment. *Cancer Nursing, 7,* 491–497.

Christman, N.J. (1990). Uncertainty and adjustment during radiotherapy. *Nursing Research, 39,* 17–20, 47.

Christman, N.J., McConnell, E.A., Pfeiffer, C., et al (1988). Uncertainty, coping and distress following myocardial infarction: Transition from hospital to home. *Research in Nursing and Health, 11,* 71–82.

Clark, C.R., Gregor, F.M. (1988). Developing a sensation information message for femoral arteriography. *Journal of Advanced Nursing, 13,* 237–244.

Cochrane, J. (1989). A comparison of nurses' and patients' perceptions of intensive care unit stressors. *Journal of Advanced Nursing, 14,* 1038–1043.

Cohen, S., Williamson, G. (1991). Stress and infectious disease in humans. *Psychological Bulletin, 109,* 5–23.

Corney, R., Everett, H., Howells, A., Crowther, M. (1992). The care of patients undergoing surgery for gynaecological cancer: The need for information, emotional support and counseling. *Journal of Advanced Nursing, 17* (6), 667–671.

Crosby, F. (1984). Job satisfaction and domestic life. In M. Lee and R. Kungo (eds.): *Management of Work and Personal Life.* NY: Praeger.

Crosby, L.J. (1988). Stress factors, emotional stress and rheumatoid arthritis disease activity. *Journal of Advanced Nursing, 13,* 452–461.

Crowe, J.M., Runions, J., Ebbesen, L., et al (1996). Anxiety and depression after acute myocardial infarction. *Heart & Lung: Journal of Acute & Critical Care, 25,* 98–107.

Curly, M.A. (1988). Effects of the nursing mutual participation of care on parentive series in pediatric intensive care unit. *Heart & Lung, 17,* 682–688.

Darwin, C.R. (1872). *The Expression of Emotions in Man and Animals.* London: John Murray.

D'Avanzo, A.D., Peters, M. (1983). Stresses of hospitalization in the elderly: Nurses' and patients' perceptions. *Journal of Advanced Nursing, 8,* 99–105.

D'Avanzo, C.E., Frye, B., and Froman, R. (1994). Stress in Cambodian refugee families. *Image: Journal of Nursing Scholarship, 26* (2), 101–105.

Davies, A. D., & Peters, M. (1983). Stresses of hospitalization in the elderly: Nurses' and patients' perceptions. *Journal of Advanced Nursing, 8,* 99–105.

DeLongis, A., Folkman, S., & Lazarus, R. (1988). The impact of daily stress on health and mood: Psychological and social resources as mediators. *Journal of Personality and Social Psychology, 54,* 486–495.

Devine, E.C., Cook, T.D. (1986). Clinical and cost-saving effects of psychoeducational interventions with surgical patients: A meta-analysis. *Research in Nursing and Health, 9,* 89–105.

Dimond, M., McCance, K., King, K. (1987). Forced residential relocation: Its impact on the well-being of older adults. *Western Journal of Nursing Research, 4,* 445–461.

Dimond, M., Caserta, M., Lund, D. (1994). Understanding depression in bereaved older adults, *Clinical Nursing Research, 31,* 253–268.

Dixon, J.P., Dixon, J.K., Spinner J. (1989). Perceptions of life-pattern disintegrity as a link in the relationship between stress and illness. *Advances in Nursing Science, 11* (2), 1–11.

Dollard, J., Miller, N. (1950). *Personality and Psychotherapy.* New York: McGraw Hill.

Dolnick, E. (1989, March/April). Scared to death. *Hippocrates,* 106–108.

Domar, D.A., Everett, L.L., Keller, M.G. (1989). Preoperative anxiety: Is it a predictable entity? *Anesthesiologist Analogue, 69,* 763–767.

Donahue, M.P. (1990). The tyranny of ethics. In J.C. McCloskey and H. Grace (eds.): *Current Issues in Nursing,* 3rd ed. St. Louis: C.V. Mosby.

Dossey, B.M., Guzzetta, C.E. (1994). Implications for biopsychosocial-spiritual concerns in cardiovascular nursing. *Journal of Cardiovascular Nursing, 8* (4), 72–88.

Dossey, B.M., Keegan, L., Guzzetta, C., Kolkmeier, L. (1995). *Holistic Nursing: A Handbook for Practice,* 2nd ed. Gaithersburg, MD: Aspen.

Doswell, W.A. (1989). Physiological responses to stress. In J.J. Fitzpatrick, R.L. Taunton, and J. Benoliel (eds.): *Annual Review of Nursing Research,* Vol. 7. New York: Springer.

Egan, E.C. (1993). Intervention and the stress-health outcome linkage: Theoretical orientations. In J.S. Barnfather and B.L. Lyon (eds.): *Stress and Coping: State of the Science and Implications for Nursing Theory, Research, and Practice.* Indianapolis: Center Nursing Press, Sigma Theta Tau International, pp. 171–183.

Elliott, G., Eisdorfer, C. (1982). *Stress and Human Health.* New York: Springer.

Emery, G., Tracy, N.L. (1987). Theoretical issues in the cognitive behavioral treatment of anxiety disorders. In L. Michelson and L. Ashcer (eds.): *Anxiety and Stress Disorders.* New York: The Guilford Press.

Erikson, E. (1963). *Childhood and Society* (rev. ed.). New York: Norton.

Erickson, H., Swain, M.A. (1982). A model for assessing potential adaptation to stress. *Research in Nursing and Health, 5,* 93–101.

Erickson, H., Tomlin, E., Swain, M.A. (1983). *Modeling and Role Modeling: A Theory and Paradigm for Nursing.* Englewood Cliffs, NJ: Prentice Hall.

Figley, C.R., McCubbin, H. (1983). *Stress and the Family, Vol. II: Coping with catastrophe.* New York: Brunner/Mazel.

Folkman, S., Lazarus, R.S. (1980). An analysis of coping in a middle-aged community sample. *Journal of Health and Social Behavior, 21,* 219–239.

Frederickson, K. (1989). Anxiety transmission in the patient with myocardial infarction. *Heart & Lung, 18,* 617–622.

Freel, M.I. (1990). Truth telling. In J.C. McCloskey and H. Grace (eds.): *Current Issues in Nursing,* 3rd ed. St. Louis: C.V. Mosby.

Freud, S. (1926). Inhibition, symptoms, and anxiety. In *Standard Edition of the Complete Psychological Works of Sigmund Freud,* Vol. 20. London: Hogarth Press.

Freud, S. (1936). *The Problem of Anxiety.* New York: W.W. Norton.

Freud, S. (1953). *The Standard Edition of the Complete Psychological Writings.* London: Hogarth Press.

Frisch, N.C., Bowman, S. (1995). Helen C. Erickson, Evelyn M. Tomlin and Mary Ann P. Swain. In J.B. George (ed.): *Nursing Theories: The Base for Professional Nursing Practice,* 4th ed. Norwalk, CT: Appleton & Lange, pp. 355–371.

Frye, B. (1991). Cultural themes in health-care decision making among Cambodian refugee women. *Journal of Community Health Nursing, 8* (1), 33–44.

Frye, B., D'Avanzo, C. (1994). Cultural themes in family stress and violence among Cambodian refugee women in the inner city. *Advanced Nursing Science, 16* (3), 64–77.

Gardner, K.G., Wheeler, E. (1987). Patients' perceptions of support. *Western Journal of Nursing Research, 9,* 115–131.

Garvin, B.J., Kennedy, C., Baker, C., Polivka, B. (1992). Cardiovascular responses of CCU patients when communicating with nurses, physicians, and families. *Health Communication, 4* (4), 291–301.

Gast, P.L., Baker, C. (1989). The CCU patient: Anxiety and annoyance to noise. *Critical Care Nursing Quarterly, 12* (3), 39–54.

Gebbie, K.M., Lavin, M. (eds.): (1975). *Classification of Nursing Diagnoses: Proceedings of the First National Conference.* St. Louis: C.V. Mosby.

Gennaro, S. (1988). Postpartal anxiety and depression in mothers of term and preterm infants. *Nursing Research, 37,* 82–85.

Gennaro, S., Brooten, D., Roncoli, M., Kumar, S. (1993). Stress and health outcomes among mothers of low birth-weight infants. *Western Journal of Nursing Research, 15,* 97–113.

Gift, A.G., Cahill, C.A. (1990). Psychophysiologic aspects of dyspnea in chronic obstructive pulmonary disease: A pilot study. *Heart & Lung, 19,* 252–257.

Gift, A.G., Moore, T., Soeken, K. (1992). Relaxation to reduce dyspnea and anxiety in COPD patients. *Nursing Research, 41,* 242–246.

Gillis, C.L. (1984). Reducing family stress during and after coronary artery bypass surgery. *Nursing Clinics of North America, 19* (l), 103–111.

Grady, K.L., Jalowiec, A., Grusk, B., et al (1992). Symptom distress in cardiac transplant candidates. *Heart & Lung, 21,* 434–439.

Graves, J.K., Ware, M.E. (1990). Parents' and health professionals' perceptions concerning parental stress during a child's hospitalization. *Child Health Care, 19,* 37–42.

Grey, M., Cameron, M., Thurber, F. (1991). Coping and adaptation in children with diabetes. *Nursing Research, 40,* 144–149.

Groer, M.W., Thomas, S., Shoffner, D. (1992). Adolescent stress and coping: A longitudinal study. *Research in Nursing and Health, 15,* 209–217.

Gupta, L., Verma, R. (1983). Psychosocial antecedents of myocardial infarction. *Medical Research, 77,* 697–701.

Gurklis, J.A., Menke, E.M. (1988). Identification of stressors and use of coping methods in chronic hemodialysis patients. *Nursing Research, 37,* 236–239, 248.

Gurklis, J.A., Menke, E. (1995). Chronic hemodialysis patients' perceptions of stress, coping, and social support. *American Nephrology Nurses' Association Journal, 22* (4), 381–389.

Guzetta, C.E. (1989). Effects of relaxation and music therapy on patients in a coronary care unit with presumptive acute myocardial infarction. *Heart & Lung, 18,* 609–616.

Haines, C., Perger, C., Nagy, S. (1995). A comparison of the stressors experienced by parents of intubated and non-intubated children. *Journal of Advanced Nursing 21,* 350–355.

Hall, J., Weaver, B.A. (1974). *Nursing of Families in Crisis.* Philadelphia: Lippincott.

Halm, M.A. (1990). Effects of support groups on anxiety of family members during critical illness. *Heart & Lung, 19,* 62–71.

Halstead, M.T., Fernsler, J. (1994). Coping strategies of long-term cancer survivors. *Cancer Nursing, 17,* 94–100.

Hayes, V.E., Knox, J. (1984). The experience of stress in parents of children hospitalized with long-term disabilities. *Journal of Advanced Nursing, 9,* 333–341.

Heatherton, T.F., Renn, R. (1995). Stress and the disinhibition of behavior. *Mind/Body Medicine, 1,* 72–81.

Henderson, B. (1964). The nature of nursing. *American Journal of Nursing, 64* (8), 62–68.

Henderson, V., Nite, G. (1978). *Principles and Practice of Nursing.* New York: Macmillan.

Henry, J.P. (1990). Stress, neuroendocrine patterns, and emotional response. In J.D. Noshpitz and R. D. Coddington (eds.), *Stressors and the Adjustment Disorders.* New York: Wiley.

Hertzman, M. (1990). Pain as stress: Relationships to treatment. In J.D. Noshpitz and R.D. Coddington (eds.): *Stressors and the Adjustment Disorders.* New York: Wiley.

Heuer, L. (1993). Parental stressors in a pediatric intensive care unit. Pediatric intensive care unit. *Pediatric Nursing, 19* (2), 128–131.

Highfield, M.F. (1992). Spiritual health of oncology patients: Nurse and patient perspectives. *Cancer Nursing, 15* (l), 1–8.

Hilbert, G.A. (1994). Cardiac patients and spouses. *Clinical Nursing Research, 3,* 243–252.

Hilton, A. (1989). The relationship of uncertainty, control, commitment and threat of recurrence to coping strategies used by women diagnosed with breast cancer. *Journal of Behavioral Medicine, 12,* 39–54.

Hjelm-Karlsson, K. (1989). Effects of information to patients undergoing intravenous pyelography: An intervention study. *Journal of Advanced Nursing, 14,* 853–862.

Holmes, T.H., Masuda, M. (1974). Life changes and illness susceptibility. In B.S. Dohrenwend and B.P. Dohrenwend (eds.): *Stressful Life Events: Their Nature and Effects.* New York: Wiley.

Holmes, T.H., Rahe, R.H. (1967). The social readjustment rating scale. *Journal of Psychosomatic Research, 11,* 213–218.

Horowitz, M.J. (1986). *Stress Response Syndromes,* 2nd ed. New York: Aronson.

Jacobson, G. (1994). The meaning of stressful life experiences in nine- to eleven-year-old children: A phenomenological study. *Nursing Research, 43,* 95–99.

Jalowiec, A. (1993). Coping with illness: Synthesis and critique of the nursing literature from 1980–1990. In J.S. Barnfather and B.L. Lyon (eds.): *Stress and Coping: State of the Science and Implications for Nursing Theory, Research and Practice.* Indianapolis: Center Nursing Press, Sigma Theta Tau International, pp. 65–83.

Jalowiec, A. (1987). *Changes in the Revised Version of the Jalowiec Coping Scale.* Unpublished manuscript, Loyola University of Chicago.

Jalowiec, A., Murphy, S.P., Powers, M. J. (1984). Psychometric assessment of the Jalowiec Coping Scale. *Nursing Research, 33* (3), 157–161.

Johnson, D.E. (1959). A philosophy of nursing. *Nursing Outlook, 7,* 198–200.

Johnson, D.E. (1980). The behavioral system model for nursing. In J.P. Riehl and C. Roy (eds.): *Conceptual Models for Nursing Practice,* 2nd ed. New York: Appleton-Century-Crofts.

Johnson, J.E. (1973). Effects of accurate expectations about sensation on the sensory and distress components of pain. *Journal of Personality and Social Psychology, 27* (2), 261–275.

Johnson, J.E., Lauver, D. (1989). Alternative explanations of coping with stressful experiences associated with physical illness. *Advanced Nursing, 11,* 39–52.

Kaempf, G., Amodei, M.E. (1989). The effect of music on anxiety. *AORN Journal, 50* (l), 112–118.

Keckeisen, M.E., Nyamathi, A. (1990). Coping and adjustment to illness in the acute myocardial infarction patient. *Journal of Cardiovascular Nursing, 5* (l), 25–33.

Kemp, C. (1985). Cambodian refugee health care beliefs and practices. *Journal of Community Health Nursing, 2,* 41–52.

Kernberg, 0. (1976). *Object Relations Theory and Clinical Psychoanalysis.* New York: Aronson.

Kiecolt-Glaser, J., Glaser, R. (1991). Stress and immune function in humans. In R. Ader, D. Felton, and N. Cohen (eds.): *Psychoneuroimmunology* (2nd ed). San Diego, CA: Academic Press.

Kim, M.J., McFarland, G.K., McLane, A. (eds.) (1984): *Classification of Nursing Diagnoses: Proceedings of the Fifth National Conference.* St. Louis: C.V. Mosby.

King, I. (1981). A *Theory for Nursing.* New York: Wiley.

Kinney, M., Guzzetta, C.E. (1989). Measuring critical defining characteristics of nursing diagnoses using magnitude estimation scaling. *Research in Nursing and Health, 12,* 373–380.

Knapp-Spooner, C., Yarchesk, A. (1992). Sleep patterns and stress in patients having coronary bypass. *Heart & Lung, 21,* 342–349.

Kobasa, S.C. (1979). Stressful life events, personality, and health: An inquiry into hardiness. *Journal of Personality and Social Psychology, 37,* 1–11.

Kongable, L.G., Buckwalter, K.C., Stolley, J.M. (1989). The effects of pet therapy on the social behavior of institutionalized Alzheimer's clients. *Archives of Psychiatric Nursing, 3* (4), 191–198.

Koss, J.D. (1990). Somatization and somatic complaint syndromes among Hispanics: Overview and ethnopsychological perspectives. *Transcultural Psychiatric Research Review, 27,* 5–29.

Krause, K. (1993). Coping with cancer. *Western Journal of Nursing Research, 15,* 31–43.

Lambert, V.A., Lambert, C.E., Klipple, G.L., Menshaw, E.A. (1989). Social support, hardiness and psychological well-being in women with arthritis. *Image: Journal of Nursing Scholarship, 21,* 128–131.

Landreville, P., Vezina, J. (1992). A comparison of daily hassles and major life events as correlates of well being in older adults. *Canadian Journal on Aging, 11,* 137–149.

Laughlin, H.P. (1967). *The Neuroses.* Woburn, MA: Long, Butterworth.

Lazarus, R.S. (1983). The costs and benefits of denial. In S. Breznitz (ed.): *Denial of Stress.* New York: International Universities Press.

Lazarus, R.S., Folkman, S. (1984). *Stress, Appraisal, and Coping.* New York: Springer.

Lederman, R.P., Lederman, E., Work, A., Jr., McCann, D.S. (1981). Maternal psychological and physiological correlates of fetal-newborn health status. *American Journal of Obstetrics and Gynecology, 139,* 956–958.

Leonard, B.J., Brust, J., Nelson, R. (1993). Parental distress: Caring for medically fragile children at home. *Journal of Pediatric Nursing, 8* (1), 22–30.

Leske, J.S. (1986). Needs of relatives of critically ill patients: A follow-up. *Heart & Lung, 15,* 189–193.

Leventhal, H., Johnson, J. (1983). Laboratory and field experiment action: Development of a theory of self-regulation. In P. Woolridge, M. Schmitt, J. Kipper, and R. Leonard (eds.): *Behavioral Science and Nursing Theory.* St Louis: C.V. Mosby, pp. 189–262.

Levin, R.F., Krainovich, B.C., Bahrenburg, E., Mitchell, C. (1989). Diagnostic content validity of the six most frequently cited nursing diagnostic categories: A construct replication. In R. M. Carroll-Johnson (ed.): *Classification of Nursing Diagnoses: Proceedings of the Eighth Conference.* Philadelphia: Lippincott.

Littlefield, V.M., Chang, A., Adams, B. (1990). Participation in alternate care: Relationship to anxiety, depression, and hostility. *Research in Nursing and Health, 13,* 17–25.

Lok, P. (1996). Stressors, coping mechanisms and quality of life among dialysis patients in Australia. *Journal of Advanced Nursing, 23,* 873–881.

Lueders-Bolwerk, C.A. (1990). Effects of relaxing music on state of anxiety in myocardial infarction patients. *Critical Care Nursing Quarterly, 13* (2), 63–72.

Lyon, B.L., Werner, J.S. (1987). Stress. In J. Fitzpatrick and R.L. Taunton (eds.): *Annual Review of Nursing Research,* Vol. 5. New York: Springer, pp. 3–23.

Mahon, S.M., Cella, D.F., Donovan, M.I. (1990). Psychosocial adjustment to recurrent cancer. *Oncology Nursing Forum, 17,* 47–54.

Malan, S. (1992). Psychosocial adjustment following an MI: Current views and nursing implications. *Journal of Cardiovascular Nursing, 6* (4), 57–70.

Manfredi, C., Pickett, M. (1987). Perceived stressful situations and coping strategies utilized by the elderly. *Journal of Community Health Nursing, 4* (2), 99–110.

Marks, I.M. (1987). *Fears, Phobias, and* Rituals. New York: Oxford University Press.

Marsden, C., Dracup, K. (1991). Effects of heart disease on patients and spouses. *American Association of Critical Care Nurses: Clinical Issues, 2* (2), 285–292.

Maslow, A. (1970). *Motivation and Personality.* New York: Harper.

Maslow, A. (1968). *Toward a Psychology of Being.* New York: Van Nostrand Reinhold.

McCleane, G.J., Watters, C.H. (1990). Preoperative anxiety and serum potassium. *Anesthesia, 45* (7), 583–585.

McCloskey, J.C., Bulechek, G.M. (eds.) (1992): *Nursing Interventions Classification* (NIC). St. Louis: Mosby-Year Book.

McCubbin, M.A. (1989). Family stress and family strengths: A comparison of single and two-parent families with handicapped children. *Research in Nursing and Health, 12,* 101–110.

McNett, S.C. (1987). Social support, threat, and coping responses and effectiveness in functionally disabled. *Nursing Research, 36* (2), 98–103.

Medich, C., Stuart, E., Deckro, J., Friedman (1991). Psychophysiologic control mechanisms in ischemic heart disease: The mind-heart connection. *Journal of Cardiovascular Nursing, 5* (4), 10–26.

Meek, S.S. (1993). Effects of slow stroke back massage on relaxation in hospice clients. *Image: Journal of Nursing Scholarship, 25,* 17–21.

Melynk, B. (1994). Coping with unplanned childhood hospitalization: Effects of informational interventions on mothers and children. *Nursing Research, 43,* 50–55.

Mercer, R.T. (1986). *First-Time Motherhood: Experiences from Teens to Forties.* New York: Springer.

Mercer, R.T., Ferketich, S.L. (1988). Stress and social support as predictors of anxiety and depression during pregnancy. *Advances in Nursing Science, 10* (2), 26–39.

Miles, M.S., Carter, M.C. (1982). Sources of parental stress in pediatric care units. *Child Health Care, 11* (2), 65–69.

Miles, M.S., Funk, S., Kasper, M. (1992). The stress response of mothers and fathers of preterm infants. *Research in Nursing and Health, 15,* 261–269.

Miller, S.P., Garrett, M., Stoltenberg, M., et al (1990). Stressors and stress management 1 month after myocardial infarction. *Rehabilitation Nursing, 15,* 306–310.

Mishel, M.H. (1981). The measurement of uncertainty in illness. *Nursing Research, 30,* 258–263.

Mishel, M.H. (1983). Adjusting the fit: Development of uncertainty scales for specific clinical populations. *Western Journal of Nursing Research, 5,* 355–370.

Mishel, M.H. (1984). Perceived uncertainty and stress in illness. *Research in Nursing and Health, 7,* 163–171.

Mishel, M.H. (1988). Uncertainty in illness. *Image: Journal of Nursing Scholarship, 4,* 225–232.

Mishel, M.H. (1990). Reconceptualization of the uncertainty in illness theory. *Image: Journal of Nursing Scholarship, 22,* 256–262.

Mishel, M.H., Braden, C. (1988). Finding meaning: Antecedents of uncertainty in illness. *Nursing Research, 37,* 98–103, 127.

Mishel, M.H., Braden, C.J. (1987). Uncertainty: A mediator between support and adjustment. *Western Journal of Nursing Research, 9,* 43–57.

Mishel, M.H., Hostetter, T., King, C., Graham, V. (1984). Predictors of psychosocial adjustment in patients newly diagnosed with gynecological cancer. *Cancer Nursing, 7,* 291–299.

Mishel, M.H., Sorenson, D.S. (1993). Revision of the Ways of Coping Checklist for a clinical population. *Western Journal of Nursing Research, 15,* 59–76.

Mollica, R., Wyshak, G., Lavelle, J. (1987). The psychological impact of war trauma and torture on southeast Asian refugees. *American Journal of Psychiatry, 144,* 1567–1572.

Moore, S.M. (1994). Psychologic distress of patients and their spouses after coronary artery bypass surgery. *AACN Clinical Issues in Critical Care Nursing, 5* (l), 59–65.

Muecke, M., Sassi, L. (1992). Anxiety among Cambodian refuge adolescents in transit and in resettlement. *Western Journal of Nursing Research, 14* (3), 267–291.

Mulvey, A., Dohrenwend, B.S. (1983). The relation of stressful life events to gender. *Issues in Mental Health Nursing, 5,* 219–237.

Murata, J. (1994). Family stress, social support, violence and son's behavior. *Western Journal of Nursing Research, 16,* 154–168.

Murphy, S.A. (1988). Mental distress and recovery in a high-risk bereavement sample three years after untimely death. *Nursing Research, 37,* 30–35.

Narayan, S.M., Joslin, D.J. (1980). Crisis theory and intervention: A critique of the medical model and proposal of a holistic nursing model. *Advances in Nursing Science, 2,* 27–39.

Neighbors, H., Jackson, J., Bowman, P., Gurin, G. (1983). Stress, coping and Black mental health. In R. Hess and H. Hermaline (eds.): *Innovations in Prevention,* Vol. 2. New York: Haworth.

Neuman, B. (1989). *The Neuman Systems Model: Applications in Nursing Education and Practice,* 2nd ed. Norwalk, CT: Appleton-Lange.

Nickel, J.T., Brown, K.J., Smith, D. (1990). Depression and anxiety among chronically ill heart patients: Age differences in risk and predictors. *Research in Nursing and Health, 13,* 87–97.

Norbeck, J.S., Anderson, N.J. (1989). Life stress, social support, and anxiety in mid- and late-pregnancy among low income women. *Research in Nursing and Health, 12,* 281–287.

North American Nursing Diagnosis Association (NANDA). (1994). *Nursing diagnoses: Definitions and classifications 1995–96*. Philadelphia: Author.

Northouse, L.L. (1989). The impact of breast cancer on patients and husbands. *Cancer Nursing, 12,* 276–284.

Nyamathi, A., Kashiwabara, A. (1988). Preoperative anxiety, its effect on cognitive thinking. *AORN Journal, 4* (1), 164–170.

Nyamathi, A., Jacoby, A., Constancia, P., Ruvevich, S. (1992). Coping and adjustment of spouses of critically ill patients with cardiac disease. *Heart & Lung, 21* (2), 160–166.

Oberle, K., Wry, J., Paul, P., Grace, M. (1990). Environment, anxiety, and postoperative pain. *Western Journal of Nursing Research, 12* (6), *745–757*.

Oberst, M.T., Scott, D. (1988). Post-discharge distress in surgically treated cancer patients and their spouses. *Research in Nursing and Health, 11,* 223–233.

Oberst, M.T., Thomas, S.E., Gass, K.A., Ward, S.E. (1989). Caregiving demands and appraisal of stress among family caregivers. *Cancer Nursing, 12,* 209–215.

Ochberg, F.M. (1991). Post-traumatic therapy. *Psychotherapy, 28,* 5–15.

Olson, J.K. (1995). Relationships between nurse-expressed empathy, patient-perceived empathy and patient distress. *IMAGE: Journal of Nursing Scholarship, 27* (4), 317–322.

O'Malley, P.A., Menke, E. (1988). Relationships of hope and stress after myocardial infarction. *Heart & Lung, 17,* 184–190.

Orem, D. (1991). *Nursing: Concepts of Practice,* 4th ed. St. Louis: C.V. Mosby.

Ouellette, S.C. (1993). Inquiries into hardiness. In L. Goldberger and S. Breznitz (eds.): *Handbook of Stress.* New York: Free Press.

Pargament, K.I., Ensing, D., Falgout, K., et al (1990). God help me I: Religious coping efforts as predictors of the outcomes to significant life events. *American Journal of Community Psychology, 18,* 793–824.

Peplau, H.E. (1952). *Interpersonal Relations in Nursing.* New York: Putnam's Sons.

Peplau, H.E. (1968). Psychotherapeutic strategies. *Perspectives in Psychiatric Care, 6,* 264–278.

Peplau, H.E. (1963). A working definition of anxiety. In S.F. Burd and M. Marshall (eds.): *Some Clinical Approaches to Psychiatric Nursing.* New York: Macmillan.

Perehudoff, B. (1990). Parents' perceptions of environmental stressors in the special care nursery. *Journal of Neonatal Nursing, 9* (2), 39–44.

Philichi, L. (1988). Supporting the parents when the child requires intensive care. *Focus on Critical Care, 15* (2), 34–38.

Post-White, J. (1993). The effects of imagery on emotions, immune function, and cancer outcome. *Mainlines, 14* (l), 18–20.

Preston, D.B., Crawford, C.O. (1990). A study of community differences in stress among the elderly: Implications for community health nursing. *Public Health Nursing, 3* (4), 225–239.

Primomo, J., Yates, B.C., Woods, N.F. (1990). Social support for women during chronic illness: The relationship among sources and types to adjustment. *Research in Nursing & Health, 13,* 153–161.

Prugh, D.G., Thompson, T. (1990). Illness as a source of stress: Acute illness, chronic illness, and surgical procedures. In J.D. Noshpitz and R.D. Coddington (eds.): *Stressors and the Adjustment Disorders.* New York: Wiley.

Quinn, J.F., Stralkauskas, A.J. (1993). Psychoimmunologic effects of therapeutic touch on practitioners and recently bereaved recipients: A pilot study. *Advanced Nursing Science, 15* (4), 13–26.

Ramsay, M.A.E. (1972). A survey of preoperative fear. *Anesthesia, 27 (4),* 396–402.

Redeker, N.S. (1993). Symptoms reported by older and middle-aged adults after coronary bypass surgery. *Clinical Nursing Research 2,* 148–159.

Reece, S.M. (1993). Social support and the early maternal experience of primiparas over 35. *Maternal-Child Nursing Journal, 21,* 91–98.

Robinson, L. (1990). Stress and anxiety. *Nursing Clinics of North America, 25* (4), 935–943.

Rohmeyer, P. (1991). *Clinical Journal on Anxiety.* Unpublished manuscript, University of Wisconsin-Eau Claire, Eau Claire, WI.

Roy, C. (1988). An explication of the philosophical assumptions of the Roy adaptation model. *Nursing Science Quarterly, 1,* 26–34.

Roy, C. (1984). *Introduction to nursing: An adaptation model,* 2nd ed. Englewood Cliffs, NJ: Prentice-Hall.

Ryan-Wenger, N.M. (1990). Development and psychiatric properties of the schoolagers' coping strategies inventory. *Nursing Research, 39,* 344–349.

Ryan-Wenger, N.M. (1989). Inadequacy of current stress-coping theory for nursing care of children. *Proceedings of the First and Second Rosemary Ellis Scholars, Retreat.* Cleveland, OH: Case Western Reserve University, pp. 159–161.

Sarason, I.G. (1985). Cognitive processes, anxiety, and the treatment of anxiety disorders. In A.H. Tuma and J.D. Maser (eds.): *Anxiety and the Anxiety* Disorders. Hillsdale, NJ: Erlbaum.

Schleifer, S.J., Keller, S., Bond, R., et al (1992). Major depressive disorder and immunity. *Archives of General Psychiatry, 46,* 81–87.

Selye, H. (1956). *The Stress of Life.* New York: McGraw-Hill.

Selye, H. (1974). *Stress without distress.* Philadelphia: Lippincott.

Sexton, D.L., Munro, B.H. (1988). Living with a chronic illness: The experience of women with chronic obstructive pulmonary disease (COPD). *Western Journal of Nursing Research, 10,* 26–44.

Shamoian, C.A. (1991). What is anxiety in the elderly? In C. Salzman and B.D. Lebowitz (eds.): *Anxiety in the Elderly: Treatment and Research.* New York: Springer.

Simington, J.A., Laing, G.P. (1993). Effects of therapeutic touch on anxiety in the institutionalized elderly. *Clinical Nursing Research, 2* (4), 438–450.

Simpson, C.J., Kellet, J.M. (1987). The relationship between pre-operative anxiety and postoperative delirium. *Journal of Psychiatric Research, 31* (4), 491–497.

Smyth, K.A., Yarandi, H. (1992). A path model of type A and type B responses to coping and stress in employed black women. *Nursing Research, 41,* 260–265.

Snyder, M. (1985). *Independent Nursing Interventions.* New York: Wiley.

Snyder, M. (1993). The influence of interventions on the stress-health outcome linkage. In J.S. Barnfather and B.L. Lyon (eds.): *Stress and Coping: State of the Science and Implications for Nursing Theory, Research and Practice.* Indianapolis: Center Nursing Press, Sigma Theta Tau International, pp. 159–170.

Snyder-Halpern, R. (1985). The effects of critical care unit noise on patient sleep cycles. *Critical Care Quarterly, 7,* 41–51.

Soehren, P. (1995). Stressors perceived by cardiac surgical patients in the intensive care unit. *American Journal of Critical Care, 4* (1), 71–76.

Sorenson, E.S. (1994). Daily stressors and coping responses: A comparison of rural and suburban children. *Public Health Nursing, 11* (1), 24–31.

Spielberger, C.D. (1971). Trait-state anxiety and motor behavior. *Journal of Motor Behavior, 3,* 265–279.

Spielberger, C.D. (1979). *Understanding Stress and Anxiety.* New York: Harper & Row.

Staats, M.L., Staats, T. (1983). Differences in stress levels, stressors and stress responses between managerial and professional males and females on the stress vector analysis—research edition. *Issues in Health Care of Women, 4,* 165–176.

Stanley, M.J., Frantz, R. (1988). Adjustment problems of spouses of patients undergoing coronary artery bypass graft during early convalescence. *Heart & Lung, 17,* 677–682.

Stark, L.J., Spirito, A., Williams, C., Guevremont, D. (1989). Common problems and coping strategies: Findings with normal adolescents. *Journal of Abnormal Child Psychology, 17,* 203–212.

Steelman, V.M. (1990). Intraoperative music therapy. *AORN Journal, 52,* 1026–1034.

Stokes, S.A., Gordon, S.E. (1988). Development of an instrument to measure stress in the older adult. *Nursing Research, 37,* 16–19.

Taylor, A., Green, D., Walkey, F. (1994/95, Dec/Jan). Stressed adults and their care. *Nursing New Zealand,* 19–21.

Taylor, C.B., Arnow, B. (1988). *The Nature and Treatment of Anxiety Disorders.* New York: The Free Press.

Thoits, P.A. (1982). Conceptual, methodological, and theoretical problems in studying social support as a buffer against life stress. *Journal of Health and Social Behaviors, 23,* 145–159.

Thompson, D.R. (1989). A randomized controlled trial of in-hospital nursing support for first time myocardial infarction patients and their partners: Effects on anxiety and depression. *Journal of Advanced Nursing, 14,* 291–297.

Thompson, J. (1991). Exploring gender and culture with Khmer refugee women: Reflections on participatory feminist research. *Advances in Nursing Science, 13* (3), 30–48.

Tichy, A.M., Braam, C.M., Meyer, T., Rattan, N. (1988). Stressors in pediatric intensive care units. *Pediatric Nursing, 14* (l), 40–43.

Tilden, V.P. (1984). The relationship of selected psychosocial variables and single status of adult during pregnancy. *Nursing Research, 33,* 102–107.

Tobey, G.Y., Schraeder, B.D. (1990). Impact of caretaker stress on behavioral adjustment of very low birthweight preschool children. *Nursing Research, 39,* 84–89.

Topf, M. (1985). Noise induced stress in hospital patients: Coping and nonauditory health outcomes. *Journal of Human Stress, 11,* 125–134.

Topf, M. (1992). Effects of personal control over hospital noise on sleep. *Research in Nursing and Health, 15,* 19–28.

Toth, J.C. (1987). Stressors affecting older versus younger AMI patients. *Dimensions of Critical Care Nursing, 3,* 147–157.

Toth, J.C. (1993). Is stress at hospital discharge after acute myocardial infarction greater in women than in men? *American Journal of Critical Care, 2* (1), 35–40.

Turk, D.C., Kerns, R.D. (1985). *The Family in Health and Illness: A Lifespan Perspective.* New York: John Wiley & Sons.

Updike, P. (1990). Music therapy for ICU patients. *Dimensions of Critical Care Nursing, 9* (l), 39–45.

Van Cleve, L. (1989). Parental coping in response to their child's spina bifida. *Journal of Pediatric Nursing, 4* (3), 172–176.

Van Schaik, E. (1989). Paradigms underlying the study of nerves as a popular illness term in Eastern Kentucky. *Medical Anthropology, 11,* 15–28.

Volicer, B.J. (1974). Patients' perceptions of stressful events associated with hospitalization. *Nursing Research, 23,* 235–238.

Volicer, B.J. (1977). Stress factors in the experience of hospitalization. In M.V. Batey (ed.): *Communicating Nursing Research,* Vol. 8. Boulder: WICHE, pp. 53–67.

Volicer, D.J., Bohannon, M. (1975). A hospital stress rating scale. *Nursing Research, 24,* 352–359.

Volicer, B.J., Burns, M. (1977). Preexisting correlates of hospital stress. *Nursing Research, 26,* 408–415.

Volicer, B.J., Volicer, L. (1977). Cardiovascular changes associated with stress during hospitalization. *Journal of Psychosomatic Research, 22,* 159–168.

Wagnild, G., Grupp, K. (1992). Major stressors among elderly health care clients. *Home Healthcare Nurse, 9* (4), 15–21.

Wallerstein J., Kelley, J. (1980). *Surviving the breakup.* NY: Basic Books.

Webster, K.K., Christman, N.J. (1988). Perceived uncertainty and coping post myocardial infarction. *Western Journal of Nursing Research, 10,* 384–401.

Wells, J., Howard, G., Nowlin, W., Vargas, M. (1986). Presurgical anxiety and postoperative pain and adjustment: Effects of a stress inoculation procedure. *Journal of Consulting Clinical Psychology, 54,* 831–835.

Werner, J.S. (1993). Stressors and health outcomes: Synthesis of nursing research, 1980–1990. In J.S. Barnfather and B.L. Lyon (eds.): *Stress and Coping: State of the Science and Implications for Nursing Theory, Research and Practice.* Indianapolis: Center Nursing Press, Sigma Theta Tau International, pp. 11–41.

White, J. (1992). Music therapy: An intervention to reduce anxiety in the myocardial infarction patient. *Clinical Nurse Specialist, 6* (2), 58–63.

White, N.E., Richter, J., Fry, C. (1992). Coping, social support, and adaptation to chronic illness. *Western Journal of Nursing Research, 14* (2), 211–224.

Whitley, G.G. (1989). Anxiety: Defining the diagnosis. *Journal of Psychosocial Nursing, 27* (10), 7–8, 10–12.

Whitley, G.G. (1992). Concept analysis of anxiety. *Nursing Diagnosis, 3* (3), 107–116.

Wineman, N.M. (1990). Adaptation to multiple sclerosis: The role of social support, functional disability, and perceived uncertainty. *Nursing Research, 39,* 294–299.

Wolff, H.G. (1953). *Stress and Disease.* Springfield, IL: Thomas.

Workshop on Alternative Medicine (1992). *Alternative Medicine: Expanding Medical Horizons.* Washington, D.C.: U.S. Government Printing Office.

Yarcheski, A., Knapp-Spooner, C. (1994). Stressors associated with coronary bypass surgery. *Clinical Nursing Research, 3,* (1), 57–68.

Younger, J. (1991). A theory of mastery. *Advances in Nursing Science, 14,* 76–89.

Younger, J. (1993). Developmental and testing of the Mastery of Stress Instrument. *Clinical Nursing Research, 14,* 76–89.

Zacharias, D.R., Gilg, C., Foxall, M. (1994). Quality of life and coping in patients with gynecological cancer and their spouses. *Oncology Nursing Forum, 21,* 1699–1706.

Zimmerman, L.M., Pierson, M.A., Marker, J. (1988). Effects of music on patient anxiety in coronary care units. *Heart & Lung, 17,* 560–566.

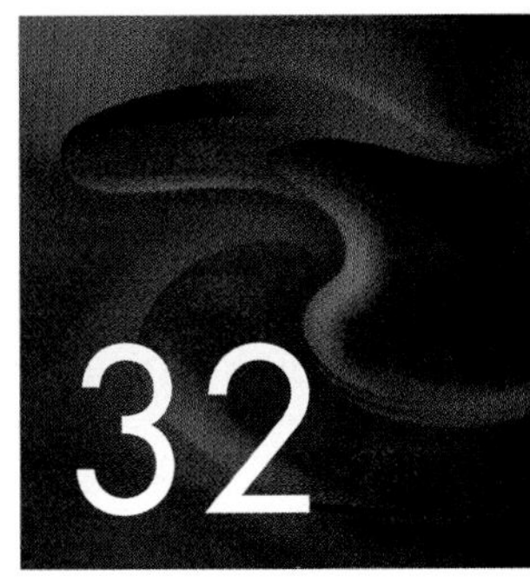

Touch 32

Sandra J. Weiss and Rosemary Campos

With a special section by Hob Osterlund

Jessie Jabar, a 2-week-old baby boy, born 6 weeks prematurely, was exposed to cocaine in the womb as a result of his mother's drug use. The nurse has assessed an erratic heart rate, rapid breathing with periods of apnea; episodes of shrill, intense crying; and fairly persistent tremors. His nursing care plan includes reducing the amount of stimulation from sights, sounds, and handling because these could increase his physiologic symptoms and behavioral distress.

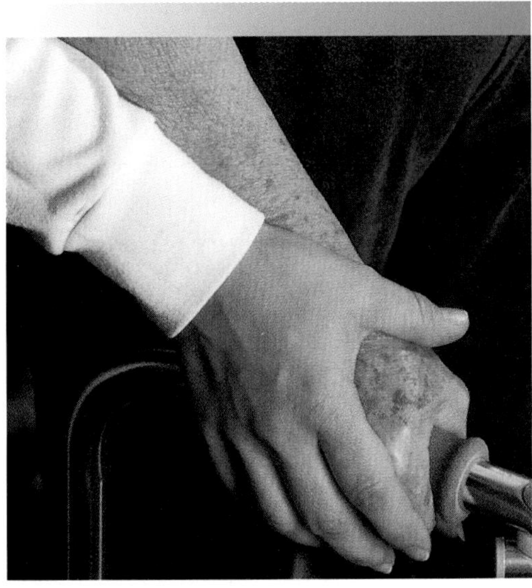

As the nurse begins to provide necessary physical care to Jessie, the nurse touches him only in the least stressful way, to avoid overstimulating his fragile nervous system. The nurse moves him very gently to clean him, for instance, never using undue pressure or abrupt actions. As much as possible, the nurse avoids touch that involves vigorous movement of the skin. The nurse also avoids touching areas of his body with multiple nerve endings and nerve pathways, such as his face and head.

Between procedures, the nurse places Jessie in a position he likes, and refrains from touching him so he can recover from the handling. The nurse further assesses how he responds to different kinds of touch, and what causes him distress. It seems Jessie is most distressed when exposed to air and when his arms and legs are flailing around. Under these conditions, he cries vigorously and his tremors are worse. As soon as the nurse completes her physical nursing care, she slowly and gently swaddles Jessie in a blanket. This action soothes him, demonstrated by his crying subsiding into whimpering, and diminution of wrinkles between his brows.

The nurse records these observations in his medical record, including the fact that Jessie responded well to soft stroking on his abdomen while his temperature was being taken. It is important to find ways of using expressive, caring touch so that Jessie experiences more than being touched only during painful or distressing procedures.

OBJECTIVES

After studying this chapter, the student will be able to:

- **understand how touch may impede or enhance a patient's health and well-being**
- **assess individual differences in response to touch**
- **assess factors influencing the effects of touch**
- **individualize touching each patient so that it is appropriate to each patient's needs for, unique attitudes toward, and tolerance for touch**
- **identify how their own attitudes and feelings about touch influence the ways they touch patients during nursing care**

Just as the nurse finishes charting, Jessie's mother enters the nursery. The nurse greets Ms. Jabar and tells her of Jessie's progress and some details of the plan of care. Ms. Jabar seems upset so the nurse encourages her to express her feelings. Ms. Jabar begins to cry, and says that a nurse on an earlier shift had said she could not touch Jessie because he was on "minimal handling precautions." The nurse puts her hand supportively on Ms. Jabar's shoulder and suggests they go to a quieter area of the nursery where they could talk. After Jessie's mother discussed her frustration and sadness, the nurse emphasizes to Ms. Jabar that her continued presence with Jessie is very important. He needs to feel her love and support, and the two of them need time together to develop their special relationship.

SCOPE OF NURSING PRACTICE

Touch is a central component of nursing care, because physical contact with patients is necessary for all physical assessments and procedures. Consider, for instance, the extensive touching required to change dressings, move or reposition a patient, provide personal hygiene care, care for an intravenous site, or give an injection. In addition, comfort measures to reassure or relax patients, such as back rubs or massage, holding the patient's hand, or placing an arm around the patient's shoulders, directly involve touching.

Touch can be task oriented or expressive. The nurse uses *task-oriented* touch in activities such as measuring blood pressure, or helping a person get dressed. In contrast, *expressive* touch is used solely to communicate feelings, either positive (characterized by a supportive, concerned, loving, or playful gesture) or negative (characterized or motivated by anger or impatience, as displayed in rough or abrupt touching). Keep in mind that touch can be perceived as negative by a patient, even when the nurse did not intend to touch the patient in a negative way. Each individual has a unique biologic disposition toward touch; that is, every individual will perceive the sensations associated with touch differently. One patient's affinity for a casual shoulder touch may be another's violation of bodily integrity.

Above and beyond the touch nurses use in caring for patients is the pivotal role they play in counseling families about the effects of touch among family members. The nature of the touch that family members use can be influential in promoting their children's health, enhancing the recovery of an ill family member, or comforting a chronically ill or dying loved one. Education and counseling of families about the significance of the touch they use is an important nursing responsibility.

KNOWLEDGE BASE

Understanding the role of touch in clinical practice stems from basic science research and clinical studies. This knowledge has been acquired from both animal and human research, and has contributed to different theories about touch and its clinical uses.

Basic Science

There are two major areas of the science underlying touch. The first area involves the neurophysiologic character of touch, as determined by a combination of five dimensions: location, intensity, action, duration, and frequency. For each of these dimensions, the specific qualities of touch that are used (e.g., strong intensity or vigorous actions) will influence the physical and psychological response of the person touched. The second area of the science involves the subjective perception of touch, regardless of its "objective" character (refer to Chapter 15 for a discussion of the terms subjective and objective).

The effects of various qualities of touch result from: (1) the ways in which they arouse the nervous system and (2) the personal and cultural meaning given to various qualities of touch. In addition, individuals have unique biologic dispositions toward touch; that is, they perceive the sensations associated with touch differently. A person's disposition includes how readily they perceive being touched, the strength of their response to touch, and their tolerance for the sensations created by the touch. These responses can be influenced by a person's genetic makeup or a particular health problem. In the case study, the nurse carefully assessed Jessie for his tolerance of her touch, then modified the dimensions of her touching to accommodate his needs.

DIMENSIONS OF TOUCH

Frequency is a *quantitative* dimension indicating the amount of touch; the other four dimensions of touch are *qualitative,* related to the quality of touching the very complex structure of skin (see Box 32–1). The major *touch receptors*—structures on the surface of cells that enable cells to respond when skin is touched—are free nerve endings, Meissner's corpuscles, Merkel's discs, hair nerve endings, Ruffini endings, and pacinian corpuscles (Fig. 32–1). These receptors interact in a variety of complex chemical and physical ways. Each varies in location, density, methods by which they are stimulated, and their role in our perception of the world. The four qualitative dimensions of touch largely determine what these receptors encounter and the messages they communicate to the brain.

Location. This dimension of touch refers to the actual area of the patient's body touched. The number of sensory receptors and nerve pathways within a body area influences its sensitivity to touch. Some areas of the body have more sensory receptors, such as the face and head, and produce clear, discrete, and sharply localized perceptions when touched (Schmidt, 1986). Other body areas with fewer receptors, such as the back or arm, yield less precise perceptions.

A second factor in location is the extent of contact (i.e., number of locations touched). Research has clearly demon-

BOX 32-1
DIMENSIONS OF TOUCH

Humans experience the sensation of touch by two primary means: quantity and quality. Quantity of touch refers to *frequency*; that is, how often touching occurs. Quality of touch determines its unique character and has four categories:

- location
- intensity
- action
- duration

The specific characteristics of touch for each of these dimensions (e.g., intense or vigorous actions) will influence the physical and psychological response of the person touched.

strated that when more areas of the body are touched, a person is more likely to have an enhanced body image (Weiss, 1990b).

Finally, the location of touch conveys distinct meanings and associations. Most individuals view the head and torso as the core of their physical being, so touching these areas will carry greater meaning than touching the arms or legs. Growing intimacy within early mother-infant relationships, for example, has been linked with progressive maternal touching of the trunk of the baby's body, rather than limbs only (Cannon, 1977).

Different body locations carry distinctly different sociocultural meanings as well, all of which influence how appropriate it is for the nurse to touch them. If a part of the patient's body carries stigma as a result of a physical defect or disfigurement, the patient, family, and even other health care workers may not feel comfortable touching that body part. They may try to avoid contact with the stigmatized body part, blocking out or denying its existence because of their own feelings of disgust

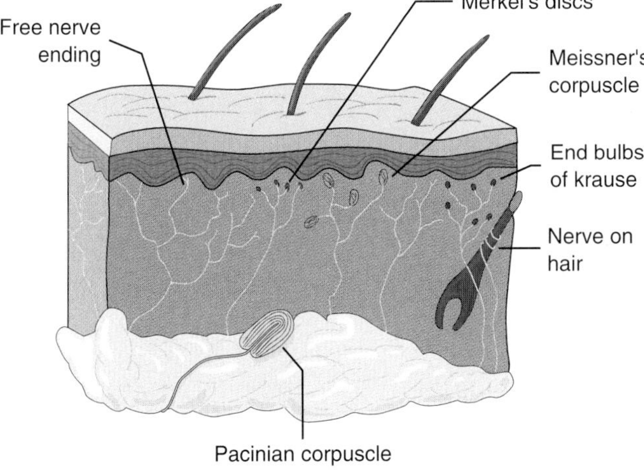

Figure 32-1. Nerve supply of the skin.

or fear. Certain skin diseases may hamper touch of the affected body part where the disease is apparent, regardless of whether the disease is contagious or not. Sexual taboos on certain body parts may also affect how these parts are touched. The buttocks, for instance, are rarely touched except by parents of young children, sexual partners, or in sports, where swatting has been culturally reinforced as an expression of a job well done.

Intensity. This dimension of touch refers to the degree to which the patient's skin is indented by the pressure of the touch. It can range from very deep to very light or barely perceptible pressure. Different degrees of intensity in a touch can result in different states of hyperexcitability in the brain's cortex. Light-intensity touch may not even be perceived and consequently elicit no response. Painfully strong intensity touch may distort the ways in which sensory receptors respond to the touch so that it is not accurately registered with the central nervous system (CNS) (Hamman and Iggo, 1984).

Action. This dimension of touch refers to the specific gesture or movement the nurse uses during touching, such as stroking, rubbing, holding, or squeezing. These actions involve a combination of pressure and stretching. Variations in these actions send three distinctive categories of messages to the brain: cutaneous, proprioceptive, and vestibular.

Cutaneous stimulation refers to stimulation of the surface receptors of the skin, as occurs when the skin surface is touched. *Proprioceptive* stimulation occurs when touch involves movement of the skin itself and nerve fiber endings (called end-organs) located in muscles, tendons, and joints. When touch involves both cutaneous and proprioceptive stimulation, the ability to perceive touch improves. *Vestibular* stimulation involves spatial movement and spatial orientation of the body. The action of lifting, for example, provokes sensations of positional change and spatial realignment. When touch involves a combination of cutaneous, proprioceptive and vestibular stimulation, it is more likely to stimulate the patient's central nervous system (Korner, 1990).

The *function* of each action also determines how touch is received. The function of touch can be described as either procedural or expressive. *Procedural touch* includes touch used in such essential nursing activities as taking a patient's blood pressure and pulse measurement, using physical restraint, or assisting with self-care activities. In contrast, *expressive touch* is nonessential contact, used solely to communicate positive or negative feelings. *Positive* expressive touch is a supportive, concerned, loving, or playful gesture toward another individual. One aspect of this is a comfort touch—touch involving empathy, the acute awareness of the feelings and emotional needs of the person being touched (Morse, 1983). *Negative* expressive touch, on the other hand, communicates feelings such as anger or impatience through rough, abrupt actions. Negative touch has been most often addressed in the literature on physical abuse in the family (e.g., Main and Stadtman, 1981; Schneider-Rosen et al, 1985), but has also been found to occur by health-care personnel (Birch, 1986).

The overt function of a touch may be procedural (task-oriented), but be imbued with expressive feelings nonetheless. This can occur when the nurse provides comfort touching during certain procedures or tasks; for example, reassuring the patient or facilitating decreased pain during a neurologic workup. The perceived intent to comfort, in this case, will be conveyed in the quality of the nurse's touch, and be experienced by the patient as a positive expression of feeling, rather than being strictly procedural. Comfort touching, such as a back massage or neck rub, may be experienced by the patient as procedural if the nurse completes it perfunctorily, however. Research bears out the validity of the nurse's intent as a critical factor in touch (Quinn, 1984).

Duration. The duration, or length of time the nurse maintains body contact, also determines how touch is interpreted by CNS receptors. Short-duration touch, like light-intensity touch, may not be sufficient to register much sensation, and longer contact may be necessary for the patient to perceive sensory stimulation. Lengthy, repetitive touching, on the other hand, may cause sensory receptors to stop responding due to repetitive motion, making it more difficult for the patient to recognize he or she is being touched at all (Hochreiter et al, 1983).

PERCEPTIONS OF TOUCH

Individuals perceive the sensations associated with touch differently. Three factors determine these individual differences: the threshold of touch perception, strength of response to touch, and tolerance for touch (see Box 32–2).

Threshold. The time it takes for a patient to realize that he or she is being touched is called the *tactile threshold.* Some patients respond to even the lightest intensity touch, consisting of brief contact with the surface of their skin, while others do not notice even very strong lengthy touch in which the nurse vigorously moves the muscles as well as the skin surface.

Strength of Response. Individuals vary in the strength of their response to touch once it is noticed. Some people may experience very potent, long-lasting behavioral and physiologic responses, while others experience minimal arousal from strong intensity, lengthy, or vigorous touch.

Tolerance. Individuals also vary in their tolerance for the sensations elicited by touch. One patient may have a strong response to touch and be able to tolerate the response to touch with no difficulty. Another patient may have a minimal response but find the sensations associated with touch intolerable. Some children protest and struggle to free themselves when handled or held, for example, and display various forms of physiologic, emotional, and behavioral hyperreactivity (Royeen, 1986). These reactions may represent attempts to escape and manage excessive arousal from touch. Lack of tolerance for touch may be caused to some degree by inadequate self-regulation of emotional and physiologic responses or lack of maternal contact at a critical age.

Differences in how patients perceive touch are also substantially influenced by genetically determined mechanisms in each person's central nervous system (Robinson, 1986). These differences can be seen in the earliest months of life (Garcia-Coll, 1990).

Illness, especially illness that impairs patient functioning or disrupts the development of the nervous system, can significantly influence a patient's threshold, strength of response, and tolerance for touch. Both aversion to and lower thresholds for touch have been noted in preterm infants, for example, like Jessie (Anderson, 1986; Beaver, 1987). One explanation for these phenomena may be that birth before term deprives the infant of maternal biorhythms that help regulate natural tactile stimulation, a part of the intrauterine environment (Rose, 1990). Children and adult patients with impaired sensory receptors from neuropathies (nerve disease), burns, or skin diseases often have negative or unusual reactions to touch as well (Nurmikko, 1991; Vinik et al, 1995). Following surgery in which nerves are severed, the patient's resulting scar tissue can be either less sensitive or acutely sensitive to touch. Conditions such as neuralgia (pain along a nerve) after a herpes outbreak can make a patient highly sensitive to the gentlest brushing movement, and unable to even tolerate wearing clothes.

BOX 32–2
FACTORS INFLUENCING PERCEPTIONS OF TOUCH

- Threshold for perceiving touch
- Strength of response to touch
- Tolerance for sensations associated with touch

Relevant Research

The majority of clinical knowledge regarding touch stems from developmental studies. These studies have yielded substantive data on the effects of touch on brain and cognitive development, as well as social development and attachment. Related studies have pursued the effects of touch with infants, including effects of parents' patterns of touch, and the effects of touch on regulation of the infant's behavior and physiology. Knowledge regarding effects of touch on adults is less extensive, but there is some information on how touch influences the therapeutic relationship, as well as psychological and physical responses to care, especially in critically ill patients.

EFFECTS OF TOUCH ON BRAIN DEVELOPMENT

Development of some areas of the brain occurs during a critical period after birth and may be somewhat unalterable after that time. During this period, certain types of input from the environment are essential for adequate organization of the brain and behavior (Huntley, 1997; Nicolelis et al, 1996). Receptors and neural pathways associated with touch sensations are the first to develop in early infancy, and an infant's primary form of stimulation is through the touch received in care. As a result, touch is central to development of the brain's "hard wiring" (the networks of nerve cells that form the foundation of learning and cognition) during this initial critical period.

Animal research indicates that early touching affects the size of the brain's cortex as well as the numbers and patterns of connections between nerve cells in the brain (Greenough, 1990). If an animal is deprived of the opportunity to touch or "cuddle" with others of its species when young, it demonstrates decreased brain size as it develops. However, if an animal experiences an enriched tactile environment early in life, later deprivation of touch does not appear to reduce brain size. These findings suggest that touch early in life may be crucial in forming a foundation to protect against the negative effects of sensory deprivation later in life.

Touch continues to influence brain structure throughout the lifespan by contributing to adjustment and maintenance of the linkages between neural pathways in the brain (Merzenich, 1990). Older animals that are given environments enriched by touch have demonstrated increased brain size (Diamond, 1990). In addition, touch helps in regaining functions damaged by brain lesions and infarcts, or peripheral nerve injury. For example, in brain-damaged monkeys, repetitive pressure and rubbing on the surface of the hand was found to stimulate generation of new neural networks in the brain in areas adjacent to those previously destroyed. These newly formed pathways in the brain then assumed the functions of the damaged areas (Kaas et al, 1983). Such findings parallel the recovery demonstrated by stroke patients in regaining functions such as speech or use of a hand as a result of intensive stimulation and physical therapy of affected limbs.

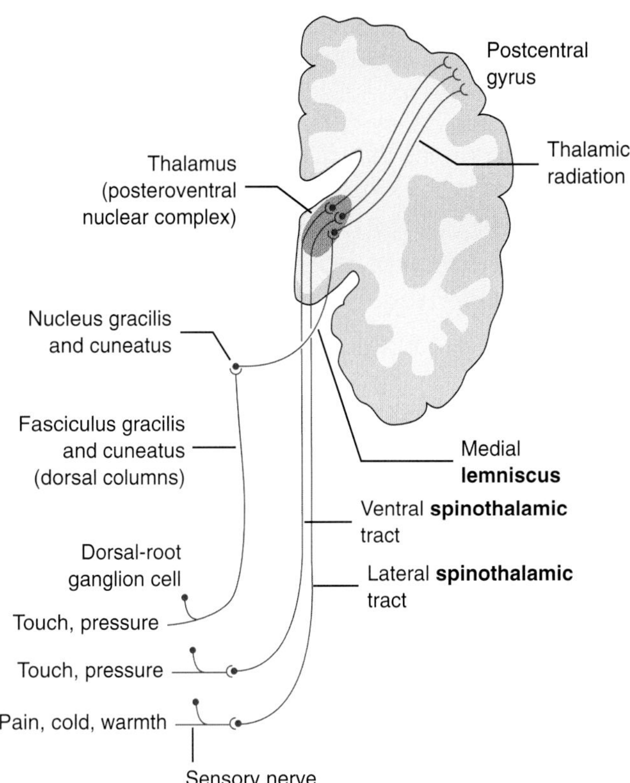

Figure 32–2. Neurologic pathways for pressure, pain, and temperature sensation.

EFFECTS OF TOUCH ON COGNITIVE DEVELOPMENT

Touch can both enhance and limit cognitive development. As mentioned earlier, cognitive development is limited to a large extent by the neural networks established early in life. These neural structures influence the ways an infant organizes information about himself or herself and the external world. To prevent potential behavioral and intellectual limitations, infant cognitive and psychomotor development can be enhanced by touch under certain circumstances (Koniak-Griffin and Ludington-Hoe, 1988; Scafidi et al, 1986).

Parents' aversion to touch or use of abusive touch with their children may be a factor in development of language difficulties and other learning disorders (Frank and Levinson, 1973) as well as disorganized behavior such as repetitive speech and behavior, anxiety, and withdrawal, especially under stress (Belsky et al, 1984; Main and Goldwyn, 1984). One explanation for these childhood problems lies in the effect of touch on two different aspects of the nervous system: the lemniscal and spinothalamic systems (Fig. 32–2). In the lemniscal system, a network of nerve fibers governs interpretation of the spatial and temporal aspects of tactile stimuli. These nerve fibers are thought to produce a discrete, precisely localized, and affectively neutral form of sensory input, which is necessary for development of images and memories. In contrast, a protective mechanism in the spinothalamic system is thought to warn or defend the organism against potential harm, eliciting movement, alertness, and negative emotional arousal. Overactivation of the protective system during certain types of touch may thus interfere with development of connections within the brain's cortex essential to effective perception and learning.

When parents of healthy children use qualities of touch that heighten CNS stimulation, the children are more likely to develop a sophisticated and accurate body image (Weiss, 1990b). These qualities of touch include stronger intensity, longer duration, greater frequency, more vigorous actions that evoke diverse sensations in muscles and tendons, and touching of body areas that have many receptors and nervous pathways. These more arousing forms of touch may help create discrete, precisely localized perceptions of the body and more effective messages to the brain regarding the body's characteristics.

The function and structure of other sensory systems are also influenced and may even be limited by the nature of early tactile experience. This occurs because of the earlier development of skin sensations. The sensory nerves for skin sensations are the first to completely myelinize in the infant—that is, to be covered with an insulating fatty sheath that aids transmission of messages within the nervous system (Turkewitz and Kenny, 1982). Infants then transfer much of the information learned through touch to visual and auditory knowledge (Pineau and Streri, 1990; Rose, 1990). For instance, very low–birth weight newborns receiving special touch interventions early in life demonstrate better auditory responses later in life than those that did not receive such touch (Helders et al, 1988).

EFFECTS OF TOUCH ON SOCIAL DEVELOPMENT AND ATTACHMENT

Social development is another area where touch affects the neural networks underlying behavior. The nature of touch that an infant receives can influence his or her later capacity for attachment, intimacy, and other social behaviors.

Deprivation and Rejection. A classic study of touch deprivation demonstrated that infant monkeys deprived of physical contact with other monkeys during their early months would form long-lasting attachments to cloth-covered, inanimate, monkey-like frames even though they provided no food (Harlow, 1958). Apparently, the monkeys preferred the cloth-covered frames to wire frames with food because the tactile sensations from the cloth provided comfort, especially during periods of stress. Another, more recent study showed that monkeys reared without the opportunity for physical contact developed abnormal behavior such as repetitive rocking or head banging, were fearful of exploration, and exhibited more self-clinging and self-touching behaviors to soothe themselves than normally reared monkeys (Suomi, 1990). As adults, these monkeys avoided social contacts or were hyperaggressive. Their sexual behavior was also abnormal, and they did not learn the mutual grooming behaviors that become a basis for later social relationships with monkey peers. Female monkeys who were physically deprived as infants also failed to provide adequate care for their infants, did not nurse properly, and were physically abusive. These monkey studies make it very clear that touching in early infancy is critical for social development (Suomi, 1997). Deprivation of touch in the second 6 months of life does not appear to have the same long-term negative consequences as does deprivation during the first 6 months of life, when touch seems to be such a central form of input (Immelmann and Suomi, 1981).

Results of human studies are consistent with those of animal studies. A classic study involved infants orphaned in the first 6 months of life cared for in institutions (Spitz, 1945). Their lack of ongoing physical and emotional nurturance from a caring adult resulted in failure to thrive, a disorder in which the infant shows disinterest in food, poor weight gain, delayed motor development, and lack of emotional expression. Infants orphaned after 6 months also were affected by the loss of physical and emotional nurturance. However, instead of failure to thrive, they exhibited intense grief reactions. Research shows that infants living in the home can also experience failure to thrive. Mothers of these infants touch their babies less during both feeding and play than other mothers do. They also use less active, vigorous touch (Polan and Ward, 1994). Other studies have indicated that children establish patterns of intimacy and affection through early touch experiences, and that these patterns persist in their subsequent interpersonal relations. The confidence or distrust in people that a child develops through initial touch experience may influence expectations for all later relationships.

How do experiences of early infancy influence socioemotional development? Staying close to an attachment figure (an adult who provides security and comfort) appears to be an innate response of all mammal infants to conditions of stress or uncertainty (Bowlby, 1988). In situations of strong fear or threat from the environment, only actual physical contact with an attachment figure appears to reassure the infant. Rejection of physical contact by an attachment figure during such times can at first lead to angry and aggressive infant behaviors, as well as abnormal responses like hairpulling, hand flapping, and repetitive speech or movements (Main and Stadtman, 1981). This may occur because the child's needs for proximity become even stronger when rejected, since his or her stress or uncertainty is further increased. When a child's needs for reassuring contact are consistently denied, he or she eventually avoids physical contact with parents when under stress. The child may actively ignore or move away from the parent if approached, or signal to be put down if picked up. This pattern of attachment behavior has been called an insecure, avoidant response to attachment needs. It is viewed as a child's strategy for shifting attention away from the attachment figure and the cues that increase his or her fears or anxiety. Instead, the child copes by focusing attention on other activities or objects that serve as distractions from the need for closeness to another person during distress.

Parental rejection of physical contact may eventually lead the infant to develop a conscious or unconscious pattern of avoiding contact with others during times of stress (Main et al, 1985). A mother's pattern of gazing at, touching, and holding her infant during routine mother-infant contact reveals her true feelings for the infant (Kaitz et al, 1992). When maternal-infant touch is very infrequent, the nurse should view it as a signal that the mother may be intolerant of physical contact or may have a problem breast- or bottle-feeding her infant (Polan and Ward, 1994). Avoidance of physical closeness within a family is often perpetuated across generations, as are patterns of physical abuse. Parents who were themselves abused may continue to use this as their primary, if not sole, method of achieving physical closeness to their loved ones.

Successful interventions for children with attachment problems whose parents have aversion to touch involve a desensitization process (Hopkins, 1987). In this process, the child gradually learns to seek out comfort through physical contact when distressed. Simultaneous therapeutic work with the parents is also required so that they can be receptive to the child's attempts to be held or stroked.

In contrast to the attachment problems just described, infants who demonstrate secure attachment behaviors have parents who use more affectionate touch when in contact with their babies, such as more tender, careful holding of the

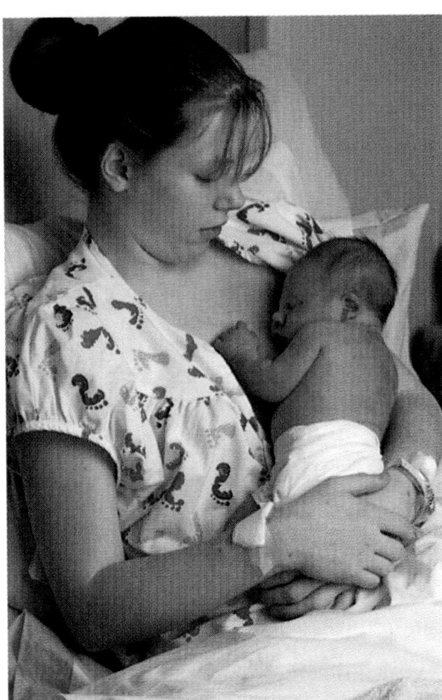

Figure 32–3. Mother and infant experiencing skin-to-skin bonding.

infant. Physical contact between mother and infant can be increased by the use of soft baby carriers and by infant massage and may result in more secure attachments for babies (Anisfeld et al, 1990; Hansen and Ulrey, 1988).

Attachment patterns developed in early childhood also seem to influence relationships in later life. For example, children who avoid physical comforting from parents seem less ready to establish new relationships with others (Main and Weston, 1981), and children who are physically abused by their parents are more physically aggressive to both peers and caregivers than are nonbattered children (Main and George, 1985). There is also a strong relationship between a parent's rejection of physical contact with his or her infant and the parent's retrospective account of being physically rejected in his or her own childhood (Main, 1990). In sum, initial tactile experiences may influence later relationships with close adults as well.

Early physical contact between parents and infants may also influence parent bonding to the infant (Fig. 32–3). This knowledge was one reason why the nurse in the case study at the beginning of the chapter wanted to assure that Jessie's mother could touch him regardless of the "minimal handling precautions." Physical contact during an early, sensitive period is often described as crucial for parental bonding even though some nursing research has not shown this to be the case for mothers or fathers (Curry, 1982; Toney, 1982; Troy, 1993).

Although further studies are warranted to better understand how early interactions influence attachment patterns, the nurse should provide every opportunity for early contact between infants and parents. Skin-to-skin contact with parents is not only preferable but beneficial in many ways. Such contact may help regulate an infant's body temperature, and enhance parental satisfaction (Affonso et al, 1993; Anderson, 1995; Legault and Goulet, 1995). However, parents and caregivers should not regard early contact as absolutely essential to the development of attachment feelings (Troy, 1993).

Parental Touch. Observation of the touch used by parents with their neonates suggests that mothers follow a certain progression of touch. This pattern of touch is the primary component of mother-infant bonding. As they become familiar with their infant, mothers move from initial fingertip and palm touching to contact with the infant's trunk and face (Cannon, 1977). Observation of fathers immediately after birth reveals that actual touching of the infant is rare, but physical closeness and gazing at the baby are common (Tomlinson et al, 1991). Even in the neonatal intensive care unit (ICU), studies have shown that fathers touch their babies less than mothers (Harrison and Woods, 1991; Thurman and Korteland, 1989). When parents touch their babies in the ICU they typically stroke, hold, or brush the baby's hands, back, or head. Studies also show that both mothers and fathers are more likely to touch their babies when alone with the infant, rather than together. And mothers are more likely to touch the infant when it is brought to the mother's room, rather than the mother going to the intensive care nursery. These findings suggest that nurses need to develop and support time alone with the infant for both mothers and fathers.

EFFECTS OF TOUCH ON PSYCHOPHYSIOLOGIC REGULATION

Touching young animals increases the optimal functioning of their physiologic systems, and establishes the patterns for how they handle physiologic arousal later in life. Maternal contact with young rat infants has been proven to reduce the infants' stress response, either by buffering normal increases in hormones or by helping to bring elevated plasma cortisol (the level of the hormone regulating metabolism in blood) resulting from stress back to homeostasis (Levine and Stanton, 1990). When separated from mothers in infancy, monkeys experience dramatic changes in autonomic nervous system (ANS) functioning. These changes may in turn create disturbances in the operation of the brain's hypothalamus as well as impairment of immune system responses (Reite and Capitanio, 1985). These disturbances are stabilized when the monkey infant is reunited with its mother and is closely held by her. Visual, olfactory, or auditory contact is not sufficient for this stabilization to occur; touch is the necessary factor (Suomi, 1990).

Maternal contact is also essential in regulating both animal and human infant physiology. For instance, a mother rat's tactile stimulation of her baby is necessary for it to achieve optimal behavioral and physiologic arousal. Maternal touch also provides specific sensory cues to the infant that trigger normal growth and development (Hofer, 1987; Schanberg et al, 1984).

A good example of how physiologic responses of mothers influence those of their infants is the close coordination of breathing patterns and sleep stages noted in mothers and infants who are in physical contact during sleep (McKenna et al, 1990). Based on this phenomenon, mother-infant *co-sleeping* has been proposed to reduce the incidence of sudden infant death syndrome (SIDS) in infants at risk.

Likewise, the physiologic effect of an infant's touch on its mother has been well documented. Infant contact with the mother's nipple is associated with lower maternal gastric levels and better maternal neuroendocrine function (Widstrom et al, 1990).

TOUCH IN HEALTH CARE

Nurses seem to touch patients more frequently than any other category of health care personnel (Barnett, 1972; Mitchell et al, 1985), with hands, arms, and shoulders receiving most touching. Nurses who report touching their patients more also demonstrate higher self-esteem, and greater use of touch in their personal lives (Schaefer, 1981). More highly educated and experienced nurses seem more inclined to touch; while nurses who feel burned out touch patients less (Estabrooks, 1989).

Multiple factors in addition to education and job satisfaction affect nurses' patterns of touch. A nurse is more likely to touch a patient when:

- the patient is in pain or frightened
- the patient responds positively to touch or reciprocates the touch
- the nurse feels compassion for the patient

A nurse is less likely to touch a patient when:

- the patient has a behavioral problem
- the patient presents a pathologic or physical risk
- the patient is seen as being responsible for his or her own health problems (such as, for instance, an alcoholic with cirrhosis)

It is interesting to note that nursing personnel report being aware when they touch patients, but studies in psychiatric and medical-surgical settings indicate that patients often are not aware that they have been touched. This suggests that nurses need to focus on the patient as well as on the procedure, trying to ensure that the patient is more aware of touch provided during nursing care.

Across health care settings, touch is often restricted to procedures or tasks related to care. The need for more "affective touching" of patients has been consistently emphasized. In fact, nurses who use touch in their interactions with patients are more favorably rated by their patients (Lewis et al, 1995). One possible reason that health care professionals may use so little expressive or affective touch is a concern that their touch will be misinterpreted by patients. Nurses identify potential misinterpretation of meaning, social mores and taboos, and comfort levels (their own as well as patients') with touch as hindrances to its use.

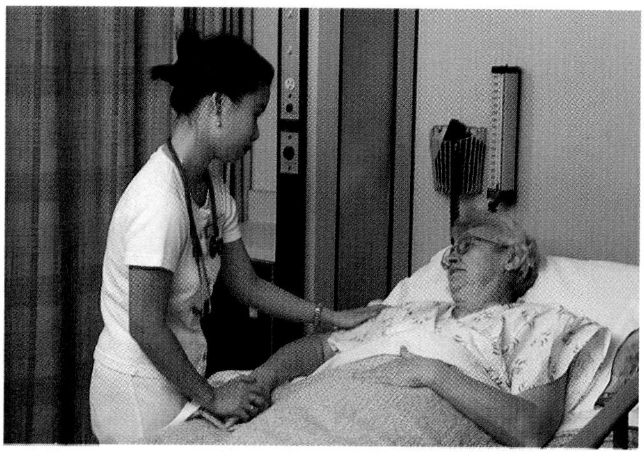

Figure 32–4. Nurse practicing therapeutic use of touch with a patient.

These concerns about how patients view touch are warranted to some degree. Interpretations regarding the meaning of touch can be very different for staff and patients. Patients may experience touch much less positively, viewing it as task oriented or controlling rather than as expressions of empathy or support.

Touch can indeed have many meanings and functions. Touch can instigate action, accomplish a task, gain attention, punish or restrain, show aggression, bring pain relief, provide physical protection, or orient a patient to reality. It can also express security, understanding, support, warmth, caring, reassurance, empathy, closeness, and willingness to be involved (Fig. 32–4). Whether the nurse's touch is understood by the patient will depend to a great extent on the context of the touching. For instance, what did the nurse's facial expression and voice communicate while touching ? What did the nurse feel when touching? These personal factors contribute to the nurse's "touching style" (Estabrooks and Morse, 1992). The particular style the nurse uses in a given situation will define the meaning of a touch.

Effects of Touch on the Therapeutic Relationship. How can touch enhance the nurse-patient relationship? Studies have found that patients who are touched on the arm or given a handshake evaluate the interaction more positively or disclose more personal information (Moore and Gilbert, 1995; Whitcher and Fisher, 1979). Exercises involving physical contact among members of group therapy sessions also seem to produce greater self-disclosure than in groups where no contact takes place.

It has also been found that patients touched by nurses exhibit more positive facial expressions, eye contact, body movements, and verbal responses toward and about the nurse than patients who are not touched (Knable, 1981); see Fig. 32–5. When nurses touch psychiatric patients, the patients' verbal interaction, rapport, and willingness to interact with the nurse can increase. Touching the arm of an elderly or con-

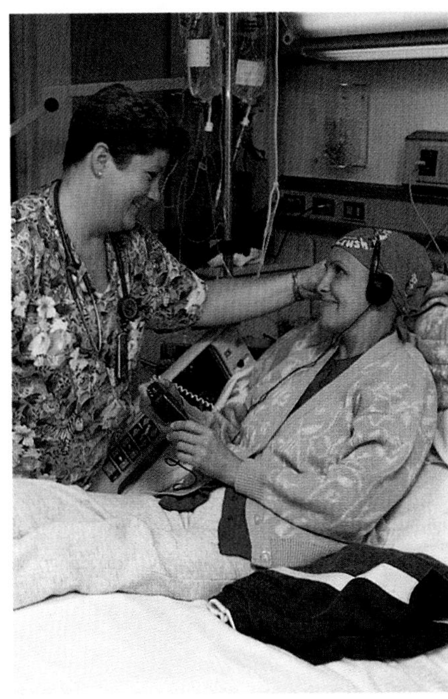

Figure 32-5. Nurse using caring touch during a procedure.

fused patient can help focus his or her attention when the nurse is making a verbal request (Langland and Panicucci, 1982). In women undergoing labor, however, the touch of partners is generally viewed as more reassuring and comforting than that of nurses and physicians (Birch, 1986).

Effects of Touch on Patients' Psychological Responses. In general, touch helps reduce psychological distress. Infants, for example, demonstrate less fussiness and emotional upset when carried more frequently by their mothers during the first 3 months of life (Hunziker and Barr, 1986). Bolstering the amount of infant holding through planned interventions combining touch and soothing verbal cues also decreases the length and amount of crying and fussiness. Verbal comfort measures alone rarely succeed in quieting or soothing emotionally distressed infants, whereas the combination of interventions appears to be quite successful (Korner, 1990). If the infant is not in distress, however, verbal interventions may be more successful than touch in maintaining a quiet state and reducing activity levels (Oehler, 1985; Weiss, 1992b).

Gentle body stroking and massage can help infants become more alert and focus more effectively on objects in their environment. These forms of affective touch also result in a quieter, more relaxed baby who is easier to comfort when distressed (Blackburn and Barnard, 1985; Field, 1987; Grossmann et al, 1985; Jay, 1982). These positive effects may depend, however, on the qualities of touch that nurses or parents use. Touch of strong intensity, more vigorous action, long duration, or contact with highly innervated areas of the body increases behavioral agitation and the corresponding potential for emotional distress in high-risk infants, such as those with congenital heart disease or pervasive developmental disorders (Weiss, 1992b, 1993). The nurse of the case presentation applied this knowledge to Jessie, the premature infant exposed to cocaine in utero. The nurse used qualities of touch to soothe Jessie and help reduce his agitation and crying, because agitation and crying can deplete needed calories and increase vulnerability to neurobehavioral problems.

Touch can also effectively reduce anxiety in adults. For instance, comforting touch administered to cardiovascular patients seems to reduce their anxiety levels (Weiss, 1990a). Gentle touch administered by nurses during preoperative teaching sessions tends to make patients less anxious about impending surgery (Whitcher and Fisher, 1979). Further, slow-stroke back massage significantly lowers women's anxiety (Longworth, 1982).

Effects of Touch on Patients' Physiologic Responses. Touch has significant effects on various physical responses as well. For example, placing the nude neonate on the mother's bare chest immediately after birth maintains the neonate's body temperature as well as taking the neonate from the mother and placing it in a heated crib (Hill and Shronk, 1979).

Touch unrelated to any procedure may also produce positive physical responses in high-risk infants. Rubbing or stroking the infant's body and extremities, or placing the hands on the infant's head or abdomen for intermittent periods have produced decreased frequency of apnea (temporary cessation of breathing), increased hematocrit, and decreased oxygen demand (indicating more effective body metabolism), increased food intake, and weight gain (Jay, 1982; Rausch, 1981). However, other studies have found no relationship between these kinds of touch and weight gain, morbidity, need for mechanical ventilation, or tolerance of oral nutrients.

In some cases, touch can actually have negative health effects on high-risk infants by disturbing homeostasis. For example, increased cortisol levels, tachycardia or bradycardia, elevated blood pressure, decreased hemoglobin oxygen saturation, and respiratory problems have all been observed in premature infants after procedural touch or other routine procedures (Als et al, 1986; Gorski et al, 1984; Gunnar et al, 1987; Harrison et al, 1990; Long et al, 1980; Medoff-Cooper, 1988; Norris et al, 1982). Studies such as these on the possible negative effects of touch have led many hospitals to adopt minimal touch policies, such as those noted in the case study. However, these detrimental responses may be associated only with procedural touching and not with expressive, interactive touch (Gorski et al, 1990). Procedures are often performed in standard ways regardless of the infant's observed reactions. Thus, the procedures per se may not be the cause of increased physiologic arousal. Instead, the quality of the touch used during procedures (i.e., touch that arouses rather than calms the infant) may be the determining factor (Weiss, 1992b). Infants with fragile nervous systems (such as Jessie Jabar) do not have the self-regulatory capacities necessary to buffer stimulation from the environment or dampen the strength of their responses. In such infants, excessive nervous system arousal can trigger life-threatening respiratory or cardiovascular problems. Thus, the nurse should use more calming, gentle touch even when performing standard procedures.

Nurses' touch influences physiologic arousal in critically ill adults as well. For example, in cardiac patients and patients in a shock-trauma unit, changes in heart rate may occur in response to nurses' pulse-taking and hand-holding (Lynch et al, 1974; Mills et al, 1976). However, some studies have found no such effects (Lynch et al, 1977; Weiss, 1990a).

In general, noninvasive nursing procedures, stroking, and massage either calm the nervous system or do not affect it at all (Fakouri and Jones, 1987; Hill, 1993; Meek, 1993, Mitchell et al, 1985; Weiss, 1990a). Evidence does not support a negative impact of touch on the physiologic responses of most adult patients.

Therapeutic Touch. Therapeutic touch is a technique involving an interaction of "energy fields" between the nurse and patient (Krieger, 1981). Human beings are considered complex fields of various life energies. In a state of health all of the individual's energies are in balance. Disease is a manifestation of disequilibrium, blockage, and/or deficits in human energy flow. In this technique, the nurse does not touch the patient but holds her or his hands 2 to 6 inches above the patient's body (Fig. 32–6). Healing energy is directed through the nurse's hands by focusing on the intent to therapeutically help the patient. This involves identifying imbalances or blockages within the patient's energy field through sensations felt in the hands, then redirecting or rebalancing the energy in those areas through a conscious intent to heal.

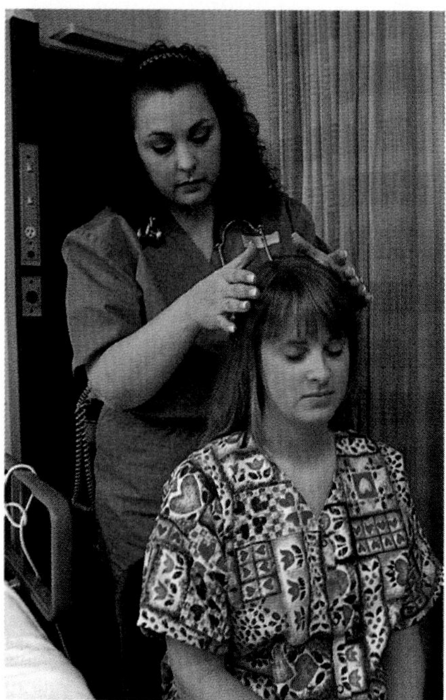

Figure 32–6. Nurse performing the therapeutic touch technique on a patient, holding her hands several inches from the patient's head.

Studies of the impact of therapeutic touch have demonstrated a number of outcomes, such as elevated serum hemoglobin (Krieger, 1975), deep relaxation (Krieger et al, 1979), decreased anxiety (Quinn, 1984; Simington and Laing, 1993), decreased headache pain (Keller and Bzdek, 1986), and accelerated wound healing (Wirth, 1990).

Measuring energy exchange through scientific means has proven difficult, and some researchers contend that effects attributed to therapeutic touch may be actually due to the perceived affection, trust, concern, or acceptance being communicated from the nurse to the patient rather than any therapeutic exchange of energy fields (Smith, 1990). The actual physiologic workings of therapeutic touch and its effects on patients remain controversial and merit further study.

The use of therapeutic touch in a clinical setting is becoming more common. An example of a program that uses a variety of approaches is presented in Box 32–3.

RELEVANT THEORY

Three primary perspectives guide our understanding of touch and its impact: holistic, humanistic, and neurophysiologic perspectives of touch (Box 32–4).

Holistic Theory

The holistic, or field, model of touch is derived from Eastern philosophies and only recently is being tested scientifically. Within the holistic matrix, touch is a "laying on of hands" through which *Prana* (a vital energy existing in healthy persons) can be intentionally directed to another person with diminished energy due to illness or injury (Kunz and Peper, 1982).

Therapeutic touch, discussed in the preceding section, is one example of an intervention stemming from the holistic perspective. In the holistic view, compassion is the essential factor in healing, not any physical attributes of touch. Compassion—or altruistic intent to help—is said to be transferred from one person's body to another through waves of energy radiated from a bioenergetic field surrounding the body.

Humanistic Theory

The humanistic model of touch derives from European philosophies of phenomenology and existentialism. The humanistic perspective differentiates mere physical handling from touch that communicates empathy or sympathy. In the humanistic view, touch is reciprocal; one is touched in turn as she or he touches another (Merleau-Ponty, 1962). This reciprocity fosters empathy or sympathy for another, as the distinction between the toucher and the touched becomes blurred. Humanists fear that if touch becomes solely functional and cognitive, lacking closeness or reciprocity, then the

BOX 32-3
HEALING TOUCH AT THE QUEEN'S MEDICAL CENTER, HONOLULU, HAWAII

Hob Osterlund, RN, MS, CHTP
Clinical Coordinator, Pain Management Services

Healing Touch (HT) is a collective of hands-on techniques that includes the work of many visionary professionals including Dolores Kreiger *(Therapeutic Touch: Accepting Your Power to Heal)*, Brugh Joy, MD *(Joy's Way)*, Barbara Brennan *(Hands of Light* and *Light Emerging)* and Janet Mentgen *(Healing Touch: A Resource for Health Care Professionals.)* At its core, HT has two basic assumptions: (1) that the human body is surrounded by and constantly interacting with an energy field, often called the "subtle body," and (2) that there is such a thing as a human energy exchange. These assumptions are based on the work of Albert Einstein, who theorized the relationship between energy and matter. In HT, a nurse or other practitioner consciously focuses on the highest healing intention for the recipient and uses the hands to relieve pain, increase relaxation, and facilitate wound healing. This intention and the work itself often bring about very positive responses by the person receiving treatment as well as by those who have witnessed the treatment.

Many medical centers are now integrating HT and therapeutic touch (TT) into their services. One such institution is The Queen's Medical Center in Honolulu, Hawaii. Since its quiet beginning in 1991, it has grown to a service assisted by four Pain Management Services nurses and 30 volunteers who collectively gave more than 3000 HT treatments to QMC inpatients in 1996; to a service supported by more than 200 employees trained in HT as well as by the medical center administration and board of trustees; to a service where a long-discussed postoperative mastectomy HT study is under way and where a research protocol for treating employees with HT for acute back injuries is nearly completed for Institutional Review Committee (IRC); and to a service that has received media attention, statewide awards, and consistent consumer praise.

The volunteer program was the brainchild of Mary Magota, RN. It was Mary who responded to a 1994 article in the Honolulu Advertiser which described the use of HT at QMC. Why not, she said, train and utilize retired nurses to do HT? The idea grew into reality quickly, as if preordained. Retired nurses, we found, were a tremendous community resource. They are often very healthy, talented, and unshakable; out of gratitude, they are eager to return their energies to the community. What better place than inpatient bedside care, where they cut their professional teeth?

One by one these nurses took Healing Touch courses and became volunteers. Soon people from other backgrounds applied to volunteer: active nurses, ministers, massage therapists, professional musicians, graduate students, even a clown and a retired navy pilot. Each brings a special perspective and style; all have in common their willingness to learn and their interest in being of service to human beings in need.

Since 1994 the number has grown from one to 30 volunteers, covering a portion of the 60 to 70 patients referred to us and who are on our daily list. Volunteers are here seven days a week. Although most of them treat patients in the afternoon, we also have two evening volunteers who stay until late at night helping patients get some rest.

RESEARCH

As part of more than 50 HT research projects going on nationally, two studies are under way at QMC. Data collection is actively occurring for the Postoperative Pain Study (POPS). The principal investigator is Diana Davids, RN, MS, CCRN; she is joined by investigators from pain management, breast health, Lokomaika'i, patient care consulting services, and others. In this study mastectomy patients are randomized into two groups: immediate treatment and delayed treatment. The immediate treatment group receives HT one day preoperatively and immediately in the postanesthesia care unit (PACU). The delayed treatment group receives HT one day postmastectomy. Pain levels and analgesia use are recorded by interview and journal for one week after surgery and will be compared to one another.

The second project is the Back Injury Treatment for Employees (BITE) study. This study creation is as a result of encouragement from the QMC Lokomaika'i or "Inner Health" medical executive committee, which has been interested in doing research on the impact of HT on employees with acute back injuries. Employees at QMC have had the option of receiving post-injury HT since 1995. The principal investigator is Hob Osterlund, RN, MS, CHTP, joined by co-investigators from employee health, risk management, pain management, nursing research, workers' compensation, the emergency department, and others.

PATIENT AND TREATER RESPONSE

A third project is for the purpose of quality assurance. This patient satisfaction questionnaire has been ongoing over the last year. To date 184 patients have been interviewed. Of these patients, 87.7% rate themselves "very satisfied" and 8.6% "satisfied." Of those who had pain prior to a treatment (134), there was an average decrease in pain of 2.9 points on a 0–10 scale. Of those who felt anxious prior to treatment (149), there was an average increase in relaxation of 2.0 points on a 1–4 scale. A total of 37% had prior knowledge about HT when they were admitted to the medical center.

When the patients are asked for further comment, many touching details are revealed. "Helped me more than morphine," "pain relief for 12 hours," "helps me deal with the frustration of being here," "feeling safe, spiritual and very relaxed," "it felt like another human being was taking my pain and discomfort away," "it's comforting, like being in heaven," "so glad Queen's offers this," and so on.

continued on next page

BOX 32-3 (cont'd)
HEALING TOUCH AT THE QUEEN'S MEDICAL CENTER

Letters of gratitude arrive every week, full of stories from patients and families about the impact of HT on their lives. One of the volunteers is moved to write poetry each week about her experiences.

Poems

Today in the hospital
A dear man's Japanese wife
and blind daughter
help me give him
a Healing Touch treatment.

I show the blind daughter where to put her hands.
She wants to feel where my hands are.
Her hands are gentle,
instinctively giving healing touch
long before I came.
She's the youngest of five daughters.

Her dad sleeps more peacefully now.

****

He is a medical doctor,
retired now,
a patient.

He watches me carefully
as I do Healing Touch.

He went to the same medical school
as my husband did.

He tells me
his grandchildren are the lights
of his life.

He thanks me
for Healing Touch.

****

Two faithful daughters
stand at his side.
He is hard of hearing
and cannot breathe well.
"Daddy,"
one tells him,
"They're here
to give you Healing Touch."
He nods approval.
When we are done
his breathing is easier.

****

"You people relax me so much.
What a gift of love you give us patients.
Thank you," she says
as she holds my hand.
Cancer has filled her body.
Later I see her walking the hall
with her devoted husband.
"I like your hat,"
I tell her.
She laughs.
"I have to try to look beautiful."
"You are very beautiful,"
I say.

****

She is frightened,
jumps out of a truck.
Hits her head.
Her once-young, vigorous,
immortal life
is gone.
She tries to find what is lost
and cries and thrashes in her bed.
God bless her.

****

Above the HT desk there is a trophy commemorating the Healing Touch program's "Spirit of Hawaii" award for "outstanding achievement and service in the spirit of our islands: from a local television station and another trophy for winning JC Penney's "Golden Rule Award" for outstanding volunteer service to the community. The latter was accompanied by a $1000 check and a congratulatory letter from Hawaii's lieutenant governor Mazi Hirono, as well as President Bill Clinton. A file of thank you letters from former patients and their loved ones bulges in the drawer. When a representative from QMC Patient Relations is asked about the impression she has of HT based on patients' comments, she says "they tell me it's an asset to QMC, one of the highlights of their hospital stay and that it made a real difference in their recovery or condition."

One special letter is from a physician describing his hospitalization and HT treatment:

> There is one program I must say something about, because it is so unique and it is so incredibly useful and broad-minded for Queen's Medical Center to support it: **Healing Touch.** I had known nothing of it before experiencing the "treatments." The release and transmission of positive healing energy is accomplished competently and

BOX 32-3 (cont'd)
HEALING TOUCH AT THE QUEEN'S MEDICAL CENTER

effectively. Without "evidence" to "prove" these effects, I am sure there are skeptics—however, they are *not* found among the recipient patients, who are universally enthusiastic in my small sampling. Nor are the skeptics among the highly skilled and caring practitioners of this art, for by its very nature it is a healing art more than western medicine can measure and document. So it is a gift, given compassionately, and received openly . . . greatly appreciated and repeatedly requested. A gift of caring Queen's to its community, patients, staff, and family. Wonderful. Thank you.

ATTRIBUTIONS OF SUCCESS

To what do we attribute this kind of response and success at The Queen's Medical Center? Many factors have contributed to the Healing Touch program, including: **Administration and Board of Trustees,** who are visionary in their support of a new paradigm in health care, truly integrating the best of curing and healing. **Volunteers,** who are of the highest caliber in their ability to provide treatments and in their motivation. They are without exception moved to offer HT because of a desire to assist their fellow human beings, and are willing to collectively offer thousands of hours to the comfort of QMC patients. **Nurses,** who have been quick to see the first-hand impact of HT on their patients. They are eager to refer appropriate patients, to be trained and to support the program. **Patients and loved ones,** who experience and witness the impact of HT. They write letters of support and praise to QMC administration, become trained themselves to treat their families and discuss their symptom relief with their doctors. **Physicians,** whose training might lead them to skepticism, have also witnessed the impact on their patients. They encourage science and research despite the difficulty measuring such concepts as intention and receptivity to same. **Hawaii's culture,** which is a collective of many cultures that have long traditions in healing modalities and an understanding of global rather than either/or thinking. **Queen's founders,** who themselves are the royalty of a culture that believes in healing in a large and integrated sense. Finally and most importantly, the success is due to the timing and universal wisdom of that which defines the oneness in us all: God, divine will, holy spirit. Whatever our culture teaches us to call it, the "it" is a great undefinable but wholly tangible **Spirit of Love.**

inherent empathy of touch will be lost (Wyschograd, 1981). From this perspective, the goal is to transform all touch, even object-oriented and utilitarian touch, into acceptance, mutuality, and genuine communication (Weber, 1990).

These humanistic views of touch are emphasized in clinical literature on reality orientation (knowing time, place and person), as well as literature on deaf, blind, semiconscious, withdrawn, and dying patients. Humanists also see touch as central to the development of trust and a genuine communication of caring in often impersonal high-technology or institutional environments (Goodykoontz, 1980; Seaman, 1982). Particularly for patients vulnerable to depersonalization and isolation (e.g., elderly, critically ill, or homeless patients), touch can be a significant means of communicating concern and emotional support.

Neurophysiologic Theory

The neurophysiologic perspective of touch stems from neuroscience and biopsychology. From this perspective, the impact of touch on the central nervous system (CNS) and the autonomic nervous system (ANS) is crucial. As noted earlier in the chapter, sensory receptors and nerve pathways provide different types of feedback to the CNS. Nerve impulse transmission to the CNS affects the heart, blood vessels, respiratory center, and systems governing muscle movement, depending on whether the impulse does not significantly affect ANS activity or affects either the sympathetic or parasympathetic division of the ANS.

Research shows that certain qualities of touch are more conducive to CNS and ANS arousal than others (Boxes 32–5 and 32–6). They include vigorous actions of long duration

BOX 32-4
CONCEPTUAL PERSPECTIVES OF TOUCH

- Holistic
- Humanistic
- Neurophysiologic

BOX 32-5
QUALITIES OF TOUCH THAT AROUSE THE NERVOUS SYSTEM

- Long duration
- Strong intensity
- Contact with body areas having many nerve endings
- Movements that stimulate deeper muscles and tissues

BOX 32-6
QUALITIES OF TOUCH THAT CALM THE NERVOUS SYSTEM

- Weak intensity
- Short duration
- Contact with body areas having few nerve endings
- Movements on skin surface only

and strong intensity that elicit skin, muscle and tissue sensations and actions that involve contact with many body areas, especially areas with many nerve endings, such as the face, hands, or feet (Weiss, 1986). The common link among qualities of touch that cause neural excitation is their ability to stimulate sensory receptors and enhance transmission across neural pathways. In contrast, the nervous system is calmed by touch that involves short duration, weak-intensity actions with little pressure, stretching, or muscle and tissue sensation. Calming touch also uses body areas having few nerve endings, such as the back, arms, or legs. The neurophysiologic perspective aims to better understand how touch may impair or foster healthy development or healing through its varied effects on the nervous system.

FACTORS AFFECTING CLINICAL DECISIONS

The nurse must consider patients' individual differences when evaluating the potential effects of touch or planning touch as a nursing intervention. Important factors include:

- Age. Sensory and neural capacities, as well as psychosocial needs, differ widely across the lifespan.
- Gender. Research seems to indicate that men and women experience touch differently.
- Cultural and family background. Cultural and family attitudes about touch will influence the amount and types of touch that a patient considers appropriate.

In addition, spirituality, ethics, financial considerations, the setting in which touch occurs, and differences in individuals' social status can affect patients' comfort with being touched.

Age

Considering a patient's age before touching is important for two reasons: age-related differences in sensory and neural capacities, and age-related differences in response to touch.

Infants and Children. Touch is especially important in infants, defining motor, emotional, and learning capacities for life. Skin sensations develop early, making input from touch a far more potent stimulus than input from other senses (Turkewitz and Kenny, 1982). Very young babies have higher thresholds for external stimuli—that is, they don't experience such stimuli readily—and so are less sensitive to touch. But infants become more sensitive to stimulation starting at about 1 month of age (Stern, 1988). As they develop and gain more control over the excitation that their brains encounter, they gain more control over their response to touch and other types of stimulation (Kopp, 1982). However, infants born prematurely or infants with underdeveloped nervous systems may be unresponsive or hypersensitive to touch (Gorski et al, 1990; Rose, 1990), like Jessie Jabar.

In infancy and the preschool years, parents usually provide most of a child's touch experience. As a child matures, however, parents often spend increasingly less time in physical contact with him or her. School-age children actually receive most of their touch from peers.

Adolescents. Adolescents also experience peer touch, but in older adolescence, touch from a girlfriend or boyfriend is most frequent, and parent touch is minimal. It has been demonstrated that teenagers sometimes use sexual behavior as a substitute for the loss of close-holding, affective parental touch (McAnarney, 1990); see Fig. 32–7.

Adults. Adults, of course, may also use sexual activity as a means of being held and cuddled. Adults acquire almost all touch from spouses or partners; if a partner is not available, interpersonal touch may be rare.

Elderly Adults. For the elderly, changes in sensory acuity (the ability to recognize or experience sounds, sights, touch) affect response to touch. Older patients may lose sensation in some areas of the body, and develop increased sensitivity and fragility due to thin skin (Fanslow, 1990). Elderly patients also have much greater difficulty than young ones in recovering their ability to feel things that they touch or recognize when they are being touched after suffering damage to brain areas governing skin sensations (Burton et al, 1990).

The need for touch does not lessen as people age. It may in fact increase due to loss of vision and hearing as well as social isolation (Vortherms, 1991). Nurses and nursing students may be less comfortable touching older patients, and describe their experience of touching the elderly in less positive ways (Tobiason, 1981)—at the same time elderly patients may desire even more touch than most patients.

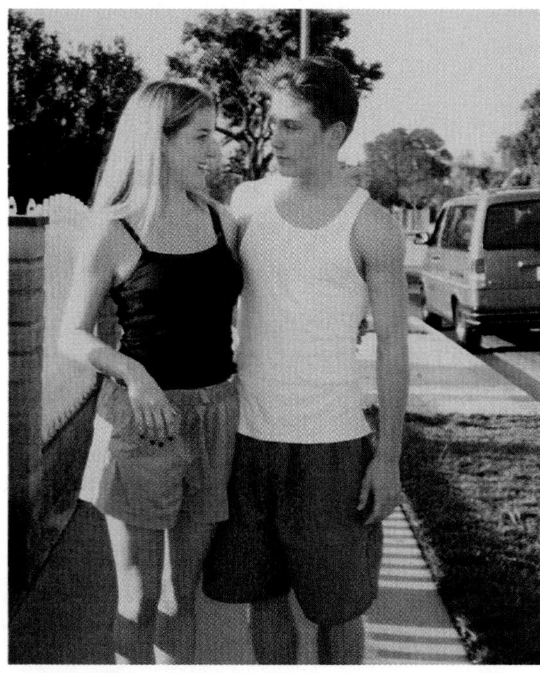

Figure 32–7. Older adolescents often fulfill their need for touch through physical contact with a girlfriend or boyfriend.

Clearly, age can have a significant impact on a person's physiologic response to touch and whether he or she receives touch at all. The effects of these developmental differences will depend upon each person's (1) own needs for physical contact and (2) ability to acquire the amount and type of touch they want.

Gender

Numerous studies have shown that males and females receive different kinds of touch, and respond differently to the touch they do receive. Females have lower thresholds for touch than males (Hofer, 1981; Maccoby and Jacklin, 1974)—that is, girls and women more readily recognize when they are touched. Men and boys require a touch of stronger intensity and duration. Animal studies have consistently shown that gender differences are biologically based to a great extent; females are more responsive than males to stimulation of the brain's somatosensory cortex (Diamond, 1990).

Paradoxically, however, touch may have a greater impact on males (Weiner et al, 1985; Weiss, 1990a). Touch seems to be a more important determinant of men's cognitive development (learning and thinking), anxiety levels, and physiologic responses (for example, vital signs). In addition, deprivation of touch has more pronounced negative effects on the development of emotional and behavioral problems in male animals than in female animals (Suomi, 1990). These gender differences persist from infancy through old age, and have been observed in various species.

Males and females also generally receive and give different amounts and types of touching at various points in their lives (Maccoby and Jacklin, 1974). For instance, women tend to receive and give more touch than men—although some studies have found that men view touch more positively than women (Weiss, 1990a; Whitcher and Fisher, 1979). American men tend to respond most positively to typical "male" touch, such as handshakes and back slaps. Women, in contrast, commonly use touch to care for, console, or comfort others.

Although these differences are not completely understood, the gender of both the person touching and the person being touched affects how the touch is perceived. In routine procedures such as bathing and in more complex ones such as catheterization, it is especially important for the nurse to consider the degree and type of touch that each patient feels comfortable with by a person of the same or opposite gender. For instance, some men feel uncomfortable being cared for and touched by another man; some women become anxious when cared for by a man. Each patient's preferences must be ascertained so that touch does not increase but reduces distress.

Individual and Family Values

Substantial differences exist between families of various cultures in their patterns of touch, and in the kinds of touch they may find helpful from nurses. Moreover, a patient's history of touch within his or her family influences his or her response to touch from nurses (Weiss, 1992b). To ensure maximum benefit from touch, the nurse needs to understand the role played by family touch in the patient's well-being, and how to best support the family through touch.

If a patient was abused as a child or perceives touch as negative, for instance, he or she may exhibit aversion or defensiveness to touch (see Box 32–7). Touching of particularly traumatized body areas may elicit specific reactions; because the nurse may not know a patient's history of physical abuse, she or he must be alert to signs of discomfort with touch.

A family may also need assistance with their touch to better help a family member. For example, the nurse may need to help parents with a preterm infant (like Ms. Jabar in the case presentation) achieve an optimal fit between their and the infant's needs for touch. Such parents may inadvertently overload the infant with touch when the infant's neural system can handle only small amounts of light-intensity touch. Or, they may be afraid to handle the infant and not touch him or her at all. In either case, the nurse can help the parents recognize their infant's cues regarding readiness for contact or need to withdraw, then develop a plan to teach the parents ways to touch the infant uniquely designed for the infant's needs.

Such individualized interventions were used by the nurse in the case presentation at the beginning of the chapter. As that nurse noted, in some situations family members may need comforting touch as much as the patient. A gentle pat on the back, a hug, or a hand squeeze may provide immeasurable support to a family member feeling overwhelmed in trying to cope with a medical crisis or deal with the grief of losing a loved one.

Finally, family members may help the nurse better understand a patient's response to touch and better plan interventions involving touch. Such insight into the patient's beliefs and preferences regarding touch can help the nurse develop a plan of care incorporating touch most effectively. The family's role is especially critical when the patient is a child, or is too ill to share his or her own wishes and views of appropriate and desirable care.

BOX 32-7
SIGNS OF POTENTIAL AVERSION TO TOUCH

Patients may exhibit many different signs of defensiveness or aversion to touch, as a result of child abuse, disease, conditioning, or culture. The nurse should be alert for:

- jumpiness
- ticklishness
- muscle tightening
- increased talkativeness
- breathing changes
- flinching
- skin mottling
- hiccuping
- arching of back or entire body
- fussiness
- abnormal sensitivity

Educational Background and Socioeconomic Status

Every society has certain standards about the appropriateness of touching others, usually based on their status. In general, higher-status persons initiate touching of lower-status persons, but not vice versa (Juni and Brannon, 1981). This pattern reflects the overarching sociopolitical climate of our society, in which convention holds that persons of more perceived power or authority tend to take the interpersonal initiative with those of less power and authority.

Some patients view nurses as authority figures, as professionals of high status. However, others may perceive nurses as being of lesser status than themselves. The nurse needs to consider the potential for such different views among patients when making judgments about when and whom to touch. In most cases, the nurse, by virtue of his or her professional status, will probably be perceived as having legitimate procedural or task-oriented reasons to touch the patient. But physical contact of a more expressive or supportive nature, even within the context of the nurse-patient relationship, may convey different meanings to different patients. It therefore warrants careful assessment.

Culture and Ethnicity

Culture and ethnicity can also influence the nature and perception of touch. For instance, in Hispanic cultures, touch tends to be frequently expressed, with men commonly hugging one another and women commonly kissing and holding hands (Monrroy, 1983). In contrast, in some Caucasian cultures (e.g., German, British), touch tends to not be a major aspect of everyday social life. Such culturally influenced patterns of touch may develop early in life, with some children reared with extensive body contact and vigorous massage and others touched very little. Different preferences for touch may then become firmly ingrained and determine how the person wishes to be touched later in life.

Cultures also vary dramatically in the use of touch and may negate specific kinds of touch. For example, some Vietnamese believe that touching a person's head may take away the spirit (Boyle and Andrews, 1989). In Thailand and Laos, it is considered rude to touch a child on the top of the head because the head is the home of the spirit. As the child's spirit is not strong, patting the top of the head may cause the child to become ill. In India it is considered rude to touch a woman (Jandt, 1995). If you were observing friends having coffee in America, you might see them touch each other once or twice an hour. If you were observing in a London coffee shop, you probably would not see them touch at all. The same observation in a French coffee shop, would include seeing friends touch each other a hundred times an hour (Jandt, 1995).

Each culture socializes its members to use and expect certain types of touch. The nurse must be sensitive to culturally appropriate use of touch to best meet each patient's needs. Talking to the family, even if not of a culture foreign to the nurse, about what is culturally appropriate may help the nurse plan appropriate touch intervention.

When language barriers prevent effective verbal communication, touch can also help nurses communicate with patients. Touch can guide patients to the right location, protect and support patients in times of crises, or soothe them when they require consolation. All of this can occur without words, as long as the person being touched seems receptive to physical contact.

Spirituality and Religious Practices

Spirituality can be defined as the striving for a higher meaning or purpose in the face of the indignities, crises, and suffering of life. For patients who are ill or dying, spiritual needs can become paramount, and nurses are often called upon to support the patient or family in their spiritual quest. Touch may provide the most tangible means of such support. Touch can communicate that the nurse is fully present and attentive more concretely than any other form of communication.

The nurse's presence and sympathy may be best communicated by simple means: holding the patient's hand, sitting next to the patient with an arm around him or her, or providing a gentle, comforting massage. The most spiritual moments may be moments of silence in which simple physical contact communicates empathy of the patient's emotional or physical suffering. For a nurse, there may be no greater privilege than providing such support in the most vulnerable moments of another human being's life.

Setting in Which Care Is Delivered

The setting in which touch occurs influences perceptions of its appropriateness or acceptability. Within hospital or clinic environments—the nurse's territory—both procedural and expressive touching may be well accepted. However, in the home care setting, the patient may feel more comfortable establishing the parameters for touching. A patient who typically uses physical contact in his or her personal interactions may feel free to touch the nurse. For another patient whose typical patterns may involve minimal or no physical contact, it may be more appropriate for the nurse to initiate touch, but only to perform a necessary nursing procedure. The home-care nurse should let the patient take the lead in defining what is acceptable touch behavior.

Being in the patient's home may also obscure professional and social boundaries. Since patients tend to feel more comfortable and empowered at home, a patient could misinterpret touch to mean that the nurse is seeking an intimate relationship. A nurse detecting signs of such misinterpretation should use touch judiciously and only in relation to specific procedures.

In certain critical care environments, two conflicting needs may influence touch. On one hand, the patient's need for touch may increase as a response to the depersonalized, technological nature of the modern health care setting. On the other hand, a seriously ill patient may be more vulnerable to the detrimental effects of touch (e.g., heart rhythm and respiratory irregularities, blood pressure elevation). The pathologic processes underlying illness, along with drug effects and intrusive medical procedures, may weaken the patient's ability to cope with neurologic stimulation, and potentiate further medical problems (Gorski et al, 1990; Oehler, 1985; Weiss, 1986). In such situations, the nurse needs to carefully monitor the effects of touch on the patient and be attuned to proper timing and the type of touch needed to maximize benefit and decrease vulnerability. (Refer back to Box 32–6 for qualities of touch that calm the nervous system.)

Ethical Considerations

Three ethical principles should guide nurses in any situation involving touch. The first two are the principles of beneficence and nonmaleficence, which mandate that all touch be done for the good of the patient, without in any way causing harm. Consider the patient who is psychologically averse to touch, or one made physiologically vulnerable to touch as a result of temperament or illness. For such patients, the nurse bears a substantial responsibility for weighing the benefits versus the costs of touch. The same positive expressive touch used to excellent effect with one patient may harm another.

Similarly, the nurse should always consider the ethics of using touch to control or restrain any agitated, confused, or aggressive patient. For instance, is the intervention truly necessary for the patient's well-being? Does the restraint not only do good, but also preclude harm? Such questions raise difficult and complex issues that have no ready answers; but we must examine them to assure the ethical use of touch for restraint or control.

The nurse must also consider the ethical principle of autonomy, or respect for the patient. This principle addresses the importance of being invited or given permission by the patient to be touched. Although this permission is assumed in most procedural health care tasks, the nurse must not take it for granted. The nurse must carefully assess for nonverbal cues in patients unable to speak (e.g., intubated patients) or move (e.g., immobilized or paralyzed patients) and solicit the family's input in making decisions about using touch beyond what is required to complete lifesaving health care measures.

Financial Considerations

Certain financial considerations apply to touch in health care. Increasingly scarce resources within health care institutions may affect the quality of touch used in nursing care; the nurse may be asked to care for too many patients, or delegate care activities to less skilled personnel. Such situations may decrease the nurse's opportunity to effectively assess the tactile needs of each patient and provide touch tailored to each patient's unique clinical profile. The health care institution may maintain that nursing time spent in comforting, supportive touch is not cost-effective. As a result, certain procedures may be discouraged, such as giving back massages or holding children while they undergo painful procedures.

There are additional dangers in such a tightened fiscal climate of performing procedural touch in a rushed, rough, or standardized manner, or using no expressive touch at all. Nurses should be aware that such policies may have direct, detrimental physical and psychological consequences for patients. It is the nurse's responsibility to advocate for quality of care by assuring that physical and emotional comfort continue to be a central component of nursing care.

FUTURE DEVELOPMENTS

The science underlying touch is still young. Further development is needed in at least three areas: developing individualized protocols, reducing patient distress, and providing family education.

Patient-tailored protocols initially involve designing and testing assessments of each patient's response to touch. These assessments would ideally include input from the patient and family, as well as nursing observations. Assessment must include the patient's history of touch, his or her patterns of touch in everyday life, attitudes toward being touched, and any temperament or disease-related factors that might influence his or her threshold, strength of response, and tolerance for touch. Based on this assessment, the nurse could then more easily develop an individualized care plan incorporating the amount and type of touch most therapeutic for the patient.

More attention must also be paid to the efficacy of touch in comforting patients and reducing their disease-, procedural-, and treatment-related pain and suffering. Stroking, massage, and holding may be both key and cost-effective in these areas, helping decrease the need for expensive analgesics and sedatives or augment these drugs' effects. As discussed earlier, animal studies clearly demonstrate how physical contact and handling buffer and deactivate the stress response. Infant care is beginning to benefit from application of this research, but these findings have been applied to a lesser extent in other age groups. Carefully conducted studies to examine the usefulness of such interventions, especially in adult populations, is sorely needed.

Nurses are in contact with families across numerous clinical arenas, and are in an excellent position to teach them about the effects of touch. These areas of education might include:

- how touch influences the healthy development of infants and children
- how to monitor and modify touch in family members vulnerable to stimulation overload, such as low–birth weight infants, patients with myocardial infarction, or children with autism
- how to aid recovery of brain function in brain-damaged patients (e.g., stroke victims) through massage and other touch interventions
- how touch can reduce physiologic arousal and emotional distress during periods of stress (see Patient Teaching box)

PATIENT TEACHING
MASSAGE

Family members providing care may use massage rather than pharmaceuticals to obtain the following outcomes: reduce nervous system arousal, enhance relaxation, and stimulate circulation.

TEACHING GOALS

The goals for this educational intervention include acquiring both knowledge and skills:

- Patient and family can describe the benefits of massage.
- Patient and family can verbalize their unique responses to the types of touch used in massage.
- Family members can provide a massage using knowledge of centering, context, and types of therapeutic touch.
- Patient and family can evaluate the effect of massage.

CONTENT

Knowledge about the benefits of massage and the types of touch used in massage is followed by demonstrations and practice.

TEACHING STRATEGIES

Focused discussion regarding:

- Benefits of massage.
- Individual feelings about touch and massage.

Demonstration and return demonstration:

- Preparing the person for massage.
- Techniques of massage.
- Attending to individual differences.
- Evaluation.

Facilitate recall:

- Provide written material on key points.
- Provide pictures of massage strokes.

Facilitate the family's ability to evaluate the effectiveness of their care and to use other methods to accomplish outcomes. Discuss measures used to evaluate the effect of massage (pulse rate, respiratory rate, self-report).

In the future, family education should be a normal aspect of planning care, whether conducted in the hospital, at discharge, or as part of community or home care. To ensure the effectiveness of such family interventions, more studies such as the one discussed in the Research Highlight: Kangaroo Care are needed.

NURSING CARE ACTIONS

The research and clinically based conclusions identified in earlier sections of this chapter guide the practices and procedures of touch used in everyday nursing care.

RESEARCH HIGHLIGHT
KANGAROO CARE

The behavioral and physiologic effects of kangaroo care (KC) as a nursing intervention were compared with infants who remained in an open-air crib (control infants). Kangaroo care involves placing a diaper-clad infant in an upright position between the mother's breasts in a skin-to-skin, chest-to-chest contact.

The study was a randomized, controlled clinical trial of 25 preterm infants in open-air cribs. The researchers recorded heart rate (HR), respiratory rate, oxygen saturation, abdominal skin temperature and state of arousal every minute using skin probes, thermistors, and observational assessments of infant facial, vocal, and body activity. Before and after KC, infants were placed on their right sides. During KC, they were placed on their abdomen upright between their mothers' breasts. Control infants were placed on their right sides throughout the assessment period.

The researchers found that the infants' skin temperature increased 0.6°C and heart rate increased an average of 8 beats per minute during KC. Infants in KC also averaged twice as much time in quiet regular sleep compared with pretest and posttest periods. KC, they confirmed, effectively decreased activity and promoted deep sleep; and no infant heat loss occurred during KC.

IMPLICATIONS FOR NURSING PRACTICE

The researchers concluded that KC:

- Is safe and beneficial for open-air crib populations.
- Does not produce physiologic instability or disruptions in either sleep or awake states.
- Has a comforting effect on both infants and mothers.
- Helps mothers further realize their unique contributions to their infant's health.

Ludington-Hoe, S.M., Thompson, C., Swinth, J., Hadeed, A.J., Anderson, G.C. (1994). Kangaroo care: research results, and practice implications and guidelines. *Neonatal Network 13* (1), 19–27.

Principles and Practices

Five general principles underlie the therapeutic use of touch in nursing practice:

- Touch is central to all nursing care.
- Touch may have therapeutic or detrimental effects.
- Touch serves as a nonverbal form of communication.
- Touch must be individualized.
- The nurse's attitude will affect both practice and perception of touch (see Box 32–8).

BOX 32-8
FIVE PRINCIPLES UNDERLYING THE THERAPEUTIC USE OF TOUCH

Five basic principles inform touch in nursing:

1. Touch is a central component of nursing care. It is the basis for nursing procedures, comfort measures, and emotional support. Too frequently, however, nurses provide care without a conscious awareness of the touch that they are using. Nurses must recognize the variety and extent of touch involved during care, so touch can be provided in the context of a thoughtful assessment and specific nursing care goal.
2. Touch can have either therapeutic or detrimental effects. The effects of touch are dependent on how well the type of touch used and the particular needs of each patient fit. Not all touch is the same, and even standardized types of touch can be experienced very differently by different patients. Touch that may be beneficial for some patients may put others at risk.
3. Touch is a language that communicates various messages. These nonverbal messages depend on its location, action, intensity, and duration, and, of course, how the patient perceives it. The moment a nurse touches a different part of the patient's body with a slightly different pressure or movement, sensory receptors are affected in new ways. These slight changes can create the potential for more or less sensitivity to touch, and for better or worse sensory relay of the touch to the brain.
4. Different patients must be touched differently. All patients' thresholds, perceptions, and reactions to touch are based on their attitudes toward touch and their vulnerability to its neurophysiologic effects. Some patients are exceptionally sensitive to even the slightest touch and have difficulty tolerating it. Such a response could be the result of abusive experiences earlier in life or some particular characteristic of their nervous system. Touching conducive to their well-being will not be the same as that appropriate for a patient with a high tolerance or need for physical contact.
5. A nurse's attitudes toward touch will affect how she touches, and how that touch is experienced by patients and family members. Nurses' own values, past experiences and cultural upbringing will all affect what is considered appropriate touching, and the boundaries of comfort when touching others. This is an often overlooked and underappreciated aspect of touching. It is imperative that all nurses be aware of their own attitudes about and comfort with touch to determine whether they are congruent with a patient's needs.

To implement these five principles, the nurse first performs a careful assessment of the patient's need for touch and what touch is most appropriate. The nurse then develops touch-specific goals and incorporates them into the plan of care. Interventions can be designed to achieve those specific goals, with periodic evaluation and modification as necessary.

ASSESSMENT

Assessment is, first and foremost, careful observation. To assess the patient's touch needs, the nurse observes three basic types of interactions: how family and friends touch the patient, how the patient responds when touched by other health care personnel, and how the patient responds to the nurse's touch.

How the patient's family normally touches him or her provides information about the kinds of touch the patient is accustomed to receiving and will accept. Keep in mind that loved ones may touch the patient differently if he or she is critically ill or attached to intimidating equipment, which may make them fearful of disrupting care and harming the patient. If this occurs, the nurse should try to determine why the family is touching differently. Unless there is a specific reason not to (as with Jessie in the case study), they should be encouraged to touch the patient frequently and spontaneously.

The nurse should also observe the patient's response to the touch of family, nurse, and other health care personnel. When touched, does the patient show or express positive or negative emotions? Does the patient withdraw from touch by moving his or her limbs or even entire body away from it? Or does he or she remain positively engaged while being touched, and even return the touch in some way, such as reaching out or hugging? What is the patient's cardiac or respiratory response during touch? If the patient is being monitored electronically for changes in vital signs, these responses will be easy to verify. In other patients, these physiologic responses may be so strong that the nurse can readily observe signs of rapid breathing or racing heartbeat. Changes in the patient's speech, including more or less speech, may also be evident, with a decided positive or negative content, and vocal changes, such as softer speech or higher pitch. The nurse needs to assess all of these signs within the context of the situation, and how all responses fit together as a whole.

The purpose of these observations is to determine whether patients want to be touched or not, and the types of touch with which they are comfortable. The nurse in the case study at the beginning of the chapter used extensive observation in her clinical decision making. This decision-making process is highlighted in the Clinical Decision Making box.

CLINICAL DECISION MAKING
TOUCH AND CARING FOR A DRUG-EXPOSED INFANT

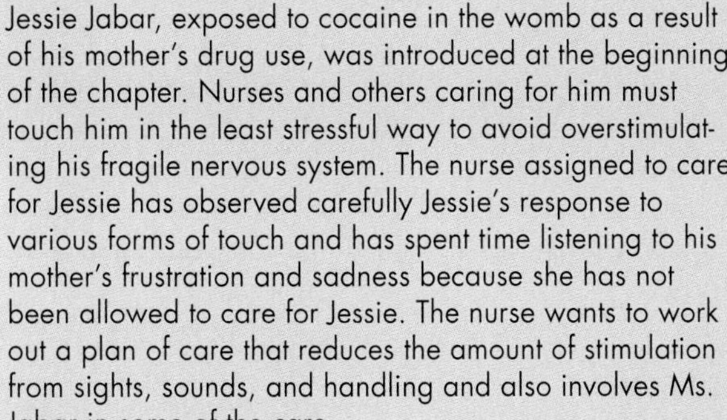

Jessie Jabar, exposed to cocaine in the womb as a result of his mother's drug use, was introduced at the beginning of the chapter. Nurses and others caring for him must touch him in the least stressful way to avoid overstimulating his fragile nervous system. The nurse assigned to care for Jessie has observed carefully Jessie's response to various forms of touch and has spent time listening to his mother's frustration and sadness because she has not been allowed to care for Jessie. The nurse wants to work out a plan of care that reduces the amount of stimulation from sights, sounds, and handling and also involves Ms. Jabar in some of the care.

RELEVANT QUESTIONS

Questions the nurse raises as clinical decision making progresses include:

- How must it feel to Jessie to be unable to control his limbs and be subjected to unexpected sounds and movements?
- What might touch from a nurse mean to Jessie? Would a routine pattern of care be best? What care is absolutely necessary?
- Could Ms. Jabar provide some of the care that required touch? If so, what preparation would she need?
- In addition to the apparent need to avoid overstimulation of Jessie's fragile nervous system, what other outcomes of care should be identified?
- How will Jessie communicate his response to care? What behaviors can be used to evaluate the effectiveness of the care plan?
- How do I feel about a mother who exposed her unborn child to cocaine and who may still be using drugs?
- Does Ms. Jabar feel guilty because of Jessie's condition? If so, will this influence her handling of Jessie? Does Ms. Jabar need help herself?
- What is Jessie's home environment?

KNOWLEDGE BASE

The nurse analyzed the following information to formulate tentative answers to the questions:

- Jessie is experiencing an erratic heart rate, rapid breathing with apneic periods, episodes of intense crying, and tremors. Past experience led the nurse to interpret these signs of physiological instability as indicators of "distress."
- In some contexts, Jessie's indicators of distress (particularly the crying and tremors) are more intense. The nurse noted the necessity for more observation to determine Jessie's unique needs.
- Ms. Jabar must have contact with Jessie to begin the bonding process.
- Touch is critical after birth because it affects brain development, cognitive functioning, social development, and attachment.
- Perceptions of touch are influenced by age, gender, and individual and family values. Even though Jessie may not have developed strong preferences yet, it is important to consider those of the mother.
- The five dimensions of touch (frequency, location, intensity, action, and duration) must be used skillfully with Jessie to avoid physical overstimulation and lack of adequate social stimulation.

CLINICAL DECISIONS

As the clinical decision-making process continues, the nurse debates key points and selects a course of action.

- The rationale for "minimal handling precautions" versus the mother's feelings about not being allowed to touch Jessie. The nurse respects the importance of the mother's caring for Jessie and decides to negotiate a role for the mother in Jessie's care. This requires careful construction of a rationale to obtain the support of other members of the health care team.
- The need for care that requires physical handling versus the distress caused by handling. The nurse reflects critically on specific patient situations and recalls Jessie's distress at being uncovered and his preferences for soft abdominal stroking. When Jessie was carefully wrapped in a blanket his brows relaxed and crying decreased. The nurse concludes that the routine plan of care will overstimulate Jessie's nervous system; instead, care must be individualized. These points of care are noted in the plan. By sharing observations and conclusions with the mother and other nurses, the nurse's practice is opened to critical reexamination and modification.
- Jessie's immediate need for skillful handling versus the long-term need for bonding with his mother. The nurse believes that Ms. Jabar is motivated to learn to handle Jessie and should be allowed to participate in his care. Ms. Jabar learns to observe Jessie's signs of distress: facial expression, crying, and tremors. The nurse then describes what she has learned about the best kinds of touch to use with Jessie, and which to avoid. Ms. Jabar goes with the nurse when care is given to Jessie so she can watch, learn, and apply various kinds of touch. The nurse and Ms. Jabar have daily conferences about Jessie's care.

The nurse may also find talking to patients themselves or their families about their comfort with touch very useful. The nurse might start the conversation with a statement like:

> We want to do everything we can to make your stay with us as positive as possible. So much of nursing care requires us to touch our patients. Some people like it, others don't. I want to care for you in a way that is most comfortable for you. Do you like to be handled gently or firmly? Do you enjoy backrubs?

Once the subject is broached, the nurse can follow up on the patient or family member's response for as much understanding and in as much detail as possible. Some people may not want to discuss this topic. If the nurse senses any hesitancy, she should not pursue the discussion further. As long as they sense the nurse's comfort with the topic, however, most patients and family members will usually readily share their own preferences and feelings.

The nursing assessment for touch must attend to the age, gender, family history, culture, and ethnicity of the individual patient. It must also include the patient's perception of his or her threshold for touch, strength of response to touch, and tolerance for touch. Each of these areas of assessment has been shown to affect the outcomes of the therapeutic use of touch.

OUTCOMES

Once the nurse has gathered enough information to make a preliminary assessment, a few outcomes for care focusing on touching the patient can be formulated. For instance, the outcome "keep oriented to time and place" could be identified in the plan of care for a patient who becomes confused. The nurse, following an assessment and conversation with family to determine the degree of touch that would be appropriate, would provide as much tender, caring touch as possible to help orient the patient to time and place.

In the situation of a baby that has frequent periods of apnea or crying following strong touch, the outcome of care would be to prevent or reduce those occurrences. The plan of care would indicate that outcome with the nursing action: "Avoid frequent touching or any vigorous stimulation of skin when providing care. The baby consistently becomes fussy and cries when touched."

Two very common outcomes of touch are reduced psychological distress and relaxation. These outcomes are significant in a wide range of nursing care situations. Reduced psychological distress can be an important outcome for a hospitalized child who feels abandoned by the parents, for a family member who has just lost a loved one, for a patient awaiting surgery, for a dying patient receiving hospice care, and for a mother experiencing a difficult labor. In each of these situations, touch can be used to reduce psychological distress. Relaxation is also an important outcome because it can promote healing as well as produce a desirable mental state. This might be an important outcome for a patient experiencing a series of stressful treatments, someone newly admitted to a hospital or a long-term care facility, an adolescent on bed rest for several weeks, or for a relative sitting next to the bed of a loved one who is unconscious.

In varying degrees, every patient health outcome is influenced by effective procedural or expressive touch. Touch is also associated with higher levels of patient satisfaction.

INTERVENTIONS

As detailed in the Knowledge Base section of this chapter, the nurse using touch as an intervention must consider:

- the five dimensions of touch (location, intensity, action, duration, frequency)
- the subjective perception of touch (threshold, strength of response, tolerance)
- individual differences (age, gender, family norms, culture, ethnicity)
- personal attitudes about touch

Touch may be required in the process of performing another nursing action or procedure. For example, touch is involved when helping a surgical patient walk shortly after completion of the surgery or when checking vital signs. Touch can also be an intervention in itself. For example, an elderly person who easily becomes confused can be helped to maintain reality orientation by the use of touch—not as a part of another nursing action but by itself. In both types of cases, the nurse should develop an intervention for the patient and family that reflects existing knowledge about touch.

The nurse must ensure that touch always conveys warmth and acceptance to the patient. The nurse can do this by being available for physical contact when sought by a patient, and by using nurturing or caring touch—not just procedural touch. These interventions may sound simple and obvious, but complex factors may come into play. For example, a nurse unaware of her or his own attitudes toward and comfort with touch may touch a patient in ways that meet her or his own needs, not the patient's needs. When caring for children who want to be cuddled and stroked during all procedures, a nurse conditioned by minimal touch in her or his own family may find it difficult to give these children the touch they need.

The challenge facing the nurse is to make the patient's well-being the top priority. Sometimes the nurse may not be able to meet the patient's needs for touch, regardless of a desire to provide the best care possible. The nurse needs to recognize and acknowledge those situations, and turn to a supervisor or coworker for help. It may be appropriate to be relieved from a specific assignment, allowing a different nurse who is a better fit with the patient's touch needs to take responsibility for care.

The nurse can ask herself or himself a few questions to better understand personal attitudes and feelings about touching. For instance: How much do I touch others? Do I want people to touch me? If so, who, when and how? Am I comfortable putting my arm around someone's shoulder or holding their hand? How would I feel if a patient hugged me? When do I feel most comfortable with touch? Least comfortable? Without a good understanding of her or his own responses to touch, a nurse will find it difficult to determine how to use touch effectively in patient care.

Procedures

The steps involved in giving a back massage are outlined in Procedure 32–1.

PROCEDURE 32-1

Giving a Back Massage

Objective

Provide relaxation, increase patient comfort, and stimulate circulation.

Terminology

- *effleurage*—long stroking motions used in giving a back massage
- *petrissage*—kneading motions used to relax muscles during the back massage

Critical Elements

Prior to administering a back massage, the care provider should assess the patient for the presence of dressings or suture lines, skin lesions, burns, arthritis, coagulation difficulties, or any other conditions that may be contraindicated when giving a back massage.

The care provider should perform a complete skin assessment prior to giving a back massage. Patients with very fragile skin (such as those on long-term steroid therapy), may need special consideration when administering a back massage, and firm kneading or stroking should be used with caution.

Patients with a history of elevated blood pressure or dysrhythmia should have vital signs assessed prior to a back massage. The stimulation received during the back massage may cause a response by the autonomic nervous system that in turn may cause a change in blood pressure or heart rate.

The ability of the patient to turn to the side or lie in a prone position may also be an influencing factor.

Lotion or oil is usually used in giving a back massage. If possible, this should be warmed prior to the back massage since the application of cold lotion can cause muscle tension. Although alcohol may cool the skin, it is also very drying and is therefore not recommended for back massages.

Always raise the bed to an appropriate height so the care provider does not experience back strain. Remember to lower the bed and leave the siderails up when the back massage is completed.

Equipment

- lotion/oil
- bath blanket

Special Considerations

The issue of touch is one that is very personal. It may be affected by such things as age, previous experience, cultural factors, and other things unknown to the care provider. Therefore the patient should always be asked whether he or she would like a back massage prior to initiating this procedure.

A back massage may be administered while giving a bath and is often done after cleansing the back. It may also be done as a method to help relax the patient at bedtime. Its use to help relax patients may help reduce the pharmacologic interventions needed for either pain or sleep at bedtime. Administering a back massage can be an effective means of administering passive exercise to the patient with limited mobility.

Nursing Interventions

Action	*Rationale*
1. Assemble equipment.	1. Promotes task organization.
2. Identify patient.	2. Provides for patient safety.
3. Explain procedure.	3. Promotes patient comfort with procedure.
4. Close door/curtain.	4. Protects patient privacy.
5. Position patient in side-lying position or prone.	5. Positions patient for back massage.
6. Fold back top linen and open patient gown to expose back.	6. Allows access to patient's back for procedure.
7. Apply lotion/oil to both hands and rub hands together.	7. Warms lotion/oil prior to application.

continued on next page

PROCEDURE 32-1 (cont'd)

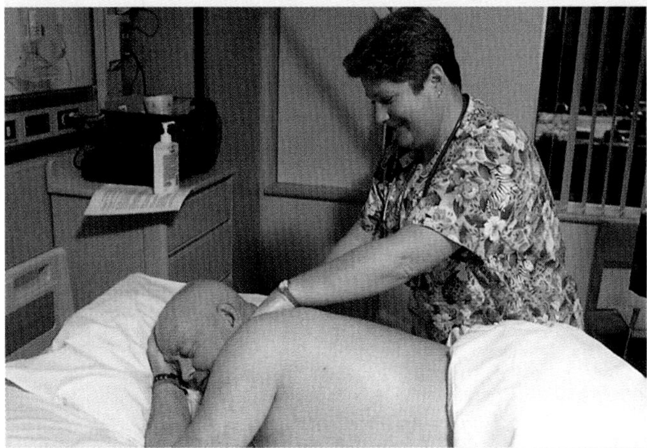

Figure 32–8. Back massage.

8. Start at sacral area and use slow effleurage strokes up central portion of back and down outer edges, including buttocks.	8. Provides relaxing movement.
9. Begin petrissage motion on area of shoulders and upper arms (Fig. 32–8).	9. Relaxes muscles in area where tension is often greatest.
10. Using smaller circular strokes, rub up back along central area and down sides, including buttocks.	10. Provides relaxation and circulatory stimulation.
11. Optional: Use gentle to moderate pressure from both hands (one hand on top of other) going up back over spinal column.	11. Provides relaxation and circulatory stimulation.
12. Continue back massage for 3 to 5 minutes.	12. Provides adequate time for patient relaxation as well as circulatory stimulation.
13. Assist patient back to position of comfort, closing gown, and replacing top linens.	13. Promotes patient comfort and warmth.
14. Discard or return supplies to appropriate place.	14. Provides for clean, organized work area.

Documentation

Record the procedure in the patient record including the patient's response as well as the care provider's assessment of the patient's skin integrity.

Elements of Patient Teaching

Instruct the patient and family about the purpose of the back massage. If the family will be doing this procedure for the patient, they must be instructed on any special considerations or limitations related to the patient's condition.

CHAPTER HIGHLIGHTS

- Touch can be task-oriented (procedural) or expressive.
- The effects of touch result from the degree to which it arouses the person's neurologic system and the personal and cultural meaning that the person applies to the various qualities of touch.
- Touch affects therapeutic relationships, psychological responses, and physiologic responses.
- Age, gender, family norms, culture, and ethnicity influence responses to touch.
- Assessment of an individual's response to the five dimensions of touch and perception of touch is critical to the use of touch as a nursing intervention.
- Touch is a powerful nursing intervention and influences the outcomes of care.
- Each nurse must be sensitive to his or her own attitudes and perceptions about touch.

REFERENCES

Affonso, D., Bosque, E., Wahlberg, V., Brady, J. (1993). Reconciliation and healing for mothers through skin-to-skin contact provided in an American tertiary level intensive care nursery. *Neonatal Network, 12,* 25–32.

Als, H., Lawton, G., Brown, E., et al (1986). Individualized behavioral and environmental care for the very low birth weight infant at high risk for bronchopulmonary dysplasia: Neonatal intensive care unit and developmental outcome. *Pediatrics, 78,* 1123.

Anderson, G.C. (1995). Touch and the kangaroo care method. In T. Field (ed.): *Touch in Early Development.* Mahwah, NJ: Lawrence Erlbaum Associates, Inc., pp. 35–51.

Anderson, J. (1986). Sensory intervention with the preterm infant in the neonatal intensive care unit. *American Journal of Occupational Therapy, 40* (1), 19–26.

Anisfeld, E., Casper, V., Nozyce, M., Cunningham, N. (1990). Does infant carrying promote attachment? An experimental study of the effects of increased physical contact on the development of attachment. *Child Development, 61* (5), 161–162.

Barnett, K. (1972). A survey of the current utilization of touch by health team personnel with hospitalized patients. *International Journal of Nursing Studies, 9,* 195–209.

Beaver, P. (1987). Premature infants' response to touch and pain: Can nurses make a difference? *Neonatal Network, 63* (3), 13–17.

Belsky, J., Rovine, M., Taylor, D. (1984). The origins of individual differences in infant-mother attachment: Maternal and infant contributions. *Child Development, 55,* 718–728.

Birch, E. (1986). The experience of touch received during labor: Postpartum perceptions of therapeutic value. *Journal of Nurse-Midwifery, 31* (6), 270–276.

Blackburn, S., Barnard, K. (1985). Analysis of caregiving events relating to preterm infants in the special care unit. In A.W. Gottfried and J.L. Gaiter (eds.): *Infant Stress Under Intensive Care.* Baltimore: University Park Press, pp. 113–129.

Boguslawski, M. (1980). Therapeutic touch: A facilitator of pain relief. *Topics in Clinical Nursing, 2,* 27–37.

Bowlby, J. (1988). *A Secure Base: Parent-child Attachment and Healthy Human Development.* New York: Basic Books.

Boyle, J., Andrews, M. (1989). *Transcultural Concepts in Nursing Care.* Glenview, IL: Scott, Foreman/Little Brown.

Burton, H., Sathian, K., Shao, D. (1990). Altered responses to cutaneous stimuli in the second somatosensory cortex following lesions of the postcentral gyrus in infant and juvenile macaques. *Journal of Comparative Neurology, 291* (3), 395–414.

Cannon, R.B. (1977). The development of maternal touch during early mother-infant interaction. *Journal of Obstetric, Gynecologic, and Neonatal Nursing, 6* (2), 28–33.

Casher, L., Dixson, B. (1967). The therapeutic use of touch. *Journal of Psychiatric Nursing, 5* (5), 442–451.

Curry, M.A. (1982). Maternal attachment behavior and mother's self-concept. The effect of early skin-to-skin contact, *Nursing Research, 31,* 73–78.

Diamond, M. (1990). Evidence for tactile stimulation improving CNS function. In K. Barnard and T.B. Brazelton (eds.): *Touch: The Foundation of Experience.* Madison, CT: International Universities Press, pp. 73–96.

Estabrooks, C. (1989). Touch: A nursing strategy in the intensive care unit. *Heart and Lung, 18* (4), 392–401.

Estabrooks, C., Morse, J. (1992). Toward a theory of touch: The touching process and acquiring a touching style. *Journal of Advanced Nursing,* 17, 448–456.

Fakouri, C., Jones, P. (1987). Relaxation Rx: Slow stroke back rub. *Journal of Gerontological Nursing, 13* (2), 32–35.

Fanslow, C. (1981). Death: A natural facet of the life continuum. In D. Krieger (ed.): *Foundations for Holistic Health Nursing Practices, the Renaissance Nurse.* Philadelphia: J.B. Lippincott, pp. 249–271.

Fanslow, C. (1983). Therapeutic touch: A healing modality throughout life. *Topics in Clinical Nursing, 3,* 72–79.

Fanslow, C. (1990). Touch and the elderly. In K. Barnard and T.B. Brazelton (eds.): *Touch: The Foundation of Experience.* Madison, CT: International Universities Press, pp. 541–557.

Field, T. (1987). Alleviating stress in ICU neonates. In N. Gunzenhauser (ed.): *Infant Stimulation.* Biscayne Bay, FL: Johnson and Johnson, pp. 121–128.

Frank, J., Levinson, H. (1973). Dysmetric dyslexia and dyspraxia. *Journal of the American Academy of Child Psychiatry, 12,* 690–701.

Garcia-Coll, C. (1990). Developmental outcomes of minority infants: A process-oriented look into our beginnings. *Child Development, 61,* 270–289.

Goodykoontz, L. (1980). Touch: Dynamic aspect of nursing care. *Journal of Nursing Care, 13* (6), 16–18.

Gorski, P., Leonard, C., Sweet, D., et al. (1984). Caregiver-infant interaction and the immature nervous system. In C.C. Brown (ed.): *The Many Faces of Touch.* Skillman, NJ: Johnson and Johnson, pp. 84–90.

Gorski, P., Huntington, L., Lewkowicz, D. (1990). Handling preterm infants in hospitals: Stimulating controversy about timing of stimulation. *Clinics in Perinatology, 1* (1), 103–112.

Greenough, W. (1990). Brain storage of information from cutaneous and other modalities in development and adulthood. In K. Barnard and T.B. Brazelton (eds.): *Touch: The Foundation of Experience.* Madison, CT: International Universities Press, pp. 97–126.

Grossman, K., Spangler, G., Suess, G., Unzer, L. (1985). Maternal sensitivity and newborn's orientation responses as related to quality of attachment in northern Germany. In I. Bretherton and E. Waters (eds.): *Growing Points of Attachment.* Monographs of the Society for Research in Child Development, Serial 209, *50,* 1–2.

Gunnar, M., Isensee, J., Fust, L. (1987). Adrenocortical activity and the Brazelton Neonatal Assessment Scale: Moderating effects of the newborn's biomedical status. *Child Development, 58* (6), 1448–1458.

Hamman, W., Iggo, A. (1984). *Sensory Receptor Mechanisms.* Singapore: World Scientific Publishing Co.

Hansen, R., Ulrey, G. (1988). Motorically impaired infants: Impact of a massage procedure on caregiver-infant interactions. *Journal of the Multihandicapped Person, 1* (1), 61–68.

Harlow, H. (1958). The nature of love. *American Psychologist, 13,* 673–685.

Harrison, L., Leeper, J., Yoon, M. (1990). Effects of early parent touch on preterm infants' heart rates and arterial oxygen saturation levels. *Journal of Advanced Nursing, 15,* 877–885.

Harrison, L., Woods, S. (1991). Early parental touch and preterm infants. *Journal of Obstetric, Gynecologic and Neonatal Nursing, 20* (4), 299–306.

Helders, P., Cats, B., van der Net, J., Debast, S. (1988). The effects of a tactile stimulation/range-finding program on the development of very low birth weight infants during initial hospitalization. *Child: Care, Health and Development, 14* (5), 341–354.

Hill, C.F. (1993). Is massage beneficial to critically ill patients in intensive care units? A critical review. *Intensive and Critical Care Nursing, 9,* 116–121.

Hill, S.T., Shronk, L.K. (1979). The effect of early parent-infant contact on newborn body temperature. *Journal of Obstetric, Gynecologic and Neonatal Nursing,* 8, 287–290.

Hochreiter, N., Jewell, M., Barber, L., Browne, P. (1983). Effect of vibration on tactile sensitivity. *Physical Therapy, 63,* 934–937.

Hofer, M. (1987). Early social relationships: A psychobiologist's view. *Child Development, 58,* 633–647.

Hofer, M. (1981). *The Roots of Human Behavior.* San Francisco: W.H. Freeman.

Hopkins, J. (1987). Failure of the holding relationship: Some effects of physical rejection on the child's attachment and his inner experience. *Journal of Child Psychotherapy, 13,* 5–17.

Huntley, G. (1997). Differential effects of abnormal tactile experience on shaping representation patterns in developing and adult motor cortex. *Journal of Neuroscience,* 17 (23), 9220–9232.

Hunziker, U., Barr, R. (1986). Increased carrying reduces infant crying: A randomized controlled trial. *Pediatrics, 77* (5), 641– 648.

Immelmann, K., Suomi, S. (1981). Sensitive phases in development. In K. Immelmann, G. Barlow, L. Petrinovich, and M. Main (eds.): *Behavioral Development: The Bielefeld Interdisciplinary Project.* New York: Cambridge University Press.

Jandt, F. (1995). *Intercultural communication.* Thousand Oaks, CA: Sage Publications, Inc.

Jay, S. (1982). The effects of gentle human touch on mechanically ventilated very-short-gestation infants (Monograph 12). *Maternal-Child Nursing Journal, 11,* 199–256.

Juni, S., Brannon, R. (1981). Interpersonal touching as a function of status and sex. *Journal of Social Psychology, 114,* 135–136.

Kaitz, M., Lapidot, P., Bronner, R., Eidelman, A.I. (1992). Parturient women can recognize their infants by touch. *Developmental Psychology, 28,* 35–39.

Kaas, J., Merzenich, M., Killackey, H. (1983). The recognition of somatosensory cortex following peripheral nerve damage in adult and developing mammals. *Annual Review of Neuroscience, 6,* 325–356.

Keller, E., Bzdek, V.M. (1986). Effects of therapeutic touch on tension headache pain. *Nursing Research, 35,* 101–106.

Knable, J. (1981). Handholding: One means of transcending barriers of communication. *Heart and Lung,* 10, 1106–1110.

Koniak-Griffin, D., Ludington-Hoe, S. (1988). Developmental and temperamental outcomes of sensory stimulation in healthy infants. *Nursing Research,* 37 (2), 70–76.

Kopp, C. (1982). Antecedents of self-regulation: A developmental perspective. *Developmental Psychology, 18* (2), 199–214.

Korner, A. (1990). The many faces of touch. In K. Barnard and T.B. Brazelton (eds.): *Touch: The Foundation of Experience.* Madison, CT: International Universities Press, pp. 269–297.

Krieger, D. (1979). The therapeutic touch: How to use your hands to help or heal. Englewood Cliffs, NJ: Prentice-Hall.

Krieger, D. (1981). *Foundations of Holistic Health: Nursing Practice.* Philadelphia: J.B. Lippincott Co.

Krieger, D. (1975). Therapeutic touch: The imprimatur of nursing. *American Journal of Nursing, 5,* 784–787.

Krieger, D., Peper, E., Ancoli, S. (1979). Searching for evidence of physiological change. *American Journal of Nursing, 4,* 660–662.

Kunz, D., Peper, E. (1982). Fields and their clinical implications. *American Theosophist, 70,* 395–440.

Langland, R.M., Panicucci, C.L. (1982). Effects of touch on communication with elderly confused clients. *Journal of Gerontological Nursing,* 8, 152–155.

Legault M., Goulet C. (1995). Comparison of kangaroo and traditional methods of removing preterm infants from incubators. *Journal of Obstetric, Gynecologic, and Neonatal Nursing, 24,* 501–506.

Leininger, M. (1978). *Transcultural Nursing: Concepts, Theories and Practices.* New York: John Wiley and Sons.

Levine, S., Stanton, M. (1990). The hormonal consequences of mother-infant contact. In K. Barnard and T.B. Brazelton (eds.): *Touch: The Foundation of Experience.* Madison, CT: International Universities Press, pp. 165–193.

Lewis, R.J., Derlega, V.J., Nichols, B., et al (1995). Sex differences in observers' reactions to a nurse's use of touch. *Journal of Nonverbal Behavior, 19,* 101–113.

Long, J., Philip, A., Lucey, J. (1980). Excessive handling as a cause of hypoxemia. *Pediatrics, 65* (2), 203–207.

Longworth, J.C.D. (1982). Psychophysiological effects of slow stroke back massage in normotensive females. *Advances in Nursing Science, 4* (4), 44–61.

Lozoff, B., Brittenham, G. (1979). Infant care: Cache or carry. *Journal of Pediatrics, 95,* 478–483.

Lynch, T.J., Flaherty, L., Emrich, C., et al (1974). The effect of human contact on the heart activity of curarized patients in a shock-trauma unit. *American Heart Journal, 88,* 160–169.

Lynch, J.J., Thomas, S.A., Paskewitz, D., et al (1977). Human contact and cardiac arrhythmia in a coronary care unit. *Psychosomatic Medicine,* 39, 188–192.

Maccoby, E., Jacklin, C. (1974). *The psychology of sex differences.* Stanford: Stanford University Press.

Macrae, J. (1979). Therapeutic touch in practice. *American Journal of Nursing,* 4, 664–665.

Main, M. (1990). Parental aversion to infant-initiated contact is correlated with the parents' own rejection during childhood: The effects of experience on signals of security with respect to attachment. In K. Barnard and T.B. Brazelton (eds.): *Touch: The Foundation of Experience.* Madison, CT: International Universities Press, pp. 461–495.

Main, M., George, C. (1985). Response of abused and disadvantaged toddlers to distress in arguments: A study in the day care setting. *Developmental Psychology, 21* (3), 407–412.

Main, M., Goldwyn, R. (1984). Predicting rejection of her infant from mother's representation of her own experience: Implications for the abused-abusing intergenerational cycle. *Child Abuse and Neglect,* 8, 203–217.

Main, M., Kaplan, N., Cassidy, J. (1985). Security in infancy, childhood and adulthood: A move to the level of representation. In I. Bretherton and E. Waters (eds.): *Growing points of attachment theory and research.* Monograph of the Society for Research in Child Development, Vol. 50, #1–2. Chicago: University of Chicago Press.

Main, M., Stadtman, J. (1981). Infant response to rejectional physical contact by the mother: Aggression, avoidance and conflict. *Journal of the American Academy of Child Psychology, 202,* 292–307.

Main, M., Weston, D. (1981). The quality of the toddlers relationship to mother and father: Related conflict behavior and the readiness to establish new relationships. *Child Development, 52,* 932–940.

McAnarney, E. (1990). Adolescents and touch. In K. Barnard and T.B. Brazelton (eds.): *Touch: The Foundation of Experience.* Madison, CT: International Universities Press, pp. 497–515.

McBride, M.R., Mistretta, C.M. (1982). Light touch thresholds in diabetic patients. *Diabetes Care, 5,* 311–315.

McKenna, J., Mosko, S., Dungy, C., McAninch, J. (1990). Sleep and arousal patterns of co-sleeping mother/infant pairs: A preliminary physiologic study with implications for the study of sudden infant death syndrome (SIDS). *American Journal of Physical Anthropology, 83* (3), 331–347.

Medoff-Cooper, B. (1988). The effects of handling on preterm infants with bronchopulmonary dysplasia. *Image, 20* (3), 132–134.

Meek, S.S. (1993). Effects of slow stroke back massage on relaxation in hospice clients. Image: *Journal of Nursing Scholarship, 25,* 17–21.

Merleau-Ponty, M. (1962). *The Phenomenology of Perception* (translated by C. Smith). New York: Humanities Press.

Merzenich, M. (1990). Development and maintenance of cortical somatosensory representations: Functional "maps" and neuroanatomical repertoires. In K. Barnard and T.B. Brazelton (eds.): *Touch: The Foundation of Experience.* Madison, CT: International Universities Press, pp. 47–72.

Mills, M., Thomas, S., Lynch, J., Katcher, A. (1976). Effect of pulse palpation on cardiac arrhythmia in coronary care patients. *Nursing Research 25,* 378–382.

Mitchell, P., Habermann-Little, B., Johnson, F., Van Inwegen-Scott, D., Tyler, D. (1985). Critically ill children: The importance of touch in a high technology environment. *Nursing Administration Quarterly, 9* (4), 38–46.

Monrroy, L. (1983). Nursing care of Raza/Latina patients. In M. Orque, B. Block, L. Monrroy (eds.): *Ethnic nursing care: A multicultural approach.* St. Louis: C.V. Mosby, pp. 115–148.

Montagu, A. (1971). *Touching: The human significance of the skin.* New York: Columbia University Press.

Moore, J., Gilbert, D. (1995). Elderly residents: Perceptions of nurses' comforting touch. *Journal of Gerontological Nursing, 21,* 6–13.

Morse, J. (1983). An ethnoscientific analysis of comfort: A preliminary investigation. *Nursing Papers: The Canadian Journal of Nursing Research, 15* (1), 6–19.

Nicolelis, L., DeOliveira, R., Lin, R., et al (1996). Active tactile exploration influences the functional maturation of the somatosensory system. Journal of Neurophysiology, *75*(5), 2192–2196.

Norris, S. Campbell, L., Brenkert, S. (1982). Nursing procedures and alterations in transcutaneous oxygen tension in premature infants. *Nursing Research, 31,* 330–336.

Nurmikko, T. (1991). Altered cutaneous sensation in trigeminal neuralgia. *Archives of Neurology, 48, 523–527.*

Oehler, J. (1985). Examining the issue of tactile stimulation for preterm infants. *Neonatal Network, 4* (3), 25–32.

Pettigrew, J. (1990). Intensive nursing care: The ministry of presence. *Critical Care Nursing Clinics of North America, 2* (3), 503–508.

Pineau, A., Streri, A. (1990). Internodal transfer of spatial arrangement of the component parts of an object in infants aged 4–5 months. *Perception, 19* (6), 95–804.

Polan H., Ward M. (1994). Role of the mother's touch in failure to thrive: A preliminary investigation. *Journal of the American Academy of Child and Adolescent Psychiatry, 33,* 1098.

Quinn, J. (1984). Therapeutic touch as energy exchange: Testing the theory. *Advances in Nursing Science, 6,* 42–49.

Rausch, P. (1981). Effects of tactile and kinesthetic stimulation in premature infants. *Journal of Obstetric, Gynecologic, and Neonatal Nursing,* 10, 34–37.

Reite, M., Capitanio, J. (1985). On the nature of social separation and social attachment. In M. Reite and T. Field (eds.): *The Psychobiology of Attachment.* New York: Academic Press, pp. 223–258.

Robinson, D. (1986). On the biological determination of personality structure. *Personality and Individual Differences, 7* (3), 435–438.

Rose, S. (1990). Perception and cognition in preterm infants: The sense of touch. In K. Barnard and T.B. Brazelton (eds.), *Touch: The Foundation of Experience.* Madison, CT: International Universities Press, pp. 299–323.

Royeen, C. (1986). The development of a touch scale for measuring tactile defensiveness in children. *American Journal of Occupational Therapy, 40* (6), 414–419.

Scafidi, F., Field, T., Schanberg, S., et al (1986). Effects of tactile/kinesthetic stimulation on the clinical course and sleep-wake behavior of preterm neonates. *Infant Behavior and Development,* 9, 91–105.

Schaefer, J. (1981). *The Relationship Between Attributes of Nurses and Their Use of Affective Touch.* Unpublished master's thesis. Seattle: University of Washington.

Schanberg, S., Evoniuk, G., Kuhn, C. (1984). Tactile and nutritional aspects of maternal care: Specific regulators of neuroendocrine functions and cellular development. *Proceedings of the Society for Experimental Biology and Medicine, 175,* 135–146.

Schmidt, R. (1986). *Fundamentals of Sensory Physiology.* New York: Springer-Verlag.

Schneider-Rosen, K., Braunwald, K, Carlson, V., Cicchetti, D. (1985). Current perspectives in attachment theory: Illustration from the study of maltreated infants. In I. Bretherton and E. Waters (eds.): *Growing points of attachment theory and research.* Monographs of the Society of Research in Child Development, Serial #209, vol. 50, #1–2.

Seaman, L. (1982). Affective nursing touch. *Geriatric Nursing, 3* (3), 162–164.

Simington, J.A., Laing, G.P. (1993). Effects of therapeutic touch on anxiety in the institutionalized elderly. *Clinical Nursing Research, 4,* 438–450.

Smith, J. (1990). Therapeutic touch: A critical appraisal. In K. Barnard and T.B. Brazelton (eds.): *Touch: The Foundation of Experience.* Madison, CT: International Universities Press, pp. 405–422.

Smutkupt, S., Barna, L.M. (1976). Impact of nonverbal communication in an intercultural setting: Thailand. *International and Intercultural Communication Annual,* 3, 130–138.

Spitz, R. (1945). Hospitalism—An inquiry into the genesis of psychiatric conditions of early childhood. *Psychoanalytic Study of the Child,* 1, 53–74.

Stern, D. (1988). Affect in the context of the infant's lived experience: Some considerations. *International Journal of Psychoanalysis, 69,* 233–238.

Suomi, S. (1990). The role of tactile contact in rhesus monkey social development. In K. Barnard and T.B. Brazelton (eds.): *Touch: The Foundation of Experience.* Madison, CT: International Universities Press, pp. 129–164.

Suomi, S. (1997). Early determinants of behavior: Evidence from primate studies. *British Medical Bulletin,* 53 (1), 170–184.

Thurman, S., Korteland, C. (1989). The behavior of mothers and fathers toward their infants during neonatal intensive care visits. *Children's Health Care, 18* (4), 247–251.

Tobiason, S. (1981). Touching is for everyone. *American Journal of Nursing,* 81, 728–730.

Tomlinson, P., Rothenberg, M., Carver, L. (1991). Behavioral interaction of fathers with infants and mothers in the immediate postpartum period. *Journal of Nurse-Midwifery, 36* (1), 232–239.

Toney, L. (1982). The effects of holding the newborn at delivery on paternal bonding. *Nursing Research,* 32, 16–19.

Troy N. (1993). Early contact and maternal attachment among women using public health care facilities. *Applied Nursing Research, 6,* 161–166.

Turkewitz, J., Kenny, P. (1982). Limitations on input as a basis for neural organization and perceptual development: A preliminary theoretical statement. *Developmental Psychobiology, 15,* 357–368.

Vinik, A., Stansberry, K., Suwanwalaikorn, S., et al (1995). Quantitative measurement of cutaneous perception in diabetic neuropathy. *Muscle and Nerve, 18,* 574–584.

Vortherms, R. (1991). Clinically improving communication through touch. *Journal of Gerontological Nursing, 1* (5), 6–10.

Weber, R. (1990). A philosophical perspective on touch. In K. Barnard and T.B. Brazelton (eds.): *Touch: The Foundation of Experience.* Madison, CT: International Universities Press, pp. 11–43.

Weiner, I., Schnabel, I., Lubow, R., Feldon, J. (1985). The effects of early handling on latent inhibition in male and female rats. *Developmental Psychobiology, 18,* 291–297.

Weiss, S. (1979). The language of touch. *Nursing Research, 28* (2), 76–80.

Weiss, S. (1986). Psychophysiologic effects of caregiver touch on incidence of cardiac arrhythmia. *Heart & Lung, 15* (5), 495–506.

Weiss, S. (1990a). Effects of differential touch on nervous system arousal of patients recovering from cardiac disease. *Heart & Lung, 19* (4), 474–480.

Weiss, S. (1990b). Parental touching: Correlates of body image in children. In K. Barnard and T.B. Brazelton (eds.): *Touch: The Foundation of Experience.* Madison, CT: International Universities Press, pp. 425–460.

Weiss, S. (1992a). The tactile environment of caregiving: Implications for health science and health care. *The Science of Caring,* 3 (2), 33–40.

Weiss, S. (1992b). Psychophysiologic and behavioral effects of tactile stimulation on infants with congenital heart disease. *Research in Nursing and Health,* 15 (2), 93–101.

Weiss, S. (1993). Familial touch and perceptual reactivity of children with severe mental illness. In L. Chafetz (ed.): *New Directions for Mental Health Services: A Nursing Perspective on Severe Mental Illness,* pp. 53–64.

Whitcher, S., Fisher, J. (1979). Multidimensional reaction to therapeutic touch in a hospital setting. *Journal of Personality and Social Psychology, 37* (1), 87–96.

Widstrom, A., Wahlberg, V., Matthlesen, A., et al (1990). Short-term effects of early suckling and touch of the nipple on maternal behavior. *Early Human Development, 21* (3), 153–163.

Willis, F., Hofmann, G. (1975). Development of tactile patterns in relation to age, sex, and race. *Developmental Psychology, 11,* 866.

Wirth, D. (1990). The effect of noncontact therapeutic touch on the healing rate of full thickness dermal wounds. *Subtle Energies,* 1, 1–20.

Wolfson, I. (1990). Therapeutic touch and midwifery. In K. Barnard and T.B. Brazelton (eds.): *Touch: The Foundation of Experience.* Madison, CT: International Universities Press, pp. 383–403.

Wyschograd, E. (1981). Empathy and sympathy as tactile encounter. *Journal of Philosophy, 6,* 25–43.

33 Sexual Health Protection and Health Promotion

Diana L. Taylor, Nancy Fugate Woods, and Judith A. Berg

OBJECTIVES

After studying this chapter, the student will be able to:

- **use a holistic framework, i.e., one that includes biopsychosocial, cultural, and lifespan dimensions in assessment and treatment of health concerns for men and women**
- **incorporate individual differences, gender, and contextual dimensions in clinical decision making**
- **implement health protection and health promotion principles specific to men's and women's health**
- **implement practice guidelines for sexual health assessment (sexual history, physical assessment) and sexual health promotion (contraception and sexually transmitted infection [STI] prevention, male/female self-examination)**
- **assess personal readiness to implement nursing care specific to men's and women's sexual health**

Lucy, age 17 and Zack, age 18, come to the health clinic to discuss sexual concerns, including pregnancy, birth control, and sexually transmitted infections (STI). Lucy tells the nurse that she and Zack have been dating for 3 months, and that lately he has been pressuring her to have sex. Lucy reports one previous sexual experience, during which she was infected with human papilloma virus (HPV). At that time, the nurse at the STI clinic told her that because of this infection she is more susceptible to other STIs.

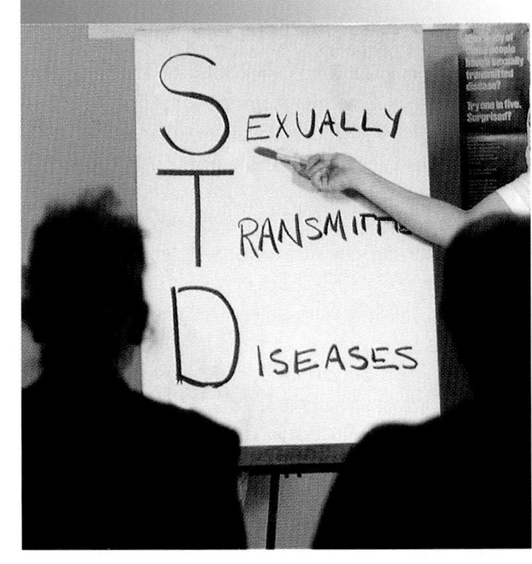

Now Lucy expresses worries about contracting acquired immunodeficiency syndrome (AIDS) or becoming pregnant. She asks for birth control counseling and information about protecting herself from acquiring sexually transmitted infections. She tells the nurse that Zack doesn't want to use a condom because he loves her and wants her to have his baby.

Lucy feels she can't talk with her parents and has moved in with her grandmother due to her parents' drug use. Now, she also finds herself unable to have a serious discussion with Zack about her fears or about her anger at him for pressuring her to have sex and ignoring her concerns.

The nurse identifies numerous health issues and also remains sensitive to Lucy's priorities. The nurse asks Lucy to return to the clinic for a follow-up exam and colposcopy necessary to determine the outcome of the treatment for HPV. She also makes separate appointments for Lucy and Zack. She assures Lucy that she will help her attain the knowledge she wants and support her in decision making.

SCOPE OF NURSING PRACTICE

Health for women and men has come to mean more than reproductive health and more than freedom from disease. Health from a perspective of individual women and men is defined in terms of attaining, retaining, and regaining an optimal sense of well-being (Fogel and Woods, 1995; Griffith-Kenney, 1986).

Women's health has traditionally been defined in reproductive terms, and men's health has been defined in terms of specific diseases. An expanded definition of women's and men's health includes (1) women's and men's health experiences across the lifespan; (2) women's and men's health in relation to the environment; and (3) the processes of attaining, maintaining, and regaining health as women and men experience it (Fogel and Woods, 1995; Woods, 1988). This conceptualization of women's and men's health considers physical, psychosocial, and sexual well-being in the context of the interpersonal, socioeconomic, political, and environmental context in which the individual operates (McBride and McBride, 1981). The interplay between health, self, body, and gender at the individual level is linked to the creation of a sense of healthiness in the body politic of society (Saltonstall, 1993).

The knowledge base in this chapter includes two content areas:

- the relationship of gender to health
- the nurse's role in sexual health protection and promotion

The interaction of gender and sexuality forms the basis for men's and women's health and illness responses as uniquely male or female. Gender is a term that refers to sexual identity, either male or female. Sexuality is an important dimension of the human personality. It is an integrated, unique expression of the self that encompasses the physiologic and psychosocial processes inherent in sexual development and sexual response (Fogel, 1990).

Gender and sexuality aspects of health cross all dimensions of nursing care for individuals across the lifespan. Every nursing encounter requires the nurse to consider the impact of gender on health and illness. For example, the married mother of two small children finds out that she has seriously high blood pressure. The blood pressure cannot be assessed or treated effectively without a broad holistic framework that includes understanding the impact of gender.

In addition, in outpatient, clinic, hospital, long-term care, and home settings, nurses implement specific practices that incorporate principles of primary, secondary, and tertiary prevention in women's and men's sexual health. These practices include counseling, educating, supporting, and direct care actions for individuals, families, partners, and communities.

KNOWLEDGE BASE

The knowledge base essential to men's and women's health must consider various biologic, psychosocial, and cultural factors related to gender, sexuality, and sexual health (Fogel, 1990). Nursing has traditionally been the health profession most concerned with the total person, and this biopsychosocial approach takes a holistic view of patients that encompasses attention to sexuality, gender, and sexual health as well as alterations in sexual health.

Sexuality

An important dimension of the human personality, sexuality is an integrated, unique expression of the self that encompasses the physiologic and psychosocial processes inherent in sexual development and response. Sexuality underlies much of who and what a person is, and is a significant aspect of identity throughout life.

Definitions and descriptions of human sexuality are varied, complex, and at times, vague. Sexuality is not just overt sexual behavior, nor is it only an anatomic assignment of gender. It is a deep, pervasive aspect of the total human personality, present in some degree from birth until life's last moment. Sexuality encompasses an individual's particular way of being male or female.

Because sexuality involves much more than sexual activity or sexual functioning, it underlies the complete range of human experience and contributes to our lives in many ways. To understand human sexuality and its expression, nurses must examine biologic, psychological, and sociocultural factors. These categories are not mutually exclusive, but rather overlap and intertwine.

Sexual Health

Defining healthy sexual functioning is difficult, because health is a value that changes, just as other social and cultural values change. Many people do not even consider what sexual health is until its absence is noted. According to the World Health Organization (WHO, 1975), sexual health is *the integration of the somatic, emotional, intellectual, and social aspects of sexual beings in ways that are positively enriching and that enhance personality, communication, and love.* Though this definition may not be compatible with all individuals' view of sexuality because of the word "love," it does have strengths. It encompasses the following elements:

- capacity to enjoy and control sexual and reproductive behavior in accordance with a social and personal ethic
- freedom from fear, shame, guilt, false beliefs, and other psychological factors that inhibit sexual response and impair sexual relationships
- freedom from organic disorders, disease and deficiencies that interfere with sexual and reproductive functions

In essence, sexual health may be considered the physical and emotional state of well-being that enables us to enjoy and act on our sexual feelings (Boston Women's Health Book Collective, 1985; Fogel, 1990).

Biologic Basis for Women's and Men's Sexual Health

The biologic basis for women's and men's sexual health begins with the genetic determination of gender at the moment of conception, when either the X or the Y chromosome in the sperm unites with the X chromosome of the female egg. The XX chromosomal combination produces a female; the XY combination, a male. The Y chromosome appears to directly influence body growth, skeletal muscle maturation, and the slower growth rate in boys; this appears to be caused by the testes-determining genes localized in the Y chromosome. The only established effect of the Y chromosome is to determine maleness (Rynerson, 1990).

In males and females, reproductive organs are located internally as well as externally. Internal organs are involved with reproduction (spermatogenesis and oogenesis), whereas the external organs function primarily in physical or sexual pleasure.

MALE REPRODUCTIVE SYSTEM

Male external reproductive organs include the penis, testes, and scrotum (Fig. 33–1); internal organs include the prostate, seminal vesicles, and bulbourethral glands (Fig. 33–2).

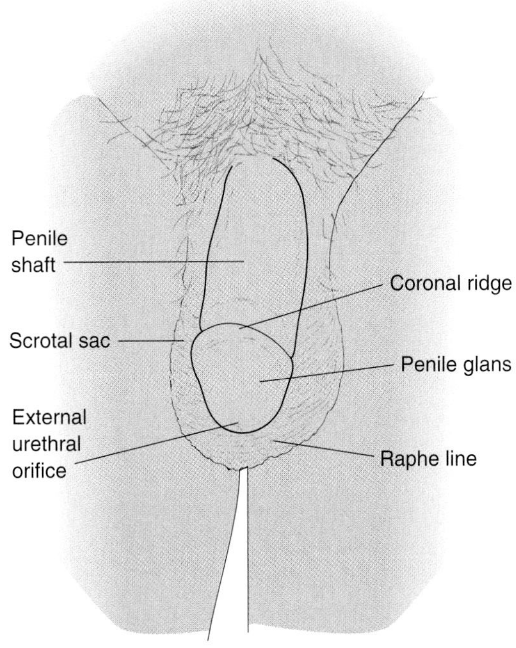

Figure 33–1. Male genitalia.

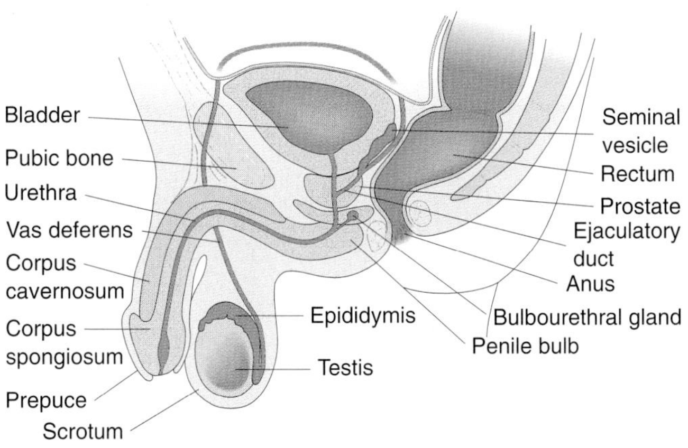

Figure 33–2. Male internal reproductive organs.

PENIS

The penis consists of two sections: the shaft and the glans. Three cylindrical bodies of erectile tissue compose the penile shaft: two corpora cavernosa and the corpus spongiosum (see Fig. 33–2). The corpora cavernosa are located dorsally; the corpus spongiosum is located ventrally and contains the urethra (Rynerson, 1990). Erectile tissue is made up of an irregular network of potential vascular spaces, which are connected to arteries and veins. These vascular spaces are empty when the penis is in the flaccid state. In response to sexual excitement, blood flows into the spaces due to arteriolar dilation and increased hydraulic pressure, producing an erection. Once orgasm has been achieved, the penis returns to a flaccid state as blood flows back out of the vascular spaces (Rynerson, 1990).

The rounded distal portion of the penis, the glans is highly sensitive due to its rich supply of nerve endings. It is covered by the foreskin, or prepuce. In many males, the foreskin is removed in a surgical procedure known as circumcision. The foreskin is normally retractable, and does not interfere with sexual pleasure. A substance known as smegma is produced under the foreskin; this has no known function.

SCROTUM AND TESTES

The scrotum is a thin sac of skin forming a pouch. The outermost layer of scrotal skin appears darker than the body and contains sweat glands. An inner layer is composed of involuntary muscle that contracts with sexual excitement, cold, or exercise; that same tissue relaxes in heat, such as in hot weather or in a hot bath. The contracting and relaxing of this inner layer of scrotal tissue serves an adaptive, protective function, because sperm are very sensitive to extreme temperatures.

The scrotal sac is partitioned into two compartments, each having a testis, epididymis, and spermatic cord. The spermatic cord, which includes the vas deferens and an abundant supply of blood vessels, nerves, and muscle fibers, supports the testis. The vas deferens is the passage through which the sperm travel from the scrotum to an ejaculatory duct.

The testes are responsible for the production of sperm and the secretion of the male hormone, testosterone. The spermatozoa are produced in the seminiferous tubules, leave the testes to mature in the epididymis, and exit the epididymis via the vas deferens. The vas enters the abdominal cavity, passes posterior to the bladder, and empties into the ejaculatory duct. Approximately 20 percent of the ejaculate comes from the vas deferens (Rynerson, 1990).

Testosterone, the male sex hormone, is produced by Leydig cells located between the seminiferous tubules in the scrotum. A dysfunction in the seminiferous tubules will not affect the production of testosterone; however, spermatogenesis depends on normal testosterone production.

INTERNAL SEX ORGANS

The prostate gland is located inferior to the bladder; it produces an alkaline prostatic fluid that is important in protecting sperm from the acidity of the vagina. Prostatic fluid makes up approximately 20 percent of the semen, or ejaculate.

Seminal vesicles are a pair of vesicles that are located posterior to the prostate. They join at the vas deferens to form the ejaculatory duct. They produce a seminal fluid that makes up about 60 percent of semen. This fluid consists of an activating principle, fructose, and prostaglandins. Activating principle transforms sperm from an immobile to a mobile state, while fructose provides the sperm energy. The prostaglandins may stimulate sufficient uterine contractions to enhance sperm migration to the fallopian tubes (Rynerson, 1990).

The bulbourethral, or Cowper's, glands are located inferior to the prostate. They secrete a small amount of a preejaculatory fluid, also alkaline in nature, that protects the sperm from the acidity in the urethra. It is possibly this protective, neutralizing action that accounts for the presence of isolated sperm from a previous ejaculate in the preejaculatory fluid (Rynerson, 1990). It was previously believed that this preejaculatory fluid had sufficient motile sperm to cause pregnancy; however, more recent research suggests that this fluid can contain human immunodeficiency virus (HIV) but not motile sperm capable of causing pregnancy (Pudney et al, 1992).

BREASTS

The male breast is a not a part of the reproductive system, but is a potentially erotic structure (Rynerson, 1990). The erectile tissue of the nipple responds to friction, sexual excitement, and cold, making it more prominent and rigid.

FEMALE REPRODUCTIVE SYSTEM

External female genitalia include the mons pubis, the labia majora and minora, the vaginal orifice, and the clitoris (Fig. 33–3). Internal reproductive organs consist of the vagina, uterus, fallopian tubes, and ovaries (Fig. 33–4).

MONS PUBIS

A mound of fatty tissue covering the pubic bone, the mons pubis becomes more accentuated with puberty and is generally covered with a fine layer of dark pubic hair. The amount and distribution of pubic hair varies widely among women.

LABIA MAJORA

The labia majora, or outer lips, are folds of skin that cover the entrance to the vagina. They are more prominent anteriorly, in the area of the mons pubis; they continue posteriorly to the anal region, where they are less distinctive and flatten to become part of the surrounding tissue. After puberty, the labia majora are covered laterally by hair. On the lateral and medial aspects of these labia, sweat and sebaceous glands are located. The labia majora provide protection for the urethra and vagina (Rynerson, 1990).

LABIA MINORA

Between the labia majora are structures known as the labia minora, or inner lips of the vagina. Anteriorly, the labia minora converge to form the hood or prepuce, over the clitoris. Posterior, and slightly deeper, is a portion of the labia minora called the frenulum, known as the lower fold of the

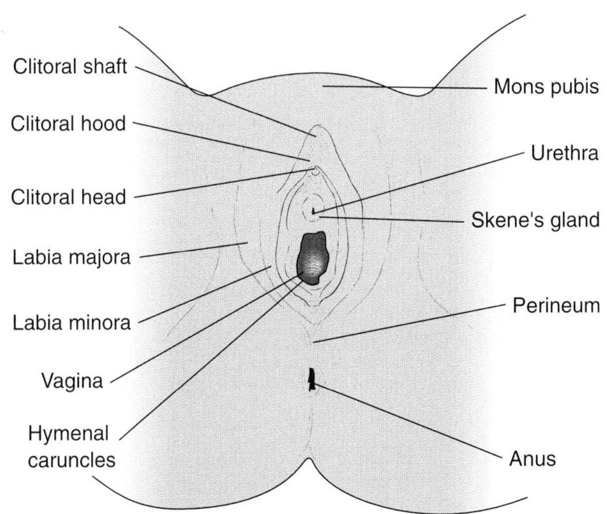

Figure 33–3. Female genitalia.

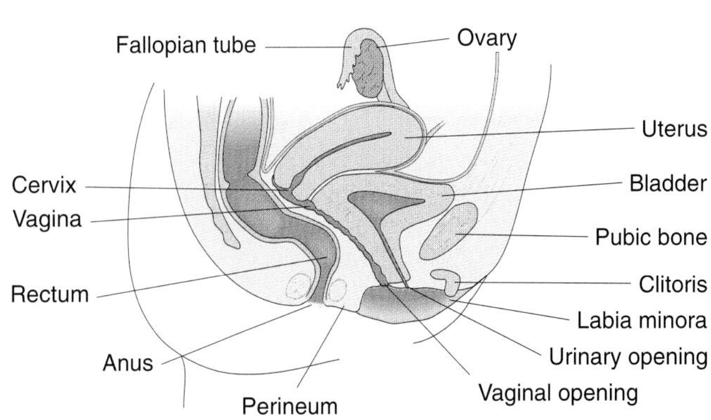

Figure 33–4. Female internal reproductive organs.

clitoris. The labia minora cover the urethral orifice, vaginal opening, and the openings of the Bartholin's glands, in addition to the clitoris. The labia minora are not covered by hair but do contain sebaceous glands that secrete some lubrication. Vascular, spongy connective tissue with many tactile nerve endings composes the labia minora, making the area very sensitive (Rynerson, 1990).

CLITORIS

The clitoris, from the Greek word meaning *key,* is a particularly sensitive and erotic area for women (Rynerson, 1990). It has two parts: the body and the glans. About ½ to 1 inch long, the clitoris is similar histologically to the penis; it is composed of erectile tissue, or corpora cavernosa. The clitoris also contains many nerves and blood vessels. When a female is sexually stimulated, the rich supply of nerves and blood vessels causes the clitoris to become engorged and serves to provide sexual pleasure. Like the penis, the clitoris produces smegma.

VAGINAL ORIFICE

The vaginal orifice, or introitus, is generally visible only when the labia majora and minora are separated. At the entrance to the vagina is a membrane called the hymen. Normally, this membrane is perforated enough to allow for menses. The hymen is visualized as an irregular narrow fold around the introitus and forms what is known as the hymenal ring. Although the hymen appears to serve no physiologic purpose, it has mythical significance to various cultures: women who possess an intact hymen are sexually inexperienced or virginal, whereas those whose hymens are torn are nonvirginal (Rynerson, 1990). Certainly, this idea is untrue, for the hymen can be broken by vigorous exercise or remain intact even with sexual intercourse.

Two sets of glands can be found in the female genitalia: Bartholin's and Skene's. Barotholin's glands are located at the posterior surface of the vaginal introitus (see Fig. 33–3) and are analogous to Cowper's glands in the male. There is debate whether these glands secrete a mucus to moisten the vagina or a fluid to afford lubrication during intercourse. The ducts leading from these glands can become clogged and form painful cysts; such cysts have the potential to develop into an abscess. Often, this cyst formation occurs secondary to a sexually transmitted infection such as gonorrhea or chlamydia. Skene's glands (paraurethral glands) are located on either side of the urethra and do not appear to have a specific purpose. However, they are also a site for possible infection and cyst formation (Rynerson, 1990).

VAGINA

The vagina is the genital opening connecting the internal and external structures. When not stimulated, the walls of the vagina collapse; with sexual excitement, they become more distended. The vagina is a multilayered structure; the innermost layer is a mucosal surface that has a rich blood supply and has estrogen receptors that are responsive to hormone levels. Premenopausally, the texture is fleshy and soft; postmenopausally, the lining becomes thin and fragile. The middle layer is composed of muscle fibers, especially during the childbearing years, allowing for contraction and expansion. The outer covering is a thin mucosa. Of note, the vagina does not contain secretory glands, and it is widely believed that the vagina does not have a rich nerve supply. If true, this could explain why vaginal sensations during intercourse may be minimal for many women (Lauver and Welch, 1990).

There appears to be some debate about whether the vagina is erotically sensitive. Predominant beliefs have held that the upper two thirds of the vagina is not particularly sensitive and that women experience orgasm only through clitoral stimulation. However, more contemporary data from case reports and direct laboratory observations support the idea of erotically sensitive areas in the vagina. The Graefenberg spot ("G spot") is identified as the area around the urethra and on the anterior vaginal wall. This area is believed by 84 percent of women in a large national survey to produce pleasurable feelings when stimulated (Davidson et al, 1989). If further research validates the existence of these sensitive areas, the idea that some women have orgasms through vaginal stimulation, or vaginal involvement in orgasms, would be supported (Lauver and Welch, 1990).

Although most women do not emit a fluid with orgasm, Belzer (1981) and Alzate and Hoch (1986) report this is a usual occurrence for some women. Some reports note that this fluid is chemically similar to prostatic fluid, while others note its similarity to urine; still others report that the nature and source of this fluid is unknown (Darling et al, 1990; Lauver and Welch, 1990).

UTERUS

Except for uterine contractions that may be noted with orgasm, the role of the uterus in sexual expression is negligible from a physiologic perspective (Rynerson, 1990). The uterus is a hollow muscular structure that houses the embryo if impregnation occurs. The uterus consists of several layers and portions. The major portion is called the body; the fundus is the uppermost portion of the uterus at the level of the fallopian tubes, while the lower portions are the isthmus and cervix, which lead into the vaginal canal. The innermost layer of the uterus, the endometrium, is made up of a rich network of glands and blood vessels that cyclically develop and then shed with menses. The next layer is primarily muscular tissue and is known as the myometrium. During menses or orgasm, these muscular fibers contract. During the birthing process, it is these muscular contractions that propel the fetus out of the uterus. The outermost layer of the uterus is called the perimetrium.

FALLOPIAN TUBES

The paired fallopian tubes lie between the uterus and the ovaries. The ovarian end of the fallopian tube does not actually connect with the ovary but has fingerlike projections in close proximity to the ovaries. These fimbriated ends, as they are called, attract the released ovum by creating wavelike motions; similarly, hairlike projections called cilia that line the fallopian tubes provide wavelike motions that afford passage through the tubes. However, the fallopian tubes serve more than to provide the route for ovum transport; it is in the uterine end of the tube that actual fertilization takes place.

OVARIES

The two ovaries have two functions: to produce the germ cells or ova, and secrete the female hormones of estrogen and progesterone. The ova do not follow a direct tubular course; rather, their release occurs by a rupturing of the wall of the ovary followed by subsequent movement out of the ovary. Like the male testes, the ovaries have numerous follicles in various stages of maturation. Approximately once every month after puberty, a follicle matures, ruptures, and releases from the ovum cell. The remaining empty follicle is labeled the corpus luteum, which produces progesterone for 12 to 14 days and then eventually decomposes in the body (Lauver and Welch, 1990).

BREASTS

Although the function of breasts is to produce milk, they are highly valued by both men and women as sexual organs (Bernhard, 1995). Breasts vary greatly in size from woman to woman, yet this variability does not appear to influence the tactile sensitivity attributed to them. The breast is made up of glandular, fibrous, and fatty tissue. The nipple especially is supplied with nervous innervation. The erectile tissue of the nipple is very responsive to cold, friction, and sexual excitement and becomes more rigid and prominent (Rynerson, 1990).

Psychosocial Basis for Women's and Men's Sexual Health

Psychosocial aspects of sexuality are even more complex than biologic ones (Rynerson, 1990). Research in this area has provided some understanding that sexuality is influenced by interacting psychological, social, cultural, and spiritual forces. Gender identity, gender role, sexual orientation, and spirituality are the psychosocial aspects of gender and sexual health presented here.

SEXUAL ORIENTATION

Sexual orientation refers to partner preference; this includes physical and emotional attraction to another person (Rynerson, 1990). Sexual orientation is thought of as existing on a continuum that extends from exclusive orientation to persons of the opposite sex (heterosexuality), through orientation to persons of both sexes (bisexuality), to exclusive orientation to persons of the same sex (homosexuality). Although there is still considerable debate about whether sexual preference is determined primarily by culture or primarily by biology (which can include prenatal development as well as genetic endowment), currently, very few authorities believe that people consciously choose to be homosexual or heterosexual.

Just where a person falls on this sexual preference continuum is not always immediately obvious to the person. Teenagers may experiment with both heterosexual and homosexual behavior. Women, in particular (many of them married or previously married with children) have reported the discovery of homosexual feelings later in life when they have enough time, confidence, and experience for self-awareness (Carlson et al, 1996). Both men and women may know that they have homosexual feelings at an early age but do not choose to act on these feelings until much later or at all.

Various studies suggest that 20 percent of all American men and women have engaged in same-sex relationships, either exclusively or in addition to heterosexual relationships (Michaels, 1995). In spite of antidiscrimination laws upholding basic rights of sexual preference, there is still a pervasive taboo about homosexuality that continues to manifest itself in a variety of forms of discrimination and homophobia (an irrational fear of homosexuality).

While there is a paucity of information on the health care needs of gay and bisexual men and women, there is general agreement among medical professionals and gay and lesbian advocacy groups that the nature and prevalence of certain health problems differ between gay, lesbian, bisexual, and heterosexual men and women. Although sexually transmitted diseases are less prevalent in lesbians than heterosexual, bisexual, and gay men and women, lesbians appear to be at higher risk for breast cancer (Bernhard, 1995). Gay men and women are more likely than men and women in the general population to attempt suicide and to have problems with alcohol and substance abuse that may reflect a higher rate of depression among these groups (Bernhard, 1995; Tewkesbury, 1995).

GENDER IDENTITY AND GENDER ROLE

Sex is the type of genitals we have—male or female; it is also something that we do with our bodies when we engage in intimate physical relations with another person. Gender is the expression of masculinity or femininity, which is a sense of self, a reflection of spirit or soul, and which is perceived by others using numerous social signals that have nothing to do with one's sex or sexual orientation.

Gender refers to responses, meanings, and cues that are socially learned and are reflections of what society visualizes as masculinity and femininity (Rynerson, 1990). *Gender identity* refers to the hard-to-define sense of "being" male or "being" female that is usually in accord with, but sometimes opposed to, physical anatomy. There is no clear agreement on how gender identity is formed, but most current theories say that gender identity is formed before birth. Gender identity can be distinguished from biologic sex, which is body linked, as it includes definitions of the self and behavior toward others. Both biologic (sex) and social learning (identity and roles) are involved in the determination of gender identity. Gender, as well as gender differences, provides a framework within which one can interpret the responses of the body (Petras, 1978).

It is only in the last four decades that science has been applied to the topic of gender identity disorders. Contemporary terms used to describe gender identity disorders include transsexualism, gender dysphoria, and transgender. *Transsexual* is a person whose gender identity is opposite to her or his biologic sex. *Gender dysphoria* is a term used to describe a person who feels trapped in a body of the opposite sex. *Transgender,* in the broadest sense, means mixing elements of both genders, sometimes both sexes. The category covers cross-dressers, transsexuals, masculine women, and feminine men. From limited studies to date, an estimated 1 to 3 percent of the world's population is defined as transgendered.

Although much literature has accumulated on the characteristics, causes, and treatment of transsexualism, no clear understanding of the nature and cause of transsexualism has yet emerged. Explanations for transsexuality include both biologic and social-learning hypotheses. The American Psychiatric Association's DSM (Diagnostic and Statistical Manual) IV defines the criteria for diagnosis of Gender Identity Disorder (GID) to include: evidence of a "strong and persistent cross-gender identification" and evidence of "persistent discomfort about one's assigned sex or a sense of inappropriateness in the gender role of that sex." Although controversy exists about the use of the DSM-IV criteria to diagnose a gender variation, the GID diagnosis has allowed insurance companies to reimburse for gender reassignment procedures and for some states to classify transsexualism as a "disability," allowing transsexuals protection under disability laws (Green, 1994). Most experts consider gender differences as a naturally occurring social variation and do not consider gender dysphoria a disability. Although transsexualism is not a form of mental illness, some people with borderline psychosis, recurrent depression, or gross personality disorder experience gender dysphoria. The International Gender Dysphoria Association has developed evaluation and treatment guidelines to adequately assess individuals with gender dysphoria (Walker et al, 1985). *Gender reassignment* (as opposed to the vernacular "sex change," which is impossible) provides medical-surgical options to allow transsexual people to live in their "correct" gender role.

Gender role is the behavior one exhibits as measured by what the particular culture regards as feminine or masculine. The term *gender role,* first used in the biomedical and developmental psychology literature in the 1950s, is used to signify all those things that a person says or does to disclose himself as having the status of a boy or man, or girl or woman, respectively (Money, 1955). There is great cultural variation as to the specific tasks or characteristics expected of women and men, but most cultures do in fact ascribe different expectations for each sex (Rynerson, 1990). Typically, gender role and gender identity is congruent; these may or may not be congruent with biologic sex.

Cultural Basis for Women's and Men's Sexual Health

Cultural and social values and attitudes shape human sexual behavior. Each society shapes, structures, and guides the sexual and gender development and expression of all its members and develops accepted patterns of expression based on the internal values, needs, and logic of the culture. These unique patterns result in wide diversity of sexual and gender-specific behavior, rules and regulations, symbols, sanctions, and taboos across societies. One example of a cultural difference is female circumcision. Female circumcision is a common practice among some African tribes but is viewed negatively in the United States. Variations in the ethnographic spectrum of human sexual expression demand a tolerance for differences (Smith, 1990).

U.S. CULTURE

In the United States sexuality is associated with genitalia, body image, and self-esteem. From birth, children are socialized to assume and develop an identity based on a gender role. Before their third birthday, most children can identify their own sex, as well as that of others, and they develop a sense of which behaviors are more appropriate for their own gender. Many children learn early in life that boys (and the activities of boys) have higher status than girls do in society. This early socialization is associated with inequities in general health as well as in sexual relationships.

U.S. CULTURE AND EXPECTATIONS OF WOMEN

Women are brought up to feel that they deserve sexual pleasure only if they look a certain way or weigh a certain amount. The dominant U.S. culture teaches men and women that sexuality and procreation are distinctly different, while still accepting fertility and sexual cycles as integrative aspects of the human experience. In general, our culture also believes in the "big bang" theory of heterosexual pleasure that holds that the thrusting of the penis into the vagina is the most pleasurable part of sexuality. Although this is true for some men and women, it is not true for all. It is only one part of sexuality and pleasure, but many people feel abnormal if they do not enjoy stereotypical sexual expression (Northrup, 1994).

The potentially pleasurable and life-enhancing effects of sex between men and women may be limited or even destroyed by the fundamentally unequal nature of their socially prescribed relationships (Doyal, 1995). Because most sexual encounters between men and women involve a process of implicit or explicit negotiation, many women are socialized to conduct these negotiations from a position of weakness or inferiority, resulting in heterosexual experiences that are neither happy nor healthy. Of course, individual men may not feel powerful or confident in their sexual interactions with women. However, the broad picture is one where men's sexual coerciveness toward women has not merely been tolerated but expected or socially sanctioned (Doyal, 1995). Socially sanctioned male dominance of heterosex can affect women's health and healthy sexual relationships on a number of different levels. Psychological distress from compulsory heterosexual intercourse will have a negative impact on women's mental health and the diseases that it can transmit.

The cultural imperative that judges a woman's worth by her attachment to a man and by her sexual attractiveness to men is pervasive in our society. Far too many women have internalized the culturally sanctioned sexual habits and needs of men as their own, when in fact male sexuality and sexual needs are probably more different and varied than empirical evidence suggests (Sabo and Gordon, 1995).

U.S. CULTURE AND EXPECTATIONS OF MEN

The socially prescribed male role is one that requires men to be "non-communicative, competitive and nongiving, and inexpressive, and to evaluate life success in terms of external achievements rather than personal and interpersonal fulfillment" (Harrison et al, 1992, p. 272). Although there is some debate over specific elements of the "traditional male role," using stereotypical standards of male sexuality and masculinity as norms to guide individual behavior and self-worth leads to both psychological and physical problems for men. Brannon (1976) has described central characteristics of the dominant male gender role in our society. First, men cannot be "sissies" (like women) and must demonstrate a sense of independence and self-reliance. Furthermore, this stereotypical male feels the need to be superior to others or more powerful than others, through violence if necessary.

Although these stereotypical concepts of male gender socialization have been heavily criticized by men's studies scholars as too simplistic and inconsistent with social reality (Carrigan et al, 1987), they provide some insight into the negative effects of traditional gender role socialization on men's health and illness. For example, when a gender role stereotype becomes the norm for defining masculinity, few men will be able to live up to its standards. This leads to feelings of inadequacy, attributions of deviance, and hypermasculine compensations such as rape and other forms of violence and aggression (Gordon, 1995). In addition, stereotypical masculine role socialization fosters behaviors such as risk taking that are harmful to men's health (Allen and Whatley, 1986; Harrison et al, 1992). This gender stereotype becomes a serious problem when used by men to their advantage to legitimate their power in relation to women (Carrigan et al, 1987). However, studies of men experiencing illness or coping with a less desirable body image have found that men have control over the process of gender role definition (Gordon, 1995), suggesting that masculinity is not conferred by nature or biology alone. Rather, men have the capacity to construct a personally satisfying male self-concept without resorting to stereotypes that are exploitative or health damaging.

Societal expectations regarding the stereotypical male sex role also exact costs on men's ability to seek and obtain health education, counseling, and preventive or curative care. The male sex-role stereotype demands that men be healthy, strong, and self-sufficient (Forrester, 1986). In an attempt to maintain a masculine self-image, men may be reluctant to admit or recognize their health needs, or to seek health care. Men's fundamental psychological needs may be the same as women's, but the fulfillment of the socially prescribed male role (inexpressive, competitive) works against the fulfillment of psychological needs (Harrison, 1984). The perceived conflict between basic psychological needs and a stereotyped male role contributes to men's increasing vulnerability to illness. For example, men are more likely than women to ignore symptoms and fail to seek health care in a timely fashion.

Because society has such profound impact upon health behaviors, including sexual health behaviors, it is no surprise that men have greater difficulty seeking care from health care providers for sexual health issues than do women. It is not uncommon to find that it is the female partner who seeks care for sexually transmitted infections rather than the male, who is more likely to experience tangible symptoms such as penile discharge or burning with urination.

Physiologic Sexual Response

Masters and Johnson (1966) first identified the human sexual response cycle as an orderly sequence of physiologic responses to sexual stimuli. They identified four phases: excitement, plateau, orgasm, and resolution. In the 1970s, Kaplan (1979) reinterpreted the sexual response cycle as phases of desire, excitement, and orgasm. Kaplan's desire phase is unique, but the excitement and orgasmic phases resemble those of Masters and Johnson. The American Psychiatric Association (APA, 1994) describes a sexual response cycle that combines those described by Masters and Johnson and by Kaplan (Fig. 33–5).

Although the phases of the sexual response cycle are the same for males and females, certain differences within these phases are specific to gender (Lauver and Welch, 1990). Notably, a common pattern in males comprises a rapid excitement phase, followed by a short plateau, orgasm, and then resolution. Females may experience one of several patterns, though three patterns are very commonly recognized. The first pattern consists of multiple orgasms with a shallow resolution period. The second pattern is composed of several peaks in the plateau phase with a longer resolution period. In this pattern, the female does not achieve total orgasm. In the third pattern, the female's sexual excitement is interrupted and followed by an intense orgasm and a rapid resolution (Lauver and Welch, 1990).

The second difference in the sexual response cycle between women and men is the refractory period. This refractory, or recovery, period follows ejaculation by the male during which he is not capable of further ejaculation (Lauver and Welch,

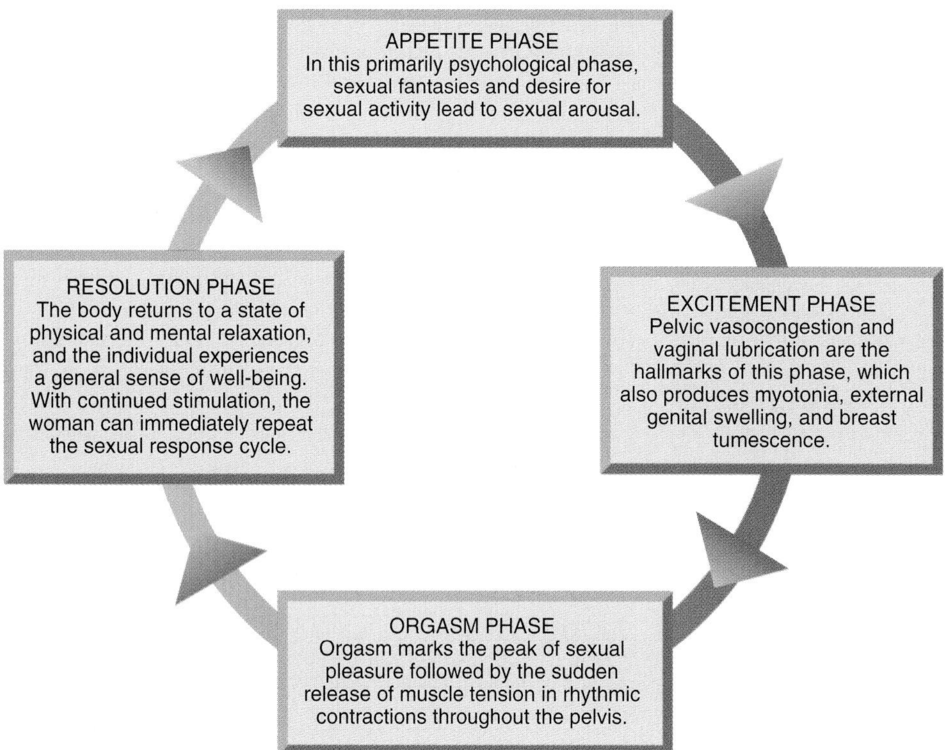

Figure 33–5. Human sexual response cycle.

1990). The female appears to have no such refractory period and may have repeated orgasms before experiencing resolution. Table 33–1 compares women's and men's sexual responses by phase.

SEXUAL EXPRESSION

Social norms shape, structure, or restrict the forms of sexual expression that are considered appropriate. Behavior that was once considered perverted is perhaps now regarded only as deviant and may in the future be looked upon as an acceptable alternative to "normal" sexual activity. In general, people are more willing to accept their own sexuality, recognizing that this is but one facet of their personalities (Lipkin and Cohen, 1992).

An understanding of what are healthy sexual expression, behavior, and function is essential to effective health promotion for men and women across the lifespan. A few of the more common types of sexual expression involving genital activities will be described here. The focus here will be on genital activities because nongenital activities can include everything from style of dress to interpersonal communications. Variations of sexual expression, such as sadomasochism, fisting, rimming, or group sex, and their definitions can be found in sexuality-specific references from organizations like Sex Information and Education Council of the U.S. (SIECUS) or the American Association of Sex Educators, Counselors and Therapists.

Masturbation refers to erotic self-stimulation, usually to the point of orgasm. Attitudes toward masturbation have shifted in the past 20 years from an attitude that masturbation is evil and harmful to an attitude that masturbation is part of healthy sexual expression or simply pleasurable. Masturbation practices begin early in life when infants explore their genitals. Often self-stimulation continues throughout life, whether or not the individual has a permanent, intimate relationship (Rynerson, 1990). Because of taboos against masturbation, people need to be reassured that masturbation can be helpful as a sexual outlet and as a means to be comfortable with one's own body.

Petting is defined as erotic stimulation of a person by a sexual partner, without actual sexual intercourse. Sometimes referred to as "foreplay" to intercourse, petting can include kissing, genital caresses, and oral-genital contact and may result in orgasm (Alexander and LaRosa, 1994). During adolescence, petting is one way to experience sexual excitement without engaging in intercourse. During adulthood, petting may be used as foreplay to intercourse or for sexual variety.

Oral-genital stimulation or "oral sex" is defined as **cunnilingus,** the act of sucking or licking vulva and clitoris, and **fellatio,** the act of sucking or licking the penis and scrotum. The prevalence of oral-genital stimulation appears to be widespread, with one study finding 80 percent of college students and nearly all adults reporting oral-genital sexual experience (Alexander and LaRosa, 1994).

Anal intercourse is another form of sexual expression for both heterosexual and gay couples. Because the anal region has no natural lubrication of its own and the anal sphincter has limited expansion, caution must be taken to avoid pain and injury. Use of condoms and water-soluble lubricants (pe-

TABLE 33-1 Physiological Changes in Human Sexual Response

Male	Female
Excitement Phase	
1. Penile erection (within 3 to 8 seconds) as phase is prolonged. 2. Thickening, flattening, and elevation of scrotal sac. 3. Partial testicular elevation and size increase. 4. Nipple erection (in about 30% of men).	1. Vaginal lubrication (within 10 to 30 seconds) as phase is prolonged. 2. Thickening of vaginal walls and labia. 3. Expansion of inner two thirds of vagina and elevation of cervix and corpus. 4. Tumescence of clitoris. 5. Nipple erection (in all women). 6. Sex flush (in about 25% of women).
Plateau Phase	
1. Increase in penile coronal circumference. 2. Testicular tumescence (50 to 100% enlarged). 3. Full testicular elevation and rotation (orgasm inevitable). 4. Purple hue to corona of penis (inconsistent). 5. Mucoid secretion (perhaps from Cowper's glands). 6. Sex tension flush (in 25% of men). 7. Carpopedal spasm. 8. Generalized muscular tension. 9. Hyperventilation. 10. Tachycardia (100 to 160 bpm). 11. Increased blood pressure (20 to 80 mmHg systolic; 10 to 40 mmHg diastolic).	1. Orgasmic platform in outer one third of vagina. 2. Full expansion of vagina. 3. Uterine and cervical elevation. 4. Discoloration of labia minora. 5. Mucoid secretion (perhaps from Bartholin's glands). 6. Withdrawal of clitoris. 7. Sex flush (in 75% of women). 8. Carpopedal spasm. 9. Muscular tension. 10. Hyperventilation. 11. Tachycardia. 12. Increased blood pressure (20 to 60 mmHg systolic; 10 to 20 mmHg diastolic).
Orgasmic Phase	
1. Ejaculation. 2. Contraction of accessory organs of reproduction (vas deferens, seminal vesicles, ejaculatory duct). 3. Relaxation of external bladder sphincter and contraction of internal bladder sphincter. 4. Contractions of penile urethra (0.8-second interval for three to four contractions). 5. Anal sphincter contractions. 6. Specific skeletal muscle contractions. 7. Hyperventilation (up to 40 breaths/minute). 8. Tachycardia (up to 180 bpm). 9. Increased blood pressure (40 to 100 mmHg systolic; 20 to 50 mmHg diastolic).	1. Pelvic response. 2. Contraction of uterus from fundus toward lower uterine segment. 3. Minimal relaxation of external cervical os. 4. Contractions of orgasmic platform (0.8-second interval for 5 to 12 contractions). 5. External rectal sphincter contraction. 6. External urethral sphincter contractions. 7. Hyperventilation (up to 40 breaths/minute). 8. Tachycardia (up to 180 bpm). 9. Increased blood pressure (30 to 80 mmHg systolic; 20 to 40 mmHg diastolic).
Resolution Phase	
1. Refractory period with rapid loss of pelvic vasocongestion. 2. Loss of penile erection is a two-stage response: 50% loss rapidly; gradual loss of rest of erection. 3. Sweating reaction (30 to 40% of men). 4. Hyperventilation. 5. Tachycardia decreases.	1. Ready return to orgasm with retarded loss of pelvic vasocongestion. 2. Loss of flush in labia minora and orgasmic platform (rapid). 3. Remainder of pelvic vasocongestion slow. 4. Loss of clitoral tumescence. 5. Sweating reaction (30 to 40% of women). 6. Hyperventilation. 7. Tachycardia decreases.

Sources: Masters and Johnson, 1966; Fogel and Woods, 1981; Woods, 1984.
From Fogel, C., Lauver, D. (eds.) (1990). *Sexual Health Promotion.* Philadelphia: W.B. Saunders, p. 49.

troleum based products weaken condoms) will allow anal intercourse to be pleasurable and free of infection transmission, inasmuch as both hepatitis B and HIV have been found to be transmitted via anal tissue.

The task of distinguishing personal truths about sexual expression from the inherited cultural distortions or from negative sexual experiences is a challenge for individual men and women as well as for health care providers. A first step is to redefine sexual expression from the perspective of the human being rather than the sexual object as well as to determine personal preferences for where, what, when, who, and how sexual expression is manifested. Understanding the wide variation in sexual expression and sexual pleasure will provide the knowledge base for nursing assessment of sexual health as well as the alterations in sexual health.

ALTERATIONS IN SEXUAL HEALTH

Sexual behavior, one of the most important of all human activities, is the process by which the species is reproduced, is the central behavior around which families are formed, and is the key component in the emotional lives of men and women. Sexual behavior is also central to a number of social and medical problems: marital difficulties and divorce; incest and family violence; the reproductive issues of infertility, sterility, contraception, unwanted/unintended pregnancy and abortion; sexually transmitted infections; as well as chronic disease management (Alexander and LaRosa, 1994).

Illness, body image concerns, and sexual abuse all have the potential to interfere with women's and men's sexual health. Although the focus of this chapter is on the nurse's role in sexual health promotion and disease prevention, it is appropriate to provide a brief overview of variations on health that may temporarily or chronically influence sexual health.

SEXUAL PROBLEMS

Because sexuality is multidimensional, many situations and factors can cause sexual problems. To determine how a particular situation or factor affects an individual's sexuality, the nurse must consider all of the components of sexuality and must keep in mind that individuals respond to events differently (Bernhard, 1995). Masters and Johnson (1970) reported that half of all married couples experienced dysfunctions at some time during their marriage.

SEXUAL DYSFUNCTION

Sexual dysfunction refers to impaired, incomplete, or lack of expression of normal human sexual desires and responses. However, these concerns become dysfunctions only when they cause subjective discomfort or distress (Bernhard, 1995).

Today we know that sexual dysfunction can result from a number of causes, whereas historically, most were thought to derive from psychological factors (Bernhard, 1995). Physical or organic factors such as chronic disease, medications, and surgery can result in sexual problems and will be discussed in a subsequent section. Relationship difficulties may trigger sexual dysfunction. Traumatic events and sexual experiences, such as incest or rape, can lead to sexual dysfunction in both men and women. Furthermore, maintenance of sexual dysfunction can be due to inadequate or inaccurate sexual knowledge or lack of effective communication between partners (Bernhard, 1995).

Sexologists and sex therapists define the principal sexual dysfunctions in men and women: inhibited sexual desire (lack of interest in sexual activity), anorgasmia (inability to achieve orgasm), vaginismus (vaginal muscle spasms that interfere with intercourse), male erectile disorder (insufficient erection to permit coitus), and premature ejaculation (ejaculation occurs before the person wishes it). Dyspareunia in women is sometimes considered a sexual dysfunction. Sex therapy, including education and counseling, is recommended for these disorders. The Diagnostic and Statistical Manual for Mental Disorders (DSM-IV) acknowledges these dysfunctions as well as sexual aversion disorder (extreme repulsion by and avoidance of almost all genital sexual contact) and female sexual arousal disorder (partial or complete failure to attain or maintain vaginal lubrication and swelling or sexual excitement) (APA, 1994). However, these dysfunctions go beyond the scope of nursing and must be treated by a health care practitioner with extensive training in sex counseling and therapy.

In women, inhibited sexual desire, or lack of interest in sexual activity, is the most common sexual dysfunction for which women seek help (Stuart et al, 1987). Women experiencing this dysfunction are less likely to express romantic love feelings for their partners and to be satisfied with their ability to listen to their partners. Although the cause is unknown, it may be caused by biologic, psychological, and relationship factors as well as high stress levels (Bernhard, 1995). Successful treatment includes psychotherapy, communication skills training, and sensate focus therapy (deliberate form of touching as a communication method). Another common sexual dysfunction in women is anorgasmia, which can be defined as primary or secondary anorgasmia. Primary anorgasmia may be caused by sexual trauma, current relationship issues, lack of education and information about sexual matters, or interpersonal concerns (Heiman and Grafton-Becker, 1989). Secondary anorgasmia is often due to psychoactive drugs, episiotomy scars, or pelvic surgery, especially oophorectomy (Bernhard, 1995). Behavioral therapy has proved successful through the use of desensitization and directed masturbation or self-pleasuring activities (Barbach, 1976, 1980).

Male erectile disorder, once known as impotence, is the persistent or recurrent partial or complete failure to attain or maintain an erection of sufficient firmness to permit coitus to be initiated or completed. Although isolated, transient episodes of inability to obtain or maintain an erection are normal and do not require assessment or intervention, a pattern that is persistent warrants intervention (Field, 1990). In erectile disorder, whatever the cause, the vascular reflex mechanism fails to pump enough blood into the cavernous sinuses of the penis to make the penis firm and erect. While the man may even feel aroused and sexually excited, his penis does not become erect. Because the erectile and ejaculatory responses are dissociable, the man may ejaculate despite a flaccid penis. The incidence of erectile disorder does not seem to be affected by sex or social class, but does increase with age. About 75 percent of men are unable to sustain an erection by age 80, whereas only 2 percent of men experience difficulty before age 40 (Karacan et al, 1983).

There are a number of theories about the causes of male erectile disorder but no one specific psychodynamic pattern has been correlated with erectile disorder. A common sequel to erectile disorder is depression and may precede or follow the erectile disorder. In addition, relationship discord may be either a precipitating or resulting factor.

Diagnosis of erectile disorder must distinguish between organic or psychological etiology. More than 100 conditions as well as certain drugs can produce erectile disorder. When the cause of the disorder is primarily organic, the onset is usually slow and insidious, whereas a psychogenic erectile disorder is characteristically sudden in onset (Field, 1990). The use of nocturnal penile tumescence (NPT) monitoring has been used to establish whether the basic neurophysiologic mechanisms involved in the erectile reflex are intact. Because the healthy male has five to six erections per night, which occur during REM sleep and are unrelated to emotional state, the results of NPT can be used to guide decisions about which studies and tests should be done to determine specific causes of erectile dysfunction.

Another common male sexual dysfunction is premature ejaculation, which may be primary or secondary. Primary premature ejaculation refers to lack of control over the ejaculatory reflex since the onset of sexual activity, whereas secondary premature ejaculation refers to the loss of control after a period of more effective sexual functioning. Reactions to premature ejaculation range from unawareness—until a frustrated partner seeks help—to guilt about the problem. This sometimes leads to avoidance of sexual encounters or to the development of erectile dysfunction (Field, 1990). Techniques employed to achieve ejaculatory control include more frequent ejaculation, variation in coital position, attempting multiple orgasm, communication strategies that prolong sexual excitement, and the "stop-start" and "squeeze" techniques (Crooks and Baur, 1983). These techniques were designed to prolong the sensations prior to orgasm, increasing the man's awareness and potential for control of ejaculation. The nurse can provide education and counseling for the couple attempting these strategies, forewarning them that results may take weeks or months.

In contrast to premature ejaculation, inhibited male orgasm is defined as the persistent or recurrent delay in or absence of orgasm in a male following a normal sexual excitement phase during sexual activity that is adequate in focus, intensity, and duration (APA, 1987). Suggested causes include marital conflict, relationship ambivalence, and environmental causes. Physiologic causes are not common but include the effects of drugs that impair the sympathetic nervous system (e.g., thioridazine and antihypertensives) and neurologic diseases such as atrophic lateral sclerosis and multiple sclerosis (Field, 1990). As with erectile dysfunction, the treatment involves behavioral reconditioning and psychotherapy or couples counseling.

Nurses who are not specially trained in sex therapy can provide basic information, education, and initial counseling to clients about basic mechanisms of sexual arousal, the phases of the sexual response cycle, the frequency of sexual dysfunction, a hopeful attitude, and information about treatment options. The nurse can also influence the client's attitude positively toward further treatment and referral for sex therapy. Problems that usually require psychotherapy and/or sex therapy include:

- clinical depression underlying the sexual complaint
- significant past psychiatric history
- problems complicated by gender confusion or dysphoria
- primary sexual dysfunction
- lack of commitment to the relationship by one or both partners
- significant secrets, such as ongoing infidelities, kept by one partner
- major difficulties in a relationship with a partner
- major family or work problems (Field, 1990)

ILLNESS

Illness can lead to changes in an individual's sexuality and sexual functioning. Short-term illnesses and long-term illnesses have different implications. Acute illnesses, such as an upper respiratory infection or diarrhea, are relatively short term (lasting from a few hours to a few weeks or months) and full restoration to health is expected. Therefore, an interruption in sexual functioning during an acute illness may not require intervention. However, chronic illness (permanent illness or disability that is stable or progressive) may require professional intervention or, at the very least, education from a health professional regarding the alteration in sexual function. Such chronic illnesses as rheumatoid arthritis, multiple sclerosis, cancer, and ulcerative colitis may have biologic, psychosocial, and cultural considerations that influence the individual's ability to adapt to altered sexuality. Moreover, pain, fatigue, and depression, which frequently accompany chronic illness, may impair sexual functioning.

Common chronic diseases that will alter sexual health and function during adulthood are musculoskeletal conditions (arthritis) and cardiopulmonary disease (coronary artery disease, emphysema) as well as disabilities (spinal cord injuries). Musculoskeletal conditions include symptoms of pain, stiffness, fatigue, and weakness (sometimes medication-induced) resulting in decreased self-esteem, anxiety, altered body image, change in role function, and social isolation, which further decreases sexual functioning (Dalton, 1990). Heart or blood vessel disease, a common cause of disease and death in middle and older adults, will impact sexual functioning. Although research-based literature (in men only) suggests modest energy expenditure during sexual activity, especially when the man uses the on-bottom coital position with a familiar partner, safety in resuming sexual activity after a myocardial infarction remains a concern of both patient and health care provider (Burke, 1990). Sexual activity in a familiar environment is not associated with increased risk of myocardial infarction (MI), especially among men with the ability to walk and subsequently climb stairs without undue increase in heart rate or development of arrhythmias or cardiac symptoms. However, many men and their partners experience fear of symptoms (chest pain), another

MI, or death as reasons for avoiding sexual activity. These fears combined with concurrent depression and anxiety associated with heart disease serve to alter sexual health. Chronic lung disease (asthma, chronic bronchitis, and emphysema) impacts sexual function through shortness of breath, easy fatigability, as well as impaired erectile function in men and anorgasmia in women (Stockdale-Wooley, 1990).

Disabilities due to trauma, disease, and congenital anomalies that affect the distal portion of the spinal cord or autonomic nervous system have the potential for affecting some aspect of the sexual response. The individual who is rendered paraplegic by disease or injury usually is at least a young adult who already has experienced physical, intellectual, psychological, and emotional stages of growth and development prior to the disability. However, the child with a congenital disability (meningomyelocele, spina bifida) has the added burdens of adapting to a disability along with the growth and development process. Although any illness can affect the spinal cord or peripheral nerves, such as diabetes or multiple sclerosis, trauma is the major cause of paralysis. Because injury to the spinal cord alters the physical, psychological, occupational, personal, and recreational aspects of daily living, nursing plays an important coordinating role in the care, counsel, and education of individuals with spinal cord disabilities. Frequently, so much physical and emotional energy has been used in the struggle to acknowledge their new selves, the disabled person may not have focused on sexual capabilities, particularly if the health professional is working with the patient within the first 12 months after the trauma (Sackett, 1990).

Pain. Pain may be present in both acute and chronic illness. Pain can have a profound effect on sexuality and sexual functioning by altering desire or by disrupting the sexual response cycle (Carter, 1990). In addition, medication used to relieve chronic pain may decrease sexual desire.

Although chronic conditions such as arthritis and cancer side effects result in pain during sexual activity, pain that is specific to sexual experience alters men's and women's sexual health. Types of pain include chronic pelvic, vulvar, or scrotal pain, or pain that is present during intercourse, masturbation, or sexual touching. In women, dyspareunia secondary to pelvic pain, vaginismus, and vulvadynia is the most common. Little is known about sexual pain conditions in men, but clinical reports suggest that men do report scrotal, urethral, and prostatic pain associated with sexual activity secondary to infection or chronic disease.

When a woman frequently experiences vaginal pain before, during, or after sexual intercourse, the condition is called dyspareunia. Approximately one in five women may suffer from this disorder at any given time, and many more experience it at some point in their lives. Dyspareunia results when there is not enough lubrication in the vaginal walls to relieve friction during heterosexual intercourse or sexual touching. It may also occur when penetration puts pressure on abnormal tissue deep within the pelvis (as with endometriosis or adhesions) (Carlson et al, 1996). Vaginismus, by contrast, is a relatively rare form of sexual pain disorder in which muscles in the outer third of the vagina (pubococcygeus muscles) involuntarily contract to prevent penetration, making sexual intercourse impossible, difficult, or painful.

Dyspareunia can occur in any woman who has intercourse without adequate stimulation, as well as in women with disorders of desire or excitement (sexual dysfunction). At certain points in a woman's life, vaginal lubrication is reduced because of hormonal changes such as lactation, menopause, or menstrual cycle phase. Pain may develop after an episiotomy or secondary to pelvic disorders such as endometriosis, pelvic inflammatory disease, adhesions, ovarian cancer, ovarian cysts, or tears in the ligaments that support the uterus (Carlson et al, 1996). Occasionally deep (but episodic) vaginal pain may occur when the penis hits the cervix during thrusting, and this can be alleviated by learning alternate sexual positions. Vaginismus by contrast seems to be a way for the body to avoid sexual contact. It is particularly common in women who experienced sexual trauma such as rape. Sexual pain occurring in both men and women may develop because of some local irritation or infection, which is further aggravated by sexual intercourse. Common causes of irritation are yeast infections; urinary tract infections; sexually transmitted diseases such as herpes or genital warts; as well as allergic reactions to spermicide or the latex in condoms or diaphragms.

Fatigue. Persons with fatigue often feel exhausted or depleted and may experience weakness. Fatigue may have a physiologic influence on sexual functioning, as well as a psychosocial influence. Physiologic changes associated with fatigue include depletion of the glycogen stores along with buildup of lactic acid and other metabolites in the muscle (Carter, 1990). These changes can lead to a reduction in muscles' ability to contract as well as an increase in muscle recovery time.

Fatigue may also be a response to some of the psychosocial processes observed in chronic illness. Alteration in self-image, reduced emotional gratification, and boredom are psychosocial issues that have the potential to contribute to fatigue. Patients who have fatigue may not be able to engage in their usual sexual activities due to an alteration in their sexual interest or due to an alteration in muscle physiology.

Depression. Depression is known to lead to a marked decrease in sexual desire (Carter, 1990). Fatigue and somatic complaints are frequently reported by depressed individuals and may interact with other dynamics to influence sexual functioning. Reactive depression, the most common form in individuals with chronic illness, may include feelings of low self-esteem, inferiority, or guilt (Carter, 1990). Patients with reactive depression may respond to treatment that includes antidepressant medications and working through feelings of loss that are associated with chronic illness. The resumption of the usual pattern of sexual functioning by the individual may be indicative of reactive depression resolution.

SEXUALLY TRANSMITTED INFECTIONS

The term *sexually transmitted infection* (STI) has replaced the term *sexually transmitted disease* (STD), which carries certain social stigma. Sexually transmitted infections are infectious disease syndromes primarily transmitted through sexual contact (Fogel, 1995). STIs can be caused by a wide variety of bacteria, viruses, protozoa, and ectoparasites. STIs cause symptoms that interrupt normal sexual function, if only temporarily. Box 33–1 lists important information about STIs.

Gonorrhea. The most commonly reported communicable disease in the United States, gonorrhea is caused by the aerobic, gram-negative diplococci *Neisseria gonorrhoeae.* The organism is transmitted almost exclusively by sexual contact. Genital-to-genital contact is the principal means of transmission; however, it also can be spread by oral-to-genital and anal-to-genital contact (Hatcher et al, 1994). Women are not uncommonly asymptomatic, and when symptoms are present, they tend to be less specific than the symptoms observed in men. Men's symptoms tend to be a penile discharge or "drip" with concomitant urethral burning and burning on urination. Women may have a purulent endocervical discharge, menstrual irregularities, and chronic or acute pelvic pain. Sometimes women experience dysuria associated with gonorrhea.

BOX 33–1
BASIC FACTS ABOUT SEXUALLY TRANSMITTED INFECTIONS

- Using condoms and spermicidal contraceptives can reduce the risk of infection.
- Persons with a new sexual partner or more than one sexual partner may be at increased risk for infection.
- If symptoms of infection are suspected, the person should avoid intercourse or instruct each male partner to use a condom.
- Any prescribed medication regimen should be completed fully. Disappearance of symptoms does not mean that the infection is cured.
- The nurse should encourage persons with suspected STI to have an examination and specific testing. Second-guessing or phone diagnosing (e.g., "I think it's what I had last year") should be avoided.
- Persons in poor general health and those with certain chronic health problems are at greater risk for infection.
- It is common for a person with one STI to have another STI as well.
- Presence of infection can interfere with the accuracy of Pap smear results.
- An infected person must inform all his or her sexual partners of the need for examination and possible treatment.
- Cleansing the genitals before and after sexual activity and postcoital urination may help prevent infection.

From Griffith-Kenney, J. (ed.) (1986). *Contemporary Women's Health: A Nursing Advocacy Approach.* Menlo Park, CA: Addison-Wesley.

Chlamydia. In the United States, genital infections caused by *Chlamydia trachomatis* (*C. trachomatis*) are the most common STIs in women. Although chlamydia is not an infection reported to the Centers for Disease Control (CDC), an estimated 3 to 4 million Americans are newly infected each year (Fogel, 1995). Chlamydial infections are thought to be a factor in the rising infertility rate among women and men in the United States. Chlamydia apparently is responsible for more severe subclinical tubal inflammation than gonorrhea, with subsequent tubal damage, despite its more benign signs and symptoms (Hatcher et al, 1994).

The major mode of transmission of chlamydia is sexual contact. Men may experience urethral burning, burning on urination, and a penile discharge. Women may experience spotting or postcoital bleeding, mucoid or purulent cervical discharge, or burning with urination (Fogel, 1995). Acute salpingitis (infection of the fallopian tubes) is the most serious complication of chlamydia infections, and past chlamydial infections are associated with an increased risk of ectopic pregnancy and tubal factor infertility in women (Hatcher et al, 1994).

Pelvic Inflammatory Disease (PID). PID most commonly involves the fallopian tubes (salpingitis) and uterus (endometritis). It rarely affects the ovaries and peritoneal surfaces. Multiple organisms can cause PID, but the most common agents are *C. trachomatis* and *N. gonorrhoeae.* Most PID is thought to result from microorganisms ascending from the vagina and endocervix to the upper genital tract (Fogel, 1995). Most frequently, this occurs at the end of menses or just after menses. Menstrual blood may act as a medium for growth of the invading microorganism, while the slightly open cervical os and absent cervical mucus during menses may explain this phenomenon (Fogel, 1995).

Symptoms of PID vary, depending on whether the infection is acute or chronic. There may be dull, cramping, and intermittent pain (subacute) or severe, persistent, and incapacitating pain (acute). Irregular bleeding (intermenstrual) or spotting may accompany the abdominal or pelvic symptoms. The feared consequences of PID are chronic pelvic pain and infertility due to the subsequent development of scar tissue and adhesions in the fallopian tubes and other structures in the abdomen.

Syphilis. One of the earliest described STIs, syphilis is caused by *Treponema pallidum,* a motile spirochete (Fogel, 1995). Transmission is thought to occur through microabrasions during sexual intercourse, kissing, biting, or oral-genital sex (Lichtman and Duran, 1990). Individuals infected with syphilis may exhibit signs of primary (ulcer or chancre at site of infection), secondary (manifestations that include rash, mucocutaneous lesions, and adenopathy), or tertiary or latent (cardiac, neurologic, ophthalmic, auditory, or gummatous lesions) stage disease (CDC, 1993). Untreated syphilis can be fatal in the tertiary stage. In 1990, syphilis reached its highest incidence since the end of World War II, with more than 50,000 new cases reported (Division of STD/HIV Prevention, 1991). This increased incidence may be attributed to drug use and to the lack of access to health care by groups at high risk for syphilis, such as drug users (Fogel, 1995). The risk to drug users, particularly injection drug users, is increased due to blood-borne pathogens acquired through shared needle use or to exposure through unprotected sexual activity (US DHHS, 1995). This risk appears to be greater in women who opt for hormonal contraception.

Human Papillomavirus (HPV) Infection. HPV infections are more commonly known as genital or venereal warts; health care providers often refer to the infection as condyloma. Health care providers are not required to report HPV infections, so the true incidence is not known. However, genital warts appeared to be the most rapidly spreading STI from the mid-1960s until the onset of the AIDS epidemic (Aral and Holmes, 1991). HPV is considered to be highly contagious, and as many as 85 percent of exposed sexual partners will develop genital warts (Fogel, 1995). In women, genital warts are most frequently seen in the posterior part of the introitus, on the vulva, vagina, anus, and cervix. In men, genital warts occur on the shaft and glans of the penis, in the urethra, on scrotal tissue, and in the anus. Genital warts range in appearance from flat-topped papules to cauliflower-like masses. The warts are often painless but may be uncomfortable, particularly when lesions are large or extensive. Specific serotypes of HPV have recently been linked to genital squamous cell carcinoma in women, particularly to cervical cancer. More than 90 percent of cervical neoplasms have been associated with these serotypes (Fogel, 1995). Papanicolaou (Pap) smears and physical examination are used to diagnose HPV infection.

Herpes Simplex Virus (HSV) Infection. This painful vesicular eruption of the skin and genital mucosa is caused by two different subtypes of HSV: herpes simplex virus 1 (HSV-1) and herpes simplex virus 2 (HSV-2). Common belief once held that HSV-1 (most commonly associated with gingivostomatitis and fever blisters) is transmitted nonsexually; HSV-2 (genital lesions), sexually. However, reflecting changing sexual mores and practices, HSV-1 is now often detected in genital lesions, and HSV-2 in fever blisters.

The initial herpetic infection characteristically produces both systemic and local symptoms that last about 3 weeks (Fogel, 1995). Women generally have a more severe clinical course than men, and first symptoms in both genders tend to be genital discomfort and neuralgic pain. Systemic symptoms appear early, peak about 72 to 96 hours after lesions appear, and then subside over a period of 72 to 96 hours. The characteristic ulcerative lesions last approximately 4 to 15 days before crusting over. The most outstanding characteristic of herpes lesions is intense discomfort.

Genital herpes may be recurrent and has no cure. Most infected persons never recognize signs suggestive of genital herpes, whereas some will have symptoms shortly after infection and then never again. A minority of the total U.S. population infected with genital herpes has recurrent episodes (CDC, 1993). Recurrences are more common in men than in women (Smith et al, 1990).

Hepatitis B (HB) Infection. Transmitted parenterally and by sexual contact (Fogel, 1995), HB infection is more contagious than HIV and is the most common STI worldwide (Cefalo and Moos, 1990). HB is a disease of the liver and often goes undetected. Of persons infected as adults, 6 to 10 percent become chronic HB virus carriers (CDC, 1993); 25 percent of chronic carriers die from primary liver cancer or cirrhosis of the liver (Fogel, 1995). Symptoms of HB include skin eruptions, urticaria, arthralgias, arthritis, lassitude, nausea, headache, fever, and mild abdominal pain (Fogel, 1995). Later stages may be marked by clay-colored stools, dark urine, abdominal pain, and jaundice may appear.

Human Immunodeficiency Virus (HIV) Infection. HIV is the cause of AIDS. Transmission of HIV occurs only through direct contact with body fluids rich in T-4 lymphocytes (Fogel, 1995). HIV has been detected in body fluids such as blood, semen, vaginal secretions, cerebrospinal fluid, urine, tears, and saliva. Only blood, semen, and vaginal secretions have been implicated in person-to-person transmission. Sexual contact and inoculation of blood are the major routes of transmission. Available data suggest that female-to-male transmission is less efficient than male-to-female transmission (O'Brien et al, 1992). AIDS now is the leading cause of death for all Americans age 25 to 44 and is perhaps the most highly gendered disease in our history; incidence is about nine times higher in men than in women (Sabo and Gordon, 1995).

Trends in the AIDS epidemic in the United States reflect dramatic shifts in its impact, including the persons affected by gender, race/ethnicity; geographic areas; and mode of transmission. HIV/AIDS is increasing significantly among women, people of color, and injection drug users. The Southern area of the country is experiencing significant increases in AIDS cases, whereas cases are decreasing in the Northeast. In addition, although AIDS was originally viewed as a condition affecting primarily gay men, recent trends show a decrease in the cases reported as a result of men who have sex with men and an increase in cases acquired through injection drug use and heterosexual contact.

Estimates based on age distribution of AIDS cases suggest that in recent years as many as half of new HIV infections may be among young people under 25 years of age. Fifty-five percent of the AIDS cases reported among young men aged 13 to 24 years were related to men who have sex with men and 10 percent were due to injection drug use. In contrast, 51 percent of the AIDS cases reported among young women 13 to 24 years were due to heterosexual contact and 17 percent were due to injecting drugs (UNAIDS, 1996).

BODY IMAGE CONCERNS

Good self-esteem and a positive self-concept are important aspects of healthy sexual functioning in both men and women. The high value that American society places on physical attractiveness (and ideal body weight) for women has a profound effect on women's self-esteem. The standards of what constitutes attractiveness are not always realistic and most often not even healthful. A youthful appearance is a requirement for physical attractiveness much more for women than for men, and the differences in attitudes toward the aging process for men and women can be detrimental to the older women's self-concept, self-esteem, and mental health. For men, physical fitness and physical prowess are values that are obtained early in life; in adulthood, men embrace strenuous games, sports, competition, and exercise as symbols of masculinity. Although there is less emphasis on weight and youthful appearance by men, there is some concern about these issues, especially as hair loss occurs, which influences self-esteem.

SEXUAL VIOLENCE

Violence against women is pervasive in our society, occurring in all socioeconomic and ethnic groups, and must be considered as a means to exert control over women (Campbell and Landenburger, 1995). Each year, in the United States, over 2 million women are assaulted by a family member and over two thirds of all violent attacks against women are committed by someone the victim knows. Women are 10 times more likely than men to be attacked by spouses, ex-spouses, partners, boyfriends, parents, or children. One in three women seeking emergency care has a history of partner violence. Abuse occurs in between 7 and 17 percent of all pregnancies, and approximately half of battered women are abused during pregnancy (Campbell and Humphreys, 1993). One in seven women visiting a doctor's office has a history of relationship violence. Violence is not limited to heterosexual relationships and has been reported between lesbian partners (Carlson et al, 1996).

Violence can be psychological, sexual, or physical and can range from sexual harassment to homicide. Regardless of which form it takes, all types of psychological, sexual, or physical abuse against women (along with rape, incest, and sexual harassment) are acts of violence in which the perpetrator asserts control or power, thereby victimizing a woman and limiting her personal freedom.

The sequelae of these victimizations include acute effects (genital and nongenital injuries, sexually transmitted infections, and pregnancy), late consequences (chronic pelvic pain and other forms of chronic pain, gastrointestinal symptoms, premenstrual symptoms, and negative health behaviors, such as sexual promiscuity), and long-term increases in the use of medical services (Koss and Heslet, 1992).

Sexual violence against women includes rape (date or acquaintance, stranger, and marital), incest, and prostitution (Campbell and Landenburger, 1995). **Rape** can involve any sexual assault—including but not limited to sexual intercourse—achieved with physical force or the threat of physical force. Motivated by the desire to dominate or humiliate, rape is an act of violence rather than an act of sexuality. Rape outside of marriage has been considered as **date** or **acquaintance rape** and **stranger rape.** Although both forms are sexual assault, women raped by a stranger are viewed as unwilling victims, whereas women experiencing date rape are often viewed as responsible for the assault. Social norms that support power differentials in gender roles have been found to lead to violence (Lloyd, 1991). If social norms ascribe to women the role of maintaining relationships, women are blamed for any abuse or sexual violence that takes place. The role and responsibility of the male as the perpetrator of abuse becomes a secondary issue. These opposing roles of initiator and gatekeeper set up an adversarial process in the intimate relationship. **Marital rape,** sexual assault within marriage or within a long-term cohabiting relationship, occurs in 10 to 14 percent of U.S. women, and almost half of all battered women are also being raped on an ongoing basis by their partners (Campbell, 1989; Campbell and Landenburger, 1995). The sexual assault laws in most states have not applied to husbands, essentially legalizing marital rape. By 1990, only 10 states still retained this exception, but the fact that in the United States it is legal for a man to rape his wife is indicative of the remnants of attitudes that condone violence against women (Campbell and Landenburger, 1995). Clearly, these social norms influence the sexual health and experiences of men and women. **Incest** is a sexual act whereby a parent or a significant person whom a child trusts abuses that trust and exerts control over a child. The legal definition of incest is usually limited to sexual intercourse between blood relatives but has been broadened to include explicit sexual contact (Finkelhor, 1980). Other forms of sexual violence and sexual oppression against women include **prostitution** and **sexual harassment.** Prostitution can be considered as both economic exploitation and sexual domination of women. The majority of prostitutes have been sexually assaulted in childhood and are often forced into prostitution by violence or by drug addiction (Hartman et al, 1987). Sexual harassment includes gender-specific verbal and nonverbal harassment; inappropriate and offensive sexual advances; and sexual bribery, coercion, and assault (Fitzgerald et al, 1988). In most cases of sexual harassment, there is a power differential between the victim and the perpetrator.

SEXUAL ASSAULT

There is an escalating epidemic of rape in the United States. All victims have psychological injury, and over half sustain physical injury in the assault (Hampton, 1995). One of every eight adult women surveyed in the National Women's Study reported that she had been the victim of at least one forcible rape sometime in her lifetime. Four in 10 rape victims have been raped more than once. At least 1.4 million women are raped each year (Hatcher et al, 1994). Data from the 1987 National Survey of Children reveal that 12.7 percent of white females, 8 percent of African American females, 1.9 percent of white males, and 6.1 percent of African American males had experienced nonvoluntary sexual intercourse by age 20 (Hatcher et al, 1994).

Sexual assault has diverse and long-lasting health consequences. It is thought that approximately 50 percent of all rapes go unreported, and the incidence of rape and sexual assault can therefore only be estimated. Since 1976, the reported rate of forcible rape has risen 38 percent. This may be due to better reporting, or to an increase in the actual rates of the offense.

In addition to sexual assault on adult women, sexual abuse of children is considered a major public health problem. There is little doubt that sexual abuse is as frequent and as damaging to the long-term development of children as is physical abuse. The National Center for Child Abuse and Neglect conservatively estimates that 100,000 children are sexually abused yearly, and that a high proportion of such cases involve the parents or other adult figures familiar to the child. Clinical reports suggest that up to half of their female patients have experienced sexual exploitation at some time in their lives.

Sexual violence in older women is a growing problem that is underreported in crime statistics and often not identified by clinicians (DeLorey and Wolf, 1993). Overcoming ageism and acknowledging the sexuality of older women are fundamental to the improved recognition of sexual violence throughout the lifespan.

Reducing the frequency of sexual abuse among women and children requires social and behavior modifications such as changing the attitudes that foster violence towards women and children, increasing the ability of women and children to avoid sexual violence by strengthening concepts of self, helping women and children acquire coping skills and the ability to defend themselves, increasing community awareness regarding sexual violence, and affirming women's control of their bodies and their responsibility to support each other in enforcing control (Sparks and Bar On, 1981).

SEXUAL HARASSMENT

Sexual harassment has been a fixture of the workplace since women first began to work outside the home. Although true epidemiologic studies do not exist, large-scale surveys of working women suggest that approximately one of every two women will be harassed at some point during their academic or working lives (Fitzgerald, 1993). Sexual harassment is an interaction between two or more people in which one person is the recipient of unwanted sexual behavior by another person (Spratlen, 1988). Though women are most commonly the victims of sexual harassment, men have reported such incidents. Data indicate that harassment is degrading, frightening, and sometimes physically violent; frequently extends over a considerable period; and can result in profound job-related, psychological, and health-related consequences (Fitzgerald, 1993).

Included under sexual harassment are a number of behaviors including gender-specific verbal and nonverbal harassment, inappropriate and offensive sexual advances, and sexual bribery (Fitzgerald et al, 1988). In most cases of sexual harassment, there is a power differential between the perpetrator and his or her victim (Campbell and Landenburger, 1995). It is the power differential in the relationship that can lead to a fear of reporting the harassment, which allows the harassment to continue. This continuing harassment, then, prohibits the necessary psychological healing of the victim.

Relevant Research

The foundation for an understanding of sexual health promotion includes a research and theory-based literature related to gender and health within a multidimensional framework of biologic, psychosocial, and cultural influences. In particular, gender differences related to health and illness are critical to sexual health and sexual health promotion practices. Nursing research has provided leadership in the understanding of the multidimensional nature of gender and health.

NURSING RESEARCH

Nursing science is built on a core of "holism" where multiple levels of inquiry can be considered and applied. This core provides the foundation for the study of men's and women's health, and nursing's scientific and research process has included an intensive study of multidimensional aspects of individuals, groups, and community as they adapt to health and illness. Not only is the unit of analysis of concern to nursing science, but so is the biopsychosocial environment or context in which the individual, family, and community resides.

In evoking a biopsychosocial framework, nursing utilizes a convenient and realistic way to visualize the diversity of factors that may be involved in women's and men's health or illness. A biopsychosocial perspective provides a model for classifying clinical and experimental findings that involve multidimensional causal factors. Further, individual or physiologic adaptation can be considered within the context of a person's personal and cultural beliefs or lifespan development. However, although a central strength of nursing is the attempt to maintain a holistic perspective, gender, sex role characteristics, and sexual health must be included in nursing practice to the same degree as other social factors (socioeconomic status, culture, and ethnicity). Viewing a patient as a whole means extending the clinical assessment beyond the genitourinary system and attending to the patient's gender or sexual identity. The clinical implication for the nurse is that health risks due to gender must be an integral part of clinical practice as those due to socioeconomic or ethnic status.

Nursing practice for men's and women's sexual health is more than discrete tasks, and includes both concepts and actions. Underlying the treatments and intervention strategies should be a system of guiding concepts relating to the practitioner, the patient, the intervention and the environment, as well as the interactions among these dimensions. Many nurse researchers and theorists (Box 33–2) have proposed conceptual models to guide nursing practice in the area of gender-specific health care delivery. Angela McBride, one of the earli-

BOX 33-2
NURSING PRACTICE MODELS FOR MEN'S AND WOMEN'S HEALTH: NURSE RESEARCHERS AND NURSING THEORISTS

- David Allen
- Joanne Hall
- Angela McBride
- Afaf Meleis
- Nola Pender
- Joan Shaver
- Patricia Stevens
- Diana Taylor
- Nancy Woods
- Allen Whatley

est theorists to write about gender and health, proposed that men's and women's health means redefining the very nature of health care so that physical, psychological, and sexual well-being are presumed to be intertwined, as well as determined by the context (interpersonal, socioeconomic, political, environmental) in which the individual operates (McBride and McBride, 1981).

The interaction of the individual or group with its environment is also of particular concern to nursing science when attempting to understand gender-specific phenomena. Nursing science has a practice and applied component that is characterized by values of humanism, personal concern, intuition, sensitivity to alternative views, and collaboration. These core concepts of nursing are also of central concern in feminist methodology and theory. Both feminists and nurses value research and practice methods that presume the integrity of the subject as a complex, perceptive individual or group of individuals. Joan Shaver's human ecological model (1985) is based upon the interaction of the individual with the environment and the influence of that interaction upon health-related behavior. Although this model improves understanding of environmental influences upon personal behavior, it does not explain the importance of the physical and sociopolitical elements of the environment that have significant impact upon the health of many women and men, especially the poor and disadvantaged. Doris Williams (1989), in her feminist critique of health promotion in the U.S., rejects the emphasis on individual behavior as the most important determinant of health.

A model of health adaptation incorporating multiple individual and environmental variables developed by Nola Pender (1982, 1987) includes polar constructs of health promotion and health protection. The domain of health protection includes individual behavior directed toward the regulation and maintenance of homeostasis and structural integrity. Health promotion is the actualization of inherent and acquired individual potential. Both health protecting and health promoting behaviors include physical, social, and self-care components. Assumptions guiding Pender's model include concepts of personal choice and self-directed behavior. The assumption of personal choice suggests that change, self-actualization, or the capacity for change exists if the individual so chooses. A second assumption supposes that individual behavior is purposeful and motivated toward a goal. Purpose can only exist if choices are available and the individual is capable of making a choice. In a revision of this model, Pender has added a component of environmental modification that includes community assessment and sociopolitical change. Environmental modification is considered along with personal change strategies for illness prevention and health promotion.

Nancy Woods also proposed an agenda for future nursing research in women's health and recommended studies that focus on adolescent, middle-aged, and elderly women; health promotion, illness prevention, and health of the chronically ill or disabled; the influence of environment on women and their health; and new research traditions that recognize biologic, psychological, social, and cultural contexts. Woods (1988) and coworkers (Taylor and Woods, 1991; Woods et al, 1993) have taken a leadership role in nursing research of women's health phenomena by identifying factors that link roles, personal relationships, social support, stressors, and coping patterns to health status in women.

Afaf Meleis (1990) recommends the use of feminist principles to approach the concept of health, proposing that health is a social rather than a personal issue, especially for women. A feminist paradigm recognizes the centrality of the person/environment interaction to health and illness and can be applied to men's health as well as women's health. Furthermore, feminist principles recognize issues of ethnicity, health access, and socioeconomic status as important to health. Feminism is a world view that values women and confronts systematic injustices based on gender. Feminism focuses on women's experiences, but there is no universal women's experience because gender is not the sole definition of women's lives (Hall and Stevens, 1991). Class, race, ethnicity, education, age, national origin, and sexual orientation characterize multiple "feminisms"; they can also provide a basis for understanding men's health. These multiple feminisms share basic principles:

- a valuing of women and a validation of women's experiences, ideas, and needs
- a recognition of the existence of ideologic, structural, and interpersonal conditions that oppress women
- a desire to bring about social change of oppressive constraints through criticism and political action (Hall and Stevens, 1991)

In the same way, men should be considered as individuals and the same ideologic, structural, and interpersonal conditions are oppressive to many men, especially gay men or men of color.

A combined nursing-feminist approach to men's and women's health emphasizes the importance of experiential analysis. Women see their lives in terms of relationships with loved ones; what happens to other people affects them. At the same time, a woman's socialization history can lead to poor health or illness. Yapko (1992) suggests that men are socialized to be "self-oriented" and women are socialized to be "other-oriented."

Throughout life, mothers advise their daughters to be good children, good wives, and good mothers, which suggests that a woman's worth is dependent on the woman's relation to other people, and not on the woman as a unique individual. Men are socialized to pursue independent goals regardless of family or relationships, whereas women suppress their individual personality and a healthy sense of their own self-worth in order to obtain approval from others. This sexist socialization can create patterns that expose women to a variety of negative experiences, such as illness symptoms and depression, and may work against individual well-being. Although these generalizations oversimplify the complexity of individual human response, the critical factor is to understand that there are differences between men and women and each individual's meaning of health and illness. Furthermore, while differences exist among men and women, a significant similarity remains; biopsychosocial, sexual, and cultural dimensions within the individual operate with the context of multiple environments (interpersonal, social, physical) to affect health.

Nursing theorists have also extended feminist frameworks to apply to men's health and have expressed a discontent with health care based on male stereotypes and role-related issues (Allen and Whatley, 1986). Allen (1985) has conceptualized men's health in terms of the health consequences resulting from the way men are socialized and postulates that a positive goal for a men's health movement would be to identify the linkages between causes of male mortality and men's lives. As a nurse scientist, Allen challenges the biomedical models of men's health and suggests that men's health and illness are related to sociopolitical and cultural processes, and not biologic givens. Allen and Whatley (1986) propose a revision of the "adaptation" models of health and illness for application to men's health. These investigators suggest that adaptation/coping models fail to question the cardiovascular disease, but when prescribed for men may reinforce male stereotypes of the powerful individualist. Allen and Whatley suggest instead that men should be included in the treatment plan with a focus on transformation of the individual, the environment, or both.

Building on these nurse theorists' and researchers' works, McBride (1993) and Woods (1995) suggest an ecologic view of women's health, a theory that can also be extended to men's health. From an ecologic view of women's health, personal factors directly influencing the health of men and women—such as food intake, energy expenditure, reproductive and sexual experiences, injury, exposures to toxic and infectious agents, and substance abuse—are closely related to the social and physical environments in which they live. Individual characteristics, such as age, genetic makeup, health-related knowledge, skills, and values, interact with contextual factors such as access to education, income, work opportunities, family and dependent care responsibilities, or housing availability and quality to influence health status. Social, cultural, and community contexts such as the prevalence of domestic and other types of violence, availability of health and social services, clean water, sanitation services, fuel, employment opportunities, transportation, food supplies, and community support organizations highly impact men's and women's health. Whereas most scientific disciplines have typically adopted a unidimensional view of health and illness, nursing theorists have advocated for a biopsychosocial and cultural framework for guiding men's and women's health. Clearly physical, psychological, and sexual well-being are intertwined in these conceptual models. In addition, nursing has been at the forefront in considering gender, ethnicity, and socioeconomic status as critical to health, illness, and nursing practice for men's and women's health (Taylor and Woods, 1996).

Relevant Theory

PSYCHOANALYTIC THEORY

The psychoanalytic theories of Freud and Erikson are basic to understanding sexuality, even though in contemporary scientific literature there is considerable questioning of their value (Rynerson, 1990). Regardless, the psychoanalytic view integrates inborn physiologic and psychological dimensions and social factors as they relate to psychosexual development. Freud believed that sexual feelings begin in infancy and change from one form to another into adulthood. He identi-

BOX 33-3
FREUD'S STAGES OF SEXUAL DEVELOPMENT

- **Oral stage:** infancy through 18 months. During this period, the oral region (the sensory area of the mouth, lips, and tongue) provides the greatest sensual satisfaction. Sucking and swallowing reduce tension and provide pleasure.
- **Anal stage:** age 18 months to 3 years. During this period, the greatest amount of sensual pleasure is obtained from the anal and urethral areas. Toilet training is a source of tension between child and parent.
- **Phallic stage:** age 3 to 5 years. The region of greatest sensual pleasure is the genital region. The Oedipal/Electra complex occurs in the later part of the phallic stage. During this stage the child "loves" the parent of the opposite sex. The parent of the same sex is considered a rival.
- **Latency stage:** age 6 to 12 years. At the beginning of the latency stage, the child is resolving the Oedipal/Electra conflict, so this is a phase of sexual latency. During this period, children form close relationships with others of their own age and sex. They direct energy to physical and intellectual quests.
- **Genital stage:** puberty to adulthood. Increased hormones stimulate sexual development. Sexual urges reawaken but are now directed outside the family.

BOX 33-4
ERIKSON'S EIGHT STAGES OF DEVELOPMENT

Stage	Task	Threat
Infant	Trust	Mistrust
Toddler	Autonomy	Shame and doubt
Preschooler	Initiative	Guilt
School age	Industry	Inferiority
Adolescent	Identity	Identity diffusion
Early adulthood	Intimacy	Isolation
Middle adulthood	Generativity	Self-absorption
Late adulthood	Integrity	Despair

fied four stages of psychosexual development (Box 33–3) that center on the early years of life (Barkauskas et al, 1994). At each stage, libido is invested in different areas of the body, which determines how the individual interacts with other people.

Psychosocial development has been explained by Erik Erikson (Barkauskas et al, 1994). Erikson suggested eight developmental stages and identified a central task and a threat to the accomplishment of that task for each developmental stage (Box 33–4). The central task for each stage is identified as a "crisis" or turning point when development must move one way; it is a time when a pair of opposite qualities are presented that must be resolved and integrated in order to proceed with ego development. Dealing with each task provides the basis for movement to the next stage.

The theories of Freud and Erikson help us to understand sexual development but impose a moralistic perspective built upon social mores of their age. Their notions of sexuality integrated with social development offered new explanations yet do not necessarily mesh with contemporary mores. In response to the need for more information about sexuality, theorists of the 1960s and 1970s provided more of the "how to" information. It was the work of Masters and Johnson that initiated enormous interest and attention in this area. Although this work has provided advancement in our understanding of sexual response, it has been criticized for taking sexuality from something of mystery to something mechanical.

FEMINIST THEORY

The self-help movement and the women's movement were born out of the 1960s' and 1970s' interest in sexuality and sexual expression, though interest in women's health had been linked to the sociopolitical movement for women's rights. The early focus of the women's health movement was primarily a reaction to the existing health care system. However, feminists agreed on neither the causes nor the solutions to women's health problems.

Three distinct approaches to improving the women's health system corresponded to the major feminist schools of thought in the U.S. in the 1970s. Radical feminists focused on self-help alternatives and organized for a totally new health care system. Socialist feminists argued for a reorganization of the financing of health care to remove the profit motive. Liberal feminists believed that more power for women in the existing system, such as more women physicians, would bring about the desired changes in women's health (Fee, 1975; Webster and Lipetz, 1986). In addition to these major philosophies, single-interest groups within the larger women's health movement focused on issues such as abortion rights, home birth, self-help clinics, and older women's health.

Largely as an outgrowth of the women's movement, alternatives to traditional male-dominated, disease-oriented systems of care are now available to women, men, and their health care providers. In the 1970s the women's health movement empowered women's health consumers through education and peer support. A key publication was the book by the Boston Women's Health Collective, *Our Bodies, Ourselves* (1971, 1976, and 1985), which served as a force for change and documentation of progress in women's health care. It was this publication, and others like it, that have tied self-awareness to sexuality and sexual health. Within the past decade, both men and women have shown increasing concern and motivation to take an active role in their own health. This is clearly evident in the proliferation of classes, magazines, and community health activities emphasizing self-care. The focus of these programs is to assist people in becoming knowledgeable partners in maintaining and promoting personal health. Wellness, disease prevention, and health promotion form the core of self-help and self-care strategies, while professional care and guidance remains a secondary process. Health care providers must maintain current knowledge of self-help resources (Box 33–5).

BOX 33-5
RESOURCES: SEXUAL HEALTH

American Association of Sex Educators and Therapists
435 North Michigan Ave., Suite 1717
Chicago, IL 60611
312-644-0828

Good Vibrations
Store and Catalog Company for sexual aids and information
1210 Valencia Street
San Francisco, CA 94110
415-974-8980 (Retail Store and Mail Order)

National Gay and Lesbian Task Force
1517 U Street NW
Washington, DC 20009
202-332-6483
800-221-7044

Sex Information & Education Council of the U.S. (SIECUS)
130 West 42nd St., Suite 2500
New York, NY 10036
212-819-9770

FACTORS AFFECTING CLINICAL DECISIONS

Research has provided some understanding that men's and women's sexual health is influenced by interacting psychological, social, cultural, spiritual, and ethical factors.

Age

Sexuality cannot be confined to a specific age or to a specific time span; rather, it must be considered a part of human development and progression throughout life. To understand the physiologic, psychological, and social aspects of human sexuality, these must be examined for each life stage. The aim is to provide the nurse with a basic understanding of what constitutes the range of sexual behavior and the characteristics of healthy sexuality during each life stage (Rynerson, 1990).

INFANTS AND CHILDREN

Infancy, from birth to 1 year, is the oral phase of development according to Freud and the stage of trust versus mistrust according to Erikson (Rynerson, 1990). It is a time for acquiring a sense of self, which forms the basis for manifestations of healthy sexuality later in life. Needs are satisfied by sucking, taking in nourishment, and by tactile exploration of objects or the skin of another person. Trust is established as the infant experiences the satisfaction of needs in a nurturing and nourishing environment. Mistrust, on the other hand, can be established when there are prolonged delays or inconsistencies in having basic needs met. It is thought that there is little inner awareness of gender differences in the infancy stage, though adults most often interact and respond with infants according to gender. Although these differences in behavior by adults may not be deliberate attempts to influence gender behavior, roles, and attitudes, they do reflect general societal attitudes that males and females differ. In the infancy stage, the infant is the passive recipient of interactions that occur (Rynerson, 1990).

The next stage of early childhood, age 1 to 3 years, is identified by Freud as the anal stage; to Erikson, it is the stage of autonomy versus shame and doubt (Rynerson, 1990). The child's sense of sexuality during this stage is manifested as self-stimulating behaviors such as touching and exploring the genitals. Shame or doubt can occur if the parents respond to this behavior by displaying discomfort or disgust because this gives the child the sense that the body is untouchable or somehow dirty. Although socialization as a male or female begins during infancy, from age 1 to 3 the child has a beginning awareness of sexual differences and sexual roles (Barkauskas et al, 1994).

The third stage of development, ages 4 to 5, is the phallic or genital stage (Freud) and the stage of initiative versus guilt (Erikson) (Rynerson, 1990). During this stage, the child's genitals increase in sensitivity, which makes the focus of pleasure in the genital area. Concomitantly, the child becomes more socially responsible and is able to give love and affection. The stage is marked by the child's beginning recognition of an identity, including a clear concept of gender, and beginning to imitate the parent of the same sex, learning more of a sex role identity, and becoming acutely aware of sexual differences. Interest in the parent of the opposite sex may become romantic and lead to conflict when the child realizes he or she cannot replace the parent of the same sex. Because the child cannot compete with this larger and more powerful rival, she or he resolves the tension by identifying with the parent of the same sex. Freud called this the Oedipal complex (Barkauskas et al, 1994).

During the middle years of childhood, ages 6 to 12, the child moves from the close ties of family to the larger world of peers, school, and neighborhood (Barkauskas et al, 1994). Socialization is primarily by peer play. Freud identified this as the latency stage, during which rapid physical development occurs, and the whole body becomes the focus of pleasure. Psychosexual development is held in abeyance. Erikson described it as the stage of industry versus inferiority (Rynerson, 1990). At this stage, the child, it is hoped, develops a sense of industriousness and accomplishment rather than a sense of inadequacy.

Gender differences are very apparent in both the third and fourth stages of development, but both physiologic and psychosocial experiences have a great impact on sexuality and the continuing development of gender identity and role. In response to queries about sex and the birth process, it is most healthy to impart to the child that males and females both receive and give love and that intercourse is pleasurable for both sexes (Rynerson, 1990). In later childhood, same-sex friendships serve many purposes, including expanding sex role behaviors, coping with physical sexual inadequacy, and initiating activities that indicate sexual preference for a partner (Rynerson, 1990). Experimentation in same-sex sexual behaviors is normal at this developmental level and may or may not be intermittent, short lived, and undisclosed.

ADOLESCENTS

Adolescence is a developmental phase that spans 10 years and begins with puberty, which refers to the hormonal and physical changes leading to maturation of reproductive capacity. Freud refers to adolescence as the genital stage in which sexual urges reawaken but are directed outside the family; oedipal issues are worked out at a different level and sensuous or affectional attachments are directed toward peers rather than toward parents. Erikson identified the stage as identity versus identity diffusion. Identity is defined as having a clear sense of gender identity as well as a sense of purpose toward becoming a contributing member of society (Rynerson, 1990). Adolescence is often viewed by adults as a time of turmoil and trouble, inasmuch as rapid physiologic changes are accompanied by conflict and anxiety and often behavior inconsistencies and mood swings.

Physiologic sexual maturation in males begins at about age 12 or later, with the enlargement of the testes and scrotum, accompanied by the development of pubic hair. Following these events are rapid increases in height and concomitant increased sensitivity in nipples and breasts, changes in body hair and musculature, and body contour changes. These alterations often cause a lack of coordination and awkwardness that is a source of embarrassment to the adolescent male. The commencement of nocturnal emissions follows the maturation of the prostate gland and seminal vesicles. Because the male sexual organs are external, they are more easily stimulated and create awareness of sexual arousal. Kinsey's studies provide the basis for understanding that adolescence is a time for rapid increase in sex drive and orgasmic capacity in the male. However, later research indicates that the heightened need for sexual gratification in males during this stage of development is a result of a combination of physiologic, cultural, and social learning influences; given cultural norms of today, male and female differences may be diminishing (Rynerson, 1990).

Females reach sexual maturity at about age 10 to 13, approximately 2 years earlier than males. During this time, females' breasts begin to develop, pubic hair appears, and growth of the uterus and vaginal canal occur. Concomitantly, there is enlargement of the labia and clitoris. Menarche, or onset of menstruation, generally occurs following the peak of the female growth spurt and is the point of complete sexual maturity (mean age for U.S. girls = 12.3 years). Female sexual organs are internal and are, therefore, less easily stimulated than are male sex organs. For this reason, there may be less awareness of sexual arousal by the adolescent female (Rynerson, 1990).

During adolescence, young men and women experiment with their sexuality and may engage in behaviors that include kissing, petting, and genital stimulation without penile penetration (Bernhard, 1995). These activities may result in orgasm by one or both partners. Some adolescents go on to participate in sexual intercourse. There is wide variation in perceptions and attitudes toward the adolescent engaging in sexual activities. Some believe that sexual experimentation is optimal for a person's development, while others believe that self-denial is character-building. Despite conflicting beliefs about adolescent sexual activity, it is known that adolescents of both sexes are engaging in intercourse at an earlier age and that more females are sexually active than in previous years (Rynerson, 1990). However, most authors do agree that for both sexes intercourse in the context of a meaningful relationship is still the norm (Rynerson, 1990). It is noted in the literature that mothers and fathers are very good at teaching and modeling sex role behaviors in relation to being men and women but do very poorly when it comes to teaching about being lovers and mates. This interesting situation may partially explain why marital relationships have a high failure rate.

Role socialization in adolescence focuses on dating as preparation for mate selection. Dating serves the purpose of freedom of choice, during which the adolescent tests out ideas about the self and opposite sex partners. These social encounters may lead to experiencing intercourse and the pleasures of heterosexual acts (Rynerson, 1990), but may also serve to provide the adolescent with experience at sorting through feelings of inadequacies in interpersonal relationships. Females appear to be particularly sensitive to these inadequacies because sensitivity, empathy, and acceptance are extremely important to them, and their frustrations, jealousies, and conflicts tend to be over friends (Rynerson, 1990). Males tend to disagree and argue about activities, property, and girlfriends.

ADULTHOOD

Healthy individuals arrive at adulthood having survived the turmoil of adolescence with at least an identity oriented toward purpose in life, gender constancy, and an idea about gender roles, however unclear these are in today's world (Rynerson, 1990). Adulthood begins at the end of adolescence when the individual is establishing himself or herself as an autonomous member of society. There are no identifiable biologic developments that mark this stage in sexuality growth.

According to Erikson, the stage of adulthood is characterized by developing intimacy, which is defined as the capacity for love and mutual devotion. It is during early adult years that capacity for full sexual expression is maximal, both in physical expression with a partner and in gender role behaviors. Primary tasks include developing satisfactory work, social relationships, and educational pursuits.

Middle adulthood, according to Erikson, is a time of generativity and productivity. Stagnation, or being in a rut, is the consequence of not assuming the developmental tasks of this life stage (Rynerson, 1990). Stage-related crises of both women and men have occupied much of the developmental literature and are most obvious in middle adulthood. Davis (1980) believes these midlife crises revolve around losses in "critical life exchange values." Physiologic changes in the process of aging and the challenges to the present value systems of youth and beauty are difficult to reconcile. Particularly for women, these physiologic changes, in partnership with gender role (equality, power, and money) issues, contribute to women's struggles.

Biologic changes in middle adulthood include a decrease in height, muscle mass, strength, and cardiac power (Fogel and Woods, 1995); these factors might have long-term consequences to health. Virtually all women who live long enough experience the menopausal transition, either naturally or as a medical event (medically or surgically). In the United States, most women experience menopause during their late 40s and early 50s; the median age is approximately 51 years. Unlike the average age at menarche, the average age at menopause has remained about the same since the Middle Ages (Fogel and Woods, 1995). Natural menopause is a gradual process with progressive increases in anovulatory cycles and eventual cessation of menses, whereas surgical removal of the uterus and ovaries or radiation or chemotherapy causes a sudden cessation of menses. The resultant loss in estrogen levels produces a number of physiologic symptoms (hot flashes, night sweats, fatigue, vaginal dryness) that have the potential to alter sexuality during this phase in womens' lives. These potential alterations might include a decrease in frequency of sexual intercourse, decrease in masturbation, and an increase in alternate forms of sexual expression, such as oral sex, physical touching, and mutual pleasuring. The effect of menopause on mood and behavior responses, such as depression and anxiety or loss of libido, is less clear; mood and behavior responses during this phase in womens' lives may be due to hormonal changes associated with menopause, normal aging processes, psychological transitions that may occur in the midlife decades, or cultural beliefs and expectations, and from dietary and lifestyle habits (Fogel and Woods, 1995).

Men do not have the same dramatic change that women experience in midlife. Rather, there is a more insidious decline in androgen-dependent tissues, which produce changes in the penis and scrotum. These physiologic changes also mean concomitant reduction in sexual response capacity, though there are individual variations in these changes.

Probably the most widely speculated about and reported means of coping with midlife issues by men is to engage in affairs. However, changes in sex role norms in society have led to more women in midlife engaging in affairs, as well. These affairs may be an attempt to bolster identity as a sexual being, find companionship, seek revenge, or to satisfy needs that have changed (Rynerson, 1990).

ELDERLY ADULTS

In adults over age 65, a number of biologic factors influence sexual expression. In females, cells of the reproductive tract and the breasts are estrogen-dependent for growth and function. The decline of estrogen production that begins at menopause is responsible for many of the changes in tissue status of older women. The ovaries, uterus, and cervix decrease in size; the vagina narrows and shortens and vaginal epithelium atrophies (surface is thin, pale, fragile, and easily traumatized); and intercourse may be painful. Often, the frequency of intercourse in this age group depends on the availability of a partner, physical health, previous sexual activity, and desire (Barkauskas et al, 1994).

Testosterone declines in older males, but this decline occurs later than the decline in estrogen in the female. Testes decrease in size and are less firm on palpation. Although sperm production either remains the same or decreases slightly, the motility and size of sperm changes. The prostate gland is enlarged and, often, secretion is impaired. The seminal fluid is reduced in both amount and viscosity. These changes do not necessarily mean a decrease in libido in the male, or a loss in satisfaction with intercourse (Barkauskas et al, 1994). However, the major age changes in sexual function include erectile ability and the change in the character of ejaculation. Penile erection is less firm and requires more stimulation and a longer time period to achieve. Once penile erection occurs and is lost without ejaculation, there may be a refractory period before a second erection can ensue (Shippee-Rice, 1990).

TABLE 33–2 Age-Related Changes in Female Sexual Response

Phase	Physiologic Change
Excitement	Delayed production of vaginal secretions and lubrication
Plateau	Reduced expansion in vaginal length and width
	Decreased uterine elevation
	Increased flaccidity of labia majora; labia do not elevate and flatten against perineum
	Decreased vasocongestion and color change in labia minora
	Decreased clitoral size after age 60
Orgasm	Decreased duration
Resolution	More rapid onset

Tables 33–2 and 33–3 list possible changes in the four phases of sexual response in aging females and males. Many of the physiologic, psychological, and social changes elders experience influence their sexuality and therefore their ability to meet such basic human needs as intimacy and self-actualization (Shippee-Rice, 1990). In two large-scale studies of sexual activity in the aged (Brecher, 1984; Starr and Weiner, 1982), the majority of individuals indicated a high level of satisfaction with their sexual activity (Shippee-Rice, 1990). Respondents held generally positive or at least accepting attitudes toward nudity, oral/genital intercourse, and masturbation. These elders continued to maintain an interest in sex that was not related to the frequency or type of sexual activity. Study participants generally felt positive about themselves and their own sexuality and believed that sexual expression is important for a continuing sense of mental and physical well-being (Shippee-Rice, 1990). These same respondents reported hand holding, hugging, and kissing to be important means of physical expression, even though the frequency of sexual intercourse decreased.

TABLE 33–3 Age-Related Changes in Male Sexual Response

Phase	Physiologic Change
Excitement	Slowed onset and progression of erection
	Decreased scrotal sac and testicular elevation
Plateau	Increased duration
	Greater increase in penile circumference due to reduced preejaculatory fluid emission
	Diminished involuntary spasms
	Decreased intensity and duration of sex flush
Orgasm	Decreased duration
	Decreased number of contractions in expelling semen
Resolution	More rapid onset
	Longer duration (may last 12 to 24 hours)

Gender, Health, and Illness

An interaction model can explain gender differences in health outcomes. That is, sex differences indirectly affect health and illness through an interaction of biologic and behavioral characteristics. This interaction model may operate in three potential pathways (Matthews, 1989):

- Gender may alter the degree of exposure to environmental factors that contribute to disease development.
- Gender may modify the individual's response to such exposure.
- Gender could modify the relationship between a specific level of a risk factor and disease development.

Furthermore, social scientists have long observed that social inequality influences the types and patterns of health and illness (Conrad and Kern, 1994).

Gender differences related to sexual health have been reported. Recent research on HIV and AIDS demonstrates some of the important concerns related to women's and men's health. Although the basic biomedical processes that underlie AIDS are likely to be the same for women and men, the psychological and physiologic reactions may differ on the basis of gender, and influence virus exposure and disease progression (Rodin and Ickovics, 1990). Furthermore, gender differences in hormones and genetics, as well as differences in social conditions, sex roles, and socioeconomic factors, are likely to influence the course of AIDS differently for women and men.

The number of AIDS cases among women has increased 600 percent since 1986 and two and a half times faster than among men (CDC, 1990). The majority of women with AIDS are of reproductive age and are either African American (52 percent) or Hispanic (20 percent). More than one third of women with AIDS had heterosexual contact with a person at risk for AIDS compared with only 2 percent of men who fit this category (Guinan and Hardy, 1987).

AIDS is on the rise among women, African Americans, and Hispanics/Latinos, and is increasing among persons becoming infected via heterosexual contact or injection drug use. Today, women account for 42 percent of the cumulative adult/adolescent AIDS cases reported worldwide and 17 percent of the cases reported in the United States (U.S. DHHS, 1995; UNAIDS, 1996).

Among women between the ages of 25 and 44, AIDS is the third leading cause of death and is increasing faster in women than in men. Paralleling the trends in the developing world, women of color clearly bear a disproportionate burden of HIV/AIDS in the United States. African American and Hispanic/Latina women, who make up 21 percent of the U.S. female population, are most severely impacted. By year-end 1995, they accounted for 56 percent and 21 percent, respectively, of the new AIDS cases reported among women (UNAIDS, 1996).

In contrast to the developing world, where over three quarters of the HIV infections among women are the result of unprotected heterosexual contact, in the United States injection drug use plays a significant role in HIV infections among women. U.S. women are as likely to become infected with HIV through injection drug use as through heterosexual intercourse. Of the new female AIDS cases reported in 1995, most were associated with injection drug use (38 percent) and heterosexual contact with a man with/or at risk of HIV infection (38 percent) (U.S. DHHS, 1995). The 1995 AIDS case rate among African American women was 59.2 per 100,000. This rate was 16 times higher than the rate for white women (3.8 per 100,000) and more than 2 times higher than the rate for Hispanic/Latina women (25.4 per 100,000). However, 47 percent of Latinas were infected through heterosexual contact compared with 34 percent of African American women.

New evidence suggests that the efficiency of HIV transmission may be greater from a man to a woman (Padian et al, 1991). In a recent study of HIV transmission in primates, rhesus monkeys who received subcutaneous progesterone implants were 7.7 times more likely to become infected with SIV (the virus in monkeys that is similar to HIV) than those monkeys that did not receive the progesterone. The findings raised strong concerns regarding the effects of two contraceptives that contain progesterone—the implant Norplant, and the injectable Depo-Provera—on HIV transmission in women. Furthermore, this study also suggests that endogenous progesterone (dominant in the post-ovulatory phase of the menstrual cycle) may be responsible for increased male-female HIV transmission due to progesterone-induced changes in the vaginal lining, vaginal pH, and cervical mucus of human beings (Marx et al, 1996). Progestational effects from lower dose monophasic and triphasic oral contraceptives have not been investigated.

Women also may die significantly sooner after an AIDS diagnosis than do men. Again, the mechanism for this differential is not clear. The likely rationale is that biopsychosocial mechanisms operate differently for women exposed to HIV, or that diagnosis and treatment occur later in the disease process due to socioeconomic factors or limited access to care.

Disease severity of other STIs is also greater for women than men, except for homosexual males. Among racial groups, the highest morbidity is seen in African Americans, the lowest in Asian, with whites in between (Lichtman and Duran, 1990). Women experience a disproportionate amount of the burden of having STIs, including the complications of sterility, numerous perinatal infections, genital tract neoplasia, and possibly death (from ectopic pregnancy, ruptured tubo-ovarian abscess, AIDS, and hepatitis B virus infection) (Fogel, 1990). Teenage and young adult women are most at risk for STIs, and are at high risk for the potential sequelae of these infections (pelvic pain, subfertility, increased risk of ectopic pregnancy, and pelvic inflammatory disease). In addition, STIs in women are often silent infections, going unrecognized until damage is done. Congenital anomalies, mental retardation, and death may occur to the offspring of women suffering from asymptomatic STIs (Cates and Alexander, 1988).

Individual and Family Values

The family is one social environment affecting men's and women's health; it has the capacity to provide either or both therapeutic and nontherapeutic experiences for individual family members. Family wellness contributes to both the individual wellness of family members and the level of wellness within the community (Pender, 1987). Like other environments (community, society, work), the family is important to the physical, mental, spiritual, and social health of individual family members.

Health values, attitudes, and behaviors are often learned within the family context where health-promoting (or health-damaging) skills are conveyed to children. Just as individuals must assume responsibility for their own health, families must also assume responsibility for the health of the family structure (Gillis et al, 1989). Aspects of the family that must be considered when attempting to influence the individual health of male and female members of the family system include socialization to gender roles, cultural values toward health, the power structure of health decision-making roles, and coping patterns during developmental transitions or illness. These factors are of particular importance in the assessment of individual health status within the multiple environments that promote sexual health and wellness. However, more complete family assessment models can be found in the writings of nurse clinicians and nurse researchers with expertise in family assessment and family interventions (Gillis et al, 1989; Wright and Leahey, 1984; Wright et al, 1990).

Although most nursing care is delivered to families during times of crisis and life transition, nurses have the opportunity to focus on the family when screening for health risks. Certainly family violence is a health risk for the individual woman and child, but the health of the family structure itself is also at risk. Chronic disease, such as hypertension or depression in a male family member, will usually increase the health risk for other family members, especially the mother or wife who must increase her caretaking responsibilities. Or, the diagnosis and treatment of breast cancer in a mother will have a major impact on her partner's and children's health.

EDUCATIONAL BACKGROUND

It is clear that a number of criteria are important to achieve and sustain good health. In addition to having a healthful physical and social environment, an adequate income, safe housing, good nutrition, and access to preventive and treatment services, men and women need to be educated and motivated to maintain healthful behaviors. Level of education has been inversely associated with poverty and illiteracy, both of which are directly related to health and health promotion activities. Economic gains for women have resulted in their independence, which furthers gender and sexual equity.

Educational level is one way of defining education; health education directed at the individual is another. Historically, health education has been viewed as biomedically oriented with the focus on compliance with prescribed medical regimens. Furthermore, the goals of health education have at times put the burden of change on the individual (victim blaming) rather than on society or on health care institutions where it belonged (Redman and Thomas, 1992). Although health education has been challenged with regard to its impact on health-related behavior and health status for individuals and groups, an increasing number of studies are providing evidence that health education can result in sustained behavioral change (Christman et al, 1992; Green, 1987; Redman, 1988; Starn and Paperny, 1990).

Critics of health education materials, especially through mass media, note that the emphasis is on individual responsibility and behavior and tends to ignore social, political, economic, and environmental factors that may profoundly influence particular illness-related behaviors. Reducing sexual violence has been identified as a public health problem that demands personal and community health approaches (Chalk and King, 1996).

Nurses must attend to the individual as well as the community needs for sexual health education. Personal self-education about current sexual health promotion is the nurse's first responsibility. Personal and professional education in sexual health promotion can begin with the use of Brash's "Toward a Model of Sexual Health for Nurses" (1990) (this model is described in Nursing Care Actions). Education beyond the individual might be community approaches to reducing sexual violence, such as educating emergency room personnel on violence assessment or developing school health education programs on anger management.

SOCIOECONOMIC STATUS

The intersections of social status and roles critically influence men's and women's health and health care providers. While the predominant focus has been on the biomedical basis for health and illness, nursing researchers and social scientists have demonstrated how health and illness are socially and economically produced and experienced in different ways by diverse groups of men and women (Olesen et al, 1997; Sabo and Gordon, 1995).

Americans' health has declined in conjunction with the deterioration of the social and economic programs that had been built during the previous decades (Friedman, 1994). Women, minority males, and children have fared the worst in the past decade. Women represent two thirds of all poor adults and 80 percent of working women are stuck in traditional "female" jobs, such as secretaries, clerical workers, and salesclerks. Most women are making less than $20,000 a year (nearly half the rate for white males), are more likely than men to live in poor housing and receive no health insurance, and twice as likely to draw no pension. American women face the worst gender-based pay gap in the developed world and the average female college graduate today will earn less than a man with no more than a high school diploma (Faludi, 1991). Furthermore, unlike other industrialized nations, the U.S. government still has no family leave and child care programs, and more than 99 percent of American private employers don't offer child care to their employees. American business has yet to make an honest effort at eradicating sex and racial discrimination. In a 1990 national poll of chief executives at Fortune 1000 companies, more than 80 percent acknowledged that discrimination impedes women and minority male progress in the workforce (Faludi, 1991). Yet, less than 1 percent of these same companies had developed plans for changing discriminatory patterns.

Disadvantaged people become ill because of poor nutrition, poor living conditions, high levels of stress, and reduced access to health care. Then, because they are ill, they may miss work or lose their jobs and may become even poorer. Combined with stigmatism due to racism, sexism, ageism, or homophobia, health outcomes will decline further. In light of this evidence, sexual health protection and sexual health promotion will not flourish when individuals are disadvantaged. Poverty restricts access to health care services, resulting in chronic disease from late or untreated STDs, unintended pregnancies, and treatment for sexual problems that reduce quality of life.

CULTURE AND ETHNICITY

Every culture guides the rate and direction of sexual development and expression of its members (Smith, 1990). An expanding volume of literature is available to assist health professionals in understanding cultures different from white, middle-class American culture as well as on the impact of culture in health and illness (Olesen et al, 1997). A cross-cultural analysis of different peoples reveals tremendous cultural diversity in sexual beliefs and practices. No two cultures are alike. Each society's sexuality is created by different values, beliefs, ideas, and environments (Smith, 1990). The practice of sexuality in a particular culture is based upon the interdependence of rules and beliefs about marriage, family, kinship, social responsibilities, and religion. Sexual behaviors and practices in Hispanic cultures are largely influenced by religious beliefs and by the high value placed upon children. Motherhood is seen by many Hispanic women as their most important social role (Paula et al, 1996). In these cultures, monogamy is encouraged and expected. Those who follow strict Roman Catholic tenets about pregnancy prevention calendar menstrual periods to calculate midcycle fertility and practice abstinence during calculated fertile times. No other contraceptive methods are permitted (Fogel and Lauver, 1990).

Orthodox Jews follow religious beliefs that forbid sexual activity during menstruation. For this group, religious laws do not allow sexual relations between husband and wife beginning with the onset of her menstrual period to the end of seven "clean" days following menstruation (Donin, 1949). Before resuming sexual activity, the Jewish woman must immerse herself in a kosher mikvah (bath) in order to be purified.

CULTURE AND SEXUALITY

In most cultures, there is an explicit and well-defined view about the nature of human sexuality. A highly individualized erotic code exists in societies that consists of signs and acts that suggest or enhance sexuality. For example, various fragrances or odors, foods, speech, postures, and behaviors symbolize eroticism in societies. Additionally, societies regulate sexual behavior of their members by explicitly defining the rights, responsibilities, and obligations of members in a sexual relationship. Culture-specific sexual practices, such as female circumcision or polygamy, are unique and specific to a particular society. Each society shapes, structures, and guides the sexual development and expression of all its members and develops a unique sexual expression that is based on the internal values, needs, and logic of the culture. Thus, there is tremendous diversity of sexual behavior, rules and regulations, symbols, sanctions, and taboos. Variations in the ethnographic spectrum of sexual behavior demand a tolerance for differences (Smith, 1990).

Because sexual matters in most societies are private, many serious problems exist with data collection and analysis of sexual practices in diverse groups (Smith, 1990). This problem has led to a very limited knowledge base.

CULTURAL DIVERSITY

There is a wide diversity within the United States among various ethnic and racial groups, as well as wide diversity of ethnic and social backgrounds within each racial group. For example, "Asians" include Japanese, Chinese, Korean, and Vietnamese. This category includes third-generation residents, recent arrivals, rural and urban populations, the highly educated, and those with limited schooling. Similar diversity exists among Hispanics, Native Americans, and African Americans. The gap in research on differences in health beliefs and attitudes between different ethnic and racial groups too often is matched by a lack of sensitivity to these issues by health providers and the health care delivery system. There is a similar lack of data on sex-race differences and how these affect the onset, course, and handling of various illnesses.

Prevention and health promotion strategies must be adapted to consider cultural beliefs and attitudes as well as gender. In many cultures, asking direct questions about personal problems and habits is considered rude and inappropriate. Therefore, assessment of the man or woman must be approached in an indirect manner or modified to accommodate the individual's reluctance for personal disclosure. In some traditional cultures and recent immigrant cultures, the family plays a central role in decision making or health advice.

HOMOSEXUALITY

A gay or lesbian lifestyle or sexual preference must be considered part of cultural diversity as it relates to health. Although population research is lacking, approximately 10 to 15 percent of the American people consider themselves gay or lesbian, which suggests that health care providers must expect that a substantial number of their patients will be in this cultural group.

Gay men and lesbian women describe negative encounters with the health care system including ostracism, invasive questioning, derogatory comments, breaches of confidentiality, shock, embarrassment, unfriendliness, pity, condescension, and fear (Stevens and Hall, 1988; Taylor and Robertson, 1994). As a result of these negative experiences in health care encounters, many gay men and lesbian women report hesitation in using health care systems and delay seeking necessary care and treatment. Due to this reluctance, gay men and lesbian women increase their risk of disease and illness because of a relative lack of medical or health-related knowledge. For example, many lesbian women believe that they are at low risk for contracting STIs and cervical cancer, and do not have regular Pap smear tests. However, by avoiding regular pelvic examinations, they do not obtain clinical breast exams and mammography, thereby increasing their risk of undetected breast cancer.

SPIRITUALITY AND RELIGIOUS PRACTICES

Religion and spirituality are not necessarily synonymous. Historically, organized religion has often been used as a tool for enforcing social values, such as the role of women and restricting sexual expression to the "sanctity of marriage." However, spirituality may provide a basis for an individual's belief system or a method of stress reduction and personal rejuvenation. According to Pender (1987), beliefs about spirituality and life are important dimensions of personal wellness, including sexual health. For example, rather than discussing the legal and socially sanctioned aspects of sexual expression, the spiritual component of sexual health promotion addresses the particular individual's belief systems within which he or she may choose to express sexuality. Certainly socialization experiences and cultural beliefs are combined with spirituality to compose an individual's beliefs about sexual health and illness. However, the contribution of spirituality is to allow an individual to operate within his or her own unique system of beliefs, rather than within the commonly recognized, legally and socially sanctioned communal system of beliefs.

Settings in Which Care Is Delivered

Women and men receive health care services in a variety of settings, usually determined by the location of their health care provider, or more commonly, by their type of insurance (or lack of insurance). Health delivery settings within traditional medical systems include practitioner offices, clinics, women's health centers, group practices, neighborhood health centers, health maintenance organizations, urgent care centers, emergency rooms, and hospitals. The diversity of health service settings is partially based upon the American free enterprise system with its emphasis on competition, fee-for-service payment, and the predominance of the private sector, which includes private practitioners, proprietary hospitals, and drug companies (Lee and Estes, 1990). Certain delivery settings may be more sensitive to gender-specific or sexual health needs (e.g., women's health centers, teen clinics), but the major problem facing both men's and women's health is the lack of comprehensive primary health care as well as access to basic health benefits.

In 1995, 40 million Americans had no health insurance coverage and 36 percent of those uninsured were children. In addition, 26 million more Americans had no insurance for substantial periods, sometimes for months. Another 83 million Americans face bankruptcy because their insurance does not protect them from catastrophic medical costs (Davis and Rowland, 1990). One quarter of all pregnant women (approximately 300,000) do not have insurance coverage for prenatal or pregnancy-related services (Freeman 1990 et al, 1990; Gerber Fried, 1990). This lack of access to prenatal care contributes to an alarming number of infant deaths and low birth weights each year. Furthermore, contraceptive services and devices are excluded from most health insurance plans.

One trend that is almost complete in some areas is the rapid growth in managed care, including the merger of services and institutions. With the financial markets driving these changes and the massive movement of capital into health care systems, for-profit managed care organizations (MCO) and other health care corporations are emerging at a rate that has already concentrated economic power in a handful of companies in some areas of the country (Shaffer, 1995). Nine of the ten largest MCOs are for-profit (Kaiser is the only nonprofit MCO), and they currently insure over half of all privately insured managed care enrollees (otherwise known as patients!). Early MCOs, such as health maintenance organizations (HMOs), attempted to reverse the financial incentives of the fee-for-service system, emphasizing primary and preventive care as well as expanding the opportunities for advanced practice nurses who filled the demand for primary care practitioners at a lower cost than physicians while maintaining high quality (Shaffer, 1995).

Managed care presents some potential threats and benefits to gender-based health care delivery in general and sexual health promotion in particular. In a market-based health care system, cost controls are the major active forces, with quality playing a minor role in health care delivery. As profits are being taken out of the system, fewer resources are available for building a new health care delivery system. Complex problems such as sexual dysfunction or sexual problems related to chronic disease are not likely to be "covered" by the for-profit MCOs. This existing bias is likely to be exacerbated by the time limitation of patient visits employed by MCOs or by the increasing numbers of patients scheduled at discounted rates. Managed care plans may refuse to enroll, or to drop providers who take care of sicker populations, such as those with cancer or AIDS.

In contrast, if MCOs use the early Kaiser HMO model that focuses on community outreach, disease prevention, and health promotion, sexual health status could improve. Although the Kaiser system has been criticized for restricting access to employed individuals, Kaiser's original focus on prevention has made them a leader in providing "health" as well as "illness" services. Kaiser has also has employed nurse practitioners as primary care providers whose educational emphasis is on disease prevention and health promotion. Sexual history taking, risk assessment, sexual health promotion, and limited intervention strategies for sexual problems are part of the advanced practice nurse's clinical education. The challenge for health care providers in these MCOs will be to integrate gender/race/class–sensitive health care and sexual health promotion into a comprehensive primary health care system.

The recent shift from institutional health care to the family has implications for sexual health promotion. As health care services continue to be shifted away from institutions and into the community, the family, and particularly women, will bear an increasing burden. Not only will women be called upon to be unpaid caregivers to disabled and/or elderly family members, they may be deterred from entering the workforce due to this role. The hidden costs to the health care system for this shift remain virtually unexplored. However, cost may include decreased access to health care due to a lack of health insurance, which has traditionally been obtained through employment. This trend, as it relates to sexual health, may influence treatment and prevention options for specific STDs, as well as sexual health protection and promotion services. For example, some delivery providers believe that pelvic inflammatory disease should be treated within a hospital setting by intravenous administration of antibiotics. The rationale for this treatment mode is to preserve reproductive capacity and to avoid the sequelae of chronic pelvic pain. By minimizing patients' access to in-house treatment (due to economics—lack of insurance or reduced coverage for in-house treatment by insurers), the adverse sequelae of PID may be increased.

As more health care services are delivered outside the hospital and in the home, nurses will need to be comfortable and competent in providing sexual health promotion to individuals and families in the home environment. Knowledge of family and home assessment will be necessary along with sexual counseling skills. Acceptance of one's own sexuality and awareness of one's biases is even more important when delivering care in the home, where the nurse is interacting with multiple family members in a noninstitutional environment.

Ethical Considerations

A number of ethical issues are involved in sexual health promotion. Included in this context are sociopolitical concerns, reproductive technologies, medicalization of men's and women's health problems, and power differentials based on race and class, as well as gender. All of these broad topic areas influence the ethical delivery of sexual health promotion and disease prevention activities, either by directly affecting access to care or by influencing individual choice.

Development and implementation of medical technology have themselves become powerful social forces. The shift to "fetus-as-patient" has led to demands by some doctors and lawyers that pregnant and laboring women should be subjected to physical regulation, forced surgery, detention, or even criminal or civil punishment for behavior deemed dangerous to the fetus. This has promoted increased use of prenatal testing and fetal heart rate monitoring despite their unproven value in reducing the morbidity and mortality of newborns (Institute of Medicine, 1989; Kaczorowski et al, 1998). These procedures have also contributed to the escalating cesarean section rate (Dildy et al, 1997). The issue of women's civil rights is polarized by forced medical treatment on the one hand and lack of access to treatment on the other.

The bodies of women, usually pregnant women, have served as the battlefield over which major constitutional cases have been fought for more than two decades (Annas, 1994). The primary fight in this century has been over abortion, and this particular issue has implications for sexual health promotion. Nurses have always been at the forefront of advocacy efforts to develop and maintain reproductive freedoms. Margaret Sanger, a nurse and the founder of the National Planned Parenthood organization, was dedicated to making contraceptive choice a woman's decision; over time, this national organization has expanded to include reproductive and sexual health care for men. Over more than a century, public health nurses have been active in family planning programs and improving access to reproductive health knowledge, especially for poor women and women of color.

Medical and reproductive technologies illustrate the social and ethical issues facing women and men in the health care delivery system. Although medical technology has solved many problems, it has also created new ones. Because of women's childbearing capacity, their exposure to technologies differs greatly from that of men. For example, the cesarean birth rate has increased from 5 percent in 1970 to 23 percent in 1988, and is expected to increase to 50 percent over the next 20 years (Belle, 1990). Although cesarean births have improved neonatal mortality (Amirikia et al, 1988; Dildy et al, 1997), they have also been associated with physical, financial, and psychological costs.

Medical management of high-risk pregnancies includes other medical technologies. Women are administered potentially dangerous experimental drugs to prolong pregnancy to a viable age for the fetus.

Scientific breakthroughs now offer reproductive alternatives to some infertile couples, single persons, postmenopausal women, women who have had chemotherapy, and fertile couples at risk of passing on a genetic disorder (IOM, 1989). However, there are serious issues ranging from who does (and who does not) get to use assisted reproductive technologies (ART), to the risks they pose to women. Technology for treating infertility has become big business, with 250 in vitro fertilization (IVF) clinics operating in 1991. Yet no government oversight of the reproductive technology industry exists, and many laboratories in which human embryos are handled are exempt from the federal inspections required of other medical laboratories (White, 1992). From in vitro fertilization and embryo transfer to genetic diagnosis of an embryo before implantation, success rates of ART are low compared with the extraordinary costs. In its most recent report, the Society for Assisted Reproductive Medicine (SART, 1996) reported 1994 outcomes and successes of 249 centers offering ART: 21 percent live birth rate for IVF, 28 percent rate for GIFT (gamete intrafallopian transfer), and 29 percent rate for ZIFT (zygote intrafallopian transfer), and transfer of frozen embryos resulted in a 15 percent delivery rate. As these technologies increase, ethical challenges increase owing to the complexity of problems raised by the conflicting ethical principles in this area of reproductive health. For instance, what should be done with the extra eggs and sperm (gametes), fertilized eggs (embryos), and frozen embryos that have not been implanted? What about the practice of aborting some fetuses during a multiple pregnancy so that one will thrive? Many of the new technologies involve an alarming degree of invasiveness and medical manipulation of women's bodies. Despite claims that ART "serves" women, the long-term effects of many of the ARTs—on women and their children—are not yet known. For those who do pursue ART, it is important for nurses to assist them and their families to become fully informed of the physical, emotional, ethical and financial burdens involved; to help them find the information they need to remain in charge of the decisions they must make; and to find the support they will need for what is frequently an arduous path (Boston Women's Health Book Collective, 1998; James, 1992).

While women are subjected to the majority of reproductive technologies, few technological efforts have focused on male fertility or infertility. Men are subjected to fewer painful or invasive procedures, and often are not considered a part of the infertility problem or a part of any solution. The focus on the "woman as the problem" has the potential to disrupt the couple's relationship. Either the male partner feels left out, or may feel that the woman is the problem and everything will be fine when she "gets fixed" (Go, 1992).

Normal events such as menstruation, childbirth, menopause, and female sexual responses continue to be "medicalized" rather than considered normative transitions. Emphasis on routine intrauterine fetal monitoring during childbirth, the lithotomy position, and other interventions occurring during childbirth continue. "Treatment" for menopause as a hormone-deficiency disease, rather than the closure of menstrual life, exposes women to other life-threatening illness such as cancer. And men certainly are not immune to medicalization of their developmental transitions or lifestyle choices. Alternate sexual preference has been considered a psychiatric disorder until only recently and midlife men are now being prescribed testosterone as a means for dealing with depressive mood changes.

Power differentials have been pointed out in relation to education, earning potential, and reproductive technologies. This differential in educational and economic opportunity limits the ability of women to access health care and to have personal choice in their own sexual health. Despite the influence of the women's movement and the self-care movement, lower socioeconomic groups (particularly women, women of color, gay men, and men of color) do not enjoy the same opportunity to access health care services as do white males.

Financial Considerations

Economic issues influence men's and women's sexual health, particularly costs related to health care that remain invisible but affect men's and women's health directly or indirectly. STIs place heavy demands on health care services and have high economic costs. The total annual expenditure for the direct care of STI patients in the United States exceeds $2 billion (McGregor et al, 1988), and it is estimated the costs of treating pelvic inflammatory disease (PID) and its sequelae alone exceed $2.6 billion annually (Centers for Disease Control, 1991).

Federal funding for shelters for battered women has been withheld, and one third of the one million battered women who seek emergency shelter each year can find none (Faludi, 1991). Although chronic diseases and the effects of poverty in minority males are disproportionate to other males, there is no organized economic effort at state or federal levels to develop prevention programs (Staples, 1995).

Generally, disease prevention and health promotion programs incur costs in the present while benefits are derived in the future (Pender, 1987). The nurse can assess how much patients are willing to spend to improve their health status when they feel well or to protect them from a health problem that has a long latency period. Emphasizing short-term as well as long-term benefits may enhance individual acceptance of prevention or promotion services. Using information about actual as well as potential effects on the individual or community may also improve acceptance. Yet the cost-effectiveness of screening is compromised by individual nonadherence to prescribed treatment regimens. Particularly, in areas of sexual health promotion, such as condom and/or other contraceptive use, the cost to the individual and to the community for nonadherence is great.

Quantifying the benefits of preventive health care services is difficult. The economic consequences of STIs are enormous and are most common in young persons, those with multiple sexual contacts, prostitutes, homosexual and bisexual men, and persons with infected sexual partners (U.S. Preventive Services Task Force, 1989). However, condom use to prevent an STI acquisition was more than twice as frequently reported when a favorable attitude was perceived by a male sexual partner (Fleisher et al, 1994). In a study of 2900 high school students in greater Miami, Florida, it was noted that the more knowledge about HIV and AIDS a respondent had, the less importance he or she placed on pregnancy prevention, and as the importance of preventing pregnancy declined, so did the frequency of condom use (Langer et al, 1994). Males who were in a steady dating relationship and perceived pregnancy prevention as more important than AIDS prevention were the most likely to report using condoms often (Langer et al, 1994).

FUTURE DEVELOPMENTS

An Expanded Knowledge Base to Guide Sexual Health Promotion

There is a need for both a conceptual and a systemic change in the knowledge base that informs health care providers about women, men, health, and illness. Sexual health promotion must be considered within this expanded model of men's and women's health. First, "women" and "men" should not be defined as a monolithic category, but as a heterogeneous group that includes men and women of color, men and women with disabilities, girls, boys, adolescents, middle-aged adults, perimenopausal women, homeless, and immigrant men and women. The knowledge base must include more of a focus than currently exists on the psychosocial issues that contextualize health problems such as racism, sexism, violence against women, gender roles, poverty, and health belief systems. This presumes an expansion of existing research methodologies and multidisciplinary research to examine the interaction of biology, psychology, and society across different cultures.

The knowledge base for men's health and women's health must progress beyond the current model of health care (aggressive cure of disease) to an expanded model of health care that includes assertive prevention of illness and promotion of health and wellness. There is a dearth of knowledge on the efficacy and accuracy of nonpharmacologic interventions that can act as health prevention or promotion strategies. Multiple forms of healing must be considered in a model that embraces a holistic approach to the individual throughout all stages of life.

An expanded theory of men's and women's health should incorporate personal, interpersonal, and developmental processes that influence individual health and well-being. Traditional theories of growth and development focus on deficiencies and are inadequate to explain gender- or culture-specific strengths. Borrowing from the work of relational and educational psychology, a new perspective of gender, culture, and health might be applied. Rather than the misogynist view of women as passive, weak, dependent, or developmentally deficient, a perspective of "mutuality in relation" would provide a framework for validating women's strengths as well as understanding men's struggles for growth and connection (Lewis and Bernstein, 1996). The label of dependency that stigmatizes women and impairs quality of health and health care can be recast as a positive quality, interdependence.

The knowledge base must also include a focus on the environment relevant to men's and women's health such as health care delivery and health care providers. Examination of the barriers to health care that men, women, and their families face is necessary so that appropriate mechanisms for service delivery can be created and utilized. New knowledge is needed on health service delivery in other cultures and the use of noninstitutional settings.

Using this expanded model of men's and women's health in the application of sexual health promotion, the nurse will recognize the important differences among and between groups of men and women. In particular, the nurse will consider diversities in age, geography (rural/urban residence), employment, occupation, educational level, social class, degree of acculturation, sexual preferences, and religious beliefs and integrate them into an individualized health promotion plan. Nurses are well prepared to focus on both health and illness, but new skills in sexual health promotion will be required. Transformative principles of communication, as described by Belenky and coworkers (1986) will improve the quality of the health care encounter for men and women.

Future Technology Developments in Men's and Women's Health

For women, new technology has brought the female condom, which provides a physical barrier that lines the vagina entirely and partially shields the perineum (Hatcher et al, 1994). The advantage to this contraceptive method is that it provides some physical barrier to contact with sexually transmitted organisms in addition to the protection afforded by the spermicide used concomitantly. Further, this method provides women the opportunity to actively protect themselves from both pregnancy and STIs. Since women now have access to pregnancy testing and to ovulation detection in the privacy of their own homes, their ability to protect themselves from unintended pregnancy or to time intercourse for fertility enhancement has markedly improved. Recent advancements in urinary incontinence treatment include vaginal weights to help women identify and strengthen pelvic floor muscles; intraurethral devices to minimize the effects of stress incontinence; a flexible ring-shaped device that laterally supports the urethra; and the continence control pad, a new external urethral occlusion device (Gartley and Saltmarche, 1997). In conjunction with Kegel exercises aimed at increasing pelvic muscles' ability to prevent urine leakage, these new technologies assist women to avoid embarrasing accidents that prevent them from engaging in sexual activity with their partners.

For men, new knowledge has expanded understanding of erectile dysfunction and increased awareness of the role that lifestyle changes can play in sexual health enhancement. Regular exercise, a low-fat diet, and smoking cessation increase a man's chances of remaining potent as he grows older (Butler et al, 1994). Treatments for erectile dysfunction have expanded to include intracorporeal injection, external vacuum devices, penile implants, and most recently prescription pharmaceuticals (e.g., Viagra) (Pfizer, 1998, Reisner, 1993). These new technologies offer an opportunity for the millions of men who suffer erectile dysfunction to restore sexual health (Greiner and Weigel, 1996), although more research is needed into pharmaceuticals usage.

New knowledge in the areas of men's and women's sexual health will have application to nursing practice. As the self-care movement in women's health expands to men and their health, more and more individuals will have a good general understanding of how their body works throughout their lives and will apply self-care practices, such as lifestyle changes that promote health. These self-care practices include sexual disease prevention through use of contraceptive devices that protect against infection, disease detection through self-examination for changes that denote vaginal or urethral infections, and sexual health promotion through communication with a sexual partner or accessing technologies or health care to remedy sexual health problems. To accommodate this quest for knowledge of self-care and new technologies by men and women, nurses must include health promotion practices in all educating sessions and provide an arena for men and women to ask questions or to answer health-related questions that might be sensitive. Further, nurses must keep abreast of research-based knowledge regarding sexual health promotion and STI prevention.

NURSING CARE ACTIONS

HEALTH PROTECTION

Health protection refers to activities that seek to protect clients from potential or actual health problems or disease. It includes three types of prevention: primary, secondary, and tertiary. *Primary prevention* refers to (1) generalized health promotion directed at sustaining or increasing the level of well-being through education; and (2) specific protection focused on decreasing the probability of encountering illness and injury. *Secondary prevention* refers to organized, direct screening efforts or education of the public to promote discovery of individuals with early stages of disease. In addition, secondary prevention is early diagnosis and prompt intervention to halt the pathologic process, thereby shortening its duration and severity and enabling the individual to regain normal function at the earliest possible point. *Tertiary prevention* occurs when a defect or disability is permanent and irreversible. Rehabilitation or restoring the individual to an optimal level of functioning within the constraints of the disability is the goal of tertiary preventive care.

HEALTH PROMOTION

Health promotion moves beyond prevention and refers to activities directed toward developing the resources of clients that maintain or enhance well-being. Health promotion behaviors are those behaviors that have the potential to maintain or improve the individual's current level of health. Examples of these behaviors include rest, exercise, adequate nutrition, weight maintenance or reduction, stress reduction, and positive interpersonal relationships. Specific sexual health protection behaviors include breast or testicular self-examination, contraception, safer sex practices, and sexual health status monitoring or surveillance.

REQUIRED COMPETENCIES

The nurse's role in promoting sexual health is built on a knowledge base that recognizes human sexuality as a biologic, psychological, social, and cultural phenomenon. Patients may require a variety of health services related to their sexual health, ranging from education to intensive therapy for complex sexual dysfunction issues. The nurse's ability to intervene at these various levels depends on her or his training. Some nurses are comfortable providing only basic educational information and sexual health assessment, whereas others have obtained more comprehensive training and are able to provide sex therapy.

Basic nursing education prepares a nurse to provide information to patients and to promote an environment in which patients feel able to express feelings and worries. However, this basic nursing education is effective only if the nurse has an accurate knowledge base, self-awareness of personal value systems and self-acceptance as a sexual being, and the ability to communicate genuinely and therapeutically with patients on sexuality issues (Fogel, 1990).

Active listening strategies and communication techniques are required for the nurse to elicit feelings and problems and to demonstrate acceptance of a client's concerns regarding issues of sexual health. A caring and concerned demeanor by itself is not a sufficient basis for providing sexual health care. The nurse also needs an accurate knowledge base from which to draw clarifying information and provide patient education. Furthermore, the nurse must have identified her or his own sexual issues and biases, to heighten sensitivity to others. Without attention to this important step, the nurse may limit the therapeutic effect of interventions by displaying attitudes or opinions that inhibit the patient from disclosing all relevant information.

Effective nursing practice is free of cultural bias and prejudice. This requires that the nurse overcome any personal cultural bias and learn to empathize with each patient's particular perspective. Nurses should strive to understand the influence of the patient's culture on sexuality. The sexual health of the patient should be promoted by individual and community education on male and female sexuality and sexual relationships, as well as a sensitive concern for the individual cultural variations in sexual behavior (Smith, 1990).

To provide effective sexual health assessment, education, and counseling, nurses first must be comfortable with their own sexuality and be aware of their sexual biases (Bernhard, 1995). As a first step in providing sexual health care, Brash (1990) suggests that the nurse (or any health care provider) focus on five statements or assertions:

- I know and accept my sexual self and my body as OK.
- I choose a sexual lifestyle that fits and satisfies me.
- I am sexually assertive.
- I am free to express masculine and feminine sides of myself.
- I am sexually competent and sexually responsible.

The second requirement for nurses is to maintain current and accurate knowledge about sexual health and the effects of various illnesses and treatments on men's and women's sexual function. The third requirement for a nurse who provides sexual health promotion is an appropriate attitude. The nurse should be comfortable in discussing sexuality and have a genuine desire to help. Specific qualities and skills in a health care provider include empathy, comfort in talking about sensitive subjects, good training, confidentiality, and a lack of embarrassment.

Sexual Health Assessment

The purpose of sexual health assessment is to assess for sexual health dysfunction and to provide an arena for sexual health promotion through discussion and education. In the event that sexual dysfunction is identified, the nurse can play an important role in beginning the process of sexual health restoration (see Box 33–5).

The nurse begins a sexual health assessment by making the patient feel comfortable and at ease. Privacy must be assured, and the patient reassured that all information elicited during the assessment will be kept strictly confidential. The nurse may want to keep notes about the visit but not record information in the patient's medical record. These measures all promote trust and foster the sharing of feelings and concerns. Adequate time must be allowed for the assessment, so that the patient or the nurse does not feel rushed or pressured.

HEALTH HISTORY

The sexual health history includes biologic, psychological, social, and cultural dimensions. Some nurses prefer to use a specific model for sexual health assessment. Fogel and colleagues (1990) describe one such model that includes specific problem areas related to sexuality and sexual functioning. Alternatively, a nurse comfortable with doing sexual assessments may prefer to individualize the assessment and gear it to the specific setting or patient situation.

Another approach is to utilize a short format of three questions, as suggested by Woods (1984) (Box 33–6). These three questions allow the nurse to gather information about the patient's usual sexual roles, view of himself or herself as a sexual being, and sexual functioning.

Whatever the assessment approach, the nurse uses active listening strategies and good communication techniques to elicit the patient's expression of feelings and problems and to demonstrate acceptance of the patient's concerns about sexual health issues. The nurse must keep in mind that a patient may be reluctant to reveal all relevant information. To encourage full disclosure, the nurse may provide a lead-in statement about why this information is important and why it is a routine part of health assessment. Alternatively, sexual health questions may naturally follow a specific question from the patient regarding a sexual issue, such as concern about possible infection. In this case, a lead-in statement may not be needed.

BOX 33-6
THREE SEXUAL HEALTH HISTORY QUESTIONS

1. Has anything (illness, pregnancy, surgery) interfered with your being a (mother/wife/husband/father/worker)?
2. Has anything (illness, medical treatment, surgery) changed the way you feel about yourself as a man or woman?
3. Has anything (surgery, medication, disease) altered your ability to function sexually?

From Woods, N. (1984). *Human Sexuality in Health and Illness*, 3rd ed. St. Louis: C.V. Mosby.

Furthermore, the nurse must not make assumptions or convey a judgmental attitude about the patient's sexual behavior, feelings, or attitudes. Examples of history questions that do not convey any assumptions or judgments on the nurse's part include "Are you sexually active at the present time . . . with a man, woman or both?" "Do you have questions or concerns about your sexual health?" and "Are you having sexual difficulties or problems that you wish to discuss?" (Bernhard, 1995).

In addition to the usual sexual history, sexual health assessment of individuals with chronic conditions should include an assessment of the sexual relationship as it existed before the onset of the chronic disease or condition. The assessment should identify adaptive and maladaptive behaviors that communicate messages of desire or rejection, foreplay and positions that are pleasing and uncomfortable, and alternative expressions of sexuality that are perceived as acceptable or deviant. An important area of psychological assessment is the identification of stimuli influencing sexual behavior, e.g., loss of ability to use traditional positions for sexual activity and previous ability to cope with pain or anxiety. The sexual history should take into account the effect of medications that may decrease desire or sexual function.

Sexual history taking specific to men and women with chronic lung disease might include questions such as "When you engage in sexual activity, do you have problems with shortness of breath?" or "How does the shortness of breath affect your ability to engage in sexual activity?" (Stockdale-Wooley, 1990). Inquiring about other similar symptoms associated with respiratory disease includes the following: coughing, wheezing, sputum, mouth odor, orthopnea/lying down, chest pain/pressure, palpitations, or anxiety. Or the nurse might ask, "What preparation(s) do you take before engaging in sexual activity?" For example, medications, nebulizers, metered dose inhaler, extension device, oxygen, breathing exercises, postural drainage, or relaxation exercises that might reduce respiratory distress or enhance sexual pleasure.

For men with spinal cord injuries, the health professional should assess objectively erectile potential. Sexual ability of men with paralysis can be predicted on the basis of several simple examinations: reflex contractions of the anal sphincter, conscious control of the anal sphincter, and presence or

BOX 33-7
ASSESSMENT FOR ABUSE

- Physical safety
- Legal needs
- Support needs and options
- Economic status
- Feelings of blame, isolation, fear, and responsibility
- Resources available
    - Immediate and future
    - Community shelters
    - Support groups and counseling
    - Legal options
    - Safety plan
    - Economic assistance

NOTE: Assessment for violence against women should be a part of every health history done by nurses for all women regardless of their point of entry to the health care system. At each contact, nurses should assess their patients on the points listed here. Assessment must take place in a private, confidential setting.
From Campbell, J., Landenburger, K. (1995). *Women's Health Care: A Comprehensive Handbook*. Thousand Oaks, CA: Sage, p. 420.

BOX 33-8
ELEMENTS OF APPROPRIATE DOCUMENTATION OF BATTERED WOMEN

HISTORY

- Description of past and present injuries
- Photographs of visible injuries
- Body map with notation of past and present injury
- Record of her description of incident, including name of her assailant
- Specific notation as to occurrence and nature of any forced sex

PHYSICAL

- Notation of complete physical exam, including neurological exam
- Notation of pelvic exam if history of forced sex
- Notation of x-ray of past and present bone injuries

NOTE: It is important that the nurse document risk for abuse, level of risk, past or present abuse, and information regarding the assailant. Both historical information and physical findings are included in documentation. This information may be essential for women involved in assault or child custody cases.
From Campbell, J., Landenburger, K. (1995). *Women's Health Care: A Comprehensive Handbook*. Thousand Oaks, CA: p. 421.

absence of sensation of the penis, scrotum, and perianal dermatomes (Sackett, 1990).

The sexual health history must also include assessment of past or present violence. Nursing assessment for violence and sexual abuse should take place for all individuals entering the health care system. Although more information is written about sexual abuse of women and women are more commonly sexual abuse victims, nurses must be alert to abuse directed toward males. The assessment should be conducted in private with confidentiality stressed. However, nurses must uphold reporting laws in states where those exist, and it is very important that nurses in these states inform patients about this reporting requirement. Fear of reprisal has important implications for patients and may influence willingness to report past or present abuse, or fear that abuse will occur in the future.

A thorough assessment gathers information on physical, emotional, and sexual trauma from violence (Box 33–7); risk for future abuse (Box 33–8); cultural background and beliefs; perceptions of the individual's relationships with others; and the individual's stated needs (Campbell and Landenburger, 1995). It is essential that the assessment be performed in private, for any individual accompanying the patient may, in fact, be the abuser. Campbell and Landenburger (1995) developed a model for categorizing individuals into three groups in terms of abuse: no risk, low risk, or moderate to high risk. This model was specifically developed for use with women; however, the principles apply to both men and women. Women with no signs of current or past abuse are considered at no risk; however, as many are hesitant to speak of concerns, future visits should include questions about whether there have been any changes in the woman's life or whether she has additional information or questions about topics brought out at previous visits (Campbell and Landenburger, 1995).

Women at low risk show no evidence of recent or current abuse. For this group, the nurse provides education that helps the woman gain perspective on her current situation and information about resources (group and individual formats) for assistance. The nurse should record the risk level, preventive measures, and teaching. Moderate to high risk assessment includes evaluation of a woman's fear for both psychological and physical abuse (Campbell and Landenburger, 1995). Risk factors for lethality (stalking, frequent harassment, threats or an escalation of threats, use of weapons or threat with weapons, excessive control and jealousy, and public use of violence) should be assessed. The determined risk level should also be documented, and any past or present physical evidence of abuse from prior or current assault must be either photographed or shown on a body map as well as described narratively (Campbell and Landenburger, 1995). As well, it is important that the assailant be identified in the record, even if the patient is not ready to make a police report at the present time.

Nursing interventions include immediate care for a woman in a potentially harmful or presently abusive situation (Box 33–9). In these instances, referral to a shelter, access to counseling, and legal resources should be discussed. Nurses need to have knowledge of available resources and shelters that might offer protection when reprisal is feared. If there is evidence of sexual assault, referral to a health care provider who is expert at collecting data after sexual assault is essential. Advanced practice certification of sexual assault nurse examiners can be obtained in most states, which provides nurses the opportunity to provide this comprehensive care to victims of sexual assault.

BOX 33-9
VIOLENCE PREVENTION: PRIMARY AND SECONDARY PREVENTION STRATEGIES

Sexual health promotion would not be complete without knowledge of violence prevention strategies. Nurses in all settings are likely to encounter individuals at risk for, or actual victims of, violence. The following section includes basic strategies for both primary and secondary prevention. Primary prevention of violence against women and men would necessarily encompass a total attitudinal change in the values of society (Campbell and Landenburger, 1995). Essential components of this change are (1) teaching boys and girls the values of interdependence; (2) teaching respect for human life; and (3) making a commitment to empathy and strength in the development of the human species regardless of sex, race, or socioeconomic status (Campbell and Landenburger, 1995).

Secondary prevention has already been undertaken in our society with the establishment of programs that encourage women and children to speak about their experiences. These programs need to be supported and expanded to include gay men, men of color, and all victims of abuse. Laws need to be developed that punish perpetrators of violence and protect victims from further abuse. Too often, abusers are ignored or given few, if any, restrictions. These same abusers go on to inflict more abuse, as we disbelieve victims or fail to recognize them. Nurses are involved with women at key times when they can be screened for the presence or absence of all forms of abuse. Nurses can be instrumental in changing public policy in general and specific health care practices, so that violence decreases in our society.

PHYSICAL ASSESSMENT

Health history questions pertinent to sexual health provide important information for the next step in sexual health assessment—physical assessment of the genitalia. This step involves two components: inspecting and palpating genital organs and obtaining various cultures and smears to rule out specific infections or diseases.

ASSESSING FEMALE PATIENTS

In women, physical assessment includes inspection and palpation of the external genitalia and speculum examination of the vagina and cervix. These procedures are followed with bimanual palpation to assess internal genitalia (vagina, cervix, uterus, fallopian tubes, and ovaries) and to evaluate pelvic support. This palpation provides information regarding size, shape, consistency, position, mobility, and tenderness of structures, as well as any nodules, masses, or other abnormalities (Wheeler, 1995).

Cultures and smears of the female cervix provide important screening information. The Pap smear is performed to screen for cervical cancer and other diseases such as those caused by the human papilloma virus (HPV). Gonorrhea, chlamydia, and herpes cultures may be performed to detect these particular diseases, and wet-mounts of vaginal discharge are performed to detect various vaginal infections.

A woman with physical disabilities may not be able to assume the traditional lithotomy position for the pelvic examination which requires her to be on her back, knees bent, legs spread apart with her feet placed in metal stirrups at the foot of the exam table (Planned Parenthood Alameda/San Francisco, 1991). Alternative positions, such as a knee-chest position or a lateral position (woman lies on her side with top leg flexed) may be more comfortable for rectal, vaginal, or perineal assessment. For greater comfort, the woman may be assisted into a V-shaped position (two assistants are needed to support the woman's legs and allow her to maintain the position) or the M-shaped position (woman lies on her back, knees bent and apart, feet resting on the exam table close to her buttocks) during the speculum and pelvic examinations (Fig. 33–6). A disabled woman is the best judge of which position will work for her and how to use assistance effectively (Planned Parenthood Alameda/San Francisco, 1991). Nurses play an important role in explaining the procedures to disabled women so that they might choose optimal positioning or suggest effective alternatives. In this role, nurses promote a partnership between patient and provider and assist in mediating barriers to health care access.

Physical assessment of individuals with musculoskeletal conditions should include determination of flexion, abduction, and external rotation to ascertain the extent of hip and hand involvement and to determine musculoskeletal pain and/or contractures in all joints (Dalton, 1990). Specific questions to be asked when assessing sexual health in individuals with arthritis have been developed by Dalton (1990, p. 332). One global question that can be applied to any chronic condition, "In what ways, if any, has your arthritis affected your sexual relationship with your spouse/partner/significant other?" Other questions to include in sexual health assessment include: "What was your sexual relationship like before you had arthritis? How has that changed?" or "Specifically, what sexual adaptations have been helpful? Exercise and rest? Increase or decrease in analgesics? Use of local lubricants? Time of day? Positions of comfort? Expressions of intimacy?"

ASSESSING MALE PATIENTS

Physical assessment of the male genitalia includes inspection of the external genitalia (penis and scrotum) and palpation of the penis, scrotum, testes, and prostate. Inspection of the penis focuses on the size and shape of the penis, location of the urinary meatus, and the texture and color of the penile skin. Inspection and palpation of the scrotum provides information about the color and texture of the skin, asymmetry of the scrotal contents (normal to have left testis lower than the right), the tone of the dartos muscle, and the ability of the muscle to contract with cold or relax with warmth. Palpation of the scrotal contents provides information about the contour and texture of the testes, the size, shape, consistency,

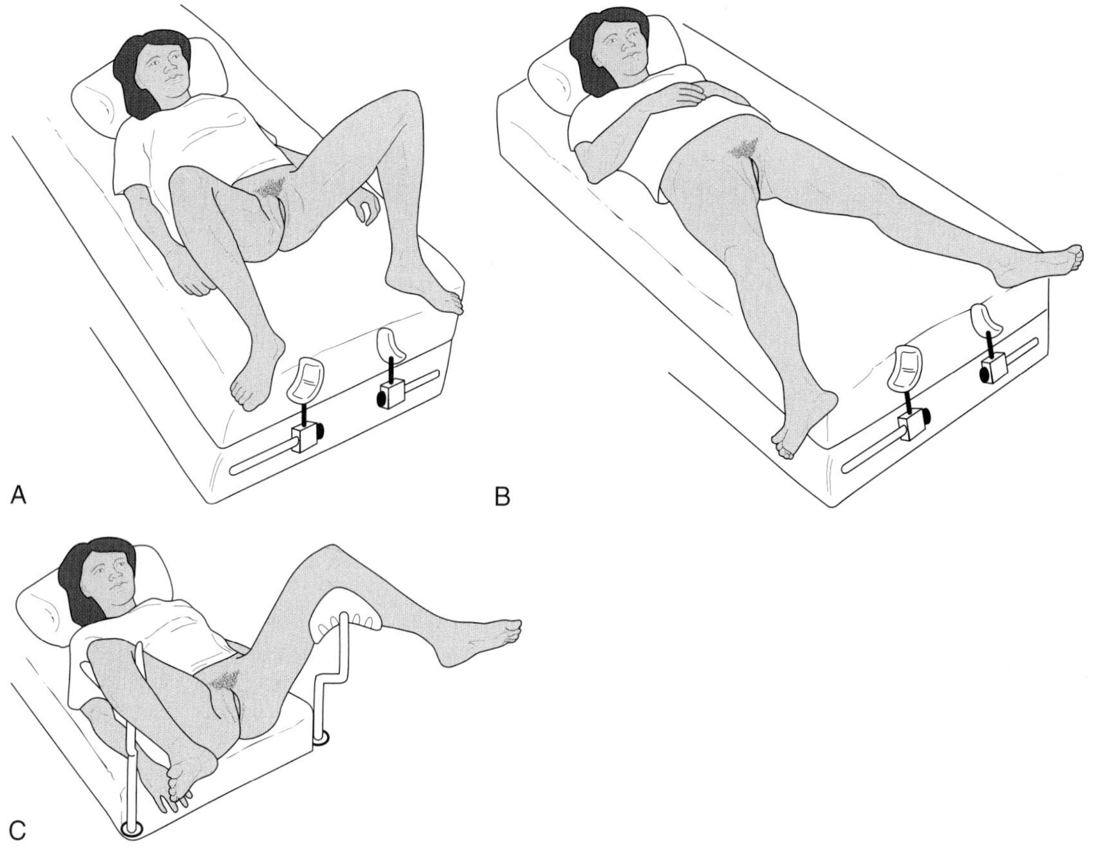

Figure 33–6. Positions for pelvic examination of females.

and tenderness of the epididymis. Palpation of the prostate gland is an important procedure for detecting early changes in the size, shape, and texture (Box 33–10) and also extent of encroachment into the rectal lumen (Box 33–11). This is one of the most important assessment measures in detecting prostate cancer.

Males experiencing symptoms of burning with urination or with ejaculation, or who have a urethral discharge, will be cultured for gonorrhea and chlamydia. In addition to urethral cultures, symptomatic men may have throat and anal cultures done, as well. Those who have been exposed to gonorrheal or chlamydial infections, but are not symptomatic, will also have cultures obtained.

BOX 33–10
ELEMENTS OF THE PROSTATE EXAMINATION

- Surface: smooth or nodular?
- Consistency: rubbery, hard, boggy, soft, or fluctuant?
- Shape: rounded or flat?
- Size: normal, enlarged, or atrophied?
- Mobility: fixed or movable?
- Sensitivity: tender or nontender?

BOX 33–11
STAGING PROSTATIC ENLARGEMENT

- Grade I: Encroaches less than 1 cm into the rectal lumen
- Grade II: Encroaches 1–2 cm into the rectal lumen
- Grade III: Encroaches 2–3 cm into the rectal lumen
- Grade IV: Encroaches more than 4 cm into the rectal lumen

Sexual Health Promotion

Sex education is a major role for the nurse in sexual health promotion. In this role, the nurse provides accurate information, dispels myths, and corrects misinformation (Fogel, 1990). The degree of information provided should match the patient's interest and developmental level. Fogel (1990) suggests limiting information to a specific topic rather than providing a more general focus. This technique is more apt to satisfy the patient's specific concerns and is better suited to achieving a preset goal, which results in a more satisfactory level of functioning. For example, during physical assessment the nurse can be describing strategies for self-examination and self-care. As the nurse inspects the male patient's penis,

CLINICAL DECISION MAKING
SEXUAL HEALTH AND A TEENAGE COUPLE

ASSESSMENT

The nurse who meets with Lucy and Zack must assess the health issues presented by this teenage couple and proceed through clinical decision-making processes. The concerns brought forth by Lucy include pregnancy protection, sexually transmitted infection protection (including AIDS protection), pressure exerted by Zack to engage in sexual intercourse and to avoid pregnancy protection, estrangement from parents and relocation to her grandmother's home, experiencing pressure to engage in sexual activity and how refusal might affect her relationship with Zack, and treatment for a sexually acquired infection (HPV). She has limited family support and is having difficulty discussing her fears with her boyfriend. Zack does not plan to use a condom should Lucy consent to sex, because he states that he wants her to be pregnant.

Nursing assessment begins when the nurse becomes aware of a client's need (Fogel et al, 1990). Because the primary source of data is the client, the nurse must provide an atmosphere in which the patient, or couple, can ask questions and discuss concerns in private. Both subjective and objective data are gathered during this phase with additional data obtained from medical records, physical examination, or laboratory tests. Contextual information about the patient's environment is obtained during the interview; in this case presentation, contextual data include the information about Lucy's living situation (with her grandmother) and the pressure she is receiving from Zack to have sex and to avoid protection from pregnancy. Since this couple appears to have differing issues, it is essential that the nurse determine who the patient is. If Lucy is the patient, then the nurse must ask Lucy if she wishes to be interviewed in private. If Zack is the patient, the same question must be directed toward him. It may be that the couple has jointly decided to be interviewed together; however, in the course of the interview, the nurse may determine that a joint interview is not productive or that the two need to be seen separately. It is within the scope of the nursing role to make that suggestion. However, the ultimate decision must be left to the patient(s). In our case, Lucy states her wish to be interviewed alone and Zack agrees to this preference.

REFLECTION

In the diagnosis phase of nursing assessment, the gathered data are assimilated and clustered into related categories or groupings (Fogel et al, 1990). This phase involves making a summary statement of the gathered data that actually define or describe the nature of the patient's health problem; this restatement must be validated by the client for accuracy. Natural groupings noted in the case presentation are pregnancy prevention, STI protection, and STI treatment, which can often be discussed simultaneously; communication issues with Lucy's parents and with Zack; and Lucy's strong feelings about the pressure that Zack is exerting on her to engage in sex and to become pregnant. It is important that the nurse ask Lucy if these are indeed the issues that she has come for help/advice about.

SETTING PRIORITIES

Each of the areas identified in the nursing diagnosis requires a specific plan of care. In the context of a busy clinic setting, it may not be realistic to address *all* of the issues presented in the case at one visit. Nurses must prioritize, with input from the patient as to priorities, and plan the care for those problems that are mutually agreed upon. A future appointment may need to be made for the remaining issues. In this case, Lucy and the nurse agree that her communication problems with Zack and her worries about the pressure he is exerting are the most important health issues to address. These receive priority, because if Lucy decides to abstain from sexual intercourse with Zack, she has no immediate need for pregnancy prevention information or STI protection. She does, however, have a very important need to obtain treatment for her sexually acquired HPV and will receive that treatment at this clinic visit.

NURSING ACTIONS

A nursing care plan for Lucy about her communication problems with Zack might include education about handling differences in sexual desire, setting limits with a partner, healthy sexual expression, plus potential gender and age differences in determining when to become sexually involved with a partner. The nursing care plan might include information about other adults in Lucy's life who could lend support and advice on these issues or a referral to individual counseling or couples counseling by a licensed professional experienced with teenagers and their problems. The nursing assessment must include directed questions that elicit any history of abuse that might be directing Lucy's worries; physical or sexual abuse must be reported to the appropriate authority and immediate intervention strategies applied. Lucy must be advised that she can call the clinic or an alternate health care provider for assistance on these issues at any time. Her limited family network makes this an essential part of the nursing care plan.

Contraceptive options and STI protection can be discussed by the nurse as part of the nursing care plan. Both verbal and written information can provide the knowledge base that Lucy needs to promote her own sexual health. She may decide to consult Zack about these important concerns, although he has demonstrated a lack of interest in allowing Lucy to protect herself from unintended pregnancy. Additionally, prescription methods and devices can be provided to Lucy by the licensed health care provider scheduled to treat her HPV infection. Coordination of these visit components is often left to the nurse.

Follow-up appointments to address remaining health care issues should be scheduled before Lucy leaves the clinic. In this way, the nurse can be assured that a follow-up plan is in place and that Lucy will have some continuity in her health care provision.

information about STI symptoms can be described (e.g., herpes lesions) or simple instructions about cleaning an uncircumcised penis can be provided. While examining the female patient, the nurse can offer her a mirror so that she might watch the examination process, and the nurse can provide information about anatomy, signs and symptoms, and personal hygiene strategies.

Although some nurses are able to provide intensive sexual therapy, referral to another trained professional for this service is the norm. In this situation, the nurse must have explored suitable options for patients with sexual concerns and should have some mechanism for collecting data as to the patient's satisfaction with the referral provider. In this way, the nurse can be assured that the referral providers suggested are, in fact, providing high-quality sexual health care. Nurses may also serve as consultants for the development of sex education programs for community groups or schools. This role provides a unique opportunity to positively influence course content that includes bio-psycho-social-cultural dimensions of human sexuality. As well, nurses may be asked to share their experience with sexual health promotion with other nurses who lack this experience or knowledge base. In this way, the nurse is able to ensure that sexual health promotion remains an important part of the nursing role.

Nurses may perform many roles in the provision of sexual health care or in sexual health promotion; however, central to these roles is the creation of an environment that is supportive of sexual health and a milieu that minimizes anxiety or guilt that patients might feel when relating their sexual thoughts, behaviors, or feelings (Fogel, 1990). Anticipatory guidance that provides patients with information about what to expect or what range of behaviors might occur can alleviate many sexual health concerns, particularly when patients might be worried about issues such as same-sex behaviors or libido concerns (hypoactive, hyperactive, or differences with partner). Validating normalcy is one of the major ways that nurses can promote sexual health, particularly when individuals express anxiety about healthy sexual expression. Fogel (1990) identified adolescence, childbirth, midlife, and as the effects of aging are felt as likely times that individuals may seek this validation of normalcy from health care providers. However, in addition to validating normalcy, the nurse must be prepared to assess for variations from normal and provide education and other intervention strategies should this be necessary.

If the nurse identifies sexual dysfunction in an individual, the primary intervention strategies to be utilized include:

- informing the client of the dysfunction
- providing verbal and written information
- providing a list of references for further reading
- providing referral sources
- coordinating a specific referral for the client

Some nurses have obtained additional training, including certification in sexual counseling, which allows them to provide more specific interventions that individuals can do while waiting for intensive therapy. Others must rely upon published self-care strategies that begin the process of remedying specific dysfunctions. All have the necessary knowledge and experience to assist the individual with obtaining professional guidance and treatment in the dysfunctional area. Nurses must know which professionals in the geographic area specialize in treatment of sexual dysfunction and should maintain a feedback system, such as written evaluations from referred individuals about the referral professionals. In this way, nurses can avoid the mistake of continuing to refer clients to professionals who are reported to be ineffective, offensive, or nonresponsive. Crucial to assisting individuals with obtaining professional help is coordination of the referral process by the nurse. Rather than handing the individual a referral list, the nurse can better facilitate the referral process by providing a referral letter that outlines specific findings or by telephoning the professional chosen by the client. This may ensure that the client has a smoother entry into professional treatment and may provide the nurse with more confidence that the client will actually obtain care for the identified dysfunction.

Sexual health promotion of the patient living with a chronic disease and his or her partner is an important function of a health professional. The nurse can make suggestions that may help the individual and his or her partner approach sexual activity more comfortably. Information may be given regarding normal sexual response as well as changes that accompany a particular chronic condition. It is important to communicate to the patient that the chronic condition does not directly decrease sexual ability or the capacity to enjoy sex. Rather, the degree of exercise intolerance associated with cardiac or respiratory disease most directly affects any limitation of sexual activity. The frequency of sexual activity is often limited, as is the frequency of other physical activities. Individuals should be encouraged to approach sexual activity as they do other physical activities, incorporating the same methods to ensure energy conservation. Sexual activity should be paced like any other activity. Choice of time of day may be important. For some, this may be midmorning—after a night's rest or morning medications. There are other modifications and adaptations a professional can suggest that may be helpful in engaging in sexual activity. The patient's partner may be encouraged to assume a more active role. Positions utilized may be a consideration. For individuals with chronic lung disease, the side-lying position and the position with the male seated (on a chair or bedside) and then straddled may be the most comfortable (Stockdale-Wooley, 1990).

The nurse can provide information about, and suggest alterations in, the contextual or situational factors to minimize cardiovascular stress with sexual activity. A teaching plan for adults (and their partners) with cardiac disease has been developed by Burke (1990). Because sexual activity and orgasm, like any physical activity, places increased demands on the cardiovascular system, individuals may want to do the following to avoid strain and promote success:

- Wait 2 or more hours after eating meals.
- Wait 2 or more hours after drinking alcohol.

- Avoid an environment that is too hot or cold.
- Be rested and relaxed.
- Have nitroglycerine available or use nitroglycerine prophylactically if sexual arousal/orgasm usually precipitates angina symptoms (Burke, 1990, pp. 365–366).

Alternative forms of sexual gratification should be encouraged if mutually pleasing and acceptable to patient and partner, inasmuch as intercourse is only one aspect of heterosexual expression. Caressing, embracing, cuddling, and open communication are other forms of expression that are less fatiguing and anxiety producing. An important factor to any adjustment to altered sexual function is a supportive spouse or partner.

TEACHING ABOUT CONTRACEPTION

Preventing an unwanted pregnancy is an important consideration in sexual health promotion. Options counseling may be provided by the nurse during a pregnancy diagnosis visit; it must start with providing the woman with an opportunity to clarify and articulate her feelings (Hatcher et al, 1994). When presenting the pregnancy test result, the nurse should allow adequate time for the woman to express her feelings and to ask questions. Integral to options counseling is assessing the woman's personal support system and suggesting that she access support and assistance from these individuals. Counseling referrals should be provided if the woman feels that this would be helpful, especially if her personal support system is limited. Nurses should encourage women to talk with their partners, family, or friends about the options available. These options include continuing the pregnancy and keeping the baby; continuing the pregnancy but placing the baby with adoptive parents; or terminating the pregnancy by either surgical or medical procedures. Women who choose either of the first two options must be given referrals for pregnancy care and should be given instructions for an optimal pregnancy (Box 33–12). Women choosing to terminate their pregnancies with surgical or medical methods should be provided with education materials about these procedures, referrals to providers, and instructions about pregnancy complications, such as miscarriage. Abortion providers and their staffs are responsible for educating women about the safety, efficacy, and potential complications of these procedures.

BOX 33-12
INSTRUCTIONS FOR AN OPTIMAL PREGNANCY

- Review the medical and family history risk factors and refer for genetic counseling, if indicated. Testing for AIDS is recommended for all women before they become pregnant.
- Plan ahead if there is a serious medical condition, such as diabetes or epilepsy
- Take a vitamin that includes folic acid 0.4 mg every day
- Avoid exposure to potentially toxic agents, including alcohol, smoking, excessive caffeine; x-ray of the abdominal area; illegal drug use; and megadose vitamins (or mega anything else)
- Do not take any medications until it has been discussed with your health care provider
- Make healthy diet a top priority
- Aim for fitness, but with moderation
- Minimize your risk for STD exposure
- Avoid body temperature elevation (do not use a hot tub or sauna. Try to avoid contagious viral illness, such as influenza)
- Avoid contact with cat fecal matter (toxoplasma infection during pregnancy can be dangerous for the fetus)
- Have a pregnancy test and see your clinician as soon as possible
- Watch for danger signs of possible pregnancy complications (abdominal pain, bleeding, unusual vaginal discharge)

From Hatcher, R. Trussell, J., Stewart, F., et al (1994). *Contraceptive Technology 1994–1996*, 16th rev. ed. New York: Irvington, pp. 469–470.

PRIMARY PREVENTION

Choosing a contraceptive method to prevent pregnancy is an important decision for both women and men. The method of choice must be effective, safe, and must fit into the individual's or couple's lifestyle. Users themselves should make the contraceptive choice based upon information provided by health professionals who are knowledgeable about the risks and benefits of all methods. Nurses are particularly positioned to provide this information because their education and training includes a sound knowledge base from which to educate and to assist in decision making. The information provided by nurses about the various contraceptive methods available must include methods descriptions, effectiveness rates, continuation rates, and failure rates. Box 33–13 summarizes how the nurse can assist patients in select appropriate contraceptive methods.

Current understanding of the results in the literature on contraceptive efficacy is summarized in Table 33–4.

SECONDARY PREVENTION

Many sexually active couples are not using effective pregnancy prevention methods. Inconsistent or incorrect use of contraceptives is reported in at least half of pregnant women receiving counseling for abortion. Because clinicians have access to a large proportion of persons at risk for unintended pregnancy, counseling regarding the use of pregnancy prevention methods could have a significant public health impact if performed effectively. Mosher (1988) estimated that approximately one third of all unwanted pregnancies and 500,000 abortions could be prevented if the proportion of women not using contraception were reduced by half.

BOX 33-13
NURSES' ROLE IN ASSISTING PATIENTS IN SELECTING A CONTRACEPTIVE METHOD

- Provide written summary of available contraceptive methods.
- Answer the patient's questions and concerns.
- Assess the patient's health history regarding:
  - Previous contraceptive use, particularly contraceptive failures
  - Previous sexually transmitted infections (STIs)
  - Pregnancy history
  - Contraindications to hormonal methods
  - Menstrual history (i.e., menstrual regularity, menstrual changes, menstrual symptoms, or perimenstrual symptoms)
- Determine personal considerations, such as:
  - Problems with previous methods
  - Preference
  - Cost
  - Religious/moral beliefs
  - Comfort with method of choice
  - Ability to use method (physical constraints, partner objections)
  - STI/human immunodeficiency virus risk
- If no medical contraindication to preferred method exists, provide education on:
  - Proper use
  - Risks/benefits
  - Possible side effects
  - Serious side effects requiring medical intervention
  - Failure rate
  - Effectiveness against STIs
- If medical contraindication to method of choice, assist the patient in selecting alternative. Provide education as to this alternative method:
  - Proper use
  - Risks/benefits
  - Possible side effects
  - Serious side effects requiring medical intervention
  - Failure rate
  - Effectiveness against STIs
- Provide emergency contact information in the event serious side effects occur.

Assessment for pregnancy prevention overlaps with intervention strategies because it is often therapeutic in itself. Assessment involves counseling the individual or couple about contraceptive method effectiveness, informed consent, and risk-benefit factors as they relate to the individual or couple's choice of pregnancy prevention method. Discussing informed consent and method effectiveness provides necessary information while discussion of risk-benefit factors assists the couple or individual in their personal decision-making process.

The effectiveness of pregnancy prevention counseling and assessment depends upon the age, developmental maturity, sex, parity, and health status of the individual, as well as on the level of training, clinical practice setting, and counseling skills of the provider (Box 33–14). Counseling for pregnancy prevention must include information about effectiveness of various methods, safety factors and side effects, and personal considerations such as cost, changing needs, pattern of sexual activity, and access to health services (Hatcher et al, 1994). Providing the adult woman with information and suggestions for individualizing her choice is usually adequate in helping her choose an appropriate pregnancy prevention method. However, for the teenager, contraceptive initiation and continuation involves multiple strategies.

BOX 33-14
SECONDARY PREVENTION IN FERTILITY CONTROL: THE NURSE'S ROLE

- Provide education to patients about reproductive physiology and fertility control options.
- Educate patients about available pregnancy testing.
- Educate patients about signs and symptoms of early pregnancy.
- Provide pregnancy testing for patients who are at risk for unintended pregnancy.
- Inform patient of result of pregnancy test.
- If pregnancy test is positive, provide complete information about pregnancy outcome options.
- If negative pregnancy test, discuss available contraceptive options.

It is not sufficient for the nurse to provide only information about contraceptive methods; rather, information must also be presented to the patient about access to pregnancy testing should there be a method failure, error in use of the chosen method, or the occurrence of worry or concern about the possibility of pregnancy. Following a pregnancy test, the nurse must be prepared to provide the patient with the result of the test and then be available to provide information about options.

TEACHING PREVENTION OF SEXUALLY TRANSMITTED INFECTIONS

Currently available preventive measures include treatment of current cases (if treatment exists), identification and treatment of all sexual partners of the infected person, and minimization of risk behaviors for contracting and transmitting STIs. Effective efforts must also go beyond the individual and involve institutional, community, and government efforts (Lichtman and Duran, 1990).

PRIMARY PREVENTION

The nurse's role in primary prevention of STIs involves educating men and women about ways to prevent acquisition of STIs and HIV/AIDS. Strategies involve behaviors that are sometimes called "safer sex" practices. These include:

- knowing one's partner
- reducing the number of partners
- practicing low-risk sex
- avoiding the exchange of body fluids (Fogel, 1995)

TABLE 33-4 Percentage of Women Experiencing a Contraceptive Failure During the First Year of Typical Use and the First Year of Perfect Use and the Percentage Continuing Use at the End of the First Year, United States

	% of Women Experiencing an Accidental Pregnancy within the First Year of Use		% of Women Continuing Use at One Year
Method (1)	*Typical Use* (2)	*Perfect Use* (3)	(4)
Chance	85	85	
Spermicides	21	6	43
Periodic Abstinence	20		67
Calendar		9	
Ovulation Method		3	
Sympto-Thermal		2	
Post-Ovulation		1	
Withdrawal	19	4	
Cap			
Parous Women	36	26	45
Nulliparous Women	18	9	58
Sponge			
Parous Women	36	20	45
Nulliparous Women	18	9	58
Diaphragm	18	6	58
Condom			
Female (Reality)	21	5	56
Male	12	3	63
Pill	3		72
Progestin Only		0.5	
Combined		0.1	
IUD			
Progesterone T	2.0	1.5	81
Copper T 380A	0.8	0.6	78
LNg 20	0.1	0.1	81
Depo-Provera	0.3	0.3	70
Norplant (6 Capsules)	0.09	0.09	85
Female Sterilization	0.4	0.4	100
Male Sterilization	0.15	0.10	100

Emergency Contraceptive Pills: Treatment initiated within 72 hours after unprotected intercourse reduces the risk of pregnancy by at least 75%.
Lactational Amenorrhea Method: LAM is a highly effective, *temporary* method of contraception.
From Hatcher, R., Trussell, J., Stewart, F., et al (1994). *Contraceptive Technology*, 16th rev. ed. New York: Irvington, p. 113.

Knowing one's partner may be the critical feature of practicing safer sex, for this knowledge may help to eliminate those partners who bring high risk of STIs. Limiting the number of sexual partners and those partners who have multiple sexual partners decreases the chances of acquiring an STI. In addition, partners should be asked about exposure to STIs and about their sexual practices, including their number of partners. Anal-genital intercourse, anal-oral contact, and anal-digital activity are considered high-risk sexual behaviors (Stone et al, 1986). Vaginal or oral intercourse should never follow anal contact without thorough washing. Furthermore, safer sex practices embrace the concept of avoiding body fluid exchange; critically important to this avoidance is whether or not male partners resist wearing condoms.

Included under the rubric of safer sex practices are mutual masturbation (as long as body fluids come in contact only with intact skin); caressing, hugging, body rubbing, massage, and hand-to-genital touching; and possibly deep kissing and oral sex (when the woman does not have her menses or a vaginal or cervical infection). It has been reported that rubber (dental) dams may provide additional safety for oral sex to women (Hatcher et al, 1994); however, studies have not been done to confirm this method of protection (Fogel, 1995).

Currently, the sole physical barrier promoted for the prevention of sexual transmission of HIV and other STIs is the condom (Stein, 1990). Nurses can help to motivate patients to use condoms by discussing condom use and effectiveness. The discussion must include accurate information about effectiveness and about how condoms are properly used (Fig. 33–7). The nurse must be sensitive to cultural barriers to condom use, as well as to other barriers, such as claims of reduction in sensation (by male and/or female partner),

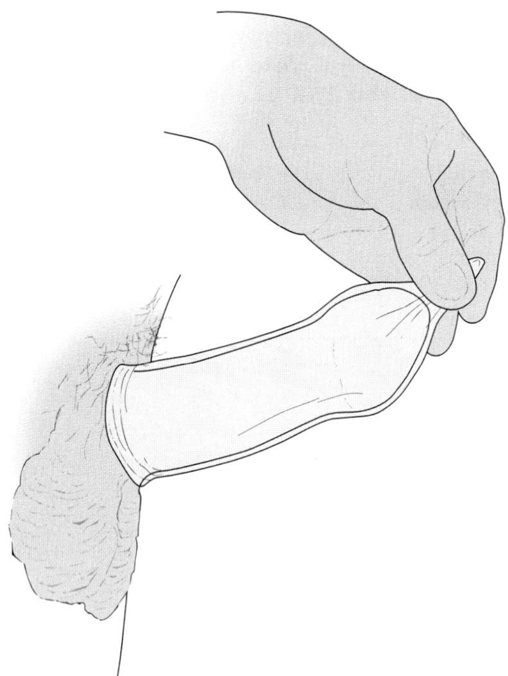

Figure 33-7. Proper use of a condom.

expense, and inconvenience. Nurses may need to assist patients to develop the social skills necessary to negotiate condom usage. This assistance may include role playing and practice sessions in which the patient is given specific language to use. An example of a lead-in question appropriate for a woman or a man might be "I would like us to talk about something that is a little embarrassing, but I think it's important for both of us. I think we should talk about safer sex." In this way, nurses can assist patients in reducing their risk of acquiring an STI while fostering the ability to confront sexual issues openly.

Selection of a contraceptive method has a direct impact on STI risk (Hatcher et al, 1994). Specifically, latex condoms and all spermicidal agents that contain nonoxynol-9 have been shown to be effective barriers to many of the bacterial and viral STIs, including gonorrhea, chlamydia, herpes, condyloma acuminatum (HPV), and HIV infections (Hatcher et al, 1994). A diaphragm that is placed properly and used with spermicide provides protection for the cervix. The contraceptive sponge, which is not presently being manufactured, is protective against gonorrhea, and possibly other STIs (Hatcher et al, 1994). Because none of these methods is completely protective against all STIs, their effectiveness can be enhanced when utilized with other safer sex practices, such as alternatives to penetrative intercourse. In combination with other risk-reducing practices (limiting number of sex partners, knowing sexual history of sexual partner, and identifying his or her risk), individuals can greatly reduce their exposure to STIs (Box 33–15).

SECONDARY PREVENTION

Nurses can minimize the patient's delay in seeking treatment by understanding the underlying reasons for the delay.

BOX 33-15
STRATEGIES FOR PREVENTING SEXUALLY TRANSMITTED INFECTIONS

- Engage in sex with one mutually faithful partner.
- Abstain from sex with any person who has lesions, rashes, or malodorous discharges from the genitals.
- Do not have intercourse with any person whose sexual history is unknown or who is at high risk for acquired immunodefiency syndrome (AIDS).
- Use condoms consistently and throughout genital contact.
- Wash and urinate before and after sexual intercourse.

From Fogel, C., Lauver, D. (eds.) (1990). *Sexual Health Promotion.* Philadelphia: W.B. Saunders.

Patients may delay seeking treatment for STIs because they believe they may be stereotyped or suffer social stigma, embarrassment, or some degree of shame during the encounter. Other patients may delay seeking treatment because of limited accessibility to health care. And still others may not seek treatment because they are unaware of the signs and symptoms of STIs. Psychosocial reactions of patients with STIs will vary, and there is little research that explains individual reactions to STIs. Clinical reports suggest a wide range of reactions, such as acceptance, hurt, disbelief, anger, and concern about long-term effects (Smith et al, 1990). To reduce the delay in treatment of STIs, nurses may need to identify and plan routine screening for individuals at higher risk. Moreover, infected individuals should be asked to identify and inform exposed partners; these partners must be encouraged to seek treatment regardless of symptomatology. Nurses may need to develop and instigate procedures by which exposed partners can obtain treatment without delay and without lengthy appointment-related procedures. By providing ease of access for partner treatment, STI transmission can be reduced.

Nurses need to assess the biopsychosocial needs of patients with STIs in a holistic way. Traditionally, patients with STIs have experienced discrimination and prejudice from health care providers. Men and women with STIs need holistic care and attention to their emotional feelings, fears, and physical comfort. They also need to be assured about the privacy and confidentiality of their medical records.

A thorough history, examination, and appropriate laboratory tests are needed to diagnose STIs. Patients with STIs may be anxious or embarrassed. Therefore, take the history prior to the exam, while the patient is dressed. Approach the patient with a nonjudgmental, objective attitude that is sensitive to the personal issues involved, but direct enough to obtain the information needed for optimum health care counseling. Elicit the history in a nonjudgmental manner, using open-ended questions, and avoid assumptions of sexual orientation. Refer, whenever possible, to all partners as partners and not by gender or stereotypical labels (e.g., husband, wife, etc.). Additional questions include type of sexual activity, number of contacts, symptomatology, and potential sites of infection (mouth, cervix, rectum, urethra). Other necessary data include any information that will influence the treatment plan, history of drug allergies, pregnancy, previously diagnosed conditions, and general health status. Menstrual cycle data should be collected to rule out pregnancy (last menstrual period [LMP], regular cycles).

During the examination, the patient's comfort, modesty, and privacy should be respected. Drape the patient for privacy and warmth. For women, the speculum should be warmed, and it is helpful to cover the metal stirrups of the examination table. A detailed explanation of the specific procedures is usually reassuring to the patient. Assure the patient of confidentiality throughout the interaction.

The patient who has an STI needs to be encouraged to seek treatment at the earliest stage of symptoms, and sexual partners also need to be evaluated. Patients and partners need to know how to follow the treatment regimen adequately; specifically, they need to know whether or not sexual abstinence may be necessary, and if so, for how long. Education is necessary for all patients so that they can respond promptly to symptoms, follow treatment instructions, refer partners for treatment, return for all follow-up appointments, practice prevention, and request periodic check-ups if their lifestyle places them at a higher risk of contracting STIs (Box 33–16).

TEACHING PATIENT SELF-EXAMINATION

The self-care movement has influenced nursing practice to the degree that nurses are routinely asked to teach self-assessment techniques. Particularly in the area of sexual health, self-assessment skills have been developed to encourage early intervention when variance from health is detected. In addition, self-assessment has been utilized as a tool to understand one's body more completely. In this way, awareness of one's own sexuality can be developed while practicing a disease prevention technique: self-examination. Teaching patients to do appropriate self-examinations can enhance the provider-patient partnership in the provision of health care (Box 33–17). When providers do not teach the patient to perform self-examinations, a valuable opportunity is missed (Misener and Fuller, 1995).

One component of self-assessment is risk screening. Traditionally, risk appraisal in health protection or prevention of disease and illness has focused on the individual, but a comprehensive risk assessment should also include the social, physical, and cultural environment.

The principle of risk screening as a method of prevention is that each person is likely to incur quantifiable health hazards

BOX 33-16
PATIENT EDUCATION FOR ALL SEXUALLY TRANSMITTED INFECTIONS

- Taking prescribed medication: how, when, things to avoid.
- Obtaining repeat cultures after treatment for test of cure: when, why, what happens at the clinic.
- Recheck: when, why, what happens at the clinic.
- Sex partners: need for medical care; need for a period of abstinence from sexual intercourse; realistic health plan, including how patient will tell partners, where patient will refer partners, when partners will go, where patient can reach nurse for additional assistance, and where nurse can reach patient if necessary.
- Future health: the need to seek medical attention immediately if any unusual bumps, sores, rashes, or discharges appear; importance of periodic return visits to clinic even if no symptoms are apparent.
- Be sure the patient leaves the clinic with no unanswered questions.

From Fogel, C., Lauver, D. (eds.) (1990). *Sexual Health Promotion*. Philadelphia: W.B. Saunders.

BOX 33-17
TEACHING SELF-ASSESSMENT TO WOMEN

The teaching of genital self-examination may be indicated for clients in the following situations:

1. Clients using barrier or intrauterine contraceptive devices. The clients need to check the placement of devices.
2. Clients who have recurring vaginal infections.
3. Clients at risk for sexually transmitted diseases.

The teaching session is initiated with a thorough presentation of the anatomy of the female genitalia and the normal appearance and feel of organs, structures, and discharge.

The following steps are recommended in teaching self-examination:

1. Find a comfortable position that will allow for viewing of the external genitalia with a mirror. A source of light from a nearby lamp is often necessary.
2. Inspect the condition of the hair and skin over the genitalia. Spread the hairs and inspect all the surfaces of the labia. Look for bumps, sores, warts, and blisters.
3. Spread the labia and look at the clitoris for bumps, blisters, sores, and warts.
4. Look at the urethral opening and the area of the Bartholin's glands for swelling or redness.
5. Insert a finger into the vagina and feel the consistency of normal tissue and get used to the plane of the vagina.
6. Insert a finger deep into the vagina and locate the cervix. Feel the os and then feel the entire surface by circling it with the finger.
7. Look carefully at the type of discharge that is on the finger when it is taken out.

Some women's self-help groups teach self-examination by vaginal speculum. This is not recommended because of the difficulty of this maneuver on oneself and because professional judgment is needed for adequate assessment.

From Barkauskas, V., Stoltenberg-Allen, K., Baumann, L., Darling-Fisher, C. (1994). *Health & Physical Assessment*. St. Louis: C.V. Mosby, p. 685.

PATIENT TEACHING
TESTICULAR SELF-EXAMINATION

The best time to do the exam is after a warm bath or shower when the scrotal skin is relaxed. Follow these steps:

1. Stand and place your right leg on an elevated surface. A tub side or toilet seat works fine.
2. Explore the surface of the right testicle by gently rolling it between the thumb and fingers of both hands. Feel for any hard lumps or nodules. The testicle should feel round and smooth.
3. Notice any enlargement of the testicle or a change in its consistency. It is normal for one testicle to be slightly larger than the other. Any major size differences should be reported to a health professional.
4. Repeat, lifting the left leg and examining your left testicle.

Call your health professional for an immediate appointment if you notice any of the following:

- Unusual lumps or nodules in the testes.
- Unexplained pain or swelling in the testes or scrotum.
- Penile discharge, or sores on your penis. Do not have intercourse without using a condom if you notice a penile discharge or sores on your penis.

From Kemper, D. (1994). *Kaiser Permanente Healthwise Handbook: A Self-Care Guide for You and Your Family.* Boise, ID: Healthwise.

as a member of a specific group; average risks can be applied once the person's characteristics are known and compared with the mortality experience of a similar population cohort (Pender, 1987). The population cohort is usually a national database that represents only mortality statistics for those diseases that have high mortality rates.

Although the assessment of health risks may be useful as one component of health protection, it must be linked to behavior-change strategies and appropriate community resources. It is unethical to assess risk levels without providing education or preventive strategies to facilitate behavior change efforts. The nurse should link risk appraisal with comprehensive lifestyle assessment that focuses on enhancing well-being and self-care as opposed to only identifying risk factors for disease (Pender, 1987). Testicular self-examination for men and breast and genital self-examination for women are specific examples of self-assessment techniques that can be taught by nurses.

TESTICULAR SELF-EXAMINATION

Testicular cancer is the most common form of cancer in men between age 15 and 40 years, accounting for approximately 5500 new cases each year and 350 deaths (American Cancer Society, 1989). This form of cancer is more common in white males. Risk factors include cryptorchidism (undescended testicle), trauma, testicular atrophy, preexisting endocrinopathies, and genetic factors (Henderson et al, 1979). The principal screening tests for testicular cancer are annual clinical examination of the testes and monthly testicular self-examination (TSE) (see Patient Teaching box).

There is little information on the sensitivity, specificity, or positive predictive value of TSE or the clinical testicular exam in asymptomatic males. Health professionals, including nurses, have done much to promote breast self-examination (BSE) in women, yet the education of young men in the desirability of monthly TSE has been largely neglected (Meadus,

RESEARCH HIGHLIGHT
COMPARISON OF TWO BREAST SELF-EXAMINATION PALPATION TECHNIQUES

There is general agreement on the importance of breast self-examination for early lump detection. But is one method of breast palpation better than another?

The researchers asking this question compared two popular approaches to breast palpation: the vertical strip (VS) and the concentric circle (CC).

The sample consisted of 34 adult women from a Veterans outpatient clinic in the Northwest. They were randomly assigned according to breast size (large or small) to one of two groups. Subjects were pretested and then taught one method of palpation.

Proficiency in the palpation technique, area covered, and number of lumps discovered were evaluated. Those doing the evaluation had an interrater reliability of 86 percent.

During the breast self-examination, the VS group covered significantly more area than the CC group. Breast size did not affect breast area covered. Lump detection using breast models did not differ between the two groups.

IMPLICATIONS FOR NURSING PRACTICE

Nurses can teach breast self-examination using either the VS or the CC pattern of palpation. This practice should be evaluated as more research is available.

From Murali, M., Crabtree, K. (1992). Comparison of two breast self-examination palpation techniques. *Cancer Nursing, 15* (4), 276–282.

PATIENT TEACHING
BREAST SELF-EXAMINATION

Establish a regular time each month to examine your breasts, such as a few days after your period when your breasts are not swollen or tender. Women who do not menstruate (after menopause and women who have had hysterectomies) can examine their breasts the first day of each month.

Most women's breast tissue has some lumps or thickening. When in doubt about a particular lump, check the other breast. If you find a similar lump in the same area on the other breast, both breasts are probably normal. Be on the lookout for a lump that feels much harder than the rest of the breast.

Have any areas of concern checked by your health professional. The important thing is to learn what is normal for you and to report changes to your doctor.

The breast self-exam takes place in two stages:

STAGE 1: IN FRONT OF THE MIRROR

Examine your breasts visually in a mirror. Few women have breasts that match exactly. It is normal for one breast to be slightly larger than the other. Learn what is normal for you.

Look at your breasts in four positions:

- standing with your arms at your sides
- standing with your hands on your hips
- standing with your arms raised overhead
- standing and bending forward

In each position, look for changes in the contour and shape of your breasts, the color and texture of the skin and nipple, and any discharge from the nipples. Squeeze the nipple of each breast gently between thumb and index finger. Look for a discharge.

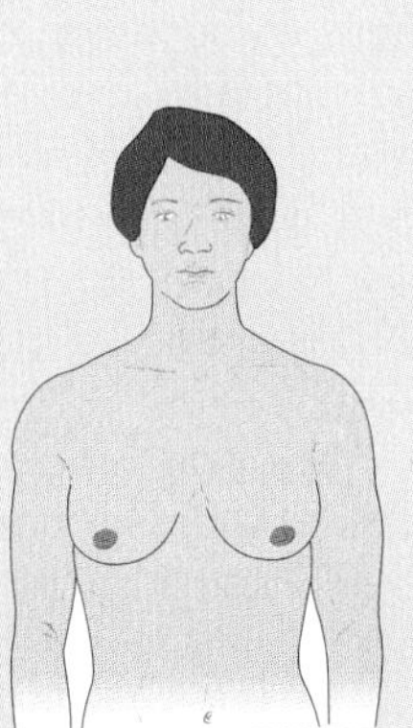

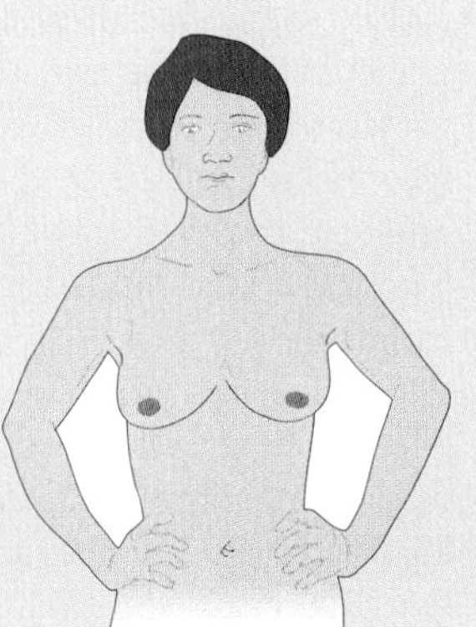

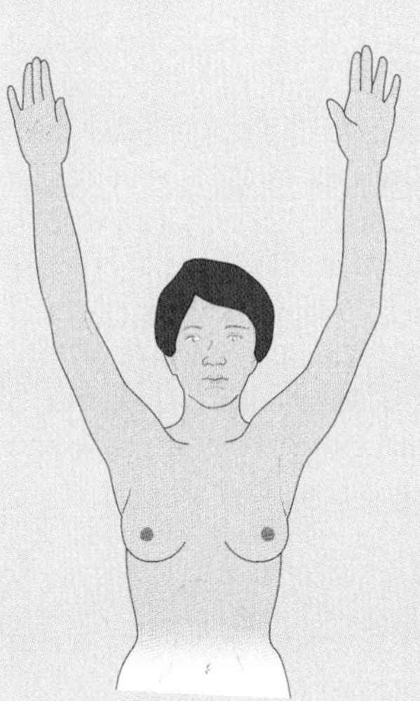

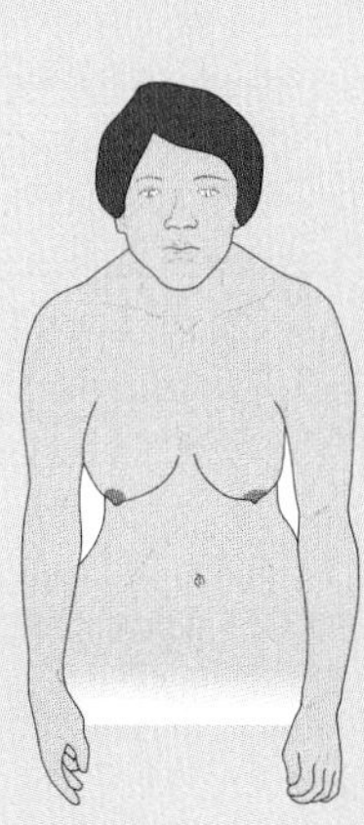

STAGE 2: LYING DOWN

To examine your left breast, place a pillow or folded towel under your left shoulder. Use your right hand to examine your left breast. If your breasts are large, lie on your right side and turn your left shoulder back flat to spread the breast tissue more evenly over your chest wall.

Use the pads of your middle three fingers to examine your breast. Move the fingers in small, dime-sized circles. Don't lift your fingers away from the skin. Use light, medium, and deep pressure in each spot to feel the full thickness of the breast tissue. You are feeling for lumps, thickening, or changes of any kind.

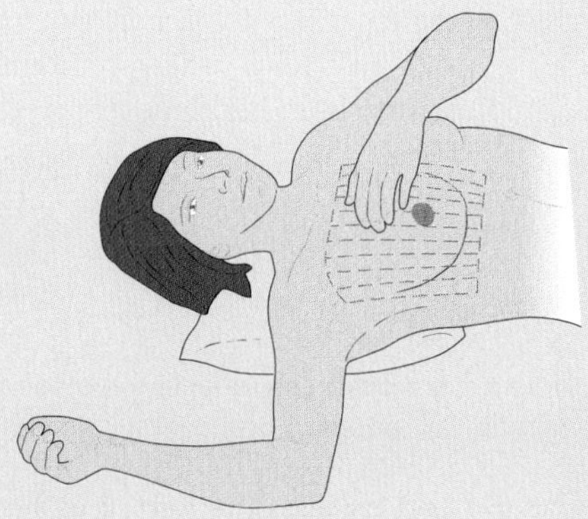

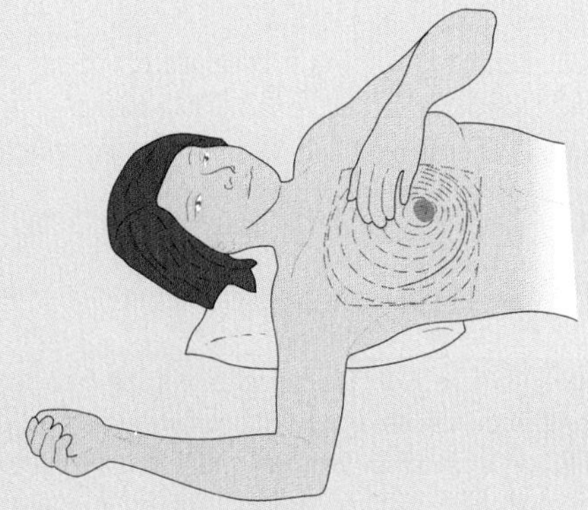

PATIENT TEACHING
BREAST SELF-EXAMINATION *Continued*

Examine your entire breast using a vertical strip pattern (see illustration). Examine all tissue from the collarbone to the armpit and from the bra line to the breastbone. Start in the armpit and work down to the bottom of the bra line. Move one finger width toward the middle and work up to the collarbone. Repeat until you have covered all the breast tissue.

Another way of doing this is to imagine that your breast is a clock. Start on the outside of the breast at 12:00, move slowly to 1:00 and then around the clock back to 12:00. Then move one inch in toward the nipple and go around the clock again.

Move the pillow or towel to the other shoulder and repeat this procedure for the other breast.

If you discover any unusual lumps, thickening, discharge from the nipple, or change of any kind, report them to your doctor immediately. Remember, most lumps are not malignant, but you will need your doctor to make a diagnosis.

If you examine your breasts monthly, you will learn what is normal for you and quickly recognize if something changes. The breast self-exam takes some practice.

From Kemper, D. (1994). *Kaiser Permanente Healthwise Handbook: A Self-Care Guide for You and Your Family.* Boise, ID: Healthwise.

1995). Delay in seeking professional help and diagnosis of testicular cancer occurs because of subtle symptoms or because many men are first diagnosed with other disorders (e.g., epididymitis, testicular trauma, hydrocele) (Bosl et al, 1981). Information on the accuracy of TSE is not available; however, research to date indicates that education about testicular cancer and self-exam may enhance knowledge and self-reported claims of TSE performance (Reno, 1988). Further study is needed to promote adherence to TSE and to document the effects of early detection on morbidity and mortality of testicular cancer (Finney et al, 1995).

BREAST SELF-EXAMINATION

Breast cancer is the leading cause of cancer deaths in women age 40 to 55. However, breast cancer is highly treatable if detected early. The components to early detection are breast self-examination, clinical breast examination, and mammography. The steps for teaching self-assessment are outlined in the Patient Teaching: Breast Self-Examination box. The clinical breast examination for early detection of breast problems is the health professional's physical exam. This exam is very similar to the self-exam, but it is performed by an experienced health professional. It is recommended every 1 to 2 years for women under 50, and every year for women over 50. A mammogram is a breast x-ray that helps to find breast tumors too small to be detected by breast self-exam and the clinical breast exam. For women over 50, a mammogram is recommended yearly. The American Cancer Society recommends that women between 40 and 50 have a mammogram every other year; the first mammogram to establish a baseline reading is recommended between age 35 and 40. Some health care providers do not agree with these guidelines and believe that mammograms have not been shown to save lives in women younger than 50 and do not recommend routine screening until age 50. However, all recommend that women with a family history of breast cancer or who have a history of a breast mass start screening at an earlier age.

Nursing has provided most of the research-based knowledge about the effectiveness of BSE as well as conducted the majority of clinical trials that test BSE methods. The Research Highlight box describes a randomized clinical trial that tested two BSE methods. This clinical trial was conducted by a nurse researcher and a clinical nurse; they collaborated on implementing an important and well-designed study of great relevance to nursing practice as well as to sexual health promotion.

SELF-EXAMINATION OF THE FEMALE GENITALIA

Encouraging women to perform self-examination of the genitalia is an important step in sexual health promotion. By encouraging women to be health experts for themselves, nurses are assisting these patients to become familiar with the normal functioning of their bodies, while promoting early intervention should variance from health be discovered.

CHAPTER HIGHLIGHTS

- This chapter focused on the relationship of gender to health with an emphasis on sexual health promotion and protection.
- The health of men and women must be evaluated from a broad perspective that includes biopsychosocial, cultural, and lifespan dimensions.
- STIs and violence are adversely affecting the health of an increasing number of people, particularly women and children.
- Sexual behaviors and attitudes are formed in the context of family, culture, race, ethnicity, religious, and social-political

values. As a result, sexual behaviors and attitudes are very diverse. The nurse must be able to accept this diversity.
- Acceptance of one's own sexuality is an important first step in being able to help patients with sexual health issues.
- Factors associated with disease and illness such as fatigue, pain, or depression can affect one's sexual health.
- Implementing sexual health promotion and health protection interventions are an important part of the scope of nursing practice.
- Educating individuals, families, and communities to be agents for their own care is another major component of the scope of nursing practice.

REFERENCES

Alexander, L., LaRosa, J. (1994). *New Dimensions in Women's Health.* Boston: Jones & Bartlett.

Allen, D. (1985). Critical social theory: Philosophical and historical dimensions of health. *Proceedings of the Forum on Doctoral Education in Nursing.* Birmingham, AL, June 1985.

Allen, D., Whatley, M. (1986). Nursing and men's health: Some critical considerations. *Nursing Clinics of North America, 21* (1), 3–13.

Alzate, H., Hoch, Z. (1986). The "G spot" and "female ejaculation": A current appraisal. *Journal of Sex and Marital Therapy, 12,* 211–220.

American Cancer Society (1989). Cancer statistics. *CA 39,* 3–20.

American Psychiatric Association (1987). *Diagnostic and Statistical Manual of Mental Disorders,* 3rd ed rev. Washington, DC: Author.

American Psychiatric Association (1994). *Diagnostic and Statistical Manual of Mental Disorders,* 4th ed. Washington, DC: Author.

Amirikia, H., Zarewych, B., Evans, T. (1988). Cesarean section: A 15-year review of changing incidence, indications, and risks. *American Journal of Obstetrics and Gynecology, 140,* 81–90.

Annas, G. (1994). *The Rights of Patients.* Carbondale, IL: Southern Illinois University Press.

Annon, J. (1976). *Behavior Treatment of Sexual Problems.* San Francisco: Harper & Row.

Aral, S., Holmes, K. (1991). Sexually transmitted diseases in the AIDS era. *Scientific American, 264,* 62–29.

Bader, J. (1985) Respite care: Temporary relief for caregivers. *Women and Health 10* (2,3), 39–52.

Barbach, L. (1976). *For Yourself: The Fulfillment of Female Sexuality.* New York: Doubleday.

Barbach, L. (1980). *Women Discover Orgasm.* New York: Free Press.

Barkauskas, V., Stoltenberg-Allen, K., Baumann, L., Darling-Fisher, C. (1994). *Health & Physical Assessment.* St. Louis: Mosby.

Bayne-Smith, M. (1996). *Race, Gender and Health.* Thousand Oaks, CA: Sage.

Belenky, M., Clinchy, B., Rule, N., Tarule, J. (1986). *Women's Ways of Knowing.* New York: Basic Books.

Belle, D. (1990). Poverty and women's health. *American Psychologist, 45,* 385–388.

Belzer, E. (1981). Orgasmic expulsions of women: A review and heuristic inquiry. *Journal of Sex Research, 17,* 1–12.

Benjamin, H. (1966). *The Transsexual Phenomenon.* New York: Julian Press.

Berer, M. (1988). Whatever happened to "a woman's right to choose?" *Feminist Review, 23,* 24–37.

Bernhard, L. (1995). Sexuality in women's lives. In C. Fogel and N. Woods (eds.): *Women's Health Care: A Comprehensive Handbook.* Thousand Oaks, CA: Sage, pp. 475–495.

Bosl, G., Vogelzang, N., Goldman, A. (1981). Impact of delay in diagnosis on clinical stage of testicular cancer. *Lancet, 2,* 970–972.

Boston Women's Health Book Collective (1985). *The New Our Bodies, Ourselves.* New York: Simon & Schuster.

Boston Women's Health Book Collective (1998). Assisted low-tech and high-tech reproductive technologies (Chapter 18). *Our Bodies, Ourselves for the New Century.* New York: Touchstone.

Brannon, R. (1976). The male sex role: Our culture's blueprint of manhood, and what it's done for us lately. In D. David and R. Brannon (eds.): *The Forty-Nine Percent Majority.* Reading, MA: Addison-Wesley, pp. 1–45.

Brash, K. (1990). Toward a model of sexual health for nurses. *Holistic Nursing Practice, 4* (4), 62–69.

Brecher, E. (1984). *Love, Sex, and Aging: A Consumer Union Report.* Boston: Little, Brown & Co.

Brody, E.M. (1985). Parent care as a normative family stress. *The Gerontologist, 25,* 19–29.

Brody, E.M. (1994). Women as unpaid caregivers. In E. Friedman (ed.): *An Unfinished Revolution: Women and Health Care in America.* New York: United Hospital Fund.

Bullough, V. (1975). Transsexualism in history. *Archives of Sexual Behavior, 4,* 561–571.

Burke, L. (1990). Cardiovascular disturbances and sexuality. In C. Fogel and D. Lauver (eds.): *Sexual Health Promotion.* Philadelphia: W.B. Saunders.

Butler, R., Lewis, M., Hoffman, E., Whitehead, E. (1994). Love and sex after 60: How to evaluate and treat the impotent older man. A roundtable discussion. *Geriatrics, 49* (10), 27–32.

Campbell, J. (1989). Women's responses to sexual abuse in intimate relationships. *Health Care for Women International, 8,* 335–347.

Campbell, J., Humphreys, J. (1993). *Nursing Care of Survivors of Family Violence.* St. Louis: C.V. Mosby, p. 157.

Campbell, J., Landenburger, K. (1995). Violence against women. In C. Fogel, and N. Woods (eds.): *Women's Health Care: A Comprehensive Handbook.* Thousand Oaks, CA: Sage, pp. 407–425.

Carlson, K., Eisenstat, S., Ziporyn, T. (1996). *The Harvard Guide to Women's Health.* Cambridge, MA: Harvard University Press, pp. 560–565.

Carrigan, T., Connell, B., Lee, J. (1987). Toward a new sociology of masculinity. In H. Brod (ed.): *The Making of Masculinities—The New Men's Studies.* Boston: Allen and Unwin, pp. 63–100.

Carter, M. (1990). Disturbances in sexuality: Illness, chronic disease, and sexuality. In C. Fogel and D. Lauver (eds.): *Sexual Health Promotion.* Philadelphia: W.B. Saunders, pp. 305–312.

Cates, Jr., W., Alexander, E. (1988). Sexually transmitted diseases and the fetus: A continuing challenge. *Annals of the New York Academy of Sciences, 549,* 1–16.

Cefalo, R., Moos, M-K. (1990). Prenatal screening for hepatitis B virus. *Current Practices, 10* (1), 1–2.

Centers for Disease Control. (1993). 1993 sexually transmitted diseases treatment guidelines. *Morbidity and Mortality Weekly Report: Recommendations and Reports, 42* (RR-14), i–102.

Centers for Disease Control. (1991, April). Pelvic inflammatory disease: Guidelines for prevention and management. *Morbidity and Mortality Weekly Report, 40,* 1–24.

Centers for Disease Control. (1990). *HIV/AIDS surveillance report.* Atlanta, GA: Author.

Chalk, R., King, P. (eds.) (1996). Violence in Families: Assessing Prevention and Treatment Programs. Washington, DC: National Academic Press.

Chester, B., Robin, R., Koss, et al (1994). Grandmother dishonored: Violence against women by male partners in American Indian communities. *Violence and Victims, 9* (3), 249–258.

Christman, N., Kirchoff, K., Oakley, M. (1992). Concrete objective information. In G. Bulechek and J. McCloskey (eds.): Nursing Interventions: Essential Nursing Treatments. Philadelphia: W.B. Saunders.

Cohen, S., Mitchell, E., Olesen, V., et al (1994). From female disease to women's health: New educational paradigms. In Dan, A. (ed.): *Reframing Women's Health: Multidisciplinary Research and Practice.* Thousand Oaks, CA: Sage.

Connell, R. (1987). *Gender and Power.* Stanford, CA: Stanford University Press.

Conrad, P., Kern, R. (1994). *The Sociology of Health and Illness,* 4th ed. New York: St. Martin's.

Cooperstock, R. (1981). A review of women's psychotropic drug use. In E. Howell and M. Ayes (eds.): *Women and Mental Health.* New York: Basic Books, pp. 131–140.

Crooks, R., Baur, K. (1983). *Our Sexuality.* Menlo Park, CA: Benjamin & Cummings.

Dalton, J. (1990). Chronic musculoskeletal symptoms and sexuality. In C. Fogel and D. Lauver (eds.): *Sexual Health Promotion.* Philadelphia: W.B. Saunders.

Darling, C., Davidson, J., Conway-Welch, C. (1990). Female ejaculation: Perceived origins, the Grafenberg spot/area, and sexual responsiveness. *Archives of Sexual Behavior, 19* (1), 29–47.

Davidson, J., Darling, C., Conway-Welch, C. (1989). The role of the Grafenberg spot and female ejaculation in the female orgasmic response: An empirical analysis. *Journal of Sex and Marital Therapy, 15* (2), 102–120.

Davis, A. (1980). Whoever said life begins at 40 was a fink or, those golden years—phooey. *International Journal of Women's Studies, 3,* 583–589.

Davis, K., Rowland, D. (1990). Uninsured and underinsured: Inequalities in health care in the United States. In P.R. Lee and C.L. Estes (eds.): *The Nation's Health,* 3rd ed. Boston: Jones & Bartlett.

DeHoff, J.B., Forrest, K.A. (1984). Men's health. In J.M. Swanson and K.A. Forrest (eds.): *Men's Reproductive Health.* New York: Springer.

DeLorey, C., Wolf, K. (1993). Sexual violence and older women. *AWHONNs Clinical Issues in Perinatal and Women's Health Nursing, 4* (2), 173–179.

Dildy, G., Clark, S., Garife, T., et al (1997). Current status of the multicenter randomized clinical trial of fetal oxygen saturation monitoring in the United States. *European Journal of Obstetrics, Gynecology, and Reproductive Biology, 72 Supplement,* 543–550.

Division of STD/HIV prevention (1991). *Sexually Transmitted Disease Surveillance, 1990* (U.S. Department of Health and Human Services, Public Health Services). Atlanta: Centers for Disease Control.

Doll, R., Peto, R. (1981). Causes of cancer: Quantitative estimates of avoidable risk of cancer in United States today. *Journal of the National Cancer Institute, 66* (6), 1191–1308.

Donin, H. (1949). *To Be a Jew: A Guide to Jewish Observance in Contemporary Life.* New York: Basic Books, Inc.

Doress, P., Siegal, D. (1987). *Ourselves Growing Older.* New York: Simon & Schuster.

Doyal, L. (1995). *What Makes Women Sick?* New Brunswick, NJ: Rutgers University Press.

Faludi, S. (1991). *Backlash: The Undeclared War Against American Women.* New York: Crown.

Fee, E. (1975). Women and health care: A comparison of theories. *International Journal of Health Services, 5* (3), 397–415.

Field, M. (1990). Psychosomatic sexual dysfunction. In C. Fogel and D. Lauver (eds.): *Sexual Health Promotion.* Philadelphia: W.B. Saunders.

Finkelhor, D. (1980). Risk factors in the sexual victimization of children. *Child Abuse and Neglect, 4,* 265–273.

Finney, J., Weist, M., Friman, P. (1995). Evaluation of two health education strategies for testicular self-examination. *Journal of Applied Behavior Analysis, 28* (1), 39–46.

Fitzgerald, L. (1993). Sexual harassment: Violence against women in the workplace. *American Psychologist, 48* (10), 1070–1076.

Fitzgerald, L., Weitzman, L., Gold, Y., Ormerod, M. (1988). Academic harassment: Sex and denial in scholarly garb. *Psychology of Women Quarterly, 12* (4), 329–340.

Fleisher, J., Senie, R., Minkoff, H., Jaccard, J. (1994). Condom use relative to knowledge of sexually transmitted disease prevention, method of birth control, and past or present infection. *Journal of Community Health, 19* (6), 395–407.

Fogel, C. (1990). Sexual health promotion. In C. Fogel and D. Lauver (eds.): *Sexual Health Promotion.* Philadelphia: W.B. Saunders, pp. 1–18.

Fogel, C. (1995). Sexually transmitted diseases. In C. Fogel and N. Woods (eds.): *Women's Health Care: A Comprehensive Handbook.* Thousand Oaks, CA: Sage, pp. 571–609.

Fogel, C., Forker, J., Welch, M. (1990). Sexual health care. In C. Fogel and D. Lauver (eds.): *Sexual Health Promotion.* Philadelphia: W.B. Saunders.

Fogel, C., Lauver, D. (eds.) (1990). *Sexual Health Promotion.* Philadelphia: W.B. Saunders.

Fogel, C., Woods, N. (1995). Midlife women's health. In C. Fogel and N. Woods (eds.): *Women's Health Care: A Com-*

prehensive Handbook. Thousand Oaks, CA: Sage, pp. 79–100.

Forrester, D. (1986). Myths of masculinity: Impact on men's health. *Nursing Clinics of North America, 21* (1), 15–23.

Freeman, H., Blendon, R., Aiken, L., et al (1990). Americans report on their access to health care. In P. Lee and C. Estes (eds.): *The Nation's Health* (3rd ed.), Boston: Jones and Bartlett, pp. 309–319.

Friedman, E. (1994). *The Unfinished Revolution: Women and Health Care in America*. New York: United Hospital Fund.

Gartley, C., Saltmarche, A. (1997). Recent advances in urinary incontinence treatment. *Menopause Management, 6* (2), 17–21.

Gerber Fried, M. (1990). *From Abortion to Reproductive Freedom: Transforming a Movement*. Boston: South End Press.

Gillis, C. Highley, B., Roberts, B., Martinson, I. (eds.) (1989). *Towards a science of family nursing*. Menlo Park, CA: Addison-Wesley.

Go, K. (1992). Recent advances in the treatment of male infertility. *Clinical Issues in Perinatal & Women's Health Nursing, 3* (2), 347–352.

Gordon, D. (1995). Testicular cancer and masculinity. In G. Sabo and D. Gordon (eds.), *Men's Health and Illness*. Thousand Oaks, CA: Sage, pp. 246–266.

Green, C. (1987). What can patient health education coordinators learn from 10 years of compliance research? *Patient Education and Counseling, 10*, 167–174.

Green, J. (1994). *Investigation into discrimination against transgendered people*. San Francisco: SF Human Rights Commission.

Greiner, K., Weigel, J. (1996). Erectile dysfunction. *American Family Physician, 54* (5), 1675–1682.

Griffith-Kenny, J. (ed.) (1986). *Contemporary Women's Health: A Nursing Advocacy Approach*. Menlo Park, CA: Addison-Wesley.

Guinan, M., Hardy, A. (1987). Epidemiology of AIDS in women in the United States. *Journal of the American Medical Association, 257*, 2039–2042.

Hall, J., Stevens, P. (1991). Rigor in feminist research. *Advances in Nursing Science, 13* (3), 16–29.

Hampton, H. (1995). Care of the woman who has been raped. *New England Journal of Medicine, 332* (4), 234–237.

Harrison, J. (1984). Warning: The male sex role may be dangerous to your health. In J. M. Swanson and K.A. Forrest (eds.): *Men's Reproductive Health*. New York: Springer.

Harrison, J., Chin, J., Ficarrotto, T. (1992). In M. Kimmel and M. Messner (eds.): *Men's Lives*, 2nd ed. New York: Macmillan, pp. 271–285.

Hartman, C., Burgess, A., McCormack, A. (1987). Pathways and cycles of runaways: A model for understanding repetitive runaway behavior. *Hospital and Community Psychiatry, 38* (3), 292–299.

Hatcher, R., Trussell, J., Stewart, F., et al (1994). *Contraceptive Technology 1994–1996*, 16th rev. ed. New York: Irvington.

Heiman, J., Grafton-Becker, V. (1989). Orgasmic disorders in women. In S. Leiblum and R. Rosen (eds.): *Principles and Practice of Sex Therapy*, 2nd ed. New York: Guilford, pp. 51–88.

Henderson, B., Benton, B., Jing, J., et al (1979). Risk factors for cancer of the testes in young men. *Cancer, 23*, 598–602.

Institute of Medicine (1989). The basic science foundations of medically assisted conception: An agenda. Washington, D.C.: Institute of Medicine and the Board on Agriculture.

James, C. (1992). The nursing role in assisted reproductive technologies. *Clinical Issues in Perinatal & Women's Health Nursing, 3* (2), 347–352.

Kaczorowski, J., Levitt, C., Hanvey, L., et al (1998). A national survey of use of obstetric procedures and technologies in Canadian hospitals: Routine or based on existing evidence? *Birth, 25*, (1), 11–18.

Kaplan, H. (1979). *Disorders of Sexual Desire*. New York: Simon & Schuster.

Karacan, I., Aslan, C., Williams, R. (1993). Diagnostic evaluation of male impotence: Problems and promises. In W. E. Fann (ed.): *Pharmacology and Treatment of Sexual Disorders*. Jamaica: SP Medical & Scientific Books.

Kolodny, R., Masters, W., Johnson, V. (1979). *Textbook of Sexual Medicine*. Boston: Little, Brown & Co.

Koss, M., Heslet, L. (1992). Somatic consequences of violence against women. *Archives of Family Medicine, 1* (1), 53–59.

Lauver, D., Welch, M. (1990). A biopsychosocial approach to sexuality: Sexual response cycle. In C. Fogel and D. Lauver (eds.): *Sexual Health Promotion*. Philadelphia: W.B. Saunders, pp. 39–52.

Langer, L., Zimmerman, R., Katz, J. (1994). Which is more important to high school students: Preventing pregnancy or preventing AIDS? *Family Planning Perspectives, 26* (4), 154–159.

Lee, P.R., Estes, C.L. (1990): *The Nation's Health*, 3rd ed. Boston: Jones & Bartlett.

Letellier, P. (1994). Gay and bisexual male domestic violence victimization: Challenges to feminist theory and responses to violence. *Violence and Victims, 9* (2), 95–106.

Lewis, J., Bernstein, J. (1996). *Women's Health: A Relational Perspective Across the Life Cycle*. Boston: Jones & Bartlett.

Lichtman, R., Duran, P. (1990). Sexually transmitted diseases. In R. Lichtman and S. Papera (eds.): *Gynecology Well-Woman Care*. Norwalk, CT: Appleton-Lange, pp. 203–248.

Lipkin, G., Cohen, R. (1992). *Effective Approaches to Patients' Behavior*. New York: Springer.

Lloyd, S. (1991). The dark side of courtship: Violence and sexual exploitation. *Family Relations, 40* (1), 14–20.

Marx, M.D., Preston, A. Spira, M. (1996). Progesterone implants enhance SIV vaginal transmission and early viral load. *Nature Medicine, 2* (10), 1084–1088.

Masters, W. (1987). Sexuality in perspective. *Trans Stud Coll Phys Philadelphia, 9, 45–57.*

Masters, W., Johnson, V. (1966). *Human Sexual Response*. Boston: Little, Brown & Co.

Masters, W., Johnson, V. (1970). *Human Sexual Inadequacy*. Boston: Little, Brown & Co.

Matthews, K. (1989). Interactive effects of behavior and reproductive hormones on sex differences in risk for coronary heart disease. *Health Psychology, 8* (4), 373–387.

McBride, A. (1986). Women's health: Where nursing and feminism converge. In J. Griffith-Kenney (ed.): *Contemporary Women's Health: A Nursing Advocacy Approach*. Menlo Park, CA: Addison-Wesley, pp. 3–10.

McBride, A., McBride, W. (1981). Theoretical underpinnings for women's health. *Women & Health, 6* (1–2), 37–55.

McBride, A. (1993). From gynecology to GYN-ecology: Developing a practice-research agenda for women's health. *Health Care for Women International, 14,* 315–325.

McGregor, J.A., French, J.I., Spencer, N.E. (1988). Prevention of sexually-transmitted diseases in women. *Journal of Reproductive Medicine, 31* (1 suppl.), 109–118.

Meadus, R. (1995). Testicular self-examination (TSE). *Canadian Nurse, 91* (8), 41–44.

Meleis, A. (1990). Being and becoming healthy: The core of nursing knowledge. *Nursing Science Quarterly, 3* (3), 107–114.

Michaels, R. (1995). *Sex in America.* Boston: Little-Brown.

Misener, T., Fuller, S. (1995). Testicular versus breast and colorectal cancer screening: Early detection practices of primary care physicians. *Cancer Practice, 3* (5), 310–316.

Money, J. (1955). An examination of some basic sexual concepts: The evidence of human hermaphroditism. *Bulletin of Johns Hopkins Hospital, 97,* 301–319.

Mosher, W. (1988). Fertility and family planning in the United States. *Family Planning perspectives, 20,* 207–217.

Murali, M., Crabtree, K. (1992). Comparison of two breast self-examination palpation techniques. *Cancer Nursing, 15* (4), 276– 282.

National Center for Health Statistics (1988). *Vital Statistics: Life Tables,* Vol. 11, Section 6. U.S. Department of Health and Human Services Publication No. 8811–47. Hyattsville, MD.

National Center for Health Statistics (1993). *Current Estimates from the National Health Interview Survey, 1992* (Series 10). Hyattsville, MD: U.S. Department of Health and Human Services.

National Research Council (1996). Understanding violence against women. *Report of the Panel on Research on Violence Against Women.* N.A. Crowell and A. Burgess (eds.). Washington, DC: National Academy Press.

Neel, J. (1990). Toward an explanation of the human sex ratio. In M. Ory and H. Warner (eds.): *Gender, Health, and Longevity: Multidisciplinary Perspectives.* New York: Springer, pp. 57–72.

Northrup, C. (1994). *Women's Bodies, Women's Wisdom.* New York: Bantam Books.

O'Brien, T., Shaffer, N., Jaffe, N. (1992). Acquisition and transmission of HIV. In M. Sande and P. Volberding (eds.): *The Medical Management of AIDS,* 3rd ed. Philadelphia: W.B. Saunders, pp. 3–17.

Olesen, V., Taylor, D., Rurek, S., Clarke, A. (1997). Strengths and strongholds in women's health research. In S. Ruzek, V. Olesen, and A. Clark (eds.): *Women's Health: Complexities and Differences.* Columbus, OH: Ohio State University Press, pp. 580–606.

Padian, N., Shibaski, S., Jewell, N. (1991). Female-to-male transmission of human immunodeficiency virus. *Journal of the American Medical Association, 266* (12), 1664–1667.

Paula, T., Lagana, K., Gonzalez-Ramirez, L. (1996). Mexican Americans. In J. Lipson, S. Dibble, P. Minarik (eds.): *Culture & Nursing Care: A Pocket Guide.* San Francisco: UCSF Nursing Press, pp. 203–221.

Pender, N. (1982; 1987). *Health Promotion in Nursing Practice.* Norwalk, CT: Appleton-Century-Crofts.

Petras, J. (1978). *The Social Meaning of Human Sexuality.* Newton, MA: Allyn & Bacon.

Pfizer (1998). Viagra (Sildenafile citrate) prescribing information. New York: Pfizer US Pharmaceuticals.

Planned Parenthood Alameda/San Francisco (1991). *Table Manners: A Guide to the Pelvic Examination for Disabled Women and Health Care Providers,* 3rd printing. San Francisco, CA: Susan Ferreyra & Katrine Hughes.

Pudney, J., Oneta, M., Mayer, K., et al (1992). Pre-ejaculatory fluid as potential vector for sexual transmission of HIV-1. *Lancet, 340* (8833), 1470.

Redman, B., Thomas, S. (1992). Patient teaching. In G. Bulechek and J. McCloskey (eds.): *Nursing Interventions: Essential Nursing Treatments.* Philadelphia: W.B. Saunders, pp. 140–150.

Redman, B. (1988). *The process of Patient Education.* St. Louis: C.V. Mosby.

Reisner, G. (1993). Impotence. *Australian Family Physician, 22* (8), 1393–1397.

Reno, D. (1988). Men's knowledge and health beliefs about testicular cancer and testicular self-examination. *Cancer Nursing, 11* (2), 112–117.

Risen, C. (1995). A guide to taking a sexual history. *The Psychiatric Clinics of North America, 18* (1), pp. 39–53.

Rodin, J., Ickovics, J. (1990). Review and research agenda as we approach the 21st century. *American Psychologist, 45* (9), 1018–1034.

Ross, C., Bird, C. (1994). Sex stratification and health lifestyle: Consequences for men's and women's perceived health. *Journal of Health and Social Behavior, 35* (2), 161–178.

Rurek, V. Olesen, and A. Clarke (eds): *Women's Health: Complexities and Differences.* Columbus: Ohio State University Press.

Rynerson, B. (1990). Sexuality throughout the life cycle. In C. Fogel and D. Lauver (eds.): *Sexual Health Promotion.* Philadelphia: W.B. Saunders, pp. 53–86.

Sabo, D., Gordon, D. (eds.) (1995). *Men's Health and Illness: Gender, Power, and the Body.* Thousand Oaks, CA: Sage.

Sabo, G., Gordon, D. (1995). Rethinking men's health and illness. In G. Sabo and D. Gordon (eds.): *Men's Health & Illness.* Thousand Oaks, CA: Sage, pp. 246–266.

Sackett, C. (1990). Spinal cord conditions and sexuality. In C. Fogel and D. Lauver (eds.): *Sexual Health Promotion.* Philadelphia: W.B. Saunders.

Saltonstall, R. (1993). Healthy bodies, social bodies: Men's and women's concepts and practices of health in everyday life. *Social Science and Medicine, 36* (1), 7–14.

Shaffer, E. (1995). Managed care: Your money or your life. *The National Women's Health Network News, 20,*(4), 1–5.

Shaver, J. (1985). A biopsychosocial view of health. *Nursing Outlook, 33* (4), 186–191.

Shippee-Rice, R. (1990). Sexuality and aging. In C. Fogel and D. Lauver (eds.): *Sexual Health Promotion.* Philadelphia: W.B. Saunders, pp. 97–116.

Smith, L. (1990). Human sexuality from a cultural perspective. In C. Fogel and D. Lauver (eds.): *Sexual Health Promotion.* Philadelphia: W.B. Saunders, pp. 87–96.

Smith, L., Lauver, D., Gray, P. (1990). Sexually transmitted diseases. In C. Fogel and D. Lauver (eds.): *Sexual Health Promotion.* Philadelphia: W.B. Saunders, pp. 459–484.

Society for Assisted Reproductive Technology (1996). Assisted reproductive technology in the United States and Canada: 1994 results generated from the ASRM/SART Registry. *Fertility & Sterility, 66*(5), 697–705.

Sparks, C., Bar On, B. (1981). *A Social Change Approach to the Prevention of Sexual Violence Toward Women.* Columbus, OH: Intrepid Clearinghouse.

Spratlen, L. (1988). Sexual harassment counseling. *Journal of Psychosocial Nursing, 26* (2), 28–33.

Stark, E. (1981). Wife abuse in the medical setting. *National Clearinghouse on Domestic Violence (No. 7)*. Washington, DC: NIMH.

Staples, R. (1995). Health among African American males. In D. Sabo and D. Gordon (eds.) *Men's Health and Illness.* Thousand Oaks, CA: Sage, p. 121.

Starn, J., Paperny, D. (1990). Computer games to enhance adolescent sex education. *Maternal-Child Nursing, 15,* 250–253.

Starr, B., Weiner, M. (1982). *Sex and Sexuality in the Mature Years.* Briarcliff Manor: Stein & Day.

Stein, Z. (1990). HIV prevention: The need for methods women can use. *American Journal of Public Health, 80,* 460–462.

Stevens, P., Hall, J. (1988). Stigma, health beliefs and experiences with health care in lesbian women. *Image: Journal of Nursing Scholarship, 20* (2), 69–73.

Stockdale-Wooley, R. (1990). Respiratory disturbances and sexuality. In C. Fogel and D. Lauver (eds.): *Sexual Health Promotion.* Philadelphia: Saunders.

Stone, K., Grimes, D., Magder, L. (1986). Primary prevention of sexually transmitted diseases. *Journal of the American Medical Association, 255* (13), 1763–1766.

Stuart, F., Hammond, D., Pett, M. (1987). Inhibited sexual desire in women. *Archives of Sexual Behavior, 16* (2), 23–33.

Taylor, D., Woods, N. (1991). *Menstruation, Health and Illness.* Washington, DC: Taylor & Francis.

Taylor, D., Woods, N. (1996). Changing women's health, changing nursing practice. *Journal of Obstetrical, Gynecological & Neonatal Nursing Clinical Issues, 25* (9).

Taylor, I, Robertson, A. (1994). The health needs of gay men: A discussion of the literature and implications for nursing. *Journal of Advanced Nursing, 20* (3), 560–566.

Tewkesbury, R. (1995). Sexual adaptations among gay men with HIV. In D. Sabo and D. Gordon (eds.): *Men's Health & Illness: Gender, Power and the Body.* Thousand Oaks, CA: Sage.

UNAIDS (1996). The HIV/AIDS situation in mid-1996: Global and regional highlights. *Joint United Nations Programme on HIV/AIDS, Fact Sheet: July 1, 1996* (pp. 2–3). Geneva, Switzerland: United Nations.

U.S. Department of Health and Human Services (DHHS), Public Health Service (PHS), Centers for Disease Control and Prevention (CDC) (1995). HIV/AIDS surveillance Report. *U.S. HIV and AIDS Cases Reported Through December 1995, Year-End Edition, 7* (2), 5–21.

U.S. Department of Public Health (1992). *Healthy People 2000: National Health Promotion and Disease Prevention Objectives.* Boston: Jones & Bartlett.

U.S. Preventive Services Task Force (1989). Counseling to prevent human immunodeficiency virus infection and other sexually transmitted diseases. In *Guide to Clinical Preventive Services: An Assessment of the Effectiveness of 169 Interventions. Report of the U.S. Preventive Services Task Force.* Baltimore: William & Wilkins, pp. 331–339.

Valverde, M. (1985). *Sex, Power & Pleasure.* Toronto, Canada: Women's Press.

Verbrugge, L., Wingard, D. (1987). Sex differentials in health and mortality. *Women and Health, 12* (2), 103–145.

Walker, P., Berger, J., Green, R., et al (1985). Standards of care: The hormonal and surgical sex reassignment of gender dysphoric persons. *Archives of Sexual Behavior, 14,* 79–90.

Webster, D., Lipetz, M. (1986). Changing definitions; changing times. *Nursing Clinics of North America, 21* (1), 89–97.

Wheeler, L. (1995). In C. Fogel and N. Woods (eds.): *Women's Health Care: A Comprehensive Handbook.* Thousand Oaks, CA: Sage, pp. 141–187.

White, G. (1992). Understanding the ethical issues in infertility nursing practice. *Clinical Issues in Perinatal & Women's Health Nursing, 3*(2), 347–352.

Williams, D. (1989). Political theory and individualistic health promotion. *Advances in Nursing Science, 12* (1), 14–25.

Wingard, D. (1982). The sex differential in mortality rates: Demographic and behavioral factors. *American Journal of Epidemiology, 115* (2), 205–216.

Woods, N. (1984). *Human Sexuality in Health and Illness, 3rd ed.* St. Louis: C.V. Mosby.

Woods, N. (1988). Women's health. In J.J. Fitzpatrick, R.L. Taunton, and J.Q. Benoliel (eds.): *Annual Review of Nursing Research, vol. 6.* New York: Springer.

Woods, N. (1995). Women and their health. In C. Fogel and N. Woods (eds.): *Women's Health Care.* Thousand Oaks, CA: Sage, pp. 1–22.

Woods, N., Lentz, M., Mitchell, E. (1993). The new woman: Health-promoting and health-damaging behaviors. *Health Care for Women International, 14* (5), 389–405.

World Health Organization (1975). *Education and Treatment in Human Sexuality: The Training of Health Professionals* (Report of a WHO Meeting, Technical Report Series, No. 572).

Wright, L., Leahey, M. (1984). *Nurses and Families: A Guide to Family Assessment and Intervention.* Philadelphia: F.A. Davis.

Wright, L., Watson, W., Bell, J. (1990). The family nursing unit: A unique integration of research, education and clinical practice. In J. Bell, W. Watson, and L. Wright (eds.): *The Cutting Edge of Family Nursing.* Calgary, Alberta: Family Nursing Unit Publications.

Yapko, M. (1992). *Free Yourself from Depression.* Emmaus, PA: Rodale Press.

34 Grief

Margaret S. Miles

OBJECTIVES

After studying this chapter, students will be able to:

- **understand the theoretical and conceptual models about grief from the social sciences and nursing literature**
- **summarize important research related to grief**
- **understand grief responses of individuals when death occurs in a family**
- **evaluate factors that influence an individual's response to death**
- **appreciate the importance of the health care team's response to bereaved families in helping them cope with the death**
- **identify specific ways in which nurses can intervene to help bereaved individuals and families in a variety of settings**

Death of a family member is an event that few individuals can avoid. Such losses can occur when one is a young child, as when a grandparent dies or a mother has a stillbirth, through old age, when the deaths of friends and family members become almost commonplace. It has been estimated that every year about 8 million Americans experience the death of an immediate family member (Osterweis et al, 1984). Grief or bereavement, which involves emotional, behavioral, cognitive, and physical responses, is the normal reaction to the difficult and stressful experience of losing someone close to us. Some consider grief a universal response because similar ways of responding to death have been reported in a wide variety of cultures, despite the fact that cultures often vary widely in their rituals surrounding grieving and burial (Miles and Demi, 1994; Osterweis et al, 1984).

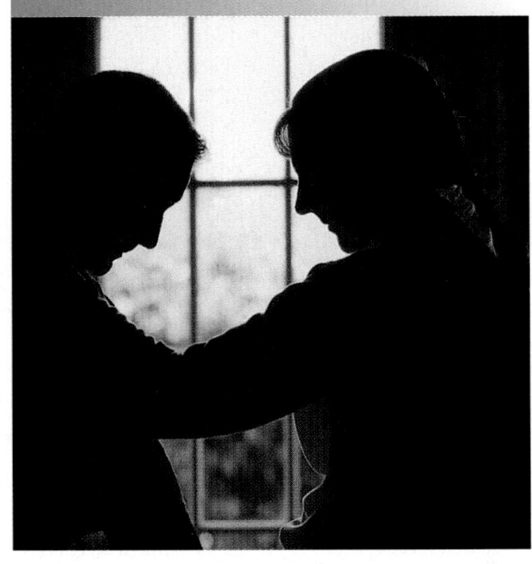

The writings of clinicians working with the bereaved and scholars studying the bereaved or conceptualizing about the grief process can sensitize us as to what it is like for an individual or family when a loved one dies. This body of knowledge can also help us as health care professionals to respond more appropriately, sensitively, and therapeutically to help the bereaved.

This chapter provides background information to help nurses understand how family members who are grieving may respond and provides the basis for nursing interventions to help them. The case presentation, using the death of an infant as the event, focuses on how various family members respond and are helped to cope with this tragic and unexpected death.

Mary Jonathan, a 25-year-old nurse, has just arrived for the morning shift in the emergency room of a small community hospital when she is alerted to the imminent arrival of an emergency involving a 4-month-old infant. Johnny was found in his crib blue and not breathing by his mother. While his father started CPR, his mother telephoned 911. The emergency rescue team that arrived continued resuscitation.

Mary is assigned to work with Johnny's parents, while her colleague, Steve, is assigned to work with the resuscitation team. Mr. and Mrs. Smithers arrive minutes behind the ambulance and are distraught, immediately asking about their baby. Knowing the situation is grim, Mary finds a private room for the parents to wait. She informs them about the efforts of the physicians, nurses, and others to try to help their baby and asks them about whom she might call to be with them. They ask for the maternal grandmother, a widow, and their minister.

After the phone calls are sensitively and carefully made, Mary again checks with the physician in charge of the code and learns that the baby is likely not going to survive. With his permission, she tells the parents what the team is continuing to try to do to help the baby, but she also forewarns them of the fact that he may not be saved. Mrs. Smithers sobs loudly and clings to her husband; Mr. Smithers remains rather stoic and grim. The nurse stays with the parents when the physician arrives and informs them that Johnny is dead. He explains that Johnny may have died of sudden infant death syndrome (SIDS), discusses the fact that we don't really know what causes SIDS, and explains to the parents the need to do an autopsy to make sure.

When the doctor leaves the room, Mary facilitates their grief response further by accepting their crying, encouraging them to share their feelings with her and with each other, and listening as they tell her about their infant son and what he meant to them. Since Mrs. Smithers does most of the crying and talking, Mary quietly turns to the father and says, "I know fathers hurt a lot too, but think they have to feel strong for the mother. How are you doing?" The father looks at his wife and then begins to sob.

Mrs. Black, the maternal grandmother, arrives and Mary tells her about the infant's problems and death. Mrs. Black becomes very distraught and sobs hysterically. Eventually, she reveals to Mary and the parents that she herself had lost a baby to what was then called "crib death" before the birth of Mrs. Smithers; she had never before told her daughter about this death. Mary helps Mrs. Black and Mrs. Smithers support each other in their mutual losses.

Mary then asks the parents and grandmother whether they want to see Johnny. The mother immediately responds affirmatively, but the father and the grandmother are more hesitant. She encourages them to each do what makes them individually feel comfortable. In the end, both parents decide to see Johnny. The sobbing mother picks him up, rocks him, and sings to him. The father, more hesitant, stands nearby. The grandmother remains in the waiting room to get her composure. Mary asks the parents if they prefer for her to leave but they ask that she stay with them during the 20-minute visit. When they put Johnny down, both parents appear calmer. The grandmother then asks if Mary would accompany her alone to see the baby. When she sees him, she sobs and tells Mary in more detail about the death of her own son over 20 years earlier.

Mary then problem solves with the parents about how to help their 3-year-old daughter, whom they left with a neighbor when the ambulance arrived. The nurse provides them information about what 3-year-olds understand about death, about how a preschooler might behave when grieving, and about the importance of including her in some of the family funeral rituals. In addition, she prepares them for some difficult decisions they will have to make about burial and funeral arrangements for their only son. When their minister arrives, she leaves them alone together for an appropriate time.

Before the parents leave, Mary gives them Johnny's clothes and blanket and a foot and hand print of their son. Mrs. Smithers expresses feelings of self-blame that she didn't get up earlier in the morning to check on her son when he didn't wake her as usual. She says she feels she could have found him struggling and saved him. Mary further explains SIDS to the parents, especially emphasizing the fact that we don't know what causes SIDS and that there is likely nothing they did or didn't do to cause the death. Mary also briefly discusses the pain and grief parents and all family members often experience for months following the death, and she gives them a pamphlet about grief and SIDS. Finally, Mary tells the parents about the SIDS parent support group and the state SIDS counseling program, alerting them to the fact that the nurses from this program will be contacting them soon. Being sensitive to how difficult leaving the hospital without their son can be, Mary accompanies them to their car. She cautions the father that he is in a state of shock and distress and that driving carefully is important. When they are gone, Mary contacts the SIDS counseling program about the death and talks to the public health nurse, Joan Hurst, who will be visiting the parents in their home.

SCOPE OF NURSING PRACTICE

The American Nurses' Association has defined nursing as the diagnosis and treatment of human responses to health problems (1980). The responses of family members and others to the death of a loved one is one of the most profound human responses nurses encounter, and nurses have traditionally reached out in various ways to help these grieving individuals and families. Helping the bereaved also fits with Henderson's view of nursing by helping individuals in their recovery from the death of a family member or friend and by facilitating healthy responses to the stresses experienced during bereavement.

Nurses work in a wide variety of settings where death occurs, either commonly or uncommonly. In some settings, such as the oncology unit, death is encountered frequently and nurses are called upon regularly to help families. A new and growing area where nurses work with dying patients and their families is home health and hospice programs. Nurses in these settings develop unique skills in approaching these grieving families. In other settings, such as the emergency room or critical care unit, where the emphasis is on saving lives, staff can view death as a failure of their abilities and may have a more difficult time in helping families. Settings such as the maternity unit are set up to rejoice in the joy of a new life; death of an infant in such a setting can be difficult for everyone involved. Nurses who work in tertiary care pediatric units also find themselves working with dying children and their grieving parents, siblings and other family members. Since death of a child is so difficult in our society, pediatric nurses have an important role in helping families at a very vulnerable period in their lives.

Nurses in all settings have a particularly important role in helping the bereaved and can make a difference. Whatever the type of loss, the responses of nurses and other health care providers, police, and emergency medical personnel toward the family are very important in their immediate and subsequent reaction. Jost and Haase (1989) interviewed bereaved parents and found that most parents indicated their experiences with health care providers at the time of death affected their grieving later—for some it positively helped them and for others negative experiences complicated their grief. Studies have identified a positive impact when nurses and other health care professionals provided follow-up contacts with bereaved families through telephone calls, home visits, groups, and return appointments to the health facility (Cohen et al, 1978; Mahon et al, 1981). A number of studies also have shown positive effects of self-help and professionally run groups for the bereaved (Murphy, 1991; Murphy et al, 1989; Vachon et al, 1980; Videka-Sherman, 1982).

Thus, individual nurses can provide sensitive and caring interventions to family members that help them cope with death and with their grief in the months following death. Nurses in institutions develop protocols that provide clear direction to all staff in how to help family members through this difficult process. Nurses have also been instrumental in starting bereavement programs within an institution or community that provide special services and follow-up to families who are grieving.

KNOWLEDGE BASE

Relevant Theory: Current Conceptualizations about Grief

Our current views about grief have been influenced by Freud's psychoanalytic writings about mourning (1915/1957). Based on his clinical work with individuals and his own losses, Freud continually struggled over his lifetime to understand mourning. He viewed grief, also referred to as mourning, as a normal reaction to the loss of a loved person, or an abstraction that has taken the place of a loved person. Mourning was considered to involve painful dejection, cessation of interest in the outside world, loss of capacity to love, inhibition of activity, and feelings of being punished. Resolution is accomplished through the slow process of reality testing in which the loss of the individual is verified and there is a gradual breaking of ties to the deceased. In a letter 9 years after the death of his daughter and 6 years after the death of her youngest son, his favorite grandson, Freud (1929/1960) poignantly discusses the long-term impact of grief from a personal perspective:

> although we know that after such a loss the acute state of mourning will subside, we also know we shall remain inconsolable and will never find a substitute. No matter what may fill the gap, even if it be filled completely, it nevertheless remains something else and actually this is how it should be. It is the only way of perpetuating that love which we do not want to relinquish.

Lindemann (1944), in his seminal paper, "Symptomatology and Management of Acute Grief," poignantly described the symptomatology of normal grief. His paper was based on psychiatric interviews with relatives of those who died in the Coconut Grove fire disaster, as well as psychoneurotic patients, relatives of deceased hospitalized patients, and relatives of servicemen who died in World War II. He described acute grief as a syndrome with both psychological and somatic symptomatology and identified five striking features of grief: somatic distress, preoccupation with thoughts of the deceased, guilt, hostility, and loss of usual patterns of behavior. The duration of normal grief is dependent on the success of the "grief work," which he described as the emancipation from the bondage to the deceased, readjustment to the environment in which the deceased is missing, and formation of new relationships. Based on his work with women whose husbands were involved in the war, Lindemann also proposed the concept of "anticipatory grief," experienced in anticipation of a loss. Lindemann's paper continues to be the most widely quoted paper on grief.

Caplan (1964), in the development of "crisis theory," proposed that grief, as well as other life events, could trigger a crisis that is generally resolved in 4 to 6 weeks. To Caplan, a crisis is a turning point for an individual and may lead to either improved or worsened health. During a crisis, the individual has a heightened desire for help and is more susceptible to the influence of others. The outcome of a crisis is determined by the balance of stressors and resources. Caplan's crisis theory, along with Lindemann's paper, erroneously gave the impression that the grief response was short-lived. However, Caplan subsequently revised his concept of grief as a single crisis to a series of crises called "life transitions," which are resolved over a much longer period of time.

Parkes, who is noted for his ongoing research and theory development in the area of widowhood, also viewed grief as a major life transition—a period of challenge and readjustment (Parkes, 1972; Parkes and Weiss, 1983). Parkes described grief as "a complex time-consuming process in which a person gradually changes his view of the world and the places and habits by means of which he orients and relates to it" (Parkes, 1970, p. 465). Grief involves a process of realization—making psychologically real an event that is not desirable and for which one does not have adequate coping (Parkes, 1972). He also described the painful emotional, behavioral, and physical manifestations of grief. This included "pangs of grief"—acute episodes of severe anxiety and psychological pain in which the lost person is strongly missed and "pining"—a persistent and obtrusive wish for the person who is gone, along with preoccupation with thoughts of the deceased. Other responses include separation anxiety, anger, guilt, depression, aimlessness, sleep disturbances, aches and pains, loss of energy, and appetite changes (Glick et al, 1974; Parkes, 1970, 1972). Parkes (1970) suggested there were several phases in the grief process: numbness, yearning and protest, disorganization, and reorganization.

Parkes and his colleagues also suggested, based on their research, that many factors influenced one's response to grief. These included past childhood experiences, personality, religious beliefs, the relationship with the deceased, the mode of death, lack of forewarning of the death, other life crises, age, socioeconomic status, and level of social support (Glick et al, 1974; Parkes, 1972; Parkes and Weiss, 1983). The collective work of Parkes and his colleagues has been extremely important in describing the manifestations of grief and in identifying risk factors related to selected mental and physical health outcomes.

During the 1960s and 1970s, Bowlby (1960, 1961) also made major contributions to the conceptualization of loss and grief through his studies on attachment. He proposed that attachment is a protective biologic mechanism that ensures the survival of the individual and the species. His astute observations of infants and young children separated from their mothers led Bowlby to identify the "separation response syndrome," in which separation from a significant other evokes behavior patterns that function to restore the lost mother. The separation response syndrome entails three phases: protest, despair, and detachment (Bowlby, 1960). Bowlby's work was important in providing insight into the experiences of attachment and loss in children and was influential in the development of programs and policies related to child care, hospitalization, and interventions with children experiencing short- and long-term losses.

Based on Freud's observation of reminiscence and compulsive repetition following a traumatic event, Horowitz considers the response to death as a general stress response syndrome (Horowitz, 1982). He suggests that a major loss requires a change in one's inner psychic models that occurs over time. During this process, painful emotional responses such as vulnerability, rage, guilt, and sadness are experienced. Because these emotional states are powerful, controls are activated to prevent unendurable anguish or "flooding." Thus, grief involves an outcry stage that is replaced by a vacillation between "denial or numbing," in which reality is avoided and blocked, and "intrusion," in which the reality is faced. As the reality and schemata are integrated, the stress response syndrome is resolved. Horowitz's model is closely related to the Diagnostic and Statistical Manual of Mental Disorders (DSM)-III diagnosis of posttraumatic stress disorders.

Worden (1982) has proposed a scheme for understanding the grief process that builds on the work of many other theorists and researchers and on his own research. Worden proposes that three "tasks of mourning" must be completed in order to resolve grief. Task I is to accept the reality of loss. Task II is to experience the pain of grief. Task III is to adjust to an environment in which the deceased is missing. Worden proposes that grieving individuals need to take action, and that grief resolution can be influenced by intervention. In addition, he also details complicated grief responses, and identifies key determinants influencing grief outcomes such as the role of the deceased, the nature of the attachment, the type of death, historical factors, personality, and social variables.

Several nurses have proposed conceptual models of grief. Demi's model (1989) builds on the work of Parkes, Caplan, and others and synthesizes grief, life transition, and stress and coping theories. Demi suggests that the bereaved experience crisis periods during bereavement, comparable to Parkes' stages of numbness and yearning, disorganization, and reorganization. The outcome of each crisis is a potential turning point that may lead to positive outcomes or to poor outcomes such as diminished health and psychosocial deterioration. Adaptation is influenced by the balance of interpersonal and sociocultural stressors and resources and individual developmental stage.

Dimond (1981), based on work with elderly widows and widowers, also proposes that adjustment to the loss of a spouse is a psychosocial transition rather than an acute crisis. She postulates that the adaptation of elderly widows and widowers depends upon the interaction of three critical factors—the adequacy of the support network, the number of other losses, and one's coping skills. Rigdon and coworkers (1987) theorized that elderly bereaved individuals have a primary responsibility to help themselves to a "new life," but also must invite others to help them to get there.

Walker and colleagues (1977) in their studies of widows and widowers also apply the concept of support networks to the crisis of bereavement. They suggest that distress is caused by a lack of fit between social and psychological needs of the individual and the individual's social network.

Miles (1984) has proposed a conceptual model, based largely on the work of Parkes, for understanding parental grief. The model describes the responses experienced by bereaved parents during three overlapping phases of grief—acute distress and shock, intense grief, and reorganization. During the phase of intense grief, parents experience deep loneliness and emptiness; feelings of helplessness that can lead to guilt, fear, and anger; depression and disorganization; cognitive changes; and physical symptoms. Miles suggests that the "search for meaning" is critical in the resolution of grief and can lead to positive outcomes, despite the tragedy and related stressors (Miles and Crandall, 1983). In addition, Miles, along with her colleague Demi, has proposed a conceptual model of parental bereavement guilt (Miles, 1984; Miles and Demi, 1983–84, 1986). They identify the process through which guilt feelings are developed in bereaved parents, identify factors that may impact on guilt responses, and propose a topology of guilt feelings. Miles' conceptualizations about parental grief were developed from observations grounded in clinical practice and were the basis of a publication used for over a decade by Compassionate Friends to help bereaved parents understand and cope with their grief (Miles, 1980).

The Grief Process

This review of some of the commonly used theories and conceptual models about grief and selected research demonstrates a number of consistent views about grief. Grief can be described as the emotional, cognitive, behavioral, and physical responses experienced by individuals coping with the death of someone with whom they had a close relationship, generally a relative or close friend (Osterweis et al, 1984).

Many authors believe there are overlapping phases in the grief process but most do not believe that grief is experienced in "stages." There is an early period of acute distress and shock including numbness, disbelief, and behavioral responses such as crying, wailing, and acting out. This numbness is thought to be protective for the bereaved, allowing them time to face the reality of the loss. However, as time passes and the bereaved is faced with living life daily without the individual who died, the intensity of the grief response often escalates. This often occurs at a time when family and friends are not longer available to support and listen to the griever.

Commonly, the manifestations of grief during this phase of intense grief have been identified to include emotional, cognitive, behavioral, and physical responses. Emotional responses include loneliness and emptiness; guilt feelings; fear and anxiety; anger, hostility, and irritability; and despair and depression. Cognitive responses include an inability to concentrate and confused thinking. Behavioral changes can include disorganization and impaired problem solving. An increased use of alcohol and drugs may be a problematic behavioral change for some bereaved individuals who are not coping well. Physical responses can include somatic symptoms such as headaches or backaches or can involve the development of a health problem such as hypertension.

The phase of reorganization is reached when the individual returns to his or her usual level of functioning in society and has more good than bad days. However, this does not mean that the pain associated with the death is gone. The pain is generally as intense as earlier in the grief process; it is just not experienced as often and the "pangs of grief" don't last as long. There are suggestions that many bereaved individuals search for a meaning in their loss during the phase of reorganization and may grow in many ways as a result of this search and the experience of having survived the death of a loved one.

The duration of grief varies with the individual, but there is now a general agreement that the experiences associated with grief involve a long-term process and can extend for months and years. With a very close relationship such as death of one's child, some aspects of grief never truly end. Although there is widespread agreement on the normalcy of many grief manifestations, there is little agreement about what constitutes complicated or abnormal grief (Demi and Miles, 1987; Worden, 1982).

Relevant Research

The body of research literature focused on grief and the bereaved is extensive, with the researchers coming from many disciplines—sociology, psychiatry, nursing, psychology, social work, and counseling. A number of nurse researchers and/or nursing research teams have done ongoing programs of research with bereaved individuals and families. A brief summary of their work related to bereavement follows. A previous review of this literature was completed in 1986 by Demi and Miles.

Ida Martinson, a pioneer in the development and evaluation of programs aimed at helping families take their dying children home to die, has followed these families for more than a decade following the child's death. A number of studies by Martinson and her colleagues have focused on the response of these families following the death (Davies et al, 1986; Martinson and Campos, 1991; Martinson et al, 1987a, 1987b, 1991; McClowry et al, 1987; Moore et al, 1988). Bereaved parents continued to experience psychological and somatic symptoms 2 years after the death of their child. Seven to nine years later, many parents and siblings still reported pain and loss and reported that an "empty space" continued to exist within the family. Long-term follow-up of siblings revealed that many siblings perceived that they matured and grew as a result of the loss, but for some the death of their brother or sister had a continuing negative impact on their lives.

Lauer and her colleagues, building on the work of Martinson, also developed a home care program for dying children using a nursing model (Lauer and Camitta, 1980; Lauer et al, 1983, 1985, 1989; Mulhern et al, 1983). They compared the adjustment of families whose children died at home and in the hospital. In general, they found that families who took their children home to die had satisfactory adjustments to the death. Siblings, in particular, adjusted better in these families because they felt included in the terminal illness and death. It must be pointed out, however, that the families who chose to take their child home to die were likely different prior to the death from the families who did not make this difficult choice.

Hogan has studied adolescent reactions to sibling death (Hogan and Balk, 1990; Hogan and Desantis, 1992; Hogan and Greenfield, 1991). In interviews with these youth, she identified an "ongoing attachment" as a persistent theme. Like

RESEARCH HIGHLIGHT
SUPPORTIVE INTERVENTIONS FOR PARENTS OF CHILDREN WHO DIED IN ACCIDENTS

The purpose of this nursing study was to develop and test a two-dimensional supportive intervention for parents of children who died in accidents.

The intervention involved informational and emotional support provided to parents in 90-minute group sessions for 6 weeks. One question this study posed was whether the intervention would be more effective in the early months following grief or later. Thus, there was an early transition group (2 to 6 months after death) and a later transition group (7 to 13 months after death).

Most parents found both aspects of the intervention equally useful. However, the early transition group focused more on their deceased child and liked the content focused on managing their emotional responses to the loss and related role changes. The later transition group focused more on coping and memories of their child as well as communication problems with other family members; they liked the content that focused on cognitive changes, and dealing with the future.

Findings indicate the helpfulness to parents of attending a semi-structured bereavement support group following sudden accidental death of a child. The findings support the notion that time since death influences the needs of parents and hence the intervention themes. Both groups indicated the need for more sessions, suggesting that support group interventions for bereaved parents are needed over a longer period of time.

Implications for Nursing Practice This study was important in delineating more clearly the supportive needs of the bereaved following sudden accidental death. The study developed and tested sound principles of intervention that could be used in guiding others who develop such bereavement support groups.

Abstracted from Murphy, S.A., Aroian, K., Baugher, R. (1989). A theory-based preventive intervention program for bereaved parents whose children have died in accidents. *Journal of Traumatic Stress, 2,* 319–334.

Martinson and colleagues, she discovered that teens with dysfunctional patterns of self-concept had higher grief symptom levels.

Miles has examined the emotional and physical responses of bereaved parents whose children died of a chronic illness, accident, or suicide. No differences in distress were found among the groups; however, parents from a lower socioeconomic status and those with higher concurrent life stressors were more distressed (Miles, 1985; Demi and Miles, 1988). Analyzing qualitative data from the same study, Miles and Demi (1991–92) found that suicide-bereaved parents reported more guilt feelings and many indicated that guilt was the most distressing aspect of their grief. Both suicide- and accident-bereaved parents reported a high level of death causation and childrearing guilt (Miles and Demi, 1983–84, 1986). In another paper, Miles and Crandall (1983) found many bereaved parents reported growth experiences as a result of their struggle to come to terms with the death of their child.

Demi also has done research related to the adjustment to widowhood following sudden death (Demi, 1978, 1984). All of the widows were still experiencing extreme emotional distress 12 to 18 months after their spouses' death. Suicide survivors did not exhibit a less satisfactory adjustment, but did exhibit more resentment and guilt. In another study, Demi and Gilbert (1987) examined the relationships between parents' and siblings' grief reactions following the death of a child. Parents' emotional distress and the level of role dysfunction was related to siblings' distress and behavior problems.

Murphy studied stress, coping, and health outcomes in survivors of the Mt. St. Helens volcano eruption disaster (Murphy, 1984, 1986, 1988; Cowan and Murphy, 1985). She found that bereaved subject's reported significantly higher levels of stress and lower levels of mental health than survivors who did not experience a death. Murphy also showed therapeutic benefits of a theory-based preventive intervention program for parents following the accidental death of a child (Murphy, 1991; Murphy et al, 1989, 1998).

Vachon and her colleagues have reported on a number of studies with widows in Canada (Vachon, 1983; Vachon et al, 1976, 1980, 1982a, 1982b; Walker et al, 1977). Most women were no longer highly distressed 2 years following the death, however deficits in social support, health, and financial problems were found in those who were still distressed.

Dimond and Lund have studied the bereaved elderly (Burks et al, 1988; Dimond, 1981; Dimond et al, 1987; Johnson et al, 1986; Lund et al, 1985, 1985–86, 1986a, 1986b, 1990). Findings from their longitudinal study of the elderly bereaved found that the small group who were still having difficulties 2 years after the death had lower self-esteem and experienced more intense feelings early in bereavement.

Nurse researchers have used qualitative research approaches to better understand the grief experience of specific populations. For example, what themes characterize the grieving process for infirm or dependent older parents experiencing the death of an adult child? Researchers (Cacace and Williamson, 1996) asked parents who had experienced the death of an adult child these three questions:

1. What has your life been like since your son/daughter died?
2. How, if in any way, would your experience have been different if the death of your child occurred in infancy or early childhood rather than in adulthood?

3. What, if anything, would you tell parents who are presently expecting or have experienced the death of an adult child?

Data analysis led to the identification of five themes:

- Personal disruption (the death was the most significant event in their life and they feel robbed of the pleasure of an adult relationship with their child)
- Unnatural survivorship (the wish to change places with the adult child who died)
- Isolation (separation from social activities)
- Reminders (visions and dreams, events, physical resemblance in other children and grandchildren)
- Coping strategies (changing relationship to grandchildren, strengthening family ties, seeking support through others as well as spiritual and diversional activities)

Grief associated with the death of a person with acquired immunodeficiency syndrome/human immunodeficiency virus (AIDS/HIV) also has the potential for some unique characteristics. Three themes in the bereavement process identified by informants whose partners had died of AIDS are: (a) identifying with the dying partner; (b) seeking support of friends and families; and (c) accepting the loss of the partner, both intellectually and emotionally (Ferrell and Boyle, 1992).

Depression has been identified as a major outcome variable in the bereavement literature. What factors influence the intensity of the depression? How is the intensity of the depression manifested in one's feeling of loss? Researchers (Dimond et al, 1994) identified four factors that influence depression in older adults during the grieving process: illness, deaths, relocation, and relationships. In general, the greater the number of illnesses, other deaths, relocations, and negative encounters, the greater the depression. Table 34–1 shows the comparison in affect between two persons with different levels of depression during the post-bereavement process.

FACTORS AFFECTING CLINICAL DECISIONS

An important advance in research has been the identification of the many factors influencing the grief process and grief

TABLE 34–1 Comparison of Post-Bereavement Comments: Two Cases

Low Depression Scores Male 73 Years Old (Mr. A)	High Depression Scores Male 73 Years Old (Mr. B)
3 weeks (T_1) and 2 months (T_2)	
Great loss; miss her terribly. No financial problems. Still working. Satisfied with daily routine. Keeping active at home with hobby. Planning to join church choir. Health, pretty good. Remarriage: maybe. Really optimistic about future.	Sorrow, sadness, loneliness; have tried not to be sad. Thinking about relocating, confused. Son very ill. Miss my wife. Difficulty sleeping, no ambition, very tired, dizzy, no appetite, spend a lot of time in bed. Visit cemetery every other day. Sometimes think I can make a new life (future), but then feel it isn't worth it.
6 months	
Lonesome. Making every effort to adapt to my situation. Participating in family Round Robin letter. Nephew's wife died (drowned) recently. A little arthritis. Remarriage: maybe (laughs), not too many want to put up with a seventy-year-old. I'm optimistic about the future.	Very lonely. Waves of partial ups and significant downs. Pain like depression, maybe nervousness and anxiety. (Moved residence—too many memories in old place.) Depressing at first; I'm adjusting to move now. Daughter is getting a divorce. I'm worried about her. My eyesight is going fast. Feel alone. Trouble sleeping. Close friend died. I think I can be happier in the future. Remarriage: not at present. Fearful of being blind and imposing that on someone else.
1 year	
Oh, everything is better; much improved. Anniversary date was very difficult. Starting to date. I'm part of life again. Haven't been sick at all. I'm looking forward to a good future.	Very traumatic. Car accident, seriously injured. New lady friend dropped me. Anniversary date very difficult, discouraged. No place in life for a single person. Sometimes I think, what's the use, there is no future.
18 months	
Some confusion over whether to remarry. Did remarry. Moved to new wife's home. Feel a little uncomfortable here. I've enjoyed the companionship. Healthy, swimming again. Lost 2 sisters recently. Still feel pain of my wife's death. Future is going to be okay, my outlook is very good.	Pretty awful. City sued me for collision with train. Still upset at lady friend dropping me. Dating, but "gun shy." No ambition. Seeing psychiatrist. On meds. Hope the future will be less lonely.
2 years	
Very enjoyable. Very productive. I have a companion. I've got so much going for me. Health is excellent. Future is bright.	Loneliness is persistent, periods of depression. Several friends have died—very disturbing. Biggest problem is loneliness. Dating—they take, but they don't give. Daughter moved out of town. Future is not very exciting. Remarriage: I don't think so.

From Dimond, M., Caserta, M., Lund, D. (1994). Understanding depression in bereaved older adults. *Clinical Nursing Research, 3* (3), 265.

outcomes. Some of the more salient factors include gender, age, role with the deceased, socioeconomic level, coping strategies, and level of social support (Demi, 1989; Osterweis et al., 1984; Parkes, 1972; Parkes and Weiss, 1983; Worden, 1982).

Gender

A number of studies have identified gender differences in response to death. Mandell and coworkers (1980) found that fathers of infants who died of SIDS expressed a limited ability to ask for help and often appeared stoic and unemotional, despite their deep pain, because of societal attitudes toward men. Other research with bereaved parents suggests that mothers report more distress than fathers. Research comparing responses of widows and widowers, however, is less conclusive. Gallagher and colleagues (1983) found that bereaved elderly widows reported more distress than widowers following the death of a spouse. However, others researchers comparing elderly widows and widowers reported differing findings (Demi, 1989). Methodologic problems with this research include the fact that many studies had very small, inadequate samples of men. Thus, the more distressed men may not be participating in research. In addition, it may be that men do not as easily reveal their feelings of distress even in research projects. It is important as a professional not to assume that a bereaved male is not experiencing as much pain as women. Many bereaved fathers, widowers, and other men have had the experience of being overlooked by professionals, family members, and friends during their period of grieving. We need to learn more about how men grieve and about their needs during this stressful time.

Age

Age is another factor that may influence one's response. Research has indicated that younger widows (Maddison and Walker, 1967; Sanders, 1980–81) and older widowers are at higher risk for problems (Rees and Lutkins, 1967). Sanders (1980–81) found that younger women who experienced the death of a spouse initially manifested greater grief intensity; however, at 18 months, a reverse trend was noted, with older spouses showing more intense grief. The elderly bereaved may be at greater risk of problems because of their already declining health and their repeated experiences with loss. Although clinicians and researchers have documented that the experience of death in childhood and adolescence has negative consequences for the child, an emerging body of literature suggests that many children can mature and grow as a result of a death in the family (Hogan and Balk, 1990; Martinson et al, 1987a). The literature on the topic of bereavement in children, however, is extensive and is beyond the scope of this chapter (Wass and Corr, 1984).

Role

The role of the deceased and the bereaved also appears to be a factor in bereavement. Two studies have found that bereaved parents reported more distress than widows and other bereaved groups (Owen et al, 1982–83; Sanders, 1979–80). It has been hypothesized that the parents have a closer attachment and greater sense of responsibility toward children than other relationships, including a spouse. Parkes also found that the greater the level of dependence a widow had with her deceased husband, the more distress reported (Parkes, 1970).

Coping Style

The coping style of the bereaved is also important. Herth (1990) found a relationship between hope and grief resolution. Not surprising, hope was higher in individuals with a longer duration of spouse illness, adequate income, good health, fewer concurrent losses, and more support from friends. Clark and coworkers (1986) found that widowers who experienced a "balanced coping strategy" including a diversity of helpful resources coped more effectively with the death of a spouse.

Socioeconomic Status

Socioeconomic status has been found to be a predictor of poor adjustment in many studies of widows. Scott and Kivett (1980) found that widowed black, older women in the rural South often had problems following the death of a spouse because of the absence of basic vital services related to financial assistance, health care, housing, and transportation. Miles identified socioeconomic status to be a predictor of distress in bereaved parents (Miles, 1985).

Social Support

Social support, particularly the number of friends and family who provide tangible and emotional help following a death has been found to be important in many studies (Parkes, 1970; Vachon et al, 1982). Davidowitz and Myrick (1984) interviewed individuals who had lost a loved one by death to determine facilitative and nonfacilitative responses. Facilitative responses tended to be nonjudgmental and nondirective, and were focused more on the individual's feelings and needs. Nonfacilitative responses included unsolicited advice, false reassurance, and directives that life must go on. Similar findings were noted by Lord (1987) who interviewed survivors of a drunk-driving accident. Attentiveness to their feelings and listening, privacy, and tangible assistance were deemed helpful, whereas inappropriate comments, prying, being told the death was "God's will," and withdrawal from family or friends were seen as unhelpful. Interviews with family members who experienced the death of a spouse or child in a motor vehicle accident indicated that being allowed to ventilate, the expression of concern, "being there," and meeting others with a similar loss were most helpful (Lehman et al, 1984).

Situational Differences

Many factors surrounding the death of a loved one may impact on both their immediate and long-term grief response. Characteristics of the final illness and/or aspects of the death event and special issues surrounding certain types of loss are important. In addition, the response of the health care team toward the individual and family can be critical.

Much of the bereavement literature suggests that sudden, unexpected death is more difficult to resolve than grief following a period of illness (Osterweis et al, 1984; Rando, 1994; Worden, 1982). Sudden death leaves the bereaved individuals stunned and in shock. There were no opportunities for preparation or for closure. Too, the financial and legal situations that can be planned for when one is terminally ill may not be in order. SIDS is particularly difficult because it involves the sudden and totally unexpected death of an infant (Nikolaisen and Williams, 1980). Sudden death also frequently occurs as a result of a vehicular or drowning accident, which leaves the survived feeling both guilty and fearful. Fear is linked to concern that another individual in the family could die of an accident too (Miles and Perry, 1985). Murder and suicide, two additional causes of sudden death, carry with them both stigma and great confusion about why the death occurred. Anger is particularly difficult with murder, and guilt appears to be particularly difficult with suicide. Accidents, suicide, and murder more frequently occur with teenagers and young adults who leave behind parents, siblings, friends, and others in the community as grievers. The death of a young adult, especially from such seemingly avoidable and violent means, is difficult for all survivors.

Death following a chronic or lingering illness allows both the bereaved and the family to prepare emotionally and legally. There are opportunities for planning and for dealing with unfinished business such as conflicts. In addition, the bereaved can begin to prepare themselves emotionally for the death, and some level of anticipatory grief may occur. On the other hand, one cannot assume that families or dying individuals were able to face the reality of the fatal illness. Many families never openly discuss the death among themselves or with the dying person, and denial about the severity of the illness may continue until death. Thus, the bereaved may be just as stunned as when there has been a sudden death. Another issue for the survivors is the fact that they may have experienced a long period of stress related to coping with the final illness. Hospitalizations, complicated care decisions, home care of the seriously ill individual, financial costs, and the related emotional strain may have been experienced for many months, even years (Strauss, 1994).

Thus, consideration should be given to the mode of death and to whether the death was sudden and unexpected, or followed a long period of illness. However, this information should never be used to make assumptions about the bereaved. It is essential that the nurse assess the bereaved individual or family to learn more about their perspective of the illness, dying, and death experiences. This can be done by providing opportunities for them to tell you their story—their view of what they experienced.

Although the death of a loved one is always a difficult experience, certain types of loss may be more difficult or problematic to survivors because of societal issues or personal expectations that surround the death (Osterweis et al, 1984; Worden, 1982). For example, women (and their partners) who experience a miscarriage often have difficulty obtaining the support they need during grief. Family and friends may not even have known about the pregnancy or the loss, and if they did, they may dismiss the loss because "it was only a miscarriage." Likewise, parents who decide to have a therapeutic abortion because of a genetic abnormality of their child may not reveal their loss to others or may meet with hostility because of their decision to abort. Parents who experience the death of a child generally experience an outpouring of support at the time of death. However, as time goes on and their grief increases, they often find that no one is able to really listen to their intense pain. Grievers who have experienced the death of a family member or significant other from suicide or murder often experience stigma and even blame from society. As a result, they may find themselves grieving alone. Children who have experienced any type of loss are vulnerable because their grief is often ignored or dismissed by adults who either deny the fact that they are in pain or don't really know how to respond to them (Wass and Corr, 1984). More recently, attention has been focused on survivors following the death of a family member or lover from AIDS. These individuals described isolation and disconnectedness as a major theme in their grief (Sowell et al, 1991).

FUTURE DEVELOPMENTS

A major concern regarding nursing intervention with the bereaved is whether this important role will remain within the domain of nursing practice. The downsizing of hospitals and other institutions, the increased acuity of patients, the shortage of staff, and the increased focus on a more medical model of care have increasingly reduced the time available for nurses to work with distressed families. In addition, there are other professionals, such as physicians, social workers, and chaplains, who are also involved in helping bereaved family members. However, nurses have a unique and important role because of their availability and closeness to the patient and family as nursing care is provided. Providing supportive care to families is as important to the nurse as it is to the family because it provides rewarding outcomes in a difficult situation.

Thus, it is vital that nurses work toward maintaining the time and skills necessary to work with grieving families at the time of death and after death occurs. Protocols should be developed in every setting that help direct the approach to families. In addition, newly graduated nurses need additional education preparation for their important role in helping bereaved families, and bereavement intervention and related topics should be ongoing topics of inservice and continuing education. Nurse educators need to see that content on grief and interventions with the bereaved is included at all levels of undergraduate nursing programs. Graduate programs should include more in-depth content regarding assessment and working with the bereaved. As managed care becomes more common, nurses can be leaders in setting up bereavement management programs within managed care systems.

NURSING CARE ACTIONS

Nurses work with grieving individuals in a wide variety of situations and settings. The principles of intervention would differ depending on the setting and the situations surrounding the death.

Assessment

The following are some general assessment guidelines to use when approaching bereaved individuals:

- What is the relationship with the individual who died? What was the level of dependence on and/or the nature of the attachment with the individual? Were there any unresolved relationship issues with the deceased prior to death? What is the meaning of the death to the bereaved individual?
- What were the circumstances surrounding the individual's illness and death? Were there any unique circumstances such as a sudden, unexpected death; an accident in which multiple family members were injured or killed; or a chronic illness that involved many years of illness and suffering; a death caused by murder, suicide, or AIDS, which can add additional burdens including stigma? What is the perception of the bereaved about the illness, period of dying, and/or death event?
- Were there any aspects of the situation that might add to the grief response of the family member such as ambivalence in the relationship with the deceased, feelings of guilt related to the cause of death or to the past relationship with the deceased, a lack of opportunity for closure with the deceased as when there is no body to verify the death, or family conflicts surrounding the death that may impede the grief process?
- What does the bereaved understand about the cause of death? Are there any confusions or unresolved issues or remaining unanswered questions?
- When did the loss/death occur? Is there any relationship between this date and the current feelings and problems? Where is the bereaved individual in terms of the grief process and the tasks of grief? Is he or she still experiencing acute distress and shock? Is he or she actively grieving and trying to cope with the loss and resultant pain?
- What is the most difficult problem for the individual at the present time (e.g., loneliness, guilt, fear of going crazy, lack of support)? Is the individual searching for meaning and trying to resolve the death and reorganize life around the loss? Are there any suggestions that the individual may be experiencing problematic grief responses that require additional counseling and help?
- How has the loss affected other family members? How is the relationship between family members? Are they grieving together or separately? What are their unique grieving patterns? Are there sources of conflict? How are the children in the family grieving and coping? Are they isolated or included?
- What is the nature of the support network for the individual and for the family as a unit at this time? How can the support network be strengthened? Is the individual finding support and meaning in their spiritual views or religious rituals? Is a bereavement group warranted and acceptable?

Intervention

Interventions with the bereaved will also differ depending on the timing and circumstances of one's encounter (see Clinical Decision Making box). The following are some general principles that can be followed in almost any situation.

Goal: Help the individual and/or family actualize the loss.

Intervention: Prepare family members for the impending pronouncement of death by providing honest information about the condition of the family member during treatment. Allow time for them to absorb the pronouncement of death. Allow family members the opportunity to see the deceased following death. Encourage them to talk about the individual who died and the death. Use correct words such as "dying" and "died", rather than "passed away" or "gone."

Goal: Help the bereaved to acknowledge and express their feelings.

Intervention: Listen with empathy. Allow the bereaved to talk about the death, the meaning of their loss, their

CLINICAL DECISION MAKING
JOHNNY'S DEATH FROM SUDDEN INFANT DEATH SYNDROME (SIDS)

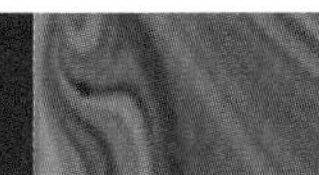

CLINICAL DECISIONS REGARDING IMMEDIATE CARE

The case study of Johnny illustrates some important unfolding clinical decisions made by his nurse, Mary. The following outline details these decisions:
Based on her awareness of the potential death of Johnny from SIDS and the devastating impact this will have on his parents, she

- Found a private room.
- Helped them to call someone to be with them (grandmother and minister).
- Stayed with them as much as they desired.

CLINICAL DECISIONS REGARDING FAMILY

Based on her awareness of the importance of preparing the parents for the infant's death and, at the same time, helping them feel everything was done, she

- Kept them informed about the fact that the medical team is trying to help their son in the best way possible.
- Told them truthfully how sick their baby was.
- With MD's permission, forewarned them about Johnny's possible death.
- Stayed with the parents when the MD came in to tell them of the child's death.
- Helped the grandmother understand what had happened when she came.

PERSONAL REFLECTIONS AND ROLE OF NURSE

Knowing that her most important role was to help this couple and the grandmother grieve over their child's death, she

- Accepted their emotional responses without judgment.
- Encouraged them to talk about what they were feeling.
- Listened to them as they talked about what Johnny meant to them.
- Gently assisted the father to share his feelings.
- Helped the grandmother to share her previously untold story of having lost a baby to SIDS years earlier.
- Helped the parents and grandmother, on their own terms, to see their baby one last time both to verify the reality of the death and to help them say their "goodbye's."

Knowing that a SIDS death often causes parents to feel guilty because they didn't prevent the death somehow, she

- Provided information about SIDS and emphasized the fact that, in most cases, we do not know what causes it and stated clearly that they were not responsible for the child's death.
- Listened to the mother's feeling of guilt and normalized guilt but again reiterated that they were not to blame.

CLINICAL DECISIONS REGARDING FUTURE CARE

Realizing that the family will have many other issues to deal with after they leave the hospital, she

- Prepared them for decisions they would have to make such as funeral and burial decisions.
- Helped them problem solve how to tell their 3-year-old about the baby's death.
- Reminded them that their decision-making capacities were inhibited and to be cautious in making decisions.
- Cautioned them about safety in driving home.
- Prepared them briefly about the grief they would experience in the months to come
- Referred them to the SIDS support group and called the SIDS counseling program to visit them.
- Sensitively gave them their baby's clothes and accompanied them to the car to reduce the pain of leaving.

emotional pain, related behavioral difficulties, communication problems with others, etc. Listening is hard work and can be painful for the helper. Nonjudgmental acceptance of the bereaved, whatever they may share, is important.

Goal: Normalize the grief process.
Intervention: Help the bereaved to understand their grief responses and to accept the universality and normality of how they are feeling (see Patient Teaching box). This can be done by providing the bereaved information about grief (verbally, books, pamphlets) and by reassuring them regarding specific responses they are experiencing. It is not unusual for the bereaved to think they are truly "going crazy" during the most acute period of grief; such reassurance, if appropriate to their situation, is often accepted with relief. Individuals who appear to be having prolonged, exaggerated, or complicated grief reactions should be referred for therapy.

Goal: Facilitate healthy coping responses.
Intervention: Reinforce positive coping efforts. Remind the bereaved individual of the importance of patience and being good to oneself during the grief process. Encourage attempts to resume normal activities. Reinforce and encourage positive ways to hold onto memories of the deceased, while letting go. Help the bereaved to organize a plan for daily activities, if needed. Discourage overdependence on drugs and alcohol.

PATIENT TEACHING
TEACHING ABOUT GRIEVING

Grieving individuals often do not understand their own emotional responses and behaviors during the grieving period. An important nursing intervention is helping them understand the scope and normality of the grief response. This can be done by discussing and normalizing aspects of grief as they are experienced by the individual, by providing written materials such as the description of grief that follows, by giving the individual a list of books about grief that are available in local libraries and bookstores, or by referring them to a bereavement support group where they can meet with others in a similar situation.

UNDERSTANDING GRIEF

The death of a relative or close friend is one of life's most painful experiences. After someone dies, we experience a long period of grieving in which we try to come to grips with the meaning that this person's death has for our own lives. At first, it's not unusual to be in a state of shock. You feel sort of numb and find it hard to believe that the death has occurred. Of course, it's also not unusual to cry a lot, become depressed, or feel angry about what has happened. All of these reactions are particularly common if the death was sudden and unexpected. Over time, however, as the reality of the death becomes more evident, most people experience a deep sense of loneliness, emptiness, and intense yearning to have the person back. This is a particularly difficult time because it is so painful. Many grieving individuals also feel a sense of helplessness that they couldn't prevent the death from occurring. This can lead to feelings of guilt related to feeling responsible in some vague way for the death, fear that someone else might die, and anger about why the death occurred. Grieving individuals also experience behavioral changes such as disorganization and difficulty in making plans or problem solving, and cognitive problems including difficulty concentrating and confused thought processes. Associated with the stress of grieving, bereaved individuals can develop physical symptoms such as headaches, sighing, appetite changes, or fatigue, or can develop health problems. Over time, these emotional responses to grief abate and are experienced with less intensity or less often. Some bereaved individuals, particularly grieving parents, say that one never actually recovers from grief. However, it should eventually be possible for the bereaved to resume normal life activities and to remember the deceased with more happiness and less pain. The bereaved are often helped by searching for a greater meaning in their loss. They may put their energies into some activity to help others or to improve society, or they may reassess their own lives and become closer to their families or to others.

Adapted from Miles, M.S. (1984). Helping adults mourn the death of a child. In H. Wass and C. Corr (eds.): *Children and Death*. Washington, D.C.: Hemisphere Publishing Co., pp. 219–241.

Goal: Assist the bereaved in communicating with, supporting, and getting support from family.

Intervention: Provide information about how grief affects a family. Listen to frustrations that arise because of the inadequate responses of family members. Facilitate the development of understanding of the potential differing responses of various family members and help the bereaved to be patient with them. Identify ways the bereaved can let family know what they need.

Goal: Identification of ways to increase the support network.

Intervention: Refer bereaved, if interested, to a bereavement self-help group. Encourage the individual to seek and accept help from among friends and coworkers.

CHAPTER HIGHLIGHTS

- The growth of home health and hospice programs has increased nurses' opportunities for working with dying patients and their families.
- Theory from many disciplines contributes to the understanding of the grief process.
- Grief involves emotional, cognitive, behavioral, and physical responses.
- There are overlapping phases in the grief process but not "stages" per se.
- Gender, age, coping style, socioeconomic status, social support, and the individual's specific situation influence an individual's grief response.
- Nursing care begins with a thorough assessment of the survivors and their responses.
- Nursing actions include: helping the individual/family actualize the loss; helping the bereaved acknowledge and express their feelings; normalizing the grief process; facilitating healthy coping responses; assisting the bereaved in communicating with, supporting, and getting support from family; and, increasing ways to increase the bereaved support network.

REFERENCES

American Nurses' Association (1980). *Nursing Policy Statement.* Kansas City, MO: Author.

Bowlby, J. (1960). Grief and mourning in infancy and early childhood. *Psychoanalytic Study of the Child, 15,* 9–52.

Bowlby, J. (1961). Processes of mourning. *International Journal of Psychoanalysis, 42,* 317–340.

Burks, V.K., Lund, D.A., Gregg, C.H., Bluhm, H.P. (1988). Bereavement and remarriage for older adults. *Death Studies, 12,* 51–60.

Cacace, M.F., Williamson, E. (1996). Grieving the death of an adult child. *Journal of Gerontological Nursing, 22* (2), 16–22.

Caplan, G. (1964). *Principles of Preventive Psychiatry.* New York: Basic Books.

Clark, P.G., Siviski, R.W., Weiner, R. (1986). Coping strategies of widowers in the first year. *Family Relations, 35,* 425–430.

Cohen, L., Zilkha, S., Middleton, J., O'Donnohue, H. (1978). Perinatal mortality: Assisting parental affirmation. *The American Journal of Orthopsychiatry, 48,* 727–731.

Cowan, M.R., Murphy, S.A. (1985). Identification of postdisaster bereavement risk predictors. *Nursing Research, 34,* 71–75.

Davidowitz, M., Myrick, R.D. (1984). Responding to the bereaved: An analysis of "helping" statements. *Death Education, 8,* 1–10.

Davies, E., Spinetta, J., Martinson, I., et al (1986). Manifestations of levels of functioning in grieving families. *Journal of Family Issues, 7,* 297–313.

Demi, A. (1978). Adjustment to widowhood after a sudden death: Suicide and non-suicide survivors compared. In M.V. Batey (ed.): *Communicating Nursing Research,* Vol. 11. Boulder, CO: Western Interstate Commission for Higher Education, pp. 91–99.

Demi, A.S. (1984). Social adjustment of widows after a sudden death. *Death Education, 8,* 91–111.

Demi, A.S. (1989). Death of a spouse. In R. Kalish (ed.): *Midlife Loss: Coping Strategies.* Newbury Park, CA: Sage, pp. 218–248.

Demi, A.S., Gilbert, C.M. (1987). Relationship of parental grief to sibling grief. *Archives of Psychiatric Nursing, 1,* 385–391.

Demi, A.S., Miles, M.S. (1986). Bereavement research. In H. Werley and H. Fitzpatrick (eds.): *Annual Review of Nursing Research, 4* (1), 105–123.

Demi, A.S., Miles, M.S. (1987). Parameters of normal grief: A Delphi study. *Death Studies, 11,* 397–412.

Demi, A.S., Miles, M.S. (1988). Suicide bereaved parents: Emotional distress and physical health problems. *Death Studies, 12,* 297–307.

Dimond, M.F. (1981). Bereavement and the elderly: A critical review with implications for nursing practice and research. *Journal of Advanced Nursing, 6,* 461–470.

Dimond, M., Caserta, M., Lund, D. (1994). Understanding depression in bereaved older adults. *Clinical Nursing Research, 3* (3), 253–268.

Dimond, M.F., Lund, D.A., Caserta, M.S. (1987). The role of social support in the first two years of bereavement in an elderly sample. *Gerontologist, 27,* 599–604.

Ferrell, J.A., Boyle, J.S. (1992). Bereavement experiences: Caring for a partner with AIDS. *Journal of Community Health Nursing, 9* (3), 127–135.

Freud, S. (1957). Mourning and melancholia. In J. Strachey (ed. and trans.): *The Standard Edition of the Complete Psychological Works of Sigmund Freud,* Vol. XIV. London: Hogarth Press, pp. 243–258. (Originally published in 1915)

Freud, S. (1960). Letter to Binswanger. In E.L. Freud (ed.): *Letters of Sigmund Freud.* New York: Basic Books, Inc, p. 386. (Originally published in 1929)

Gallagher, D.E., Breckenridge, N.J., Thompson, L.W., Peterson, J.A. (1983). Effects of bereavement on indicators of mental health in elderly widows and widowers. *Journal of Gerontology, 38,* 565–571.

Glick, L.O., Weiss, R.S., Parkes, C.M. (1974). *The First Year of Bereavement.* New York: John Wiley and Sons.

Herth, K. (1990). Relationship of hope, coping styles, concurrent losses, and setting to grief resolution in the elderly widow(er). *Research in Nursing and Health, 13,* 109–117.

Hogan, N., DeSantis, L. (1992). Adolescent sibling bereavement: An ongoing attachment. *Qualitative Health Research, 2,* 159–177.

Hogan, N.S., Balk, D.E. (1990). Adolescent reactions to sibling death: Perceptions of mothers, fathers, and teenagers. *Nursing Research, 39,* 103–106.

Hogan, N.S., Greenfield, D.B. (1991). Adolescent sibling bereavement symptomatology in a large community sample. *Journal of Adolescent Research, 6,* 97–112.

Horowitz, M.J. (1982). Stress response syndromes and their treatment. In L. Goldberger and S. Breznitz (eds.): *Handbook of Stress: Theoretical and Clinical Aspects.* New York: The Free Press.

Johnson, R.J., Lund, D.A., Dimond, M.R. (1986). Stress, self-esteem and coping during bereavement among the elderly. *Social-Psychology-Quarterly, 49,* 273–279.

Jost, K.E., Haase, J.E. (1989). At the time of death: Help for the child's parents. *Children's Health Care, 18,* 146–152.

Lauer, M.E., Camitta, B.M. (1980). Home care for dying children: A service model. *Journal of Pediatrics, 62,* 106–113.

Lauer, M.E., Mulhern, R.K., Bohne, J.B., Camitta, B.M. (1985). Children's perceptions of their sibling's death at home or hospital: The precursors of differential adjustment. *Cancer Nursing, 8,* 21–27.

Lauer, M.E., Mulhern, R.K., Schell, M.J., Camitta, B.M. (1989). Long-term follow-up of parental adjustment following a child's death at home or hospital. *Cancer, 63,* 988–994.

Lauer, M.E., Mulhern, R.K., Wallskog, J.M., Camitta, B.M. (1983). A comparison study of parental adaptation following a child's death at home or in the hospital. *Pediatrics, 71,* 107–112.

Lehman, D.R., Ellard, J.H., Wortman, C.B. (1986). Social support for the bereaved: Recipients' and providers' perspectives on what is helpful. *Journal of Consulting and Clinical Psychology, 54,* 438–446.

Lindemann, E. (1944). Symptomatology and management of acute grief. *American Journal of Psychiatry, 101,* 141–148.

Lord, J.H. (1987). Survivor grief following a drunk-driving crash. *Death Studies, 11,* 413–435.

Lund, D.A., Caserta, M.S., Dimond, M. (1986a). Gender differences through two years of bereavement among the elderly. *The Gerontologist, 26,* 314–320.

Lund, D.A., Caserta, M.S., Dimond, M.F., Gray, R.M. (1986b). Impact of bereavement on the self-conceptions of older surviving spouses. *Symbolic Interaction, 9,* 235–244.

Lund, D.A., Caserta, M.S., Vank-Pelt, J., Gass, K.A. (1990). Stability of social support networks after later-life spousal bereavement. *Death Studies, 14,* 53–73.

Lund, D.A., Dimond, M., Caserta, M.S., et al (1985–86). Identifying elderly with coping difficulties after two-year bereavement. *Omega, 16,* 213–244.

Lund, D.A., Dimond, M.F., Juretich, M. (1985). Bereavement support groups for the elderly: Characteristics of potential participants. *Death Studies, 9,* 309–321.

Mahon, C.K., Perez, R.H., Ratliff, M., Schreiner, R.L. (1981). Neonatal death: Parental evaluation of the NICU experience. *Issues in Comprehensive Pediatric Nursing, 5,* 279–292.

Maddison, D., Walker, W. (1967). Factors affecting the outcome of conjugal bereavement. *British Journal of Psychiatry, 113,* 1057–1067.

Mandell, F., McAnulty, E., Reece, R.M. (1980). Observations of paternal response to sudden unanticipated infant death. *Pediatrics, 65,* 221–225.

Martinson, I.M., Campos, R.G. (1991). Adolescent bereavement: Long term responses to a sibling's death from cancer. *Journal of Adolescent Research, 6,* 54–69.

Martinson, I.M., Davies, E.B., McClowry, S.G. (1987a). The long-term effect of sibling death on self-concept. *Journal of Pediatric Nursing, 2,* 227–235.

Martinson, I.M., Davies, E.B., McClowry, S. (1991). Parental depression following the death of a child. *Death Studies, 15,* 259–267.

Martinson, I., Kersey, J., Nesbitt, M. (1987b). Children's adjustment to the death of a sibling from cancer. *Advances in Thanatology, 6,* 1–7.

McClowry, S.G., Davies, E.B., May, K.A., et al (1987). The empty space phenomenon: The process of grief in the bereaved family. *Death Studies, 11,* 361–374.

Miles, M.S. (1980). *The grief of parents. . . . When a child dies.* Compassionate Friends, Inc., P.O. Box 1347, Oak Brook, IL 60521.

Miles, M.S. (1984). Helping adults mourn the death of a child. In H. Wass and C. Corr. (eds.): *Children and Death.* Washington, D.C.: Hemisphere Publishing Co, pp. 219–241.

Miles, M.S. (1985). Emotional symptoms and physical health in bereaved parents. *Nursing Research, 34* (2), 76–81.

Miles, M.S., Crandall, E.K. (1983). The search for meaning and its implication for growth in bereaved parents. *Health Values: Achieving High Level Wellness, 7* (1), 19–23.

Miles, M.S., Demi, A.C. (1986). Guilt in Bereaved Parents. In T. Rando (ed.): *Parental Loss of a Child: Clinical and Research Considerations.* Champaign, IL: Research Press.

Miles, M.S., Demi, A.C. (1991–92). Guilt in parents bereaved by accident, suicide, and chronic disease. *Omega, 24,* 203–215.

Miles, M.S., Demi, A. (1994). Historical and contemporary theories of grief. In I.B. Corless, B.B. Germino, and M. Pittman (eds.): *Dying, Death, and Bereavement: Theoretical Perspectives and Other Ways of Knowing.* Boston: Jones and Bartlett Publishers, pp. 83–106.

Miles, M.S., Demi, A. (1983–84). Toward the development of a theory of bereavement guilt. *Omega, 14* (4), 299–314.

Miles, M.S., Perry, K. (1985). Parental response to the sudden accidental death of a child. *Critical Care Quarterly, 8,* 73–84.

Moore, I.D., Gillis, C.L., Martinson, I. (1988). Psychosomatic manifestations of bereavement in parents two years after the death of a child with cancer. *Nursing Research, 37,* 104–107.

Mulhern, R.K., Lauer, M.E., Hoffmann, R.G. (1983). Death of a child at home or in the hospital: Subsequent psychological adjustment of the family. *Pediatrics, 71,* 743–747.

Murphy, S.A. (1984). Stress levels and health status of victims of a natural disaster. *Research in Nursing and Health, 7,* 205–215.

Murphy, S. (1986). Perceptions of stress, coping, and recovery one and three years after a natural disaster. *Issues in Mental Health Nursing, 8,* 63–77.

Murphy, S. (1988). Mental distress and recovery in a high-risk bereavement sample three years after untimely death. *Nursing Research, 37,* 30–35.

Murphy, S. (1991). Preventive intervention following accidental death of a child. *Image: Journal of Nursing Scholarship, 22,* 174–179.

Murphy, S., Aroian, K., Baugher, R. (1989). A theory-based preventive intervention program for bereaved parents whose children have died in accidents. *Journal of Traumatic Stress, 2,* 319–334.

Murphy, S., Johnson, C., Cain, K.C., Gupta, A.D., Dimond, M., and Lohan, J. (1998). Broad-spectrum group treatment for parents bereaved by the violent deaths of their 12- to 28-year old children: A randomized clinical trial. *Death Studies, 22,* 209–235.

Nikolaisen, S.M., Williams, R.A, (1980). Parents' view of support following the loss of their infant to Sudden Infant Death Syndrome. *Western Journal of Nursing Research, 2,* 593–601.

Osterweis, M., Solomon, F., Green, M. (eds.): (1984). *Bereavement: Reactions, Consequences, and Care.* Washington, D.C.: National Academy Press.

Owen, G., Fulton, R., Markusen, E. (1982–83). Death at a distance: A study of family survivors. *Omega, 13,* 191–225.

Parkes, C.M. (1970). The first year of bereavement: A longitudinal study of the reaction of London widows to the death of their husbands. *Psychiatry, 33,* 444–467.

Parkes, C.M. (1972). *Bereavement: Studies of grief in adult life.* New York: International Universities Press.

Parkes, C.M., Weiss, R.S. (1983). *Recovery from Bereavement.* New York: Basic Books.

Rando, T.A. (1994). Complications in mourning traumatic death. In I.B. Corless, B.B. Germino, and M. Pittman (eds.): *Dying, Death, and Bereavement: Theoretical Perspectives and Other Ways of Knowing.* Boston: Jones and Bartlett Publishers, pp. 253–272.

Rees, W.J., Lutkins, S. (1967). Mortality of bereavement. *British Medical Journal, 14,* 13–16.

Rigdon, I.S., Clayton, B.C., Dimond, M. (1987). Toward a theory of helpfulness for the elderly bereaved: An invitation to a new life. *Advances in Nursing Science, 9,* 32–43.

Sanders, C.M. (1979–80). A comparison of adult bereavement in the death of a spouse, child, and parent. *Omega, 10,* 303–323.

Sanders, C.M. (1980–81). Comparison of younger and older spouses in bereavement outcome. *Omega, 11,* 217–232.

Scott, J.P., Kivett, V.R. (1980). The widowed, black, older adult in the rural south: Implications for policy. *Family Relations, 29,* 83–90.

Sowell, R.L., Bramlett, M.H., Gueldner, S.H., et al (1991). The lived experience of survival and bereavement following the death of a lover from AIDS. *Image, 23,* 89–94.

Strauss, A. (1994). Chronic illness, the health care system, AIDS, and dying. In I.B. Corless, B.B. Germino, and M. Pittman (eds.): *Dying, Death, and Bereavement: Theoretical Perspectives and Other Ways of Knowing.* Boston: Jones and Bartlett Publishers, pp. 15–30.

Vachon, M. (1983). Predictors of bereavement outcome. *Medical Aspects of Human Sexuality, 17,* 194.

Vachon, M.L.S., Formo, A., Freedman, K., et al (1976). Stress reactions to bereavement. *Essence, 1,* 23.

Vachon, M.L.S., Freedman, K., Formo, A., et al (1977). The final illness in cancer: The widow's perspective. *Canadian Medical Association Journal, 117,* 1151–1154.

Vachon, M.L.S., Lyall, W.A.I., Rogers, J., et al (1980). A controlled study of self-help intervention for widows. *American Journal of Psychiatry, 137,* 1380–1384.

Vachon, M.L.S., Rogers, J., Lyall, A., et al (1982a). Predictors and correlates of adaptation to conjugal bereavement. *American Journal of Psychiatry, 139,* 998–1002.

Vachon, M.L.S., Sheldon, A.R., Lancee, W.J., et al (1982b). Correlates of enduring distress patterns following bereavement: Social network, life situation and personality. *Psychological Medicine, 12,* 783–788.

Videka-Sherman, L. (1982). Effects of participation in a self-help group for bereaved parents: Compassionate Friends. *Prevention in Human Services, 1,* 69–77.

Walker, M., MacBride, A., Vachon, M.L.S. (1977). Social support networks and the crisis of bereavement. *Social Science & Medicine, 11,* 35–41.

Wass, H., Corr, C. (eds.) (1984). *Children and Death.* Washington, D.C.: Hemisphere Publishing Co.

Worden, J.W. (1982). *Grief Counseling and Grief Therapy.* New York: Springer Publishing Company.

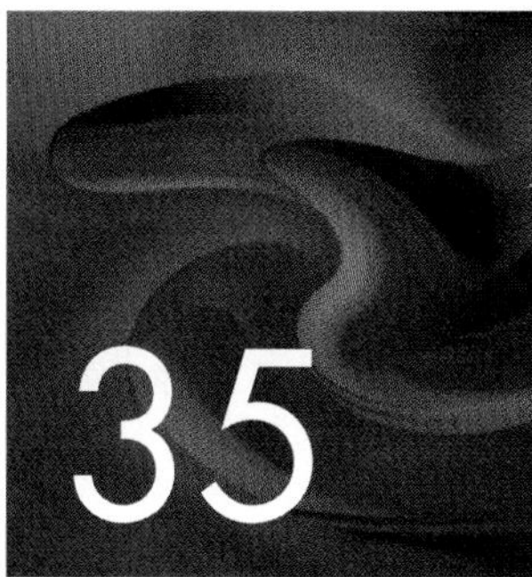

Care of the Dying 35

Margaret S. Miles, Lori J. Andreas, and Beth P. Black

Tom is a 45-year-old self-employed carpenter with cancer of the pancreas. Tom and Diane have two girls, Jane and Jennifer, who are in their early teens. Tom was diagnosed with cancer of the pancreas 2 years earlier and, against all odds for his diagnosis, he not only survived but actually did very well for 2 years. Now, however, the cancer has spread throughout his body and he was recently told by his doctor that he had only a few months to live.

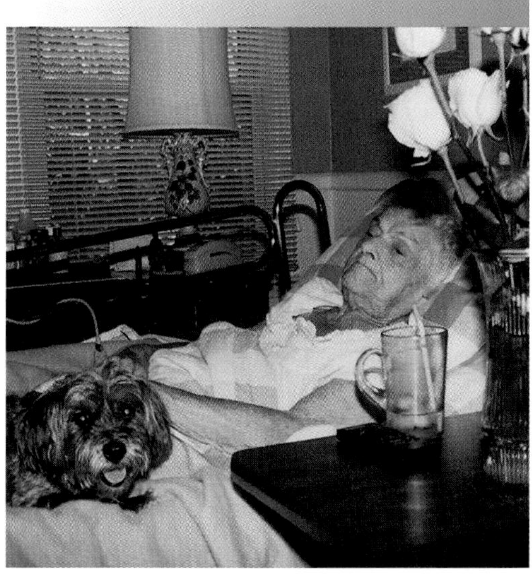

Tom was referred to the hospice program for care and support for him and his family. Maureen, the hospice nurse assigned to him, met with Tom and his wife to assess his physical and psychosocial needs and that of the family. Maureen learned that Tom has a biliary drain that his wife irrigates twice a day when she also changes his dressing. He is in a great deal of pain and is on fentanyl patches, as well as continuous release oral morphine every 12 hours as needed. He is very thin and weak but continues to walk around the house and get to the bathroom. He particularly likes to sit in the family room and look out over his garden and yard.

Diane informed Maureen that Tom's family are Eastern Europeans who immigrated to this country just before he was born. The family was very poor and Tom grew up feeling he didn't get his due share in life. He is presently alienated from his extended family and sees Diane and his children as his only family support. Tom was also described as stubborn and independent. This is reflected in his occupation as a self-employed carpenter who struggled alone to make a go of his business.

Tom has coped with his illness in the past through denial, avoidance, hard work, and anger. His present anger about his illness reflects an ongoing layer of anger that was always present in his life. On the other hand, Tom has a strong sense of humor and often switches from anger to humor in coping with situations. Tom is now more open about his illness and prognosis, although he still vacillates between talking about fighting "this thing" and making it, and

OBJECTIVES

After studying this chapter, students will be able to:

- **base nursing actions on an understanding of the physiology of dying and related symptoms that may be manifested in the dying person**
- **understand the various ways to conceptualize how individuals cope with their dying**
- **be familiar with selected research related to care of the dying**
- **identify specific ways nurses can intervene to help an individual who is dying and his or her family**
- **implement a family-centered approach to care of the dying**
- **evaluate factors that influence an individual and family's response to dying**

about preparing himself and his family for his death. He shares with the nurse and his wife his worry about what will happen to the family when he is gone.

Diane was the youngest daughter in her middle-class family. Although her parents are now deceased, she has three sisters. However, her most supportive sister is also battling cancer. Another sister is helpful with the children but they are not close. Her oldest sister has so many problems of her own that she is usually not supportive. Diane is a very emotional person who freely expresses her feelings but who also tends to get highly anxious worrying about everything that is or could go wrong. She is not a good planner or problem solver and often runs into difficulty for not thinking things out carefully.

The family has no savings, owes many bills, and has no health insurance. Now that Tom can no longer work, Diane is working two part-time jobs to try to keep the family bills paid and food on the table. They have missed several payments on their home and the financial situation is a major concern of both Tom and Diane.

Jennifer and Jane are very special to both parents, who try to give them everything they can despite their financial constraints. The girls are busy with studies, school activities, and friends. Although they are not always present in the room during the nurses' visits, Maureen is aware that they are watching and listening to what is going on from their nearby bedroom. They seem genuinely concerned about their father.

SCOPE OF NURSING PRACTICE

Nurses have an extremely important role in the care of the dying and their families in a wide variety of settings. Nurses are the primary caretakers for dying patients during hospitalization. They provide care on a 24-hour-a-day basis and often establish strong and therapeutic relationships with the patient and family. Increasingly nurses are involved with the patient and family as caregivers in the home through hospice and home health programs. In providing care in the home, they are the most consistent health care provider helping the family. They develop and implement the plan of care and they teach the family how to be caregivers. Nurses also direct the care given to the elderly who die in nursing homes. They have an important role in helping staff in these units meet the needs of dying residents, and in working with families faced with terminal illness. In the case of acute illness and sudden death, nurses are very involved in the emergency department setting or the critical care unit both in attempts to save life and in offering support to the family after death. Nurses are also the most consistent caregivers to infants and children in neonatal and intensive care and other pediatric units and, in this capacity, interact frequently to help their parents. The care provided to patients and families by nurses in these many settings is vitally important in helping them cope with the dying and death and in helping them grieve in the months to come.

Care of individuals who are dying and their families is encompassed in Henderson's definition of nursing (1978) in which she states that the nurse assists individuals, sick or well, in the performance of activities contributing toward health or a peaceful death. In this era of home care and family involvement, Henderson's definition would most certainly also refer to assisting families in caring for the dying. The American Nurses' Association social policy statement (1995) also encompasses care of the dying and their families as an important role of nurses. The American Nurses' Association Code for Nurses (1985) and their five position statements regarding nurses and end of life decisions (1996) are other important documents that delineate the role of the nurse in caring for dying patients.

Caring for the dying and their families takes intense and sensitive skills in both the physiologic domain of care and in the psychosocial realm of caring. Providing nursing care to a dying patient as well as the family is an art, a science, and a challenge. Working with or knowing individuals who are dying or who have died is difficult for everyone because it taps into our own anxiety about whether or when we might be faced with illness and death ourselves. These opportunities to work with dying patients and their families challenge nurses to confront their own attitudes, beliefs, and feelings about death and may raise many questions about life and death and about one's role as a nurse.

KNOWLEDGE BASE

Physiologic Domain

A patient with a serious health problem or terminal illness is considered to be dying when, despite maximal existing therapeutic effort, clear and convincing evidence exists showing that the progression of the life-threatening illness is inevitably leading to a natural physiologic dying process that culminates in death (Williams and Berry, 1996). Theories and research about the physiologic changes that occur in the dying process are sparse. One of the best reviews about the physiology of dying has been written by Martinson and Neelon (1994). They note that dying is not a simple isolated phenomenon but involves a series of complex interrelated cellular changes that occur over time and are closely related to the underlying disease processes. Some symptoms that may occur around the time of death include respiratory distress, respiratory infections, generalized sepsis, decreased urine output, mottled skin, and changes in temperature. The heart rate may be high with an irregular pulse, respirations may be more rapid with periods of apnea, and blood pressure may fall. Some patients become agitated and distressed, while others show decreased mental alertness, sleepiness, or apathy.

Regardless of the disease process, however, death usually results from failure of the brain, lungs, and/or heart. Death occurs when the brain, for a variety of reasons, ceases to operate effectively in controlling breathing, heart action, or arterial muscular tone; when the lungs are unable to supply adequate air for gas exchange with the bloodstream allowing for adequate oxygenation of the tissues in vital organs; and/or when the heart or blood vessels are unable to maintain adequate circulation to the tissues. Because of the current technological advances, cardiopulmonary function can be supported for long periods and may alter the course of dying. However, cardiopulmonary failure is the most common final cause of death. Thus, symptoms related to cardiac function and breathing are the most common final experiences, particularly rapid Cheyne-Stokes respirations caused by a decrease in circulation time between the lungs and the brain (Durham and Weiss, 1997; Martinson and Neelon, 1994). Nurses caring for dying patients have an important role in managing and minimizing the symptoms associated with dying. These include problems associated with pain, fatigue, elimination, nausea and vomiting, nutrition and hydration, and respiratory distress (Corless, 1994; Martinson and Neelon, 1994) (see section on Nursing Care Actions).

Psychosocial Domain

The diagnosis of a terminal illness is thought to be a highly stressful event for the individual and the family. It marks a transition from one state, that of living and life, toward another of dying and death. Individuals who are dying feel two competing demands. One is to live every day to the fullest. The other is to prepare for the end of life as it is known, and the severing of temporal relationships. What is it like to have a terminal illness and to undergo the dying process? How do individuals respond emotionally and behaviorally when faced with their own death? Unfortunately, after more than two decades of interest in this topic, we still have limited research about the psychosocial aspects of dying. There is however much rich insight in the professional clinical literature and in books written by the dying and their families to help us develop broad views.

One of the most popular models for thinking about the dying experience is that developed by Kubler-Ross in the late 1960s. In her book *On Death and Dying* (1969), she reflected on her interviews with dying patients and suggested that dying individuals experience five emotional responses from time of diagnosis until death: denial, anger, bargaining, depression, and acceptance. Although she did not contend that these emotions occurred in a sequential progression, she did imply that acceptance was the final goal that could be attained with support from others. The model was popularized by the lay and professional press because it was written from the heart, simple and clear, and insightful, and was timely in helping the nation confront previously buried feelings about death. Unfortunately, these responses were interpreted as a stage formula for assessing and helping the dying and the concepts were applied in a rigid manner. Most clinicians working with dying patients and scholars writing about responses to death now suggest that one's response to dying is much too complicated to be captured by her stage theory of death (Germain, 1980; Kastenbaum, 1991). In addition, factors such as one's personality, communication patterns, physiologic responses to the illness, reactions to medications, and influence of the health care system are not easily captured by her model of dying. Most professionals working with the dying would strongly support the view that dying individuals have a myriad of emotional and behavioral responses to dying (Shneidman, 1984). These responses, rather than occurring in some staged order, ebb and flow from day to day and minute to minute.

Still, denial, as described by Kubler-Ross and others, may be one of the most universal reactions to the knowledge of a fatal diagnosis and to one's impending death (Becker, 1973; Kastenbaum, 1991; Weisman, 1972). There are many facets to denial—denial of one's diagnosis, denial of the significance of the diagnosis including one's own feelings, and denial of one's prognosis and impending death. Although most dying individuals eventually move beyond denial to some understanding of their situation, some simply do not have the opportunity to move beyond denial because of lack of information or lack of support, or because they have difficulty facing the reality of their own death. Denial may be quite adaptive if one has a long-term, painful terminal illness. This posture of denial may help a person live one day at a time. Denial also may be linked to hope, another response described by Kubler-Ross and others. Hope may include hope for a cure or it may be hope for a day without pain or an opportunity to live long enough to meet some expectation of importance.

Acceptance, the other end of the Kubler-Ross model, may actually be much less common than she suggested. This is especially true in the 1990s because of the many treatment options available that give those with a terminal illness ongoing hope for a treatment that may make them better. Weisman (1972) suggested that individuals fluctuate between acceptance and denial, like a kaleidoscope with fragments constantly rearranging into new patterns. Acceptance can be confused with depression or fatalistic resignation, responses that also include withdrawal and solitude. An individual with a true acceptance of dying may experience a feeling of having concluded a full and rich life, or, through spiritual insights, may feel prepared for the ending of life on this earth.

Anger is another common response to dying. Dying individuals frequently have bouts of anger about their plight—the pain, weakness, frustration, loss of control, loss of all that they have and have known, and the unfairness of it all. Fear poses another troublesome and difficult response to dying. Persons who are dying may fear the process of dying more than death itself. Norman Cousins, writing in his autobiographical book,

Anatomy of an Illness (1979), noted that he and his fellow patients, all seriously ill, experienced fears related to not being able to function normally again, incapacitation, adding to the burden of the family, suffering undue pain, being abandoned, not being told everything or not being included in decisions, and a morbid fear of intrusive technology.

Several authors with extensive experience in working with dying patients suggest that dying is a uniquely individual experience and suggest that responses to dying are related to one's personality style and way of coping throughout life (Nuland, 1993; Pattison, 1967; Shneidman, 1984; Weisman, 1972). Shneidman (1984) suggests that individuals tend to die as they lived, especially in the difficult moments of their lives. Thus, individuals who were deniers may deny their fatal prognosis. Individuals who were angry throughout their lives may express a great deal of anger when dying. Those who are fatalistic will view their illness fatalistically. Others, however, suggest that individuals may grow and change personally and spiritually as they are coping with their own terminal illness and death. Nuland (1993) notes, "every life is different from any other that has gone before it, and so is every death" (p. 3).

An individual's responses are undoubtedly related to the progression of his or her underlying illness (Strauss, 1994). Pain, nausea, loss of hair, fatigue, weakness, and drugs all affect and alter responses to dying (Martinson and Neelon, 1994; Preston and McCorkle, 1995). Not only do these symptoms cause suffering, they also lead to a loss of ability to carry out activities of daily living and to an overall loss of control. These responses require nursing care that is focused on both the physical and the psychological needs of the individual patient.

Emotional and behavioral responses are also related to how the dying person is treated by others. Glaser and Strauss in the 1960s (1965) found that both families and health care professionals often tried to shield information about terminal illness from dying individuals. But the dying person often figured out how sick they were by observing their own bodily decline and the responses of family and health care professionals toward them. These communication barriers, described in the 1960s, can still exist today when questions are responded to by evasion, silence, changing the subject, untruthful responses, or painful clichés. Thus an important need of dying persons is interaction with significant others and genuine communication, including responses that are genuine, caring, reflective, truthful and that enhance their own problem solving. Cousins (1979, p. 154) noted, in describing feelings of depersonalization experienced by himself and fellow hospitalized patients:

> And there was the utter void created by the longing—reducible, unremitting, pervasive—for warmth of human contact. A warm smile and an outstretched hand were valued even above the offerings of modern science, but the latter were far more accessible than the former.

Recently, Mullins (1996) identified that patients with acquired immunodeficiency syndrome (AIDS) wanted most from the nurse to be treated as an individual.

Research on the Role of Nurses in Caring for the Dying

On the one hand, it is acknowledged that there is a cultural context for death and that individuals have some freedom to shape their dying role; on the other hand the notion of the "good death" is implicit in conversations about death and dying. Interest in the notion of cultural scripts for dying has led to research regarding nursing care of dying patients and their families. One study by Hunt (1992) asked the question about what nurses view as a "good death." Nurses in their study reported the following as important:

- physical symptom control
- patients and family openly accepting the diagnosis and prognosis
- presentation of hope and desire to live
- keeping mobile and "fighting back"
- enjoyment of life to the end
- a peaceful death

Nurses gave priority in their caregiving to physical symptom control and keeping the patient mobile. They struggled to balance the realistic acceptance of death with the will to live. They implemented this struggle by being vague about the length of a terminal phase and encouraging patients to "fight back" as long as possible. Indulgence and choice were encouraged in aspects of living—whatever the patient enjoyed. Efforts to prolong life when death was near were not valued.

Another study examined the practice of expert staff oncology nurses when caring for dying patients (Rittman et al, 1997). Four themes or patterns were identified as important to these nurses:

- knowing the patient and stage of illness
- preserving hope
- easing the struggle
- providing privacy

Irrespective of the intensity of their relationship with the patient and family, these four standards of care were maintained.

In another study (Steeves et al, 1994), nursing care was described as involving three interrelated goals:

- maintaining the values of the health care establishment by monitoring, acting on the patient's behalf, and protecting patients
- "being there" for patients, being with the dying patient, and becoming part of the patients' families
- reconciling health care values and the experience of patients as characterized by teaching and telling the truth

McClement and Degner (1995) completed an exploratory, descriptive study to identify expert nursing behaviors in the care of dying adults in the intensive care unit. Ten nurses, nominated as experts in the care of dying adults, were interviewed. Behaviors found to be important were responding after death has occurred, responding to the family, responding to anger, responding to colleagues, providing comfort care, and enhancing personal growth.

One unique study examined the nursing behaviors from the perspective of patients (Mullins, 1996). This descriptive study involved 46 individuals between the ages of 18 and 55 years with human immunodeficiency virus (HIV) and AIDS. The participants were interviewed using the Caring Behaviors Assessment tool. The subjects indicated "treat me as an individual" as the highest scoring item on the tool. Other items indicated their desire to have nurses who gave knowledgeable, competent care and who were available when needed, and who treated them with respect and accepted them and their feelings without judgment.

These and many other studies indicate that nurses caring for dying patients and their families have values and beliefs that guide their goals in providing care. A strong theme in these studies is the importance of providing expert nursing care in the context of a therapeutic relationship that respects and accepts the individual.

FACTORS AFFECTING CLINICAL DECISIONS

Age and Developmental Stage

Individuals can die at any age. Death claims infants, children, teenagers, young adults, the middle-aged, and the elderly. The dying person's age is an important factor affecting both their response and the response of others toward them. Because of a sense of "timeliness" of death, the death of an infant, child, or teenager is difficult for everyone to understand and accept, whereas the death of someone who is old is more easily understood and accepted. Likewise, death is experienced differently by a 3-year-old than by someone who is 88.

ELDERLY ADULTS

Societal attitudes toward death are ones of more acceptance when the elderly die. However, as our lifespan increases, so does our view about when one is old . . . 70s, 80s, 90s! Death in the elderly is acceptable, to some extent, because their contributions to society have been fulfilled. They have decreased social responsibility—their children are reared, they have retired from work, and their contributions are made or not made. Some elderly, however, still have a highly important social role in the family as the family elder, support person, babysitter, or financial advisor. Others have been completely isolated from family by distance, cognitive decline, or social problems.

Although it is more acceptable to die when one is old, society prefers to think of the old dying suddenly with their "boots on." Thoughts such as the following depict this attitude: "When my dad died unexpectedly at 80 years of age after he had spaded his garden, I thought this is how he would have wanted to go . . ." However, what happens generally is a long period of gradual deterioration and decline with increasing physical and mental incapacity. Issues for the elderly facing death include coping with deteriorated health and pain, losing contact with friends and family, the death of the spouse, family members, and friends, the loss of home or residence, and intense loneliness. Weisman (1972) noted:

> Of everyone who must face death, it is often the aged, those who live the longest, who have the most difficulty in finding serene and secure circumstances in which to complete life. Not only must they endure an accumulation of physical illness, but they endure an accumulation of economic, social, and emotional problems that are inherent in extended survival itself.

Attitudes of the elderly themselves toward death reflect contrasting views (Kastenbaum, 1991). One view is that dealing with death is an important developmental stage for the elderly. They have experienced the death of many peers, are less concerned about the needs of survivors, and have fewer desires for additional life experiences. Some anticipate death by talking about it, are ready to join others who have died, and plan for it by giving away belongings. Death may be viewed as preferable to progressively deteriorating physical health along with an inability to be useful and concern about becoming a burden to others. The other view of death and the elderly is that the elderly fear death because they are so close to it. This view suggests that few people, even the very aged, willingly accept death without a quiver of regret or remorse or without remnants of the struggle to survive. A very old person, accustomed to life, may find it very difficult to accept death.

Nurses working with the elderly who are dying are challenged to help them cope with their fragile, diminishing health, while at the same time helping them feel good about themselves and about their lives. The elderly without family particularly need a relationship with a nurse to help them with dying. Nurses also may be called upon to help the families of the elderly to meet the needs of their family member and to deal with their own feelings and fatigue as caregivers.

MIDDLE-AGED ADULTS

Societal attitudes toward death in the middle years vary according to the dying person's developmental age and role (Kastenbaum, 1991). The middle years encompass a broad span of life from middle adulthood through to the retirement years. During the retirement years, responsibilities have lessened but this is the time to reap the benefits of one's hard work and to enjoy family and grandchildren. The caregiving and nurturing role of grandparents is particularly important in many families. Thus, death is unacceptable, because it robs the individual and family of rewards of life as well as important supportive roles in the family. In the working years, death is not welcome because responsibilities at work are still great, and one's contributions may not be completed. In the early middle age years when one is a childrearing parent, the individual still has an important societal role in rearing children along with other ongoing responsibilities. This is particularly salient today when many individuals in their middle adult years are bearing and rearing children. The death of a parent with dependent children is a particularly poignant loss for all involved. Nurses work with middle-aged dying adults in a wide variety of settings. Their roles include caring for and supporting the patient, while at the same time helping the family to cope and grieve.

YOUNG ADULTS AND ADOLESCENTS

Death of a young adult or adolescent is difficult to accept in our society. Youth are considered at the threshold of adult life, leaving behind much that is unfulfilled. Furthermore, young adults and adolescents are considered vital, energetic, and full of life. Death is even more difficult when you realize that most of the deaths in this age are sudden and tragic: homicide, suicide, violent accidents.

C.W. Guisewell (1980, p. 2A) summarized poignantly how society views death of youth:

> People go to funerals of ones whom they have known with a variety of emotions. Sometimes, when the end has come after long and inhuman suffering, it is relief that is felt—even gratitude. Sometimes there is a kind of reflective joy in the memory of a long life fruitfully spent and peacefully concluded in its natural time. These feelings can be felt in spite of one's selfish sense of loss.
>
> But the mourners at a funeral for someone young wear an expression of perplexity and anger. The thing is wrong, unjust. Whatever consolation is offered, whatever assurances their respective faiths may provide, there is a pervasive sense of wrongness about it all . . . .

Developmentally, adolescents see themselves as immortal. They are "now" oriented and easily deny death. On the surface, they fear death the least because they are too busy to spend time with thinking about death. Also, at this age, most youth can be reasonably sure of a full life ahead and death is a remote possibility. On the other hand, the major cause of death of teens and young adults is sudden death related to their own behaviors (Cairns and Cairns, 1994). Automobile accidents are the primary cause of death, with suicide second and homicide third. African American youth, especially boys, may have a fatalistic vision of their future due to the high incidence of homicide deaths in many ghetto areas.

When an adolescent has a terminal illness, it is difficult for his or her parents, siblings, extended family, and health care team. For the adolescent, the main goal is to live every moment until death occurs. Thus, they may want to continue doing whatever is possible and often want to try any treatment to gain a reprieve. Although adolescents may appear to be denying the reality of their situation, as death nears they often want to talk about it with close friends, staff, or parents. Sometimes, however, staff and parents have a hard time being open and honest with such adolescents—wanting to protect them from the harsh reality and keep up their hope. Adolescents have been known to protect their parents from knowing about their feelings and fears because they are sensitive to the pain and anxiety the parents are experiencing. Strains between the adolescent and parents can occur when parents overprotect and the adolescent needs to become increasingly independent despite a terminal illness.

Nurses have an important role in caring for terminally ill adolescents. Teens may develop close relationships with nursing staff and reach out for support and honest answers. An especially important role for the nurse is to help the teen or young adult find some meaning in his or her life, however short it was. Care of the dying adolescent or young adult can be challenging for nursing staff and may be particularly difficult for young nurses who can easily identify themselves or their friends with the teen or young adult who is dying.

CHILDREN

In our culture and society, we do not in any way accept the idea that a child can die. As a result, parents, family, friends, and staff all feel frustrated, confused, and angry when a child dies. Children are at the beginning of life, representing innocence, joy, and happiness, and they should not suffer. To be confronted with a dying child is indeed a challenge to the meaning of life and to our views that children should be healthy, happy, and long lived. Yet, children do die—chronic illness, infectious diseases, and fatal accidents are some of the common causes of death in childhood.

Adults often think that dying children do not understand death, and parents as well as health care staff often have a hard time communicating honestly with them. Although the barriers for talking with dying children honestly about their illness and prognosis have been reduced for cancer and other chronic illnesses, children with HIV/AIDS may still experience lack of disclosure from parents due to the stigma involved with the diagnosis of HIV (Lipson, 1993). HIV is associated with taboo sexual and drug-related behaviors, although children with HIV generally acquire it through blood products, perinatal transmission, or sexual abuse.

Parents are the pivotal figures to talk with the dying child, but need much support and help themselves to do this. The nurse has an important role in helping parents understand the child's needs and identifying how to communicate honestly with their child. However, as with adolescents, younger children also may try to protect parents and may turn to nursing staff to share their feelings and concerns. When working with a dying child, it is important for the nurse to observe behavior, listen to feelings, and sit with the child in silence. If you do this, children will tell you verbally or nonverbally of their concerns, fears, and needs. The younger the child, the more the concern may be shared in hidden ways: stories, pictures, play activities, indirect questions. Positive religious images such as views about heaven, God, Jesus, and meeting others who have died, and the belief that their lives had meaning are important ingredients that help them cope.

Most of all, children, like adults, need reassurance from their nurse, doctor, and family that they will not suffer or be abandoned and left alone. A letter written by a 13-year-old boy who died of leukemia beautifully summarizes the needs of the dying child. This letter was written to the editor of a newspaper in the 1970s and published in a column written by Saul Kapel, M.D. (1974):

> I am a 13-year-old boy. I am dying. I write this to you who are and will become nurses and doctors in the hope that by sharing my feelings with you you may someday be better able to help those who share my experience.
>
> But no one likes to talk about such things. In fact, no one likes to talk much at all. Doctoring and nursing must be advancing, but I wish it would hurry. The dying person is not yet seen as a person and thus cannot be communicated with as such. He is a symbol of what every human fears and what we each know . . . .
>
> But for me, fear is today and dying now. You slip in and out of my room, give me medication and check my blood pressure. Is it because you are insecure or just a human being that I sense your fright? Why are you afraid?
>
> I am the one who is dying. I know you feel insecure, don't know what to say, don't know what to do. But please believe me, if you care, you can't go wrong. Just admit that you care. This is really what we search for. We may ask for whys and wherefores, but we really don't want answers.
>
> Don't run away. Wait. All I want to know is that there will be someone to hold my hand when I need it. I'm afraid. Death may be routine to you, but it is new to me. You may not see me as unique, but I've never died before. To me once is unique.
>
> You whisper about my youth, but when one is dying, is he really so young any more? I have lots I wish we could talk about. It really would not take much of your time, because you are in here quite a bit anyway.
>
> If only we could be honest—both admit of our fears, touch one another. If you really care, would you lose so much of your professionalism if you even cried with me just person to person? Then it might not be so hard to die in a hospital with friends and relatives close by.

This essay poignantly describes the need of a child for honest and caring communication.

The care of a child who is dying is complex, stressful, and demanding. The nurse must confront his or her own feelings about children and death, meet many challenges in helping the parents deal with their intense grief, and provide complicated psychosocial and physical care to the child. As noted by Davies and Eng (1993), such care requires significant attention to the nurses' own personal needs and responses, while maintaining and developing one's professional role as a nurse. Providing quality care to the dying child and the child's family can be extremely rewarding. Many nurses who do confront the issues involved with care of dying children grow immensely as a person and a professional.

Individual and Family Values

Because most individuals, in one way or another, are tied to a family, the dying and death of an individual is a family matter (Leahey and Wright, 1987). Our family involves the collection of individuals with whom we live and/or have a close and ongoing relationship. Obviously, death of one family member causes a response in the entire family system. The hospice movement with its emphasis on home caregiving of the dying individual by family members forced us to focus on the family's response to and needs related to death in a very intensive and holistic and challenging fashion. One of the issues that evolved was a redefinition of the family because not all dying individuals had a traditional family or were in contact with their families. This particularly occurred with the HIV epidemic in the gay community. Their "families" were often their partners and close friends.

Families in our society, because of the increased lifespan of the elderly and the distance that often separates family members, may have had little experience with death in their own lives. Children often have little preparation about death in their family and, when death occurs, may be shielded from the experience rather than being included as a full member of the family facing a part of life that cannot ultimately be avoided. Thus, when confronted with death for the first time, families can find the experience difficult and challenging.

In addition, we have to consider the cultural, spiritual, educational, and historical backgrounds of families with which we are working. These factors influence styles of communication, values underlying treatment decisions, ability to confront death openly, rituals surrounding death and grief, and ways of grieving individually and collectively. For example, the family's communication patterns and ways of coping with distressful feelings influence how and with whom one communicates. Some families are very open in their communication patterns, with open sharing and discussion of events and feelings. Open families would tend to more easily talk about an impending death and process their feelings collectively. Other families may have limited or rigid communication rules and taboos about death. However, even open families may have a taboo or difficulties in openly discussing the death of a family member. Each family brings their own experiences with death to the present situation.

The HIV/AIDS epidemic stimulated research regarding the process of accepting death (Brown and Powell-Cope, 1993; Siegl and Morse, 1994; Powell-Cope, 1995). These studies highlight the complexity of the experiences of having a family member die. They also support the conclusion that it is not a linear process. Family members saw the loss of a family member as a major life transition requiring new coping strategies. Coping strategies include taking one day at a time, living fully in the present, actualizing future dreams, and keeping reality at a tolerable level.

An intergenerational and systems perspective provides a useful framework when working with families. This perspective suggests that each member of a family and the family as a whole system are affected by the illness and death of a family member. Furthermore, the intergenerational family should be considered as well as the nuclear family. Nowhere is this more evident than when families are called upon to make end-of-life decisions (Degner, 1995). An example is the family of an elderly man with Alzheimer's who is critically ill. The immediate family includes his elderly wife and three adult children who are called upon to make a decision about whether to stop treatment. In this case, the children are middle aged and live across the country. Making this decision is complicated by the fact that the mother is too distressed and wants the children to decide. The children are strangers to each other, having lived apart for years and having developed their own values and beliefs. Furthermore, they each have a unique and different relationship with their father. One sibling wants to stop treatment and let her father die in peace without more suffering. Another sibling wants treatment to continue at all cost. The third sibling is unable to decide and wavers back and forth. How this family resolves these issues and decides will have an impact on their family system for the remainder of their lives. The critical care nurse working with this family has a critical role in helping the family understand the severity of their husband/father's condition, share their grief, establish communication with each other, and make a decision that will help them heal and recover as a family.

In viewing death and dying within a family system perspective, the role of the dying person in the context of the family also must be considered. If the father whose employment is the main source of income is dying, the family may face issues regarding their financial security in the future. If a mother caring for children is dying, the family will be concerned about who is going to care for the children.

When a parent dies leaving behind young children, the responses and needs of the children are important to consider. However, it is difficult to face the idea that a child will suffer grief. As a result, adults may pretend children don't understand, don't know what happened, and therefore don't have feelings. The younger the child, the more this happens. In addition, surviving parents often have difficulty dealing with their children because of their own grief (Siegel et al, 1990). Increasingly, however, parents, families, health care professionals, educators, counselors, ministers, and others are trying to identify and meet the needs of a child when a parent is seriously ill or has died. Nurses have an important role in helping children and their parents deal with death. Interventions such as helping parents communicate honestly with the children, and guiding them in how to help the children understand the illness and death, to facilitate the sharing of feelings, and to help the children cope with their grief are useful in helping families deal with death.

Spirituality

Religious and spiritual beliefs are important issues for individuals who are coping with dying and for their families (Attig, 1995; Reed, 1987). At no time are individuals confronted more directly with their views about life and about death than when they are dying. Religion is a system of beliefs and the accompanying rituals and behaviors that interpret one's experiences and define proper conduct (Numbers and Amundsen, 1986). There are thousands of religious groups in the world and thus numerous complex and rich ways that individuals may view life and death. Some religious groups help one to accept death and embrace it, as with the focus on heaven as a peaceful place where one will be reunited with loved ones who have died, or reincarnation, which gives a sense of continued life in another form. Some religions create fear, as with the image of hell and fire as punishment. Other religions have ways of helping individuals avoid thoughts of death, as by focusing on prayer and rituals that seek a miracle cure with no acknowledgment of the possibility that one may not get the miracle and may die. Religious groups also have taboos and norms related to illness care, to dying, and to death. It is important to elicit from the individual or the family any specific needs related to religious beliefs.

Not all individuals adhere to a formal religion. Spirituality, on the other hand, is a dimension within every person that involves the deeper sense of self, the drive toward belonging and openness and love, and that search for the meaning of life and the forces that influence life (Reed, 1987). Thus, for all dying individuals of all ages the search for meaning in one's death and in one's life through relationships with others and through religion and spirituality is an important element of coping with death (Attig, 1995; Frankl, 1963). Nurses, with their close relationship to dying patients, often have the opportunity to help them with their spiritual search and to reinforce the religious meaning of their death.

Spirituality is also an important issue for families (Numbers and Amundsen, 1986). Some families adhere to beliefs that support continuation of treatment even with an obvious terminal condition because of the belief that only God is in charge of life and death. Other religious beliefs may limit the amount and type of medical treatments that can be agreed upon. Nurses must understand and respect the wide variety of religious backgrounds and spiritual beliefs they may encounter in families they are caring for. Most important is for nurses to be aware of their own beliefs and values, and not to impose personal beliefs on families in this time of crisis.

Culture and Ethnicity

The cultural background of the dying person and the family is a fundamental and important aspect of their being and behaving. Ethnicity refers to one's belonging in a particular social group with its own unique cultural and social system (Specter, 1996). Culture refers to the broader aspects of ethnicity. There are hundreds of ethnic groups and cultures in the United States alone. It is becoming increasingly important to recognize, understand, and accept individuals from widely diverse cultures as we provide nursing care. Unfortunately, there has been limited research about how different cultural groups respond to the dying process. Much of what we know comes from clinical observations and experiences coupled with anthropological and cultural research of a broader nature. Despite this lack of information, it is essential that the nurse caring for the dying patient consider the following issues when assessing patients:

- What do the patient and family identify as their ethnic or cultural heritage? To what extent are they embedded in this heritage?
- How do they, from the perspective of this heritage, perceive the family and its roles when dealing with illness and death?
- What, if any, are the religious or spiritual aspects of this heritage that may be important in coping with dying and death?
- How does this cultural or ethnic group, and this family in particular, view illness, treatment decisions, dying, death, and grief? How do individuals in this ethnic group cope with pain and suffering, and how does that fit with the patient and family in particular? What are their beliefs and practices? Are there any culturally prescribed or important rituals, customs, or needs that should be met for the patient or the family?
- What do patients and families from this ethnic or cultural group expect from health care professionals, particularly nurses and doctors?
- What resources are available in the community to help families from this ethnic or cultural group should their need for help become evident?

Type of Death and Setting

Responses to death and dying are also influenced by the type of death experienced, particularly whether the death is perceived as expected or sudden death (Kastenbaum, 1991). Death following a chronic illness or lifelong health problem usually involves a trajectory of gradual decline as evidenced by increasing complications, pain, and suffering (Strauss, 1994). This often involves such conditions as cancer, chronic heart disease, pulmonary disease including emphysema, progressive neurologic disorders including multiple sclerosis, and HIV/AIDS. Families of individuals dying following a chronic illness often grieve at the time of diagnosis and when symptoms reappear. Over time, they may experience anticipatory grief as they psychologically prepare themselves for the death (Rolland, 1990). Many feelings, including anger, guilt, fear, sadness, and depression, are associated with anticipatory grief (Rando, 1986). However, despite their long-term experience in coping with a chronic illness, families experience much uncertainty and lingering hope. Thus, death is not always expected or anticipated. Because of denial, difficulty accepting the illness and prognosis, or inadequate communication with the health care team, some families may not openly face the reality of the illness and may not talk about it. Daly and her colleagues (1996) found that the chronically critically ill who are admitted to the hospital often do not have do-not-resuscitate orders in their medical record. This was particularly true for those who are younger or are married.

Patients dying of a chronic illness may die in any setting, including an intensive care unit, general or specialized hospital unit, or nursing home, and nurses have a primary and critical role in caregiving in all settings. Nurses on hospital units are the most consistent and ever present health caregiver involved with the patient and family. Nurses in home health and hospice nursing are the critical link between the patient and family and the health care system.

Increasingly, patients dying of a chronic illness are sent home to die. The care of dying patients, whether at home or in an institution, has improved greatly with the advent of hospice programs of care.

Hospice

Hospice programs for care of the dying patient and his family have increased in number since the 1970s and are available in almost all areas of the country. These programs care for terminally ill patients of all ages from infants to the frail elderly. The principles of hospice care include open communication about death and dying, a focus on living fully and completely until death, death with dignity, adequate pain and comfort measures, and family-centered care (Corless, 1994; Martinson, 1995). Home care of dying patients allows the family to have the satisfaction of helping their loved one to die within the family home and of being in control of this care. Stresses associated with home care include dealing with intense symptom distress and dealing with the terminal event. Many hospice programs include inpatient respite care programs. Hospice care can also be provided in institutional settings by ensuring that hospice principles of care, particularly the focus on comfort measures rather than curative treatment, are carried out. Researchers have compared the costs of home care with hospital care. One such study (Birenbaum and Clarke-Steffen, 1992) provides an excellent conceptualization of costs of care. It is not surprising that home care costs are lower than hospital care costs. Yet, cost alone should not be the deciding factor about where care is provided.

Death also occurs suddenly, in accidents, homicide, and suicide, and following acute illness or surgery. Most sudden deaths occur in the emergency department or an intensive care unit (ICU). McClement and Degner (1995) point out the important role of the nurse in these situations, both in caring for the dying person and in helping the family. Expert nursing behaviors include providing physical and psychological care that reduces discomfort and creating a peaceful, dignified bedside scene. Nurses also help the family face the reality of the death, respond to their need for information, and support them in their grief. Family needs are particularly important because sudden death leaves the survivors stunned and highly distressed. There is no time to say goodbye, to make plans, to prepare oneself, and the grief that follows is difficult for everyone. Nurses responsibilities include maintaining family involvement with their family member who is dying or has died, keeping the family informed about the prognosis, pro-

RESEARCH HIGHLIGHT
PEDIATRIC HOSPICE CARE

In the 1970s, Ida Martinson and her colleagues, concerned about the way dying children were cared for in hospitals, conducted a demonstration study comparing the experiences of children dying in the hospital with those of children dying at home (Martinson, 1986). The program involved a program of education and support for families enabling them to care for their child at home for as long as they wished, coupled with an individualized program of support from volunteer nurses or health care agencies. The results of the demonstration project showed that families were able to manage the pain and other symptoms of their dying children, they were positive about their ability to be with their child and be in control of their child's care, and the dying children appreciated being able to remain with the family. Subsequently, other studies have reported positive experiences and outcomes of home care for the dying child (Lauer et al, 1983; Martinson, 1995). This includes parental satisfaction and adjustment and positive responses of siblings. In addition, hospice care has been found to be less costly (Martinson, 1995).

International nursing studies also have shown similar positive findings (Martinson, 1995). Recently a study conducted in Greece also supported the findings of Martinson and others (Papadatou et al, 1996). This study indicated that none of the families regretted their decision, while three of the five who opted for hospital care did have regrets. The mothers indicated the importance of availability of a physician and the presence and support of other health care team members, the availability of information and reassurance through regular telephone communication, the availability of medications at home, and someone to help with household chores.

Collectively, these studies conclude that caring for the terminally ill child at home is a desired alternative to hospitalization for some families. What is not known is what factors influence families to choose home care of a dying child, and what might be different about families who are unable to make this difficult decision.

As a result of Martinson's work and subsequent studies, home care of dying children has become a common program of care both in the United States and internationally. However, the care and support of professionals, including nurses, is an important component of such care. Home care for dying children is now commonly carried out through general hospice programs, specialized pediatric hospices, and home health programs of care.

viding nonjudgmental emotional support, and helping the family begin to share their grief (McClement and Degner, 1995). Nurses in critical care settings also often help families with difficult decisions about use of respirators, do-not-resuscitate orders, organ donation, autopsies, and funeral decisions that are complicated and emotionally intense.

Ethical Considerations

The rapid development of health care technology of today's hospital continues to create new problems and challenges. Many of these issues revolve around complex and difficult end-of-life decisions. These include decisions about whether or not to apply treatment that might temporarily prolong life and decisions to terminate treatments in the terminally ill that will end life. Such decisions are especially common regarding use of respirators, dialysis, and artificial nutrition and hydration, although many other treatments may be involved (Degner, 1995)

Nurses become involved in these end-of-life decisions in many settings. It is a responsibility of all nurses to help inform the public and their patients about the Patient Self-Determination Act, passed in 1991 (ANA, 1996) (see Box 35–1). This federal law applies to all health care institutions receiving Medicaid funds and requires that all individuals receiving medical care must be given written information about their rights, under state law, to make decisions about medical care, including the right to accept or refuse medical or surgical treatment. Individuals also must be given information about their rights to formulate advance directives such as living wills and durable powers of attorney for health care. Advance directives are legal forms, commonly called "living wills," which state what medical treatment an individual chooses to accept or refuse in the event that he or she is unable to make these decisions and is mortally ill (see Box 35–2). A durable power of attorney for health care appoints a proxy or agent, usually a relative or trusted friend, to make health decisions when one is unable to do so for oneself. It has broader applications than a living will. These directives are ideally completed when one is healthy, but nurses and others have a responsibility to determine whether they are completed and currently reflect the patient's choices whenever an individual is admitted to a health care institution.

BOX 35–1
POSITION STATEMENTS OF THE AMERICAN NURSES' ASSOCIATION ON END-OF-LIFE DECISIONS

- Assisted Suicide
- Foregoing Nutrition and Hydration
- Nursing and the Patient Self-Determination Acts
- Nursing Care and Do-Not-Resuscitate Decisions
- Promotion of Comfort and Relief of Pain in Dying Patients

American Nurses' Association (1996). Position Statements on Nurses and End of Life Decisions. Washington, DC.

RESEARCH HIGHLIGHT
GUIDELINES FOR SUPPORTING FAMILIES IN DECISION MAKING ABOUT LIFE-SUSTAINING CARE

Tilden and colleagues (1995), based on their research interviews with family members of patients without advance directives, developed guidelines for how to include and support families in decision making about life-sustaining technology. The guidelines include:

- offering effective communication that is timely, frequent, coordinated, and ongoing
- providing family-centered care that includes clarifying family membership and identifying the family spokesperson
- meeting with individual family members separately and with the family as a unit, facilitating the expression of grief
- assisting the family to reach consensus in making treatment decisions while keeping the focus on what the patient would have wanted
- continuing to give quality care to the dying family member with attention to comfort and dignity

Data from this study reflect the benefits of encouraging advanced planning for serious illness. As advances in medical technology lead to ever more "negotiable" deaths, the need grows for improved planning and enhanced communication relative to withdrawal of life-sustaining treatments.

Helping families of dying patients deal with difficult treatment decisions is another major role of the nurse (Degner, 1995; Jezewski, 1994). Decisions may be complicated when the person who is dying is unconscious, is no longer competent, or, as in the case of children, is not considered capable of making such decisions. In these situations the responsibility for decision falls on the surrogate decision maker, usually the spouse or parent or individual named as the power of attorney for health. Knowing the previous values and wishes of the adult patient is extremely helpful in making these decisions. With children, however, the decision making is complicated because one usually does not know what the infant or child would have wanted. The emotional distress of parents and others, and the desire to keep a child alive even when the burden of treatments is high and the ultimate outcome is known to be poor makes resuscitation and treatment decisions difficult (Fleishman et al, 1994).

BOX 35-2
ADVANCE DIRECTIVES: SOME DEFINITIONS

Advance directive: A set of directions that one gives in writing about the health care desired or not desired should one ever lose the ability to make decisions for oneself. Advance directives can be made through a living will or by naming someone who knows one's wishes as one's health care power of attorney.

Living will: A document that tells others what you do and do not want in terms of health care if you become terminally ill or incurably sick or are in a persistent vegetative state from which you will not recover. You can direct your doctor not to use heroic treatments that would delay your dying or to stop treatments if they have been started.

Health Care Power of Attorney: In a legal document, you name a person to make medical care decisions for you if you later become unable to decide yourself. This person is called your "health care agent." You can also say what medical treatments you would and would not want.

Nurses, particularly in ICUs, sometimes face ethical dilemmas concerning unclear or conflicting do-not-resuscitate (DNR) orders (ANA, 1996; Jezewski, 1994). DNR decisions should be made by the patient or the family if the patient is incapacitated in cooperation with the attending physician. The decisions must be recorded in the medical record, and reviewed and updated periodically to reflect changes in the patient's condition.

Likewise, the decision to withhold medically provided nutrition and hydration should be made by the patient or surrogate along with the health care team. Like all other interventions, medically provided hydration and nutrition, provided by nasogastric or gastrostomy tubes, may or may not be justified in the terminally or mortally ill. Ethical dilemmas occur when it is uncertain whether the provision of nutrition in this manner is more beneficial or burdensome. As with all other interventions, the anticipated benefits must outweigh the anticipated burdens for the intervention to be justifiable (ANA, 1996). Whether treatments are continued or discontinued or not started, the major role of the nurse is to keep the patient as comfortable as possible and to preserve dignity. Nevertheless, these complicated treatment decisions affect the nurse professionally and personally. If a nurse believes that her moral integrity is compromised by her professional responsibility to carry out a particular order for a patient, she should acknowledge her dilemma and transfer responsibility to another nurse. Many hospitals have ethics committees that can help nurses and family members with difficult decisions.

Increasingly a concern about issues surrounding assisted suicide has entered the political realm of debate (Daly et al, 1997; Tolle, 1997). Assisted suicide involves the act of aiding another person in ending his or her own life. The issue of assisted suicide reflects our values and beliefs as a society. Although numerous discussions and analyses in both the lay and professional press have critiqued the morality of as-

RESEARCH HIGHLIGHT
A CLINICAL TRIAL TO IMPROVE END-OF-LIFE DECISIONS

A controlled trial to improve end-of-life decision making and reduce the frequency of a mechanically supported, painful and prolonged process of dying in patients who were terminally ill was recently published (SUPPORT investigators, 1995). This 2-year prospective study involved 4301 patients in Phase I. Findings confirmed substantial shortcomings in the communication, frequency of aggressive treatment, and other problematic characteristics of hospital death, with few physicians aware of their patients preferences.

Phase II was a 2-year controlled clinical trial with 4804 patients and their physicians. For the clinical trial, patients were randomized into an intervention and control group. The intervention involved providing the physicians estimates of the likelihood of 6-month survival daily as well as other periodic data about outcomes and disabilities. Also, a specially trained nurse had multiple contacts with the patient, family, physician, and hospital staff to elicit preferences, improve understanding of outcomes, encourage attention to pain control, and facilitate care planning and patient-physician communication. Surprisingly, the intervention failed to improve care or patient outcomes. While the intervention nurses talked with most patients and/or families and communicated directly with the physicians as well as documenting patient preferences in the medical record, this information was not adequately used by physicians in making end-of-life care decisions for their patients. This suggests the need for nurses to more clearly identify their role and responsibility with patients and family and with their physicians regarding end-of-life decisions. There is certainly a need for greater professional and societal attention to this important problem.

sisted suicide, strong arguments continue to exist for and against it (Daly et al, 1997). The debate has entered the legal arena. On June 26, 1997, the Supreme Court decided to allow, rather than stifle, public debate on physician-assisted suicide. As noted by Chief Justice William Rehnquist, "Throughout the nation, Americans are engaged in an earnest and profound debate about the morality, legality, and practicality of physician-assisted suicide. Our holding permits this debate to continue, as it should in a democratic society."

Because of nurses' intense and close association with dying patients and their families, nurses must be knowledgeable about all of the legal and moral aspects of assisted suicide, especially as the issue is debated in the courts and weighed in state elections. The laws related to assisted suicide will vary from state to state, and will change over time as laws are challenged and changed. Of utmost importance is being aware of our responsibilities related to the issue of assisted suicide, particularly if it becomes legalized. Assisted suicide calls on nurses to think about their own moral values as well as the ethical principles of the profession. The ethical principles of respect for person, autonomy, beneficence, nonmaleficence, veracity, confidentiality, fidelity, and justice make assisted suicide a complicated moral issue for nurses. Some argue that the nursing duty of beneficence and the obligation to respect the autonomy of competent persons is a strong consideration in justifying assisted suicide (Daly et al, 1997). Others argue that reverence for life prohibits us from any acts that will bring about a death that would not otherwise occur (Daly et al, 1997). Other arguments against assisted suicide include creating an expectation among the terminally ill that they should minimize the burden on the family by choosing this option, abuse of vulnerable populations such as the elderly or those with diminished cognition, and slowing of efforts to improve the care of the dying.

Because of the complexity of the issues involved and the possible legalization of assisted suicide in some states, both the American Nurses' Association and the National League for Nursing have appointed task forces to explore the issues surrounding assisted suicide. The ANA has a position paper on assisted suicide (1996). The National League for Nursing has

RESEARCH HIGHLIGHT
CONFLICT REGARDING DO-NOT-RESUSCITATE STATUS

Jezewski (1994) completed a grounded theory study designed to describe the conflict experienced by critical care nurses during the process of consenting to do-not-resuscitate (DNR) status, as well as the strategies used in an attempt to prevent, minimize, and/or resolve these conflicts. Twenty-two critical care nurses were interviewed using a semi-structured in-depth interview.

Conflicts were both intrapersonal, inner conflict in coming to terms with a DNR decision, and interpersonal, conflict among family, patients, and staff involved in consenting to a DNR status. Nurses often saw themselves as a culture broker in trying to reduce these conflicts. They used advocacy, negotiation, mediation, and sensitivity to the patients' and families' needs. The authors conclude that critical care nurses play an active and important role in assisting patients and families with DNR decisions.

put out a paper, "Life-Terminating Choices: A Framework for Nursing Decision-Making" (May et al, 1997), which explores the issues surrounding assisted suicide for the individual nurse and the profession. Assisted suicide is and will continue to be an issue of utmost importance to nurses.

FUTURE DEVELOPMENTS

Over the past two decades, a number of influences have impacted on the care of the dying and bereaved. Prior to the 1960s and 1970s, dying patients were often not declared as terminally ill, painful treatments were continued when no longer effective, pain management was grossly inadequate, and there was little communication between the dying patient, the health care team, and the family about the impending death. Bereaved family members were given little help or support immediately after the death or over the long duration of their bereavement. During the 1960s and 1970s, sociologists, philosophers, and psychologists, along with professionals such as nurses, doctors, social workers, and ministers, became interested in the way death was covered up in our society and concerned about the way dying patients were treated (Benoliel, 1994). The efforts of these pioneering men and women led to the publication of important articles and books on death and grief, research related to the topic, and the inclusion of content related to death, dying, and grief in educational programs at all levels and in other settings such as churches. In addition, the hospice concept was imported from England to provide more humane care to dying patients and many support groups were started to provide assistance to individuals with terminal illness and to their families. Thus, the care of dying patients and their families has improved drastically in all settings.

Because of the increased capabilities to provide highly technological and pharmacologic treatments to individuals with serious illness, future developments related to death and dying will revolve around complicated end-of-life decisions. It will be important to continue to find effective approaches to helping individuals and families deal with end-of-life decisions. A related need is for nurses to help the public face issues related to death and end-of-life decisions and make plans regarding death while still healthy. Although there have been many educational programs regarding advance directives, Nolan and Bruder (1997) report that the number of patients choosing to write these documents remains low. Lack of understanding how or why to complete these documents, difficulty accepting death, and concerns about premature death or abandonment are factors that reduce their usefulness.

There is a strong need to know more about the symptom distress associated with dying and to develop and test interventions to reduce discomfort. When life-sustaining treatments are refused, the patient and family's concerns turn to issues related to the quality of comfort care for the patient.

The need for improved quality care to the dying has been highlighted by the recent debates about legalizing assisted suicide (Tolle, 1997). It has been argued that a strong impetus for legalized assisted suicide is the absence of clear direction in how we care for dying patients. The role of professionals, including nurses, regarding patient-requested assisted suicide will continue to be debated into the next decade (ANA, 1996).

A relatively new and growing issue that has complicated end-of-life care relates to health care financing, Medicare and Medicaid regulations, and managed care, resulting in increasing questions about what kinds of treatment for the terminally ill will be supported and about the financing of end-of-life care. For example, the Medicare hospice program allows 6 months of hospice care for an elderly person with a clear terminal condition. However, the program was developed based on a model for care of individuals with cancer where the course of illness and dying may be more accurately predicted. The program rules become problematic when the elderly person has other chronic but less predictable conditions such as heart disease.

Another major challenge that we are facing is learning how to give care to dying persons and their families from cultures and with religious beliefs that differ from the mainstream culture. Over the next decade, the number and type of ethnic minorities in our country will increase greatly. We know very little about how different ethnic groups cope with death, dying, and grief. More research is needed in this area and for cultural guidelines that deal with broad issues to enhance sensitivity to cultures different from our own.

NURSING CARE ACTIONS

Holistic nursing care to the dying patient must encompass both the physiologic and psychosocial domain of care (Corless, 1994). To ensure that medical and nursing care remains appropriate to the needs of each person, care at the end of life for all patients and their families must be individualized by considering how the individuals are coping and responding to their decline in health in the context of their unique personality and life experiences. As noted earlier, the symptoms associated with dying are diverse and depend on the underlying disease process. Interventions should address these symptoms with the goal of maximizing the comfort, decreasing the discomfort, and promoting the dignity and cognition of the dying patient. Symptoms of most concern include pain, fatigue, elimination, nausea and vomiting, nutrition and hydration, and respiratory distress (Corless, 1994; Martinson and Neelon, 1994).

Managing Pain

Effective pain control is a prerequisite for effective control of other physical and ultimately, psychosocial and spiritual symptoms in terminal patients. Uncontrolled pain in the terminally ill patient can result in hopelessness, depression, anger, fatigue and isolation, and the patient is unable to rest and sleep adequately. Unfortunately, control of pain remains inadequate and the public continues to be concerned about dying in pain. Inadequate pain management may be due to an inadequate understanding of the pain response and of pain management, and may also be related to attitudes regarding use of narcotics in our present drug culture. The key to intervention requires the treatment of the patient's total pain experience: physical, psychosocial, social, spiritual, and financial (Dalton and Fenerstein, 1988). Palliative care concepts leading to successful opioid analgesic therapy include keeping the treatment simple, preventing side effects, and assessing the patient's response frequently (Corless, 1994).

Pain can be divided into two broad categories: somatic/visceral (nociceptive) and neuropathic (deafferentation). These types of pain differ in their etiology, symptoms, and response to analgesics. Somatic/visceral pain arises from direct stimulation of afferent nerves due to tumor involvement of skin, soft tissue, or viscera. Somatic pain is often described as dull or aching and is well localized. Visceral pain tends to be poorly localized and is often referred to dermatomal sites distant from the source of pain. Common causes of somatic pain include bone and soft tissue metastases. Common causes of visceral pain include liver metastases causing capsular distension and biliary, bowel, or ureteral obstruction. Neuropathic pain results from injury to peripheral nerves rather than stimulation of nerve endings. Common causes of neuropathic pain include tumor invasion of the brachial or lumbosacral plexus, spinal nerve compression, herpes zoster infection or surgical interruption of nerves. Neuropathic pain is described as sharp, burning or shooting and is associated with paresthesias and dysesthesias (Cherney, 1998).

Assessment of pain in the dying patient is critical to facilitating optimal comfort. Pain assessment and management should be based on an understanding of the individual's personality and responses to treatment, coping style, and emotional response to dying (Cherney, 1998; Dalton and Fenerstein, 1988). Pain assessment involves doing a thorough assessment of the severity, pattern, duration, characteristics, and location of the pain. The nurse must elicit a thorough pain history including past and present pain experiences, prior and current medications, and the response to these medications, including time to onset of peak effect, duration of action, and side effects. An important aspect of the pain history is ascertaining the patient's pain relief goals. Ongoing pain assessments should be done at regular intervals and focus on intensity, quality, duration, and location. A 0 to 10 numeric scale to rate pain intensity (0 = no pain; 10 = worst pain imaginable) may be useful. In addition, it is vital to evaluate the effect of pain on the patient's mood, sleep patterns, eating, mobility, and activities of daily living. An important aspect of pain assessment is determining whether sleeping patterns are restful or are a coping response due to pain.

Many dying patients experience increased pain over time. Analgesic requirements may increase in the last week of life, and especially in the last 24 hours of life (Coyle et al, 1990). Thus, there is no optimal dose of pain medication that will help all patients. The proper dose is the dose that is effective in reducing pain and suffering (ANA, 1996). Pain medications should be given on a routine basis as well as added medication if the pain is not reduced adequately. Tolerance to pain medications may require high doses of medications to maintain adequate pain control. The ANA position statement on promotion of comfort and relief of pain in dying patients indicates that aggressive efforts to relieve pain in dying patients are an obligation of the nurse, who should not hesitate to use full and effective doses of pain medication (ANA, 1996). The increasing titration of medication to achieve control of pain, even at the expense of life, thus hastening death secondarily, is ethically justified. Thus, an important goal for pain management is to find the drug, the dose, and the route that is optimal for the patient. Titration of narcotics with frequent reevaluation and assessment is of most importance to maintain adequate comfort level (Bruera et al, 1990).

A wide variety of drugs can be given for pain management. The drug of choice depends on the type of pain being experienced by the patient, the effectiveness of a given drug or combination of drugs, and the level of side effects induced by the drugs. Opiates are a particularly effective class of drugs for pain management (Payne, 1998). When converting from one opiate to another, equianalgesic doses may be used to assure effective conversion.

Morphine is generally a very effective opiate for pain and is given in a variety of dosages and routes. There is a concentrated immediate release tablet and liquid solution. The liquid morphine is particularly useful for someone who is having difficulty swallowing because it can be dropped in the mouth and will be absorbed. Short-acting morphine is usually given about every 2 to 4 hours. One successful pain management program includes use of sustained-release morphine every 12 hours with supplemental short-acting morphine every 2 to 4 hours. The dose of the sustained-release morphine should be increased when the patient needs more than two or three doses of breakthrough medications a day. The breakthrough dose should be one third of the sustained-release dose.

Fentanyl transdermal patches represent the most recent addition to opioid pain management (Payne 1998). This is a rectangular transparent medicated patch that is applied to the skin, usually in the area of the upper chest. The patch provides a continuous systemic delivery of fentanyl, a potent opioid analgesic, for 72 hours. In addition to analgesia, alterations in mood, euphoria and dysphoria, and drowsiness commonly occur. Thus, fentanyl may increase the patient's tolerance for pain and decrease the perception of suffering. Fentanyl patches are often used in conjunction with other pain medications for breakthrough pain.

Oxycodone, a semisynthetic narcotic with an action similar to morphine, provides both analgesia and sedation. Oxycodone comes in tablets and liquid solution. It can be used as

PATIENT TEACHING
FOCUSING ON FAMILY NEEDS IN THE CARE OF THE DYING

The family is frequently the focus of teaching when caring for a dying person. The family needs to be prepared for pain management, providing good physical care, and attending to the dying person's and their own psychological health.

In the situation with Tom and Diane, the hospice nurse (Maureen) teaches Diane about the pain response, the purpose of pain medications, how to assess Tom's pain, and how to alter pain medications as needed. A related teaching objective is to prepare Diane to assess possible side effects from the pain medication, i.e., constipation, nausea and vomiting, and drowsiness. Included in this objective is information on preventing constipation through the use of stool softeners and dietary changes that increase the bulk in his diet.

As Diane is providing physical care to Tom, Maureen teaches her how to irrigate the catheter and change the dressings associated with his biliary drain. Attention is focused on preventing infection by use of aseptic wound care and frequent good hand washing. Maureen gives Diane some clues about teaching her daughters these procedures. She also demonstrates these techniques and observes Diane's techniques before moving on to another part of the teaching plan.

Maureen also provides Diane with written instructions and procedures because she knows that Diane is under stress and may not remember everything she was taught.

Maureen also assesses Tom's pain and physical condition on each visit, making certain Diane is able to implement care to achieve desired outcomes. She also calls in between visits to provide support and answer questions.

a single entity and may be considered in patients who are nauseated from other opiates.

Parenteral administration of opiates is not usually used unless oral medications cannot be given or are not effective. Opiates can be administered by either intravenous or subcutaneous route. Continuous (basal) administration with a delivery mechanism that can accommodate bolus injection is optimal to manage pain.

The prevention of side effects is critical to effective opioid analgesia. Nausea and constipation are the most common side effects. Other side effects include sedation, confusion, myoclonic jerks, seizure, and respiratory depression. Sedation and respiratory depression are often linked with narcotic use; however, it is more likely that the sedation and respiratory depression are more a consequence of the dying process than induced by narcotics, particularly very late in advanced illness.

Although drug therapies are the primary treatments for pain, patients with difficult or specialized pain problems may require alternative treatments. Decisions about the potential usefulness of these procedures should be made in consultation with pain management specialists. Low invasive procedures include application of heat or cold massage, transcutaneous electrical nerve stimulation (TENS) to areas of focal pain, trigger point injections, and acupuncture. These have little associated morbidity and are relatively inexpensive. In addition, behavioral techniques such as biofeedback, hypnosis, relaxation, imagery, music therapy or psychotherapy can be used. These can be very helpful to patients with episodic pain, pain related to specific activities, and pain in patients in whom loss of self-control is a distressing component of their pain.

Procedures of moderate invasiveness include nonneurolytic nerve blocks with local anesthetics or steroids, neurolytic blocks of peripheral, central or sympathetic nerves, or intrathecal and epidural administration of opioids with or without local anesthetics. These procedures pose more significant risks of complications, may require hospitalization, and are expensive. Procedures of high invasiveness include neurolytic blocks of the neuraxis, implantation of spinal cord stimulators, and neurodestructive procedures such as cordotomy, thalamotomy, and hypophysectomy. These are rarely indicated, carry considerable risk, and are expensive.

Successful pain management in the terminally ill child poses an enormous challenge to the health provider (Eland, 1989; Kachoyenos and Zollo, 1995). Although children of any age can and do experience severe pain, a child's ability to communicate will depend on his age, cognitive level, and social experience (Miles and Neelon, 1989). Young children may not have the conceptual skills or vocabulary to describe, quantitate, or localize pain. In addition they may not be willing to communicate their feelings to health care providers directly because of fear of injections. School-age children have more sophisticated cognitive abilities, social maturity, and communication skills to assist caregivers in assessing pain. However, they may have reservations about opioid analgesics for fear of becoming addicted. Assessment of pain in children is complicated and must involve attention to behavioral, physiologic, and psychological responses. Coffman and colleagues (1997) found that the pain indicators nurses most frequently use with children include physiologic changes such as increased heart, respiratory, and blood pressure rate; behaviors such as irritability and crying; and neuromuscular responses such as tenseness and rigidity, squirming, and drawing up the legs. In addition, the verbal responses of children are used. While children develop a rich and diverse vocabulary for describing pain as they mature, children of all ages can effectively use a rating scale such as the Oucher to rate their pain (Beyer, 1989). Parents play a critical role in pain management with the dying child. They have an important role in pain assessment, are knowledgeable about the most effective means of pain management, and are able to evaluate outcomes effectively. Pain management in children needs to follow the same principles as for adults. A child should not die in pain. The child needs to have adequate and effective medications that will reduce or stop pain. Like adults, they may need doses of narcotics that exceed the recommended dosage for routine use. In addition, distraction, guided imagery, relaxation, and other comfort measures may reduce the pain response in children.

Pain management in the elderly presents special challenges. The elderly are an at-risk group for the undertreatment of pain because of inappropriate beliefs about their pain sensitivity, pain tolerance, and ability to use opioids. Elderly patients, like other adults, require aggressive pain assessment and management. It has been estimated that the prevalence of pain in those older than 60 years of age (250 per 1000) is double that in those younger than 60 (125 per 1000) (Crook et al, 1984). Cognitive impairment and delirium, common among the sick elderly, pose serious barriers to pain assessment. Also a high prevalence of visual, hearing, and motor impairments in the elderly impede the use of traditional pain assessment tools. Thus, as with children, nurses need to assess behavioral, psychological, and physiologic responses of the elderly. Opioids are effective for the management of pain in most terminally ill elderly patients. In the elderly, Cheyne-Stokes respiratory patterns are not unusual during sleep and should not prompt the discontinuation of opioid analgesia. Elderly people tend to be more sensitive to the analgesic effects of opioids, experiencing higher peak effect and longer duration of pain relief (Kaiko, 1980).

Managing Fatigue

Fatigue, described by Piper (1989) as an overwhelming sustained sense of exhaustion and decreased capacity for physical and mental work, can be a major quality of life problem for the dying (Lichter, 1990). The actual mechanisms that produce fatigue are largely unknown (Piper, 1989). However, some of them include accumulation of metabolites caused by physical decline and cell destruction; changes in energy expenditure from the disease, anorexia, anemia, infection, and fever; changes in activity and rest patterns such as decreased mobility and increased physical dependence; and as a side effect of the overall disease process as well as drugs such as opioids, tranquilizers, and antidepressants (Piper, 1989). Interventions for the treatment of fatigue include frequent assessment and counseling with the patient and family as to how to pace and select activities, allow for rest periods, arrange for uninterrupted sleep, and set attainable goals. Medications can increase appetite and lead to gains in weight and strength in persons with advanced cancer.

Enhancing Elimination

Elimination is an important consideration in the care of the dying. Incontinence may occur secondary to the terminal illness or related to decreased cognitive status. Keeping the patient dry is important to prevent skin breakdown. The use of special diapers developed for adults who are incontinent is extremely useful. In addition, an indwelling catheter may be warranted if the patient cannot get out of bed, is uncomfortable using the diapers, or is not able to empty the bladder. There may be a decreased output of urine with some terminal conditions. In addition, due to the stasis of urine or use of a catheter, coupled with a compromised immune system, bladder infections may occur.

Constipation in the terminally ill patient is a common problem related to the use of opioids to manage pain. Neuroleptics, antidepressants, antihistamines, and other drugs can compound the problem. Immobility and decreased fluid and dietary intake also contribute to constipation. Untreated constipation may cause nausea and loss of appetite; it leads to abdominal distension, pain, and ultimately intestinal obstruction. Constipation must be aggressively prevented with a daily bowel regimen that includes a bowel stimulant, stool softener, increased fluids, and high fiber intake. It is important to keep track of bowel movements and make sure the patient has a bowel movement at least every two to three days. Use of suppositories, Therevac mini enemas, or manual disimpaction may be needed periodically.

Controlling Nausea and Vomiting

Nausea and vomiting are distressing symptom management problems for the terminally ill patient. Nausea and vomiting can be induced by a variety of clinical states such as slowing of the gastrointestinal system functions or tumor growth. The use of opiates for pain management is a common cause of nausea.

Nausea and vomiting related to medication can usually be controlled by adjusting the type, dose, or route of administration of medications. In addition, antacids or ulcer medications, such as ranitidine, given on a regular basis may help. Other interventions for the relief of nausea include pharmacologic treatment with antiemetics. Prochlorperazine, chlorpromazine, and haloperidol are effective antiemetics. Metoclopramide and scopolamine are other pharmacologic agents successfully used for the relief of nausea and vomiting. Relaxation, guided imagery, and distraction have been found to be effective in the control of symptoms. Other nursing interventions include small frequent snacks if the patient is able to tolerate food and fluids. The snacks should consist of foods and fluids that sound good to the patient. More often clear liquids are best tolerated. Oral care is extremely important when the patient is experiencing nausea and vomiting.

Vomiting caused by bowel obstruction is a common and distressing outcome of malignancies, particularly those within or metastatic to the peritoneal cavity (Ripamonti, 1994). This complication may arise at any time, but is more likely during the advanced stages of disease. The onset of obstruction is rarely an acute event. Symptoms gradually worsen until they become continuous, and their presence and intensity depends on the level involved. The symptoms, which are almost always present, are intestinal colic, abdominal distension with pain, visible peristalsis, anorexia, hepatomegaly, and vomiting. Vomiting can be intermittent or continuous. Bowel obstruction is a serious complication that necessitates decision making by the physician, nurse, patient, and family about whether to proceed with surgery or use some other palliative procedure, such as percutaneous gastrostomy, to relieve the symptoms.

Promoting Adequate Nutrition and Hydration

Terminally ill individuals commonly experience a slow or rapid decline in their interest in eating. Nutrition and fluids should be offered to the dying person in small amounts as often as they wish to try to eat. Food and fluids, however, should never become an issue between the patient and caregiver. Declines in eating and drinking are a normal part of the dying process. In a thoughtful essay about hydration in dying patients, Zerwekh (1997), an experienced hospice nurse and community health clinical nurse specialist, noted that we should expect a patient with advanced terminal illness who is within days of death to develop a fluid deficit. The patient typically drinks less because of an inability to swallow, nausea, loss of appetite, decreased energy, emotional withdrawal, and a reduced level of consciousness. The patient also may lose fluids from bleeding, vomiting, diarrhea, and other problems associated with the illness. This process is commonly called *terminal dehydration*. Signs include dry skin and mucous membranes, postural hypotension, low urine output, reduced tissue perfusion, and thickened secretions. The process involves multiple, complex physiologic changes that are an expected part of the dying process. The benefits of dehydration for the dying patient include concentrated urine with smaller volumes, decreased vomiting and nausea, diminished oral and airway secretions, less stool including diarrhea, and less edema and ascites. It has been hypothesized that the blood changes subsequent to terminal dehydration produce a natural analgesia in the last days of life. According to Zerwekh (1997), providing artificial hydration to dying patients may do more harm than good.

Artificial hydration and nutrition, nourishment and fluids provided by nasogastric or gastrostomy tubes or intravenous or central lines, are life-sustaining medical therapies with attendant risk and benefits, especially for the terminally ill. A recent review completed by the American Hospice Physicians addressed the clinical efficacy of artificial hydration and nutrition in relation to eight terminal diseases: end-stage heart, renal, lung, neurologic diseases, liver failure, cancer, immune system failure, bone marrow failure. With the exception of immune system failure, there is at present no convincing evidence of benefit from aggressive artificial hydration and nutrition in the dying process (Williams and Berry, 1996).

There are risks and burdens associated with artificial nutrition and hydration in the terminally ill patient. Advanced illness may be associated with malabsorptive states, and artificial nutrition can cause nausea and vomiting and may precipitate diarrhea or impactions. If the patient has a nasogastric or percutaneous enteral gastrotomy tube, local irritation around the tube, systemic infection, or aspiration can occur. With total parenteral nutrition, electrolyte imbalances can occur and phlebotomy carries risks of infection. With increased hydration, the patient may experience copious oral and airway secretions, causing increased respiratory distress. There may also be a risk of pulmonary edema and for some patients a persistence or worsening of edema and/or ascites. There will be larger urine volumes, increasing problems with incontinence. Dying individuals also may suffer from the intrusive procedures required to place and monitor tubes and lines in the body. Furthermore, they may experience embarassment related to the increased caregiving required by family members or the nurse (Zerwekh, 1997).

Some insist that fluids must be provided to all terminally ill patients to prevent "suffering." However, the concept of suffering from dehydration is from the perspective of the healthy person. The physiology of living, according to Zerwekh (1997) is very different from the physiology of dying. That terminally ill patients don't suffer as a result of dehydration was reported in a survey of hospice nurses by Andrews and Levine (1989). They found that 82 percent of hospice nurses disagreed with the statement "dehydration is painful." In addition, another hospice nurse researcher, Smith (1995) reported a high comfort level in a small group of hospice patients who were severely dehydrated and near death. Others have reported that the dying who are dehydrated do not experience thirst (Zerwekh, 1997).

One symptom that the dying who are dehydrated may experience is dry mouth. This may be caused by many other aspects of their illness and treatment. Discomfort from dry mouth should be relieved with sips of a favorite beverage, if possible, ice chips, popsicles, hard candies, or gauze soaked in ice water. Good mouth care is essential to prevent problems. Swabbing the mouth or gentle suctioning may be necessary to remove secretions. Brush the gums, teeth, and tongue with a soft toothbrush. Moisture enhancing solutions can be helpful, whereas drying agents such as alcohol, peroxide, and betadine should be avoided. Applying ointment to the lips will prevent cracking and drying.

When evaluating the benefits and burdens of artificial nutrition and hydration at the end of life, the question should be asked if the provision of nutrition and hydration will affect the length of the patient's life. The interventions comprising artificial hydration and nutrition may be indicated in the course of a terminal disease process as a therapeutic trial directed toward well-defined, realistic, achievable goals.

The amount of fat stores of the dying patient largely determines the length of life. Once fat stores are exhausted, protein stores are tapped, and rapidly progressive weakness ensues. From a normally nourished state, death due to depletion of calorie stores occurs in about 70 days. The relationship of the duration of dehydration and survival is uncertain. Factors include reduced fluid requirements due to metabolic changes and compensatory mechanisms and water production from the burning of fat. Of utmost importance is consideration of the effect of artificial nutrition and hydration on the quality of life on the dying patient (ANA, 1996).

Decisions about use of artificial nutrition and hydration do not lie with the nurse. Rather, they are made by the patient and family in conjunction with the physician. As medical therapies, artificial nutrition and hydration should be instituted only after obtaining proper informed consent. However, nurses have a major role in influencing these decisions directly or through their support of the patient and family. The nurse assesses the physiologic and psychological status of the patient, and determines the views of the patient and the family. Home health and hospice nurses, with their personalized contact with the patient in the home, have a major role in helping the patient and family with these issues. It is often the home health or hospice nurses' recommendations based on their assessments that are followed by attending physicians. One of the most difficult areas of decision in this realm has to do with stopping artificial nutrition in a terminally ill patient. It is more difficult to withdraw a treatment than to decide not to use it. However, the same principles of burden and benefit apply to decision making about withdrawing treatment.

It is vital that the nurse caring for dying patients be aware of the position statement of the American Nurses Association on Foregoing Nutrition and Hydration (1996). This position statement clarifies issues related to benefits and burdens, and clarifies the moral code for nurses in this realm. Of utmost importance is the focus on identifying the patient's own wishes in regard to decisions about initiating or stopping artificial nutrition and hydration.

Managing Respiratory Distress

Respiratory distress, shortness of breath and dyspnea are common symptoms in the terminally ill. Respiratory distress occurs in approximately 29 to 74 percent of patients with terminal cancer and also occurs in the terminally ill patient with other diseases such as end-stage cardiac disease, emphysema, and other pulmonary diseases. Other conditions such as anemia and neuromuscular disease are associated with dyspnea at the end of life. Respiratory distress often occurs as part of the terminal events in the dying process.

Dyspnea is a subjective uncomfortable awareness of difficulty in breathing (Wasserman and Casaburi, 1988). It is important to ask the patient or family about the degree of dyspnea and the associated distress. The nurse also assesses dyspnea or respiratory distress by observing the depth and rate of respirations, the color of the person's skin, the amount of respiratory effort, and facial changes such as pursing of the lips or flaring of the nostrils.

Medications can decrease the effort of breathing and reduce dyspnea. The administration of bronchodilators, theophylline, and corticosteroids can help relieve dyspnea and may be administered in an attempt to manage respiratory distress. Morphine is an effective medication to help decrease dyspnea by suppressing respiration and also providing sedation. Studies suggest that morphine was able to decrease the intensity of dyspnea without statistically modifying the oxygen saturation level in the blood, the respiratory rate, or overall exchange of air (Bruera et al, 1990). Administration of oxygen may also reduce respiratory distress. The use of oxygen and nebulized morphine has had some therapeutic benefit in terminally ill AIDS and chronic obstructive pulmonary disease patients.

Dyspnea is perceived as one of the most devastating symptoms by the patient and family. As a result, patients can experience intense anxiety or depression (Gift, 1990). To decrease psychological discomfort associated with dyspnea, an antidepressant or antianxiety drug may be ordered. Benzodiazepines such as lorazepam are particularly effective. In addition, opiates given to treat dyspnea also provide a sedative and calming effect that can help. Relaxation and psychophysical techniques have been found helpful in relieving dyspnea (Gift et al, 1992). Using individualized relaxation tape recordings during times of panic when dyspnea occurs has a calming and therapeutic effect. Other psychophysiologic techniques include meditation, visual imagery, and yoga. Fresh air and fans are simple interventions that can be helpful. Energy conservation, activity modification including advanced planning, and decrease in activities are also practical interventions.

Addressing Psychosocial Aspects of Care

Care of the dying patient also must focus on psychosocial aspects of care. This includes maintaining function and encouraging autonomy for as long as possible. Thus, dying patients should be encouraged to ambulate and engage in favorite activities to the extent possible, and to have visitors to the extent desired. The individual coping pattern of the individual is respected and the person is helped to find a search for meaning (Frankl, 1963) in his or her final days. The dignity of the individual should be maintained by completing invasive and embarassing procedures in privacy and with an attitude of acceptance. Clean bedclothes, sponge baths or showers, and skin care are important in increasing comfort and positive feelings. Aggressive care, such as cardiopulmonary resuscitation or intravenous fluids, should not be initiated unless specifically desired by the patient. There should be opportunities for the individual to talk with the nurse and/or with family members about feelings and worries associated with dying. Spiritual needs should be evaluated with referrals, if necessary, to the chaplain or family minister or rabbi. Most importantly, most patients want assurance that they will not be isolated or die alone.

Family Care

Nursing care of the dying patient always involves care of the family. Nurses work closely with the family in plan-

CLINICAL DECISION MAKING
A CASE STUDY IN HOME CARE OF THE DYING

SITUATION

Tom has reached the point with his cancer that he now has peritoneal and hepatic involvement with significant ascites (accumulation of fluid in the peritoneal cavity) and edema (the body tissues contain an excessive amount of tissue fluid). His pain is severe although it can be managed with the fentanyl patch and liquid morphine. Diane has had to quit her jobs and devote herself to his care. She tells Maureen, the hospice nurse, that she is concerned that Tom is not eating and has even stopped taking juices and ice chips. There is a steady decline in his physical state with progressive weakness; he is very drowsy and sleeps most of the time. Diane is worried about her husband dying of dehydration and starvation. She asks about whether they should be giving him a feeding tube or intravenous fluids.

CLINICAL QUESTIONS

As Maureen listens to Diane's observations and concerns, she considers these clinical questions:

- What might be the physiologic basis for Tom to stop eating and drinking?
- What is likely to happen to him in the near future as a result of his illness and nutritional status?
- What might some of the issues be for Diane regarding Tom and eating?
- What would be the benefits and burdens of artificial nutrition and/or hydration for Tom?
- How should Tom be involved in discussing these issues?
- What are some of the ways of approaching a discussion with Tom and Diane about his present health status and prognosis?

DECISION MAKING

Maureen thinks about these questions in the context of the care plan already established with Diane's and Tom's input. The main objective of that plan is to assist Diane provide excellent care to Tom including pain management and physical care.

Another goal of that plan is encouraging Tom to remain as active as he can, despite his fatigue. Maureen helps Diane understand the need to be active and independent for as long as possible. She problem solves with Maureen and Tom about what he would like to do on a daily basis and helps them develop a schedule that combines activity and rest throughout the day.

One of Maureen's goals is to help Tom cope with his illness, to make him feel as important as she can, and to help him see ways in which his life had importance and meaning. To accomplish this, Maureen allows time to listen to his feelings about his illness and impending death. She also encourages Tom to talk about his life and then points out the positives of what he has achieved or done for others, particularly his wife and daughters, Jane and Jennifer.

Maureen's nursing care of Jane and Jennifer focuses on establishing trust with them, sensitively helping them to ask their questions or share their concerns, letting them know what is being done for their dad, reinforcing their importance to their father, and helping them see how they can help their dad.

Maureen is aware that as Tom's condition deteriorates, she will have to prepare Tom, Diane, Jane, and Jennifer for his dying. This involves knowledge of what to anticipate, what to do, whom to call, and information about the hospice social worker and chaplain. She knows that she and other members of the hospice team will help the family express their grief.

Maureen provides Diane with information about the benefits and burdens of artificial nutrition for Tom. With Diane's agreement, Maureen sets up a clinical conference with the hospice team and Maureen to reach a decision about artificial nutrition. The complex nature of the decision to provide or not to provide artifical nutrition to Tom leads Maureen to conclude that it warrants an interdisciplinary perspective.

ning the care for the patient and in helping the family implement the care, to the extent desired and possible. Nurses also help the family cope with their distress related to the dying process, to share their feeling of grief and loss, and to identify ways of communicating within the family about the death. Nurses have an important role in helping the family anticipate what will happen to the patient as the dying process unfolds and in knowing what to do at the time of death. This is especially important when the patient is being cared for at home.

Nurses have a vital role in helping families grieve at the time of death, because no matter how much the death was anticipated, it only becomes real when it occurs. Many institutions and all hospices have bereavement care programs for reaching out to families after death.

Care After Death

Nurses are generally involved in helping families at the time of and following death. They are also responsible for helping the patient during the final hours and preparing the body after death. Every agency and institution has procedures that need to be followed during and following the death of a patient.

In the final hours, it is important to provide comfort measures, especially those that involve gentle touch, adequate pain and antianxiety medications, and mouth care. It is important to maintain a calm and peaceful environment for the patient. If the family is providing care, the nurse helps the family understand how to care for the patient and what to

BOX 35-3
ORGANIZATIONS CONCERNED ABOUT CARE OF THE DYING

Choice in Dying
200 Varick Street
New York, NY 10014-4810
212-366-5540 or 1-800-989-9455
cid@choices.org

Hospice Association of America
228 Seventh Street SE
Washington, DC 20003
202-546-4739

Hospice Nurses Association
211 North Whitfield Street
Medical Center East, Suite 375
Pittsburgh, PA 15206-3031
412-361-2470
hnafan@usa.pipeline.com

expect regarding the terminal event. Death may occur peacefully with only a moderate amount of physical distress, or it may be accompanied by intense physical distress such as acute respiratory distress, bleeding, or convulsions. The nurse can usually anticipate the amount and type of distress and help the family be prepared. Usually the patient will be in a semiconscious state near the end of life, but may still hear, as it is thought that hearing may be the last sense to go. Thus, the family may wish to talk to the dying person, play favorite music, pray, or read from religious books.

At the time of death, secretions should be wiped from the mouth. The head of the bed is placed down, the eyes closed, and a towel placed under the chin to help close the mouth. Tubes are removed unless the patient is going to have an autopsy or is a medical examiner's case. The body may be prepared by a gentle washing. It is not uncommon for the patient to be incontinent of urine or stool so the genital area should be cleaned. After the body is prepared, the family may want to have time alone with the deceased.

In home care, the family is instructed to call the hospice or home health nurse when the patient is dying or has died. The nurse declares the patient as deceased and calls the physician. The nurse also helps the family with their grief and helps them to call the funeral home. In the hospital, the physician is called to declare the patient as deceased. The family, if they are not present, is called. The body is not removed until the family has arrived and has fulfilled their need to be with the deceased, as this is an important time for grieving and closure. The body is then taken, usually by the nursing staff, to the morgue until the funeral home representative arrives. Sometimes an autopsy may be conducted if the family agrees and the physician is interested in learning more about the cause of death. Cases of sudden death or unexplained death as well as suicide and murder become cases for the medical examiner or coroner. In these cases, the body is first taken to the county or state medical examiner's office before being released to the family.

CHAPTER HIGHLIGHTS

- Care of the dying patient and family involves a complex array of interventions that focus on both the physical and psychosocial dimensions of care.
- Control of pain and other physical symptoms is essential.
- Supporting the patient and family through their transition is also critical.
- Although care of dying patients is a challenge for the nurse, it also can be rewarding both personally and professionally.
- Excellent care is invaluable to both the patient who is in the process of dying and to the family who is left with their memories and their grief.
- Professional nursing organizations have developed position papers and guidelines to assist nurses with complex issues such as assisted suicide.

REFERENCES

American Nurses' Association (1985). *Code for Nurses with Interpretive Statements.* Kansas City, MO: Author.

American Nurses' Association (1995). *Nursing: A Social Policy Statement.* Washington, DC.

American Nurses' Association (1996). *Position Statements on Nurses and End of Life Decisions.* Washington, D.C.: Author.

Andrews, M., Levine, A. (1989). Dehydration in the terminal patient: Perception of hospice nurses. *American Journal of Hospice Care, 6,* 31–34.

Attig, T. (1995). Respecting the spirituality of the dying and bereaved. In I.B. Corless, B.B. Germino, and M. Pittman (eds.): *A Challenge for Living: Dying, Death, and Bereavement.* Boston: Jones and Bartlett Publishers, pp. 117–130.

Becker, E. (1973). *The Denial of Death.* New York: The Free Press.

Benoliel, J.Q. (1994). Death and dying as a field of inquiry. In I.B. Corless, B.B. Germino, and M. Pittman (eds.): *Dying, Death, and Bereavement: Theoretical Perspectives and Other Ways of Knowing.* Boston: Jones and Bartlett Publishers, pp. 15–30.

Beyer, J.E. (1989). The Oucher: A pain intensity scale for children. In S.G. Funk, E.M. Tornquist, M.T. Champagne, et al (eds.): *Key Aspects of Comfort: Management of Pain, Fatigue, and Nausea.* New York: Springer Publishing Company, pp. 65–71.

Birenbaum, L.K., Clarke-Steffen (1992). Terminal care costs in childhood cancer. *Pediatric Nursing, 18* (3), 285–288.

Brown, M.A., Powell-Cope, G. (1993). Themes of loss and dying in caring for a family member with AIDS. *Research in Nursing and Health, 16,* 179–191.

Bruera E., MacMillian K., Pither J., MacDonald R.N. (1990). Effects of morphine on the dyspnea of terminal cancer patients. *Journal of Pain and Symptom Management, 5,* 341–344.

Cairns, R.B., Cairns, B.D. (1994). *Lifelines and Risks: Pathways of Youth in Our Time.* New York: Cambridge University Press.

Cherney, N.I. (1998). Cancer pain: Principles of assessment. In A. Beyer, R.K. Portenoy, and D.E. Weissman (eds.), *Principles and Practices of Supportive Oncology.* Philadelphia: Lippincott-Raven. 3–59.

Coffman, S., Alvarez, Y., Pyngolil, M., et al (1997). Nursing assessment and management of pain in critically ill children. *Heart and Lung, 26,* 221–228.

Corless, I.B. (1994). Dying well: Symptom control within hospice care. In J.J. Fitzpatrick and J.S. Stevenson (eds.): *Annual Review of Nursing Research, Vol. 12.* New York: Springer Publishing Company.

Cousins, N. (1979). *The Anatomy of an Illness as Perceived by the Patient.* New York: W.W. Norton & Company.

Coyle, N., Adelhardt, J., Foley, K.M., Portenoy, R.K. (1990). Character of terminal illness in the advanced cancer patient: Pain and other symptoms during the last four weeks of life. *Journal of Pain and Symptom Management, 5,* 83–93.

Crook, J., Rideour, E., Browne, G. (1984). The prevalence of pain complaints in a general population. *Pain, 18,* 299–324.

Dalton, J., Fenerstein, M. (1988). Biobehavioral factors in cancer pain. *Pain, 33,* 137–147.

Daly, B.J., Berry, D., Fitzpatrick, J.J., et al (1997). Assisted suicide: Implications for nurses and nursing. *Nursing Outlook, 45,* 209–214.

Daly, B.J., Gorecki, J., Sadowski, A., et al (1996). Do-not-resuscitate practices in the chronically critically ill. *Heart and Lung, 25,* 310–317.

Davies, B., Eng, B. (1993). Factors influencing nursing care of children who are terminally ill: A selective review. *Pediatric Nursing, 19,* 9–13.

Degner, L.F. (1995). Treatment decision making. In I.B. Corless, B.B. Germino, and M. Pittman (eds.): *A Challenge for Living: Dying, Death, and Bereavement.* Boston: Jones and Bartlett Publishers, pp. 3–16.

Durham, E., Weiss, L. (1997). How patients die. *American Journal of Nursing, 97* (12), 41–46.

Eland, J.M. (1989). Pharmacologic management of pain. In B. Martin (ed.): *Pediatric Hospice Care: What Helps.* Los Angeles: Children's Hospital.

Fleishman, A.R., Nolan, K., Dubler, N.N., et al (1994). Caring for gravely ill children. *Pediatrics, 94,* 433–439.

Frankl, V. (1963). *A Man's Search for Meaning: An Introduction to Logotherapy.* New York: Washington Square Press.

Germain, C.P. (1980). Nursing the dying: Implications of Kubler-Ross' Staging Theory. *Annals of the American Academy of Political and Social Science, 447,* 46–58.

Gift, A.G. (1990). Dyspnea. *Nursing Clinics of North America, 25,* 955–965.

Gift, A.G., Moore, T., Soeken, K. (1992). Relaxation to reduce dyspnea and anxiety in COPD patients. *Nursing Research, 41,* 242–246.

Glaser, B.G., Strauss, A.L. (1965). *Awareness of Dying.* Chicago: Aldine.

Guisewell, C.W. (1980). Small voices pierce death's veil. *Kansas City Star,* April 30, 1980, p. 2A.

Henderson, V. (1978). The concept of nursing. *Journal of Advanced Nursing, 3,* 113–130.

Hunt, M. (1992). "Scripts" for dying at home—displayed in nurses', patients' and relatives' talk. *Journal of Advanced Nursing, 17,* 1297–1302.

Jezewski, M.A. (1994). Do-not-resuscitate status: Conflict and culture brokering in critical care units. *Heart and Lung, 23,* 458–465.

Kachoyenos, M.K., Zollo, M.B. (1995). Ethics in pain management of infants and children. *Maternal-Child Nursing Journal, 20,* 142–147.

Kaiko, R.F. (1980). Age and morphine analgesia in cancer patients with post operative pain. *Clinical Pharmacology and Therapeutics, 28,* 823–826.

Kapel, S. (1974). Dying boy's letter pleads for empathy. *Kansas City Times,* March 8, 1974.

Kastenbaum, R. (1991). *Death, Society, and Human Experience.* NY: Merrill.

Kubler-Ross, E. (1969). *On Death and Dying.* New York: Macmillan.

Lauer, M.E., Mulhern, R.K., Wallskog, J.M., Camitta, B.M. (1983). A comparison study of parental adaptation following a child's death at home or in the hospital. *Pediatrics, 1,* 107–112.

Leahey, M., Wright, L.M. (1987). *Families and Life-Threatening Illness.* Springhouse, PA: Springhouse Corporation.

Lichter, I. (1990). Weakness in terminal illness. *Palliative Medicine, 4,* 73–80.

Lipson, M. (1993). What do you say to a child with AIDS? *Hastings Center Report, 23,* 6–12.

Martinson, I.M., Moldow, D.G., Armstrong, G.D., et al (1986). Home care for children dying of cancer. *Research in Nursing and Health, 9,* 11–16.

Martinson, I.M. (1995). Pediatric hospice care. *Annual Review of Nursing Research 13,* 195–214.

Martinson, I., Neelon, V. (1994). Physiological characteristics of dying and death. In I.B. Corless, B.B. Germino, and M. Pittman (eds.): *Dying, Death, and Bereavement: Theoretical Perspectives and Other Ways of Knowing.* Boston: Jones and Bartlett Publishers, pp. 15–30.

May, B., Anthony, A.L., Neil, R.M., and Todd, B. (1997). Life-terminating choices: A framework for nursing decision making. *Nursing and Health Care Perspectives, 18,* (4), 198–204.

McClement, S.E., Degner, L.F. (1995). Expert nursing behaviors in care of the dying adult in the intensive care unit. *Heart and Lung, 24,* 408–419.

Miles, M.S., Neelon, V. (1989). Approaches to pain in infants and children: A discussion. In S.G. Funk, E.M. Tornquist, M.T. Champagne, et al (eds.): *Key Aspects of Comfort: Management of Pain, Fatigue, and Nausea.* New York: Springer Publishing Company, pp. 105–117.

Mullins, I.L. (1996). Nursing caring behaviors for persons with acquired immunodeficiency syndrome/human immunodeficiency virus. *Applied Nursing Research, 9,* 18–23.

Nolan, M.T., Bruder, M. (1997). Patients' attitudes toward advance directives and end-of-life treatment decisions. *Nursing Outlook, 45,* 204–208.

Nuland, S.B. (1993). *How We Die.* New York: Alfred A. Knopf.

Numbers, R., Amundsen, D.W. (1986). *Caring and Curing: Health and Medicine in the Western Religious Traditions.* New York: Macmillan Publishing Company.

Papadatou, D., Yfantopoulos, J., Kosmidis, H.V. (1996). Death of a child at home or in hospital: Experiences of Greek mothers. *Death Studies, 20,* 215–235.

Pasero, C.L., McCaffrey, M. (1997). Breakthrough pain with the fentanyl patch. *American Journal of Nursing, 97* (12), 18–20.

Pattison, M. (1967). The experience of dying. *American Journal of Psychotherapy, 21,* 32–43.

Payne, R. (1998). Pharmacologic management of pain. In A. Beyer, R.K. Portenoy, and D.E. Weissman. *Principles and Practices of Supportive Oncology.* Philadelphia: Lippincott-Raven. 61–75.

Piper, B.F. (1989). Fatigue: Current bases for practice. In S.G. Funk, E.M. Tornquist, M.T. Champagne, et al (eds.): *Key Aspects of Comfort: Management of Pain, Fatigue, and Nausea.* New York: Springer Publishing Company, pp. 187–198.

Powell-Cope, G.M. (1995). The experiences of gay couples affected by HIV infection. *Qualitative Health Research, 5* (1), 36–62.

Preston, F., McCorkle, R. (1995). Philosophy, principles and politics of symptom management for the terminally ill. In I.B. Corless, B.B. Germino, and M. Pittman (eds.): *A Challenge for Living: Dying, Death, and Bereavement.* Boston: Jones and Bartlett Publishers, pp. 17–36.

Rando, T. (1986). *Loss and Anticipatory Grief.* Lexington, Kentucky: Lexington Books.

Reed, P. (1987). Spirituality and well-being in terminally ill hospitalized adults. *Research in Nursing and Health, 10,* 334–344.

Ripamonti, C. (1994). Management of bowel obstruction in advanced cancer patients. *Journal of Pain and Symptom Management, 9,* 193–200.

Rittman, M., Paige, P., Rivera, J., et al (1997). Phenomenological study of nurses caring for dying patients. *Cancer Nursing, 20* (2), 115–119.

Rolland, J.S. (1990). Anticipatory loss: A family systems developmental framework. *Family Process, 29,* 229–244.

Shneidman, E.S. (ed.) (1984). *Death: Current Prospectives.* Mountain View, CA: Mayfield Publishing Company.

Siegel, K., Raveis, V.H., Bettes, B., et al (1990). Perceptions of parental competence while facing the death of a spouse. *American Journal of Orthopsychiatry, 70, 567–576.*

Siegel, D., Morse, J.M. (1994). Tolerating reality: The experience of parents of HIV positive sons. *Social Science and Medicine, 38,* (7):959–971.

Smith, S.A. (1995). Patient induced dehydration: Can it ever be therapeutic? *Oncology Nursing Forum, 22,* 1487–1491.

Specter, R.E. (1996). *Cultural Diversity in Health and Illness,* 4th ed. Stamford, CT: Appleton & Lange.

Steeves, R., Cohen, M.Z., Wise, C.T. (1994). An analysis of critical incidents describing the essence of oncology nursing. *ONF Supplement, 21* (8), 19–25.

Strauss, A. (1994). Chronic illness, the health care system, AIDS, and dying. In I.B. Corless, B.B. Germino, and M. Pittman (eds.): *Dying, Death, and Bereavement: Theoretical Perspectives and Other Ways of Knowing.* Boston: Jones and Bartlett Publishers, pp. 15–30.

SUPPORT investigators. A controlled trial to improve care for seriously ill hospitalized patients: The study to understand prognoses and preferences for outcomes and risks of treatment. *Journal of the American Medical Association, 274,* 1591–1598.

Tilden, V., Tolle, S., Garland, M., Nelson, C. (1995). Decisions about life-sustaining treament: Impact of physicians behaviors on the family. *Archives of Internal Medicine, 155,* 633–638.

Tolle, S.W. (1997). *How Oregon's Physician-Assisted Suicide Law Spurs Improvements in End-of-Life Care.* Grantmakers Concerned with End of Life Care, 888 Seventh Avenue, New York, NY: 10106.

Wasserman, K., Casaburi, R. (1988). Dyspnea: Physiological and pathophysiological mechanisms. *Annual Review of Medicine, 39,* 503–515.

Weisman, A.D. (1972). *On Dying and Denying: A Psychiatric Study of Terminality.* New York: Behavioral Publications, Inc.

Williams, C., Berry, Z. (1996). Artificial hydration and nutrition in the terminally ill. Paper presented at the annual assembly of American Academy of Hospice and Palliative Medicine, June 13, 1996. Snowbird, UT:

Zerwekh, J.V. (1997). Do dying patients really need IV fluids? *American Journal of Nursing, 97,* 26–31.

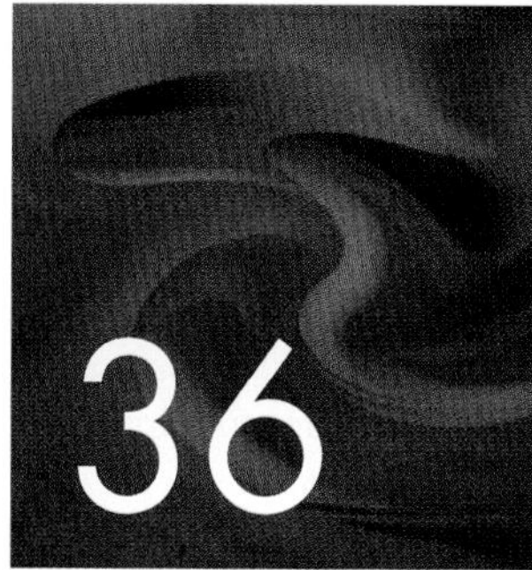

Health Promotion and Self-Care

36

Katherine Crabtree and Julia Brown

Mrs. Walker, a 45-year-old office manager and divorced mother, has come to the clinic of her health maintenance organization for a health checkup after a free workplace screening revealed that her blood pressure was high. Today her blood pressure is slightly elevated, as it has been on two previous visits. She has no other signs or symptoms of hypertension, her heart rate and rhythm are normal, and she reports she is in good health and takes no medication. She attributes her high blood pressure to stress from her job and family life. She works 60 hours a week while caring for two teenage sons and her father, who is recovering from a recent stroke. She worries about the rising cost of college tuition for her sons, and the costs of caring for her father. She would like to retire at age 65 and travel.

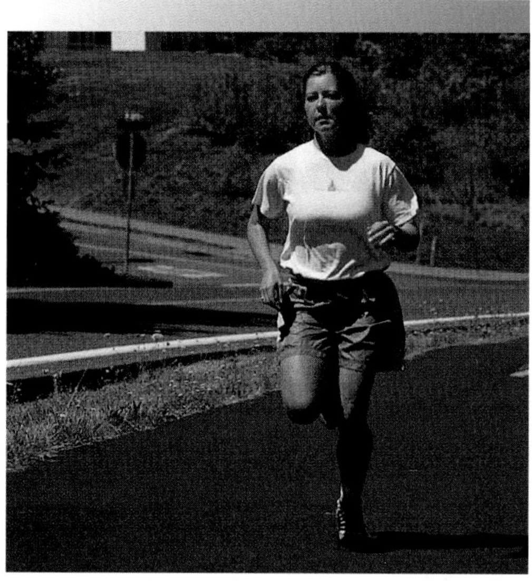

Mrs. Walker's family history reveals that her mother died of a heart attack at age 55. Her father has been treated for hypertension for many years and suffered a stroke at age 67. Mrs. Walker's own lifestyle involves health risks. She has smoked two packs of cigarettes a day for the past 22 years, and she consumes a moderate amount of alcohol. The family diet is high in calories and animal fat, a source of cholesterol, and she and her sons eat at fast food restaurants frequently. She does not exercise regularly. She says she enjoys camping with her sons, but they have not been hiking or camping for the past 6 months. Instead, her sons play video games after school and watch sports on television every weekend for hours at a time. Mrs. Walker expresses a desire to change the family's sedentary lifestyle.

OBJECTIVES

After studying this chapter, students will be able to:

- **assess an individual's health habits for health promotion, disease prevention, and self-care**
- **use a holistic framework for developing a health promotion plan of care**
- **analyze their own health behaviors in terms of serving as a role model for others**
- **modify patient education strategies to incorporate factors associated with health education outcomes**
- **participate in health screening activities**

SCOPE OF NURSING PRACTICE

What is health promotion, what is self-care, and of what concern are they to nurses? Health promotion has been defined as the performance of activities and practices to prevent disease and enhance health. Self-care refers to the activities that individuals handle themselves to prevent disease, promote health, limit illness, and restore functioning. These activities may be based on technical knowledge and skills derived from a wide array of professional and lay sources, but the "generic attribute of self-care is its nonprofessional, nonbureaucratic, nonindustrial character" (Levin and Idler, 1983, p. 181).

Health promotion programs take many forms, depending on how health is defined. Programs are more restricted in scope when health is defined as the absence of physical disease than when a broader definition is accepted. Most nurses subscribe to a broad view of health as encompassing the individual's functioning in the biologic, psychological, and social spheres. That definition closely resembles the one adopted by the World Health Organization (WHO), which designates health as "a state of complete physical, mental, and social well-being, not merely the absence of disease or infirmity" (1948). Broad views of health call for comprehensive programs including a wide variety of preventive, health protective, and health promoting measures. In 1978, WHO affirmed a goal of *Health for All by the Year 2000* (see Box 36–1).

In the United States, health promotion efforts have been directed to all five areas listed in the WHO charter, but the major focus has been on the development of personal skills for healthier living. One reason for this emphasis is the "do-it-yourself" propensity of the American people, expressed in the field of health as self-care. Self-care has always been the main form of primary health care (Wolinsky, 1980). In the 1970s a movement arose among laypersons to expand self-care into areas that at that time were controlled by professionals. This movement was fueled by disillusion with professional medicine, fear of illnesses induced by medical treatment, and the desire of people to reclaim personal control over their lives and health (DeFriese et al, 1989).

Although some health professionals today may oppose this trend, most approve a more active role for Americans in their own health care (U.S. DHHS, 1990). In nursing, self-care is believed to be the cornerstone of health promotion, and a major nursing goal is to encourage it. In nursing practice textbooks, nurses are urged to foster self-care in patients by providing information about nutrition, sleep, exercise, stress management, sexuality, psychological well-being, personal safety, and environmental management (Hill and Smith, 1985; Pender, 1996; Steiger and Lipson, 1985).

Another reason for our individualistic orientation to health promotion lies in the link found by social epidemiologists between particular individual behaviors and illnesses, such as between smoking and lung cancer (Belloc and Breslow, 1972; Breslow and Somers, 1977). Consequently, many health scientists since the 1970s have concluded that the best way to improve the health of the American people is for laypersons to adhere to healthy lifestyles (Fuchs, 1974). In 1979, the Surgeon General of the United States, Dr. Julius Richmond, listed objectives for a healthier America by 1990 in his report *Healthy People*. He said these objectives could be reached through preventive health services, health protection, and, especially, health promotion through personal behavior. Estimating that 50 percent of the mortality from the 10 leading causes of death in 1976 had been due to unhealthy behavior or lifestyle, the Surgeon General strongly recommended the development of health programs to help Americans make behavioral changes (U.S. DHEW, 1979, p. 10); see Box 36–2.

Why should health promotion and self-care be matters of concern for nurses? First, health promotion and self-care have been designated as the major ways to achieve the goal of *Health for All by the Year 2000* for the American people. Second, the efforts and cooperation of laypersons and health professionals alike will be required to achieve that goal. Third, nurses can exert a strong influence on the outcome, for they serve as role models, teachers, and advocates for better health. Fourth, because of nursing's philosophical commitment to

BOX 36-1
HEALTH PROMOTION AND THE WORLD HEALTH ORGANIZATION (WHO)

Recognizing the importance of health promotion for achieving its goal of *Health for All by the Year 2000*, WHO issued a Charter of Health Promotion in 1986. This charter specified five general areas of focus:

- building healthy public policy
- creating environments supportive to health
- strengthening community actions
- developing personal skills for healthier living
- reorienting health services (Salmon, 1987, p. 75)

Because of different needs, WHO's various member nations have placed different emphases on the curative, preventive, and health-promoting components of their programs to achieve health for their populations. Poorer nations have addressed basic needs such as food and sanitation, treatment of common diseases and injuries, and control of infectious diseases. More affluent nations such as the United States have addressed such problems, but to a lesser degree. Two infectious diseases, acquired immunodeficiency syndrome (AIDS) and tuberculosis, have recently reached epidemic proportions, and require programs of prevention and treatment. However, the major health problems associated with affluence, industrialization, and urban life are chronic conditions such as heart disease, cancer, stroke; environmental pollution; accidents and injuries; substance abuse; psychological stress; neglect and violence resulting from weakened family and social ties. Given these problems, affluent nations in their plans for *Health for All* have emphasized the prevention of chronic disease, health protection and health promotion.

BOX 36-2
HEALTH PROMOTING, PROTECTION, AND PREVENTION SERVICES OBJECTIVES

Since 1979, the nation's objectives have been revised, and progress monitored. In his 1990 report, *Healthy People 2000: National Health Promotion and Disease Prevention Objectives,* Surgeon General Louis Sullivan reaffirmed that "the individual is both the starting point and the ultimate target of the campaign toward Healthy People 2000" (U.S. DHHS, 1990, p. 85). He listed three major health goals for the nation:

- increase the span of healthy life for Americans
- reduce health disparities among Americans because of educational, political, or economic disadvantage
- provide access to preventive services for all Americans

Again, as in 1979, disease prevention, health protection, and health promotion were the recommended means to attain these goals. Preventive services included screening, counseling, immunization, and antibiotic treatments for individuals. Health protection strategies included environmental or regulatory measures providing protection for large population groups. All the listed health promotion activities referred to "lifestyle" or individual behaviors such as exercise, nutrition, the use of tobacco, alcohol and drugs, family planning, mental health, violence, and physical and mental abuse.

Most of the programs developed to date have assigned responsibility for health to the individual, and have been designed to help individuals change their behaviors to reduce health risk, particularly for heart problems, cancer and stroke (Salmon, 1987). Change may be induced by individuals working alone (self-care), in a group, or with a professional. Change may also involve large-scale educational attempts to change the lifestyles of whole communities or populations-at-risk.

holistic health and wellness, health promotion and the furthering of self-care are central components of the nurse's role. This is true whether the nurse works in a traditional setting such as a hospital or clinic, or in the broader community as a nurse practitioner, midwife, school nurse, camp counselor, occupational health nurse, or consultant to private or public agencies. To perform their roles adequately and to meet the challenge, nurses will need to make full use of the existing knowledge and technology for health promotion.

KNOWLEDGE BASE

Nurses influence health promotion and self-care behaviors by serving as role models, teachers, and community advocates. The primary interventions are empowerment and education strategies designed to (1) reduce risk factors associated with disease, and (2) facilitate voluntary adaptation of those behaviors conducive to health. Effective implementation of these interventions requires the nurse to integrate theory and research from a number of disciplines including epidemiology, nursing, psychology, sociology, and health services. There are many ways this interdisciplinary knowledge base could be organized. For the purpose of the chapter, it is organized with a focus on its application in nursing practice:

- identification and assessment of risk factors
- behaviors affecting health
- community-based outcome research
- interventions with an individual focus
- nursing theory

The research base is extensive; only classical and a sampling of typical studies are presented.

IDENTIFICATION AND ASSESSMENT OF RISK FACTORS

Epidemiologists have made major contributions to the understanding of the natural history of a disease and of factors that contribute to the risk or likelihood of developing a disease. The basic questions addressed by this discipline include:

- What are the health problems of a given population?
- What causes a specific disease, impairment, or health problem?
- How is that problem distributed in the population?
- Why is that problem more prevalent among certain people under certain conditions at certain times?

Answers to these questions are sought by studying the natural history of a disease or health problem, linking agent, host, and environment. The **agent** is what causes the problem, whether biological, chemical, physical, nutritional, or other. The **host** is the person, with particular genetic, psychological, sociocultural characteristics, and particular lifestyle. The **environment** is both physical and social. (These concepts are discussed in Chapter 6.) By discovering the agent and the host and environmental characteristics that contribute to a health problem, the epidemiologist opens the way for developing effective interventions. By plotting the rate, spread, and distribution of problems among a population, the epidemiologist identifies the major health problems and groups at risk who would most benefit from interventions.

These interventions include treatment, but the primary goal of epidemiologists is to **prevent** the further spread of the illness throughout the population. Prevention may be at the primary, secondary or tertiary level. Primary prevention refers to interventions preventing the emergence of pathology; secondary prevention refers to detecting and treating a condition in early stages; and tertiary prevention involves limiting disability once the problem occurs. (Table 36–1 provides more complete definitions of these and other terms.)

This emphasis on prevention makes epidemiology relevant for health promotion. Some health professionals consider

TABLE 36-1 Definitions of Common Terms

Epidemiology	The study of the determinants and distribution of disease and health problems in populations
Primary prevention	Intervention before pathologic changes have begun, accomplished by specific protection strategies and general health promotion
Secondary prevention	The detection and treatment of a disease or health problem in its presymptomatic or early stages, thereby curing the condition, or at least slowing its course and limiting disability
Tertiary prevention	Intervention to limit disability, restore functioning, and rehabilitate persons with impairments
Risk factors	Characteristics or behaviors associated with an increased likelihood of developing a health problem or disease. Some risk factors such as the personal behavior of smoking are modifiable. Others such as age, gender or inherited genetic predispositions are not modifiable
Salutogenesis	The forces maintaining, restoring, or enhancing health and well-being, such as a person's general outlook on life, the feeling that events are predictable and manageable, and that sufficient resources are available to meet the demands of stressors

only primary prevention to be relevant to health promotion, and others, both primary and secondary prevention. Many nurses, however, view health promotion as involving all forms of prevention, both activities by well persons to retain or improve their health and activities by ill persons or persons with chronic conditions to aid recovery or improve functioning.

IDENTIFICATION OF RISK FACTORS

For health promotion and disease prevention, epidemiologists have identified many of the agents and risk factors for major diseases, both acute and chronic. They have examined the part that personal behaviors play in causing specific diseases, such as the effect of smoking on lung cancer, or the effects of physical inactivity, smoking, and diets high in calories and saturated fats on cardiovascular disease (see Box 36–3). For example, the Framingham Study indicated that smoking and physical inactivity contributed to cardiovascular disease, although not as significantly as high blood pressure (Morisky et al, 1986). That study, initiated in the 1950s, followed the health status of more than 5000 healthy adults in Framingham, Massachusetts, and their descendants over two generations. Recently, the study of cardiovascular risk factors has been extended to children and adolescents. The findings of the Framingham Study have helped identify the long-term effects of hypertension and other modifiable risk factors (smoking, poor nutrition, elevated cholesterol, and lack of exercise) on morbidity (illness) and mortality (death) rates from stroke and heart disease.

BOX 36-3
RANKING RISK FACTORS FOR CANCER

According to a 1996 report from the Harvard School of Public Health, nearly two thirds of cancer deaths in the United States are attributed to tobacco use, poor diet, obesity, and sedentary lifestyle. The percentage of cancer deaths linked to specific risk factors is as follows:

Tobacco use	30%
Poor diet/obesity	30%
Sedentary lifestyle	5%
Occupational factors	5%
Family history of cancer	5%
Viruses and other biologic agents	5%
Perinatal factors, growth	5%
Reproductive factors	5%
Alcohol use	3%
Socioeconomic status	3%
Environmental pollution	2%
Ionizing or ultraviolet radiation	2%
Prescription drugs and medical procedures	1%
Salt, food additives, contaminants	1%

Perhaps the most classical study for health promotion is the Alameda Study. In this study, data on the health habits and social relations of almost 6900 residents of Alameda County, California, were collected in 1965 and again a decade later (see Box 36–4).

These findings about the importance of everyday self-care practices for better health and longer life attracted much public attention. The National Health Interview Surveys (NHIS) of 1977, 1983, 1985, and 1990 collected data on the health

BOX 36-4
THE ALAMEDA STUDY

Unlike most of their predecessors, the investigators in the Alameda Study did not seek to explain why people succumb to cancer, heart disease, or other specific diseases or health problems. Instead, they examined the influence of certain ways of living on physical health status and mortality. The health status in 1965, health status a decade later, and long-term survival were all better for participants who:

- had never smoked
- abstained or used alcohol in moderation
- maintained desirable weight
- exercised
- slept 7–8 hours a night
- ate breakfast regularly
- did not snack

It was estimated that a 45-year-old man who practiced 6 or 7 of these habits could expect to live 11 years longer than a 45-year-old man with 3 or fewer good habits (Breslow and Enstrom, 1980; Breslow and Somers, 1977).

RESEARCH HIGHLIGHT
POPULAR VIEWS OF HEALTH

RESEARCH PROBLEM

Nursing practice is influenced by the definitions of health that nurses use. If a nurse's view of health is not compatible with that of the consumer, the end result may be conflicting goals and minimal adherence to the treatment plan.

SUMMARY OF STUDY

The purpose of this study was to identify the meaning of health by adult consumers and to determine potential differences in meaning associated with gender, age, and education. The definitions of health were analyzed according to the health levels/subcategories of Smith (1983); and Woods (1989).

Sixty-five adults (44 women and 21 men) ranging from 18 to 73 years of age served as subjects. Educational preparation ranged from completing high school through completing college. The participants were recruited in public places to participate in the study. Data were collected using a questionnaire designed to obtain adults' views on the meaning of health.

The data analysis showed significant differences in the meaning of health based on gender and education. There were no significant differences associated with age. Both men and women ranked self-concept, fitness, and role performance high. Men ranked body image and clinical definitions higher. Women ranked health promotion, social involvement and harmony higher than men did. High school graduates ranked body image and self-actualization higher. Fitness was ranked higher by those with college education.

IMPLICATIONS FOR NURSING PRACTICE

Consumers view health in broader terms than clinical measurements. Consumers also hold different meanings of health. Nurses must consider each consumer's health views and goals and assist them toward attainment of **their** goals.

From Kenney, J.W. (1992). The consumer's view of health. *Journal of Advanced Nursing, 17,* 829–834.

habits of the general U.S. population age 18 years and older. These surveys basically confirmed the Alameda findings and demonstrated that although many adults have healthy habits, many do not, particularly persons in more economically and socially disadvantaged groups (Schoenborn, 1986). The results suggest a need to develop more effective health promotion strategies, especially for minority groups with morbidity and mortality rates above the national average.

The focus of research such as the studies just described has been on avoiding or preventing specific health disorders or illness generally. Most of these researchers have defined health, in keeping with the biomedical model, as the absence of disease or health problems. They may distinguish degrees of illness or disability but not degrees of wellness. This emphasis on pathogenesis (the process where microorganisms cause disease) has proved very useful in controlling disease, but can offer little understanding of the forces maintaining and enhancing health. Terris (1975) has therefore proposed an epidemiology of health that would distinguish differing degrees of wellness among persons who are free from disease, as reflected in growth and development, physical fitness, intellectual functioning, capacity for performance, zest and vitality, and a sense of comfort and well-being. The knowledge base for this epidemiology of health is as yet undeveloped. Perhaps the current interest in wellness and health enhancement may accelerate its development (see Research Highlight: Popular Views of Health).

RESEARCH ON HEALTH SCREENING (ASSESSMENT OF RISK FACTORS)

The U.S. Preventive Services Task Force in 1989 published up-to-date recommendations based on results from research on screening tests. To be cost-effective, screening tests should be accurate, sensitive, and specific. A sensitive test misses no cases, and results in no false-negative diagnoses that might delay treatment and jeopardize health and life. It also detects early-stage disease so that prompt treatment can reduce its severity and improve its outcome. A specific test identifies only true cases, and results in no false-positive diagnoses that might bring about unnecessary worry; uncomfortable, expensive but unneeded treatments; and perhaps ineligibility for health insurance. Vision and hearing screening tests are effective, often detecting conditions that can be remedied and thus improving quality of life. Hypertension, also, can be detected and treated early enough to make a significant difference in length and quality of life. However, other widely adopted screening tests (e.g., fecal occult blood tests) are not cost-effective, yielding few true cases and resulting in many false-positive findings that require extensive and costly follow-up tests to determine if disease is present. The most recent recommendations for health screening are shown in Figure 36–1. These recommendations are listed in the *Clinician's Handbook of Preventive Services* (U.S. DHHS, 1998), the most widely used single guide to health promotion services.

Several issues raised by screening may be illustrated by the case of human immunodeficiency virus (HIV), the cause of acquired immunodeficiency syndrome (AIDS). Screening involves a preliminary test (enzyme-linked immunosorbent assay [ELISA]) and a confirmatory test (Western blot). A positive reading, whether true or false, conveys social stigma and has financial consequences, so individuals may seek anonymous testing as a protection. Patients who have been exposed to the virus should be counseled to obtain follow-up testing at 6 weeks, 12 weeks, and 6 months after exposure because the

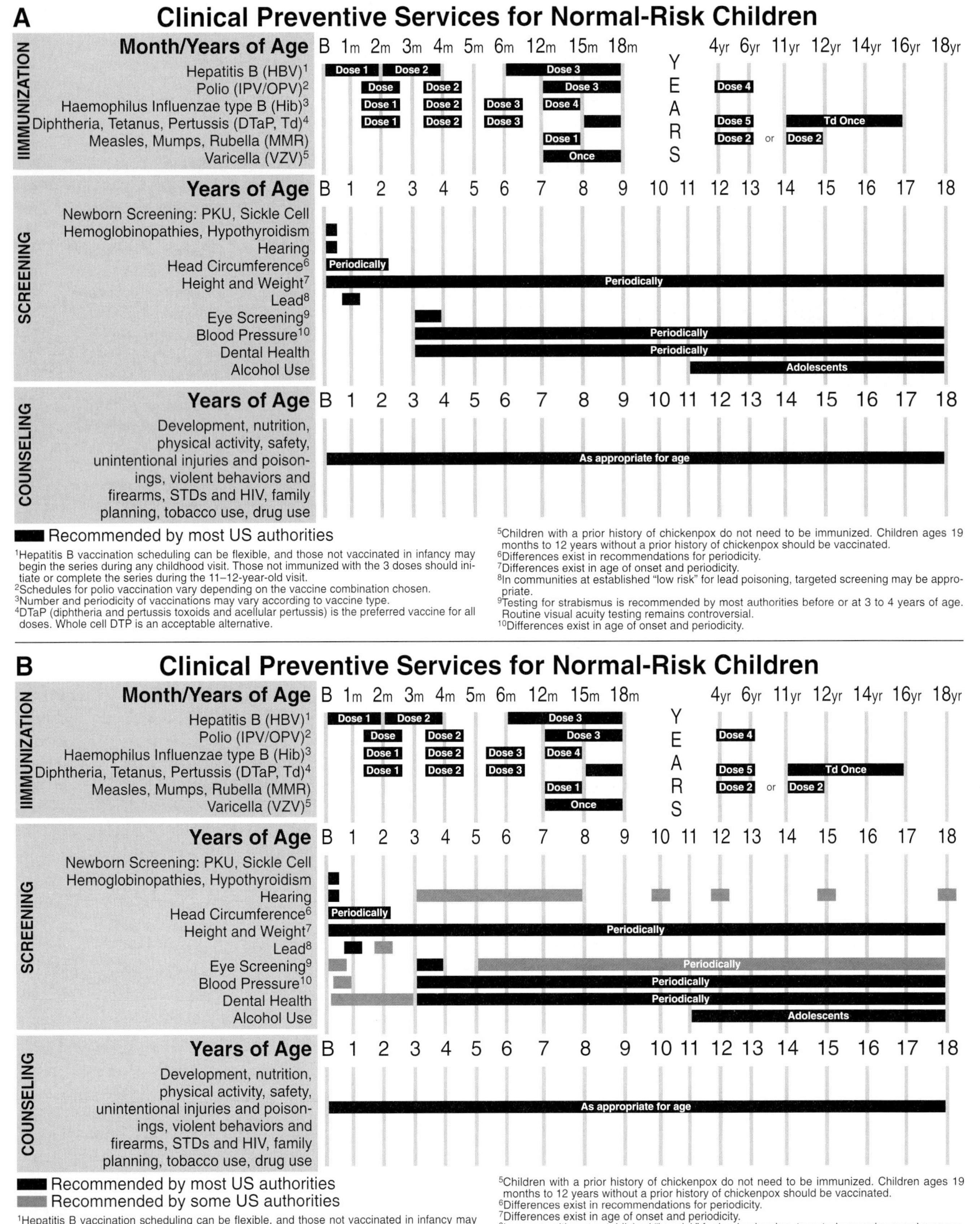

Figure 36-1. Recommended preventive care timelines for children and adults. (From U.S. Dept. of Health and Human Services [1998]. *Clinician's Handbook of Preventive Services.* Rockville, MD: Author.)

C Clinical Preventive Services for Normal-Risk Adults

Years of Age 18 25 30 35 40 45 50 55 60 65 70 75

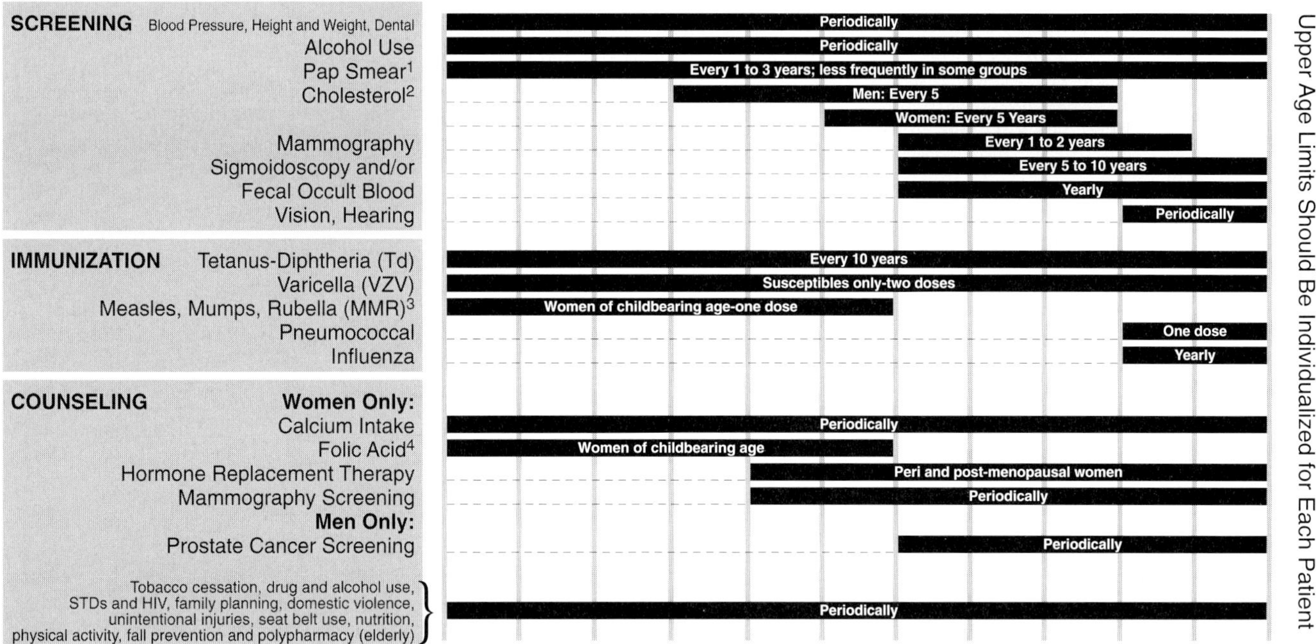

■ Recommended by most US authorities

[1]There is no upper age limit for Pap smears, but regular testing in women over age 65 may be discontinued in those who have had regular screening with consistently normal results. Pap smears are not necessary in women who have undergone a hysterectomy in which the cervix was removed for reasons other than cervical cancer or its precursors.

[2]Some authorities recommend initiating screening at age 19. Screening at less frequent intervals may be reasonable in low risk individuals, including those with previously normal levels.

[3]MMR need only be given to women of childbearing age who lack documented evidence of immunization and are capable of becoming pregnant.

[4]Folic acid 0.4 mg per day is recommended for women of childbearing age who are capable of becoming pregnant.

D Clinical Preventive Services for Normal-Risk Adults

Years of Age 18 25 30 35 40 45 50 55 60 65 70 75

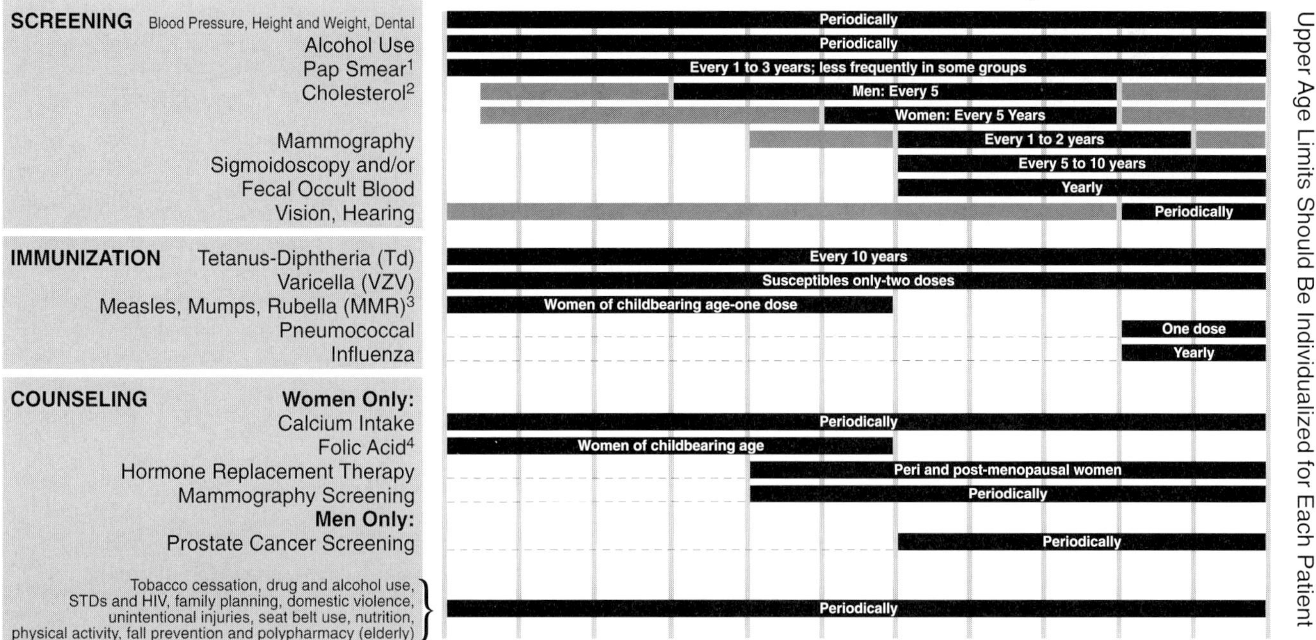

■ Recommended by most US authorities

■ Recommended by most US authorities

[1]There is no upper age limit for Pap smears, but regular testing in women over age 65 may be discontinued in those who have had regular screening with consistently normal results. Pap smears are not necessary in women who have undergone a hysterectomy in which the cervix was removed for reasons other than cervical cancer or its precursors.

[2]Some authorities recommend initiating screening at age 19. Screening at less frequent intervals may be reasonable in low risk individuals, including those with previously normal levels.

[3]MMR need only be given to women of childbearing age who lack documented evidence of immunization and are capable of becoming pregnant.

[4]Folic acid 0.4 mg per day is recommended for women of childbearing age who are capable of becoming pregnant.

Figure 36-1. *Continued*

time between exposure and conversion to a positive test varies. They should also be counseled regarding their personal risk factors such as unprotected sexual intercourse, sharing of needles among intravenous drug users, or other exposure to blood or body fluids of someone who is HIV positive. Health care workers are at risk because they are exposed to patients' body fluids. They have therefore been directed by the Centers for Disease Control to take universal precautions with all patients in that HIV status is often unknown. (See Chapter 18 for more information on personal safety.)

Finally, some applied research evaluates health-screening tests performed by laypersons on themselves, often at the urging of a nurse or other health practitioner. Testicular self-examination among men is one example. Breast self-examination among women is another. Although definitive studies on the efficacy of these practices have yet to be done, there is some evidence that survival is better for women who performed breast self-examination regularly before diagnosis (Morrison, 1991). Still, breast self-examination has been criticized as being too insensitive and irregular, resulting in extensive workups in too many cases that later prove to be benign. For detection of very small tumors, mammography is considered superior to palpation whether performed by women on themselves or by health professionals. Mammography is not infallible either, and is inaccessible to many women because of expense. Until more information is available, the most prudent course would probably be to combine, wherever possible, regular breast self-examination with mammography and periodic examinations by a health professional.

Behaviors Affecting Health

SALUTOGENIC VIEW OF HEALTH BEHAVIOR

The sociologist A. Antonovsky has proposed a **salutogenic** approach to health. This approach examines the forces and process by which health and well-being are created, maintained, restored, or enhanced. This is in contrast to a pathogenic approach, which focuses on causes of disease. (See Table 36–1 for a definition of salutogenesis.) In his research on menopausal women in Israel, Antonovsky was surprised to find that 29 percent of a group of concentration camp survivors showed moderately good physical and mental health despite the horrors of the camp, their years as displaced persons, and then their adjustment as immigrants to a country that witnessed three wars! This dramatic finding led Antonovsky to formulate his salutogenic model of health to "unravel the mystery of health" (Antonovsky, 1979, 1987). The question addressed was "how do people manage to stay healthy?" rather than "How do people become ill?" (see Box 36–5).

BOX 36-5
THE SALUTOGENIC MODEL

According to the salutogenic model, health is assessed on a continuum, ranging from "health-ease," or optimal wellness, at one end to "dis-ease" at the other end. Over a lifetime, a person shifts back and forth along this continuum, sometimes approaching the "wellness" and sometimes the "disease" end. The person's position is determined less by stressful events than by the way he or she handles the tension created by those events. In turn, the way tension is managed depends on the person's "resistance resources" and "sense of coherence."

RESISTANCE RESOURCES

- genetic inheritance
- intelligence
- knowledge
- ego strength
- coping skills
- social supports
- material resources
- stable system of values and beliefs
- emergency care
- preventive health orientation

SENSE OF COHERENCE

- person's general outlook on life
- feeling that life makes sense, that events are not arbitrary but rather are predictable and manageable
- confidence that a person's resources are sufficient to meet the demands posed by stressors, and that demands are challenges, worthy of effort
- faith that events are under some sort of control, even if not a person's own

A person with a weak sense of coherence is unlikely to manage tension successfully when resistance resources are scarce, and therefore is more likely to become ill. Which particular disease develops is a result of environment, constitutional makeup, and personal susceptibility. In contrast, a person with a strong sense of coherence is able to mobilize existing resistance resources, manage tension effectively, and resist health breakdown. Successful coping enhances the ability to deal with subsequent stressors, and reinforces the sense of coherence so that the person continues to move toward the healthy end of the continuum and optimal wellness.

The wellness-oriented salutogenic model has been recommended to nurses as a viable alternative to the disease-oriented biomedical model for guiding practice, research, and education (Sullivan, 1989). Use of the framework would change practice by strengthening the involvement of nurses in wellness-enhancing aspects of health promotion. Nurses would assess patients' health potential (e.g., resistance resources and level of coherence) as well as sickness potential (e.g., risk factors). Nurses would direct interventions toward fostering a strong sense of competence in their patients, and toward maximizing their patients' resources by providing knowledge, services, and techniques for managing tension effectively. Such interventions should promote both current health and the ability to maintain health during future stressful situations.

HEALTH BELIEF MODEL

The health belief model (HBM) was developed by Rosenstock in the 1950s to explain why people do or do not seek preventive health care such as immunizations and screening to detect disease. The original version of the model contained five elements:

- the individual's beliefs regarding **seriousness** of a particular health condition
- personal **susceptibility** to that condition
- benefits from taking recommended actions
- barriers to that action
- presence of a trigger or **cue** to take action (Rosenstock, 1966, 1974)

It was predicted that those individuals would be more likely to take a preventive action (e.g., perform regular breast self-examination) when they:

- experienced a cue to do so (a media message recommending breast self-examination)
- felt susceptible to the condition (breast cancer)
- believed that the condition was serious (life-threatening)
- believed that the benefits of taking the action (early detection and treatment with increased chance of survival) outweighed the barriers (lack of confidence in one's ability to detect tumors, and costs in time, effort and convenience)

The major components of the HBM are shown in Table 36–2.

Over the years, the HBM has been extended in the hope of improving its predictive capacity for a broader range of health behaviors. Many demographic, psychological, and social factors have been added, including age, sex, social class, ethnicity, personality, peer pressure, social support, knowledge of disease, and previous care experiences. Despite these changes, the ability of the model to predict health behaviors is modest, and the best predictors remain the individual's perceptions of benefits and barriers (Janz and Becker, 1984). Today, criticisms center on the model's failure to place sufficient importance on environmental and other factors outside the individual's control.

Nevertheless, the HBM has exerted an enormous influence on practice in the field of prevention. Using the model, nurses and other health professionals can discover their patients' beliefs about the worth and cost of particular health actions. They may then tailor interventions to the needs of specific individuals, target groups, or populations (Becker et al, 1977). For example, practitioners might offer patients alternative programs and they can choose the one they personally consider most beneficial and least costly. Or, practitioners might emphasize different benefits of health behaviors for different populations. Thus, for adolescents who do not feel susceptible to heart disease, improved appearance and strength might be emphasized as benefits of exercise; for older adults who do feel susceptible, prevention of heart disease might be stressed. As a third example, practitioners might seek to change patients' perceptions that discourage preventive measures or healthy behaviors. They might attempt this either directly through education and persuasion, or indirectly through environmental and structural changes to eliminate barriers. Possible structural changes include extending clinic hours or offering programs at readily accessible neighborhood sites such as schools or shopping malls.

TABLE 36–2 Basic Components of the Health Belief Model to Use for Assessment and Intervention with Patients

Perceived susceptibility	Belief in personal vulnerability to the health threat
Perceived seriousness	Belief that the health threat is likely to have severe personal consequences
Benefits	Belief that personal action or treatment is preventive, effective
Barriers (cost, inconvenience, etc.)	Belief that personal barriers to action can be overcome
Cues to action (environmental or internal)	Action triggered by event, or role model

The HBM has most often been used to explain behaviors used to avoid health problems or detect disease in an asymptomatic stage. It has seldom been used to explain why some healthy people exercise, eat special foods, or engage in other health-enhancing behaviors in a quest for "high-level wellness."

COGNITIVE-BEHAVIORAL PSYCHOLOGY APPROACHES TO HEALTH PROMOTION

Through its theories of learning and human behavior, the discipline of psychology has contributed much to our understanding of the factors involved in habit formation and behavior change. This understanding is vital to the development of strategies for eliminating unhealthy habits and establishing healthy behaviors in the interests of disease prevention and health promotion. The cognitive-behavioral psychology approach to health promotion combines behavioral principles from classical (automatic or reflexive response) and operant (instrumentally learned skeletal response) conditioning, with cognitive elements (thoughts, beliefs, and attitudes) to explain and predict individual health behavior and to guide interventions for behavior change. Behavior that has a negative impact on health is viewed as the way a person has **learned** to cope with the demands of the physical and social environment. Because the behavior is learned, it may also be changed or unlearned by applying learning principles.

Nurses and other professionals have often applied principles of cognitive-behavioral psychology in programs designed to change people's unhealthy or maladaptive behaviors, such as overeating or smoking. The baseline data for designing, monitoring, and evaluating the outcome of a behavior change program are provided by analyzing the stimulus or **antecedents (A)** of the problem behavior, the **behavior** response **(B),** and the **consequences (C).** A log kept by the patient helps in the development of an effective program by uncovering the **ABCs** of the behavioral pattern. A log also alerts the patient to internal and external cues that stimulate or reinforce the behavior, and to the consequences of that behavior (Watson and Tharp, 1989). Such awareness makes it easier for the patient to carry out a self-management program to achieve long-term control over the problem behavior.

An example of an ABC is a person who begins drinking excessive alcohol after work. Analysis of the situation might show that the individual was experiencing stress from intense job insecurity (A), used alcohol to reduce the feeling of stress (B), and found that the consumption of alcohol decreased performance at work and thus increased job insecurity (C). Another common example is the person who eats to the point of excessive weight gain. On analysis the person may learn that the overeating (B) is associated with a sense of loneliness (A). The increased weight gain resulted in withdrawal from social situations (C), thus increasing the feeling of loneliness.

Behavior may be changed by modifying the stimulus, the behavior, or the consequences. The stimuli for unhealthy behavior may be eliminated, whereas stimuli enhancing healthy behavior may be increased. The behavior response may be changed by "behavioral rehearsal" or the systematic practice of performance. The technique of mental imagery in which a person pictures him/herself performing the behavior in a variety of circumstances may also help.

In the situation of stress in the work place, the individual may accept the situation as necessary given the economy but decide to use exercise to reduce the feeling of stress. The individual may go to the gym immediately after work to reduce the stress. Or the person may decide that working in another setting is less stressful and change jobs. In the situation of overeating, the person may handle the sense of loneliness by joining a reading club or a craft group, etc. The person may also use mental imagery (picturing how they wanted to look) as another means of avoiding overeating until the sense of loneliness was not so strong. Pregnant women use imagery to handle the stress of pregnancy. They picture the baby after birth and imagine the good times ahead.

The consequences may be manipulated by providing or withholding rewards and by establishing aversive consequences. The most commonly used strategy is self-reward or positive self-reinforcement, in which the individual rewards him/herself with verbal praise or some tangible good following satisfactory performance of the desired behavior. Self-reward has proved effective in a number of studies involving weight reduction (Kanfer and Gaelick, 1986). Another helpful technique is to minimize the unpleasant consequences of performing the behavior; for example, do not exercise in a setting where one feels conspicuous or embarrassed. People are more likely to repeat behavior associated with a pleasant outcome. Finally, by learning the technique of self-management, individuals can monitor and evaluate their behavior, and then reinforce themselves for healthy behavior while withholding rewards for undesired behavior (Karoly and Kanfer, 1982). Nurses can help patients learn these strategies to change their behavior and improve their health.

STRESS AND COPING

Stress is a pervasive phenomenon, and is associated with illness and disease, so stress management is an important component of health promotion. The cognitive theory of stress and coping developed by Lazarus and his associates (Lazarus and Folkman, 1984) is the prevailing theory used to guide stress management. The theory holds that people, when faced with problems, may cope by addressing either the problems directly, or the stress evoked by the problem. Sometimes people cope with stress in healthy ways and sometimes in unhealthy ways such as smoking, drinking, overeating, or using drugs. Stress management programs try to help people replace unhealthy behaviors with adaptive, healthy forms of coping. (For more information on stress and coping, see Chapter 31.)

LOCUS OF CONTROL

The concept of **locus of control** refers to an individual's belief regarding whether outcomes of events depend on one's own actions or depend on fate, chance or powerful others (Rotter, 1966). According to this theory, people who believe that their health results from their own actions engage in preventive care and health-promoting behaviors to a greater extent than people who believe their health results from factors outside their control. However, the research to date has indicated that locus of control has only a modest effect on health behavior.

SELF-EFFICACY

Self-efficacy, or personal belief in one's ability to perform a specific behavior, is a central concept in Bandura's (1986) social cognitive theory. Bandura hypothesizes that persons are more likely to perform a behavior if they feel confident in their ability to perform and if they see the behavior as leading to a desirable outcome. With regard to health-promoting behaviors (e.g., weight control), persons with a weak sense of self-efficacy may not attempt to change despite belief in the benefits of change. Persons with a strong sense of self-efficacy are more likely to sustain their change efforts despite obstacles. Some studies support this hypothesis, linking self-efficacy with the health-promoting behaviors of exercise, weight control, and smoking cessation. Because of its potential value for health promotion and self-care, interventions to enhance self-efficacy are presently being designed and tested. Using relaxation techniques as a means of reducing stress is one such intervention. It builds on people's belief in their ability to do something to improve their situation. Natural childbirth is another intervention linked with self-efficacy.

These psychological theories, along with many others, have guided health promotion efforts with varying effectiveness. Regardless of the theory used, several researchers have independently reached the conclusion that behavior change occurs in stages. Prochaska and coworkers (1992) identified five stages during which the person:

- receives information about the benefits of change
- actively considers the need to change
- makes a commitment to change and prepares for change
- changes behavior
- maintains the new behavior

To be most effective, strategies used by nurses and other practitioners should be tailored to the patient's particular stage of behavior change.

This model by Prochaska and coworkers currently permeates the clinical literature in all areas of health behavior change. They have also translated their model into lay terms for individuals seeking to help themselves. The book for the general public is *Changing for Good* (Prochaska et al, 1994).

All of these theories of human behavior have been applied by nurses to health promotion efforts with individual patients. However, continued systematic inquiry is needed to refine these theories and develop more effective ways to help patients adopt and sustain healthy lifestyles.

BOX 36–6
HEALTH PROMOTION PROGRAM STRATEGIES

Suggested strategies for health promotion programs include education, technology, legislation and regulation, taxation, and persuasion through the use of incentives. Education enables people to make personal choices that result in healthier consequences both for themselves and others. Technology has produced health-promoting products such as low-fat foods, seat belts, anti-lock brakes, and automatic inflatable airbags for cars. Technology has also facilitated the psychological techniques of behavior modification, biofeedback, and hypnosis used to help people lose weight, quit smoking, or reduce stress

Legislation and regulation at local, state, and federal levels can enforce health precautions and eliminate health hazards in industries, health care facilities, public agencies, and the environment. Examples include fluoridation of water supplies; building and fire codes; regulation of food and drugs; pasteurization of milk; standards for air, water, and soil quality; the screening of newborns for phenylketonuria; and needle exchange programs to prevent human immunodeficiency virus (HIV) transmission. Taxation and taxation credits may be used to discourage unhealthy conditions and encourage healthy situations. "Sin taxes" may be levied on cigarettes and alcohol to discourage their use. Tax deductions may be available for firms offering health programs to employees, and for companies that develop vehicles using cleaner fuels and thereby reducing air pollution levels. Incentives may be used to induce specific behaviors. For example, lower health insurance premiums may be offered to nonsmokers and nondrinkers, or subsidies may be offered to tobacco farmers who switch to the cultivation of new crops.

Community-Based Health Promotion Interventions

Some research on health promotion and self-care has focused on the determinants of health behavior and principles of change; other research has tested the effectiveness of interventions that apply those principles to reduce unhealthy behavior and foster healthy behavior (see Box 36–6). The Stanford Five-City Project (Farquhar et al, 1985) and the Multiple Risk Factor Intervention Trials (Multiple Risk Factor Research Group, 1982) were two large-scale experimental studies that tested the feasibility and cost-effectiveness of community health education programs in preventing cardiovascular disease by reducing risk factors.

STANFORD FIVE-CITY PROJECT

In this study (Farquhar et al, 1985), two communities received the experimental treatment (the education program) and three control communities did not. The program was comprehensive and continued over a decade. Health messages about smoking, overweight, high blood pressure, and high cholesterol levels were disseminated through the media, community organizations, self-help clinics, and in restaurants, cafeterias, workshops, and grocery stores. Trained group leaders conducted classes in community colleges, schools, hospitals, churches, and other voluntary and nonprofit organizations. Incentive-based competitions were held.

The change in risk factors was measured through surveys conducted before and during the course of the intervention in the experimental and control communities. Cardiovascular disease rates were assessed through continuous community surveillance of fatal and nonfatal heart attacks and stroke. Preliminary analyses of the data revealed that residents in the two intervention communities increased their exercise, reduced their tobacco use, and lowered their cholesterol levels. As a result, similar comprehensive community-based demonstration projects have been initiated in Minnesota and Rhode Island, and by the World Health Organization in 16 different countries.

MULTIPLE RISK FACTOR INTERVENTION TRIAL (MRFIT)

The MRFIT (Multiple Risk Factor Research Group, 1982) evaluated an intervention to reduce cardiovascular disease among middle-aged men with no evidence of the disease, but at high risk because of their serum cholesterol, blood pressure, and smoking. About 13,000 high-risk candidates from 22 different clinical sites were enrolled in the trial and randomly assigned to one of two groups. One group received information and behavioral interventions for the risk factors of diet, exercise, elevated cholesterol, smoking, and hypertension. The other group was referred to customary courses of health care. Subjects in both the intervention and the usual-community-care group were found to change their behavior and reduce their cardiovascular risk. At long-term follow-up, 10.5 years later, it was found that subjects had tended to maintain their dietary behavior for lowering cholesterol, but to resume smoking. Those men who did not resume smoking reduced their risk for death from coronary heart disease.

Individual-Focused Health Promotion Interventions

SELF-CARE PROGRAMS

There is general consensus that certain self-care behaviors for health promotion (e.g., no smoking, alcohol only in moderation, seat belt use) have a positive influence on individual health and on population morbidity and mortality rates. There also is little argument about the safety of health programs that promote nutritional eating habits and moderate exercise. (High levels of exercise can be hazardous, being linked to infertility, damage to the immune system, cancer and premature aging). Besides being safe, such programs can be effective in altering individual lifestyles, at least temporarily. Thus, the programs of AT&T, Johnson & Johnson, and Blue Cross of Indiana all succeeded in increasing employees' exercise levels, reducing their blood pressure, and lowering their cholesterol levels (Conrad, 1987). Short-term success at modifying behavior has also been demonstrated with behavioral conditioning, group discussion, counseling, hypnosis, interpersonal communication, and self-analysis (McKinlay, 1974). However, long-term studies are needed to determine whether such programs produce permanent changes in the behavior of individuals.

While these health promotion programs are considered safe and can be effective in changing risk behaviors at least for the short run, their effectiveness in preventing future illness, improving the health of the individual, or lengthening life expectancy is not known. For instance, cholesterol reduction is almost universally recommended. Yet the data from the most sophisticated test to date (MRFIT) clearly showed that:

> modifying dietary, exercise, and other health behaviors has minimal benefits. Data on the impact of elevated cholesterol on middle-aged men not already at high risk for a heart attack, on women, and on the elderly are minimal or nonexistent. The long-term effects of cholesterol-lowering drugs are unknown. And those high-risk individuals who do lower their cholesterol appear to die more from noncoronary causes (Goldstein, 1993, p. 153).

A model constructed to calculate the benefits of a lifelong program of dietary cholesterol reduction determined that persons at low risk (defined in terms of blood pressure, smoking history, and high-density lipoprotein level) "could expect to live from 3 days to 3 months longer, and those at high risk would gain from 18 days to 12 months" (Becker, 1993, p. 2). Clearly, more research is needed to clarify the health effects of modifying lifestyles.

ATTITUDES OF PROVIDERS AND LAYPERSONS

With regard to self-care, laypersons hold more positive views than health professionals. At least one survey has suggested that the public believes self-care in general is helpful (Green, 1985). Users of nonprescription drugs and home remedies quite consistently report satisfaction (Brown and Marcy, 1991). Health professionals are more divided in their opinion. Some view self-medication as dangerous, others as a waste of money, still others as useful for minor, self-limiting illnesses. Wilkinson and colleagues (1987) reported that a panel of physicians judged that 21 percent of the self-care actions taken by 340 laypersons for minor symptoms were potentially harmful, and 10 percent inappropriate. Professional opposition is common to the use of unconventional remedies for chronic or life-threatening diseases such as arthritis and cancer. The safety of herbal remedies is frequently questioned because some have been shown to be toxic, some interact with prescribed drugs, and others are of unknown toxicity (Spoerke, 1980; Der Marderosian, 1980). Even the use of vitamins and dietary supplements is controversial (Nishiwaki and Bouchard, 1989).

However, there are no firm data by which to decide whether self-care is any less safe than professional care, for professional care itself is not without danger. Iatrogenic or negative side effects are estimated to occur in 20 percent of all professional interventions. We can only guess about the effectiveness of self-care when it is extended to areas of diagnosis and treatment previously under professional control. Research will be needed to determine the risks of false positives and false negatives in self-diagnosis, and of improper or overmedication in self-treatment (Levin et al, 1976), and people will have to decide how to trade off possible damage for the presumed psychological and economic benefits of self-care. How effective self-care is in reducing the use of services is still another question requiring research.

Nursing Theory

Nursing has contributed to the knowledge base for health promotion and self-care through its conceptual, empirical, and clinical work about the meaning of health and the means to achieve it. (See Chapter 2, The Nature of Nursing Knowledge, for a discussion of nursing theory.). Four nursing theories are particularly relevant to the health promotion and self-care knowledge base. These theories have stimulated research and guided practice.

SMITH'S FOUR LEVELS OF HEALTH

Smith's conceptualization of health (1983) has probably enjoyed the most acceptance among nurses. Smith identifies four levels of health—clinical health, functional health, adaptive health, and eudaemonistic health—which build on each other. **Clinical health,** defined as the absence of clinical signs and symptoms, is the basic level. It frees individuals to pursue the second level of **functional health,** or the fulfillment of usual work and social roles. When individuals are also able to respond to change in their environments and maintain their health despite new stresses, they have attained the third level or **adaptive health.** Finally, successful adaptation to the environment frees individuals to engage in activities that promote zest for living and self-actualization, thus reaching the fourth and highest level of **eudaemonistic health.** Eudaemonistic health is the state of optimal or positive well-being.

Smith's model assumes that any activity or intervention which helps a person move up through these levels of health is health promotive. Her broad definition of health also implies expansion of the nurse's role to include assisting patients, whether ill or well, to achieve better health and well-being. For such interventions to be meaningful, the nurse will need to assess patients' conceptions of health, health risks and practices, and personal health goals.

OREM'S SELF-CARE DEFICIT THEORY

Many proponents of health promotion and self-care in nursing have taken Orem's (1985, 1991) theory of nursing as a point of departure. Orem (1991, p. 184) defines health as "a state of a person . . . characterized by soundness or wholeness of developed human structures and bodily and mental functioning." She distinguishes health from "well-being," which is the individual's perceived condition of existence and experience of contentment and self-actualization. Orem assumes that individuals are responsible for their own health, and that self-care is essential for achieving health and well-being. The nurse's role is to assess the patient's self-care abilities (knowledge and skill) rather than the patient's attainment of the desired health outcomes. If necessary, nurses should provide resources to meet patients' needs during their periods of "self-care deficit," while teaching them skills to care for themselves (Denyes, 1988; Hartweg, 1990, Simmons, 1990).

WOODS'S SELF-CARE STRATEGIES

Woods (1989) has tried to relate Orem's self-care deficit theory more directly to health-promoting behavior. By combining Orem's theory with Smith's model of health, Woods has been able to devise self-care strategies for each level of health. For example, individuals may promote their clinical health by screening for early detection of illness, monitoring symptoms, and using medications and over-the-counter preparations judiciously. They may function normally at work and in social roles by adopting "normalization" strategies (such as the use of prostheses). Their adaptive health may be promoted by stress self-management, and their eudaemonistic health by self-care strategies that promote fitness and harmony.

PENDER'S HEALTH PROMOTION MODEL

Pender's (1996) approach to the field of health promotion is somewhat different. She is interested in explaining behavior, such as exercise, undertaken to increase wellness (self-actualization or eudaemonistic health). She believes that the forces that motivate wellness behavior are quite different from those that motivate behavior to prevent illness. On the assumption that beliefs and attitudes are the primary determinants of behavior, Pender's health promotion model incorporates the selected variables of the health belief model along with situational factors and self-efficacy.

Pender's initial Health Promotion Model (HPM) is shown in Figure 36–2. The HPM is a framework for integrating nursing and behavioral science perspectives on factors influencing health promotion and disease protection behaviors. It is a competence or approach-oriented model that does not include fear or threat as a motivator for health behavior. Publication of the first model led to additional research testing various components of the model. This research led Pender to revise the model to include three new factors: activity-related affect, commitment to a plan of action, and immediate competing demands and preferences. The Revised Health Promotion Model (RHPM) is shown in Figure 36–3.

The key headings are defined to aid in understanding the RHPM. Individual characteristics and experiences refer to those unique prior experiences that affect an individual's later actions. Behavior-specific cognitions and affect are those factors thought to be of major motivational significance. Pender believes these variables can be changed through nursing interventions. The behavioral outcome is the commitment to a health-promoting plan of action. The model indicates that unless the individual encounters a competing demand that cannot be avoided or a competing preference that is not resisted, the health-promoting behavior will occur.

Pender's model has been criticized for being more relevant to white middle-class persons than other groups. Yet it remains a very popular model within nursing.

Specific nursing actions associated with the RHPM are presented later in this chapter.

CRITIQUE OF NURSING THEORIES

If the knowledge base for nursing practice in health promotion is to grow, theoretical models such as those described above need further refinement and testing. The existing models have been criticized on two counts. First, they omit some factors presumed to influence health behavior such as self-esteem and social support (Duffy, 1988). Second, the strategies derived from these models for promoting self-care and healthy behaviors appear to be more appropriate for middle-class Americans than for persons of lower socioeconomic status, or from certain ethnic groups and age categories. For example, the heavy reliance on cognitive/educational interventions may be more effective with a well-educated individual who values learning. It is particularly important in the case of such populations, and of

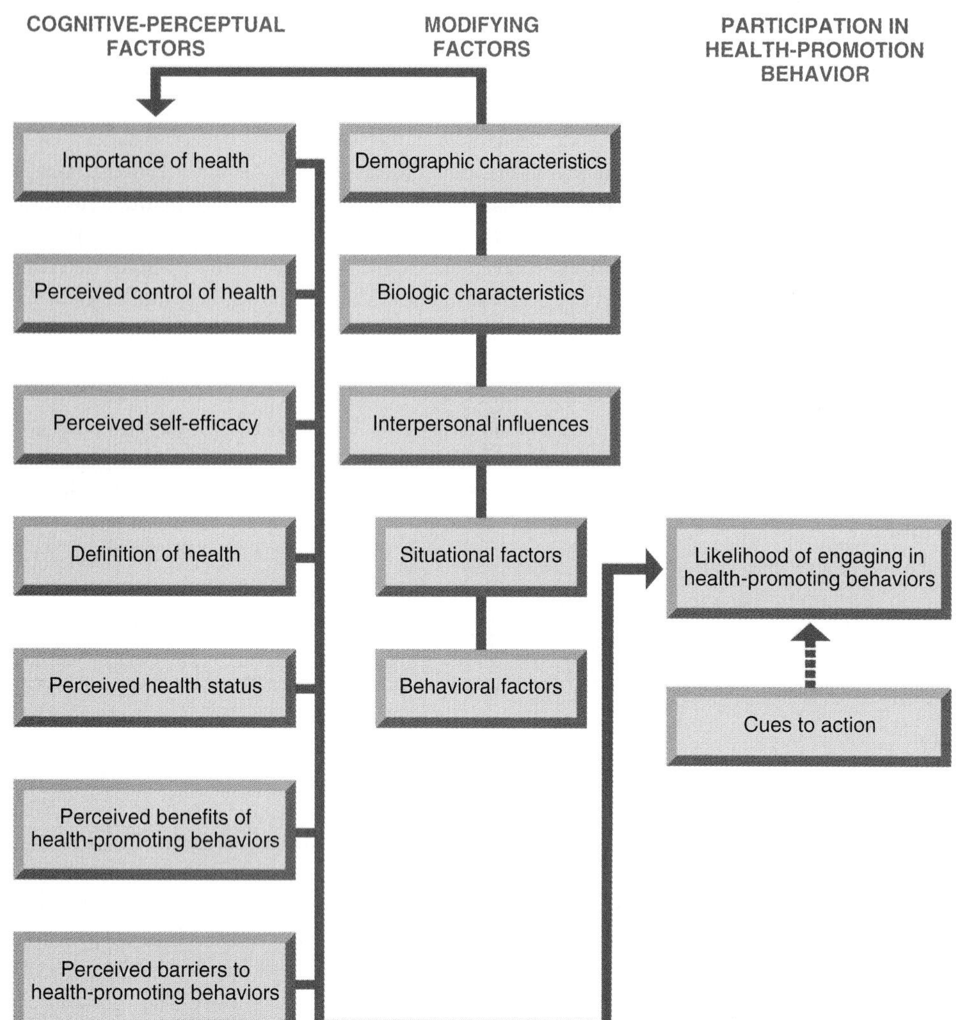

Figure 36–2. Health promotion model. (From Pender, N.J. [1996]. *Health Promotion in Nursing Practice,* 3rd ed. Stamford, CT: Appleton & Lange.)

all other individuals who find self-care difficult, that strategies to improve and maintain health be based on a more comprehensive view of health promotion than self-care and individual responsibility for lifestyles.

Milio (1976, 1981) has presented one such view. Her public health approach emphasizes the social context of health promotion. She argues that the health of a population depends on customary personal choice-making. Individuals tend to choose those options that they believe cost less and deliver more of what they have been socialized to value. The range of available choices, however, is limited by the financial resources of the individuals and their communities. It is also limited by the decisions of organizations, both public and private, as they decide which programs to fund and which ones not to fund. Government decisions concerning the allocation, distribution, and price of goods and services, policies about food, housing, energy, employment, transportation, and antipollution enforcement all affect the daily choices of individuals regarding diet, residence, exercise, and pace of life.

Milio contends that health-damaging options are often less expensive, more attractively packaged and more accessible than health-promoting options. To make healthy choices, individuals must often resist the pressures of advertising and the temptations of our prevailing American lifestyle, and act differently than their peers. For health promotion programs to be effective in improving the health of the population, the range of available options must be broadened, particularly for low-income groups, and it must be made easier for all people to choose healthy over health-damaging alternatives. For example, a local effort to teach healthful nutrition might be supplemented by a program to make healthful low-cost foods available. This would require changes in the structure of community, public, and private organizations. At the present time many services are fragmented, with different agencies offering different components of the service. A person may be required to go to one agency for education regarding nutrition and to another to obtain assistance in obtaining the low-cost foods. Similarly, to expand the range of options for the national population, changes would be required in the decisions and policies of the federal government and large corporations. In Milio's view, morbidity and mortality rates cannot be substantially decreased or the health of the population substantially improved by educational/persuasion efforts focusing on the individual alone; societal resources and the cooperative efforts of major organizations and government agencies are also necessary. One way to fulfill the responsibilities stated in

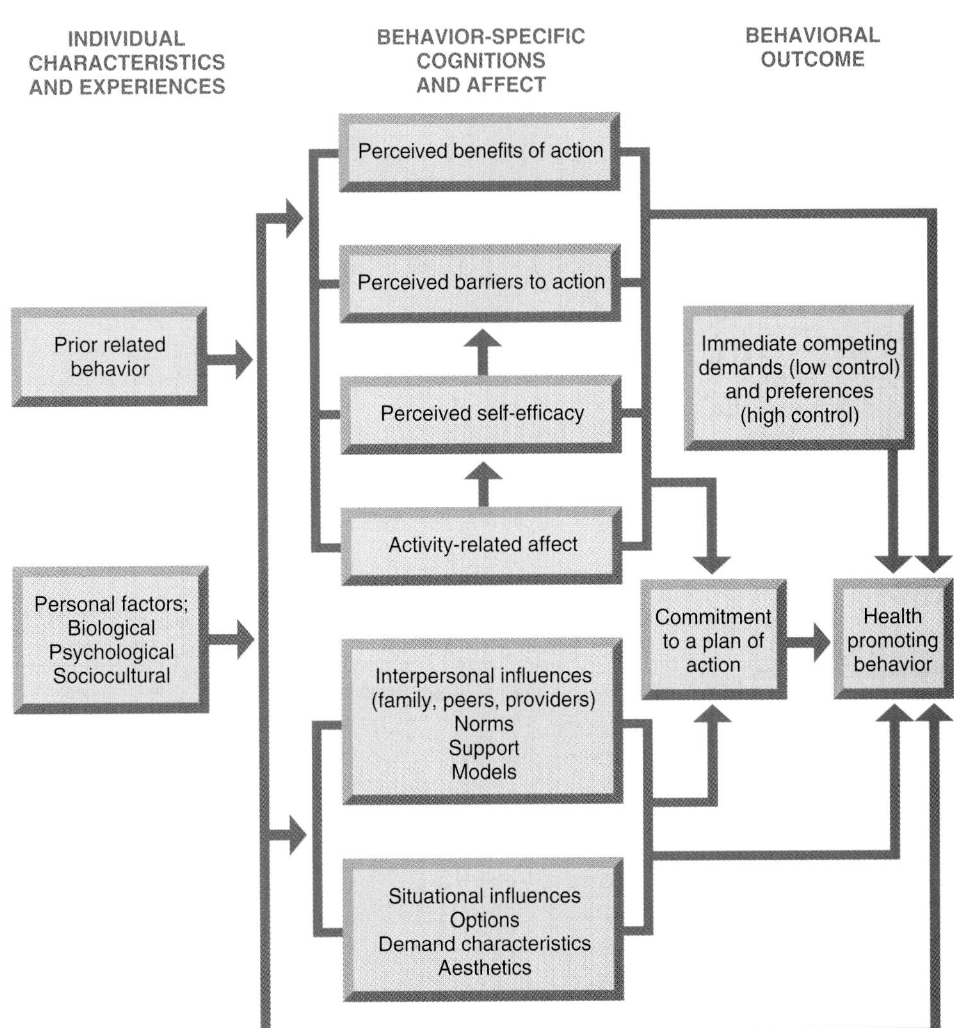

Figure 36–3. Revised health promotion model. (From Pender, N.J. [1996]. *Health Promotion in Nursing Practice,* 3rd ed. Stamford, CT: Appleton & Lange.)

its Social Policy Statement (see Chapter 1) is for nurses and nursing organizations to participate actively in promoting, formulating, and implementing such policies.

FACTORS AFFECTING CLINICAL DECISIONS

Individuals differ in their health promotion and self-care practices, according to their health perceptions and attitudes, physical condition, and psychological and personality characteristics. These personal characteristics, in turn, are affected by sociodemographic factors such as gender, age, family factors, socioeconomic status, culture and ethnic background, and religious affiliation (Fig. 36–4).

Gender

We know that women in this country practice self-care more than men because they:

- historically have supplied the bulk of health care for their families
- express more favorable attitudes toward self-care
- are more likely to self-medicate and use alternative and unorthodox forms of health care
- have been exhorted by the feminist movement to regain control of their health from the male-dominated medical establishment by diagnosing and treating themselves (Green, 1985; Levin and Idler, 1983; Stacey and Olesen, 1993)

Pregnancy, Papanicolaou (Pap) smear, and cholesterol screening kits are commercially available, as are over-the-counter medications for conditions such as vaginitis.

Besides practicing more self-care than men, women also perform more health promotion activities (except for exercise). More women than men, in all age and education categories, report practicing five or six of the Alameda "good" health habits (Schoenborn, 1986; Wilson and Elinson, 1981). Women smoke less, drink less, use illicit narcotics less, and have better eating habits. Over recent decades, gender differences in smoking behavior have dwindled as the percentage of men who smoke has decreased, and the percentages of young girls and women who smoke have increased. Today, over 28 percent of men and nearly 24 percent of women

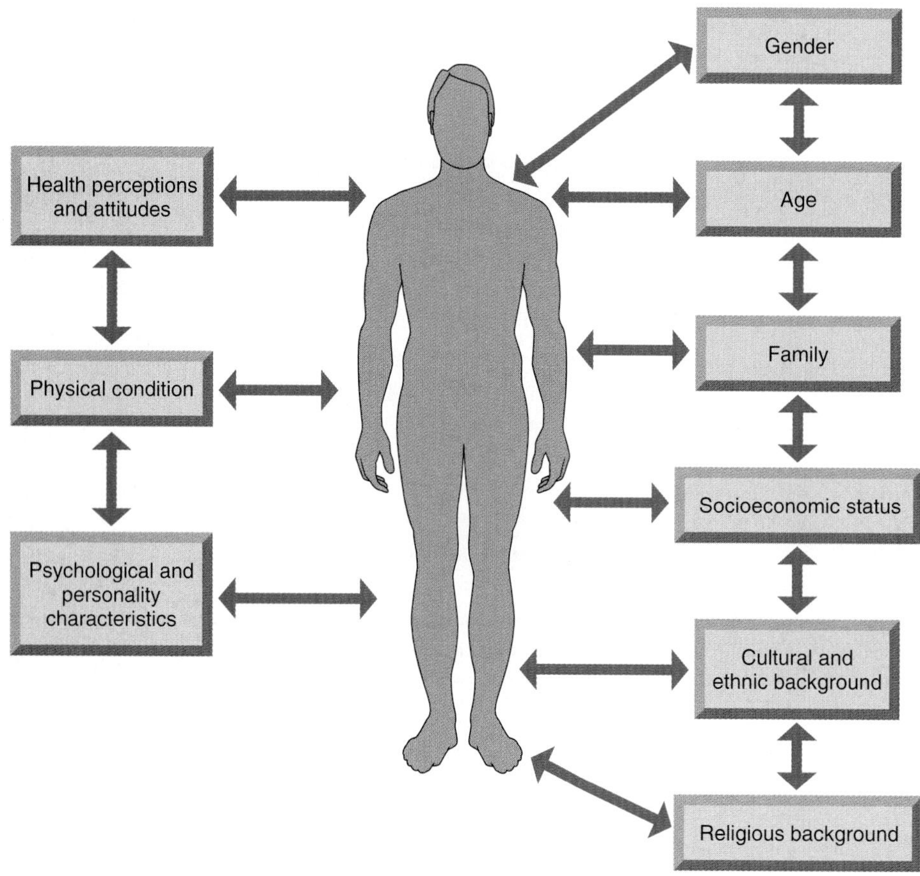

Figure 36-4. Factors affecting health promotion and self-care.

smoke (CDC, 1993). Because of this change in women's smoking behavior, lung cancer has surpassed breast cancer as the leading cause of cancer in American women.

Women use alcohol and illicit drugs less than men do (Lex, 1991). Because more men than women use drugs, and also because substance abuse is less likely to be diagnosed in women, treatment programs have traditionally focused on the needs of men. Due to lack of treatment, many women with drug problems continue to take drugs, and if they become pregnant, their fetuses may be harmed.

Women, generally, have better eating habits than men. Gender differences first appear in adolescence, perhaps less because of a concern for health than from concern for appearance. Concern for appearance provides strong motivation, especially for women, to eat diets low in calories and cholesterol, and high in fruits and vegetables (Cockerham et al, 1988a, 1988b; Hayes and Ross, 1987). However, concern for body appearance may at times lead to the adoption of unhealthy eating habits. When appearance norms conflict with good health habits, women's health suffers. Currently, our society considers the ideal body shape to be thin. This standard pressures females, especially, to diet beginning in preadolescent years and continuing throughout life. In one study, 45 percent of the girls age 7 to 13 wanted to be thinner, and 37 percent were already dieting. It has been estimated that 90 percent of the patients with eating disorders are female, that 1 of every 100 adolescent girls has anorexia nervosa, and that the incidence of bulimia is somewhere between 1.3 and 4 percent. Rolls and coworkers (1991) suggest that restricted eating may be a phase in the typical development of young women in Western culture, requiring treatment only if protracted or carried to such an extreme as to pose serious and life-threatening consequences.

Exercise is an important health-promoting activity in which men surpass women. In 1985, the National Health Interview Survey reported that over 44 percent of American males versus nearly 39 percent of American females were "regularly active," but that most did not engage in "appropriate exercise" (Caspersen et al, 1986). It should also be noted that exercise may involve health hazards when carried to extremes, or when steroids are used to build muscles and achieve strength and endurance.

In other areas of health promotion and protection, women are more active than men. Women engage in less risk-taking behavior than men as shown by lower death rates for lung cancer, motor vehicle accidents, cirrhosis of the liver, bronchitis, emphysema and asthma, suicide, and homicide (Nathanson, 1977). Women also perform more gender-specific preventive care (e.g., breast self-examination, prenatal and postnatal care, contraception) than do men (e.g., testicular examinations). Finally, women also use more preventive services that require professional intervention, such as dental and physical checkups and immunizations (Harris and Guten, 1979; Nathanson, 1977). This difference may result from socialization patterns that lead women to acknowledge vulnerability, or from the predominant medical model which historically has singled out women for special professional attention, especially during childbearing and childrearing.

Age

Most of the existing research has found no differences among age groups in the practice of self-care conducted without direct contact with a professional. This holds both for self-diagnosis and for self-medication using home remedies or nonprescribed medications for curative or health-promoting purposes (Brown and March, 1991). For example, from 44 to 66 percent of adults, and up to 66% of all adolescents and children currently use some form of vitamin or mineral supplement (Muncie and Sobal, 1987).

Older persons appear to have better health-promoting habits than younger persons. They follow more of the Alameda "good" practices (Breslow and Enstrom, 1980; Wilson and Elinson, 1981). Their nutrition is better, they drink less alcohol, use drugs less, and smoke less (Cockerham et al, 1988a, 1988b; Hayes and Ross, 1987; Lee and Markides, 1991; Lex, 1991). Only about 8 percent of people over age 74 years smoke, in contrast to just over 30 percent of people age 15 to 44 (CDC, 1993). A larger proportion—almost 52 percent—of persons age 18 to 29 exercise regularly versus 32 percent of people age 65 and above, but only 10 percent of the younger group, and 7.5 percent of the older group meet the Public Health Service's criteria for "appropriate" physical activity (Casperson et al, 1986; Cockerham et al, 1988b; Hayes and Ross, 1987).

Clearly all age groups might improve their health promotion practices, but the payoffs for behavioral change appear especially great for younger Americans. Poor health practices early in life set a foundation for adult illness, whereas positive health practices tend to persist into adulthood and exert a positive effect on later health and longevity (Belloc and Breslow, 1972; Perry et al, 1985). Although adolescence presents a unique opportunity to maximize optimal health-promoting behavior, it also poses a challenge to health educators. Adolescents often know the rules for healthy living, but fail to practice them. In one large survey of 11,000 students in grades 8 through 10, a majority of the students reported drinking alcohol, using drugs and tobacco, and being careless in avoiding injury (Medical News and Perspectives, 1988). Adolescents do not perceive such high-risk health behaviors as a problem for themselves because they tend to feel invincible. They worry more about immediate health problems affecting appearance such as acne than about preventing heart or other serious disease in the distant future (Feldman et al, 1986).

Health education programs for adolescents are more likely to be effective in producing positive and persisting behavioral changes if programs:

- involve more personal interaction among students, peers, parents, family members, and teachers
- secure parental support and participation
- present the health message in a dramatic and entertaining way (Cresanta et al, 1986)

Kaiser Permanente, a major health insurance company, has developed two educational plays with music, dance, and songs to encourage audience participation. "Professor Bodywise" dramatizes the consequences of unhealthy behavior and encourages grade school children to adopt healthy behavior. "Secrets" speaks out about safe sex, and the transmission of HIV disease and AIDS. These plays have been well received by students at a number of schools in the Northwest, and have significantly increased adolescents' awareness of their health behavior.

There is more controversy about the cost-effectiveness of health promotion programs for elderly persons. Research findings present conflicting pictures of the relation between the health practices of the elderly and their health status. Nevertheless, nurses and other health professionals appear committed to offering health promotion programs for the elderly on the assumption that these may result, if not in longer life, at least in improved functional ability and a better quality of life. Thus, Moyer (1981) and O'Neal (1982) both urge nurses to extend self-care educational efforts to the aged in institutions, hospitals, and the community. These efforts might include:

- health talks on radio reading services for the visually impaired
- discussions in church groups and garden clubs
- health messages for preretirement programs at industrial firms or municipal agencies
- participation in community-based fitness programs
- programs in community senior citizen housing or recreation centers

Nurses might deliver these services on a consultative basis, or persuade agencies or businesses to sponsor the programs for public relations reasons.

Individual and Family Values

Both marital status and parenthood have a positive effect on health, as indicated by significantly higher mortality rates of unmarried persons and nonparents. The benefit is particularly great for men. In part, this linkage may be attributed to a "selection factor"—those individuals who are healthier are more likely to marry and have children. But the linkage also may be due in part to the genuinely benign influence of marital and parental roles, involving routines, norms of responsibility, social control, and social support, both received and given. Social support provides meaning to life, buffers the strains of life events and environmental stressors, reduces social isolation, and inhibits suicide and other self-destructive acts. Both a sense of responsibility toward family members and restrictions imposed by other family members discourage negative health behavior and encourage health-promoting behavior. Thus, data from a national sample have indicated that married individuals and parents maintain more orderly lifestyles, take fewer risks, engage in less substance abuse, have significantly better eating habits, but are less likely to exercise than their counterparts (Cockerham et al, 1988a; Hayes and Ross, 1987; Umberson, 1987).

The above should not be construed to indicate that all families have healthy lifestyles. Clearly, there are dysfunctional families as shown by the incidence of child and spouse abuse, as well as alcoholism and drug addiction among parents. In other families, spouses and parents may behave in ways that adversely affect their own and their children's psychological and physical health. Some of these families hold alternative views about health and health professionals may disagree with them. These families may refuse vaccinations, object to fluoridation, and self-medicate in ways that health professionals consider to be ineffective or dangerous. In such situations, the nurse may be caught between fear of alienating the family and the professional responsibility of advising the family of potential harm from use of the alternative treatment itself or from its interaction with traditional therapies.

EDUCATIONAL BACKGROUND

Persons with more education express more favorable attitudes toward self-care, and self-medicate more than persons with less education. They also engage in more health promotive behavior. According to a National Health Survey, persons with more than 12 years of education reported five or six favorable "Alameda" health practices more frequently than persons with less than 12 years of education. Those with more education tend to

- exercise more
- eat more nutritionally balanced diets
- smoke less
- have more dental and physical checkups
- use seat belts (Cockerham et al, 1988b; Grunberg et al, 1991)

SOCIOECONOMIC STATUS

Education is a better predictor of health habits than occupational status or income, except when income dips below the poverty level. Lack of resources and opportunities make it harder for the poor to acquire knowledge about healthy ways of living, or to act upon that knowledge once acquired. To adopt healthier lifestyles, the poor need a favorable community infrastructure meeting their basic needs for food, shelter, clean air, clean water, and safety. They also need:

- day care facilities to free parents to seek jobs
- centers to provide immunization, maternity, and family planning services
- transportation into and out of the area
- advocates to help them obtain food stamps and food, find housing, and cope with the welfare, health, and judicial systems

The unhealthy lifestyle of persons in poverty is reflected in:

- less prenatal care and poorer pregnancy outcomes
- higher rates of infant mortality
- higher rates of growth retardation (16 percent)
- more injuries
- higher rates of obesity (37 percent of women are overweight)
- greater tendency toward high blood pressure

The poor smoke more, exercise less (32 percent of the poor engage in no leisure time physical activity), and use preventive measures less often than more affluent Americans. Forty percent of their children have untreated dental caries; and in 1987 only 22 percent of low-income women over age 40 had ever had a breast examination or mammogram (U.S. DHHS, 1990).

CULTURE AND ETHNICITY

An individual's health behavior is largely the product of social and cultural norms, the beliefs and values of the society and particular ethnic group to which he or she belongs. To that extent that the cultural beliefs and customs of minority ethnic groups differ from those of the larger society, their members' health problems and health behaviors may also be expected to differ.

The health of ethnic minority groups in our society is generally poorer than that of the overall U.S. population. We do not know how much this health difference is due to economic factors, and how much to the effect of cultural influences on health practices. The limited information available on the self-care, disease prevention, and health promotion practices of our major ethnic populations is summarized below, together with a listing of their major health problems. All generalizations based on these population profiles of blacks, Hispanics and Native Americans should be treated with caution. There are many subgroups within these populations with different lifestyles, and there are many individual exceptions as well. Chapter 6 contains information about other ethnic groups. Specific data about other groups can also be obtained from government publications such as *Health, United States, 1994* and *Healthy People 2000.*

Blacks. In the United States, blacks have higher rates of cancer, stroke, hypertension, diabetes, and homicide (U.S. DHHS, 1990), and a higher mortality rate from disease than whites (Ransford, 1986). The prevalence of AIDS among blacks is triple, and the incidence of low birth weight and infant mortality is roughly double the rates among whites (Reeb et al, 1987).

The relatively unfavorable health status of blacks results in part from their high incidence of poverty. Roughly one third of all blacks in this nation are "poor" (U.S. DHHS, 1990) and thereby prone to the problems associated with poverty: poor nutrition, poor housing, poor public facilities, much violence and crime, a dangerous environment, lack of support and a lack of access to health care services.

A second reason for the higher than average mortality and morbidity rates of blacks may lie in their personal health habits, and insufficient use of routine preventive measures. Thus, a higher percentage of blacks smoke (29.2 percent) than of whites (25.5 percent) (CDC, 1993). Black women are less likely to exercise, or maintain a favorable weight. In the period 1976–80, 44 percent of black women aged 20 to 74 were overweight (U.S. DHHS, 1990). Blacks are less likely to immunize their children against polio and measles, or to obtain vision tests for them. They visit dentists less often, and develop more periodontal disease. They seek fewer family planning services. Lack of prenatal care, along with stress and family problems, contribute to the relatively high rates of intrapartum (labor) complications among black women and of low birth weight in their infants (Reeb et al, 1987). It is imperative to remember that the statistics do not provide insight into causes of behavior. The statistics only tell "what is" and not "why." For example, the higher incidence of smoking could be linked to culture, to community, to economic status, or to educational level. The point of the statistics is the identification of people at risk and of risky health behaviors.

Black women have made one significant advance in positive health behavior, so recent it has not yet been reflected in mortality data. According to the 1986 National Health Interview Survey, black women are now, in contrast to earlier years, **more** likely than white women to obtain a Pap test or a breast examination (Duelberg, 1992). It is not known whether changes in the medical care system or special educational projects led to this change in behavior. Unfortunately, the change has not extended to poor elderly black women who use public hospitals. They continue to have breast and cervical cancers diagnosed at late stages, when treatment is less successful (Mandelblatt et al, 1991).

These, then, are some of the health problems and risky health behaviors of blacks that might be targeted by nurses and other health professionals for intervention efforts in the interests of health protection and promotion. Although nurses as individuals can do little to change some factors contributing to poor health status such as a person's socioeconomic status, they can work with local community health groups and social services to make health care equally accessible in all communities, and to target interventions to specific health risks they face.

Hispanics. This term covers several different cultural groups, including Cubans, Puerto Ricans, and Mexican-Americans; Mexican-Americans comprise by far the largest number. Health data for the "Hispanic population" are sometimes gathered from all these groups and pooled; at other times data obtained from Mexican-Americans are generalized to other Spanish-speaking groups. In either instance, ignoring the differences among the groups makes the data difficult to interpret. In reporting the health data in this section we will specify the particular group studied when that information is available, and use the term *Hispanic* only when the source of the information did not designate a particular group.

Diabetes is more prevalent among Hispanics, especially in older age groups, and possibly more severe, with higher mortality rates. According to the Hispanic Health and Nutrition Examination Survey (HHANES) the age-adjusted prevalence of self-reported diabetes for Hispanics in the early 1980s was nearly 7 percent for men and almost 8 percent for women, compared with rates of nearly 3 percent and 4 percent, respectively, in the total United States population (Perez-Stable et al, 1989).

Hispanics are also at greater risk for tuberculosis (prevalence is 10.3 per 100,000), elevated blood pressure, obesity (39 percent of Mexican-American women ages 20 to 74 are overweight), and growth retardation among children from low-income families. In 1988, growth retardation was evidenced in 13 percent of Hispanic children under 1 year of age, and 16 percent for children age 1 year (U.S. DHHS, 1990). The overall cancer mortality rate is lower among Mexican-Americans than other whites, according to studies conducted in Colorado, New Mexico, Los Angeles, and Texas. Mexican-Americans contract more stomach, liver, and gallbladder cancers, but fewer lung, colon, breast, and prostate cancers (Martin and Suarez, 1987).

To some extent, behavior patterns may account for these rates. The high rates of diabetes and obesity may be related to eating habits and relatively low physical activity levels. Lung cancer rates may be low because Hispanics have traditionally smoked less than other whites or blacks (Greenberg et al, 1987). A recent surge in smoking, particularly among younger males, will doubtless increase cancer and cigarette-linked diseases in the near future (Marcus and Crane, 1985).

The failure of many Hispanics to use preventive services accounts for other health problems (Andersen et al, 1981). Growth retardation in children may be due to lack of prenatal care. The higher mortality of Mexican-American women for cervical cancer may be explained by diagnosis at a later stage of the disease. Clearly there is a need to promote free or low-cost screening programs for this population (Martin and Suarez, 1987).

Hispanics fail to use preventive services because of lack of accessibility to care (almost 22 percent lack medical insurance), lack of education, and economic barriers. Some writers seek an explanation in certain cultural characteristics that have been attributed to Mexican-Americans, and by extension, to Hispanics generally. These characteristics are lack of future orientation, recklessness, machismo, and reluctance to accept personal responsibility (Weaver, 1973). It should be remembered, however, that Mexican-Americans do not comprise a monolithic community, and there is great variation in lifestyle among them. Furthermore, to generalize from Mexican-Americans to other Hispanic groups is questionable.

Native Americans, Alaskans. In the 1980s, the leading cause of death for Native Americans as for the general U.S. population, was diseases of the heart. This was followed by accidents, and then malignant neoplasms (tumors). However, Native Americans are at less risk than other Americans for heart disease or cancer. They are at greater risk for tuberculosis (the age-adjusted mortality rate was 400 percent higher), alcoholism, diabetes, accidents, homicide, pneumonia and influenza, suicide (28 percent greater), and communicable diseases such as mumps, dysentery, hepatitis, venereal disease, and measles (U.S. DHHS, 1990, 1991). The great increase in the prevalence of non–insulin-dependent diabetes mellitus among Native Americans has been attributed to the interplay between genetic factors and the adoption of the lifestyle of white Americans. Changes in total caloric intake, in specific nutrients, and in activity levels may have led to an increase in obesity and triggered metabolic changes culminating in diabetes (Szathmary et al, 1987).

The Native American birth rate is the highest of any population subgroup in this country, at nearly 28 births per 1000 in 1985–1987. Dramatic improvements in maternal and infant health have been noted in recent years, with the maternal mortality rate down from nearly 83 per 1,000,000 live births in 1959 to just under 9 in 1985–1987, and the infant mortality rate down from almost 63 per 1000 births to just under 10. However, infant deaths after 28 days exceed those of the general population (U.S. DHHS, 1991). Among Native American children, ear infections are common, and anemia afflicts one fourth of all Alaskan children (Levitan and Johnson, 1975).

The problems of ethnic and minority group members are related to patterns of health behavior that may be targeted for interventions by concerned health professionals. However, existing health promotion programs may be inappropriate and ineffective for minorities since they were often developed by and for white middle-class Americans. Inattention to basic health necessities (food, shelter, safety, sanitary facilities) sabotages the success of well-intended efforts. Health programs for minorities should address these issues along with specific problems of accidents and injuries, alcoholism and suicide, nutrition, obesity, diabetes, and prenatal care.

SPIRITUALITY AND RELIGIOUS PRACTICES

Religious beliefs and practices have relevance for health promotion and disease prevention by reason of their prescriptions and restrictions for diet and lifestyle. Religions holding that the body is a prison from which the soul is liberated at death as some Christian religions do, may consider health-promoting activities unimportant. Religions proclaiming that the body is the temple of the soul may provide strong directives for the personal lives of believers (Dwyer et al, 1990; Troyer, 1988). These may result in distinctive lifestyles with regard to dietary practices, smoking and drinking habits, sexual contacts, hygiene, marital stability, occupation and hence socioeconomic status, and place of residence (e.g., rural versus urban). Sometimes these lifestyle prescriptions are health promoting from the perspective of the health professional, and sometimes not. Some religious groups discourage certain actions such as vaccination considered health protective or promoting by health professionals, and some may not accept modern public health principles or medical treatment. (Information on specific health-related religious practices is provided in Chapter 6.)

The extent to which individual members will adhere to these directives depends on the depth of their commitment, frequency of church attendance, and extent of social interaction with other believers (Dwyer et al, 1990). For example, the Seventh Day Adventists, Mormons, Amish, and Hutterites differ in their lifestyles from the dominant society. They all tend to live in communities of believers. The Seventh Day Adventists are usually vegetarian, and do not smoke, drink tea, coffee, or alcohol. The Mormons avoid smoking and stimulants, but eat meat in moderation. The agricultural Amish eat meat, drink tea and coffee, but strongly discourage alcohol and tobacco. The agricultural Hutterites eat meat, drink tea and coffee, but drink alcohol in moderation. All four of these groups have lower rates of cancer than the general population. These lower rates pertain mainly to cancers associated with smoking, which all of the groups oppose. In all four groups the incidence of breast cancer is higher than average (Troyer, 1988).

According to some scholars, the differences in the mortality and morbidity rates of religious groups are due not solely to their particular health practices, but also to the social support afforded by their social networks, and by the sense of belonging that individuals derive from a community of believers. It is to this support and sense of belonging that religion's protective power against suicide has been attributed (Pescosolido and Georgianna, 1989).

Finally, where there is a concentration of members of a particular religious group, the health consequences of that religion may extend beyond its own adherents to the community-at-large (Dwyer et al, 1990). For example, non-Mormons in Utah also enjoy a lower incidence of cancer than the national average. Their cancer morbidity may be decreased because of diminished exposure to secondary smoke.

Setting

Health promotion and self-care activities take place in every setting. In the acute care setting, the nurse provides health education specific to the patient's needs from admission to discharge. For example, the nurse may teach the presurgical patient the deep-breathing, coughing, and turning exercises known to prevent postoperative respiratory or circulatory complications. At discharge the nurse may teach the patient and family about the medications the patient will take after discharge. In the home setting, the nurse is always alert to potential health hazards and educates the family regarding these. For example, throw rugs on a hardwood floor might be a hazard for an elderly person using a walker. In the ambulatory setting, the nurse attends to the whole person and not just the precipitating health problem. Increasingly the nurse uses databases to identify potential health problems and intervene appropriately. For example, a 45-year-old woman may be in the ambulatory surgical unit for a minor surgical procedure. The nurse could use this as an opportunity to review health screening recommendations and identify those the woman needs to attend to such as mammography.

Ethical Considerations

Self-care and health promotion appeal to many Americans because they reflect the basic American cultural values of independence and self-reliance. Many people believe that making choices and acting on their own behalf strengthen problem-solving skills, increase self-esteem, provide a sense of competence and empowerment, and give them control over many aspects of their lives. However, there is a darker side (Becker, 1993), found in a number of troubling ethical, moral, practical, and financial issues, including:

- Who should decide on matters of health?
- Can and will Americans assume personal responsibility for their health?
- Does the emphasis on individual health promotion and self-care divert attention from the environmental, genetic, social, political, and economic factors affecting health?

WHO SHOULD DECIDE ON MATTERS OF HEALTH AND HEALTH CARE?

Should individuals themselves, professionals, or some third party have the final say about **when** care is necessary and **what** that care should consist of? Probably most laypersons would agree that people themselves should have the greatest say in decisions regarding their own health, but with certain qualifications regarding conditions and circumstances. These qualifications indicate a greater or lesser willingness to share the decision-making power with health professionals. A few laypersons would rely almost entirely on self-care and keep professional help to a minimum (Boston Women's Health Book Collective, 1975; DeFriese et al, 1989). Others consider self-care only a supplement to professional care and welcome expert advice and help. Still others have little confidence in self-care and would rely almost entirely on professional care.

Most health professionals today approve individual decision-making and self-care when it's in line with professional recommendations. They reserve control over the more serious disorders, difficult diagnoses and complicated procedures, citing reasons of safety. They do not oppose self-treatment by laypersons for minor, self-limiting conditions (such as the common cold or warts), and for persistent or resistant chronic conditions when medical treatment has been ineffective (such as some back problems). Self-treatment for such conditions eases the work burden of professionals, decreases excessive use of formal health services, and helps to contain health care costs.

Health promotion advocates almost always bow to the expert opinion of health professionals, and believe that laypersons should do the same. This tendency has grown as health professionals have become more involved in health promotion programs. Finally, in recent years, the health promotion movement has increasingly involved third parties (insurance companies, commercial firms, hospitals, marketing organizations, and corporate systems) as their power to make decisions regarding health has expanded. This third-party involvement is changing the character of health promotion. Cost containment is being emphasized and not the potential for improving people's health (Goldstein, 1992; Milio, 1988). How to balance cost and quality in a market-driven health care system will be a major issue for policy makers.

The ethical dilemma involved here is who should make decisions on health matters. To what extent should individuals make decisions for themselves, and when should professionals step in to ensure safety and optimize health outcomes? Is health more important than independence? Or finally, should a third party that develops health products and services, manages care, or pays the bill be permitted to make the decisions?

Should an individual suffering from severe mental illness be free to accept or reject treatment? Should a person suffering from epilepsy be restricted for treatment to the drugs and surgical procedures most physicians trained in Western medicine use? Or should the individual be free to explore other treatments, such as the ketogenic diet developed at Harvard?

WILL AMERICANS ASSUME PERSONAL RESPONSIBILITY FOR THEIR HEALTH?

How ready people are to accept responsibility for their health, and therefore practice self-care and health promotion, depends in part on their beliefs about the etiology of health and illness. Some are not ready since they believe that illness is caused by forces outside their control. Persons ready to accept personal responsibility for health believe in free will, and that people **choose** whether to act in healthy or unhealthy ways (Goldstein, 1992). Americans most likely to believe this are young, white, middle-class, better educated, employed, and relatively healthy (Goldstein, 1992). Poor people are less likely to accept responsibility and practice health promotion, for in reality, they have fewer choices than middle-class individuals.

But it isn't only the poor who find it difficult to make healthy choices, because at-risk behavior is bound to our culture and social structure (McKinlay, 1974). Thus, at-risk behavior for heart problems (such as the competitive, aggressive, hurried behavior characterizing the Type A personality) is often justified by values, beliefs, and norms of our dominant culture, and abundantly rewarded. As another example, some American businesses and industries (e.g., the food and tobacco industries) expend enormous resources promoting at-risk behaviors by linking them to popularity, attractiveness, and courage. They hire entertainers and other culture heroes of our society to endorse smoking, drinking, and fast driving.

The emphasis on personal responsibility for health, with its tie to basic values, tends to give health promotion a moralistic tone. So also does the fact that the at-risk behaviors that most American health promotion programs seek to eliminate or control (drinking, smoking, overeating, and sexual intercourse) are pleasurable activities, historically receiving moral disapproval. As Goldstein puts it, "the potential for moralizing and punitive reactions in it is great" (1992, p. 143). There is a danger of "victim-blaming," of creating stigma and personal guilt in individuals with unhealthy lifestyles (Becker, 1993; Conrad, 1987; Goldstein, 1992). They may be judged lazy, lacking in willpower, reckless, or otherwise faulty, and blamed for failing to exercise, lose weight, quit smoking, reduce their cholesterol, or learn to use health services "properly." People who become ill may be blamed on the presumption that their problems are self-inflicted by something they should not have done (e.g., smoked, ate a high-fat diet) or something they failed to do (e.g., did not exercise regularly). The following ethical issues are involved:

- Are behavior changes made simply to improve health, or to obtain conformity to a moral standard?
- To what extent should health workers be agents of social regulation?
- Is it ethical to attempt behavior control at all, especially if it is to enforce a particular type of conformity?

Health promotion and self-care offer the benefits of fostering competence, independence and a sense of control, as well as preventing illness and improving health. However, individual responsibility for health may also become a burden if people are blamed for their own ill health and required to pay for their own care. This view would limit access to care and compromise the principles of equity and right to health care.

DOES AN EMPHASIS ON HEALTH PROMOTION AND SELF-CARE DIVERT ATTENTION FROM THE ENVIRONMENTAL, GENETIC, SOCIAL, POLITICAL, AND ECONOMIC FACTORS AFFECTING HEALTH?

An emphasis on health promotion and self-care does not minimize the importance of attending to the environmental, genetic, social, political, and economic factors affecting health. This would certainly not be the case if the WHO guidelines for health promotion were to be implemented in their entirety. If that were the case, there would be efforts directed toward:

- public policy and community action
- ecological and environmental issues
- eliminating inequities in health and living conditions
- reorienting health services to promote health
- changing personal lifestyles

In the United States, however, the major emphasis has not been this inclusive, instead focusing on one aspect of health promotion and self-care—the development of personal skills for healthier living (Salmon, 1987). In this approach, people are seen as free agents able to solve their health problems through personal transformation, and illness may be attributed to personal failings (Becker, 1993; Conrad, 1987; Crawford, 1977). Health efforts focus on changing the individual's behavior and psychological state. For instance, illness in the workplace may be attributed to laziness about using protective gear, to genetic susceptibility, or to psychological maladjustment. Accordingly, the overstressed worker is offered biofeedback, psychological counseling, or transcendental meditation to manage stress. The structure of incentives and sanctions that reward stress-generating behavior, the organization of work, and management style remain unchanged. Environmental changes may be limited to labeling the nutritional content of cafeteria foods or instituting a no-smoking policy.

The individualistic approach tends to obscure the social causes of disease. This approach also ignores the fact that large-scale structural changes have historically been the major factors in improving the health of populations. These changes included:

- rising standards of living
- decreased poverty
- better education
- emergence of social welfare programs
- public health measures that provided better sewer systems, sanitary water supplies, and more sanitary food production and distribution

Health problems resulting from social structure factors require group efforts for resolution (Becker, 1993). For example, problems of pollution and workplace exposure to carcinogenic substances can only be dealt with through group efforts resulting in government policy, legislation and regulation by agencies such as the Occupational Safety and Health Administration (OSHA).

Financial Considerations

What are the economic consequences of self-care and health promotion? Health promotion and self-care have won the support of many organizations for economic reasons, either for profit or for the desire to contain health costs. Many commercial enterprises and private health corporations have capitalized on the huge market for health-related products and services. They sell kits for self-diagnosis of blood pressure, cholesterol, and other problems, drugs and devices for self-treatment, and an abundance of paraphernalia and programs to improve fitness and control weight. Magazines and books targeting health concerns advertise the commercially available products and services, and give advice on fitness and nutrition. The companies have profited considerably, and the magazines and books have gained wide readerships.

Other organizations turn to individual-oriented health promotion programs and self-care for reasons of cost containment. Administrators of health care facilities hope these programs will check health costs by reducing the number of visits to medical practitioners, the use of expensive technology, and unnecessary diagnostic tests (Abosede, 1984). Employers in industrial and business firms hope the programs, by improving the health of employees, will both enhance worker productivity through decreased absenteeism and sick leave, and reduce health care costs paid in the form of employee benefits. (Today, employers pay 30 percent of the American health care bill.)

Judging the success of these programs is difficult because hard data are scarce, and the existing evidence is conflicting. The costs of preventing some diseases can exceed the costs of medical treatment when interventions are directed to large numbers of people, only a few of whom would have become sick (Russell, 1986). On the other hand, self-care for upper respiratory infections has been found to be cost-effective (Zapka and Averill, 1979), as has exercise for reducing risks for coronary heart disease (Hatziandreu et al, 1988). In another study, persons using self-care visited physicians less often and stayed fewer days in hospital than other persons (Fleming et al, 1984). We may conclude that cost containment is a promising but unproven benefit of health promotion.

Cost containment is a worthy goal, and profit-making is an American way of life. Still there are hidden dangers when the bottom line for health promotion becomes economics. The efficacy, quality, and safety of the commercially available health products and services are often unknown, and unregulated. They may lack health benefit or even be dangerous. Health appraisals by employers may result in job discrimination based on lifestyle if they are used for personnel purposes of recruitment, job placement, promotion, retention, and early retirement. There is a punitive, coercive element in an employer's raising insurance premiums for employees who engage in at-risk behavior such as smoking. There is a danger that health promotion programs will be substituted for environmental or organizational changes.

All of these situations have ethical as well as financial implications. Should employers intrude on the private life of employees, by inquiring into their off-work behaviors of smoking, exercise, diet, and blood pressure control? When allocating resources between efforts at prevention and treatment of illness, to what extent should cost-effectiveness take precedence over alleviation of suffering? How far may the government go in regulating the production of goods and services in a free enterprise economy? When health conflicts with the economic issues of productivity or employment, what compromises are reasonable and ethically acceptable?

FUTURE DEVELOPMENTS

Health promotion activities in the immediate future will continue to be shaped by the nation's health needs, the extent of progress toward national and state health objectives, and the press for cost containment. As for current progress, the Surgeon General (U.S. DHHS, 1990) estimates that 50 percent of the 226 measurable objectives for 1990 have been achieved, 25 percent have not, and the others cannot be evaluated due to a lack of data. Clearly, a system to monitor progress is needed.

There has been substantial progress in immunization, and in the control of infectious disease, high blood pressure, accidental injury, smoking, and use of alcohol and other drugs. Progress has lagged in the areas of pregnancy and infant health, nutrition, fitness and exercise, family planning, sexually transmitted diseases, and occupational safety and health. Health promotion efforts in those areas are expected to increase in order to avoid expensive high-technology treatments for health problems developing later. Again in the interest of cost containment, many programs will be directed toward changing behaviors associated with the major health problems of cardiovascular disease, injuries, and cancer. Lamm (1991) has estimated that the annual costs of those problems are, respectively, $135, $100, and $70 billion.

Effects of Health Promotion and Self-Care on the Health Care Delivery System

Depending on their motivation, advocates of self-care and health promotion may push for different changes in the health care system, ranging from matters of access and equity to the nature of the patient-practitioner relationship.

Among those persons advocating health promotion and self-care for economic reasons, some claim that health is not a right but a duty, which should be enforced by economic sanctions. They argue that the virtuous should not be taxed to provide care for those who persist in unhealthy habits, that the latter are responsible for their own illness, and should therefore pay their own bills (Becker, 1993; Crawford, 1977; Levin et al, 1976). The opposing viewpoint is linked to a view of social justice that emphasizes equity in access and services. It is also linked to the position that we have a responsibility to those less fortunate. An argument can also be put forward that sometimes risky health behaviors begin at a time when the behavior is not known to have a negative consequence for later health. Many people became addicted to nicotine before it was known to be associated with cancer.

A desire to limit the control health care providers have over access to health care has motivated some Americans to advocate health promotion and self-care. That motivation bears implications for health professionals and their roles. When the health care provider is in control, the patient usually assumes a passive, dependent role. The patient is given a set of options determined by the provider. The patient can reject the options, but that usually results in the loss of access to health care. Americans advocating health promotion, self-care, and personal responsibility for one's health see the provider as a consultant or partner in decision making. As a consultant or partner, providers would have to learn to accept more assertive, self-confident, and knowledgeable patients, and provide more dignified care. By relinquishing their monopoly on knowledge, and spending more time sharing that knowledge with their patients, health professionals should provide better quality of care. To achieve such a partnership in the patient-practitioner relationship, professional education would have to change significantly. The Kellogg Foundation and the Pew Health Professions Commission are two influential national groups calling for such changes.

Focus on Individual Behavior

In general, health promotion efforts in the near future will continue to focus on changing the health behaviors of individuals, rather than on changing the social, economic or political structure. But greater effort will be directed to groups or whole communities as the way to reach more people and influence health practices of families and subsequent generations. The particular form these health programs will take will depend on current knowledge about the relation of behavior to health.

Research will improve and expand our knowledge about why people do or do not control their weight, smoke, eat a nutritious diet, exercise, engage in risky sexual behavior; and about why the same behavior may affect the health of various individuals differently. Basic research may focus on:

- combined effects of heredity, environment, and lifestyle on health
- biochemistry of the brain
- relationships of the psychoneuroimmunologic and endocrine systems
- interaction of human physiologic and psychological systems

Greater understanding of these systems and processes will enable professionals to better identify the specific risk factors of particular individuals and to tailor prescriptions to optimize their health.

Applied research will center on developing various strategies to change behavior, and on testing their effectiveness with different populations and under different conditions. Some research may examine the circumstances under which one strategy (e.g., education, behavior modification, economic incentives) is more appropriate than another (McGinnis, 1982). Another promising area for research concerns the fit of the strategy to the stage of the behavior. For example, most youths experiment at smoking, but only a minority proceed to become chronic smokers. A different strategy may be needed to block the transition from experimentation to regular smoking than to help confirmed smokers quit.

Social and Economic Changes

The future of health promotion in our nation will be affected not only by development of its science base through research, but also by changes in the social and economic structure of our society (McGinnis, 1982). These changes include nontraditional family structures, policies regarding access to and payment for health care, and advances in technology. Reforms in the health care delivery system will encourage health promotion programs and self-care. Economic incentives for health promotion are likely to expand (for example, health insurers may cover costs incurred to stay healthy). New technologies to promote health will develop. Thus, communication systems will link health professionals and patients in widely dispersed geographic areas. More homes will have computerized interactive video systems, enabling people to have access to professional consultation. People will be able to transmit their personal medical histories and physiologic data through technology (e.g., x-rays and ECGs sent via phone lines, computers, and fax machines) to a health expert, to secure professional evaluation, and to obtain an order for a prescription or other treatment.

Support for these and other strategies to help achieve the nation's health goals may be provided by coalitions developed by private organizations and government at all levels. Creative experiments with innovative health promotion projects in the private sector may result in demonstration programs. In some instances such as with immunization programs the government may provide resources to assist in the implementation and evaluation of these programs. If successful, these programs may then be adopted across the nation.

However, business and industry don't always act in the best interests of workers and consumers, and often value profits over serving the nation's health needs responsibly (Milio, 1988). The government is therefore expected to use tax incentives to induce the food and advertising industries to promote the marketing of healthy products. The government is also expected to increase health and safety regulations in schools, workplaces, and recreational areas, and to increase its regulation of commercial health products and services to ensure their safety, efficacy, and quality.

In the future greater attention may be paid to health promotion among the disadvantaged and other high-risk groups. Recognizing that much of the federally funded research has to date been conducted with white males, our government has directed the National Institutes of Health to seek and fund more research on women and minorities. The expansion of the knowledge base in these areas will provide insight about new ways to promote health.

The extent to which Americans will actively support health promotion and self-care programs will depend on the importance they assign to these benefits, beliefs, and attitudes, as well as on the safety and effectiveness of these programs in improving the health of the American public. The public's decisions on the allocation of resources between individual-oriented health promotion efforts and alternative group approaches such as policy development, government regulation, and community efforts will depend on their judgment of the relative cost-effectiveness of these various techniques. It will also depend on the importance they assign to control of environmental and workplace hazards, improved standards of living, and the need for structural reforms in our health care system. But underlying all these decisions and deliberations are the ethical issues of individual freedom and behavior control in a democratic society, regulation of industry and business in a free enterprise society, and the question regarding whose good is being served.

Health for All by the Year 2000

To attain the goal of *Health for All by the Year 2000*, individuals, families, communities, organizations, industries, and government must be actively engaged in preventing illness and promoting health, while containing health care costs. Health promotion strategies for accomplishing this goal are education, technology, legislation, regulation, taxation, and persuasion through the use of incentives. Self-care also provides a means of achieving health promotion goals while maintaining individual autonomy and reducing costs.

Education of Health Professionals

Finally, the education of health professionals will also change. At present health professionals are trained to emphasize disease detection and cure. In the future, they must also learn the intricacies of prevention and health promotion, and nontraditional alternatives for enhancing health. They must know how to develop community-based health promotion programs, and train lay workers in schools and industry to implement these programs. Instruction in these skills will probably become a standard part of the curriculum for the health worker of tomorrow.

NURSING CARE ACTIONS

History shows that the nursing profession has emphasized its role in health promotion and disease prevention. Florence Nightingale, in 1893, spoke of nursing as putting a person in the best possible condition for nature to restore or preserve health. The 1923 Goldmark Report emphasized the need for public health nursing as an adjunct to hospital nursing. In 1955, Virginia Henderson defined nursing as assisting the individual, sick or well, in the performance of those activities contributing to health. The 1970 Commission for the Study of Nursing and Nursing Education verified that nursing involved the care of patients on a continuum from "well" to "acutely ill." The first Social Policy Statement published by the American Nurses' Association (1980) states that all nurses are responsible for the inclusion of preventive nursing as part of generalized and specialized practice.

But because nurses were part of a health care system that emphasized the treatment of illness, a typical nurse had neither time nor encouragement for health promotion activities. Today, the radical changes taking place in the private sector health care system are changing that. The evolving health care system is market driven and emphasizes cost containment, outcomes from care, and empowered consumers with a sense of responsibility for their own health. The system is moving from an emphasis on the treatment of disease to an emphasis on health promotion, disease prevention, and management of chronic illness. These changes are exciting developments for nursing. All nurses will be spending more time in health promotion activities. In addition new roles for nurses that emphasize health promotion and self-care such as the telephone triage and advice nurse and the care manager nurse are rapidly developing.

Nursing care actions for health promotion and self-care include:

- implementing strategies for health promotion at the individual and group level
- implementing strategies for disease prevention at the individual and group level
- incorporating primary prevention, secondary prevention, and tertiary prevention strategies appropriately into every patient encounter (Table 36–3)

These strategies require competencies in five areas:

- assessment
- advocacy
- education and counseling
- care management
- role modeling

Health Assessment

Chapter 15, Patient Assessment, includes a description of the subjective and objective data collected as part of a nursing assessment. The assessment of an individual and family for either health promotion or disease prevention builds on that assessment. The health promotion assessment explores patterns in lifestyle based on relationships among health status and beliefs, environment, and behavior. The disease prevention assessment explores the prevalence of risk factors associ-

TABLE 36–3 Examples of Nursing Care Actions by Level of Prevention

Level of Prevention	Nursing Care Actions
Primary prevention	• Immunization • General health education • Well-baby examination • Community assessment • Seat belt education • Parenting classes
Secondary prevention	• Smoking cessation clinic • Weight reduction clinic • Screening surveys • Abuse avoidance training • Exercise class for obese people after acute injury • Interventions to prevent complications, e.g., pressure ulcers and respiratory problems following surgery
Tertiary prevention	• Referral to self-help groups, e.g., Reach to Recovery • Patient/family teaching on assessing for complications, e.g., signs and symptoms of insulin shock and diabetic coma • Patient/family teaching on health promotion during recovery, e.g., proper diet, exercise, and stress reduction techniques for a patient recovering from myocardial infarction

ated with a specific disease. Many health promotion assessments include disease prevention assessment. The outcomes of the assessment are agreement between the individual and the nurse regarding the individual's health status; positive health-related behaviors and beliefs; risky health behaviors; and motivation to change.

FRAMEWORKS FOR HEALTH ASSESSMENT OF INDIVIDUALS

Tanner (1991) identifies these three components of a health promotion assessment:

- **Health history and physical assessment.** The health history includes assessment of the current and previous state of physical health, psychosocial health, and the health of the family of origin (see Chapter 15.) The sexual history is considered relevant and includes psychosocial development, quality of relationships within the family, attitudes of family members about sexual behavior, and conflicts regarding sexual behavior. Individuals known to be at risk for acquiring and spreading sexually transmitted diseases should be assessed to determine knowledge of safe sexual practices and symptoms of sexual diseases. Suggested questions for a sexual health history are included in Chapter 33.
- **Health-promoting behaviors.** The most common health-promoting behaviors are nutritional practices, sleep, physical activity, and stress management. The easiest way to conduct a nutritional assessment is to ask the individual to record accurately normal eating habits in an "eating diary." The diary should include antecedents and consequences of eating to identify emotional and social triggers associated with eating. The information in the diary can be compared with normal or average daily requirements and an appropriate plan developed for the individual. Chapter 22 contains further information about nutritional assessment. Physical exercise can be assessed in the same way. The individual can maintain an exercise diary recording all routine physical activity over the course of a week. The record should indicate the type of activity, length of time performed, and the heart rate if known. Response to the activity should also be recorded. The individual's activity level can be compared with appropriate norms and a plan for an ideal activity level developed. Stress management is the third set of health-promoting behaviors. Exposure to stress can be assessed through a variety of means. Chapter 31 provides examples of stress assessment tools and techniques for reducing stress. Health promotion includes identification of effective means of handling stress such as the use of progressive relaxation techniques, meditation, leisure activities, and adequate sleep (see Chapter 25 regarding assessment of sleep).
- **Health-protecting behaviors.** Part of health promotion assessment is identifying the behaviors the individual engages in that protect or maintain health. The individual should be interviewed regarding areas including tobacco use, alcohol and chemical substance use, and exposure to environmental hazards and injury. Information regarding their knowledge and attitudes regarding smoking, alcohol, and drug use should also be obtained. The exposure to environmental hazards such as chemical sprays or lifting heavy objects should be assessed. Exposure to accidental injury should also be assessed. For example, does the individual wear a seat belt when riding in an automobile? Are guns kept in the home stored properly?

The assessment should note the resources that enhance the individual's health promotion behaviors (such as a family that takes time to read and discuss health information) as well as those forces that may be deterrents to health promotion behaviors (such as working in a setting where smoking is the norm).

Pender (1996) provides another framework for the assessment of health. It is a holistic approach based on the use of different tools for different areas of the assessment. The beginning student should be familiar with this approach to health assessment but cannot be expected to implement this complex a health assessment. The assessment includes these nine areas:

- **Functional health patterns.** This component of the assessment includes data regarding the individual's health status, beliefs, and behaviors. It includes but is not limited to areas such as nutrition, elimination, rest and sleep, self-concept, role relationships, sexuality, stress tolerance, exercise level, spiritual strength, and health perception.
- **Physical fitness evaluation.** This component of the assessment includes data regarding (1) cardiorespiratory endurance (the ability of the respiratory and circulatory systems to efficiently adjust and recover from exercise); (2) muscular strength and endurance; (3) body composition (percentage of body fat); and (4) flexibility (the ability to move muscles and joints through their minimum range of motion).
- **Nutritional assessment.** This component of the assessment includes four types of data: (1) data regarding height, weight and skinfold thickness (anthropometric data); (2) biochemical data from blood and urine that could identify problems such as elevated blood cholesterol and glucose; (3) clinical examination data that might suggest malnutrition; and (4) the individual's dietary patterns.
- **Health risk appraisal.** The health risk appraisal is an attempt to identify an individual's risk for developing a particular disease by synthesizing and analyzing risk factors based on age, genetics, biologic characteristics, personal health habits, lifestyle, and environment. An individual's risk is determined by comparison with the average risk for a group with similar characteristics. The accuracy of this approach has been questioned

because it may not account for all the factors associated with the development of a disease.

- **Life stress review.** Stress can be assessed through many different techniques. Some well-established tools are described in Chapter 31, Stress and Anxiety.
- **Spiritual health assessment.** A holistic approach to health assessment includes spiritual health because spiritual beliefs can affect one's interpretation of events. The assessment is more than asking about membership in a particular religion. It explores the meaning of life by assessing the individual's relationships with a higher being, with self, and with others.
- **Social support systems.** The concept of social support and its assessment are discussed in Chapter 29, Social Support.
- **Health beliefs review.** This component of the assessment explores health-specific and behavior-specific beliefs. Health-specific beliefs include areas such as intrinsic motivation for health behavior and perceived health care competence. Behavior-specific beliefs include areas such as the perception of positive outcomes and barriers associated with exercise and the emotional support for exercise provided by others.
- **Lifestyle assessment.** This component of the assessment is a thoughtful review of the individual's health habits. All aspects of the individual's life must be considered.

Assessment of these nine areas provides the basis for developing an individually tailored health promotion and disease protection plan.

HEALTH ASSESSMENT OF THE FAMILY

The family is the primary social structure in which health behaviors, beliefs, and values are learned and reinforced. Assessment of the family is critical to successful implementation of health promotion strategies.

A health-promoting family assessment contains four essential components:

- listening to the family
- engaging in participatory dialogue
- recognizing patterns
- envisaging action and positive change (Hartrick et al, 1994)

Listening involves gaining an understanding of the family story as the family experiences it. Participatory dialogue is used to elicit perceptions of the different members of the family. The nurses poses questions but family members are also encouraged to ask questions. As a picture of the family's health experience forms, the family and nurse identify the recurrent patterns and themes that may influence health and health behaviors. As the assessment continues, the family moves its focus from deficits to potentials. This enables the family with the assistance of the nurse to make informed health choices.

The literature contains an array of tools for assessing the health of a family. Pender (1996) recommends that any tool selected for family assessment cover the following topics:

- **Nutrition**—What do family members know about nutrition? What are their eating practices? Do they value healthy eating?
- **Physical activity**—Do family members engage in physical exercise together? Do they have exercise equipment in the home? What activities characterize time together?
- **Stress control and management**—Does the family spend time together relaxing and laughing? Is emotional expression encouraged? Do family members minimize stressful demands on each other?
- **Health responsibility**—Does the family have a plan for preventive health care, such as an immunization schedule? Do family members discuss news items regarding health? Do family members feel a sense of responsibility for the health of the family?
- **Family resilience and resources**—Do family members have a common sense of purpose in life? Do family members offer support to each other? Is there a sense of togetherness?
- **Family support**—Do family members visit regularly? Is the family involved in community affairs? Do family members praise each other?

The family health assessment complements the individual assessment. The two must be viewed as interactive (one affects the other and vice versa).

HEALTH ASSESSMENT OF THE COMMUNITY

It is important to mention health assessment of the community even though the beginning student will not be expected to be competent in this aspect of nursing practice. Whereas in the past, an assessment was done **on** the community, it is now done **with** the community. The assessment is a systematic effort to define needs, opportunities and resources involved in implementing community health promotion programs. There are many frameworks for a community health assessment. In general, the assessment includes information about the people, the geographic setting and environment, the social systems in place, and the health-related resources. The assets as well as the limitations are noted.

Advocacy

Advocacy is the act of informing and supporting a person, family, or community to make the best decision possible. An advocate does not make a decision for another but instead promotes and accepts the right of the other to make the decision.

Advocacy at the individual and family level involves:

- Sharing appropriate information in an unbiased manner so the individual can evaluate it without preconceived ideas. This requires the nurse to be aware of personal biases and to set them aside while assisting the individual or family. It also requires the nurse to review any information shared with the person for biases held by the author of the material.

- Assisting the individual in developing decision-making skills suitable for the health problem. This can be done through storytelling, using examples of individuals dealing with a similar health problem (the neighbor who quit smoking); talking a situation through with the individual and pointing out aspects of his or her decision making; presenting situations and asking the individual to state how he or she would handle it; or role playing.
- Supporting the individual after a decision has been reached. This requires the nurse to facilitate the individual's involvement in self-help groups such as Alcoholics Anonymous or Reach to Recovery (for women recovering from breast amputation); providing feedback so individuals can take pleasure in their progress; strengthening internal motivation by linking the new health behavior to other goals and values the person holds; and identifying coping strategies to use when motivation falters.

Advocacy also takes place at the community level. The skills required at this level of advocacy differ from those used in working with an individual or family. At the community level the nurse must:

- Be assertive on behalf of the individuals in that community.
- Take risks and seize opportunities to present information on behalf of others.
- Be able to state the issues clearly and briefly and with supporting facts.
- Identify cost-effective solutions to the issues identified.
- Be willing to work until the issue is resolved.
- Have knowledge about the private and public sector resources and political structures.

There are no prescriptions for advocacy. The nurse must understand the importance of advocacy and determine how to implement that nursing care action with the specific individual or family.

Education and Counseling

HEALTH EDUCATION

Health education is the core of all health promotion and disease prevention interventions. Yet teaching in and of itself does not assure health promotion behaviors. It is imperative that individuals have knowledge, but as Pender's RHPM shows, there are many other factors associated with implementing health promotion behaviors.

What specific factors identified through research seem to explain the willingness to implement health-promoting behaviors? What, in addition to education, influences changing a lifestyle? Theorists interested in answering that question analyzed their own work to identify the primary determinants of a behavior change. Fishbein and colleagues (as cited in Pender, 1996, p. 46) list these eight factors as significant:

- **Intention:** The person has made a commitment to perform the behavior.
- **Environmental constraints:** No external conditions or circumstances exist that make it impossible for the behavior to occur.
- **Ability:** The person has the skills necessary to perform the behavior.
- **Anticipated outcomes:** The person believes that the advantages (benefits) of performing the behavior outweigh the disadvantages (costs); the person has a positive attitude toward performing the behavior.
- **Norms:** The person perceives more social pressure to perform the behavior than not perform the behavior.
- **Self-standards:** The person perceives performance of the behavior as more consistent than inconsistent with his or her self-image.
- **Emotion:** The person's emotional reaction to performing the behavior is more positive than negative.
- **Self-efficacy:** The person perceives that he or she has the capabilities for performing the behavior under a number of different circumstances.

This list can be used in structuring nursing care actions. The educational intervention would include attention to these eight factors as well as to the specific knowledge, skill, or attitude being taught (see Patient Teaching box). Self-help groups attribute some of their effectiveness to attending to factors such as those listed.

Relapse to former behaviors does occur even with highly motivated individuals. The nurse can present the likelihood of a relapse occurring by describing the implementation of health promoting behaviors as having a circular pattern in which the original behavior does occur periodically. This approach prevents the individual from feeling guilty or a failure when a relapse does occur. In structuring health promotion interventions, the nurse can use strategies such as the following to maintain motivation:

- Early in the process emphasize the negative consequences of risky behavior and the benefits of positive health behaviors. Make the illustrations clearly applicable to the individual or individuals in the group. Do not generalize.
- Request a financial deposit that is returned when the desired health-promoting behaviors are demonstrated.
- Have the individual develop response strategies to implement when tempted to relapse. For example, people trying to quit smoking might find themselves wanting a cigarette. If they know this is likely to occur

PATIENT TEACHING
GUIDING HEALTH BEHAVIOR CHANGE: A CASE EXAMPLE

The nurse explains to Mrs. Walker that exercise reduces the risk for heart disease and stroke by helping control blood pressure, improve serum lipids, control weight, reduce stress, and promote a sense of psychological well-being. Exercise also helps prevent bone loss that occurs with aging (osteoporosis).

Next the nurse describes the American College of Sports Medicine recommendations for walking a minimum of 20 to 30 minutes three to five times per week at 70 percent of maximal heart rate to maintain cardiovascular fitness. The optimal preventive effect of exercise on cardiovascular disease is achieved by burning 2000 calories per week, which translates into walking about 1 hour a day (Paffenbarger et al, 1984). For weight control, exercise should be performed 4 or 5 times a week.

The nurse and Mrs. Walker negotiate a contract setting realistic short-term goals and providing for evaluation as goals are revised. Mrs. Walker agrees to start slowly by exercising 20 minutes, 3 times a week, and gradually increases the frequency, duration, and intensity of exercise. She is more likely to succeed by concentrating on one behavior and gradually advancing physical demands. The contract specifies a reward for successfully performing the exercise. This reward (e.g., a subscription to a favorite magazine) is something valued and selected by the client. Finally, the contract specifies the nurse's responsibility for helping Mrs. Walker acquire the information and skills needed for changing her behavior. This includes teaching Mrs. Walker how to check her pulse, determine her appropriate target heart rate, prevent injuries, and monitor signs and symptoms associated with exercise that warn when to quit exercising.

Mrs. Walker is taught how to monitor her pulse to see if she is achieving her target heart rate, and to provide feedback on her progress. Target heart rate is calculated using the formula

$$(220 - \text{client's age}) \times .70$$

An aerobic rate is 70 percent of the maximal heart rate. Using this formula, Mrs. Walker's target heart rate would be 123.

The nurse encourages Mrs. Walker to keep an exercise log and review it with her periodically. The log serves as a means of self-reinforcement by documenting improvement. By recording thoughts, sensations and feelings as well as exercise frequency, duration, and intensity, the log permits an analysis of the antecedents (A) or stimuli, behavior (B), and consequences (C) of the exercise program, and of the situations leading to lapses. The nurse can then develop better strategies to avoid risky situations and prevent lapses.

After a couple of weeks, Mrs. Walker reports difficulty in maintaining her exercise routine. To help Mrs. Walker reach her goal of greater consistency, the nurse teaches her the techniques of self-management and problem-solving. She suggests Mrs. Walker:

- incorporate physical exercise into her daily routine
- climb stairs instead of taking the elevator
- choose forms of recreation that involve the entire family in physical exercise
- vary the type of exercise according to the time of day, weather, setting, availability of equipment and facilities
- find other people with whom to exercise
- join a walking club or a health club, or
- resort to walking in a mall with its controlled climate, security, and convenience

Once Mrs. Walker is well established in her exercise program, the nurse suggests adding a nutritional component to her health promotion program. Mrs. Walker's diet is high in fat, sugar, sodium, and calories, as is typical of the diet of many Americans. Mrs. Walker is overweight, as are 29 percent of women, 16 percent of men, and increasing numbers of children and adolescents in the United States (U.S. DHHS, 1990, p. 21). In planning the nutrition program, the nurse repeats the process used in designing the exercise program for Mrs. Walker. The exercise and weight reduction programs are then mutually reinforcing.

Finally, because Mrs. Walker is concerned about the health of her sons as well as of herself, the nurse points out that by changing her own lifestyle, Mrs. Walker is serving as a role model for healthier behavior. She suggests additionally that Mrs. Walker might contract with her sons for exercise. She might resume her camping and hiking activities with them to reduce their sedentary pursuits. In these ways, health promotion becomes a family project, integrated into family lifestyle and deriving strength from group support.

and have a response in mind, such as calling a friend committed to helping them stay cigarette-free, they are likely to avoid a relapse.

Some health promotion educational materials are based on fear (e.g., "Stop smoking or develop lung cancer!") as an effective motivator. Early cancer and AIDS education materials used fear as a motivator. However, both the research literature and experience of clinicians indicate that fear appeals have inconsistent effects (Damrosch, 1991). The nurse should use fear appeals cautiously, perhaps combining **low-level** fear appeals with educational materials and other motivational suggestions.

Chapter 13, Patient Teaching, contains information on patient and family teaching that is applicable to teaching

Health-Style: A Self-Test

All of us want good health. But many of us do not know how to be as healthy as possible. Health experts now describe *life-style* as one of the most important factors affecting health. In fact, it is estimated that as many as seven of the ten leading causes of death could be reduced through common-sense changes in life-style. That's what this brief test, developed by the Public Health Service, is all about. Its purpose is simply to tell you how well you are doing to stay healthy. The behaviors covered in the test are recommended for most Americans. Some of them may not apply to people with certain chronic diseases or disabilities, or to pregnant women. Such people may require special instructions from their physicians.

Cigarette Smoking

If you never smoke, enter a score of 10 for this section and go to the next section on *Alcohol and Drugs.*

	almost always	sometimes	almost never
1. I avoid smoking cigarettes.	2	1	0
2. I smoke only low tar and nicotine cigarettes *or* I smoke a pipe or cigars.	2	1	0
Smoking score:	______		

Alcohol and Drugs

	almost always	sometimes	almost never
1. I avoid drinking alcoholic beverages *or* I drink no more than one or two drinks a day.	4	1	0
2. I avoid using alcohol or other drugs (especially illegal drugs) as a way of handling stressful situations or the problems in my life.	2	1	0
3. I am careful not to drink alcohol when taking certain medicines (for example, medicine for sleeping, pain, colds, and allergies), or when pregnant.	2	1	0
4. I read and follow the label directions when using prescribed and over-the-counter drugs.	2	1	0
Alcohol and drugs score:	______		

Eating Habits

	almost always	sometimes	almost never
1. I eat a variety of foods each day, such as fruits and vegetables, whole grain breads and cereals, lean meats, dairy products, dry peas and beans, and nuts and seeds.	4	1	0
2. I limit the amount of fat, saturated fat, and cholesterol I eat (including fat on meats, eggs, butter, cream, shortenings, and organ meats such as liver).	2	1	0
3. I limit the amount of salt I eat by cooking with only small amounts, not adding salt at the table, and avoiding salty snacks.	2	1	0
4. I avoid eating too much sugar (especially frequent snacks of sticky candy or soft drinks).	2	1	0
Eating habits score:	______		

Exercise and Fitness

	almost always	sometimes	almost never
1. I maintain a desired weight, avoiding overweight and underweight.	2	1	0
2. I do vigorous exercises for 15 to 30 minutes at least three times a week (examples include running, swimming, brisk walking).	3	1	0
3. I do exercises that enhance my muscle tone for 15 to 30 minutes at least three times a week (examples include yoga and calisthenics).	2	1	0
4. I use part of my leisure time participating in individual, family, or team activities that increase my level of fitness (such as gardening, bowling, golf, and baseball).	2	1	0
Exercise/fitness score:	______		

Stress Control

	almost always	sometimes	almost never
1. I have a job or do other work that I enjoy.	2	1	0
2. I find it easy to relax and express my feelings freely.	2	1	0
3. I recognize early, and prepare for, events or situations likely to be stressful for me.	2	1	0
4. I have close friends, relatives, or others whom I can talk to about personal matters and call on for help when needed.	2	1	0
5. I participate in group activities (such as church and community organizations) or hobbies that I enjoy.	2	1	0
Stress control score:	______		

Safety

	almost always	sometimes	almost never
1. I wear a seat belt while riding in a car.	2	1	0
2. I avoid driving while under the influence of alcohol and other drugs.	2	1	0
3. I obey traffic rules and the speed limit when driving.	2	1	0
4. I am careful when using potentially harmful products or substances (such as household cleaners, poisons, and electrical devices).	2	1	0
5. I avoid smoking in bed.	2	1	0
Safety score:	______		

Figure 36–5. Health style: A self-test. (From National Health Information Clearinghouse, Washington, D.C.)

health promotion and self-care behaviors. The preceding material is a supplement to that content.

HEALTH COUNSELING

The nurse who has incorporated health promotion and disease prevention into everyday practice takes every opportunity to counsel patients and families about personal risk factors. Glynn and Manley (cited in U.S. DHHS, 1994) provide this example of health counseling for smoking cessation:

- Provide services in a smoke-free environment.
- Take every opportunity to ask about smoking ("Do you smoke?" "How much do you smoke?" "Are you interested in stopping smoking?")

Health-Style: A Self-Test *(continued)*

What Your Scores Mean to You

Scores of 9 and 10
Excellent! Your answers show that you are aware of the importance of this area to your health. More important, you are putting your knowledge to work for you by practicing good health habits. As long as you continue to do so, this area should not pose a serious health risk. It's likely that you are setting an example for your family and friends to follow. Because you got a very high test score on this part of the test, you may want to consider other areas where your scores indicate room for improvement.

Scores of 6 to 8
Your health practices in this area are good, but there is room for improvement. Look again at the items you answered with "Sometimes" or "Almost never." What changes can you make to improve your score? Even a small change can often help you achieve better health.

Scores of 3 to 5
Your health risks are showing! Would you like more information about the risks you are facing and about why it is important for you to change these behaviors? Perhaps you need help in deciding how to successfully make the changes you desire. In either case, help is available.

Scores of 0 to 2
Obviously, you were concerned enough about your health to take the test, but your answers show that you may be taking serious and unnecessary risks with your health. Perhaps you are unaware of the risks and what to do about them. You can easily get the information and help you need to improve, if you wish. The next step is up to you.

Where Do You Go from Here

Start by asking yourself a few frank questions: *Am I really doing all I can to be as healthy as possible? What steps can I take to feel better? Am I willing to begin now?* If you scored low in one or more sections of the test, decide what changes you want to make for improvement. You might pick that aspect of your life-style where you feel you have the best chance for success and tackle that one first. Once you have improved your score there, go on to other areas.

If you already have tried to change your health habits (to stop smoking or exercise regularly, for example), don't be discouraged if you haven't yet succeeded. The difficulty you have encountered may be due to influences you've never really thought about—such as advertising—or to a lack of support and encouragement. Understanding these influences is an important step toward changing the way they affect you.

There's help available. In addition to personal actions you can take on your own, there are community programs and groups (such as the YMCA or the local chapter of the American Heart Association) that can assist you and your family to make the changes you want to make. If you want to know more about these groups or about health risks, contact your local health department or the National Health Information Clearinghouse. There's a lot you can do to stay healthy or to improve your health—and there are organizations that can help you. Start a new "health-style" today!

For assistance in locating specific information on these and other health topics, write to the National Health Information Clearinghouse:

National Health Information Clearinghouse
P.O. Box 1133
Washington, DC 20013

Figure 36-5. *Continued*

- Assess the patient's smoking status using a brief, self-administered questionnaire (the same questions as listed above) that can become part of the patient's record.
- Put a sticker on the chart of a patient who smokes as a reminder to keep track of smoking cessation interventions.
- Advise every smoker to stop. Be clear in your message and make it personal.
- Assist the patient to stop by setting a quit date, providing self-help materials, providing motivational materials, offering access to techniques such as nicotine gum or patch, signing a stop-smoking contract, and providing information of self-help groups and clinics.
- Follow-up with a phone call in 7 days and a visit 1 to 2 weeks later.

The *Clinician's Handbook of Preventive Services* (1994) provides guides to counseling for a variety of risky behaviors. Box 36–7 lists principles of effective patient education and counseling developed by the U.S. Preventive Services Task Force.

BOX 36-7
U.S. PREVENTATIVE SERVICES TASK FORCE PATIENT EDUCATION/COUNSELING STRATEGIES

1. Frame the teaching to match the patient's perceptions.
2. Fully inform patients of the purposes and expected effects of interventions and when to expect these effects.
3. Suggest small changes rather than large ones.
4. Be specific.
5. It is sometimes easier to add new behaviors than to eliminate established behaviors.
6. Link new behaviors to old behaviors.
7. Use the power of the profession.
8. Get explicit commitments from the patient.
9. Use a combination of strategies.
10. Involve office staff.
11. Refer.
12. Monitor progress through follow-up contact.

From U.S. Preventive Services Task Force (1996). Patient Education/Counseling Strategies. In *Guide to Clinical Preventive Services,* 2nd ed. Washington, D.C.: U.S. Department of Health and Human Services, Chap iv.

Care Management

Nurses are being assigned to manage the care of individuals and groups. In that role the nurse is expected to keep individ-

CLINICAL DECISION MAKING
FACILITATING HEALTHY BEHAVIORS

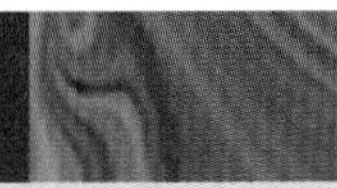

Mrs. Walker makes a routine visit to her company's occupational health nurse. She is concerned because she doesn't feel as healthy as she would like and knows that she should do something to lose weight.

SELF-REFLECTION

The nurse is pleased with this sign of motivation from Mrs. Walker because she has been concerned about Mrs. Walker's health status. Aware of her own negative feelings about people who continue to smoke, the nurse first makes a conscious effort to set those attitudes aside and to focus on Mrs. Walker and her situation.

KNOWLEDGE BASE

Primary and secondary prevention are a major part of the occupational health nurse's role. This involves health education, nutrition counseling, disease prevention programs such as smoking cessation, physical examinations, case-finding, and screening surveys. The nurse knows that a holistic approach is necessary when helping an individual such as Mrs. Walker make a lifestyle change. Mrs. Walker's health perceptions and attitudes, physical condition, psychological and personality characteristics, gender, age, family, community, work environment, socioeconomic status, culture and ethnic background, and religious background will all influence her efforts at health promotion.

From her record the nurse notes that Mrs. Walker exhibits many of the classic risk factors for cardiovascular disease. Her family history and age are risks that cannot be changed. However, her excess weight, hypertension, smoking, lack of exercise, and stress at work can be modified, although change will require effort. In discussing these risk factors with Mrs. Walker, the nurse draws on her familiarity with the Health Belief Model to clarify her client's beliefs and values, and her readiness and commitment to change her behavior. The discussion serves as a trigger to action for Mrs. Walker because she has been contemplating the need to change her health habits ever since her father's stroke. Mrs. Walker says she is not yet willing to give up smoking, but would like to increase her exercise and reduce her weight.

After a thorough history taking and physical examination rules out contraindications to exercise, the nurse and Mrs. Walker devise a health promotion plan, starting with an exercise program. Mrs. Walker will focus on exercise first and weight reduction later.

CLINICAL QUESTIONS

Mrs. Walker is at high risk for cardiovascular disease, the leading cause of death in the United States. What are the risk factors and which can be modified? How might the nurse help Mrs. Walker to develop a health promotion plan to lessen her chance of a heart attack? What type of exercise plan is safe and feasible for a sedentary person such as Mrs. Walker? What behaviors should the nurse encourage her to monitor for progress? Is her family supportive of Mrs. Walker's plan to reduce her weight? Will her family value her need for time for exercise? The nurse also knows the likelihood that Mrs. Walker will have a relapse from her diet and exercise regimens and wants to prepare her for that so she does not feel guilty when it happens.

PLAN OF CARE

The nurse and Mrs. Walker decide to meet weekly to monitor progress and continue to add to Mrs. Walker's knowledge base through health education. These sessions will also be used to develop Mrs. Walker's decision-making skills as they relate to health promotion and disease prevention. In addition, Mrs. Walker will select a fellow worker who is on an exercise regimen as a role model and advocate. She will also consider joining the self-help group for employees motivated to improve their overall health status through eliminating risky health behaviors.

Finally, the nurse asks Mrs. Walker to determine the progress she would like to make in an exercise program. Mrs. Walker is to think about this and return the next week with her goals. The nurse will then develop a contract with Mrs. Walker specifying what she will do and what the nurse will do, along with the rewards for her when she meets her goals.

uals independent as long as possible and to the extent possible. This requires the nurse to think in terms of health promotion, disease prevention, and symptom control. As care manager the nurse allocates resources and provides services within a cost-effective framework.

To serve as a care manager the nurse must understand health as well as illness and be able to use health assessment as the basis for an effective health-promoting plan of care. The role of care manager is likely to be the primary role for nursing within the health care system. The beginning nursing student will not implement this role but should understand it as one model of practice.

Role Modeling

THE NURSE AS ROLE MODEL

Learning by observing the behavior of another is a very powerful technique. For example, the individual who is considering stopping smoking will be influenced by others who have or have not stopped smoking. It is for this reason that the nurse must be a role model for health promotion and disease prevention behaviors. The patient will be less positively influenced by a nurse demonstrating unhealthy behaviors than by a nurse demonstrating healthy behaviors. It is more difficult for a nurse who smokes than one who does not smoke to assist a patient to stop smoking. The same statement can be made for any other health-promoting behavior.

The "Health Style: A Self-Test," from the National Health Information Clearinghouse, is provided for the reader to use to assess her or his ability to serve as a role model (Fig. 36–5).

OTHERS AS ROLE MODELS

Others can be used as role models as an intervention for health promotion. In implementing this intervention, the nurse should consider the following questions:

- Is there a role model with whom the person can identify (e.g., gender, age, ethnicity)?
- Can the person be involved in selecting a role model (e.g., a sponsor from a self-help group)?
- Can the person be given enough time to observe the desired behavior and the important aspects of the behavior?
- Does the person have the necessary knowledge and skills to perform the behavior?
- Does the person perceive the rewards for imitating the desired behavior?
- Does the person have time to mentally and physically rehearse the desired behavior?

If the answer to the majority of these questions is "yes," role modeling as an intervention is likely to be effective.

CHAPTER HIGHLIGHTS

- Health promotion and self-care are concepts fundamental to nursing practice.
- Research has led to the formulation of several models of health promotion and disease prevention.
- Research has documented the positive outcomes from health promotion interventions.
- The knowledge base for health promotion strategies is interdisciplinary, drawing heavily from the fields of epidemiology, sociology, psychology, and nursing.
- Nursing care actions include assessment, advocacy, education and counseling, care management, and role modeling. These actions are implemented at the individual, family, and community level. They are part of primary prevention, secondary prevention, and tertiary prevention nursing care actions. The focus for the beginning nursing student is assessment of the individual and health education for the individual. Yet health promotion for the individual cannot be separated from the family and community. Therefore, information of those aspects of health promotion and self-care is included.

REFERENCES

Abosede, O.A. (1984). Self-medication: An important aspect of primary care. *Social Science and Medicine, 19* (7), 699–703.

Andersen, R., Lewis, S.Z., Giachello, A.L., et al (1981). Access to medical care among the Hispanic population of the southwestern United States. *Journal of Health and Social Behavior, 22,* 78–89.

Antonovsky, A. (1979). *Health, Stress, and Coping.* San Francisco: Jossey-Bass.

Antonovsky, A. (1987). *Unraveling the Mystery of Health.* San Francisco: Jossey-Bass.

Bandura, A. (1986). *Social Foundations of Thought and Action: A Social Cognitive Theory.* Englewood Cliffs, NJ: Prentice-Hall.

Becker, M.H. (1993). A medical sociologist looks at health promotion. *Journal of Health and Social Behavior, 34,* 1–6.

Becker, M.H., Haefner, D.F., Kasl, S.V., et al (1977). Selected psychosocial models and correlates of individual health-related behaviors. *Medical Care, 15,* 27–46.

Belloc, N.B., Breslow, L. (1972). Relationship of physical health status and health practices. *Preventive Medicine, 1,* 409–421.

Boston Women's Health Book Collective. (1975). *Our Bodies, Ourselves: A Book by and for Women,* 2nd ed. New York: Simon and Schuster.

Breslow, L., Enstrom, J.E. (1980). Persistence of health habits and their relationship to mortality. *Preventive Medicine, 9,* 469–483.

Breslow, L.B., Somers, A.R. (1977). The lifetime health-monitoring program. *New England Journal of Medicine, 296,* 601–608.

Brown, J.S., Marcy, S.A. (1991). The use of botanicals for health purposes by members of a prepaid health plan. *Research in Nursing and Health, 14,* 339–350.

Caspersen, C.J., Christenson, G.M., Pollard, R.A. (1986). Status of the 1990 physical fitness and exercise objectives—Evidence from NHIS 1985. *Public Health Reports, 101* (6), 587–592.

Centers for Disease Control (1993). Cigarette smoking among adults—United States, 1991. *Morbidity & Mortality Weekly Report, 42* (12), 230–233.

Cockerham, W.C., Kunz, G., Lueschen, G. (1988a). Social stratification and health lifestyles in two systems of health care delivery: A comparison of the United States and West Germany. *Journal of Health and Social Behavior, 29,* 113–126.

Cockerham, W.C., Kunz, G., Lueschen, G. (1988b). On concern with appearance, health beliefs, and eating habits: A reappraisal comparing Americans and West Germans. *Journal of Health and Social Behavior, 29,* 265–270.

Conrad, P. (1987). Wellness in the workplace: Potentials and pitfalls of worksite health promotion. *Milbank Quarterly, 65* (2), 258–275.

Crawford, R. (1977). You are dangerous to your health: The ideology and politics of victim blaming. *International Journal of Health Services, 7* (4), 663–680.

Cresanta, J.L., Hyg, M.S., Burke, G.L., et al (1986). Prevention of atherosclerosis in childhood. *Pediatric Clinics of North America, 33* (4), 835–859.

Damrosch, S. (1991). General strategies for motivating people to change their behavior. *Nursing Clinics of North America, 26* (4), 833–844.

DeFriese, G.H., Woomert, A., Guild, P.A., et al (1989). From activated patient to pacified activist: A study of the self-care movement in the United States. *Social Science and Medicine, 29* (2), 195–204.

Denyes, M.J. (1988). Orem's model used for health promotion: Directions from research. *Advances in Nursing Science, 11* (1), 13–21.

Der Marderosian, A.H. (1980). Controversies concerning herbal remedies. *American Druggist, 182,* 35–39.

Duelberg, S.I. (1992). Preventive health behavior among black and white women in urban and rural areas. *Social Science and Medicine, 34,* 191–198.

Duffy, M.E. (1988). Determinants of health promotion in midlife women. *Nursing Research, 37,* 358–362.

Dunnell, K., Cartwright, A. (1972). *Medicine Takers, Prescribers and Hoarders.* London: Routledge & Kegan Paul.

Dwyer, J.W., Clarke, L.L., Miller, M.K. (1990). The effect of religious concentration and affiliation on county cancer mortality rates. *Journal of Health and Social Behavior, 31,* 185–202.

Farquhar, J.W., Fortmann, S.P., Maccoby, N., et al (1985). The Stanford five-city project: Design and methods. *American Journal of Epidemiology, 122,* 323–334.

Feldman, W., Hodgson, C., Corber, S., Quinn, A. (1986). Health concerns and health related behaviors of adolescents. *Journal of Canadian Medical Association, 134,* 489–493.

Fleming, G.V., Giachello, A.L., Andersen, R.M., Andrade, P. (1984). Self-care: Substitute, supplement or stimulus for formal medical care services? *Medical Care, 22,* 950–966.

Fuchs, V.R. (1974). *Who Shall Live? Health, Economics and Social Choice.* New York: Basic Books.

Goldstein, M.S. (1992). *The Health Movement: Promoting Fitness in America.* New York: Macmillan.

Green, K. (1985). Consumer views of selfcare: Promise or panacea. *Journal of the Royal Society of Health, 2, 65–67.*

Greenberg, M.A., Wiggins, C.L., Kutvirt, D.M., Samet, J.M. (1986). Cigarette use among Hispanic and non-Hispanic white school children, Albuquerque, New Mexico. *American Journal of Public Health, 77,* 621–622.

Grunberg, N.E., Winders, S.E., Wewers, M.E. (1991). Gender differences in tobacco use. *Health Psychology, 10,* 143–153.

Harris, D.M., Guten, G. (1979). Health-protective behavior: An exploratory study. *Journal of Health and Social Behavior, 20,* 17–29.

Hartrick, G., Lindsey, A.E., Hills, M. (1994). Family nursing assessment: Meeting the challenge of health promotion. *Journal of Advanced Nursing, 20,* 85–91.

Hartweg, D.L. (1990). Health promotion self-care within Orem's general theory of nursing. *Journal of Advanced Nursing, 15,* 35–41.

Hatziandreu, E.I., Kaplan, J.P., Weinstein, M.C., et al (1988). A cost-effectiveness analysis of exercise as a health promotion activity. *American Journal of Public Health, 78,* 1417–1421.

Hayes, D., Ross, C.E. (1987). Concern with appearance, health beliefs, and eating habits. *Journal of Health and Social Behavior, 28,* 120–130.

Hill, L., Smith, N. (1986). *Self Care Nursing.* Englewood Cliffs, NJ: Prentice-Hall.

Janz, N.K., Becker, M.H. (1984). The health belief model: A decade later. *Health Education Quarterly, 11,* 1–47.

Kanfer, F.H., Gaelick, L. (1986). Self-management methods. In F.H. Kanfer and A.P. Goldstein (eds.): *Helping People Change,* 3rd ed. New York: Pergamon Press, pp. 283–345.

Karoly, F.H., Kanfer, F.H. (eds.) (1982). *Self-Management and Behavior Change: From Theory and to Practice.* Elmsford, NY: Pergamon Press.

Lamm, R.D. (1990). Health care as economic cancer. In R.D. Lamm: *The Brave New World of Health Care.* Denver, CO: Center for Public Policy and Contemporary Issues, University of Denver, pp. 55–70.

Lazarus, T.S., Folkman, S. (1984). *Stress, Appraisal, and Coping.* New York: Springer Publishing Company.

Lee, D.J., Markides, K.S. (1991). Health behaviors, risk factors, and health indicators associated with cigarette use in Mexican Americans: Results from the Hispanic HANES. *American Journal of Public Health, 81,* 859–864.

Levin, L.S., Idler, E.L. (1983). Self-care in health. *Annual Review of Public Health, 4,* 181–201.

Levin, L.S., Katz, A.H., Holst, E. (1976). *Self-Care: Lay Initiatives in Health.* New York: Prodist.

Levitan, S.A., Johnson, W.B. (1976). *Indian Giving.* Baltimore: The Johns Hopkins University Press.

Lex, B.W. (1991). Some gender differences in alcohol and polysubstance users. *Health Psychology, 10,* 121–132.

Mandelblatt, J., Andrews, H., Kerner, J., et al (1991). Determinants of late stage diagnosis of breast and cervical cancer: The impact of age, race, social class, and hospital type. *American Journal of Public Health, 81, 646–649.*

Marcus, A.C., Crane, L.A. (1985). Smoking behavior among US Latinos: An emerging challenge for public health. *American Journal of Public Health, 75,* 169–172.

Martin, J., Suarez, L. (1987). Cancer mortality among Mexican Americans and other Whites in Texas, 1969–80. *American Journal of Public Health, 77,* 851–853.

McGinnis, J.M. (1982). Future directions of health promotion. In R.B. Taylor, J.R. Ureda, and J.W. Denham (eds.): *Health Promotion: Principles and Clinical Applications.* Norwalk, CT: Appleton-Century-Crofts, pp. 405–428.

McKinlay, J.B. (June, 1974). A case for refocusing upstream: The political economy of illness. Applying behavioral science to cardiovascular risk. *Proceedings of the American Heart Association Conference.* Seattle, Washington, pp. 7–17.

Medical News & Perspectives (1988). Even "knowing better" about smoking, other health risks, may not deter adolescents. *JAMA, 260* (11), 1512–1513.

Milio, N. (1976). A framework for prevention: Changing health-damaging to health-generating life patterns. *American Journal of Public Health, 66,* 435–439.

Milio, N. (1988). The profitization of health promotion. *International Journal of Health Services, 18, 573–585.*

Milio, N. (1981). Promoting Health Through Public Policy. Philadelphia: F.A. Davis Co.

Milio, N. (1977). Self-care in urban settings. *Health Education Monographs, 5* (2), 135–144.

Morisky, D.E., McCarthy, W.J., Kite, E.A. (1986). Targeting primary prevention programs to high-risk populations. *Advances in Health Education and Promotion, 1* (Pt. A), 23–64.

Morrison, A.S. (1991). Is self-examination effective in screening for breast cancer: *Journal of the National Cancer Institute, 83* (4), 226–227.

Moyer, N.C. (1981). Health promotion and the assessment of health habits in the elderly. *Topics in Clinical Nursing, 3* (1), 51–58.

Multiple Risk Factor Intervention Trial Research Group (1982). Multiple risk factor intervention trial. Risk factor changes and mortality results. *JAMA, 248* (12), 1465–1477.

Muncie, H.L., Sobal, J. (1987). The vitamin-mineral supplement history. *Journal of Family Practice, 24* (4), 365–368.

Nathanson, C. (1977). Sex roles as variables in preventive health behavior. *Journal of Community Health, 3,* 142–155.

Nelson, E.C., Simmons, J.S. (February, 1983). Health promotion—the second public health revolution: Promise or threat? *Family & Community Health,* 1–15.

Nishiwaki, R., Bouchard, C. (1989). Combating nutrition quackery: The San Bernardino County experience. *American Journal of Public Health, 79,* 652–653.

O'Neal, D.J., III (1982). Promotion of health in the family. *Journal of Gerontological Nursing, 8,* 146–148.

Orem, D.E. (1985). *Nursing: Concepts of Practice,* 3rd ed. New York: McGraw-Hill.

Orem, D.E. (1991). *Nursing: Concepts of Practice,* 4th ed. St. Louis: C.V. Mosby.

Paffenbarger, R.S., Jr., Hyde, R.T., Wing, A.L., Steinmetz, C.H. (1984). A natural history of athleticism and cardiovascular health. *JAMA, 252* (4), 491–495.

Pender, N.J. (1996). *Health Promotion in Nursing Practice,* 3rd ed. Stamford, CT: Appleton & Lange.

Perez-Stable, E.J., McMillen, M.M., Harris, M.I., et al (1989). Self-reported diabetes in Mexican Americans: HHANES 1982–84. *American Journal of Public Health, 79,* 770–772.

Perry, C.L., Griffin, G., Murray, D.M. (1985). Assessing needs for youth health promotion. *Preventive Medicine,* 14, 379–393.

Pescosolido, B.A., Georgianna, S. (1989). Durkheim, suicide, and religion. *American Sociological Review, 54,* 33–48.

Prochaska, J.O., Norcross, J.C., Fowler, J.L., et al (1992). Attendance and outcome in a work site weight control program: Processes and stages of change as process and predictor variables. *Addictive Behaviors, 17,* 35–45.

Prochaska, J.O., Norcross, J.C., Di Clemente, R. (1994). *Changing for Good.* New York: Avon Books.

Ransford, H.E. (1986). Race, heart disease worry and health protective behavior. *Social Science and Medicine, 22,* 1355–1362.

Reeb, K.G., Graham, A.V., Zyzanski, S.J., Kitsono, G.C. (1987). Predicting low birthweight and complicated labor in urban black women: A biopsychosocial perspective. *Social Science and Medicine, 25,* 1321–1327.

Rolls, B.J., Federoff, I.C., Guthrie, J.F. (1991). Gender differences in eating behavior and body weight regulation. *Health Psychology, 10,* 133–142.

Rosenstock, I. (1966). Why people use health services. *Milbank Memorial Fund Quarterly, 44,* 94–127.

Rosenstock, I.M. (1974). Historical origins of the Health Belief Model. *Health Education Monographs, 2,* 328–335.

Rotter, J.B. (1966). Generalized expectancies for internal versus external control of reinforcement. *Psychology Monograms, 80,* 1028.

Russell, L.B. (1986). *Is Prevention Better than Cure?* Washington, D.C.: The Brookings Institution.

Salmon, J.W. (1987). Dilemmas in studying social change versus individual change: Considerations from political economy. In Wingspread Conference, *Conceptual Issues in Health Promotion.* Racine, Wisconsin, pp. 70–80.

Schiller, P.L., Levin, J.S. (1983). Is self-care a social movement? *Social Science and Medicine, 17* (18), 1345–1352.

Schoenborn, C.A. (1986). Health habits of U.S. adults, 1985: The "Alameda 7" revisited. *Public Health Reports, 101,* 571–580.

Sehnert, K.W. (November-December, 1980). A course for activated patients. *Social Policy,* 40–46.

Simmons, S.J. (1990). The health-promoting self-care system model: Directions for nursing research and practice. *Journal of Advanced Nursing, 15,* 1162–1166.

Smith, J.A. (1983). *The Idea of Health: Implications for the Nursing Professional.* New York: Teachers College, Columbia University.

Spoerke, D.G., Jr. (1980). *Herbal Medications.* Santa Barbara, CA: Woodbridge Press Publishing Co.

Stacey, M., Olesen, V. (1993). Introduction (women, men and health). *Social Science and Medicine, 35,* 1–5.

Steiger, N., Lipson, J. (1985). *Self-Care Nursing: Theory and Practice.* Bowie, MD: Brady Corporation.

Sullivan, G.C. (1989). Evaluating Antonovsky's Salutogenic Model for its adaptability to nursing. *Journal of Advanced Nursing, 14,* 336–342.

Syme, S.L. (1984). Social support and risk reduction. *Mobius, 4* (3), 44–54.

Szathmary, E.J.E., Ritenbaugh, C., Goodby, C.M. (1987). Dietary change and plasma glucose levels in an Amerindian population undergoing cultural transition. *Social Science and Medicine, 24,* 791–804.

Tanner, E.K. (1991). Assessment of a health-promotive life style. *Nursing Clinics of North America,* 26 (4), 845–854.

Terris, M. (1975). Approaches to an epidemiology of health. *American Journal of Public Health, 65,* 1037–1045.

Troyer, H. (1988). Review of cancer among 4 religious sects: Evidence that life-styles are distinctive sets of risk factors. *Social Science and Medicine, 26,* 1007–1017.

Umberson, D. (1987). Family status and health behaviors: Social control as a dimension of social integration. *Journal of Health and Social Behavior, 28,* 306–319.

U.S. Department of Health, Education and Welfare (1979). *Healthy People: The Surgeon General's Report on Health Promotion and Disease Prevention* (DHEW [PHS] Publication No. 79-555071). Washington, D.C.: U.S. Government Printing Office.

U.S. Department of Health and Human Services (1990). *Healthy People 2000: National Health Promotion and Disease Prevention Objectives* (DHHS [PBS] Publication No. 91-50212). Washington, D.C.: U.S. Government Printing Office.

U.S. Department of Health and Human Services (1991). *Trends in Indian Health 1990* (DHHS [PHS, IHS]). Rockville, MD.

U.S. Preventive Services Task Force (1989). *Guide to Clinical Preventive Services: An Assessment of the Effectiveness of 169 Interventions.* Baltimore: Williams & Wilkins.

U.S. Public Health Service (1998). *Clinician's Handbook of Preventive Services.* 2nd ed. McLean, VA: International Medical Publishing.

Watson, D.L., Tharp, R.G. (1989). *Self-Directed Behavior,* 5th ed. Pacific Grove, CA: Brooks/Cole Publishing Company.

Weaver, J.L. (1973). Mexican American health care behavior: A critical review of the literature. *Social Science Quarterly, 54,* 85–102.

Wilkinson, I.F., Darby, D.N., Mant, A. (1987). Self-care and self-medication: An evaluation of individuals' health care decisions. *Medical Care, 25,* 965–978.

Wilson, R.W., Elinson, J. (1981). National survey of personal health practices and consequences: Background, conceptual issues, and selected findings. *Public Health Reports, 96,* 218–225.

Wolinsky, F.D. (1980). *The Sociology of Health.* Boston, MA: Little, Brown.

Woods, N. (1989). Conceptualizations of self-care: Toward health-oriented models. *Advances in Nursing Science, 12* (1), 1–13.

World Health Organization (1948). Constitution of the World Health Organization. In *Basic Documents.* Geneva: World Health Organization.

Zapka, J., Averill, B.W. (1979). Self-care for colds: A cost-effective alternative to upper respiratory infection management. *American Journal of Public Health, 69,* 814–816.

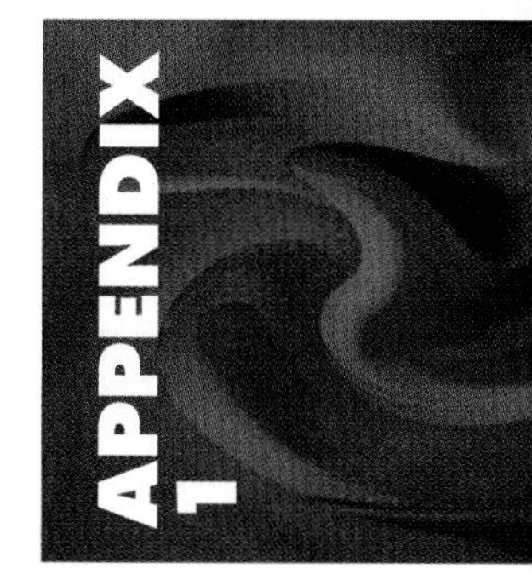

NANDA Nursing Diagnoses

This list represents the NANDA-approved nursing diagnoses for clinical use and testing (1994).

Activity Intolerance
Activity Intolerance, Risk for
Adaptive Capacity: Intracranial, Decreased
Adjustment, Impaired
Airway Clearance, Ineffective
Anxiety
Aspiration, Risk for

Body Image Disturbance
Body Temperature, Risk for Altered
Breastfeeding, Effective
Breastfeeding, Ineffective
Breastfeeding, Interrupted
*Breathing Pattern, Ineffective

Caregiver Role Strain
Caregiver Role Strain, Risk for
Communication, Impaired Verbal
Community Coping, Ineffective
Community Coping, Potential for Enhanced
Confusion, Acute
Confusion, Chronic
Constipation
Constipation, Colonic
Constipation, Perceived

Decisional Conflict (Specify)
*Decreased Cardiac Output
Defensive Coping
Denial, Ineffective
Diarrhea
Disorganized Infant Behavior
Disorganized Infant Behavior, Risk for
Disuse Syndrome, Risk for
Diversional Activity Deficit
Dysfunctional Ventilatory Weaning Response (DVWR)
Dysreflexia

Energy Field Disturbance
Environmental Interpretation Syndrome, Impaired

*Family Coping: Compromised, Ineffective
*Family Coping: Disabling, Ineffective
Family Coping: Potential for Growth
Family Process: Alcoholism, Altered
Family Processes, Altered
Fatigue
Fear
*Fluid Volume Deficit
Fluid Volume Deficit, Risk for
*Fluid Volume Excess

Gas Exchange, Impaired
*Grieving, Anticipatory
*Grieving, Dysfunctional
Growth and Development, Altered

Health Maintenance, Altered
Health Seeking Behaviors (Specify)
Home Maintenance Management, Impaired
Hopelessness
Hyperthermia
Hypothermia

Incontinence, Bowel
Incontinence, Functional
Incontinence, Reflex
Incontinence, Stress
Incontinence, Total
Incontinence, Urge
*Individual Coping, Ineffective
Infant Feeding Pattern, Ineffective
Infection, Risk for
Injury, Risk for

*Knowledge Deficit (Specify)

Loneliness, Risk for

*Diagnoses revised by small work groups at the 1994 Biennial Conference on the Classification of Nursing Diagnoses; changes approved and added in 1996.

Management of Therapeutic Regimen: Community, Ineffective
Management of Therapeutic Regimen: Families, Ineffective
Management of Therapeutic Regimen: Individual, Effective
Management of Therapeutic Regimen (Individuals), Ineffective
Memory, Impaired

Noncompliance (Specify)
Nutrition: Less than Body Requirements, Altered
Nutrition: More than Body Requirements, Altered
Nutrition: Risk for More than Body Requirements, Altered

Oral Mucous Membrane, Altered
Organized Infant Behavior, Potential for Enhanced

*Pain
*Pain, Chronic
Parental Role Conflict
Parent/Infant/Child Attachment, Risk for Altered
Parenting, Altered
Parenting, Risk for Altered
Perioperative Positioning Injury, Risk for
Peripheral Neurovascular Dysfunction, Risk for
Personal Identity Disturbance
Physical Mobility, Impaired
Poisoning, Risk for
Post-Trauma Response
Powerlessness
Protection, Altered

Rape-Trauma Syndrome
Rape-Trauma Syndrome: Compound Reaction
Rape-Trauma Syndrome: Silent Reaction
Relocation Stress Syndrome
Role Performance, Altered

Self Care Deficit
- Bathing/Hygiene
- Dressing/Grooming
- Feeding
- Toileting

*Self Esteem, Chronic Low
*Self Esteem Disturbance
*Self Esteem, Situational Low
Self Mutilation, Risk for
Sensory/Perceptual Alterations (Specify) (Visual, Auditory, Kinesthetic, Gustatory, Tactile, Olfactory)
Sexual Dysfunction
Sexuality Patterns, Altered
Skin Integrity, Impaired
Skin Integrity, Risk for Impaired
Sleep Pattern Disturbance
Social Interaction, Impaired
Social Isolation
Spiritual Distress (Distress of the Human Spirit)
Spiritual Well-Being, Potential for Enhanced
Suffocation, Risk for
Sustain Spontaneous Ventilation, Inability to
Swallowing, Impaired

Thermoregulation, Ineffective
*Thought Processes, Altered
Tissue Integrity, Impaired
Tissue Perfusion, Altered (Specify Type) (Renal, Cerebral, Cardiopulmonary, Gastrointestinal, Peripheral)
Trauma, Risk for

Unilateral Neglect
Urinary Elimination, Altered
Urinary Retention

*Violence, Risk for: Self Directed or Directed at Others

---

*Diagnoses revised by small work groups at the 1994 Biennial Conference on the Classification of Nursing Diagnoses; changes approved and added in 1996.

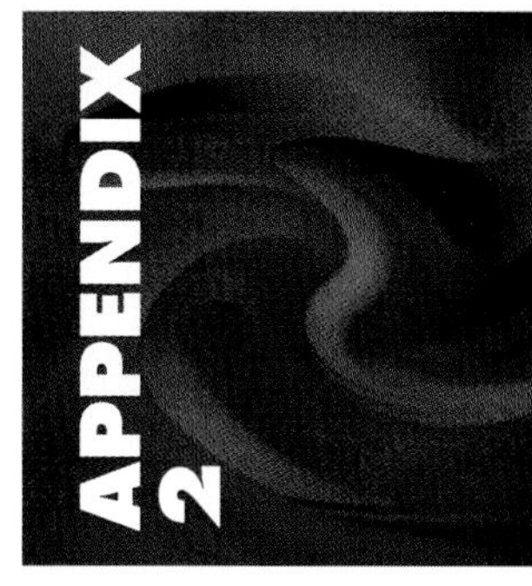

Abbreviations and Terminology

(Compiled by Charold Baer, RN, PhD)

Abbreviations

Abbreviation	Meaning
abd.	abdomen
a.c.	before meals (ante cibum)
ACTH	adrenocorticotropic hormone
ADH	antidiuretic hormone
ad lib	as desired
Adm.	administration
AMA	against medical advice
aq.	water (aqua)
ASHD	arteriosclerotic heart disease
ausc	auscultation
A-V	arteriovenous, atrioventricular
A&W	alive and well
BBB	bundle branch block
b.i.d.	twice a day (bis in die)
BM	bowel movement
BMR	basal metabolic rate
BP	blood pressure
BPH	benign prostatic hypertrophy
BSA	body surface area
BUN	blood urea nitrogen (test of kidney function)
C1, C2	first, second cervical vertebra
C_{σ}	creatinine clearance (test of kidney function)
Ca	calcium, cancer
CBC, c.b.c.	complete blood count
cc.	cubic centimeter, 1/1000 liter
cc	chief complaint
CCU	coronary care unit
CHF	congestive heart failure
Cl	chloride
cm.	centimeter (1/100 meter)
CNS	central nervous system
CO_2	carbon dioxide
COPD	chronic obstructive pulmonary disease
CSF	cerebrospinal fluid
CT	computed axial tomography
cu	cubic
CVA	cerebrovascular accident
D_5W	5% dextrose in water
Dx	diagnosis
DC	discontinue
D&C	dilation and curettage
diff.	differential blood count (numbers of all types of blood cells)
DOA	dead on arrival
DOE	dyspnea on exertion
DTs	delirium tremens (confusion, hallucinations, incoherence—due to alcoholic withdrawal)
DTR	deep tendon reflex
ECG	electrocardiogram
EEG	electroencephalogram
EENT	eyes, ears, nose, throat
EKG	electrocardiogram
EMG	electromyogram
ER	emergency room
FBS	fasting blood sugar
Fe	iron
FH	family history
FUO	fever of undetermined origin
GC	gonorrhea
GFR	glomerular filtration rate (kidney function test)
GI	gastrointestinal
Gm, gm	gram
Grav. 1,2,3	first, second, third pregnancy
GTT	glucose tolerance test
gtt.	drops (guttae)
GU	genitourinary
GYN	gynecologic
H	hydrogen
Hct, hct	hematocrit
HEENT	head, eyes, ears, nose, throat
Hg	mercury
HGB, hgb	hemoglobin
HPI	history of present illness
h.s.	at bedtime (hora somni)
ICU	intensive care unit
I & D	incision and drainage
IM	intramuscular (injection)
I & O	intake and output
IPPB	intermittent positive pressure breathing (asthma and emphysema therapy)
IV	intravenous (injection)
IVP	intravenous pyelogram, IV push
K	potassium
kg	kilogram (1000 grams)
KUB	kidney, ureter, and bladder (abdominal x-ray)
L	liter
L1, L2	first, second lumbar vertebra
LLL	left lower lobe

continued

Abbreviations *Continued*			
Abbreviation	**Meaning**	**Abbreviation**	**Meaning**
LLQ	left lower quadrant	Pro time	prothrombin time (test of blood clotting)
LMP	last menstrual period	Pt	patient
LP	lumbar puncture	PVC	premature ventricular contraction
LUL	left upper lobe	q	every
LUQ	left upper quadrant	qd	every day (quaque die)
mEq	milliequivalent (measurement of the concentration of a solution)	qh	every hour (quaque hora)
		q.i.d.	four times daily (quater in die)
mEq/L	milliequivalent per liter	qns	quantity not sufficient
mg	milligram (1/1000 gram)	RBC	red blood count or red blood cell (corpuscle)
MI	myocardial infarction (heart attack)	RLL	right lower lobe
ml, mL	milliliter (1/1000 liter)	RLQ	right lower quadrant
mm	millimeter (1/1000 meter; .039 inch)	RML	right middle lobe
mu	millimicron (1/1000 micron or 1/1,000,000 mm)	R/O	rule out
µg	microgram (1/1,000,000 gram)	RUL	right upper lobe
Na	sodium	RUQ	right upper quadrant
NG	nasogastric	Rx	treatment, prescription
NPO	nothing by mouth (nil per os)	S1, S2	first, second sacral vertebra or sacral nerve
O_2	oxygen	S-A	sinoatrial
OB	obstetrics	SC	subcutaneous (injection)
OD	right eye (oculus dexter)	SH	social history
OS	left eye (oculus sinister)	S.O.B.	shortness of breath
PAC	premature atrial contractions	soln.	solution
Para 1,2,3	unipara, bipara, tripara (number of viable births)	stat.	immediately (statim)
		T1, T2	first, second thoracic vertebra
PAT	paroxysmal atrial tachycardia	t.i.d.	three times daily (ter in die)
p.c.	after meals (post cibum)	TPR	temperature, pulse, respiration
PCO_2	carbon dioxide pressure	UA	urinalysis
PERRLA	pupils equal, round, react to light, and accommodate	UCHD	usual childhood diseases
		URI	upper respiratory infection
pH	hydrogen ion concentration (measure of acidity)	UTI	urinary tract infection
PID	pelvic inflammatory disease	VD	venereal disease
PMI	point of maximal impulse	VO	verbal order
p.o., PO	orally (per os)	WBC	white blood count; white blood cell
PO_2	oxygen pressure	WD	well-developed
prn	as required (pro re nata)	WN	well-nourished

Medical Terminology: Prefixes

Prefix	Meaning	Prefix	Meaning
a	no, not, without	in	in, not
ab	away from	infra	below
ad	toward	inter	between
ambi	both	intra	within
an	no, not, without	macro	large
ana	up	mal	bad
ante	forward, before	mesa	middle
anti	against	meta	beyond, change
auto	self	micro	small
bi	two	neo	new
brady	slow	pan	all
cata	down	para	near
circum	around	per	through, by
con	with, together	peri	surrounding
contra	against	poly	many
de	from, lack of	post	after, behind
dia	complete, through	pre	before
dis	to free or undo	pro	before
dys	bad, painful	pseudo	false
ecto	outside	re	back
em	in	retro	behind
endo	within, inner	semi	half
epi	above, upon	sub	under
eu	good	super	above
ex	out, away from	sym	together
exo	outside, outer	syn	together
extra	in addition	tachy	fast
hemi	half	trans	across
hyper	above, excessive	ultra	beyond, excess
hypo	below, deficient		

Medical Terminology: Suffixes

Suffix	Meaning	Suffix	Meaning
-ac	pertaining to	-or	one who
-al	pertaining to	-orrhagia	bursting forth of blood
-algia	pain	-orrhaphy	suture
-ar	pertaining to	-orrhea	flow, discharge
-ary	pertaining to	-orrhexia	rupture
-blast	embryonic	-osis	condition
-cele	hernia	-ostomy	make a new opening
-centesis	surgical puncture	-otomy	to cut into
-clysis	irrigation, washing	-ous	pertaining to
-coccus	berry shaped	-pathy	disease
-crit	to separate	-penia	deficiency
-drome	to run	-pexy	fixation
-ectasis	stretching, dilatation	-physis	to grow
-ectomy	to excise	-plasia	formation, development
-er	one who	-plasm	growth, formation
-fusion	to pour	-plasty	surgical repair
-genesis	condition of producing	-poiesis	formation
-grade	to go	-ptosis	drooping, prolapse
-gram	record	-ptysis	spitting
-graph	instrument for recording	-sclerosis	hardening
-graphy	process of recording	-scope	instrument to visually examine
-ia	condition, process	-spasm	sudden violent involuntary contraction
-ic	pertaining to	-stalsis	constriction
-ist	one who specializes in	-stasis	to stop, control
-itis	inflammation	-stenosis	tightening, narrowing
-logy	process of studying	-therapy	treatment
-lysis	to break	-tic	pertaining to
-malacia	softening	-tome	instrument to cut
-megaly	enlargement	-tomy	process of cutting
-meter	to measure	-tresia	opening
-odynia	pain	-tripsy	surgical crushing
-oid	pertaining to	-trophy	development
-ole	little	-ule	little
-oma	tumor	-y	process, condition
-opsy	to view		

Medical Terminology: Combining Forms

Combining Form	Meaning	Combining Form	Meaning
acu/o	sharp	mult/i	many
alb/o	white	myc/o	fungus
anis/o	unequal	nat/i	birth
anter/o	front	ne/o	new
bi/o	life	necr/o	death
bol/o	to throw or cast off	nect/o	to bind, connect
carcin/o	cancer	norm/o	rule, order
chlor/o	green	null/i	none
chrom/o	color	onc/o	mass, tumor
chron/o	time	path/o	disease
cis/o	to cut	pex/o	fixation
cyan/o	blue	phil/os	love, attraction to
dextr/o	right	physi/o	nature
dipl/o	double	plas/o	development
dist/o	far	poster/o	back
dors/o	back	prot/o	first
duct/o	to carry or lead	proxim/o	near
ectop/o	misplaced	py/o	pus
electr/o	electricity	pyr/o	fire, fever
eosin/o	rosy, dawn colored	radi/i	rays
erythr/o	red	sarc/o	flesh
furc/o	forking, branching	scop/o	examination
gen/o	beginning	secti/o	to cut
gnos/o	knowledge	seps/o	infection
granul/o	granules	sinistr/o	left
heter/o	different	somn/o	sleep
hist/o	tissue	son/o	sound
hom/o	same	staphyl/o	clusters, grapes
inguin/o	groin	strept/o	twisted chains
is/o	equal	thel/o	nipple-like
kinesi/o	movement	the/o	to put or place
later/o	side	therm/o	heat
leuk/o	white	tom/o	to cut
lith/o	stone, calculus	top/o	place, position
medi/o	middle	tr/i	three
melan/o	black	un/i	one
mon/o	single	ventr/o	belly side
morph/o	shape, form	viscer/o	internal organs
mort/o	death	xanth/o	yellow
muc/o	mucus		

The Hematologic System

Combining Form	Meaning
agglutin/o	clumping
bas/o	base
cyt/o	cell
fibrin/o	fibrin
hemat/o	blood
hem/o	blood
immun/o	safe
kary/o	nucleus
lymph/o	lymph
myel/o	bone marrow
neutr/o	neutral
nucle/o	nucleus
poikil/o	varied, irregular
reticul/o	network
sanguin/o	blood
sider/o	iron
spher/o	globe, round
splen/o	spleen
thromb/o	clot
thym/o	thymus

Suffix	Meaning
-cyte	cell
-cytosis	condition of cells
-emia	blood condition
-globin	protein
-globulin	protein
-pheresis	removal
-philia	attraction for
-phoresis	transmission
-poiesis	formation

The Musculoskeletal System			
Combining Form	**Meaning**	**Combining Form**	**Meaning**
acetabul/o	acetabulum	lord/o	curve, swayback
acr/o	extremity	lumb/o	lower back
acromi/o	shoulder	mandibul/o	lower jaw bone
ankyl/o	stiff	maxill/o	upper jaw bone
aponeur/o	aponeurosis	metacarp/o	hand bones
arthr/o	joint	metatars/o	foot bones
articul/o	joint	my/o	muscle
axill/o	armpit	olecran/o	elbow
brachi/o	arm	oste/o	bone
burs/o	bursa	patell/o	kneecap
calcane/o	heel	pelv/i	pelvis
carp/o	wrist bones	perone/o	fibula
caud/o	toward the tail	phalang/o	fingers, toes
cephal/o	head	pod/o	foot
cervic/o	neck	pub/o	pubis
chir/o	hand, foot	rachi/o	spinal column
chondr/o	cartilage	radi/o	radius
clavicul/o	clavicle	rhabdomy/o	skeletal muscle
coccyg/o	coccyx	sacr/o	sacrum
condyl/o	condyle	scapul/o	scapula
crani/o	skull	scoli/o	crooked, bent
dactyl/o	fingers, toes	spin/o	spine
fasci/o	fascia	spondyl/o	vertebrae
femor/o	femur	stern/o	sternum
fibr/o	fibers	submaxill/o	lower jaw bone
fibul/o	fibula	syndesm/o	ligament
humer/o	humerus	synovi/o	synovia
ili/o	ilium	tars/o	ankle, instep bones
ischi/o	ischium	ten/o	tendon
kyph/o	humpback	thorac/o	chest
lamin/o	lamina	tibi/o	tibia
leiomy/o	smooth muscle	uln/o	ulna
ligament/o	ligament	vertebr/o	vertebrae

The Musculoskeletal System	
Prefix	**Meaning**
amphi-	on both sides
Suffix	**Meaning**
-clast	to break
-porosis	passage
Other Structures	
diaphysis	epiphysis
fontanelle	foramen
trochanter	tubercle
tuberosity	vertebral arch
xyphoid process	suture
intervertebral disk	manubrium

The Nervous System

Combining Form	Meaning	Cranial Nerves	
algesi/o	excessive sensitivity	I	Olfactory
cephal/o	head	II	Optic
cerebell/o	cerebellum	III	Oculomotor
cerebr/o	cerebrum	IV	Trochlear
dur/o	dura mater	V	Trigeminal
encephal/o	brain	VI	Abducens
esthesi/o	feeling	VII	Facial
gangli/o	ganglion	VIII	Auditory
gli/o	glue	IX	Glossopharyngeal
leps/o	seizure	X	Vagus
mening/o	meninges, membrane	XI	Spinal Accessory
myel/o	spinal cord	XII	Hypoglossal
narc/o	sleep		
neur/o	nerve		
phas/o	speech		
plex/o	network		
pont/o	pons		
tax/o	coordination, order		
thalam/o	thalamus		
ventricul/o	ventricle		

Suffix	Meaning
-asthenia	lack of strength
-paresis	slight paralysis
-plegia	paralysis

The Cardiovascular System

Combining Form	Meaning
aneurysm/o	aneurysm
angi/o	vessel
aort/o	aorta
arteri/o	artery
arteriol/o	arteriole
ather/o	plaque
atri/o	atrium
cardi/o	heart
coron/o	heart
ox/i (y)	oxygen
phleb/o	vein
sphygm/o	pulse
steth/o	chest
valv/o	valve
vas/o	vessel
ven/o	vein
ventricul/o	ventricle
venul/o	venule

The Respiratory System

Combining Form	Meaning
adenoid/o	adenoids
aer/o	air
alveol/o	alveolus
anthrac/o	coal dust
bronch/o	bronchus
bronchiol/o	bronchiole
epiglott/o	epiglottis
laryng/o	larynx
lob/o	lobe
myx/o	mucus
nas/o	nose
orth/o	straight
ox/i (y)	oxygen
pector/o	chest
pharyng/o	pharynx
phren/o	diaphragm
phon/o	voice
pleur/o	pleura
pne/o	breath
pneum/o	air
pneumon/o	lung
pulmon/o	lung
rhin/o	nose
sinus/o	sinus
spir/o	breath
thorac/o	chest
tonsill/o	tonsils
trache/o	trachea

Suffix	Meaning
-capnia	carbon dioxide
-osmia	smell, odor
-pnea	breathing
-thorax	pleural cavity

The Renal System

Combining Form	Meaning
albumin/o	protein
azot/o	urea, nitrogen
bacteri/o	bacteria
cali/o	calyx
cortic/o	cortex
cyst/o	urinary bladder
glomerul/o	glomerulus
medull/o	medulla
nephr/o	kidney
noct/i	night
olig/o	scanty
py/o	pus
pyel/o	renal pelvis
ren/o	kidney
ur/o	urine
ureter/o	ureters
urethr/o	urethra
vesic/o	urinary bladder

Suffix	Meaning
-uria	urine

Fluids and Electrolytes

Combining Form	Meaning
glyc/o	sugar
calci/o	calcium
dips/o	thirst
dextr/o	sugar
kal/i	potassium
natr/o	sodium
gluc/o	sugar
hydr/o	water
chlor/o	chloride
vol/o	volume
magnesi/o	magnesium
cellul/o	cell

The Reproductive System

Combining Form	Meaning
amni/o	amnion, sac for embryo
andr/o	male
balan/o	glans penis
bartholin/o	Bartholin's glands
cervic/o	cervix
chori/o	chorion
colp/o	vagina
culd/o	cul-de-sac
cry/o	cold
crypt/o	hidden
epididym/o	epididymis
episi/o	vulva
gon/o	seed
gravid/o	pregnancy
gynec/o	woman, female
hyster/o	uterus
lact/o	milk
mamm/o	breast
mast/o	breast
men/o	menses
metr/o-metri/o	uterus
oo/o	egg, ovum
oophor/o	ovary
orchid/o-orchi/o	testis
ov/o	egg
ovari/o	ovary
par/o	bear
perine/o	perineum
prostat/o	prostate gland
salping/o	fallopian tube
sperm/o	spermatozoa
spermat/o	spermatozoa
syphil/o	syphilis
test/o	testis
uter/o	uterus
vagin/o	vagina
vas/o	vessel, duct
vesicul/o	seminal vessels
vulv/o	vulva

Suffix	Meaning
-para	to bear
-tocia	labor
-cyesis	pregnancy
-arche	beginning
-partum	birth, labor

The Sensory Systems

Integumentary System

Combining Form	*Meaning*
acanth/o	thorny, spiny
adip/o	fat
caus/o	burn
cutane/o	skin
derm/o	skin
dermat/o	skin
diaphor/o	sweat
erythem/o	flushed, redness
hidr/o	sweat
hist/o	tissue
kerat/o	horny, hard
lip/o	fat
onych/o	nail
pachy/o	thick
seb/o	sebum
squam/o	scale
trich/o	hair
ungu/o	nail
xer/o	dry

Optical System

Combining Form	*Meaning*
ambly/o	dull, dim
aque/o	water
blephar/o	eyelid
cor/o	pupil
core/o	pupil
corne/o	cornea
conjunctiv/o	conjunctiva
cycl/o	ciliary, body of eye
dacry/o	tear
dacryocyst/o	lacrimal sac
dacryoaden/o	tear gland
glauc/o	grey
ir/o	iris

Optical System *Continued*

Combining Form	*Meaning*
irid/o	iris
kerat/o	cornea, horny
lacrim/o	tear
mi/o	smaller
ocul/o	eye
ophthalm/o	eye
phot/o	light
presby/o	old age
pupill/o	pupil
retin/o	retina
scler/o	sclera
vitre/o	glassy

Suffix	***Meaning***
-opia	vision
-tropia	to turn

Auditory System

Combining Form	*Meaning*
acou/o	hearing
audi/o	hearing
aur/i	ear
aur/o	ear
cerumin/o	cerumin
myring/o	eardrum
ot/o	ear
staped/o	stapes
tympan/o	eardrum

Suffix	***Meaning***
-emphraxis	blockage
-cusis	hearing
-phonia	sound

The Digestive System

Combining Form	Meaning
abdomin/o	abdomen
amyl/o	starch
an/o	anus
appendic/o	appendix
bilirubin/o	bilirubin
bucc/o	cheek
cec/o	cecum
celi/o	belly
cheil/o	lip
chol/e	bile
cholescyst/o	gall bladder
choledoch/o	common bile duct
cib/o	meals
col/o	colon
dent/o	tooth
duoden/o	duodenum
emesis	vomitus
enter/o	intestines (small)
esophag/o	esophagus
gastr/o	stomach
gingiv/o	gums
gloss/o	tongue
hepat/o	liver
herni/o	hernia
ile/o	ileum
jejun/o	jejunum
labi/o	lip
lapar/o	abdomen
lingu/o	tongue
lip/o	fat
odont/o	tooth
omphal/o	navel
or/o	mouth
palat/o	palate
pancreat/o	pancreas
peps/ia	digestion
peritone/o	peritoneum
phag/o	to eat, swallow
pharyng/o	throat, pharynx
proct/o	rectum
sial/o	saliva
sialaden/o	salivary glands
sigmoid/o	sigmoid
splen/o	spleen
steat/o	fat
stomat/o	mouth

Suffix	Meaning
-ase	enzyme
-iasis	condition
-prandial	meal

Endocrine System

Combining Form	Meaning
aden/o	gland
adren/o	adrenal glands
cortic/o	cortex
crin/o	secrete
estr/o	female
parathyroid/o	parathyroid
ster/o	solid structure
thym/o	thymus
thyroid/o	thyroid
toxic/o	poison

Psychiatric Terms

Combining Form	Meaning	Suffix	Meaning
ment/o	mind	-mania	madness, abnormal preoccupation
phren/o	mind	-phobia	fear of
psych/o	mind		
schiz/o	split		

Term	Term
acrophobia	narcolepsy
algophobia	panophobia
androphobia	paranoia
agnosia	schizophrenia
agoraphobia	chromophobia
hydrophobia	gynephobia
amentia	monophobia
amnesia	noctiphobia
aphonia	acrocyanosis
autism	agraphia
catalepsy	decerebration
dementia	dromolepsy
egomania	neurosis
hyperkinesis	psychosis
megalomania	prodrome
necromania	
pyromania	

Units of Measurement

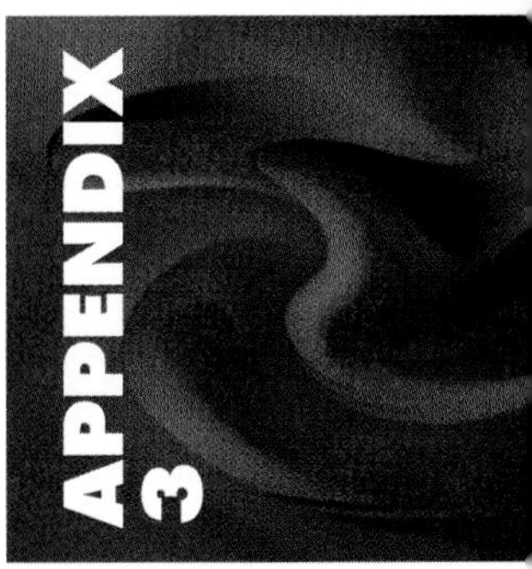

SI Units (Système International d'Unités or International System of Units)

SI Base Units

Quantity	*Name*	*Symbol*
Length	meter	m
Mass	kilogram	kg
Time	second	s
Electric current	ampere	A
Temperature	kelvin	K
Luminous intensity	candela	cd
Amount of a substance	mole	mol

Some SI-Derived Units

Quantity	*Name of derived unit*	*Symbol*
Area	square meter	m^2
Volume	cubic meter	m^3
Speed, velocity	meter per second	m/s
Acceleration	meter per second squared	m/s^2
Mass density	kilogram per cubic meter	kg/m^3
Concentration of a substance	mole per cubic meter	mol/m^3
Specific volume	cubic meter per kilogram	m^3/kg
Luminescence	candela per square meter	cd/m^3

SI-Derived Units with Special Names

Quantity	*Name*	*Symbol*	*Expressed in terms of other units*
Frequency	hertz	Hz	s^{-1}
Force	newton	N	$kg \cdot m \cdot s^2$ or $kg \cdot m/s^2$
Pressure	pascal	Pa	$N \cdot m^{-2}$ or N/m^2
Energy, work, amount of heat	joule	J	$kg \cdot m^2 \cdot s^{-2}$ or $N \cdot m$
Power	watt	W	$J \cdot s$ or J/s
Quantity of electricity	coulomb	C	$A \cdot s$
Electromotive force	volt	V	W/A
Capacitance	farad	F	C/V
Electrical resistance	ohm	Ω	V/a
Conductance	siemens	S	A/V
Inductance	henry	H	Wϕ/A
Illuminance	lux	lx	ln/m^2
Absorbed (radiation) dose	gray	Gy	J/kg
Dose equivalent (radiation)	sievert	Sv	J/kg
Activity (radiation)	becquerel	Bq	s^{-1}

Prefixes and Multiples Used in SI

Prefix	*Symbol*	*Power*	*Multiple or portion of a multiple*
tera	T	10^{12}	1,000,000,000,000
giga	G	10^9	1,000,000,000
mega	M	10^4	1,000,000
kilo	k	10^3	1,000
hecto	h	10^2	100
deca	da	10^1	10
unity			1
deci	d	10^{-1}	0.1
centi	c	10^{-2}	0.01
milli	m	10^{-3}	0.001
micro	μ	10^{-6}	0.000001
nano	n	10^{-9}	0.000000001
pico	p	10^{-12}	0.000000000001
femto	f	10^{-15}	0.000000000000001
atto	a	10^{-18}	0.000000000000000001

Metric System

Masses

Table		Grams		Grains
1 Kilogram	=	1000.0	=	15,432.35
1 Hectogram	=	100.0	=	1,543.23
1 Decagram	=	10.0	=	154.323
1 Gram	=	1.0	=	15.432
1 Decigram	=	0.1	=	1.5432
1 Centigram	=	0.01	=	0.15432
1 Milligram	=	0.001	=	0.01543
1 Microgram	=	10^{-6}	=	15.432×10^{-6}
1 Nanogram	=	10^{-9}	=	15.432×10^{-9}
1 Picogram	=	10^{-12}	=	15.432×10^{-12}
1 Femtogram	=	10^{-15}	=	15.432×10^{-15}
1 Attogram	=	10^{-18}	=	15.432×10^{-18}

Arabic numbers are used with masses and measures, as 10 g, or 3 ml, etc. Portions of masses and measures are usually expressed decimally. 10^{-1} indicates 0.1; 10^{-6} = 0.000001; etc.

Weights and Measures

Length

Millimeters (mm)	Centimeters (cm)	Inches (in.)	Feet (ft)	Yards (yd)	Meters (m)
1.0	0.1	0.03937	0.00328	0.0011	0.001
10.0	1.0	0.3937	0.03281	0.0109	0.01
25.4	2.54	1.0	0.0833	0.0278	0.0254
304.8	30.48	12.0	1.0	0.333	0.3048
914.40	91.44	36.0	3.0	1.0	0.9144
1000.0	100.0	39.37	3.2808	1.0936	1.0

Volume (Fluid)

Milliliters (ml)	U.S. Fluid Drams (fl ʒ)	Cubic Inches (in.^{3})	U.S. Fluid Ounces (fl ℥)	U.S. Fluid Quarts (qt)	Liters (L)
1.0	0.2705	0.061	0.03381	0.00106	0.001
3.679	1.0	0.226	0.125	0.00391	0.00369
16.3866	4.4329	1.0	0.5541	0.0173	0.01639
29.573	8.0	1.8047	1.0	0.03125	0.02957
949.332	256.0	57.75	32.0	1.0	0.9463
1000.0	270.52	61.025	33.815	1.0567	1.0

Arabic numbers are used with masses and measures, as 10 g, or 3 ml, etc. Portions of masses and measures are usually expressed decimally. For practical purposes, 1 cm^3 (cubic centimeter) is equivalent to 1 ml (milliliter) and 1 drop (gtt) of water is equivalent to a minim (m).
1 gallon = 4 quarts = 8 pints = 3.785 liters.
1 pint = 473.16 ml.

Weight

Grains (gr)	Grams (g)	Apothecaries' Ounces (℥)	Avoirdupois Pounds (lb)	Kilograms (kg)
1.0	0.0648	0.00208	0.0001429	0.000065
15.432	1.0	0.03215	0.002205	0.0001
480.0	31.1	1.0	0.06855	0.0311
7000.0	453.5924	14.583	1.0	0.45354
15432.358	1000.0	32.15	2.2046	1.0

1 microgram (μg) = 0.0001 milligram.
1 mg = 1 milligram = 0.001 g; 1000 mg = 1 g.

Apothecaries' Weight

20 grains = 1 scruple	3 scruples = 1 dram
8 drams = 1 ounce	12 ounces = 1 pound

Avoirdupois Weight

27.343 grains = 1 dram	16 drams = 1 ounce
16 ounces = 1 pound	100 pounds = 1 hundredweight
2000 pounds = 1 short ton	2240 pounds = 1 long ton
1 oz troy = 480 grains	1 oz avoirdupois = 437.5 grains
1 lb troy = 5760 grains	1 lb avoirdupois = 7000 grains

Circular Measure

60 seconds = 1 minute	60 minutes = 1 degree
90 degrees = 1 quadrant	4 quadrants = 360 degrees = circle

Cubic Measure

1728 cubic inches = 1 cubic foot	27 cubic feet = 1 cubic yard
2150.42 cubic inches = 1 standard bushel	268.8 cubic inches = 1 dry (U.S.) gallon
1 cubic foot = about four-fifths of a bushel	128 cubic feet = 1 cord (wood)

Dry Measure

2 pints = 1 quart	8 quarts = 1 peck	4 pecks = 1 bushel

Liquid Measure

16 ounces = 1 pint	4 quarts = 1 gallon	2 barrels = 1 hogshead (U.S.)
1000 milliliters = 1 liter	31.5 gallons = 1 barrel (U.S.)	1 quart = 0.946 liter
4 gills = 1 pint	2 pints = 1 quart	

Barrels and hogsheads vary in size. A U.S. gallon is equal to 0.8327 British gallon; therefore, a British gallon is equal to 1.201 U.S. gallons. 1 liter is equal to 1.0567 quarts.

Linear Measure

1 inch = 2.54 centimeters	40 rods = 1 furlong	8 furlongs = 1 statute mile
12 inches = 1 foot	3 feet = 1 yard	5.5 yards = 1 rod
1 statute mile = 5280 feet	3 statute miles = 1 statute league	

Troy Weight

24 grains = 1 pennyweight	20 pennyweights = 1 ounce	12 ounces = 1 pound

Used for weighing gold, silver, and jewels.

Household Measures* and Weights

Approximate equivalents: 60 gtt = 1 teaspoonful = 5 ml = 60 minims = 60 grains = 1 dram = ⅛ ounce.

1 teaspoon = ⅛ fl. oz = 1 dram	16 teaspoons (liquid) = 1 cup
3 teaspoons = 1 tablespoon	12 tablespoons (dry) = 1 cup
1 tablespoon = ½ fl. oz = 4 drams	1 cup = 8 fl. oz
1 tumbler or glass = 8 fl. oz; 1 pint	

*Household measures are not precise. For instance, a household teaspoon will hold 3 to 5 ml of liquid. Therefore, household equivalents should not be substituted for medication prescribed by the physician. *Note:* Traditionally, the word "weights" is used in these tables, but "masses" is the correct term.

Conversion Rules and Factors

To convert units of one system into another, multiply the number of units in column I by the equivalent factor opposite that unit in column II.

Weight

1 attogram	= 15.432 × 10^{-18} grains
1 femtogram	= 15.432 × 10^{-15} grains
1 picogram	= 15.432 × 10^{-12} grains
1 nanogram	= 15.432 × 10^{-9} grains
1 microgram	= 15.432 × 10^{-6} grains
1 milligram	= 0.015432 grain
1 centigram	= 0.15432 grain
1 decigram	= 1.5432 grains
1 decagram	= 154.323 grains
1 hectogram	= 1543.23 grains
1 gram	= 15.432 grains
1 gram	= 0.25720 apothecaries' dram
1 gram	= 0.03527 avoirdupois ounce
1 gram	= 0.03215 apothecaries' or troy ounce
1 kilogram	= 35.274 avoirdupois ounces
1 kilogram	= 32.151 apothecaries' or troy ounces
1 kilogram	= 2.2046 avoirdupois pounds
1 grain	= 64.7989 milligrams
1 grain	= 0.0648 gram
1 apothecaries' dram	= 3.8879 grams
1 avoirdupois ounce	= 28.3495 grams
1 apothecaries' or troy ounce	= 31.1035 grams
1 avoirdupois pound	= 463.5924 grams

Volume (Air or Gas)

1 cubic centimeter (cm^3)	= 0.06102 cubic inch
1 cubic meter (m^3)	= 35.314 cubic feet
1 cubic meter	= 1.3079 cubic yards
1 cubic inch ($in.^3$)	= 16.3872 cubic centimeters
1 cubic foot (ft^3)	= 0.02832 cubic meter

Capacity (Fluid or Liquid)

1 milliliter	= 16.23 minims
1 milliliter	= 0.2705 fluid dram
1 milliliter	= 0.0338 fluid ounce
1 liter	= 33.8148 fluid ounces
1 liter	= 2.1134 pints
1 liter	= 1.0567 quarts
1 liter	= 0.2642 gallon
1 fluid dram	= 3.697 milliliters
1 fluid ounce	= 29.573 milliliters
1 pint	= 473.1765 milliliters
1 quart	= 946.353 milliliters
1 gallon	= 3.785 liters

Time

1 millisecond	= one-thousandth (0.001) of a second
1 second	= 1/60 of a minute
1 minute	= 1/60 of an hour
1 hour	= 1/24 of a day

Temperature

Given a temperature on a Fahrenheit scale: to convert it to degrees Celsius, subtract 32 and multiply by 5/9. Given a temperature on a Celsius scale: to convert it to degrees Fahrenheit, multiply by 9/5 and add 32. Degrees Celsius are equivalent to degrees Centigrade.

Pressure

To Obtain	*Multiply*	*By*
lb/sq in.	atmospheres	14.696
lb/sq in.	in. of water	0.03609
lb/sq in.	ft of water	0.4335
lb/sq in.	in. of mercury	0.4912
lb/sq in.	kg/sq meter	0.00142
lb/sq in.	kg/sq cm	14.22
lb/sq in.	cm of mercury	0.1934
lb/sq ft	atmospheres	2116.8
lb/sq ft	in. of water	5.204
lb/sq ft	ft of water	62.48
lb/sq ft	in. of mercury	70.727
lb/sq ft	cm of mercury	27.845
lb/sq ft	kg/sq meter	0.20482
lb/cu in.	gm/ml	0.03613
lb/cu ft	lb/cu in.	1728.0
lb/cu ft	gm/ml	62.428
lb/U.S. gallon	gm/L	8.345
in. of water	in. of mercury	13.60
in. of water	cm of mercury	5.3543
ft of water	atmospheres	33.95
ft of water	lb/sq in.	2.307
ft of water	kg/sq meter	0.00328
ft of water	in. of mercury	1.133
ft of water	cm of mercury	0.4461
atmospheres	ft of water	0.02947
atmospheres	in. of mercury	0.03342
atmospheres	kg/sq cm	0.9678
bars	atmospheres	1.0133
in. of mercury	atmospheres	29.921
in. of mercury	lb/sq in.	2.036
mm of mercury	atmospheres	760.0
g/ml	lb/cu in.	27.68
g/sq cm	kg/sq meter	0.1
kg/sq meter	lb/sq in.	703.1
kg/sq meter	in. of water	25.40
kg/sq meter	in. of mercury	345.32
kg/sq meter	cm of mercury	135.95
kg/sq meter	atmospheres	10332.0
kg/sq cm	atmospheres	1.0332

Flow Rate

To Obtain	*Multiply*	*By*
cu ft/hr	cc/min	0.00212
cu ft/hr	L/min	2.12
L/min	cu ft/hr	0.472

Parts per Million

Conversion of parts per million (ppm) to percent:
1 ppm = 0.0001%, 10 ppm = 0.001%, 100 ppm = 0.01%, 1000 ppm = 0.1%, 10,000 ppm = 1%, etc.

Energy

1 foot pound = 1.35582 joules
1 joule = 0.2389 Calorie (kilocalorie)
1 Calorie (kilocalorie) = 1000 calories = 4184 joules
A large Calorie, or kilocalorie, is always written with a capital C.

pH

The pH scale is simply a series of numbers stating where a given solution would stand in a series of solutions arranged according to acidity or alkalinity. At one extreme (high pH) lies a highly alkaline solution, which may be made by dissolving 4 g of sodium hydroxide in water to make a liter of solution; at the other extreme (low pH) is an acid solution containing 3.65 g of hydrogen chloride per liter of water. Halfway between lies purified water, which is neutral. All other solutions can be arranged on this scale, and their acidity or alkalinity can be stated by giving the numbers that indicate their relative positions. If the pH of a certain solution is 5.3, it falls between gastric juice and urine on the above scale, is moderately acid, and will turn litmus red.

Tenth-normal HCl	−1.00	
Gastric juice	*1.4	Litmus is red in this acid range.
Urine	*6.0	
Water	7.0—Neutral	
Blood	7.35–7.45	
Bile	*7.5	Litmus is blue in this acid range.
Pancreatic juice	8.5	
Tenth-normal NaOH	13.00	

*These body fluids vary rather widely in pH; typical figures have been used for simplicity. Urine samples obtained from healthy individuals may have pH anywhere between 4.7 and 8.0.

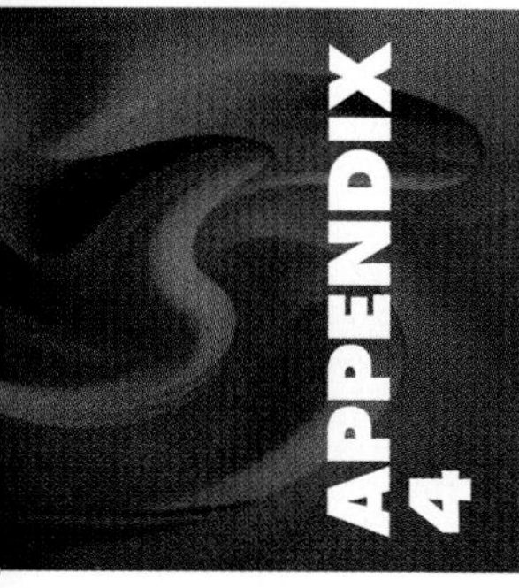

Reference Laboratory Values

(From Conn, R.B., Borer, W.Z., & Snyder, J.W. [1997]. Current Diagnosis Vol. 9. Philadelphia: W.B. Saunders.)

Reference Values for Hematology

	Conventional Units	SI Units
Acid hemolysis (Ham test)	No hemolysis	No hemolysis
Alkaline phosphatase, leukocyte	Total score 14–100	Total score 14–100
Cell counts		
Erythrocytes		
Males	4.6–6.2 million/mm^3	4.6–6.2 × 10^{12}/L
Females	4.2–5.4 million/mm^3	4.2–5.4 × 10^{12}/L
Children (varies with age)	4.5–5.1 million/mm^3	4.5–5.1 × 10^{12}/L
Leukocytes, total	4500–11,000/mm^3	4.5–11.0 × 10^9/L
Leukocytes, differential counts*		
Myelocytes	0%	0/L
Band neutrophils	3–5%	150–400 × 10^6/L
Segmented neutrophils	54–62%	3000–5800 × 10^6/L
Lymphocytes	25–33%	1500–3000 × 10^6/L
Monocytes	3–7%	300–500 × 10^6/L
Eosinophils	1–3%	50–250 × 10^6/L
Basophils	0–1%	15–50 × 10^6/L
Platelets	150,000–400,000/mm^3	150–400 × 10^9/L
Reticulocytes	25,000–75,000/mm^3 (0.5–1.5% of erythrocytes)	25–75 × 10^9/L
Coagulation tests		
Bleeding time (template)	2.75–8.0 min	2.75–8.0 min
Coagulation time (glass tube)	5–15 min	5–15 min
D-Dimer	<0.5 μg/mL	<0.5 mg/L
Factor VIII and other coagulation factors	50–150% of normal	0.5–1.5 of normal
Fibrin split products (Thrombo-Welco test)	<10 μg/mL	<10 mg/L
Fibrinogen	200–400 mg/dL	2.0–4.0 g/L
Partial thromboplastin time (PTT)	20–35 s	20–35 s
Prothrombin time (PT)	12.0–14.0 s	12.0–14.0 s
Coombs' test		
Direct	Negative	Negative
Indirect	Negative	Negative
Corpuscular values of erythrocytes		
Mean corpuscular hemoglobin (MCH)	26–34 pg/cell	26–34 pg/cell
Mean corpuscular volume (MCV)	80–96 μm^3	80–96 fL
Mean corpuscular hemoglobin concentration (MCHC)	32–36 g/dL	320–360 g/L
Haptoglobin	20–165 mg/dL	0.20–1.65 g/L
Hematocrit		
Males	40–54 mL/dL	0.40–0.54
Females	37–47 mL/dL	0.37–0.47
Newborns	49–54 mL/dL	0.49–0.54
Children (varies with age)	35–49 mL/dL	0.35–0.49
Hemoglobin		
Males	13.0–18.0 g/dL	8.1–11.2 mmol/L
Females	12.0–16.0 g/dL	7.4–9.9 mmol/L

Reference Values for Hematology *Continued*

	Conventional Units	SI Units
Newborns	16.5–19.5 g/dL	10.2–12.1 mmol/L
Children (varies with age)	11.2–16.5 g/dL	7.0–10.2 mmol/L
Hemoglobin, fetal	<1.0% of total	<0.01 of total
Hemoglobin A_{1C}	3–5% of total	0.03–0.05 of total
Hemoglobin A_2	1.5–3.0% of total	0.015–0.03 of total
Hemoglobin, plasma	0.0–5.0 mg/dL	0.0–3.2 μmol/L
Methemoglobin	30–130 mg/dL	19–80 μmol/L
Erythrocyte sedimentation rate (ESR)		
Wintrobe		
Males	0–5 mm/h	0–5 mm/h
Females	0–15 mm/h	0–15 mm/h
Westergren		
Males	0–15 mm/h	0–15 mm/h
Females	0–20 mm/h	0–20 mm/h

*Conventional units are percentages; SI units are absolute counts.

Reference Values* for Clinical Chemistry (Blood, Serum, and Plasma)

	Conventional Units	SI Units
Acetoacetate plus acetone		
Qualitative	Negative	Negative
Quantitative	0.3–2.0 mg/dL	30–200 μmol/L
Acid phosphatase, serum (thymolphthalein monophosphate substrate)	0.1–0.6 U/L	0.1–0.6 U/L
ACTH (see corticotropin)		
Alanine aminotransferase (ALT, SGPT), serum	1–45 U/L	1–45 U/L
Albumin, serum	3.3–5.2 g/dL	33–52 g/L
Aldolase, serum	0.0–7.0 U/L	0.0–7.0 U/L
Aldosterone, plasma		
Standing	5–30 ng/dL	140–830 pmol/L
Recumbent	3–10 ng/dL	80–275 pmol/L
Alkaline phosphatase (ALP), serum		
Adult	35–150 U/L	35–150 U/L
Adolescent	100–500 U/L	100–500 U/L
Child	100–350 U/L	100–350 U/L
Ammonia nitrogen, plasma	10–50 μmol/L	10–50 μmol/L
Amylase, serum	25–125 U/L	25–125 U/L
Anion gap, serum, calculated	8–16 mEq/L	8–16 mmol/L
Ascorbic acid, blood	0.4–1.5 mg/dL	23–85 μmol/L
Aspartate aminotransferase (AST, SGOT), serum	1–36 U/L	1–36 U/L
Base excess, arterial blood, calculated	0 ± 2 mEq/L	0 ± 2 mmol/L
β-Carotene, serum	60–260 μg/dL	1.1–8.6 μmol/L
Bicarbonate		
Venous plasma	23–29 mEq/L	23–29 mmol/L
Arterial blood	21–27 mEq/L	21–27 mmol/L
Bile acids, serum	0.3–3.0 mg/dL	0.8–7.6 μmol/L
Bilirubin, serum		
Conjugated	0.1–0.4 mg/dL	1.7–6.8 μmol/L
Total	0.3–1.1 mg/dL	5.1–19.0 μmol/L
Calcium, serum	8.4–10.6 mg/dL	2.10–2.65 mmol/L
Calcium, ionized, serum	4.25–5.25 mg/dL	1.05–1.30 mmol/L
Carbon dioxide, total, serum or plasma	24–31 mEq/L	24–31 mmol/L
Carbon dioxide tension (P_{CO_2}), blood	35–45 mmHg	35–45 mmHg
Ceruloplasmin, serum	23–44 mg/dL	230–440 mg/L
Chloride, serum or plasma	96–106 mEq/L	96–106 mmol/L
Cholesterol, serum or EDTA plasma		
Desirable range	<200 mg/dL	<5.20 mmol/L
LDL cholesterol	60–180 mg/dL	1.55–4.65 mmol/L
HDL cholesterol	30–80 mg/dL	0.80–2.05 mmol/L

continued

Reference Values* for Clinical Chemistry (Blood, Serum, and Plasma) *Continued*

	Conventional Units	SI Units
Copper	70–140 μg/dL	11–22 μmol/L
Corticotropin (ACTH), plasma, 8 AM	10–80 pg/mL	2–18 pmol/L
Cortisol, plasma		
8:00 AM	6–23 μg/dL	170–630 nmol/L
4:00 PM	3–15 μg/dL	80–410 nmol/L
10:00 PM	<50% of 8:00 AM value	<50% of 8:00 AM value
Creatine, serum		
Males	0.2–0.5 mg/dL	15–40 μmol/L
Females	0.3–0.9 mg/dL	25–70 μmol/L
Creatine kinase (CK), serum		
Males	55–170 U/L	55–170 U/L
Females	30–135 U/L	30–135 U/L
Creatine kinase MB isoenzyme, serum	<5% of total CK activity <5% ng/mL by immunoassay	<5% of total CK activity <5% ng/mL by immunoassay
Creatinine, serum	0.6–1.2 mg/dL	50–110 μmol/L
Estradiol-17β, adult		
Males	10–65 pg/mL	35–240 pmol/L
Females		
Follicular phase	30–100 pg/mL	110–370 pmol/L
Ovulatory phase	200–400 pg/mL	730–1470 pmol/L
Luteal phase	50–140 pg/mL	180–510 pmol/L
Ferritin, serum	20–200 ng/mL	20–200 μg/L
Fibrinogen, plasma	200–400 mg/dL	2.0–4.0 g/L
Folate, serum	3.0–18.0 ng/mL	6.8–41.0 nmol/L
erythrocytes	145–540 ng/mL	330–1220 nmol/L
Follicle-stimulating hormone (FSH), plasma		
Males	4–25 mU/mL	4–25 U/L
Females, premenopausal	4–30 mU/mL	4–30 U/L
Females, postmenopausal	40–250 mU/mL	40–250 U/L
γ-Glutamyltransferase (GGT), serum	5–40 U/L	5–40 U/L
Gastrin, fasting, serum	0–110 pg/mL	0–110 mg/L
Glucose, fasting, plasma or serum	70–115 mg/dL	3.9–6.4 nmol/L
Growth hormone (hGH), plasma, adult, fasting	0–6 ng/mL	0–6 μg/L
Haptoglobin, serum	20–165 mg/dL	0.20–1.65 g/L
Insulin, fasting, plasma	5–25 μU/mL	36–179 pmol/L
Iron, serum	75–175 μg/dL	13–31 μmol/L
Iron binding capacity, serum		
Total	250–410 μg/dL	45–73 μmol/L
Saturation	20–55%	0.20–0.55
Lactate		
Venous whole blood	5.0–20.0 mg/dL	0.6–2.2 mmol/L
Arterial whole blood	5.0–15.0 mg/dL	0.6–1.7 mmol/L
Lactate dehydrogenase (LD), serum	110–220 U/L	110–220 U/L
Lipase, serum	10–140 U/L	10–140 U/L
Lutropin (LH), serum		
Males	1–9 U/L	1–9 U/L
Females		
Follicular phase	2–10 U/L	2–10 U/L
Midcycle peak	15–65 U/L	15–65 U/L
Luteal phase	1–12 U/L	1–12 U/L
Postmenopausal	12–65 U/L	12–65 U/L
Magnesium, serum	1.3–2.1 mg/dL	0.65–1.05 mmol/L
Osmolality	275–295 mOsm/kg water	275–295 mOsm/kg water
Oxygen, blood, arterial, room air		
Partial pressure (PaO_2)	80–100 mmHg	80–100 mmHg
Saturation (SaO_2)	95–98%	95–98%
pH, arterial blood	7.35–7.45	7.35–7.45
Phosphate, inorganic, serum		
Adult	3.0–4.5 mg/dL	1.0–1.5 mmol/L
Child	4.0–7.0 mg/dL	1.3–2.3 mmol/L

Reference Values* for Clinical Chemistry (Blood, Serum, and Plasma) *Continued*

	Conventional Units	SI Units
Potassium		
Serum	3.5–5.0 mEq/L	3.5–5.0 mmol/L
Plasma	3.5–4.5 mEq/L	3.5–4.5 mmol/L
Progesterone, serum, adult		
Males	0.0–0.4 ng/mL	0.0–1.3 mmol/L
Females		
Follicular phase	0.1–1.5 ng/mL	0.3–4.8 mmol/L
Luteal phase	2.5–28.0 ng/mL	8.0–89.0 mmol/L
Prolactin, serum		
Males	1.0–15.0 ng/mL	1.0–15.0 μg/L
Females	1.0–20.0 ng/mL	1.0–20.0 μg/L
Protein, serum, electrophoresis		
Total	6.0–8.0 g/dL	60–80 g/L
Albumin	3.5–5.5 g/dL	35–55 g/L
Globulins		
$Alpha_1$	0.2–0.4 g/dL	2.0–4.0 g/L
$Alpha_2$	0.5–0.9 g/dL	5.0–9.0 g/L
Beta	0.6–1.1 g/dL	6.0–11.0 g/L
Gamma	0.7–1.7 g/dL	7.0–17.0 g/L
Pyruvate, blood	0.3–0.9 mg/dL	0.03–0.10 mmol/L
Rheumatoid factor	0.0–30.0 IU/mL	0.0–30.0 kIU/L
Sodium, serum or plasma	135–145 mEq/L	135–145 mmol/L
Testosterone, plasma		
Males, adult	300–1200 ng/dL	10.4–41.6 nmol/L
Females, adult	20–75 ng/dL	0.7–2.6 nmol/L
Pregnant females	40–200 ng/dL	1.4–6.9 nmol/L
Thyroglobulin	3–42 ng/mL	3–42 μg/L
Thyrotropin (hTSH), serum	0.4–4.8 μIU/mL	0.4–4.8 mIU/L
Thyrotropin-releasing hormone (TRH)	5–60 pg/mL	5–60 ng/L
Thyroxine (FT_4), free, serum	0.9–2.1 ng/dL	12–27 pmol/L
Thyroxine (T_4), serum	4.5–12.0 μg/dL	58–154 nmol/L
Thyroxine-binding globulin (TBG)	15.0–34.0 μg/mL	15.0–34.0 mg/L
Transferrin	250–430 mg/dL	2.5–4.3 g/L
Triglycerides, serum, after 12-hr fast	40–150 mg/dL	0.4–1.5 g/L
Triiodothyronine (T_3), serum	70–190 ng/dL	1.1–2.9 nmol/L
Triiodothyronine uptake, resin (T_3RU)	25–38%	0.25–0.38
Urate		
Males	2.5–8.0 mg/dL	150–480 μmol/L
Females	2.2–7.0 mg/dL	130–420 μmol/L
Urea, serum or plasma	24–49 mg/dL	4.0–8.2 nmol/L
Urea nitrogen, serum or plasma	11–23 mg/dL	8.0–16.4 nmol/L
Viscosity, serum	1.4–1.8 × water	1.4–1.8 × water
Vitamin A, serum	20–80 μg/dL	0.70–2.80 μmol/L
Vitamin B_{12}, serum	180–900 pg/mL	133–664 pmol/L

*Reference values may vary, depending on the method and sample source used.

Reference Values for Clinical Chemistry (Urine)

	Conventional Units	SI Units
Acetone and acetoacetate, qualitative	Negative	Negative
Albumin		
Qualitative	Negative	Negative
Quantitative	10–100 mg/24 hr	0.15–1.5 μmol/day
Aldosterone	3–20 μg/24 hr	8.3–55 nmol/day
δ-Aminolevulinic acid (δ-ALA)	1.3–7.0 mg/24 hr	10–53 μmol/day
Amylase	<17 U/hr	<17 U/hr
Amylase/creatinine clearance ratio	0.01–0.04	0.01–0.04
Bilirubin, qualitative	Negative	Negative
Calcium (regular diet)	<250 mg/24 hr	<6.3 nmol/day
Catecholamines		
Epinephrine	<10 μg/24 hr	<55 nmol/day
Norepinephrine	<100 μg/24 hr	<590 nmol/day
Total free catecholamines	4–126 μg/24 hr	24–745 nmol/day
Total metanephrines	0.1–1.6 mg/24 hr	0.5–8.1 μmol/day
Chloride (varies with intake)	110–250 mEq/24 hr	110–250 mmol/day
Copper	0–50 μg/24 hr	0.0–0.80 μmol/day
Cortisol, free	10–100 μg/24 hr	27.6–276 nmol/day
Creatine		
Males	0–40 mg/24 hr	0.0–0.30 mmol/day
Females	0–80 mg/24 hr	0.0–0.60 mmol/day
Creatinine	15–25 mg/kg/24 hr	0.13–0.22 mmol/kg/day
Creatinine clearance (endogenous)		
Males	110–150 mL/min/1.73 m^2	110–150 mL/min/1.73 m^2
Females	105–132 mL/min/1.73 m^2	105–132 mL/min/1.73 m^2
Cystine or cysteine	Negative	Negative
Dehydroepiandrosterone		
Males	0.2–2.0 mg/24 hr	0.7–6.9 μmol/day
Females	0.2–1.8 mg/24 hr	0.7–6.2 μmol/day
Estrogens, total		
Males	4–25 μg/24 hr	14–90 nmol/day
Females	5–100 μg/24 hr	18–360 nmol/day
Glucose (as reducing substance)	<250 mg/24 hr	<250 mg/day
Hemoglobin and myoglobin, qualitative	Negative	Negative
Homogentisic acid, qualitative	Negative	Negative
17-Hydroxycorticosteroids		
Males	3–9 mg/24 hr	8.3–25 μmol/day
Females	2–8 mg/24 hr	5.5–22 μmol/day
5-Hydroxyindoleacetic acid		
Qualitative	Negative	Negative
Quantitative	2–6 mg/24 hr	10–31 μmol/day
17-Ketogenic steroids		
Males	5–23 mg/24 hr	17–80 μmol/day
Females	3–15 mg/24 hr	10–52 μmol/day
17-Ketosteroids		
Males	8–22 mg/24 hr	28–76 μmol/day
Females	6–15 mg/24 hr	21–52 μmol/day
Magnesium	6–10 mEq/24 hr	3–5 mmol/day
Metanephrines	0.05–1.2 ng/mg creatinine	0.03–0.70 mmol/mmol creatinine
Osmolality	38–1400 mOsm/kg water	38–1400 mOsm/kg water
pH	4.6–8.0	4.6–8.0
Phenylpyruvic acid, qualitative	Negative	Negative
Phosphate	0.4–1.3 g/24 hr	13–42 mmol/day
Porphobilinogen		
Qualitative	Negative	Negative
Quantitative	<2 mg/24 hr	<9 μmol/day
Porphyrins		
Coproporphyrin	50–250 μg/24 hr	77–380 nmol/day
Uroporphyrin	10–30 μg/24 hr	12–36 nmol/day
Potassium	25–125 mEq/24 hr	25–125 mmol/day

Reference Values for Clinical Chemistry (Urine) *Continued*

	Conventional Units	SI Units
Pregnanediol		
Males	0.0–1.9 mg/24 hr	0.0–6.0 μmol/day
Females		
Proliferative phase	0.0–2.6 mg/24 hr	0.0–8.0 μmol/day
Luteal phase	2.6–10.6 mg/24 hr	8–33 μmol/day
Postmenopausal	0.2–1.0 mg/24 hr	0.6–3.1 μmol/day
Pregnanetriol	0.0–2.5 mg/24 hr	0.0–7.4 μmol/day
Protein, total		
Qualitative	Negative	Negative
Quantitative	10–150 mg/24 hr	10–150 mg/day
Protein/creatinine ratio	<0.2	<0.2
Sodium (regular diet)	60–260 mEq/24 hr	60–260 mmol/day
Specific gravity		
Random specimen	1.003–1.030	1.003–1.030
24-Hour collection	1.015–1.025	1.015–1.025
Urate (regular diet)	250–750 mg/24 hr	1.5–4.4 mmol/day
Urobilinogen	0.5–4.0 mg/24 hr	0.6–6.8 μmol/day
Vanillylmandelic acid (VMA)	1.0–8.0 mg/24 hr	5–40 μmol/day

Index

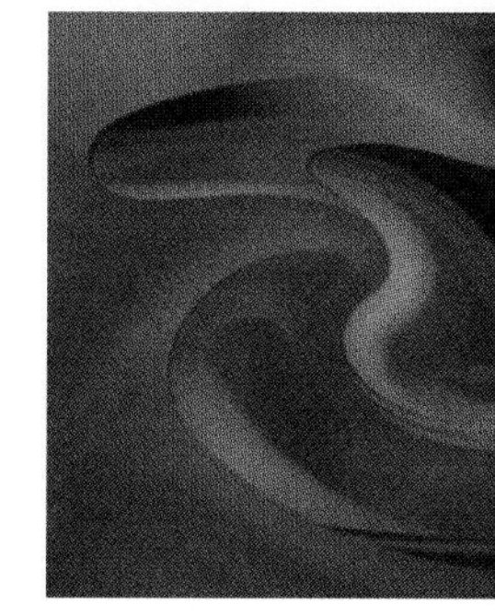

Note: Page numbers in *italics* indicate illustrations; those followed by t indicate tables; those followed by b indicate boxed and display text; and those followed by p indicate procedures.

INTERNET RESOURCES

Nursing Organizations

Academy of Medical-Surgical Nurses
www.amsn.inurse.com

American Academy of Ambulatory Care Nurses
aaacn.inurse.com

American Academy of Nurse Practitioners
www.aanp.org

American Association of Critical-Care Nurses
www.aacn.org

American Association of Diabetes Educators
www.aadenet.org

American Association of Neuroscience Nurses
www.aann.org

American Association of Nurse Anesthetists
www.aana.com

American Association of Occupational Health Nurses
www.aaohn.org

American Association of Spinal Cord Injury Nurses
www.epva.org

American College of Nurse Practitioners
www.nurse.org/acnp

American Nephrology Nurses' Association
www.anna.inurse.com

American Nurses' Association
www.ana.org

American Society of Peri-Anesthesia Nurses
www.aspan.org

American Society of Plastic and Reconstructive Surgical Nurses
www.asprsn.inurse.com

American Thoracic Society Nursing Assembly
www.thoracic.org/nur

Association of Nurses in AIDS Care
www.anacnet.org/aids

Association of Operating Room Nurses
www.aorn.org

Association for Professionals in Infection Control and Epidemiology
www.apic.org

Association of Women's Health, Obstetric, and Neonatal Nurses
www.awhonn.org

Dermatology Nurses Association
www.dna.inurse.com

Emergency Nurses Association
www.ena.org

National Association of Orthopaedic Nurses
www.naon.inurse.com

National League for Nursing
www.nln.org

National Student Nurses' Association
www.nsna.org

Oncology Nursing Society
www.ons.org

Sigma Theta Tau International
http://stti-web.iupui.edu

Society of Gastroenterology Nurses and Associates, Inc.
www.sgna.org

Society of Urologic Nurses and Associates
www.suna.inurse.com

WorldWide Nurse
www.wwnurse.com

Wound, Ostomy and Continence Nursing Society
www.wocn.org

Community Organizations and Other Resources

Alternative and Complementary Therapies

Alternative Medicine
http://galaxy.tradewave.com/galaxy/Medicine/therapeutics/Alternativw-Medicine.html

Alternative Medicine (Health a-to-z)
www.healthatoz.com/categories/AM.htm

American Holistic Nurses Association
www.ahna.org

American Massage Therapy Association
www.amtamassage.org

Complementary Therapies
www.wholenurse.com

Healing Touch International, Inc.
www.healingtouch.net

Nurses Certification Program in Interactive Imagery
http://members.aol.com//NCPII/NCPII.html

The Wellness Center
www.newfrontiers.com/wellness

Cancer/Death and Dying

American Brain Tumor Association
www.abta.org

American Cancer Society
www.cancer.org

Breast Cancer Information Clearing House
http://nysernet.org/bcic

Canadian Cancer Society (National Office)
www.cancer.ca

CDC's Tobacco Information and Prevention Source Page
www.cdc.gov/nccdphp/osh/tobacco.htm

Choice in Dying
www.choices.org

Funeral and Memorial Societies of America
www.funerals.org

Hospice Association of America
www.nahc.org

Leukemia Society of America
www.leukemia.org

National Cancer Institute
www.nih.gov/nci

NCI's CancerNet
www.nci.nih.gov

National Hospice Organization
www.nho.org

National Ovarian Cancer Coalition
www.ovarian.org

The Quitnet
www.quitnet.org

Rory Foundation
www.roryfoundation.org

Susan G. Komen Breast Cancer Foundation
www.komen.org

Cardiovascular and Hematologic Problems

American Association of Blood Banks
www.aabb.org

American Heart Association
www.american heart.org

American Heart Association Women's Website
www.women.americanheart.org

Heart Information Network
www.heartinfo.org

Mended Hearts, Inc.
www.mendedhearts.org

National Hemophilia Foundation
www.hemophilia.org

Diabetes Mellitus

American Diabetes Association
www.diabetes.org

American Dietetic Association
www.eatright.org

CDC-Diabetes Home Page
www.cdc.gov/nccdphp/ddt/ddthome.htm

National Institute of Diabetes and Digestive and Kidney Disease
www.niddk.nih.gov

Elderly/Gerontology

Alcohol Rehab for the Elderly
www.hmc.net

Alzheimer's Association
www.alz.org

American Association of Retired Persons
www.aarp.org

American Federation for Aging Research
www.afar.org

National Institute on Aging
www.nih.gov.nia

Eye and Ear Problems

American Foundation for the Blind
www.afb.org

American Speech-Language-Hearing Association
www.asha.org

Deafness Research Foundation
www.drf.org

Eye Bank Associations of America
www.restoresight.org

Meniere's Network of the Ear Foundation
www.theearfound.org

Self-Help for Hard of Hearing People
www.shhh.org

Gastrointestinal Problems

American Anorexia/Bulimia Association, Inc.
members.aol.com/amanba/index.html

American Liver Foundation
www.liverfoundation.org

Crohn's and Colitis Foundation of America
www.ccfa.org

Healthy Weight
www.healthyweight.com

Immunologic Problems/Infection Control and Prevention

AIDS Treatment Data Network
www.aidsnyc.org

Allergy, Asthma, & Immunology Online
http://allergy.mcg.edu

American Academy of Allergy, Asthma, and Immunology
www.aaaai.org

Centers for Disease Control and Prevention
www.cdc.gov

HIV/AIDS Surveillance Report
Centers for Disease Control and Prevention
www.cdc.gov/nchstp/hiv__aids/stat

Immune Deficiency Foundation
www.primaryimmune.org

Infectious Disease WebLink
http://pages.prodigy.net/pdeziel/

Latex Allergy Homepage
http://allergy.mcg.edu/physician/ltxhome.html

National AIDS Treatment Advocacy Project
www.natap.org

National Center for Infectious Diseases
www.cdc.gov/ncidod/ncid.htm

National Foundation for Infectious Diseases
www.nfid.org

The Safer Sex Page
www.safersex.org

Musculoskeletal Problems

Ankylosing Spondylitis Association
www.spondylitis.org

Arthritis Foundation
www.arthritis.org

Backpain Hotline—Texas Back Institute
www.texasback.com

National Institute of Arthritis and Musculoskeletal and Skin Diseases
www.nih.gov/niams

Neurologic Problems and Rehabilitation

American Paralysis Association
www.apacure.com

Amyotrophic Lateral Sclerosis Association
www.alsa.org

Epilepsy Foundation of America
www.efa.org

Epilepsy Ontario
epilepsyontario.org

Huntington's Disease Society of America
dsa.mgh.harvard.edu

Migraine Resource Center
www.migrainehelp.com

National Headache Foundation
www.headaches.org

National Multiple Sclerosis Society
www.nmss.org

National Stroke Organization
www.stroke.org

Parkinson's Disease Foundation
www.parkinsons-foundation.org

Reproductive Health Problems

All About Menopause
www.menopause.org

Atlanta Reproductive Health Center
www.ivf.com/endohtml.html

Bair PMS Home Page
www.bairpms.com

Center for Human Reproduction
www.centerforhumanreprod.com

Endometriosis Association
www.endometrios.org

Planned Parenthood Federation of America, Inc.
www.ppfa.org

The Safer Sex Page
www.safersex.org